Disorders of Voluntary Muscle

Disorders of
Voluntary Muscle

EDITED BY

Sir John Walton
TD, MA, MD, DSc, FRCP

Warden, Green College, Oxford; Honorary Consultant
Neurologist, Oxford District and
Regional Health Authorities

Former Professor of Neurology and Dean of Medicine,
University of Newcastle upon Tyne

FIFTH EDITION

CHURCHILL LIVINGSTONE
EDINBURGH LONDON MELBOURNE AND NEW YORK 1988

CHURCHILL LIVINGSTONE
Medical Division of Longman Group UK Limited

Distributed in the United States of America by Churchill
Livingstone Inc., 19 West 44th Street, New York, N.Y.
10036, and by associated companies, branches and
representatives throughout the world.

First edition 1964
Second edition 1969
Third edition 1974
Fourth edition 1981
Fifth edition 1988

ISBN 0-443-03882-1

British Library Cataloguing in Publication Data
Walton, Sir John, 1922–
  Disorders of voluntary muscle. —
  5th ed.
  1. Striated muscle — Diseases
  I. Title
  616.7'4   RC925

Library of Congress Cataloging in Publication Data
Disorders of voluntary muscle/edited by Sir John Walton. —
5th ed.
  p.   cm.
  Includes bibliographies and index
  1. Muscles — Diseases.   2. Neuromuscular diseases.
I. Walton, John Nicholas.
  [DNLM: 1. Muscular Diseases.   2. Neuromuscular
Diseases.]
RC925.D535 1988
616.7'4 — dc19   87-27626
                                         CIP

Printed at The Bath Press, Avon

Preface to the Fifth Edition

When, in 1981, I wrote the preface to the fourth edition of this book, I remarked that there had been so many developments in the field of neuromuscular disease that extensive alterations and modifications in the structure of the volume had become necessary. The book was then reset in a completely different format from that of the first three editions and much rewriting and rearrangement was undertaken: completely new chapters on parasitic disorders and drug-induced neuromuscular disorders were added. Since 1981 developments have proceeded apace and in late 1983 Churchill Livingstone decided to seek the advice of an independent referee, distinguished in the field of neuromuscular disease (not a contributor) upon how best the fifth edition should be revised and reconstructed in order to deal with new knowledge and the changing emphasis in clinical practice and research which had emerged since the fourth edition was prepared and published. In the light of that opinion and the views expressed by reviewers I decided that a number of major changes would be appropriate in the fifth edition. While the overall organisation of the book into four major sections on Normal Structure and Function, Pathology, Clinical Problems and Electrodiagnosis remains much the same, the opening chapter on anatomy and physiology is substantially shorter than in the last edition; the chapters on the pathology and clinical manifestations of peripheral nerve disease have been combined into a single brief overview included for differential diagnostic purposes; new chapters on immunology, the pathophysiology of excitation in skeletal muscle, on medical and psychological and on orthopaedic management have been included; disorders associated with myotonia are reviewed in a separate chapter from the muscular dystrophies and the neuromuscular complications of malignancy no longer require a separate chapter, being subsumed under miscellaneous neuromuscular disorders; a new section on avian myopathy has been added to the much revised chapter on neuromuscular disease in animals; and finally consideration of electrodiagnosis, now covered in only three chapters, has been completely reorganised. I hope that in consequence of these changes the book will prove even more useful than in the past as a work of reference and that the very extensive updating of all of the chapters, many of which have been totally rewritten, will mean that it is well up-to-date even in the exciting and rapidly changing field of neuromuscular disease. In the course of this revision, very many illustrations have been replaced and many new ones have been added, some from other publications but very many original; where appropriate, acknowledgements to original sources are given either in the captions to the illustrations or at the end of individual chapters.

Inevitably, as in previous editions, the reader will find evidence of some duplication and overlap between different chapters in that many diseases, and particularly the muscular dystrophies and spinal muscular atrophies, are commented upon in several chapters but from different points of view and with varying emphasis upon their clinical, pathological, biochemical and physiological characteristics. This has proved necessary in order that each individual chapter can stand as a comprehensive essay upon the topic to which it is devoted; I hope and believe that as a result the book will be no less useful, and may even be more so, as a work of reference.

Sadly, since publication of the last edition, two much-valued contributors, Dr J. A. R. Lenman and Professor E. Zaimis, have died and will be greatly missed. I wish to thank most sincerely Dr J. C. Brown, Dr B. F. Fell, Dr R. A. Henson, Professor R. J. Johns, Dr D. M. Lewis, Professor A. J. McComas, Dr H. M. Price, Dr R. M. A. P. Ridge, Sir Peter Tizard, Dr R. L. van de Velde and Dr C. B. Wynn-Parry for their contributions to previous editions. We welcome as new contributors Dr R. L. Barchi, Professor E. A. Barnard, Dr S. M. Chou, Dr M. J. Cullen, Professor R. H. T. Edwards, Dr I. T. Ferguson, Professor C. S. B. Galasko, Professor P. Harper, Professor

J. B. Harris, Dr D. N. Landon, Dr R. P. Lisak, Mrs. R. McKerrell, Dr C. Sewry, Dr I. S. Schofield and Dr C. R. Slater. As in the past, much new material from other publications has been reproduced or referred to (and fully acknowledged) in this edition and I wish to express my gratitude and appreciation to the authors, editors and publishers concerned for allowing us to include this material. And I am especially grateful to the staff of Churchill Livingstone, to Mrs. Heather Russell, who has given invaluable editorial help, and to my secretary, Miss Rosemary Allan, for their patient and willing cooperation and for their forbearance during the production of this edition.

Oxford, 1988   J. W.

Preface to the First Edition

The last fifteen years have seen a world-wide awakening of interest in diseases of muscle and during this period several outstanding books upon this subject have been published. At first sight, therefore, a new text-book devoted to this group of disorders may seem to be superfluous. However, the excellent work on *Diseases of Muscle* by Adam, Denny Brown and Pearson, now in its second edition, approaches the subject primarily from the pathological standpoint, while the three-volume work on *Structure and Function of Muscle* edited by Geoffrey Bourne, consists of a series of comprehensive essays of encyclopaedic scope, invaluable for reference by the research worker but perhaps too weighty for the general reader. Furthermore, the volume on *Neuromuscular Disorders*, embodying the proceedings of the 1958 meeting of the Association for Research in Nervous and Mental Disease, is primarily a commentary upon research in this field, while the recent work *Muscular Dystrophy in Man and Animals* edited by Bourne and Golarz, surveys only the problem of muscular dystrophy.

In designing the present volume, therefore, it has been my aim and that of the other twenty-four contributors, each an acknowledged expert in the field, to give an up-to-date and comprehensive yet concise view of disorders of muscle from several standpoints. The book is aimed primarily at the clinician, whether he be a general physician, paediatrician or neurologist, a post-graduate student studying for a higher examination or any doctor wishing to expand his knowledge of this group of disorders. The first section of the book is devoted to a consideration of modern views of the structure and function of muscle, the second to the changes, both structural and biochemical, which may occur in disease, and the third contains a series of essays on the clinical and genetic aspects of muscle disease in man with a chapter describing the related disorders which occur in animals; the final section deals with electrical methods of investigation of muscular disease. Throughout, references are given not only to original sources of information but also to current research.

In the preparation of this volume I am indebted to the contributors; I am sure that many of them, like myself, are grateful for the help they have obtained from previous publications, pre-eminent among which are the four volumes to which I have referred above. More detailed acknowledgements of sources of material contained in this volume are given, where necessary, at the end of individual chapters. I wish personally to thank Mr J. Rivers, Mr A. S. Knightley and the staff of J. and A. Churchill Ltd for all the patience and understanding they have shown during the process of publication and, as always, I am deeply indebted to my secretary, Miss Rosemary Allan, for her unfailing willingness and efficiency.

Newcastle upon Tyne, 1964   J. W.

Contributors

Raymond D. Adams
AM, MD, DSc, MD
Former Senior Neurologist and Chief of
Neurology Service, Massachusetts General
Hospital; Emeritus Bullard Professor of
Neuropathology, Harvard Medical School,
Boston, Massachusetts, USA

Zohar Argov
MD
Department of Neurology, Hadassah University
Hospital, Jerusalem, Israel

Karl-Erik Åström
MD, PhD
Professor of Neurology, King Saud University,
Riyadh, Kingdom of Saudi Arabia

Robert L. Barchi
MD, PhD
David Mahoney Professor of Neuroscience and
Professor, Departments of Neurology,
Biochemistry and Biophysics, University of
Pennsylvania School of Medicine, Philadelphia,
Pennsylvania, USA

Eric A. Barnard
PhD, FRS
Director, MRC Molecular Neurobiology Unit,
University of Cambridge Medical School,
Cambridge, UK

D. D. Barwick
MB, FRCP(Edin)
Consultant Neurologist (Clinical
Neurophysiology), Regional Neurological Centre,
Newcastle General Hospital; Clinical Lecturer in
Neurology, University of Newcastle upon Tyne,
UK

R. Bradley
MSc, BVetMed, MRCVS, MRCPath, MIBiol
Head of the Department of Pathology, Central
Veterinary Laboratory, New Haw, Weybridge,
UK

Walter G. Bradley
DM, FRCP
Professor and Chairman, Department of
Neurology, University of Vermont College of
Medicine, Burlington, Vermont, USA

Malcolm J. Campbell
MB BS, FRCP
Consultant Neurological Physician, Bristol Royal
Infirmary; Frenchay Hospital, Bristol, UK

S. M. Chou
MD, PhD
Head, Neuropathology Section, Cleveland Clinic
Foundation; Former Professor & Director of
Neuropathology Laboratory, West Virginia
University Medical Center, West Virginia, USA

Christian Coërs
MD
Emeritus Professor of Neurology, Brussels
University, Belgium

M. J. Cullen
MA, DPhil
Senior Research Associate, Muscular Dystrophy
Research Laboratories, Regional Neurological
Centre, Newcastle General Hospital, Newcastle
upon Tyne, UK

S Currie
MA, MD, BChir, FRCP
Consultant Neurologist, St James's University

Hospital; Clinical Lecturer, University of Leeds, UK

Victor Dubowitz
BSc, PhD, MD, FRCP, DCH
Professor of Paediatrics, University of London; Co-Director, Jerry Lewis Muscle Research Centre; Honorary Consultant Physician, Hammersmith Hospital, London, UK

R. H. T. Edwards
PhD, FRCP
Professor of Medicine and Head of the University Department of Medicine, University of Liverpool, UK

Alan E. H. Emery
MD, PhD(Johns Hopkins), DSc, FRCP, FRS(Edin)
Emeritus Professor of Human Genetics, Medical School, University of Edinburgh, UK

Andrew G. Engel
MD
William L. McKnight Professor of Neuroscience, Mayo Medical School; Consultant in Neurology, Mayo Clinic, Minnesota, USA

P. R. W. Fawcett
BSc, MB, BS, MRCP
Consultant Clinical Neurophysiologist, Regional Neurological Centre, Newcastle General Hospital; Clinical Lecturer in Neurology, University of Newcastle upon Tyne, UK

Iain T. Ferguson
MD, FRCPE
Consultant Neurologist, Southmead Hospital; Honorary Lecturer, University of Bristol, UK

John B. Foster
MD, FRCP
Reader in Neurology, University of Newcastle, Consultant Neurologist, Newcastle General Hospital and Northern Regional Health Authority, Newcastle upon Tyne, UK

C. S. B. Galasko
MB, MSc, ChM, FRCS(Eng), FRCS(Edin)
Professor of Orthopaedic Surgery, University of Manchester; Honorary Consultant Orthopaedic Surgeon, Salford Health Authority, Manchester, UK

David Gardner-Medwin
MD, FRCP
Consultant Paediatric Neurologist, Newcastle General Hospital, Newcastle upon Tyne, UK

J. Gergely
MD, PhD
Director, Department of Muscle Research, Boston Biomedical Research Institute; Biochemist, Massachusetts General Hospital; Associate Professor, Harvard Medical School, Massachusetts, USA

Peter S. Harper
DM, FRCP
Professor and Consultant in Medical Genetics, University of Wales College of Medicine, Cardiff, UK

John B. Harris
BPharm, PhD, FIBiol
Professor of Experimental Neurology in the University of Newcastle; Director, Muscular Dystrophy Laboratories, Regional Neurological Centre, Newcastle General Hospital, Newcastle upon Tyne, UK

P. Hudgson
MB, BS, FRCP, FRACP
Consultant Neurologist, Northern Region and Newcastle Health Authorities; Senior Lecturer in Neurology, University of Newcastle; Clinical Director, Muscular Dystrophy Research Laboratories, Newcastle General Hospital, Newcastle upon Tyne, UK

Huw A. John
BSc, PhD
Research Fellow, Institute of Animal Genetics, University of Edinburgh, UK

K. W. Jones
BSc, PhD
Reader, Genetics Department, University of Edinburgh, UK

Byron A. Kakulas
AO, MD(Hon Athens), MD(WA), FRACP, FRCPath, FRCPA
Professor of Neuropathology, University of Western Australia; Medical Director, Neuromuscular Foundation and Institute of Western Australia; Head of the Department of

Neuropathology, Royal Perth Hospital, Western Australia

D. N. Landon
MB BS, BSc, LRCP, MRCS
Reader in Neurocytology, University Department of Clinical Neurology, Institute of Neurology, London, UK

The late J. A. R. Lenman
MB, ChB, FRCP(Edin), FRS(Edin)
Former Reader in Neurology, Dundee University; Honorary Consultant Neurologist, Tayside Area Health Board, Dundee

Paul D. Lewis
MD, DSc, MRCP, FRCPath
Reader in Histopathology, Royal Postgraduate Medical School, Hammersmith Hospital, London, UK

R. P. Lisak
MD
Professor and Chairman, Department of Neurology, Wayne State University of Medicine: Chief of Neurology, Harper-Grace Hospital; Neurologist-in-Chief, Detroit Medical Center, Michigan, USA

F. L. Mastaglia
MD, FRACP, FRCP
Professor of Neurology, University of Western Australia; Consultant Neurologist, Queen Elizabeth II Medical Centre, Perth, Western Australia

R. E. McKerrell
MA, VetMB, MRCVS
Wellcome Laboratory for Comparative Neurology, Department of Clinical Veterinary Medicine, University of Cambridge, UK

Christopher Pallis
DM, FRCP
Reader Emeritus in Neurology, Royal Postgraduate Medical School, London, UK

R. J. T. Pennington
PhD, DSc, FRSE
Former Member of the Medical Research Council External Scientific Staff; Honorary Reader in Neurochemistry, University of

Newcastle; Honorary Senior Neurochemist, Regional Neurological Centre, Newcastle upon Tyne, UK

Ian S. Schofield
MB, BS, BMed Sci, MRCP
Consultant Neurophysiologist, Regional Neurological Centre, Newcastle upon Tyne, UK

Caroline Sewry
MD, PhD
Lecturer, Jerry Lewis Muscle Research Centre, Royal Postgraduate Medical School, Hammersmith Hospital, London, UK

J. A. Simpson
MD, FRCP, FRCP(Edin), FRCP(Glas), FRS(Edin)
Emeritus Professor of Neurology, University of Glasgow; former Physician in Charge, Department of Neurology, Institute of Neurological Sciences, Glasgow, UK

C. R. Slater
PhD
Senior Lecturer in Clinical Science, Department of Neurology, University of Newcastle upon Tyne, UK

P. K. Thomas
DSc. MD, FRCP
Professor of Neurology in the University of London at the Royal Free Hospital School of Medicine and the Institute of Neurology, London, UK

D. W.-Wray
MA, MSc, DPhil
Senior Lecturer in Pharmacology, Royal Free Hospital School of Medicine, University of London, UK

Sir John Walton
TD, MA, MD, DSc, FRCP(Lond), Dr de'l Univ(Hon) (Aix-Marseille), DSc(Hon) (Leeds), DSc(Hon) (Leicester), MD(Hon) Sheffield, Hon FACP, FRCP(Hon) (Edin), FRCP(Hon) (Canada)
Warden, Green College, Oxford; Honorary Consultant Neurologist, Oxford District and Regional Health Authorities; Former Professor of Neurology and Dean of Medicine, University of Newcastle upon Tyne, UK

Contents

The anatomy and physiology of the motor unit

INTRODUCTION

Skeletal muscle fibres are innervated by motor neurones which have cell bodies lying within the central nervous system and axons extending peripherally to the muscles. A single motor neurone and the many muscle fibres uniquely innervated by it are known as a *motor unit*. Because a nerve impulse in a motor neurone normally elicits the contraction of all the muscle fibres it innervates, the motor unit is the elementary unit of neuromuscular function; under normal circumstances, all voluntary muscle contractions result from the activation of a number of complete motor units.

Each motor unit consists of a large number of cells, the anatomical and physiological properties of which are closely matched so that the unit as a whole is specialised in order to do a particular kind of work. This matching results largely from interactions between nerve and muscle which continue throughout life to promote both the formation and the maintenance of a well-integrated yet still adaptable neuromuscular system.

In this chapter, we first describe the basic features of the cells that make up motor units and their role in the generation of voluntary movements. We then indicate some of the ways in which these cells interact throughout life so that in spite of major changes resulting from varied patterns of use, ageing, injury or disease, the motor unit remains functionally adequate.

ANATOMICAL ORGANISATION OF THE MOTOR UNIT

Nerve

The activity of the motor unit is coordinated by the *motor neurone* (Fig. 1.1). The *cell body* of the motor neurone contains the nucleus and the intracellular organelles associated with protein synthesis, viz. the ribosomes and rough endoplasmic reticulum (the Nissl substance of neurohistology). Neural inputs to motor neurones are made at synapses located either on the cell body or on the many elongated *dendrites* which extend from it.

Nerve impulses arising in the motor neurone are carried to the muscle fibres by a single *motor axon*. The axonal cytoplasm contains a prominent cytoskeleton. This is composed primarily of two types

of proteinaceous fibres, *neurofilaments* and *microtubules* (Alberts et al 1983). Neurofilaments are a neurone-specific form of 10 nm diameter 'intermediate filament'. Like the other keratin-related proteins of this class, they form extremely stable intracellular fibres which are thought to provide the mechanical rigidity necessary to maintain the elongated form of the axon. Microtubules are much more dynamic structures found in almost all cells. Each microtubule is a helical polymer, 25 nm in diameter, of the protein tubulin. The main role of microtubules in axons appears to be to provide a track along which membrane-bound vesicles move carrying material between the cell body and the periphery (see below).

Surrounding each axon is an insulating *myelin* sheath formed of many layers of plasma membrane of the *Schwann cells*, a type of glial cell. Each Schwann cell is typically about 1 mm long, so a motor axon innervating distal limb muscles may be associated with several hundred Schwann cells. A gap in the myelin sheath, the *node of Ranvier*, is present at the boundary between adjacent Schwann cells. Each individual axon, together with its associated Schwann cells, is surrounded by a connective tissue sheath. This consists of a mesh-like *basal lamina* together with

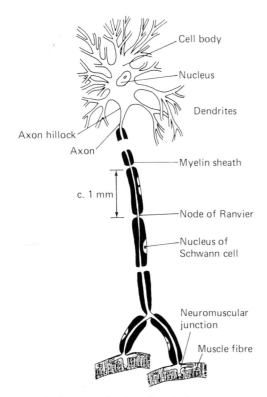

Fig. 1.1 A diagrammatic view of a spinal motor neurone. The cell body and its dendrites lie within the spinal cord. The single axon emerges from the enlarged axon hillock and lies mainly outside the cord. Schwann cells wrapped around the axon form the myelin sheath which is interrupted at the nodes of Ranvier. At the neuromuscular junction the axon loses its myelin and branches to form the presynaptic terminal

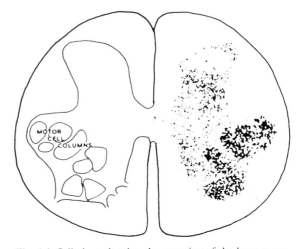

Fig. 1.2 Cell chart showing the grouping of the large motor neurones in the anterior horns of the spinal cord. The outlines of the columns of motor neurones innervating individual muscles, determined from the study of polio patients, are shown on the left (from Sharrard 1955, by courtesy of H. A. Sissons: Disorders of Voluntary Muscle, 3rd edn.)

associated fibrous components of the extracellular matrix including collagen and elastin.

The spinal motor neurones innervating an individual muscle lie in a more or less well-defined 'column', two or three segments long, within the anterior horn of the spinal cord (Romanes 1940, 1941, Sharrard 1955) (Fig. 1.2). The columns for more proximal muscles tend to lie medial to those supplying more distal muscles although there is a good deal of overlap. The motor axons leave the spinal cord at discrete points where they gather together to form the ventral roots, each root containing axons destined for many muscles. Motor axons of the ventral roots join with sensory axons of the dorsal roots to form the *peripheral nerves*. A cross-section of a peripheral nerve (Fig. 1.3) reveals that the myelinated axons normally consist of two distinct populations with respect to size. The largest axons, some 8–20 μm in diameter in man, include the alpha motor axons that innervate the muscle fibres of the motor units, and the sensory afferents from the specialised intrafusal muscle fibres of the muscle spindles and the Golgi tendon organs (see below). The smallest axons, 1–8 μm in diameter, include the gamma motor axons that innervate the intrafusal muscle fibres and small sensory axons.

In the periphery, the axons destined for a single

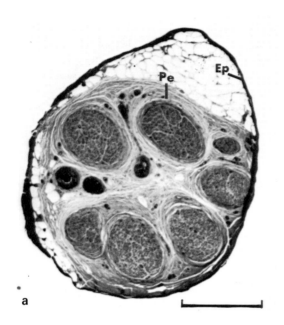

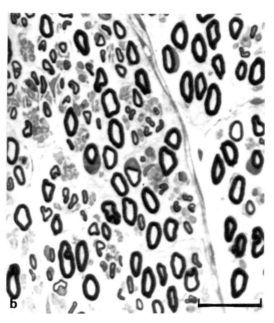

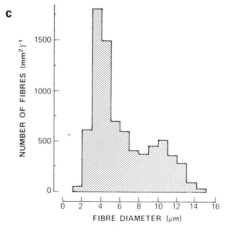

Fig. 1.3 The structure of peripheral nerve (human sural nerve). a. Low power view of transverse section showing fascicles, epineurium (Ep) and perineurium (Pe). Scale bar = 0.5 nm   b. Higher power view showing large and small diameter myelinated axons. Scale bar = 25 μm   c. Frequency distribution of myelinated nerve fibre diameters (after Asbury & Johnson 1978)

muscle come together and separate from the main trunk to form a well-defined muscle nerve. In most muscle nerves, about half of the myelinated axons are motor and half sensory (Boyd & Davey 1968). Until such a nerve reaches its target muscle, the axons rarely branch. Within the muscle, extensive branching at the nodes of Ranvier leads to the formation of numerous intra-muscular nerve bundles from which individual axons split off to innervate each muscle fibre.

Peripheral nerves are surrounded by a tough connective tissue sheath, the *epineurium*. Within the nerve, axons are grouped into fascicles, each surrounded by a further sheath, the *perineurium* (Fig. 1.3a).

Muscle

Each motor neurone innervates a large number of *skeletal muscle* fibres (Fig. 1.4), all contained within the same muscle. In man most motor units contain 100–1000 muscle fibres but some may have as many as 10 000 (Cooper 1966). Individual muscle fibres are usually between 10 and 100 μm in diameter and between a few millimetres and several centimetres long. In the light microscope, muscle fibres exhibit transverse striations. These result from alternating arrays of two types of longitudinally oriented contractile filaments. The *thin filaments* are composed mainly of the protein *actin* while the *thick filaments* are based on *myosin*. The repeating unit, from the centre of one group of thin filaments to the centre of the next group, is the *sarcomere*, and is usually 2.5–3.5 μm long. Muscle contraction results from an interaction between the thin filaments and molecular 'cross-bridges' protruding from the thick filaments. This interaction generates a force which causes the filaments to slide past each other, making the muscle fibre shorten or develop tension. The details of muscle fibre ultrastructure are described in Chapter 2.

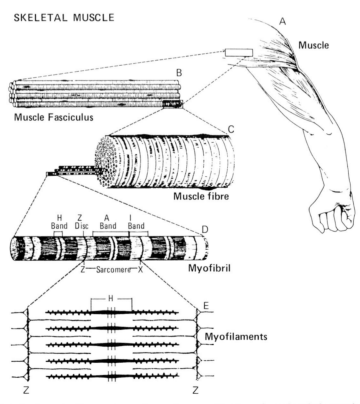

Fig. 1.4 Organisation of skeletal muscle. Progressing, at increasing magnifications, from the whole muscle (A) , to a fascicle (B) and a single muscle fibre (C). At the sub-cellular level, the muscle fibre contains myofibrils (D) which are bundles of contractile filaments (E) (after Bloom & Fawcett 1968)

Muscle fibres arise during development by the fusion of numerous myogenic cells and therefore contain many nuclei within a common cytoplasm. There are usually about a hundred nuclei per millimetre of muscle fibre. Each muscle fibre is contained within a stocking-like layer of extracellular matrix, the *basal lamina*, strengthened with fibres of collagen. Closely associated with each muscle fibre, lying within the basal lamina sheath, are numerous *satellite cells*. During muscle growth or regeneration, the satellite cells divide and apparently provide a supply of new muscle-forming cells. The number of satellite cells associated with a given muscle fibre varies, but is usually between 1% and 10% of the number of myonuclei. The ends of each muscle fibre are connected to the tendons by an elaboration of the connective tissue sheath, joined to the fibre at the *myo-tendinous junction*.

Muscle fibres are grouped within the muscles into fascicles, each with its own vascular supply and connective tissue sheath (*perimysium*). Fascicles vary greatly in size, but in man typically contain about a thousand fibres. Each fascicle contains fibres belonging to a number of motor units, and these are extensively intermixed. Indeed, in most normal muscles, it is rare for a muscle fibre to lie adjacent to another fibre from the same motor unit (Edström & Kugelberg 1968). Although they are widely dispersed, the fibres of an individual motor unit generally occupy only a part of the total muscle cross-section. The muscle as a whole is enclosed in a tough *epimysium*.

Several distinct classes, or 'types', of muscle fibre are present in most muscles, each of which is characterised by a functionally interrelated set of properties which suit it for a particular form of contraction (see below). An important principle of motor unit organisation is that all the fibres of any one motor unit have very similar properties. Thus each motor unit can itself be considered as being of a particular type, to be used in a characteristic way, appropriate to its functional properties.

Neuromuscular junction

Nerve impulses are transmitted to an individual muscle fibre at a highly specialised site of contact, the *neuromuscular junction*, also referred to as the *motor end-plate* (Fig. 1.5). At these junctions, the nerve action potential causes the release of a chemical transmitter, acetylcholine, which acts on specialised proteins in the membrane of the muscle fibre to initiate an action potential in the muscle fibre. This, in turn, leads to the rapid activation of the contractile apparatus of the muscle cell (see Ch. 3 for details of the process of neuromuscular transmission).

In mammalian muscle fibres, a single neuromuscular junction about 25–50 μm long is normally present, approximately equidistant from the fibre ends. As a motor axon makes contact with the muscle, it forms a number of fine unmyelinated terminal branches. These branches are accommodated in depressions ('gutters') in a dome of specialised cytoplasm and capped by extensions of the terminal Schwann cells. With the electron microscope (see Ch. 2), it can be seen that the plasma membrane of the axon terminal remains separated from that of the postsynaptic membrane of the muscle fibre by a gap of about 50 nm and a single layer of specialised synaptic basal lamina.

The postsynaptic membrane is thrown into numerous tight folds, about 1 μm deep, initially recognised with the light microscope and referred to as the 'subneural apparatus' (Couteaux 1960). Within the synaptic region, a number of functionally important molecules are present in high density, including acetylcholine receptors, voltage-dependent Na^+ channels and the enzyme acetylcholinesterase (see below and Ch. 3 for further details). In recent years, the use of methods which allow these components to be visualised has shown how closely their distribution is matched to the regions of contact with the motor axon terminal and to each other (Fig. 1.5). Beneath the postsynaptic membrane is an accumulation of a number of components of the cytoskeleton (Froehner 1986) and a cluster of 5–10 myonuclei. These subsynaptic components may help to maintain the local high concentration of synaptic molecules.

Sensory structures

In addition to the cells of the motor unit proper, each muscle contains sensory structures which convey information about muscle length and tension to the central nervous system (Kuffler et al 1984). The cell bodies of the sensory neurones associated with these structures are located in the

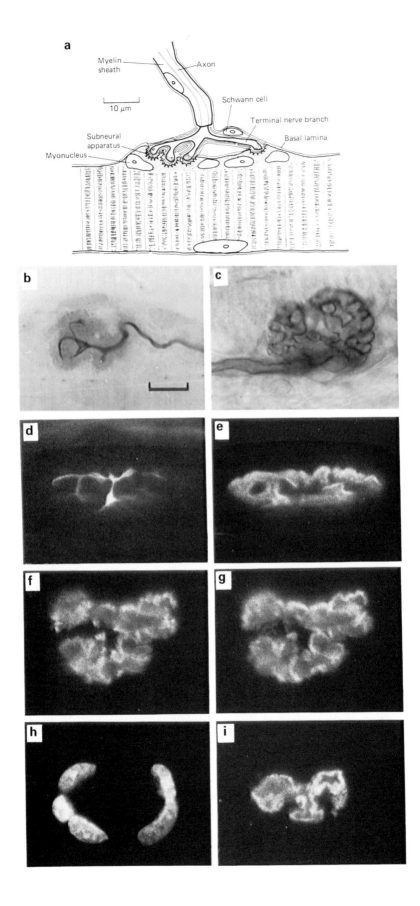

a

Myelin sheath

Axon

Schwann cell

Terminal nerve branch

Basal lamina

10 μm

Subneural apparatus

Myonucleus

dorsal root ganglia. From here they send one process centrally to make synaptic contact with as many as 300–400 spinal motor neurones, while their peripheral axon forms the sensory afferent.

Muscle spindles consist of a bundle of four to six specialised *intrafusal muscle fibres*. The endings of sensory axons make contact with these fibres and generate nerve impulses when the length of the muscle changes. Two types of sensory neurone innervate each spindle: large-diameter Group IA afferents form *primary endings* near the centre of each intrafusal fibre and smaller Group II afferent axons make less elaborate *secondary endings*. The two types of ending and the structures asssociated with them are generally specialised to allow them to respond either to the absolute length of the muscle or to changes in that length. The intrafusal fibres also receive motor innervation from small *gamma motor neurones*. While contraction of these fibres generates little tension, it serves to keep the spindle taut when the muscle contracts and thus allows the sensory ending to respond to stretch over a range of muscle lengths. The discharge from the spindle afferents is relayed directly to the ipsilateral spinal motor neurones innervating the muscle in which the spindle is found.

Golgi tendon organs are located at the ends of the muscle fibres. Each tendon organ is formed from a common tendon to which a number of muscle fibres are attached. The sensory nerve ending wraps around this tendon and responds when tension is generated by contraction of any of the muscle fibres ending on it. The discharge from a Golgi tendon organ is also 'fed' to the ipsilateral alpha motor neurones where it is inhibitory.

FUNCTIONAL ORGANISATION OF THE MOTOR UNIT

Motor neurone

The dexterity typical of voluntary movements in mammals requires the precise control of the motor

units in each muscle. The nerve impulses that trigger motor unit contraction arise as a result of the combined effects of as many as 10 000 excitatory and inhibitory synaptic inputs impinging on each motor neurone. These inputs originate from higher levels in the central nervous system, interneurones within the spinal cord, and sensory neurones innervating muscle, joints and skin (Kuffler et al 1984, Kandel & Schwartz 1985).

Motor neurones have a resting membrane potential of between -60 and -70 mV. Propagated action potentials are generated only when the membrane potential is reduced to a threshold level of about -50 mV. A typical excitatory synaptic input generates a postsynaptic depolarisation of less than 250 μV. As a result, action potentials are generated only when a large number of different excitatory inputs discharge more or less synchronously (spatial summation) or a smaller number of inputs discharge at a high frequency so that the individual synaptic potentials sum (temporal summation). Inhibitory synaptic inputs also exhibit spatial and temporal summation, but their effect is primarily to decrease the electrical resistance of the cell membrane and to stabilise the membrane potential at a value near to the resting potential. In the spinal motor neurone, the inhibitory input probably causes an increase in K^+ conductance, leading to a small hyperpolarisation, and in Cl^--conductance.

When the net effect of excitatory and inhibitory inputs is a depolarisation which exceeds the threshold, a regenerative, Na^+-dependent action potential is generated at the *axon hillock*, the site of origin of the motor axon (Fig. 1.1). This region is particularly sensitive to depolarisation because it has a very high local density of the voltage-sensitive Na^+ channels which are responsible for the regenerative nature of the action potential (Kandel & Schwartz 1985). This property is shared with action potential generating regions in other cells such as the node of Ranvier of myeli-

Fig. 1.5 The neuromuscular junction: a. the principal cellular and sub-cellular components; b. silver stain shows the axon and its terminal branches (human); c. the myelin is stained with Sudan black and the postsynaptic region with a histochemical reaction for AChE (rat); d & e. two views of a rat junction in which the nerve is stained with an antibody to neurofilament protein (d) and the AChR with a fluorescent conjugate of alpha-bungarotoxin(fl-BgTx) (e); f & g. two views of another rat junction in which the AChE is stained with a fluorescent antibody (f) and the AChR with fl-BgTx (g); h & i. views of a human junction in which the cluster of myonuclei have been stained with a fluorescent dye (h) and the AChR with fl-BgTx (i). The scale bar in b = 10 μm and applies to frames b-i

nated axons and the postsynaptic membrane of the neuromuscular junction.

Motor axon

The motor axon and the Schwann cells associated with it act together as a functional unit, the physiological behaviour of the axon being determined as much by the presence of the myelin as by the basic properties of the axonal membrane. In unmyelinated axons, impulses propagate continuously; the ionic currents generated by activity in one region spread along the axon and excite the adjacent nerve membrane. The speed of nerve impulse propagation is determined by the rate at which such currents can depolarise the membrane to the threshold for action potential generation. This is limited both by the resistance to the flow of current through the axoplasm and the amount of current taken up in charging the large electrical capacitance of the plasma membrane. In larger diameter unmyelinated axons, because the longitudinal resistance to current flow is less, impulses are conducted faster than in smaller axons (Hursh 1939).

In a myelinated axon, the insulation afforded by the myelin sheath restricts the flow of current across the membrane and greatly reduces the membrane's effective capacitance. As a result, most of the current entering the axon in an active region leaves the axon by crossing the naked membrane at the nodes of Ranvier. To take advantage of this situation, voltage-dependent Na^+ channels are normally concentrated in the nodal membrane but are largely absent in the internodal region (Waxman & Ritchie 1985). The net effect is that the nerve impulse 'jumps' rapidly from one node to the next ('saltatory' conduction) and the overall conduction velocity is much faster than that for an unmyelinated axon of the same size.

The velocity of action potential propagation in myelinated axons is influenced by several structural factors. As in unmyelinated axons, the larger the diameter of the axon the greater the conduction velocity. In addition, increasing the thickness of the myelin sheath improves its insulating properties and this, too, speeds conduction. On biophysical grounds, Rushton (1951) pointed out that there should be an optimal ratio between the

diameter of the axon and the external diameter of the myelin sheath, and that this ratio should be the same irrespective of the actual size of the nerve fibre. In practice, for large axons this is true, and the ratio is approximately 0.7 (Gasser & Grundfest 1939).

Conduction velocity is also influenced by the distance between successive nodes of Ranvier, as this determines the length of the 'jumps' taken by the nerve impulse. In general, internodal length is proportional to axon diameter (Fig. 1.6a), although the constant of proportionality is not the same in all nerves (Bradley 1974): action potentials in larger-diameter nerve fibres therefore move in longer jumps. However, because current spreads

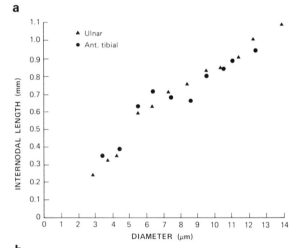

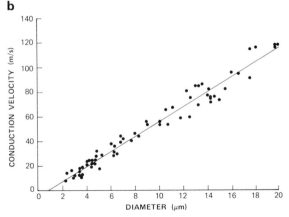

Fig. 1.6 Properties of myelinated axons. a. Internodal length is directly related to nerve fibre diameter (data from Vizoso 1950 for human ulnar and anterior tibial nerves). b. Action potential conduction velocity is similarly related to fibre diameter (after Hursh 1939)

more rapidly in larger axons, the time taken for each jump is roughly constant (about 15 μs for limb nerves). The combined effect of all these relationships is that there is a direct proportionality between action potential conduction velocity and nerve fibre diameter in myelinated nerves (Fig. 1.6b), as in unmyelinated ones, although for somewhat different reasons. For most myelinated axons, the constant of proportionality is 6 m/s/μm diameter (Hursh 1939).

It follows from what has been said above, that action potentials in large myelinated axons may travel at more than 100 m/s whereas those in the smaller axons travel at about 6–60 m/s. As the main peak of the action potential lasts about 1 ms, it may 'occupy' a distance of up to 100 mm (equivalent to about 100 internodes) in a large-diameter axon. Thus, although the process of excitation moves discontinuously from node to node, the resulting potential change travels more smoothly.

Axonal transport of material. As in most cells, the synthesis of macromolecules in motor neurones occurs in the vicinity of the nucleus. An important feature of the motor neurone is that the synthesis of new proteins occurs only in the cell body. To enable proteins, as well as other new membrane components and mitochondria, to reach the axon and its terminals, specialised transport mechanisms are present within the axon (Grafstein & Forman 1980, Alberts et al 1983).

Two mechanisms of axonal transport have been discovered. One operates at a rate of about 1 mm/day ('slow' transport) and represents the rate of synthesis and 'extrusion' of new components of the axonal cytoplasm. These include the main elements of the cytoskeleton and many soluble cytoplasmic proteins. The second mechanism is much faster (100–400 mm/day) and involves the movement of membrane-bound vesicles containing the transported substances along the axonal microtubules. This process now appears to be mediated by mechano-protein cross-links between the vesicles and the microtubules which are probably analogous in their operation to the myosin cross-bridges in muscle (Miller & Lasek 1985). This 'fast' transport also operates in a retrograde direction, conveying to the cell body

material which enters the axoplasm at the terminal.

Neuromuscular junction

At the neuromuscular junction, both the nerve and muscle cells are highly specialised to carry out the process of neuromuscular transmission, which is described in detail by Wray in Chapter 3. Within the axon terminal, the neurotransmitter acetylcholine (ACh) is synthesised from choline and acetylCoA in a reaction catalysed by the enzyme choline acetyltransferase (ChAT; EC 2.3.1.6). Up to 90% of the total active ChAT in muscle is located within the nerve terminals; it is transported there from its site of synthesis in the cell body.

The resting concentration of choline in cholinergic neurones is much higher than typical concentrations for plasma or interstitial fluid and is maintained at such a high level, partly because there is a continual turnover of phospholipids in cells and partly because cholinergic neurones possess a high-affinity uptake system for the accumulation of free choline from the interstitial fluid. At times of accelerated ACh synthesis, as during high levels of synaptic activity, the uptake of choline is enhanced so that the choline released by hydrolysis of ACh in the synaptic cleft (see below) can be reutilised. The details of ACh release are considered in Chapter 3.

The postsynaptic surface of the muscle cell is also highly differentiated. Of most immediate significance to neuromuscular transmission is the presence of a high density of ACh receptors (AChR). On binding ACh, these complex membrane proteins form an ion channel which allows a net entry of positive ions into the muscle fibre, thus generating a local depolarisation, the *end-plate potential*. As at the motor axon hillock and the node of Ranvier, a high density of voltage-dependent Na+ channels is present in the muscle fibre membrane at the neuromuscular junction (Angelides 1986) and allows the end-plate potential to generate a muscle fibre action potential.

Acetylcholine is released from the nerve terminal in packets of several thousand molecules. In normal circumstances, several hundred such packets· are released by a single nerve impulse.

This is considerably more transmitter than is necessary to bring the muscle fibre to the action potential threshold. As a result of this high *safety factor*, the process of neuromuscular transmission is normally very reliable, even during repetitive activity when the amount of transmitter released may decline slightly (Elmqvist & Quastel 1965).

The activity of the ACh released by a nerve impulse is terminated by hydrolysis by the enzyme acetylcholinesterase (AChE; EC 3.1,1,7) and by diffusion out of the synaptic cleft. AChE is a highly polymorphic enzyme and numerous forms exist in skeletal muscle (Massoulié & Bon 1982). Most of the functionally significant AChE is located, not in the muscle fibre itself, but in the synaptic basal lamina (McMahan et al 1978). Because the synaptic gap is very narrow, most of the ACh released from the nerve is able to reach and bind to AChR before it can be hydrolysed by the intervening AChE. However, as individual ACh molecules dissociate from AChR, they are generally broken down before they are able to bind a second time. Drugs that block AChE activity allow individual ACh molecules to bind repeatedly and thus prolong the synaptic currents that flow as a result of ACh action.

Skeletal muscle

An action potential generated at the neuromuscular junction propagates towards the ends of the muscle fibre at a velocity of about 5 m/s. The wave of depolarisation is carried to the interior of the muscle fibre by tubular invaginations of the plasma membrane, the transverse tubules (or *T-tubules*). Depolarisation of the T-tubules causes the release of Ca^{2+} from the extensive *sarcoplasmic reticulum* (SR), a specialised form of endoplasmic reticulum, into the cytoplasm. When the concentration of free Ca^{2+} in the vicinity of the contractile filaments reaches about $10^{-6}M$ (it is normally about $10^{-8}M$), interaction between myosin cross-bridges and the thin filaments can take place and contraction ensues. The cyclic making and breaking of actin–myosin cross-bridges, which accounts for contraction, is powered by the hydrolysis of ATP in a reaction catalysed by ATPase activity associated with the myosin cross-bridges. The interaction between thick and thin

filaments comes to an end and the muscle relaxes when the Ca^{2+} released into the cytoplasm is reaccumulated by the SR. (See Ch. 2 and Ch. 4 for further details of the ultrastructural and molecular basis of muscle contraction.)

Isometric contractions. Most experimental studies of muscle contraction are made with the ends of the muscle rigidly fixed so that shortening does not occur. In these *isometric* conditions the response to a single muscle fibre action potential is a *twitch*, an increase in tension which rises to a peak in less than 100 ms and decays slightly more slowly. If the muscle is stimulated repetitively at a frequency greater than about 5 Hz, successive twitches sum and a greater maximum tension is produced than in a single twitch. As the frequency of stimulation is increased to about 50–200 Hz, the individual responses 'fuse' to form a *tetanus*, a smooth and rapid increase in tension rising to a stable plateau (Fig. 1.7). At still higher frequencies there is no further increase in peak tension, although the rate of rise of tension may continue to increase (Harris & Wilson 1971).

The characteristics of the isometric response depend not only on the contractile events themselves, but also on the high degree of elasticity associated with the muscle. This elasticity, which is effectively in series with the contractile appar-

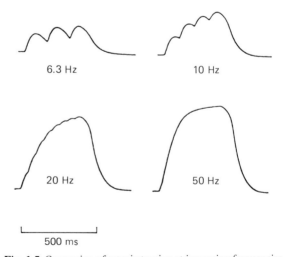

Fig. 1.7 Generation of tetanic tension at increasing frequencies of stimulation. Rat soleus muscle stimulated at 6.3, 10, 20 and 50 impulses/s (adapted from Buller A J Disorders of voluntary muscle, 3rd edn. Fig. 2.1)

atus, is present both in the tendons and connective tissue sheaths, and within the sarcomeres themselves. If it were possible to remove all of the elasticity from the muscle, a muscle action potential would result in the prompt generation of all the tension the contractile component could bear. Repetitive stimulation would merely prolong the period of tension and would have no effect on the amount of tension recorded. As it is, the series elasticity must be stretched before the full tension generated by the contractile component can be recorded.

Hill (1949) considered the amount of tension a muscle could bear at any moment (as opposed to the amount that could be recorded) as a measure of the intensity of the 'active state'. In a single twitch, the active state lasts for only a few ms. (In a mammalian muscle it may not even be fully expressed after a single action potential.) Because it takes a relatively long time to stretch the elastic component, the active state begins to decline as the tension is still rising. With repetitive stimulation, the active state is prolonged, the elastic component becomes more fully stretched, and more tension is recorded. At the appropriate frequency, the developed tension reaches the maximum that the contractile component can generate: this maximal tetanic tension is often referred to as 'P$_o$' and in mammalian muscle is typically 5–10 times greater than the tension in a twitch.

The absolute amount of tension generated in a contraction is proportional to the number of inter-filament cross-bridges that can be made. This depends in turn on two structural features of the muscle. The first is the cross-sectional area of the contractile material: in general, most of the bulk of the muscle fibre is occupied by the thick and thin filaments which are very regularly spaced; as a result, the total tension a muscle can generate is closely related to its total cross-sectional area.

The magnitude of the contraction is also dependent on the length of the muscle. This property may be studied by constructing a length–tension diagram as shown in Fig. 1.8. First the passive tension, which results solely from the elastic component, is measured in the unstimulated muscle at different muscle lengths. Next the total tension during a maximal tetanic contrac-

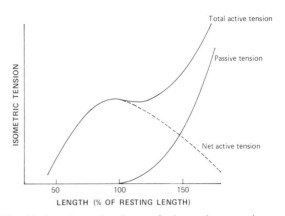

Fig. 1.8 Length–tension diagram for isometric contractions. Passive tension is measured in the unstimulated muscle. Total active tension is the tension generated during maximal tetanic stimulation at each length. Net active tension, the difference between the two other curves, is the tension generated by the contractile component itself

tion is measured at a variety of muscle lengths. This tension represents the sum of both elastic and contractile components. When the passive tension is subtracted from the total tension ('net active tension'), the tension generated by the contractile component itself is obtained. This curve shows that a muscle can generate its maximal active tension only over a narrow range of lengths. The optimal length, at which the muscle generates the greatest tension, is that at which the thin filaments just completely overlap the region of the thick filaments that bears the cross-bridges, and thus permits the maximum number of cross-bridge interactions to occur (Gordon et al 1966).

Isotonic contractions. If an active muscle is allowed to shorten against a constant load, the contraction is said to be isotonic. The rate of shortening is maximal when no load is being lifted but decreases as the load is increased (Aidley 1978). Pure isometric or isotonic contractions rarely occur in the body: most contractions are hybrids involving both load-bearing and short-ening; moreover many are 'eccentric', a term applied to the condition where a muscle is stretched while it is still developing tension. Eccentric contractions are probably used primarily to stabilise a limb in a rigid position. Although in most circumstances they involve relatively small 'stretches', they result in the rapid onset of fatigue and may be damaging (Edwards et al 1981). They are poorly understood, and the features that allow elongation without causing major damage have not been well studied.

MOTOR UNIT SPECIALISATION AND PATTERNS OF USE

Muscle fibre diversity

Mammalian motor units contract at different speeds (Close 1972). In most muscles, two distinct classes or 'types' of unit can be distinguished: 'slow-twitch' or Type I, and 'fast-twitch' or Type II (Fig. 1.9). The precise speed of contraction varies greatly from animal to animal; e.g. in a mouse, a typical fast motor unit reaches its peak tension (T_c) after a single stimulus in about 6 ms, whereas in a cat T_c is typically 25 ms and in man about 35 ms. The T_c of slow units in these species is typically 20 ms, 75 ms and 90 ms respectively. In man, and possibly in several other species, the differentiation of motor units into fast-twitch and slow-twitch is rather arbitrary because in most muscles there is a continuum of motor unit twitch

speeds rather than two distinct populations (Freund 1983). Muscles which have a marked predominance of one type of muscle fibre are themselves either fast or slow. As slow muscles tend to be reddish in appearance, because of their large myoglobin content, the terms 'slow, red' and 'fast, white' have entered the scientific vocabulary.

Two factors are chiefly responsible for determining the speed of contraction of an individual muscle fibre. The first is the particular species of contractile proteins present (Pette & Vrbová 1985). Both actin and myosin, as well as most of the regulatory proteins associated with them, exist in several closely related 'isoforms' (see Ch. 4). Myosin has been most carefully studied in this respect; distinct isoforms exist in fast and slow muscle fibres, as well as in fetal and neonatal muscles. Because the ATPase activity of slow myosin is less than that of fast, appropriate histochemical methods for the demonstration of ATPase activity can distinguish fast from slow fibres. More recently, monoclonal antibodies specific for the different myosin isoforms have come to be used for the same purpose.

While the contractile proteins present determine the speed of contraction, the speed of relaxation — and hence the frequency of repetitive stimulation a muscle fibre can 'follow' — is largely determined by the rate of calcium uptake into the SR. Fast fibres have more extensive SR than slow fibres (Eisenberg & Kuda 1976) and are much richer in the Ca^{2+}–Mg^{2+} ATPase that is responsible for Ca^{2+} uptake (Pette & Vrbová 1985).

Fast and slow muscle fibres have also long been known to differ in their patterns of energy metabolism. Slow-twitch muscle fibres rely on oxidative mechanisms for the generation of energy whereas fast-twitch fibres rely on glycolysis, either on its own ('fast, glycolytic' or Type IIB fibres) or in combination with oxidative mechanisms ('fast, oxidative-glycolytic' or Type IIA fibres). In keeping with these patterns, slow-twitch fibres have more mitochondria and are more highly vascularised than fast-twitch fibres (Eisenberg & Kuda 1976).

Closely related to the pattern of energy metabolism is the ability of the muscle to sustain contraction. Whereas muscle fibres with oxidative

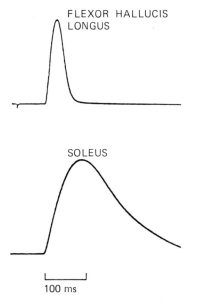

Fig. 1.9 Isometric twitches in a fast (flexor hallucis longus) and a slow (soleus) muscle of the cat (from Buller & Lewis 1963)

metabolism are able to produce substantial tension for some minutes ('fatigue-resistant'), those utilising glycolytic pathways fatigue rapidly in the face of sustained stimulation ('fatiguable'). Because metabolic and contractile properties are normally closely coupled in individual muscle fibres, histochemical procedures which demonstrate the activity of mitochondrial enzymes, such as succinate dehydrogenase, show higher activity in those fibres with low myosin-ATPase activity while procedures for enzymes of glycolysis, such as phosphorylase, show greater activity in high-ATPase fibres.

The general correlation between the speed of contraction of a muscle and the metabolic properties of its muscle fibres suggested to Henneman and his colleagues that individual motor units might be composed of fibres of a single metabolic type (Henneman & Olsen 1965, Wuerker et al 1965). This was subsequently elegantly confirmed by a number of studies (Edström & Kugelberg 1968, Burke et al 1973, Nemeth et al 1981). These all demonstrated that, whether one considers molecules related to the speed of contraction or to energy metabolism, all the muscle fibres in a given motor unit are essentially identical. Thus the motor unit itself may be considered to be 'fast, fatiguable', 'slow, fatigue-resistant' or to be of an intermediate type.

Fatigue of muscles. It is a common experience that sick people complain of feeling 'tired', 'weak' or 'fatigued', but it is clear that these expressions do not always refer to muscle fatigue itself. In the normal healthy person, however, muscle 'fatigue' usually follows a period of extremely strenuous activity, or a period of continuous low-level activity. We may therefore define fatigue as the condition in which muscles fail to maintain tension, or fail to develop constant tension, in response to stimulation at a constant frequency. The stimulus may be imposed or generated voluntarily.

Muscle fatigue in healthy people does not result from a failure of neuromuscular transmission or from a failure of the action potential mechanism in nerve or muscle, because the relevant safety factors are too high. Rather, fatigue arises either from a failure of excitation–contraction coupling

(Edwards et al 1977) or from a depletion of energy resources (Dawson et al 1978). These two alternatives are not mutually exclusive, but Fitch & McComas (1985) have presented compelling evidence that, at least during relatively high rates of stimulation (electrical stimulation of the nerve at 20 Hz or maximal voluntary contractions lasting 90 s), the dominant factor is the depletion of energy resources.

Vascular supply. The different patterns of energy metabolism of fast and slow motor units require that the microcirculation is appropriately organised. Ranvier (1874) is credited with being the first to observe that red muscles have a higher capillarity than white, a feature now documented by many others. As a result of the higher capillarity, blood flow through the predominantly slow soleus muscle of the cat during normal standing (approximately 50 ml/100 g per min) is much higher than through the gastrocnemius (approximately 14 ml/100 g per min) (Hilton et al 1970). In mixed muscles, blood flow at rest tends to be proportional to the number of slow fibres. As muscle activity increases, blood flow increases to become proportional to the number of fast muscle fibres, and particularly the fast oxidative–glycolytic fibres (Laughlin & Armstrong 1982). This increase in blood flow does not result simply from the selective dilatation of small blood vessels to fast fibres; blood supply to the viscera is decreased and cardiac output is also increased.

In some quadrupeds, there is a clear segregation of slow motor units into those muscles that are involved with posture, such as soleus, and fast motor units into those muscles concerned with rapid movements, such as extensor digitorum longus. In humans, the extent of such segregation is not so clear. None the less, there is great variation in the proportions of the various muscle fibre types in human muscles and it is reasonable to assume that this is of functional significance.

Motor neurone diversity

Motor neurones, as well as muscle fibres, show considerable diversity of form and function. One of the most important properties to show variation is the size of the cell body. The functional significance of cell size derives from its electrical conse-quences; the resistance of a cell is inversely related to its size. A given synaptic current therefore generates a larger voltage change in a small cell than in a large one. For a given intensity of excit-atory synaptic input to the 'pool' of motor neurones innervating a single muscle, small cells are more likely to reach threshold than large ones (Kernell 1966, Burke 1967). By the same token, a given inhibitory input has a more powerful effect on a small cell than on a large one. This effect of cell size on excitability influences the order in which motor units are recruited as the strength of muscle activation is increased (see below) as well as the order in which they 'drop out' as activation decreases (see summary by DeLuca 1985).

Low threshold motor neurones, presumed to be relatively small in size, also have relatively small-diameter axons. Because action potential conduc-tion velocity is inversely related to axon diameter (see above) action potentials generated in low-threshold neurones are conducted more slowly than those in high-threshold neurones. Further-more, action potentials in 'slow' motor neurones, but not in 'fast', are followed by a characteristic 'after-hyperpolarisation' which prolongs the 'refractory period' during which another action potential cannot be generated (Eccles et al 1958). Thus, the motor neurones innervating 'fast' and 'slow' muscle fibres have distinctive functional properties and are themselves 'fast' and 'slow', although in a different sense to the muscle fibres they innervate.

The presynaptic terminals of fast and slow motor neurones differ in structural complexity: those of fast neurones have more terminal branches and synaptic boutons than those of slow neurones (Korneliussen & Waerhaug 1973, Ogata & Yamasaki 1985). The functional significance of these structural differences is not yet known.

Matching of nerve and muscle properties

Not surprisingly, the functional properties of the motor neurone and muscle fibres comprising a given motor unit are carefully matched. Slowly contracting motor units are innervated by low-threshold motor neurones, the axons of which conduct relatively slowly. The long after-hyper-

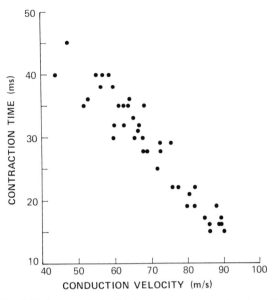

Fig. 1.10 Inverse relationship between the contraction time of a motor unit (the time to peak tension of an isometric twitch) and the conduction velocity of the motor axon in the first superficial lumbrical muscle of the cat (data from Appelber & Emonet-Dénand 1967)

polarisation in these neurones helps to ensure that the frequency of firing is relatively low. In contrast, rapidly contracting units are innervated by relatively high-threshold motor neurones with rapidly conducting action potentials which can occur in high-frequency bursts. As a result, when a large number of motor units is studied, there is a close correlation between motor axon conduction velocity and contraction speed (Fig. 1.10).

A second important aspect of nerve–muscle matching is that 'large' motor neurones innervate 'large' motor units. More strictly, the tension generated by motor units innervated by high-threshold, rapidly conducting motor neurones is generally greater than that generated by units innervated by low-threshold, slowly conducting neurones (see below).

Patterns of motor unit use

The strength of muscle contraction can be increased by the central nervous system in two ways: either by changing the number of active motor units ('recruitment') or by altering the frequency of firing so that successive twitches begin to sum and the tension generated by individual units increases ('frequency coding') (Freund 1983).

Recruitment order. In a given set of circumstances, the order in which motor units are recruited is relatively constant and related to their 'size', as defined by the amount of tension they generate. As a muscle is activated from rest, the first units to be recruited are usually the weakest. As increasing strength of contraction is called for, larger and larger units are recruited. As a result of this pattern of excitation, each newly recruited unit adds a roughly constant proportion of the background contractile strength (Fig. 1.11). The orderly recruitment of motor units according to their size ('size principle') has been considered in detail by Henneman and his colleagues (Henneman et al 1965) and has been shown to apply in many, although perhaps not all (Sica & McComas 1971, Wyman et al 1974) situations. In any case, the precise order in which motor units are recruited is not rigidly fixed. In muscles in which a range of movements is possible, the

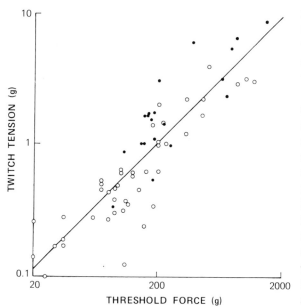

Fig. 1.11 Direct relationship between the threshold force at which a particular motor unit is normally excited and the twitch tension of the motor unit, determined in the first dorsal interosseous muscle of man. Open and filled circles are results from two experiments on the same subject (from Milner-Brown et al 1973)

particular order of recruitment may depend on the movement being made (Denier van der Gon et al 1982), probably as a consequence of differing descending inputs to the motor neurones for each different class or direction of movement.

Although the order in which motor units are recruited is fixed for a particular movement, the absolute tension at which recruitment occurs depends very much on the speed with which the movement is made. As the speed increases, the threshold for all units falls, with the result that large units are used transiently when it is necessary to develop tension rapidly (Freund 1983).

Firing patterns. Many early studies (reviewed by Freund 1983) pointed to differences in the firing patterns of motor neurones. Eccles and his colleagues showed that, in cats, the motor neurones innervating postural muscles such as the soleus were active in quiet standing and inhibited when the flexors were excited (Eccles et al 1958). Burke and his colleagues showed that, even in mixed muscles, slow units were active during quiet standing and that during movement, when fast units were activated, slow units were inhibited (Burke et al 1970). This was an important observation because it indicated that the pattern of activity of a motor unit is related to its functional type regardless of the particular muscle it is in.

During activity, the firing patterns of fast and slow motor units differ considerably. In general, slow motor neurones discharge continuously at a frequency of about 10–20 Hz. In contrast, fast motor neurones usually discharge in short, high-frequency (up to 100 Hz) bursts. Hennig & Lømo (1985) made a detailed study of the relationship between firing patterns and motor unit tension in fast and slow muscles of the rat. They found that the slow motor units of the soleus muscle fired more or less continuously at about 20 Hz, at which rate they generate 50–80 % of their maximal tetanic force. Similarly, fast motor units, when active, fired at a mean frequency of about 80 Hz at which rate they, too, generate 50–80 % of their maximal force. In units of both types, small changes in frequency of activation lead to substantial changes in tension. These results show that the firing pattern of a motor neurone is well matched to the contractile properties of the muscle fibres it innervates.

The distinctions between slow and fast motor units, involving excitation threshold, pattern of activity, contractile speed and pattern of energy metabolism, suit them to distinctive physiological roles. Slow-twitch units are easily activated. Through their reliance on abundantly available energy stores of carbohydrate and fat, in combination with a good oxygen delivery system, they are able to maintain tension for prolonged periods. However, they lack the ability to contract rapidly. They are thus well suited for the moderate but continuous contractions required to maintain posture and in prolonged exertion. By contrast, fast-twitch units are specialised for explosive, short-term activity where considerable loads are to be borne and their energy source, glycogen, is rapidly available but relatively quickly exhausted.

The central control of motor unit activity is beyond the scope of this chapter. Clearly, the activity of sensory receptors in the muscle, joints and skin, the interneurones and recurrent motor axon collaterals in the spinal cord, and descending pathways from higher centres all influence the pattern of motor unit activation (see, e.g, Kuffler et al 1984).

MOTOR UNIT PLASTICITY

So far, we have considered the motor unit as if the properties of its cells, and the relationships between them, were fixed. In most biological systems, including the neuromuscular system, functional interrelationships are maintained by the interplay of numerous dynamic interactions: this gives the overall system the advantage of adaptability. There are two main ways in which the performance of the neuromuscular system adapts to changes in conditions: one is through alterations in the patterns of motor unit activation by the central nervous system and is beyond the scope of this chapter; the other is through changes in the properties of the units themselves. In the rest of this chapter, we consider how the properties of motor units vary during development, the nature and limits of their adaptability in the mature individual, the response of the motor unit

to injury and, finally, how the adaptive potential of the motor unit helps to reduce the functional impact of the loss of motor units during ageing.

Development of the motor unit

The formation of the neuromuscular system, although a continuous process, can be divided into two distinctive phases: in the first, the various cells that give rise to nerve and muscle interact to form a system that is immature, but none the less functional; in the second phase this immature system undergoes numerous transformations which shape the fully mature motor units. The cell–cell interactions involved in the first phase precede the development of a functional system; by contrast, the events of the second phase depend critically on how the system is used.

Early events. Motor neurones are among the first nerve cells to be 'born' (Jacobson 1978). Like other newly formed neurones, they migrate away from the basal surface of the neural epithelium and lodge in the marginal zone of the ventrolateral quadrant of the developing spinal cord. Soon afterwards, the motor axon grows away from the neuraxis towards the muscles. In limb regions, the motor axons from several segments contribute to the formation of the plexuses. Within the plexus, the relative positions of the axons change so that those destined for anatomically related muscles come together. When this happens, the target muscles have not yet formed. This supports the view, derived from a variety of experiments (Lance-Jones & Landmesser 1980), that the factors governing the formation of the main divisions of the peripheral nerves are independent of the muscles themselves.

Skeletal muscles arise from the myotomal cells of the segmented embryonic somites (Alberts et al 1983). As development proceeds, some of these cells become fibroblasts; others, although still dividing, become committed to making muscle. Apparently as a result of environmental cues, cells from this myogenic line eventually stop dividing and become post-mitotic *myoblasts*. The formation of muscle fibres begins with the alignment and subsequent fusion of myoblasts so that their nuclei come to occupy a common cytoplasm. The multinucleated cells thus formed are called *myotubes*.

Soon after myotubes form, the pattern of protein synthesis coded by their nuclei changes dramatically. Particularly notable is the appearance of the proteins which make up the contractile filaments, metabolic proteins such as creatine kinase, integral membrane proteins such as the acetylcholine receptor, and the various components of the basal lamina. Although the expression of the different genes for these various proteins is not inextricably linked, during normal development their products appear as a closely associated cohort that accounts for the coordinated appearance of muscle properties.

Motor axons are present in muscle-forming regions of the embryo before myotubes first appear. Myotubes become innervated very soon (less than one day) after they first appear (Bennett & Pettigrew 1974). Although this early innervation is very immature, activity in the nerve is almost immediately able to elicit muscle contraction and to exert an important influence on subsequent muscle development.

The first axon to innervate each muscle fibre does so at a discrete spot apparently chosen at random along the length of the still very short (<1 mm) muscle fibre. This axon is soon joined at the same spot by the terminals of several other axons, each of which becomes able to elicit muscle contraction. This early state of *polyneuronal innervation* stands in marked contrast to the adult condition in which each muscle fibre is innervated by a single axon (Bennett 1983, Purves & Lichtman, 1985).

As muscle fibres are being innervated, approximately one-half of the motor neurones that were initially produced, die. The extent of this cell death is greatly influenced by the amount of muscle available for innervation. Removing limb buds before innervation causes nearly all the motor neurones to die, whereas enlarging the bulk of muscle 'rescues' substantial numbers of neurones which would normally die. As there is very little indication that growing motor neurones ever innervate the 'wrong' muscle, motor neurone death seems designed to ensure the survival of appropriate *numbers* of neurones, rather than to eliminate qualitative errors of connectivity.

Maturation of the motor unit. Many properties of nerve and muscle cells change dramatically during the first few weeks after initial nerve–muscle contacts form. The dendrites of the motor neurones increase in extent and complexity and many synapses form on them, while other synapses are lost from the region of the axon hillock (Ronnevi & Conradi 1974). The motor axon increases in diameter and length, and myelin forms as individual Schwann cells wrap themselves around the axon (Geren 1954, Ribchester 1986): this results in an increase in the speed of conduction of nerve impulses and in the frequency with which they can be generated and propagated.

Newly innervated muscle fibres grow rapidly in length and girth and begin to express the properties that mark them as belonging to a particular 'type'. Increase in length is accompanied by continued fusion of myogenic cells, derived, it is thought, from satellite cells (Ontell 1979). Muscle growth depends critically on the integrity and activity of the nerve supply. Denervation during muscle formation arrests growth (Harris 1981) and may lead to death of muscle fibres that have already formed (Jaros & Johnstone 1983).

The mature pattern of muscle fibre innervation arises during this period by the gradual elimination of supernumary nerve–muscle contacts (Fig. 1.12). This process, which lasts several weeks and is enhanced by activity (Hopkins & Brown 1984), determines the sets of muscle fibres that make up the adult motor units. As the redundant innervation is lost, the terminal of the 'sole-surviving' axon at each neuromuscular junction expands and takes on its adult form (Slater 1982). Extensive folding of the muscle fibre surface occurs, as does an increase in the metabolic half-life of the acetylcholine receptors in the muscle membrane and an increase in the speed of operation of the ionic channels associated with them (Ribchester 1986). These events fail to occur if the nerve is cut at an early stage in development, suggesting that maturation of the junction requires a continuing interaction between nerve and muscle cells.

The 'type-specific' properties of fully mature muscle fibres, such as the speed of contraction and the molecular factors that underlie it, develop during the first few weeks after birth in laboratory

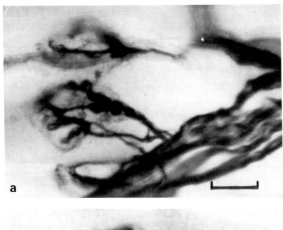

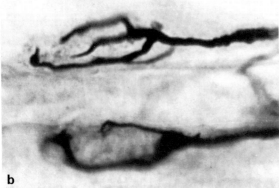

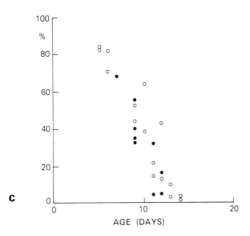

Fig. 1.12 Loss of polyaxonal innervation of muscle fibres during development (mouse). a. Multiple axons innervate most muscle fibres one week after birth (silver stain). b. A single, more robust axon innervates most muscle fibres by two weeks of age. c. Time course of the loss of polyaxonal innervation in the mouse soleus muscle, determined both by physiological and anatomical criteria (experimental details in Slater 1982). Scale bar = 10 µm

mammals (Buller et al 1960a, Close 1964). Several factors seem to govern the expression of these properties: one is the pattern of activity imposed by the nerve (see below). However, some recent studies indicate that muscle fibres may express type-specific properties at a very early stage in development, and that selective innervation by motor neurones of an appropriate type may occur (Thompson 1986).

Neural control of muscle fibre properties

The influence of innervation on muscle properties persists into adulthood (Pette & Vrbová 1985). A dramatic demonstration of this is the atrophy of muscle which follows paralysis resulting from immobilisation or denervation (see below). Although the alterations in motor unit properties which accompany specialised training are more modest, they, too, reflect the response of motor unit properties to changing use. Between these extremes lie modifications of motor unit properties which are associated with recovery from injury or disease.

Much of our current thinking about the nature of the effect of innervation on the properties of mature muscle stems from a series of animal experiments in which the nerve supply to predominantly fast and slow muscles was cut and then surgically redirected, so that the 'fast' nerve reinnervated the 'slow' muscle and vice versa. Effective 'cross reinnervation' was accompanied by a change in the speed of contraction of each muscle so that it came to resemble that of the muscle of the opposite type (Fig. 1.13) (Buller et al 1960b). These changes in the speed of contraction are now known to reflect alterations of many muscle fibre properties including the myosin isoforms, metabolic enzyme profiles and the extent of vascularisation (Pette & Vrbová 1985).

In contrast to the changes in muscle that occur in these experiments, the motor neurones retain their characteristic type-specific properties: thus the after-hyperpolarisation and relatively slow conduction velocity of 'slow' motor neurones are preserved even when they innervate what had been a fast muscle (Kuno et al 1974). This suggests an important generalisation concerning the plasticity of the mature motor unit: whereas

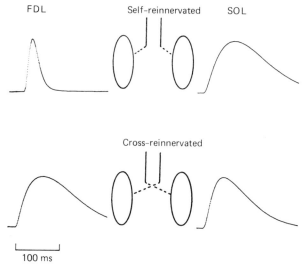

FDL   Self-reinnervated   SOL

Cross-reinnervated

100 ms

Fig. 1.13 Transformation of twitch speed following cross-reinnervation in the cat. (Top line) Twitches of the fast flexor hallucis longus (FDL) and the slow soleus (SOL) muscles, reinnervated by their own nerves. (Bottom line) Twitches of the same muscles after their nerve supplies had been experimentally crossed (adapted from Buller 1972)

In contrast, it is now well established that the amount and pattern of muscle activity, whether elicited by nerve impulses or by direct electrical stimulation of denervated muscles, has profound effects on many muscle fibre properties (Pette & Vrbová 1985). In general, if muscles are stimulated directly or through the nerve with a pattern of activity characteristic of slow motor units (e.g. continuous 10 Hz), their properties come to resemble those of slow units, whereas stimulation with short, high-frequency bursts, characteristic of fast units, induces the properties of fast units. Detailed analysis of this transformation has shown that while the pattern of activity influences many type-specific muscle properties, these do not all change at the same rate. Changes in the proteins of energy metabolism and calcium sequestration can be detected within a week, when the earliest slowing of the contractile response is seen, but changes in the contractile proteins, and myosin isoforms in particular, do not occur until some weeks later.

the type-specific properties of muscle fibres can be modified by the nerve, those of the motor neurones themselves are much more stable and are probably independent of the particular type of muscle fibre they innervate.

The nature of the neural influence on muscle. Two distinct views have emerged over the years to explain how motor nerves exert long-term control over the muscles they innervate. The first is that nerves exert a 'trophic' influence on muscle, most clearly seen in the maintenance of muscle bulk, which is mediated by chemical messengers released from the nerves which act on the muscle. The second view is that muscles alter their properties in response to changes in the pattern and amount of their own activity, which is normally imposed on them by their innervation. Strong evidence for control of target tissues by one 'trophic' substance, nerve growth factor, has emerged from studies of those parts of the peripheral nervous system that derive from the neural crest (Purves & Lichtman 1985). While much work is currently under way to determine whether or not similar factors may account for nerve–muscle interactions, no clear picture has yet emerged.

Effects of training on motor unit properties

Although mature muscle fibres are capable of nearly complete transformation from one fibre type to another in experimental situations, extremes of imposed activity have to be used that lie well beyond what is possible during normal voluntary movement. Nevertheless the intense training programmes undertaken by top-class athletes can induce significant modifications of motor unit properties.

Broadly speaking, training programmes are usually aimed at increasing either endurance or maximum power, but usually not both. For endurance training, activities such as long-distance running are pursued, in which the muscles work against relatively modest loads but undergo considerable changes in length. This predominantly isotonic exercise leads to an increase in the rate of oxygen utilisation and is accompanied by an increase in the content of mitochondria and the density of capillaries around the muscle fibres. In general, however, even very rigorous and prolonged endurance training leads to relatively little change in muscle fibre diameter or in the proportion of slow to fast fibres, as determined by the intensity of myofibrillar ATP-ase activity (Ingjer 1979, Larsson & Ansverd 1985).

To increase strength, it is necessary to increase the cross-sectional area of muscle. Weight training involves exertion against heavy loads with relatively little length change. This predominantly isometric activity increases muscle fibre diameter and, hence, capacity for generating force. In experimental circumstances, increasing the load on a particular muscle, even if it is denervated, leads to what is known as 'compensatory hypertrophy' (Gutmann et al 1971). It appears to be a general principle that tension on muscles, however imposed, leads to hypertrophy.

Hormonal effects on muscle

Endocrinologists have often reported that a number of factors other than activity may influence muscle development. For example, certain highly specialised muscles such as the levator ani in quadrupeds, develop only in the presence of an adequate level of testosterone. In other circumstances, however, endocrine disturbances are either without effect on muscle, or they affect muscle growth, rather than muscle fibre production or differentiation (see Hudgson & Hall 1982).

In contrast, there is compelling evidence that the level of circulating thyroid hormones is a significant determinant of muscle differentiation. It has been known for many years that hypothyroidism in both man and animals results in a slowing of the muscle twitch (Wilson & Walton 1959, Gold et al 1970). It now appears that hypothyroidism results in the transformation of fast-twitch muscle fibres, expressing fast forms of myosin and troponin, into muscle fibres expressing slow forms of these proteins (Johnson et al 1980, Dhoot & Perry 1981). Moreover, Nwoye & Mommaerts (1981) reported that the subunit composition of lactate dehydrogenase was also susceptible to the effects of changes in thyroid status. Hyperthyroidism results in the transformation of slow into fast muscle fibres but, in the rat at least, the transformation is incomplete and results primarily from a change in the capacity of the muscle fibres to utilise oxidative rather than glycolytic metabolic pathways (Nwoye & Mommaerts 1981).

While the effects of hypothyroidism are dependent on an intact nerve supply, and can be blocked by surgical denervation (Johnson et al 1980), it is not clear whether the thyroid hormones act directly on muscle fibres or indirectly, via the regulation of growth hormone levels and the somatomedins (Butler-Browne et al 1984, Whalen et al 1985).

RESPONSE OF THE MOTOR UNIT TO DAMAGE

The greatest test of the motor unit's ability to respond to changing circumstances comes when injury or disease causes damage to the nerve or muscle cells. The regenerative capacity of peripheral nerve and skeletal muscle is highly developed and allows many forms of damage to be adequately compensated. Although traumatic injury may lead to simultaneous damage of nerve and muscle, some injuries and many diseases have a more selective effect and it is useful to consider the response to damage of nerve and muscle separately.

Nerve section

When a peripheral nerve is severed, a characteristic sequence of events is initiated, both in the nerve and in the muscle, which promote effective reinnervation. An appreciation of these events forms the basis for interpretation of less complete nerve damage, such as occurs in the early stages of anterior horn cell disorders.

Nerve degeneration. When a peripheral axon is cut its distal segment degenerates. The first part of the axon to break down is the synaptic terminal; the more proximal portion of the isolated axon segment breaks down more slowly (Miledi & Slater 1970). Axonal degeneration is accompanied by proliferation of Schwann cells within the basal lamina tube surrounding each nerve fibre and their temporary transformation into phagocytes which play an important part in removing axonal debris.

Nerve regeneration. Within a few days after

damage, axonal sprouts begin to emerge from the proximal stump. If the basal lamina tubes remain intact, as when the nerve has been crushed, they provide a direct channel for axonal growth. If, however, the nerve is cut and the ends retract, the growing sprouts may wander aimlessly for weeks. The rate of axonal regeneration is usually close to that of the slow component of axonal transport, about 1 mm/day, presumably because it depends on the assembly of a new cytoskeletal framework. Axonal growth usually continues unabated until the axons reach an appropriate target, even if this takes months.

A number of changes, known collectively as *chromatolysis*, occur in the cell body of the motor neurone following axonal damage (Kandel & Schwartz 1985). These include a dispersal of the protein-synthetic apparatus of the cell, and a peripheral movement of the nucleus. In addition, the after-hyperpolarisation of 'slow' motor neurones is reduced (Kuno et al 1974) and many of the synaptic inputs to the motor neurone are withdrawn. These changes are associated with an altered pattern of protein synthesis by the cell body, presumably related to the changing demands associated with growth (Kandel & Schwartz 1985). Many of these changes are reversed if the regenerating axon makes functional contact with a muscle.

Denervation effects on muscle. Within a few days of nerve section, a sequence of events is initiated in the muscle fibres which brings them to a state of great sensitivity to the effects of regenerating axons (Kuffler et al 1984). The resting membrane potential falls from about -75 mV to about -60 mV, approaching the threshold for action potential generation. (This is one of the factors which account for the spontaneous *fibrillation* of denervated muscle fibres.) In addition, denervated muscles become highly sensitive to acetylcholine. This *denervation supersensitivity* results from the appearance of acetylcholine receptors in regions of the muscle fibre surface not associated with the neuromuscular junction, a condition which resembles that of embryonic muscle fibres (Diamond & Miledi 1962). Recent studies show that another component of the surface of embryonic muscle fibres, N-

CAM (nerve-cell adhesion molecule), also appears after denervation of mature muscle (Sanes et al 1986). It seems likely that these components favour the formation of new synaptic contacts by regenerating axons.

On a longer time scale, denervation leads to profound muscle fibre atrophy. This results from alterations in the normal balance of synthesis and breakdown of many muscle constituents, often increasing the rate of turnover of muscle components as well as tipping the balance in favour of net loss.

Reinnervation of muscle. Regenerating motor axons usually reinnervate denervated muscle fibres at the site of the original neuromuscular junction. This tendency appears to be related to the presence of an accumulation of N-CAM and of factors in the synaptic basal lamina that induce the growing axon tip to differentiate into a presynaptic terminal (Sanes et al 1978).

Neuromuscular transmission is usually restored within a day or two after the arrival of the regenerating axon. Although the safety factor of transmission is initially low, it returns nearly to normal over a period of several weeks, in parallel with maturation of the nerve terminal structure and the loss of any aberrant nerve sprouts that may have formed.

Reinnervation is very effective if it occurs soon after nerve damage, but it becomes less so as the time between damage and the arrival of the growing nerve at the muscle increases (Gutmann & Young 1944). In man, it may take many months after injuries far from the muscle before nerves reach their targets, by which time it may have become impossible for fully effective reinnervation to occur. Even when effective synaptic contacts are restored after damage, their functional significance depends on the accuracy of reinnervation. If the nerve has been cut through, the axons may enter basal lamina tubes destined for inappropriate muscles; because regenerating motor nerves appear to have little ability to distinguish between different muscles, reinnervation of an inappropriate muscle may ensue. There is apparently no mechanism for the correction of such an error of regeneration which may render the reinnervation worse than useless.

Restoration of muscle properties after reinnervation. Effective reinnervation of muscle is followed by reversal of the effects of denervation. Resting potential returns to normal, extrajunctional sensitivity to acetylcholine is lost and, with time, the muscle fibres regain their original dimensions. Because direct electrical stimulation of denervated muscles can prevent or reverse most of the changes associated with denervation (Lømo 1976), it seems that the loss of muscle activity has a key role in the induction of denervation-induced changes. At the same time, a number of observations suggest that there may be significant consequences of denervation other than paralysis.

Partial denervation. Diseases of the motor neurone often result in the death of a fraction of the cells innervating a given muscle. The presence of denervated muscle fibres scattered throughout the muscle appears to promote the outgrowth of sprouts from the surviving axons, either at the nodes of Ranvier or from the axon terminal itself, and the reinnervation of the denervated muscle fibres with which they make contact (Hopkins & Brown 1984).

An important consequence of this response is that new muscle fibres are added to the surviving motor units. Often, the properties of such added fibres will not be appropriate to their new nerve supply. In time, however, the activity pattern of the new innervation will cause them to come to match the rest of the muscle fibres in the unit. The result of this process is that distinctive clusters of muscle fibres of similar type appear. This *fibre type grouping* is often a useful indication of a neurogenic disturbance.

Muscle injury

A number of events can cause muscle fibres to degenerate: some of the most obvious are mechanical trauma and primary myopathic disease such as the muscular dystrophies. It is often the case that destruction of the muscle fibres leaves a substantial number of satellite cells intact; as long as this number is large enough, muscle regeneration can occur and in favourable cases can largely restore the lost tissue. As with damage to peripheral nerves, survival of intact basal lamina sheaths does much to aid regeneration of muscle and its subsequent reinnervation.

Muscle degeneration. Any event which leads to a breakdown of the permeability barrier to inorganic ions presented by the muscle fibre plasma membrane will result in muscle fibre damage. In the case of small lesions, the damage may involve only a part of the muscle fibre's length but often the whole cell breaks down. It is likely that a common step in the breakdown of muscle fibres, which may be triggered by a variety of events, is the entry of calcium into the cell and the activation of intracellular calcium-dependent proteases and phospholipases.

When the vascular supply to a damaged mammalian muscle remains substantially intact, muscle fibre breakdown is accompanied within a day or two by an invasion of phagocytic cells originating in the blood. These cells cross the intact basal lamina sheaths and ingest muscle fibre debris. Within a few days, the bulk of this debris has been disposed of and the phagocytic cells have departed. In other circumstances, especially when the vascular supply is damaged and access of phagocytic cells is impaired, the removal of debris may take much longer.

Muscle regeneration. Even before muscle fibre breakdown is complete, satellite cells within the basal lamina sheath begin to divide, producing the myogenic progeny that will form new muscle fibres. In favourable experimental circumstances in mammals, the original population of muscle fibre nuclei can be replaced within a few days, the new cells promptly fusing to form myotubes within the basal lamina tube. If the nerve supply remains intact, these myotubes become innervated within a day or two. After two to three weeks, they have grown to the size of normal muscle fibres (Harris et al 1975).

The rapid and complete regeneration of damaged muscle cells depends on several factors. If an insufficient number of satellite cells survive damage, regeneration is not possible. If the basal lamina tubes are disrupted, as in experiments in which the muscle is 'minced' or in severe trauma, the cellular events leading to new muscle fibre formation are spatially disorganised, and regeneration is much less effective. If reinnervation is prevented or delayed, the regenerated muscle fibres fail to grow after their initial formation but may survive until effective nerve regeneration can occur.

Regeneration of the neuromuscular junction

When muscle fibres regenerate within the original basal lamina sheath, the specialised features of the neuromuscular junction are rapidly reconstructed. Although the formation of mature postsynaptic specialisations takes several weeks during normal development, it can occur within a few days during muscle regeneration in adult mammals. This is true even if damage to the nerve results in the absence of the nerve terminal during the regeneration process (Jirmanová & Thesleff 1972, Slater & Allen 1985).

The basal lamina has a key role in promoting rapid and effective restoration of functional innervation. The involvement of synaptic basal lamina in the recognition and reinnervation of original synaptic sites by regenerating axons has already been mentioned. In addition, surviving basal lamina promotes the formation of synaptic folds and the accumulation of AChR at original synaptic sites on regenerating muscle fibres, even if the nerve supply and Schwann cells have been destroyed (McMahan & Slater 1984).

Changes in muscle innervation in old age

There is strong evidence that the number of motor units declines in old age (Campbell et al 1973, McComas et al 1973) (Fig. 1.14). This loss of motor units results from the death of motor neurones, for reasons that are not understood. In contrast to muscle, there is no mechanism for the replacement of neurones. The sporadic death of motor neurones leaves muscle fibres denervated and evokes sprouting of the surviving motor neurones in a manner similar to that already discussed in the context of partial denervation.

Initially, the surviving neurones take over the denervated fibres. The motor units increase in size and the transformation of the properties of the reinnervated fibres leads to increasing fibre-type grouping. As the number of surviving motor

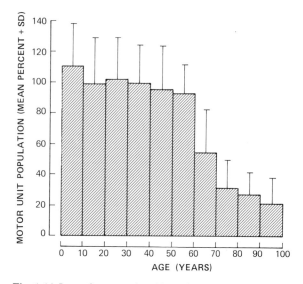

Fig. 1.14 Loss of motor units with age in humans. The estimated number of motor units in various muscles in humans at different ages, relative to the overall mean number found in normal subjects from 0 to 60 years (from McComas et al 1973)

neurones falls, they become unable to reinnervate all the denervated muscle fibres. As a result, both the delicacy of control and, eventually, overall strength, are lost. Ultimately, some muscles may become completely denervated.

CONCLUSION

We are able to use our muscles to create an almost infinite variety of movements, differing in speed, force and direction. Because motor commands from the central nervous system can take the form of action potentials only in the motor axons, this variety depends critically on the patterns of connections of those axons with the muscle fibres. Although each motor neurone controls a set of muscle fibres with very similar properties, motor units vary from those specialised for relatively slow, maintained contractions of limited force to those specialised for fast but brief and powerful efforts. Because the speed of action potential propagation in the motor axon and the contractile properties of the muscle fibres in each motor unit are closely related to the excitability of the motor neurone, the set of motor units innervating a muscle has an inherent functional order which ensures that increasing demand is met with smoothly graded contractions over a wide range of speeds and forces.

The matching of properties between the motor neurone, its associated Schwann cells, and the muscle fibres it innervates arises during development as a result of a complex set of poorly understood cell–cell interactions. One component of these interactions is the pattern of activity of the motor unit itself, which has an important influence on the development of the specific properties of the muscle fibres in the mature motor unit. The survival into adulthood of the sensitivity of muscle fibres to the way they are used endows the mature motor unit with the ability to adapt its properties to meet changing demands.

After damage to the motor unit, many cellular activities which have an important role in development are reactivated. These allow the regeneration of damaged motor axons and muscle fibres, and reinnervation of muscle fibres denervated as a consequence of motor neurone death. Although the extent of functional recovery after certain forms of damage can be impressive, there are very definite limits: motor neurones themselves cannot be replaced and there appears to be no peripheral mechanism to correct the reinnervation of inappropriate muscles by the wayward growth of regenerating axons.

The many interacting relationships between the cells within individual motor units and between the motor units of individual muscles provide an important background against which the details of any disorder of voluntary muscle may be viewed.

REFERENCES

Aidley D J 1978 The physiology of excitable cells, 2nd edn. Cambridge University Press, Cambridge

Alberts B, Bray D, Lewis J, Raff M, Roberts K, Watson J D 1983 Molecular biology of the cell. Garland, New York

Angelides K J 1986 Fluorescently labelled Na+ channels are localized and immobilized to synapses of innervated muscle fibers. Nature 321: 63–66

Appelberg B, Emonet-Dénand F 1967 Motor units of the first superficial lumbrical muscle of the cat. Journal of Neurophysiology 30: 154–160

Asbury A K, Johnson P C 1978 Pathology of peripheral nerve. W B Saunders, Philadelphia

Bennett M R 1983 Development of neuromuscular synapses. Physiological Reviews 63: 915–1048

Bennett M R, Pettigrew A G 1974 The formation of synapses in striated muscle during development. Journal of Physiology (London) 241: 515–545

Bloom W, Fawcett D W 1968 A textbook of histology, 9th edn. W B Saunders, Philadelphia

Boyd I A, Davey M R 1968 Composition of peripheral nerves. Livingstone, Edinburgh

Bradley W G 1974 Disorders of peripheral nerves. Blackwell Scientific Publications, Oxford

Buller A J 1972 The neural control of some characteristics of skeletal muscle. In: Downman C B B (ed) Modern trends in physiology, 1. Butterworth, London, p 72–85

Buller A J, Eccles J C, Eccles R M 1960a Differentiation of fast and slow muscles in the cat hind limb. Journal of Physiology (London) 15: 399–416

Buller A J, Eccles J C, Eccles R M 1960b Interaction between motorneurones and muscles in respect of the characteristic speeds of their responses. Journal of Physiology (London) 150: 417–439

Buller A J, Lewis D M 1963 Factors affecting the differentiation of mammalian fast and slow muscle fibres.

In: Gutmann E, Hnik P (eds) The effect of use and disuse on neuromuscular functions. Publishing House of the Czechoslovak Academy of Sciences, Prague, p 149–159

Burke R E 1967 Motor unit types of the cat triceps surae muscle. Journal of Physiology (London) 193: 141–160

Burke R E, Jankowska E, tenBruggencate G 1970 A comparison of peripheral and rubrospinal input to slow and fast twitch motor units of triceps surae. Journal of Physiology (London) 207: 709–732

Burke R E, Levine D N, Tsairis P, Zujac F E 1973 Physiological types and histochemical profiles in motor units of the cat gastrocnemius. Journal of Physiology (London) 234: 723–748

Butler-Browne G S, Herlicoviez D, Whalen R G 1984 Effects of hypothyroidism on myosin isozyme transitions in developing rat muscle. FEBS Letters 166: 71–75

Campbell M J, McComas A J, Petito F 1973 Physiological changes in ageing muscles. Journal of Neurology, Neurosurgery and Psychiatry 36: 174–182

Close R 1964 Dynamic properties of fast and slow skeletal muscles of the rat during development. Journal of Physiology (London) 173: 74–95

Close R 1972 Dynamic properties of mammalian skeletal muscle. Physiological Reviews 52: 129–197

Cooper S 1966 Muscle spindles and motor units. In: Andrew B L (ed) Control and innervation of skeletal muscle. University of St. Andrews, p 9–16

Couteaux R 1960 Motor end plate structure. In: Bourne G H (ed) Structure and function of muscle, Vol. I. Academic Press, New York, p 337

Dawson M J, Gadian D G, Wilkie D R 1978 Muscle fatigue investigated by phosphorus nuclear magnetic resonance. Nature (London) 247: 861–866

DeLuca C J 1985 Control properties of motor units. Journal of Experimental Biology 115: 125–136

Denier van der Gon J J, Gielen C C A M, ter Haar Romeny

B M 1982 Changes in recruitment threshold of motor units in the human biceps muscle. Journal of Physiology (London) 328: 28P

Dhoot G K, Perry S V 1981 Effect of thyroidectomy on the distribution of the fast and slow forms of troponin I in rat soleus muscle. FEBS Letters 133: 225–229

Diamond J, Miledi R 1962 A study of foetal and new-born rat muscle fibres. Journal of Physiology (London) 162: 393–408

Eccles J C, Eccles R M, Lundberg A 1958 The action potentials of the alpha motoneurones supplying fast and slow muscles. Journal of Physiology (London) 142: 275–291

Edstrőm L, Kugelberg E 1968 Histochemical composition, distribution of fibres and fatiguability of single motor units. Journal of Neurology, Neurosurgery and Psychiatry 31: 424–433

Edwards R H T, Hill D K, Jones D A, Merton P A 1977 Fatigue of long duration in human skeletal muscle after exercise. Journal of Physiology (London) 272: 769–778

Edwards R H T, Mills K R, Newham D J 1981 Greater low frequency fatigue produced by eccentric rather than concentric muscle contractions. Journal of Physiology (London) 317: 17P

Eisenberg B R, Kuda A M 1976 Discrimination between fiber populations in mammalian skeletal muscle using ultrastructural parameters. Journal of Ultrastructural Research 54: 76–88

Elmqvist D, Quastel D M J 1965 A quantitative study of end-plate potentials in isolated human muscle. Journal of Physiology (London) 178: 505–529

Fitch S, McComas A 1985 Influence of human muscle length on fatigue. Journal of Physiology (London) 272: 769–778

Freund H J 1983 Motor unit and muscle activity in voluntary motor control. Physiological Reviews 63: 387–436

Froehner S C 1986 The role of the postsynaptic cytoskeleton in AChR organization. Trends in Neuroscience 9: 37–41

Gasser H S, Grundfest H L 1939 Axon diameters in relation to the spike dimensions and the conduction velocity in mammalian A fibres. American Journal of Physiology 127: 393–414

Geren B 1954 The formation from the Schwann cell surface of myelin in the peripheral nerves of chick embryos. Experimental Cell Research 7: 558–562

Gold H K, Spann J F, Braunwald E 1970 The effect of alterations in the thyroid state on the intrinsic contractile properties of isolated rat skeletal muscle. Journal of Clinical Investigation 49: 849–854

Gordon A M, Huxley A F, Julian F J 1966 The variation in isometric tension with sarcomere length in vertebrate muscle fibres. Journal of Physiology (London) 184: 170–192

Grafstein B, Forman D S 1980 Intracellular transport in neurons. Physiological Reviews 60: 1167–1283

Gutmann E, Young J Z 1944 Reinnervation of muscle after various periods of atrophy. Journal of Anatomy 78: 15–43

Gutmann E, Schiaffino S, Hanzlikova V 1971 Mechanism of compensatory hypertrophy in the skeletal muscle of the rat. Experimental Neurology 31: 451–464

Harris A J 1981 Embryonic growth and innervation of rat skeletal muscles. I. Neural regulation of muscle fibre numbers. Philosophical Transactions of the Royal Society of London (Biology) 293: 257–314

Harris J B, Wilson P 1971 Mechanical properties of dystrophic mouse muscle. Journal of Neurology, Neurosurgery and Psychiatry 34: 512–520

Harris J B, Johnson M A, Karlsson E 1975 Pathological responses of rat skeletal muscle to a single subcutaneous injection of a toxin isolated from the venom of the Australian tiger snake, Notechis scutatus scutatus. Clinical and Experimental Pharmacology and Physiology 2: 383–404

Henneman E, Olsen C B 1965 Relations between structure and function in the design of skeletal muscles. Journal of Neurophysiology 28: 581–598

Henneman E, Somjen G, Carpenter D O 1965 Functional significance of cell size in spinal motoneurons. Journal of Neurophysiology 28: 560–580

Hennig R, Lømo T 1985 Firing patterns of motor units in normal rats. Nature (London) 314: 164–166

Hill A V 1949 The abrupt transition from rest to activity in muscle. Proceedings of the Royal Society of London (Biology) 136: 399–420

Hilton S M, Jeffries M G, Vrbová G 1970 Functional specialisation of the vascular bed of the soleus muscle. Journal of Physiology (London) 206: 543–562

Hopkins W G, Brown M C 1984 Development of nerve cells and their connections. Cambridge University Press, Cambridge

Hudgson P, Hall R 1982 Endocrine myopathies. In: Walton J N, Mastaglia F L (eds) Skeletal muscle pathology. Churchill Livingstone. Edinburgh, p 393–408

Hursh J B 1939 Conduction velocity and diameter of nerve fibers. American Journal of Physiology 127: 131–139

Ingjer F 1979 Effects of endurance training on muscle fibre ATP-ase activity, capillary supply and mitochondrial content in man. Journal of Physiology (London) 294: 419–432

Jacobson M 1978 Developmental neurobiology, 2nd edn. Plenum, New York

Jaros E, Johnstone D 1983 Effect of denervation upon muscle fibre number in normal and dystrophic (dy/dy) mice. Journal of Physiology (London) 343: 104P

Jirmanová I, Thesleff S 1972 Ultrastructural study of experimental degeneration and regeneration in the adult rat. Zeitung für Zellforschung und Mikroskopische Anatomie 131: 77–97

Johnson M A, Mastaglia F L, Montgomery A G, Pope B, Weeds A G 1980 Changes in myosin light chains in the rat soleus after thyroidectomy. FEBS Letters 110: 230–235

Kandel E R, Schwartz J H 1985 Principles of neuroscience, 2nd edn. Elsevier, New York

Kernell D 1966 Input resistance, electrical excitability and size of ventral horn cells in cat spinal cord. Science (New York) 152: 1637–1640

Korneliussen H, Waerhaug O 1973 Three morphological types of motor nerve terminals in the rat diaphragm, and their possible innervation of different muscle fiber types. Zeitschrift für Anatomie und Entwicklungsbiologie 140: 73–84

Kuffler S W, Nicholls J G, Martin A R 1984 From neuron to brain, 2nd edn. Sinauer, Sunderland, Massachusetts

Kuno M, Miyata Y, Muños-Martinez E J 1974 Properties of fast and slow motoneurones following motor reinnervation. Journal of Physiology (London) 242: 273–288

Lance-Jones C. Landmesser L 1980 Motoneurone projection patterns in the chick hind limb following early partial reversals of the spinal cord. Journal of Physiology (London) 302: 581–602

Larsson L, Ansverd T 1985 Effects of long-term physical training and detraining on enzyme histochemical and functional skeletal muscle characteristics in man. Muscle and Nerve 8: 714–722

Laughlin M H, Armstrong R B 1982 Muscular blood flow distribution patterns as a function of running speed in rats. American Journal of Physiology 243: 296–306

Lømo T 1976 The role of activity in the control of membrane and contractile properties of skeletal muscle. In: Thesleff S (ed) Motor innervation of muscle. Academic Press, London, p 289–321

McComas A J, Upton A R M, Sica R E P 1973 Motoneurone disease and ageing. Lancet ii: 1477–1480

McMahan U J, Sanes J R, Marshall L M 1978 Cholinesterase is associated with the basal lamina at the neuromuscular junction. Nature (London) 271: 172–174

McMahan U J, Slater C R 1984 Influence of basal lamina on the accumulation of acetylcholine receptors at synaptic sites in regenerating muscle. Journal of Cell Biology 98: 1453–1473

Massoulié J, Bon S 1982 The molecular forms of cholinesterase and acetylcholinesterase in vertebrates. Annual Reviews of Neuroscience 5: 57–106

Miledi R, Slater C R 1970 On the degeneration of rat neuromuscular junctions after nerve section. Journal of Physiology (London) 207: 507–528

Miller R H, Lasek R J 1985 Cross-bridges mediate anterograde and retrograde transport along microtubules in squid axoplasm. Journal of Cell Biology 101: 2181–2193

Milner-Brown H S, Stein R B, Yemm R 1973 The orderly recruitment of human motor units during voluntary isometric contractions. Journal of Physiology (London) 230: 359–370

Nemeth P M, Pette D, Vrbová G 1981 Comparison of enzyme activities among single muscle fibres within defined motor units. Journal of Physiology (London) 311: 489–495

Nwoye L, Mommaerts W F H M 1981 The effects of thyroid status on some properties of rat fast-twitch muscle. Journal of Muscle Research and Cell Motility 2: 307–320

Ogata T, Yamasaki Y 1985 The three-dimensional structure of motor endplates in different fiber types of rat intercostal muscle. Cell and Tissue Research 241: 465–472

Ontell M 1979 The source of 'new' muscle fibers in neonatal muscle. In: Mauro A (ed) Muscle regeneration. Raven Press, New York, p 137–146

Pette D, Vrbová G 1985 Neural control of phenotypic expression in mammalian muscle fibres. Muscle and Nerve 8: 676–689

Purves D, Lichtman J W 1985 Principles of neural development. Sinauer, Sunderland, Massachusetts

Ranvier L 1874 De quelques faits relatifs á l'histologie et á la physiologie des muscles striés. Archives Physiologie Normale et Pathologique 6: 1–15

Ribchester R R 1986 Molecule, nerve and embryo. Blackie, Glasgow

Romanes G J 1940 Cell columns in the spinal cord of the human foetus of fourteen weeks. Journal of Anatomy (London) 75: 145–152

Romanes G J 1941 The development and significance of the cell columns in the ventral horn of the cervical and upper thoracic spinal cord of the rabbit. Journal of Anatomy (London) 76: 112–130

Ronnevi L-O, Conradi S 1974 Ultrastructural evidence for spontaneous elimination of synaptic terminals on spinal motorneurones in the kitten. Brain Research 80: 335–339

Rushton W A H 1951 A theory of the effects of fibre size in medullated nerve. Journal of Physiology (London) 115: 101–122

Sanes J R, Marshall L M, McMahan U J 1978 Reinnervation of muscle fiber basal lamina after removal of myofibers. Journal of Cell Biology 78: 176–198

Sanes J R, Schachner M, Covault J 1986 Expression of several adhesive macromolecules (N-CAM, L1, J1, NILE, uvomorulin, laminin, fibronectin, and a heparan sulfate proteoglycan) in embryonic, adult and denervated adult skeletal muscle. Journal of Cell Biology 102: 420–431

Sharrard W J W 1955 The distribution of the permanent paralysis in the lower limb in poliomyelitis. Journal of Bone and Joint Surgery 38B: 540–558

Sica R E P, McComas A J 1971 Fast and slow twitch units in a human muscle. Journal of Neurology, Neurosurgery and Psychiatry 34: 113–120

Slater C R 1982 Post-natal maturation of nerve-muscle junctions in the hindlimb muscles of the mouse. Developmental Biology 94: 11–22

Slater C R, Allen E G 1985 Acetylcholine receptor distribution on regenerating mammalian muscle fibers at sites of mature and developing nerve-muscle junctions. Journal de Physiologie (Paris) 80: 238–246

Thompson W 1986 Changes in the innervation of mammalian skeletal muscle fibers during postnatal development. Trends in Neuroscience 9: 25–28

Vizoso A D 1950 The relationship between internodal length and growth in human nerves. Journal of Anatomy (London) 82: 110–134

Waxman S G, Ritchie J M 1985 Organization of ion channels in the myelinated nerve fiber. Science (New York) 228: 1502–1507

Whalen R G, Toutant M, Butler-Browne G S, Watkins S C 1985 Hereditary pituitary dwarfism in mice affects skeletal and cardiac myosin isozyme transitions differentially. Journal of Cell Biology 101: 603–609

Wilson J, Walton J N 1959 Some muscular manifestations of hypothyroidism. Journal of Neurology, Neurosurgery and Psychiatry 22: 320–324

Wuerker R B, McPhedran A M, Henneman E 1965 Properties of motor units in a heterogeneous pale muscle (m. gastrocnemius) of the cat. Journal of Neurophysiology 28: 85–89

Wyman R J, Waldron I, Wachtel G M 1974 Lack of fixed order of recruitment in cat motoneuron pools. Experimental Brain Research 20: 101–114

The ultrastructure of the motor unit

INTRODUCTION

This chapter describes the ultrastructure of the motor unit, and concentrates in particular on the muscle fibres and their modifications from one type of unit to another. The structure of muscle is exactly tuned to its function, and slight differences in activity from muscle to muscle and from fibre to fibre are associated with subtle differences in their fine structure. When electron micrographs are examined it is important to remember that they have been obtained from a functioning dynamic tissue and represent more than the flat two-dimensional image that they are usually taken to portray.

The basic ultrastructure of the skeletal muscle fibre was largely established during the 1950s and 1960s. In the last decade there has been a resurgence of interest in filling in the details of its fine structure, using new techniques such as immunolabelling to identify the location of many of the minor proteins. At the time of writing, much of this new information is only now being fitted into the general body of information about the motor unit and in this chapter coverage is limited to those features that are accepted to be a normal part of the structure of nerve and muscle.

INNERVATION OF THE MOTOR UNIT

The motor units of all postcranial skeletal muscles receive their innervation from motor neurones in lamina IX of the ventral grey columns of the spinal medulla. These cells have a bimodal size distribution, with mean diameters of 20 and 40–50 μm (Van Buren & Frank 1965), and the fibres to which they give rise show a similarly bimodal diameter distribution, both in the ventral spinal roots and in the distal branches close to the muscles supplied (Boyd & Davey 1968). Within the major nerve trunks these motor nerve fibres constitute only a minor proportion of the total fibre population, but this rises to more than 50% within the nerves to individual muscles. The large fibre population has diameters of between 12 and 20 μm, diminishing to 10–15 μm in the distal branches. This population consists of alpha fibres, which innervate fast motor units exclusively, and beta fibres which are distributed both to slow motor units and to some of the intrafusal myofibres of the muscle spindles. The tapering of individual fibres is associated with a substantial degree of branching within the major nerve trunks (Gilliatt 1966, Wray 1969) and further branching occurs within the muscle. As each motor end-plate in mature mammalian muscle receives only a single motor nerve terminal, each motor neurone is connected through its branching axon to several muscle fibres, the two elements constituting a single motor unit.

The nerves to individual limb muscles of mammals usually enter their deep surfaces in company with a major component of the arterial supply to that muscle and there divide into a number of minor branches which ramify and further subdivide within the central region of the muscle belly. The bundles of nerve fibres comprising each branch are enclosed by perineurial sheaths continuous with that of the parent nerve, the number of layers of perineurial cells diminishing progressively so that the finest branches consist of a single myelinated nerve fibre within a unilamellar sheath. At the neuromuscular junction the axon loses its myelin sheath and further divides into a small terminal arborisation in close contact with the surface membrane of the muscle cell, the region of contact being covered on its external surface by an extension of the Schwann cell sheath. This Schwann cell covering does not, however, provide an effective seal between the extracellular space at the interface between nerve and muscle and the endomysium and there is thus a potential portal of entry into the endoneurium of the parent nerve for extraneous materials of large molecular weight; this has been shown to be freely permeable to tracers such as horseradish peroxidase, which are excluded by the perineurial sheath.

THE NEUROMUSCULAR JUNCTION

The nerve axons of the motor unit terminate at specialised regions of the muscle fibres. The combination of the axon terminal (with its associated Schwann cell), with the postsynaptic membrane and postsynaptic sarcoplasm, constitutes the neuromuscular junction (Fig. 2.1). The physiology of electrical transmission at the junction will be covered in detail in Chapter 3 and we deal here only with its fine structure.

The most conspicuous components of the axon terminal are the synaptic vesicles and mitochondria, but there are also coated vesicles, dense-coated vesicles, vacuoles, microtubules, neurofilaments, lysosomes and glycogen granules (Fig. 2.2). The relative abundance of the different terminal constituents tends to vary within any one junction, from junction to junction, with the age of the junction and with its neural activity. Stereological studies have shown that in human and rat axon terminals the mitochondria generally occupy about 15% of the terminal volume and that there are on average 50–70 synaptic vesicle profiles per μm^2 of terminal (Engel & Santa 1971, Engel et al 1976). The diameter of the vesicles is 45–60 nm; they contain acetylcholine and ATP, and are coated with synapsin 1, a synapse-specific phosphoprotein. The synaptic vesicles tend to cluster towards the side of the terminal facing the myofibre and concentrate in small groups close to the presynaptic membranes. These 'active zones' (Couteaux & Pecot-Dechauvassine 1970) are considered to be the sites of acetylcholine release from the synaptic vesicles. Elegant time-resolved freeze-fracture studies of frog muscle have shown that the P face of the presynaptic membrane contains many exocytotic dimples 5 ms after being stimulated (Heuser et al 1979, Heuser & Reese 1981). The dimples, which appear immediately adjacent to the active zones, are thought to represent the points of fusion of the synaptic vesicles with the presynaptic membrane. In fast-twitch frog muscle fibres the active zones are

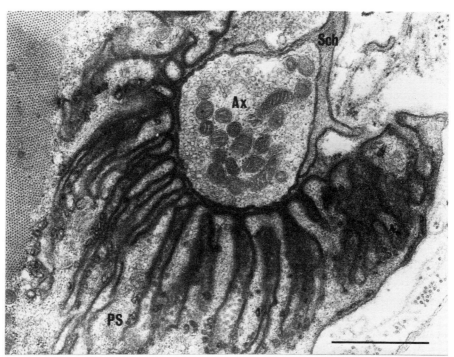

Fig. 2.1 Transverse section through a neuromuscular junction in a human quadriceps muscle which has been stained for acetylcholinesterase to highlight the membrane topography. Ax = axon terminal, Sch = Schwann cell process, PS = postsynaptic sarcoplasm. Scale = 1 μm (Micrograph kindly donated by Dr. Tim Walls)

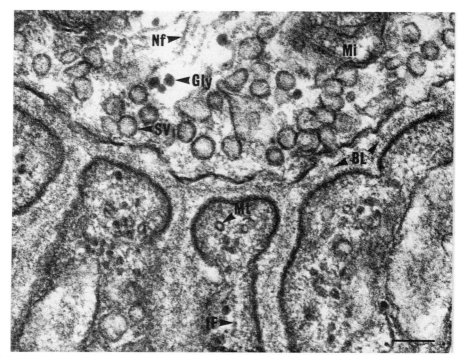

Fig. 2.2 Higher magnification view of a neuromuscular synapse. Note the clustering of the synaptic vesicles (SV) in zones facing the crests of the postsynaptic folds. The postsynaptic membrane is thickened at the crests and for a short distance into the clefts. Nf = neurofilament, Mi = mitochondrion, Gly = glycogen, BL = basal lamina, Mt = microtubule, IF = intermediate filament. Rat soleus muscle. Scale = 0.1 μm

linear and are regularly spaced such that each zone is situated opposite the cleft between two folds of the postsynaptic membrane (see Ch. 3, Fig. 3.2). In mammals where the neuromuscular junction is less elongated and more convoluted than in the frog, the active zones are shorter and less regularly dispersed.

The pre- and postsynaptic membranes at the neuromuscular junction are separated by a space 60–80 nm wide. It is into this synaptic space that acetylcholine is released when the nerve axon is stimulated. Within the synaptic space there is a basal lamina (Fig. 2.2) which is continuous at the edge of the junction with the basal laminae of both muscle fibre and the Schwann cell covering the axon terminal. It has become apparent over recent years that the basal lamina of the neuromuscular junction plays an important part in junction development and regeneration (see review by Sanes & Chiu 1983). This role must be dependent on unique properties of its molecular components, some of which are common to the remainder of the basal lamina and others are not. One important component is acetylcholinesterase (Fig. 2.1) for which the junctional basal lamina must contain specific binding sites. Other unique components are an antigen which reacts with antisera raised against muscle membrane collagen and another which reacts with antisera raised against lens capsule basement membrane (Sanes & Hall 1979). Fibronectin, laminin and collagen IV are common to both junctional and extrajunctional basal lamina, but collagen V is found only in extrajunctional areas (Sanes 1982).

The postsynaptic membrane is deeply folded in such a way that the postsynaptic surface is considerably enlarged and the volume of the synaptic space is increased. Stereological measurements on human intercostal muscle and rat limb muscle show that the area ratio of the postsynaptic to presynaptic membranes is of the order of 10:1 (Engel & Santa 1971, Engel et al 1976). The clefts tend to be longer (~1.5 μm) in human end-plates than in rat end-plates (~1.0 μm), and in fast twitch fibres than slow twitch fibres (Padykula & Gauthier 1970). Figure 2.3 is a scanning electron micrograph showing the topography of the muscle surface at a mouse end-plate after removal of the nerve terminal. The synaptic clefts are variable in

length and width and seem to have no preferred orientation. The complexity of the folding of the postsynaptic membrane is further displayed in Figure 2.4 where the membrane at a human neuromuscular junction has been sectioned face on.

The postsynaptic membrane appears thicker and more electron–dense at the crests of the folds and for a short distance into the clefts (Fig. 2.2). Electron microscopic autoradiography using labelled α-bungarotoxin has shown that these denser areas are the sites of highest concentration of the acetylcholine receptor (Fertuk & Salpeter 1974, Barnard et al 1975). Rosenbluth (1974) showed that the membranes contained particles 6–12 nm in diameter with a 10–15 nm spacing, giving a concentration of 10 000 granules per μm^2. This figure is in accord with electrophysiological and autoradiographic estimates of acetylcholine receptor packing density.

The structure and different forms of the acetylcholine receptor have attracted much scientific attention during the last 10 years. It is known to be a pentameric protein made from four types of subunit, $\alpha_2\beta\gamma\delta$, arranged around a central ion channel. The subunits span the postsynaptic membrane and when acetylcholine binds to the two α-subunits the channel opens and the endplate current is initiated. The primary sequences of all four subunits have been elucidated by recombinant DNA techniques, and recently the structural basis of the difference between fetal and adult forms of the receptor has also been defined (Mishina et al 1986).

Cytoskeletal elements, microtubules and intermediate filaments, are found in the sarcoplasm adjacent to the postsynaptic membrane (Fig. 2.2). Quick-freeze and deep-etch techniques have revealed details of the subsynaptic cytoskeleton (Heuser & Salpeter 1979, Hirokawa & Heuser 1982). The receptor–containing area of membrane is in contact with a meshwork of fine filaments which constitute the 'fuzzy' layer in conventional transmission electron micrographs (Fig. 2.2); these fine filaments are in turn in contact with the network of intermediate filaments and microtubules. No immunoelectron-microscopy has yet been done in this area but immunocytochemistry at the light microscope level has revealed β-actin

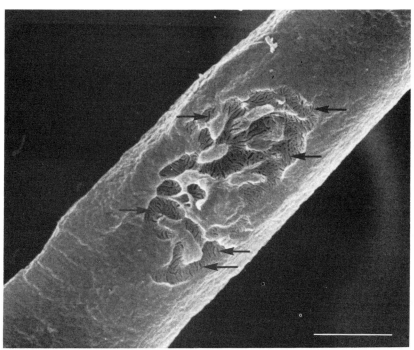

Fig. 2.3 The surface of a muscle fibre from which the axon terminal and basal lamina has been stripped by 6N HCl thus exposing the clefts (arrows) in the postsynaptic gutters. Fifteen-day-old mouse. Scale = 5 μm (Scanning electron micrograph kindly donated by Dr K. Kitaoka, Ehime University, Japan)

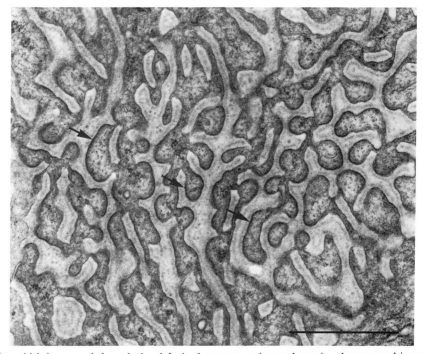

Fig. 2.4 A section which has passed through the clefts in the postsynaptic membrane in a human quadriceps muscle showing the complexity of the folding. Thickened membranes (arrows) correspond to the ACh-receptor containing areas. Scale = 1 μm

(Hall et al 1981), vinculin, α-actinin and filamin (Bloch & Hall 1983).

THE MYOFIBRE

Basal lamina

The basal lamina is the thin (20–30 nm) outermost coating of the muscle fibre; it ensheathes the entire muscle fibre including its symphysis with the axon terminals at the neuromuscular junctions and its union with the tendons at the myotendinous junctions. The basal lamina is secreted by the muscle fibre itself, unlike the collagen fibrils immediately adjacent to it, which are of fibroblastic origin. This thin layer of collagen fibrils (the reticular lamina) in combination with the basal lamina, constitutes the basement membrane described by nineteenth-century histologists and named the 'sarcolemma' by Bowman (1840), a term now often used wrongly as a synonym for the plasmalemma (plasma membrane).

At the ultrastructural level the basal lamina is usually described as 'amorphous', although 'finely filamentous' would be more accurate. Its main constituents are filamentous proteins, but these are so slender as to be hardly resolvable by present-day conventional transmission microscopy of thin sections. Between the basal lamina and the underlying plasma membrane there is an electron-lucent layer, 10–15 nm wide, which corresponds to the glycocalyx of other cell types (Fig. 2.5). This 'gap' is traversed by very fine bridges which run from the plasma membrane into the basal lamina. These connecting bridges presumably result in the plasma membrane and the basal lamina moving together during muscle contraction, the movement of the myofibrils being transmitted to the fibre surface by the intermediate filament system (see below). Furthermore, the myofibrils of closely adjacent myofibres are frequently seen in very close register, with the Z lines at corresponding levels, implying that there is a third level of linkage connecting basal lamina to basal lamina, as well as those connecting basal lamina to plasma membrane and plasma membrane to myofibril. The nature of this third connection has yet to be elucidated.

Chemically, the major protein of the basal lamina is collagen type IV (Bailey et al 1979).

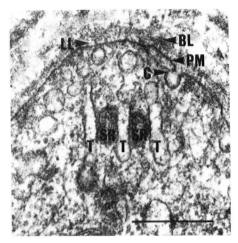

Fig. 2.5 Part of the periphery of a regenerating human muscle fibre. BL = basal lamina (lamina densa), LL = lamina lucida, PM = plasma membrane (Plasmalemma), C = caveola, T = T tubule, SR = sarcoplasmic reticulum. Scale = 0.5 μm

Immunofluorescent antibody staining has localised acetylcholinesterase to the basal lamina of the neuromuscular junction, while fibronectin and laminin are found in both junctional and extra-junctional areas (McMahan et al 1978, Sanes 1982). (Acetylcholinesterase is also found at the myotendinous junction although the significance of this is still uncertain.) Further specialisation of the junctional basal lamina is implied by its binding of a fluorescein-labelled lectin (Sanes & Cheney 1982) indicating that there are synapse-specific carbohydrates. Collagen V is found in the basement membrane, but in the collagen fibrils of the reticular layer, not the basal lamina.

The role of the basal lamina in the physiology of skeletal muscle is still only poorly understood. Work on other tissues, in particular blood capillaries and renal glomeruli, has attributed two functions to the basal lamina: as a semipermeable filter and as a supporting structure. The basal lamina of muscle allows the inward passage of 12 nm ferritin molecules but not a colloidal gold–horseradish peroxidase complex of 20–25 nm diameter, suggesting that it may act as a diffusion barrier for large molecules (Oldfors & Fardeau 1983). It does not, on the other hand, appear to prevent the passage of material expelled from pathological muscle into the extracellular space (Cullen & Mastaglia 1982).

The best evidence for the basal lamina as a supporting structure is seen in muscle which is regenerating. The basal lamina is remarkably resistant to noxious agents and persists as an 'empty tube' when the necrotic fibre debris is removed by phagocytes. Regeneration involves the fusion of satellite cell-derived myoblasts within the basal lamina tubes to form multinucleate myotubes. The myotubes are aligned in parallel with the longitudinal axis of the basal lamina tubes with which they make direct contact. While the myoblasts and myotubes appear to make use of the basal lamina as a support or guide when it is present (Vracko & Benditt 1972), regeneration can occur in its absence, e.g. in explanted muscle cultured in vivo in which new myotubes will grow out of, and away from, the original lamina (Bischoff 1975).

The basal lamina also appears to have an important influence in regeneration of the neuromuscular synapse, in guiding regrowth of axons of denervated fibres back to the original site of the end-plate, and in localising the accumulation of acetylcholine receptors on regenerated myofibres, also at the original site. Sanes et al (1978), using denervated frog cutaneous pectoralis muscle, damaged the myofibres so that they and their nerve terminals degenerated, and only the basal lamina sheath remained; muscle regeneration was prevented by X-irradiation. Axons regenerating into the region contacted the basal lamina almost exclusively at the original synaptic sites and, within the terminals, the synaptic organelles lined up opposite periodic specialisations in the basal lamina. When reinnervation was prevented while the myofibres were allowed to grow back, they developed accumulations of acetylcholine receptors selectively localised to the original synaptic site (Burden et al 1979). It seems from these two pieces of work that specific molecules within the junctional basal lamina attract the axon and also influence the differentiation of the postsynaptic membrane.

Plasmalemma

The outer surface of the muscle fibre is covered by a plasmalemma or cell membrane. This is itself related externally to the basal lamina component of the sarcolemma, from which it is separated by a 20 nm electron-lucent gap corresponding to the glycocalyx of the surface membrane which lacks contrast in conventionally stained electron micrographs. Like other cell membranes, the muscle plasmalemma consists of a proteolipid bilayer, the latter component being comprised of neutral lipid, phospholipids, and cholesterol esters and cholesterol; the proportion of the last is reported to be highest in slow-twitch fibres (Fischbeck et al 1982). Apart from the proteins which contribute to its intrinsic structure, the plasmalemma also contains a number of particulate proteins serving a range of specialised functions: these include the acetylcholine receptor and other receptor molecules, transport channels for a range of ionic species, ATPases associated with metabolically driven ionic pumps, and transport proteins for glucose and amino acids.

Specialised regions of the plasmalemma occur at the neuromuscular junction and the myotendinous junction, and these will be discussed in detail elsewhere. Over the remainder of the fibre it possesses a relatively uniform ultrastructure and, at resting length, a smooth external contour indented at intervals by myosatellite cells (see p. 58), which on contraction is thrown into fine circumferential folds. This surface element of the plasmalemma is in direct continuity with an extensive system of subsurface caveolae via a series of 20–40 nm pores (Fig. 2.6) and many of these are in turn connected to the transverse tubular system. The pores are scattered in a semi-regular fashion over the surface of the myofibre, and in human muscle number between 12 and 20 μm^2 (Schmalbruch 1979a, Bonilla et al 1981), but it has been reported that both their numbers and their distribution can be altered by hypoxia in vivo and by delayed fixation (Schmalbruch 1985, Lee et al 1986). The caveolae make a substantial contribution to the total plasmalemmal area, estimated to amount to 47% in sectioned (Mobley & Eisenberg 1975), and up to 80% in freeze-fractured frog muscle fibres (Dulhunty & Franzini-Armstrong 1975). The most superficial element of cytoplasm subjacent to the surface portions of the plasmalemma between the caveolae shows an increase in electron density in conventional sectioned preparations (Fig. 2.6) which in chicken slow-twitch fibres is associated with a peripheral layer of the structural protein, vinculin (Shear & Bloch 1985).

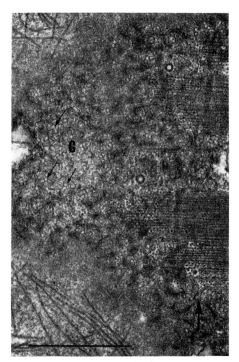

Fig. 2.6 A transmission micrograph of a longitudinal section which shaves the surface of a human myofibre. The superficial sarcoplasm is packed with lobulated sub-surface caveolae (C). They are connected to the plasmalemma by small round pores (small arrows), and are continuous with the tubules of the T system (large arrow). Scale = 1 μm

Freeze-fracture studies of skeletal muscle have revealed that the muscle-cell plasmalemma contains numerous intramembranous particles, occurring either singly or as aggregates (Ellisman et al 1976), the majority of the basic units having mean diameters of about either 6 or 10 nm. The 10 nm particles occur on both the P and E faces of the membrane and it has been claimed that in cultured chick myotubes up to 50% of these may represent sodium/potassium-ATPase molecules (Pumplin & Fambrough 1983). Change in the numbers and distribution of these 10 nm particles has been claimed to occur in both denervated and dystrophic muscle (Schotland et al 1981), but the values reported for normal muscle also vary widely (Yoshioka & Okuda 1977, Ketelsen 1980, Schotland et al 1981), and their numbers have also been reported to decrease during prolonged hypoxia (Schmalbruch 1980).

The 6 nm particles always occur on the P face of the plasmalemma and characteristically form rectangular arrays of up to 100 individual particles. In both human and animal muscle these 6 nm particle arrays are found almost exclusively on the type II, fast-twitch fibres (Rash & Ellisman 1974, Rash et al 1974, Schmalbruch 1979a, Shafiq et al 1979, Schotland et al 1981), with their highest incidence in a band 0.5–1 mm from the margin of the neuromuscular junction. 6 nm particle arrays are absent from the majority of slow-twitch fibres and from human fetal muscle (Schmalbruch 1979a), and appear relatively late in the development of fast-twitch fibres (Hudson et al 1982). Experimental denervation of fast fibres does not appear to affect either the numbers or sizes of their particle arrays, at least in the short term (Ellisman & Rash 1977, Tachikawa & Clementi 1979), but in the rat innervation is required for the development of square arrays up to 30 days postnatal (Sirken & Fischbeck 1985), and experimental reinnervation of slow muscle by a fast-muscle nerve has been shown to induce development of 6 nm particle arrays with a similar density and distribution to those found in normal fast-twitch fibres (Ellisman et al 1978). Neonatal tenotomy, in which function is impaired without loss of innervation, also slows the development of square arrays (Sirken & Fischbeck 1985). Square arrays are reported to be greatly reduced or absent in the plasmalemmae of myofibres in Duchenne dystrophy (Peluchetti et al 1985, Wakayama et al 1985) (see Ch. 8).

Myofibril

Some 80% of the mass of striated muscle fibres is composed of the myofilaments, and these are organised into compact longitudinally orientated bands, the myofibrils. The latter are usually described to be polygonal in cross-section with a maximum diameter of 1–2 μm, and to be unbranched with a length equivalent to that of the myofibre as a whole. Each myofibril is composed of serially repeating segments of identical structure known as sarcomeres, and the fairly exact lateral alignment of these with their neighbours in adjacent myofibrils is responsible for the characteristic transverse striations of the myofibre as a whole. This generalised image of the myofibril is subject to considerable variations between fibre

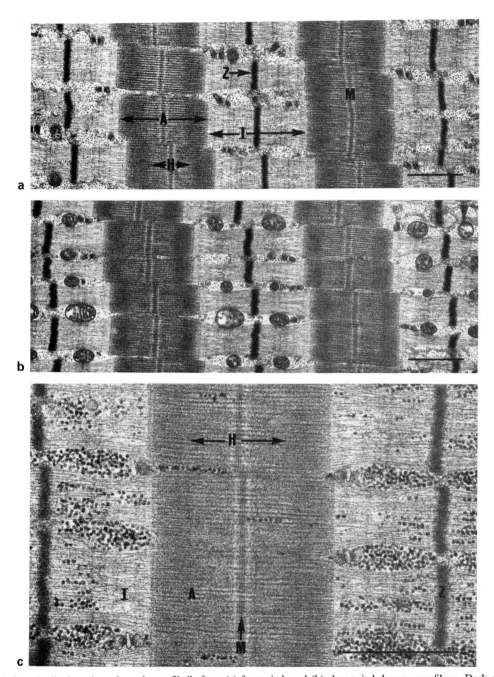

Fig. 2.7 Longitudinal sections through myofibrils from (a) fast-twitch and (b) slow-twitch human myofibres. Dark A bands (A) alternate with pale I bands (I), the latter bisected at their mid-points by dense narrow Z lines (Z). The parallel thick filaments which compose the A band are linked at their mid-points by a narrow transverse stripe, the M line (M). The thin I filaments interdigitate with the thick A-band filaments, and their central ends are marked by the presence of a central paler region of the A band, the H zone (H). Note the broader M and Z lines and more numerous mitochondria in the slow-twitch fibre. A detailed view of a single fast-twitch sarcomere is shown in (c). The dense granules within and between the myofibrils are glycogen. Scale = 1 μm

types in individual species, and between species and phyla. These relate not only to the degree to which individual myofibrils can be distinguished as separate entities, a function of the extent to which they are enveloped by SR, the myofibrils of fast-twitch fibres being more clearly defined than those of slow fibres, particularly in the region of the A band (see below), a difference which permits fibres to be differentiated into Fibrillenstruktur and Felderstruktur fibres respectively by light microscopy (Kruger 1952, Gray 1958), but also to their geometry, the transverse sections of many myofibrils deviating widely from the normal polygonal shape to form flat ribbons 1–2 μm thick and many tens of microns wide. Myofibrils are also not infrequently branched, a tendency which increases in muscle disease.

Each sarcomere along the length of the myofibrils consists of a dense central 'A' (anisotropic) band 1.5–1.6 μm long, flanked by two paler 'I' (isotropic) bands of variable longitudinal dimension, depending upon the state of shortening of the fibre (Fig. 2.7). The A band is crossed at its mid-point by a dark narrow transverse line, the 'M' line (Mittelschreibe), bordered by a paler band of variable width, the 'H' zone (Hellerband). The A band is composed of a regular hexagonal array of filaments 15–18 nm in diameter and tapering gently at either end (Fig. 2.8a,b), the principal constituent of which is the protein 'myosin'. The pale I bands on either side of the A band are divided at their mid-point by a narrow dense line, the Z line (Zwischenscheibe) or Z disc. The I band is also constructed of parallel filaments which vary in length from 1.0 to 1.35 μm in different vertebrate species: they are considerably more slender, with a diameter of 7 nm, and are less regular in their arrangement than those of the A band. Each I filament consists of paired α-helices of chains of a globular protein 'actin' in combination with a second globular protein 'troponin', and a long-chain protein 'tropomyosin'. At the Z line the I filaments of the two halves of one I band form regular square lattices and have a common attachment to the dense matrix material of the Z line (Fig. 2.8a,b). The Z lines mark the longitudinal boundaries of the individual sarcomeres, each of which consist of one A band and two half I bands (Fig. 2.7). The

free ends of the I filaments interdigitate between the elements of the hexagonal A-band lattice, each I filament occupying the centre of a triangular space between three adjacent A filaments (Fig. 2.8b). Contraction of the myofibre is brought about by the shortening of sarcomeres that make up its constituent myofibrils, and this is accomplished by a sliding movement of the I filaments towards the centre of the A band: at its physiological limit this process results in the extinction of the I and H bands, the latter representing the portion of the A-filament lattice unoccupied by I filaments, and apposition of the Z discs to the ends of the A bands. During relaxation following a contraction this sliding movement is reversed until the normal resting length of the sarcomere of between 2.5 and 3.0 μm has been restored. The possible mechanisms responsible for the generation of force required to produce the inward movement of the I filaments are discussed below.

A band. The A filaments which compose the anisotropic band of the sarcomere have a remarkably constant length of between 1.5 and 1.6 μm in a wide range of vertebrate species, the precise value depending upon the method of tissue preparation employed, and a value of 1.57 μm has been obtained from frozen sections of human muscle (Sjostrom & Squire 1977). Each filament carries a series of regularly arranged side projections, cross-bridges, from their tapered tips to approximately 80 nm from their mid-points to leave a smooth 160 nm long central zone spanning the M line: this has become known as the pseudo-H zone or bare zone. The individual myosin molecules which compose the A filaments are rod-shaped, 170 nm long, two-stranded alpha helices 2 nm in diameter bearing two pear-shaped heads 19 nm by 4.5 nm at one end (Fig. 2.8c) (Elliott & Offer 1978). Each myosin molecule is a hexamer comprised of two 'heavy' chains of about 200 000 daltons, and four 'light' chains of 20 000 daltons each. The two heavy chains wind around each other in a coiled coil of α-helices to form the tail of the molecule, and then fold separately to produce the two heads. The light chains are of two chemically distinct classes and one of each class is associated with each head (Craig & Knight

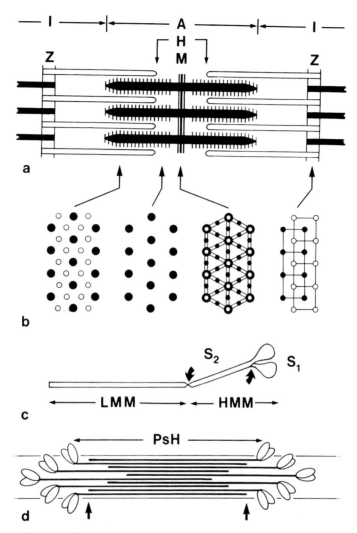

Fig. 2.8 a & b. Diagrammatic views of the structure of the sarcomere. The A band (A) is composed of a hexagonal lattice of thick filaments with tapered ends, linked together by M-line bridges (M) at their midpoints. The central bare zone of each filament is flanked by longer terminal regions which carry a regular series of lateral projections. The I filaments of each half I band (I) are attached to the Z discs (Z) in a regular square array, and interdigitate with the A-band filaments to form a second hexagonal lattice. The interval between the central ends of the two sets of I filaments constitutes the H zone (H). Representative cross-sectional appearances are illustrated in (b). c. A schematic view of the myosin molecule. The rod-shaped shaft of the light meromyosin (LMM) component is joined by a more flexible section to heavy meromyosin (HMM), which consists of a straight shaft (the S_2 subunit) and two pear-shaped heads (the S_1 subunits). The sites on the molecule susceptible to enzymic attack are indicated by curved arrows. d. A diagram of the antiparallel packing of the individual myosin molecules at the centre of an I filament. The heads project from the surface of the filament, and the smooth region between the most central pair of heads is the 'pseudo-H zone'. The somewhat shorter region of overlap of the shafts of the molecules is marked by arrows. Reproduced from Landon (1982) with permission from the editors and publishers

1983), and those of fast muscle appear to differ from those of slow muscle, a difference which is reflected in their actomyosin ATPase activities. The shaft of this molecule can be dissected into two components by tryptic digestion to yield: (1) a straight length of two chain alpha helices approximately 90 nm long with a molecular weight of 150 000 known as light meromyosin (LMM); (2) a shorter, more massive portion consisting of the remaining part of the shaft and its two attached heads, heavy meromyosin (HMM), having a molecular weight of around

350 000. The heads, which alone possess actin binding and ATPase activity, may be separated from the helical component by papain digestion (Lowey et al 1969) to give the S1 (heads) and S2 (shaft) subunits of HMM (Fig. 2.8c). The shafts of the individual myosin molecules have been shown by Huxley (1963) to stack together to form the shaft of the A filament, and in such a manner that the paired heads lie on its surface, with the myosin molecules in each half of one A filament arrayed with opposite polarities, the heads pointing towards the two ends of the filament. The region of overlap of the two arrays of LMM tails from each half gives rise to the central bare zone (Fig. 2.8d). X-ray diffraction studies have demonstrated that the myosin heads are arranged round the A filaments in a semi-regular helix (Craig & Offer 1976a), with pairs of heads on opposite sides of the shaft at intervals of 14.3 nm, each successive pair being rotated by 120 degrees about the axis of the shaft relative to its nearest neighbours, to give an overall axial repeat of 43.0 nm (Huxley & Brown 1967). It has been suggested that the HMM component of the molecule interacts only weakly with the shafts of adjacent myosin molecules, and that its junction with LMM may act as a flexible joint, permitting the HMM component of each myosin molecule to lie at a variable angle to the shaft (Huxley 1969, Lowey et al 1969, Trinick & Elliott 1979).

The pseudo-H zone of the A band shows a number of transverse striations, of which a central dense band and a pair flanking it at 22 nm to either side are the most prominent, and together constitute the histological M line (Fig. 2.8a). With some methods of preparation the A bands of slow twitch fibres show an additional pair of less dense lines at 43.7 nm from the centre of the A filament, to give a five-banded M line (Sjostrom & Squire 1977). Studies of the three-dimensional structure of the M line have shown that its constituent bands represent the positions of substantial cross-bridges which link each A filament to its six nearest neighbours in a hexagonal array (Fig. 2.8b). When the M-line region of the A band is viewed in transverse section each of these bridges shows a thickening at its mid-point, and these have been interpreted to indicate the existence of a set of short small-diameter (4–5 nm) longitudinally orientated 'M filaments' midway between each A filament (Fig. 2.8b). A model structure of a three-banded M line incorporating these components has been described by Knappeis & Carlsen (1968), the main features of which have been confirmed by Luther & Squire (1978). The M line is presumed to stabilise the transverse and longitudinal order of the thick filament lattice of the A band, and in muscles which do not have M lines the thick filaments are in general in less good register (Page 1965). A number of non-myosin M proteins have been isolated, but their locations and function within the intact M line are at present unknown: examples are a 160 000 dalton component which has been ascribed a structural role in the M cross-bridges (Chowrashi & Pepe 1979), and the MM isoenzyme of creatine kinase (Wallimann et al 1979).

A number of other non-myosin proteins are now known to be located in the A band, and the most abundant and the best characterised of these is C protein. It is an elongated monomer lacking any helical component, 35 nm in length, with a molecular weight of 140 000 daltons (Offer et al 1973). It has been shown to bind tightly to both the LMM and S2 portions of myosin at physiological ionic strength, but not to the myosin heads, and thus does not interfere with either its ATPase or actin-binding properties. Antibody-staining studies have shown that C protein is bound strongly and solely to seven narrow stripes in the mid-zone of the cross-bridge region of the A band, and that these have the same 43 nm repeat as the underlying myosin backbone of the thick filament (Pepe & Druker 1975, Craig & Offer 1976b). The function of the C protein is not known, but it has been suggested to have a role in regulating the assembly of the myosin molecules into thick filaments. Another non-myosin protein, H protein, has been isolated from crude preparations of C protein, and has been found to be restricted to a narrow band in the inner region of the cross-bridge zone, two 43 nm repeats central to the inner edge of the region containing C protein (Craig & Megerman 1979); other proteins, so far uncharacterised, are thought to be located in the distal (D) cross-bridge zone.

I band. The major component of the thin myofilaments which characterise the I bands of the sarcomeres is the protein 'actin'. Its monomeric form (G actin) is a globular molecule 5.46 nm in diameter with a molecular weight of 45 000 daltons. The monomers are assembled into a filamentous polymer (F actin) which is a right-handed two-stranded helix 6–7 nm in diameter, so twisted that 13–15 actin molecules are required for every full rotation of the helix, the units of the two strands being staggered relative one to another by one half period (Fig. 2.9). The grooves on either side of the twin chains of actin molecules are occupied by a second I-filament protein, 'tropomyosin'. This is a rod-shaped molecule 38.5 nm long containing a left-handed alpha helix with a molecular weight of 63 000 daltons. These units are assembled end-to-end to form a pair of continuous spiral strands running the length of the I filament (Cohen et al 1971, Ebashi 1980). Each tropomyosin molecule is attached to exactly seven

actin monomers, and it is this relationship rather than the more variable pitch of the actin helix which defines the functional unit of the I filament. I filaments vary in length from 1.0 to 1.35 μm in various animal species, but within any one species have a constant and well-defined length (Huxley 1963, Sjostrom & Squire 1977). At the distal ends of the sarcomere the I filaments end in the Z line in a regular square 22 nm array, and at their central ends penetrate the hexagonal lattice of the A band where each occupies a trigonal point between three adjacent thick filaments to form a second interlocking hexagonal lattice. The affinity of the I filaments for myosin has been demonstrated by treating I bands isolated from homogenised muscle with the S_1 subfragments of HMM (Huxley 1963): the individual filaments become 'decorated' with regularly arranged arrow heads of Sl subunits at intervals of 35–37 nm. These arrow heads are always directed towards the free ends of the filaments, demonstrating that they are struc-

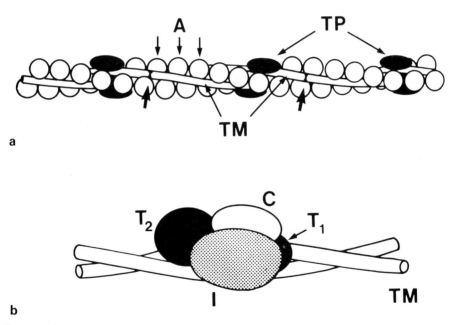

Fig. 2.9 a. A diagrammatic representation of a portion of an I filament. Two chains of globular actin molecules (A) are wound in a right-handed helix, the two grooves between them containing rod-shaped molecules of tropomyosin (TM) assembled end-to-end to produce a second double helix. A third, more or less globular protein troponin (TP), is attached to a specific binding site on each tropomyosin molecule and is thus located at regular intervals along the I filament. Broad arrows indicate the points of contact of individual tropomyosin molecules.   b. An enlarged view of the subcomponents of the troponin complex attached to the tropomyosin double helix stripped of its actin helices. T_1 binds the complex to the tropomyosin molecule: T_2 links it to the C and I subunits, which have calcium-binding and inhibitory functions respectively. Redrawn after Ebashi (1980), and reproduced from Landon (1982) with permission from the editors and publishers

turally polarised, with the polarity reversing on the two sides of the Z line.

The I bands of longitudinally sectioned muscle often show regular transverse striations with a period of approximately 40 nm (Huxley 1967), and a similar periodicity has been detected in X-ray diffraction images of unfixed muscle (Huxley & Brown 1967). Studies using antibody staining (Pepe 1966, Ohtsuki et al 1967) have shown that these cross-striations represent the location of a third I-filament protein, 'troponin' (Ebashi et al 1968). This has a molecular weight of around 80 000 daltons and a roughly globular structure composed of three major subunits: 'troponin C', the Ca^{2+}–binding component which confers Ca^{2+} sensitivity to the actomyosin complex; 'troponin I' with an inhibitory function; and 'troponin T', responsible for binding the complex to a specific point on each tropomyosin molecule in the grooves of the actin helix (Fig. 2.9), to give the observed periodicity of 38.5 nm along the I filaments (Ohtsuki 1975, 1979). Each of the subcomponents of troponin is polymorphic with specific variants related to myofibre type (Perry & Dhoot 1980). The properties of troponin have been reviewed by Ebashi (1980) and its role in the regulation of muscular contraction is outlined below. In addition to the fine cross-banding attributable to the regular attachments of the troponin complexes, the I band also usually shows one or more broader transverse bands, the N lines. The most constant is the N_1 line which lies close to the Z disc at the point at which the I filaments become organised into a regular square array (see below). A second N_2 line may also be visible some 0.2–0.3 μm further into the I band (Page 1968, Franzini-Armstrong 1970). The function of the N lines is unknown, but they appear to represent material linking the I filaments together in the transverse plane and may in part be composed of the 500 000 dalton protein 'nebulin'. Another very large protein 'titin' with a molecular weight of about 1×10^6 daltons is also found in the I band. Nebulin and titin may also be components of the thin elastic filaments which are thought to connect the A filaments to the Z disc (Wang 1982).

Z disc. The Z line or disc is an optically and electron-dense transverse structure which divides each I band at its mid-point, and constitutes the boundary between adjacent sarcomeres. Electron micrographs of sections cut at a shallow angle to the plane of the disc show that the filaments of each half I band lose their apparently haphazard arrangement immediately adjacent to the disc, and become organised into a regular 22 nm square array, the square lattices so formed on the two surfaces of the disc being offset one from another by 50% along each axis (Fig. 2.8a). Each individual I filament is therefore positioned opposite the centre of a square formed by the ends of four filaments from the I band of the opposite side of the disc. In the plane of the disc itself the two lattices combine to create a small regular square lattice of half the period (Fig. 2.10a). Longitudinal sections show that the terminal 20–30 nm portions of the I filaments thicken as they approach the disc, and acquire increased electron density which merges with that of the amorphous dense material of the Z disc itself. Within the thickness of the disc the ends of the I filaments interdigitate (Fig. 2.10b); the extent of the overlap varies with myofibre type, slow-twitch fibres having Z discs of approximately twice the thickness (90–100 nm) of those of fast-twitch fibres (40–50 nm).

The appearances described above are those usually seen following conventional aldehyde fixation, but where the primary fixative is osmium tetroxide, as was almost invariably the case before the introduction of glutaraldehyde, the fine structure of the disc shows certain consistent differences (Fardeau 1969a,b, Landon 1969, 1970b, MacDonald & Engel 1971). The lattice period of the disc is increased to 15.5 nm and its axes are rotated so that they lie at 45 degrees to those of the I-filament arrays of the adjacent I bands and also present a characteristic 'woven' appearance (Reedy 1964). In longitudinal sections the I filaments of the opposed sarcomeres no longer interdigitate, and appear to be linked by short oblique Z filaments to their nearest neighbours in the next sarcomere (Fig. 2.11). A number of models of Z-disc structure have been proposed. The earliest of these were necessarily based upon observations of osmium tetroxide-fixed tissue, and invoked the existence of 'Z filaments' (Knappeis & Carlsen 1962), a 'Z membrane' (Franzini-Armstrong &

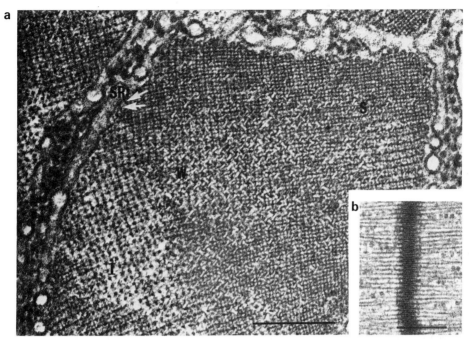

Fig. 2.10 a. A transverse section through the Z-line region of a rat myofibre fixed with glutaraldehyde during the course of a tetanic contraction. The plane of section passes through the end of the I band (I), where the I filaments form a regular square array with a 22 nm period, and also through the Z-disc lattice, part of which (S) shows the small square 11 nm lattice characteristic of unstimulated glutaraldehyde fixed tissue, and part of the larger woven lattice (W) with its axes at 45 degrees to those of the small and large square lattices, usually associated with primary fixation in osmium tetroxide (see text). Note the short filaments (arrows) connecting the Z disc to the sarcoplasmic reticulum (SR). b. Illustrates the appearance of a glutaraldehyde-fixed, fast-twitch Z line in longitudinal section. Scale = 0.25 μm

Porter 1964), and looping actin filaments (Kelly 1967) to account for the linking elements between the I filaments of adjacent sarcomeres seen in longitudinal sections. These models are not readily compatible with the Z-disc structure found in glutaraldehyde–fixed tissue and various alternative models have been proposed (Landon 1970b, MacDonald & Engel 1971, Rowe 1971, 1973, Kelly & Cahill 1972, Ullrick et al 1977), some of which have placed more emphasis on the non-filamentous components of the disc, while others invoke more ingenious looping configurations. The merits and weaknesses of these various proposals have been reviewed elsewhere (Squire 1981, Landon 1982, O'Brien & Dickins 1983).

Most explanations of the mechanisms underlying the process of muscular contraction assign the Z disc an entirely passive role as an anchor upon which the I filaments of adjacent sarcomeres may pull, and through which the tension they generate is transmitted to the attachments of the myofibre. In the intact fibre each sarcomere acts as a closed-volume system and it is well established that shortening is accompanied by an appropriate increase in the transverse diameter of the A band, brought about by an increase in the inter-A-filament spacing (Elliott et al 1963, Brandt et al 1967). There is also evidence from fine structural studies of fixed tissue (Reedy 1967, Franzini-Armstrong 1973), and X-ray diffraction studies on living muscle (Elliott et al 1967), that the I-filament spacing in the zone of the ordered square array adjacent to the Z disc also increases with sarcomere shortening. Experiments in which rat muscles were fixed with glutaraldehyde during the course of a tetanic contraction (Landon 1970c) have confirmed that the I-filament spacing increases in contracted muscles, and have shown that the fine square lattice characteristic of muscles fixed with aldehydes is converted wholly or in part to the larger woven form normally seen during primary osmium tetroxide fixation

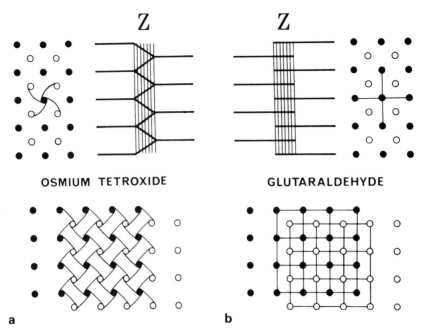

Fig. 2.11 A diagrammatic view of the internal structure of the Z disc seen in longitudinal and transverse section following (a), osmium tetroxide and (b), glutaraldehyde primary fixation. Transected I filaments arising from one side of the disc are represented by open circles, those from the other by closed circles. The dense matrix of the disc is indicated by vertical hatching. Reproduced from Landon (1982) with permission from the editors and publishers

(Fig. 2.10a). The observations suggest that the Z disc undergoes transitory and reversible changes in both its radial dimensions and internal structure during the course of muscular contraction in vivo, and it has been proposed that the fine square and coarse woven lattices represent alternative and interconvertible forms of Z-disc structure which correspond to the relaxed and contracted states of the sarcomere respectively (Landon 1970c). It is not known whether these changes are active components of the contractile process, as envisaged in the theory of contraction proposed by Ullrick (1967), or whether they are a passive corollary of the process of sarcomere shortening as has been suggested by Davey (1976), enabling the I filaments to maintain optimal geometrical alignment for the transmission of tension as the sarcomere shortens.

The close similarity of the appearance of the 40 nm orthorhombic lattice of negatively stained isolated tropomyosin crystals to the large woven lattice of the Z disc prompted suggestions that tropomyosin in a somewhat similar crystalline form could constitute the backbone of the disc,

the I filaments being attached to the corners of each square by means of their individual tropomyosin double helices (Huxley 1963). It was subsequently demonstrated that none of the polymorphic forms of tropomyosin known have a symmetry that can be manipulated to fit the Z lattice without distorting the basic pattern of their internal connections (Caspar et al 1969), and that only minor amounts of tropomyosin can be demonstrated within the disc by immunostaining (Endo et al 1966), or by chemical extraction (Stromer et al 1967, 1969). The protein α-actinin (Ebashi et al 1964), which has a strong cross-linking affinity for actin (Briskey et al 1967), has since been shown to be localised to the lattice region of the Z disc (Masaki et al 1967, Schollmeyer et al 1974), and to contribute approximately 50% of its mass (Suzuki et al 1976). It is an asymmetrical rod-shaped molecule, 4 × 40 nm, which appears to be a homodimer of a 100 000 dalton polypeptide chain (Suzuki et al 1976, Singh et al 1977): it is believed to cross-link the interpenetrating ends of the I filaments within the disc, and it has been suggested that it may also be responsible for imposing consistent 'polarity' on the I filaments emerging from the two faces of the disc. A number of other proteins have been extracted from Z lines, including a 55 000 dalton protein isolated from chicken muscle by Ohashi & Maruyama (1980). This is distinguishable both immunologically and in its amino-acid composition from both α-actinin and desmin; it is located exclusively in the Z discs and, when precipitated from solution, yields crystals having a square lattice structure of similar dimensions to the fine square Z lattice. It is yet to be determined whether it has a structural role within the disc. Abnormalities of Z-disc structure, including the Z-line 'streaming' and 'nemaline bodies', are described in Chapter 8.

Leptomeres

The myofibres of a number of vertebrate species have been reported to contain transversely banded fibrous bodies which have been variously termed 'leptomeres', 'leptomeric fibrils', 'striated bodies' and 'microladders' (Ruska & Edwards 1957, Mair & Tomé 1972). They appear to consist of bundles of fine filaments bound together at regular intervals by cross bands of dense matrix material, with a periodicity reported to range from 120 to 200 nm. They may occur anywhere within the myofibre, and with any orientation, but are chiefly found within the cytoplasm immediately beneath the plasmalemma and are often, but by no means always, associated with the margin of a Z disc of a superficial myofibril. Leptomeres are most abundant in skeletal or cardiac muscle fibres which have become modified for special functions, e.g. the intrafusal myofibres of the muscle spindles (Katz 1961, Gruner 1961, Landon 1966, Scalzi & Price 1971), and the fibres of cardiac conducting tissue (Page et al 1969, Viragh & Challice 1969, Bogusch 1975). The function and significance of leptomeres is not known, although they have been ascribed a mechanical role in some situations (Thornell et al 1976).

Muscle contraction

Certain of the links in the chain of events which lead to the contraction of the myofibrils and the generation of force are well understood, but others have still to be elucidated. Events at the neuromuscular junction are discussed in preceding and subsequent chapters. After generation of the action potential at the end-plate and its spread across the surface membrane, depolarisation enters and passes along the T tubules to trigger release of calcium ions from the SR. Various proposals have been made as to how this electrical signal initiates the release of chemical energy, but the issue is still not resolved. In contrast, much more is known about how chemical energy is transformed into mechanical work when a muscle contracts, and some theories of muscle contraction are outlined below. The history of many of these ideas has been reviewed by Needham (1971).

The sliding filament model of muscle contraction was suggested independently by H. E. Huxley & Hanson (1954) and by A. F. Huxley & Niedergerke (1954) on the basis of electron microscopy and the results of X-ray diffraction. It was proposed that contraction was the result of two sets of filaments sliding between each other, with an increase in their overlap but no change in the length of the individual filaments. During the last 30 years the sliding-filament model has become generally accepted but it does not, by itself, reveal how the force to move the filaments is generated. A possible explanation for this was suggested by the observations by H. E. Huxley (1957) of cross-bridges projecting from the surface of the A filaments towards the I filaments. It was subsequently proposed that these cross-bridges could provide the necessary physical link between the two sets of filaments and that the sliding force was produced by a change in conformation of the cross-bridges while they were attached to the I filament. Since 1957 enormous effort has been put into attempts to test the validity of the 'cross-bridge theory' and to clarify the molecular details of the mechanism. Various schemes have been proposed (A. F. Huxley 1957, 1974, H. E. Huxley 1969, A. F. Huxley & Simmons 1971); for details of these and other models the reader is referred to the reviews by Squire (1981) and Craig (1986).

In the A. F Huxley & Simmons (1971) model, itself a development of H. E. Huxley's (1957) hypothesis, the attachment of the cross-bridges (myosin heads) to the I filament (actin) sites is considered to be a transient event resulting in co-operative hydrolysis of ATP, to be followed by detachment of the myosin heads, the energy released powering a force-generating movement of the cross-bridges. Serial repetition of this process, each cross-bridge engaging a succession of actin monomers along an adjacent I filament in a ratchet-like manner, would drive the I-filament array deeper into the A band and thereby cause the sarcomere to shorten.

The key role of the calcium ions, released from the SR when the muscle fibre is stimulated, is to remove the block which prevents interaction between the A and I filaments in relaxed muscle. During activation troponin C responds to the local rise in calcium ion concentration by changing its tertiary structure and, via troponin T, causes tropomyosin to move in the groove between the paired actin helices, thereby removing the obstacle which has previously prevented interaction between the cross-bridges and the active sites on the thin filaments. This hypothesis is known as the 'steric blocking' model, and has gained wide acceptance in recent years. During relaxation, calcium ions are actively sequestered by the SR, thus reducing their concentration within the myofibril lattice; this results in a reverse shift of the troponin and tropomyosin molecules, and thus inactivation, by reblocking, of the cross-bridge binding sites. The regulation of muscle contraction by calcium and the roles of the non-actin and non-myosin proteins have been reviewed by Ebashi (1980).

The cross-bridge theory of muscle contraction has not gone unchallenged; e.g. McClare (1971) attacked it on thermodynamic principles and formulated an alternative 'molecular machine' in which the myosin molecules exist in a long-lived excited state after hydrolysing ATP. The existence of such a state has not been verified but it has proved to be unnecessary as working thermodynamic cross-bridge models have since been formulated (Tregear & Marston 1979). Another alternative model suggested that electrostatic repulsive forces between the thick and thin filaments caused the sarcomeres to expand laterally and thus to shorten in order to maintain constant volume (Spencer & Worthington 1960, Elliott et al 1970). A variant of this idea invokes dynamic outward expansion of the Z discs as the driving force responsible for fibre shortening (Ullrick 1967). These theories are, however, incompatible with the observation that in skinned fibres the myofibrils are contractile although the interfilament distance does not appear to increase with shortening (Matsubara & Elliott 1972). The cross-bridge theory has been vigorously debated for some 30 years and so far has largely withstood the assaults of its critics (Tregear & Marston 1979).

Mitochondria

The mitochondria of skeletal muscle are irregularly shaped closed sacs, with walls composed of two proteolipid membranes; the outer provides the organelle with a continuous smooth external contour, while the inner is thrown into a series of flat folds, the cristae, which partly sub-divide the central cavity. In skeletal muscle the cristae usually have the shape of flat plates, but zig-zag forms can be found occasionally in normal muscle, and concentric and branched cristae may occur in a number of myopathic conditions. The space enclosed by the inner membrane contains a moderately electron-dense finely granular matrix, within which are scattered small dense calcium-containing granules and occasional larger spherical osmiophilic lipid droplets.

The inner and outer mitochondrial membranes differ substantially in both their chemical composition and biological properties. The outer membrane closely resembles other cellular membranes in structure, consisting of protein and lipid in approximately equal proportions, and shows little specific enzyme or transport activity; the inner membrane possesses a greatly increased proportion of protein, reflecting the presence of enzymes responsible for electron transport and oxidative phosphorylation, as well as numerous transport systems involved in the movement of substrates, metabolic intermediates and adenine nucleotides between the cytoplasm and the mitochondrial matrix, which itself contains a further battery of enzymes.

The space between the membranes, often called the intramembrane space, is the site of some enzymic activity and may also contain organic paracrystalline inclusions. Two varieties of these have been identified (Hammersen et al 1980, Stadhouders 1981): the more common is the 'parking lot' or type 1 inclusion which has a distinctive and complex structure (Fig. 2.12a) with a highly variable appearance in micrographs dependent upon its orientation relative to the plane of section (Schmalbruch 1983); the other, type 2, crystals are dense rectangular or elongated rhomboidal bodies (Fig. 2.12b) with an internal structure which is a fine regular lattice (Morgan-Hughes et al 1977). The type 1 crystals tend to occupy and distend that part of the intramembrane space which forms the core of the mitochondrial cristae, whereas the type 2 crystals usually lie between the inner and outer membranes, often in chains which displace the matrix and cristae to the ends of the mitochondrion, and to short segments between adjacent crystals (Fig. 2.12b); however, type 1 crystals can also on occasion be found in an intramural position and small type 2 crystals within the cristae.

The composition and functional significance of the paracrystalline inclusions are unknown, and although there appear to be structural similarities between the type 1 crystals and isolated cytochrome c oxidase crystals (Maniloff et al 1973, Landon 1982), Bonilla et al (1975) were unable to obtain electron histochemical evidence that they possess cytochrome oxidase activity. There appears to be no relationship between either type of crystalloid and any particular class of myofibre; both may be found within a single fibre and, rarely, within a single mitochondrion (D. N. Landon unpublished observations).

Paracrystalline inclusions may be found occasionally in normal human muscle of all ages (Hammersen et al 1980) and they are a regular feature of the myopathology of a number of disease states (DiMauro 1979, Carafoli & Roman 1980, Stadhouders 1981, Morgan-Hughes 1982), not all of which may involve a primary disturbance of mitochondrial function (Engel & Dale 1968, Chou 1969, Fardeau 1970). They may also be induced experimentally by ischaemia (Hanzlikova & Schiaffino 1977, Heine & Schaeg 1979), and by the administration of mitochondrial poisons including the uncoupling agent 2,4–dinitrophenol (Melmed et al 1975, Sahgal et

al 1979), and the respiratory chain inhibitor diphenyleneiodonium (Byrne et al 1982).

The mitochondria of skeletal muscle are situated both between the myofibrils and as aggregations beneath the plasmalemma. The latter are more prominent in type I, slow-twitch fibres, particularly in small rodents, and are greatly accentuated in certain human metabolic disorders, to give rise to the 'ragged-red' fibres seen in frozen sections stained with the Gomori trichrome technique. In mammalian muscles in general, mitochondrial content is inversely related to body size (Gauthier & Padykula 1966); and in human muscle the fibres of children contain, on average, a higher mitochondrial volume fraction (4.5%) than those of adults (3.4%) (Jerusalem et al 1975), and those of men (5.2%) more than those of women (4.1%) (Hoppeler et al 1973). The majority of the intermyofibrillar mitochondria are located adjacent to the Z lines of the sarcomeres, appearing in longitudinal sections as relatively inconspicuous, paired profiles at the level of each half I band, with the remainder orientated longitudinally between the myofibrils. Transverse sections taken close to the plane of the Z line show that the paired profiles represent mitochondria which partly or completely encircle each myofibril like a bracelet. In several mammalian species the mitochondria which surround individual myofibrils, particularly those in type I and type IIA fibres, can be shown to be parts of extensively branched 'mega' mitochondria which form continuous networks across the transverse dimension of the fibre (Fig. 2.12c) (Gauthier & Padykula 1966, Gauthier 1969, Schiaffino et al 1970, Rambourg & Segretain 1980), and are also connected to the longitudinal chains of intermyofibrillar mitochondria.

Quantitative studies of animal muscle have demonstrated substantial and consistent differences in the volume fractions of mitochondria in different myofibre types. The mitochondrial volume fractions of guinea pig red (soleus) and white (vastus) fibres are 5% and 1.9% respectively (Eisenberg et al 1974, Eisenberg & Kuda 1975), and similar figures have been obtained in studies of the rat soleus (6.6%) and medial gastrocnemius (2.1%) muscles (Stonnington & Engel 1973, Davey & Wong 1980), and for the red (4.9%) and white

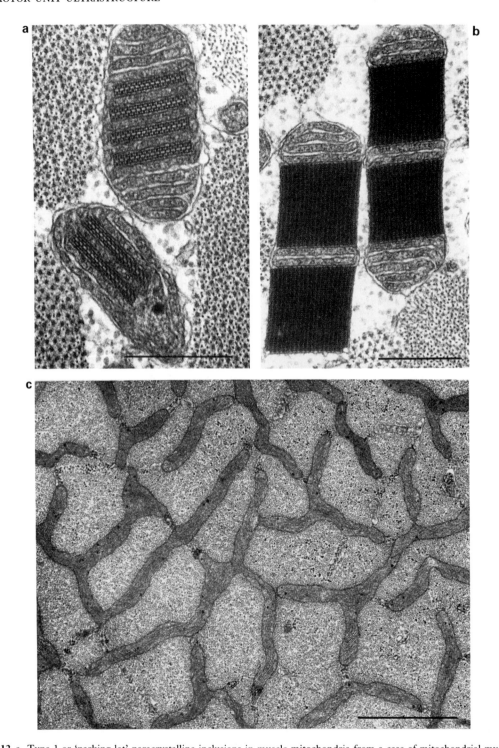

Fig. 2.12 a. Type 1 or 'parking lot' paracrystalline inclusions in muscle mitochondria from a case of mitochondrial myopathy. The crystals lie within the cristae in the intramembrane space.   b. Type 2 paracrystalline inclusions from the same case. They are more dense, with a fine regular internal structure always distinguishable from that of the type 1 crystals, and usually, as in this example, lie between the inner and outer membranes of the mitochondrion, displacing the matrix and cristae to its ends, and to small segments between adjacent crystals.   c. A transverse section through the 1 band region of a myofibre from the soleus muscle of a rat, illustrating the massive and extensively branched mitochondria (M) characteristic of slow red muscle fibres. Scales = 5 μm

(1.6%) fibres of the cat gastrocnemius (Kamien-iecka & Schmalbruch 1980). Fast red (type IIA) fibres generally possess larger individual mito-chondrial profiles than either slow (type I) or fast glycolytic (type IIB) fibres, but their orientation is predominantly longitudinal in contrast with the transverse orientation of the majority of the mito-chondria in the slow type I fibres (Eisenberg & Kuda 1976). Quantitative fine structural studies of human muscle have confirmed the histochemi-cal observation that there are greater numbers of mitochondria in type I than in type II fibres (Shafiq et al 1966, Ogata & Murata 1969, Eisen-berg 1983), and differences in the numbers and sizes of mitochondrial profiles have been used to identify myofibre types in human biopsies (Payne et al 1975).

Mitochondrial volume fraction has been shown to increase in the muscle of trained human subjects (orienteers) by Hoppeler et al (1973), and in long-distance runners when compared with untrained controls (Friden et al 1984). Compari-sons of distance runners with weight lifters have shown opposing trends in mitochondrial volume fraction when compared with controls, runners showing a generalised increase in all fibre types, but greatest in type I fibres, and weight lifters a loss of mitochondrial volume fraction in all except type IIA fibres (Prince et al 1981). In a study of the effects of training on sedentary middle-aged men, mitochondrial fraction increase was shown to be restricted to fibre types I and IIA (Sjostrom et al 1982b).

Internal membrane systems

Sarcoplasmic reticulum. The sarcoplasmic reticulum (SR) is a meshwork of membrane-bound tubules and cisternae which ensheath the myofibrils and abut upon the T-system tubules. There is, however, no membrane continuity with the T system, nor any communication with the extracellular space. The greater part of the SR is in the form of tubules which are organised roughly parallel to the longitudinal axis of the muscle fibre and which, in mammalian muscle, are divided by the T tubules into two intercommunicating systems, one lying over the A band and the other over the I band (Fig. 2.13). The longitudinal

tubules over the I band are less regularly organ-ised than those over the A band, probably because they share the space between the myofibrils with mitochondria and also have to withstand longitu-dinal compression during contraction of the muscle fibres. Where the SR tubules approach the T tubules they fuse circumferentially to form two transversely orientated terminal cisternae, one on either side of each T tubule (Fig. 2.14). This arrangement of two elements of the SR sand-wiching one T-system tubule is known as a 'triad'.

For convenience of nomenclature the SR is commonly divided into the longitudinal tubules and the terminal cisternae. An alternative more functional division is into free SR and junctional SR, the latter being the part of the terminal cisterna which faces the T tubule. The free SR is highly specialised as a calcium pump, while the junctional SR is in some way adapted to receive signals from the T system which control its capacity to accumulate calcium. The SR is the main calcium storage and release site in the muscle fibre. When the fibre is relaxed the SR maintains a Ca^{2+} concentration gradient of at least 1:1000 across its membrane (Hasselbach 1979). It is able to achieve this because the free SR membrane is very richly endowed with Ca^{2+} transport ATPase, which in rabbit muscle makes up 50–70% of all the SR membrane protein (Meissner & Fleischer 1971, Sarzala et al 1975). The ATPase molecules are concentrated in the cytoplasmic leaflet of the SR membrane, making the membrane highly asymmetrical. The P faces of freeze-fracture replicas of SR membranes contain abundant 8.5 nm intramembranous particles, and on the outer surface there are equally numerous particles 4 nm high which are the extramembranous tails of the intramembranous particles. Their packing is irregular (Franzini-Armstrong 1983) but they have an overall density of about 16 000 per μm^2 (Jilka et al 1975). It is thought that these particles represent a major portion of the ATPase molecule which projects from the membrane into the water phase of the sarcoplasm (Martonosi 1982).

As well as being composed of a membrane which is highly specialised as a calcium pump, the interior of the SR contains large quantities of a calcium-binding protein, calsequestrin. Calseques-trin is confined to the terminal cisternae of the SR

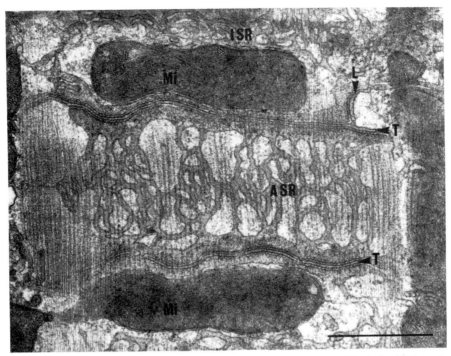

Fig. 2.13 Longitudinal section showing the division of the sarcoplasmic reticulum by the T tubules (T) into elements adjacent to the A band (ASR) and those adjacent to the I band (ISR). Note the longitudinal branch (L) to the T tubule. Mi = Mitochondrion. Mouse diaphragm muscle. Scale = 1 μm

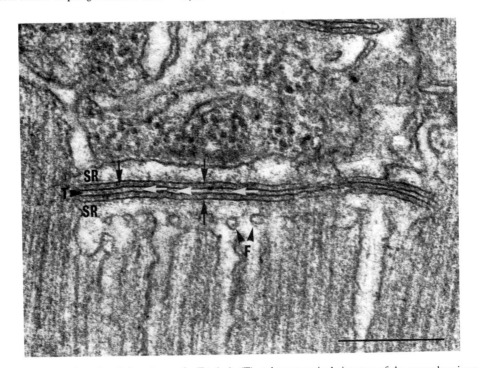

Fig. 2.14 Longitudinal section of a triad made up of a T tubule (T) and two terminal cisternae of the sarcoplasmic reticulum (SR). Note the feet (black arrows) which can appear as blocks, pillars or laminae. Note also the lamina (white arrows) in the lumen of the T tubule. F = fenestrations in the SR. Rat EDL muscle. Scale = 0.5 μm

where it sometimes appears as a granular electron-dense material in electron micrographs (MacLennan & Holland 1975). Isolated SR forms a heterogeneous mixture of 'light' and 'heavy' SR, of which the heavy fraction is derived from the terminal cisternae: it contains the calsequestrin and is composed of both free and junctional SR; the light fraction is composed entirely of free SR.

The amount of SR contained by a muscle fibre varies from muscle to muscle and from species to species. Published figures for the volume fraction range from <1.0% in the cat soleus and gastrocnemius (Schmalbruch 1979b) to >9% in the rat EDL (Davey & Wong 1980). In general, within any one species the fast–twitch glycolytic fibres contain approximately twice the volume of SR found in the slow-twitch oxidative fibres. The minimum interval after which a muscle contraction can be repeated is dependent upon the speed with which the free calcium ions can be sequestered by the SR following their release; the membrane surface area is therefore probably a more physiologically significant parameter than the contained volume. Published figures for the surface density of SR in mammalian muscle range from 0.09 μm^2 per μm^3 fibre in human slow-twitch fibres (Eisenberg 1983) to 4.59 μm^2 per μm^3 fibre in the fast-twitch fibres of the rat gastrocnemius (Stonnington & Engel 1973). Within any one species the fine structural parameter that correlates most strongly with the myofibre type is the surface density of the terminal cisternae (Eisenberg 1983).

There is a small subcomponent of the SR which is usually overlooked in the standard texts. This forms a tight band around the Z lines of the myofibrils: the tubules are narrower (30–50 nm) than other SR tubules, and can be difficult to identify in longitudinal sections, but show up clearly in transverse sections which pass through the plane of the Z line (Fig. 2.15). Short filamentous bridges link the SR to the Z line (Fig. 2.10a) to give the appearance of a mechanically stable structure. One may speculate that this part of the SR constitutes an anchor for the whole meshwork and prevents any major longitudinal displacement during contraction of the myofibrils. It is of interest that this association between the Z line and SR is present from a very early stage of

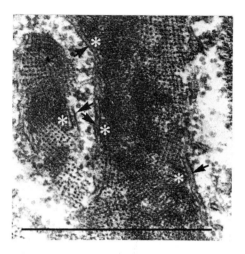

Fig. 2.15 Transverse section through the Z line of human triceps muscle showing the close apposition of a narrow SR tubule (arrows) to those areas corresponding to the exact centre of the Z line (asterisks). Scale = 1.0 μm

myofibril development (Walker et al 1975), implying that the SR collar must grow in conjunction with the myofibril as new filaments are added to its periphery. Whether this band of SR is linked to the intermediate filaments of desmin which link adjacent Z lines is not clear.

T system. The transverse tubular system or T system is a network of fine extensions of the plasma membrane which penetrates the muscle fibre and acts as a pathway for the inward propagation of the action potential. In man and other mammals the tubules of the T system skirt the myofibrils at the level of the A- and I-band junctions, two per sarcomere (Fig. 2.13). Although the greater part of the T system follows a transverse course, there are also occasional longitudinal elements linking these transverse tubules (Fig. 2.13). The peripheral connections of the T tubules to the plasma membrane may be direct or via caveolae.

T tubules are flattened in profile and, at their outer surfaces, measure 25–35 nm in the direction of the fibre axis and 90–130 nm perpendicular to it (Cullen et al 1984). The dimensions of the tubules seem to be fairly constant, although experimental modification of the tonicity of the extracellular fluid can cause swelling or shrinkage (Davey & O'Brien 1978). The volume of the muscle fibre occupied by the T system is extremely small: it varies with the type of myofibre but generally falls within the range 0.1–0.5% (Eisenberg 1983), the volume in fast glycolytic fibres being approximately twice that of slow oxidative fibres; this is due to a difference in the relative spacing of the tubules, not in their dimensions (Cullen et al 1984). More physiologically significant is the surface area of the T system per unit volume of the myofibre (surface density). This has a range in value of approximately 0.06–0.4 μm^2 per μm^3 muscle fibre, with the value for the fast glycolytic fibres being again approximately twice that of the slow oxidative fibres.

The T tubule is usually considered to be hollow and in diagrammatic representations is normally depicted as an empty tube (e.g. Fig. 55 in Schmalbruch 1985). However, in glutaraldehyde-fixed material a thin central lamina can often be resolved within the tubule lumen (Fig. 2.14). The significance of this structure and whether it corresponds to the tannic-acid-binding material described by Bonilla (1977) is uncertain. It is unusual to observe any larger structures within the T tubules of healthy muscle but, in stressed or diseased muscle, cellular debris can sometimes be seen in expanded tubules (Libelius et al 1979, Kelly et al 1986) as though they are acting as channels or gutters through which intracellular debris can escape to the extracellular space. This housekeeping role of the T system is probably of minor significance in healthy muscle where exocytosis appears to occur mainly via the plasma membrane.

The triad. The three-component complex formed by a transverse tubule flanked by two SR terminal cisternae is termed a triad (Fig. 2.14). The triads are inconspicuous elements of the muscle fibre but their fine structure has received considerable attention, as the site at which the electrical signal propagated along the T tubule is converted into a signal for Ca^{2+} release from the SR, thus occupying a central role in the contractile function of skeletal muscle. Although the triad is the most common form of association between the T system and SR in mammalian muscle, other combinations are also seen. Dyads, where the T tubule is flanked by the SR on only one side, often

occur in slow-twitch fibres and e.g. about 10% of associations in the rat soleus muscle are dyads (Cullen et al 1984). In contrast, pentads (two T tubules, three terminal cisternae) are the commonest naturally occurring associations seen in some particularly fast-contracting muscles (Revel 1962). Pentads and other multiple complexes are also common in atrophic, immature and regenerating fibres (Fig. 2.5). Peripheral couplings, where the SR receives its signals directly from the plasma membrane, are often seen in immature muscle and also in the primitive chordate, *Amphioxus*, which has no T system.

At the triad the apposed membranes of the T tubule and terminal cisterna are separated by a junctional gap of 11–14 nm. This gap is spanned by a double row of periodic densities or 'feet' (Franzini-Armstrong 1980). These originate on the SR side of the gap and in some views appear to make contact with the membrane of the T tubule. The appearance of the feet is variable. In attempting to devise a model of the structure of the feet, Franzini-Armstrong & Nunzi (1983) defined three basic appearances dependent on the plane of section: they could appear elongated in a plane parallel to the adjacent SR and T-tubule membranes; as a single dense column touching both membranes; or they could form a column with a hollow centre. Feet of the latter appearance have been called 'pillars' (Eisenberg & Gilai 1979) or 'bridges' (Somlyo 1979). On the basis of a comparison of the appearance of triads in tissue prepared by a range of different methods, Franzini-Armstrong & Nunzi were able to propose a model in which the feet cross the entire junctional gap, have lateral extensions at their midpoint and a central less dense core. In a more recent study of the three-dimensional substructure of the feet on freeze-dried heavy SR vesicles, Ferguson et al (1984) have found that they are composed of four subunits, and that in the double rows along the triads the feet do not abut corner to corner but are offset by half a subunit. A slightly different model of the feet has been described by Saito and his colleagues (Saito et al 1984) who examined tannic-acid-stained and negatively stained preparations of isolated terminal cisternae: they observed a chequer-board lattice of alternating square-shaped feet and spaces between them. The feet were

20 nm on each side with a centre-to-centre spacing of 40 nm and extended 12 nm from the surface of the junctional face of the SR membrane.

Freeze-fracture studies of the triad have shown that the cytoplasmic leaflet of the T-tubule component of the triad contains clusters of four particles repeating at regular intervals, and these lie opposite alternate sites of foot attachment. The cytoplasmic leaflet of the junctional SR is crowded with particles but the luminal leaflet is flat and has either a few small particles or very small pits (Franzini-Armstrong & Nunzi 1983). This is in contrast to the free SR where the tightly packed 8.5 nm particles (Ca^{2+} transport ATPase) do not leave pits on the luminal face.

Despite the detailed knowledge which has been obtained of the structure of the triad, the physiological events which occur during transmission of the signal for Ca^{2+} release from the SR are still obscure. One hypothesis, based on the observation that the number of pillars (feet) increases following stimulation, suggests that the pillars undergo a molecular reorganisation when the T tubule is depolarised. It is proposed that this produces a transient electrical coupling between the T tubule and terminal cisternae of the SR; depolarisation of the terminal cisternae then allows the release of the Ca^{2+} (Eisenberg 1983). An alternative hypothesis invokes a capacitance effect by which charge movement occurring in the membrane of the T tubule produces a tenfold increase in Ca^{2+} permeability in the SR (Schneider & Chandler 1973, Adrian & Almers 1976). It is suggested that there is a voltage sensor in the T-tubule membrane (Chandler et al 1976) and that there are shifts of macromolecular dipoles within the adjacent membranes (Adrian 1978). In the model proposed by Chandler et al (1976) it is suggested that each charge particle is associated with one foot; however, it has been found that muscle fibres showing different amounts of charge movement show no corresponding difference in the distribution of the junctional feet (Cullen et al 1984, Dulhunty et al 1984). Considerable research effort has gone into identifying a physiological role for the junctional feet in excitation–contraction coupling. The possibility should be borne in mind, however, that their role is mechanical, serving to bind the SR to the T

system and preventing their separation during the dimensional changes associated with contraction and relaxation.

There has recently been considerable interest in the possibility that the excitatory signal is transmitted across the junctional gap by chemical means. Experiments with skinned frog muscle fibres have shown that inositol triphosphate (IP_3) induces release of calcium from the SR, and that blockers of IP_3 also blocked the calcium transients associated with excitation (Vergara et al 1985). IP_3 is known to release calcium from the endoplasmic reticulum (ER) in other tissues (Berridge & Irvine 1984), and it is suggested by Vergara's group that it might act in a homologous way in skeletal muscle. The results of further work in this area will be of great interest.

The only structural feature of the triad which has been found to have a close quantitative relationship with the observed range of activation properties of skeletal muscle is the density of 'indentations' in the terminal cisternae of the SR. The indentations are arranged in a row in the terminal cisterna parallel with the T tubule (Rayns et al 1975), and there is a close correlation between the number of indentations and the amount of asymmetrical charge movement (Dulhunty et al 1983). There is also a close correlation between the fall in amount of charge movement and the numbers of indentations after denervation of rat EDL muscle fibres. In the soleus, where there is no change in charge movement after denervation, there is no change in the number of indentations, and this has been advanced as strong evidence for a functional link between the two during excitation–contraction coupling (Dulhunty et al 1984). Comparison of the freeze-fracture images published by Dulhunty and her co-workers (1983, 1984) with thin-sectioned material shows that the 'indentations' correspond to the fenestrations which mark the separation between the terminal cisternae and the longitudinal tubules of the SR (Fig. 2.14). These are 50–60 nm removed from the junctional SR where one might expect the initial steps of excitation–contraction coupling to occur. Although the indentations themselves are unlikely to be the sites of the initial interaction between T tubule and SR, they may well be closely associated with charge movement, and Dulhunty and her colleagues (1984) suggest that they may mark sites of calcium release.

Cytoskeleton

Eukaryotic cells, including muscle, contain three major cytoskeletal networks: F-actin or actin-like microfilaments (6 nm diameter), intermediate filaments (10–12 nm) and microtubules (25 nm). Because of its role in cell differentiation, motility and intracellular movement, the cytoskeleton has become a major area of interest in cell biology (see Porter 1984). In mature skeletal muscle, by far the greatest part of the F actin resides in the I filaments of the myofibrils, but it is also found in the Z lines (Lazarides 1980) and the stress fibres (Ishikawa et al 1969). The intermediate filaments are composed of a heterogeneous group of proteins:

in muscle, 'desmin' (skeletin) is probably the major component (Tokuyasu et al 1983) but others including 'vimentin', 'synemin' and 'epinemin' have also been described (Lawson 1983, Wang & Ramirez-Mitchell 1983). The intermediate filaments form bands which link the Z lines of adjacent myofibrils (Fig. 2.16), and also link Z lines of peripheral myofibrils to the plasma membrane. Some intermediate filaments run circumferentially around the myofibrils, and others parallel with their long axes (Wang & Ramirez-Mitchell 1983). It has been proposed that the attachment of the intermediate filaments to the plasma membrane is via molecules of 'spectrin', 'vinculin' or 'ankyrin', which in turn link to an integral membrane protein (Pardo et al 1983).

The microtubules, composed of α- and β-tubulin, are in general aligned parallel with the longitudinal axis of the muscle fibres, but others

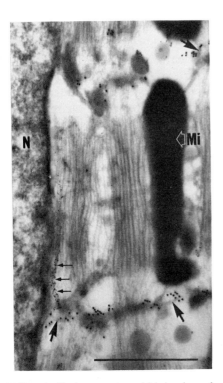

Fig. 2.16 Longitudinal cryosection which has been double-stained with 15 nm immunogold conjugated anti-desmin to identify the intermediate filaments (large arrows) and 5 nm immunogold conjugated anti-tubulin to identify the microtubules (small arrows). Mi = mitochondrion, N = myonucleus. Scale = 1.0 μm (Micrograph kindly donated by Dr. Simon Watkins, Harvard University, Boston)

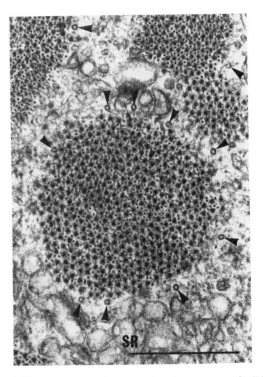

Fig. 2.17 Transverse section through an immature myofibril in regenerating rat muscle. Note the microtubules (arrows) closely surrounding the myofibril. SR = sarcoplasmic reticulum. Scale = 0.6 μm (Micrograph kindly donated by Dr. Sanjay Sesodia, Pasteur Institute, Paris)

spiral around the myofibrils. Microtubules and intermediate filaments are prominent in immature myotubes but become less conspicuous in mature myofibres. Growing myofibrils are closely surrounded by microtubules (Fig. 2.17); experiments in which interdigitating microtubule–myosin arrays were observed following the addition of taxol to chick myoblast cultures, have led to the suggestion that, during myofibrillogenesis, microtubules provide a scaffolding or substrate along which myosin monomers polymerise and are delivered as myosin filaments to the myofibril periphery (Antin et al 1981). Other evidence that microtubules play a part in the development of the myofibrils has come from experiments on cultured myotubes in which the microtubules were depolymerised by the addition of colcemide or cytochalasin and the myofibrils became greatly distorted (Holtzer et al 1975). Evidence for involvement of intermediate filaments in the morphogenesis of the myofibril is, to date, much less clear: the subunit composition of the intermediate filaments is known to change during the maturation of chick myotubes (Bennett et al 1979), and changes in location and organisation of the filaments during development have been described by Tokuyasu and his colleagues (Tokuyasu et al 1985).

Ultrastructure and histochemical fibre type

Attempts have been made by several groups of workers to correlate ultrastructural differences between muscle fibres with their histochemically defined fibre type: types I, IIA and IIB (slow-twitch oxidative, fast-twitch oxidative/glycolytic and fast-twitch glycolytic respectively). Electron-microscopic identification of defined fibre types would have potential use in obtaining ultrastructural correlates of known physiological or biochemical differences. This has been achieved quite successfully in animal muscles (Eisenberg et al 1974, Eisenberg & Kuda 1975, 1976, Schmalbruch 1979b), but the results obtained from human muscle have been more equivocal.

The features which have been most often measured are the Z-line and M-line widths, and mitochondrial and sarcotubular volume fractions. Reports of Z-line widths have varied widely between different studies, from values of 69 nm (type I), 58 nm (IIA) and 56 nm (IIB) obtained by Prince et al (1981), to 128 nm (type I), 104 nm (IIA) and 88 nm (IIB) obtained by Sjostrom et al (1982b). The differences reflect the problems of measuring Z-line widths in thin sections due to the difficulty of defining the physical limits of the structure. There is, however, general agreement that Z lines are broadest in type I fibres and narrowest in type IIB fibres.

The M line (Fig. 2.7) consists of three or five parallel lines of transverse M bridges (Knappeis & Carlsen 1968), the outer pair of which show considerable variation in staining intensity (Cullen & Weightman 1975). Using ultrathin frozen sections Sjostrom and his colleagues (1982a, b) have shown that only type I fibres display all five lines strongly; type IIA fibres have three strong central and two weak outer lines, and IIB fibres have only three central lines.

The mitochondrial content of muscles differs in men and women, and also varies with the extent to which a muscle is exercised (Hoppeler et al 1973). In general, however, oxidative fibres have a higher content than glycolytic fibres. Sjostrom's group (Angquist & Sjostrom 1980, Sjostrom et al 1982b) obtained volume fraction values of 5.6% (type I), 4.0% (IIA) and 2.8% (IIB) in the vastus lateralis muscle. In contrast Eisenberg (1983) measured only 1.14% in the fast fibres in the same muscle, with 3.03% in the slow fibres.

Several animal studies have shown an up to twofold difference in the volume of SR (Eisenberg & Kuda 1975, 1976, Schmalbruch 1979b) and of the T system (Luff & Atwood 1971, Cullen et al 1984) in fast fibres compared with slow. This relationship also seems to hold in man where Eisenberg (1983) has obtained values of 1.22% and 1.94% for the volume of SR in slow and fast fibres respectively in the quadriceps muscle, and values of 0.13% and 0.28% for the volumes of the T system in the same muscle.

To date, no single ultrastructural feature has been found which can be used reliably to distinguish muscle fibre type. (Sjostrom's group consider the M-line structure to be a reliable criterion but for those examining routine biopsy material this is impractical because of the high degree of standardisation required to obtain reproducible results — see p. 550 of Sjostrom et al 1982b). The difficulty stems from the fact that features such as Z-line width, and mitochondrial and SR volume, show continuous variation with overlap between values for defined fibre types (Schmalbruch 1985). Accuracy may be improved by using more than one feature but, whereas the identification may be reliable at either end of the continuum, fibres showing intermediate values are still difficult to type. Sjostrom and his colleagues (1982b) examined the human anterior tibialis and vastus lateralis muscles, using the M-line structure as the criterion of fibre type, and found that 83% of fibres were identified correctly using Z-line width, but that mitochondrial content was a much less reliable indicator, correlating with M-line width in only 37% of fibres.

Other myofibre constituents

In mature adult muscle the myofibrils, mitochondria, SR and T systems occupy most of the visible space in the myofibres. However, there are other constituents of the cytoplasm, minor in terms of space occupied but nevertheless having important roles in its metabolism: these are the fuels (glycogen and neutral lipid) and the organelles involved in synthesis and breakdown of the cell's various components (ribosomes, rough endoplasmic reticulum, Golgi apparatus and lysosomes).

Particles of *glycogen* can be seen in most muscle fibres, although they are scarce in a muscle which has just undergone prolonged exercise. The particles are 25–30 nm in diameter and are usually located around the I band (Fig. 2.18) but, in fibres in which they are plentiful, they may form regularly spaced rows in parallel with the A filaments. Fast-twitch fibres usually contain more glycogen particles than the slow-twitch fibres, but there is great variation in glycogen content among fibre types, and also within the same fibre type, and Essen & Henriksson (1974) reported a seven-fold variation in both slow-twitch and fast-twitch fibres in man.

Droplets of neutral *lipid* are usually found in close association with mitochondria. They represent approximately one-quarter of the total lipid in human muscle, most of the remainder being the phospholipid of the various membrane systems

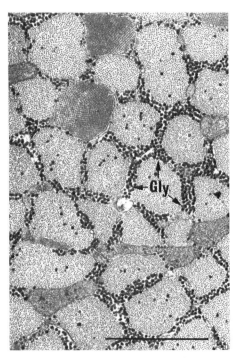

Fig. 2.18 Transverse section through the I band of a human fast-twitch fibre showing the accumulation of glycogen (Gly) between the myofibrils. Scale = 1 μm

(Waku 1977). Stereological measurements of the volume fraction occupied by lipid droplets in human muscle fibres have yielded a range of values from 0.12% (Jerusalem et al 1975) to 0.36% (Cullen & Weightman 1975). Lipid droplets are more common in slow-twitch oxidative fibres, but probably never constitute more than 1% of their volume in healthy muscle. Prince and his co-workers (1981) measured the lipid volume of slow-twitch oxidative, fast-twitch oxidative-glycolytic and fast-twitch glycolytic fibres separately and reported values of 0.66%, 0.22% and 0.15% respectively.

The organelles involved in protein synthesis are, not surprisingly, most conspicuous in developing or regenerating muscle fibres. *Ribosomes*, on which the events of protein synthesis are catalysed, are distributed throughout the cytoplasm (Fig. 2.19a). They are composed of a complex of RNA and protein and are slightly smaller (15–20 nm) than glycogen particles. *Polyribosomes* consist of a set of ribosomes spaced along a single messenger RNA molecule (Fig. 2.19a).

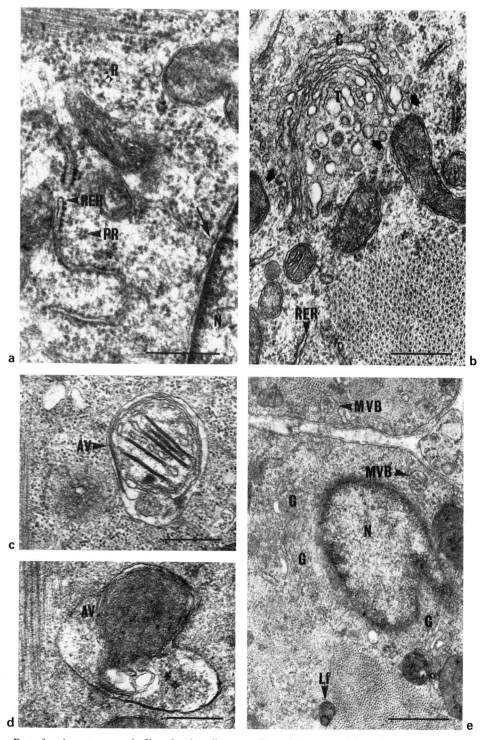

Fig. 2.19 a. Part of an immature muscle fibre showing ribosomes (R), polyribosomes (PR) and rough endoplasmic reticulum (RER). Note the continuity of the membranes of the endoplasmic reticulum and nuclear envelope (arrow). N = nucleus. b. Golgi apparatus in an immature myofibre showing cis (C) and trans (T) faces, with Golgi vesicles (arrows) being shed at the periphery. RER = rough endoplasmic reticulum. c. An autophagic vacuole (AV) containing a degenerate mitochondrion in a mouse soleus muscle. d. An autophagic vacuole (AV) containing a mitochondrion and cytoplasmic debris in a case of motor neurone disease. Scale (a–d) = 0.5 μm e. The perinuclear area of an immature myofibre showing Golgi apparatus (G), multivesicular bodies (MVB) and a small lipofuscin granule (Lf). N = nucleus. Scale = 1.0 μm

The endoplasmic reticulum, which is in continuity with the outer membrane of the nuclear envelope (Fig. 2.19a), is a complex system of interconnecting tubules and cisternae. In skeletal muscle the smooth endoplasmic reticulum, the sarcoplasmic reticulum, has become specialised for the binding and release of calcium ions. In *rough endoplasmic reticulum* (RER) the cytoplasmic surface of the membrane is studded with ribosomes and polyribosomes (Fig. 2.19a) with the larger (60s) subunit attached to the membrane and the smaller (40s) subunit distal to it. It is a major site of protein synthesis. Some of the proteins synthesised by the RER are moved via transfer vesicles to the *Golgi apparatus*, a stack of membrane-bound flattened cisternae (Fig. 2.19b). Each stack has two distinct sides: a usually convex 'cis' or forming face, and a usually concave 'trans' or maturing face. Within the Golgi apparatus macromolecules are modified, sorted and packaged for secretion or for delivery to other organelles. Golgi vesicles (~50 nm diameter) are shed from the periphery of the flattened cisternae. Golgi membrane systems are rare in mature muscle, being occasionally seen subsarcolemmally close to the nuclei, but like the ribosomes and RER are more conspicuous in developing muscle.

In liver parenchymal cells, and other metabolically active tissues, acid phosphatase and other lysosomal enzymes are concentrated in the most superficial cisternae of the 'trans' face, and in coated vesicles nearby. This suggests that primary *lysosomes* originate from the Golgi apparatus. It is not clear whether this is also the case in skeletal muscle where structures indistinguishable from the SR have been found to stain for lysosomal enzymes. For a summary of the evidence for an SR origin for primary lysosomes in muscle, the reader is referred to the review by Bird & Roisen (1986). Whatever the source of the primary lysosomes, their fate is to form secondary lysosomes by fusion with a membrane-bound substrate: this may be extracellular material in an endosome or intracellular material which has been wrapped prior to digestion. The autophagic vacuoles (Fig. 2.19c, d) thus formed are heterogeneous in size and appearance but can frequently be seen to contain mitochondrial remains or glycogen. Multivesicular bodies (Fig. 2.19e) are secondary lysosomes which are thought to be involved in membrane recycling. Myelin figures and lipofuscin granules are late-stage products of lysosomal digestion. Each of these various types of lysosome is comparatively rare in healthy muscle where the turnover of organelles is low, but they become much more common in diseased muscle and in old age (Ch. 8). The cellular source of the membranes which wrap and isolate the contents of the secondary lysosomes is controversial: they may be derived from the T system (Libelius et al 1979, Engel & Banker 1986) or, by homology with other classes of cell, from the SR (Christie & Stoward 1977, Cullen & Mastaglia 1982).

Myonuclei

The myofibre is a multinucleate syncytium which arises during ontogeny from the fusion of successive generations of mononuclear myoblasts/satellite cells. Each individual myofibre contains between 40 and 120 nuclei per mm of length, slow-twitch red fibres containing on average three times the nuclear population of white fast-twitch fibres (Burleigh 1977, Schmalbruch & Hellhammer 1977), and a 10 cm fibre may therefore contain upwards of 4000 nuclei in total. All intrinsic nuclei of skeletal muscle are diploid (Lash et al 1957, Strehler et al 1963, Bischoff & Holtzer 1969), with the corollary that they are incapable of synthesising DNA or of mitosis once incorporated into the myofibre. The mass of sarcoplasm which each nucleus is able to sustain appears to have a finite upper limit (Moss 1968), and work-induced hypertrophy of mature muscle is accompanied by an increase in the total content of nuclei within each fibre, obtained from the proliferation and fusion of its associated satellite cells (see p. 58), and not by a shift towards polyploidy of existing nuclei, as has been reported to be the case in hypertrophied human cardiac myocytes (Adler & Costabell 1975).

Most of the nuclei of normal mature myofibres are located superficially immediately beneath the plasmalemma. In relaxed muscle they are smooth ellipsoidal structures, approximately 10 μm long and 2.5 μm wide, with their long axis parallel to that of the fibre. In contracted muscle they develop an undulant profile with a series of ridges and grooves at right angles to the fibre axis. They therefore appear to have a defined location within the superficial zone of the myofibre, and are there surrounded by a small aggregation of sarcoplasm which normally contains one or two small stacks of Golgi membranes, some small elements of rough endoplasmic reticulum and a few mitochondria, and glycogen. Granules of lipofuscin, when present, are also usually located in the perinuclear cytoplasm.

In normal active skeletal muscle the intrinsic myonuclei usually show well-dispersed chromatin and have two nucleoli (Fig. 2.20a). In fibres which have undergone long-term denervation atrophy

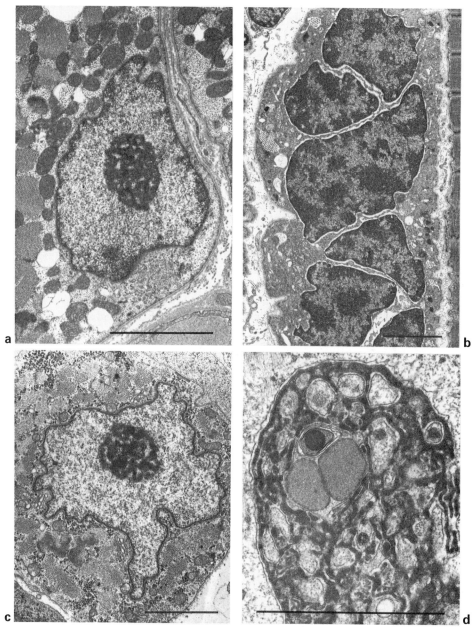

Fig. 2.20 Examples of the differing appearances of myonuclei: a. a normal nucleus with a rim of heterochromatin and a prominent nucleolus, lying in the superficial sarcoplasm beneath the plasmalemma; b. the nuclei of an atrophied fibre with condensed 'tigroid' heterochromatin; c. a nucleus in a developing myofibre having an irregular profile, dispersed chromatin and a massive nucleolus with conspicuous nucleonemata; d. part of a collapsed pyknotic nucleus from a denervated atrophying fibre. Scale = 3 μm

the nuclei become smaller, spherical and accumulate in small groups, and these changes are accompanied by disappearance of the nucleoli and condensation of their nucleoplasm into conspicuous dense clumps of heterochromatin attached to the nuclear envelope (Fig. 2.20b). The nuclei of growing or regenerating myofibres, on the other hand, are characterised by increase in size, an overall irregularity of outline in transverse section, and have fully dispersed chromatin and one or more large nucleoli containing prominent nucleonemata (Fig. 2.20c). In the more acute stages of fibre atrophy or degeneration from any cause, numbers of nuclei may undergo pyknosis, which is characterised by loss of volume, with condensation of the chromatin and collapse of the nuclear envelope, to produce a shrunken convoluted structure (Fig. 2.20d and Ch. 8). Further degeneration results in fragmentation of the collapsed nuclear envelope and its destruction by lysosomal activity.

Satellite cells

Myosatellite cells are a population of small, flattened mononucleate cells found in close apposition to the surface membrane of striated muscle fibres and beneath their basal laminae (Mauro 1961, Muir et al 1965, Campion 1984). They appear to be evenly distributed along the length of the myofibres (Muir 1970, Schultz 1979), but not necessarily entirely at random, as they are found more frequently in close association with intrinsic myonuclei than would occur by chance (Teravainen 1970, Ontell 1974), and they also commonly occur in increased numbers adjacent to the sole plates of neuromuscular junctions (perisynaptic satellite cells, Kelly 1978). Increased numbers of myosatellite cells are also found in association with the polar intracapsular regions of intrafusal myofibres in muscle spindles (Landon 1966). Myosatellite cells are considered to be a persisting population of myoblastic stem cells, the source of additional myofibre nuclei during the hypertrophic phase of muscle growth (Ishikawa 1966, Church 1969, Moss & Leblond 1971), and the source of the cells responsible for the regenerative repair of damaged muscle fibres in situ (Reznik 1969, 1970), in reimplanted minced muscle (Snow 1979), and in muscle cells cultured in vitro (Bischoff 1979).

The myosatellite cells lie beneath the myofibre basal lamina in a matching depression in the fibre surface (Fig. 2.21), and this close relationship, and the inclusion of the cell within the overall contour of the fibre, ensures that myosatellite cells can be identified with confidence only by the use of electron microscopy (Mauro 1961). They have, however, been identified in living frog muscle fibres by means of interference contrast optics (Lawrence & Mauro 1979), and their distinctive nuclear morphology allows a proportion to be identified in stained plastic sections (Ontell 1974). The numbers of myosatellite cells associated with each fibre declines with increase in age in mammals, including man (Allbrook et al 1971, Gibson & Schultz 1983); 10% of the 'myonuclei' are satellite cells in young human subjects, with the numbers falling to 2–3% in the normal muscle of adults. Myosatellite cell numbers increase in denervated muscle (Hess & Rosner 1970, Aloisi et al 1973, Ontell 1975, McGeatchie & Allbrook 1978, Schultz 1978, Murray & Robbins 1982, Snow 1983), in mildly traumatised muscle (Teravainen 1970) and in many muscle diseases (Shafiq et al 1967, Mair & Tomé 1972, Chou & Nonaka 1977, Lipton 1979, Wakayama & Schotland 1979). Myosatellite cells can be liberated from mature animal muscle fibres for study in vitro by enzymatic destruction of the basal laminae (Bischoff 1974); a quantitative method for obtaining myogenic cells from adult human muscle has been described by Yasin et al (1977).

The fine structure of myosatellite cells reflects their supposed stem-cell function (Fig. 2.21). Their nuclei contain conspicuous masses of clumped peripheral heterochromatin (Conen & Bell 1970, Schmalbruch 1985), lack nucleoli and are usually asymmetrically placed towards one pole of their fusiform cytoplasm (Franzini-Armstrong 1979). The perinuclear cytoplasm contains a few small mitochondria, and occasional stacks of rough endoplasmic reticulum and Golgi membrane systems; they may also contain glycogen, collections of phospholipid and lipofuscin granules in older human subjects. Paired centrioles also occur in this region, and one is occasionally associated with a longitudinal cilium lying embedded within the adjacent cytoplasm (Muir 1970, Conen & Bell 1970, Mair & Tomé 1972). The apposed plasma membranes of the myosatellite cell and the

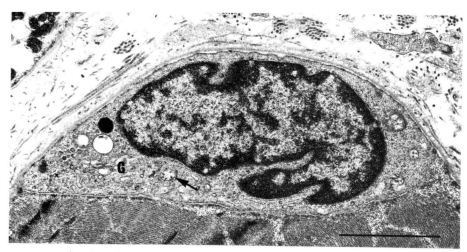

Fig. 2.21 A transverse section through a myosatellite cell lying beneath the basal lamina of a human muscle fibre. The nucleus is indented, and contains conspicuous clumped heterochromatin. The cytoplasm is characterised by numerous free ribosomes, Golgi vesicles (G) and contains the shaft of a cilium (arrow). Scale = 2 μm

myofibre are characteristically marked by numbers of attached pinocytotic vesicles, and over most of their region of apposition have a uniform separation of around 15 nm; this is occasionally increased by the presence of lamellated phospholipid material between the two cells, and narrowed by the presence of adhaerens-type junctions. Myosatellite cells seldom, if ever, contain organised arrays of myofilaments, and cells containing myofibrils in a similar satellite position can be shown by serial sectioning to be developing satellite myotubes (Landon 1970a, Ontell 1977).

THE MYOTENDINOUS JUNCTION

Muscle fibres usually taper as they approach their associated tendon and in the tapered zone become folded and ridged (Fig. 2.22a). In the area of attachment, finger-like projections of the fibres overlap and attach to collagenous projections of the tendon. The complex subdivision of the fibres results in a greatly increased surface area for attachment, and this extra membrane has been calculated to be 32 times that of the fibre cross-sectional area in the frog sartorius muscle (Eisenberg & Milton 1984).

At the myotendinous junction the myofibrils terminate in a Z-line-like material which may occupy the length of a sarcomere or more. This dense material is filamentous, contains α-actinin

(Trotter et al 1983) and closely approaches the cytoplasmic face of the plasma membrane which itself appears thickened. Fine filaments project from the outer face of the plasma membrane across the lamina lucida and insert into the basal lamina (lamina densa). It has been suggested that these 'spines' transmit force from the muscle fibre to the basal lamina and thence to the closely attached collagen fibrils (Fig. 2.22b) of the tendon (Korneliussen 1973). Force transmission at the myotendinous junction is unimpaired after detergent extraction of the plasma membrane. The fine filaments running from the cytoplasmic dense material to the basal lamina persist after the detergent treatment, suggesting that in intact fibres they run through the hydrophobic centre of the plasma membrane which in itself plays no significant part in the transmission of tension (Trotter et al 1981).

The collagen fibrils close to the myotendinous junction are more ordered than those in the endomysium away from the junction, although their mean diameter of 30 nm is unchanged (Fig. 2.22b). This contrasts with the tendon itself in which the fibrils range in diameter from 20 to 250 nm (Moore 1983).

Chiquet & Fambrough (1984a, b) have recently isolated and characterised a secretory protein, 'myotendinous antigen', which is found at the points of insertion of muscle into tendon. The appearance of 'myotendinous antigen' during

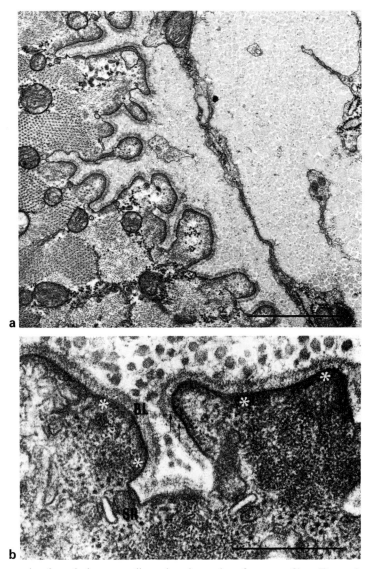

Fig. 2.22 a. Transverse section through the myotendinous junction region of a rat myofibre. The surface area of the fibre is greatly increased by irregular folds and ridges. The adjacent collagen fibrils have a wide range of diameters typical of a tendon. Scale = 1 μm   b. The plasma membrane at a myotendinous junction. Note the electron-dense plaques (asterisks) below the membrane and the filaments (arrows) crossing the lamina lucida to the basal lamina (BL). Note also the sarcoplasmic reticulum cisterna (SR) extending feet to the plasma membrane. Scale = 0.5 μm

limb morphogenesis, and its distribution in adult muscle, are compatible with it being involved in attaching muscle fibres to tendon fascicles.

An unexplained feature of myotendinous junctions is that they display acetylcholinesterase activity (Couteaux 1953, Zelena 1965). Nishikawa (1981) stained several different rat muscles for AChE activity at the light and electron microscopy level, and found that the activity was in the basal lamina, that it was higher in newborn than adult animals, and in slow fibres than fast fibres, and that it persisted for a time when a muscle was denervated but later declined as the fibres atrophied.

MUSCLE DEVELOPMENT

Mammalian striated muscle arises from cells in the metamerically segmented paraxial myotomes of the embryonic somatic mesoderm, differentiation following a proximo-distal and cephalo-caudal progression. The cells of the more medial parts of the myotomes differentiate in situ to give rise to the axial muscles of the trunk, while the more lateral and ventral migrate outwards into the somatopleuric mesoderm to form the muscles of the limbs and body wall. In the human embryo, condensations of mesenchyme are detectable at the sites of future muscle masses in the limb buds at the sixth week of gestation, and by the eighth week the primordia of the majority of the individual muscles are clearly defined. These anlage are composed of groups of small myotubes, multinucleate syncytia consisting of a central chain of rounded nuclei enclosed by a peripheral shell of amphiphilic cytoplasm bearing the first traces of cross-striation, lying within a loose stroma of connective tissue. Ultrastructurally the myotubes are characterised by central columns of nuclei containing prominent nucleoli, and syncytial cytoplasm rich in ribosomes, sarcotubular membranes, glycogen granules, lipid droplets and small myofibrils. The myotubes occur in small clusters separated by a reticulum of angular mesenchymal fibroblasts in a structureless matrix, and each is closely related to a number of less differentiated myogenic cells (Kelly & Zacks 1969). These consist of true mononucleate myoblasts — rounded cells containing small dense nuclei lacking nucleoli, and with cytoplasm rich in free ribosomes and large undulating cisterns of rough endoplasmic reticulum — and multinucleated myofilament-containing cells which represent the initial stage in the formation of the next generation of myotubes (see below); both varieties lie within the basal lamina of the established myotube, against which they abut. Only the mononucleate cells show evidence of mitosis, and it has been proposed that a proportion of myoblast divisions is 'critical' or 'quantal' (Holtzer 1970), in that one or both of the daughter cells are thereafter irrevocably committed to differentiation and fusion, either with other post-mitotic myoblasts to form

a new myotube, or with an existing myotube to add to its complement of nuclei and cytoplasm (see below). Studies of muscle regeneration in vitro have shown that the switch from proliferation to fusion requires a minimal density of cells, and appears to be promoted by the accumulation of a high-molecular-weight diffusible polypeptide within the culture medium (Konigsberg 1971). The shift into the post-mitotic phase is signalled by a prolongation of the Gl portion of the mitotic cycle (Konigsberg et al 1978), and initiation of the synthesis of muscle-specific proteins (Stockdale & Holtzer 1961). A small proportion of the mononucleate cells associated with the myotubes shows evidence of proliferation of rough endoplasmic reticulum from the nuclear envelope and the presence of a rudimentary nucleolus attached to the peripheral heterochromatin, and these structural modifications may be associated with the onset of prefusion differentiation in 'postquantal' cells.

Myoblast fusion has been observed by light-microscopic time–lapse photography (Cooper & Konigsberg 1961), but convincing fine structural images of the process are rare. Focal breakdown of the adjacent membranes of laterally aligned chick myoblasts in tissue culture has been observed by Shimada (1971), and this appeared to lead to the formation of cytoplasmic bridges between the cells which subsequently coalesced by breakdown of the residual portions of the membranes into vesicles. Lipton & Konigsberg (1972) described fusion in tissue-cultured quail muscle in which a single initial pore created by a small focal area of membrane fusion expanded by lateral extension without further membrane breakdown until fusion was complete. Discontinuous lengths of paired membranes between areas of cytoplasm containing differing patterns of myofibril content can be seen in transverse sections of muscle fibres regenerating in vivo: such appearances presumably represent incomplete stages of fusion. The individual contributions of fused myogenic cells to their joint cytoplasm have been identified by Ross et al (1970) on the basis of their differing content of ribosomes.

Once myotube formation has been initiated at the site of a future muscle their numbers increase rapidly: in the small mammals most studied experimentally, this continues until the second or third postnatal week (Kelly & Zacks 1969), and in man until at least the fourth postnatal month (Montgomery 1962) and possibly until the fifth decade (Adams & DeReuck 1973). This process of myotube hyperplasia is accompanied, and eventually succeeded, by a more prolonged phase of fibre hypertrophy extending throughout the growing period of the animal, in which the individual fibres increase in diameter and nuclear content and also in length to keep pace with the increasing dimensions of the trunk and limb segments within which they lie. The source of the additional myotubes which appear during the hyperplastic phase of muscle growth has been the subject of controversy in the past, some histologists favouring the idea that the increase in numbers is obtained from the splitting of pre-existing myotubes (MacCallum 1898, Cuajunco 1942), others that the new myotubes arise from the fusion of a continuously proliferating population of myogenic stem cells (Schwann 1839). Modern studies of the fine structure of muscle development, both in vivo and in vitro, have clearly demonstrated that the latter view is correct. Rows of mononucleate myoblasts become aligned along the length of pre-existing myotubes, and there fuse to form slender flattened multinucleated bands closely adherent to their more developed neighbour (Fig. 2.23a). Their nuclei possess prominent nucleoli, and the cytoplasm contains numerous free polysomes, Golgi membrane systems, some rough endoplasmic reticulum and thin bundles of thick and thin myofilaments organised into myofibrils. A striking feature of the interface between the new myotube and its more mature neighbour is the presence of finger or keel-like projections from the surface of the former, which lie within reciprocal invaginations of the cell membrane and cytoplasm of the older myotube (Kelly & Zacks 1969, Landon 1970a, 1971). The projections extend deep into the substance of the established myotube and are frequently found in close proximity to its nuclei (Fig. 2.23a), and the surfaces of both the invading and invaded cells bear 'coated' uptake vesicles. Quantitative studies (Landon 1971) have shown that these contacts achieve their greatest morpho-

logical complexity at the earliest stages of differentiation of the new myotubes, as judged by their content of myofibrils, and it has been suggested that the phenomenon may be associated with the transfer of morphogenetic information (Landon 1982). More subtle sites of intercellular contact in the form of 'gap junctions' have been reported to be widespread among the myogenic cells at early stages of muscle differentiation (Kelly & Zacks 1969, Rash & Staehelin 1974) and Rash & Fambrough (1973) have proposed that the appearance of gap junctions, and the concomitant increase in the electrical coupling of the cells in contact, are a normal prelude to cell fusion.

Continued differentiation of the secondary myotubes is associated with increase in their diameter, nuclear number and myofilament content, and with their separation from the primary myotubes (Landon 1971, Ontell 1979). The last is frequently accompanied by the appearance of columns of myoblasts interposed between the adjacent primary and secondary myotubes, and within their common basal lamina; these are the progenitors of the tertiary and later generations of myotubes, and there is evidence that such cells preferentially associate with the smallest, and thus by inference the least mature, of the existing myotube pair (Kelly & Zacks 1969). The new myotube resulting from their fusion will thus lie alongside, and differentiate in association with a secondary myotube in a similar manner to that described for the primary and secondary generations (Fig. 2.23b). Proliferation of new myotubes is accompanied by the concurrent maturation of established myotubes to myofibres, with migration of the nuclei to a peripheral subplasmalemmal position, synthesis of contractile proteins and their assembly into larger and more numerous myofibrils, maturation of the sarcotubular system and the establishment of a neuromuscular synapse.

Primitive myofibrils make an early appearance in the post-fusion development of mammalian myotubes and have been reported to be present in pre-fusion myoblasts in chicken muscle (Stockdale & Holtzer 1961). Slender organised bundles of I filaments attached to small dense bodies occur first in the more superficial parts of the myotube cytoplasm (Heuson-Stiennon 1965), coincidentally with the appearance of the first small regular

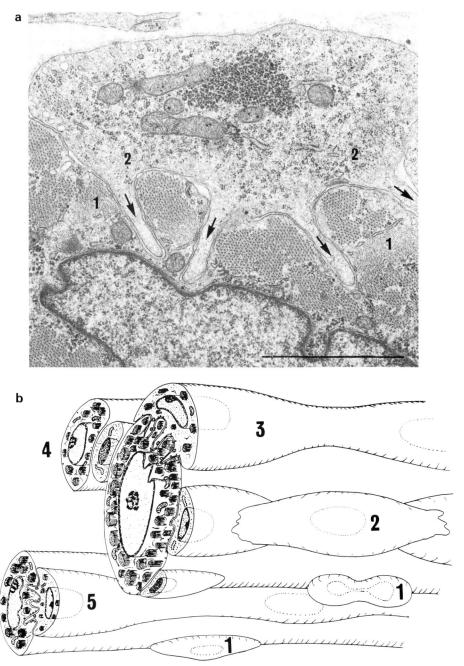

Fig. 2.23 a. A transverse section through a developing rat muscle illustrating the characteristic contacts between two generations of developing myotubes. The younger myotube (2) possesses numerous processes on its deep surface (arrows) which penetrate matching clefts into the substance of its more mature neighbour (1). Scale = 2 μm   b. A schematic illustration of the events associated with the production of new myotubes during the hyperplastic phase of myogenesis. Mononucleate myoblasts (1) adherent to the surface of pre-existing myotubes proliferate and differentiate to form chains of overlapping spindle-shaped cells (2). These then fuse, and the resulting nascent myotube (3) starts to synthesise contractile proteins and develops a close morphological relationship with the surface of its more mature neighbour. This contact is lost with further differentiation (4), and the two myotubes become separated by proliferation of myoblasts between their opposed surfaces. Repetition of these processes (5) gives rise to successive generations of new myotubes. Reproduced from Landon (1982) with permission from the editors and publishers

arrays of A filaments (Dessouky & Hibbs 1965, Fischman 1967); the latter are apparently synthesised in situ by long spiral polysomes which are closely associated with the peripheral filaments of each nascent A band (Allen & Pepe 1965, Larson et al 1973). Other filamentous components of the early developing myotube are the actin filaments of stress fibres which form a discontinuous feltwork beneath the plasmalemma, and randomly orientated 10 nm filaments (Ishikawa et al 1968), composed of 'desmin' (Lazarides & Balzer 1978); these diminish as the myofibrils increase in size and density (Bennett et al 1979) but some persist in the vicinity of the Z disc of the mature fibre and may assist in controlling the transverse alignment of the myofibrils (Thornell et al 1980).

The two components of the sarcotubular system, the transverse tubules and the sarcoplasmic reticulum, can be identified from the earliest stages of myotube differentiation, and appear to develop simultaneously (Ezerman & Ishikawa 1967, Schiaffino & Margreth 1969), the T tubules from invaginations of the surface membrane, and the sarcoplasmic reticulum from outgrowths of the rough endoplasmic reticulum of the early myotube. An extensive branched system of T tubules develops within the subplasmalemmal cytoplasm, from which branches penetrate between the myofibrils where they make triadic contacts with elements of the sarcoplasmic reticulum (Walker & Schrodt 1968, Kelly 1971, 1980). In the rat the sarcoplasmic reticulum has become organised into cylindrical segments by the second postnatal week, alternately in register with the A and I bands of successive sarcomeres, and triadic junctions have developed between the T tubules and the terminal cisterns of the reticulum at their interfaces opposite the junction of each A and I band. The differences in the extent and arrangement of the sarcoplasmic reticulum in fast- and slow-twitch fibres visible in adult muscle develops rather later in postnatal life (Luff & Attwood 1971), concurrently with their acquisition of mature contractile properties.

The hypertrophic phase of muscle growth, during which established fibres increase in both diameter and length, is associated with an increase in the numbers of their contained nuclei. It is now clear that this increase is brought about by the fusion of mononucleate cells with the growing fibres, and that this population of stem cells can be identified with the satellite cells (see p. 58). Satellite cells divide continuously throughout the period of active myogenesis (Hellmuth & Allbrook 1973) and it has been shown by radioautography (Moss & Leblond 1970, 1971) that a substantial proportion of the labelled daughter nuclei become incorporated into the myofibres as true muscle nuclei. Similar results have been obtained by implanting clonal cultures of labelled myoblasts into normal muscles of the original donor (Lipton & Schultz 1979). During the most active phase of myogenesis approximately 50% of the products of satellite cell divisions failed to fuse with myofibres (Hellmuth & Allbrook 1973) thereby maintaining a constant satellite cell population equivalent to approximately one-third of the numbers of true myonuclei (Schultz 1974). With cessation of growth, satellite cell numbers decline to about 5% of the total number of myofibre nuclei in small animals and to 2% in man.

The increase in fibre diameter associated with postnatal growth of the myofibres is largely attributable to an increase in the numbers of their contained myofibrils. These have a bimodal diameter distribution in growing muscle, and it has been suggested that myofibrils may have an optimum maximum diameter of 1–1.2 μm, and that when this value is exceeded they proliferate by subdivision (Goldspink 1970). Fine structural appearances compatible with this hypothesis are common, both during postnatal growth (Goldspink 1970) and in muscles responding to release from immobilisation (Shear 1975) or undergoing work hypertrophy (Goldspink & Ward 1979). These take the form of longitudinal clefts partly subdividing large myofibrils in the regions of their A and I bands, and areas of disorganisation at the Z disc; Goldspink (1970, 1971) has suggested that such division may be caused by an imbalance of mechanical forces during contraction.

Growth in length of individual myofibres is achieved by the addition of extra sarcomeres (Close 1964, 1972), with a small contribution from a reduction in the extent of the overlap of the thick and thin myofilaments at resting length as growth proceeds (Goldspink 1968), resulting in an increase in mean sarcomere length. Studies in which markers have been inserted into growing muscles (Kitiyakara & Angevine 1963) and autoradiographic experiments using isotope-labelled precursors of myofilament proteins (Williams & Goldspink 1971), have shown that the additional sarcomeres are incorporated into the ends of the growing myofibre at its osseous or tendinous insertions. Other workers have failed to confirm these findings (Crawford 1954, MacKay & Harrop 1969) and Schmalbruch (1985) has proposed an alternative mechanism in which sarcomere formation occurs along the length of the myofibril at foci of Z-disc damage of the kind observed in human muscle fibres subject to excessive 'eccentric' contraction (Fridén et al 1984). Immobilisation of growing mouse muscle at shortened length has been shown to result in a decrease in the rate of addition of sarcomeres (Williams & Goldspink

1971, 1973), normal numbers being recovered when the restriction to movement is removed. A similar adjustment of sarcomere numbers to functional length has been shown by Tabary et al (1972) to occur in the adult cat.

ACKNOWLEDGEMENTS

The authors wish to acknowledge their gratitude to Mr B. C. Young and Mr J. M. Walsh for their expert technical assistance in preparing material used to illustrate this chapter, to Mrs J. P. Humphreys for preparing the typescript, and to the editors and publishers referred to in figure captions for their permission to include material from previous publications in this chapter.

REFERENCES

Adams R D, DeReuck J 1973 Metrics of muscle. In: Kakulas B A (ed) Basic research in myology. Excerpta Medica, Amsterdam, vol I, p 3

Adler C-P, Costabel U 1975 Cell number in human heart in atrophy, hypertrophy, and under the influence of cytostatics. In: Fleckenstein A, Rona G (eds) Recent advances in studies on cardiac structure and metabolism, Vol 6. Pathophysiology and morphology of myocardial cell alteration. University Park Press, Baltimore, p 343–355

Adrian R H 1978 Charge movement in the membrane of striated muscle. Annual Reviews of Biophysics and Bioengineering 7: 85–112

Adrian R H, Almers W 1976 Charge movement in the membrane of striated muscle. Journal of Physiology 254: 339–360

Allbrook D B, Han M F, Hellmuth A E 1971 Population of muscle satellite cells in relation to age and mitotic activity. Pathology 3: 233–243

Allen E R, Pepe F A 1965 Ultrastructure of developing muscle cells in the chick embryo. American Journal of Anatomy 116: 115–148

Aloisi M, Mussini I, Schiaffino S 1973 Activation of muscle nuclei in denervation and hypertrophy. In: Kakulas B A (ed) Basic research in myology. Excerpta Medica, Amsterdam, vol I, p 338–342

Angquist K-A, Sjostrom M 1980 Intermittent claudication and muscle fibre fine structure. Morphometric data on mitochondrial volumes. Ultrastructural Pathology 1: 461–470

Antin P B, Forry-Schandies S, Friedman T M, Tapscott S J, Holtzer H 1981 Taxol induces postmitotic myoblasts to assemble interdigitating microtubule-myosin arrays that exclude actin filaments. Journal of Cell Biology 90: 300–308

Bailey A J, Shellswell G B, Duance V C 1979 Identification and change of collagen types in differentiating myoblasts and developing chick muscle. Nature 278: 67–68

Barnard E A, Dolly J O, Porter C W, Albuquerque E 1975 The acetylcholine receptor and the ionic conductance modulation system of skeletal muscle. Experimental Neurology 48: 1–28

Bennett G S, Fellini S A, Toyama Y, Holtzer H 1979 Redistribution of intermediate filament subunits during skeletal myogenesis and maturation in vitro. Journal of Cell Biology 82: 577–584

Berridge M J, Irvine R F 1984 Inositol triphosphate, a novel second messenger in cellular signal transduction. Nature 312: 315–321

Bird J W C, Roisen F J 1986 Lysosomes in muscle: developmental aspects, enzyme activities, and role in protein turnover. In: Engel A G, Banker B Q (eds) Myology. McGraw-Hill, New York, p 745

Bischoff R 1974 Enzymatic liberation of myogenic cells from adult rat muscle. Anatomical Record 180: 645–662

Bischoff R 1975 Regeneration of single skeletal muscle fibers in vitro. Anatomical Record 182: 215–236

Bischoff R 1979 Tissue culture studies on the origin of myogenic cells during muscle regeneration in the rat. In: Mauro A (ed) Muscle regeneration. Raven Press, New York, p 13–29

Bischoff R, Holtzer H 1969 Mitosis and the processes of differentiation of myogenic cells in vitro. Journal of Cell Biology 41: 188–200

Bloch R J, Hall Z W 1983 Cytoskeletal components of the vertebrate neuromuscular junction: vinculin, α-actinin and filamin. Journal of Cell Biology 97: 217–223

Bogusch G 1975 Electron microscopic observations on leptomeric fibrils and leptomeric complexes in the hen and pigeon heart. Journal of Molecular and Cellular Cardiology 7: 733–745

Bonilla E 1977 Staining of transverse tubular system of skeletal muscles by tannic acid-glutaraldehyde fixation. Journal of Ultrastructure Research 58: 162–165

Bonilla E, Schotland D L, DiMauro S, Aldover B 1975

Electron cytochemistry of crystalline inclusions in human skeletal muscle mitochondria. Journal of Ultrastructure Research 51: 404–408

Bonilla E, Fischbeck K, Schotland D L 1981 Freeze-fracture studies of muscle caveolae in human muscular dystrophy. American Journal of Pathology 104: 167–173

Bowman W 1840 On the minute structure and movements of voluntary muscle. Philosophical Transactions of the Royal Society of London, p 457–501

Boyd I A, Davey M R 1968 Composition of peripheral nerves. Livingstone, Edinburgh

Brandt P W, Lopez E, Reuben J P, Grundfest H 1967 The relationship between myofilament packing density and sarcomere length in frog striated muscle. Journal of Cell Biology 33: 255–263

Briskey E J, Seraydarian K, Mommaerts W F H M 1967 The modification of actomyosin by α actinin. II. The interaction between α actinin and actin. Biochimica et Biophysica Acta 133: 424–434

Burden S J, Sargent P B, McMahan U J 1979 Acetylcholine receptors in regenerating muscle accumulate at original synaptic sites in the absence of the nerve. Journal of Cell Biology 82: 412–425

Burleigh I G 1974 On the cellular regulation of growth and development in skeletal muscle. Biological Reviews 49: 267–320

Burleigh I G 1977 Observations on the number of nuclei within the fibres of some red and white muscles. Journal of Cell Science 23: 269–284

Byrne E, Hayes D J, Morgan-Hughes J A, Clark J B 1982 Some effects of experimentally induced mitochondrial lesions on the function and metabolic content of rat muscle. Proceedings of the Vth International Congress on Neuromuscular Diseases, Marseille 1982, (Abst) 35:3

Campion D R 1984 The muscle satellite cell: a review. International Review of Cytology 87: 225–251

Carafoli E, Roman I 1980 Mitochondria and disease. Molecular Aspects of Medicine 3: 295–429

Caspar D L D, Cohen C, Longley W 1969 Tropomyosin: crystal structure, polymorphism and molecular interactions. Journal of Molecular Biology 41: 87–107

Chandler W K, Rakowski R F, Schneider M F 1976 Effects of glycerol treatment and maintained depolarization on charge movement in skeletal muscle. Journal of Physiology 254: 284–316

Chiquet M, Fambrough D M 1984a Chick myotendinous antigen. I. A monoclonal antibody as a marker for tendon and muscle morphogenesis. Journal of Cell Biology 98: 1926–1936

Chiquet M, Fambrough D M 1984b Chick myotendinous antigen. II. A novel extracellular glycoprotein complex consisting of large disulphide-linked subunits. Journal of Cell Biology 98: 1937–1946

Chou S M 1969 'Megaconial' mitochondria observed in a case of chronic polymyositis. Acta Neuropathologica (Berlin) 12: 68–89

Chou S M, Nonaka I 1977 Satellite cells and muscle regeneration in diseased human skeletal muscle. Journal of the Neurological Sciences 34: 131–145

Chowrashi P K, Pepe F A 1979 M-band proteins: evidence for more than one component. In: Pepe F A, Sanger J W, Nachmias V T (eds) Motility in cell function. Academic Press, New York p 419–422

Christie K N, Stoward P J 1977 A cytochemical study of acid phosphatases in dystrophic hamster muscle. Journal of Ultrastructure Research 58: 219–234

Church J C T 1969 Satellite cells and myogenesis; a study in the fruit bat web. Journal of Anatomy 105: 419–438

Close R I 1964 Dynamic properties of fast and slow skeletal muscles of the rat during development. Journal of Physiology (London) 173: 74–95

Close R I 1972 Dynamic properties of mammalian skeletal muscles. Physiological Reviews 52: 129–197

Cohen C, Caspar D L D, Parry D A D, Lucas R M 1971 Tropomyosin crystal dynamics. Cold Spring Harbor Symposium on Quantitative Biology 36: 205–216

Conen P E, Bell C D 1970 Study of satellite cells in mature and fetal human muscle and rhabdomyosarcoma. In: Mauro A, Shafiq S A, Milhorat A T (eds) Regeneration of striated muscle and myogenesis. Excerpta Medica, Amsterdam, p 194–217

Cooper W G, Konigsberg I R 1961 Dynamics of myogenesis in vitro. Anatomical Record 140: 195–205

Couteaux R 1953 Particularités histochimique des zones d'insertion du muscle strié. Comptes rendus des séances de la Société de Biologie 147: 1974–1976

Couteaux R, Pecot-Dechauvassine M 1970 Vesicules synaptiques et poches au niveau des 'zones actives' de la jonction neuromusculaire. Comptes rendus hebdomadaires des séances de l'Académie des sciences D 271: 2346–2349

Craig R 1986 The structure of the contractile filaments. In: Engel A G, Banker B Q (eds) Myology. McGraw-Hill, New York, p 73

Craig R, Offer G 1976a Axial arrangement of crossbridges in thick filaments of vertebrate skeletal muscle. Journal of Molecular Biology 102: 325–332

Craig R, Offer G 1976b The location of C-protein in rabbit skeletal muscle. Proceedings of the Royal Society of London B 192: 451–461

Craig R, Megerman J 1979 Electron microscope studies on muscle thick filaments. In: Pepe F A, Sanger J W, Nachmias V T (eds) Motility in cell function. Academic Press, New York, p 91–102

Craig R, Knight P 1983 Myosin molecules, thick filaments and the actin-myosin complex. In: Harris J R (ed) Electron microscopy of proteins. Macromolecular structure and function, vol 4, p 97–203

Crawford G N C 1954 An experimental study of muscle growth in the rabbit. Journal of Bone and Joint Surgery 36: 294–303

Cuajunco F 1942 Development of the human motor end plate. Carnegie Institute, Washington publications 541. Contributions to Embryology 30: 127–152

Cullen M J, Weightman D 1975 The ultrastructure of normal human muscle in relation to fibre type. Journal of the Neurological Sciences 25: 43–56

Cullen M J, Mastaglia F L 1982 Pathological reactions of skeletal muscle. In: Mastaglia F L, Walton J N (eds) Skeletal muscle pathology. Churchill Livingstone, Edinburgh, p 88–139

Cullen M J, Hollingworth S, Marshall M W 1984 A comparative study of the transverse tubular system of the rat extensor digitorum longus and soleus muscles. Journal of Anatomy 138: 297–308

Davey D F 1976 The relation between Z-disk lattice spacing and sarcomere length in sartorius muscle fibres from *Hyla cerulea*. Australian Journal of Experimental Biological and Medical Science 54: 441–447

Davey D F, O'Brien G M 1978 The sarcoplasmic reticulum and T-system of rat extensor digitorum longus muscles exposed to hypertonic solutions. Australian Journal of Experimental Biology and Medical Science 56: 409–419

Davey D F, Wong S Y P 1980 Morphometric analysis of rat extensor digitorum longus and soleus muscles. Australian Journal of Experimental Biology and Medical Science 58: 213–230

Dessouky D A, Hibbs R G 1965 An electron microscope study of the development of the somatic muscle of the chick embryo. American Journal of Anatomy 116: 523–566

DiMauro S 1979 Metabolic myopathies. In: Vinken P J, Bruyn G W (eds) Handbook of clinical neurology. North Holland, Amsterdam, vol. 41, p 175–234

Dulhunty A F, Franzini-Armstrong C 1975 The relative contribution of folds and caveolae to the surface membrane of frog skeletal muscle fibres at different sarcomere lengths. Journal of Physiology (London) 250: 513–539

Dulhunty A F, Gage P W, Valois A A 1983 Indentations in the terminal cisternae of slow- and fast-twitch muscle fibres from normal and paraplegic rats. Journal of Ultrastructure Research 84: 50–59

Dulhunty A F, Gage P W, Valois A A 1984 Indentations in the terminal cisternae of denervated rat extensor digitorum longus and soleus muscles. Journal of Ultrastructure Research 88: 30–34

Ebashi S 1980 Regulation of muscle contraction. Proceedings of the Royal Society of London B 207: 259–286

Ebashi S, Ebashi F, Maruyama K 1964 A new protein factor promoting contraction of actomyosin. Nature 203: 645–646

Ebashi S, Kodama A, Ebashi F 1968 Troponin. I. Preparation and physiological function. Journal of Biochemistry (Tokyo) 64: 465–477

Eisenberg B R 1983 Quantitative ultrastructure of mammalian skeletal muscle. In: Peachey L D, Adrian R H (eds) Handbook of physiology, section 10: Skeletal muscle. American Physiological Society, Bethesda, p 73–112

Eisenberg B R, Kuda A M, Peter J B 1974 Stereological analysis of mammalian skeletal muscle. I Soleus muscle of the adult guinea pig. Journal of Cell Biology 60: 732–754

Eisenberg B R, Kuda A M 1975 Stereological analysis of mammalian skeletal muscle. II White vastus muscle of the adult guinea pig. Journal of Ultrastructure Research 51: 176–187

Eisenberg B R, Kuda A M, 1976 Discrimination between fiber populations in mammalian skeletal muscle by using ultrastructural parameters. Journal of Ultrastructure Research 54: 76–88

Eisenberg B R, Gilai A 1979 Structural changes in single muscle fibers after stimulation at a low frequency. Journal of General Physiology 74: 1–16

Eisenberg B R, Milton R L 1984 Muscle fiber termination at the tendon in the frog's sartorius: a stereological study. American Journal of Anatomy 171: 273–284

Elliott A, Offer G 1978 Shape and flexibility of the myosin molecule. Journal of Molecular Biology 123: 505–519

Elliott G F, Lowy J, Worthington C R 1963 An X-ray and light diffraction study of the filament lattice of striated muscle in the living state and rigor. Journal of Molecular Biology 6: 295–305

Elliott G F, Lowy J, Millman B M 1967 Low angle X-ray diffraction studies of living striated muscle during contraction. Journal of Molecular Biology 25: 31–45

Elliott G F, Rome E M, Spencer M 1970 A type of contraction hypothesis appplicable to all muscles. Nature 226: 400–417

Ellisman M H, Rash J E, Staehelin L A, Porter K R 1976 Studies of excitable membranes — II. A comparison of specializations at neuromuscular junctions and nonjunctional sarcolemmas of mammalian fast and slow twitch muscle fibers. Journal of Cell Biology 68: 752–774

Ellisman M H, Rash J E 1977 Studies of excitable membranes. III. Freeze-fracture examination of the membrane specializations at the neuromuscular junction and in the non-junctional sarcolemma after denervation. Brain Research 137: 197–206

Ellisman M H, Brooke M H, Kaiser K K, Rash J E 1978 Appearance in slow muscle sarcolemma of specializations characteristic of fast muscle after reinnervation by a fast muscle nerve. Experimental Neurology 58: 59–67

Endo M, Nonomura Y, Mosaki T, Ohtsuki I, Ebashi S 1966 Localization of native tropomyosin in relation to striation patterns. Journal of Biochemistry (Tokyo) 60: 605–608

Engel A G, Dale A J D 1968 Autophagic glycogenosis of late onset with mitochondrial abnormalities: light and electronmicroscopic observations. Proceedings of the Mayo Clinic 43: 233–279

Engel A G, Santa T 1971 Histometric analysis of the ultrastructure of the neuromuscular junction in myasthenia gravis and in the myasthenic syndrome. Annals of the New York Academy of Sciences 183: 46–63

Engel A G, Tsujihata M, Lindstrom J M, Lennon V A 1976 The motor end-plate in myasthenia gravis and in experimental autoimmune myasthenia gravis. A quantitative ultrastructural study. Annals of the New York Academy of Sciences 274: 60–79

Engel A G, Banker B Q 1986 Ultrastructural changes in diseased muscle. In: Engel A G, Banker B Q (eds) Myology. McGraw-Hill, New York, p 909

Essen B, Henriksson J 1974 Glycogen content of individual muscle fibers in man. Acta Physiologica Scandinavica 90: 645–647

Ezerman E B, Ishikawa H 1967 Differentiation of the sarcoplasmic reticulum and the T-system in developing chick skeletal muscle. Journal of Cell Biology 35: 405–420

Fardeau M 1969a Ultrastructure des fibres musculaires squelettiques. La Presse Médicale 77: 1341–1344

Fardeau M 1969b Etude d'une nouvelle observation de 'nemaline myopathy'. II. Données ultrastructurales. Acta Neuropathologica (Berlin) 13: 250–266

Fardeau M 1970 Ultrastructural lesions in progressive muscular dystrophies: a critical study of their specificity. In: Canal N, Scarlato G, Walton J N (eds) Muscle diseases. Excerpta Medica, Amsterdam, p 98–108

Ferguson D G, Schwartz H W, Franzini-Armstrong C 1984 Subunit structure of junctional feet in triads of skeletal muscle. A freeze-drying rotary shadowing study. Journal of Cell Biology 99: 1735–1742

Fertuk H C, Salpeter M M 1974 Localization of acetylcholine receptor by ^{125}I-labelled, α-bungarotoxin binding at mouse motor endplates. Proceedings of the National Academy of Sciences USA 71: 1376–1378

Fischbeck K H, Bonilla E, Schotland D L 1982 Freeze-fracture analysis of plasma membrane cholesterol in fast- and slow-twitch muscles. Journal of Ultrastructure Research 81: 117–123

Fischman D A 1967 An electron microscope study of myofibril formation in embryonic chick skeletal muscle. Journal of Cell Biology 32: 557–575

Franzini-Armstrong C 1970 Details of the I-band structure as revealed by the localization of Ferritin. Tissue and Cell 2: 327–338

Franzini-Armstrong C 1973 The structure of a simple Z line. Journal of Cell Biology 58: 630–642

Franzini-Armstrong C 1979 A description of satellite and

invasive cells in frog sartorius. In: Mauro A (ed) Muscle regeneration. Raven Press, New York, p 233–238

Franzini-Amstrong C 1980 Structure of sarcoplasmic reticulum. Federation Proceedings 39: 2403–2409

Franzini-Armstrong C 1983 Disposition of Ca ATPase in SR membrane from skeletal muscle. Journal of Cell Biology 97:260a

Franzini-Armstrong C, Porter K R 1964 The Z disc of skeletal muscle fibrils. Zeitschrift für Zellforschung und mikroskopische Anatomie 61: 661–672

Franzini-Armstrong C, Nunzi G 1983 Junctional feet and particles in the triads of a fast-twitch muscle fibre. Journal of Muscle Research and Cell Motility 4: 233–252

Fridén J 1984 Changes in human skeletal muscle induced by long-term eccentric exercise. Cell and Tissue Research 236: 365–372

Fridén J, Sjostrom M, Ekblom B 1984 Muscle fibre type characteristics in endurance trained and untrained individuals. European Journal of Applied Physiology 52: 266–271

Gauthier G F 1969 On the relationship of ultrastructural and cytochemical features to colour in mammalian skeletal muscle. Zeitschrift für Zellforschung und mikroskopische Anatomie 95: 462–482

Gauthier G F, Padykula H A 1966 Cytological studies of fiber types in skeletal muscle. Journal of Cell Biology 28: 333–354

Gibson M C, Schultz E 1983 Age-related differences in absolute numbers of skeletal muscle satellite cells. Muscle and Nerve 6: 574–580

Gilliatt R W 1966 Axon branching in motor nerves. In: Andrew B L (ed) Control and innervation of skeletal muscle. Thomson, Dundee, p 53–60

Goldspink G 1968 Sarcomere length during postnatal growth of mammalian muscle fibres. Journal of Cell Science 3: 539–548

Goldspink G 1970 The proliferation of myofibrils during muscle fibre growth. Journal of Cell Science 6: 593–604

Goldspink G 1971 Changes in striated muscle fibres during contraction and growth with particular reference to myofibril splitting. Journal of Cell Science 9: 123–137

Goldspink G, Ward P S 1979 Changes in rodent muscle fibre types during post-natal growth, undernutrition and exercise. Journal of Physiology 296: 453–469

Gray E G 1958 The structures of fast and slow muscle fibres in the frog. Journal of Anatomy 92: 559–562

Gruner J-E 1961 La structure fine du fuseau neuromusculaire humain. Revue Neurologique 104: 490–507

Hall Z W, Lubit B W, Schwartz J H 1981 Cytoplasmic actin in postsynaptic structures at the neuromuscular junction. Journal of Cell Biology 90: 789–792

Hammersen F, Gidlof A, Larsson J, Lewis D H 1980 The occurrence of paracrystalline mitochondrial inclusions in normal human skeletal muscle. Acta Neuropathologica (Berlin) 49: 35–41

Hanzlikova V, Schiaffino S 1977 Mitochondrial changes in ischaemic skeletal muscle. Journal of Ultrastructure Research 60: 121–133

Hasselbach W 1979 The sarcoplasmic calcium pump. A model of energy transmission in biological membranes. Topics in Current Chemistry 78: 1–56

Heine H, Schaeg G 1979 Origin and function of 'rod-like' structures in mitochondria. Acta Anatomica (Basel) 103: 1–10

Hellmuth A E, Allbrook D 1973 Satellite cells as the stem cells of skeletal muscle. In: Kakulas B A (ed) Basic research in myology. Excerpta Medica, Amsterdam, p 343–345

Hess A, Rosner S 1970 The satellite cell bud and myoblast in denervated mammalian muscle fibers. American Journal of Anatomy 129: 21–40

Heuser J E, Salpeter S R 1979 Organization of acetylcholine receptors in quick-frozen, deep-etched and rotary-replicated Torpedo postsynaptic membrane. Journal of Cell Biology 82: 150–173

Heuser J E, Reese T S, Dennis M J, Jan Y, Jan L, Evans L 1979 Synaptic vesicle exocytosis captured by quick freezing and correlated with quantal transmitter release. Journal of Cell Biology 81: 275–300

Heuser J E, Reese T S 1981 Structural changes after transmitter release at the frog neuromuscular junction. Journal of Cell Biology 88: 564–580

Heuson-Stiennon J A 1965 Morphogenèse de la cellule musculaire striée, etudiée au microscope électronique. I Formation des structures fibrillaires. Journal de Microscopie 4: 657–678

Hirokawa N, Heuser J E 1982 Internal and external differentiations of the postsynaptic membrane at the neuromuscular junction. Journal of Neurocytology 11: 487–510

Holtzer H 1970 Proliferation and quantal cell cycles in the differentiation of muscle, cartilage and red blood cells. In: Padykula H A (ed) Gene expression in somatic cells. Academic Press, New York, p 69–88

Holtzer H, Croop J, Dienstman S, Ishikawa H, Somlyo A P 1975 Effects of cytochalasin B and colcemid on myogenic cultures. Proceedings of the National Academy of Sciences USA 72: 513–517

Hoppeler H, Luthi P, Claassen H, Weibel E R, Howald H 1973 The ultrastructure of the normal human skeletal muscle: a morphometric analysis on untrained men, women and well trained orienteers. Pfluegers Archiv für die gesamte Physiologie des menschen und der tiere 344: 217–232

Hudson C S, Dyas B K, Rash J E 1982 Changes in number and distribution of orthogonal arrays during postnatal muscle development. Developmental Brain Research 4: 91–101

Huxley A F 1957 Muscle structure and theories of contraction. Progress in Biophysical Chemistry 7: 255–318

Huxley A F 1974 Muscular contraction. Journal of Physiology 243: 1–43

Huxley A F, Niedergerke R 1954 Interference microscopy of living muscle fibres. Nature 173: 971–973

Huxley A F, Simmons R M 1971 Proposed mechanism of force generation in striated muscle. Nature 233: 533–538

Huxley H E 1957 The double array of filaments in cross-striated muscle. Journal of Biophysical and Biochemical Cytology 3: 631–648

Huxley H E 1963 Electron microscopic studies on the structure of natural and synthetic protein filaments from striated muscle. Journal of Molecular Biology 7: 281–308

Huxley H E 1967 Recent X-ray diffraction and electron microscope studies of striated muscle. Journal of General Physiology 50: 71–83

Huxley H E 1969 The mechanism of muscle contraction. Science 164: 1356–1366

Huxley H E, Hanson J 1954 Changes in the cross striations

of muscle during contraction and stretch and their structural interpretation. Nature 173: 973–976

Huxley H E, Brown W 1967 The low-angle X-ray diagram of vertebrate striated muscle and its behaviour during contraction and rigor. Journal of Molecular Biology 30: 383–434

Ishikawa H 1966 Electron microscopic observations of satellite cells with special reference to the development of mammalian skeletal muscle. Zeitschrift für Anatomie und Entwicklungsgeschichte 125: 43–63

Ishikawa H, Bischoff R, Holtzer H 1968 Mitosis and intermediate sized filaments in developing skeletal muscle. Journal of Cell Biology 38: 538–555

Ishikawa H, Bischoff R, Holtzer H 1969 The formation of arrowhead complexes with heavy meromyosin in a variety of cell types. Journal of Cell Biology 43: 312–328

Jerusalem F, Engel A G, Peterson H A 1975 Human muscle fiber fine structure: morphometric data on controls. Neurology (Minneapolis) 25: 127–134

Jilka R L, Martonosi A N, Tillack T W 1975 Effect of purified $(Mg^{2+} + Ca^{2+})$ activated ATPase of sarcoplasmic reticulum upon the passive Ca^{2+} permeability and ultrastructure of phospholipid vesicles. Journal of Biological Chemistry 250: 7511–7524

Kamieniecka Z, Schmalbruch H 1980 Neuromuscular disorders with abnormal mitochondria. In: Bourne G H, Danielli J F (eds) International Review of Cytology vol 65. Academic Press, New York, p 321–357

Katz B 1961 The terminations of the afferent nerve fibre in the muscle spindle of the frog. Philosphical Transactions of the Royal Society of London B 243: 221–240

Kelly A M 1971 Sarcoplasmic reticulum and T tubules in differentiating rat skeletal muscle. Journal of Cell Biology 49: 335–344

Kelly A M 1978 Perisynaptic satellite cells in the developing and mature rat soleus muscle. Anatomical Record 190: 891–903

Kelly A M 1980 T tubules in neonatal rat soleus and extensor digitorum longus muscles. Developmental Biology 80: 501–505

Kelly A M, Zacks S I 1969 The histogenesis of rat intercostal muscle. Journal of Cell Biology 42: 135–153

Kelly D E 1967 Models of muscle Z-band fine structure based on a looping filament configuration. Journal of Cell Biology 34: 827–840

Kelly D E, Cahill M A 1972 Filamentous and matrix components of skeletal muscle Z-disks. Anatomical Record 172: 623–642

Kelly F J, McGrath J A, Goldspink D F, Cullen M J 1986 A morphological/biochemical study on the actions of corticosteroids on rat skeletal muscle. Muscle and Nerve 9: 1–10

Ketelsen U-P 1980 Quantitative freeze-fracture studies of human skeletal muscle cell membranes under normal and pathological conditions. In: Angelini C, Danieli G A, Fontanari A (eds) Muscular dystrophy research: advances and trends. Excerpta Medica, Amsterdam, p 79–87

Kitiyakara A, Angevine D M 1963 A study of the pattern of post embryonic growth of m. gracilis in mice. Developmental Biology 8: 322–340

Knappeis G G, Carlsen F 1962 The ultrastructure of the Z disc in skeletal muscle. Journal of Cell Biology 13: 323–335

Knappeis G G, Carlsen F 1968 The ultrastructure of the M-line in skeletal muscle. Journal of Cell Biology 38: 202–211

Konigsberg I R 1971 Diffusion-mediated control of myoblast fusion. Developmental Biology 26: 133–152

Konigsberg I R, Sollman P A, Mixter L O 1978 The duration of the terminal G^1 of fusing myoblasts. Developmental Biology 63: 11–26

Korneliussen H 1973 Ultrastructure of myotendinous junctions in myxine and rat. Specializations between the plasma membrane and the lamina densa. Zeitschrift für Anatomie und Entwicklungsgeschichte 142: 91–101

Kruger P 1952 Tetanus und Tonus der quergestriebten Skelettmuskeln der Wirbeltiere und des Menchen. Akademischer Verlag, Liepzig

Landon D N 1966 Electron microscopy of muscle spindles. In: Andrew B L (ed) Control and innervation of skeletal muscle. Thomson, Dundee, p 96–111

Landon D N 1969 The fine structure of the Z disc of rat striated muscle. Journal of Anatomy 106: 172p

Landon D N 1970a Observations on the morphogenesis of rat skeletal muscle. Journal of Anatomy 107: 385–387p

Landon D N 1970b The influence of fixation upon the fine structure of the Z-disk of rat striated muscle. Journal of Cell Science 6: 257–276

Landon D N 1970c Change in Z-disk structure with muscular contraction. Journal of Physiology 211: 44–45p

Landon D N 1971 A quantitative study of some of the fine structural features of developing myotubes in the rat. Journal of Anatomy 110: 170–171p

Landon D N 1982 Skeletal muscle—normal morphology, development and innervation. In: Mastaglia F L, Walton J N (eds) Skeletal muscle pathology. Churchill Livingstone, Edinburgh, p 1–87

Larson P F, Fulthorpe J J, Hudgson P 1973 The alignment of polysomes along myosin filaments in developing myofibrils. Journal of Anatomy 116: 327–334

Lash J W, Holtzer H, Swift H 1957 Regeneration of mature skeletal muscle. Anatomical Record 128: 679–698

Lawrence T, Mauro A 1979 Identification of satellite cells in vitro in frog muscle fibers by Nomarski optics. In: Mauro A (ed) Muscle regeneration. Raven Press, New York, p 275–284

Lawson D 1983 Epinemin: a new protein associated with vimentin filaments in non-neural cells. Journal of Cell Biology 97: 1891–1905

Lazarides E 1980 Intermediate filaments as mechanical integrators of cellular space. Nature 283: 249–256

Lazarides E, Balzer D R 1978 Specificity of desmin to avian and mammalian muscle cells. Cell 14: 429–438

Lee R E, Poulos A C, Mayer R F, Rash J E 1986 Caveolae preservation in the characterization of human neuromuscular disease. Muscle and Nerve 9: 127–137

Libelius R, Jirmanova I, Lundquist I, Thesleff S, Barnard E A 1979 T-tubule endocytosis in dystrophic chicken muscle and its relation to muscle fiber degeneration. Acta Neuropathologica (Berlin) 48: 31–38

Lipton B H 1979 Skeletal muscle regeneration in muscular dystrophy. In: Mauro A (ed) Muscle regeneration. Raven Press, New York, p 31–40

Lipton B H, Konigsberg I R 1972 A fine structural analysis of the fusion of myogenic cells. Journal of Cell Biology 53: 348–364

Lipton B H, Schultz E 1979 Developmental fate of skeletal muscle satellite cells. Science 205: 1292–1294

Lowey S, Slayter H S, Weeds A G, Baker H 1969 Structure of the myosin molecule. I Subfragments of myosin by enzymic degradation. Journal of Molecular Biology 42: 1–29

Luff A R, Atwood H L 1971 Changes in the sarcoplasmic reticulum and transverse tubular system of fast and slow skeletal muscles of the mouse during post-natal development. Journal of Cell Biology 51: 369–383

Luther P, Squire S 1978 Three-dimensional structure of the vertebrate muscle M-region. Journal of Molecular Biology 125: 313–324

MacCallum J B 1898 On the histogenesis of the striated muscle fibre and the growth of the human sartorius muscle. Johns Hopkins Hospital Bulletin 9: 208–215

McClare C W F 1971 Biochemical machines. Maxwell's demon and living organisms. Journal of Theoretical Biology 30: 1–34

MacDonald R D, Engel A G 1971 Observations on organization of Z-disk components and on rod-bodies of Z-disk origin. Journal of Cell Biology 48: 431–437

McGeatchie J, Allbrook D 1978 Cell proliferation in skeletal muscle following denervation or tenotomy. Cell and Tissue Research 193: 259–267

MacKay B, Harrop T J 1969 An experimental study of the longitudinal growth of skeletal muscle in the rat. Acta Anatomica (Basel) 72: 38–49

MacLennan D H, Holland P C 1975 Calcium transport in sarcoplasmic reticulum. Annual Review of Biophysics and Bioengineering 4: 377–404

McMahan U J, Sanes J R, Marshall L M 1978 Cholinesterase is associated with the basal lamina at the neuromuscular junction. Nature 271: 172–174

Mair W G P, Tomé F M S 1972 Atlas of the ultrastructure of diseased human muscle. Churchill Livingstone, Edinburgh

Maniloff J, Vanderkooi G, Hayashi H, Capaldi R A 1973 Optical analysis of electron micrographs of cytochrome oxidase membranes. Biochemica et Biophysica Acta 298: 180–183

Martonosi A N 1982 Regulation of cytoplasmic calcium concentration by sarcoplasmic reticulum. In: Schotland D L (ed) Disorders of the motor unit. John Wiley, New York, p 565–583

Masaki T, Endo M, Ebashi S 1967 Localization of 6s component of alpha actinin at the Z-band. Journal of Biochemistry (Tokyo) 62: 630–632

Matsubara I, Elliott G F 1972 X-ray diffraction studies on skinned single fibres of frog skeletal muscle. Journal of Molecular Biology 72: 657–669

Mauro A 1961 Satellite cell of skeletal muscle fibres. Journal of Biophysical and Biochemical Cytology 9: 493–495

Meissner G, Fleischer S 1971 Characterization of sarcoplasmic reticulum from skeletal muscle. Biochimica et Biophysica Acta 241:356–378

Melmed C, Karpati G, Carpenter S 1975 Experimental mitochondrial myopathy produced by in vivo uncoupling of oxidative phosphorylation. Journal of the Neurological Sciences 26: 305–318

Mishina M, Takai T, Imoto K, Noda M, Takahashi T, Numa S, Methfessel C, Sakmann B 1986 Molecular distinction between fetal and adult forms of muscle acetylcholine receptor. Nature 321: 406–411

Mobley B A, Eisenberg B R 1975 Sizes of components in frog skeletal muscle measured by methods of stereology. Journal of General Physiology 66: 31–45

Montgomery R D 1962 Growth of human striated muscle. Nature 195: 194–195

Moore M J 1983 The dual connective tissue system of rat soleus muscle. Muscle and Nerve 6: 416–422

Morgan-Hughes J A 1982 Mitochondrial myopathies. In: Mastaglia F L, Walton J N (eds) Skeletal muscle pathology. Churchill Livingstone, Edinburgh, p 309–339

Morgan-Hughes J A, Darveniza P, Kahn S N, Landon D N, Sherratt R M, Land J M, Clark J B 1977 A mitochondrial myopathy characterized by a deficiency in reducible cytochrome b. Brain 100: 617–640

Moss F P 1968 The relationship between the dimensions of the fibres and the number of nuclei during normal growth of skeletal muscle in the domestic fowl. American Journal of Anatomy 122: 555–564

Moss F P, Leblond C P 1970 Nature of dividing nuclei in skeletal muscle of growing rats. Journal of Cell Biology 44: 459–462

Moss F P, Leblond C P 1971 Satellite cells as the source of nuclei in muscles of growing rats. Anatomical Record 170: 421–436

Muir A R 1970 The structure and distibution of satellite cells. In: Mauro A, Shafiq S A, Milhorat A T (eds) Regeneration of striated muscle and myogenesis. Excerpta Medica, Amsterdam, p 91–100

Muir A R, Kanji A H M, Allbrook D B 1965 The structure of satellite cells in skeletal muscle. Journal of Anatomy 99: 435–444

Murray M A, Robbins N 1982 Cell proliferation in denervated muscle: identity and origin of the dividing cells. Neuroscience 7: 1823–1833

Needham D M 1971 Machina carnis. Cambridge University Press, Cambridge

Nishikawa M 1981 Histo- and cytochemistry of acetylcholinesterase activity at the myotendinous junctions in skeletal muscles of rats. Acta Histochemica et Cytochemica 14: 670–686

O'Brien E J, Dickens M J 1983 Actin and thin filaments. In: Harris J R (ed) Electron microscopy of proteins. Macromolecular strucutre and function, vol 4, p 1–95

Offer G, Moss C, Starr R 1973 A new protein of the thick filaments of vertebrate skeletal myofibrils. Extraction purification and characterization. Journal of Molecular Biology 74: 653–676

Ogata T, Murata F 1969 Cytological features of three fiber types in human striated muscle. Tohoko Journal of Experimental Medicine 99: 225–245

Ohashi K, Maruyama K 1980 A new structural protein located in the Z-line of chicken skeletal muscle. In: Ebashi S, Maruyama K, Endo M (eds) Muscle contraction its regulatory mechanisms. Japanese Scientific Societies Press, Tokyo, p 497–505

Ohtsuki I 1975 Distribution of troponin components in the thin filament studied by immunoelectron microscopy. Journal of Biochemistry (Tokyo) 77: 633–639

Ohtsuki I 1979 Molecular arrangement of troponin-T in the thin filament. Journal of Biochemistry (Tokyo) 86: 491–497

Ohtsuki I, Masaki T, Nonomura Y, Ebashi S 1967 Periodic distribution of troponin along the thin filament. Journal of Biochemistry (Tokyo) 61: 817–819

Oldfors A, Fardeau M 1983 The permeability of the basal lamina at the neuromuscular junction. An ultrastructural study of rat skeletal muscle using particulate tracers. Neuropathology and Applied Neurobiology 9: 419–432

Ontell M 1974 Muscle satellite cells. Anatomical Record 178: 211–228

Ontell M 1975 Evidence of myoblastic potential of satellite cells in denervated muscles. Cell and Tissue Research 160: 345–353

Ontell M 1977 Neonatal muscle: an electron microscopic study. Anatomical Record 189: 669–690

Ontell M 1979 The source of 'new' muscle fibers in neonatal muscle. In: Mauro A (ed) Muscle regeneration. Raven Press, New York, p 137–146

Padykula H A, Gauthier G F 1970 The ultrastructure of the neuromuscular junctions of mammalian red, white, and intermediate skeletal muscle fibers. Journal of Cell Biology 46: 27–41

Page E, Power B, Fozzard H A, Meddoff D A 1969 Sarcolemmal evaginations with knob-like or stalked projections in purkinje fibers of the sheep's heart. Journal of Ultrastructure Research 28: 288–300

Page S G 1965 A comparison of the fine structure of frog slow and twitch muscle fibres. Journal of Cell Biology 26: 477–497

Page S G 1968 Fine structure of tortoise skeletal muscle. Journal of Physiology 197: 709–715

Pardo J V, Siliciano J D, Craig S W 1983 A vinculin-containing cortical lattice in skeletal muscle: transverse lattice elements ('costameres') mark sites of attachment between myofibrils and sarcolemma. Proceedings of the National Academy of Sciences USA 80: 1008–1012

Payne C M, Stern L Z, Curless R G, Hannapel L K 1975 Ultrastructural fiber typing in normal and diseased human muscle. Journal of the Neurological Sciences 25: 99–108

Peluchetti D, Mora M, Protti A, Cornelio F 1985 Freeze-fracture analysis of the muscle fiber plasma membrane in Duchenne dystrophy. Neurology 35: 928–930

Pepe F A 1966 Some aspects of the structural organization of the myofibril as revealed by antibody-staining methods. Journal of Cell Biology 28: 505–525

Pepe F A, Drucker B 1975 The myosin filament. III. C-protein. Journal of Molecular Biology 99: 609–617

Perry S V, Dhoot G K 1980 Biochemical aspects of muscle development and differentiation. In: Goldspink D F (ed) Development and specialization of skeletal muscle. Cambridge University Press, Cambridge, p 51–64

Porter K R 1984 The cytomatrix: a short history of its study. Journal of Cell Biology 99: 3s–12s

Prince F P, Hikida R S, Hagerman F C, Staron R S, Allen W H 1981 A morphometric analysis of human muscle fibers with relation to fiber types and adaptations to exercise. Journal of the Neurological Sciences 49: 165–179

Pumplin D W, Fambrough D M 1983 (Na$^+$ + K$^+$)-ATPase correlated with a major group of intramembrane particles in freeze-fracture replicas of cultured chick myotubes. Journal of Cell Biology 97: 1214–1225

Rambourg A, Segretain D 1980 Three-dimensional electron microscopy of mitochondria and endoplasmic reticulum in the red muscle fiber of the rat diaphragm. Anatomical Record 197: 33–48

Rash J E, Fambrough D 1973 Ultrastructural and electrophysiological correlates of cell coupling and cytoplasmic fusion during myogenesis in vitro. Developmental Biology 30: 166–186

Rash J E, Ellisman M H 1974 Studies of excitable membranes. I. Macromolecular specializations of the neuromuscular junction and the nonjunctional sarcolemma. Journal of Cell Biology 63: 567–586

Rash J E, Staehelin L A 1974 Freeze-cleave demonstration of gap junctions between skeletal myogenic cells in vitro. Developmental Biology 36: 455–461

Rash J E, Ellisman M H, Staehelin L A, Porter K R 1974 Molecular specializations of excitable membranes in normal, chronically denervated, and dystrophic muscle fibers. In: Milhorat A T (ed) Exploratory concepts in muscular dystrophy II. Excerpta Medica, Amsterdam, p 271–291

Rayns D G, Devine C E, Sutherland C L 1975 Freeze-fracture of membrane systems in vertebrate muscle. I. Striated muscle. Journal of Ultrastructure Research 50: 306–321

Reedy M K 1964 The structure of actin filaments and the origin of the axial periodicity in the I substance of vertebrate striated muscle. Proceedings of the Royal Society of London B 160: 458–460

Reedy M K 1967 Personal communication, quoted by Elliott, Lowy and Millman 1967

Revel J P 1962 The sarcoplasmic reticulum of the bat cricothyroid muscle. Journal of Cell Biology 12: 571–588

Reznik M 1969 Thymidine ^{3}H uptake by satellite cells of regenerating skeletal muscle. Journal of Cell Biology 40: 568–571

Reznik M 1970 Satellite cells, myoblasts and skeletal muscle regeneration. In: Mauro A, Shafiq S A, Milhorat A T (eds) Regeneration of skeletal muscle, and myogenesis. Excerpta Medica, Amsterdam, p 133–156

Rosenbluth J 1974 Structure of amphibian motor-end plate. Evidence for granular component projecting from the outer surface of the receptive membrane. Journal of Cell Biology 62: 755–766

Ross K F A, Jans D E, Larson P F et al 1970 Distribution of ribosomal RNA in fusing myoblasts. Nature 226: 545–547

Rowe R W 1971 Ultrastructure of the Z-line of skeletal muscle fibers. Journal of Cell Biology 51: 674–685

Rowe R W 1973 The ultrastructure of Z-disks from white, intermediate, and red fibers of mammalian striated muscle. Journal of Cell Biology 57: 261–277

Ruska H A, Edwards G A 1957 A new cytoplasmic pattern in striated muscle fibres and its possible relation to growth. Growth 21: 73–88

Sahgal V, Subramani V, Hughes R, Shah H, Singh H 1979 On the pathogenesis of mitochondrial myopathies: an experimental study. Acta Neuropathologica (Berlin) 46: 177–183

Saito A, Seiler S, Chu A, Fleischer S 1984 Preparation and morphology of sarcoplasmic reticulum terminal cisternae from rabbit skeletal muscle. Journal of Cell Biology 99: 875–885

Sanes J R 1982 Laminin, fibronectin and collagen in synaptic and extrasynaptic portions of muscle fiber basement membrane. Journal of Cell Biology 93: 442–451

Sanes J R, Marshall L M, McMahan U J 1978 Reinnervation of muscle fiber basal lamina after removal of myofibers. Differentiation of regenerating axons at original synaptic sites. Journal of Cell Biology 78: 176–198

Sanes J R, Hall Z W 1979 Antibodies that bind specifically to synaptic sites on muscle fiber basal lamina. Journal of Cell Biology 83: 357–370

Sanes J R, Cheney J M 1982 Lectin binding reveals a synapse-specific carbohydrate in skeletal muscle. Nature 300: 646–647

Sanes J R, Chiu A Y 1983 The basal lamina of the neuromuscular junction. Cold Spring Harbor Symposium on Quantitative Biology 48: 667–678

Sarzala M G, Pilarska M, Zubrzycka E, Michalak M 1975 Changes in the structure, composition and function of sarcoplasmic reticulum membrane during development. European Journal of Biochemistry 57: 25–34

Scalzi H A, Price H M 1971 The arrangement and sensory innervation of the intrafusal fibers in the feline muscle spindle. Journal of Ultrastructure Research 36: 375–390

Schiaffino S, Margreth A 1969 Coordinated development of the sarcoplasmic reticulum and T-system during postnatal differentiation of rat skeletal muscle. Journal of Cell Biology 41: 855–875

Schiaffino S, Hanzlikova V, Pierobon S 1970 Relations between structure and function in rat skeletal muscle fibers. Journal of Cell Biology 47: 107–119

Schmalbruch H 1979a 'Square arrays' in the sarcolemma of human skeletal muscle fibres. Nature 281: 145–146

Schmalbruch H 1979b The membrane systems in different fibre types of the triceps surae muscle of cat. Cell and Tissue Research 204: 187–200

Schmalbruch H 1980 Delayed fixation alters the pattern of intramembrane particles in mammalian muscle fibers. Journal of Ultrastructure Research 70: 15–20

Schmalbruch H 1983 The fine structure of mitochondrial abnormalities in muscle diseases. In: Scarlatto G, Cerri C (eds) Mitochondrial pathology in muscle diseases. Piccin, Padua, p 41–56

Schmalbruch H 1985 Skeletal muscle. Handbook of microscopic anatomy, vol 2, Pt 6. Springer-Verlag, Berlin

Schmalbruch H, Hellhammer U 1977 The number of nuclei in adult rat muscles with special reference to satellite cells. Anatomical Record 189: 169–176

Schneider M, Chandler W K 1973 Voltage dependent charge movement in skeletal muscle: a possible step in excitation-contraction coupling. Nature 242: 244–246

Schollmeyer J V, Goll D E, Stromer M H, Dayton W, Singh I, Robson R 1974 Studies on the composition of the Z-disk. Journal of Cell Biology 63:303a

Schotland D L, Bonilla E, Wakayama Y 1981 Freeze-fracture studies of muscle plasma membrane in human muscular dystrophy. Acta Neuropathologica (Berlin) 54: 189–197

Schultz E 1974 A quantitative study of the satellite cell population in post-natal mouse lumbrical muscle. Anatomical Record 180: 589–596

Schultz E 1978 Changes in satellite cells of growing muscle following denervation. Anatomical Record 190: 299–312

Schultz E 1979 Quantification of satellite cells in growing muscle using electron microscopy and fiber whole mounts. In: Mauro A (ed) Muscle regeneration. Raven Press, New York, p 131–135

Schwann T 1839 Mikroskopische Untersuchungen uber die Uebereinstimmung in der Struktur und dem Wachsthum der Thiere und Pflanzen. Reimer, Berlin

Shafiq S A, Gorycki M A, Goldstone L, Milhorat A T 1966 Fine structure of fiber types in normal human muscle. Anatomical Record 156: 283–302

Shafiq S A, Gorycki M, Milhorat A T 1967 An electron microscopic study of regeneration and satellite cells in human muscle. Neurology (Minneapolis) 17: 567–574

Shafiq S A, Leung B, Schutta H S 1979 A freeze-fracture study of fibre types in normal human muscle. Journal of the Neurological Sciences 42: 129–138

Shear C R 1975 Myofibril proliferation in developing skeletal muscle. In: Bradley W G, Gardner-Medwin D, Walton J N (eds) Recent advances in myology. Excerpta Medica, Amsterdam, p 364–373

Shear C R, Bloch R J 1985 Vinculin in subsarcolemmal densities in chicken skeletal muscle: localization and relationship to intracellular and extracellular structures. Journal of Cell Biology 101: 240–256

Shimada Y 1971 Electron microscope observations on the fusion of chick myoblasts in vitro. Journal of Cell Biology 48: 128–142

Singh I, Goll D E, Robson R M, Stromer M H 1977 N- and C- terminal amino acids of purified alpha actinin. Biochimica et Biophysica Acta 491: 29–45

Sirken S M, Fischbeck K H 1985 Freeze-fracture studies of denervated and tenotomized rat muscle. Journal of Neuropathology and Experimental Neurology 44: 147–155

Sjostrom M, Squire J M 1977 The fine structure of the A-band in cryo-sections. Journal of Molecular Biology 109: 49–68

Sjostrom M, Kidman S, Henriksson-Larsen K, Angquist K-A 1982a Z- and M-band appearance in different histochemically defined types of human skeletal muscle fibres. Journal of Histochemistry and Cytochemistry 30: 1–11

Sjostrom M, Angqvist K-A, Bylund A-C, Friden J, Gustavsson L, Shersten T 1982b Morphometric analysis of human muscle fiber types. Muscle and Nerve 5: 538–553

Snow M H 1979 Origin of regenerating myoblasts in mammalian skeletal muscle. In: Mauro A (ed) Muscle regeneration. Raven Press, New York, p 91–100

Snow M H 1983 A quantitative ultrastructural analysis of satellite cells in denervated fast and slow muscles of the mouse. Anatomical Record 207: 593–604

Somlyo A V 1979 Bridging structures spanning the junctional gap at the triad of skeletal muscle. Journal of Cell Biology 80: 743–750

Spencer M, Worthington C R 1960 A hypothesis of contraction in striated muscle. Nature 187: 388–391

Squire J 1981 The structural basis of muscular contraction. Plenum, New York

Stadhouders A M 1981 Mitochondrial ultrastructural changes in muscular diseases. In: Busch H F M, Jennekens F G I, Scholte H R (eds) Mitochondria and muscular diseases. Mefar, Netherlands, p 113–132

Stockdale F E, Holtzer H 1961 DNA synthesis and myogenesis. Experimental Cell Research 24: 508–520

Stonnington H H, Engel A G 1973 Normal and denervated muscle. A morphometric study of fine structure. Neurology (New York) 23: 714–724

Strehler B L, Konigsberg I R, Kelley J E T 1963 Ploidy of myotube nuclei developing in vitro as determined with a recording double beam micro-spectrophotometer. Experimental Cell Research 32: 232–241

Stromer M H, Hartshorne D J, Rice R V 1967 Removal and reconstruction of Z-line material in striated muscle. Journal of Cell Biology 35: 623–628

Stromer M H, Hartshorne D J, Mueller H, Rice R V 1969 The effects of various protein fractions on Z- and M- line reconstruction. Journal of Cell Biology 40: 167–178

Suzuki A, Goll D E, Singh I, Allen R E, Robson R M, Stromer M H 1976 Some properties of purified skeletal muscle alpha actinin. Journal of Biological Chemistry 251: 6860–6870

Tabary J C, Tabart C, Tardieu C, Tardieu G, Goldspink G 1972 Physiological and structural changes in the cat's soleus muscle due to immobilization at different lengths by plaster casts. Journal of Physiology 224: 231–244

Tachikawa T, Clementi F 1979 Early effects of denervation on the morphology of junctional and extrajunctional sarcolemma. Neuroscience 4: 437–451

Teravainen H 1970 Satellite cells of striated muscle after compression injury so slight as not to cause degeneration of the muscle fibres. Zeitschrift für Zellforschung und Mikroskopische Anatomie 103: 320–327

Thornell L-E, Sjostrom M, Andersson K-E 1976 The relationship between mechanical stress and myofibrillar organization in heart purkinje fibres. Journal of Molecular and Cellular Cardiology 8: 689–695

Thornell L-E, Edstrom L, Eriksson A, Henrikson K-G, Angquist K-A 1980 The distribution of intermediate filament protein (skeletin) in normal and diseased human skeletal muscle. Journal of the Neurological Sciences 47: 153–170

Tokuyasu K T, Dutton A H, Singer S J 1983 Immunoelectromicroscopic studies of desmin (skeletin) localization and intermediate filament organization in chicken skeletal muscle. Journal of Cell Biology 96: 1727–1735

Tokuyasu K T, Maher P A, Singer S J 1985 Distributions of vimentin and desmin in developing chick myotubes in vivo. II. Immunoelectronmicroscopic study. Journal of Cell Biology 100: 1157–1166

Tregear R T, Marston S B 1979 The crossbridge theory. Annual Reviews of Physiology 41: 723–736

Trinick J, Elliott A 1979 Electron microscopic studies of thick filaments from vertebrate skeletal muscle. Journal of Molecular Biology 131: 133–136

Trotter J A, Corbett K, Avner B P 1981 Structure and function of the murine muscle-tendon junction. Anatomical Record 201: 293–302

Trotter J A, Eberhard S, Samora A 1983 Structural domains of the muscle tendon junction. I. The internal lamina and the connecting domain. Anatomical Record 207: 573–591

Ullrick W C 1967 A theory of contraction for striated muscle. Journal of Theoretical Biology 15: 53–69

Ullrick W C, Toselli P A, Saide J D, Phear W P C 1977 Fine structure of the vertebrate Z-disc. Journal of Molecular Biology 115: 61–74

van Buren J M, Frank K 1965 Correlation between the morphology and potential field of a spinal motor nucleus in the cat. Electroencephalography and Clinical Neurophysiology 19: 112–126

Vergara J, Tsien R Y, Delay M 1985 Inositol 1,4,5-triphosphate: a possible chemical link in excitation-contraction coupling in muscle. Proceedings of the National Academy of Science USA 82: 6352–6356

Viragh S Z, Challice C E 1969 Variation in filamentous and fibrillar organization and associated sarcolemmal structures in cells of the normal mammalian heart. Journal of Ultrastructure Research 28: 321–334

Vracko R, Benditt E P 1972 Basal lamina: the scaffold for orderly cell replacement. Observations on regeneration of injured skeletal muscle fibres and capillaries. Journal of Cell Biology 55: 406–419

Wakayama Y, Schotland D L 1979 Muscle satellite cell populations in Duchenne dystrophy. In: Mauro A (ed) Muscle regeneration. Raven Press, New York, p 121–130

Wakayama Y, Okayasu H, Shibuya A, Kumagai T 1985 Duchenne dystrophy: reduced density of orthogonal array subunit particles in muscle plasma membrane. Neurology 34: 1313–1317

Waku K 1977 Skeletal muscle. In: Snyder F (ed) Lipid metabolism in mammals. Plenum, New York, p 189

Walker S M, Schrodt G R 1968 Triads in skeletal muscle fibers of 19-day fetal rats. Journal of Cell Biology 37: 564–569

Walker S M, Schrodt G R, Currier F J, Turner E V 1975 Relationship of the sarcoplasmic reticulum to fibril and triadic junction development in skeletal muscle fibers of fetal monkeys and humans. Journal of Morphology 146: 97–128

Wallimann T, Pelloni G, Turner D C, Eppenberger H M 1979 Removal of the M-line by treatment with Fab' fragments of antibodies against MM-creatine kinase. In: Pepe F A, Sanger J W, Nachmias V T (eds) Motility in cell function. Academic Press, New York, p 415–417

Wang K 1982 Myofilamentous and myofibrillar connections: role of titin, nebulin and intermediate filaments. In: Pearson M L, Epstein H F (eds) Muscle development. Cold Spring Harbor Laboratory, p 439–452

Wang K, Ramirez-Mitchell R 1983 A network of transverse and longitudinal intermediate filaments is associated with sarcomeres of adult vertebrate skeletal muscle. Journal of Cell Biology 96: 562–570

Williams P E, Goldspink G 1971 Longitudinal growth of striated muscle fibres. Journal of Cell Science 9: 751–767

Williams P E, Goldspink G 1973 The effect of immobilization on the longitudinal growth of striated muscle fibres. Journal of Anatomy 116: 45–55

Wray S H 1969 Innervation ratios for large and small limb muscles in the baboon. Journal of Comparative Neurology 137: 227–250

Yasin R, Van Beers G, Nurse K C E, Al-Ani S, Landon D N, Thompson E J 1977 A quantitative technique for growing human skeletal muscle in culture starting from mononucleated cells. Journal of the Neurological Sciences 32: 347–360

Yoshioka M, Okuda R 1977 Human skeletal muscle fibers in normal and pathological states; freeze-etch replica observations. Journal of Electron Microscopy (Tokyo) 26: 103–110

Zelena J 1965 Development of acetylcholinesterase activity at muscle junctions. Nature 205: 295–296

Neuromuscular transmission

INTRODUCTION

Many of the processes involved in neuromuscular transmission are well understood (see e.g. Katz 1966, Hubbard 1973). When the motor nerve is stimulated, an action potential travels along the nerve as far as the nerve terminal where the transmitter, acetylcholine (ACh) is released. ACh then travels across the synaptic cleft to the postsynaptic membrane causing a local depolarisation in the muscle fibre. This in turn triggers a propagated action potential in the muscle fibre, leading to muscle contraction. ACh is meanwhile hydrolysed to choline by the enzyme acetylcholinesterase (EC 3.1.1.7). Choline is taken up by nerve terminals and used to resynthesise ACh via the enzyme choline acetyltransferase (EC 2.3.1.6) (MacIntosh & Collier 1976).

Concerning the release process, depolarisation associated with the nerve terminal action potential causes voltage-dependent calcium channels in the nerve membrane to open briefly. This allows calcium ions to enter nerve terminals, leading to ACh release in distinct multimolecular packets (for review see Baker 1977, Ginsborg & Jenkinson 1976).

ACh released by nerve stimulation combines with specific acetylcholine receptors on the postsynaptic membrane. This causes end-plate channels to open transiently, leading to a large brief ionic current via the channels and consequent depolarisation in the muscle fibre (for reviews see, e.g. Wray 1980, Hille 1984). The ACh receptor (AChR) and its associated channel is a protein, the amino acid structure of which has recently been determined (e.g. Noda et al 1983b).

Nerve endings are found in surface depressions of the muscle membrane (synaptic 'gutters' or

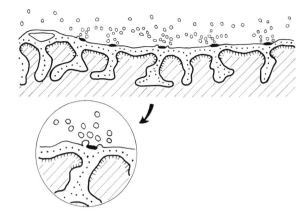

Fig. 3.1 Schematic diagram of frog neuromuscular junction (Porter & Barnard 1975) traced from micrographs by Couteaux & Pecot-Dechavassine (1968). Vesicles can be seen in the nerve terminal aligned in stacks near the thickenings (dense bars) in the presynaptic membrane (Birks et al 1960a, b, Heuser et al 1974). The striations on the postsynaptic membrane represent its 'thickened' zone, rich in ACh receptors. Dotted lines show the acetylcholinesterase present throughout the cleft. The inset shows fusion of vesicles with the presynaptic membrane at either side of the presynaptic thickening. After being released from the nerve terminal, ACh binds first to receptors located conveniently at the crests of the folds, and then probably diffuses into the fold depths where it is hydrolysed

'troughs'). The nerve terminal is separated by a gap of about 50 nm from the postsynaptic membrane which is highly folded (Fig. 3.1). Specific histochemical staining (reviewed by e.g. Bowden & Duchen 1976) has shown that the acetylcholinesterase enzyme is present throughout the cleft, including the folds. This location of the enzyme was confirmed by autoradiographic studies using radiolabelled diisopropylfluorophosphonate (DFP) (see e.g. Barnard 1974).

The aim of this chapter is to provide an up-to-date summary of present understanding of neuromuscular transmission, without trying to replace a standard textbook or more detailed technical review. The above mechanisms will be discussed, especially where relevant to known neuromuscular disorders.

PRESYNAPTIC EVENTS

Active zones

Thickenings of the nerve terminal membrane usually occur opposite the mouths of the postsynaptic folds. Membrane-bound vesicles (about

50 nm in diameter) are aligned in stacks around these thickenings (Fig. 3.1). Vesicles appear to touch or fuse with the axolemma on either side of the thickenings. These observations led to the suggestion that ACh is released at such areas: 'active zones' (e.g. Heuser 1976). The active zone membrane, when examined by freeze-fracture electron microscopy, consists of particles (each of width about 11 nm) arranged in parallel double rows (Fig 3.2). For frog neuromuscular junctions, which have elongated nerve terminals, rows of active zone particles are located at right angles to the longitudinal axis of the terminal, opposite the sites of the postsynaptic folds (e.g. Heuser et al 1974). For mammalian muscles, which have less elongated nerve terminals, active zones continue to follow the sites of postsynaptic folds, but they are shorter and less regularly spaced (e.g. Fukunaga et al 1982, 1983).

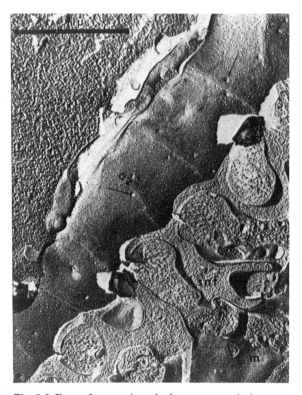

Fig. 3.2 Freeze-fracture view of a frog nerve terminal membrane fixed during nerve stimulation (Heuser et al 1974). Parallel rows of particles are seen at active zones (e.g. az). Circular dimples (arrows to some) beside the active zones probably represent vesicles fusing with membrane, presumably to discharge ACh by exocytosis. Subneural fold, snf; muscle fibre, m

As ACh release appears to occur close to the active zone particles (circular dimples in Fig. 3.2), it has been suggested that these membrane-spanning particles are the voltage-dependent calcium channels which open when the nerve terminal is depolarised (Heuser et al 1974, Pumplin et al 1981).

End-plate potentials and miniature end-plate potentials

Much useful insight into neuromuscular transmission has been gained by recording voltages intracellularly with fine-tipped glass microelectrodes inserted into single muscle cells. Many of the classic papers are collected in the source book by Cooke & Lipkin (1972). The potential difference between inside and outside the muscle cell ('membrane potential') is usually about -70 mV in resting muscle. In unstimulated muscle fibres, if the microelectrode is placed in an end-plate region, small potential changes are observed (Fatt & Katz 1952) — the miniature end-plate potential (mepp) (Fig. 3.3A). These mepps occur spontaneously and at random (approx one per second), each mepp having a small amplitude (0.5–1 mV), which is insufficient to trigger action potentials in muscle fibres. The mepp comes about by the release of a single multimolecular packet of ACh

from the nerve terminal. The ACh then acts postsynaptically to produce the observed electrical changes in the muscle fibre.

When the nerve is stimulated, many such packets of ACh are released almost simultaneously from the nerve terminal (Katz 1966). The depolarisation produced in the muscle fibre at the end-plate by this ACh (see Introduction) is known as the end-plate potential (epp) (Fig. 3.3B). The number of packets released for each single nerve stimulus is usually called the quantal content, m. As *each* packet produces a response of magnitude corresponding to the mepp amplitude, the epp amplitude is, therefore, the quantal content times the mepp amplitude. Thus if the mepp and epp amplitudes are measured, the quantal content can be found (For corrections to this method of calculation, and for other methods of obtaining quantal content, see e.g. Martin 1966.) Quantal content for human muscle is about 60 (Lambert & Elmqvist 1971).

Detailed statistical analysis has shown that the *single* packet of ACh released spontaneously to produce a mepp contains on average the same number of ACh molecules as are found in *each* of the packets released almost simultaneously by nerve stimulation to form an epp (del Castillo & Katz 1954a, Martin 1966).

A mepp and an epp differ in the number of packets of ACh involved, but otherwise have many features in common. Thus both mepps and epps follow a similar time course (Fig. 3.3) and both respond similarly to drugs such as neostigmine and tubocurarine (Fatt & Katz 1952).

The number of ACh molecules released in a single packet is remarkably constant and unaffected by most drugs, by changes in ionic environment or by osmotic changes. The *amplitude* of the mepp is determined mainly by the number of ACh molecules in a packet and by the postsynaptic action of the ACh. As the former is relatively constant, the mepp amplitude is largely determined by the postsynaptic action of ACh, which can be readily varied by postsynaptically acting drugs such as tubocurarine. On the other hand, the *frequency* of random release of packets of ACh can be easily and markedly affected by factors which change the presynaptic conditions. So, e.g. mepp frequency is increased by a rise in the

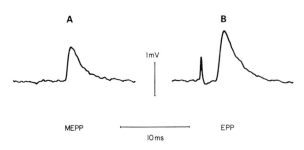

Fig. 3.3 Intracellular recordings using microelectrodes at end-plate regions of mouse diaphragm muscle (23°C) (Peers & Wray, unpublished data) (A) Spontaneously occurring miniature end-plate potential. (B) End-plate potential evoked by nerve stimulation. The narrow spike preceding the epp is caused by the brief pulse used to stimulate the nerve.

The epp is normally much larger in amplitude than the mepp, and so the epp would normally trigger an action potential in the muscle fibre causing muscle contraction and the expulsion of the microelectrode. Therefore, in B above, the epp has been reduced in amplitude by tubocurarine so that it is below threshold for stimulating an action potential

osmolarity of the bathing solution (for further discussion see Ginsborg & Jenkinson 1976).

Calcium ion influx

In solutions containing low Ca^{2+} concentrations, epp amplitudes are reduced. Analysis of such epps to find the number of packets released per nerve stimulus (i.e. the quantal content) shows that epp amplitudes are reduced because the quantal content is reduced (del Castillo & Katz 1954a). In other words, Ca^{2+} ions act presynaptically to affect the number of packets of ACh released.

Provided that Ca^{2+} ions are present in the bathing solution, depolarisation of nerve terminals, *however caused*, is effective in inducing Ca^{2+} entry and release of ACh. So, e.g. increasing the K^+ ion concentration of the bathing solution will depolarise cells. This depolarisation at the nerve terminal leads to an increase in release of packets of ACh which can be recorded as an increase in mepp frequency (Liley 1956). Alternatively, nerve terminals can be depolarised by passing current pulses from a nearby extracellular electrode and this again leads to ACh release (Liley 1956). Sodium ions themselves are not responsible for release, as ACh is also released using such current pulses in the absence of sodium ions (Katz & Miledi 1969a).

For ACh release to occur, Ca^{2+} ions must be present externally during nerve terminal depolarisation. Thus nerve stimulation in Ca^{2+}-free solution completely abolishes ACh release. In such Ca^{2+}-free solutions, short pulses of Ca^{2+} ions can be applied externally via a microelectrode at different times in relation to the time of a depolarising pulse. In this way it was shown that ACh release occurs only when Ca^{2+} ions are present externally during the period of the depolarisation and for a very short time afterwards (Katz & Miledi 1967a). During the period of depolarisation, the nerve terminal membrane becomes transiently more permeable to Ca^{2+} ions, allowing Ca^{2+} entry into the nerve terminal. Intracellular free Ca^{2+} concentration is normally very low (about 0.1 μM) (Baker 1977), while the physiological concentration of extracellular *free* Ca^{2+} is about 2 mM.

Intracellular presynaptic recordings cannot be made at the small terminals of the skeletal neuromuscular junction. However, Ca^{2+} currents can be studied indirectly, especially when K^+ currents are eliminated by suitable drugs (Penner & Dreyer 1986). Regenerative Ca^{2+} action potentials can be produced in skeletal muscle nerve terminals, particularly when solutions containing high Ca^{2+} concentrations are used (Katz & Miledi 1969a). The squid giant synapse has large presynaptic terminals and this allows the direct intracellular presynaptic recording of such Ca^{2+} action potentials (Katz & Miledi 1969b). It is to be emphasised that Ca^{2+} action potentials do not occur under normal physiological conditions.

It might be expected that, as the Ca^{2+} ion is positively charged, making the inside of the nerve terminal *very* positive would electrostatically repel Ca^{2+} entry. This is in fact found to be the case: very large experimentally induced presynaptic depolarisations in the squid giant synapse (about 200 mV) prevent Ca^{2+} entry, even though the depolarisation itself has made the presynaptic membrane permeable to Ca^{2+} ions (Katz & Miledi 1967b, Llinas et al 1981). Similar results are found at frog (Katz & Miledi 1977a, Dudel 1983) and crayfish (Dudel et al 1983) neuromuscular junctions. These experiments shed light on the process of Ca^{2+} ion entry. However, presynaptic depolarisation under *normal* physiological conditions at nerve terminals is not large enough to cause electrostatic repulsion of Ca^{2+} ions.

Direct recording of Ca^{2+} currents is possible at the squid giant synapse (Llinas et al 1976, 1981, Augustine et al 1985b). From such recordings it was shown that the Ca^{2+} permeability rises at the beginning of a depolarising pulse, and falls back to normal after the pulse. These Ca^{2+} permeability changes do not take place instantaneously, but rather have time constants of the order of milliseconds.

Furthermore, increase in Ca^{2+} concentration inside presynaptic terminals during nerve depolarisation has been detected for the squid giant synapse. For this, compounds sensitive to Ca^{2+} ion (aequorin or arsenazo III) were injected into nerve terminals. Aequorin emits light in the presence of Ca^{2+} ions (Llinas et al 1972, Llinas & Nicholson 1975), while Ca^{2+} ions also affect light transmission through preparations containing arsenazo III (Miledi & Parker 1981, Charlton et al 1982, Augustine et al 1985a).

Current through *individual* Ca^{2+} channels has not been observed electrophysiologically at the small presynaptic terminals of the skeletal neuromuscular junction. However, currents produced by single voltage-dependent Ca^{2+} channels have now been observed in other neurones and in heart muscle membranes using the 'patch clamp' technique (see below) (e.g. Tsien 1983, Reuter 1983, Reuter et al 1985). In heart muscle, for instance, each Ca^{2+} channel opens for about 1 ms. The frequency of Ca^{2+} channel opening increases when the membrane is suddenly depolarised, leading to an increase in overall Ca^{2+} current. There appear to be several types of voltage-dependent Ca^{2+} channels (e.g. Nilius et al 1985, Nowycky et al 1985, Penner & Dreyer 1986). Furthermore, biochemical investigations have led to the isolation of the Ca^{2+} antagonist receptor of Ca^{2+} channels from, e.g. skeletal muscle transverse tubules (Borsotto et al 1984, Curtis & Catterall 1984). Further work is leading to an understanding of the subunit structure of this glycoprotein.

Acetylcholine release

Intracellular action of calcium ions. The fact that Ca^{2+} ions cause release of transmitter has been shown directly for the squid giant synapse. A pulse of Ca^{2+} ions injected via a microelectrode into the nerve terminal of the synapse causes transmitter release (Miledi 1973, Miledi & Parker 1981, Charlton et al 1982).

Following a brief depolarisation of motor nerve terminals, there is a time interval ('synaptic delay') of at least 0.5 ms (20 °C) before the epp appears (Katz & Miledi 1965). This delay does not arise because of the time taken for the ACh to diffuse across the synaptic cleft to the postsynaptic membrane, nor because of the time taken for the ACh to act on the postsynaptic membrane (see End-plate response, below). Thus the synaptic delay occurs presynaptically by a delay in the release of ACh following the brief depolarisation of the nerve terminal.

This presynaptic delay is made up from two steps, at least in the squid giant synapse. First, following presynaptic depolarisation, there is a

delay before Ca^{2+} channels open and Ca^{2+} current starts to flow into the nerve. Secondly, once Ca^{2+} current has started to flow, there is a further delay (approximately 0.2 ms) before transmitter is released (Llinas et al 1981). During the latter very short delay, Ca^{2+} ions which enter the nerve terminal via Ca^{2+} channels must travel to an intracellular binding site and then cause release. The Ca^{2+} channels (active zone particles) therefore must be situated very near to intracellular Ca^{2+} binding sites and to release sites (see Active zones above).

The number of packets of ACh released by nerve stimulation increases steeply and non-linearly ($\alpha[Ca]^n$, n=3 to 4) with increasing extracellular calcium concentration [Ca] (Fig. 3.4), before eventually reaching a plateau (see Cull-Candy et al 1980 for further references). The entry of Ca^{2+}

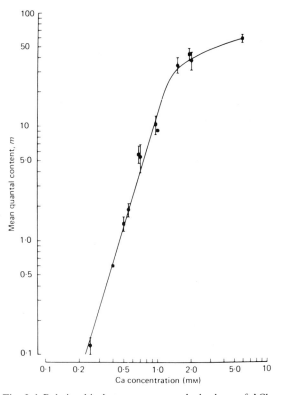

Fig. 3.4 Relationship between nerve-evoked release of ACh (quantal content) and extracellular Ca^{2+} concentration in normal human intercostal muscle (24°C). The initial part of the curve is steep and non-linear (release proportional to $[Ca]^{3.3}$) with increasing calcium concentration, [Ca], and appears linear in this figure only because logarithmic scales have been used for the axes (after Cull-Candy et al 1980)

into the nerve terminal during the epp is proportional to the extracellular Ca^{2+} concentration (see e.g. Silinsky 1985): a graph of ACh release against intracellular Ca^{2+} concentration during the epp might therefore also be expected to have a shape similar to that of Fig. 3.4. The non-linear release curve has been interpreted to imply 'co-operation' between three or four Ca^{2+} ions to cause release (Dodge & Rahamimoff 1967), and such co-operation probably occurs intracellularly. When the release versus Ca^{2+} concentration curve (Fig. 3.4) reaches an eventual plateau, this probably comes about by saturation of the intracellular action of Ca^{2+}, not by a saturation of Ca^{2+} entry via the channels (Silinsky 1985).

The curve of ACh release versus Ca^{2+} concentration is shifted to the right by Mg^{2+} ions (Jenkinson 1957, see Silinsky 1985 for further references). Mg^{2+} ions act as a competitive antagonist to Ca^{2+} ions in causing release of ACh. The site of competition is probably at the external surface of the Ca^{2+} channel, because if Mg^{2+} is delivered intracellularly, it does not inhibit release (Kharasch et al 1981). In addition, large (2–3 mM) concentrations of ionised Mg^{2+} are normally found intracellularly (Baker 1972), and this would probably have produced a block of release if the Mg^{2+} ions had acted inside the nerve terminal.

Although Ca^{2+} is necessary for initiating transmitter release, the actual level of release may also be independently modulated by the potential of the presynaptic membrane (Llinas et al 1981, Dudel 1983, Dudel et al 1983). It appears that entry of a fixed amount of Ca^{2+} ions may become more effective in producing transmitter release as the nerve terminal is depolarised, although the effect may be small (Augustine et al 1985b); potential-sensitive proteins in the membrane may be involved. Further evidence for potential-dependent effects comes from studies of the time course of release. After a nerve impulse, packets of ACh are not released simultaneously, but are distributed in time (Fig. 3.5) after a minimum delay. It appears that the minimum delay is also controlled directly by the potential of the presynaptic membrane (Datyner & Gage 1980, Dudel 1984a, b).

For unstimulated spontaneous release (mepps),

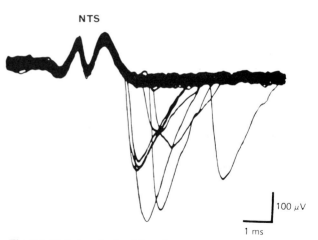

NTS

100 µV

1 ms

Fig. 3.5 Variations in the delay when release occurs following nerve stimulation. Responses were detected by an extracellular microelectrode placed very near to the end-plate in a mouse diaphragm muscle. Recordings were made in solutions containing high Mg^{2+} and low Ca^{2+} concentrations to reduce release. Usually, stimulation of the nerve under these conditions gave either a failure to release ACh, or the release of one packet of ACh. The release of a single packet of ACh occurs with a variable delay and this has been shown by superimposing the results of many nerve stimuli. Downward deflections: end-plate responses; NTS: nerve terminal action potential (Datyner & Gage 1980)

it is likely that intracellular free Ca^{2+} is also involved in causing release of packets of ACh (e.g. Hubbard 1973). Under resting conditions, where voltage-dependent Ca^{2+} channels in the membrane are not open, the mepp frequency is not very dependent on extracellular Ca^{2+} concentration. Since intracellular Ca^{2+} concentration is low, the resting frequency of release is also low. Intracellular free Ca^{2+} can be increased by agents causing the release of Ca^{2+} from bound intracellular stores, such as mitochondria. Poisoning the mitochondria with agents such as ruthenium red causes the release of free Ca^{2+} and, as expected, a marked increase in mepp frequency (see Alnaes & Rahamimoff 1975 for further references).

Vesicles or gates. The vesicles found in nerve terminals (see Active zones and Fig. 3.1) contain ACh and are roughly constant in size. Electrophysiological recordings have shown that ACh is released in 'packets' (see End-plate potentials and miniature end-plate potentials), each of a fairly constant number of ACh molecules, leading to approximately constant mepp amplitudes. It was natural to suggest that a 'packet' of ACh is released when a vesicle fuses with the cytoplasmic membrane, rapidly discharging its contents by exocytosis (del Castillo & Katz 1955, Hubbard & Kwanbunbumpen 1968, Katz 1978). Constancy of the amount of ACh released in a packet would arise because of constancy of size of the vesicles. Convincing evidence for exocytosis is now available from electron microscopy of freeze-fractured membranes. The presynaptic membrane becomes marked with circular dimples if terminals are fixed while packets of ACh are being secreted (Heuser et al 1974) (Fig. 3.2). The dimples usually occur alongside the rows of particles forming the active zones, and may be caused by the exocytosis of vesicles of ACh. Further support for the vesicular release theory (see e.g. Ceccarelli & Hurlbut 1980 for further references) comes from studies using black widow spider venom and lanthanum ions. Both these agents cause a large release of ACh followed by virtually complete depletion of vesicles, at which point secretion of ACh is almost completely abolished.

Approximately 10^4 ACh molecules are *released* into the synaptic cleft during the action of a single 'packet' of transmitter at the skeletal neuromuscular junction (Fletcher & Forrester 1975, Kuffler & Yoshikami 1975, Miledi et al 1983a). Synaptic vesicles probably *contain* about this number of ACh molecules (e.g. Miledi et al 1980, 1982a), suggesting that the whole content of a vesicle is released as a packet. Thus there is considerable evidence for the vesicular theory.

However, the vesicular theory has been under attack in recent years from a number of angles. An alternative theory suggests that ACh is released directly from the cytoplasm via some membrane gate (see Tauc 1982 for further references). It is known that free ACh is found in the cytoplasm, where it is synthesised from choline using the enzyme choline acetyltransferase (MacIntosh & Collier 1976). Experiments were done mainly on the electric organs of the ray *Torpedo*. After nerve stimulation, the level of free (cytoplasmic) ACh is reduced whereas the level of bound (vesicular) ACh is unchanged (Israel & Dunant 1979). Furthermore, the extent of this reduction in cytoplasmic ACh corresponds to the extent of ACh released from the terminal (Dunant et al 1980,

Israel & Lesbats 1981, Dunant & Israel 1985). In addition experiments using radiolabelled precursors of ACh have shown that *newly* synthesised ACh (produced in the cytoplasm) is preferentially released (Potter 1970). Thus ACh appears to be released from the cytoplasm. One possibility is that ACh is very rapidly transferred from cytoplasm to vesicles and then rapidly released. However, most of the vesicles contain ACh which exchanges only slowly with cytoplasmic ACh (e.g. Marchbanks 1968, MacIntosh & Collier 1976, Corthay et al 1982) and so it appears that ACh is released *directly* from the cytoplasm.

This apparent release of ACh from the cytoplasm poses a serious difficulty for the vesicular theory. At the frog neuromuscular junction, bound (vesicular) ACh is released as well as free (cytoplasmic) ACh (Miledi et al 1982a), making the situation more complex.

If ACh is released directly from the cytoplasm, how is the approximate constancy of a packet of ACh produced? A channel may open in the nerve terminal membrane for a short fixed time, allowing a number of ACh molecules to pass through it. However, this is unlikely as, for such a channel, the number of ACh molecules released would vary with temperature and nerve terminal membrane potential and this was not found (Cohen & Van der Kloot 1983, Van der Kloot & Cohen 1984). Possibly a *very small number* of 'active vesicles', placed at strategic points at active zones, may rapidly exchange ACh with the cytoplasm and release ACh by exocytosis (Israel et al 1979, Zimmerman 1979), thus producing constancy of the packet of ACh released.

Proponents of the non-vesicular theory of ACh release have suggested that the function of the vesicles is instead to take up intracellular Ca^{2+} ions following Ca^{2+} entry and then later to expel these ions by exocytosis (Tauc 1982). In summary, it is probably fair to say that it is still not clear whether packets of ACh are released from active vesicles or alternatively directly from the cytoplasm in some way.

Continuous molecular leakage. At rest, ACh is released spontaneously in packets to form mepps as mentioned previously. In addition, ACh is released spontaneously by continuous molecular leakage from nerve terminals. The amount of ACh released under resting conditions to produce mepps can be calculated. This latter amount of ACh is found to be only a few per cent of the total resting ACh released when measured by chemical means (e.g. Fletcher & Forrester 1975). Thus the vast majority of spontaneous release is by 'non-quantal' molecular leakage. A large fraction of the molecular leakage occurs from nerve terminals (Miledi et al 1982b). This 'non-quantal' release produces very little postsynaptic effect, because it leads to only a very low average ACh concentration (6–30 mM) at the postsynaptic membrane. It has been detected electrophysiologically, since application of tubocurarine removes the small depolarisation (<1 mV) produced by this ACh in the presence of an acetylcholinesterase inhibitor (Katz & Miledi 1977b, 1981, Vyskocil & Illes 1978, Smith 1984).

The factors influencing 'non-quantal' release of ACh are not well understood. Non-quantal release continues in the absence of Ca^{2+} ions (Vizi & Vyskocil 1979). The end-plate potential is composed purely of quantal release and therefore depolarisation of the nerve terminal by an action potential leading to the epp does not cause an increase in non-quantal release; neither does depolarisation by high K^+ ion concentration. This is surprising, as simple molecular leakage might be expected to be affected by the nerve terminal membrane potential for the positively charged quaternary ACh ion.

Facilitation and depression

Transmitter release depends on the frequency of nerve stimulation (e.g. del Castillo & Katz 1954b, Ginsborg & Jenkinson 1976, Silinsky 1985). In normal Ca^{2+} solutions (where many packets of ACh are released per nerve impulse) if the nerve is repetitively stimulated, successive epps generally decline in amplitude (Fig. 3.6, top trace). This 'depression' comes about because successively fewer packets of ACh are released per nerve impulse. On the other hand, under conditions where only a small number of packets of ACh are released (for instance in low Ca^{2+} solutions or in the Lambert–Eaton myasthenic syndrome, see Sites of presynaptic drug action, below) successive

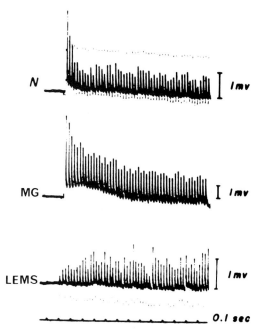

Fig. 3.6 Intracellular recordings of epps evoked by 40 Hz nerve stimulation for human intercostal muscle in vitro. N: normal muscle with tubocurarine (2 μg/ml) in the bath; MG: myasthenia gravis patient, no tubocurarine; LEMS: Lambert–Eaton myasthenic syndrome patient with tubocurarine (0.2 μg/ml). Approximate equality of epp amplitudes in this figure comes about because a relatively high concentration of tubocurarine was used in normals (N) for which transmission was not already clinically impaired (Lambert & Elmqvist 1971, reproduced with permission from the New York Academy of Sciences)

epps generally increase in size during a train of nerve stimuli ('facilitation') (Fig. 3.6, lower trace). Again, the mechanism is a presynaptic effect; there is a progressive increase in the number of packets of ACh released. Facilitation is short lasting: the interval between successive nerve stimuli must be less than a few hundred milliseconds for the effect to be seen.

During both facilitation and depression, the amount of Ca^{2+} ion entry into the nerve terminal *per nerve impulse* does not change — at least in the squid giant synapse where such Ca^{2+} currents can be measured (Miledi & Parker 1981, Charlton et al 1982). Similarly, intracellular Ca^{2+} concentration (as detected by Ca^{2+} sensitive dyes) increases by the same amount each time the nerve is stimulated in the train. There is an increase in intracellular Ca^{2+} concentration lasting for several seconds even after a single nerve stimulation. Since ACh release is a highly non-linear function of intracellular Ca^{2+} concentration (see above), a fixed increase in intracellular Ca^{2+} concentration produced by a nerve impulse would be more effective in releasing ACh when added to residual intracellular Ca^{2+} from an earlier nerve impulse (Katz & Miledi 1968, Rahamimoff 1968). Therefore, summation of intracellular Ca^{2+} levels in the nerve terminal during a train may produce facilitation. Other later steps in the release process (e.g. exocytosis of vesicles) do not themselves appear to contribute facilitatory effects, as the amplitude of subsequent epps is not affected by presence or absence of ACh release for the first nerve stimulus (del Castillo & Katz 1954b).

For normal Ca^{2+} concentrations where quantal release is high, during high-frequency nerve stimulation there is probably a depletion of ACh available for release (e.g. Martin 1966, Ginsborg & Jenkinson 1976). Therefore ACh release decreases throughout the train (even though there is an underlying increase in intracellular residual Ca^{2+}) and depression of epp amplitude is seen. When quantal content is low, ACh depletion does not occur and then facilitation can be observed.

Electrophysiologists usually record epps either in low Ca^{2+} solutions without tubocurarine or in normal solutions with tubocurarine to prevent triggering of action potentials. It now seems clear that, although the phenomenon of ACh depletion can lead to depression, tubocurarine itself can also produce depression (Bowman 1980, Magleby et al 1981, Gibb & Marshall 1984). The drug does this by acting presynaptically, causing a reduction in quantal release during the high-frequency nerve stimulation.

For facilitation to occur, nerve impulses must follow each other in less than a few hundred milliseconds. However, after much longer intervals between stimuli a qualitatively different facilitatory effect can be seen — 'post-tetanic potentiation' (e.g. Hubbard 1963, Magleby 1973a,b, Magleby & Zengel 1975a,b). This latter effect can be detected most clearly after high-frequency nerve stimulation followed by a longer period of rest: nerve stimulation then causes greater ACh release than before the train. In contrast to facilitation, post-tetanic potentiation can be detected for periods up to minutes after such repetitive

nerve stimulation. The resting frequency of mepps is also increased during this period (Miledi & Thies 1971, Lev-Tov & Rahamimoff 1980, Zengel & Magleby 1981). Post-tetanic potentiation is a more complex process than facilitation, and is possibly caused by a longer-term increase in the *total* Ca^{2+} intracellular concentration, irrespective of the source of the Ca^{2+} (e.g. channels, pumps or internal stores). So, for instance, Ca^{2+} entry via channels during high-frequency nerve stimulation is not necessary: post-tetanic potentiation still occurs after nerve stimulation in calcium-free solutions (Misler & Hurlbut 1983). The increased total Ca^{2+} concentration may produce longer-term changes in the terminal, affecting proteins concerned with secretion (Silinsky 1985).

Finally, a further process has recently been discovered by which repetitive nerve stimulation increases ACh release. This process has been termed 'augmentation' and is intermediate in duration between facilitation and post-tetanic potentiation (Magleby & Zengel 1976a,b,c, 1982).

Sites of presynaptic drug action

Aminopyridines. The duration of the nerve terminal action potential is prolonged by 4-amino-pyridine (4-AP) or 3,4-diaminopyridine (3,4-DAP) (Lundh & Thesleff 1977, Lundh et al 1977a, Meves & Pichon 1977, Molgo et al 1977, 1979, 1980, Illes & Thesleff 1978, Kenyon & Gibbons 1979, Thesleff 1980). These drugs probably act mainly by blocking electrically operated K^+ channels involved in the action potential. The prolongation in depolarisation thereby produced at the nerve terminal allows more Ca^{2+} ions to enter the terminal than normal, leading to an increased quantal ACh release following nerve stimulation; correspondingly, the epp amplitude is greatly increased. Spontaneous quantal release (i.e. mepps) is in general not affected by 4-AP or 3,4-DAP, as action potentials are not involved in the generation of mepps. Both drugs have recently proved useful in the treatment of the Lambert–Eaton myasthenic syndrome (LEMS) which is a presynaptic disorder of neuromuscular transmission often associated with small-cell lung carcinoma (see below) (Lambert & Elmqvist 1971, Lundh et al 1977b, Murray & Newsom-Davis

1981, Murray et al 1984). Both drugs can also act on the central nervous system to produce convulsions, but 3,4-DAP is less convulsant and is therefore preferred.

LEMS IgG. Many drugs are now available acting on voltage-dependent Ca^{2+} channels (e.g. Gilman et al 1985). These 'calcium antagonists' have powerful actions on heart and blood-vessel calcium channels, but seem to be ineffective as antagonists of Ca^{2+} channels at nerve-terminal membranes of the skeletal neuromuscular junction (Gotgilf & Magazanik 1977, Nachshen & Blaustein 1979, Publicover & Duncan 1979, Bregestovski et al 1980, but see Penner & Dreyer 1986). However, it has recently been found that IgG antibodies present in the plasma of LEMS patients act on skeletal muscle nerve terminals, probably as antagonists of voltage-dependent Ca^{2+} channels (Lang et al 1981, 1983, 1984a, Prior et al 1985).

In biopsied muscle from LEMS patients, there is a reduced release of ACh following a single nerve stimulation: the quantal content of the epp is reduced to a few packets (Lambert & Elmqvist 1971, Cull-Candy et al 1980). This can lead to failure to trigger muscle action potentials; hence muscle twitch tension is reduced. High-frequency nerve stimulation leads to a progressive increase in ACh release; this is the phenomenon of facilitation associated with a low initial quantal content (Fig. 3.6, see above). Along with the progressive increase in epp amplitudes at high-frequency nerve stimulation, action potentials can be triggered progressively in more muscle fibres and so muscle tension increases during the high-frequency train. As a result, the patient's strength improves during continuous exercise.

To show the autoimmune nature of the syndrome, the IgG fraction was taken from plasma of LEMS patients and injected daily into mice (Lang et al 1981, 1983, Prior et al 1985). The epps produced in these mice were then measured and their quantal content determined. It was found that such injections of LEMS IgG caused a reduction in quantal content in the mice. Furthermore, measurements of high-frequency trains of epps in mice showed either facilitation or less marked depression than usual (Fig. 3.7). This showed that the main electrophysiological features of the syndrome could be transferred to mice via the IgG

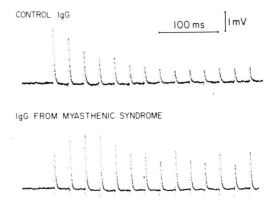

Fig. 3.7 Intracellular recordings of epps evoked by 40 Hz nerve stimulation for mouse diaphragm muscle in vitro. Upper trace: mouse injected with control IgG; lower trace: mouse injected with LEMS IgG. Tubocurarine was present in the bath at concentrations of 3.3 and 2.4 μg/ml respectively. As in Fig. 3.6, approximate equality of amplitudes arises because a higher tubocurarine concentration was used for controls (Newsom-Davis et al 1982)

fraction, strongly suggesting an autoimmune basis for the disorder. Consistent with this, immunosuppressive therapy (using azathioprine and prednisolone) and plasma exchange (which should reduce antibody levels) have both proved effective in the treatment of LEMS patients (Newsom-Davis & Murray 1984).

As mentioned above, the site of action of the IgG antibody is likely to be the voltage-dependent Ca^{2+} channel at the nerve terminal (Fukunaga et al 1982, 1983, Lang et al 1984b, 1985, Wray et al 1984, 1987, Roberts et al 1985). LEMS IgG probably causes the loss of function of these channels, leading to decreased Ca^{2+} entry following nerve terminal depolarisation, thereby reducing quantal ACh release.

Botulinum neurotoxin. This toxin is produced by strains of *Clostridium botulinum* and it can lead to fatal poisoning when present in foodstuffs. The toxin acts at nerve terminals of the skeletal neuromuscular junction (Sellin 1985). It binds to the nerve terminal membrane and then travels to the inside of the nerve terminal where it produces its action (Simpson 1980, Dolly et al 1984). The toxin does not affect Ca^{2+} entry into nerve terminals (Gundersen et al 1982), but acts intraterminally to reduce the effect of Ca^{2+} in promoting release. Following nerve stimulation, the quantal content of the epp is therefore reduced (Harris & Miledi

1971, Cull-Candy et al 1976). Probably because of this reduced quantal content, facilitation of epp amplitudes occurs in high-frequency trains of epps. Quantal spontaneous release (i.e. mepps) is determined by intraterminal processes and this form of release is also reduced by the toxin: there is a marked reduction in mepp frequency (Thesleff 1982, Tse et al 1982, 1986, Kim et al 1984, Dolly et al 1985). However, it is still not understood where precisely the toxin acts inside the nerve terminal to produce these effects. The process of vesicle exocytosis itself may be directly impaired by the toxin, leading to reduction in quantal content.

Hemicholinium-3. As mentioned in the Introduction, choline is used for the resynthesis of ACh within the nerve terminal by choline acetyltransferase (MacIntosh & Collier 1976). Choline is found in the extracellular fluid and is transported into the nerve terminal by a specific carrier mechanism in the membrane. Hemicholinium-3 (HC-3) inhibits this choline transport system, leading to a decrease in ACh synthesis and hence a decrease in total and 'bound' (vesicular) ACh levels (Potter 1970, Gundersen et al 1981, Dolezal & Tucek 1983, Veldsema-Currie et al 1984). Continuous nerve stimulation at high frequency or continuous exposure to high [K⁺] solutions leads to a gradual decrease in the rate of release of ACh (Elmqvist & Quastel 1965). This decrease in ACh release occurs by a reduction in the number of ACh molecules per packet released. Hemicholinium-3 is one of the few drugs to affect the size of the packet; on the other hand, the quantal content of the epp is unchanged by HC-3. The overall result is a gradual decrease in both mepp and epp amplitudes during continuous high-frequency nerve stimulation. At high concentrations there is, in addition, an immediate postsynaptic action of HC-3 to decrease ACh sensitivity (Martin & Orkand 1961, Thies & Brooks 1961).

POSTSYNAPTIC EVENTS

End-plate response

The postsynaptic events generating epps following nerve stimulation are as follows (see e.g. Katz

1966, Ginsborg & Jenkinson 1976). As mentioned in the Introduction, ACh causes channels to open briefly and current flows via these channels. This 'end-plate current' (epc) flowing into the muscle cell causes a depolarisation so initiating the epp at the end-plate region (Fig. 3.8). When the end-plate current has subsided, the remaining depolarisation of the epp then decays more slowly by a purely passive process determined by the passive electrical properties of the membrane.

The spontaneous release of a single packet of ACh leads to a similar but smaller event, the miniature end-plate potential (mepp). A correspondingly smaller current flows via the postsynaptic channels: the 'miniature end-plate current' (mepc). The mepc has a similar time course to the epc. The current flowing across the end-plate membrane during the action of ACh (the epc or mepc) can be measured experimentally by the voltage-clamp technique (Fig. 3.9).

During the time that end-plate channels are open, ions flow down their concentration and electrical gradients. Clamping the inside of the muscle fibre at less negative voltages (i.e. depolarisation) decreases the electrical gradient and hence the end-plate current is also decreased in amplitude (Fig. 3.10). Further depolarisation eventually reduces the epc amplitude to zero. The membrane

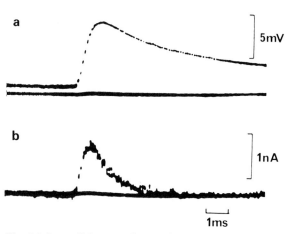

Fig. 3.8 Intracellular recordings at frog end-plate. Upper trace: end-plate potential; lower trace: end-plate current in the same fibre. The end-plate current normally leads to depolarisation, producing the end-plate potential. In the lower record, potential changes have been eliminated experimentally using the voltage clamp technique (see Fig. 3.9) (after Takeuchi & Takeuchi 1959)

potential where this happens is known as the reversal potential and is usually in the range −15 to 0 mV. The actual value of the reversal potential is determined by concentration gradients and permeabilities of only those ions which flow through the channels. The concentrations of Na⁺ and K⁺ ions were found to affect the reversal

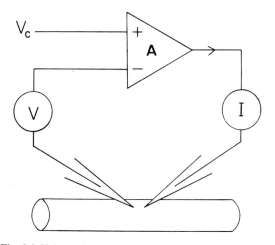

Fig. 3.9 Voltage clamp technique. Two microelectrodes are inserted into the muscle fibre near each other at the end-plate region. One microelectrode records the intracellular voltage (V) while the other passes current (I) into or out of the muscle fibre. Electronic circuitry (amplifier, A) controls the current passed by the latter electrode so that the intracellular voltage is held constant ('clamped') at voltage V_c. Postsynaptic currents induced by ACh can be measured under these clamped conditions since such currents are then equal to the current passed into the fibre by one of the microelectrodes. Passive changes involving charging the capacitance of the membrane cannot occur under these conditions

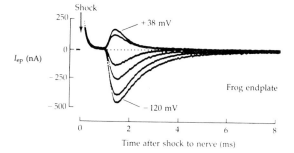

Fig. 3.10 End-plate currents measured by the voltage clamp technique. Recordings of current (Iep) were made at various membrane potentials from −120 mV (bottom trace) in steps to +38 mV (top trace). The end-plate current is reduced to zero at about 0 mV (Magleby & Stevens 1972, Hille 1984)

potential whereas the concentration of Cl⁻ ions did not (Takeuchi & Takeuchi 1960). Therefore, the end-plate channels are permeable to Na⁺ ions (usually flowing inwards) and K⁺ ions (usually flowing outwards) but not to Cl⁻ ions.

There are important differences between the epp and the muscle action potential triggered by the epp. The epp can only be recorded locally in a region around the end-plate with an amplitude falling off passively within a mm or so from the postsynaptic region (Fatt & Katz 1951); this is unlike the action potential, which is a propagated response throughout the whole fibre. Secondly, the epp is continuously graded: the amplitude varies with the amount of ACh liberated by the nerve terminal or with a change in the postsynaptic sensitivity to the depolarising action of ACh; this is in contrast to the action potential which is an all-or-nothing regenerative event. Thirdly, channels are opened chemically (i.e. by ACh) at the end-plate (Anderson & Stevens 1973) while the channels producing the action potential are opened by electrical changes in membrane potential (Hodgkin & Huxley 1952a,b,c,d, Hille 1984). Action potentials involve the opening firstly of channels specific for Na⁺ ions, and these channels can be blocked selectively by tetrodotoxin (Narahashi et al 1964), which has no effect at the end-plate channels. During the action potential, after a delay, channels specific for K⁺ ions open, and these channels can be blocked with 4-aminopyridine or tetraethylammonium (see Hille 1984). An individual channel at the end-plate, when opened by ACh, becomes permeable to both Na⁺ and K⁺ ions. Thus the chemically operated channels at the end-plate differ from the Na⁺ and K⁺ channels involved in the action potential (Kordas 1969, Dionne & Ruff 1977, Wray 1980).

The effects of ACh released by the nerve impulse can be mimicked fairly well by applying a short pulse of ACh locally: this can be done by the iontophoretic technique. For this, ACh is electrically ejected from an ACh-filled micropipette placed near the postsynaptic membrane (Krnjevic & Miledi 1958). The end-plate response to nerve stimulation is fairly similar to that for iontophoretically applied ACh (Fig. 3.11). Unlike nerve-stimulated release there is almost no appreciable delay in the onset of the response after suitable iontophoretic application (Katz & Miledi 1965). This lack of delay for iontophoretic application comes about because ACh reacts rapidly with postsynaptic receptors while the delay for nerve-stimulated release occurs presynaptically (see Acetylcholine release, above).

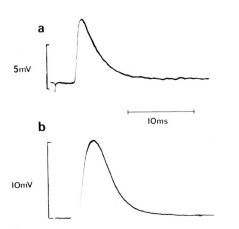

Fig. 3.11 Intracellular recordings for rat diaphragm muscle (24–25°C): a. end-plate potential following nerve stimulation; initial small deflection; nerve stimulation; b. end-plate response following a 1 ms application of ACh by the iontophoretic techniques. The break in the trace immediately before the response corresponds to the iontophoretic pulse (after Krnjevic & Miledi 1958, with permission from Macmillan)

Sensitivity to iontophoretically applied ACh is limited to around the end-plate region in normal muscle fibres (Miledi 1960a). However, some days after denervation, muscle fibres develop sensitivity to iontophoretically applied ACh over their whole length (Axelsson & Thesleff 1959, Miledi 1960b). This is because 'extrajunctional' receptors and their associated channels appear throughout the length of the muscle fibre after denervation.

Single channels

Patch clamp recording. It is now possible to record directly the tiny current flowing through a single ion channel (Neher & Sakmann 1976a, Sakmann & Neher 1983, Hille 1984). For this technique, a rather blunt glass microelectrode or 'pipette' (tip diameter about 1 μm), filled with an agonist such as ACh, is placed in contact with a small patch of membrane (Fig. 3.12). The current flowing through this very small patch of membrane can be recorded. It is found that ACh and other depolarising drugs produce tiny rectangular pulses of current.

The amplitude, i, of each pulse is fairly constant (Fig. 3.12) and equal to a few pA. The conductance of the channel can be found by applying

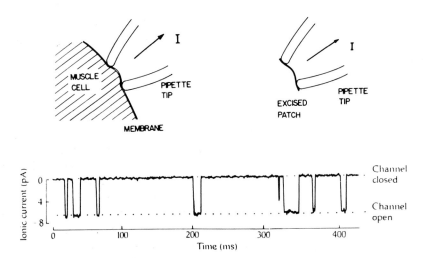

Fig. 3.12 Upper left: the patch clamp method of recording current (I) flowing through a small area (about 1 μm in diameter) of membrane of a cell. The pipette tip is tightly sealed against the outer face of the membrane. Upper right: withdrawal of pipette from the cell can result in a patch of membrane continuing to be attached to the pipette. Currents can be recorded across this excised patch of membrane. The effects on the excised membrane of known changes in ionic and drug concentration can therefore be investigated. Lower trace (Hille 1984): current flowing across an excised patch of membrane (cultured rat myotube, 23°C) showing brief openings of single channels in response to ACh. Note the constant amplitude of each current pulse but the variable open time

Ohm's Law, knowing the voltage V_m, across the membrane: conductance, $\gamma = i/V_m$. With i in amps and V_m in volts, the units of conductance are Siemens (S) (1 pS = 10^{-12} Siemens).

Channels appear to have at least two states: an open conducting state and a closed state. Under constant experimental conditions, the duration of the open state (i.e. the duration of each current pulse) varies (Fig. 3.12). Channels in the open state appear to 'decay' to the closed state under much the same physical laws as those governing radioactive decays. To be precise, there is a constant probability per unit time for *each* single channel open state to 'decay' to the closed state, independent of when the channel opened in the first place (e.g. Colquhoun & Hawkes 1983). For radioactive decay, this law leads to the well-known exponential loss of radioactivity. Analogously to this, channel open times also follow an exponential distribution (Fig. 3.13), at least as a first approximation. The *mean* open time at approximately 22 °C and for normal resting potentials is found to be about 1 ms for muscle end-plate channels when ACh is the agonist.

The patch clamp technique has found wide applications for a range of different channels (e.g. voltage-sensitive Na^+, K^+ and Ca^{2+} channels; Hille 1984). The noise levels in this type of recording depend on how well the membrane is sealed to the rim of the glass pipette: the better the seal, the lower the noise. Applying suction to the electrode improves the seal, producing a high leakage resistance or 'gigaseal' (Horn & Patlak 1980, Hamill et al 1981, Sakmann & Neher 1984). The method finds immediate application to cultured cells, where good membrane–pipette seals can be formed. For non-cultured muscle cells, pre-treatment with collagenase and other enzymes has been used to improve the seal.

Noise analysis. *Direct* recording of the individual pulses of current produced by single channel opening is not possible by conventional *intracellular* microelectrode techniques, because such individual current pulses are normally too small to detect by this method. However, before the advent of patch recording, much had already been learnt *indirectly* about the properties of channels by intracellular recording methods using the technique of noise analysis (Katz & Miledi 1970, 1972, 1977c, Anderson & Stevens 1973, Colquhoun 1975, 1979, 1981, Rang 1975, Neher & Stevens 1977, Wray 1980). For this technique, ACh is applied continuously at an end-plate, either in the bath or iontophoretically, while current flowing at the end-plate is measured by the voltage clamp technique using intracellular microelectrodes. The collision of ACh molecules with receptors is a random process leading in turn to random opening of channels: the number of channels open at any one time, therefore, is not a constant. This creates fluctuations in the current flowing across the end-plate membrane. These current fluctuations produced by ACh (or other agonists) can be detected: the current recording at high amplification becomes more 'noisy' in the presence of ACh (Fig 3.14). This noise can be analysed to give indirect information about the underlying single channel currents. More specifically, the mean current, i, passed by a single channel, the mean open time, τ, and the mean number of channels opened per second (frequency of channel opening, n) can be obtained.

To extract this information from the noise, the variance $\bar{I}^2$ of the noise produced by ACh must first be measured, as well as the mean overall current flowing through the end-plate, I. The

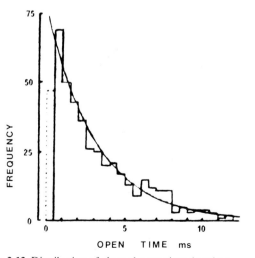

Fig. 3.13 Distribution of channel open time durations. Recordings were made from the frog neuromuscular junction in the presence of 50 nM ACh (membrane potential −80 mV, temperature 8°C). The distribution is fitted with a single exponential curve (after Colquhoun & Hawkes 1983)

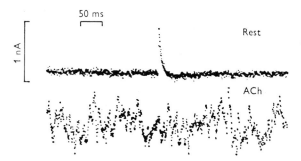

Fig. 3.14 Currents measured at a frog end-plate in a voltage clamped fibre (-100 mV, 8°C). The upper trace shows control current, including a spontaneously occurring mepc. The lower trace shows the increase in noise produced by the application of ACh (Anderson & Stevens 1973)

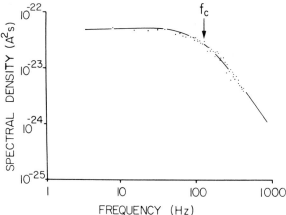

Fig. 3.15 Power spectrum of ACh-induced current noise at a voltage clamped rat muscle (-70 mV, 24°C). Spectral density is plotted against frequency on log-log axes. The theoretical 'Lorentzian' curve (Anderson & Stevens 1973) is shown and fits the experimental points well. The half power frequency, f_c, is 134 Hz, leading to a channel open time of 1.2 ms (Gwilt & Wray, unpublished data)

single channel current, i, is then calculated from $i = \bar{I}^2/I$. Values found by this method for single channel current are usually a few pA and of the same order of magnitude as found in patch clamp studies.

The mean channel open time, τ, can be obtained by analysis of the frequency components present in the noise variance (the 'power spectrum') (Anderson & Stevens 1973). The experimental power spectrum can usually be fitted by the theoretical 'Lorentzian' curve as shown in Fig. 3.15. The 'half-power frequency', f_c, at which the spectrum falls to one-half maximum, is related to the channel open time by $\tau = 1/(2\pi f_c)$. Hence, when the power spectrum is fitted to the theoretical curve, the channel open time can be found. Values calculated by this method for mean open time agree with those found in patch clamp studies.

The analysis described thus far has been on fluctuations, or noise, in the current recorded by the voltage clamp technique. Useful information can also be obtained using a single intracellular microelectrode to record membrane potential in unclamped fibres (Katz & Miledi 1972). In this case, continuous application of ACh produces an overall depolarisation, while single channels each produce a tiny depolarisation. Random opening of channels again produces noise, this time in the recorded voltage. Analysis of the voltage noise and its variance ($\bar{E}^2$) proceeds analogously to that for current noise. Information is obtained on the size of the depolarisation produced by a single channel

opening (a), the time constant for decay of the single channel depolarisation, τ_v, and channel opening frequency, n. For instance, for the action of ACh on cat muscle (37 °C) one finds a single channel depolarisation (a) of about 0.1 μV (Wray 1981b).

The time constant for decay of single channel depolarization (τ_v) obtained from voltage noise is different from the channel open time (τ). The voltage blip produced by a single channel arises as follows. The underlying current pulse first charges the membrane: when the channel closes, the depolarisation then decays passively (just as happens for an epp or mepp) with a time constant approximately equal to the membrane time constant. Thus the time constant (τ_v) for decay of each single-channel voltage blip, found in voltage noise analysis, is equal to the membrane time constant or a good approximation to it (e.g. Wray 1981b). This compares with current noise analysis, where the time constant obtained is the channel open time (τ).

Finally, having determined a and τ_v, one can calculate n, the frequency of channel opening, from $n = \bar{E}^2/(a^2 \tau_v)$. Typically, 1–2 μM ACh applied to cat muscle at 37 °C leads to the opening of around 3×10^8 channels per second (Wray 1981b).

Single channel properties. Open time and conductance of the end-plate channel activated by ACh have been extensively measured by both noise analysis and patch recording (Katz & Miledi 1972, Anderson & Stevens 1973, Ben-Haim et al 1975, Dreyer & Peper 1975, Dreyer et al 1976a, Colquhoun et al 1977, Cull-Candy et al 1979, Wray 1980, 1981b, Sakmann & Neher 1983, Hille 1984). The open time depends strongly on temperature: e.g. the normal mean open time of about 1 ms at 22 °C is increased to about 3 ms when the temperature is lowered by 10 °C (at a membrane potential of −75 mV). The open time also depends strongly on membrane potential — as membrane potential is hyperpolarised by 50 mV, channel open time increases by about 50% (at 19 °C). On the other hand, the conductance of the channel opened by ACh varies little with temperature or membrane potential, having values usually in the range 20–40 pS for normal end-plates.

From the above values of channel conductance and open time (at room temperature and normal membrane potential), one finds that each channel, while open, passes a quantity of charge equal to about 2×10^{-15} coulombs, equivalent to the passage of about 10^4 univalent ions.

Useful information can be obtained from knowing the size of the depolarisation produced by a single channel opening, a. Thus for cat muscle (37 °C) a is 0.1 μV (see previous section), which compares with a mepp amplitude of about 0.5 mV: thus the single channel depolarisation is some three orders of magnitude smaller than the mepp. This suggests that a mepp is produced by the synchronous opening of several thousand ion channels, therefore implicating the simultaneous action of several thousand ACh molecules on the postsynaptic receptors.

An important discovery by Anderson & Stevens (1973) was that, at 8 °C, the open time of a single channel was found to be identical to the decay constant of mepcs or epcs, even at different membrane potentials. The decay of both mepcs and epcs is therefore determined by the rate of closing of the channel. Thus, after the nerve is stimulated, any ACh which has not bound to receptors must disappear (by hydrolysis and diffusion) from the synaptic cleft in a time much less

than the channel open time. At higher temperatures (22 °C), epc decay is somewhat slower than the channel open time (by a factor of 1.4) (Katz & Miledi 1973a, Colquhoun et al 1977). Therefore, at higher temperatures, some ACh remains in the cleft after some channels have closed, and continues to open channels, so prolonging the epc slightly.

ACh is normally removed from the synaptic cleft by rapid hydrolysis via the enzyme acetylcholinesterase which is present in the cleft in roughly equimolecular numbers to the number of ACh receptors (Barnard et al 1971, Porter et al 1973). The ACh receptor and the acetylcholinesterase are distinct molecules (Changeux 1975). The effect of the acetylcholinesterase enzyme is made clear after it has been inhibited with a drug such as neostigmine: then one finds that the mepcs are prolonged about sixfold, while the channel open time, from noise analysis, is unchanged (Katz & Miledi 1973a). In this case, ACh molecules persist in the synaptic cleft, and so can act repeatedly, causing channels to open. The prolongation of end-plate currents by acetylcholinesterase inhibitors leads in turn to the well-known increase in amplitude and prolongation of epps and mepps.

For the extrajunctional channels found in denervated muscle (see End-plate response), noise analysis and patch recording show that the open time of the channels is three to five times longer than that of normal end-plate channels, while the conductance of the channels is about 70% of normal (Dreyer et al 1976a,b, Neher & Sakmann 1976b). Channel open time and conductance for denervated muscle have similar temperature and membrane potential dependence to that for normal end-plate channels.

Recent improvements in patch clamp recording techniques have shown further features of the single channel pulses of current. During the open state of the end-plate channel, there are *brief* interruptions of shut periods (Fig. 3.16a): the channel appears to 'flicker' briefly to a shut state (Colquhoun & Sakmann 1981, Sakmann & Neher 1984, Colquhoun & Sakmann 1985). During the flicker, agonist appears to remain bound to the receptor. When the channel eventually closes at the end of the current pulse, the agonist then

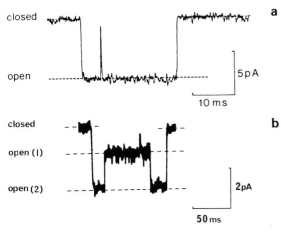

Fig. 3.16 Single channel patch clamp recordings during applications of ACh. a. The open channel current is interrupted by a brief flicker to the closed state (frog endplate) (Sakmann & Neher 1984, reproduced with permission from the *Annual Review of Physiology*) b. The open channel current has at least two different open conductance levels or 'states', (1) and (2) cultured 'rat myoballs' (after Hamill & Sakmann 1981, reproduced with permission from Macmillan)

finally dissociates. There then follows a much longer shut state before agonist again binds to the receptor to re-open the channel.

Another recent finding (at least for channels in cultured muscle cells) is the discovery that there is more than one open state of the channel, each state having a different conductance (Fig. 3.16b) (Hamill & Sakmann 1981, Trautmann 1982, Auerbach & Sachs 1983, Sachs 1983, Takeda & Trautmann 1984, Colquhoun & Sakmann 1985). The same channel appears to exhibit transitions between at least two open conductance states. It is not clear whether multiple conductance states are also found at normal muscle end-plate channels.

Conductances obtained by the patch clamp method are about 40% higher than values found by noise analysis in the same cells. This could be because noise analysis gives *mean* results, thereby averaging over flickerings and any multiple conductance states (Fenwick et al 1982).

The acetylcholine receptor

Considerable progress in understanding the acetylcholine receptor (AChR) has come about by the use of neurotoxins found in certain snake venoms (Lee 1972). These neurotoxins bind specifically and almost irreversibly to the acetylcholine receptor, preventing its reaction with ACh. This action accounts for the paralysing effect resulting from the venom of such snakes. One of the most useful toxins is α-bungarotoxin (α-BuTX) obtained from the snake *Bungarus multicinctus*. The toxin can be labelled with a radioactive, fluorescent or enzyme marker without appreciable loss of activity. When such labelled toxin is bound to receptors, the resulting complex then leads to ready detection of AChR (for reviews see e.g. Dolly 1979, Barnard 1979, Dolly & Barnard 1984). Much work has been carried out on the receptor-rich electric organs of the fish *Electrophorus* and *Torpedo*. Mammalian muscle has also been investigated, although this is more difficult experimentally because of the less rich distribution of receptors.

Localisation. Electron microscope autoradiography of muscles pretreated with radioactively labelled α-BuTX has shown that AChR is mainly found on the crests of the postsynaptic folds of the motor end-plate (Fig. 3.1) at a density of about 25 000 receptors per μm^2 (Barnard et al 1975, Porter & Barnard 1975, 1976, Fertuck & Salpeter 1976, Matthews-Bellinger & Salpeter 1978). The total number of α-BuTX binding sites per muscle end-plate is in the range $3–9 \times 10^7$.

Labelling by a peroxidase conjugate of α-BuTX has shown that some binding sites also appear to exist on the presynaptic membrane (Bender et al 1976, Engel et al 1977b, Lentz et al 1977); thus AChRs could also be present presynaptically. The *quantitative* extent of these binding sites cannot be readily assessed by peroxidase-labelled α-BuTX. However, the extent of presynaptic binding must be quite small, as the more quantitative (but less sensitive) technique using radiolabelled α-BuTX does not lead to detection of presynaptic binding. Indeed, removal of the nerve terminal before binding with [³H]α-BuTX did not measurably affect binding. Therefore, any presynaptic AChR sites were below the error limit of the radiolabelled technique, and numbers of AChR (if present) are likely to be less than 10% of the number of postsynaptic receptors.

Isolation. The AChR has been isolated from muscles by the following technique (Dolly 1979,

Dolly & Barnard 1984). Membrane proteins, including the AChR, are brought into solution with a detergent (in the presence of protease inhibitors to prevent AChR degradation). For purification, the AChR is then absorbed on to α-toxin immobilised on a gel. The AChR can then be eluted from the column by application of a high concentration of carbachol. Variations in these methods exist, e.g. monoclonal antibodies directed against the AChR may be used in the column instead of the α-toxin (Lennon et al 1980, Momoi & Lennon 1982).

After purification, the AChR retains its ability to bind nicotinic cholinoceptor agonists and antagonists. This binding can be detected and made quantitative as the rate of binding of $[^3H]\alpha$-BuTX to the isolated AChR is, as expected, found to be retarded by the presence of such agonists or antagonists (Barnard et al 1977, see Dolly 1979 for further references).

Molecular structure. Muscle AChR is an acidic glycoprotein, composed of subunits which can be dissociated using sodium dodecyl sulphate gel electrophoresis. The molecular weights of these dissociated subunits, termed α, β, γ, δ are approximately 40–45, 49–53, 53–56, 57–68 kilodaltons respectively for muscle (Dolly & Barnard 1984), and rather similar for fish (Raftery et al 1980). The AChR in muscle and fish exists normally as a pentamer: $\alpha_2 \beta\gamma\delta$. The α subunit contains the ACh binding site: thus it is likely that the pentameric AChR has two ACh binding sites (for reviews see Karlin 1980, Changeux 1981, Conti-Tronconi & Raftery 1982).

The ion channel is an integral part of the pentameric AChR. Evidence for this has been obtained by inserting purified AChR from fish into lipid bilayers. Agonists such as ACh act on these reconstituted receptors causing increases in membrane permeability, similar to that expected from channel openings (Changeux et al 1979, Wu & Raftery 1979, Lindstrom et al 1980, Nelson et al 1980, Huganir & Racker 1982, Miller 1982). Indeed, patch recording from such reconstituted receptors shows that the channels can have the expected values of open time and conductance (Tank & Miller 1983).

The pentameric receptor/channel complex spans the membrane with the five subunits comprising

a 'rosette' around the central pore/channel which is formed between them (Fig. 3.17) (e.g. Kistler et al 1982, Brisson & Unwin 1985). Following binding of ACh molecules to the recognition sites, the whole AChR pentamer probably undergoes a conformational change causing the channel to open.

Exciting progress has taken place recently on the molecular structure of the AChR. Complete amino-acid sequences have been obtained for each subunit of the AChR obtained from fish electric organ and muscle (Noda et al 1982, 1983a, b, c, Sumikawa et al 1982, Claudio et al 1983, Devilliers-Thiery et al 1983, Takai et al 1984, 1985, Tanabe et al 1984, Kubo et al 1985, Shibahara et al 1985). To obtain these sequences, mRNA was taken from muscle or electric organs and used to produce cloned DNA corresponding to that

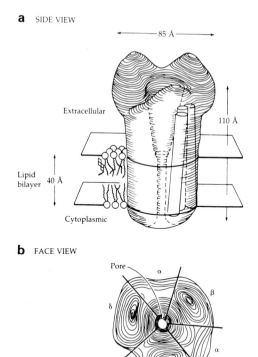

Fig. 3.17 Three-dimensional structure of the acetylcholine receptor, based on electron microscopy and X-ray diffraction. a. Side view of receptor in relation to the lipid bilayer of the plasma membrane. Cylinders represent α-helices of the peptide chains. b. Face view of AChR with tentative arrangement of subunits around the central pore (Kistler et al 1982, Hille 1984, reproduced with permission from the Biophysical Society)

responsible for the synthesis of AChR subunit protein. The sequence of this DNA was then found and hence the amino-acid sequence of the corresponding subunit protein could be deduced.

Subunits consist of 437–501 amino acids, allowing calculation of true protein molecular weights. Carbohydrate (4%) is also present (Vandlen et al 1979), leading to a calculated total molecular weight of approximately 278 kilodaltons for the fish AChR (Dolly & Barnard 1984). There is considerable amino-acid sequence homology between subunits in the same species, and also between different species.

Knowing the amino-acid structure, one can make reasonable predictions concerning the secondary structure. For each subunit there are probably at least five or six α-helices long enough

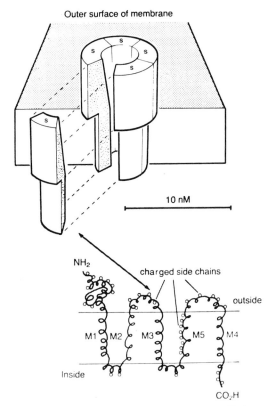

Fig. 3.18 Tentative model of secondary structure. Each subunit (s) consists of a single polypeptide chain composed of α-helices (M1–M5) spanning the membrane. The subunits fit together as shown in the figure to form the receptor channel complex (after Stevens 1985). Other tentative models have the polypeptide chain spanning the membrane seven times instead of five (Criado et al 1985)

to span the membrane (Fig. 3.18) (Finer-Moore & Stroud 1984, Guy 1984, Criado 1985).

Each subunit probably has a similar structure, spanning the membrane and fitting together to form a channel down the middle (Fig. 3.17, 3.18). One α-helix (M5, see Fig. 3.18) has polar residues on one side and non-polar residues on the other and may possibly form the channel lining, each subunit contributing its M5 helix as a lining. Further work is needed to clarify this very tentative picture. From a knowledge of the size of ions able to pass through the channel, it seems that the central pore has an internal diameter of about 0.65 nm at its narrowest, during its open state (Adams et al 1980, Dwyer et al 1980).

A further use of cloned DNA for AChR subunits has been to measure specific mRNA levels in muscle fibres. This assay is based on the fact that specific mRNA for an AChR subunit binds to the corresponding cloned DNA. In this way it was found that denervation causes a large increase in AChR subunit mRNA in the muscle fibre. This reflects an increase in synthesis of AChR which underlies the increase in number of receptors throughout the membrane of denervated muscle (see End-plate response) (Merlie et al 1984, Klarsfeld & Changeux 1985). Similar techniques have been applied to show that AChR-subunit mRNA in innervated fibres is more abundant near synapses, corresponding to synthesis of receptors there (Merlie & Sanes 1985).

Function. Progress in understanding the function of the AChR has been made recently by using the cloned DNA for the receptor subunits. Corresponding mRNA can be produced in the laboratory from cloned DNA, and is specific for the synthesis of each subunit. When this specific mRNA is injected into frog oocytes, the latter cell translates the mRNA into functional protein (Mishina et al 1984, 1985, Sakmann et al 1985, Takai et al 1985). AChR is produced in the oocyte membrane, provided mRNA corresponding to *all four* subunits are injected into the same oocyte. In support of this, the oocyte then binds α-BuTX and produces a rapid depolarisation when ACh is applied, and this is blocked by tubocurarine. The underlying ion channels also have the expected reversal potential, open time and conductance.

Furthermore, isolation of this synthesised AChR shows a similar subunit structure as for native AChR. Similar results had previously been obtained using non-specific extracts of mRNA from muscle and electric organ injected into oocytes (Sumikawa et al 1981, Barnard et al 1982, Miledi & Sumikawa 1982, Miledi et al 1982c, 1983b).

Recent interesting work has involved the synthesis in oocytes of hybrid AChRs composed of subunits from different species (Sakmann et al 1985). When mRNA for the δ subunit of calf AChR was injected into oocytes together with mRNA for the α, β, γ subunits of *Torpedo* AChR, hybrid AChR channels were formed in the oocyte. Calf, *Torpedo* and hybrid channels all had similar conductance and ionic selectivity. The channel open time was much longer for calf AChR than for *Torpedo*. The hybrid channel open time (and its voltage sensitivity) resembled that for calf AChR, and this suggests that the δ subunit plays a key role in determining channel open time.

Further progress has been made using mutant cloned DNA for the α-subunit (Mishina et al 1985). The corresponding specific mutant mRNA was injected into the oocyte together with normal specific mRNA for the other three subunits. The effect of known changes in amino-acid sequence of the α-subunit could be investigated to determine associated changes in the function of the AChR in the oocyte. For instance, deleting certain amino acids in each of the regions M2, M3, M4 and M5 did not affect binding of agonist, but did prevent the channel from opening. This would be expected if these membrane-spanning α-helices intimately surround the channel and hence are concerned with its function. Changes in certain regions of the amino-acid chain which are on the intracellular face had no effect on receptor function. Changes in the portion of the amino-acid chain between the N-terminus and the M1 chain reduced agonist binding, consistent with the idea that the ACh binding site is in this extracellular region.

Antibodies against acetylcholine receptor

Studies using antibodies against the acetylcholine receptor have proved valuable for two main reasons. Firstly, they have provided an understanding of the neuromuscular disease myasthenia gravis (MG), and secondly they have led to a better understanding of the structure and function of the ACh receptor itself.

Approximately 90% of patients with myasthenia gravis possess antibodies against the acetylcholine receptor (e.g. Lindstrom et al 1976b). The fact that such antibodies can lead to the symptoms of myasthenia gravis was first shown by injecting purified AChR into rabbits (Patrick & Lindstrom 1973; for reviews see Newsom-Davis 1982, Vincent 1983, Lindstrom 1985). Production of antibody in these animals directed against the receptor led to muscle weakness. This 'animal model' of the disorder is usually referred to as experimental autoimmune myasthenia gravis (EAMG). Furthermore, passive transfer of AChR antibody (from MG patients or EAMG animals) to animals also leads to muscle weakness (Lindstrom et al 1976a, Toyka et al 1977, 1978). Interestingly, monoclonal antibodies against the AChR can also transfer impairment of neuromuscular transmission to animals (e.g. Lennon & Lambert 1980, Burres et al 1981, Dwyer et al 1981, Tzartos 1984).

For both MG patients and EAMG animals, there is decreased binding of α-bungarotoxin at end-plates, indicative of loss of receptors from the postsynaptic membrane (Fambrough et al 1973, Heinemann et al 1978, Ito et al 1978, Reiness & Weinberg 1978, Stanley & Drachman 1978, Drachman 1983). This loss of receptors comes about, both in MG and chronically in EAMG, by antibodies cross-linking the receptors. Receptors are then internalised and hence degraded faster than normal. Normal end-plate receptors are usually degraded with a half-life of about one week. Another mechanism of receptor loss is by complement-mediated lysis of the postsynaptic membrane (Engel et al 1977a, Sahashi et al 1978).

The loss of AChRs leads to a reduction in postsynaptic sensitivity in MG and EAMG (e.g. Elmqvist et al 1964, Green et al 1975, Rash et al 1976), underlying the reduced amplitudes of epps and mepps. The size of the packet of ACh released from MG nerve terminals is at least as large as for normal terminals (Cull-Candy et al 1979). The decrease in epp amplitude by receptor loss leads to failure of many muscle fibres to trigger an action potential and therefore muscle weakness is produced.

During high-frequency nerve stimulation, for both normal and MG muscle, there is depression of ACh release (Fig. 3.6). In normal muscles, although such depression of release occurs, the resulting epps remain large enough to trigger muscle action potentials. However, in MG, because of the overall reduction in postsynaptic responses, epps during high-frequency trains fall below the threshold for triggering muscle action potentials. Thus muscle weakness becomes more severe during high frequency nerve stimulation in MG patients (Lambert & Elmqvist 1971).

Noise analysis of muscle from MG patients and from EAMG animals shows that channel open time and channel conductance are similar to normal values (Cull-Candy et al 1979, Alema et al 1981). Therefore those channels which remain functional in MG and EAMG appear to have normal properties, at least in this respect (but see Albuquerque et al 1981).

Polyclonal and especially monoclonal antibodies have provided useful information about the normal ACh receptor. For instance, some (but not all) antibodies raised against one subunit cross-react with other subunits, providing support for the idea of extensive amino acid sequence similarity between subunits (Tzartos & Lindstrom 1980; for further references see Tzartos 1984, Lindstrom 1985). Moreover, certain antibody preparations cross-react with AChR from several species, implying partial similarities in the amino-acid sequence and structure between species. Other antibodies do not cross-react, and hence are raised against specific determinants not found on other species. These findings of a high degree of homology were confirmed by the full amino-acid sequencing discussed above.

The effect of acute binding of antibody on receptor *function* has been studied by measuring mepps, ACh sensitivity and noise in muscles, and by measuring $^{22}Na^+$ or thallium flux in reconstituted lipid vesicles containing AChR (Albuquerque et al 1976, Bevan et al 1977, 1978, Harvey et al 1978, Lindstrom et al 1981, 1983, Dolly et al 1982, 1983, Lerrick et al 1983, Donnelly et al 1984, Lacey et al 1985, Wan & Lindstrom 1985). Such acute exposures to antibody do not allow sufficient time for appreciable AChR degradation to occur and effects are due to pharmacological blocking of receptors. The *site* of binding of the antibody can be found by studying possible interference by the antibody with binding of agonists and antagonists at the receptor (Lindstrom 1976, Fulpius et al 1980, James et al 1980, Gomez et al 1981, Lennon & Lambert 1981, Mochly-Rosen & Fuchs 1981, Donnelly et al 1984, Whiting et al 1985a,b). For instance, block of α-bungarotoxin binding probably indicates antibody binding near to (but not necessarily at) the ACh binding site. Antibody preparations (from EAMG animals and MG patients) have a wide range of specificities and either (i) block the binding of ACh to its binding site on the AChR, or (ii) prevent channels opening by binding away from the ACh binding site, or (iii) bind away from the ACh binding site without loss of function. The majority of EAMG and MG antibodies fall in category (iii). Many of these latter antibodies compete amongst themselves for a well-defined structural region of the AChR — the 'main immunogenic region' (MIR), which is probably located on the α-subunit (e.g. Lindstrom 1985, Tzartos & Lindstrom 1980). Thus the vast majority of antibodies found in MG patients do not cause direct, acute block of receptors. The antibodies in category (ii) above are especially interesting because they may be interfering with the step(s) between ACh binding and subsequent channel opening, possibly by binding to the channel itself. Those channels which remain functional have normal channel open time and conductance (Dolly et al 1982, Lacey et al 1985). These antibodies (especially monoclonals) should prove useful in correlating the molecular structure of the receptor with its function.

An interesting recent development has been the use of monoclonal antibodies raised against synthetic short chain peptides of about 10 amino acids. These peptides are synthesised to be of the same sequence as small portions of the known amino-acid sequence found in AChR. For instance, antibodies raised or reacting against the C-terminus region bind intracellularly, showing that this terminus is located intracellularly (Fig. 3.18) (Lindstrom et al 1984, Neumann et al 1984, Ratnam & Lindstrom 1984, Young et al 1985).

The N-terminus is located extracellularly, and thus the amino-acid chain spans the membrane an odd number of times (perhaps five or seven times). Other portions of the amino-acid chain present on the intracellular face have also been mapped in this way (Criado et al 1985, LaRochelle et al 1985). The site of ACh binding is also being explored using antibodies raised against specific amino acids which may be involved in ACh binding (e.g. Plumer et al 1984), but this approach is still in its early stages.

Channel-blocking drugs

As described above, agonists such as ACh cause channels to open. Certain drugs, such as local anaesthetics, appear to block these open channels (Katz & Miledi 1975, Adams 1977, Ruff 1977, Neher & Steinbach 1978, Ogden et al 1981; for reviews see e.g. Wray 1980, Dreyer 1982). They interact with the open channel, causing the channel conductance to fall to zero. When the channel-blocking drug leaves its binding site, the channel is thought to revert back to its open state with agonist still bound. The open channel may then either shut as agonist dissociates or it may first encounter repeated blockings by the drug (Fig. 3.19).

Channel-blocking drugs lead to characteristic changes in, e.g. end-plate currents (Kordas 1970, Beam 1976). Following initial opening of the channel by nerve-released ACh, channels become rapidly blocked by such drugs. This rapid initial block of channels in turn causes epcs to initially decay more rapidly than normal. Later dissociation of blocking drug from the channel causes channels to transiently re-open, producing a slower tail of epc decay: a two-component epc is produced (Fig. 3.20b). For certain channel-blocking drugs, the dissociation rate is so slow that the 'tail' cannot be detected: the epc then consists of a single component decay which is more rapid than normal (Fig. 3.20c).

Although the rate of dissociation of different

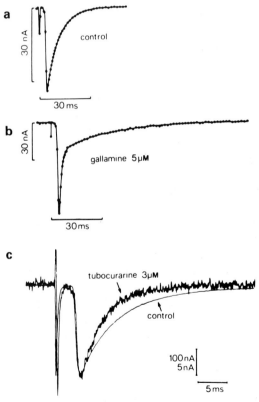

Fig. 3.20 Action of channel-blocking drugs on the epc. Besides their competitive action, gallamine and tubocurarine also block open channels. The figures (Dreyer 1982) show epcs at frog end-plates (11–12°C). Epcs normally decay exponentially (a). Gallamine induces a two-component decay (b) (Colquhoun & Sheridan 1981). Tubocurarine produces a single component epc with a faster exponential decay (c) (Colquhoun et al 1979)

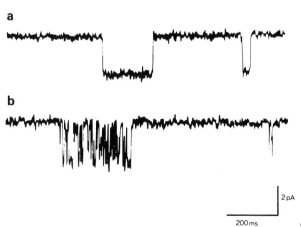

Fig. 3.19 The effect of the channel-blocking drug benzocaine. Patch clamp recordings were made of single channel currents induced by ACh in denervated frog muscle (9°C): a. in the absence of benzocaine; b. in the presence of benzocaine. Repeated channel blockings can be seen in the lower trace. (Ogden et al 1981, reproduced with permission from Macmillan)

channel-blocking drugs varies widely, the rate of binding of these drugs to the channel is usually rather similar. One possibility is a simple plugging of the open channel by the drug molecule. The extent of channel block increases with the concentration of channel-blocking drug and with the number of open channels available for block.

Besides local anaesthetics, a wide range of drugs have been found which block open channels. Some examples are histrionicotoxin (Albuquerque et al 1974), atropine (Adler et al 1978), mecamylamine (Wray 1981a, Varanda et al 1985), tubocurarine (Katz & Miledi 1978, Colquhoun et al 1979), gallamine (Colquhoun & Sheridan 1981), certain antibiotics (e.g. clindamycin and lincomycin) (Fiekers et al 1979, 1983) and some barbiturates (Adams 1976) as well as agonists themselves (Adams & Sakmann 1978, Sine & Steinbach 1984, Ogden & Colquhoun 1985).

Neuromuscular blocking drugs

Neuromuscular blocking drugs in use by anaesthetists to obtain muscle relaxation during surgical operations are of two types: competitive antagonists and depolarising agonists.

Competitive antagonists. Drugs in the category of competitive antagonist, of which tubocurarine is the classic example (Jenkinson 1960), act by combining reversibly with the ACh-binding site on the receptor. They do not themselves cause channels to open at the neuromuscular junction, but prevent ACh from triggering channel opening. Increasing the concentration of ACh in the cleft (e.g. by using an anticholinesterase such as neostigmine) can overcome the competitive block. More recently, relatively rapidly acting competitive antagonists such as vecuronium (Marshall et al 1980, 1983) and atracurium (Hughes & Chapple 1981, Payne & Hughes 1981) have been introduced for use during anaesthesia.

Besides the action of tubocurarine as a competitive antagonist, the drug can also block open channels (see above). However, the main effect of the drug under conditions encountered clinically is mainly competitive. So, e.g. tubocurarine at micromolar concentrations does not markedly affect the channel open time and epc decay rate

at normal resting potentials, but simply reduces the frequency of channel opening induced by agonists such as ACh (Katz & Miledi 1972, Colquhoun et al 1979). This competitive mechanism underlies the well-known shift in dose-response curves by tubocurarine. On the other hand, channel block becomes more important at hyperpolarised potentials and at higher agonist concentrations.

Agonists. Depolarising blocking drugs (such as suxamethonium and decamethonium) are agonists at the neuromuscular junction. They act at AChRs to cause channels to open and this in turn produces a depolarisation at the end-plate region (Zaimis & Head 1976, Zaimis & Wray 1981). The action is similar to that of ACh in the presence of inhibitors of acetylcholinesterase to prevent ACh breakdown (Burns & Paton 1951, Wray 1981b) (Fig. 3.21). At drug concentrations found clinically (around 1 μM) and for many minutes, depolarisation is well maintained, at least for cat and man. This maintained depolarisation causes inactivation of the electrically operated Na^+ channels (not the AChR channels) responsible for action potentials (see End-plate response); hence, no action potentials can be triggered and paralysis results.

During the application of depolarising drugs at micromolar concentrations, the depolarisation wanes rather slowly (Fig. 3.21). Throughout this period, channels continue to be opened by the agonist. The frequency of opening of channels can be followed by noise analysis and this is also shown in Fig. 3.21. The number of channels opened per second by the agonist also falls quite slowly. The process of inactivation of receptor function during prolonged agonist application is known as desensitisation (e.g. Elmqvist & Thesleff 1962, Nastuk et al 1966, Rang 1975, Ginsborg & Jenkinson 1976). It can thus be seen that at this low concentration, desensitisation occurs slowly (Paton & Waud 1962). Similar slow desensitisation is also seen for suberyldicholine, suxamethonium and decamethonium at a concentration of 1 μM. Therefore the end-plate remains sensitive to agonists for many minutes: blockade of neuromuscular transmission does not occur by this slow process of desensitisation of ACh receptors at

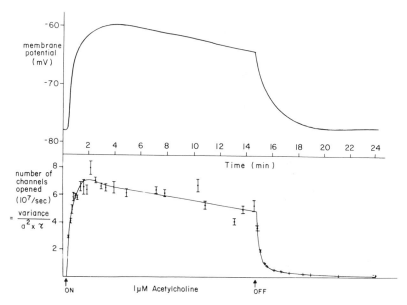

Fig. 3.21 Prolonged exposure to ACh. Upper trace: membrane potential; lower trace: frequency of opening of channels obtained from the noise variance. Recordings were made during application of ACh (1 μM) to cat tenuissimus muscle (38°C) in the presence of eserine to prevent hydrolysis of ACh (Wray 1978b, 1981b)

these concentrations. The maintained depolarisation itself will normally be sufficient to produce neuromuscular blockade by inactivating action potentials.

The fact that some desensitisation does occur (albeit slowly) during exposure to depolarising drugs is indicated also by the fact that repeated applications of decamethonium produce progressively smaller depolarisations (Burns & Paton 1951). Futhermore, desensitisation proceeds at a faster rate for higher agonist concentrations (e.g. Katz & Thesleff 1957, Wray 1981b). Such concentrations are probably found when ACh is applied locally by iontophoresis, leading to more rapid desensitisation (Axelsson & Thesleff 1958). Of course, if the ACh receptors are inactivated (desensitised) by depolarising drugs, they will also be unable to respond to nerve-released ACh and block of transmission would again be produced. During *prolonged* doses of depolarising drugs, sufficient desensitisation may occur for the mechanism of the block to change from that due to depolarisation to that due to desensitisation; and this might be the mechanism of the so-called 'dual block' (Zaimis 1953). For certain species (e.g. rat, see Zaimis & Head 1976) the end-plate is normally

rather insensitive to depolarising drugs so that small depolarisations are produced and higher concentrations of blocking drug are needed to produce neuromuscular blockade. The mechanism of blockade at such higher concentrations may then be due throughout to desensitisation for such species.

Recently the phenomenon of desensitisation has been studied by the patch clamp method (Sakmann et al 1980). In the presence of agonist, desensitised channels have long, closed, silent periods, then they open in bursts before closing again (Fig. 3.22). The bursts themselves are arranged in clusters, with even longer closed silent periods separating them. Desensitisation itself is a little-understood process whereby the receptor/channel complex appears to revert to at least two kinds of inactive conformational states.

Noise analysis and patch clamp recording have shown that channel open time differs markedly for different agonists (Katz & Miledi 1973b, Colquhoun et al 1975, 1977, Dreyer et al 1976b, Neher & Sakmann 1976a,b). The mean channel open times are: suberyldicholine: 1.6–3.3 ms; ACh: 1.1 ms; acetylmonoethylcholine: 0.66 ms; carbachol: 0.3–0.4 ms; decamethonium: 0.5 ms; nicotine: 0.22 ms;

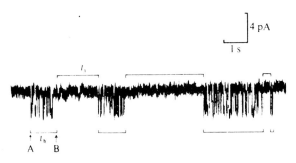

Fig. 3.22 Bursts of single channel openings followed by long silent periods occur for 'desensitised' receptors. The recording was made from denervated frog muscle by the patch clamp technique using 10 μM ACh (11°C). Note the slow time scale so that individual openings are barely resolved. The arrows (A,B) indicate onset and cessation of a single channel burst, duration t_b, (t_1: interval between bursts) (Sakmann et al 1980, reproduced with permission from Macmillan)

acetylthiocholine: 0.12 ms (20°C, −75 mV). On the other hand, the single channel conductance is approximately the same value as for ACh for each of these agonists. The variation in channel open time suggests that agonist remains attached to the receptor while the channel is open.

At concentrations which produce neuromuscular block (about 1 μM), the depolarising drugs ACh, suberyldicholine, suxamethonium and decamethonium all produce large depolarisations of about 20 mV for cat muscle (37°C) (Wray 1978a). Such a depolarisation is large enough to cause depolarisation block. Channel open time (and hence the depolarisation produced by a single channel opening, a) varies widely between these agonists. The overall depolarisation of 20 mV produced in cat muscle is similar for each of these drugs because the smaller the single channel depolarisation, a, the larger the channel opening frequency turns out to be, at least for this muscle at this concentration.

Besides acting at the ACh−binding site to cause channels to open, agonists can also block open channels (see Channel-blocking drugs). This kind of block has been reported for suberyldicholine, carbachol, ACh and decamethonium. Except for suberyldicholine, channel block occurs at high concentrations and is, therefore, unlikely to be important in experiments and clinical procedures carried out at about 1 μM. Furthermore, channel block by ACh itself is unlikely to contribute during the action of ACh released by nerve stimulation.

CONCLUSION

The cohesive picture of neuromuscular transmission described in this chapter has been built up over several decades. This picture provides a sound basis for understanding disorders of human neuromuscular transmission, such as myasthenia gravis and the Lambert–Eaton myasthenic syndrome.

However, much remains to be clarified at normal neuromuscular junctions. For instance, very little is known about the functioning of voltage-dependent Ca^{2+} channels on the presynaptic membrane, or about how Ca^{2+} causes release of ACh. The origin of the packets of ACh is still debated. On the postsynaptic side, it is not yet clear on the molecular level how ACh causes channels to open. Exciting progress on these questions can be anticipated over the coming years, and this should prove useful both scientifically and clinically.

ACKNOWLEDGEMENTS

I am most grateful to C. Peers for his unfailing help and for useful criticism and comments throughout the preparation of this chapter. I would also like to thank A. Vincent & D. J. Withington-Wray for their comments on the manuscript.

REFERENCES

Adams P R 1976 Drug blockade of open end-plate channels. Journal of Physiology 260: 531

Adams P R 1977 Voltage jump analysis of procaine action at frog end plates. Journal of Physiology 268: 291

Adams P R, Sakmann B 1978 Decamethonium both opens and blocks endplate channels. Proceedings of the National Academy of Sciences USA 75: 2994

Adams D J, Dwyer T M, Hille B 1980 The permeability of end plate channels to monovalent and divalent cations. Journal of General Physiology 75: 493

Adler M, Albuquerque E X, Lebeda F J 1978 Kinetic analysis of end-plate currents altered by atropine and scopolamine. Molecular Pharmacology 14: 514

Albuquerque E X, Kuba K, Daly J 1974 Effect of histrionicotoxin on the ionic conductance modulator of the cholinergic receptor: A quantitative analysis of the end-plate current. Journal of Pharmacological and Experimental Therapeutics 189: 513

Albuquerque E X, Lebeda F J, Appel S H, Almon R, Kauffmann F C, Mayer R F, Narahashi T, Yeh J Z 1976 Effects of normal and myasthenic serum factors on innervated and chronically denervated mammalian muscles. Annals of the New York Academy of Sciences 274: 475

Albuquerque E X, Warnick J E, Mayer R F, Eldefrawi A T, Eldefrawi M E 1981 Recent advances in the molecular mechanisms of human and animal models of myasthenia gravis. Annals of the New York Academy of Sciences 377: 496

Alemà S, Cull-Candy S G, Miledi R, Trautmann A 1981 Properties of end-plate channels in rats immunized against acetylcholine receptors. Journal of Physiology 311: 251

Alnaes E, Rahamimoff R 1975 On the role of mitochondria in transmitter release from motor nerve terminals. Journal of Physiology 248: 285

Anderson C R, Stevens C F 1973 Voltage clamp analysis of acetylcholine produced end-plate current fluctuations at frog neuromuscular junction. Journal of Physiology 235: 655

Auerbach A, Sachs F 1983 Flickering of a nicotinic ion channel to a subconductance state. Biophysical Journal 42: 1

Augustine G J, Charlton M P, Smith S J 1985a Calcium entry into voltage-clamped presynaptic terminals of squid. Journal of Physiology 367: 143

Augustine G J, Charlton M P, Smith S J 1985b Calcium entry and transmitter release at voltage-clamped nerve terminals of squid. Journal of Physiology 369: 163

Axelsson J, Thesleff S 1958 The desensitizing effect of acetylcholine on mammalian motor end-plate. Acta Physiologica Scandinavica 43: 15

Axelsson J, Thesleff S 1959 A study of supersensitivity in denervated mammalian skeletal muscle. Journal of Physiology 147: 178

Baker P F 1972 Transport and metabolism of calcium ions in nerves. Progress in Biophysical and Molecular Biology 24: 177

Baker P F 1977 Calcium and the control of neurosecretion. Scientific Progress, Oxford 64: 95

Barnard E A 1974 Neuromuscular junction — enzymatic destruction of acetylcholine. In: Hubbard J I (ed) The peripheral nervous system. Plenum, New York, p 201

Barnard E A 1979 Visualization and counting of receptors at the light and electron microscope levels. In: O'Brien R D (ed) The receptors, a comprehensive treatise. Plenum, New York, Vol 1: 247

Barnard E A, Wieckowski J, Chiu T H 1971 Cholinergic receptor molecules and cholinesterase molecules at mouse skeletal muscle junction. Nature 234: 207

Barnard E A, Dolly J O, Porter C W, Albuquerque E X 1975 The acetylcholine receptor and the ionic conductance modulation system of skeletal muscle. Experimental Neurobiology 48: 1

Barnard E A, Coates V, Dolly J O, Mallick B 1977 Binding of α-bungarotoxin and cholinergic ligands to acetylcholine receptors in the membrane of skeletal muscle. Cell Biology International Reports 1: 99

Barnard E A, Miledi R, Sumikawa K 1982 Translation of exogenous messenger RNA coding for nicotinic acetylcholine receptors produces functioning receptors in Xenopus oocytes. Proceedings of the Royal Society B215: 241

Beam K G 1976 A quantitative description of end-plate currents in the presence of two lidocaine derivatives. Journal of Physiology 258: 301

Bender A N, Ringel S P, Engel W K, Vogel Z, Daniels M P 1976 Immunoperoxidase localization of alpha bungarotoxin: a new approach to myasthenia gravis. Annals of the New York Academy of Sciences 274: 20

Ben-Haim D, Dreyer F, Peper K 1975 Acetylcholine receptor: modification of synaptic gating mechanism after treatment with a disulfide bond reducing agent. Pflugers Achives 355: 19

Bevan S, Kullberg R W, Heinemann S F 1977 Human myasthenic sera reduce acetylcholine sensitivity of human muscle cells in tissue culture. Nature 267: 263

Bevan S, Kullberg R W, Rice J 1978 Acetylcholine induced conductance fluctuations in cultured human myotubes. Nature 273: 469

Birks R, Huxley H E, Katz B 1960a The fine structure of the neuromuscular junction of the frog. Journal of Physiology 150: 134

Birks R, Katz B, Miledi R 1960b Physiological and structural changes at the amphibian myoneural junction in the course of nerve degeneration. Journal of Physiology 150: 145

Borsotto M, Barhanin J, Norman R I, Lazdunski M 1984 Purification of the dihydropyridine receptor of the voltage-dependent Ca^{2+} channel from skeletal muscle transverse tubules using $(+)$ [^{3}H] PN200–110. Biochemical and Biophysical Research Communications 122: 1357

Bowden R E M, Duchen L W 1976 The anatomy and pathology of the neuromuscular junction. In: Zaimis E (ed) Handbook of experimental pharmacology XLII Neuromuscular junction. Springer-Verlag, Berlin, p 23

Bowman W C 1980 Prejunctional and postjunctional cholinoceptors at the neuromuscular junction. Anaesthesia and Analgesia 59: 935

Bregestovski P D, Miledi R, Parker I 1980 Blocking of frog endplate channels by the organic calcium antagonist D600. Proceedings of the Royal Society B211: 15

Brisson A, Unwin P N T 1985 Quaternary structure of the acetylcholine receptor. Nature 315: 474

Burns B D, Paton W D M 1951 Depolarization of the motor end-plate by decamethonium and acetylcholine. Journal of Physiology 115: 41

Burres S A, Crayton J W, Gomez C M, Richman D P 1981 Myasthenia induced by monoclonal anti-acetylcholine receptor antibodies: clinical and electrophysiological aspects. Annals of Neurology 9: 563

Ceccarelli B, Hurlbut W P 1980 Vesicle hypothesis of the release of quanta of acetylcholine. Pharmacological Reviews 60: 396

Changeux J P 1975 The cholinergic receptor protein from fish electric organ. In: Iverson L L, Iverson S D, Snyder S H (eds) Handbook of psychopharmacology. Plenum, New York, Vol 6, p 235

Changeux J P 1981 The acetylcholine receptor: An 'allosteric' membrane protein. Harvey Lectures 75: 85

Changeux J P, Heidmann T, Popot J L, Sobel A 1979 Reconstitution of a functional acetylcholine regulator under defined conditions. Federation of European Biochemical Societies Letters 105: 181

Charlton M P, Smith S J, Zucker R S 1982 Role of presynaptic calcium ions and channels in synaptic facilitation and depression at the squid giant synapse. Journal of Physiology 323: 173

Claudio T, Ballivet M, Patrick J, Heinemann S 1983 Nucleotide and deduced amino acid sequences of torpedo californica acetylcholine receptor γ subunit. Proceedings of the National Academy of Sciences, USA 80: 1111

Cohen I S, Van der Kloot W 1983 Effects of low temperature and terminal membrane potential on quantal size at frog neuromuscular junction. Journal of Physiology 336: 335

Colquhoun D 1975 Mechanisms of drug action at the voluntary muscle endplate. Annual Review of Pharmacology 15: 307

Colquhoun D 1979 The link between drug binding and response: theories and observations. In: O'Brien R D (ed) The receptors: A comprehensive treatise. Plenum, New York, Vol 1: 93

Colquhoun D 1981 How fast do drugs work? Trends in Pharmacological Sciences 2: 212

Colquhoun D, Dionne V E, Steinbach J H, Stevens C F 1975 Conductance of channels opened by acetylcholine-type drugs in muscle end-plate. Nature 253: 204

Colquhoun D, Large W A, Rang H P 1977 An analysis of the action of false transmitter at the neuromuscular junction. Journal of Physiology 266: 361

Colquhoun D, Dreyer F, Sheridan R E 1979 The actions of tubocurarine at the frog neuromuscular junction. Journal of Physiology 293: 247

Colquhoun D, Sakman B 1981 Fluctuations in the microsecond time range of the current through single acetylcholine receptor ion channels. Nature 294: 464

Colquhoun D, Sheridan R E 1981 The modes of action of gallamine. Proceedings of the Royal Society B211: 181

Colquhoun D, Hawkes A G 1983 The principles of the stochastic interpretation of ion-channel mechanisms. In: Sakmann B, Neher E (eds) Single channel recording. Plenum, New York, ch 9, p 135

Colquhoun D, Sakmann B 1985 Fast events in single-channel currents activated by acetylcholine and its analogues at the frog muscle end-plate. Journal of Physiology 369: 501

Conti-Tronconi B M, Raftery M A 1982 The nicotinic cholinergic receptor: correlation of molecular structure with functional properties. Annual Review of Biochemistry 51: 491

Cooke I, Lipkin Jr M 1972 Cellular neurophysiology: a source book. Holt, Rinehart and Winston, New York

Corthay J, Dunant Y, Loctin F 1982 Acetylcholine changes underlying transmission of a single nerve impulse in the presence of 4-aminopyridine in Torpedo. Journal of Physiology 325: 461

Couteaux R, Pecot-Dechavassine M 1968 Particularites structurales de sarcoplasme sous-neural. Comptes rendues Hebdomadaires des Seánces de l'Académie des Sciences 266: 8

Criado M, Sarin V, Fox J L, Lindstrom J 1985 Structural localization of the sequence 235–242 of the nicotinic acetylcholine receptor. Biochemical and Biophysical Research Communications 128: 864

Cull-Candy S G, Lundh H, Thesleff S 1976 Effects of botulinum toxin on neuromuscular transmission in the rat. Journal of Physiology 260: 177

Cull-Candy S G, Miledi R, Trautmann A 1979 End-plate currents and acetylcholine noise at normal and myasthenic human end-plates. Journal of Physiology 287: 247

Cull-Candy S G, Miledi R, Trautmann A, Uchitel O D 1980 On the release of transmitter at normal, myasthenia gravis and myasthenic syndrome affected human end-plates. Journal of Physiology 299: 621

Curtis B M, Catterall W A 1984 Purification of the calcium antagonist receptor of the voltage-sensitive calcium channel from skeletal muscle transverse tubules. Biochemistry 23: 2113

Datyner N B, Gage P W 1980 Phasic secretion of acetylcholine at a mammalian neuromuscular junction. Journal of Physiology 303: 299

Del Castillo J, Katz B 1954a Quantal components of the end-plate potential. Journal of Physiology 124: 560

Del Castillo J, Katz B 1954b Statistical factors involved in neuromuscular facilitation and depression. Journal of Physiology 124: 574

Del Castillo J, Katz B 1955 Local activity at a depolarized nerve-muscle junction. Journal of Physiology 128: 396

Devilliers-Thiery A, Giraudat J, Bentaboulet M, Changeux J P 1983 Complete mRNA coding sequence of the acetylcholine binding α- subunit of Torpedo marmorata acetylcholine receptor: a model for the transmembrane organization of the polypeptide chain. Proceedings of the National Academy of Sciences USA 80: 2067

Dionne V E, Ruff R L 1977 Endplate current fluctuations reveal only one channel type at frog neuromuscular junction. Nature 266: 263

Dodge Jr F A, Rahamimoff R 1967 Co-operative action of Ca^{2+} ions in transmitter release at the neuromuscular junction. Journal of Physiology 193: 419

Dolezal V, Tucek S 1983 The synthesis and release of acetylcholine in normal and denervated rat diaphragms during incubation in vitro. Journal of Physiology 334: 461

Dolly J O 1979 Biochemistry of acetylcholine receptors from skeletal muscle. In: Tipton K F (ed) Physiological and pharmacological biochemistry, Vol. 26. University Park Press, Baltimore, ch 6, p 257

Dolly J O, Gwilt M, Mehraban F, Wray D 1982 Action on end-plate channels of antibodies against pure acetylcholine receptors from muscle. Journal of Physiology 336: 56P

Dolly J O, Mehraban F, Gwilt M, Wray D 1983 Biochemical and electrophysiological properties of antibodies against pure acetylcholine receptor from vertebrate muscles and its subunits from Torpedo in relation to experimental myasthenia. Neurochemistry International 5: 455

Dolly J O, Barnard E A 1984 Nicotinic acetylcholine receptors: an overview. Biochemical Pharmacology 33: 841

Dolly J O, Black J, Williams R S, Melling J 1984 Acceptors for botulinum neurotoxin reside on motor nerve terminals and mediate its internalization. Nature 307: 457

Dolly J O, Lande S, Wray D 1985 A population of miniature end-plate potentials unaffected by botulinum neurotoxin at mouse motor nerve terminals. Journal of Physiology 365: 80P

Donnelly D, Mihovilovic M, Gonzalez-Ros J M, Ferragut J A, Richman D, Martinez-Carrion M 1984 A non-cholinergic site directed monoclonal antibody can impair agonist-induced ion flux in Torpedo californica acetylcholine receptor. Proceedings of the National Academy of Sciences USA 81: 7999

Drachman D B 1983 Myasthenia gravis: immunobiology of a receptor disorder. Trends in Neurosciences 6: 446

Dreyer F 1982 Acetylcholine receptor. British Journal of Anaesthesia 54: 115

Dreyer F, Peper K 1975 Density and dose-response curve of

acetylcholine receptors in frog neuromuscular junction. Nature 253: 641

Dreyer F, Muller K-D, Peper K, Stertz R 1976a The M. omohyoideus of the mouse as a convenient mammalian muscle preparation. Pflugers Archives 367: 115

Dreyer F, Walther Chr, Peper K 1976b Junctional and extrajunctional acetylcholine receptors in normal and denervated frog muscle fibres: noise analysis experiments with different agonists. Pflugers Archives 366: 1

Dudel J 1983 Transmitter release triggered by a local depolarization in motor nerve terminals of the frog: role of calcium entry and of depolarization. Neuroscience Letters 41: 133

Dudel J 1984a Control of transmitter release at frog's motor nerve terminals I. Dependence on amplitude and duration of depolarization. Pflugers Archives 402: 225

Dudel J 1984b Control of quantal transmitter release at frog's motor nerve terminals II. Modulation by de- or hyperpolarizing pulses. Pflugers Archives 402: 235

Dudel J, Parnas I, Parnas H 1983 Neurotransmitter release and its facilitation in crayfish muscle VI. Release determined by both intracellular calcium concentration and depolarization of the nerve terminal. Pflugers Archives 399: 1

Dunant Y, Corthay J, Eder L, Loctin F 1980 Acetylcholine changes during nerve impulse transmission. Analysis with a rapid freezing device. In: Taxi J (ed) Ontogenesis and functional mechanisms of peripheral synapses. Elsevier/ North Holland, Amsterdam

Dunant Y, Israel M 1985 The release of acetylcholine. Scientific American 252: 40

Dwyer T M, Adams D J, Hille B 1980 The permeability of the end plate channel to organic cations in frog muscle. Journal of General Physiology 75: 469

Dwyer D S, Kearney J F, Bradley R J, Kemp G E, Oh S J 1981 Interaction of human antibody and murine monoclonal antibody with muscle acetylcholine receptor. Annals of the New York Academy of Sciences 377: 143

Elmqvist D, Thesleff S 1962 Ideas regarding receptor desensitization at the motor end-plate. Revue Canadienne de Biologie 21: 229

Elmqvist D, Hoffman W W, Kugelberg J, Quastel D M J 1964 An electrophysiological investigation of neuromuscular transmission in myasthenia gravis. Journal of Physiology 174: 417

Elmqvist D, Quastel D M J 1965 Presynaptic action of hemicholinium at the neuromuscular junction. Journal of Physiology 177: 463

Engel A G, Lambert E H, Howard F M 1977a Immune complexes (IgG and C3) at the motor end-plate in myasthenia gravis. Ultrastructural and light microscopic localization and electrophysiologic correlations. Mayo Clinic Proceedings 52: 267

Engel A G, Lindstrom J M, Lambert E H, Lennon V A 1977b Ultrastructural localization of the acetylcholine receptor in myasthenia gravis and in its experimental autoimmune model. Neurology (Minneapolis) 27: 307

Fambrough D M, Drachmann D B, Satyamurti S 1973 Neuromuscular junction in myasthenia gravis: decreased acetylcholine receptors. Science 182: 293

Fatt P, Katz B 1951 An analysis of the end-plate potential recorded with an intracellular electrode. Journal of Physiology 115: 320

Fatt P, Katz B 1952 Spontaneous subthreshold activity at motor nerve endings. Journal of Physiology 117: 109

Fenwick E M, Marty A, Neher E 1982 Sodium and calcium channels in bovine chromaffin cells. Journal of Physiology 331: 599

Fertuck H C, Salpeter M M 1976 Quantitation of junctional and extrajunctional acetylcholine receptors by electron microscope autoradiography after ^{125}I-α-bungarotoxin binding at mouse neuromuscular junctions. Journal of Cell Biology 69: 144

Fiekers J F, Marshall I G, Parsons R L 1979 Clindamycin and lincomycin alter miniature end-plate current decay. Nature 281: 680

Fiekers J F, Henderson F, Marshall I G, Parsons R L 1983 An electrophysiological study of lincomycin and clindamycin at the neuromuscular junction. Comparative effects on endplate currents and quantal content. Journal of Pharmacological and Experimental Therapeutics 227: 308

Finer-Moore J, Stroud R M 1984 Amphipathic analysis and possible formation of the ion channel in an acetylcholine receptor. Proceedings of the National Academy of Sciences USA 81: 155

Fletcher P, Forrester T 1975 The effect of curare on the release of acetylcholine from mammalian motor nerve terminals and an estimate of quantum content. Journal of Physiology 251: 131

Fukunaga H, Engel A G, Osame M, Lambert E H 1982 Paucity and disorganization of presynaptic membrane active zones in the Lambert-Eaton myasthenic syndrome. Muscle and Nerve 5: 686

Fukunaga H, Engel A G, Lang B, Newsom-Davis J, Vincent A 1983 Passive transfer of Lambert-Eaton myasthenic syndrome with IgG from man to mouse depletes the presynaptic active zones. Proceedings of the National Academy of Sciences USA 80: 7636

Fulpius B W, Miskin R, Reich E 1980 Antibodies from myasthenic patients that compete with cholinergic agents for binding to nicotinic receptors. Proceedings of the National Academy of Sciences USA 77: 4326

Gibb A J, Marshall I G 1984 Pre- and post-junctional effects of tubocurarine and other nicotinic antagonists during repetitive stimulation in the rat. Journal of Physiology 351: 275

Gilman A G, Goodman L S, Rall T W, Murad F 1985 Goodman and Gilman's Pharmacological basis of therapeutics 7th edn. Macmillan, New York

Ginsborg B L, Jenkinson D H 1976 Transmission of impulses from nerve to muscle. In: Zaimis E (ed) Handbook of experimental pharmacology, XLII Neuromuscular junction. Springer-Verlag, Berlin, p 229

Gomez C M, Richman D P, Burres S A, Arnason B G W, Berman P W, Fitch F W 1981 Monoclonal hybridoma antiacetylcholine receptor antibodies: antibody specificity and effect of passive transfer. Annals of the New York Academy of Sciences 377: 96

Gotgilf M, Magazanik L G 1977 Action of calcium channel blocking agents (verapamil, D-600 and manganese ions) on transmitter release from motor nerve endings of frog muscle. Neurophysiology 9: 415

Green D P L, Miledi R, Perez de la Mora M, Vincent A 1975 Acetylcholine receptors. Philosophical Transactions of the Royal Society B270: 551

Gundersen C B, Jenden D J, Newton M W 1981 β-bungaro-toxin stimulates the synthesis and accumulation of acetylcholine in rat phrenic nerve diaphragm preparations. Journal of Physiology 310: 13

Gundersen C B, Katz B, Miledi R 1982 The antagonism between botulinum toxin and calcium in motor nerve terminals. Proceedings of the Royal Society B216: 369

Guy R 1984 A structural model of the acetylcholine receptor channel based on the partition energy and helix packing calculations. Biophysical Journal 45: 249

Hamill O P, Sakmann B 1981 Multiple conductance states of single acetylcholine receptor channels in embryonic muscle cells. Nature 294: 462

Hamill O P, Marty A, Neher E, Sakmann B, Sigworth F J 1981 Improved patch-clamp techniques for high resolution current recording from cells and cell-free membrane patches. Pflugers Archives 391: 85

Harris A J, Miledi R 1971 The effect of type D botulinum toxin on frog neuromuscular junction. Journal of Physiology 217: 497

Harvey A L, Robertson J G, Barkas T, Harrison R, Lunt G G, Stephenson F A, Campbell M J, Teague R H 1978 Reduction of acetylcholine sensitivity of chick muscle in culture by myasthenia gravis serum. Clinical and Experimental Immunology 34: 411

Heinemann S, Merlie J, Lindstrom J 1978 Modulation of acetylcholine receptor in rat diaphragm by anti-receptor sera. Nature 274: 65

Heuser J 1976 Morphology of synaptic vesicle discharge and reformation at the frog neuromuscular junction. In: Thesleff S (ed) Motor innervation of muscle. Academic Press, London, p 51

Heuser J E, Reese T S, Landis D M D 1974 Functional changes in frog neuromuscular junctions studied with freeze fracture. Journal of Neurocytology 3: 109

Hille B 1984 Ionic channels of excitable membranes. Sinauer, Massachusetts USA

Hodgkin A L, Huxley A F 1952a Currents carried by sodium and potassium ions through the membrane of the giant axon of Loligo. Journal of Physiology 116: 449

Hodgkin A L, Huxley A F 1952b The components of membrane conductance in the giant axon of Loligo. Journal of Physiology 116: 473

Hodgkin A L, Huxley A F 1952c The dual effect of membrane potential on sodium conductance in the giant axon of Loligo. Journal of Physiology 116: 497

Hodgkin A L, Huxley A F 1952d A quantitative description of membrane current and its application to conductance and excitation in nerve. Journal of Physiology 117: 500

Horn R, Patlak J 1980 Single channel currents from excised patches of muscle membrane. Proceedings of the National Academy of Sciences USA 77: 6930

Hubbard J I 1963 Repetitive stimulation at the mammalian neuromuscular junction, and the mobilization of transmitter. Journal of Physiology 169: 641

Hubbard J I 1973 Microphysiology of vertebrate neuromuscular transmission. Physiological Reviews 53: 674

Hubbard J I, Kwanbunbumpen S 1968 Evidence for the vesicle hypothesis. Journal of Physiology 194: 407

Huganir R L, Racker E 1982 Properties of proteoliposomes reconstituted with acetylcholine receptor from Torpedo californica. Journal of Biological Chemistry 257: 9372

Hughes R, Chapple D J 1981 Pharmacology of atracurium: a new competitive neuromuscular blocking drug. British Journal of Anaesthesia 53: 31

Illes P, Thesleff S 1978 4-aminopyridine and evoked transmitter release from motor nerve endings. British Journal of Pharmacology 64: 623

Israel M, Dunant Y 1979 On the mechanism of acetylcholine release. In: Tucek S (ed) Progress in brain research. The cholinergic synapse. Elsevier, Amsterdam 49: 125

Israel M, Dunant Y, Manaranche R 1979 The present status of the vesicular theory. Progress in Neurobiology 13: 237

Israel M, Lesbats B 1981 Continuous determination by a chemiluminescent method of acetylcholine release and compartmentation in Torpedo electric organ synaptosomes. Journal of Neurochemistry 37: 1475

Ito Y, Miledi R, Vincent A, Newsom-Davis J 1978 Acetylcholine receptors and end-plate electrophysiology in myasthenia gravis. Brain 101: 345

James R W, Kato A C, Rey M J, Fulpius B W 1980 Monoclonal antibodies directed against the neurotransmitter binding site of nicotinic acetylcholine receptor. FEBS Letters 120: 145

Jenkinson D H 1957 The nature of the antagonism between calcium and magnesium ions at the neuromuscular junction. Journal of Physiology 138: 434

Jenkinson D H 1960 The antagonism between tubocurarine and substances which depolarize the motor end plate. Journal of Physiology 152: 309

Karlin A 1980 Molecular properties of nicotinic acetylcholine receptors. In: Cotman C W, Poste G, Nicolson G (eds) Cell Surface Reviews 6: 191

Katz B 1966 Nerve, muscle and synapse. McGraw-Hill, USA

Katz B 1978 The release of the neuromuscular transmitter and the present state of the vesicular hypothesis. In: Porter R (ed) Studies in neurophysiology. Cambridge University Press

Katz B, Thesleff S 1957 A study of the 'desensitization' produced by acetylcholine at the motor end-plate. Journal of Physiology 138: 63

Katz B, Miledi R 1965 The measurement of synaptic delay, and the time course of acetylcholine release at the neuromuscular junction. Proceedings of the Royal Society B161: 483

Katz B, Miledi R 1967a The timing of calcium action during neuromuscular transmission. Journal of Physiology 189: 535

Katz B, Miledi R 1967b A study of synaptic transmission in the absence of nerve impulses. Journal of Physiology 192: 407

Katz B, Miledi R 1968 The role of calcium in neuromuscular facilitation. Journal of Physiology 195: 481

Katz B, Miledi R 1969a Spontaneous and evoked activity of motor nerve endings in calcium Ringer. Journal of Physiology 203: 689

Katz B, Miledi R 1969b Tetrodotoxin-resistant electrical activity in presynaptic terminals. Journal of Physiology 203: 459

Katz B, Miledi R 1970 Membrane noise produced by acetylcholine. Nature 226: 962

Katz B, Miledi R 1972 The statistical nature of the acetylcholine potential and its molecular components. Journal of Physiology 224: 665

Katz B, Miledi R 1973a The binding of acetylcholine to receptors and its removal from the synaptic cleft. Journal of Physiology 231: 549

Katz B, Miledi R 1973b The characteristics of 'end-plate noise' produced by different depolarizing drugs. Journal of Physiology 230: 707

Katz B, Miledi R 1975 The effect of procaine on the action of acetylcholine at the neuromuscular junction. Journal of Physiology 249: 269

Katz B, Miledi R 1977a Suppression of transmitter release at the neuromuscular junction. Proceedings of the Royal Society B196: 465

Katz B, Miledi R 1977b Transmitter leakage from motor nerve endings. Proceedings of the Royal Society B196: 59

Katz B, Miledi R 1977c The analysis of end-plate noise- a new approach to the study of acetylcholine/receptor interaction. In: Thesleff S (ed) Motor innervation of muscle. Academic Press, New York, p 31

Katz B, Miledi R 1978 A re-examination of curare action at the motor end-plate. Proceedings of the Royal Society B203: 119

Katz B, Miledi R 1981 Does the motor nerve impulse evoke 'non-quantal' transmitter release? Proceedings of the Royal Society B212: 131

Kenyon J L, Gibbons W R 1979 4-aminopyridine and the early outward current of sheep cardiac purkinje fibres. Journal of General Physiology 73: 139

Kharasch E D, Mellow A M, Silinsky F M 1981 Intracellular magnesium does not antagonize calcium-dependent acetylcholine secretion. Journal of Physiology 314: 255

Kim Y I, Lomo T, Lupa M T, Thesleff S 1984 Miniature end-plate potentials in rat skeletal muscle poisoned with botulinum toxin. Journal of Physiology 356: 587

Kistler J, Stroud R M, Klymkowsky M W, Lalancette R A, Fairclough R M 1982 Structure and function of an acetylcholine receptor. Biophysical Journal 37: 371

Klarsfeld A, Changeux J-P 1985 Activity regulates the levels of acetylcholine receptor α-subunit mRNA in cultured chicken myotubes. Proceedings of the National Academy of Sciences USA 82: 4558

Kordas M 1969 The effect of membrane polarization on the time course of the end plate current in frog sartorius muscle. Journal of Physiology 204: 493

Kordas M 1970 The effect of procaine on neuromuscular transmission. Journal of Physiology 209: 689

Krnjevic K, Miledi R 1958 Acetylcholine in mammalian neuromuscular transmission. Nature 182: 805

Kubo T, Noda M, Takai T et al 1985 Primary structure of δ subunit precursor of calf muscle acetylcholine receptor deduced from cDNA sequence. European Journal of Biochemistry 149: 5

Kuffler S W, Yoshikami D 1975 The number of transmitter molecules in a quantum: an estimate from iontophoretic application of acetylcholine at the neuromuscular synapse. Journal of Physiology 251: 465

Lacey G, Newsom-Davis J, Vincent A, Whiting P, Wray D 1985 The effect of monoclonal antibodies on the function of mouse acetylcholine receptor. British Journal of Pharmacology 85: 214P

Lambert E H, Elmqvist D 1971 Quantal components of end-plate potentials in the myasthenic syndrome. Annals of the New York Academy of Sciences 183: 183

Lang B, Newsom-Davis J, Vincent A 1981 Autoimmune aetiology for myasthenic (Eaton-Lambert) syndrome. Lancet ii: 224

Lang B, Newsom-Davis J, Prior C, Wray D 1983 Antibodies to nerve terminals: an electrophysiological study of a human myasthenic syndrome transferred to mouse. Journal of Physiology 344: 335

Lang B, Molenaar P C, Newsom-Davis J, Vincent A 1984a Passive transfer of Lambert Eaton myasthenic syndrome in mice: decreased rates of resting and evoked release of acetylcholine from skeletal muscle. Journal of Neurochemistry 42: 658

Lang B, Newsom-Davis J, Prior C, Wray D 1984b Effect of passively transferred Lambert-Eaton myasthenic syndrome antibodies on the calcium sensitivity of transmitter release in the mouse. Journal of Physiology 357: 28P

Lang B, Newsom-Davis J, Peers C, Wray D 1985 Mechanism of action of human autoantibodies interfering with acetylcholine release in the mouse. Journal of Physiology 365: 79P

LaRochelle W J, Wray B E, Sealock R, Froehner S C 1985 Immunochemical demonstration that amino acids 360–377 of the acetylcholine receptor gamma-subunit are cytoplasmic. Journal of Cell Biology 100:684

Lee C Y 1972 Chemistry and pharmacology of polypeptide toxins in snake venoms. Annual Review of Pharmacology 12:265

Lennon V A, Lambert E H 1980 Myasthenia gravis induced by monoclonal antibodies to acetylcholine receptors. Nature 285:238

Lennon V A, Thompson M, Chen J 1980 Properties of nicotinic acetylcholine receptors isolated by affinity chromatography on monoclonal antibodies. Journal of Biological Chemistry 255:4395

Lennon V A, Lambert E H 1981 Monoclonal autoantibodies to acetylcholine receptors: evidence for a dominant idiotype and requirement of complement for pathogenicity. Annals of the New York Academy of Sciences 377:77

Lentz T L, Mazurkiewicz J E, Rosenthal J 1977 Cytochemical localization of acetylcholine receptors at the neuromuscular junction by means of horseradish peroxidase-labelled α-bungarotoxin. Brain Research 132:423

Lerrick A J, Wray D, Vincent A, Newsom-Davis J 1983 Electrophysiological effects of myasthenic serum factors studied in mouse muscle. Annals of Neurology 13:186

Lev-Tov A, Rahamimoff R 1980 A study of tetanic and post-tetanic potentiation of miniature end-plate potentials at the frog neuromuscular junction. Journal of Physiology 309:247

Liley A W 1956 The effects of presynaptic polarization on the spontaneous activity at the mammalian neuromuscular junction. Journal of Physiology 134:427

Lindstrom J M 1976 Immunological studies of acetylcholine receptors. Journal of Supramolecular Structures 4:389

Lindstrom J M 1985 Immunobiology of myasthenia gravis, experimental autoimmune myasthenia gravis and Lambert-Eaton syndrome. Annual Review of Immunology 3:109

Lindstrom J M, Engel A G, Seybold M E, Lennon V A, Lambert E H 1976a Pathological mechanisms in experimental autoimmune myasthenia gravis. II Passive transfer of experimental autoimmune myasthenia gravis in rats with anti-acetylcholine receptor antibodies. Journal of Experimental Medicine 144:739

Lindstrom J M, Seybold M E, Lennon V A, Whittingham S, Duane D D 1976b Antibody to acetylcholine receptor in myasthenia gravis. Neurology 26:1054

Lindstrom J M, Anholt R, Einarson B, Engel A, Osame M, Montal M 1980 Purification of acetylcholine receptors, reconstitution into lipid vesicles and study of agonist-induced cation channel regulation. Journal of Biological Chemistry 255:8340

Lindstrom J M, Tzartos S, Gullick W 1981 Structure and function of the acetylcholine receptor molecule studied using monoclonal antibodies. Annals of the New York Academy of Sciences 377:1

Lindstrom J M, Tzartos S, Gullick W, Hochschwender S, Swanson L, Sargent P, Jacob M, Montal M 1983 Use of monoclonal antibodies to study acetylcholine receptors from electric organs, muscle and brain and the autoimmune response to receptor in myasthenia gravis. Cold Spring Harbour Symposia in Quantitative Biology 48:89

Lindstrom J M, Criado M, Hochschwender S, Fox J L, Sarin V 1984 Immunochemical tests of acetylcholine receptor subunit models. Nature 311:573

Llinas R, Blinks J R, Nicholson C 1972 Calcium transient in presynaptic terminal of squid giant synapse: detection with aequorin. Science, New York 176:1127

Llinas R, Nicholson C 1975 Calcium role in depolarization-secretion coupling: an aequorin study in squid giant synapse. Proceedings of the National Academy of Sciences USA 72:187

Llinas R, Steinberg I Z, Walton K 1976 Presynaptic calcium currents and their relation to synaptic transmission: voltage clamp study in squid giant synapse and theoretical model for the calcium gate. Proceedings of the National Academy of Sciences USA 73:2918

Llinas R, Steinberg I Z, Walton K 1981 Relationship between presynaptic calcium current and postsynaptic potential in squid giant synapse. Biophysical Journal 33:323

Lundh H, Thesleff S 1977 The mode of action of 4-aminopyridine and guanidine on transmitter release from motor nerve terminals. European Journal of Pharmacology 42:411

Lundh H, Leander S, Thesleff S 1977a Antagonism of the paralysis produced by botulinum toxin in the rat. Journal of Neurobiology 32:29

Lundh H, Nilsson O, Rosen I 1977b 4-aminopyridine — a new drug tested in the treatment of Eaton-Lambert syndrome. Journal of Neurology, Neurosurgery and Psychiatry 40:1109

MacIntosh F C, Collier B 1976 Neurochemistry of cholinergic terminals. In: Zaimis E (ed) Handbook of experimental pharmacology, XLII Neuromuscular junction. Springer-Verlag, Berlin, p 99

Magleby K L 1973a The effect of repetitive stimulation on facilitation of transmitter release at the frog neuromuscular junction. Journal of Physiology 234:327

Magleby K L 1973b The effect of tetanic and post-tetanic potentiation on facilitation of transmitter release at the frog neuromuscular junction. Journal of Physiology 234:353

Magleby K L, Stevens C F 1972 The effect of voltage on the time course of end-plate currents. Journal of Physiology 223:151

Magleby K L, Zengel J E 1975a A dual effect of repetitive stimulation on post-tetanic potentiation of transmitter release at the frog neuromuscular junction. Journal of Physiology 245:163

Magleby K L, Zengel J E 1975b A quantitative description of tetanic and post-tetanic potentiation of transmitter release at the frog neuromuscular junction. Journal of Physiology 245:183

Magleby K L, Zengel J E 1976a Augmentation: a process that acts to increase transmitter release at the frog neuromuscular junction. Journal of Physiology 257:449

Magleby K L, Zengel J E 1976b Long term changes in augmentation, potentiation and depression of transmitter release as a function of repeated synaptic activity at the frog neuromuscular junction. Journal of Physiology 257:471

Magleby K L, Zengel J E 1976c Stimulation-induced factors which affect augmentation and potentiation of transmitter

release at the neuromuscular junction. Journal of Physiology 260:687

Magleby K L, Pallotta B S, Terrar D A 1981 The effect of (+)-tubocurarine on neuromuscular transmission during repetitive stimulation in the rat, mouse and frog. Journal of Physiology 312:97

Magleby K L, Zengel J E 1982 A quantitative description of stimulation-induced changes in transmitter release at the frog neuromuscular junction. Journal of General Physiology 80:613

Marchbanks R M 1968 Exchangeability of radioactive acetylcholine with the bound acetylcholine of synaptosomes and synaptic vesicles. Biochemical Journal 106:87

Marshall I G, Agoston S, Booij L H D J, Durant N N, Foldes F F 1980 Pharmacology of Org NC45 compared with other non-depolarizing blocking drugs. British Journal of Anaesthesia 52:113

Marshall I G, Gibb A J, Durant N N 1983 Neuromuscular and vagal blocking actions of pancuronium bromide, its metabolites, and vecuronium bromide (Org NC45) and its potential metabolites in the anaesthetized cat. British Journal of Anaesthesia 55:703

Martin A R 1966 Quantal nature of synaptic transmission. Physiological Reviews 46:51

Martin A R, Orkand R K 1961 Postsynaptic action of HC-3 on neuromuscular transmission. Federation Proceedings 20:579

Matthews-Bellinger J, Salpeter M M 1978 Distribution of acetylcholine receptors at frog neuromuscular junctions with a discussion of some physiological implications. Journal of Physiology 279:197

Merlie J P, Isenberg K E, Russel S D, Sanes J R 1984 Denervation supersensitivity in skeletal muscle: analysis with a cloned cDNA probe. Journal of Cell Biology 99:332

Merlie J P, Sanes J R 1985 Concentration of acetylcholine receptor mRNA in synaptic regions of adult muscle fibres. Nature 317:66

Meves H, Pichon Y 1977 The effects of internal and external 4-aminopyridine on the potassium-currents in intracellularly perfused squid giant axons. Journal of Physiology 268:511

Miledi R 1960a Junctional and extra-junctional acetylcholine receptors in skeletal muscle fibres. Journal of Physiology 151:24

Miledi R 1960b The acetylcholine sensitivity of frog muscle fibres after complete or partial denervation. Journal of Physiology 151:1

Miledi R 1973 Transmitter release induced by injection of calcium ions into nerve terminals. Proceedings of the Royal Society B183:421

Miledi R, Thies R 1971 Tetanic and post-tetanic rise in frequency of miniature end-plate potentials in low-calcium solutions. Journal of Physiology 212:245

Miledi R, Molenaar P C, Polak R L 1980 The effect of Lanthanum ions on acetylcholine in frog muscle. Journal of Physiology 309:199

Miledi R, Parker I 1981 Calcium transients recorded with arsenazo III in the presynaptic terminal of the squid giant synapse. Proceedings of the Royal Society B212:197

Miledi R, Sumikawa K 1982 Synthesis of cat muscle acetylcholine receptors by Xenopus oocytes. Biomedical Research 3:390

Miledi R, Molenaar P C, Polak R L 1982a Free and bound acetylcholine in frog muscle. Journal of Physiology 333:189

Miledi R, Molenaar P C, Polak R L, Tas J W M, Van der

Laaken T 1982b Neural and non-neural acetylcholine in the rat diaphragm. Proceedings of the Royal Society B214:153

Miledi R, Parker I, Sumikawa K 1982c Properties of acetylcholine receptors translated by cat muscle mRNA in Xenopus oocytes. The EMBO Journal 1:1307

Miledi R, Molenaar P C, Polak R L 1983a Electrophysiological and chemical determination of acetylcholine release at the frog neuromuscular junction. Journal of Physiology 334:245

Miledi R, Parker I, Sumikawa K 1983b Recording of single γ-aminobutyrate- and acetylcholine-activated receptor channels translated by exogenous mRNA in Xenopus oocytes. Proceedings of the Royal Society B218:481

Miller C 1982 Reconstitution of ion channels in planar lipid bilayers: a five year progress report. Communications in Molecular and Cellular Biophysics 1:413

Mishina M, Kurosaki T, Tobimatsu T, et al 1984 Expression of functional acetylcholine receptor from cloned cDNAs. Nature 307:604

Mishina M, Tobimatsu T, Imoto K, et al 1985 Localization of functional regions of acetylcholine receptor α-subunit by site-directed mutagenesis. Nature 313:364

Misler S, Hurlbut W P 1983 Post-tetanic potentiation of acetylcholine release at the frog neuromuscular junction develops after stimulation in Ca^{2+}-free solutions. Proceedings of the National Academy of Sciences USA 80:315

Mochly-Rosen D, Fuchs S 1981 Monoclonal anti-acetylcholine-receptor antibodies directed against the cholinergic binding site. Biochemistry 20:5920

Molgo J, Lemeignan J, Lechat P 1977 Effects of 4-aminopyridine at the frog neuromuscular junction. Journal of Pharmacology and Experimental Therapeutics 203:653

Molgo J, Lemeignan M, Lechat P 1979 Analysis of the action of 4-aminopyridine during repetitive stimulation at the neuromuscular junction. European Journal of Pharmacology 53:307

Molgo J E, Lundh H, Thesleff S 1980 Potency of 3,4-diaminopyridine and 4-aminopyridine on mammalian neuromuscular transmission and the effect of pH changes. European Journal of Pharmacology 61:25

Momoi M Y, Lennon V A 1982 Purification and biochemical characterization of nicotinic acetylcholine receptors of human muscle. Journal of Biological Chemistry 257:12757

Murray N M F, Newsom-Davis J 1981 Treatment with oral 4-aminopyridine in disorders of neuromuscular transmission. Neurology (NY) 31:256

Murray N M F, Newsom-Davis J, Karni Y, Wiles C M 1984 Oral 3,4-diaminopyridine in the treatment of the Lambert Eaton myasthenic syndrome. Journal of Neurology, Neurosurgery and Psychiatry 47:1052

Nachshen D A, Blaustein M P 1979 The effects of some 'calcium antagonists' on calcium influx in presynaptic nerve terminals. Molecular Pharmacology 16:579

Narahashi T, Moore J W, Scott W R 1964 Tetrodotoxin blockage of sodium conductance increase in lobster giant axons. Journal of General Physiology 47:965

Nastuk W L, Manthey A A, Gissen A J 1966 Activation and inactivation of postjunctional membrane receptors. Annals of the New York Academy of Sciences 137:999

Neher E, Sakmann B 1976a Single channel currents recorded from membrane of denervated frog muscle fibres. Nature 260:799

Neher E, Sakmann B 1976b Noise analysis of drug induced voltage clamp currents in denervated frog muscle fibres. Journal of Physiology 258:705

Neher E, Stevens C F 1977 Conductance fluctuations and ionic pores in membranes. Annual Review of Biophysics and Bioengineering 6:345

Neher E, Steinbach J H 1978 Local anaesthetics transiently block currents through single acetylcholine-receptor channels. Journal of Physiology 277:153

Nelson N, Anholt R, Lindstrom J, Montal M 1980 Reconstitution of purified acetylcholine receptors with functional ion channels in planar lipid bilayers. Proceedings of the National Academy of Sciences USA 77:3057

Neumann D, Fridkin M, Fuchs S 1984 Anti-acetylcholine receptor response achieved by immunization with a synthetic peptide from the receptor sequence. Biochemical and Biophysical Research Communications 121:B73

Newsom-Davis J 1982 Autoimmune diseases of neuromuscular transmission. Clinics in Immunology and Allergy 2:405

Newsom-Davis J, Murray N, Wray D et al 1982 Lambert-Eaton myasthenic syndrome: electrophysiological evidence for a humoral factor. Muscle and Nerve 5:S17

Newsom-Davis J, Murray N M F 1984 Plasma exchange and immunosuppressive drug treatment in the Lambert-Eaton myasthenic syndrome. Neurology 34:480

Nilius B, Hess P, Lansman J B, Tsien R W 1985 A novel type of cardiac calcium channel in ventricular cells. Nature 316:433

Noda M, Takahashi H, Tanabe T et al 1982 Primary structure of α-subunit precursor of Torpedo californica acetylcholine receptor deduced from cDNA sequence. Nature 299:793

Noda M, Takahashi H, Tanabe T et al 1983a Primary structures of β- and δ-subunit precursors of Torpedo californica acetylcholine receptor deduced from cDNA sequences. Nature 301:251

Noda M, Takahashi H, Tanabe T et al 1983b Structural homology of Torpedo californica acetylcholine receptor subunits. Nature 302:528

Noda M, Furutani Y, Takahashi H, et al 1983c Cloning and sequence analysis of calf cDNA and human genomic DNA encoding α-subunit precursor of muscle acetylcholine receptor. Nature 305:818

Nowycky M C, Fox A P, Tsien R W 1985 Three types of neuronal calcium channel with different calcium agonist selectivity. Nature 316:440

Ogden D C, Siegelbaum S A, Colquhoun D 1981 Block of acetylcholine-activated ion channels by an uncharged local anaesthetic. Nature 289:596

Ogden D C, Colquhoun D 1985 Ion channel block by acetylcholine, carbachol and suberyldicholine at the frog neuromuscular junction. Proceedings of the Royal Society B225:329

Paton W D M, Waud D R 1962 Drug-receptor interactions at the neuromuscular junction. In: De Reuck A V S (ed) Curare and curare-like agents. Ciba Foundation Study Group. Churchill, London, No 12 p 34

Patrick J, Lindstrom J 1973 Autoimmune response to acetylcholine receptor. Science 180:871

Payne J P, Hughes R 1981 Evaluation of atracurium in anaesthetized man. British Journal of Anaesthesia 53:45

Penner R, Dreyer F 1986 Two different presynaptic calcium currents in mouse motor nerve terminals. Pflugers Archiv 406:190

Plumer R, Fels G, Maelicke A 1984 Antibodies against preselected peptides to map functional sites on the acetylcholine receptor. Federation of European Biochemical Societies Letters 178:204

Porter C W, Barnard E A, Chiu T H 1973 The ultrastructural localization and quantitation of cholinergic receptors at the mouse end-plate. Journal of Membrane Biology 14:383

Porter C W, Barnard E A 1975 The density of cholinergic receptors at the end-plate postsynaptic membrane: ultrastructural studies in two mammalian species. Journal of Membrane Biology 20:31

Porter C W, Barnard E A 1976 Ultrastructural studies on the acetylcholine receptor at the motor end plates of normal and pathologic muscles. Annals of the New York Academy of Sciences 274:85

Potter L T 1970 Synthesis, storage and release of [^{14}C] acetylcholine in isolated rat diaphragm muscles. Journal of Physiology 206:145

Prior C, Lang B, Wray D, Newsom-Davis J 1985 Action of Lambert Eaton myasthenic syndrome IgG at mouse motor nerve terminals. Annals of Neurology 17:587

Publicover S J, Duncan C J 1979 The action of verapamil on the rate of spontaneous release of transmitter at the frog neuromuscular junction. European Journal of Pharmacology 54:119

Pumplin D W, Reese T S, Llinas R 1981 Are the presynaptic membrane particles the calcium channels? Proceedings of the National Academy of Sciences USA 78:7210

Raftery M A, Hunkapiller M W, Strader C D, Hood L E 1980 Acetylcholine receptor: complex of homologous subunits. Science 208:1454

Rahamimoff R 1968 A dual effect of calcium ions on neuromuscular facilitation. Journal of Physiology 195:471

Rang H P 1975 Acetylcholine receptors. Quarterly Reviews of Biophysics 7:283

Rash J E, Albuquerque E X, Hudson C S, Mayer R F, Sattersfield 1976 Studies on human myasthenia gravis: electrophysiological and ultrastructural evidence compatible with antibody attachment to acetylcholine receptor complex. Proceedings of the National Academy of Sciences USA 73:4584

Ratnam M, Lindstrom J 1984 Structural features of the nicotinic acetylcholine receptor revealed by autoantibodies to synthetic peptides. Biochemical and Biophysical Research Communications 122:1225

Reiness C G, Weinberg C B 1978 Antibody to acetylcholine receptor increases degradation of junctional and extrajunctional receptors in adult muscle. Nature 274:68

Reuter H 1983 Calcium channel modulation by neurotransmitters, enzymes and drugs. Nature 301:569

Reuter H, Porzig H, Kokubun S, Prod'hom B 1985 1,4-dihydropyridines as tools in the study of Ca^{2+} channels. Trends in Neurosciences 8:396

Roberts A, Perera S, Lang B, Vincent A, Newsom-Davis J 1985 Paraneoplastic myasthenic syndrome IgG inhibits ^{45}Ca^{2+} flux in a human small cell carcinoma line. Nature 317:737

Ruff R L 1977 A quantitative analysis of local anaesthetic alteration of miniature end-plate currents and end-plate current fluctuations. Journal of Physiology 264:89

Sachs F 1983 Is the acetylcholine receptor a unit-conductance channel? In: Sakmann B, Neher E (eds) Single channel recording. Plenum, New York, p 365

Sahashi K, Engel A G, Lindstrom J M, Lambert E H, Lennon V A 1978 Ultrastructural localization of immune complexes (IgG and C3) at the end plate in experimental autoimmune myasthenia gravis. Journal of Neuropathology and Experimental Neurology 37:212

Sakmann B, Patlak J, Neher E 1980 Single acetylcholine-activated channels shows burst-kinetics in the presence of desensitizing concentrations of agonist. Nature 286:71

Sakmann B, Neher E 1983 Single channel recording. Plenum, New York

Sakmann B, Neher E 1984 Patch clamp techniques for studying ionic channels in excitable membranes. Annual Review of Physiology 46:455

Sakmann B, Methfessel C, Mishina M, Takahashi T, Takai T, Kurasaki M, Fukuda K, Numa S 1985 Role of acetylcholine receptor subunits in gating of the channel. Nature 318:538

Sellin L C 1985 The pharmacological mechanism of botulism. Trends in Pharmacological Sciences 6:80

Shibahara S, Kubo T, Perski H, Takahashi H, Noda M, Numa S 1985 Cloning and sequence analysis of human genomic DNA encoding γ subunit precursor of muscle acetylcholine receptor. European Journal of Biochemistry 146:15

Silinsky E M 1985 The biophysical pharmacology of calcium-dependent acetylcholine secretion. Pharmacological Reviews 37:81

Simpson L L 1980 Kinetic studies on the interaction between botulinum toxin type A and the cholinergic neuromuscular junction. Journal of Pharmacological and Experimental Therapeutics 212:16

Sine S M, Steinbach J H 1984 Agonists block currents through acetylcholine receptor channels. Biophysical Journal 46:277

Smith D O 1984 Acetylcholine storage release and leakage at the neuromuscular junction of mature adult and aged rats. Journal of Physiology 347:161

Stanley E F, Drachman D B 1978 Effect of myasthenic immunoglobulin on acetylcholine receptors of intact mammalian neuromuscular junctions. Science 200:1285

Stevens C F 1985 AChR structure: a new twist in the story. Trends in Neurosciences 79:1

Sumikawa K, Houghton M, Emtage J S, Richards B M, Barnard E A 1981 Active multi-subunit ACh receptor assembled by translation of heterologous mRNA in Xenopus oocytes. Nature 292:862

Sumikawa K, Houghton M, Smith J C, Richards B M, Barnard E A 1982 The molecular cloning and characterization of cDNA coding for the α- subunit of the acetylcholine receptor. Nucleic Acids Research 10:5809

Takai T, Noda M, Furutani Y et al 1984 Primary structure of γ subunit precursor of calf-muscle acetylcholine receptor deduced from the cDNA sequence. European Journal of Biochemistry 143:109

Takai T, Noda M, Mishina M et al 1985 Cloning, sequencing and expression of cDNA for a novel subunit of acetylcholine receptor from calf muscle. Nature 315:761

Takeda K, Trautmann A 1984 A patch clamp study of the partial agonist actions of tubocurarine on rat myotubes. Journal of Physiology 349:353

Takeuchi A, Takeuchi N 1959 Active phase of frog's end-plate potential. Journal of Neurophysiology 22:395

Takeuchi A, Takeuchi N 1960 On the permeability of end-plate membrane during the action of transmitter. Journal of Physiology 154:52

Tanabe T, Noda M, Furutani Y et al 1984 Primary structure of β subunit precursor of calf muscle acetylcholine receptor deduced from cDNA sequence. European Journal of Biochemistry 144:11

Tank D W, Miller C 1983 Patch-clamped liposomes: recording reconstituted ion channels. In: Sakmann B, Neher E (eds) Single channel recording. Plenum, New York

Tauc L 1982 Nonvesicular release of neurotransmitter. Physiological Reviews 62:857

Thesleff S 1980 Aminopyridines and synaptic transmission. Neuroscience 5:1413

Thesleff S W 1982 Spontaneous transmitter release in experimental neuromuscular disorders of the rat. Muscle and Nerve 5:S12

Thies R E, Brooks V B 1961 Postsynaptic neuromuscular block produced by hemicholinium no. 3. Federation Proceedings 20:569

Toyka K V, Birnberger K L, Anzil A P, Schlegel C, Besinger U, Struppler A 1978 Myasthenia gravis: further electrophysiological and ultrastructural analysis of transmission failure in the mouse passive transfer model. Journal of Neurology, Neurosurgery and Psychiatry 41:746

Toyka K V, Drachman D B, Griffin D E et al 1977 Myasthenia gravis. Study of humoral immune mechanisms by passive transfer to mice. New England Journal of Medicine 296:125

Trautmann A 1982 Curare can open and block ion channels associated with cholinergic receptors. Nature 298:272

Tse C K, Dolly J O, Hambleton P, Wray D, Melling J 1982 Preparation and characterization of homogeneous neurotoxin type A from Clostridium botulinum. Its inhibitory action on neuronal release of acetylcholine in the absence and presence of β-bungarotoxin. European Journal of Biochemistry 122:493

Tse C K, Wray D, Melling J, Dolly J O 1986 Actions of β-bungarotoxin on spontaneous release of transmitter at muscle end-plates treated with botulinum toxin. Toxicon 24:123

Tsien R W 1983 Calcium channels in excitable cell membranes. Annual Reviews of Physiology 45:351

Tzartos S J 1984 Monoclonal antibodies as probes of the acetylcholine receptor and myasthenia gravis. Trends in Biochemical Sciences 9:63

Tzartos S J, Lindstrom J M 1980 Monoclonal antibodies used to probe acetylcholine receptor structure: localization of the main immunogenic region and detection of similarities between subunits. Proceedings of the National Academy of Sciences USA 77:755

Van der Kloot W, Cohen I S 1984 Temperature effects on spontaneous and evoked quantal size at the frog neuromuscular junction. Journal of Neuroscience 4:2200

Vandlen R L, Wu W C-S, Eisenbach J C, Raftery M A 1979 Studies of the composition of purified Torpedo californica acetylcholine receptor and of its subunits. Biochemistry 18:1845

Varanda W A, Aracava Y, Sherby S M, VanMeter W G, Eldefrawi M E, Albuquerque E X 1985 The acetylcholine receptor of the neuromuscular junction recognizes mecamylamine as a noncompetitive antagonist. Molecular Pharmacology 28:128

Veldsema-Currie R D, Labruyere WTh, Langemeijer M W E 1984 Depletion of total acetylcholine by hemicholinium-3 in isolated rat diaphragm is less in the presence of dexamethasone. Brain Research 324:305

Vincent A 1983 Acetylcholine receptors and myasthenia gravis. Clinics in Endocrinology and Metabolism 12:57

Vizi E S, Vyskocil F 1979 Changes in total and quantal release of acetylcholine in the mouse diaphragm during activation and inhibition of membrane ATPase. Journal of Physiology 286:1

Vyskocil F, Illes P 1978 Electrophysiological examination of transmitter release in non-quantal form in the mouse diaphragm and the activity of membrane ATPase. Physiologia Bohemoslovaca 27:449

Wan K K, Lindstrom J M 1985 Effects of monoclonal antibodies on the function of acetylcholine receptors purified from Torpedo californica and reconstituted into vesicles. Biochemistry 24:1212

Whiting P, Vincent A, Newsom-Davis J 1985a Monoclonal antibodies to Torpedo acetylcholine receptor. Characterization of antigenic determinants within the cholinergic binding site. European Journal of Biochemistry 150:533

Whiting P J, Vincent A, Newsom-Davis J 1985b Monoclonal antibodies to the human acetylcholine receptor. Biochemical Society Transactions 13:116

Wray D 1978a Frequency of opening of channels by depolarizing drugs. Journal of Physiology 284:149P

Wray D 1978b End-plate voltage noise during prolonged application of acetylcholine in cat tenuissimus muscle. Journal of Physiology 278:4P

Wray D 1980 Noise analysis and channels at the postsynaptic membrane of skeletal muscle. Progress in Drug Research 24:9

Wray D 1981a The action of mecamylamine at the postsynaptic channels of cat skeletal muscle: noise analysis. British Journal of Pharmacology 74:248P

Wray D 1981b Prolonged exposure to acetylcholine: noise analysis and channel inactivation in cat tenuissimus muscle. Journal of Physiology 310:37

Wray D, Prior C, Newsom-Davis J, Lang B 1984 Site of action of Lambert-Eaton myasthenic syndrome antibodies at mouse nerve terminals. IUPHAR 9th International Congress of Pharmacology Proceedings 2:349

Wray D, Peers C, Lande S, Lang B, Newsom-Davis J 1987 Interference with calcium channels in the Lambert-Eaton myasthenic syndrome. Annals of the New York Academy of Sciences (in press)

Wu WC-S, Raftery M A 1979 Carbamylcholine-induced rapid cation efflux from reconstituted membrane vesicles containing purified acetylcholine receptor. Biochemical and Biophysical Research Communications 89:26

Young E F, Ralston E, Blake J, Ramachandran J, Hall Z W, Stroud R M 1985 Topological mapping of acetylcholine receptor: evidence for a model with five transmembrane segments and a cytoplasmic COOH-terminal peptide. Proceedings of the National Academy of Sciences USA 82:626

Zaimis E 1953 Motor end-plate differences as a determining factor in the mode of action of neuromuscular blocking substances. Journal of Physiology 122:238

Zaimis E, Head S 1976 Depolarizing neuromuscular blocking

drugs. In: Zaimis E (ed) Handbook of experimental pharmacology, XLII Neuromuscular junction. Springer-Verlag, Berlin, p 365

Zaimis E, Wray D 1981 General physiology and pharmacology of neuromuscular transmission. In: Walton J (ed) Disorders of voluntary muscle, 4th edn. Churchill Livingstone, p 76

Zengel J E, Magleby K L 1981 Changes in miniature end-plate potential frequency during repetitive nerve stimulation in the presence of Ca^{2+}, Ba^{2+} and Sr^{2+} at the frog neuromuscular junction. Journal of General Physiology 77:503

Zimmerman H 1979 Commentary: vesicle recycling and transmitter release. Neuroscience 4: 1773

Biochemical aspects of muscular structure and function

INTRODUCTION*

All cells of the organism utilise more or less the same metabolic pathways to use chemical energy — more precisely, free energy as discussed below — that is available in foodstuff to produce adenosine triphosphate (ATP) which then serves as the immediate energy source for various cell functions. What distinguishes muscle from many other tissues is the close relationship between the energy transducing and energy utilising systems; we have known for about 50 years that one component of the contractile machinery — myosin — is also the enzyme (myosin ATPase, EC 3.6.1.32) that hydrolyses ATP and that in the process the transduction of chemical into mechanical energy is achieved.

In this chapter the emphasis is on those structures, components and processes that are characteristic of muscle and relate to contraction, relaxation and their control. Some structural and physiological aspects are covered in Chapters 1 and 3, and features of the cell membrane in Chapter 10. Many excellent textbooks of biochemistry provide a general background to metabolic pathways, protein structure and membrane architecture. Two recent texts (Alberts et al 1983, Darnell et al 1986) orientated towards cell biology

---

* Readers interested in obtaining more information on topics covered in this chapter and on related matters may wish to consult the following: Needham 1971, Jolesz & Sreter 1981, Squire 1981, Morales et al 1982, Gergely & Seidel 1983, Huxley & Faruqi 1983, Webb & Trentham 1983, Harrington & Rodgers 1984, Leavis & Gergely 1984, Martonosi 1984, Pette 1984, Amos 1985, Eisenberg & Hill 1985, Frieden 1985, Gillis 1985, Inesi 1985, Cooke 1986, El-Saleh et al 1986a, Engel & Banker 1986, Hibberd & Trentham 1986, Pollard & Cooper 1986.

may be especially useful for readers interested in obtaining, or as the case may be, brushing up on, an integrated picture.

ENERGY METABOLISM

Carbohydrate metabolism

General. Glucose entering the muscle cell is either used immediately or is stored in the form of glycogen which is broken down according to the energy requirements of the muscle. The breakdown may occur, depending on the conditions, either essentially anaerobically — i.e. without oxygen — going as far as lactic acid, or it may continue with the participation of oxygen to complete the breakdown to CO_2 and water. In muscles where sudden demands on energy may arise, the anaerobic pathway is predominant and the lactic acid formed is carried by the blood stream to the liver where it is partly oxidised, partly resynthesised to glycogen (Cori 1941). In other muscles, such as cardiac muscle, where there is a slower but steady activity, the complete oxidative breakdown plays a greater part.

Anaerobic glycogen metabolism. The breakdown of glycogen involves the enzyme phosphorylase, the reaction being:

Glycogen + phosphate → glucose-1-phosphate

Phosphorylase is itself a complex enzyme system,

the structure, function and regulation of which have been clarified through extensive research taking its origin in the work of the Coris (Cori & Cori 1945). As it now appears, phosphorylase can exist in an inactive form, phosphorylase b, and an active form, phosphorylase a (see e.g. Fischer et al 1971, Krebs 1972) (Fig. 4.1). The $b \rightarrow a$ transformation is effected by ATP-dependent phosphorylation catalysed by phosphorylase kinase (EC 2.7.1.38), while the reconversion of phosphorylase a to b is catalysed by phosphorylase phosphatase (EC 3.1.3.17). Phosphorylase kinase contains four different kinds of subunits, one of which has been identified (Cohen et al 1978) with the ubiquitous Ca^{2+}-binding protein, calmodulin, which participates in the regulation of numerous cellular processes (for a review see Klee & Vanaman 1982). The calmodulin subunit of phosphorylase kinase is presumably the site of binding of the activating Ca^{2+} which is released from the sarcoplasmic reticulum (see below) when muscle contraction is initiated. Phosphorylase kinase also exists in an active and an inactive form, and, again, inactivation is brought about by phosphorylation, catalysed in this case by a cyclic adenosine monophosphatase-(AMP)-dependent protein kinase. The production from ATP of cyclic AMP — now recognised as a key mediator in many regulatory processes (see e.g. Robison et al 1971, Bitensky & Gorman 1973) — is catalysed by an enzyme, adenylate cyclase (EC 4.6.1.1), which is under the influence of hormones (glucagon) and

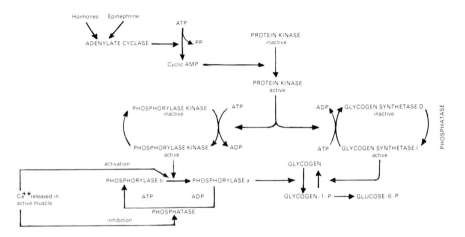

Fig. 4.1 Simplified scheme of regulation of glycogen phosphorylase and synthetase system. For details see text

neurohumoral agents (e.g. adrenaline). The regulation of the phosphorylase system also involves phosphatase inhibitors which are subject to control by a cAMP-dependent kinase (Cohen 1978, 1985).

The conversion of glucose into glycogen depends on a distinct enzyme system — glycogen synthetase (or glycogen (starch) synthase, EC 2.4.1.11) — involving UTP and the coenzyme uridine diphosphate glucose (UDPG) (Leloir & Cardini 1962). Glycogen synthetase also exists in two interconvertible forms of differing activity, D and I. In contrast to phosphorylase, in this case the phosphorylated form is inhibited, and the enzymes that catalyse the phosphorylation and dephosphorylation process are subject to control by intermediates in the breakdown of glycogen as well as by ATP and cyclic AMP (see Cohen 1978, 1985).

ATP synthesis. The reaction involving glyceraldehyde-3-phosphate oxidation and NAD* in the breakdown scheme of glycogen leads to the esterification of a phosphate residue; eventually it is transferred to adenosine diphosphate (ADP) to form ATP. The phosphate residue that participated in the phosphorolytic breakdown of glycogen also ends up as ATP, through the pyruvate kinase (EC 2.7.1.40) reaction. Thus in the anaerobic breakdown of one glucose unit of glycogen there is a net formation of three molecules of ATP. If glucose were the starting material, only two moles of ATP would be formed from glucose because of the ATP requirement in the formation of glucose-1-phosphate via the hexokinase (EC 2.7.1.1) reaction.

Glyceraldehyde phosphate, as already mentioned, reduces NAD. Under anaerobic conditions the reduction of NAD has to be reversed through its reaction with pyruvic acid resulting in the formation of lactic acid and the reoxidised form of NAD. The glycolytic process, therefore, does not involve a net change in the state of oxidation or reduction.

Aerobic metabolism. The anaerobic path of the breakdown of carbohydrates is linked to the oxidative pathway at the point of pyruvate. If there is oxidative breakdown of pyruvate the NADH formed in the reduction of glyceraldehyde phosphate is not used to form lactate by reducing pyruvate but reacts with dihydroxyacetone phosphate to form glycerol-3-phosphate (G3P) or with oxaloacetate to form malate. The latter or G3P can enter the mitochondria to regenerate dihydroxyacetone phosphate and NADH (G3P or malate shuttle).

Krebs cycle. The reaction sequence — catalysed by enzymes located in the mitochondria — leading to the complete breakdown of pyruvic acid to CO_2 and H_2O is known as the Krebs cycle or tricarboxylic acid cycle, the latter name taking its origin from the organic acids, containing three carboxyl groups, that participate in the cycle. Pyruvate is oxidised to acetate, forming a derivative with coenzyme A (CoA), acetyl-CoA. The latter interacts with an intermediate of the Krebs cycle, oxaloacetic acid, to form citric acid. In the complex sequence of reactions following this condensation both NAD and flavin-containing coenzymes are reduced and the removal of two molecules of CO_2 and water results in the complete breakdown of the acetate residue that entered the cycle, and in the regeneration of the oxaloacetic acid.

Terminal electron transport and oxidative phosphorylation. Coenzymes reduced in the operation of the citric acid cycle are finally reoxidised through a long chain of reactions catalysed by a chain of enzymes whose active groups are flavins, coenzyme Q, and iron-containing compounds, the cytochromes. In addition, non-haem Fe and Cu are involved. These enzymes form what is known as the respiratory chain and are localised in the mitochondria. They undergo cyclic reduction and reoxidation, with the formation of three ATPs for each pair of electrons. It is now clear that the energy derived from the flow of electrons is converted to a proton gradient between the matrix of the mitochondrion and the space between the external and internal mitochondrial membrane. The osmotic and electric energy of the proton gradient is then channelled into the formation of ATP from ADP and inorganic phosphate

* NAD, nicotinamide adenine dinucleotide, is the name of the coenzyme related to the vitamin nicotinic acid.

(Mitchell 1977). The detailed mechanism of the formation of osmotic into chemical energy is still being debated (see also Hill 1977 (energy transduction), Jencks 1980, 1983). There are indications that the energy is required to release tightly bound ATP which would be spontaneously formed from P_i and ADP (Boyer 1977). The energy derived from electron flow can also be used — instead of synthesising ATP — either to drive electrons backwards or for the transport of various ions. Interaction between oxidative phosphorylation and muscle contraction is established by virtue of the fact that with a tightly coupled physiologically operating oxidation–phosphorylation system, the formation of ADP in muscle contraction, by furnishing an acceptor for phosphorylation, may serve as a regulating link between the energy-conserving and energy-producing process.

Fatty acid oxidation

The oxidation of fatty acids is an important source of energy in both skeletal and cardiac muscle (Fritz et al 1958). Detailed modern enzymatic studies of the breakdown of fatty acids (Lynen & Ochoa 1953, Green 1954), the hydrolytic product of neutral fats, have fully confirmed the ideas expressed by Knoop as early as 1904 on the basis of results obtained on whole animals. Accordingly, fatty acids are broken down by the repeated pair-wise removal of carbon residues starting at the COOH end of the fatty acid molecule and leading to the formation of an acetate residue or propionic acid residue, in even or odd-numbered fatty acids, respectively. Actually, both the acetate and propionate residue appear to be linked to the coenzyme CoA mentioned earlier in connection with the operation of a citric acid cycle. Acetyl-CoA enters the citric acid cycle in exactly the same way as that formed from the oxidation of pyruvic acid and originating in glucose. Propionyl-CoA is converted into succinate, another intermediate in the citric acid cycle, by a path involving an ATP-dependent carboxylation (Flavin & Ochoa 1957). It should be added that the further flow of electrons involved in the reoxidation of the reduced NAD and NADP is the same as that in the metabolism of carbohydrates discussed above.

High-energy compounds

General. ATP belongs to a class of phosphate compounds known as high-energy phosphates. This statement means that in the reaction of ATP with water, which is catalysed by various enzymes, a relatively large amount of free energy is liberated. Free energy is the type of energy that is available for doing useful work or driving a reaction that would not occur spontaneously. The various phosphate compounds can, broadly speaking, be grouped into two classes, high- and low-energy compounds, depending on the amount of energy that becomes available for work upon cleaving the phosphate bond. The concept that phosphate bonds are carriers in energy transformation and biosynthesis was originally proposed by Lipmann (1941). In the class of high-energy compounds we have ATP, acetyl phosphate, 1-phosphoglycerol-3-phosphate, phosphoenolpyruvate, creatine phosphate; low-energy phosphates are glycerol-1-phosphate, glucose-6-phosphate, fructose-6-phosphate, glucose-1-phosphate.

The difference between the two classes of compounds is often somewhat blurred because the actual amount of free energy available depends on the concentration of the reactants and products of the reaction, and the so-called standard free energy of reaction ($\Delta F°$), usually listed in tables, refers to a hypothetical state when all the reactants are present in the concentration of 1 mole per litre. A useful way of thinking about this so-called standard free-energy change of a reaction is in terms of the relationship of standard free-energy change with the equilibrium constant (K) of the reaction, given by

$$\triangle G° = - RT \ln K$$

Typical $\triangle G°$ values for high-energy compounds are about 40 kJ/mol and for low-energy compounds 10–20 kJ/mol. The actual free energy available, $\triangle G$, depends on the concentration (or more precisely activity) of the reactants and products; it is related to $\triangle G°$ by the following equation

$$\triangle G = \triangle G° + RT \ln$$

$$\frac{\text{(product of concentrations of products)}}{\text{(product of concentrations of reactants)}}$$

Thus for the hydrolysis of ATP,

$$\triangle G = \triangle G^\circ + RT \ln \frac{(ADP)(P_i)}{(ATP)},$$

where

$$\triangle G^\circ = -RT \ln \frac{(ADP)_{eq}(P_i)_{eq}}{(ATP)_{eq}} = -RT \ln K,$$

the subscript 'eq' referring to the concentrations at equilibrium.

In considering biological energy transduction involving macromolecular systems, as in the case of muscle, some useful distinctions can and should be made among various types of free-energy definitions. The recent papers by Hill and his colleagues (Hill & Simmons 1976, Eisenberg & Hill 1985) as well as Tanford (1983) and Jencks (1980, 1983) should be consulted in this context.

Reactions of ATP. Both the bond between the terminal and the middle phosphate and that between the middle phosphate and that nearest to the ribose ring of ATP are of a high-energy character. There are several enzyme systems, phosphotransferases, in the cell which provide essentially equi-energetic transfer of phosphate from one compound to another. One is the so-called creatine kinase (EC 2.7.3.2), which catalyses the reaction:

$$CrP + ADP \rightleftharpoons Cr + ATP$$

Another enzyme present in muscle, myokinase or adenylate kinase (EC 2.7.4.3) catalyses the transfer of phosphate from ATP to AMP resulting in the formation of two ADP molecules, thus making, by the reverse reaction, further utilisation of energy available.

In addition to the reactions of ATP involving transfer of phosphates, there are enzymes in muscle that lead to the deamination of the purine ring. No evidence exists that ATP itself can be deaminated, but both ADP and AMP can serve as substrates of deaminase. Furthermore, in vivo it seems that the NH_2 group attached to the purine ring of the ATP molecule undergoes rapid exchange. This exchange, however, is not a simple reversal of the deamination reaction but seems to proceed by a pathway involving adenylosuccinate (Newton & Perry 1960).

Energetics of muscle contraction

Views on the ultimate source of the energy released by muscle in the course of contraction have undergone considerable changes over the years. The lactic acid era gave way to phosphagen, as creatine phosphate was originally called, particularly under the weight of evidence adduced by Lundsgaard (1930) showing the disappearance of creatine phosphate from exhausted muscle, even under conditions when no lactic acid appeared (for an historical review see Needham 1971). In the middle 1950s, doubts were cast on the immediate participation of ATP and CrP in the elementary event of muscle contraction (Mommaerts 1954, 1955, Fleckenstein et al 1954), but it has now been shown quite convincingly that 0.5–0.6 μmole of ATP are hydrolysed per gram of muscle during a single contraction (Cain et al 1962). Fenn (1923, 1924) showed more than 50 years ago that the total energy output of the muscle is increased as it shortens to do work (see also Mommaerts 1970). Hill (1949) originally partitioned the energy released by muscle during contraction into three terms, one corresponding to activation, another to shortening, and a third to mechanical work. The existence of a heat term which is dependent only on shortening appears doubtful in the light of recent work (Hill 1946a, b, c, d, Wilkie 1966). The correlation of each of these terms with chemical changes has been the subject of research in several laboratories (Cain et al 1962, Mommaerts et al 1962, Carlson et al 1963, Marechal & Mommaerts 1963).

There is good evidence for extra breakdown of CrP and ATP corresponding to work done (see e.g. Kushmerick & Davies 1969). The precise relationship between chemical change, activation heat and shortening heat has yet to be established (Gilbert et al 1971, 1972). Comparison of mechanical work and thermal and chemical changes has been complicated by the fact that different investigators use different experimental material. In a stimulated muscle the sum of work done and heat liberated (enthalpy) can be accounted for in terms of the enthalpy changes of known chemical reactions if the contraction phase, relaxation and recovery are included. Over shorter periods, however, at the beginning of contraction there may be discrepancies between thermal, mechanical and chemical measurements. This has led to the concept of unexplained energy or enthalpy. The shift between chemical change and energy liberation may involve redistribution among various cross-bridge states (see below) and energy changes associated with calcium release from, and binding to, the sarcoplasmic reticulum, troponin and parvalbumin. (For a detailed discussion see Kushmerick 1983, Woledge et al 1985, Homsher 1986.) The application of NMR techniques (see below) to whole isolated muscles, or whole limbs in vivo, or the use of single fibres combined with sophisticated recording techniques, caged ATP, i.e. ATP releasable by laser illumination and isotopic compounds (see Hibberd & Trentham 1986), will undoubtedly bring further clarification to the problem.

Metabolism and activity. As discussed above, the immediate source of energy for muscle contraction is ATP. The major moiety in equilibrium with it in striated muscle is creatine phosphate. The various pathways that produce ATP, anaerobic or aerobic in character and utilising substrates are determined by the nature of the muscle and its activity. Fast muscle fibres are predominant in 'white muscles'; they are characterised by predominantly anaerobic metabolism and contain only a small number of mitochondria (see Ch. 7). Fibres rich in mitochondria are in the majority in slow 'red muscles' and also account for some fibres of fast-twitch muscle. These fibres can carry out oxidative metabolism utilising either carbohydrates or fats.

High-speed contraction requiring considerable amounts of energy depends first on the use of the preformed high-energy phosphate stores, viz. creatine phosphate; when they are exhausted, anaerobic breakdown of glycogen becomes the main source of energy. Extended medium-level activity depends on oxidative metabolism of either carbohydrates or fats. After the disappearance of the muscle glycogen store, the carbohydrate substrate would be glucose, carried to the muscles by the circulation, or fatty acids also derived from plasma (Hultman et al 1986). The use of glycogen or glucose is more efficient than that of fatty acids in terms of the number of ATPs produced per oxygen molecule consumed. Other factors that determine the choice of the substrate include the rate of their uptake and, in the case of fatty acids, the rate of triglyceride hydrolysis. (For a review on the integration of anaerobic and aerobic pathways as well as of various fuel systems see Hochachka 1985.)

Whereas earlier work on the metabolism of muscles relied on muscle biopsies and the biochemical analysis of samples so obtained, more recently ^{31}P nuclear magnetic resonance studies have opened up new ways of analysing muscle metabolism, permitting continuous monitoring of the metabolic state of the muscle. The use of NMR for imaging, for which ^{1}H nuclei are important, is outside the scope of this chapter.

For metabolic studies on muscle — particularly in man — most of the NMR work has been done with ^{31}P, a naturally occurring isotope of phosphorus, and to some extent with ^{13}C spectra. Recent reports indicate the usefulness of two-dimensional ^{1}H magnetic resonance for the study of human muscle extracts with the promise of distinguishing metabolites in normal and diseased muscles (Venkatasubramanian et al 1986). Topical magnetic resonance studies permit the detection of signals over a well-defined muscle area with the use of ^{31}P. Changes in ATP, phosphocreatine and other phosphorylated compounds can be detected as muscles contract and, utilising the change in the position of some peaks, information can be obtained about the intracellular pH of muscle. NMR is useful, not only for detecting changes in concentration of metabolites but, with the use of so-called saturation transfer, the rate of exchange of phosphorus between two compounds, e.g. phosphocreatine and ATP, can be measured. For details on these topics a number of reviews are available (Dawson & Wilkie 1984, Edwards et al 1985, Dawson 1986, Radda 1986a, b).

Fatigue. The study of muscle metabolism, both in its conventional form utilising muscle biopsy as well as the more recent technique of NMR including the topical magnetic resonance version, have thrown new light on this problem. The decline in force associated with fatigue is regarded as being dependent on metabolic changes in muscle as well as on alterations in the activation of contraction. In the intact organism a central component has also to be considered: i.e., alterations of stimuli originating in the brain. The biochemical approach is particularly suited to studying the first two factors. Fatigue is clearly correlated with decrease in phosphocreatine and pH and an increase in inorganic phosphate (Dawson et al 1978). These changes can be readily studied with the use of topical magnetic resonance instruments on human volunteers.

Decreases in ATP and increases in ADP occur only in extreme exhaustion of muscle which could be produced only by electrical stimulation. According to Dawson (1986) (see also Wilkie 1986) the accumulation of phosphate and particularly its mono-anionic form is most closely correlated with the decline of force. It should be borne in mind that, as the products of creatine phosphate and ATP accumulate, the free energy available from the hydrolysis of the ATP which is available for contraction also decreases (cf. Wilkie 1986). Recent work on isolated skinned muscle fibres (Hibberd et al 1985), to be discussed below, suggests that inorganic phosphate is able to decrease force development by shifting some of the equilibria involving intermediates in the myosin- or actomyosin-catalysed ATPase cycle. In NMR studies in repetitively stimulated anaerobic frog muscle, glycolysis is activated during each contraction but comes to a rapid halt, despite the fact that P-containing metabolites have not returned to their resting values (Dawson et al 1980). Similar data have been obtained on human forearms in vivo (see Dawson & Wilkie 1984, Dawson 1986) during ischaemia while glycolysis can still be increased during maximum voluntary contraction. Thus, the authors conclude, increased glycolytic rate associated with contraction is not governed by phosphorylated metabolites (which is the theory which has been held by many investigators) but may be related to the Ca^{2+} release that triggers contraction and also activates phosphorylase. It should be recalled that although enzymes of glycogen metabolism are well characterised in vitro, complex interactions in whole muscle may lead to behaviour of an enzyme not readily explained (see e.g. Constable et al 1986). The interaction between oxidative and glycolytic metabolism during exercise, its variation from

individual to individual and its dependence on training is illustrated by the work of Chance and his colleagues (Chance et al 1986).

Repeated stimulation of muscle not only affects changes in metabolites but also shows changes in membrane properties resulting in reduced velocity of propagation of depolarisation and changes in the frequency dependence in the response to stimulation (Bigland-Ritchie & Woods 1984, Edwards 1984, Milner-Brown & Miller 1986, Metzger & Fitts 1986). It has been suggested that a reactive mechanism is at work in the intact organism resulting in a lower firing frequency of neurones just high enough to obtain maximum force development relaxation (Bigland-Ritchie et al 1986). Details of the biochemical mechanisms underlying these processes are yet to be fully explored.

The application of biochemical and NMR studies to a number of muscle diseases has shown great promise. For details the reader is referred to published reviews (Edwards 1984, Edwards et al 1985, Dawson & Wilkie 1984, Radda 1986a, b) as well as Chapter 13.

MYOFIBRILLAR PROTEINS

Myosin

Extraction, solubility. Myosin accounts for about half of the myofibrillar proteins (Hanson & Huxley 1957, Yates & Greaser 1983). It can be extracted from muscle at about pH 6.5 with minimal contamination by actin. Raising the pH and prolonging the time of extraction leads to the extraction of both actin and myosin in the form of actomyosin, which is discussed in more detail below. The solubility of myosin increases with ionic strength: about 0.6 M is the ionic strength used for extraction. Myosin is insoluble at ionic strengths less than 0.2 M when formation of aggregates occurs. This property is used for the precipitation or, as it is often somewhat loosely termed, crystallisation, of myosin (Szent-Györgyi 1945).

Structure, subunits. Myosin, a highly asymmetrical hexameric molecule, is among the largest proteins that have been well characterised. It contains two heavy chains, $M_r \sim 220\,000$, and four light chains, $M_r \sim 20\,000$. The carboxyl-terminal portions of the two heavy chains form an α-helical coiled coiled rod while the N-terminal portions of each chain appear as separate globular structures clearly shown by electron microscopy following rotary shadowing (Lowey et al 1969); these are the so-called heads of the myosin molecule (Fig. 4.2). Each head contains an ATP binding site, where the hydrolysis of ATP to ADP and phosphate takes place to yield the energy for muscle contraction, and an actin binding site.

Early work (Gergely 1950, 1953, Perry 1951, Mihalyi & Szent-Györgyi 1953, Gergely et al 1955) has shown that myosin can be cleaved into smaller fragments without loss of ATPase activity and the ability to interact with actin (Fig. 4.2). Cleavage of the heavy chains by trypsin or chymotrypsin produces a two-headed N-terminal fragment: heavy meromyosin (HMM), that contains part of the rod, and light meromyosin (LMM) (Szent-Györgyi 1953), representing about two-thirds of the rod including its C-terminus. Further digestion of HMM yields the smaller subfragment 1 (S-l) (Mueller & Perry 1962) corresponding to single myosin heads and a coiled-coil fragment (S-2) (Lowey 1964, Lowey et al 1966) linking the myosin head with the LMM portion. S-2, obtainable in a long and short form (Highsmith et al 1977, Weeds & Pope 1977, Sutoh et al 1978), corresponds to the part of the cross-bridge that connects the body of the thick filament with the myosin head and has an important role as a transmitter of force generated at the head–actin interface. Alternatively, the S-2 portion may itself play a part in force generation (Harrington 1979, Ueno & Harrington 1981, Harrington & Rodgers 1984).

Under carefully controlled conditions of digestion, S-1 can be further broken down into smaller fragments that remain non-covalently held together without loss of ATPase activity. The main fragments of the heavy chain obtained by tryptic or chymotryptic digestion starting at the N-terminus have been referred to as the 25 kDa, 50 kDa and 20 kDa peptides (Balint et al 1978). Recently a fragment has been obtained that contains the C-terminal 10 kDa portion of the 50 kDa fragment and the 20 kDa C-terminal part of S-1 (Chaussepied et al 1986a). Separation of these fragments on sodium dodecasulphate- (SDS)-containing polyacrylamide gels has made it possible to locate binding sites for ATP and actin and to locate various residues of functional significance within the myosin head (see below).

Light chains. The two light chains associated with each myosin head belong to two different chemically distinguishable classes. A variety of techniques and a combination of such techniques, including electron microscopy, antibody reactions and cross-linking, have helped to localise the light chains in the myosin head. It appears that light chains extend for a considerable distance along the myosin head, their N-terminus being close to the head–rod junction (Winkelmann & Lowey 1985, Yamamoto et al 1985). This is not surprising, considering the structural homology between the myosin light chains and Ca-binding proteins such as troponin C and calmodulin (see below), the structure of which, recently elucidated by X-ray crystallography (Sundaralingam et al 1985a, Herzberg & James 1985), has been shown to be far more elongated than envisaged earlier.

In fast skeletal muscle, the light chains have been named 'DTNB light chains' and 'alkali light chains'. The nomenclature is based on the fact that one light chain of 18 000 daltons can be dissociated by treatment with Ellman's thiol reagent (5,5′-dithio bis-2-nitrobenzoic acid (DTNB)) without significant loss of ATPase activity (Gazith et al 1970, Weeds & Lowey 1971). Further alkali treatment liberates two light chains, which have apparent molecular weights on SDS gels of about 25 000 and 16 000, and which are

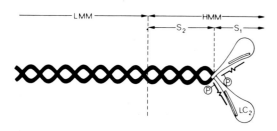

Fig. 4.2 Schematic representation of a myosin molecule showing points (broken lines) at which limited proteolysis results in formation of stable fragments. The head regions contain two kinds of light chains, one phosphorylatable. Heavy lines are intertwined α-helices. The model is not drawn to scale. For details see text. Copied with permission from Kendrick-Jones & Scholey (1981)

termed A1 and A2. The three chains have distinctive chemical features, although there are common sequences in the alkali light chains (Weeds 1969, Weeds & Frank 1972). On the basis of the sequence studies the true molecular weight of A1 is 21 000. Based on the electrophoretic mobility on SDS-containing polyacrylamide gels, the three light chains have been designated LC_1, LC_2 and LC_3, in order of increasing rates of mobility. LC_2 is the DTNB light chain and LC_1 and LC_3 correspond to A1 and A2, respectively. Myosin slow-twitch muscle contains only two main types of light chains, the mobilities of which are similar to, but distinguishable from, those of LC_1 and LC_2 respectively, of fast-muscle myosin (Lowey & Risby 1971, Sarker et al 1971, Frank & Weeds 1974). Cardiac muscle myosin also contains light chains corresponding to LC_1 and LC_2, but there are differences between those found in atria and those in the ventricles. The latter seem to be identical with those of slow skeletal myosin; the atrial light chains differ in mobility from both fast and slow skeletal muscle light chains (Bandman 1985, Barton & Buckingham 1985).

Light chains in the LC_2 mobility class (fast, slow, skeletal, cardiac) seem to be related in their ability to undergo phosphorylation by a kinase (Pires et al 1974, Yagi et al 1978), the activator of which is the ubiquitous Ca-binding protein calmodulin (see Klee & Vanaman 1982). These light chains are also known as P chains. A light chain that can undergo phosphorylation has been implicated in the regulation of smooth muscle contraction (Sherry et al 1978, Hartshorne & Siemankowski 1981). A regulatory role for LC_2 in cardiac muscle has also been suggested (Malhotra et al 1979), but the possible role of LC_2 has not been fully established in skeletal muscle. Its phosphorylation and dephosphorylation in vivo during contraction and relaxation respectively, have been reported (Barany & Barany 1980), and in vitro the effect on the mechanical properties of fibres has been observed (see e.g. Cooke & Stull 1981, Persechini et al 1985).

Myosin isozymes. In the broadest sense all myosins exhibiting different functional and structural features may be regarded as isozymes. Thus various forms found in fast and slow skeletal, cardiac and smooth muscles are isozymes. In a narrower sense, myosin molecules differing in their subunit composition but found in the same type of muscle have been regarded as isozymes. The fact that in fast-muscle myosin the sum of A1 + A2 is two per molecule although they occur in a ratio of about 1.4:0.6 suggests that some myosin molecules contain pairs of either A1 or A2 (Sarkar 1972). The existence of such homodimers has been shown by Holt & Lowey (1977) with the use of antibodies specific for one or the other light chain. Evidence for heterodimer molecules containing one A1 and one A2 has been obtained with the use of electrophoresis under non-dissociating conditions in pyrophosphate-containing gels where myosin separates into three bands corresponding to the $(A1)_2$, A1A2 and $(A2)_2$ species, in order of increasing mobility (Hoh 1978, d'Albis et al 1979, Lowey et al 1979). Electrophoresis under non-dissociating conditions has also shown the existence of myosin isozymes in cardiac muscle; here, however, the differences reside in the heavy chains. Two heavy chains, referred to as α and β, have been identified as giving rise to ββ, αβ and αα moieties, in order of increasing mobility, also known as V_3, V_2 and V_1 isozymes, respectively (Hoh et al 1978, Lompre et al 1981).

Genetic basis of myosin isoforms. The identification of various isoforms of myosin subunits and the clarification of their relationship has been greatly aided by advances both in protein and DNA sequencing, as well as immunological and DNA cloning techniques. Thus the β chain of cardiac muscle myosin appears to be identical with the heavy chain of slow skeletal muscle myosin, being the products of the same gene (Lompre et al 1984, Sinha et al 1984). Distinct genes code for the fast myosin heavy chains found in IIA and IIB type fibres (Nadal-Ginard et al 1982). The DTNB-light chain is coded for by a gene distinct from that coding for both alkali-light chains; in the latter case the transcription of a single gene leads by alternative initiating sites and splicing to two messenger RNAs, the translation of which produces two distinct light chains (Nabeshima et al 1984, Periasamy et al 1984, Robert et al 1984, 1986). Alternative splicing mechanisms (for a general reference see Leff et al 1986, Padgett et al 1986) have an important role in the production of a number of isoforms of various muscle proteins (e.g. troponin T — Medford et al 1984, tropomyosin — Ruiz-Opazo et al 1985). Differences in proteins may also arise from posttranslational modifications of the peptide chain, e.g. methylation of lysine and histidine residues in fast adult myosin heavy chains (Kuehl & Adelstein 1970, Huszar 1975)

ATPase activity. Myosin is not only a structural component of muscle but also an enzyme able to hydrolyse the terminal phosphate of ATP, producing ADP and inorganic phosphate, as first shown by Engelhardt & Ljubimova (1939). This reaction is greatly stimulated by Ca^{2+} and much less by Mg^{2+} ions (Szent-Györgyi 1945). Actin greatly increases the ATPase activity of myosin in the presence of Mg^{2+}. As discussed above, ATPase activity is entirely restricted to the heavy meromyosin fraction (Szent-Györgyi 1953, Gergely et al 1955) and can be recovered in the even smaller HMM-S-1 fragments.

The ATPase activity of myosin in fast muscle is considerably higher than that of myosin in slow muscles (Barany et al 1965, Sreter et al 1966). Barany (1967) has shown that, in general, good correlation exists between the ATPase activity of myosin and the speed of shortening of the muscle from which it has been isolated, independently of the species or the type of muscle (smooth or striated). Myosin of slow muscles shows considerable lability at pH 9, not present in myosin of fast muscles (Sreter et al 1966, Seidel 1967). Differences in ATPase activity between various myosins are mainly attributable to the differences in the heavy chains, as shown by experiments with hybrid myosins containing subunits from cardiac and fast skeletal myosins (Wagner 1981). Kinetic analysis of the ATPase reaction led to attribution of rate differences to the ADP dissociation step (Marston & Taylor 1980, Siemankowski & White 1984, Rosenfeld & Taylor 1984). Native fast-type myosin isozymes (Pastra-Landis et al 1983) and S-1 isozymes containing either A1 or A2 light chains (Wagner et al 1979) also showed only small differences at ionic strengths below the physiological level.

The work of Lymn & Taylor (1970, 1971) laid the foundations for our current views of the mechanisms of myosin-catalysed ATP hydrolysis and its acceleration by actin. They showed that the hydrolysis of ATP involves a rapid step resulting in the formation of tightly, but non-covalently bound products which are in equilibrium with bound ATP:

$$M + ATP \rightleftharpoons MATP \rightleftharpoons M^\star ATP \rightleftharpoons M^{\star\star}ADP.P_i \xrightarrow{slow} M^\star ADP.P_i \to product.$$

One or two asterisks indicate different conformations of myosin or states in the complexes, some detectable by optical or electron spin resonance spectroscopy (see Gergely & Seidel 1983, Webb & Trentham 1983). The equilibrium between the bound forms of ATP and ADP + P_i is shifted by a factor of 10^5–10^6 towards ATP, compared with the equilibrium between free ATP and ADP + P_i. This is a simplified scheme — more details will be added below in discussing the hydrolytic cycle in the presence of actin and its relation to the mechanical cross-bridge cycle. This is of importance for energetic coupling of ATP hydrolysis to mechanical work in muscle.

Functionally important regions. During the past few years there has been considerable interest in assigning various functional aspects of the myosin head to the peptides derived from it by limited proteolysis and in attempting to locate them in the three-dimensional structure. Thus the 25 k N-terminal portion has been shown to be involved in interaction with ATP, as is the 50 kDa central peptide of S1. Chemical cross-linking has led to the identification of actin-binding regions in the 50 kDa and 20 kDa region. The sulphydryl groups, whose modification by thiol reagents affects the ATPase activity of myosin and whose reactivity is in turn influenced by the nucleotide–protein interaction, have been localised in the 20 kDa segment (Elzinga & Collins 1977, Balint et al 1978). The so-called SH1 thiol has been useful as a site for binding optical and magnetic probes to myosin; these will be referred to below. While earlier studies (Reisler et al 1974, Wells & Yount 1979) suggested that the two thiol groups are in close proximity to the nucleotide binding site, recent work (Tao & Lamkin 1981, Perkins et al 1984) has furnished evidence that there is a considerable distance between the thiol groups and the nucleotide binding site. Thus the trapping of the nucleotide at its binding site (Wells & Yount 1979) resulting from cross-linking of the two thiol groups, cannot, in view of the distance between thiols and the binding site, be due to mechanistic immobilisation of the nucleotide but would have to be attributable to a conformational change induced at some distance from the site of cross-linking.

Domains. The fact that a number of proteolytic enzymes produce similar fragments within the myosin head has led to the idea that these fragments are not merely segments of the primary structure separated by regions of high proteolytic susceptibility but, rather, are more or less independently folded regions, so-called domains, within the three-dimensional structure of the myosin head (Harrington & Rodgers 1984). The domain concept (see Applegate & Reisler 1983, Mornet et al 1981, 1984) has gained some support from partial renaturation of isolated fragments of the head (Muhlrad & Morales 1984, Muhlrad et al 1986). The idea of domains in the myosin head will require further confirmation eventually obtainable when the three-dimensional structure is obtained by X-ray diffraction methods, which is now within the realm of possibility in view of the recent crystallisation (Rayment & Winkelmann 1984, Winkelmann et al 1985) of the S-1 portion of myosin. If independently folding domains exist, they are rather close to each other so that the formation of cross-linking between side-chains located in different putative domains is possible (Mornet et al 1985, Chaussepied et al 1986, Lu et al 1986b). Moreover, both ATP binding (Szilagyi et al 1979, Mahmood & Yount 1984, Okamoto & Yount 1985) and actin binding (Mornet et al 1981, Chen et al 1985) may involve sites in more than one domain. Studies of this nature will produce useful information on the interaction of various regions within the myosin head. Data have also been accumulating on distances between a number of points in the myosin molecule utilising energy transfer between chromophores attached to residues whose location is known in the primary structure. On the basis of such data tentative three-dimensional maps of

the myosin head and its relation to actin have been suggested and have been used to interpret the mechanism of energy transduction in the myosin head (Morales et al 1982, Botts et al 1984). The combination of electron microscopy and labelling of chemically identifiable residues on the myosin head with avidin appears to hold promise for visualising topographical relations (Sutoh et al 1984, 1986, Yamamoto et al 1985, Wakabayashi et al 1986).

Relation of myosin to myofilaments. As shown in Chapter 2, the electron microscope picture of a myofibril shows that myosin filaments have a diameter of about 10 nm. A myosin filament is a bundle of many myosin molecules per cross-section; the rigid rod-like part of the myosin molecules makes up the body of these filaments and the enzymatically active globular end would correspond to the bridges seen in electron micrographs between myosin and actin filaments. (For details of thick filament structure see Squire 1981.) At low ionic strength, myosin forms regular aggregates with the sidewise apposition of the rod-like part of the myosin molecules, and the globular ends appear on the side of the aggregates. The formation of the aggregates proceeds in two directions leaving a central zone free of lateral projections quite reminiscent of the appearance of the thick filaments of myofibrils seen in electron micrographs of muscle itself (Huxley 1963).

Electron-microscopic and X-ray data suggest that the cross-bridges on the myosin aggregates and thick filaments are arranged on the surface in a helical fashion, the rod portions forming the core at levels separated by 14.3 nm (Huxley & Brown 1967, Huxley 1969). The amino-acid sequence of the rod portion of the myosin heavy chain exhibits a pattern of hydrophobic and polar residues characteristic of α-helical coiled coiled structures first suggested by Crick (1953). There is a seven-residue repeat and hydrophobic residues are flanked by two and three polar ones in the sequence. This kind of sequence was first detected in tropomyosin (Hodges et al 1972, Sodek et al 1972). There is also a 28-residue repeat pattern (see McLachlan & Karn 1982, McLachlan 1984) producing alternate clusters of positive and negative charges. The spatial separation of these charges in the helix is 14.3 nm, making it possible to stabilise the interacting adjacent rods shifted by 14.3 nm. This interaction would thus play an important part in the assembly of the thick filaments, where a 14.3 nm axial repeat with helix repeats of 42.9 nm in vertebrate striated muscle has long been established (Huxley & Brown 1967). These spacings give rise to the X-ray diffraction pattern of muscle which has recently been studied with techniques capable of resolving changes on a millisecond time scale (Huxley & Faruqi 1983). The original estimate of the number of cross-bridges on each level was two, and it was suggested that the two are diametrically opposed (Huxley & Brown 1967). However, evidence has been accumulating in favour of a thick filament structure in which there are three myosin cross-bridges on successive levels separated by 14.3 nm (Fig. 4.3) (Ip & Heuser 1983, Kensler & Stewart 1983, Varriano-Marston et al 1984, for a review of earlier work see Squire 1981).

The idea that the myosin molecule contains hinges permitting segmental flexibility (Huxley 1969) has played an important part in relating information on the molecular structure of myosin, and thick filament ultrastructure, to theories of contraction. Electron-microscopic and physico-chemical evidence and the loci of proteolytic susceptibility suggest regions of flexibility at the junction of the globular heads and the rod (S-1/S-2) and within the rod itself at the junction of S-2 and light meromyosin (cf. Fig. 4.2) (Mendelson et al 1973, Thomas et al 1975, Highsmith et al 1977, Elliott & Offer 1978, Sutoh et al 1978, for reviews see Gergely & Seidel 1983, Harrington & Rodgers 1984). However, alternative views on overall flexibility rather than localised hinges have also been proposed (Hvidt et al 1982, 1984).

Actin

Polymerisability. The discovery of actin by Straub (1942) in Szent-Györgyi's laboratory showed that what in the early literature had been described as myosin was actually a complex of two proteins, myosin and actin. Actin itself can be extracted from acetone-dried muscle powder with distilled water. It is present in the watery extract as a globular protein — G-actin. Its molecular weight on the basis of its amino-acid sequence is 41 785 (Elzinga et al 1973).

Although G-actin was originally thought of as a spherical protein, three-dimensional reconstructions of electron micrographs of actin filaments combined with myosin subfragment-1 (decorated filaments) suggested over a decade ago (Moore et al 1970) that actin monomers are somewhat asymmetrical. More details of the actin structure emerged from electron-microscopic studies of actin sheets (Aebi et al 1981, Smith et al 1983) and from X-ray diffraction studies of crystals of the actin-DNase I complex (Suck et al 1981, Kabsch et al 1985). Both approaches led to an actin molecule containing two more or less globular domains separated by a cleft, and the dimensions deduced from the X-ray studies are $6.7 \times 4.0 \times 3.7$ nm.

On addition of various salts, conventionally about 0.1 M for monovalent cations and about 1 mM for divalent cations, a G-actin solution undergoes a drastic change: its viscosity increases and it exhibits birefringence of flow, suggesting the presence of large asymmetrical molecules. These are so-called F-actin (for fibrous actin) particles produced through polymerisation of the globular units (Straub 1942). Polymerisation is probably of importance in the process by which actin filaments are laid down in vivo, but it is unlikely (Martonosi et al 1960b) that the polymer-isation–depolymerisation cycle plays a significant part in the mechanism of muscle contraction (see e.g. Hayashi 1967). Structural and chemical aspects of polymerisation are discussed below. F-actin forms filaments in vitro for vertebrate muscle 10 μm or longer, in contrast to actin filaments in

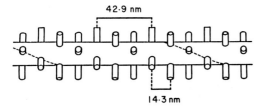

Fig. 4.3 Schematic representation of a three-stranded myosin thick filament, the model currently favoured for vertebrate muscle (see text). The helically arranged projections represent myosin heads. Copied with permission from Offer (1974)

vivo which have a length of 1 μm per half sarcomere (Page & Huxley 1963). The factors that limit the length of actin filaments in vivo have not been identified, although the involvement of other proteins associated with the filament, e.g. tropomyosin and β actinin, has been suggested (Maruyama 1965 a, b).

G-actin contains tightly bound Ca^{2+} or Mg^{2+}, $K_{ass} \sim 10^5 M^{-1}$ (Strzelecka-Golaszewska 1973, Strzelecka-Golaszewska et al 1978, Frieden et al 1980), or even $10^8 M^{-1}$ (Konno & Morales 1985) and ATP, $K_{ass} \sim 10^8$–10^{10} M^{-1} (Waechter & Engel 1977, Neidl & Engel 1979), 1 mol of each per mole of actin. In the G, but not in the F, form both the metal and nucleotide can undergo rapid exchange with added divalent cations or nucleotides respectively (Martonosi et al 1960a, Barany et al 1962, Martonosi 1962, Drabikowski & Strzelecka-Golaszewska 1963, Iyengar & Weber 1964, Oosawa et al 1964). (For a discussion of the relationship between ATP and nucleotide binding sites see Hegyi et al 1986.) It appears likely that both the bound metal and nucleotide are necessary in G-actin to stabilise its tertiary structure — removal of either leads to the irreversible denaturation of the protein and the loss of polymerisability (Nagy & Jencks 1962, Lehrer & Kerwar 1972, Frieden et al 1980), although under special conditions polymerisability and binding to myosin can be preserved (Kasai et al 1964).

Mechanism of polymerisation. The polymerisation of actin is accompanied by the hydrolysis of the bound ATP (Straub & Feuer 1950, Mommaerts 1952) and ADP remains tightly bound while the phosphate is released. Polymerisation stops when the actin monomer concentration drops below the so-called critical concentration, as first shown by Oosawa and colleagues (Oosawa et al 1959, Asakura et al 1960, Oosawa & Asakura 1975). ATP hydrolysis continues after polymerisation has stopped, and the rate of this steady-state hydrolysis, which involves the exchange of G-ADP units in the filament for G-ATP units in solution, depends upon the ionic conditions (Wegner & Engel 1975, Hill 1980, Pollard & Mooseker 1981, Wegner & Neuhaus 1981, Wegner 1982a). It has now been established that actin monomers attach and detach at the ends of the filaments, which

exhibit polarity as shown by the formation of arrowheads on addition of myosin subfragment 1 or HMM. Although attachment and detachment occur at both ends of the filaments, monomers attach preferentially to the barbed end of the filament, while detachment is favoured at the pointed end (Woodrum et al 1975, Hayashi & Ip 1976, Kondo & Ishiwata 1976).

The first step in the polymerisation process is the formation of nuclei consisting of three to four monomers (see Frieden 1985, Pollard & Cooper 1986). Several recent studies have addressed the possibility of G-actin undergoing changes before formation of nuclei. Rich & Estes (1976), in studying the susceptibility of actin to enzymatic proteolysis, discovered a new monomer form that was generated by the addition of KCl to subcritical concentrations of G-actin. The new form, although clearly monomeric and containing bound ATP, showed a decreased susceptibility to digestion, which is characteristic of F-actin. They concluded that this novel actin represented a conformationally distinct form of monomer that precedes nucleation. A conformational change preceding nucleation is also associated with polymerisation induced by Mg binding (Frieden et al 1980, Gershmann et al 1984, Selden et al 1986) and is distinguishable by spectroscopic techniques (see Frieden & Patane 1985, Cartier et al 1986).

Whereas earlier models of polymerisation implied a tight coupling between ATP hydrolysis and incorporation of a monomeric actin into the filament, newer models consider the existence of ATP–actin subunits in the filament with either random hydrolysis of ATP or hydrolysis at the boundary between the central portion of the actin filament containing ADP–actin subunits and a terminal region containing ATP–actin (also referred to as a 'cap', Carlier et al 1984). The continuous addition of monomers at one end and the removal at the other requires steady hydrolysis of ATP (treadmilling) (Wegner & Engel 1975, Hill 1980, Hill & Kirschner 1982, Wegner 1982a, Seeve & Wegner 1986) in the steady state too. For a more detailed discussion of this problem see Pollard & Cooper (1986) and references therein.

A variety of factors indigenous to muscle tissue have a regulatory role in actin polymerisation and depolymerisation. Thus, in addition to the above-mentioned mono- and divalent cation-induced actin polymerisation, several other muscle proteins including myosin (Kikuchi et al 1969), tropomyosin (Wegner 1982b), and β-actinin (Hama et al 1965, Maruyama 1971, Kawamura & Maruyama 1972) can affect the rate or extent of polymerisation. In addition to these muscle proteins, the recent interest in non-muscle actins has led to the discovery of an ever-increasing list of intracellular proteins involved in actin assembly and disassembly. These include proteins that affect either the nucleation (e.g. profilin) (Carlsson et al 1977) or the elongation stage (e.g. capping protein) (Isenberg et al 1980) of filament formation and may or may not be sensitive to intracellular Ca^{2+} concentrations. Several recent reviews have provided descriptions of these agents and the mechanisms of their actions on actin. In many instances, a variety of effects may be understood in terms of a factor's preferential binding to the pointed or barbed end of the filaments (see Hitchcock-DeGregori 1980, Schliwa 1981, Craig & Pollard 1982, Korn 1982).

Functionally important amino-acid residues in actin. The smaller domain of actin revealed by X-ray crystallography (see above) is thought to contain the N-terminal part of the actin molecule, while the C-terminal part would be in the larger one (Mornet & Ue 1984, Kabsch et al 1985, Hambly et al 1986). The detailed assignment of functional sites — including myosin and tropomyosin binding — will have to await the establishment of a higher-resolution near-atomic model in which the tertiary structure of the actin polypeptide chain can be defined. In the meantime a considerable body of information is accumulating that identifies individual amino-acid residues likely to be involved in various functional roles. Of the five Cys residues in actin (Elzinga & Collins 1972), three can be labelled in the native molecule (Lusty & Fasold 1969) without affecting its polymerisability or ATP-binding characteristics. Cys 374, which is adjacent to the COOH-terminal phenylalanyl residue, is the most reactive. In addition to its selective reaction with Cu^{2+} (Lehrer et al 1972), it can be labelled with a variety of SH-directed optical (Cheung et al 1971, Leavis & Lehrer 1974, Ando & Asai 1979, Tao & Cho 1979,

Taylor et al 1981) or spin probes (Stone et al 1970, Burley et al 1971, 1972, Thomas et al 1979). The work of Tao & Cho (1979), for example, in which acrylamide was used to quench the fluorescence of Cys-374-bound AEDANS*, has provided evidence that this thiol group is located in a region of the molecule that is partly covered in the F-form of actin. Taylor et al (1981) utilised donor and acceptor molecules attached to this residue to study intersubunit energy transfer in actin filaments. The reactivity of Cys 374 increases upon the combination of actin with HMM subfragment 1, suggesting either the proximity of the group to the myosin heads or at least some coupling between the region of actin containing Cys 374 and that directly involved in myosin binding (Duke et al 1976). Chemical cross-linking experiments have also provided indications for the participation of Cys 374 and Lys 191 in actin–actin interactions that may be involved in polymerisation (Elzinga & Phelan 1984, Sutoh 1984). Hegyi et al (1986) have identified, using a photo-activatable analogue of ATP, residues (Lys 336, Trp-356) likely to be involved in — or close to — the nucleotide binding site. The fact that cross-linking to the Trp residue takes place in G-, but not in F-actin suggests that a conformational change in this region takes place upon polymerisation.

Another residue in actin that functions as an internal probe is Tyr 69, located near the single N-methylhistidine residue in the protein. Tyr 69 is selectively nitrated by tetranitromethane, and changes in the absorption of light at 425 nm by the resulting nitrotyrosyl residue suggest that it may be somehow involved in the polymerisation process (Elzinga & Collins 1972).

A study by Lu & Szilagyi (1981) has provided insight into the surfaces of the protein involved in polymerisation. They measured differences in the reactivities of the various lysines on the protein surface in F- vs. G-actin and found that polymerisation reduced the reactivities of several, viz. Lys 61, 68, 113 and 283. The decrease in reactivity can be explained if the affected residues are located in the area of contact between monomers, although one cannot rule out conformational changes in the

---

* (acetamidoethyl) aminonaphthalene-1-sulphonate

protein. An intriguing observation in this work was that Lys 335 exhibited a substantial increase in reactivity in the polymerised form of actin, although it decreased again if actin was complexed with either myosin subfragment 1 of tropomyosin, suggesting possible conformational change in actin induced by tropomyosin incorporated into the filament. Modification of another lysine residue — 237 — (El-Saleh et al 1986b) leads to changes in the Ca^{2+}-sensitivity of the actin–myosin interaction (see below).

Isoforms. Actins isolated from various sources including non-muscular contractile systems (Korn 1982, Vanderkerckhove & Weber 1984, Robert et al 1986) have similar chemical structures. Different actins, even in the same organism, are encoded by distinct members of a multigene family. Amino-acid replacements in actin are of a very conservative nature, i.e. preserving the character (charge, hydrophobicity) of the residue, even if species far from each other on the evolutionary scale are compared. Differences in the amino-acid sequence of actins in different cell types, skeletal muscle, cardiac muscle, brain and platelets, have been found in the same organisms. Gel electrophoretic differences among actins depend on a few residues at the N terminus; although the differences correlate with certain broad groupings, the full genetic variety is not revealed by this technique but requires sequence analysis on the protein or gene level. Knowledge of differences between closely related proteins may lead to new insights in the delineation of proteins in diseased muscles.

Actin filament structure and relation to myofilaments. Electron-microscopic studies by Hanson & Lowy (1963) revealed that F-actin is a helical structure made up of subunits. Actin filaments directly isolated from muscle also have the same basic structure. Different actins, even in the same organism, are coded for by members of a multigene family. The participation of other proteins in the thin filaments found in muscle, including tropomyosin and troponin, are discussed below. The original model envisaged a twisted two-strand structure of spherical subunits. The fitting of the bilobar structure of the actin subunits, revealed by the X-ray work referred to above, has not been solved unequivocally.

The best fit of the bilobar monomer structure derived from X-ray crystallography into the F-actin helical structure was obtained by aligning the monomers with their own axis approximately at right angles to the helix axis (Egelman 1985, Trinick et al 1986) (Fig. 4.4). An alternative model with the actin monomer being orientated nearly parallel to the filament axis has also been proposed (Fowler & Aebi 1983, Smith et al 1983, 1984). It would seem, then, that there is a developing consensus favouring the first model although the details of the monomer–monomer contacts and location of the two actin lobes with respect to the filament axis have not been fully resolved. The F-actin filament, once formed, exhibits considerable flexibility; bending motions were first demonstrated by the quasi-elastic laser light-scattering experiments of Fujime and colleagues (Fujime 1970, Fujime & Ishiwata 1972, Ishiwata & Fujime 1972), and later by electron microscopy (Takebayashi et al 1977), fluorescence polarisation of labelled filaments (Yanagida & Oosawa 1978), saturation transfer EPR of spin-labelled filaments (Thomas et al 1979), and by direct dark-field microscopic visualisation of filaments labelled with a fluorescent probe (Nagashima & Asakura 1980). The correlation times characterising these motions range from seconds to

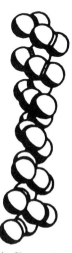

Fig. 4.4 Model of actin filament based on a bilobar structure of G-actin monomers. Copied with permission from Egelman et al (1983)

nanoseconds; the motions may involve whole filaments, subunits within filaments, or segments within subunits. In the case of labels, particularly for faster motions, it becomes difficult to distinguish between motions attributable to the protein and those of the probe itself relative to its attachment site. Addition of tropomyosin and troponin in the absence of Ca^{2+} results in a more rigid filament; however, the addition of Ca^{2+} restores the flexibility to the level of the pure actin filament (Fujime & Ishiwata 1972, Ishiwata & Fujime 1972). In addition to the bending motions along the filament, fluctuations also appear to occur in the twist of the actin helix up to 10 degrees in the azimuthal angle between adjacent monomer units (Egelman et al 1982).

Actomyosin

Natural actomyosin–reaction with ATP. As mentioned above, the early work on fibrous muscle proteins was done on solutions which according to our present knowledge would be considered to be the combination of actin and myosin, viz. actomyosin. The striking physical changes that took place on adding ATP to what then was still called myosin (Needham et al 1941) became interpreted in the light of subsequent discoveries as a dissociation of actomyosin by ATP into actin and myosin (Szent-Györgyi 1945). The discovery and isolation of the pure proteins, myosin and actin, made it possible to study their combination.

Reconstituted actomyosin. On mixing myosin and actin there is a considerable increase in viscosity and birefringence of flow, both being reversed on addition of ATP. This was interpreted as the dissociation of actomyosin into actin and myosin (Szent-Györgyi 1945) and could be confirmed on the basis of light-scattering measurements and ultracentrifuge experiments (Gergely 1956, Weber 1956).

Most of the physicochemical studies on actomyosin were carried out at high ionic strength (0.6) because of the problems of solubility. On the other hand, it is at lower ionic strength (of the order of 0.05 to 0.15), more closely corresponding to that prevailing in the muscle cell itself, that the

most interesting properties of the actin–myosin interaction come to light. Under these conditions myosin ATPase (EC 3.6.1.32) is changed into what we might call the actomyosin enzyme characterised by a high rate even in the presence of Mg in contrast to the inhibition of the myosin enzyme (Szent-Györgyi 1945). Thus actin acts as a powerful modifier of the ATPase activity of myosin, immediately suggesting interesting possibilities from the point of view of physiological regulation of energy release. It should be noted that, for quantitative studies on myosin–actin interaction, active fragments of myosin (HMM and HMM-S-1) have been widely used because complications arising out of the aggregation of myosin molecules are thereby avoided.

Until recently it was generally accepted that in actin-activated myosin ATPase activity the hydrolysis of ATP occurs following the dissociation of actomyosin and results in the formation of an $ADP.P_i$–myosin complex (Lymn & Taylor 1970, 1971, Taylor 1979). The high rate of reaction would be due to the rapid dissociation of the products. More recently, Eisenberg and his colleagues have produced evidence to show that hydrolysis of ATP also takes place on undissociated actin–myosin complexes and that myosin complexes with ATP and $ADP.P_i$ are in rapid equilibrium with the corresponding actomyosin complexes (Chalovich & Eisenberg 1982, Stein et al 1984, 1985). No consensus has been reached on the precise number of intermediate complexes. This has led to a distinction between a four-state model — with one ATP complex and one $ADP.P_i$ complex for myosin and similar complexes for actomyosin — and a six-state model containing two more $ADP.P_i$ complexes, one for myosin and one for actomyosin (see Rosenfeld & Taylor 1984, Stein et al 1985).

Another problem of interest is the identification of the chemical complex that corresponds to the tension-generating — or strong-binding — state. It appears that tension generation requires the dissociation of P_i. Studies on single fibres utilising 'caged' ATP, i.e. a form of inactive ATP that can be activated by laser irradiation, (for a review see Hibberd & Trentham 1986), suggest that following dissociation a short-lived ADP complex is released which is capable of reversible binding of P_i. Studies of this type also show that the P_i interferes with tension development (Hibberd et al 1985, Webb et al 1986).

Myofibrils, glycerol-extracted, and skinned fibres. In addition to the study of actomyosin after reconstitution, studies on systems of somewhat higher complexity have also yielded interesting results. Glycerol-extracted muscle fibres or fibre bundles (Szent-Györgyi 1949) or myofibrils contain actomyosin in their essentially undisturbed configuration. However, these preparations do not contain the excitatory mechanism of the intact cells, nor do they contain the energy supply necessary for contraction. It was found, however, that on the addition of ATP single glycerinated fibres contract, or, depending on the experimental conditions, develop tension. Another useful system was introduced by Natori (1954): the skinned fibre, the sarcolemma of which is mechanically removed. Myofibrils exhibit ATPase activity that has the characteristic feature of Mg^{2+} activation observed on reconstituted and natural actomyosin, and their contraction results in a readily observable syneresis.

Regulatory proteins: Ca^{2+} dependence

Ca^{2+} requirement of actin–myosin interaction. Bozler (1954) and, independently, Watanabe (1955) found that ethylenediaminotetra-acetic acid (EDTA), a chelating agent, inhibits the ATP-induced contraction of glycerinated fibres; the Mg-ATPase activity of myofibrils was also found to be inhibited by EDTA (Perry & Grey 1956). The basis of the action of EDTA on myofibrils and actomyosin at low ionic strength (Ebashi 1961, Weber & Winicur 1961) as well as of the inhibitory effect of higher concentrations of ATP on actomyosin superprecipitation (Weber 1959) is the removal of free Ca^{2+} ions which appear to be essential for the interaction of actin and myosin. Particularly helpful in this area was the introduction of the use of EDTA analogues (Ebashi et al 1960). One of these analogues, EGTA*, has a higher affinity to Ca^{2+} than to Mg^{2+}, thus eliminating the complications arising from the simul-

---

* EGTA: 1,2-bis (2-dicarboxymethylaminoethoxy)-ethane

taneous binding of both divalent cations present in most of the systems under study.

It was first shown by Ebashi & Ebashi (1964) that the Ca^{2+} (or EGTA) sensitivity depends on the presence of protein factors other than actin and myosin. Natural actomyosin from striated muscle, unless subjected to special purification procedures (Schaub et al 1967), contains these sensitising factors whereas reconstituted actomyosin made with highly purified actin is insensitive to EGTA. The EGTA-sensitising factors have been resolved into several components and are usually referred to as the regulatory proteins of the myofibril. They consist of tropomyosin — a protein that has been known and characterised for many years but which until recently has lacked a role — and troponin (discovered later), a term coined by Ebashi and his colleagues (Ebashi et al 1964, Ebashi & Kodama 1965, 1966, Ebashi et al 1969). Troponin is now recognised to be a complex of three protein components (Greaser & Gergely 1971, 1973). These proteins, as discussed below, are components of the thin actin filaments. Details of regulatory mechanisms that primarily depend on myosin, viz. the already-mentioned mechanism based on Ca^{2+}-dependent myosin phosphorylation in smooth muscle and that prevalent in various lower species (e.g. molluscs) involving a regulatory light chain and direct Ca^{2+} binding to myosin (see Lehman & Szent-Györgyi 1975, Kendrick-Jones & Scholey 1981), are beyond the scope of this chapter.

Tropomyosin. Tropomyosin can be extracted from an ethanol-treated muscle preparation (Bailey 1948). It shows a very strong tendency to aggregation at lower ionic strength and its true physical characteristics can be obtained only by increasing the ionic strength. Tropomyosin consists of two subunits, each having a molecular weight of about 33 000, which can be separated under denaturing conditions (Woods 1967). Tropomyosin is notable for its high α-helical content. In this respect it is very similar to the light meromyosin fraction of myosin (Cohen & Szent-Györgyi 1957), and the two subunits are arranged in a coiled-coil fashion (Cohen & Holmes 1963). Tropomyosin is characterised by a very high proportion of polar amino-acid residues, which may account for its tendency to be a stubborn contaminant of actin preparations. Various methods have been developed to obtain actin free of tropomyosin (Drabikowski & Gergely 1962, Spudich & Watt 1971). Vertebrate striated muscle tropomyosin preparations contain two different subunits (α and β) distinguishable by their electrophoretic mobility on SDS-polyacrylamide gels that form αα and αβ dimers (Yamaguchi et al 1974). The ratio of the two kinds of subunits differs in different types of muscle (e.g. only α is found in heart muscle, and the ratio of α:β also varies according to the fibre type (Cummins & Perry 1978) or the stage of ontological development (Roy et al 1979). The aggregation of tropomyosin at low ionic strength can occur both in the form of true three-dimensional crystals and so-called paracrystalline aggregates (Caspar et al 1971, Cohen et al 1971). Various forms are observed in the electron microscope that greatly contribute to our understanding of the size and shape of the molecules and the factors responsible for the interaction among the molecules. The amino-acid sequence of the tropomyosin subunits has been established (Stone et al 1974, Stone & Smillie 1978). The hydrophobic (non-polar) residues are alternately separated by three and two polar residues. This pattern, as discussed above for the myosin rod, results in the formation of the hydrophobic ridges on each of the two helices and the interaction of these hydrophobic regions forms the basis of the coiled-coil structure. Crick (1953) originally proposed such a 'knobs-into-holes' pattern for interacting α-helices. The helix–helix interaction in tropomyosin is further stabilised by ionic interactions among polar residues (Stone et al 1974, Parry 1975).

A wealth of detailed information has accumulated about tropomyosin (see Leavis & Gergely 1984) which cannot be discussed in full detail. A few important points, however, that contribute to our understanding of structural and functional features of tropomyosin are worth singling out. Notwithstanding the apparently uniform helical structure, there are variations in the stability of the molecule along its length. This differing flexibility (see Privalov 1982, Phillips et al 1986) may play an important part in the structural changes that tropomyosin may undergo in its regulatory

role (see below). The region around the single SH group of β-tropomyosin (Cys 190) shows greater temperature dependence than the rest of the molecule, which is reflected in the behaviour of fluorescent pyrene derivatives attached to its Cys 190 (Betcher-Lange & Lehrer 1978, Lehrer et al 1981).

The availability of the amino-acid sequence has made it possible to interpret the postulated end-to-end interaction of TM molecules, which may be the structural basis for some of the co-operative effects in the thin filament. Equally important is a 7-fold repeat of pairs of regions of acidic residues in the primary structure of tropomyosin which may correspond to 7 pairs of actin binding sites (McLachlan & Stewart 1976). The zones in each pair would be turned by 90 degrees relative to each other, representing on and off states in vivo (see below), and switching would involve a quarter turn of tropomyosin. Phillips et al (1986) find evidence for 7 single sites and offer a different interpretation, discussed below.

Finally, mention should be made of the genetic basis, already alluded to earlier, of variety in forms of tropomyosin, both from one species to another and also within the same organism. Some of the diversity is due to the presence of distinct genes encoding different chains, viz. α and β, and to multiple products derived from the same gene by means of alternative splicing (Ruiz-Opazo et al 1985, Flach et al 1986, Nadal-Ginard et al 1986).

Troponin. Tropomyosin alone does not account for the Ca^{2+} requirement of actomyosin ATPase activity. Ebashi & Ebashi (1964) initially assumed that a 'native tropomyosin' did exist, but now it is well established that another moiety, troponin, is also involved (Ebashi & Kodama 1965, 1966, Ebashi & Endo 1968).

Subunits. Troponin was at first considered to be a homogeneous protein and various molecular weights have been suggested (see e.g. Hartshorne & Dreizen 1972). The work of Hartshorne and his colleagues (Hartshorne & Mueller 1968, Hartshorne et al 1969) and Schaub & Perry (1969) has shown that troponin can be separated into at least two components. Greaser & Gergely (1971), by applying SDS polyacrylamide gel electrophoresis, have shown that three components, with molecular weights of 37 000, 24 000 and 20 000, are necessary for reconstruction of troponin activity. This activity is defined as the conferring of Ca^{2+} sensitivity on actomyosin in the presence of tropomyosin. The three troponin components are referred to in decreasing order of molecular weight as TnT, TnI and TnC (Greaser et al 1972), the letters indicating that the three separate components have the ability to combine with tropomyosin, inhibit actomyosin ATPase regardless of the presence of Ca^{2+} (cf. Wilkinson et al 1972), and bind Ca^{2+}, respectively. The three troponin subunits occur in a 1:1:1 ratio, there being one troponin complex for each tropomyosin molecule. The amino-acid sequence of the subunits has been determined (TnC: Collins et al 1973, 1977, TnI: Wilkinson & Grand 1975; TnT: Pearlstone et al 1976); and the molecular weights are 18 000, 21 000 and 30 503 for TnC, TnI and TnT, respectively.

Ca^{2+} binding. When Ca^{2+} activates the actin–myosin interaction it binds to troponin via the TnC subunit. There are four Ca-binding sites in a TnC molecule, falling into two classes differing in their binding constants (Potter & Gergely 1974): about $2.5 \times 10^{7} M^{-1}$ and $4 \times 10^{5} M^{-1}$. The higher affinity sites competitively bind Mg^{2+} ($K = 5 \times 10^{3}$ M^{-1}); the other two are specific for Ca^{2+}. The affinity of TnC for Ca^{2+} is enhanced upon interaction with TnI, either in the TnC–TnI complex or in whole troponin. Effects of this interaction are also reflected in other physicochemical properties that have been studied in various laboratories, suggesting conformational changes induced in TnC by other subunits and vice versa. (For details see Leavis & Gergely 1984.)

An important relationship between TnC and the family of proteins first found in fish muscle able to bind Ca^{2+} — parvalbumin or muscle Ca^{2+}-binding proteins — and more recently discovered in muscles of higher species (Lehky et al 1974) has emerged. Parvalbumin differs from the myofibril-bound TnC in that it is free in the cytoplasm; its molecular weight is about half that of TnC. X-ray diffraction and amino-acid sequence studies have suggested certain repeating features within the parvalbumin molecules, attributable to gene duplication or triplication (Kretsinger 1972). Two Ca^{2+}-binding sites have been identified, each involving a 'loop' flanked by a pair of α helices (Kretsinger & Nockolds 1973). Kretsinger and his colleagues predicted that there would be similarities between parvalbumin and TnC, and Collins and his colleagues (Collins et al 1973) showed that extensive homologies exist between the amino-acid sequences of TnC and parvalbumin. By comparison with the parvalbumin sequence there are four regions that would be probable candidates for the four Ca^{2+}-binding sites in TnC referred to above. Structural homologies between the light chains of myosin and parvalbumin and TnC have also been found (Collins 1974, Weeds & McLachlan 1974). Interestingly, with the exception of the regulatory light chain in molluscan muscle (see below), none of the other light chains contains a specific Ca^{2+}-binding site (see e.g. Bagshaw & Kendrick-Jones 1979).

From studies of the interaction of Ca^{2+} with enzymatically and chemically (cyanogen Br) produced fragments of TnC (Drabikowski et al 1977, Leavis et al 1978, Weeks & Perry 1978) it appears that the high-affinity sites are in the C-terminal half of the molecule (sites III and IV) while the low-affinity Ca^{2+}-specific sites (I and II) are in the α-terminal half. Ca^{2+}-binding to sites III and IV produces major conformational changes in the structure of TnC, while the changes occurring upon binding to site I and II are more subtle (Potter et al 1976, Levine et al 1977, Seamon et al 1977, Johnson et al 1978). Yet it appears that the binding of Ca^{2+} to the latter (Ca^{2+}-specific) sites plays a crucial part in the regulation of actin–myosin interaction (Potter & Gergely 1974) which is also reflected in the kinetics of Ca^{2+} exchange (Johnson et al 1979). One of the important developments concerning the regulatory system of striated muscle has been the crystallisation of TnC and the determination of its structure by X-ray diffraction (Herzberg & James 1985, Sundaralingam et al 1985). TnC turns out to be a dumb-bell-shaped molecule: two globular regions, each containing two Ca^{2+}-binding sites, are connected by a nine-turn single α-helix; it is much more extended than the models previously considered (see Kretsinger & Barry 1975, Leavis

& Gergely 1984). The overall length of the molecule is 7.5 nm. The spatial separation of the two domains of TnC, with a single α-helix forming the connection, raises interesting questions concerning the interaction between the two domains and with regard to interactions with the other subunits and actin. We return to this question below (page 137).

Other subunits. Structural information available on the other two subunits is of a less direct nature. Studies on the interaction among the subunits, actin and tropomyosin, utilising electron microscopy, antibodies and fragments involved in protein–protein interactions, however, shed some light on the structures of the proteins involved while also furnishing data of potential importance for understanding their function. Suggestions for the structure of troponin T have been derived from electron micrographs of troponin in combination with tropomyosin (Ohtsuki 1979, Flicker et al 1982, Phillips et al 1986). These studies have suggested that troponin T is a rather elongated structure; its C-terminus forms a globular head with TnC and TnI which in its complex with tropomyosin is close to the cysteine 190 of the latter. The C-terminal portion of TnT appears as a tail that extends somewhat beyond the C-terminus of tropomyosin. Thus in the thin filament troponin T would interact with the N-terminus of the adjacent tropomyosin as well (Fig. 4.5). In view of the fact that the regions of TnC that interact with TnI are 4–5 nm apart according to the new structural information, it is likely that troponin I also has a rather elongated shape. An answer to these questions will have to await more detailed structural studies on troponin I and troponin T.

Structural change and subunit interactions. In the meantime, information about distances within subunits and between subunits can be obtained from energy-transfer measurements utilising various acceptor and donor groups (Wang & Cheung 1986). Such studies also afford insight into changes that occur when Ca^{2+} binds to troponin C. A variety of studies utilising optical probes as well as nuclear magnetic resonance, electron paramagnetic resonance and cross-linking techniques have led to the conclusion that the first event in the chain that triggers muscle contraction is the conformational change in the N-terminal part that contains the Ca^{2+}-specific sites of troponin C. Studies with proteolytic fragments of TnC (Leavis et al 1978) have shown that a stretch of the primary structure of Tn encompassing residues 89–100 is of crucial importance in the activation of actomyosin ATPase (Grabarek et al 1981) and exhibits Ca^{2+}-dependent binding to TnI. Optical and paramagnetic probes attached to the -SH group in this region show a response to Ca^{2+}-binding at the triggering sites (Grabarek et al 1983, Wang et al 1983, Rosenfeld & Taylor 1985). Changes also occur in the subunits interacting with troponin C. This is well documented for troponin I (see e.g. Strasburg et al 1985) whereas changes in troponin T are less easily demonstrable. (For details of interactions among the subunits see Leavis & Gergely 1984.)

Phosphorylation. Phosphorylation of the TnI and TnT subunits has been reported (Cole & Perry 1975, England 1976, Moir et al 1977). Their functional role is at present not clear except that in the cardiac system, phosphorylation of TnI in vitro (Ray & England 1976) and in the perfused heart (Solaro et al 1976) decreases Ca^{2+} sensitivity and could act as part of a negative feedback system. No functional role has been assigned to the phosphorylation of tropomyosin (Mak et al 1978).

Additional myofibrillar proteins

A number of myofibrillar proteins have been described, but their function and location have not been completely elucidated. It is also not clear in every case whether one is really dealing with a new protein or whether previously known proteins appear in modified form.

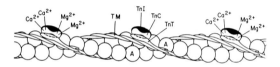

Fig. 4.5 Schematic representation of regulated thin filament. Note that actin monomers are represented as simple globular units. (For a more realistic actin structure, see Fig. 4.4.) Tropomyosin molecules are shown as coiled-coil helices; troponin subunits are drawn to suggest currently accepted structural features (see text). Copied with permission from Moss et al (1986)

α-Actinin, desmin, and β-actinin. These proteins have amino-acid compositions similar to that of actin (Ebashi et al 1964, Ebashi & Ebashi 1965, Maruyama 1965b). α-Actinin, which appears to be a highly asymmetrical rod-like molecule (Suzuki et al 1976, see also Pollard & Cooper 1986) is located in the Z band as shown by antibody labelling (Masaki et al 1967). The ability of α-actinin to cross-link F-actin (Maruyama & Ebashi 1965) may play a part in linking the actin filaments in the Z band. Since immunochemical techniques have revealed the presence of tropomyosin in the I band but not in the Z band (Pepe 1966) the disease of muscle — nemaline myopathy — in which rod-like bodies appear to be connected with the Z bands (Shy et al 1963, Price et al 1965) requires reinterpretation in molecular terms. Originally the rod-like bodies were thought to consist of tropomyosin but this now seems unlikely and the presence of α-actinin in these structures has been demonstrated (Sugita et al 1974).

Desmin (M_r 50 000), another constituent of the Z band, has been identified as the subunit of the so-called 10 nm filaments (Granger & Lazarides 1978). Filaments in the 10 nm class have been found in a variety of cells and are considered part of the so-called cytoskeleton (see Goldman et al 1979). For additional proteins, including vimentin, vinculin, spectrin and ankyrin, involved in anchoring actin filaments and the Z band to the muscle cell membrane see Lazarides & Capetanaki (1986) and Pollard & Cooper (1986).

β-Actinin may be a capping protein of actin (cf Maruyama 1965a,b, Pollard & Copper 1986) suppressing the elongation of actin filaments at their pointed end (Maruyama et al 1977, Funatsu & Ishiwata 1985).

Thick filament proteins.

M-line constituents. The identity of the M-line protein (Morimoto & Harrington 1972), which would play a part in linking the thick filaments in the middle of the sarcomere (Pepe 1972), has been considerably clarified. The presence of creatine kinase in the M line has been demonstrated (Turner et al 1973). In addition to a 165 kDa M protein (Masaki & Takaiti 1974, Trinick & Lowey 1977) there is also a 185 kDA protein, myomesin (Grove et al 1984), forming part of connecting

bridges between thick filaments (Strehler et al 1983, Wallimann et al 1983). The functional role of the presence of creatine kinase — separating a small fraction of the total creatine content — remains to be elucidated. For a review see Wallimann & Eppenberger (1985).

Other thick filament proteins. The C protein may have a structural role in the architecture of the thick filaments (Offer 1972, Offer et al 1973) and in regulating the interaction of myosin crossbridges with actin (Starr & Offer 1978). Additional components associated with thick filaments are X and H proteins (Starr & Offer 1983, Bennett et al 1985) which, together with the C protein, are associated with distinct transverse structures identifiable with specific antibodies. Their function remains to be established.

Continuous filaments. It has been suggested that fibrillin and connectin filaments are running from Z band to Z band across the entire sarcomere (Guba et al 1968). Such filaments have also been described by Hoyle and his colleagues (Hoyle 1967, Hoyle et al 1973). Connectin (Maruyama et al 1977), the main constituent of elastic protein filaments in muscle, appears to be identical with titin, a large myofibrillar protein (Wang et al 1983). A related protein is nebulin (for reviews see Wang 1982, Maruyama 1986). According to a recent report (Horowits et al 1986) repeat X-irradiation of a skinned rabbit fibre selectively destroys nebulin and titin, leading to disorganisation of sarcomeres, and interferes with force development. Moreover, recent speculation (Wood et al 1987) has connected a possible defect in nebulin biosynthesis with the genetic basis of Duchenne muscular dystrophy. Undoubtedly these findings will generate continued interest in the connectin–titin/nebulin system.

SARCOPLASMIC RETICULUM

Introduction

The key role of the free Ca^{2+} $[Ca^{2+}]_i$ concentration control of contraction in regulating the state of muscle activity or relaxation is well established. $[Ca^{2+}]_i$ itself is controlled by the transverse tubule (T tubule)/sarcoplasmic reticulum (SR) system, the anatomy of which is discussed in Chapter 2. In relaxed muscle $[Ca^{2+}]$ is kept at $\sim 0.01\ \mu M$, $\sim 10^5$ times lower than that in plasma, while activation requires $[Ca^{2+}] > 10\ \mu M$. The abrupt change in free $[Ca^{2+}]$ at the onset of contraction accomplished by release from the Ca store within the SR and return to the resting value is attributable to the ATP-dependent Ca^{2+} pump located in the SR. It should be noted that the low intracellular $[Ca^{2+}]$ in a resting muscle could not be maintained solely by the SR having a finite capacity, in view of the influx of Ca^{2+} due to the large gradient between the extracellular and intracellular space. Recent reports indicate that an ATP-dependent Ca^{2+}-pump is located in the plasma membrane and the T tubules (Brandt et al 1980, Hidalgo et al 1983, Mickelson et al 1985), which may fulfil the role of similar enzymes in other types of cells, including those in cardiac muscle. (For a review see Carafoli 1985.)

Work on the biochemistry of the mechanism of control of contraction and relaxation started with the studies of Marsh (1951, 1952) and Bendall (1952). This led to the discovery of the so-called relaxing factor, the relation of which to intracellular membranes was first recognised by Ebashi and his colleagues (Kumagai et al 1955, Ebashi 1957). They also identified ATPase activity with the so-called Kielley–Meyerhof enzyme (Kielley & Meyerhof 1948, 1950). These particulate preparations contain fragments of the sarcoplasmic reticulum that form closed vesicles. For a review of the early work see Weber (1966), Tada et al (1978), Hasselbach (1979).

Ca^{2+}-uptake, ATPase and phosphorylation

In the presence of ATP there is considerable Ca^{2+} uptake by fragments of the sarcoplasmic reticulum, and this process is promoted by a number of anions such as oxalate, phosphate and pyrophosphate (Ebashi 1961, Hasselbach & Makinose 1961, Ebashi & Lipmann 1962, Martonosi & Feretos 1964). The splitting of ATP is the energy source for the active transport of Ca^{2+} into the interior of the sarcoplasmic reticulum. Ca^{2+}-accumulation in the presence of a precipitant has been demonstrated electron-microscopically in situ in the terminal cisternae of the reticulum (Costantin et al 1965, Pease et al 1965) and in vesicles of fragmented sarcoplasmic reticulum (Ikemoto et al 1968). A value of 2.0 for the $\Delta Ca/\Delta ATP$ ratio is most likely under physiological conditions (see Hasselbach 1979). A change in the Ca^{2+} affinity of the protein appears to be correlated with the translocation of Ca^{2+} from the low-concentration outside compartment into the high-concentration interior (Ikemoto 1976). This is an important feature of current models of Ca^{2+} transport (Jencks 1980, 1983, Tanford 1983, 1984, Eisenberg & Hill 1985).

Demonstration of the Ca^{2+}-dependent formation of an acid-stable phosphorylated enzyme from ATP (Yamamoto & Tonomura 1967) implied in the ADP–ATP exchange described earlier (Ebashi & Lipmann 1962, Hasselbach & Makinose 1963) has opened up the way to the elucidation of the mechanism of an ATPase-coupled Ca^{2+}-transport process. The calcium pump can run in reverse, i.e. ATP is synthesised on the efflux of calcium from a Ca^{2+}-loaded vesicle (Makinose 1971, Makinose & Hasselbach 1971). This synthesis of ATP involves the formation of the phosphoprotein intermediate from inorganic phosphate.

Proteins

Ca^{2+}-pumping ATPase. The ATPase moiety has a molecular weight of about 100 000 and contains the sites at which phosphorylation occurs (Martonosi 1969). The spherical particles seen in electron micrographs of negatively stained preparations have been attributed to this component (Migala et al 1973, Thorley-Lawson & Green 1973, Stewart & MacLennan 1974). It also contains three types of Ca^{2+}-binding sites (Ikemoto 1975). Phosphorylation occurs at an aspartic acid residue (Bastide et al 1973). The state of some of the -SH groups of the ATPase protein appears to be influencing the activity. Conversely, the -SH groups fall into certain classes on the basis of their reactivity to thiol reagents; moreover, these reactivities change depending on the occupancy of various Ca^{2+} binding sites (Ikemoto et al 1978, see also Tada et al 1978).

The amino-acid sequence of the Ca-ATPase of the sarcoplasmic reticulum (SR), work on which was started several years ago by protein sequencing techniques, has now been deduced from the nucleotide sequence of the ATPase gene. There seem to be two distinct genes encoding the Ca^{2+}-ATPases of fast- and slow-twitch muscle SR; the highly homologous cardiac and slow-twitch muscle SR Ca^{2+}-ATPase may be products of the same gene resulting from alternative splices (Brandl et al 1986). The first reported sequence (MacLennan et al 1985) that led to a proposed three-dimensional structure embedded in the membrane appears to have been that of the skeletal slow-twitch muscle enzyme (Brandl et al 1986). The sequences are largely consistent with previous partial sequence studies and tentative connectivities established on the basis of accessibility of the SR ATPase to proteolytic enzymes. Based on the primary structure of the protein transmembranous α-helices, luminal connecting loops and cytoplasmic segments corresponding to ATP-binding, phosphorylated, calcium-binding and transducing regions or domains have been identified. It would seem that the path of calcium transported by the enzyme is surrounded by five α-helices and attempts have been made to incorporate these structural features into models of ATP-coupled Ca-transport (Tanford 1983, MacLennan et al 1985, Brandl et al 1986). The detailed three-dimensional structure will eventually have to be based on X-ray crystallography. Progress has been achieved in studies on a two-dimensional crystalline array of the Ca^{2+}-pump protein both in situ and in isolated vesicles (Castellani & Hardwicke 1983, Dux & Martonosi 1983). Three-dimensional image reconstruction of electron micrographs of these crystalline structures has led to the delineation of the overall shape of the transport enzyme and to renewed interest in, and speculation about, the possible existence of dimers that may form a functional unit of the transport enzyme (Castellani et al 1985, Franzini-Armstrong & Ferguson 1985, Taylor et al 1986). Studies on these two-dimensional crystals also afford support for the generally held view that the mechanism of Ca^{2+}-transport involves cyclic alternation between two main states of the enzyme, usually referred to as E1 and E2 or E and E*. Chemically, these states are characterised by differing affinities for Ca^{2+} and differing reactivities with respect to phosphorylation by ATP on

the one hand and inorganic phosphate on the other. Conditions that lead to the stabilisation of putative states, E1 and E2 respectively, result in changes detectable in the pattern of interaction among monomeric units in the two-dimensional lattice (Dux et al 1985). A somewhat simplified scheme incorporating the essential features of the ATP-dependent Ca^{2+}-transport system (DeMeis & Vianna 1979) is given below. For additional details see Inesi (1985).

$$E_1 \rightleftharpoons Ca_2.E_1 \rightleftharpoons Ca_2.E_1.ATP \rightleftharpoons Ca_2.E{\sim}P$$
$$\updownarrow \qquad\qquad\qquad\qquad\qquad\qquad\qquad \updownarrow$$
$$E_2 \rightleftharpoons E_2.P_i \rightleftharpoons E_2\text{-}P \rightleftharpoons Ca_2.E_2{\sim}P$$

Calsequestrin is another protein capable of binding Ca^{2+} (MacLennan & Wong 1971, Ikemoto et al 1971, 1972). It possesses numerous (~ 50) but rather low-affinity ($K \sim 10^3 M^{-1}$) Ca-binding sites per molecule ($M_r \sim 44\,000$). Its role in Ca^{2+} storage is supported by recent evidence showing its localisation in the terminal cisternae of the sarcoplasmic reticulum. These are the regions that are in close contact with the T-tubule system which, as discussed above, is involved in transmission of the depolarisation of the plasma membrane to the interior of the muscle, resulting in the release of Ca^{2+} from the sarcoplasmic reticulum on excitation.

Other proteins include a proteolipid and a high-affinity Ca^{2+}-binding protein (Ostwald & MacLennan 1974), but their functional and structural role has yet to be determined. Phospholamban was originally described as a protein with a molecular weight of 22 000 present in cardiac sarcoplasmic reticulum (Tada et al 1974, 1975). The true molecular weight of phospholamban is 6000 based on amino-acid sequence data (Fujii et al 1986, Simmerman et al 1986). It appears to be present in the SR membrane as a pentamer; a preliminary model (Simmerman et al 1986) places the C termini inside the membrane with the N termini disposed on the cytoplasmic side of the membrane. Phospholamban has also been found in slow skeletal muscle fibres (Jorgensen & Jones 1986). It can be phosphorylated by a cyclic AMP-dependent or a calmodulin-dependent protein kinase, and in view of the reported stimulation of calcium transport by the kinase (Tada et al 1974) a regulatory role for phospholamban as a mediator of the effect of catecholamines in cardiac muscle has been suggested; calmodulin-dependent phosphorylation has also been reported (LePeuch et al 1979, for a detailed discussion see Tada & Inui 1983).

Lipid–protein interaction. Early experiments showing that phospholipase destroys the ATPase and relaxing activity of elements of the sarcoplasmic reticulum (Ebashi 1957) pointed to the involvement of phospholipids in its structure and function. Phospholipase-C-treated fragments of the sarcoplasmic reticulum that have lost their ATPase and Ca^{2+}-accumulating ability again become active on the addition of phospholipids (Martonosi 1963, Martonosi et al 1968). It is now clear that the sarcoplasmic reticulum represents a membrane-bound enzyme system carrying out the ATPase-linked Ca^{2+}-transport function.

Although many details of the protein–lipid interaction remain to be elucidated, it is apparent that replacement of SR or lipids with another lipid moiety determines many properties of the ATPase-transport protein. The ATPase activity depends on certain properties of the lipid moiety (Warren et al 1974) and temperature-induced changes in the motion of the ATPase reflect changes in the fluidity of the lipid (Inesi et al 1973, Hidalgo et al 1976, 1978). A variety of studies indicate that there is a correlation between the Ca^{2+}-dependent dephosphorylation of the phosphoprotein, the mobility of the protein, and the fluidity of the membrane (see Martonosi 1984).

Proteins associated with the T-tubule/SR junction. Recent studies have shown the presence of several proteins in the fraction rich in those portions of sarcoplasmic reticulum that form the junction with T tubules (Costello et al 1986, Kawamoto et al 1986). It is thought that the 300 kDa protein, referred to as the spanning protein, establishes contact with the T-tubule membrane, suggesting identification with the structural element discernible in electron micrographs and termed 'feet', and that each of these 'feet' consists of four dimers of the 300 kDa subunits (see Franzini-Armstrong & Nunzi 1983 and the references therein). Additional proteins

identified in the junctional region are the enzymes aldolase (fructose-bisphosphate aldolase, EC 4.1.2.13) and glyceraldehyde-3-phosphate dehydrogenase (EC 1.2.1.12), the roles of which in the interaction between T tubules and SR have not been established (Kawamoto et al 1986).

Calcium release

Whereas the mechanism of Ca^{2+}-uptake into the SR has been to a large extent clarified, the processes related to the coupling of plasma membrane depolarisation to Ca^{2+}-release, the so-called excitation–contraction coupling, has been more resistent to elucidation. The first step in the physiological mechanism of Ca^{2+} release, it is generally believed, involves some change in the T-tubule/SR junctional region related to the charge movement demonstrated some years ago (Schneider & Chandler 1973, Kovacs et al 1979; for a review see Schneider 1981). The link between this charge movement to the induction of changes in the SR membrane may, according to various suggestions (Volpe et al 1986), be mediated by the actual movements of proteins by electrical currents or by some chemical process involving either Ca^{2+} — more likely in cardiac than in skeletal muscle (Fabiato & Fabiato 1979) — or, as more recent evidence suggests (Somlyo et al 1985, Vergara et al 1985, Volpe et al 1985, Ochs 1986; see, however, Somlyo 1985 for a cautionary note regarding striated muscle) phosphorylated inositol derivatives. The latter have been implicated as chemical messengers in various cellular processes (Berridge & Irvine 1984).

The difficulty of studying Ca^{2+}-release in vitro has been partly ascribable to the lack of systems that can be safely regarded as in vitro models of the triggering of the in situ intact T-SR complex. One criterion should be whether or not the speed at which Ca^{2+} is released in vitro is comparable with that involved in the physiological process, viz. 60–140 s^{-1}. Various methods used in vitro for the induction of Ca^{2+} release — drugs (caffeine, halothane) — interact extravesicularly and depolarisation is achieved by ion replacement under conditions that minimise osmotic effects (Ikemoto et al 1984). The T tubule plays an increased part in the Ca^{2+} release from the SR induced by ionic replacement (depolarisation). This has been shown in vitro on vesicular preparations from which the T-tubular elements were or were not removed (Ikemoto et al 1984) and on single fibres devoid of the plasma membrane and in which the T system had been inactivated (Donaldson 1986). In contrast, Ca^{2+} release induced by increased Ca^{2+} or by drugs such as caffeine or quercitin does not involve the T system.

Many studies are being aimed at identifying elements within the SR that respond to the process initiated in the T-tubule/SR junction. Such elements, often referred to as channels, are proteins inserted into the SR lipid membrane; studies directed at the identification of these channels at the protein chemistry level are still in a fairly early stage. Measurements of single channels for key fractions of SR incorporated into lipid membranes produce useful information on the response to factors such as Ca^{2+}, Mg^{2+} or ATP that may be involved in the physiological regulation of Ca^{2+} efflux (Smith et al 1986; for a comprehensive review on Ca^{2+} channels see Coronado 1986). Undoubtedly methods involving techniques of molecular genetics and the use of specific antibodies including monoclonals are likely to lead to further progress in this area.

EFFECT OF CHANGES IN ACTIVITY AND INNERVATION

Starting with the work of Eccles and his colleagues (Eccles et al 1958, Buller et al 1960), several authors have reported that when a fast muscle is cross-reinnervated by a nerve that originally supplied a slow muscle, it acquires properties characteristic of a slow muscle; reciprocal changes take place in a slow muscle that has been cross-reinnervated by a fast muscle nerve. Changes in contractile speed are accompanied by corresponding changes in both the myosin ATPase activity (Buller et al 1969, Bárány & Close 1971) and the protein subunit pattern (Sreter et al 1974, Weeds et al 1974). Changes have also been observed in the pattern of metabolic enzymes (Dubowitz 1967, Romanul & Van Der Meulen 1967, Guth et al 1968, Weeds et al 1974) and in the activity of the sarcoplasmic reticulum.

The work of Salmons & Vrbová (1969) shows that, even with undisturbed nerve–muscle connec-

tions, changes in physiological parameters can be brought about if the pattern of neural activity reaching the muscle is changed. When the motor nerve is stimulated continuously over a period of weeks, imposing on the fast muscle a pattern of activity similar to that normally reaching a slow muscle, a marked slowing of the time course of isometric contraction and relaxation ensues. Such stimulation also produces changes in the subunit pattern of myosin, the ATPase activity of myosin, the staining pattern of LMM paracrystals, and the Ca^{2+} uptake of the sarcoplasmic reticulum. The changes correspond to an essentially complete fast–slow transformation. The biochemical changes in myosin are paralleled by changes in the histochemical ATPase reaction, as well as by changes in the glycolytic oxidative enzyme pattern (Sreter et al 1973, Pette et al 1973, Romanul et al 1974, Salmons & Sreter 1976, Heilmann & Pette 1979).

Changes in various components on chronic stimulation do not take place synchronously (see Jolesz & Sreter 1981, Pette 1984, Swynghedauw 1986). This has been documented in many studies. Changes in metabolic enzymes and in components of the sarcoplasmic reticulum occur rather early and changes in myosin light chains precede those in the heavy chains. The latter process has been documented in detail (Brown et al 1983). Perhaps the earliest changes, within the first few days (Klug et al 1983, Leberer & Pette 1986) occur in the cytoplasmic Ca^{2+}-binding protein, parvalbumin, found in fast muscle (see Celio & Heizmann 1982). Studies on changes in the RNA level and their products suggest involvement of translational control in fibre transformation (Heilig & Pette 1982, Pluskal & Sreter 1983).

The change-over in the muscle type is attributable to the transformation of the existing fibres by the switching on of normally inactive genes and the switching off of those that had been active, rather than to the destruction of the original fibre population and its replacement by new fibres. Depending on the actual conditions of stimulation, degeneration–regeneration processes involving the formation of new fibres may also contribute to fast-to-slow muscle conversion (Maier et al 1986). Early in the course of the transformation of fast muscle, antibodies against both fast and slow myosins react with the same fibre

(Rubinstein et al 1978), while in normal fast muscle only the antibody against fast myosin reacts (Arndt & Pepe 1975, Weeds et al 1975). After complete transformation, again only one type of antibody reacts — that reacting with slow myosin. The same conclusion has been reached from SDS-gel electrophoretic studies on single fibres showing the transient presence of both fast- and slow-type myosin light chains (Pette & Schnez 1977). As has recently been shown, myosin transitions in chronic stimulation do not involve embryonic isozymes (Hoffman et al 1985). Low-frequency (10 Hz) intermittent stimulation has been shown to lead to Type IIB to IIA fibre transformation (Mabuchi et al 1982), suggesting that IIB fibres undergoing fast-to-slow transformation may go through a transitional IIA stage (see also Pette 1984). Other interventions leaving the nerve–muscle connection intact are also able to change the muscle type, as judged by histochemical and biochemical criteria. Thus, sectioning of the peroneal nerve caused changes in the ipsilateral soleus from slow to fast type (Guth & Wells 1976). Removal of the gastrocnemius and soleus muscle in the rat caused the ipsilateral plantaris to change from the relatively fast to the slow type (Samaha & Theis 1976).

Clearly, the fact that the changes in the activity pattern, with an undisturbed nerve–muscle connection, can alter the physiological and biochemical properties of a muscle raises many interesting questions concerning the so-called trophic effects of the motor nerve (Gutmann 1976, Jolesz & Sreter 1981, see also Ch. 1).

THEORIES OF CONTRACTION AND RELAXATION

Sliding model

It is well established that myosin and actin are localised in distinct filaments in the myofibril. Furthermore, during contraction the length of the individual filaments does not change, but rather their relative position, which leads to what is summed up in the term 'sliding' or 'interdigitating' model of muscle contraction (Hanson & Huxley 1955, Huxley 1960). The classic experiments of Gordon et al (1966) on single fibres, establishing a direct relationship between overlap

speed of shortening independent of overlap, not only support the sliding filament model but also the concept of independent force generators (see the thoughtful analysis of A. F. Huxley 1974, 1979) identifiable with actin–myosin links in the overlap zone.

Molecular mechanisms

The question arises, how does the interaction between actin and myosin located in different structural elements lead to tension development and to shortening of the sarcomere? X-ray work on living muscle points to the movement of the bridges projecting from the myosin filaments as the molecular event underlying contraction (Huxley & Brown 1967). Pepe's work (1966, 1967a, b) with the use of antibody staining techniques has revealed considerable changes within the thick filament structure during shortening, indicative of flexibility in some part — presumably the rod portion — of the myosin molecule. Flexibility of the rod portion would also account for the fact that the interaction between myosin and actin filaments results in the production of constant force per cross-bridge and the separation among filaments increases with decreasing sarcomere length (see Huxley 1968, 1969). As mentioned above, various lines of experimental evidence support such flexibility in myosin. While most authors consider a direct interaction between the nearly globular portions (subfragment-1) of myosin and actin as the key to contraction, a less direct type — perhaps longer range — interaction involving electrostatic and Van der Waals forces has also been suggested (Pollack 1983). The arrowhead structures resulting from the interaction of HMM or S-1 with actin (Huxley 1963) can be explained in terms of a regular attachment of the individual myosin heads to the actin globules, each head making a precise angle with the actin filament axis (Moore et al 1970). It appeared reasonable to assume that the tendency of the myosin heads to align themselves on actin in this fashion represents an important driving force in the mechanism of muscle contraction.

It has generally been assumed that the basis of force development and contraction is a rotation of the myosin heads attached to actin with respect to the filament axis. Force development would — at the molecular level — be due to the stretching of an elastic structure, forming part either of myosin or of the myosin–actin interface (Huxley 1974, 1979). Many current models place the elastic element in the S-2 portion of myosin, which is the connecting link between the rod portion and the myosin heads.

The rotating-head model implies that attachment of the head occurs in a specific orientation and that force development is associated with a rotation into another orientation, the latter being the thermodynamically favoured one also to be found in rigor. A difficulty, not fully resolved, has arisen owing to the fact that many attempts to detect intermediate orientations of probes rigidly attached to the myosin heads in fibres devoid of sarcolemma (skinned fibres) have failed. With some fluorescent dyes (Yanagida 1981, Nagano & Yanagida 1984, Yanagida 1985) as probes, and with paramagnetic spin labels on myosin (Thomas & Cooke 1980, Cooke et al 1982b) only one attached state with rigor-like orientation could be detected. On the other hand, a rhodamine probe, also on the same thiol group on the myosin head, did reveal a state other than rigor or detached (relaxed) in the presence of ADP or under conditions corresponding to activation of a fibre (Borejdo et al 1982, Burghardt et al 1984). Energy-transfer measurements leading to an estimate of the distance between a point (thiol group of light chain 1) on the myosin head attached to actin and another point on actin (Cys 374) also show two attached states in a system simulating contraction (Bhandari et al 1985). X-ray diffraction studies (see Huxley & Faruqi 1983) on contracting intact muscles show that under isometric conditions up to 90% of the myosin heads are close to the actin filaments, but the so-called layer line pattern indicates azimuthal disorder.

Time-resolved (on the millisecond time scale) diffraction patterns show that on activation the first changes are attributable to structural changes in the thin filaments, followed in about 15 ms by changes indicative of myosin-head attachment and, after a further similar lag period, tension development takes place. The earliest changes have been interpreted (Huxley et al 1982) as being related to the activation process; they suggest that the lag between changes indicative of myosin

attachment to actin and tension development is due to the formation of cross-bridges that at first do not develop tension — i.e. weak attachment. Tension appears as these bridges enter a strongly attached state capable of tension development. Huxley & Kress (1985) have proposed a model of the attached cross-bridge that would develop tension over only about 4 nm of its 12 nm total excursion. This model may reconcile some apparent discrepancies between EPR and X-ray measurements with regard to the fraction of rigidly attached cross-bridges in an active muscle. It would also provide some explanation for the apparent lack of intermediate orientations in attached states. (For details see Huxley & Kress 1985, Cooke 1986.)

The precise mode of the force generation by muscle has not been settled (Fig. 4.6). A. F. Huxley (1957) originally proposed a mechanism in which thermal energy stored in some portion of the connecting bridges played an important part.

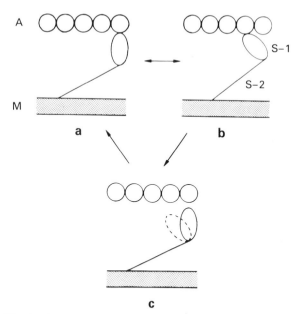

Fig. 4.6 Model of interaction of the myosin head with actin based on Huxley (1969), Huxley & Simmons (1971). a. Attachment of myosin to actin, b. tilting of myosin head, c. detachment produced by ATP followed by its hydrolysis. On the basis of in vitro kinetic studies the myosin species present in (a) + (b) carries the ADP-P product complex. The attached head may oscillate between positions (a) and (b). Whether the dissociated myosin head can oscillate between the perpendicular or tilted position or whether it is locked in the perpendicular position is not finally settled. For details see text

A later proposal (Huxley & Simmons 1971) based on very rapid mechanical transients involved attachment of myosin heads to actin via elastic connections, with the possibility of a tension-dependent equilibrium among several stable positions. Eisenberg & Hill (1978) located the elasticity in the bond between the myosin head and actin and assumed a rigid connecting link. The details of the way in which various intermediate stages in the hydrolysis of ATP can be correlated with configurational states on the myosin head with respect to actin are currently under investigation in several laboratories. Recent studies using a photoactivatable ATP (caged ATP) appear promising (see Hibberd & Trentham 1986). The original mathematical analysis given by Huxley (1957) accounted for a number of mechanical and energetic features of muscle. More recent developments in muscle energetics and mechanics and our knowledge of the details of the molecular apparatus have prompted refinements in the theoretical models such as those by T. L. Hill and his colleagues (Hill 1977, Eisenberg & Hill 1985) describing in terms of statistical mechanics, thermodynamics and kinetics the actin–myosin nucleotide system and serving as a framework for future theoretical and experimental interpretations.

Harrington and his colleagues have been concerned, over the years, with the possible role of the S-2 portion of myosin in force generation rather than serving as a passive string. They have proposed an α-helix random coil phase-change-like transformation as the basis of contractile force generation. These views are backed by experiments showing increased proteolytic sensitivity in the putative hinge region of S-2 under conditions of fibre activation by ATP (see Harrington 1979, Harrington & Rodgers 1984, Ueno & Harrington 1981, 1986a,b and references in the later two papers). If S-2 is the site of force generation, the path of energy transduction from ATP hydrolysis in the remote head region remains to be elucidated.

The work of Yanagida et al (1985) has raised some problems for the conventional view that the free energy of ATP is transduced into mechanical work within the span of the stretch of a single cross-bridge. These authors calculate a distance of >60 nm over which movement occurs as a result of the hydrolysis of a single ATP molecule. In these experiments unloaded relative movement of thick and thin filaments takes place, so that direct conversion of energy could not be determined.

Regulation

The key role of Ca^{2+} in the regulation of the actin–myosin in vitro interaction has been discussed above, together with the role of the sarcoplasmic reticulum in the modulation of the free sarcoplasmic Ca^{2+} concentration during contraction and relaxation. The question remains of how the in vivo interaction of Ca^{2+} with the contractile apparatus fits the picture. There is the (by now classic) physiological evidence that injection of Ca^{2+} into muscle cells produces contraction (Heilbrunn & Wiercinski 1947). Podolsky & Constantin (1964), working on muscle stripped of its outer membrane, could by local application of Ca^{2+} elicit contraction which, owing to the presence of Ca-accumulating reticular elements, spontaneously gave way to relaxation.

Activation by Ca^{2+} would correspond to the removal of the inhibitory effect of the tropomyosin–troponin system in the interaction of actin and myosin observed in vitro. The molecular basis of this process appears to lie in a movement, deduced from X-ray and combined electron-microscopic and optical diffraction studies, of the tropomyosin molecules located in the grooves of the actin filaments into positions where they would not interfere with the attachment of myosin heads (Haselgrove 1972, Huxley 1972, Spudich et al 1972, Parry & Squire 1973). Although questions raised by Seymour & O'Brien (1980) concerning the possibility of direct contact between myosin and tropomyosin, which is essential in a straightforward steric blocking model, have in part been answered (Amos 1981, Taylor & Amos 1981, O'Brien et al 1983), the precise details of the structure of the thin filament, including the spatial relation between tropomyosin-binding and myosin-binding sites, has not been fully resolved (Toyoshima & Wakabayashi 1984 a, b, Amos 1985). The importance of movement in the activation process of tropomyosin or some equivalent structural change in the thin filament has received further support by X-ray diffraction studies mentioned above (Kress et al 1986). Biochemical studies have raised some challenges to the simple steric blocking model in that there is considerable evidence to show that the switch from relaxation to contraction, which in vitro is brought about by adding Ca^{2+}, is not accompanied by a drastic change in the binding of myosin or active myosin fragments to actin (Chalovich et al 1981, Chalovich & Eisenberg 1982), leading to the view that the regulation of contraction involves a change in one of the kinetic steps of the actin-myosin cycle rather than a simple shift in the equilibrium. The biochemical data have been interpreted in terms of the existence of weakly and strongly attached cross-bridges and regulation would involve a shift in distribution among these (see Hill 1983, Eisenberg & Hill 1985). Brenner and his colleagues (Brenner et al 1982) found evidence for the existence of cross-bridges in relaxed muscle at low ionic strength from high-velocity stretch. Brenner et al (1984) noted differences in the X-ray diffraction pattern between relaxed muscle at low ionic strength and muscle in rigor. As mentioned above, Huxley and his colleagues (Huxley & Kress 1985, Kress et al 1986) also postulated weakly attached cross-bridges that do not generate tension and it remains to be seen whether these correspond to those deduced from in vitro studies and from stretch–velocity dependent stiffness measurements (for a discussion see Irving 1985).

The idea of co-operativity in the thin filament was first expressed by A. Weber and her colleagues some 15 years ago. The original co-operative model involved seven actins attached to one tropomyosin molecule and envisaged spreading of the effects of myosin binding within one tropomyosin–actin heptamer as well as providing a basis for the ability of Ca^{2+} bound to the troponin complex to affect more than one actin. More recently, Hill and his colleagues introduced a co-operative model involving nearest-neighbour interactions between tropomyosin molecules in the thin filament using the Ising formalism (Hill et al 1980). This model is capable of explaining the high degree of co-operativity observed in studies on binding of myosin S-1 to actin in the absence of Ca^{2+} (Greene & Eisenberg 1980), which could not be accounted for by assuming only the cooperativity based on the sevenfold interaction within a tropomyosin domain. Tropomyosin–tropomyosin interactions have also

been used to explain the variation of actin-activated S-1 ATPase as a function of S-1 concentration (Lehrer & Morris 1984). Studies with optical probes attached to troponin have not been fully interpretable in a simple manner based on the Hill–Ising model (Trybus & Taylor 1981, Greene 1986). In terms of the ATPase activity of regulated actin-activated myosin there are three states: inhibited, low activity, and high, or potentiated, activity. The relationship of these states to structurally distinguishable states is not fully understood. A simpler on–off scheme with respect to activity was connected with two sets of binding sites for actin on tropomyosin (Stewart & McLachlan 1975). More recent studies discussed above (Phillips et al 1986) suggest one set of binding sites, with three functionally different binding modes.

Further studies are required to produce a better understanding of how changes in actin–tropomyosin interaction, and in strength of interaction among various troponin components and in the interaction of troponin with tropomyosin and actin (Potter & Gergely 1974, Tao et al 1987, see also Leavis & Gergely 1984, El-Saleh et al 1986a), lead to changes in the various kinetic steps of the actin–myosin interaction cycle.

CONCLUSION

This brief survey of the biochemical features of muscle and their relation to structural problems is of necessity incomplete, but it should give an impression of the complexity of the processes involved. It clearly shows that a large number of sites exist at which defects may lead to serious disturbances of muscle function. Further elucidation of the gaps in our knowledge of the normal function of muscle is, therefore, of crucial importance for the understanding of the manifold disorders that are the subject of this volume.

ACKNOWLEDGEMENT

The preparation of this manuscript was supported by grants from the NIH (HL-5949, HL-07266) and the Muscular Dystrophy Association.

REFERENCES

Aebi U, Fowler W E, Isenberg G, Pollard T D, Smith P R 1981 Crystalline actin sheets: their structure and polymorphism. Journal of Cell Biology 91:340

Alberts B, Bray D, Lewis J, Raff M, Roberts K, Watson J D 1983 Molecular biology of Ca++. Garland Publishing, New York

Amos L A 1985 Structure of muscle filaments studied by electron microscopy. Annual Review of Biophysics and Biophysical Chemistry 14:291

Ando T, Asai H 1979 Conformational change in actin filament induced by the interaction with heavy meromyosin: effects of pH, tropomyosin and deoxy-ATP. Journal of Molecular Biology 129:265

Applegate D, Reisler E 1983 Protease-sensitive regions in myosin subfragment 1. Proceedings of the National Academy of Sciences (USA) 80:7109

Arndt I, Pepe F 1975 Antigenic specificity of red and white muscle myosin. Journal of Histochemistry and Cytochemistry 23:159

Asakura S, Kasai M, Oosawa F 1960 The effect of temperature on the equilibrium state of actin solutions. Journal of Polymer Science 44:35

Bagshaw C R, Kendrick-Jones J 1979 Characterization of homologous divalent metal ion binding sites of vertebrate and molluscan myosins using electron paramagnetic resonance spectroscopy. Journal of Molecular Biology 130:317

Bailey K 1948 Tropomyosin: A new asymmetric protein component of the muscle fibril. Biochemical Journal 43:271

Balint M, Wolf I, Tarcsafvi A, Gergely J, Sreter F 1978 Location of SH-1 and SH-2 in the heavy chain segment of heavy meromyosin. Archives of Biochemistry and Biophysics 190:793

Bandman E 1985 Myosin isoenzyme transitions in muscle development, maturation and disease. International Review of Cytology 97:97

Bárány M 1967 Activity of myosin correlated with speed of muscle shortening. Journal of General Physiology 50:197

Bárány M, Finkelman F, Therattil-Antony T 1962 Studies on the bound calcium of actin. Archives of Biochemistry and Biophysics 98:28

Bárány M, Bárány K, Reckard T, Volpe A 1965 Myosin of fast and slow muscles of the rabbit. Archives of Biochemistry and Biophysics 109:185

Bárány M, Close R I 1971 The transformation of myosin in cross-reinnervated rat muscle. Journal of Physiology 213:458

Bárány M, Bárány K 1980 Phosphorylation of the myofibrillar proteins. Annual Review of Physiology 42:275

Barton J R, Buckingham M E 1985 The myosin alkali light chain proteins and their genes. Biochemical Journal 231:249

Bastide F, Meissner G, Fleischer S, Post R L 1973 Similarity of the active site of phosphorylation of the ATPase for transport of sodium and potassium ions in kidney to that for transport of calcium ions in the sarcoplasmic reticulum of muscle. Journal of Biological Chemistry 248:8385

Bendall J R 1952 Effect of the 'Marsh Factor' on the shortening of muscle fibre models in the presence of adenosine triphosphate. Nature 170:1058

Bennett P, Starr R, Elliott A, Offer G 1985 The structure of C-protein and X-protein molecules and a polymer of X-protein. Journal of Molecular Biology 184:297

Berridge M J, Irvine R F 1984 Inositol trisphosphate, a novel second messenger in cellular signal transduction. Nature (London) 312:315

Betcher-Lange S, Lehrer S S 1978 Pyrene excimer fluorescence in rabbit skeletal αα tropomyosin labelled with N-(1-pyrene) maleimide. Journal of Biological Chemistry 253:3757

Bhandari D G, Trayer H R, Trayer I P 1985 Resonance energy transfer evidence for two attached states of the actomyosin complex. Federation of European Biochemical Societies 187:160

Bigland-Ritchie B, Woods J J 1984 Changes in muscle contractile properties and neural control during human muscle fatigue. Muscle and Nerve 7:691

Bigland-Ritchie B R, Dawson N J, Johansson R S, Lippold O C J 1986 Reflex origin for the slowing of motoneurone firing rates in fatigue of human voluntary contractions. Journal of Physiology 379:451

Bitensky M W, Gorman R E 1973 Cellular responses to cyclic AMP. Progress in Biophysics and Molecular Biology 26:409

Borejdo J, Assulin O, Ando T, Putnam S 1982 Crossbridge orientation in skeletal muscle measured by linear dichroism of an extrinsic chromophore. Journal of Molecular Biology 158:391

Botts J, Takashi R, Torgerson P, Hozumi T, Muhlrad A, Mornet D 1984 On the mechanism of energy transduction in myosin subfragment 1. Proceedings of the National Academy of Sciences (USA) 81:2060

Boyer P F 1977 Oxidative phosphorylation and photophosphorylation. Annual Review of Biochemistry 46:955

Bozler E 1954 Relaxation in extracted muscle fibers. Journal of General Physiology 38:149

Brandl C J, Green N M, Korczak B, MacLennan D H 1986 Two Ca²⁺ ATPase genes: homologies and mechanistic implications of deduced amino acid sequences. Cell 44:597

Brandt N R, Caswell A H, Brunschwig J–P 1980 ATP-energized Ca²⁺ pump in isolated transverse tubules of skeletal muscle. Journal of Biological Chemistry 255:6290

Brenner B, Schoenberg M, Chalovich J M, Green L E, Eisenberg E 1982 Evidence for cross-bridge attachment in relaxed muscle at low ionic strength. Proceedings of the National Academy of Sciences (USA) 79:7288

Brenner B, Yu L C, Podolsky R J 1984 X-ray diffraction evidence for cross-bridge formation in relaxed muscle fibers at various ionic strengths. Biophysical Journal 46:299

Brown W E, Salmons S, Whalen R G 1983 The sequential replacement of myosin subunit isoforms during muscle type transformation induced by long term electrical stimulation. Journal of Biological Chemistry 258:14686

Buller A J, Eccles J C, Eccles R M 1960 Interactions between motor neurones and muscles in respect of the characteristic speeds of their responses. Journal of Physiology 150:417

Buller A J, Mommaerts W F H M, Seraydarian K 1969 Enzymatic properties of myosin in fast and slow twitch muscles of the cat following cross-innervation. Journal of Physiology 205:581

Burghardt T P, Tidswell M, Borejdo J 1984 Crossbridge order and orientation in resting single diglycerinated muscle fibres studied by linear dichroism of bound rhodamine labels. Journal of Muscle Research and Cell Motility 5:657

Burley R, Seidel J C, Gergely J 1971 The stoichiometry of the reaction of the spin labeling of F actin and the effect of orientation of spin labeled F actin filaments. Archives of Biochemistry and Biophysics 146:597

Burley R, Seidel J C, Gergely J 1972 The effect of divalent metal binding on the electron spin resonance spectra of spin labeled actin. Evidence for a spin-spin interaction involving Mn^{2+}. Archives of Biochemistry and Biophysics 150:792

Cain D F, Infante A A, Davies R E 1962 Chemistry of muscle contraction. Nature 196:214

Carafoli E 1985 Biochemistry of plasma membrane calcium transporting systems. In: Martonosi A (ed) The enzymes of biological membranes. Plenum Press, New York, p 235

Carlier M F, Pantaloni D, Korn E D 1984 Steady state length distribution of F-actin under controlled fragmentation and mechanism of length redistribution following fragmentation. Journal of Biological Chemistry 259:9987

Carlier M, Pantaloni D, Korn E D 1986 The effects of Mg^{2+} at the high affinity and low affinity sites on the polymerization of actin and associated ATP hydrolysis. Journal of Biological Chemistry 261:10785

Carlson F D, Hardy D J, Wilkie D R 1963 Total energy production and phosphocreatine hydrolysis in the isotonic twitch. Journal of General Physiology 46:851

Carlsson L, Nystrom L-E, Sundkvist I, Markey F, Lindberg J 1977 Actin polymerizability is influenced by profilin, a low molecular weight protein in non-muscle cells. Journal of Molecular Biology 115:465

Caspar D L D, Cohen C, Longley W 1971 Tropomyosin: crystal structure polymorphism and molecular interactions. Journal of Molecular Biology 41:87

Castellani L, Hardwicke P 1983 Crystalline structure of sarcoplasmic reticulum from scallop. Journal of Cell Biology 97:557

Castellani L, Hardwicke P M D, Vibert P 1985 Dimer ribbons in the three-dimensional structure of sarcoplasmic reticulum. Journal of Molecular Biology 185:579

Celio M R, Heizmann C W 1982 Calcium-binding protein parvalbumin is associated with fast contracting muscle fibres. Nature 297:504

Chalovich J M, Chock P B, Eisenberg E 1981 Mechanism of action of troponin-tropomyosin inhibition of actomyosin ATPase activity without inhibition of myosin binding to actin. Journal of Biological Chemistry 256:575

Chalovich J M, Eisenberg E 1982 Inhibition of actomyosin ATPase activity by troponin-tropomyosin without blocking the binding of myosin to actin. Journal of Biological Chemistry 257:2432

Chance B, Leigh J S Jr, Kent J, McCully K 1986 Metabolic control principles and ^{31}P NMR. Federation Proceedings 45:2915

Chaussepied P, Mornet E, Audemard E, Derancourt J, Kassab R 1986a Abolition of ATPase activities of skeletal myosin subfragment 1 by a new selective proteolytic cleavage within the 50 kilodalton heavy chain segment. Biochemistry 25:1134

Chaussepied P, Mornet E, Kassab R 1986b Nucleotide trapping at the ATPase site of myosin subfragment 1 by a new interthiol crosslinking. Proceedings of the National Academy of Sciences (USA) 83:2037

Chen T, Applegate D, Reisler E 1985 Crosslinking of actin to myosin subfragment 1 in the presence of nucleotides. Biochemistry 24:5620

Cheung H, Cooke R, Smith L 1971 The G-actin-F-actin transformation as studied by the fluorescence of bound dansyl cysteine. Archives of Biochemistry and Biophysics 142:333

Cohen C 1985 Hormones, second messengers and the reversible phosphorylation of proteins: an overview. BioEssays 2:63

Cohen C, Szent-Györgyi A G 1957 Optical rotation and helical polypeptide chain configuration in α proteins. Journal of the American Chemical Society 79:248

Cohen C, Holmes K C 1963 X-ray diffraction evidence for α helical coiled coils in native myosins. Journal of Molecular Biology 6:423

Cohen C, Caspar D L D, Parry D A D, Lucas R M 1971 Tropomyosin crystal dynamics. Cold Spring Harbor Symposia on Quantitative Biology 36:205

Cohen P 1978 The role of cyclic AMP-dependent protein kinase in the regulation of glycose metabolism in mammalian skeletal muscle. In: Horecker B L, Stadtman E R (eds) Current topics in cell regulation 1. Academic Press, New York, p 117

Cohen P, Burchell A, Foulkes G, Cohen P T W, Vanaman T C, Nairn A C 1978 Identification of the Ca^{2+}-dependent modulator protein of the fourth sub-unit of rabbit skeletal phosphorylase kinase. Federation of European Biochemical Society Letters, 92:287

Cole H A, Perry S V 1975 The phosphorylation of troponin 1 from cardiac muscle. Biochemical Journal 149:525

Collins J H 1974 Homology of myosin light chains, troponin C and parvalbumin deduced from comparison of their amino acid sequences. Biochemical and Biophysical Research Communications 58:301

Collins J H, Potter J D, Horn M, Wilshire G, Jackman N 1973 Structural studies on rabbit skeletal muscle troponin C: evidence for gene replications and homology with calcium binding proteins from carp and hake muscle. Federation of European Biochemical Society Letters 36:268

Collins J H, Greaser M, Potter J D, Horn M 1977 Determination of the amino acid sequence of troponin C from rabbit skeletal muscle. Journal of Biological Chemistry 252:6356

Constable S H, Favier R J, Holloszy J O 1986 Exercise and glycogen depletion; effects on ability to activate muscle phosphorylase. Journal of Applied Physiology 60:1518

Cooke R 1986 The mechanism of muscle contraction. CRC Critical Reviews in Biochemistry 21:53

Cooke R, Stull J T 1981 Myosin phosphorylation: a biochemical mechanism for regulating contractility. In: Dowben R M, Shay J W (eds) Cell and muscle motility, vol 1. Plenum Press, New York, p 99

Cooke R, Crowder M S, Thomas D D 1982a Orientation of spin labels attached to cross-bridges in contracting muscle fibers. Nature (London) 300:776

Cooke R, Franks K, Stull, J T 1982b Myosin phosphorylation regulates the ATPase activity of permeable skeletal muscle fibers. Federation of European Biochemical Societies 144:33

Cori C F 1941 Phosphorylation of glycogen and glucose. Biological Symposia 5:131

Cori G T, Cori C F 1945 The enzymatic conversion of phosphorylase a to b. Journal of Biological Chemistry 158:321

Coronado R 1986 Recent advances in planar phospholipid bilayer techniques for monitoring ion channels. Annual Review of Biophysics and Biophysical Chemistry 15:259

Costantin L, Franzini-Armstrong C, Podolsky R 1965 Localization of calcium accumulating structures in striated muscle fibers. Science 147:158

Costello B, Chadwick C, Saito A, Chu A, Maurer A, Fleischer S 1986 Characterization of the junctional face membrane from terminal cisternae of sarcoplasmic reticulum. Journal of Cell Biology 103:741

Craig S W, Pollard T D 1982 Actin binding proteins. Trends in Biochemical Sciences 7:88

Crick F H C 1953 The packing of α helices: simple coiled coils. Acta Crystallographica 6:689

Cummins P, Perry S V 1978 Troponin I from human skeletal and cardiac muscles. Biochemical Journal 171:251

d'Albis A, Pantaloni C, Bechett J J 1979 An electrophoretic study of native myosin isozymes and their subunit content. European Journal of Biochemistry 99:297

Darnell J E, Lodish H, Baltimore D 1986 Molecular cell biology. Scientific American Books, New York

Dawson M J 1986 The relation between muscle function and metabolism studied by ³¹P NMR spectroscopy. In: Chen S, Ho C (eds) NMR in biology and medicine. Raven Press, New York p 185

Dawson M J, Gadian D G, Wilkie D R 1978 Muscular fatigue investigated by phosphorus nuclear magnetic resonance. Nature (London) 274:861

Dawson M J, Gadian D G, Wilkie D R 1980 Studies of the biochemistry of contracting and relaxing muscle by the use of ³¹P n.m.r. in conjunction with other techniques. Philosophical Transactions of the Royal Society London (B) 289:445.

Dawson M J, Wilkie D R 1984 Muscle and brain metabolism studied by ³¹P nuclear magnetic resonance. In: Baker P (ed) Recent advances in physiology. Churchill Livingstone, Edinburgh, p 247

DeMeis L, Vianna A L 1979 Energy interconversion by the Ca²⁺-dependent ATPase of the sarcoplasmic reticulum. Annual Review of Biochemistry 48:275

Donaldson S K B 1986 Peeled mammalian skeletal muscle fibers. Journal of General Physiology 86:501

Drabikowski W, Gergely J 1962 The effect of the temperature of extraction on the tropomyosin content in actin. Journal of Biological Chemistry 237:3412

Drabikowski W, Strzelecka-Golaszewska H 1963 The exchange of actin-bound calcium with various bivalent cations. Biochimica et Biophysica Acta 71:486

Drabikowski W, Grabarek Z, Barylko B 1977 Degradation of the TnC component of troponin by trypsin. Biochimica et Biophysica Acta 490:216

Dubowitz V 1967 Cross-innervated mammalian skeletal muscle. Histochemical, physiological and biochemical observations. Journal of Physiology 193:481

Duke J, Takashi R, Eu K, Morales M F 1976 Reciprocal reactivities of specific thiols when actin binds to myosin. Proceedings of the National Academy of Sciences (USA) 73:302

Dux L, Martonosi A 1983 Two dimensional arrays of proteins in sarcoplasmic reticulum and purified Ca²⁺ −ATPase vesicles treated with vanadate. Journal of Biological Chemistry 258:2599

Dux L, Taylor K A, Ting-Beall H P, Martonosi A 1985 Crystallization of the Ca²⁺-ATPase of sarcoplasmic reticulum by calcium and lanthanide ions. Journal of Biological Chemistry 260:11730

Ebashi S 1957 Kielley-Meyerhof's granules and the relaxation of glycerinated muscle fibers. In: Conference on the Chemistry of Muscle Contraction. Igaku Shoin, Tokyo p 89

Ebashi S, 1972 Separation of troponin into three components. Journal of Biochemistry 72:787

Ebashi S, Ebashi F, Fujie Y 1960 The effect of EDTA and its analogues on glycerinated muscle fibers and myosin adenosine triphosphatase. Journal of Biochemistry 47:54

Ebashi S, Lipmann F 1962 Adenosine triphosphate linked concentration of calcium ions in a particulate fraction of rabbit muscle. Journal of Cell Biology 14:389

Ebashi S, Ebashi F, 1964 A new protein component participating in the superprecipitation of myosin B. Journal of Biochemistry 55:604

Ebashi S, Ebashi F, Maruyama K 1964 A new protein factor promoting contraction of actomyosin. Nature 203:645

Ebashi S, Ebashi F 1965 α-actinin: a new structural protein from striated muscle I. Preparation and action on actomyosin ATP interactions. Journal of Biochemistry 58:7

Ebashi S, Kodama A 1965 A new protein factor promoting aggregation of tropomyosin. Journal of Biochemistry 58:107

Ebashi S, Kodama A 1966 Interaction of troponin with F actin in the presence of tropomyosin. Journal of Biochemistry 59:425

Ebashi S, Endo M, 1968 Calcium ion and muscle contraction. Progress in Biophysics and Molecular Biology 18:123

Ebashi S, Endo M, Ohtsuki I 1969 Control of muscle contraction. Quarterly Review of Biophysics 2:351

Eccles J C, Eccles R M, Lundberg A 1958 The action potentials of the α motor neurones supplying fast and slow muscle. Journal of Physiology 142:275

Edwards R H T 1984 New techniques for studying human muscle function, metabolism and fatigue. Muscle and Nerve 7:599

Edwards R H T, Griffiths R D, Cady E B 1985 Topical magnetic resonance for the study of muscle metabolism in human myopathy. Clinical Physiology 5:95

Egelman E H, Francis N, DeRosier D 1982 F-actin is a helix with a random variable twist. Nature (London) 298:131

Egelman E H, Francis N, DeRosier D 1983 Helical disorder and the filament structure of F-actin are elucidated by the angle-layered aggregate. Journal of Molecular Biology 166:605

Eisenberg E, Hill T L 1978 A crossbridge model of muscle contraction. Progress in Biophysics and Molecular Biology 13:55

Eisenberg E, Hill T L 1985 Muscle contraction and free energy transduction in biological systems. Science 227:999

Elliot A, Offer G 1978 Shape and flexibility of the myosin molecule. Journal of Molecular Biology 123:505

El-Saleh S C, Warber K D, Potter J D 1986a The role of tropomyosin-troponin in the regulation of skeletal muscle contraction. Journal of Biological Chemistry 7:387

El-Saleh S C, Potter J D, Solaro R J 1986b Alteration of actin-tropomyosin interaction in 2,4-pentanedione-treated rabbit skeletal myofibrils. Journal of Biological Chemistry 261:14646

Elzinga M, Collins J H 1972 The amino acid sequence of rabbit skeletal muscle actin. Cold Spring Harbor Symposia on Quantitative Biology 37:1

Elzinga M, Collins J H, Kuehl W M, Adelstein R S 1973 The complete amino acid sequence of rabbit skeletal muscle actin. Proceedings of the National Academy of Sciences (USA) 70:2687

Elzinga M, Collins J H 1977 Amino acid sequence of a myosin fragment that contains SH-1, SH-2 and $N^{\tau-}$ methylhistidine. Proceedings of the National Academy of Sciences (USA) 74:4281

Elzinga M, Phelan J J 1984 F-actin is intermolecularly crosslinked by N,N′ -p-phenylenedimaleimide through lysine-191 and cysteine-374. Proceedings of the National Academy of Sciences (USA) 812:6599

Engel A G, Banker B Q (eds) 1986 Myology, basic and clinical. McGraw-Hill, New York

Engelhardt W A, Ljubimova M N 1939 Myosins and adenosinetriphosphatase. Nature 144:668

England P 1976 Studies on the phosphorylation of the inhibitory sub-unit of troponin during modification of contraction in perfused heart. Biochemical Journal 160:295

Fabiato A, Fabiato F 1979 Calcium and cardiac excitation-contraction coupling. Annual Review of Physiology 41:473

Fenn W O 1923 A quantitative comparison between the energy liberated and the work performed by isolated sartorius muscle. Journal of Physiology 58:175

Fenn W O 1924 The relation between the work performed and the energy liberated in muscular contraction. Journal of Physiology 58:373

Fischer E H, Heilmeyer L M G Jr, Haschke R H 1971 Phosphorylase and the control of glycogen degradation. In: Horecker B L, Stadtman E R (eds) Current topics in cell regulation, vol IV. Academic Press, New York, p 211

Flach J, Lindquester G, Berish S, Hickman K, Devlin R 1986 Analysis of tropomyosin cDNAs isolate from skeletal and smooth muscle mRNA. Nucleic Acids Research 14:9193

Flavin M, Ochoa S 1957 Metabolism of propionic acid in animal tissues I. Enzymatic conversion of propionate to succinate. Journal of Biological Chemistry 229:965

Fleckenstein A, Janke J, Davies R E, Krebs H A 1954 Chemistry of muscle contraction. Nature 174:1081

Flicker P F, Phillips G N, Jr, Cohen C 1982 Troponin and its interactions with tropomyosin. Journal of Molecular Biology 162:495

Fowler W E, Aebi U 1983 A consistent picture of the actin filament related to the orientation of the actin molecule. Journal of Cell Biology 97:264

Frank G, Weeds A G 1974 The amino acid sequence of some alkali light chains of rabbit skeletal muscle myosin. European Journal of Biochemistry 44:317

Franzini-Armstrong C, Nunzi G 1983 Junctional feet and particles in the triads of a fast-twitch muscle fibre. Journal of Muscle Research and Cell Motility 4:233

Franzini-Armstrong C, Ferguson D G 1985 Density and disposition of Ca^{2+}-ATPase in sarcoplasmic reticulum membrane as determined by shadowing techniques. Biophysical Journal 48:607

Frieden C 1985 Actin and tubulin polymerisation: the use of kinetic methods to determine mechanism. Annual Review of Biophysics and Biophysical Chemistry 14:189

Frieden C, Lieberman D, Gilbert H R 1980 A fluorescent probe for conformational changes in skeletal muscle G-actin. Journal of Biological Chemistry 255:8991

Frieden C, Patane K 1985 Differences on G-actin containing bound ATP or ADP: The Mg^{2+}-induced conformational change requires ATP. Biochemistry 24:4192

Fritz I B, Davis D G, Holtrop R H, Dundee H 1958 Fatty acid oxidation by skeletal muscle during rest and activity. American Journal of Physiology 194:379

Fujii J, Kodama M, Tada M, Toda H, Sakiyama F 1986 Characterization of structural unit of phospholamban by amino acid sequencing and electrophoretic analysis. Biochemical and Biophysical Research Communications 138:1044

Fujime S 1970 Quasi-elastic light scattering from solutions of macromolecules II. Doppler broadening of light scattered from solutions of semi-flexible polymers, F-actin. Journal of the Physical Society of Japan 29:751

Fujime S, Ishiwata S 1972 Dynamic study of F-actin by quasielastic scattering of laser light. Journal of Molecular Biology 62:251

Funatsu T, Ishiwata S 1985 Characterization of β-actinin: A suppressor of the elongation at the pointed end of thin filaments in skeletal muscle. Journal of Biochemistry (Japan) 98:535

Gazith J S, Himmelfarb S, Harrington W F 1970 Studies on the sub-unit structure of myosin. Journal of Biological Chemistry 245:15

Gergely J 1950 Relation of ATPase and myosin. Federation Proceedings. Federation of American Societies for Experimental Biology 9:176

Gergely J 1953 Studies on myosin-adenosine triphosphatase. Journal of Biological Chemistry 200:543

Gergely J 1956 The interaction betwen actomyosin and adenosine triphosphate. Light scattering studies. Journal of Biological Chemistry 220:917

Gergely J, Gouvea M A, Karibian D 1955 Fragmentation of myosin by chymotrypsin. Journal of Biological Chemistry 212:165

Gergely J, Seidel J 1983 Conformational change and molecular dynamics of myosin. In: Peachey L E, Adrian R H (ed) Skeletal muscle, Handbook of Physiology. American Physiological Society, Bethesda, p 257

Gershman L C, Newman J, Seldon L A, Estes J E 1984 Bound cation exchange affects true lag phase in actin polymerisation. Biochemistry 23:2199

Gilbert C, Kretzschmar K M, Wilkie D R 1972 Work and phosphocreatine splitting during muscular contraction. Cold Spring Harbor Symposia on Quantitative Biology 37:613

Gilbert C, Kretzschmar M, Wilkie D R, Woledge R C 1971 Chemical change and energy output during muscular contraction. Journal of Physiology 218:163

Gillis J M 1985 Relaxation of vertebrate skeletal muscle. A synthesis of the biochemical and physiological approaches. Biochimica et Biophysica Acta 811:1985

Goldman R D, Milsted A, Schloss J A, Starger J, Yerna M J 1979 Cytoplasmic fibers in mammalian cells: cytoskeletal and contractile elements. Annual Review of Physiology 41:703

Gordon A M, Huxley A F, Julian F J 1966 The variation in isometric tension with sarcomere lengths in vertebrate muscle fibers. Journal of Physiology 184:170

Grabarek A, Drabikowski W, Leavis P C, Rosenfeld S S, Gergely J 1981 Proteolytic fragments of troponin C. Journal of Biological Chemistry 256:13121

Grabarek Z, Grabarek J, Leavis P C, Gergely J 1983 Cooperative binding to the Ca^{2+}-specific sites of troponin C in regulated actin and actomyosin. Journal of Biological Chemistry 258:14098

Granger D L, Lazarides E 1978 The existence of an insoluble Z disc scaffold in chicken skeletal muscle. Cell 15:1253

Greaser M, Gergely J 1971 Reconstitution of troponin activity from three protein components. Journal of Biological Chemistry 244:4226

Greaser M, Gergely J 1973 Purification and properties of the components from troponin. Journal of Biological Chemistry 248:2125

Greaser M, Yamaguchi M, Brekke C, Potter J, Gergely J 1972 Troponin subunits and their interactions. Cold Spring Harbor Symposia on Quantitative Biology 37:235

Green D E 1954 Fatty acid oxidation in soluble systems of animal tissues. Biological Reviews 29:330

Greene L E 1986 Cooperative binding of myosin subfragment one to regulated actin as measured by fluorescence changes of troponin I modified with different fluorophores. Journal of Biological Chemistry 26:1279

Greene L E, Eisenberg E 1980 Cooperative binding of myosin subfragment-1 to the actin-troponin-tropomyosin complex. Proceedings of the National Academy of Sciences (USA) 77:2616

Grove B K, Kurer V, Lehner Ch, Doetschman T C, Perriard J-C, Eppenberger H M 1984 A new 185 000 dalton skeletal muscle protein detected by monoclonal antibodies. Journal of Cell Biology 98:518

Guba F, Harsanyi V, Vajda E 1968 The muscle protein fibrillin. Acta Biochimica et Biophysica Acadamiae Scientiarum Hungaricae 3:353

Guth L, Watson P K, Brown W C 1968 Effects of cross reinnervation on some chemical properties of red and white muscles of rat and cat. Experimental Neurology 20:52

Guth L, Wells J B 1976 Physiological and histochemical properties of the soleus muscle after denervation of its antagonists. Experimental Neurology 51:310

Hama H, Maruyama K, Noda H 1965 Direct isolation of F actin from myofibrils and its physicochemical properties. Biochimica et Biophysica Acta 102:149

Hambly B D, Barden J A, Miki M, Dos Remedios C 1986 Structure and functional domains on actin. BioEssays 4:124

Hanson J, Huxley H E 1955 The structural basis of contraction in striated muscle. Symposium of the Society of Experimental Biology 9:228

Hanson J, Huxley H E 1957 Quantitative studies on the structure of cross-striated myofibrils II. Investigations by biochemical techniques. Biochimica et Biophysica Acta 23:250

Hanson J, Lowy J 1963 The structure of F actin and of elements isolated from muscle. Journal of Molecular Biology 6:46

Harrington W F 1979 Origin of the contractile force in skeletal muscle. Proceedings of the National Academy of Sciences (USA) 76:5066

Harrington W F, Rodgers M E 1984 Myosin. Annual Review of Biochemistry 53:35

Hartshorne D J, Mueller H 1968 Fractionation of troponin into two distinct proteins. Biochemical and Biophysical Research Communications 31:647

Hartshorne D J, Theiner M, Mueller H 1969 Studies on troponin. Biochimica et Biophysica Acta 175:320

Hartshorne D J, Dreizen P 1972 Studies on the subunit composition of troponin. Cold Spring Harbor Symposia on Quantitative Biology 37:255

Hartshorne D J, Siemankowski R F 1981 Regulation of smooth muscle actomyosin. Annual Review of Physiology 43:519

Haselgrove J C 1972 X-ray evidence for a conformational change in the actin-containing filaments of vertebrate striated muscle. Cold Spring Harbor Symposia on Quantitative Biology 37:341

Hasselbach W 1979 The sarcoplasmic calcium pump. A model of energy transduction. In: Biological membranes. Current Topics in Chemistry 78:1

Hasselbach W, Makinose M 1961 Die calciumpumpe der erschlaffungs grana des muskels und ihre abhangigheit von der ATP spaltung. Biochemische Zeitschrift 333:518

Hasselbach W, Makinose M 1963 Uber den mechanismus des calcium transportes durch die membranen des sarkoplasmiatchen reticulums. Biochemische Zeitschrift 339:94

Hayashi T 1967 Reactivities of actin as a contractile protein. Journal of General Physiology 50:119

Hayashi T, Ip W 1976 Polymerization polarity of actin. Journal of Mechanochemistry and Cell Motility 3:163

Hegyi G, Szilagyi L, Elzinga H 1986 Photoaffinity labeling of the nucleotide binding site of actin. Biochemistry 25:5793

Heilbrunn L V, Wiercinski F J 1947 The action of various cations on muscle protoplasm. Journal of Cellular and Comparative Physiology 29:15

Heilig A, Pette D 1983 Changes in transcriptional activity of chronically stimulated fast twitch muscle. Federation of European Biochemical Societies 51:211

Heilmann C, Pette D 1979 Molecular transformations in sarcoplasmic reticulum of fast twitch muscle by electro-stimulation. European Journal of Biochemistry 93:437

Herzberg O, James M N G 1985 Structure of the calcium regulatory muscle protein troponin-C at 2.8A resolution. Nature (London) 313:653

Hibberd M G, Dantzig J A, Trentham D R, Goldman Y E 1985 Phosphate release and force generation in skeletal muscle fibers. Science 228:1317

Hibberd M G, Trentham D R 1986 Relationships between chemical and mechanical events during muscular contraction. Annual Review of Biophysics and Biophysical Chemistry 15:119

Hidalgo C, Ikemoto N, Gergely J 1976 Role of phospholipids in the Ca-dependent ATPase of the sarcoplasmic reticulum. Enzymatic and electron spin resonance studies with phospholipid replaced membrane. Journal of Biological Chemistry 250:7219

Hidalgo C, Thomas D D, Ikemoto N 1978 Effect of the lipid environment on protein motion and enzymatic activity of the sarcoplasmic reticulum Ca ATPase. Journal of Biological Chemistry 253:6879

Hidalgo C, Gonzalez M E, Lagos R 1983 Characterization of the Ca^{2+} or Mg^{2+} ATPase of transverse tubule membranes isolated from rabbit skeletal muscle. Journal of Biological Chemistry 258:13937

Highsmith S, Kretzschmar K M, O'Konski C T, Morales M F 1977 Flexibility of the myosin rod, light meromyosin and myosin subfragment 2 in solution. Proceedings of the National Academy of Sciences (USA) 74:4986

Hill A V 1949 Work and heat in a muscle twitch. Proceedings of the Royal Society, Series B, 136:220

Hill A V 1964a The effect of load on the heat of shortening of muscle. Proceedings of the Royal Society, Series B, 159:297

Hill A V 1964b The efficiency of mechanical power development during muscular shortening and its relation to load. Proceedings of the Royal Society, Series B, 159:319

Hill A V 1964c The effect of tension in prolonging the active state in a twitch. Proceedings of the Royal Society, Series B, 159:589

Hill A V 1964d The variation of total heat production in a

twitch with velocity of shortening. Proceedings of the Royal Society, Series B, 159:596

Hill T L 1977 Free energy transduction in biology. The steady-state kinetic and thermodynamic formalism. Academic Press, New York

Hill T L 1980 Bioenergetic aspects and polymer length distribution in steady state head to tail polymerization of actin or microtubules. Proceedings of the National Academy of Sciences (USA) 77:4803

Hill T L 1983 Two elementary models for the regulation of skeletal muscle contraction by calcium. Biophysical Journal 44:383

Hill T L, Simmons R M 1976 Free energy levels and entropy production in muscle contraction and in related solution systems. Proceedings of the National Academy of Sciences (USA) 73:336

Hill T L, Eisenberg E, Greene L 1980 Theoretical model for the cooperative equilibrium binding of myosin subfragment 1 to the actin-troponin-tropomyosin complex. Proceedings of the National Academy of Sciences (USA) 77:3186

Hill T L, Kirschner M W 1982 Bioenergetics and kinetics of microtubule and actin filament assembly-disassembly. International Review of Cytology 78:1

Hitchcock-DeGregori S E 1980 Actin assembly. Nature (London) 288:437

Hochachka P W 1985 Fuels and pathways as designed systems for support of muscle work. Journal of Experimental Biology 115:149

Hoffman R K, Gambke B, Stephenson L W, Rubinstein N A 1985 Myosin transitions in chronic stimulation do not involve embryonic isozymes. Muscle and Nerve 8:796

Hoh J F Y 1978 Light chain distribution of chicken skeletal muscle myosin isoenzymes. Federation of European Biochemical Society Letters 90:297

Hoh J F Y, McGrath P A, Hale P T 1978 Electrophoretic analysis of multiple forms of rat cardiac myosin: Effects of hypophysectomy and thyroxine replacement. Journal of Molecular and Cellular Cardiology 10:1053

Holt J C, Lowey S 1977 Distribution of alkali light chains in myosin: isolation of isozymes. Biochemistry 16:4398

Homsher E 1986 The energetics of contraction. In: Engel A G, Banker B Q (eds) Myology. McGraw-Hill, New York, p 497

Horowits R, Kempner E S, Bisher M E, Podolsky R J 1986 A physiological role for titin and nebulin in skeletal muscle. Nature (London) 323:160

Hoyle G 1967 Diversity of striated muscle. American Zoologist 7:435

Hoyle G, McNeil P A, Selverston A I 1973 Ultrastructure of barnacle giant muscle fibers. Journal of Cell Biology 56:74

Hultman E, Spriet L L, Soderlund K 1986 Biochemistry of muscle fatigue. Biomedica et Biochimica Acta 45:S-97

Huszar G 1975 Tissue-specific biosynthesis of ε-N-monomethyllysine and ε-N-trimethyllysine in skeletal and cardiac muscle myosin: A model for the cell-free study of post-translational amino acid modifications in proteins. Journal of Molecular Biology 94:311

Huxley A F 1957 Muscle structure and theories of contraction. Progress in Biophysics 7:255

Huxley A F 1974 Muscular contraction: review lecture. Journal of Physiology 243:1

Huxley A F 1979 Reflections on muscle. University of Liverpool Press, Liverpool

Huxley A F, Simmons R M 1971 Proposed mechanism of force generation in striated muscle. Nature 233:533

Huxley H E 1960 Muscle cells. In: Brachet J, Mirsky A E (eds) The cell, vol. IV. Academic Press, New York p. 365

Huxley H E 1963 Electron microscope studies on the structure of natural and synthetic protein filaments from striated muscle. Journal of Molecular Biology 7:281

Huxley H E 1968 Structural difference between resting and rigor muscle. Evidence from intensity changes in the low angle equatorial X-ray diagram. Journal of Molecular Biology 37:3542

Huxley H E 1969 The mechanism of muscle contraction. Science 164:1356

Huxley H E 1972 Structural changes in the actin- and myosin-containing filaments during contraction. Cold Spring Harbor Symposia on Quantitative Biology 37:361

Huxley H E, Brown W 1967 The low angle X-ray diagram of vertebrate striated muscle and its behaviour during contraction and rigor. Journal of Molecular Biology 1:30

Huxley H E, Faruqi A R, Kress M, Bordas J, Koch M H J 1982 Time resolved X-ray diffraction studies of the myosin layer-line reflections during muscle contraction. Journal of Molecular Biology 158:637

Huxley H E, Faruqi A R 1983 Time-resolved x-ray diffraction studies on vertebrate striated muscle. Annual Review of Biophysics and Bioengineering 12:381

Huxley H E, Kress M 1985 Crossbridge behaviour during muscle contraction. Journal of Muscle Research and Cell Motility 6:163

Hvidt S, Neatler F H M, Greaser M L, Ferry J D 1982 Flexibility of myosin rod determined from dilute solution viscoelastic measurements. Biochemistry 21:4064

Hvidt S, Chang T, Yu H 1984 Rigidity of myosin and myosin rod by electric birefringence. Bipolymers 23:1283

Ikemoto N 1975 Transporting and inhibitory Ca^{2+}-binding sites on the ATPase enzyme isolated from sarcoplasmic reticulum. Journal of Biological Chemistry 250:7219

Ikemoto N 1976 Behaviour of the Ca^{2+}-transport sites linked with the phosphorylation reaction of ATPase purified from the sarcoplasmic reticulum. Journal of Biological Chemistry 251:7275

Ikemoto N, Sreter F A, Nakamura A, Gergely J 1968 Tryptic digestion and localization of Ca-uptake and ATPase activity in fragments of sarcoplasmic reticulum. Journal of Ultrastructure Research 23:216

Ikemoto N, Bhatnagar G, Gergely J 1971 Fractionation of solubilized sarcoplasmic reticulum. Biochemical and Biophysical Research Communications 44:1510

Ikemoto N, Bhatnagar G, Nagy B, Gergely J 1972 Interaction of divalent cations with the 55000 dalton protein component of the sarcoplasmic reticulum. Studies of fluorescence and circular dichroism. Journal of Biological Chemistry 247:7835

Ikemoto N, Morgan J, Yamada S 1978 Controlled conformational states of the Ca^{2+}-transport enzyme of sarcoplasmic reticulum. Journal of Biological Chemistry 253:8027

Ikemoto N, Antoniu B, Kim D H 1984 Rapid calcium release from the isolated sarcoplasmic reticulum is triggered via the attached transverse tubular system. Journal of Biological Chemistry 259:13151

Inesi G 1985 Mechanism of calcium transport. Annual Review of Physiology 47:573

Inesi G, Millman M, Eletr S 1973 Temperature induced transitions of function structure in sarcoplasmic reticulum membranes. Journal of Molecular Biology 81:483

Ip W, Heuser J 1983 Direct visualization of the myosin crossbridge helices on relaxed rabbit psoas thick filaments. Journal of Molecular Biology 171:105

Irving M 1985 Weak and strong crossbridges. Nature (London) 316:292

Isenberg G, Aebi U, Pollard T D 1980 An actin-binding protein from regulated actin filament polymerization and interactions from Acanthamoeba regulates actin filament polymerization and interactions. Nature (London) 288:455

Ishiwata S, Fujime S 1972 Effect of calcium ions on the flexibility of reconstituted thin filaments of muscle studied by quasi-elastic scattering of laser light. Journal of Molecular Biology 68:511

Iyengar M R, Weber H H 1964 The relative affinities of nucleotides to G actin and their effects. Biochimica et Biophysica Acta 86:543

Jencks W P 1980 The utilization of binding energy in coupled vectorial processes. Advances in Enzymology 51:75

Jencks W P 1983 What is a coupled vectorial process? Current Topics in Membrane and Transport 19:1

Johnson J D, Collins J H, Potter J D 1978 Dansylaziridine-labelled troponin C. A fluorescent probe of Ca^{2+}-binding for the Ca^{2+}-specific regulatory sites. Journal of Biological Chemistry 253:6451

Johnson J D, Charlton S C, Potter J D 1979 A fluorescence stopped-flow analysis of Ca^{2+}-exchange with troponin C. Journal of Biological Chemistry 254:3497

Jolesz F, Sreter F A 1981 Development, innervation and activity pattern induced changes in skeletal muscle. Annual Review of Physiology 43:531

Jorgensen A O, Jones J R 1986 Localization of phospholamban in slow but not fast canine skeletal muscle fibers. An immunocytochemical and biochemical study. Journal of Biological Chemistry 261:3775

Kabsch W, Mannherz H G, Suck D 1985 Three-dimensional structure of the complex of actin and DNase I at 4.5A resolution. European Molecular Biology Organization Journal 4:2113

Kasai M, Nakano F, Oosawa F 1964 Polymerization of actin free from nucleotides and divalent cations. Biochimica et Biophysica Acta 94:494

Kawamoto R M, Brunschwig J-P, Kim K C, Caswell A H 1986 Isolation, characterization and localization of the spanning protein from skeletal muscle triads. Journal of Cell Biology 103:1405

Kawamura M, Maruyama K 1972 Length distribution of F-actin transformed from Mg-polymer. Biochimica et Biophysica Acta 267:422

Kendrick-Jones J, Scholey J M 1981 Myosin linked regulatory systems. Journal of Muscle Research and Cell Motility 2:347

Kensler R W, Stewart M 1983 Frog skeletal muscle thick filaments are three-stranded. Journal of Molecular Biology 96:1797

Kielley W W, Meyerhof O 1948 Studies on adenosinetriphosphate of muscle. II. A new magnesium-activated adenosinetriphosphatase. Journal of Biological Chemistry 176:591

Kielley W W, Meyerhof O 1950 Studies on adenosinetriphosphatase of muscle III. The lipoprotein nature of the magnesium-activated adenosine triphosphatase. Journal of Biological Chemistry 183:391

Kikuchi M, Noda H, Maruyama K 1969 Interaction of actin within H-meromyosin at low ionic strength. Journal of Biochemistry (Japan) 65:945

Klee C B, Vanaman T C 1982 Calmodulin. Advances in Protein Chemistry 35:213

Klug G, Wiehrer W, Reichmann H, Leberer E, Pette D 1983 Relationships between early alterations in parvalbumins, sarcoplasmic reticulum and metabolic enzymes in chronically stimulated fast twitch muscle. Pflugers Archives 399:280

Kondo H, Ishiwata S 1976 Uni-directional growth of F-actin. Journal of Biochemistry (Japan) 79:159

Konno K, Morales M F 1985 Exposure of actin thiols by the removal of tightly held calcium ions. Proceedings of the National Academy of Sciences (USA) 82:7904

Korn, E D 1982 Actin polymerization and its regulation by proteins from nonmuscle cells. Physiological Reviews 62:672

Kovacs L, Rios E, Schneider M E 1979 Calcium transients and intra-membrane charge movement in skeletal muscle fibers. Nature 279:391

Krebs E G 1972 Protein kinases. In: Horecker B L, Stadtman E R (eds) Current Topics in Cell Regulation. Academic Press, New York, p 99

Kress M, Huxley H E, Faruqi A R, Hendrix J 1986 Structural changes during activation of frog muscle studied by time-resolved X-ray diffraction. Journal of Molecular Biology 188:325

Kretsinger R H 1972 Gene triplication deduced from the tertiary structure of a muscle calcium binding protein. Nature 85:240

Kretsinger R H, Nockolds C E 1973 Carp muscle calcium binding protein II. Structure determination and general description. Journal of Biological Chemistry 248:3313

Kretsinger R H, Barry C D 1975 The predicted structure of the calcium-binding component of troponin. Biochimica et Biophysica Acta 405:40

Kuehl W M, Adelstein R S 1970 The absence of 3-methylhistidine in red, cardiac and fetal myosins. Biochemical and Biophysical Research Communications 39:956

Kumagai H, Ebashi S, Takeda F 1955 Essential relaxing factor in muscle other than myokinase and creatine phosphokinase. Nature 176:166

Kushmerick M J, Davies R E 1969 The chemical energetics of muscle contraction II. The chemistry, efficiency and power of maximally working sartorius muscles with an appendix-free energy and enthalpy of ATP hydrolysis in the sarcoplasm. Proceedings of the Royal Society, Series B, 174:315

Kushmerick M J 1983 Energetics of muscle contraction. In: Peachey L D, Adrian R H, Geiger S R (eds) Handbook of physiology. American Physiological Society, Bethesda p 189

Lazarides E, Capetanaki Y G 1986 The striated muscle cytoskeleton: expression and assembly in development. In: Emerson C, Fischman D, Nadal-Ginard B, Siddiqui M A Q (eds) Muscular biology of muscle development. Alan R. Liss, New York, p 749

Leavis P C, Lehrer S S 1974 A sulfhydryl- specific fluorescent label, S-mercuric-N-dansylcysteine. Titrations of glutathione and muscle proteins. Biochemistry 13:3042

Leavis P C, Rosenfeld S, Gergely J, Grabarek Z, Drabikowski W 1978 Proteolytic fragments of troponin C. Localization of high and low affinity Ca^{2+}-binding sites and interactions with troponin I and troponin T. Journal of Biological Chemistry 253:5452

Leavis P C, Gergely J 1984 Thin filament proteins and thin

filament-linked regulation of vertebrate muscle contraction. CRC Critical Reviews in Biochemistry 16:235

Leberer E, Pette D 1986 Neural regulation of parvalbumin expression in mammalian skeletal muscle. Biochemical Journal 235:67

Leff S E, Rosenfeld M G, Evans R M 1986 Complex transcriptional units: diversity in gene expression by alternative RNA processing. Annual Reviews of Biochemistry 55:1091

Lehky P L, Blum H E, Stein E A, Fischer E H 1974 Isolation and characterization of parvalbumins from the skeletal muscle of higher vertebrates. Journal of Biological Chemistry 249:4332

Lehman W, Szent-Györgyi A G 1975 Regulation of muscle contraction. Distribution of actin control and myosin control in the animal kingdom. Journal of General Physiology 66:1

Lehrer S S, Kerwar G 1972 The intrinsic fluorescence of actin. Biochemistry 11:1211

Lehrer S S, Nagy B, Gergely J 1972 The binding of copper to actin without loss of polymerizability. The involvement of the rapidly reacting SH groups. Archives of Biochemistry and Biophysics 150:164

Lehrer S S, Graceffa P, Betteridge D 1981 Conformational dynamics of tropomyosin in solution: evidence for two conformational states. Annals of the New York Academy of Sciences 366:285

Lehrer S S, Morris E 1984 Comparison of the effects of smooth and skeletal tropomyosin on skeletal actomyosin subfragment 1 ATPase. Journal of Biological Chemistry 259:2070

Leloir L F, Cardini L E 1962 UDPG-glycogen transglucosylase. In: Boyer P D, Lardy H, Myrback K (eds) Enzymes, vol V. Academic Press, New York, p 317

LePeuch C J, Halech J, Demaille J G 1979 Concerted regulation of cardiac sarcoplasmic reticulum calcium transport by cyclic adenosine monophosphate dependent and calcium-calmodulin-dependent phosphorylations. Biochemistry 18:5150

Levine B A, Mercola D, Coffman D, Thornton J M 1977 Calcium binding by TnC. A proton magnetic resonance study. Journal of Molecular Biology 115:743

Lipmann F 1941 Metabolic generation and utilization of phosphate bound energy. Advances in Enzymology 1:99

Lompre A M, Mercadier J J, Wismewsky C, Bouveret P, Pantaloni C, d'Albis A, Schwartz K 1981 Species and age dependent changes in the relative amount of cardiac myosin isoenzymes in mammals. Developmental Biology 84:286

Lompre A M, Nadal-Ginard B, Mahdavi B 1984 Expression of the cardiac ventricular α and β myosin heavy chain gene is developmentally and hormonally regulated. Journal of Biological Chemistry 259:6437

Lowey S 1964 Meromyosin substructure: isolation of a helical sub-unit from heavy meromyosin. Science 145:597

Lowey S, Goldstein L, Luck S 1966 Isolation and characterization of a helical sub-unit from heavy meromyosin. Biochemische Zeitschrift 345:248

Lowey S, Risby D 1971 Light chains from fast and slow muscle myosin. Nature 234:81

Lowey S, Slayter H S, Weeds A G, Baker H 1969 Substructure of the myosin molecule I. Subfragments of myosin by enzymic degradation. Journal of Molecular Biology 42:1

Lowey S, Benfield P A, Silberstein L, Lang L M 1979 Distribution of light chains in fast skeletal myosin. Nature (London) 282:522

Lu R C, Szilagyi L 1981 Change of reactivity of lysine residues upon actin polymerization. Biochemistry 20:5914

Lu R C, Moo L, Wong A G 1986 Both the 25-kDa and 50-kDa domains in myosin subfragment 1 are close to the reactive thiols. Proceedings of the National Academy of Sciences (USA) 83:6392

Lundsgaard E 1930 Untersuchungen uber muskelkontraktionen ohne milchsaurebildung. Biochemische Zeitschrift 217:162

Lusty C J, Fasold H 1969 Characterisation of sulfhydryl groups of actin. Biochemistry 8:2933

Lymn R W, Taylor E W 1970 Transient state phosphate production in the hydrolysis of nucleoside triphosphates by myosin. Biochemistry 9:2975

Lymn R W, Taylor E W 1971 Mechanism of adenosine triphosphate hydrolysis by actomyosin. Biochemistry 10:4617

Lynen F, Ochoa S 1953 Enzymes of fatty acid metabolism. Biochimica et Biophysica Acta 12:299

Mabuchi K, Szvetko D, Pinter K, Sreter F A 1982 Type 2B to 2A fiber transformation in intermittently stimulated rabbit muscle. American Journal of Physiology 242:C373

Lymn R W, Taylor E W 1970 Transient state phosphate production in the hydrolysis of nucleoside triphosphates by myosin. Biochemistry 9:2975

Mabuchi K, Szvetko D, Pinter K, Sreter F A 1982 Type 2B to 2A fiber transformation in intermittently stimulated rabbit muscle. American Journal of Physiology 242:C373

McLachlan A D 1984 Structural implications of the myosin amino acid sequence. Annual Review of Biophysics and Bioengineering 13:167

McLachlan A D, Stewart M 1976 The 14-fold periodicity in α-tropomyosin and the interaction with actin. Journal of Molecular Biology 103:271

McLachlan A D, Karn J 1982 Periodic charge distributions in the myosin rod amino acid sequence match cross-bridge spacings in muscle. Nature (London) 299:226

MacLennan D H, Wong P T S 1971 Isolation of a calcium-sequestering protein from sarcoplasmic reticulum. Proceedings of the National Academy of Sciences (USA) 68:1231

MacLennan D H, Brandl C J, Korczak B, Green N M 1985 Amino acid sequence of a Ca^{2+} + Mg^{2+}-dependent ATPase from rabbit muscle sarcoplasmic reticulum deduced from its complementary DNA sequence. Nature (London) 316:6030

Mahmood R, Yount R G 1984 Photochemical probes of the active site of myosin. Irradiation of trapped 3'-0-(4-benzoyl) benzoyl-adenosine 5'-triphosphate labels the 50-kilodalton heavy chain tryptic peptide. Journal of Biological Chemistry 259:12956

Maier A, Gambke B, Pette D 1986 Degeneration-regeneration as a mechanism contributing to the fast to slow conversion of chronically stimulated fast-twitch rabbit muscle. Cell and Tissue Research 244:635

Mak A, Smillie L B, Barany M 1978 Specific phosphorylation at serine 283 of a tropomyosin from rabbit skeletal and cardiac muscle. Proceedings of the National Academy of Sciences (USA) 75:3588

Makinose M 1971 Calcium efflux-dependent formation of ATP from ADP and orthophosphate by the membranes of the sarcoplasmic reticulum vesicles. Federation of European Biochemical Society Letters 12:269

Makinose M, Hasselbach W 1971 ATP synthesis by the reverse of the sarcoplasmic reticulum pump. Federation of European Biochemical Society Letters 12:271

Malhotra A, Huang S, Bhan A 1979 Subunit function in cardiac myosin: effect of removal of LC$_2$ (18 000 M$_r$) on enzymatic properties. Biochemistry 18:461

Marechal G, Mommaerts W F H M 1963 The metabolism of phosphocreatine during an isometric tetanus in the frog sartorius muscle. Biochimica et Biophysica Acta 69:53

Marsh B B 1951 A factor modifying muscle syneresis. Nature 167:1065

Marsh B B 1952 The effects of adenosine triphosphate on the fibre volume of a muscle homogenate. Biochimica et Biophysica Acta 9:247

Marston S B, Taylor E W 1980 Comparison of the myosin and actomysoin ATPase mechanisms of the four types of vertebrate muscles. Journal of Molecular Biology 139:573

Martonosi A 1962 The specificity of the interaction of ATP with G actin. Biochimica et Biophysica Acta 57:163

Martonosi A 1963 The activating effect of phospholipids on the ATPase activity and calcium uptake of fragmented sarcoplasmic reticulum. Biochemical and Biophysical Research Communications 13:273

Martonosi A 1969 The protein composition of sarcoplasmic reticulum membranes. Biochemical and Biophysical Research Communications 36:1039

Martonosi A 1984 Mechanisms of Ca^{2+} release from sarcoplasmic reticulum of skeletal muscle. Physiological Reviews 64:1240

Martonosi A, Gouvea M A, Gergely J 1960a The interaction of C-labelled adenine nucleotides with actin. Journal of Biological Chemistry 235:1700

Martonosi A, Molino C, Gergely J 1960b The binding of divalent cations to actin. Journal of Biological Chemistry 235:1700

Martonosi A, Feretos R 1964 Sarcoplasmic reticulum I. The uptake of calcium by sarcoplasmic reticulum fragments. Journal of Biological Chemistry 239:648

Martonosi A, Donley J, Halpin R A 1968 Sarcoplasmic reticulum III. The role of phospholipids in the adenosine triphosphatase activity of Ca^{2+} transport. Journal of Biological Chemistry 243:61

Maruyama K 1965a A new protein factor hindering network formation of F actin in solution. Biochimica et Biophysica Acta 94:208

Maruyama K 1965b Some physico-chemical properties of β-actinin. Actin factor isolated from striated muscle. Biochimica et Biophysica Acta 102:542

Maruyama K 1971 A study of β-actinin, myofibrillar protein from rabbit skeletal muscle. Journal of Biochemistry (Japan) 69:369

Maruyama K 1986 Connectin, an elastic filamentous protein of striated muscle. International Review of Cytology 104:81

Maruyama K, Ebashi S 1965 α-actinin. A new structural protein from striated muscle. II. Action on actin. Journal of Biochemistry 58:13

Maruyama K, Matsubara S, Natori R et al 1977 Connectin, an elastic protein of muscle, characterization and function. Journal of Biochemistry 82:317

Masaki T, Endo M, Ebashi S 1967 Localization of 6S component of α-actinin at Z-band. Journal of Biochemistry (Tokyo) 62:630

Masaki T, Takaiti O 1974 M-protein. Journal of Biochemistry (Tokyo) 75:367

Medford R M, Nguyen H T, Destree A T, Summers E, Nadal-Ginard B 1984 A novel mechanism of alternative RNA splicing for the developmentaly regulated generation of troponin T isoforms from a single gene. Cell 38:409

Mendelson R A, Morales M F, Botts J 1973 Segmental flexibility of the S-1 moiety of myosin. Biochemistry 12:2250

Metzer J M, Fitts R H 1986 Fatigue from high- and low-frequency muscle stimulation: role of sarcolemma action potentials. Experimental Neurology 93:320

Mickelson J R, Beaudry T M, Louis C F 1985 Regulation of skeletal muscle sarcolemmal ATP-dependent calcium transport by calmodulin and cAMP-dependent protein kinase. Archives of Biochemistry and Biophysics 242:127

Migala A, Agostini B, Hasselbach W 1973 Tryptic fragmentation of the calcium transport system in the sarcoplasmic reticulum. Zeitschrift für Naturforschung 28:178

Mihalyi E, Szent-Györgyi A G 1953 Trypsin digestion of muscle proteins III. Adenosinetriphosphatase activity and actin-binding capacity of the digested myosin. Journal of Biological Chemistry 201:211

Milner-Brown H S, Miller R G 1986 Muscle membrane excitation and impulse propagation velocity are reduced during muscle fatigue. Muscle and Nerve 9:367

Mitchell P 1977 Vectorial chemiosmotic processes. Annual Review of Biochemistry 46:966

Moir A J G, Cole H A, Perry S V 1977 The phosphorylation sites of troponin T from white skeletal muscle and the effects of interaction with troponin C on their phosphorylation by phosphorylase kinase. Biochemical Journal 161:371

Mommaerts W F H M 1952 The molecular transformation of actin. III. The participation of nucleotides. Journal of Biological Chemistry 198:469

Mommaerts W F H M 1954 Is adenosine triphosphate broken down during a single muscle twitch? Nature 174:1081

Mommaerts W F H M 1955 Investigation of the presumed breakdown of adenosine triphosphate and phosphocreatine during a single muscle twitch. American Journal of Physiology 182:585

Mommaerts W F H M 1970 What is the Fenn effect? Naturwissenchaften 57:326

Mommaerts W F H M, Seraydarian K, Marechal G 1962 Work and chemical changes in isotonic muscle contraction. Biochimica et Biophysica Acta 57:1

Moore P B, Huxley H E, DeRosier D J 1970 Three dimensional reconstruction of F actin, thin filaments and decorated thin filaments. Journal of Molecular Biology 50:279

Morales M F, Borejdo J, Botts J, Cooke R, Mendelson R A, Takashi R 1982 Some physical studies of the contractile mechanism in muscle. Annual Review of Physical Chemistry 33:319

Morimoto K, Harrington W F 1972 Isolation and physical chemical properties of an M-line protein from skeletal muscle. Journal of Biological Chemistry 247:3052

Mornet D R, Bertrand P, Pantel E, Audemard E, Kassab R 1981 Structure of the actin–myosin interface. Nature (London) 292:301

Mornet D, Ue K 1984 Proteolysis and structure of skeletal muscle actin. Proceedings of the National Academy of Sciences (USA) 81:3680

Mornet D, Ue K, Morales M F 1984 Proteolysis and the

domain organization of myosin subfragment 1. Proceedings of the National Academy of Sciences (USA) 1:736

Mornet D, Ue K, Morales M F 1985 Stabilization of a primary loop in myosin subfragment 1 with a fluorescent crosslinker. Proceedings of the National Academy of Sciences (USA) 82:1658

Moss R L, Allen J D, Greaser M L 1986 Effects of partial extraction of troponin complex upon the tension-pCa relation in rabbit skeletal muscle. Further evidence that tension development involves cooperative effects within the thin filament. Journal of General Physiology 87:751

Mueller H, Perry S V 1962 The degradation of heavy meromyosin by trypsin. Biochemical Journal 85:431

Muhlrad A, Morales M F 1984 Isolation and partial renaturation of proteolytic fragments of the myosin head. Proceedings of the National Academy of Sciences (USA) 81:1003

Muhlrad A, Kasprzak A A, Ue K, Ajtai K, Burghardt T P 1986 Characterization of the isolated 20 kDa and 50 kDa fragments of the myosin head. Biochimica et Biophysica Acta 869:128

Muntener M, Rowlerson A M, Berchtold M W, Heizmann C W 1987 Changes in the concentration of the calcium-binding parvalbumin in cross-reinnervated rat muscles. Journal of Biological Chemistry 262:465

Nabeshima Y, Kurajama-Fuji Y, Muramatsu M, Ogata K 1984 Alternative transcription and two modes of splicing result in two myosin light chains from one gene. Nature (London) 308:1984

Nadal-Ginard B, Medford R M, Nguyen H T et al 1982 Structure and regulation of a mammalian sarcomeric myosin heavy chain gene. In: Pearson M L, Epstein H F (eds) Muscle development. Cold Spring Harbor Laboratories, Cold Spring Harbor, p 143

Nadal-Ginard B, Breitbart R E, Strehler E E, Ruiz-Opazo N, Periasamy M, Mahdavi V 1986 Alternative splicing: a common mechanism for the generation of contractile protein diversity from single genes. In: Emerson C, Fischman D, Nadal-Ginard B, Siddiqui M A Q (eds) Molecular biology of muscle development. UCLA Symposium on Molecular and Cellular Biology, vol 29. Alan R. Liss, New York, p 387

Nagashima H, Asakura S 1980 Dark-field light microscopic study of the flexibility of F-actin complexes. Journal of Molecular Biology 136:169

Nagano H, Yanagida T 1984 Predominant attached state of myosin cross-bridges during contraction and relaxation at low ionic strength. Journal of Molecular Biology 177:769

Nagy B, Jencks W P 1962 Optical rotatory dispersion of G-actin. Biochemistry 1:987

Natori R 1954 The property and contraction process of isolated myofibrils. Jikei Medical Journal. 1:119

Needham D M 1971 Machina carnis. University of Cambridge Press, Cambridge

Needham J, Chen S L, Needham D M, Lawrence A S G 1941 Myosin birefringence and adenylpyrophosphate. Nature 147:766

Newton A A, Perry S V 1960 The incorporation of ^{15}N into adenine nucleotides and their formation from inosine monophosphate by skeletal muscle preparations. Biochemical Journal 74:127

Niedl C, Engel J 1979 Exchange of ADP, ATP and 1:N6-ethenoadenosine 5′-triphosphate at G-actin. European Journal of Biochemistry 101:163

O'Brien E J, Couch J, Johnson G R P, Morris E P 1983 In:

dos Remedios C, Barden J A (eds), Structure of actin and the thin filament, In actin. Academic Press, Sydney, p 3

Ochs R S 1986 Inositol trisphosphate and muscle. Trends in Biochemical Sciences 11:388

Offer G 1972 C-protein and the periodicity in the thick filaments of vertebrate skeletal muscle. Cold Spring Harbor Symposia on Quantitative Biology 37:87

Offer G 1974 The molecular basis of muscular contraction. In: Bull A T, Lagnado J R, Thomas J O, Tipton K F (eds) Companion to biochemistry. Longmans, London, p 623

Offer G, Moos C, Starr R 1973 A new protein of the thick filaments of vertebrate skeletal myofibrils. Journal of Molecular Biology 74:653

Ohtsuki I 1979 Molecular arrangement of troponin T in the thin filament. Journal of Biochemistry (Tokyo) 86:491

Okamoto Y, Yount R G 1985 Identification of an active site peptide of skeletal myosin after photoaffinity labelling with N-(4-azido-2-nitrophenyl)-2-aminoethyl diphosphate. Proceedings of the National Academy of Sciences (USA) 82:1575

Oosawa F, Asakura S, Hotta K, Imai N, Ooi T 1959 G-F transformation of actin as a fibrous condensation. Journal of Polymer Science 37:323

Oosawa F, Kasai M 1971 Actin. In: Timasheff S, Fasman G (eds) Subunits in biological systems. Marcel Dekker, New York, p 5, 261

Oosawa F, Asakura S 1975 Thermodynamics of the polymerization of protein. Academic Press, London

Ostwald T J, MacLennan D H 1974 Isolation of a high affinity calcium-binding protein from sarcoplasmic reticulum. Journal of Biological Chemistry 249:974

Padgett R, Grabowski P J, Konarska M M, Seiler S, Sharp P A 1986 Splicing of messenger RNA precursors. Annual Review of Biochemistry 55:1119

Page S, Huxley H E 1963 Filament lengths in striated muscle. Journal of Cell Biology 19:369

Parry D A D 1975 Analysis of the primary sequence of α-tropomyosin from rabbit skeletal muscle. Journal of Molecular Biology 98:519

Parry D A D, Squire J M 1973 Structural role of tropomyosin in muscle regulation. Analysis of X-ray diffraction patterns from relaxed and contracting muscles. Journal of Molecular Biology 75:33

Pastra-Landis S C, Huiatt T, Lowey S 1983 Assembly and kinetic properties of myosin light chain isozymes from fast skeletal muscle. Journal of Molecular Biology 170:403

Pearlstone J R, Carpenter M R, Johnson P, Smillie L B 1976 Amino acid sequence of tropomyosin binding component of rabbit skeletal muscle troponin. Proceedings of the National Academy of Sciences (USA) 73:1902

Pease D C, Jenden D J, Howell J N 1965 Calcium uptake in glycerol-extracted rabbit psoas muscle fibres. Journal of Cellular and Comparative Physiology 65:141

Pepe F A 1966 Some aspects of the structural organisation of the myofibril as revealed by antibody-staining methods. Journal of Cell Biology 28:505

Pepe F A 1967a The myosin filament. I. Structural organisation from antibody staining observed in electron microscopy. Journal of Molecular Biology 27:203

Pepe F A 1967b The myosin filament II. Interaction between myosin and actin filaments observed during antibody staining in fluorescent and electron microscopy. Journal of Molecular Biology 27:227

Pepe F A 1972 The myosin filament: immunochemical and

ultrastructural approaches to molecular organisation. Cold Spring Harbor Symposia on Quantitative Biology 37:97

Periasamy M, Strehler E E, Garfinkel L I, Gubits R M, Ruiz-Opazo N, Nadal-Ginard B 1984 Fast skeletal muscle myosin light chains 1 and 3 are produced from a single gene by a combined process of differential RNA transcription and splicing. Journal of Biological Chemistry 259:13595

Perkins W J, Weiel J, Grammer J, Yount R G 1984 Introduction of a donor-acceptor pair by a single protein modification. Journal of Biological Chemistry 259:8786

Perry S V 1951 The adenosinetriphosphatase activity of myofibrils isolated from skeletal muscle. Biochemical Journal 48:257

Perry S V, Grey T C 1956 A study of the effects of substrate concentration and certain relaxing factors on magnesium-activated myofibrillar adenosine triphosphatase. Biochemical Journal 64:184

Persechini A, Stull J T, Cooke R 1985 The effect of myosin phosphorylation on the contractile properties of skinned rabbit skeletal muscle fibers. Journal of Biological Chemistry 260:7951

Pette D 1984 Activity induced fast to slow transition in mammalian muscle. Medicine and Science in Sports and Exercise 16:517

Pette D, Smith M E, Staudte H W, Vrbová G 1973 Effects of long-term electrical stimulation on some contractile and metabolic characteristics of fast rabbit muscle. Pflügers Archiv für die gesamte Physiologie des Menschen und der Tiere 338:257

Pette D, Schnez U 1977 Co-existence of fast and slow type myosin light chains in single muscle fibers during transformation as induced by long-term stimulation. Federation of European Biochemical Society Letters 83:128

Phillips G N, Fillers J P, Cohen C 1986 Tropomyosin crystal structure and muscle regulation. Journal of Molecular Biology 192:111

Pires E, Perry S V, Thomas M A W 1974 Myosin light chain kinase. A new enzyme from striated muscle. Federation of European Biochemical Society Letters 41:292

Pluskal M, Sreter F A 1983 Correlation between protein phenotype and gene expression in adult rabbit fast twitch muscles undergoing a fast to slow fiber type transformation in response to electrical stimulation in vivo. Biochemical and Biophysical Research Communications 113:325

Podolsky R J, Costantin L L 1964 Regulation by calcium of the contraction and relaxation of muscle fibres. Federation Proceedings. Federation of American Societies for Experimental Biology 23:933

Pollack G H 1983 The cross-bridge theory. Physiological Reviews 63:1049

Pollard T D, Mooseker M S 1981 Direct measurement of actin polymerization rate constants by electron microscopy of actin filaments nucleated by isolated microvillus cores. Journal of Cell Biology 80:654

Pollard T D, Cooper J A 1986 Actin and actin binding protein. A critical evaluation of mechanism and function. Annual Review of Biochemistry 55:987

Potter J D, Gergely J 1974 Troponin, tropomyosin and actin interactions in the Ca^{2+} regulation of muscle contraction. Biochemistry 13:2697

Potter J D, Seidel J C, Leavis P, Lehrer S S, Gergely J 1976 The effect of Ca^{2+}-binding on troponin C. Changes in spin label mobility, extrinsic fluorescence and SH reactivity. Journal of Biological Chemistry 251:7551

Price H M, Gordon J M, Pearson C M, Munsat T C, Blumberg J M 1965 New evidence for excessive accumulation of Z band material in nemaline myopathy. Proceedings of the National Academy of Sciences (USA) 54:1398

Privalov P L 1982 Stability of proteins. Proteins which do not present a single cooperative system. Advances in Protein Chemistry 35:1

Radda G K 1986a The use of NMR spectroscopy for the understanding of disease. Science 233:640

Radda G K 1986b Control of bioenergetics: from cells to man by phosphorus nuclear magnetic resonance spectroscopy. Biochemical Society Transactions 14:517

Ray K P, England P J 1976 Phosphorylation of the inhibitory subunit of troponin and its effect on the calcium dependence of cardiac myofibril adenosine triphosphatase. Federation of European Biochemical Societies 70:11

Rayment I, Winkelmann D A 1984 Crystallization of myosin subfragment 1. Proceedings of the National Academy of Sciences (USA) 81:4378

Reisler E, Burke M, Himmelfarb S, Harrington W F 1974 Spacial proximity of two essential SH groups of myosin. Biochemistry 13:3837

Rich S A, Estes J E 1976 Detection of conformational changes in actin by proteolytic digestion: evidence for a new monomeric species. Journal of Molecular Biology 104:777

Robert B, Barton P, Alonso S et al 1986 The structure and organization of actin and myosin genes and their expression in mouse striated muscle. In: Emerson C, Fischman D, Nadal-Ginard B, Siddiqui M A Q (eds) Molecular biology of muscle development. Alan Liss, New York, p 487

Robert B, Daubas P, Akimenko M A, Cohen A, Garner I, Guenet J L, Buckingham M E 1984 A single locus in the mouse encodes both myosin light chains 1 and 3; a second locus corresponds to a related pseudogene. Cell 39:129

Robinson G A, Butcher R W, Sutherland E W 1971 Cyclic AMP. Academic Press, New York

Romanual F C, Van der Meulen J P 1967 Slow and fast muscles after cross innervation. Archives of Neurology 17:387

Romanul F C A, Sreter F A, Salmons S, Gergely J 1974 The effect of a changed pattern of activity on histochemical characteristics of muscle fibers. In: Milhorat A T (ed) Exploratory concepts in muscular dystrophy. Elsevier, Amsterdam, p 344

Rosenfeld S S, Taylor E W 1984 The ATPase mechanism of skeletal and smooth muscle acto-subfragment 1. Journal of Biological Chemistry 259:11908

Rosenfeld S S, Taylor E W 1985 Kinetic studies of calcium binding to regulatory complexes from skeletal muscle. Journal of Biological Chemistry 260:252

Roy R, Sreter F A, Sarkar S 1979 Changes in tropomosin sub-units and myosin light chains during development of chicken and rabbit striated muscle. Developmental Biology 69:15

Rubinstein N, Mabuchi K, Pepe F, Salmons S, Sreter F 1978 Use of type-specific antimyosins to demonstrate the transformation of individual fibers in chronically stimulated rabbit fast muscles. Journal of Cell Biology 79:252

Ruiz-Opazo, N, Weinberger J, Nadal-Ginard B 1985 Comparison of α tropomyosin sequences from smooth and striated muscle. Nature (London) 315:67

Salmons S, Sreter F A 1976 Impulse activity in the transformation of skeletal muscle type. Nature 263:30

Salmons S, Vrbová G 1969 The influence of activity on some contractile characteristics of mammalian fast and slow muscle. Journal of Physiology 201:535

Samaha F J, Theis W H 1976 Actomyosin changes in muscle with altered function. Experimental Neurology 51:310

Sarkar S 1972 Stoichiometry and sequential removal of light chains of myosin. Cold Spring Harbor Symposia on Quantitative Biology 37:14

Sarkar S, Sreter F A, Gergely J 1971 Light chains of myosins from fast, slow and cardiac muscles. Proceedings of the National Academy of Sciences (USA) 68:946

Schaub M C, Hartshorne D J, Perry S V 1967 The adenosine triphosphatase activity of desensitised actomyosin. Biochemical Journal 104:263

Schaub M C, Perry S V 1969 The relaxing protein system of striated muscle. Resolution of the troponin complex into inhibitory and calcium ion sensitising factors and their relationship to tropomyosin. Biochemical Journal 115:993

Schliwa M 1981 Proteins associated with cytoplasmic actin. Cell 25:57

Schneider M F 1981 Membrane charge movement and depolarization-contraction coupling. Annual Review of Physiology 43:507

Schneider M F, Chandler W K 1973 Voltage dependent charge movement in skeletal muscle: a possible step in excitation-contraction coupling. Nature 242:244

Seamon K B, Hartshorne D J, Bothner-by A A 1977 Ca^{2+} and Mg^{2+} conformations of TnC as determined by ^1H and ^{19}F nuclear magnetic resonance. Biochemistry 16:4039

Seidel J C 1967 Studies on myosin from red and white skeletal muscles of the rabbit. II. Inactivation of myosin from red muscle under mild alkaline conditions. Journal of Biological Chemistry 242:5623

Selden L A, Gershman L C, Estees J E 1986 A kinetic comparison between Mg-actin and Ca-actin. Journal of Muscle Research and Cell Motility 7:215

Selve N, Wegner A 1986 Rate of treadmilling of actin filaments in vitro. Journal of Molecular Biology 187:627.

Seymour J, O'Brien E J 1980 The position of tropomyosin in muscle thin filaments. Nature 283:680

Sherry J M F, Gorecka A, Aksoy M O, Dabrowska R, Hartshorne D J 1978 Roles of calcium and phosphorylation in the regulation of the activity of gizzard myosin. Biochemistry 17:4411

Shy G M, Engel W K, Somers J E, Wanko T 1963 Nemaline myopathy: new congenital myopathy. Brain 86:793

Siemankowski R F, White H D 1984 Kinetics of the interaction between actin, ADP, and cardiac myosin-Sl. Journal of Biological Chemistry 259:5045

Simmerman H K B, Collins J H, Theibert J L, Wegener L R, Jones R L 1986 Sequence analysis of phospholamban. Identification of phosphorylation sites and two major structural domains. Journal of Biological Chemistry 261:13333

Sinha A M, Friedman D J, Nigro J M. Jakovcic S, Rabinowitz M, Umeda P K 1984 Expression of rabbit ventricular α-myosin heavy chain messenger RNA sequences in atrial muscle. Journal of Biological Chemistry 259:6674

Smith J S, Coronado R, Meissner G 1986 Single channel measurements of the calcium release channel from skeletal muscle sarcoplasmic reticulum. Journal of General Physiology 88:573

Smith P R, Fowler W E, Pollard T E, Aebi U 1983 Structure of the actin molecule determined from the electron micrographs of crystalline actin sheets with a tentative alignment of the molecule in the actin filament. Journal of Molecular Biology 167:641

Smith P R, Fowler W E, Aebi U 1984 Towards an alignment of the actin molecule within the actin filament. Ultramicroscopy 13:113

Sodek J, Hodges R S, Smillie L B, Jurasek L 1972 Amino-acid sequence of rabbit skeletal tropomyosin and its coiled-coil structure. Proceedings of the National Academy of Sciences (USA) 69:3800

Solaro R J, Moir A J G, Perry S V 1976 Phosphorylation of troponin I and the inotropic effect of adrenalin in the perfused rabbit heart. Nature (London) 262:615

Somlyo A P 1985 The messenger across the gap. Nature (London) 316:298

Somlyo A V, Bond M, Somlyo A P, Scarpa A 1985 Inositol-triphosphate lnsP₃ induced calcium release and contraction in vascular smooth muscle. Proceedings of the National Academy of Sciences (USA) 82:5231

Spudich J A, Huxley H E, Finch J T 1972 Regulation of skeletal muscle contraction II. Structural studies of the interaction of the tropomyosin-troponin complex with actin. Journal of Molecular Biology 72:619

Spudich J A, Watt S 1971 The regulation of rabbit skeletal muscle contraction I. Biochemical studies of the interaction of the tropomyosin-troponin complex with actin and the proteolytic fragments of myosin. Journal of Biological Chemistry 246:4866

Squire J 1981 The structural basis of muscle contraction. Plenum Press, New York

Sreter F A, Gergely J, Luff A L 1974 The effect of cross reinnervation on the synthesis of myosin light chains. Biochemical and Biophysical Research Communications 56:84

Sreter F A, Gergely J, Salmons S, Romanul F 1973 Synthesis by fast muscle of myosin light chains characteristic of slow muscle in response to long-term stimulation. Nature 241:17

Sreter F A, Seidel J C, Gergely J 1966 Studies on myosin from red and white skeletal muscle of the rabbit. I. adenosine triphosphate activity. Journal of Biological Chemistry 241:5772

Starr R, Offer G 1978 Interaction of C protein with heavy meromyosin and subfragment 2. Biochemical Journal 71:813

Starr R, Offer G 1983 H-protein and X-protein. Two new components of the thick filaments of vertebrate skeletal muscle. Journal of Molecular Biology 170:675

Stein L A, Chock P B, Eisenberg E 1984 The rate limiting step in the actomyosin adenosinetriphosphatase cycle. Biochemistry 23:1555

Stein L A, Greene L E, Chock P B, Eisenberg E 1985 Rate-limiting step in the actomyosin adenosinetriphosphatase cycle: studies with myosin subfragment 1 crosslinked to actin. Biochemistry 24:1357

Stewart M, McLachlan A D 1975 Fourteen actin-binding sites on tropomyosin? Nature (London) 257:331

Stewart P S, MacLennan D H 1974 Surface particles of sarcoplasmic reticulum membranes. Structural features of the ATPase. Journal of Biological Chemistry 249:985

Stone D B, Prevost S C, Botts J 1970 Studies on spin labeled actin. Biochemistry 9:3937

Stone D, Smillie L B 1978 The amino acid sequence of

rabbit skeletal α-tropomyosin. The NH$_2$- terminal half and complete sequence. Journal of Biological Chemistry 253:1137

Stone D, Sodek J, Johnson P, Smillie L B 1974 Tropomyosin: Correlation of amino acid sequence and structure. In: Biro N A (ed) Proteins of the contractile system vol. 31. Proceedings of the IX Federation of European Biochemical Society Meeting. Akad. Kiado, Budapest, p 125

Strasburg G M, Leavis P C, Gergely J 1985 Troponin C mediated calcium sensitive changes in the conformation of troponin I detected by pyrene excimer fluorescence. Journal of Biological Chemistry 260:366

Straub F B, 1942 Actin. In: Studies for the Institute of Medical Chemistry. University of Szeged, Vol. II p 3

Straub F B, Feuer G 1950 Adenodinetriphosphate: the functional group of actin. Biochimica et Biophysica Acta 4:455

Strehler E E, Carlsson E, Eppenberger H M, Thornell L E 1983 Ultrastructural localization of M-band proteins in chicken breast muscle as revealed by combined immunochemistry and ultramicrotomy. Journal of Molecular Biology 166:141

Strzelecka-Golaszewska H 1973 Relative affinities of divalent cations to the site of the tight Ca-binding in G-actin. Biochimica et Biophysica Acta 310:60

Strzelecka-Golaszewska H, Prochniewicz E, Drabikowski W 1978 Interaction of actin with divalent cations II. Characterization of protein metal complexes. European Journal of Biochemistry 88:229

Suck D, Kabsch W, Mannherz H G 1981 Three dimensional structure of the complex of skeletal muscle actin and bovine pancreatic DNase I at 6A resolution. Proceedings of the National Academy of Sciences (USA) 78:4319

Sundaralingam M, Bergstrom R, Strasburg G, Rao S T, Roychowdhury P 1985 Molecular structure of troponin C from chicken skeletal muscle at 3-angstrom resolution. Science 227:945

Sutoh K 1984 Actin–actin and actin–deoxyribonuclease I contact sites in the actin sequence. Biochemistry 23:1942

Sugita H, Masaki T, Ebashi S, Pearson C 1974 Staining of nemaline rod by fluorescent antibody against 10s-actin. Proceedings of the Japan Academy 50:237

Sutoh K, Sutoh K, Karr T, Harrington W F 1978 Isolation and physicochemical properties of a high molecular weight subfragment 2 of myosin. Journal of Molecular Biology 126:1

Sutoh K, Yamamoto K, Wakabayashi T 1984 Electron microscopic visualization of the SH 1 thiol of myosin by the use of an avidin–biotin system. Journal of Molecular Biology 178:323

Sutoh K, Yamamoto K, Wakabayashi T 1986 Electron microscopic visualization of the ATPase site of myosin by photoaffinity labeling with a biotinylated photoreactive ADP analog. Proceedings of the National Academy of Sciences (USA) 83:212

Suzuki A, Goll D E, Singh I, Allen R E, Robson R M, Stromer M H 1976 Some properties of purified skeletal α-actinin. Journal of Biological Chemistry 251:6860

Swynghedauw B 1986 Developmental and functional adaptation of contractile proteins in cardiac and skeletal muscles. Physiological Reviews 66:710

Szent-Györgyi A 1945 Studies on muscle. Acta Physiologica Scandinavica, Suppl XXV

Szent-Györgyi A 1949 Free energy relations and contraction of actomyosin. Biological Bulletin, Marine Biological Laboratory, Woods Hole, Mass 96:140

Szent-Györgyi A G 1953 Meromyosins, the sub-units of myosin. Archives of Biochemistry 42:305

Szilagyi L, Balint M, Sreter F A, Gergely J 1979 Photoaffinity labelling with an ATP analog of the N-terminal peptide of myosin. Biochemical and Biophysical Research Communications 87: 936

Tada M, Kirchenberger M A, Repke D I, Katz A M 1974 The stimulation of calcium transport in cardiac sarcoplasmic reticulum by adenosine 3′–5′ monophosphate dependent protein kinase. Journal of Biological Chemistry 249:6174

Tada M, Kirchenberger M A, Katz A 1975 Phosphorylation of a 22 000 dalton component of the cardiac sarcoplasmic reticulum by adenosine 3′:5′-monophosphate dependent protein kinase. Journal of Biological Chemistry 250:2640

Tada M, Inui M 1983 Regulation of calcium transport by the ATPase-phospholamban system. Journal of Molecular and Cellular Cardiology 15:565

Tada M, Yamamoto T, Tonomura Y 1978 Molecular mechanism of active calcium transport by sarcoplasmic reticulum. Physiological Reviews 58:1

Takebayashi T, Morita T, Oosawa F 1977 Electron microscopic investigation of the flexibility of F-actin. Biochimica et Biophysica Acta 492:357

Tanford C 1983 Mechanism of free energy coupling in active transport. Annual Review of Biochemistry 52:379

Tanford C 1984 Twenty questions concerning the reaction cycle of the sarcoplasmic reticulum calcium pump. CRC Critical Reviews in Biochemistry 17:123

Tao T, Cho J 1979 Fluorescence lifetime quenching studies on the accessibilies of actin sulfhyldryl sites. Biochemistry 18:2759

Tao T, Lamkin M 1981 Excitation energy transfer studies on the proximity between Sh1 and the adenosine-triphosphatase site in myosin subfragment 1. Biochemistry 20:5051

Tao T, Gong B-J, Leavis P C 1987 Troponin-I as a molecular switch in calcium regulation of skeletal muscle contraction: Resonance energy transfer and site-specific photocrosslining sites. Biophysical Journal 51:27a

Taylor D L, Reidler J, Spudich J A, Stryer L 1981 Detection of actin assembly by fluorescence energy transfer. Journal of Cell Biology 89:362

Taylor E W 1979 Mechanism of actomyosin ATPase and the problem of muscle contraction. Critical Reviews in Biochemistry 6:103

Taylor K A, Amos L A 1981 A new model for the geometry of the binding of myosin crossbridges to muscle thin filaments. Journal of Molecular Biology 147:297

Taylor K A, Dux L, Martonosi A 1986 Three-dimensional reconstruction of negatively stained crystals of the Ca^{2+}-ATPase from muscle sarcoplasmic reticulum. Journal of Molecular Biology 187:417

Thomas D D, Seidel J C, Hyde J S, Gergely J 1975 Motion of the S-1 segment in myosin: Its proteolytic fragments and its supramolecular complexes: saturation transfer electron spin resonance. Proceedings of the National Academy of Sciences (USA) 72:1729

Thomas D D, Seidel J C, Gergely J 1979 Rotational dynamics of spin labelled F actin in the submillisecond time range. Journal of Molecular Biology 132:257

Thomas D D, Cooke R 1980 Orientation of spin labeled myosin heads in glycerinated muscle fibers. Biophysical Journal 32:981

Thorley-Lawson D A, Green N M 1973 Studies on the location and orientation of proteins on the sarcoplasmic reticulum. European Journal of Biochemistry 40:403

Toyoshima C, Wakabayashi T 1984a Three-dimensional image analysis of the complex of thin filaments and myosin molecules from skeletal muscle. IV. Reconstitution from minimal- and high-dose images of the actin–tropomyosin–myosin subfragment-I complex. Journal of Biochemistry (Japan) 97:219

Toyoshima C, Wakabayashi T 1984b Three-dimensional image analysis of the complex of thin filaments and myosin molecules from skeletal muscle. V. Assignment of actin in the actin–tropomyosin–myosin subfragment-1 complex. Journal of Biochemistry (Japan) 97:245

Trinick J, Lowey S 1977 M-protein from chicken pectoralis muscle: isolation and characterization. Journal of Molecular Biology 113:343

Trinick J, Cooper J, Seymour J, Egelman E H 1986 Cryo-electron microscopy and three dimensional reconstruction of actin filaments. Journal of Microscopy 86:349

Trybus K M, Taylor E W 1981 Kinetic studies of the cooperative binding of subfragment 1 to regulated actin. Proceedings of the National Academy of Sciences (USA) 77:7209

Turner D C, Walliman T, Eppenberger H 1973 A protein that binds specifically to the M-line of skeletal muscle is identified as the muscle form of creatine kinase. Proceedings of the National Academy of Sciences (USA) 70:702

Ueno H, Harrington W F 1981 Conformational transition in the myosin hinge upon activation of muscle. Proceedings of the National Academy of Sciences (USA) 78:6101

Ueno H, Harrington W F 1986a Temperature dependence of local melting in the myosin subfragment 2 region of the rigor crossbridge. Journal of Molecular Biology 190:59

Ueno H, Harrington W F 1986b Local melting in the subfragment 2 region of myosin in activated muscle and its correlation with contractile force. Journal of Molecular Biology 190:69

Vanderkerckhove J, Weber K 1984 Chordate muscle actins differ distinctly from invertebrate muscle actins. Journal of Molecular Biology 179:391

Varriano-Marston E, Franzini-Armstrong C, Haselgrove J C 1984 The structure and disposition of crossbridges in deep-etched fish muscle. Journal of Muscle Research and Cell Motility 5:351

Venkatasubramanian P N, Arus C, Bárány M 1986 Two-dimensional protein magnetic resonance of human muscle extracts. Clinical Physiology and Biochemistry 4:285

Vergara J, Tsien R Y, Delay M 1985 Inositol 1,4,5-triphosphate: A possible chemical link in excitation–contraction coupling in muscle. Proceedings of the National Academy of Sciences (USA) 82:6352

Volpe P, Salviati G, DiVirgilio F, Pozzan T 1985 Inositol 1,4,5-trisphosphate induces calcium release from sarcoplasmic reticulum of skeletal muscle. Nature (London) 316:347

Volpe P, DiVirgilio F, Pozzan T, Salviati G 1986 Role of inositol 1,4,5-triphosphate in excitation–contraction coupling in skeletal muscle. Federation of European Biochemical Societies 197:1

Waechter F, Engel J 1977 Association kinetics and binding constants of nucleoside triphosphates with G actin. European Journal of Biochemistry 74:227

Wagner P D 1981 Formation and characterization of myosin hybrids containing essential light chains and heavy chains from different muscle myosins. Journal of Biological Chemistry 256:2493

Wagner P D, Slater C S, Pope B, Weeds A G 1979 Studies on the actin activation of myosin subfragment 1 isoenzymes and the role of myosin light chains. European Journal of Biochemistry 99:385

Wakabayashi T, Tomioka A, Toyoshima C, Tokunaga M, Sutoh K, Yamamoto K 1986 Three dimensional structure of the thin filament and its complex with myosin subfragment: Location of functional sites of actin and myosin. Proceedings of the XIth International Congress on Electron Microscopy, Kyoto, p 1813

Wallimann T, Doetschman T C, Eppenberger H M 1983 Novel staining pattern of skeletal muscle M-lines upon incubation with antibodies against MM-creatine kinase. Journal of Cell Biology 96:1772

Wallimann T, Eppenberger H M 1985 Localization and function of M-line-bound creatine kinase. In: Shay J W (ed) Cell and muscle motility, vol 6. Plenum Press, New York p 239

Wang C-K, Cheung H C 1986 Proximity relationship in the binary complex formed between troponin I and troponin C. Journal of Molecular Biology 191:509

Wang C-L, Leavis P C, Gergely J 1983 Kinetics of Ca^{2+} interactions between the two classes of sites of troponin C. Journal of Biological Chemistry 258:9195

Wang K 1982 Myofilamentous and myofibrillar connections: role of titin, nebulin and intermediate filaments. In: Pearson M L, Epstein H F (ed) Muscle development: Molecular and cellular control. Cold Spring Harbor Laboratories, Cold Spring Harbor, p 439

Waren G B, Toon P A, Birdshall N J M, Lee A G, Metcalfe J C 1974 Reconstitution of a calcium pump using defined membrane components. Proceedings of the National Academy of Sciences (USA) 71:622

Watanabe S 1955 Relaxing effects of EDTA on glycerol treated muscle fibers. Archives of Biochemistry and Biophysics 45:559

Webb M R, Trentham D R 1983 Chemical mechanism of myosin catalyzed ATP hydrolysis. In: Peachey L E, Adrian R H (eds) Skeletal muscle. Handbook of physiology. American Physiological Society, Bethesda, p 173

Webb M R, Hibberd M G, Goldman Y E, Trentham D R 1986 Oxygen exchange between Pi in the medium and water during ATP hydrolysis mediated by skinned fibers from rabbit skeletal muscle. Evidence for Pi binding to a force-generating state. Journal of Biological Chemistry 261:15557

Weber A 1956 The ultracentrifugal separation of L-myosin and actin in an actomyosin sol under the influence of ATP. Biochimica et Biophysica Acta 19:345

Weber A 1959 On the role of calcium in the activity of adenosine 5'- triphosphate hydrolysis by actomyosin. Journal of Biological Chemistry 234:2764

Weber A 1966 Energized calcium transport and relaxing factors. In: Sanadi D R (ed) Current topics in bioenergetics Vol 1. Academic Press, New York, p 203

Weber A, Winicur S 1961 The role of calcium in the superprecipitation of actomyosin. Journal of Biological Chemistry 236:3198

Weeds A G 1969 Light chains of myosin. Nature 223:1362

Weeds A G, Frank G 1972 Structural studies on the light chains of myosin. Cold Spring Harbor Symposia on Quantitative Biology 37:9

Weeds A G, Lowey S 1971 Substructure of the myosin molecule II. The light chains of myosin. Journal of Molecular Biology 61:701

Weeds A G, McLachlan A D 1974 Structural homology of myosin alkali light chains, troponin C and carp calcium binding protein. Nature 252:646

Weeds A G, Pope B 1977 Studies on the chymotryptic digestion of myosin. Effects of divalent cations on proteolytic susceptibility. Journal of Molecular Biology 111:129

Weeds A G, Hall R, Spurway N C S 1975 Characterisation of myosin light chains from histochemically identified fibers of rabbit psoas muscle. FEBS Letters 49:320

Weeds A G, Trentham D R, Kean C J C, Buller A J 1974 Myosin from cross-reinnervated cat muscles. Nature 247:135

Weeks R A, Perry S V 1978 Characterisation of a region of the primary sequence of troponin C involved in calcium ion dependent interaction with troponin I. Biochemical Journal 173:449

Wegner A, Engel J 1975 Kinetics of the cooperative association of actin to actin filament. Biophysical Chemistry 3:215

Wegner A, Neuhaus J-M 1981 Requirement of divalent cations for fast exchange of actin monomers and actin filament subunits. Journal of Molecular Biology 153:681

Wegner A 1982a Treadmilling of actin at physiological salt concentration. Journal of Molecular Biology 161:607

Wegner A 1982b Kinetic analysis of actin assembly suggests that tropomyosin inhibits spontaneous fragmentation of actin filaments. Journal of Molecular Biology 161:217

Wells J A, Yount R G 1979 Active site trapping of nucleotide by crosslinking 2 sulfydryls in myosin subfragment 1. Proceedings of the National Academy of Sciences (USA) 76:4966

Wilkie D R 1966 Muscle. Annual Review of Physiology 28:17

Wilkie D R 1986 Muscular fatigue: effects of hydrogen ions and inorganic phosphate. Federation Proceedings 45:2921

Wilkinson J M, Grand R J A 1975 The amino acid sequence of TnI from rabbit skeletal muscle. Biochemical Journal 149:493

Wilkinson J M, Perry S V, Cole H A, Trayer I P 1972 The regulatory proteins of the myofibril. Separation and biological activity of the components of inhibitory factor preparations. Biochemical Journal 127:215

Winkelmann D A, Lowey S 1985 Probing myosin head structure with monoclonal antibodies. Journal of Molecular Biology 188:595

Winkelmann D A, Mekeel H, Rayment I 1985 Packing analysis of crystalline myosin subfragment-1. Implications for the size and shape of the myosin head. Journal of Molecular Biology 181:487

Woledge R C, Curtin N A, Homsher E 1985 Energetic aspects of muscle contraction. Monograph of the Biological Society No. 49. Academic Press, Orlando

Wood D S et al 1987 Is nebulin the defective gene product in Duchenne muscular dystrophy? New England Journal of Medicine 316:107

Woods E F 1967 Molecular weight and sub-unit structure of tropomyosin B. Journal of Biological Chemistry 242:2859

Woodrum D T, Rich S A, Pollard T D 1975 Evidence for biased bidirectional polymerization of actin filaments using heavy meromyosin prepared by an improved method. Journal of Cell Biology 67:231

Yagi K, Yazawa M, Kakiuchi S, Ohshima M, Uenishi K 1978 Identification of an activator protein for myosin light chain kinase as the Ca^{2+}-dependent modulator protein. Journal of Biological Chemistry 253:1338

Yamaguchi M, Greaser M, Cassens R G 1974 Interactions of troponin sub-units with different forms of tropomyosin. Journal of Ultrastructure Research 33:48

Yamamoto T, Tonomura Y 1967 Reaction mechanism of the Ca^{2+}-dependent ATPase of sarcoplasmic reticulum from skeletal muscle. Journal of Biochemistry 62:558

Yamamoto K, Tokunaga M, Sutoh K, Wakabayashi T, Sekine T 1985 Location of the SH group of the alkali light chain on the myosin head as revealed by electron microscopy. Journal of Molecular Biology 183:287

Yanagida T 1981 Angles of nucleotides bound to cross-bridges in glycerinated muscle fiber at various concentrations of ε-ATP, ε-ADP and ε-AMPPNP detected by polarized fluorescence. Journal of Molecular Biology 146:539

Yanagida T 1985 Angle of active site of myosin heads in contracting muscle during sudden length changes. Journal of Muscle Research and Cell Motility 6:43

Yanagida T, Oosawa F 1978 Polarized fluorescence from ε-ADP incorporated into F-actin in a myosin-free single fiber: conformation of F-actin and changes induced in it by heavy meromyosin. Journal of Molecular Biology 126:507

Yanagida T, Arata T, Oosawa F 1985 Sliding distance of actin filament induced by a myosin crossbridge during one ATP hydrolysis cycle. Nature 316:366

Yates L D, Greaser M L 1983 Quantitative determination of myosin and actin in rabbit skeletal muscle. Journal of Molecular Biology 168:123

Pathological changes in disorders of skeletal muscle as studied with the light microscope

INTRODUCTION

Myopathology comprises all known structural changes and functional derangements of muscle and also the scientific study of the causes and mechanisms of its diseases. It deals primarily with the muscle fibre and its tendinous attachments, for these represent the only unique component of the musculature. All other structural elements of muscle, namely the connective tissue sheathing, the blood vessels and the various neural elements, are shared by many other tissues. These latter at times bear the brunt of primary pathological processes within muscle, but when this happens the muscular abnormality is usually part of a more widespread or systemic disease.

The myopathologist assumes responsibility for describing the changes in muscle fibres in disease and for distinguishing them from such deviations from the normal state as occur, e.g. in maturational delay, ageing or stress. These changes are of importance in verifying clinical diagnoses, in correlating structural changes with physiology and chemistry, in explaining symptoms, in understanding disease processes, and in formulating reasonable hypotheses as to the aetiology and pathogenesis of disease.

We shall endeavour here to describe only the most frequently observed morphological changes in muscle fibres and to discuss their nature and significance. By assembling these reactions into morphological syndromes we hope to provide the clinical myologist with a kind of 'language' by which he can speak of and conceptualise disease processes. We are well aware that the mere listing of a series of pathological reactions is highly artificial. In the living cell pathogenetic mechanisms and reaction patterns do not exist in isolation but interact in a most intricate fashion. Moreover, the types of change to be described below are linked only in a general way to specific diseases. Although one type of structural alteration may be especially prominent in one disease (e.g. nemaline bodies in nemaline myopathy) there are no cellular changes that are absolutely pathognomonic of one disease. In other words, any one of the following histological changes will be found in several different diseases. It will be obvious to the reader that the muscle fibre, like other cells, reacts in steriotyped ways, and that these ways and the range of its reaction patterns are limited.

In this volume the pathology of muscle will be presented in two chapters: this one, on general reactions as viewed by light microscopy, and a second one (Ch. 8) which will contain an account of important ultrastructural changes. The various constellations of morphological change and their spatial and temporal ordering, which constitute the pathology of specific diseases, will be referred to in the chapters devoted to these diseases.

TECHNOLOGIES IMPORTANT TO MYOPATHOLOGY

A century of research on the pathological changes in muscle, utilising light microscopy, has yielded a wealth of information, and in more recent years the transmission electron microscope (TEM) has provided new insight into the morphological basis of muscle disease. High-power resolution has enabled pathologists to perceive previously unknown types of reaction and the fine details of others already known. For the first time ultra-structural changes in the muscle fibre could be correlated with abnormalities of nuclear and cyto-plasmic elements (Mair & Tomé 1972, Åström & Adams 1980, see also Ch. 8) The critical analysis of these ultrastructural changes is of importance in myopathology. However, one should realise there is no fundamental difference between light and electron microscopy. Both are used to examine alterations in sections of fixed tissue at powers of magnification beyond that of the unaided eye. The pathologist must be prepared to adopt whichever of these methods is

appropriate for the problem at hand. Light microscopy of stained sections will remain the method of choice for most diagnostic work and research in myopathology, for it is easy to use and can be employed at a wide range of magnifications, including that of low power for surveying large fields. TEM is needed only for the study of membranes, tubular structures, muscle filaments and mitochondria.

Histochemical methods for the demonstration of particular enzymes have also shed light on a number of obscure aspects of disease (Dubowitz 1985). The phosphorylase technique has confirmed the deficiency of this enzyme in McArdle's disease. The use of the ATPase tech-nique has permitted the subdividing of individual motor units into fast phasic and slower tonic types and has shown that the type II fibres atrophy more readily with disuse and the type I fibres are earlier affected in myotonic dystrophy and certain other congenital myopathies. Histochemical typing has been particularly useful in disclosing the group atrophy of partial denervation after there has been collateral regeneration of nerve fibres (see Ch. 7).

Radionuclide and fluorescent tagging of molecules in the end-plate and within the muscle fibre have also been added to the technical arma-mentarium of the myopathologist, especially when combined with electron microscopy. This method has been particularly useful in diseases such as myasthenia gravis, which previously had an uncer-tain morphological basis. Scanning electron microscopy, freeze-fracturing and morphometric techniques have also been applied to the muscle fibre.

SOME FEATURES OF NORMAL MUSCLE THAT ARE OF IMPORTANCE TO PATHOLOGISTS

In order to understand the possible pathological reactions of the muscle fibre, certain of its anatom-ical properties must be kept in mind.

First, there is the biological fact that the human organism is born with nearly all the muscle fibres it is destined to have (some new fibres continue to form in the postnatal period according to Adams & DeReuck 1973). Their formation from myoblasts, which fuse to form myotubes and then differentiate into the thin but fully constructed fibres, takes place mostly during intrauterine life. The principal postnatal change in childhood is the rapid growth of each fibre by the addition of new myofilaments. As far as we know, fibres, once formed in early life, must survive the lifetime of the human organism, and, if totally destroyed, are never restored. Premature senescence conceivably might sometimes be the basis of disease.

Second, there is the enormous size and multi-nucleation of the muscle cell or fibre. No other cell in the animal organism approaches it in dimensions. Some muscle cells attain a width of 0.1 mm and a length of many centimetres. There are thousands of nuclei in a single cell, and each nucleus controls only a small region of the fibre. This fact, and its great length in proportion to width, allow certain muscle diseases to destroy only one segment of the fibre, leaving the rest intact and ready to regenerate, like a cut earthworm, from the surviving sound portions. The surviving segment may thus become separated from its nerve supply, which normally joins the muscle fibre near its equator.

A third anatomical fact relates to the complex structure of the muscle cell. Within its irritable cytoplasmic membrane (sarcolemma) are contained the myofibrils with their thick and thin myofilaments composed of myosin, actin, tropomyosin and meromyosin; these account both for the characteristic striations and for the contractile process. In addition, in the intervening sarcoplasm, are the endoplasmic reticulum (in a specific distribution with respect to the Z discs), the mitochondria and other organelles, with their rich content of enzymes, the myoglobin and globules of fat and glycogen. Some of these subcellular structures, such as striated myofibrils, do not occur in other cells and it might be expected that certain diseases peculiar to muscle depend on an affinity between them and the noxious agents to which the musculature is susceptible.

A fourth histological peculiarity is the investment of each muscle fibre by a thin sheath of connective tissue. This sheath is composed of delicate strands of reticulin and in places contains collagenous and elastic tissue; heavier bands of these same tissues constitute the perimysium which envelops fascicles, thus offering support and serving also to coordinate the contracting forces of aggregates of fibres. This arrangement, while mechanically advantageous, may nevertheless at times be detrimental for, in the event of an inflammatory reaction, hyperplasia of these connective tissue sheaths, or oedema, the muscle fibres may be compressed or deprived of blood supply should blood vessels be simultaneously occluded. Ischaemia may also result from diseases which directly affect the blood vessels.

A fifth histological fact derives from the close relationship between nerve and muscle. In no other organ is there found such a highly specialised functional zone between nerve fibre and parenchymal cell, nor is such an evident trophic influence exerted by the nervous system. Indeed, the muscle cell cannot survive independently for more than a few months or years. The intricacies of this control become manifest in many diseases which paralyse the groups of muscle fibres that are governed by single motor neurones. These diseases constantly remind us that all movement consists of the combined contraction of motor units which are activated and regulated by nerves and sensory end-organs lying within muscle. These motor functions depend on segmental and suprasegmental influences which converge on the anterior horn cells and are conveyed to the muscle fibre via their axons and myoneural junctions. The latter are of central importance and consist of the branching nerve fibre ending (telodendrion) and a heavily-nucleated, specialised part of the muscle fibre (the end-plate). Conduction of the nerve impulse across this junction is effected by acetylcholine which is liberated from the synaptic vesicles of the nerve ending, and the intensity and duration of its action is modified by the cholinesterase and by certain cations (see Ch. 3). These chemical substances may be quantitatively altered by derangements of the endocrine organs, liver and kidneys.

The last and perhaps least understood histological structures, from the pathological viewpoint, are the tendon fibrils. These latter attach to each end of the muscle cell, and the power of muscular contraction is transmitted through them to the skeleton, resulting in movement.

The aforementioned histological qualities are

common to all the hundreds of millions of muscle fibres that constitute the musculature. However, it must not be assumed that all the fibres possess identical structure merely because they look alike. Indeed, a number of differences between the fibres of different muscles throughout the body and between those of any one muscle have been recognised, e.g., it has been shown that the large fibres (type II or 'white fibres') possess a rich content of phosphorylase, and the thin ones (type I or 'red fibres') a great abundance of oxidative enzymes (Dubowitz 1985). Fibres of the latter type also have a larger ratio of capillaries to muscle cell. Fibres also vary with respect to their content of myoglobin, glycogen and fat, upon which depend some of the well-known differences in colour. Moreover, the disposition of connective tissue and blood vessels varies in different muscles, accounting for greater or lesser vulnerability to ischaemia. Then there are the relationships between the numbers of nerve and muscle fibres, revealed in the size of the motor units; these ratios vary greatly, being as low as 1 : c 30 for the external ocular muscles and as high as 1 : c 1500 for the gastrocnemius. Finally, there are subtle differences between muscles with respect to their physiological behaviour (Ch. 1). All these and other differences undoubtedly underlie the highly individual topography of many human muscle diseases as well as the distribution of biochemical disturbances and the action of pharmacological agents.

When considering the volumetric aspects of the muscle fibre in man and animals one must know something about the maturational aspects and the effects of age. Each muscle possesses fibres of a certain size and these vary in different epochs of life. Beginning at birth, fibres (ranging from 7 to 14 μm in diameter) gradually grow until late adolescence or early adult life. During adult years the variations in fibre size between individual muscles are considerable. Those of the ocular muscles average 17.5–20 μm in diameter, the forearm and lower leg muscles 50–60 μm in diameter, and the glutei, paravertebral, and shoulder muscles 70–85 μm, depending on the physical condition of the subject. However, the range in size of fibres within any muscle is wide; in heavy muscles it is from 10–15 μm up to 100 μm.

Groups of fibres below 40 μm in diameter are nearly always pathological.

In later life there is a loss of some fibres and a gradual increase in range of size of residual ones, at least until advanced years when diameters again diminish (Halban 1894, Wohlfart 1942, Banker et al 1957, Greenfield et al 1957, Sissons 1965). However, in most instances, especially in the younger age group, data are based on too few cases to serve as a reliable guide in pathological diagnosis. More precise data concerning the biometrics of human muscle at all ages are to be found in the article by Moore et al (1971). The most rapid growth occurs in the first years of life with a plateau being reached by adulthood, and there is a slight decline in the senile period.

Augmentation in volume during growth is presumably attributable to the action of growth hormone, and atrophy after pituitary destruction (Simmonds' disease) is probably the negative effect. At puberty the male sex hormone stimulates muscle fibre growth. Thereafter the masculine fibre exceeds the feminine one in volume as well as strength and endurance, particularly in certain muscles such as the biceps brachii. After castration of the male the fibre size reverts to its prepubertal dimension (Papanicolau & Falk 1938). Cortisone also causes atrophy and probably interferes with normal growth (see p. 163).

Concerning that aspect of muscle fibre volume related to the trophic influence of the nerve fibre, it appears that the degree of activation of muscle by the nerve impulses governs the size of the muscle fibre. The muscle fibre atrophies when activated poorly (disuse atrophy) and hypertrophies when activated excessively (work hypertrophy). This influence of activity is also true for the heart muscle fibre. The source of the neurotrophic factor has puzzled investigators. There is no doubt that complete denervation causes a much greater degree of atrophy than complete disuse, as when a tendon is cut. Thus, lack of nerve contact does more than merely halt muscle work; presumably the additional trophic influence comes through the neuromuscular junction. On the basis of studies of embryonic muscle, Drachman (1965) suggested that acetylcholine is the neuronal trophic substance.

For a time there was disagreement as to whether muscle activity resulted in an increased number of fibres (numerical increase) or an increase in size of existing fibres (volumetric increase). Morpurgo (1897) and others finally confirmed the latter mechanism. Similarly, in underuse atrophy (whether from isolating a spinal segment, splinting a limb or cutting a tendon) a volumetric, not a numerical, reduction occurs over a period of weeks but seldom exceeds 25–30% of normal (contrasting with the 75–80% loss of bulk in denervation atrophy). As stated above, histochemical studies reveal a greater reduction in the type II white, phosphorylase-rich fibres, the ones involved principally in fast-twitch or phasic reactions. In work hypertrophy, a volumetric increase occurs only if the muscle is required to overcome ever-increasing resistance per unit of time. Thus hypertrophy seems to be proportional to the intensity of contraction and not to duration of effort. By such a training programme, Denny-Brown (1961) succeeded in increasing the range in size of soleus fibres in the dog from 38–87 μm to 51–93 μm. Enlargement was accompanied by an increased number of myofibrils per fibre (1087–1206 in the control, compared with 1679–2063 in the conditioned animal) and in the amount of sarcoplasm. Data are lacking on myofibril counts in disuse atrophy, but presumably their number is decreased.

Inanition and cachexia are said to induce volumetric changes not differing essentially from those of disuse. Indeed, it is not clear in most studies of cachexia whether the operative factor was inactivity, cachexia, denervation, some other effect of disease or even age. Marin & Denny-Brown (1962) in a survey of 12 cases of cachexia, all except two of whom had malignant tumours, stressed the thinning of fibres and granulo-fatty degeneration. However, such studies have not taken account of changes in muscle associated with activity and age (see Tomlinson et al 1969).

PATHOLOGICAL CHANGES IN STRIATED MUSCLE FIBRES

Changes in volume, number and shape

An important parameter of disease in skeletal muscle is volumetric change without qualitative alteration in structure. This may take the form of diminution in size of individual fibres (hypoplasia or atrophy) or an increase (hyperplasia or hypertrophy). Alterations of size may affect all fibres or those of one enzymatic type only. The recognition of the latter change is possible only when a morphometric analysis is made on histochemically stained preparations (Brooke & Engel 1969a, b, c, d, Johnson et al 1973a, b).

Atrophy

Denervation atrophy. If deprived of innervation, muscle fibres atrophy at a standard rate (Fig. 5.1*). In several species of animals, including man, volumetric decrease proceeds at an even pace over a period of 120 days to a point where the muscle weight is only 20–30% of normal, i.e. 70–80% reduction. As the vessels and connective tissues undergo only slight changes and retain their natural appearance and bulk (they make up 10–25% of muscle weight), this means that the sarcous substance is reduced to about 5–10% of its normal volume. The denervated muscle fibre loses volume, as a fibre normally does during inactivity. Reinnervation at this stage restores fibre bulk and strength of contraction. However, if regrowth of nerve does not occur within a few months or a year or more, the thin fibres pass a point of no return and degenerate. It is as if muscle fibres were removed as being useless to the body.

Under the light microscope the atrophic fibres appear excessively nucleated (Fig. 5.1c), as the normal number of nuclei are crowded into a smaller volume of sarcoplasm. The nuclei are at first slightly enlarged and the residual myofibrils are intact. As atrophy increases, the undulating course of the thin fibres (a change due to retraction of excised tissue), when observed in longitudinal sections, may give an illusion of segmental interruption in continuity and agglutination of sarcolemmal nuclei. Gradually the muscle nuclei shrink and acquire a deep basophilia. Clumps of these dark nuclei may persist after all visible sarcoplasm has vanished.

---

* Unless otherwise noted, all figures in Chapter 5 are phase micrographs from sections of osmicated, epon-embedded material, which have been stained with paraphenylene diamine.

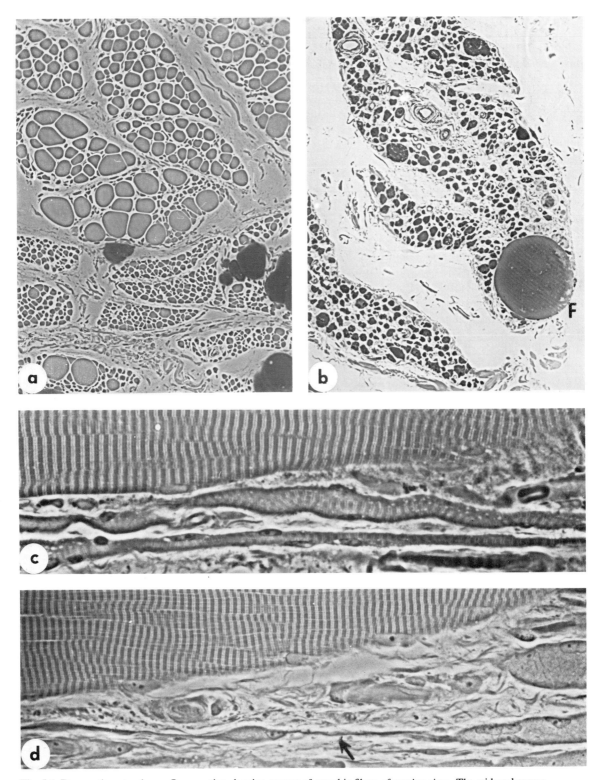

Fig. 5.1 Denervation atrophy. a. Cross-section showing groups of atrophic fibres of varying sizes. The widened spaces between the fibres contain connective tissue and a few fat cells (black), ×220. b. Cross-section showing advanced degree of atrophy. Shrunken fascicles of fibres are separated by connective tissue. F = fat cell, ×220. c. Two longitudinally cut atrophic fibres with preserved striation. Note the relative increase of sarcolemmal nuclei in the thinner fibre at bottom of picture, ×1180. d. An atrophic fibre is reduced to a thin thread (arrow), ×735

Electron-microscopic studies of denervation in animals (Pellegrini & Franzini 1963, Pellegrini & Franzini-Armstrong 1969) and in man (Afifi et al 1966, Shafiq et al 1967, Szliwowski & Drachman 1975) demonstrate a loss of myofilaments in the periphery of myofibrils, a gradual reduction in the number of myofibrils, and possibly a selective degeneration of I bands and Z lines.

Following denervation in animals there is concomitant breakdown of myofibrils, an increase of hydrolytic enzymes, and of lysosome-like elements (Pellegrini & Franzini 1963). The latter findings suggest that sarcoplasmic material is being digested within autophagic vacuoles. However, the question whether the breakdown of myofibrils is taking place inside or outside the lysosomal system has not been settled (Bird 1975).

Hyaline and vacuolar degeneration, fibrosis and fat-cell replacement are reported to occur within a few months in denervated muscle of animals, yet in man thin fibres may survive for years. Usually it is in isolated, large fibres that the degenerative changes are most conspicuous, as though the innervated fibres had suffered injury (Fig. 5.2d). This dystrophic aspect of denervation atrophy occurs at a variable interval, differing possibly from one animal to another and in different muscles in any one animal. Its nature remains uncertain, and even the exhaustive studies of Gutmann (1962) did not clarify our understanding of it.

These degenerative changes also introduce a practical problem in pathological diagnosis, that of differentiating atrophy from dystrophy. After many years of denervation, when numerous muscle fibres have been replaced by fat and fibrous tissue, distinction between the late stages of these two processes becomes increasingly uncertain; even when many fibres remain, distinction may still be difficult. In the chronic neuropathies, e.g. Charcot–Marie–Tooth disease (Fig. 5.2d), there are scattered giant fibres among surviving units, giving an overall impression of random fibre enlargement and atrophy. Further, some of the large fibres show central nucleation, hyalinisation, and often degeneration and phagocytosis, suggesting a dystrophic process. Haase & Shy (1960) believed these changes to be primary. We would insist, however, that their observations did no more than

draw attention to late secondary changes common to all denervated fibres and did not imply either that there is a primary myopathic element in these diseases or, conversely, that dystrophies are due to denervation (see Drachman et al 1967). Part of the confusion relates to the reaction of muscle fibres with residual intact innervation. They undergo hypertrophy, sometimes to a striking degree, so that if one makes a graph of their diameters, the usual symmetrical Gaussian curve is now replaced by one with two or three peaks. Schwartz et al (1976) have suggested that longitudinal splitting of muscle fibres caused by overload of poorly innervated hypertrophic fibres can also account for some of the 'myopathic' changes in denervation atrophy.

When all of the muscle fibres suffer denervation atrophy simultaneously, as may occur in poliomyelitis or acute polyneuritis, the atrophic process is randomly distributed throughout the muscle (Fig. 5.1b). However, even in this circumstance some fibres are thinner than others. It often happens, however, that the disease singles out one axon or nerve cell at a time, as in one of the progressive polyneuropathies or in motor neurone disease. Atrophy then expresses itself in a pattern determined by the distribution of the motor units (Fig. 5.1a). It is here that fibre-type grouping is most informative.

The residual fibres of sound units rapidly increase in size, many coming to exceed $100 \mu m$ in diameter (Adams 1968). The work hypertrophy of partly denervated muscle, expressed also in increased anabolic activity and decreased catabolism (Goldberg 1967), is one explanation of gigantism in muscle fibres.

Reinnervation of muscle fibres after denervation is further described on page 198.

There are, then, two standard pathological pictures of denervation atrophy — that of diffuse atrophy of all motor units (Fig. 5.1b) and the multiple, successive atrophy of single units (Fig. 5.1a). In both, the fascicular atrophy expresses itself as groups of uniformly small fibres with dark clustered nuclei and only slight change in the connective tissue. One of the main difficulties is the differentiation of diffuse denervation from disuse atrophy, cachexia, and senility. Whereas generalised denervation atrophy, when

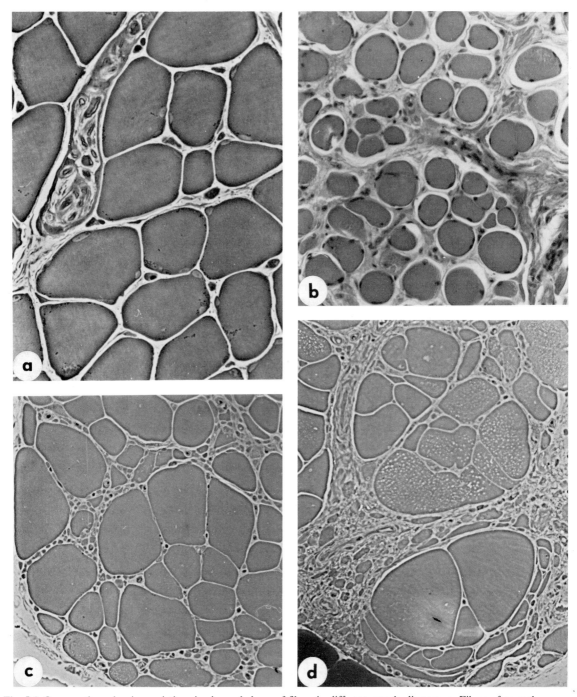

Fig. 5.2 Cross-sections showing variations in size and shape of fibres in different muscle diseases. a. Fibres of normal polygonal shape but of reduced diameter from a case of nemaline myopathy. A normal nerve twig is seen in the upper, left part of the figure, ×545. b. Section of thigh muscle in Duchenne dystrophy showing rounded shape and variation in diameter of muscle fibres. Endomysial connective tissue is relatively increased due to disappearance of muscle fibres. H and E, ×200. c. Fibres of rounded shape and a variation of their diameters from case of polymyositis. Interstitial spaces contain inflammatory cells, ×200. d. Dystrophic aspect of denervation atrophy illustrated by a section from a case of Charcot–Marie–Tooth disease. Group atrophy is seen in lower part of picture. Vacuolation in some fibres, especially the larger ones, is a sign of degeneration, ×220

advanced, is obvious enough, its earlier stages, with muscle fibres only moderately reduced in volume, may be indistinguishable from the changes of disuse and cachexia. Here one must appeal for final proof of denervation to histochemical stains of muscle to show large fields of one type of reinnervated fibres ('type-grouping') or to anatomical and physiological examination of the nerve or spinal cord. Moreover, some of the necrotising myopathies affect compact groups of fibres which, upon regeneration, may present as islands of atrophic fibres, simulating the muscle atrophy of motor unit disease.

Motor neurone diseases and chronic neuropathies. Denervation atrophy of the muscle fibre is seen most clearly in these two categories of neurological disease.

The motor neurone diseases, now that poliomyelitis has been virtually eliminated in the occidental world, stand as the prime examples of a slowly progressive atrophy of groups of muscle fibres supplied by single anterior horn cells. As these cells degenerate one or a few at a time over a period of weeks to years, the degree of muscle fibre atrophy is wide ranging. Some groups of fibres are only slightly smaller than normal (best seen in histochemical preparations) whereas others are reduced to mere clusters of shrunken sarcolemmal nuclei; many motor units fall between these two extremes. Furthermore, some of the intact units, by undergoing work hypertrophy, result in adding even greater variation in motor unit sizes.

The neurological maladies included in this category of motor neurone diseases are usually subdivided into the hereditary and acquired types. The hereditary forms are exemplified by Werdnig–Hoffmann disease but there are several other types that evolve more slowly and begin at a later age (cf. Emery 1971). The acquired types include progressive muscular atrophy, amyotrophic lateral sclerosis and progressive bulbar palsy. As a general rule the early-onset types of motor neurone disease tend to be of genetic origin while the late adult forms are idiopathic and acquired.

A textbook on muscle diseases is not the place for a detailed description of the pathology of these diseases. Suffice it to say that, for reasons which

are still obscure, the anterior horn cells and the motor nuclei of the lower brain stem undergo gradual atrophy, lose Nissl bodies and accumulate lipofuscin as the distal parts of their axons degenerate. Finally, the cell dies, only rarely exciting a neurophagic reaction. The process is so slow that few if any degeneration products of the axon and myelin sheath are to be found in specimens of nerve. Occasionally one sees that the affected nerve cell is slightly rounded and pale but not to the degree seen in classic central chromatolysis. A notable feature of some of the familial types of motor neurone disease is the presence of amorphous cytoplasmic formations. In the Guamanian type of ALS and Parkinson-dementia complex, some of the anterior horn cells contain neurofibrillary tangles. In amyotrophic lateral sclerosis the upper motor neurones are similarly involved.

In the many types of chronic sensorimotor neuropathy, such as that described originally by Charcot, Marie and Tooth, the pattern of muscle denervation tends to differ from that seen in motor neurone diseases. The latter single out individual motor units, whereas in the former the affected nerve fibres are destroyed in a different pattern and there are broad fields of markedly atrophic muscle fibres, all in more or less the same stage of atrophy; in other areas all the muscle fibres (in many adjacent units) are normal or hypertrophied. Probably this difference relates to the topography and temporal order of axonal degeneration. Wohlfart (1949) believed that the muscle spindle fibres became more atrophic in the neuropathies, reflecting a combined degeneration of both motor and sensory neurones. The motor neurones then exhibited the typical central chromatolysis of axonal injury.

Hypoplasia (hypotrophy) of muscle is another cause of small fibres. It has been known for many years that some children from birth or from an early age are weak and hypotonic ('floppy'), have retarded motor development, poor reflexes and generally thin skeletal muscles. With advancing age, strength and muscle size may slowly increase, but the musculature is always relatively subnormal. Biopsy or chance autopsy may reveal a universal smallness of normally structured muscle fibres, as though some factor essential to maturation and growth were lacking. The ailment differs from the hypoplasia resulting from the lack of normal development of motor neurones (see Zelena 1962).

Walton (1957) called the condition 'benign congenital hypotonia'; eventually, the children he studied recovered almost completely. Further study of patients with congenitally weak, hypotonic muscles shows them to be suffering from a heterogeneous group of diseases. Using modern histological techniques, especially histochemical staining and electron microscopy, myopathologists have been able to distinguish several well-defined entities (Table 5.1). In one such disease (myotubular myopathy) it has been suggested that the fibres have retained their fetal character, i.e. their development has been arrested (see p. 193). In other cases the size of the fibres is not reduced, however, and as the bulk of the muscles is diminished, there is probably a reduced number of fibres.

Some of the congenital hypotonias such as central core disease, nemaline myopathy, and the mitochondrial myopathies are distinguished additionally by special morphological features of the fibres, and these features have become the basis of a new subdivision (cf. Table 5.1). Nevertheless, further study has shown that there are many combinations of these structural alterations or organelles (Bethlem et al 1978); hence, any one type of change is non-specific (Brooke et al 1979, Fardeau 1984).

Clearly, many more observations are needed before nosology can be established, the relations between the different conditions clarified, and the significance of the structural changes and their functional equivalents ascertained.

Other causes of congenital and neonatal hypotonia and hypoplasia of muscle include well-known entities such as Werdnig–Hoffmann's infantile spinal atrophy (Pearn & Wilson 1973, Dubowitz 1975), congenital forms of muscle dystrophy (Banker et al 1957, Gubbay et al 1966, Zellweger et al 1967), dystrophia myotonica (Dyken & Harper 1973, Zellweger & Ionasescu, 1973), myasthenia gravis (McLean & McKone 1973, Whiteley et al 1976), neonatal myasthenia gravis (Namba et al 1970), acid maltase deficiency (Engel 1970a, Engel et al 1973) and polymyopa-

Table 5.1 Congenital hypotonia: some reported causes

Benign congenital hypotonia	Walton (1957)
Central core disease (p. 178)	Shy & Magee (1956); Isaacs et al (1975); Saper & Itabashi (1976); Radu et al (1977); Patterson et al (1979); Frank et al (1980)
Myotubular myopathy (p. 193)	Spiro et al (1966); Sher et al (1967); Campbell et al (1969); PeBenito et al (1978); Schochet et al (1972); Edström et al (1982); Bill et al (1979)
Type I fibre hypotrophy and central nuclei	Engel et al (1968); Kinoshita et al (1975a)
Congenital fibre type disproportion	Dubowitz (1985); Brooke (1974); Clancy et al (1980)
Congenital neuromuscular disease and external ophthalmoplegia	Bender & Bender (1977)
Nemaline myopathy (p. 184)	Shy et al (1963); Conen et al (1963); Kuitunen et al (1972); Sreter et al (1976)
Megaconial and pleoconial ('mitochondrial') myopathies	Shy et al (1966, see also p. 187)
Multicore disease	Engel et al (1971); Heffner et al (1976); Lake et al (1977); Bonnette et al (1974)
Congenital neuromuscular disorders with rods, cores, miniature cores and focal loss of cross-striations	Bethlem et al (1978)
Fingerprint body myopathy	Engel et al (1972); Fardeau et al (1976); Curless et al (1978b)
Reducing-body myopathy	Brooke & Neville (1972); Tomé & Fardeau (1975)
Sarcotubular myopathy	Jerusalem et al (1973)
Lysis of myofibrils in type I fibres	Cancilla et al (1971)
Neuromuscular disease with trilaminar muscle fibres	Ringel et al (1978)
Zebra body myopathy	Lake & Wilson (1975)
Target fibre disease	Schotland (1967)
Arthrogryposis multiplex	Banker et al (1957)
Congenital myopathy with subsarcolemmal masses	Sahgal & Sahgal (1977)
Diaphragmatic paralysis with type I fibre atrophy	De Reuck et al (1977)
Congenital neuromuscular disease with type I fibre hypotrophy, ophthalmoplegia and myofibril degeneration	Sugie et al (1982)

thies with developmental brain abnormalities and brain damage (Fenichel 1967, Curless et al 1978a).

The diseases listed in Table 5.1 and in the

above list do not exhaust the conditions that seem to interfere with muscular development. Mongolism and the other chromosomal trisomy states are associated with thinness of muscle and hypotonia. In Werner's disease, which includes weight loss, weakness, baldness, cataracts, greying of hair, wrinkling of skin, diabetes and arteriosclerosis, the muscles are thin and feeble. The reduction of the fibre girth is presumably related to an undefined endocrine or metabolic defect. The Willi-Präder syndrome (amentia, hypotonia, hypogonadism and obesity) and several other metabolic and developmental diseases of the nervous system of childhood are associated with poorly developed musculature.

Other conditions with small muscle fibres. Small, diffusely basophilic fibres with large, heavily stained sarcolemmal nuclei and sparse myofibrils represents a regenerative process (p. 199). This is particularly prominent after an attack of paroxysmal myoglobinuria (see Fig. 5.7d), in polymyositis (see Fig. 5.7b, c), and in the Duchenne type of progressive muscular dystrophy. In still other diseases, small fibres seem to preserve their eosinophilia, myofibrillar structure and natural nucleation without any indication of the cause of their atrophy. This is as striking in the muscular dystrophies and in some cases of polymyositis as is hypertrophy, with its tendency to central nucleation (Fig. 5.2c).

In Cushing's disease and with chronic corticosteroid therapy (Müller & Kugelberg 1959, Perkoff et al 1959) there is proximal weakness of limb muscles, particularly of the thighs. Random biopsies reveal an atrophic myopathy. Such muscles are notably abnormal because of the presence of many thin fibres 10–30 μm in diameter with normal-appearing sarcoplasm and myofibrils and a relative increase in sarcolemmal nuclei, many of which are centrally located. Only a few degenerating fibres may be seen and the interstitial tissue and vessels are unaltered. In addition, there are clear central zones, impoverished of myofibrillar material, in a few of the fibres. The pathological picture can be distinguished from denervation atrophy only with difficulty, save for the fact that type IIa fibres are selectively involved.

Enlargement of muscle fibres. In evaluating hypertrophy in transverse sections prepared for light miscroscopy, only those fibres in which the myofibrils are visible should be measured. In biopsied material many fibres are slightly swollen, rounded and with vitreous sarcoplasm, attributable to contraction bands or to physical alterations induced by incision. They are most prominent at the cut surfaces of the specimens. The occurrence of fibres of similar appearance, scattered throughout the specimen, is also a well-recognised feature of early Duchenne dystrophy. This appearance is due to localised areas of hypercontraction of muscle fibres associated with increased sarcoplasmic calcium (Cullen & Fulthorpe 1975).

True enlargement or hypertrophy of muscle fibres may result from the operation of several factors. As mentioned above, excessive activity increases the diameter of fibres (work hypertrophy). Within hours or days, the anabolic activities of overworked muscle increase in proportion to the catabolic processes; within a few weeks the transverse diameters are augmented by as much as 30% and the number of myofibrils by as many as 600. There are probably also more myofilaments in each myofibril. In muscles which have been partially denervated, the healthy innervated ones show a similar hypertrophy, probably also a result of overwork. The muscle fibres of the acromegalic and pituitary giant are also larger than normal. Some degree of enlargement also occurs in the uninjured parts of fibres undergoing regeneration after segmental necrosis.

Of more obscure nature is the enlargement of muscle fibres in certain forms of muscular dystrophy: this enlargement may precede the first hint of degeneration. In the more advanced stages of muscular dystrophy, where there has been considerable loss of fibres, some of those remaining surpass the normal fibres in size, probably as a result of work hypertrophy. Studies of mouse dystrophy, where the hypertrophy is prevented by denervation, bear out this supposition that it is a reaction of intact fibres to overwork.

Changes in shape of muscle fibres. Well-fixed and embedded microscopic sections of normal skeletal muscle, cut transversely, reveal the polygonal shape of the fibres (Fig. 5.2a). Together they form a virtual mosaic. It would seem that intramuscular pressures impart this angularity, for the fibres becomes manifestly more rounded or sharply angulated when their number is depleted by disease (Fig. 5.2). Nevertheless, this is not a complete explanation, because partial denervation and atrophy do not efface the angularity. Contraction bands, biopsy trauma, and early necrosis all cause swelling and rounding of the fibres.

Once segments of muscle fibres have been destroyed, especially if the sarcolemma is breached, regeneration by budding and by the fusion of liberated myoblasts results in the uninjured fibre seeming to have split. Although this may be seen in healthy muscle, as a consequence of minor injury, it is a special feature of all the necroses of muscle. Not infrequently, five or six regenerating 'shoots' occupy the same region to form a compact bundle. The latter appearance may be misinterpreted as indicating denervation atrophy of a part of a motor unit. This type of regeneration may be the basis of a slight increase in the total number of fibres in a muscle with advancing age (Adams & DeReuck 1973).

Focal necrosis, sequestration and extrusion of necrotic remnants from autophagic vacuoles (Fig. 5.3, 5.5d) can also result in altered structure; there are indentations of the surface and localised splitting of fibres (Swash et al 1978, Swash & Schwartz 1977).

Changes in numbers of fibres. Disappearance of fibres. In the strict sense, numerical reduction of the normal complement of fibres within a muscle is the most incontrovertible evidence of a primary myopathic process. It implies, essentially, a destruction of whole fibres and, if severe, results in a proportionate weakening of contractile power. In contrast, denervation and disuse atrophy are for a long time manifested only by volumetric reduction in fibre size.

The biological factor(s) responsible for any given muscle acquiring a certain average complement of muscle fibres is unknown. As remarked elsewhere, the size of the fibre population in each muscle is subject to individual variations. One suspects that hyperplasia or hypoplasia (also called hypotrophy), may be the result of many developmental anomalies. This aspect of myopathology is relatively unexplored.

Assuming that segmental necrosis is regularly followed by regeneration and restoration of fibre structure in such diseases as paroxysmal idiopathic myoglobinuria and idiopathic polymyositis, one wonders why this regenerative process fails in muscular dystrophy. Certainly this would be expected if the necrosis involved the muscle fibre in its entirety, so that no regeneration could occur. Perhaps repeated segmental necrosis such as occurs in polymyositis and muscular dystrophy eventually exhausts the recuperative powers. This feature of necrotising diseases of muscle has been difficult to study.

Denervation in itself, if reinnervation is prevented, leads to the eventual disappearance of the atrophic fibres (Fig. 5.1d). The part played by injury is not known but it seems to hasten the process in animals.

The most extreme degrees of numerical depletion are seen only in the advanced stages of a dystrophic muscular disease.

Changes in dystrophic fibres. This brings us to one of the most important problems in myopathology — the sequence of changes leading to fibre death in the muscular dystrophies.

Atrophy of fibres in haphazard distribution with normal-sized and large ones, and a decrease in the number of fibres, constitute the common picture of all the muscular dystrophies. Muscle dystrophy of Duchenne type is the one most often discussed because the changes in volume, shape and number of fibres (Fig. 5.2b) and degeneration are so striking. The latter, and some regenerative changes, are more prominent than those seen in the other dystrophies. Enlargement of fibres is prominent and, in our experience, accounts more often for the early enlargement (hypertrophy) of muscle in Duchenne dystrophy than does infiltration of fat cells (pseudo-hypertrophy). It is difficult to determine which, if any, of these changes are primary and which ones are the most significant.

In childhood Duchenne dystrophy, the prominent segmental necrosis and abortive regeneration

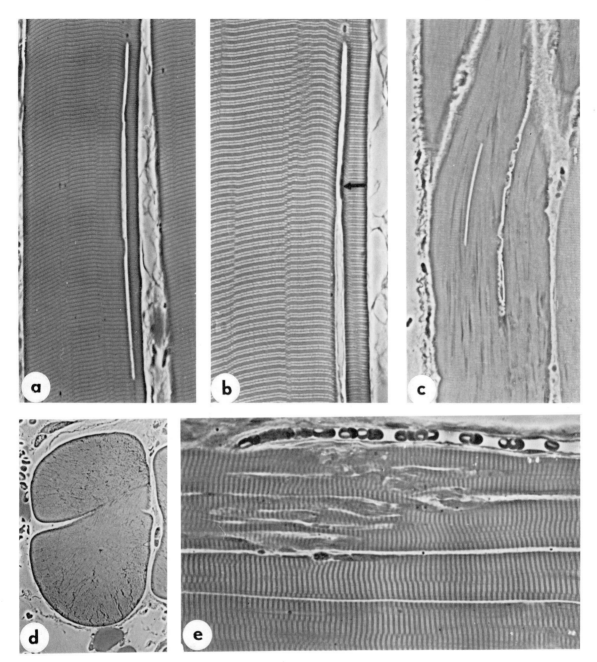

Fig. 5.3 Four longitudinal and one cross-section illustrating splitting of muscle fibres. a. Longitudinal splitting after focal necrosis, which has partly divided a fibre into a thick and thin portion in the plane of sectioning, ×350. b. Higher magnification of previous figure showing that the split contains a capillary. Note also the sarcolemmal nucleus in the thin portion facing the cleft (arrow), ×700. c. Split containing capillary penetrating from interstitial spaces, ×450. d. Cross-section showing partial splitting of fibre, ×545. e. Splitting and indentations of fibre after a focal necrosis, which has remodelled the surface of the fibre, ×700

probably explain the relatively rapid pace of the disease. Although rarely approaching in severity that which occurs in polymyositis or paroxysmal myoglobinuria, it exceeds that seen in all other types of dystrophy. Other pathological findings are: (1) vitreous and swollen appearance of many muscle fibres associated with localised areas of hypercontraction, a change which seems not invariably to progress to phagocytosis; (2) forking or branching of fibres; (3) central nucleation; (4) nuclear chains; (5) sarcoplasmic basophilia; (6) enlargement of sarcolemmal nuclei with prominent nucleation; (7) infiltration of fat cells and increase in endomysial connective tissue.

The interrelationships of these histological changes and their significance remain uncertain. We do not know whether the small fibres result from abiotrophy or represent the end-stage of segmental necrosis and regeneration. Because regenerating fibres in other diseases eventually resume normal size, whereas those in muscular dystrophy remain small, this clearly indicates that the regeneration is abnormal or abortive. Forking or branching of thin fibres, emphasised by Wohl-fart (1955) as a frequent process in the muscular dystrophies, could also be a regenerative response to segmental injury. This view is supported by the occurrence of the same phenomenon in chronic polymyositis. Small fibres with even, homogeneous basophilia (easily distinguished from the basophilic mottling of the crush artefact), an increase in number and size of sarcolemmal nuclei, and prominent nucleolation and sparsity of myofibrils, represent a regenerative reaction to injury of the muscle fibre and are secondary to the necrotic process. Enlargement and central nucleation are in some way associated, for the inward migration of nuclei is more frequent in all conditions which induce hypertrophy. Whether enlargement is due to a work hypertrophy of healthy surviving fibres or is the primary change in dystrophy has not been settled. Studies of the earliest stages in Duchenne dystrophy, where the overall diameter of the muscle fibre is increased, favour the idea of Erb (1891), that enlargement is an early primary change (see Bell & Conen 1967, Watkins & Cullen 1982). Rarely, as in some cases of the late Becker type of dystrophy described by Walton & Gardner-Medwin (1968), remarkable

muscle hypertrophy may precede the degenerative stage by several years. Denervation causes it to disappear in both human (Tyler 1950) and in mouse dystrophy (Banker & Denny-Brown 1959).

Electron-microscopic studies of the dystrophic muscle fibre (Lapresle et al 1965, Fardeau 1970, Mair & Tomé 1972, and Ch. 9) have done little more than add details to the known pathology without elucidating the nature of the basic process. More recently, Cullen & Fulthorpe (1975) concluded that the central process in Duchenne dystrophy is the formation of localised contraction clumps due to focal increase in sarcoplasmic calcium. Mokri & Engel (1975) found focal wedge-shaped lesions (with the base towards the surface of the fibre) and disruptions in the overlying sarcolemmal membrane. They suggest that these gaps are focal disintegrations of the sarcolemma and are the initial change in the dystrophic fibre (p. 174).

The end-stage of all dystrophic muscle diseases is the disappearance of muscle fibres which presumably causes the progressive paralysis. Muscle is ultimately reduced to fat and connective tissue and might even be unrecognisable were it not for the presence of scattered surviving fibres and spindles.

Fibrosis may be secondary to loss of fibres, and fat cell infiltration to the reduced number and volume of fibres. The degenerating muscle cell itself is never transformed into a fibroblast or fat cell. There is no pathological evidence of injury to nerve cells, to nerve fibres, or to intramuscular blood vessels.

Because all the muscular dystrophies are genetically determined, one must continue to search for the ways in which the abnormal gene causes degeneration of the muscle fibre. The primary change still eludes the pathologist. Is fibre necrosis the essential pathological step, or may fibres merely waste away? Perhaps both the atrophic and necrotic processes proceed in parallel, the latter being only the expression of the more intense phase of the atrophic one. Our own observations of chronic end-stage polymyositis reveal nearly all the changes considered characteristic of dystrophy. Thus, one may conclude that many of the alterations believed to be specific for dystrophy relate more to the chronicity of the disease than to its type. It is only by systematic study of large numbers of variably affected muscles at different stages of the disease that some of these problems can be settled.

It is a conventional practice to group the following conditions under the heading of muscle dystrophy: early and late, X-linked types (Duchenne and Becker); facioscapulohumeral (Landouzy–Dejerine); limb-girdle (Erb) and distal varieties; myotonic (Steinert) and various forms of progressive ophthalmoplegia, with or without dysphagia. The features that these diseases share as a group are their genetic origin, primary involvement of striated muscles, and slow progressivity and chronicity. However, there are also many differences in the clinical pattern of muscle involvement, life profile of the disease and other features. The slowly advancing adolescent and adult types (facioscapulohumeral, limb-girdle and distal forms) exhibit relatively little necrosis of muscle fibres and, at any one stage, the afore-mentioned variations in fibre size and central nucleation, fibrosis, and fat infiltration are very variable from one disease to another in any given muscle. Most conspicuously different are the muscle fibres in myotonic dystrophy, where necrosis is a rarity, rows of centrally positioned nuclei are more marked than in any other dystrophies, and spiral annulets (ringbinden) and peripheral masses of sarcoplasm filled with unorganised myofibrils, are striking features (see Fig. 5.10). Also, in myotonic dystrophy non-muscular tissues are more clearly involved: there may be testicular atrophy, cataracts, loss of hair follicles, and a mild degree of mental retardation. The mitochondrial changes in the muscle fibres of the ocular and oculopharyngeal forms are also indicative of separate disease processes (see p. 187).

Destructive (necrotic) lesions

Lethal injury to cells signifies a disturbance of homeostasis so severe that the cell cannot maintain its integrity. Its death is followed by a series of processes including autolysis, phagocytosis with removal of dead cytoplasmic elements, and repair. Mechanisms for maintaining cellular integrity and repair of injury, are, of course, very complex but all are dependent upon circulation and energy, i.e. availability of ATP. It is possible that lack of oxygen, substrate and enzymes might lead to necrosis. Viewed in another way, it would seem that under conditions of disease the nutritional and metabolic needs of the fibre exceed the supply of substrates.

The most extreme form of myonecrosis follows severe ischaemia where all or part of the muscle fibres, without regard to their contractile activity, are destroyed. In addition, the interstitial tissues undergo necrosis or at least injury. However, there are lesser degrees of substrate deficiency, where the degree of activity becomes a factor. An example is McArdle's disease, where the muscle fibre functions adequately and remains sound under conditions of minimal activity, but suffers injury and even destruction during exertion, because of its inability to mobilise its reserve of glycogen.

When the problem of myonecrosis is examined in greater detail, one may observe at least four types: (1) a focal destruction of the muscle fibre in a small, circumscribed zone (subfibre), that does not extend to the whole cross-sectional area of the fibre at any point; (2) segmental necrosis of the entire transverse diameter, usually over a span of several sarcomeres, and with preservation of the adjacent basement membrane; (3) regional tissue necrosis of muscle fibres as well as of interstitial tissue, such as occurs with occlusion of an artery and, less commonly, venous stasis, trauma, intense inflammation, injection of chemical agents; (4) contraction clots.

Focal subfibre destruction. We will define focal subfibre necrosis as a destruction of sarcoplasmic elements in a small zone, which does not involve a complete cross-sectional area of a muscle fibre (Fig. 5.4, 5.5). In focal subfibre degeneration, the continuity of the fibre is not disrupted; myofibrils are intact lateral to the lesion (Fig. 5.4a). The necrotic material is not removed by invading macrophages as in segmental necrosis, but is enclosed and digested by autolytic enzymes within membrane-bound vacuoles (secondary lysosomes). Adjacent autophagic vacuoles may merge (Fig. 5.4a and 5.4b), forming larger lesions which may be situated at the surface near the sarcolemma or deeper within the fibre. Larger lesions often extend in a longitudinal direction over many sarcomeres (Fig. 5.4c). The end-products are either extruded into the extracellular space or converted into lipofuscin granules which remain within the fibre (Fig. 5.4d). Muscle fibres seem unable to repair themselves completely after focal destruction, and unlike segmental necrosis myoblasts play no part (Schutta et al 1969). The affected fibres are indented, split, subdivided and their borders serrated, as if 'motheaten' (Figs. 5.3 and 5.5). The remodelling after focal necrosis may possibly weaken the affected fibres but apparently does not destroy them.

Segmental necrosis of muscle fibres. Partial destruction may occur in muscle fibres in which uninjured parts are able to repair the necrotic segment. This phenomenon, segmental necrosis, occurs in many diseases and hence is a fundamental, though non-specific, reaction.

The zone of altered sarcoplasm may be limited to as little as one or two sarcomeres but more often 20–30 sarcomeres or more are destroyed (Fig. 5.6). Very occasionally the lesion extends along the entire length of the fibre. Usually the altered sarcous substance has a highly refractile vitreous appearance and appears brightly eosinophilic or acidophilic in the common stains. The fragility of the coagulated sarcoplasm is shown by its tendency to fracture, particularly in the tranverse plane, revealing Bowman's discs. This appearance, while clearly abnormal, may be difficult to distinguish from artefact due to crushing or cutting of fibres, which is always prominent in biopsy material, and from contraction bands or sarcoplasmic clumps (Fig. 5.8). For this reason one should always search for infiltration of leucocytes and signs of myophagia (Fig. 5.6), which corroborate the ante mortem nature of at least part of the morphological change under consideration.

Regardless of the cause of the fibre necrosis (a point of fundamental importance), after a few days the necrotic parts of the fibre become heavily infiltrated with pleomorphic histiocytes (Fig. 5.6c), some of which continue to divide within the fibre. Many sarcolemmal nuclei in the injured segments are shrunken and pyknotic.

The electron microscopy of segmental necrosis

has shown destruction of all organelles and myofilaments, which are converted to amorphous debris; myelin-like bodies, vacuoles and other non-specific changes, evidence surely of a profound disturbance of the intrinsic metabolic mechanism of the muscle fibre, may also be seen. The plasma membrane is usually destroyed over the affected segments, whereas the basement membrane tends to be preserved.

Two experimental studies of acute necrosis are of particular interest. Price et al (1964) in cold injury noted contraction bands, which progressed to retraction clots, and the various membranous structures within the fibre were variably susceptible to injury. Mitochondria were the most sensitive organelles, but all others also degenerated rapidly. Stenger et al (1962), in a study of ischaemic lesions in dog muscle, also saw early alterations in membranous structures. However, in contrast to Price et al, they found that the myofibrils were most resistant, maintaining their integrity as a kind of skeleton up to 24 h after ischaemia. Later there was dissolution of I bands and degeneration of Z lines but, even at this stage, the A bands, H discs and M lines showed 'striking preservation of structure'.

Among human studies of segmental necrosis, the findings of which differ little from those in experimental animals, may be mentioned those of Schutta et al (1969), Kahn & Meyer (1970), Ghatak et al (1973) and Martinez et al (1973).

Emphasis here has been placed on the alterations of the muscle fibre, but invariably there are changes in the interstitial tissue and blood vessels. Endomysial fibroblasts adjacent to the necrotic segments enlarge, but actual proliferation does not occur unless there is collapse of several muscle fibres and, even then, it is not prominent. The cellularity of small vessels increases and the adventitial cells and pericytes are prominent. All these changes are of the type seen in cell necrosis in other organs and may be regarded as secondary. Incomplete regeneration, leaving a reduced population of muscle fibres, results in fibrosis, narrowing of the lumens of blood vessels and an increase in lipocytes.

In single episodes of segmental necrosis, regeneration is remarkably complete and, within a few weeks, the muscle appears to be completely

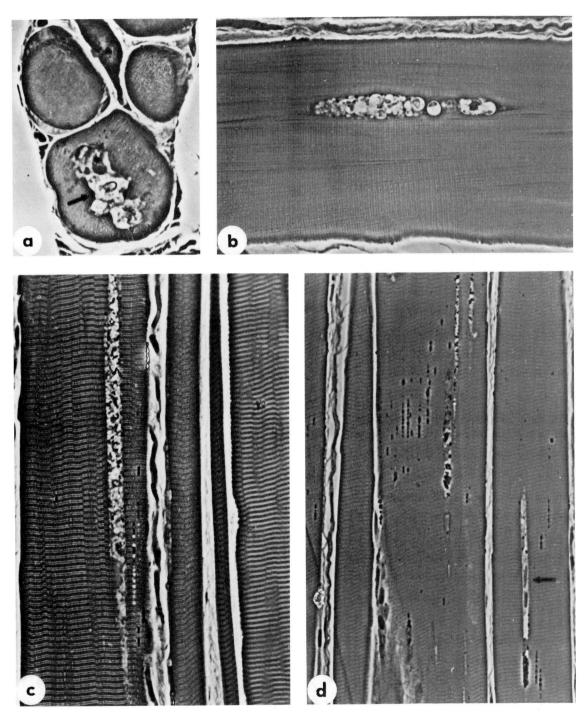

Fig. 5.4 Focal subfibre necrosis. a. Cavity with debris in central part of fibre (arrow) resulting from a confluence of smaller, autophagic vacuoles, ×545. b. Autophagic vacuoles have merged, forming a longitudinal cavity in a muscle fibre, ×700. c. Focal necrosis that has resulted in an elongated cavity, which extends over many sarcomeres in this longitudinal section, ×545. d. Fibre in the centre with two longitudinal cavities containing remnants of degenerative products. The longitudinal rows of lipofuscin bodies in this fibre indicate the location of former autophagic cavities. The split in the fibre to the right (arrow) contains capillary and connective tissue, which shows that it is connected with the interstitial space, ×350

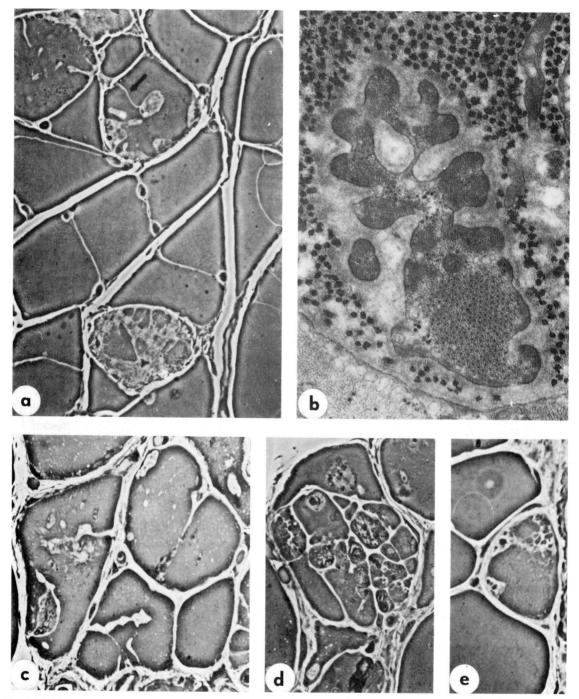

Fig. 5.5 Disfiguration of muscle fibre after focal necrosis. a. The fibre in the lower part of the figure is split into smaller components, which are embedded in connective tissue. In the upper part of the figure, a centrally located vacuole in a fibre communicates with the outside through a thin channel (arrow), ×700. b. Fragment of a muscle fibre with scalloped borders. It contains only one myofibril (or part thereof). Electron micrograph, ×42 400. c. Communication between autophagic vacuoles and interstitial space resulting in splitting of fibres, ×545. d. A fibre is split into many smaller parts, ×700. e. peripheral destruction giving the muscle fibre a 'moth-eaten' appearance, ×545

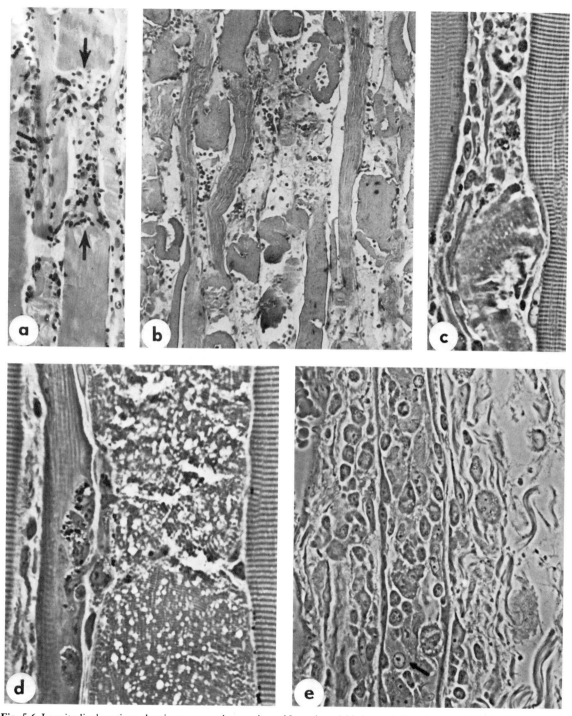

Fig. 5.6 Longitudinal sections showing segmental necrosis. a. Necrosis and histiocyte infiltration are visible in sharply dermarcated, collapsed segment of a muscle fibre from a case of polymyositis (arrows). Hyperplastic sarcolemmal nuclei in the fibre to the left (arrow) reflect regeneration. This is an example of isomorphic muscle necrosis and regeneration. H and E, ×360. b. Severe destruction with fragmentation of fibres, oedema and infiltration of cells in specimen from case of alcoholic myopathy, ×200. c, d, e. From another case of polymyositis. c. Necrotic segment is invaded by macrophages. The swollen retraction cap has indented adjacent fibres, which are normal, ×545. d. The wide fibre in the centre is necrotic but has not been invaded by macrophages. The thin fibre to the left contains four macrophages, ×545. e. Necrotic segment containing macrophages and myelocytes (arrow). The latter have large nuclei with nucleoli. The fibre is surrounded by inflammatory cells, ×545

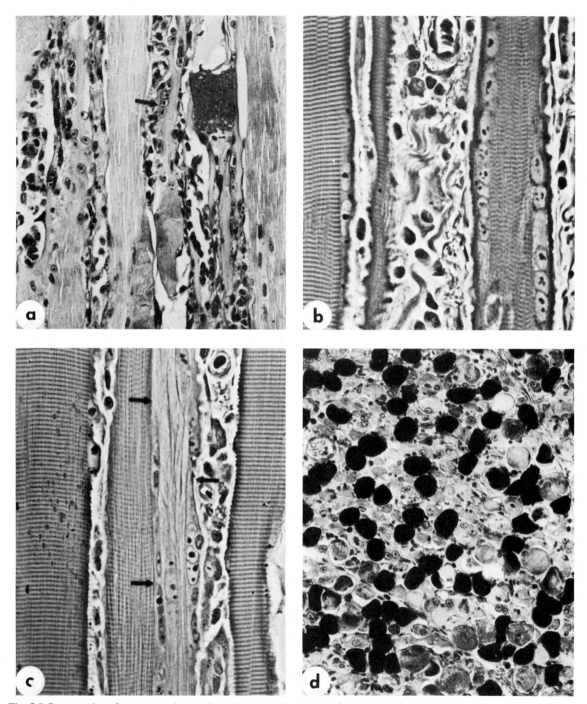

Fig. 5.7 Regeneration after segmental necrosis. a. A longitudinal section from a case of alcoholic myopathy showing a thin regenerating fibre, which contains rows of hyperplastic sarcolemmal nuclei (arrow). The sarcoplasm is bluish in the section, which was stained with H and E. To the right is a necrotic fibre, ×240. b, c. Longitudinal sections from a case of polymyositis. b. A regenerating fibre to the right of the midline with rows of hyperplastic nuclei with prominent nucleoli. Interstitial tissue with blood vessels and inflammatory cells is in the centre, ×545. c. Regenerating fibre (arrows) containing collections of large nuclei with prominent nucleoli and single myofibrils, which appear to have recently formed, ×545. d. Cross-section of gastrocnemius muscle from case of Meyer-Betz's paroxysmal rhabdomyolysis with myoglobinuria. The dark figures have survived injury and the pale ones with nucleolated sarcolemmal nuclei are regenerating. PTH-stain, ×225

restored. The regenerative process can be readily followed in lesions of different age. Surviving sarcolemmal nuclei enlarge and, once outside the sarcolemma, proliferate (Fig. 5.7). The nuclei at the junction of the healthy and necrotic segments also increase in number and size. The large size and prominence of the nucleoli of the myoblast nuclei distinguish them from histiocytes (Fig. 5.6e). Single, isolated muscle cells (myoblasts) may be seen in mitosis, but once these cells fuse to form myotubes, further division ceases. Regeneration of muscle fibre after segmental necrosis will be described further on page 199.

Severe segmental necrosis of striated muscle, while occurring in many muscle diseases, for practical reasons may be reduced to two groups.

Zenker's degeneration. This is the best known of the primary necroses of muscle. It may complicate many infective diseases, such as typhoid fever, and has been observed often in muscles such as rectus abdominis, the thigh adductors, diaphragm, biceps brachii, pectoralis major and gastrocnemius. Portions of single fibres or groups of fibres undergo vitreous or waxy degeneration. However, more typically, large numbers of adjacent fibres occupying a broad field seem to have been affected simultaneously. This feature, together with the relative sparing of the endomysium and blood vessels, the lack of inflammation, and the regular sequence of myophagia and regeneration, identify this so-called toxic, necrotic process.

The cause of Zenker's degeneration is not understood. The common incrimination of a toxin is too ambiguous to satisfy the discriminating student of muscle disease. Its occurrence in both bacterial and viral diseases suggests metabolic failure under conditions of stress.

Rhabdomyolysis with myoglobinuria. Extensive necrosis of muscle fibres from any cause, even if only one or two muscles are involved (as in crush injury) results in liberation of myoglobin, contractile proteins, enzymes, potassium and other elements into the bloodstream. The low renal threshold of this muscle pigment permits it to appear in the urine within a few hours. Aciduria favours the formation of myoglobin casts and often leads to tubular, 'lower nephron' nephrosis, which may be fatal.

In the idiopathic or Meyer-Betz (1911) syndrome segmental necrosis of muscle fibres may follow either unusual exertion or an infection. In biopsies, portions of many fibres are seen to contain altered sarcoplasm in various stages of disintegration. This sarcoplasm may appear waxy or fragmented or may take the form of strands or coagulated amorphous, flocculated masses. Myofibrillar structure is lost within a few hours; the sarcous material is eosinophilic in haematoxylin and eosin and reddish in phosphotungstic acid stains. Histochemical methods demonstrate an increase in bound lipids and phosphatides. Unlike McArdle's disease, in which myonecrosis and myoglobinuria may also occur after strenuous exercise, no excess of glycogen is present in either normal or diseased fibres. A peculiar property of the degenerating sarcoplasm is its affinity for calcium, which it binds within hours. The latter is easily detected even in the haematoxylin-eosin stains by a deep bluish basophilia of the calcium-protein precipitate. If the patient survives, as more than 75% do, the necrotic remnants are phagocytosed and brisk regenerative activity follows within a few days (Fig. 5.7d). The muscle may be restored to a normal state although, in several cases, clumps of sarcolemmal nuclei with little or no sarcoplasm about them and a mild replacement fibrosis, remain.

It is now known that the syndrome of myoglobinuria may have many different causes (Gabow et al 1982, Rowland 1984). As was stated above, it may be prominent in some cases of McArdle's disease, due to a deficiency of phosphorylase (Pearson et al 1961), and in phosphofructokinase and carnitine palmityl transferase deficiencies (DiMauro & Melis-DiMauro 1973, Hostetler et al 1978, Reza et al 1978). More recently other enzymatic defects have been shown to be involved in recurrent episodes of myoglobinuria (DiMauro et al 1982, 1983). Intense physical exertion in untrained subjects can also lead to necrosis of muscle fibres. When affected muscle fibres lie in a tight compartment such as that in the pretibial region of the leg, the entire muscle mass may undergo ischaemic necrosis (anterior tibial syndrome). The violent activity of severe convulsions and crushing of muscle in accidental injury may have similar effects. Haff disease, an epidemic myoglobinuria due to a virus or toxin, has been noted in Eastern Europe. In acute alcoholic myopathy, muscle necrosis (Fig. 5.6b) and myoglobinuria may develop after prolonged periods of drinking (Hed et al 1962, Ekbom et al 1964). In exceptional circumstances the condition is accompanied by renal failure and/or heart failure. Perkoff et al (1966) found that, during an alcoholic debauch, there may be a failure of lactic acid production under conditions of ischaemic work like that which occurs in McArdle's disease. Among other toxins with a lethal effect upon segments of muscle fibres may be mentioned the poison of Malayan sea snakes, heroin, when administered intravenously (Kendrick et al 1977), phencyclidine (Cogen et al 1978) and other drugs (Cadnapaphornchai et al 1980).

In polymyositis (Fig. 5.6c–e) one important component of the pathology is necrosis of muscle fibres. This change appears, in serial sections, to bear a topographical relationship to foci of inflammatory cells. Myoglobinuria with renal failure has been described in a few cases of polymyositis (Sloan et al 1978); myoglobin may be detected in the sera of patients with acute polymyositis before therapy (in 74.1% of the cases of Kagen 1977).

The muscle fibre may also show segmental necrosis in trichinosis and toxoplasmosis. The organisms penetrate the fibre and may be harboured for long periods. The trichina causes segmental necrosis of some fibres but becomes encysted in others. Eosinophilic and neutrophilic leucocytes and histiocytes are seen in the necrotic sarcoplasm and in the endomysial tissue. The cysts ultimately calcify. Toxoplasma pseudocysts lie inertly in the muscle fibre. On rupture, however, muscle fibre necrosis occurs with an inflammatory response.

Rhabdomyolysis with myoglobinuria may also occur in viral and bacterial infections and in the toxic shock syndrome. Approximately one-quarter of the published reports of myoglobinuria refer to patients who are said to have muscular dystrophy; however, as Berenbaum et al (1953) and Pearson et al (1957) point out, this chronic myopathy does not possess the usual features of muscular dystrophy, and is more likely to be a consequence of recurrent segmental necrosis of muscle fibres.

This use of the term 'dystrophy' only attests to the fact that it has many different meanings in myology. Some pathologists use it to refer to any process that leads ultimately to cell death, even the terminal phase of denervation atrophy (Lapresle et al 1965).

Progressive muscular dystrophy, particularly of the childhood Duchenne type, has been proposed as a special type of necrotising segmental myopathy where successive injuries of scattered fibres ultimately lead to their death. However, the myopathological findings do not fully support this hypothesis, because the relation of the necrotic process to atrophy and hypertrophy with central nucleation remains to be settled.

Segmental necrosis may, of course, occur without myoglobinuria. This means only that the necrotising process is less acute and severe, involving usually only single or small groups of fibres, as in muscular dystrophy (Pearce & Walton 1962). Acute destruction of at least 200 g muscular tissue, according to Berenbaum et al (1953), is required to produce measurable myoglobinuria. Lesser degrees of destruction are undetectable, either in blood or urine. Recurrent muscle fibre destruction will eventually lead to chronic wasting and atrophy.

Finally, it should be pointed out that pathogenesis is surely different in the many diseases leading to segmental necrosis. After all, necrosis is the end stage of various toxic, ischaemic, inflammatory, and metabolic processes. One may expect different sequences in different diseases.

Focal destruction of muscle tissue. Here, necrosis of muscle fibres is but a part of a more extensive lesion involving interstitial tissue and blood vessels. The reaction to muscle fibre necrosis is the same as that described above, but is accompanied by vigorous proliferation of endomysial fibroblasts, vascular reactions, and sometimes inflammation.

Vascular injury to muscle is the most thoroughly studied of the various types of focal destruction of muscular tissue. It may be caused either by venous or arterial occlusion or haemorrhage. Arterial occlusion has a variable pathological influence on different muscles, according to the pattern of distribution or arrangement of vessels (different for each muscle). The net effect is infarct necrosis (pan-necrosis of muscle fibres, supporting tissues and small vessels) with the conventional reactive changes. Lesser degrees of ischaemia may, however, injure muscle fibres out of proportion to the connective tissue, and it is these effects which have been described inadequately. Venous occlusion, which adds an element of congestion and often of haemorrhage, has a more devastating effect than arterial occlusion, at least in some muscles. Swelling and oedema and hydropic change in the fibres may be prominent. Infarct necrosis resembles the more diffuse necroses but differs with respect to the prominent reactions of endomysial and perimysial connective tissues and blood vessels. Nevertheless, the characteristic hallmark of this type of disease is always the focal lesion in the artery or vein. The vascular lesion may be atherosclerosis with thrombosis, bland or septic embolism, polyarteritis nodosa or some other type of vasculitis, such as giant-cell arteritis or phlebitis. The problem in pathology is satisfactory visualisation of the vascular lesion, which is often separated topographically from the myopathic change. Polyarteritis nodosa, a condition which involves the intramuscular vessels with striking regularity, is the lesion most frequently sought in muscle biopsies and fortunately is often easily identified by the concurrence of infarct necrosis, haemorrhage and denervation atrophy (secondary to lesions of the peripheral nerves) even when typical necrotising arteritis is not seen.

Trauma also elicits various combinations of necrosis of muscle fibres, interstitial tissue and blood vessels.

Regeneration after vascular or traumatic necrosis is described on page 199.

Contraction bands. Various pathogenic agents, but most particularly incision and other types of trauma, can excite contraction of myofibrils. This reaction, which may involve only a short segment of the fibre (Fig. 5.8) has been noted in humans and studied, particularly, in experimental animals (see Adams 1975, for full description and bibliography). It is known that any type of external irritation of a certain degree — e.g. from touching, probing, electrical stimulation, heat and cold — may be a sufficient stimulus (Fig. 5.8a). The ensuing changes may be reversible, but

prolonged irritation above a certain strength produces extreme degrees of contraction, visible as alterations of sarcous substance. The affected segment of a fibre may have a 'shredded' appearance, with dark bands alternating with lighter areas in which striation is still visible (Fig. 5.8b). In more severe lesions the dark bands are separated from lighter areas which contain amorphous material, fragments, and what seems to be fluid (Fig. 5.8b, c). The dark bands, called retraction bands or clots, consist of material which appears to be coagulated. They usually lie perpendicular to the long axis of the fibre.

Contraction clots do not occur in smooth muscles or in regenerating and immature fibres, which lack myofibrils (Speidel 1938). They are evidently caused by myofibrillar contractions severe enough to produce internal ruptures and 'clotting'.

At the border of a zone of injury a retraction cap may appear on the severed end of the unaffected part of the fibre (Fig. 5.8d, e), causing a swelling which can indent adjacent fibres (Speidel 1939). Probably this cap helps to seal the severed end, thus preventing leakage of sarcoplasm.

One or two days after injury, the segment with retraction clots will be invaded by macrophages which remove the necrotic fragments. The 'cleaned' region is then repaired in the usual fashion and the integrity of the fibre is restored. However, it is possible that healing may be incomplete and that the broken fibre ends freely in the connective tissue (Fig. 5.8d).

Manipulations during biopsy procedures may produce contraction bands. Certain fixatives will likewise produce such reactions in biopsies, especially if the specimen was not attached to a clamp or a stick. It is possible that certain diseased muscles are more irritable and prone to contraction bands than others.

Contraction clots occur, not only after trauma, but also in the course of disease, especially polymyositis (Fig. 5.8e, f) and in Duchenne dystrophy (Cullen & Fulthorpe 1975).

Degenerative lesions

Degeneration is here defined as any condition that alters special elements of the structure and impairs the function of the muscle fibre, but does not lead

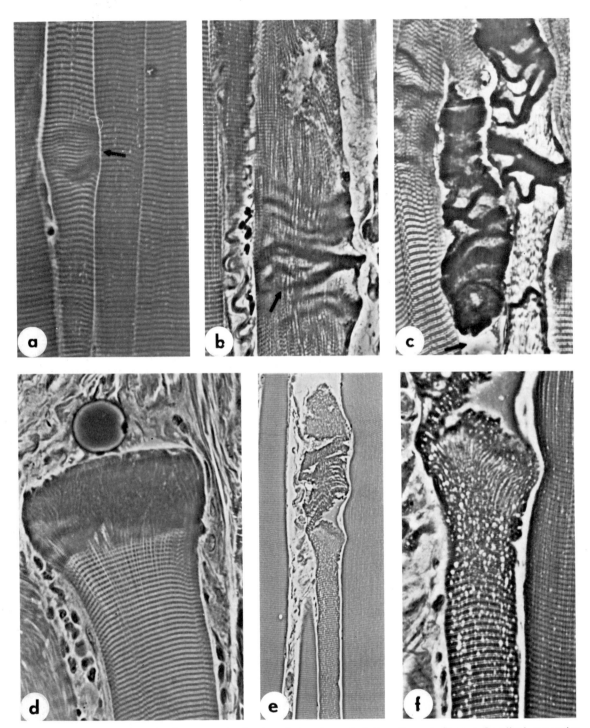

Fig. 5.8 Longitudinal sections showing contraction bands and clots due to irritation of muscle fibres. a. Localised contraction node (arrow) — probably a reversible change, ×500. b. 'Shredded' appearance of the fibre on the left side (arrow) representing a moderate degree of irritation; striation is still visible in the lighter areas between the dark bands. The fibre shows severe damage due to contraction. Contracted material is condensed into dark bands, ×500. c. Contraction bands and localised disruption (arrow) of sarcous substance. ×600. d. Retraction cap at end of severed fibre in a case of subacute polymyositis. Above the cap is connective tissue and one fat cell. A few inflammatory cells are seen to the left of the fibre, ×545. e. A fibre showing the following changes (from bottom to top): vacuolation, retraction cap, necrosis, ×220. f. Retraction cap and vacuolation seen at higher magnification. The swollen cap has indented an adjacent fibre, ×600

to necrosis. Unlike subfibre necroses, such lesions of a muscle fibre have several different features: selective loss of organelles, disturbance of architecture, disfiguration of organelles and inclusions of structured and non-structured elements. These changes will, somewhat arbitrarily, be subdivided into three groups.

Degeneration of single organelles

Destruction of sarcolemmal membrane. Alterations in the surface membrane of diseased muscle fibres have been thought by a number of investigators to be the cause of fibre degeneration (Schmalbruch 1975, Mokri & Engel 1975, Jerusalem 1976, Rowland 1976, Appel & Roses 1977, Pickard et al 1978, Bradley & Fulthorpe 1978, Carpenter & Karpati 1979.) Some of these claims were based on the visualisation of actual defects in the sarcolemma; others, using freeze-fracture techniques, showed an alteration consisting of a depletion in the number of orthogonal particle arrays (Schotland et al 1980, Osame et al 1981). Such defects are said to allow influx of calcium which leads to destruction of the fibre (Engel & Biesecker 1982, Engel et al 1984).

The problem here is to make sure that the visualised defects are not artefactual. In many instances they overlie contraction bands; others are along the margins of the biopsy specimen and could be caused by the biopsy procedure itself. It is also possible that the sarcolemmal defect may be one aspect of fibre necrosis, i.e. secondary to the necrotising process. However, the claim of a sarcolemmal defect need not be invalidated by uncertainty as to the morphological evidence. There could be a physiological abnormality in the membrane, even if it is structurally intact. For example, it could be abnormally permeable, especially in the myotonic myopathies (Appel & Roses 1983, Rüdel & Lehman-Horn 1985). At present, in our opinion, it is not possible to determine whether in any muscle disease the primary abnormality lies in the sarcolemma per se (Lucy 1980).

Selective destruction of myofibrils and myofilaments. Depletion of myofilaments and the reduction in size of remaining fibrils occur in atrophy of various causes. Glycogen usually fills widened spaces beneath the sarcolemma and between remaining myofibrils.

Non-fibrillar areas at the periphery of muscle fibres may have the appearance of clear, rather homogeneous zones under the light microscope. These so-called sarcoplasmic masses (see Fig. 5.10) have been seen in many diseases but are especially prominent in myotonic dystrophy, where they form concentric zones around a core of normal-looking myofibrils (see p. 180 and Fig. 5.10a, b). A sarcoplasmic mass contains not only sarcoplasm but also glycogen granules, normal and degenerating mitochondria, tubules and other organelles and often some residual (or newly created) myofilaments and myofibrils, which may have an abnormal orientation, occasionally into spiral annulets — so-called ringbinden (Schröder & Adams 1968). Sarcolemmal nuclei are increased in number, are in disarray and the cytoplasmic enzyme content of the fibrillar sarcoplasmic mass is enriched.

Patchy loss of myofibrils in type I fibres may feature in certain diseases, such as the congenital myopathy described by Cancilla et al (1971).

In contrast to complete disappearance of myofibrils and filaments, a selective destruction of parts of filaments has also been reported. Thus, lysis of myosin has been claimed to occur in various human muscle diseases (Yarom & Shapira 1977, Sher et al 1979). Partial destruction of myofilaments has also been observed under experimental conditions. For instance, Stenger et al (1962) found in the experimental animal a disruption and dissolution of thin filaments in the I band and granular degeneration of the Z line. The A bands and H discs were well preserved.

Depletion of mitochondria. The number of mitochondria is normally adjusted to the functional demands placed on the muscle fibre and may vary within wide limits. Continuous destruction and removal of mitochondria appear to be part of a constant, normal turnover in every living fibre. Depletion of mitochondria may be part of a pathological process. Accurate assessment of number and volume can be made reliably, but has not been attempted systematically in any of the myopathies.

Destruction of nuclei. Pyknosis of nuclei undoubtedly occurs in relation to segmental necrosis. However, it is hard to assess this parameter of disease in light-microscopic sections of muscle in human disease. The relation of nuclear necrosis to changes in surrounding organelles has not been established. Definite destruction is seen only in zones of segmental necrosis or in tissue necrosis. Darkness of staining and clusters or chains of nuclei are observed in ageing muscle fibres and in myotonic dystrophy.

Disarray of the architecture of the muscle fibre. A striking quality of the normal fibre, as seen under the microscope, is its regular structure. The observer especially notes how the thick and thin myofilaments interdigitate and form repetitive patterns in the sarcomeres, each separated by the straight Z lines. The filaments are embedded in sarcoplasm, which in the electron microscope lacks structure and is very lightly stained. Although the sarcoplasm seems amorphous, the normal structure and function of muscle are dependent not only upon the organisation of the myofilaments, but also upon the precise molecular composition and architecture of the sarcoplasm in which they are embedded. Filaments and sarcoplasm must constitute an integrated functional and morphological unit.

It seems reasonable, therefore, that different types of injury or genetic abnormality result in similar disturbances of the architecture of the fibre.

Streaming of the Z line. The Z line, which is normally straight and of even thickness, appears in some preparations to 'stream' into the adjacent sarcomeres. Isolated instances of streaming in otherwise normal fibres usually represent either an artefact or a normal phenomenon; streaming is not, in itself, a reliable indicator of disease. However, one cannot dismiss the possibility that in some cases it signifies an early pathological disturbance of molecular architecture. For this reason it must always be evaluated in the context of other findings and measured quantitatively (Meltzer et al 1976).

Disarray of myofibrils. This is an abnormality of striation, in which the normal, regular pattern of striation is disturbed irregularly, giving an appearance of smudging. Such changes have been seen in a number of different diseases. They have also been seen in normal subjects, although less commonly than the streaming of Z lines (Meltzer et al 1976). Our illustration (Fig. 5.9a) is from a case of Pompe's disease (adult form).

Central core formation. As first noted by Shy & Magee (1956) in a rare type of myopathy, each muscle fibre contains one or more zones of a dense, amorphous, relatively hyalinised sarcous substance. In the longitudinal plane these foci are shaped like thin cylinders. In Gomori's trichrome stain (in which myofibrils normally have a reddish colour) the myofibrils in the cores are condensed, i.e. more tightly packed, and bluish. Under polarised light or phase contrast microscopy the dense zones are seen to contain myofibrils with preserved cross-striation. The cores react positively to the PAS stain and negatively for phosphorylase and oxidative enzymes (Engel et al 1961, Seitelberger et al 1961).

Electron microscopy of cores has revealed such features as condensation of myofibrils, irregularity of Z lines, reduced numbers of mitochondria, and sarcotubular formations (Afifi et al 1965, Gonatas et al 1965, Dubowitz & Roy 1970). Neville & Brooke (1973) claimed that the cores may be either structureless (disorganised as described above) or structured, with normal striation. Even in the latter case, however, they found that the core was in a state of contraction, which seems at least in part to reflect some disturbance of functional state. Hence the difference between the two groups may be more a matter of degree than a qualitative difference.

This peculiar disfigurative change is believed to be determined by a genetic factor, for it has been seen in successive generations. Its significance has not been determined. Shy & Magee (1956) and Engel et al (1961) argued convincingly that the consistency of the change favours its being the mark of a distinctive disease. However, a similar core effect occurs occasionally in normal or denervated muscle (see below and Fig. 5.9c, d).

Apart from this curious alteration the only other morphological abnormality is excessive variation in size of the muscle fibres. The diameter of the fibres of the large limb muscles may come to an

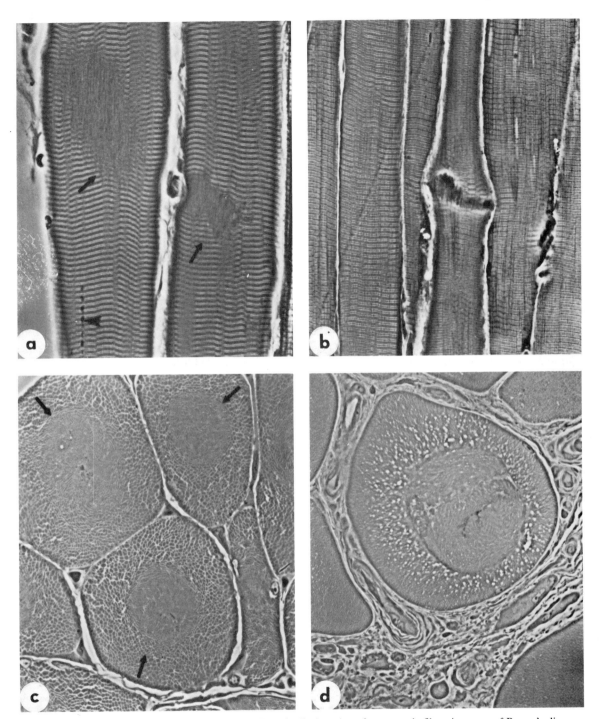

Fig. 5.9 Disarray of architecture of muscle fibres. a. Longitudinal section of two muscle fibres in a case of Pompe's disease showing smudging of normal striation within irregularly shaped areas (arrows). The row of lipofuscin granules (arrowhead) indicates the location of a former autophagic vacuole, ×545. b. Minicore of a type seen in 'multicore disease'. The fibre is swollen at the site of the change, ×545. c. Central cores or targets (arrows) in a case of denervation atrophy. The condensed myofibrils in the centre are surrounded by a peripheral zone with normal-looking myofibrils, ×545. d. A hypertrophic fibre from a case of Charcot–Marie–Tooth disease containing a central core or target of compacted myofibrils. The latter are surrounded by a zone of vacuolar degeneration. The connective tissue in the lower part of the fibre contains some thin, atrophic fibres, ×545

average of 80 μm or more (slightly more than average) but some fibres attain a size of 240 μm. Little or no degeneration or fibre loss may be found and there is no explanation for the mild persistent weakness noted in some cases. Sarcolemmal nuclei remain in their customary position and there is no cellular reaction to the central condensation of protoplasm.

Target fibres. The term 'target fibre' (Engel 1961) refers to the ringed or bull's eye appearance of certain muscle fibres viewed in transverse histochemical sections. A dark, inner core consists of a compaction of myofibrils, which lack the cross-striations and the mitochondrial oxidative enzyme activity usually found in myofibrils. The core is surrounded by a densely stained area and an outer zone of normal myofibrils. The targets may, like central cores, extend longitudinally over many sarcomeres. Biopsy and freezing of unfixed fibres seems to favour their occurrence. In osmium-stained sections the fibrils in the target zones appear homogenised and condensed (Fig. 5.9c, d). Target fibres are most often seen in denervation atrophy (Mittelbach 1966) but may also occur in other conditions. Engel (1961) noted target fibres in 60% of muscle biopsies in denervating diseases, but also in several cases of periodic paralysis.

The morphology of central cores and target zones is similar; they may be expressions of the same pathogenetic mechanism, as yet unknown.

Minicores. These structures were first described by Engel et al (1971) in what they called multicore disease (see Table 5.1 and p. 179). They differ from the cores of central core disease in that they are shorter (Fig. 5.9b), more heavily stained in osmicated preparations and more numerous. A single fibre may contain many minicores. Electron microscopy shows mostly a disorganisation of tissue and very little destruction.

Striated annulets (ringbinden, ring bundles, anneaux des fibrilles). This curious disorientation of the most peripheral (subsarcolemmal) myofibrils, from their longitudinal orientation to one of encircling the shaft of the fibre, was described long ago. Although observed many times in exper-

imental animals, most descriptions are based on human material.

It is our impression that two types of ring bundles can be identified. In type I the fibre is sructurally normal except for the disorientation of a peripheral packet of myofibrils, which encircle those longitudinally arranged (Fig. 5.10c). Sarcolemmal nuclei are in the usual position with reference to the myofibrils, in that their long axes are parallel to one another. No islands of clear sarcoplasm are present.

In Type II the sarcoplasm, especially peripheral, lacks myofibrils or retains only scattered disorganised ones (Fig. 5.10a) (Schröder & Adams 1968). Occasionally a packet of circular myofibrils is seen deep in the sarcoplasm. Some fibres may have lost all their myofibrils. The electron microscope reveals actin and myosin filaments, Z bands, and endoplasmic reticulum, without any semblance of organisation. Such ring bundles, according to Schröder & Adams (1968) represent a profound derangement of contractile elements, presumably due to a failure in the biosynthetic processes of the cells. Thus, it happens that a sarcoplasmic mass (region of sarcoplasm devoid of myofibrils) and myofibrillar derangement may or may not coincide. In some specimens, nearly every fibre shows clear zones of sarcoplasm, but no ring bundles.

The significance of these myofibrillar disruptions has long been disputed. Whereas Schäffer (1893) assumed them to be artefacts induced by incision and by the action of strong fixatives on irritable muscle, causing outright rupture of peripheral myofibrils, a view with which we earlier concurred (Adams et al 1953). Heidenhain (1918), Wohlfart (1951) and Greenfield et al (1957) insisted that they are a valid ante-mortem sign of disease.

The position we would now take is that the type I ring bundles are probably artefactual. This type of change may be found in biopsies from cases of pseudotetany, tetanus, myotonia, and many other conditions. It is probably not significant, being caused by the biopsy procedure, for it is rarely seen in post-mortem material from younger persons. On the other hand, the type II ring bundles seem part of an intrinsic pathological process. It is in myotonic dystrophy (Fig. 5.10a)

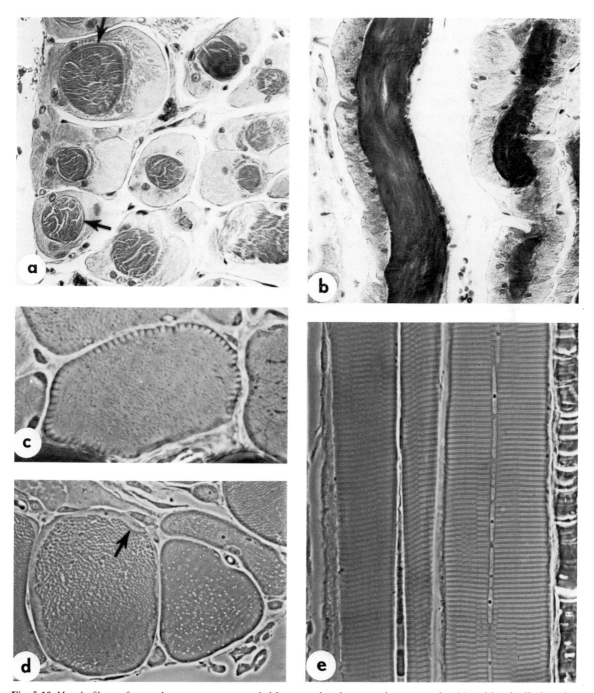

Fig. 5.10 Muscle fibres of normal appearance surrounded by sarcoplasmic masses in cross-section (a) and longitudinal section (b) from a case of myotonic dystrophy. Arrows point to ring bundles of Type II (see text). Lillie's allochrome, ×435 and 340. c. Ring bundles of Type I (see text), ×870. d. Sarcoplasm at periphery of fibre (arrow) devoid of myofibrils resulting from previous destruction, ×545. e. 'Rowing' (chains) of centrally located sarcolemmal nuclei in hypertrophic fibre in ageing muscle, ×545

that they are found so regularly (Heidenhain 1918) as to have been accepted with sarcoplasmic masses (Wohlfart 1951) as typical of this disease. The view that they are not due to fixatives has been established by their demonstration under polarised light in unfixed fresh frozen tissue (Engel 1962b). Wohlfart (1955) also noted an increasing incidence of ring bundles with age, especially in eye muscles and, as already mentioned, listed them among senile changes (see also Hübner 1977).

Other alterations in muscle fibres. We include here non-destructive modifications of parts of the fibre resulting in malformations of organelles (e.g. mitochondria), the proliferation of organelles, accumulation of substances (e.g. glycogen) and the formation of new structures.

Biochemical inclusions. Glycogen, a normal component of muscle, increases when there is a deficiency of certain enzymes, usually genetically determined, necessary for intracellular metabolism of carbohydrates. This may lead to abnormal accumulations of glycogen granules beneath the sarcolemma and between myofibrils. Some such accumulations are surrounded by newly formed membranes; others lie free in the sarcoplasm. The techniques usually employed by pathologists distort the natural appearance of glycogen stores in muscle, for much of the glycogen is water-soluble and removed during fixation, and in haematoxylin and eosin-stained sections only clear vacuoles remain. This appearance differs from that of periodic paralysis only by the greater degree of vacuolisation. Fortunately, carmine and PAS stains usually show some remaining glycogen, even when special fixatives have not been used. Glycogen granules are most readily studied in electron micrographs of osmium-stained sections.

The striated muscle fibre regularly exhibits change in at least three glycogenoses, Cori's Type II, IV, and V (Ch. 25). In the best-known of these diseases, Type II of Cori, now known as Pompe's disease, in which skeletal muscles, heart and other organs are involved in various combinations owing to a deficiency of α-1–4 glucosidase, fine aggregates of glycogen accumulate in the centre of the fibre, displacing the myofibrils (Fig. 5.11 and 5.12). As glycogen accumulates it obliterates the myofibrillar structure, leaving the fibre a nondescript bag containing rows of longitudinally oriented vacuoles, rounded basophilic refractile bodies and granules. Some impregnated fibres enlarge to as much as twice their normal size. The peripherally placed sarcolemmal nuclei usually look normal. Every muscle is involved and hence biopsy diagnosis is usually easy. Weakness and hypotonia are presumably ascribable to loss of contractile efficiency in the glycogen-impregnated fibres.

The characteristic abnormality in Type V, McArdle's disease, is absence or reduction of phosphorylase in muscle fibres (Pearson et al 1961). The accumulation of glycogen, the failure of the fibres to contract and to relax under conditions requiring strenuous work, and even the patchy necrosis, are all secondary. In severe cases blebs, filled with granulated material, are seen around the margins. In cross-sections such blebs may encircle two-thirds of the fibre, and in longitudinal sections they take the form of spindles, measuring up to 200 μm in length (Fig. 5.11a, b). Myofibrils are pressed away from the sarcolemma and the 'thickened' appearance of the latter is due to a thin band of sarcoplasm, which remains between it and the glycogen. Usually the sarcolemmal nuclei remain unaltered. Here and there single fibres disappear and are replaced by connective tissue. However, this does not prove that glycogen deposit alone results in necrosis. The mild progressive myopathy accounts for the persistent weakness noted in some cases.

Further chemical and pathological studies of this group of diseases are needed. Its boundaries are far from clear. Some cases of physiological contracture induced by exercise which we have studied have no defect of phosphorylase, therefore some other enzymatic defect was responsible. Tarui et al (1965), Satoyoshi & Kowa (1967), Layzer et al (1967) and Layzer & Rowland (1971) demonstrated contracture in patients with phosphofructokinase and phosphohexoseisomerase deficiency and other defects of glycogen breakdown are now known (Ch. 25).

Normal muscle contains droplets of lipid. They are seen as tiny vacuoles in frozen sections but are best studied with Sudan fat stains or in electron micrographs.

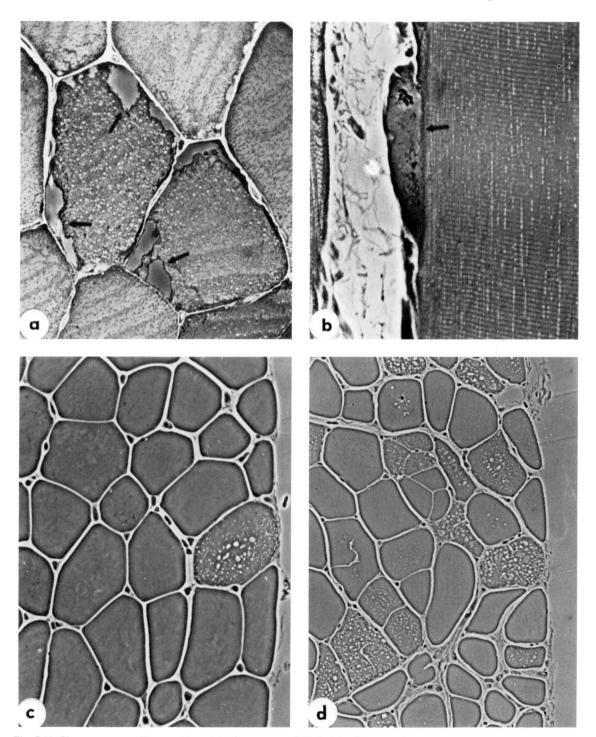

Fig. 5.11 Glycogen storage diseases: (a) and (b) from a case of McArdle's disease. a. Glycogen accumulated peripherally in two cross-sectioned fibres (arrows). The collections have a homogeneous, greyish appearance, ×545. b. Longitudinal section showing subsarcolemmal collection of glycogen (arrow), ×545. (c) and (d) from a case of the adult form of Pompe's disease. c. At an earlier stage of the disease only one fibre (shown) in many blocks of the biopsy appeared to be affected, i.e. was vacuolated, ×350. d. In a second biopsy, taken several years later, many fibres are vacuolated. The unaffected fibres have a normal appearance, ×220

A lipid-storage disease is based on an enzymatic defect which prevents the utilisation of fatty acids and causes an abnormal accumulation of lipid. A deficiency of carnitine is one important cause of lipid aggregates in skeletal muscle. In routine microscopic preparations the lipid appears as vacuoles within the sarcoplasm (Engel & Angelini 1973). The broader subject of 'lipid storage myopathies' has been reviewed by Angelini (1976, 1984) and Bradley et al (1978).

Lipid inclusions of other types have also been found. Examples are cases of ceroid lipofuscinosis (Haltia et al 1973, Carpenter et al 1977) and Fabry's disease (Tomé et al 1977). Carpenter et al consider the study of skin and muscle biopsy material under the electron microscope to be a reliable procedure for the diagnosis of all forms of lipofuscinosis.

Inclusions of formed elements. We include here structured elements, which have little or no resemblance to the organelles of normal muscle. Some probably originate in organelles which, in the course of degeneration, become distorted beyond recognition. Others may represent de novo formations.

Nemaline bodies (Fig. 5.13) were first seen in a new type of myopathy, termed nemaline myopathy because of the presence of thread- or worm-like particles beneath the sarcolemma (Conen et al 1963, Shy et al 1963). In this condition the rod-shaped structures (about 0.3–0.7 μm in diameter and 1.5–5.0 μm in length) occur singly or in aggregates, often arranged irregularly or in palisades and usually without reference to the axis of the fibre (Fig. 5.13a, b). When single and situated deep within the fibre, the rods are orientated parallel to the myofibrils. Under the electron microscope these bodies have some resemblance to Z lines. This has led to the postulation of a disorder of the muscle protein of which Z line material is believed to be composed.

Although the rod-shaped bodies identify this disease, there are usually other changes as well, such as smallness of many fibres, greater than normal variation in size and some degenerative features (Sreter et al 1976). Necrosis of fibres and phagocytosis was prominent in the cases described by Price et al (1965), but not in others.

These findings correlate with the clinical finding of weakness, hypotonia and slender muscles, corresponding in this respect to congenital hypoplasia or other congenital myopathies. In later life, some fibre loss occurs in proximal limb and trunk muscle. The specificity of nemaline bodies is negated by the fact that they are found (in smaller numbers) in other human muscle diseases and in experimental animals (Fig. 5.13c, d). Nemaline bodies have also been found in the heart muscle of two sisters with fatal cardiomyopathy, one of whom also had such bodies in skeletal muscle but no clinical sign of myopathy (Meier et al 1984).

Cytoplasmic bodies may be seen with the light microscope (Engel 1962a, Adams & Rebeiz 1966) but are best observed under the electron microscope. They are spherical bodies with an average diameter of 4 μm. Their centre is dense and homogeneous, whereas the peripheral zone contains radiating, fine fibrils. They appear to be composed of a collection of contracted myofilaments (Engel 1962a, Kinoshita et al 1975b, Cullen & Fulthorpe 1975) but it is possible that they also contain material derived from Z discs (MacDonald & Engel 1969). Cytoplasmic bodies are nonspecific and have been found in many different diseases.

Tubular aggregates, structures that are best seen with the electron microscope (Ch. 8), are groups of tightly packed, longitudinally orientated tubules, that lie among the myofibrils and cause little, if any, destruction of cytoplasmic elements. They probably represent a new growth of membranes derived, in our opinion, from the SR system. Tubular aggregates appear regularly in all types of periodic paralysis (Dyken et al 1969, Bradley 1969, Engel et al 1970, Meyers et al 1972, Schiffer et al 1976) but have been seen in a variety of unrelated conditions.

So-called honeycomb structures, zebra bodies, filamentous, fingerprint and reducing bodies, and laminated bodies (Payne & Curless 1976) have been observed in patients with muscular symptoms. Some of them are said to be characteristic of specific diseases and in some instances the disease has been named after the specific body (Table 5.1). Their significance is unknown. It seems unlikely that they figure in the pathogenesis of any particular disease.

Cylindrical spirals — unique intramuscular

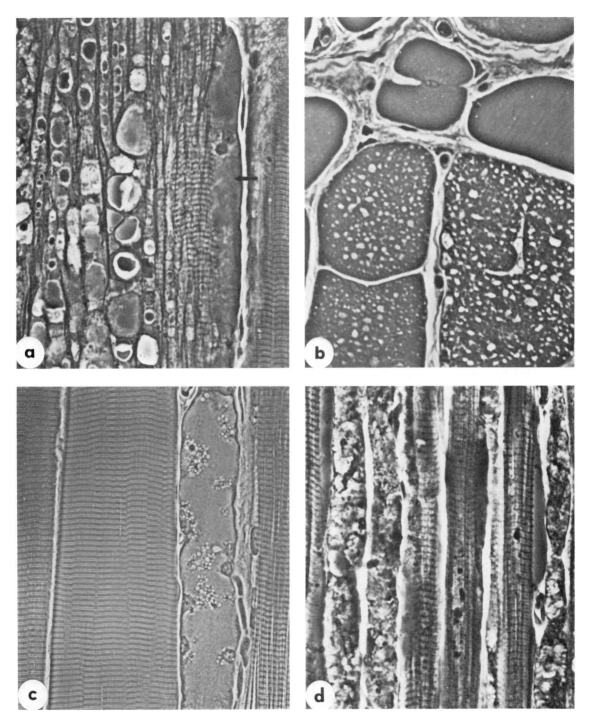

Fig. 5.12 Pompe's disease: (a), (b), and (c) are from an adult case (same biopsy as in Fig. 5.11 (c) and (d)). a. Longitudinal section of a severely affected fibre in which vacuoles of glycogen and debris (lysosomal) are located between a few remaining intact myofibrils. Glycogen has also accumulated beneath the sarcolemma (arrow), ×545. b. Characteristic vacuolation in cross-section. Partial splitting of fibre in the upper part of the picture is due to previous focal necrosis, ×545. c. Longitudinal section showing severe destruction in a fibre, which contains fluid and macrophages. Adjacent fibre appears normal, ×545. d. Longitudinal section from infantile case of Pompe's disease. There is vacuolation and severe destruction of fibres. Note also subsarcolemmal bags with glycogen, ×545

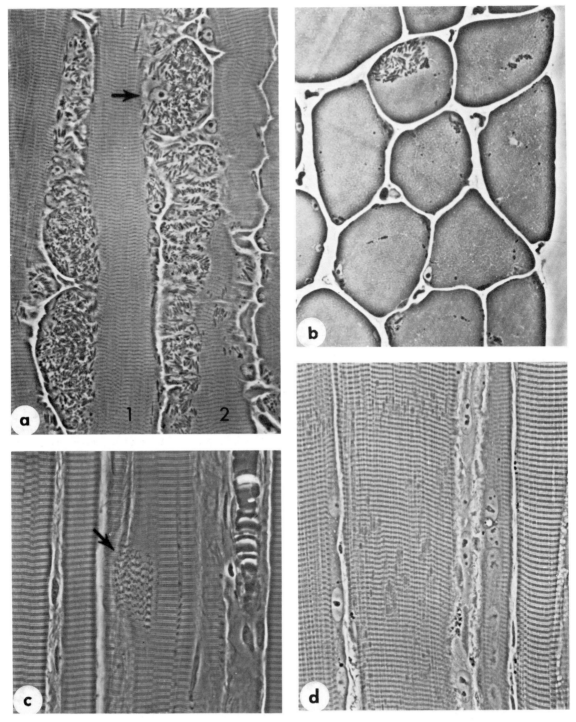

Fig. 5.13 Nemaline bodies. A case of nemaline myopathy is illustrated in longitudinal (a) and cross (b) sections. a. Fibre no. 1 contains three huge subsarcolemmal aggregates of nemaline bodies. The two rounded collections on the left side are separated from each other by a cleft. A sarcolemmal nucleus (arrow) is visible in the third collection in the upper right part of the fibre. Fibre no. 2 has a large collection in its left side. Nemaline bodies within these masses have a haphazard orientation. Those in the interior of the fibres tend to have a longitudinal direction. Except for the collections of rod-like bodies the muscle fibres appear to be unaffected, ×545. b. Nemaline bodies seen in one large collection in one fibre and singly or in smaller groups in others, ×640. c. Longitudinal section of muscle in spinal atrophy showing local swelling of fibre with rod-like bodies, ×700. d. Rod-like bodies scattered in a muscle fibre in a case of polymyositis, ×545

bodies — can be seen in the light microscope as elongated rod-like structures beneath the sarcolemmal membrane of type II fibres. In the electron microscope they appear as laminated cylinders. There is no common denominator among the cases in which they have been seen (Carpenter et al 1979, Bove et al 1980, Gibbels et al 1984).

Mitochondrial abnormalities. It was first proposed by Luft et al (1962) that a meaningful association may exist between clinical symptoms and the abnormal structure and function of mitochondria in skeletal muscles. The concept of 'mitochondrial myopathy' has since become firmly entrenched in the literature and is the source of some confusion. Logically it should mean that a disturbance in mitochondrial structure is the mechanism whereby a muscle fibre becomes diseased. However, abnormal mitochondria may also represent a secondary or compensatory reaction. Thus, in severely degenerated muscles, impairment of oxidation or 'respiratory control' may be secondary to the degenerative process (Peter et al 1970). It is also conceivable that a pathogenetic factor, operating inside or outside the muscle, may cause degenerative changes in mitochondria and in other parts of the muscle fibre as a collateral 'epiphenomenon': in other words, these changes are signs of, but not a cause of, disease (Askanas et al 1978). Even when primary, a mitochondrial change is not always associated with myopathy, and need not have led to fibre degeneration. Indeed, in some cases of reported 'mitochondrial myopathy' the patient had at most only a general feeling of fatigue, e.g., in the case described by Luft et al (1962) the clinical picture was dominated by non-muscular symptoms, and there was no destructive change in the muscle fibres. (Light microscopy in this case was carried out by one of us, KEÅ.) Finally, one should remember that biopsies are taken more often from skeletal muscles than from other organs. Hence, interest may be focused on the muscles so that more universal affections are overlooked. It is known, in fact, that in some cases of so-called mitochondrial myopathy abnormalities are found not only in muscle mitochondria but also in other organs.

Mitochondrial disease, rather than myopathy, would be a more appropriate eponym in such cases.

Abnormal appearance of mitochondria has been noted in many other disease entities, such as muscular dystrophy, which have no disturbance of the cellular respiratory system. The changes seem here to be secondary and of no pathogenetic significance. Apart from such cases there remain many reports of clinical cases — beginning with that of Luft et al (1962) — from which the true picture of mitochondrial disease has developed.

Classification of these diseases must ultimately be based upon the recognition of underlying enzymatic defects in energy metabolism rather than upon clinical and pathological findings, which are non-specific (Morgan-Hughes 1982, DiMauro et al 1985, Ch. 25 in this volume). From a clinical point of view, however, it is of value to know that mitochondrial abnormalities may occur in certain more or less well-defined syndromes (which can be grouped as outlined below), and that muscle biopsy may be a useful diagnostic tool in certain of these unexplained syndromes (Morgan-Hughes et al 1982). With the exception of the first group the following ones are heterogeneous; furthermore, there may be some overlapping between them:

(1) Hypermetabolism of non-thyroid origin. Only two patients have been described, the first by Luft et al (1962) and the second by Afifi et al (1972) and by DiMauro et al (1976).

(2) Pure myopathies. This group contains cases with affections in the limb girdle and, to a lesser degree, other skeletal muscles. In some cases a similar mitochondrial myopathy has been associated with disorders of other organs (Larsson et al 1964, Hülsmann et al 1967, Fisher & Danowski 1969, Spiro et al 1970a, Hudgson et al 1972, Shibasaki et al 1973, Worsfold et al 1973, Rawles & Weller 1974, Black et al 1975, Sengers et al 1975, Bender & Engel 1976, Schotland et al 1976, Kamieniecka 1976, Morgan-Hughes et al 1977, Bradley et al 1978, Hayes et al 1984).

(3) Ophthalmoplegic myopathies (Ch. 15). The Kearns–Sayre syndrome was described as a clinical entity in 1958 by Kearns & Sayre and by Kearns in 1965. Mitochondrial changes in this

syndrome have been noted by Carroll et al (1976) in their cases 1, 3, 4 and by Berenberg et al (1976).

Progressive external ophthalmoplegia, first described by von Graefe in 1856, was identified as a myopathy by Kiloh & Nevin (1951). Mitochondrial changes were noted by DiMauro et al (1973), Sulaiman et al (1974), Carroll et al (case 2) (1976), Reske-Nielsen et al (1976) and Johnson et al (1983).

Mitochondrial abnormalities have also been seen in muscles in cases of oculopharyngeal muscular dystrophy by Julien et al (1974) and by Couturier et al (1981). This hereditary disease was first described by Taylor in 1915 and was recognised as a myopathy by Victor et al in 1962.

(4) Syndromes with disordered function of the CNS, skeletal muscles and other organs. This is a heterogeneous group of diseases, many of which start at an early age and lead to profound disability and early death. Symptoms include retarded growth, myoclonic seizures, dementia, cerebellar ataxia, weakness, exercise intolerance, salt craving and lactic acidosis. Mitochondrial changes in the muscle fibres have also been observed in Leigh's subacute necrotising encephalomyelopathy (Kinoshita et al 1978, Willems et al 1977); Menkes' trichopoliodystrophy (French et al 1972, Ghatak et al 1972); the hepatorenal syndrome of Zellweger (Goldfischer et al 1973); progressive poliodystrophy or Alpers' disease (Suzuki & Rapin 1969, Prick et al 1983); a syndrome of encephalopathy, lactic acidosis and stroke-like episodes (Pavlakis et al 1984) and a syndrome of myoclonic epilepsy with ataxia, dementia and hearing loss (Spiro et al 1970b, Tsairis et al 1973, Fukuhara et al 1980b, Fitzsimons et al 1981, Rosing et al 1985).

A miscellany of other cases with mitochondrial changes in muscles and/or other organs have been described by van Wijngaarden et al (1967), van Biervliet et al (1977), Spiro et al (1970b), Hackett et al (1973), Tarlow et al (1973), Tsairis et al (1973); Shapira et al (1975), Hart et al (1977), Askanas et al (1978), Skoglund (1979), DiMauro et al (1980), Kobayashi et al (1982) and Morgan-Hughes et al (1982, 1984).

Because the pathology in muscle is the same in all, a single description will suffice for all groups. In all the muscle diseases called mitochondrial, the specific pathological alteration is not easily seen with the light microscope. In exceptional cases the sarcolemma is separated from the myofibrils by granular material, which proves on electron microscopy to represent groups of mitochondria. The mitochondria-laden fibres react intensely to stains for oxidative enzymes, and they have been called 'ragged-red fibres' because of the red appearance of the mitochondrial aggregates in Gomori-stained sections (Olson et al 1972 and Ch. 7).

Under the electron microscope the mitochondria are usually found to be enlarged with an abnormal, often bizarre appearance. They contain stacks of parallel lamellae, concentric rings of membranes, paracrystalline bodies and granular material (Ch. 8).

The abnormal mitochondria are usually increased in number and may form large aggregates at the periphery of fibres. Many affected fibres are of normal size and shape and are otherwise of normal appearance except for frequent and characteristic collections of glycogen and fat within the fibres, which may raise the possibility of storage disease. Nevertheless, destruction of fibres may occur, especially in cranial muscles. As the number of fibres diminishes there is replacement by interstitial fibrous tissue and lipocytes. In contrast, trunk and limb muscles in such cases are hardly affected, if at all.

Autopsy examinations have shown that the central nervous system is not involved in the progressive external ophthalmoplegia of von Graefe, Kiloh and Nevin (Beckett & Netsky 1953, Schwartz & Liu 1954) nor in the oculopharyngeal form of Taylor (Rebeiz et al 1969). Likewise, one member of such a family with facioscapulohumeral myopathy had no signs of disease in the central nervous system except for an acute infarct (Bradley et al 1978). Of particular interest in the latter case is that the mitochondrial changes were restricted to the skeletal muscles. These data support the conclusion that muscular changes and symptoms in this group of diseases are of myogenic and not of neurogenic origin. On the other hand, a spongiform encephalopathy has been found in autopsied cases of the Kearns–Sayre syndrome (Kearns & Sayre 1958, Daroff et al 1966, Castaigne et al 1971, Berenberg et al 1976).

In this syndrome abnormal mitochondria have been noted, not only in skeletal muscles, but also in other organs, such as the Purkinje cells of the cerebellum (Gonatas et al 1967). The lesions in the central nervous system explain symptoms such as ataxia, mental retardation and abnormal electroencephalographic patterns, which are common in the Kearns–Sayre syndrome.

With regard to pathogenesis, one can only speculate that abnormality of one or several genes (hereditary or acquired) may result in deficiency of one or several mitochondrial enzymes and/or impairment of the function of the respiratory chain in forming ATP. Multiple gene damage could explain the combinations of symptoms resulting from dysfunction of skeletal muscles and other organs. It is possible that morphological changes in the mitochondria are only secondary, i.e. that they represent an attempt on the part of muscle cells to compensate for the deficiency of a mitochondrial enzyme. Lactic acidosis in blood and accumulation of glycogen and fat in muscles with abnormal mitochondria also reflect a functional disturbance of the muscle fibres' oxidative functions.

Vacuoles may be seen as small holes in muscle fibres, but fine details regarding their contents, surrounding membranes, if any, and relationship to the sarcotubular system are demonstrable only with the electron microscope (see Ch. 8).

Vacuolation ('hydropic degeneration' in the classical literature) is another non-specific feature. The expression 'vacuolar myopathy' has little meaning, because the associated changes are so heterogeneous, and many different causes and pathogenetic mechanisms are involved.

True vacuoles are surrounded by membranes. The latter are probably formed from the normal membranous structures which occupy much of the volume of the muscle fibres (see Ch. 2). Probably most of the membranes around vacuoles come from the T tubules and the sarcoplasmic reticulum (Bird 1975). Other less likely sources are the Golgi apparatus, which is small in muscle fibres, and the perinuclear membranes.

Following focal necrosis (see Fig. 5.4 and p. 167), the degenerate material is walled off from the remainder of the fibre by a membrane, which forms an autophagic vacuole (also called a secondary lysosome). The sequestered material is digested by autolytic enzymes. End-products in the vacuoles are eventually extruded into the extracellular space, but some products may remain as lipofuscin bodies (Fig. 5.4d; see also Figs. 35–37 and 50d in Åström & Adams 1980).

Autophagic vacuoles have also been called 'rimmed vacuoles' (Dubowitz & Brooke 1973, Fukuhara et al 1980a) or 'lined vacuoles' (Carpenter et al 1978) as they appear to be lined with basophilic material in sections which have been stained with haematoxylin and eosin. They have been seen in different muscle diseases but are especially prominent in Pompe's disease (Fig. 5.11 and 5.12), periodic paralysis syndromes (Fig. 5.14), chloroquine-induced myopathy (Engel 1973), oculopharyngeal muscular dystrophy (Rebeiz et al 1969, Little & Perl 1982, Martin et al 1982) and in inclusion body myositis (Chad et al 1982, Danon et al 1982, Mikol et al 1982).

Multifocal hydropic change in muscle fibres is characteristic of familial hypokalaemic periodic paralysis (Fig. 5.14). In this disease as many as one-quarter of all muscle fibres may be vacuolated. The vacuoles range in size from less than five to more than 25 μm, and in many places several may seem to have coalesced. Their longitudinal dimension varies from five to 200 μm, and one fibre may contain vacuoles at several non-aligned points. The myofibrils and sarcoplasm, being displaced laterally, must curve around the vacuoles. Within the cleared zone a fine precipitated material, which stains with carmine and in the periodic-acid–Schiff (PAS) reaction, may be seen.

In some cases, biopsies taken between attacks have disclosed entirely normal muscle structure. However, the idea that the vacuolisation occurs only during attacks is patently refuted by the finding of severe vacuolar change in patients who have not suffered a manifest attack of even mild weakness for 20 years. Such instances indicate that this morphological change may be the principal finding in a late, chronic, progressive stage of this myopathy. Such pronounced vacuolisation led to necrosis of single muscle fibres in the family studied by Gruner & Porte (1959). Many attacks of paralysis, then, seem to initiate a mild

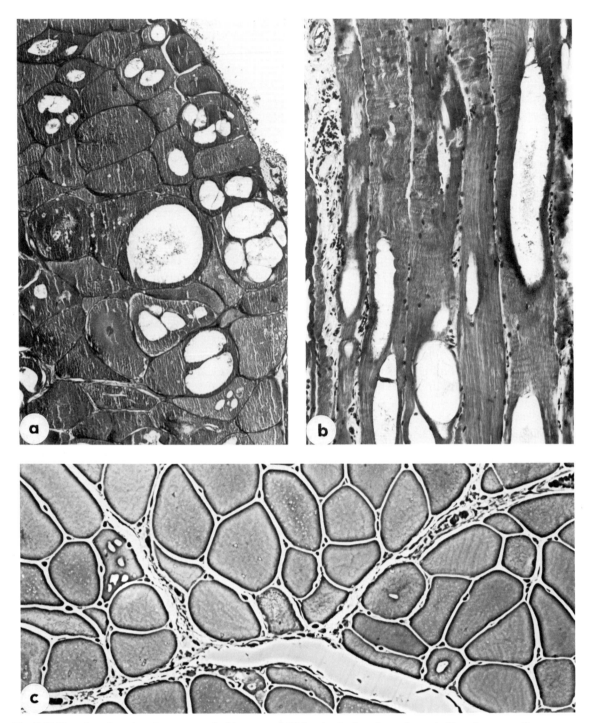

Fig. 5.14 Vacuoles of varying sizes are seen in (a) cross and (b) longitudinal sections of muscle fibres in a case of hypokalaemic periodic paralysis. Large vacuoles have expanded some muscle fibres leaving only a thin rim of muscle tissue at the periphery. H and E, ×225. c. Lesser degree of vacuolation noted in biopsy from a case of hyperkalaemic periodic paralysis, ×295

progressive myopathy. The necrotic segments of the fibre may be restored, after phagocytotic removal, by regeneration. Incomplete restoration of damaged fibres may lead to a slightly reduced population of muscle fibres and mild endomysial fibrosis. The creation of communications between vacuoles and the extracellular space, with indentation of the surface membrane, will result in remodelling and splitting of fibres (Engel 1970b).

A similar vacuolar change is said occasionally to accompany the paralysis of hyperaldosteronism and the normokalaemic periodic paralysis described by Tyler et al (1951), and by Poskanzer & Kerr (1961).

The paramyotonia of Eulenberg and the related adynamia episodica hereditaria of Gamstorp (1956), where transient paralysis may be induced by potassium and is relieved by a high dietary intake of carbohydrate, might be regarded as the obverse of hypokalaemic periodic paralysis. Multifocal vacuolisation has been observed (Fig. 5.14c), but only rarely, as might be expected, for the water content of the fibre is said to be reduced. Drager et al (1958) noted zones of clear sarcoplasm, devoid of myofibrils in some muscle fibres in their cases of paramyotonia and Gamstorp (1956) observed similar alterations in one of her three cases of hereditary episodic adynamia, together with ring bundles, which are more often seen in myotonic dystrophy.

The cause and pathogenesis of the vacuoles in periodic paralysis have been widely discussed. Shy et al (1961) demonstrated intracellular oedema by direct measurement. The associated reduction in serum potassium is presumably caused by a movement of this cation into the muscle fibre, but no explanation has been found for the migration of either potassium or water. The paralysis which follows the biochemical change cannot be ascribed to the mechanical effect of the vacuolisation per se, for loss of function greatly exceeds that to be expected if all the vacuolated muscle fibres were powerless to contract. It is more likely that paralysis is due to a change in the electrical properties of the sarcolemma or its inward extension into the transverse tubule, or in the SR system (Shy et al 1961, Engel 1970b).

The vacuoles then, must be regarded as a consequence of the disease and not a cause of the paralytic attacks. With regard to the origin of these vacuoles, Shy et al (1961) postulated that they are formed from dilatations and coalescence of SR tubules. Engel (1970b) traced the earliest stage of vacuolisation to proliferation and dilatation of SR and T systems. The mature vacuoles were found to be in communication with the extracellular space via the T tubules.

As stated above, a small part of the glycogen in the muscle fibres is normally enclosed in membrane-bound vacuoles where it is broken down by lysosomal enzymes (acid maltase). Deficiency of this enzyme in Pompe's disease (Hers 1963) leads to accumulation of glycogen in membrane-bound bags (Engel 1970a, Engel et al 1973). This is an example of the so-called lysosomal diseases (Hers 1965); it is characterised by two types of lysosomal vacuoles — the glycogen-filled vacuoles and the autophagic vacuoles with debris, which were described on page 189 (Figs. 5.11 and 5.12). Lysosomes with glycogen have also been seen in debrancher deficiency glucogenosis (Cornelio et al 1984).

Multiple small vacuoles occur in various other conditions (Fig. 5.15). We have seen them, inter alia, in denervation atrophy and polymyositis. Of particular interest was one of our patients with Charcot–Marie–Tooth's disease, in whose muscle we found late dystrophic changes of denervation (Fig. 5.2d), target phenomena (Fig. 5.9d) and multiple vacuoles (Figs. 5.9d and 5.15a). Electron microscopy showed that the vacuoles were membrane-bound and had the appearance of lysosomes.

Crescent formations. The term 'thyroid myopathy', confirming an association of disease of the thyroid gland with disorders of muscle, came to medical attention through the original reports of Hoffmann (1893) and Debré & Semelaigne (1935). Most textbooks also refer to an article by Askanazy (1898), which described and illustrated a widespread necrotising myopathy in cases of thyrotoxicosis. His findings, however, have never been corroborated. Probably, Askanazy's cases were complicated by infection and other disease processes, which could have caused a Zenker's type of necrosis. Only in ophthalmic Graves' disease have consistent structural alterations been

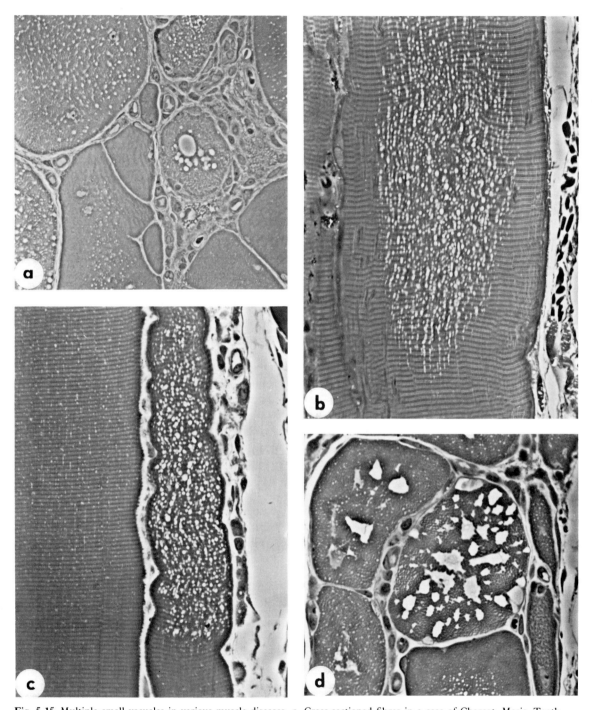

Fig. 5.15 Multiple small vacuoles in various muscle diseases. a. Cross-sectioned fibres in a case of Charcot–Marie–Tooth disease containing many small vacuoles, surrounded by a membrane. They are seen mostly in large fibres and are most numerous in the central regions of fibres. Compare this Figure with those in Figs. 5.2 (d) and 5.9 (d), which are from the same patient, ×545. b. Longitudinal section from a case of neurogenic atrophy showing many small vacuoles in the central part of the fibre, ×545. c. Longitudinal section of muscle fibre in a case of polymyositis (same as (d)); note vacuolation near zone of necrosis (not shown in the picture), ×545. d. Cross-section of muscle from a case of polymyositis showing vacuolation of fibres, ×545

found. In the eye muscles, infiltration of fat cells is the most obvious change, but degeneration of muscle fibres, a variable regenerative reaction and infiltration of lymphocytes and mononuclear histiocytes also occur. Conventional histological stains have not usually disclosed any definitive muscular lesion in either thyrotoxic myopathy or hypothyroidism, apart from a slight volumetric decrease in the former and an increase in the latter. In one specimen (from a 71-year-old woman, who died in myxoedemic coma without ever having received thyroid treatment), Åström et al (1961) discovered accumulations of mucoid material within some skeletal muscle fibres. McKeran et al (1980) claim that glycogen storage and a mitochondrial disorder are features of hypothyroid myopathy (1980).

The paper by Asbøe-Hansen et al (1952) on 'crescent formation', deserves special comment. In all 10 cases of exophthalmic goitre, in nine out of 10 cases of thyrotoxicosis without exophthalmos, and in one out of seven cases of myxoedema, these authors found in muscle biopsy sections curious deposits of semi-lunar or crescent form (in cross-sections) or spindle form (in longitudinal sections) beneath the sarcolemma. The myofibrils were pushed aside. Demonstration of these deposits required a basic lead acetate fixative. Water solubility and extractability by hyaluronidase, and the staining properties of the material suggested that it contained mucopolysaccharide. No other worker has seen these crescents, nor have we been able to find them, using the same method of fixation and staining. Their occurrence in both hyper- and hypothyroidism, two diseases of almost diametrically opposite functional and biochemical properties, must raise some doubts as to whether they reflect a basic pathological process. Clearly, these myopathies merit further study.

Nuclear alterations. Nuclear number and position within the fibre have already been mentioned in several contexts. Atrophy or hypoplasia of fibres results in a population of nuclei that is larger in proportion to the volume of visible sarcoplasm without an actual increase in numbers. In addition, in muscle hypertrophy the nuclei are more widely spaced (and sometimes central in position) without an actual change in number.

True nuclear hyperplasia probably signifies necrosis with regeneration in most instances; in the earlier phases of this process the nuclei enlarge and acquire a prominent nucleolus (Fig. 5.7).

One special form of hyperplasia is that in which there are rows or chains of sarcolemmal nuclei ('rowing phenomenon'; see Fig. 5.10e). Usually the end of one nucleus touches the end of the adjacent one and as many as 15–20 nuclei lie like this. The nuclei tend to be small and hyperchromatic. This phenomenon is seen most consistently in myotonic dystrophy, with disorganisation of myofibrils and sarcoplasmic masses, but it occurs to a lesser degree in many other diseases and in ageing muscle. In the latter, as well as in denervation atrophy, extreme atrophy may reduce the muscle fibre to a bag of pyknotic nuclei so tightly clustered as to resemble, in haematoxylin-eosin stains, a particle of calcium.

Intranuclear inclusions have been described in several conditions. Nuclei in cases of oculopharyngeal muscular dystrophy may contain tubular filaments with an outer diameter of 7–8 nm (Tomé & Fardeau 1980, Martin et al 1982, Coquet et al 1983). Another type of filament is seen in inclusion body myositis (see below). Some of the inclusions within nuclei prove on electron-microscopic examination simply to be caused by infolding of the nuclear membrane. Invaginations with cytoplasmic elements have been seen in myotonic dystrophy and congenital myotonia (Schröder & Adams 1968) and in other myopathies. It has also been noted that sarcolemmal nuclei may contain nemaline-like bodies (Jenis et al 1969, Engel 1975).

Arrested development of muscle fibres

Spiro et al (1966) described the case of a 12-year-old boy with a congenital, progressive muscle disease. The resemblance of the muscle fibres in biopsies to the myotubular stage of development persuaded them that an arrest in development had occurred — a kind of muscle retardation. Since then 70–80 similar cases have been reported under names such as myotubular, centronuclear and pericentronuclear myopathy (see Table 5.1 for references).

The muscle fibres are usually fairly thin, but

they are never as small as true embryonal fibres. Most nuclei are centrally situated and surrounded by a clear rim. A few fibres show mild degeneration and discrete alterations of internal architecture. Loss of fibres is not seen. Histochemical studies suggest that, in many cases, central nucleation is confined to small type I fibres (Engel et al 1968).

The idea of arrest of muscle development in the fetus is interesting. It recalls the earlier suggestion of Krabbe (1949) that the weak, hypotonic child with the amyotonia congenita syndrome of Oppenheim (1900) might be suffering from a congenital muscular hypoplasia.

Senile and non-specific changes

In studies of skeletal muscle tissue it is important to know that surveys of the musculature, in random post-mortem examinations, have disclosed a surprising number of instances of single fibre necrosis and phagocytosis and aggregates of lymphocytes. Wallace et al (1958) and Pearson (1959) confirmed that this type of change is common in autopsy material, where death was sudden and traumatic or due to some disease not known to affect the muscle fibres or endomysial tissue. These findings indicate that minor muscle fibre injury is continually occurring during everyday life. The pathologist must exercise caution in accepting such changes as indicating specific muscle diseases.

Our own studies of seven muscles from 134 random autopsies (Moore et al 1971) revealed in late life a high incidence (over 80%) of group atrophy and single-fibre atrophy and of nuclear aggregates, especially in leg muscles, and a lesser number of specimens with more extensive necrosis of fibres and vacuolisation.

Pigmentary atrophy, the homologue of brown atrophy of heart muscle, seems to be a reliable index of ageing, although similar impregnation of sarcoplasm near muscle nuclei by lipofuscin accompanies vitamin E deficiency, even in relatively young animals. A longitudinal row of lipofuscin deposits may also be a residue of previous focal destruction (see p. 167 and Fig. 5.4d).

Regarding other aspects of ageing, few facts are available. Assuming that nearly all the muscle fibres in the human organism were formed before birth and that all natural, postnatal modifications of structure consist essentially of growth, i.e. increase in size, the fate of such long-enduring fibres becomes a matter of great interest. Do old muscle fibres, like old neurones, ultimately waste away and disappear? Is there a sequence of disfigurative change which might constitute a 'senile myopathy'? We believe that both questions may be answered affirmatively. The range of fibre size increases in the ageing muscle because of increasing numbers of isolated small fibres. Tightly agglutinated knots of dark sarcolemmal nuclei, probably the terminal phase of the atrophic process, and group atrophy, probably attributable to senile loss of motor nerve cells, are also present, especially in leg muscles.

Fibre wasting, with loss of myofibrils and lipfuscin increase, has been noted in normal eye muscles in late life, and was called senescent atrophy (Rebeiz et al 1969). Moreover, in the ocular muscles peripheral myofibrils disappear, leaving faintly fibrillar sarcoplasmic masses; ringbinden occur in some fibres and increase with each decade of life, as first pointed out by Wohlfart (1955) and confirmed by Hübner (1977).

Inflammation

In essence, the problem here is how certain viruses, microbes, fungi, protozoa, and parasites (Clostridia, Trichinae, Cysticercae, Toxoplasmas, sarcocysts), the toxins they elaborate, or the autoallergic inflammation which they trigger, can affect the muscle fibres (Mastaglia & Ojeda 1985). Some organisms, such as Trichinae, exhibit an almost specific affinity for sarcoplasm (Ch. 18). However, the most frequent and puzzling of the inflammatory diseases of muscles are not those caused by visible organisms but those of so-called idiopathic polymyositis (Ch. 16). As shown by Walton & Adams (1958), nearly half the latter cases bear some relation to one or other of the connective tissue diseases, and associated dermatitis is common.

The relatively benign course of the disease, in many instances, has prevented an extensive study of post-mortem material. Biopsies of muscle have tended to yield only an incomplete idea of the pathological process. Thus, sections often give negative findings in the face of active disease, or reveal only one element of the process.

One component of the myopathology of this condition is necrosis of muscle fibres, which may be widespread in the severe and acute cases. More often, segments of single fibres are destroyed (Fig. 5.6). In less severe lesions, it is often the peripheral fibres of fasciculi that bear the brunt of the affection. Some of the surviving fibres, especially in cases of lupus erythematosus, are vacuolated. Once destroyed, the necrotic parts of the muscle fibre are removed by macrophages and the regenerative cycle described below begins. Necrosis may recur, and the terminal phases of the lesion result in atrophy of fibres, loss of fibres and fibrosis.

Aggregates of inflammatory cells (lymphocytes, mononuclear leucocytes, plasma cells) constitute the most obvious component of the lesion. Without this finding the diagnosis is always in doubt (the mere presence of aggregates of histiocytes (myophagia) should not be mistaken for it (Walton & Adams 1958)). The inflammatory cells must bear a relationship to some component(s) of the muscle fibres. However, because of the haphazard and incomplete sampling of lesions by the average biopsy, necrosis of muscle may be the only change, or inflammatory cell infiltration may appear to stand alone. The manner in which the myonecrosis, focal inflammation and connective tissue reaction are related can be demonstrated only in serial sections. In a study of the stereology of the lesion, segmental necrosis was invariably seen to be contiguous to a focus of perivenous lymphocytes and monocytes (J. J. Rebeiz, B. A. Kakulas and R. D. Adams, unpublished observations). Occlusion of arteries or veins is not found in adult cases except in rare instances, where a vasculitis such as polyarteritis has complicated the picture, or in lupus erythematosus, where thrombo-embolic lesions may have occurred. Some of the childhood cases of dermatomyositis have a special attribute: the major pathological feature is inflammation of vessels and thrombosis leading to infarction of muscle tissue, small peripheral nerves and other organs such as the gastrointestinal tract (Banker & Victor 1966, Banker 1975, Carpenter & Karpati 1981, Crowe et

al 1982). The lesions should be viewed as consequences of the operation of a single factor which varies in extent and intensity. The details of the early phases of the injury are unknown.

The cause of idiopathic polymyositis is indeterminate (Ch. 17). Case reports of virus-like inclusions in nuclei and/or sarcoplasm are reviewed in Chapter 8.

Inclusion body myositis is a form of polymyositis that differs from the idiopathic form and from dermatomyositis in several respects and may represent a distinct clinicopathological entity (Yunis & Samaha 1971). An association with collagen vascular disease may exist, however (Chad et al 1982, Lane et al 1985). The first case was described by Adams et al in 1965. Chou (1968) found myxovirus-like particles in nuclei and cytoplasm in muscle biopsies from a 16-year-old youth with polymyositis. Pathological changes appear especially in the limb muscles (Carpenter et al 1978, Carpenter & Karpati 1981, Mikol et al 1982, Danon et al 1982). Characteristic rimmed vacuoles are best seen in frozen sections. Other light-microscopic findings are: inclusion bodies in nuclei and/or cytoplasm, atrophy, necrosis and regeneration of single muscle fibres, inflammatory cells between fibres but no vascular changes. Electron microscopy reveals the most characteristic finding: aggregates of filaments with a diameter of 14–18 nm in the cytoplasm and, less commonly, in the nuclei of muscle fibres. Cytoplasmic bodies, whorls of membrane fragments and abnormal mitochondria are non-specific findings. The filaments may be proteinaceous, rather than viral as originally suggested (Yunis & Samaha 1971).

Myopathies without established changes in muscle fibres

There are many clinically recognisable diseases of muscle with a severe and often fluctuant course, sometimes fatal, in which the pathologist can identify no characteristic specific change in the muscle fibres per se. Some such diseases, such as tetanus with its fatal neurogenic and myogenic spasms, and acute botulism, have revealed nothing of their nature after careful study under the light microscope. Furthermore, there are some diseases of muscle, such as the myopathies of hyper- and hypothyroidism, of Addison's disease, of renal acidosis and in Milkman's disease, where pathological study has been too limited to assess the morphological status of the fibre.

Generalised spasms of unknown type, vaguely grouped as the 'stiff-man syndrome', have not been fully elucidated clinically, electromyographically or pathologically. At times this disease may seem localised in onset, but it is soon evident that other muscles share the abnormality.

In myasthenia gravis, the primary abnormality is at the neuromuscular junction (Santa et al 1972), specifically at the acetylcholine receptors on the motor end-plate (Bender et al 1976). Doubts still exist concerning pathological changes within the fibres themselves. Whereas, in many fatal cases of this disease, the only visible change is the mild disuse atrophy, in others isolated necrosis of single muscle fibres and a few aggregates of lymphocytes and monocytes have been found. When unusually prominent, as they may rarely be, the question of polymyositis or of Zenker's necrosis secondary to the terminal infection or a myopathy associated with neoplasia (e.g. malignant thymoma) always arises. In a few cases, as also noted by others, there has been unmistakable evidence of group atrophy, indicative of denervation. The occasional collections of lymphocytes in muscle in such cases (so-called lymphorrhages) help to confirm the autoimmune nature of the process.

Mass lesions in muscle

Tumours of muscle. As is true of all highly specialised postmitotic cells, the muscle fibre seldom undergoes neoplastic transformation; when it does, the tumour is usually highly malignant.

Muscle neoplasms are conventionally divided into two categories (van Unnik 1982): those that are primary, i.e. arising from a constituent element of muscle, usually the muscle cell itself; and those that are secondary, arising in some other organ and extending to muscle by direct invasion or by metastasis.

According to the histogenetic classification of tumours there are two types of tumour derived from myoblastic tissue. These are the rhabdomyoma and the rhabdomyosarcoma. Theoretically, such tumours could originate from primitive mesodermal elements that normally differentiate into myoblasts and myocytes or by the dedifferentiation of mature muscle cells. Stout (1946), in an historically important study, subdivided the rhabdomyosarcoma group into four types: the embryonal cell sarcoma; the botryoides (see below); the alveolar sarcoma; and the pleomorphic sarcoma. The granular cell myoblastoma was another type described but has proved to be a tumour of non-myoblastic origin and is no longer included in the group. Other tumours of muscle taking origin from supporting stroma (connective tissue), fat cells, blood vessels and nervous elements also occur; but, as they do not differ from similar tumours in other organs, they will not be considered here.

The rhabdomyoma is a rare tumour of adult life, more frequent in males, with a tendency to localise in the mediastinum, pharynx, larynx and tongue. The cells are large with abundant cytoplasm and uniform vesicular nuclei. In some of them myofibrils can be seen with visible striations and under the electron microscope there are recognisable Z bands and glycogen.

More frequent is the cardiac rhabdomyoma, a tumour which is found in infants, often in association with tuberous sclerosis.

The embryonal rhabdomyosarcoma is one of the more frequent soft tissue tumours of childhood, again mainly localised in the head and neck regions but also in the genito-urinary tract. Because of the grape-like appearance of the gross lesion it has been called botryoides. Its extremely variable cytological composition includes spindle-shaped cells, some with fibrillar and striated structures which help in its identification. The tumour is highly malignant, often recurring after local excision and spreading to regional nodes. Chemotherapy and radiation after excision has improved the survival rate.

The alveolar rhabdomyosarcoma is also a tumour of childhood and tends to involve the muscles of the extremities. The tumour cells are single or multinucleated and in places form islands separated by fibrous septae, hence the term 'alveolar'. In many specimens the tumour cells are so immature that cytological diagnosis is difficult.

The pleomorphic rhabdomyosarcoma, unlike

the alveolar type, is a tumour of both children and adults of both sexes. It has its greatest incidence in the fifth and sixth decades. It tends to arise in limb muscles, usually of the legs. This tumour accounts for about 10–15% of soft tissue tumours. Stout (1946) emphasised its extremely malignant character. In his series of 121 cases, of which 108 received surgical and radiation therapy, only four were symptom-free at five years but the outcome has improved with more radical surgery and modern methods of therapy (Pack & Ariel 1958).

The only symptom is usually the mass within the muscle. It may grow slowly over years or become quite aggressive with early metastases. The gross characteristics are well described by Pack & Ariel (1958), who remarked on its variable appearance. Usually it is a poorly circumscribed intramuscular mass. It may be yellow, pink or dark red depending on the amount of congestion, haemorrhage and necrosis. The cells are of four types according to Stout (1946): (1) large, rounded cells with one or several central nuclei and a strongly acidophilic cytoplasm; (2) strap-shaped cells with two or more nuclei arranged in tandem and a striated cytoplasm; (3) racquet-shaped cells with a nucleus in the expanded end; (4) giant cells with peripherally arrayed vacuoles separated by strands of cytoplasm (spider-web cells). It is the abundant acidophilic cytoplasm and delicate short fibrils in haphazard arrangement that are most diagnostic. Myofilaments can be demonstrated in electron-microscopic preparations (Fig. 5.16).

Non-neoplastic masses. Tumours originating in cells of the interstitial tissue (fibroblasts, endothelial cells, lipocytes, histiocytes) rarely arise in skeletal muscle. Very occasionally, however, haemangiomas, myxomas, lipomas and fibromas are found. Skeletal muscles may also be infiltrated by local cancerous lesions; less often they have metastases within them (Doshi & Fowler 1983).

Non-neoplastic masses comprise a relatively small group of disorders, even though their clinical presentation is often perplexing.

Rupture of a muscle tendon is recognised by its onset (a snap during exertion) and by the typical gross deformity in the profile of a muscle with weakening of its force. Reports on the pathology

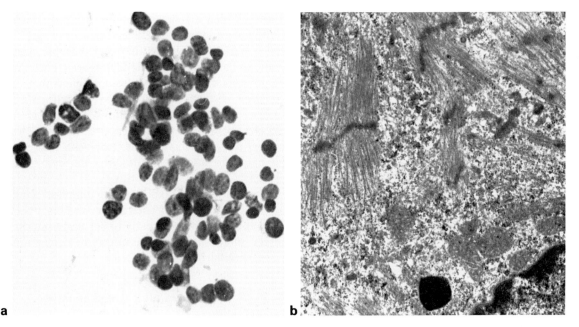

a   b

Fig. 5.16 Rhabdomysarcoma from temporal region of six-year-old child. a. Cytological specimen shows collection of rounded undifferentiated tumour cells, some of which are in mitotic division. No striations visible. H and E ×625. b. Bundles of myofilaments and Z lines are seen in cytoplasm of tumour cell. Part of nucleus and fat globule in lower right corner. Electron micrograph, ×8000 (Courtesy of Dr Peter Collins)

have been meagre. Biopsy may reveal only normal muscle or zones of injured muscle fibres replaced by connective tissue.

After extensive destruction of muscle tissue, whether from infarction, haemorrhage, or inflammation, the regenerating muscle fibres and connective tissue may produce one or more firm lumps in the muscle. During contraction they become hard, but still have more or less the feel of normal muscle. The mass rarely reaches enormous proportions. We have observed more than a dozen cases of this type. Operation revealed a network of interlacing strands of connective tissue and regenerating muscle cells. The appearance was not that of a malignant tumour and the health of the patients and the remainder of their musculature were normal several years later. This type of lesion may follow a mild injury and the enlarging muscle may raise fears of pseudohypertrophic muscular dystrophy. Probably some such pseudotumours represent a desmoid reaction. The latter most often occurs in the rectus abdominis of the post-parturient woman, and consists of large masses of hyperplastic connective tissue engulfing muscle fibres.

Another similar problem is an inflammatory pseudohypertrophy of muscles. This may involve the sternomastoid and anterior scalene muscles which become swollen and painful, first on one side, then on the other. Great overgrowth of connective tissue, giant muscle fibres measuring up to 200 μm in diameter, and atrophic fibres are mixed with infiltrations of inflammatory cells, remnants of necrotic fibres and cellular blood vessels. This condition seems to be a form of so-called localised myositis and is a benign inflammatory pseudotumour without excessive proliferation of connective tissue (Heffner et al 1977, Ho et al 1979). Certainly, idiopathic polymyositis may begin locally as a painful inflammatory mass before the development of generalised disease (Heffner & Barron 1981).

Finally, a persistent and tender lump in a muscle can be due to some type of localised spasm or possibly to an intramuscular rupture. Here one becomes involved in the confusing problem of differentiating 'fibrositis' and myositis from emotional tension with tender spots in muscles. Over the years we have received biopsy material from cases in which the only finding was an extreme state of contraction of fibres resembling artefactual change. One cannot always be sure that the offending lump was sampled in the biopsy. These cases deserve more thorough clinical, physiological and pathological study.

RESTORATION OF MUSCLE FIBRES AFTER DENERVATION AND INJURY

Experimentally induced muscle destruction and repair has been studied in animals for more than 100 years and the observations of the early workers were at times remarkably detailed, extensive and accurate. Almost everything we know about muscle repair derives from experimental studies.

Lesions have been produced in innumerable ways, e.g. by mechanical injury of all kinds, heating, freezing, electricity and other means. Most have been unpredictable in size and location because the injury was inflicted imprecisely. Cellular reactions have been difficult to interpret because destruction involved, to a variable degree, different elements of muscle. There is a need for studies in which precise lesions of known dimension have been produced in predetermined locations. Another major drawback in the analysis has been that most microscopic examinations have sampled only a few brief phases of a continuous process. Conclusions concerning the complete sequence have had to be extrapolated from a series of static pictures. The work of Speidel (1938, 1939) is an exception because it was carried out on living animals (tadpoles). However, he made no attempt to describe the cytological events.

Observations on experimental animals, which go back to the work of Sherrington and his school, have also contributed greatly to our understanding of the motor unit and the effects of denervation upon skeletal muscle fibres.

Restoration of fibres after denervation and reinnervation

Thin, denervated striated muscle fibres (p. 157) regain their normal size if reinnervated within a certain time interval. The mode of restoration depends upon how reinnervation is accomplished.

Denervated muscle fibres may have been reinnervated in one of two ways. In the first, the central part of the damaged nerve grows out and its axons re-establish connections with the same muscle fibres which had been denervated originally. In a favourable case there are no losses of nerve and muscle fibres and the motor units are restored completely. Reinnervation of this type is likely to occur especially if the nerve was incompletely severed (as in crush injury) and the lesion was situated distally, near the corresponding muscle. This type of reinnervation is less likely if the nerve was completely severed and the lesion was located proximally; it does not occur at all after injury to motor cell bodies and roots. Secondly, denervation of scattered motor units in a muscle allows collateral reinnervation from adjacent axons. This results in a regrouping of muscle fibres, so that fewer neurones and axons serve the same number of muscle fibres. This regrouping is seen especially in chronic neuropathies and in motor neurone disease.

Kugelberg et al (1970) showed that the muscle fibres within one motor unit (which are histochemically uniform) are normally scattered, so that the fibres on a cross-section of muscle appear to be isolated from each other, forming a checkerboard-like pattern. Thus, primary denervation of one motor unit results in atrophy of scattered muscle fibres and not in compact group atrophy, as was formerly believed. Only successive episodes of denervation of several motor units, after collateral reinnervation has regrouped the fibres, may result in typical group atrophy (called neurogenic atrophy): then the affected fibres in a given cluster are of the same histochemical type, because they belong now to one motor unit. In conclusion, neurogenic atrophy and reinnervation may result in various rearrangements of muscle fibre patterns, which are best studied in histochemical preparations.

Muscle fibres permanently deprived of innervation ultimately degenerate through a series of stages described on page 159.

Regeneration after destruction of fibres

Regeneration after a necrotising lesion of muscle is fundamentally different from that which follows denervation. In the latter case the atrophic fibre is thin but retains its general shape and internal structure and has all the necessary metabolic machinery for renewed growth after reinnervation. On the other hand, the fibre with segmental destruction (p. 168) has lost continuity and is usually broken into two or more pieces. Regeneration after necrosis involves multiplication of nuclei, creation of new sarcoplasm and organelles, and fusion and alignment into an integrated unit (Fig. 5.7).

The regenerative power of muscle after segmental necrosis is tremendous. After an acute attack of rhabdomyolysis with myoglobinuria one can see in repeated biopsies that the devastating destruction of muscle fibres is followed by swift removal of necrotic sarcoplasm and complete reconstitution of muscle within three to four weeks.

However, if an entire fibre is destroyed, there would seem to be no possibility of a new one being formed from pluripotential mesodermal cells, a process which for the most part ceases before birth. Regeneration after destruction can take place only if parts of the affected fibre remain intact.

Two types of regeneration occur after segmental necrosis — 'continuous' and 'discontinuous'. In continuous regeneration, or 'budding', the regeneration begins at the healthy end of a severed fibre. Sarcolemmal nuclei migrate into the junctional zone, and myoblasts that have migrated outside the fibre may fuse with it (Sloper & Pegrum 1967). The nuclei are large, with prominent nucleoli, and the surrounding cytoplasm is stained bluish in haematoxylin-eosin preparations because of increased ribonucleoprotein. Aggregates of nuclei may resemble multinucleated giant cells (muscle giant cells).

In many instances, one finds evidence that the regenerative process results in a series of muscle sprouts, sometimes forming a compact cluster of 5–6 or more. In cross-section they fit together like the pieces of a mosaic. The parent fibre, from which they have formed, is usually enlarged. The ends of these shoots are difficult to follow; some end in connective tissue, probably rendering their contractile force ineffective.

In 'discontinuous' or 'embryonal' regeneration, mononuclear myoblasts lying free in the tissue align in a single row, fuse and form a myotube, which will grow and mature into a fibre of adult type. This formation of new segments is reminiscent of the original creation of muscle in fetal life (Sloper & Partridge 1980).

Once a myotube forms, the new fibre can be traced through several stages (Fig. 5.7). At an early stage, the rows of heavily nucleated myocytes are surrounded by RNA-rich, slightly basophilic sarcoplasm and a small complement of thick, non-striated protomyofibrils. Later, the thin new fibres are distinguished from normal ones only by their smaller size, the faint basophilia of their sarcoplasm, their smaller complement of large myofibrils (protofibrils), the large size and central position of their nuclei with prominent nucleoli and increased numbers of ribosomes and microtubules. Later, the nuclei become peripheral and the myofibrils increase in number. The fibre may thus reconstitute itself completely within a few weeks. On the other hand, the regenerative process may stop short: the new muscle nuclei then undergo degeneration and the sarcoplasm withers.

The origin of the myoblasts is still disputed. The peri-endomysial connective tissue can be excluded as a source (Walker 1963). Most are known to originate within the muscle fibre. There are two hypothetical explanations of their origin: one is that they are derived from sarcolemmal nuclei (Hay 1971, Reznik 1969, 1973); the other is that they come from satellite cells (Church 1969). We favour the former view, that near an injured region sarcolemmal nuclei with some cytoplasm envelop themselves with membrane, become sequestered from the remainder of the fibre (Reznik 1969) and appear as satellite cells (Mauro 1961), i.e. cells that are situated between the basement membrane and the sarcolemma of the fibre. The satellite cells then divide and the daughter cells develop into myoblasts, which migrate outside the fibre. The alternative hypothesis postulates that the satellite cells are created during fetal life and exist in normal adult muscle (Schmalbruch & Hellhammer 1976) although as a dormant reserve. Awakened by injury, they divide and give rise to myoblasts.

The effectiveness of regeneration depends upon whether or not the scaffolding of basement membrane and supporting tissues remains intact and the basic pathological process subsides. Preservation of these structures is needed for so-called isomorphic regeneration, in which the orientation of regenerating fibres parallels that of the original fibres. The sarcolemma usually disappears over necrotic segments and its destruction probably facilitates the migration of phagocytes into the softened, necrotic muscle, and of satellite cells out of the fibre. The removal of dead tissue is a prerequisite for swift and complete repair.

Isomorphic regeneration with more or less complete reconstitution of muscle is usually seen after segmental necrosis, where supporting tissues are relatively uninjured. Fibroblastic and vascular reactions are minimal. Only in trauma, haemorrhage, infection, infarction and other crude injury does one see complete disorientation of regenerating fibres and vigorous proliferation of fibroblasts and vessels. This so-called anisomorphic regeneration can give rise to a kind of tumefaction of muscle — a local pseudotumour (see p. 198).

Repeated biopsies have shown that some degenerative lesions, such as vacuoles in periodic paralysis and tubular aggregates, are reversible, but how these structures disappear and the affected fibres reconstitute themselves is not known.

CONCLUSIONS

Following injury, the muscle fibre reacts in many respects like other living cells in the body. However, the range of its structural alterations is larger than those of any other cell in the body, and there are a number of modifications that are unique because of the special features of its anatomy and physiology, discussed in the Introduction.

These structural changes are not to be taken as the equivalents of disease. The clinician must realise that a full definition of the pathology of a disease comprises many parameters other than morphological ones. It should include: (1) all the visible structural changes in muscle; (2) their topography in the entire muscular system; (3) the presence or absence of involvement of cardiac muscle and non-muscular tissues (nervous system, eye, skin, connective tissues etc.); and (4) the chronology of the changes, best expressed by the sequence of the functional disorders they produce during life. The myopathologist with access to a small specimen from only one muscle, obtained in a single instant in the life-profile of a disease, cannot be depended upon even to provide the first component in the array of data necessary for the diagnosis of disease. To ascertain the topography of a disease in muscle a complete post-mortem study must be made; alternatively, as is more often the case, this must be determined by clinical examination and physiological testing. The same is true of data concerning involvement of other tissues. The chronology can be assessed only from the history of the illness or successive examinations.

One should also realise that structural changes in muscle fibres usually, if not always, are secondary effects of a more fundamental abnormality, which can be revealed only by molecular biological, biochemical or immunological methods. These secondary structural changes together constitute a heterogeneous group. Some of them are a direct consequence of the original defect. For example, the primary defect in McArdle's disease — deficiency of the enzyme myophosphorylase — causes morphological changes resulting from excessive accumulation of glycogen under the sarcolemma and between myofibrils. Likewise, one can conjecture that a primary genetic error in the production of protein may lead to the appearance of abnormal structures such as nemaline bodies and tubular aggregates. Other changes in muscle fibres are more strictly reparative and compensatory reactions, which have the purpose of reducing the damaging effect of the original injury, and of repairing defects after damage. In the mitochondrial myopathies, the overgrowth of mitochondria appears to represent an attempt on the part of the muscle fibres to compensate for deficiencies of various respiratory enzymes.

Newer histological techniques permit the structural changes in skeletal muscles to be described in greater detail and new types of reaction patterns to be discovered. In addition, one must expect that other methodological developments will enable the myopathologist to discern hitherto undescribed morphological alterations and to improve the definition of those already known. More important, one can look forward to a more complete understanding of their nature and their relationship to causative factors. Without doubt, the principal problems with regard to aetiology and pathogenesis for most muscle diseases remain to be solved. Essential for the solution of these problems are, first, a clear definition of structural changes at all stages of evolution of the disease and second, an understanding of their pathogenesis, meaning and interrelationship.

ACKNOWLEDGEMENTS

We thank Mr L. Cherkas for help with the photography. This study was supported in part by Grant N.S. 07596 from the National Institute of Neurological Diseases and Stroke.

REFERENCES

Adams R D 1968 The giant muscle fibre; its place in myopathology. In: Locke S (ed) Modern neurology: Papers in tribute to D Denny-Brown. Little Brown, Boston, p 225

Adams R D 1975 Diseases of muscle: A study in pathology, 3rd edn. Harper and Row, Maryland

Adams R D, Denny-Brown D, Pearson C M 1953 Diseases of muscle: A study in pathology, 1st edn. Hoeber, New York

Adams R D, Kakulas B A, Samaha F A 1965 A myopathy with cellular inclusions. Transactions of the American Neurological Association 90:213

Adams R D, Schroeder M 1966 Histopathologie der Myotonischen Erkrankungen. In: Kuhn E (ed) Progressive Muskeldystrophie, Myotonie, Myasthenie Symposium. Springer-Verlag, New York, p 191

Adams R D, DeReuck J 1973 Metrics of muscle. In: Kakulas B A (ed) Basic research in myology. Proceedings of the second international congress on muscle diseases, vol 1. Excerpta Medica, Amsterdam, p 3

Afifi A K, Smith J W, Zellweger H 1965 Congenital nonprogressive myopathy: central core disease and nemaline myopathy in one family. Neurology (Minneapolis) 15:371

Afifi A K, Aleu F P, Goodgold J, Mackay B 1966 Ultrastructure of atrophic muscle in amyotrophic lateral sclerosis. Neurology (Minneapolis) 16:475

Afifi A K, Ibrahim Z M, Bergman R A et al 1972 Morphologic features of hypermetabolic mitochondrial disease. A light microscopic, histochemical and electron microscopic study. Journal of the Neurological Sciences 15:271

Angelini C 1976 Lipid storage myopathies. A review of the metabolic defect and of treatment. Journal of Neurology (Berlin) 214:1

Angelini C 1984 Heterogeneity of lipid storage myopathies. In: Serratrice G, Cros D, Desnuelle C, Gastaut J-L, Pellessier J-F, Pouget J, Schiano A (eds) Neuromuscular diseases. Raven Press, New York

Appel S H, Roses A D 1977 Membranes and myotonia. In: Rowland L P (ed) Pathogenesis of human muscular dystrophies. Excerpta Medica, Amsterdam, p 747

Appel S H, Roses A D 1983 The muscular dystrophies. In: Stanbury J B, Wyngaarden J B, Gredricksson D S, Goldstein L, Brown M S (eds) The metabolic basis of inherited disease, 5th edn. McGraw-Hill, New York

Asbøe-Hansen G, Iversen K, Wichman B 1952 Malignant exophthalmos: muscular changes and thyrotropin content in serum. Acta Endocrinologica 11:376

Askanas V, Engel W K, Britton D E, Adornato B T, Eiben R M 1978 Reincarnation in cultured muscle of mitochondrial abnormalities. Archives of Neurology 35:801

Askanazy M 1898 Pathologisch-anatomische Beiträge zur Kenntniss des Morbus Basedowii, inbesondere uber die dabei aufretende Muskelerkrankung. Deutsche Archiv für Klinische Medizin 16:118

Åström K E, Kugelberg E, Müller R 1961 Hypothyroid myopathy. Archives of Neurology 5:472

Åström K E, Adams R D 1980 The pathologic reactions of the skeletal muscle fibre. In: Ringel S P, Klawans H L (eds) Handbook of clinical neurology: Diseases of muscle. Elsevier, New York

Banker B Q 1975 Dermatomyositis of childhood. Ultrastructural alterations of muscle and intramuscular blood vessels. Journal of Neuropathology and Experimental Neurology 34:66

Banker B Q, Victor M, Adams R D 1957 Arthrogryposis multiplex due to congenital muscular dystrophy. Brain 80:210

Banker B Q, Denny-Brown D 1959 A study of denervated muscle in normal and dystrophic mice. Journal of Neuropathology and Experimental Neurology 18:517

Banker B Q, Victor M 1966 Dermatomyositis (systemic angiopathy) of childhood. Medicine 45:261

Beckett R S, Netsky M G 1953 Familial ocular myopathy and external ophthalmoplegia. Archives of Neurology and Psychiatry 69:64

Bell C D, Conen P E 1967 Change in fibre size in Duchenne muscular dystrophy. Neurology (Minneapolis) 17:902

Bender A N, Engel W K 1976 Light-cored dense particles in mitochondria of a patient with skeletal muscle and myocardial disease. Journal of Neuropathology and Experimental Neurology 35:46

Bender A N, Ringel S P, Engel W K 1976 The acetylcholine receptor in normal and pathologic states. Immune peroxidase visualisation of alpha-bungarotoxin binding at a light and electron microscopic level. Neurology (Minneapolis) 26:477

Bender A N, Bender M B 1977 Muscle fibre hypotrophy with intact neuromuscular junctions. A study of a patient with congenital neuromuscular disease and ophthalmoplegia. Neurology (Minneapolis) 27:206

Berenbaum M C, Birch C A, Moreland J D 1953 Paroxysmal myoglobinuria. Lancet 1:892

Berenberg R A, Pellock J M, DiMauro S et al 1976 Lumping or splitting? 'Ophthalmoplegia-plus' or Kearns-Sayre syndrome. Annals of Neurology 1:37

Bethlem J, Arts W F, Dingemans K P 1978 Common origin of rods, cores, miniature cores, and focal loss of cross-striations. Archives of Neurology 35:555

Bill P L A, Cole G, Proctor N S F 1979 Centronuclear myopathy. Journal of Neurology, Neurosurgery and Psychiatry 42:548

Bird J W 1975 Skeletal muscle lysosomes. In: Dingle J T, Dean R T (eds) Lysosomes in biology and pathology, vol 4. North Holland, Amsterdam, p 75

Black J T, Judge D, Demers L, Gordon S 1975 Ragged-red fibres. A biochemical and morphological study. Journal of the Neurological Sciences 26:479

Bonnett H, Roelofs R, Olson W H 1974 Multicore disease: report of a case with onset in middle age. Neurology (Minneapolis) 24:1039

Bove K E, Iannaccone S T, Hilton P K, Samaha F 1980 Cylindrical spirals in a familial neuromuscular disorder. Annals of Neurology 7:550

Bradley W G 1969 Ultrastructural changes in adynamia episodica hereditaria and normokalemic familiar periodic paralysis. Brain 92:379

Bradley W G, Fulthorpe J J 1978 Studies of sarcolemmal integrity in myopathic muscle. Neurology (Minneapolis) 28:670

Bradley W G, Tomlinson B E, Hardy M 1978 Further studies of mitochondrial and lipid storage myopathies. Journal of the Neurological Sciences 35:201

Brooke M H 1974 Congenital fibre type disproportion. In: Kakulas B A (ed) Clinical studies in myology. Proceedings of the second international congress on muscle diseases, vol 2. Excerpta Medica, Amsterdam, p 147

Brooke M H, Engel W K 1969a The histographic analysis of human muscle biopsies with regard to fibre types. 1. Adult male and female. Neurology (Minneapolis) 19 221

Brooke M H, Engel W K 1969b The histographic analysis of human muscle biopsies with regard to fibre types. 2. Disease of the upper and lower motor neuron. Neurology (Minneapolis) 19:378

Brooke M H, Engel W K 1969c The histographic analysis of human muscle biopsies with regard to fibre types. 3. Myopathies, myasthenia gravis, and hypokalemic periodic paralysis. Neurology (Minneapolis) 19:469

Brooke M H, Engel W K 1969d The histographic analysis of human muscle biopsies with regard to fibre types. 4. Children's biopsies. Neurology (Minneapolis) 19:591

Brooke M H, Neville H E 1972 Reducing body myopathy. Neurology (Minneapolis) 22:829

Brooke M H, Carroll J E, Ringel S P 1979 Congenital hypotonia revisited. Muscle and Nerve 2:84

Cadnapaphornchai P, Taher S, McDonald F D 1980 Acute drug-associated rhabdomyolysis: An examination of its diverse renal manifestations and complications. American Journal of Medical Science 280:66

Campbell M J, Rebeiz J J, Walton J N 1969 Myotubular, centronuclear or peri-centronuclear myopathy? Journal of the Neurological Sciences 8:425

Cancilla P A, Kalyanaraman K, Verity M A, Munsat T, Pearson C M 1971 Familial myopathy with probable lysis of myofibrils in Type 1 fibres. Neurology (Minneapolis) 21:579

Carpenter S, Karpati G, Andermann F, Jacob J C, Andermann E 1977 The ultrastructural characteristics of the abnormal cytosomes in Batten-Kufs' disease. Brain 100:137

Carpenter S, Karpati G, Heller I, Eisen A 1978 Inclusion

body myositis: A distinct variety of idiopathic inflammatory myopathy. Neurology (Minneapolis) 28:8

Carpenter S, Karpati G 1979 Duchenne muscular dystrophy. Plasma membrane loss initiates muscle cell necrosis unless it is repaired. Brain 102:147

Carpenter S, Karpati G, Robitaille Y, Melmed C 1979 Cylindrical spirals in human skeletal muscle. Muscle and Nerve 2:282

Carpenter S, Karpati G 1981 The major inflammatory myopathies of unknown cause. Pathology Annual 16:2205

Carroll J E, Zwillich C, Weil J V, Brooke M H 1976 Depressed ventilatory response in oculocraniosomatic neuromuscular disease. Neurology (Minneapolis) 26:140

Castaigne P, Laplane D, Escourolle R, Augustine P, de Recondo J, Martinez Lage G J, Villaneuva Eusa J A 1971 Ophthalmoplégie externe progressive avec spongiose des noyaux du tronc cérébral. Revue Neurologique (Paris) 124:454

Chad D, Good P, Adelman L, Bradley W G, Mills J 1982 Inclusion body myositis associated with Sjögren's syndrome. Archives of Neurology (Chicago) 39:186

Chou S M 1968 Myxovirus-like structures and accompanying nuclear changes in chronic polymyositis. Archives of Pathology 86:649

Church J C T 1969 Satellite cells and myogenesis; a study in the fruit bat web. Journal of Anatomy 105:419

Clancy R R, Kelts K A, Oehlert J W 1980 Clinical variability in congenital fiber type disproportion. Journal of the Neurological Sciences 46:257

Cogen F C, Rigg G, Simmons J L, Domino E F 1978 Phencyclidine-associated acute rhabdomyolysis. Annals of Internal Medicine 88:210

Conen P E, Murphy E G, Donohue W C 1963 Light and electron microscopic studies of 'myogranules' in a child with hypotonia and muscle weakness. Canadian Medical Association Journal 89:983

Coquet M, Vallat J M, Vital C et al 1983 Nuclear inclusions in oculopharyngeal dystrophy. An ultrastructural study of six cases. Journal of the Neurological Sciences 60:151

Cornelio F, Bresolin N, Singer P A, DiMauro S, Rowland L P 1984 Clinical varieties of neuromuscular disease in debrancher deficiency. Archives of Neurology (Chicago) 41:1027

Couturier J C, Carrier H, Brunon A M, Davidas J L, Bady B 1981 La myopathie oculo-pharyngée (à propos d'une observation familiale). Lyon Médicale 245:109

Crowe W E, Bove K E, Levinson J E, Hilton P K 1982 Clinical and pathogenetic implications of histopathology in childhood polydermatomyositis. Arthritis and Rheumatism 25:126

Cullen M J, Fulthorpe J J 1975 Stages in fibre breakdown in Duchenne muscular dystrophy. Journal of the Neurological Sciences 24:179

Curless R G, Nelson M B, Brimmer F 1978a Histological patterns of muscle in infants with developmental brain abnormalities. Development Medicine and Child Neurology 20:159

Curless R G, Payne C M, Brimmer F M 1978b Fingerprint body myopathy: a report of twins. Developmental Medicine and Child Neurology 20:793

Danon M J, Reyes M G, Perurena O, Masdeu J C, Manaligod J R 1982 Inclusion body myositis. A corticosteroid-resistant idiopathic inflammatory myopathy. Archives of Neurology (Chicago) 39:760

Daroff R B, Solitaire G B, Pincus J H, Glaser G H 1966 Spongiform encephalopathy with chronic progressive external ophthalmoplegia. Central ophthalmoplegia mimicking ocular myopathy. Neurology (Minneapolis) 16:161

Debré R, Semelaigne G 1935 Syndrome of diffuse muscular hypertrophy in infants causing athletic appearance; its connection with congenital myxedema. American Journal of Diseases of Children 50:1351

Denny-Brown D 1961 Experimental studies pertaining to hypertrophy, regeneration and degeneration. Research Publications of the Association for Research in Nervous and Mental Disease 38:147

De Reuck J, Hooft C, DeCoster W, van den Bossche, Cuvelier C 1977 A progressive congenital myopathy. Initial involvement of the diaphragm with type 1 muscle fibre atrophy. European Neurology 15:217

DiMauro S, Melis-DiMauro P M 1973 Muscle carnitine palmityl transferase deficiency and myoglobinuria. Science 182:929

DiMauro S, Schotland D L, Bonilla E, Lee C P, Gambetti P, Rowland L P 1973 Progressive ophthalmoplegia, glycogen storage and abnormal mitochondria. Archives of Neurology 29:170

DiMauro S, Bonilla E, Lee C P et al 1976 Luft's disease. Further biochemical and ultrastructural studies of skeletal muscle in the second case. Journal of the Neurological Sciences 27:217

DiMauro S, Mendell J R, Sahenk Z, Bachman D, Scarpa A, Scofield R M, Reiner C 1980 Fatal infantile mitochondrial myopathy and renal dysfunction due to cytochrome-c-oxidase deficiency. Neurology (Minneapolis) 30:795

DiMauro S, Miranda A F, Olarte M, Friedman R, Hays A P 1982 Muscle phosphoglycerate mutase deficiency. Neurology (Minneapolis) 32:584

DiMauro S, Dalakas M, Miranda A F 1983 Phosphoglycerate kinase (PGK) deficiency: Another cause of recurrent myoglobinuria. Annals of Neurology 13:11

DiMauro S, Bonilla E, Zeviani M, Nakagawa M, DeVivo D C 1985 Mitochondrial myopathies. Annals of Neurology 17:521

Doshi R, Fowler T 1983 Proximal myopathy due to carcinomatous metastases in muscle. Journal of Neurology, Neurosurgery and Psychiatry 46:358

Drachman D 1965 Pharmacological denervation of skeletal muscle in chick embryos treated with botulinus toxin. Transactions of the American Neurological Association 90:241

Drachman D B, Murphy S R, Nigam M P, Hills J R 1967 Myopathic changes in chronically denervated muscles. Archives of Neurology 16:14

Drager G A, Hammill J F, Shy G M 1958 Paramyotonia congenita. Archives of Neurology and Psychiatry 80:1

Dubowitz V 1975 Infantile spinal muscular atrophy. In: Vinken P J, Bruyn G W (eds) Handbook of clinical neurology: System disorders and atrophies, vol 22. North Holland, Amsterdam, p 81

Dubowitz V 1985 Muscle biopsy: A modern approach. 3rd edn. Baillière Tindall, London

Dubowitz V, Roy S 1970 Central core disease of muscle: clinical, histochemical and electron microscopic studies of an affected mother and son. Brain 93:133

Dyken P R, Harper P S 1973 Congenital dystrophia myotonica. Neurology (Minneapolis) 23:465

Dyken M, Zeman W, Rausche T 1969 Hypokalemic periodic paralysis. Neurology (Minneapolis) 19:691

Edström L, Wroblewski R, Mair W G P 1982 Genuine myotubular myopathy. Muscle and Nerve 5:604

Ekbom K, Hed R, Kirstein L, Åström K E 1964 Muscular affections. Archives of Neurology 10:440

Emery A E H 1971 The nosology of the spinal muscular atrophies. Journal of Medical Genetics 8: 481–495

Engel A G 1970a Acid maltase deficiency in adults: studies in four cases of a syndrome which may mimic muscular dystrophy or other myopathies. Brain 93:599

Engel A G 1970b Evolution and content of vacuoles in primary hypokalemic periodic paralysis. Mayo Clinic Proceedings 45:774

Engel A G 1973 Vacuolar myopathies: multiple etiologies and sequential structural studies. In: Pearson C M, Mostofi F K (eds) The striated muscle. Williams and Wilkins, Baltimore, p 301

Engel A G, Gomez M R, Groover R V 1971 Multicore disease. Mayo Clinic Proceedings 46:666

Engel A G, Angelini C, Gomez M R 1972 Fingerprint body myopathy, a newly recognised congenital muscle disease. Mayo Clinic Proceedings 47:377

Engel A G, Angelini C 1973 Carnitine deficiency of human skeletal muscle with associated lipid storage myopathy: a new syndrome. Science 173:899

Engel A G, Gomez M R, Seybold M E 1973 The spectrum and diagnosis of acid maltase deficiency. Neurology (Minneapolis) 23:95

Engel A G, Biesecker G 1982 Complement activation in muscle fiber necrosis: Demonstration of the membrane attack complex of complement in necrotic fibers. Annals of Neurology 12:289

Engel A G, Arahata K, Biesecker G 1984 Mechanism of muscle fiber destruction. In: Serratrice G, Cros D, Desnuelle C, Gastaut J-L, Pellissier J-F, Pouget J, Schiano A (eds) Neuromuscular diseases. Raven Press, New York

Engel W K 1961 Muscle target cells: A newly recognized sign of denervation. Nature 191:389

Engel W K 1962a The essentiality of histo- and cytochemical studies of skeletal muscles in the investigation of neuromuscular disease. Neurology (Minneapolis) 12:778

Engel W K 1962b Chemocytology of striated annulets and sarcoplasmic masses in myotonic dystrophy. Journal of Histochemistry and Cytochemistry 10:229

Engel W K 1975 Abundant nuclear rods in adult-onset rod disease. Journal of Neuropathology and Experimental Neurology 34:119

Engel W K, Foster J B, Hughes B P, Huxley H E, Mahler R 1961 Central core disease — An investigation of a rare muscular abnormality. Brain 84:167

Engel W K, Gold G N, Karpati G 1968 Type 1 fibre hypotrophy and central nuclei. A rare congenital muscle abnormality with a possible experimental model. Archives of Neurology 18:435

Engel W K, Bishop D W, Cunningham G G 1970 Tubular aggregates in type 11 muscle fibres; ultrastructural and histochemical consideration. Journal of Ultrastructure Research 31:507

Erb W 1891 Dystrophia muscularis progressiva; Klinische und pathologisch-anatomische Studien. Deutsche Zeitschrift für Nervenheilkunde 1:13

Fardeau M 1970 Ultrastructural lesions in progressive muscular dystrophies. A critical study of their specificity. In: Canal N, Scarlatti G, Walton J N (eds) Muscle diseases. International Congress Series No 199. Excerpta Medica, Amsterdam, p 98

Fardeau M, Tomé F M, Derambure S 1976 Familial fingerprint body myopathy. Archives of Neurology 33:724

Fardeau M 1984 Relevance of morphologic studies in the classification and pathophysiology of congenital myopathies. In: Serratrice G, Cros D, Desnuelle C, Gastaut J- L, Pellissier J-F, Pouget J, Schiano A (eds) Neuromuscular diseases. Raven Press, New York

Fenichel G M 1967 Abnormalities of skeletal muscle maturation in brain-damaged children. Developmental Medicine and Child Neurology 9:419

Fisher E R, Danowski T S 1969 Mitochondrial myopathy. Journal of Clinical Pathology 51:619

Fitzsimons R, Clifton-Bligh P, Wolfenden W 1981 Mitochondrial myopathy and lactic acidemia with myoclonic epilepsy, ataxia and hypothalamic infertility: a variant of Ramsay-Hunt syndrome? Journal of Neurology, Neurosurgery and Psychiatry 44:79

Frank J P, Harati Y, Butler I J, Nelson T E, Scott C I 1980 Central core disease and malignant hyperthermia syndrome. Annals of Neurology 7:11

French J H, Sherard E S, Lubell H, Brotz M, Moore C L 1972 Trichopoliodystrophy. 1 Report of a case and biochemical study. Archives of Neurology 26:229

Fukuhara N , Kumamoto T, Tsubaki T 1980a Rimmed vacuoles. Acta Neuropathologica (Berlin) 51:229

Fukuhara N, Tokiguchi S, Shirakawa K, Tsubaki T 1980b Myoclonus epilepsy associated with ragged-red fibres (mitochondrial abnormalities): Disease entity or syndrome? Journal of the Neurological Sciences 47:117

Gabow P A, Kaehny W D, Kelleher S P 1982 The spectrum of rhabdomyolysis. Medicine (Baltimore) 61:141

Gamstorp I 1956 Adynamia episodica hereditaria. Acta Paediatrica Scandinavica (Suppl 108) 45:1

Ghatak N R, Hirano A, Poon T P, French J H 1972 Trichopoliodystrophy II. Pathological changes in skeletal muscle and nervous system. Archives of Neurology 26:60

Ghatak N R, Erenberg G, Hirano A, Golden G S 1973 Idiopathic rhabdomyolysis in children. Journal of the Neurological Sciences 20:253

Gibbels E, Henke U, Schadlich H J, Haupt W F, Fiehn W 1984 Cylindrical spirals in skeletal muscle: a further observation with clinical, morphological, and biochemical analysis. Muscle and Nerve 6:646

Goldberg A F 1967 Protein synthesis in tonic and phasic skeletal muscles. Nature 216:1219

Goldfischer S, Moore C L, Johnson A B et al 1973 Peroxisomal and mitochondrial defects in the cerebro-hepato-renal syndrome. Science 182:62

Gonatas N K, Perez M C, Shy G M, Evangelista I 1965 Central 'core' disease of skeletal muscle. Ultrastructural and cytochemical observations in two cases. American Journal of Pathology 47:503

Gonatas N K, Evangelista I, Martin J 1967 A generalised disorder of nervous system, skeletal muscle and heart resembling Refsum's disease and Hurler's syndrome. Part 2 (Ultrastructure). American Journal of Medicine 42:169

Greenfield J G, Shy G M, Alvord E C, Berg L 1957 An atlas of muscle pathology in neuromuscular diseases. Livingstone, Edinburgh

Gruner J, Porte A 1959 Les lésions musculaires de paralysie périodique familiale. Revue Neurologique 101:501

Gubbay S S, Walton J N, Pearce G W 1966 Clinical and pathological study of a case of congenital muscular dystrophy. Journal of Neurology, Neurosurgery and Psychiatry 29:500

Gutmann E 1962 The denervated muscle. Publishing House of Czechoslovak Academy of Science, Prague

Haase G R, Shy G M 1960 Pathological changes in muscular biopsies from patients with peroneal muscular atrophy. Brain 83:631

Hackett T N Jr, Bray P F, Ziter F A, Nyhan W L, Creer K M 1973 A metabolic myopathy associated with chronic lactic acidemia, growth failure and nerve deafness. Journal of Pediatrics 83:426

Halban J 1894 Die Dicke der quergestreiften Muskelfasern und ihre Bedeutung. Anatomische Hefte 3:267

Haltia M, Rapola J, Santavuori P 1973 Infantile type of so-called neuronal ceroid-lipofuscinosis. Histological and electron microscopic studies. Acta Neuropathologica (Berlin) 26:157

Hart Z W, Chang C H, Perrin E V, Neerunjun J A, Ayyar R 1977 Familial poliodystrophy, mitochondrial myopathy and lactic acidemia. Archives of Neurology 34:180

Hay E P 1971 Skeletal muscle regeneration. New England Journal of Medicine 284:1033

Hayes D J, Lecky B R F, Landon D N, Morgan-Hughes J A, Clark J B 1984 A new mitochondrial myopathy: biochemical studies revealing a deficiency in the cytochrome b, c, complex (complex III) of the respiratory chain. Brain 107:1165

Hed R, Lundmark C, Fahlgren H, Orell S 1962 Acute muscular syndrome in chronic alcoholism. Acta Medica Scandinavica 171:585

Heffner R, Cohen M, Duffner P, Daigler G 1976 Multicore disease in twins. Journal of Neurology, Neurosurgery and Psychiatry 39:602

Heffner R R Jr, Armbrustmacher V W, Earle K M 1977 Focal myositis. Cancer 40:301

Heffner R R, Barron S A 1981 Polymyositis beginning as a focal process. Archives of Neurology (Chicago) 38:439

Heidenhain M 1918 Ueber progressive Veränderungen der Muskulatur bei Myotonia atrophica. Beitrage zu Pathologische Anatomie und zu Allgemeine Pathologie 64:198

Hers F L 1963 Alpha-glucosidase deficiency in generalized glycogen storage disease (Pompe's disease). Biochemical Journal 86:11

Hers F L 1965 Inborn lysosomal diseases. Progress in Gastroenterology 48:625

Ho K L, Konno E T, Chason J L 1979 Focal myositis of the neck. Human Pathology 10:353

Hoffmann J 1893 Ueber chronische spinale muskelatrophie im Kindesalter auf familiärer Basis. Deutche Zeitschrift für Nervenheilkunde 3:427

Hostetler K Y, Hoppel C L, Romine J S, Sipe J C, Gross S R, Higginbottom P A 1978 Partial deficiency of muscle carnitine palmityltransferase with normal ketone production. New England Journal of Medicine 298:553

Hübner G 1977 Ringbinden der quergestreiften Muskulatur. Ein Beitrag zur Aussagekraft derartiger Struktur an einem unausgewählten Sektionsmaterial. Acta Neuropathologica (Berlin) 38:27

Hudson P, Bradley W G, Jenkinson M 1972 Familial 'mitochondrial' myopathy. A myopathy associated with disordered oxidative metabolism in muscle fibres. Part 1. Clinical, electrophysiological and pathological findings. Journal of the Neurological Sciences 16:343

Hülsmann W C, Bethlem J, Meijer A E F H, Fleury, Schellens J P M 1967 Myopathy with abnormal structure and function of muscle mitochondria. Journal of Neurology, Neurosurgery and Psychiatry 30:519

Isaacs H, Heffron J J, Badenhorst M 1975 Central core disease. A correlated genetic, histochemical, ultramicroscopic and biochemical study. Journal of Neurology, Neurosurgery and Psychiatry 38:1177

Jenis E H, Lindquist R R, Lister R C 1969 New congenital myopathy with crystalline intranuclear inclusions. Archives of Neurology 20:281

Jerusalem F 1976 Hypotheses and recent findings concerning aetiology and pathogenesis of the muscular dystrophies. Journal of Neurology 213:155

Jerusalem F, Engel A G, Gomez M R 1973 Sarcotubular myopathy. A newly recognised, benign, congenital, familial muscle disease. Neurology (Minneapolis) 23:897

Johnson M A, Polgar J, Weightman D, Appleton D 1973a Data on distribution of fibre types in thirty-six human muscles. An autopsy study. Journal of the Neurological Sciences 18:111

Johnson M A, Sideri G, Weightman D, Appleton D 1973b A comparison of fibre size, fibre type constitution and spatial fibre type distribution in normal human muscle and in muscle from cases of spinal muscular atrophy and from other neuromuscular disorders. Journal of the Neurological Sciences 20:345

Johnson M A, Turnbull D M, Dick D J, Sherratt H S A 1983 A partial deficiency of cytochrome c oxidase in chronic progressive external ophthalmoplegia. Journal of the Neurological Sciences 60:31

Julien J, Vital C, Vallat J M, Le Blanc M 1974 Oculopharyngeal muscular dystrophy. A case with abnormal mitochondria and 'fingerprint' inclusions. Journal of the Neurological Sciences 21:165

Kagen L J 1977 Myoglobinemia in inflammatory myopathies. Journal of the American Medical Association 237:1448

Kahn L B, Meyer J S 1970 Acute myopathy in chronic alcoholism. A study of 22 autopsy cases with ultrastructural observations. American Journal of Clinical Pathology 53:516

Kakulas B A 1966 In vitro destruction of skeletal muscle by sensitized cells. Nature 210:1115

Kamieniecka Z 1976 Myopathies with abnormal mitochondria. A clinical, histological and electro-physiological study. Acta Neurologica Scandinavica 55:57

Kearns T P, 1965 External ophthalmoplegia, pigmentary degeneration of the retina and cardiomyopathy: a newly recognized syndrome. Transactions of the American Ophthalmologic Society 63:559

Kearns T P, Sayre G P 1958 Retinitis pigmentosa, external ophthalmoplegia and complete heart block; unusual syndrome with histologic study in one of two cases. Archives of Ophthalmology 60:280

Kendrick W C, Hull A R, Knochel J P 1977 Rhabdomyolysis and shock after intravenous amphetamine administration. Annals of Internal Medicine 86:381

Kiloh I G, Nevin S 1951 Progressive dystrophy of the external ocular muscles. Brain 74:9

Kinoshita M, Satoyoshi E, Matsuo N 1975a 'Myotubular myopathy' and type I fibre atrophy in a family. Journal of the Neurological Sciences 26:575

Kinoshita M, Satoyoshi E, Suzuki Y 1975b Atypical myopathy with myofibrillar aggregates. Archives of Neurology 32:417

Kinoshita M, Suzuki Y, Matsuo N, Aoki F, Hajikano H 1978 'Ragged-red' fibers in Leigh's syndrome. Clinical Neurology 18:108

Kobayashi Y, Miyabayashi S, Takada G, Narisawa K, Tada K, Yamamoto T Y 1982 Ultrastructural study of the childhood mitochondrial myopathic syndrome associated with lactic acidosis. European Journal of Pediatrics 139:25

Krabbe K 1949 Les lèsions embryonnaires à la lumière des défectuosités mammaires et pectorales de la syndactylie et de la microdactylie. Acta Psychiatrica et Neurologica 24:539

Kugelberg E, Edström L, Abbruzzese M 1970 Mapping of motor units in experimentally reinnervated rat muscle. Journal of Neurology, Neurosurgery and Psychiatry 33:319

Kuitunen P, Rapola J, Noponen A L, Donner M 1972 Nemaline myopathy. Report of 4 cases and review of the literature. Acta Paediatrica Scandinavica 61:353

Lake B D, Wilson J 1975 Zebra body myopathy. Clinical, histochemical and ultrastructural studies. Journal of the Neurological Sciences 24:437

Lake B D, Cavanagh N, Wilson J 1977 Myopathy with minicores in siblings. Neuropathology and Applied Neurobiology 3:159

Lane R J M, Fulthorpe J J, Hudgson P 1985 Inclusion body myositis: a case with associated collagen vascular disease responding to treatment. Journal of Neurology, Neurosurgery and Psychiatry 48:270

Lapresle J, Fardeau M, Milhaud M 1965 Étude des ultrastructures dans les dystrophies musculaires progressives. Proceedings of the Fifth International Congress of Neuropathology. International Congress Series No 100. Excerpta Medica, Amsterdam, p 602.

Larsson L E, Linderholm H, Müller R, Ringqvist T, Sörnäs R 1964 Hereditary metabolic myopathy with paroxysmal myoglobinuria due to abnormal glycolysis. Journal of Neurology, Neurosurgery and Psychiatry 27:361

Layzer R B, Rowland L P, Ranney H M 1967 Muscle phosphofructokinase deficiency. Archives of Neurology 17:512

Layzer R B, Rowland L P 1971 Cramps. New England Journal of Medicine 285:31

Little B W, Pearl D P 1982 Oculopharyngeal muscular dystrophy. An autopsied case from the French-Canadian kindred. Journal of the Neurological Sciences 53:145

Lucy J A 1980 Is there a membrane defect in muscle and other cells? British Medical Bulletin 36:187

Luft R, Ikkos D, Palmieri G, Ernster L, Afzelius B 1962 A case of severe hypermetabolism of nonthyroid origin with a defect in the maintenance of mitochondrial respiratory control. A correlated clinical, biochemical and morphological study. Journal of Clinical Investigation 41:1776

Macdonald R D, Engel A G 1969 The cytoplasmic body: another structural anomaly of the Z disc. Acta Neuropathologica (Berlin) 14:99

Mair W G P, Tomé F M S 1972 Atlas of the ultrastructure of diseased human muscle. Williams and Wilkins, Baltimore

Marin O, Denny-Brown D 1962 Changes in skeletal muscle associated with cachexia. American Journal of Pathology 41:23

Martin J-J R, Ceuterick C M, Mercelis R J 1982 Nuclear inclusions in oculopharyngeal muscular dystrophy. Muscle and Nerve 5:735

Martinez A J, Hooshmand H, Faris A A 1973 Acute alcoholic myopathy: Enzyme histochemistry and electron microscopic findings. Journal of the Neurological Sciences 20:245

Mastaglia F L, Ojeda V J 1985 Inflammatory myositis: part 1 and 2. Annals of Neurology 17:215,3

Mauro A 1961 Satellite cell of skeletal muscle fibres. Journal of Biophysical and Biochemical Cytology 9:493

McKeran R O, Slavin G, Ward P, Paul E, Mair W G P 1980 Hypothyroid myopathy. A clinical and pathological study. Journal of Pathology 132:35

McLean W T, McKone R C 1973 Congenital myasthenia gravis in twins. Archives of Neurology 29:223

Meier C, Voellmy W, Gertsch M, Zimmermann A, Geissbuhler 1984 Nemaline myopathy appearing in adults as cardiomyopathy. Clinicopathological study. Archives of Neurology (Chicago) 41:443

Meltzer H Y, Kuncl R W, Click J, Yang V 1976 Incidence of Z band streaming and myofibrillar disruptions in skeletal muscle from healthy young people. Neurology (Minneapolis) 26:853

Meyer-Betz F 1911 Beobachtungen an einem eigenartigen mit Muskellähmungen verbundenen Fall von Hämoglobinurie. Deutsche Archiv für Klinische Medizin 85:127

Meyers K R, Gilden D H, Rinaldi F J, Hansen J L 1972 Periodic muscle weakness, normokalemia, and tubular aggregates. Neurology (Minneapolis) 22:269

Mikol J, Felten-Papaiconomou A, Ferchal F, Perol Y, Gautier B, Haguenau M, Pepin B 1982 Inclusion body myositis: clinicopathological studies and isolation of an adenovirus type 2 from muscle biopsy specimen. Annals of Neurology 11:576

Mittelbach F 1966 'Die Begleitmyopathie bei neurogenen Atrophien'. Monographien aus dem Gesamtgebiet der Neurologie und Psychiatrie. Heft 113. Springer, Heidelberg

Mokri B, Engel A G 1975 Duchenne dystrophy: electron microscopic findings pointing to a basic or early abnormality in the plasma membrane of the muscle fibre. Neurology (Minneapolis) 25:1110

Moore M J, Rebeiz J J, Holden M, Adams R D 1971 Biometric analyses of normal skeletal muscle. Acta Neuropathologica (Berlin) 19:51

Morgan-Hughes J A, Darveniza P, Kahn S N et al 1977 A mitochondrial myopathy characterized by a deficiency in reducible cytochrome b. Brain 100:617

Morgan-Hughes J A 1982 Defects of the energy pathways of skeletal muscle. In: Matthews W B, Glaser G H (eds) Recent advances in clinical neurology, vol III. Churchill Livingstone, Edinburgh

Morgan-Hughes J A, Hayes D J, Clark J B, Landon D N, Swash M, Stark R J, Rudge P 1982 Mitochondrial encephalomyopathies. Biochemical studies in two cases revealing defects in the respiratory chain. Brain 105:553

Morgan-Hughes J A, Hayes D J, Clark J B 1984 Mitochondrial myopathies. In: Serratrice G, Cros D, Desnuelle C, Gastaut J-L, Pellissier J-F, Pouget J, Schiano A (eds) Neuromuscular diseases. Raven Press, New York

Morpurgo B 1897 Ueber Activitäts-Hypertrophie der willkürlichen Muskeln. Virchows Archiv für Pathologische Anatomie 150:522

Müller R, Kugelberg E 1959 Myopathy in Cushing's syndrome. Journal of Neurology, Neurosurgery and Psychiatry 22:314

Namba T, Brown S B, Grob D 1970 Neonatal myasthenia gravis: report of two cases and review of the literature. Pediatrics 45:488

Neville H E, Brooke M H 1973 Central core fibres: structured and unstructured. In: Kakulas B A (ed) Basic research in myology. Proceedings of the Second

International Congress on Muscle Diseases, vol I. Excerpta Medica, Amsterdam, p 497

Olson W, Engel W K, Walsh G O, Einaugler R 1972 Oculocraniosomatic neuromuscular disease with 'ragged-red' fibres. Archives of Neurology 26:193

Oppenheim H 1900 Ueber allgemeine und localisierte Atonie der Muskulatur (Myatonia) in frühen Kindesalter. Monatschrift für Psychiatrie und Neurologie 8:232

Osame M, Engel A G, Rebouche C J, Scott R E 1981 Freeze-fracture electron microscopic analysis of plasma membranes of cultured muscle. Neurology (Minneapolis) 31:972

Pack G T, Ariel I M 1958 Tumors of the soft somatic tissues. A clinical treatise. P Hoeber, New York

Papanicolau G N, Falk E A 1938 General muscular hypertrophy induced by androgenic hormone. Science 87:238

Patterson V H, Hill T R G, Fletcher P J H, Heron J R 1979 Central core disease. Clinical and pathological evidence of progression within a family. Brain 102:581

Pavlakis S G, Phillips P C, DiMauro S, DeVivo D C, Rowland L P 1984 Mitochondrial myopathy, lactic acidosis and stroke like episodes (MELAS): a distinctive clinical syndrome. Annals of Neurology 16:481

Payne C M, Curless R G 1976 Concentric laminated bodies. Ultrastructural demonstration of muscle fibre type specificity. Journal of the Neurological Sciences 29:311

Pearce G W, Walton J N 1962 Progressive muscular dystrophy: the histopathological changes in skeletal muscle obtained by biopsy. Journal of Pathology and Bacteriology 83:535

Pearn J H, Wilson J 1973 Acute Werdnig-Hoffman disease. Acute infantile spinal muscular atrophy. Archives of Diseases in Childhood 48:425

Pearson C M 1959 The incidence and type of pathological alterations observed in muscle in a routine autopsy survey. Neurology (Minneapolis) 9:757

Pearson C M, Beck W S, Blahd W H 1957 Idiopathic paroxysmal myoglobinuria. Archives of Internal Medicine 99:376

Pearson C M, Rimer D G, Mommaerts W F H M 1961 A metabolic myopathy due to absence of muscle phosphorylase. American Journal of Medicine 30:502

PeBenito R, Sher J H, Cracco J B 1978 Centronuclear myopathy: clinical and pathologic features. Clinical Pediatrics 17:259

Pellegrini C, Franzini C 1963 An electron microscopic study of denervation atrophy in red and white skeletal muscle fibres. Journal of Cell Biology 17:327

Pellegrini C, Franzini-Armstrong C 1969 Recent contributions of electron microscopy to the study of normal and pathological muscle. International Review of Experimental Pathology 7:139

Perkoff G T, Silber R, Tyler F H, Cartwright G E, Wintrobe M M 1959 Myopathy due to the administration of therapeutic amounts of 17-hydroxycorticosteroids. American Journal of Medicine 26:891

Perkoff G T, Hardy P, Velez-Garcia E 1966 Alcoholic myopathy. New England Journal of Medicine 274:1277

Peter J B, Stempel K, Armstrong J 1970 Biochemistry and electron microscopy of mitochondria in muscular and neuromuscular diseases. In: Canal N, Scarlato G, Walton J N (eds) Muscle diseases. Proceedings of an International Conference on Muscle Diseases. International Congress Series No 199. Excerpta Medica, Amsterdam, p 228

Pichard N A, Gruemer H-D, Verrill H L, Isaacs E R, Robinow M, Nance W E, Myers E C, Goldsmith B 1978 Systemic membrane defect in the proximal muscular dystrophies. New England Journal of Medicine 299:841

Poskanzer D, Kerr D N S 1961 A third type of periodic paralysis with normokalemia and favourable response to sodium chloride. American Journal of Medicine 31:328

Price H M, Howes E L, Blumberg J M 1964 Ultrastructural study of muscle fibres injured by cold. 1. The acute degenerative changes. Laboratory Investigation 13:1264

Price H M, Gordon G B, Pearson C M, Munsat T L, Blumberg J M 1965 New evidence for excessive accumulation of Z-band material in nemaline myopathy. Proceedings of the National Academy of Sciences USA 54:1398

Prick M J J, Gabreels F J M, Trijbels J M F et al 1983 Progressive poliodystrophy (Alpers' disease) with a defect in cytochrome aa3 in muscle: a report of two unrelated patients. Clinical Neurology and Neurosurgery 85:57

Radu H, Rosu-Servu A M, Ionescu V, Radu A 1977 Focal abnormalities in mitochondrial distribution in muscle. Acta Neuropathologica (Berlin) 39:25

Rawles J M, Weller R O 1974 Familial association of metabolic myopathy, lactic acidosis and sideroblastic anemia. American Journal of Medicine 56:891

Rebeiz J J, Caulfield J B, Adams R D 1969 Oculopharyngeal dystrophy — a presenescent myopathy. In: Progress in neuro-ophthalmology. International Congress Series No 176. Excerpta Medica, Amsterdam, p 12

Reske-Nielsen E, Lou H C, Lowes M 1976 Progressive external ophthalmoplegia. Evidence for a generalised mitochondrial disease with a defect in pyruvate metabolism. Acta Ophthalmologica 54:553

Reza M J, Kar N C, Pearson C M, Kark R A P 1978 Recurrent myoglobinuria due to muscle carnitine palmityl transferase deficiency. Annals of Internal Medicine 88:610

Reznik M 1969 Origin of myoblasts during skeletal muscle regeneration. Electron microscopic observations. Laboratory Investigation 20:353

Reznik M 1973 Current concepts of skeletal muscle regeneration. In: Pearson C M, Mostofi F K (eds) The striated muscle. Williams and Wilkins, Baltimore, p 185

Ringel S P, Neville H E, Duster M C, Carroll J E 1978 A new congenital neuromuscular disease with trilaminar muscle fibres. Neurology (Minneapolis) 28:282

Rosing H S, Hopkins L C, Wallace D C, Epstein C M, Weidenheim K 1985 Maternally inherited mitochondrial myopathy and myoclonic epilepsy. Annals of Neurology 17:228

Rowland L P 1976 Pathogenesis of muscular dystrophies. Archives of Neurology 33:315

Rowland L P 1984 Myoglobinuria. Canadian Journal of Neurological Sciences 11:1

Rüdel R, Lehman-Horn F 1985 Membrane changes in cells from myotonia patients. Physiological Reviews 65:310

Sahgal V, Sahgal S 1977 A new congenital myopathy. A morphological, cytochemical and histochemical study. Acta Neuropathologica (Berlin) 37:225

Santa T, Engel A G, Lambert E H 1972 Histometric study of neuromuscular junction ultrastructure. 1. Myasthenia gravis. Neurology (Minneapolis) 22:71

Saper J R, Itabashi H H 1976 Central core disease — a congenital myopathy. Diseases of the Nervous System 37:649

Satoyoshi E, Kowa H 1967 A myopathy due to glycolytic abnormality. Archives of Neurology 17:248

Schäffer J 1893 Beiträge der Histologie und Histogenese der quergestreiften Muskelfasern des Menschen und einiger Wierbelthiere. Sitzungsgeschichte der Kaiserlichen Akademie der Wissenschaft in Wien; matematische-naturwissenschaftiche Classe 102:1

Schiffer D, Giordana M T, Monga G, Mollo F 1976 Histochemistry and electron microscopy of muscle fibres in a case of congenital paramyotonia. Journal of Neurology 211:125

Schmalbruch H 1975 Segmental fibre breakdown and defects of the plasmalemma in diseased human muscles. Acta Neuropathologica (Berlin) 33:129

Schmalbruch H, Hellhammer U 1976 The number of satellite cells in normal human muscle. Anatomical Record 185:279

Schochet S S Jr, Zellweger H, Ionasescu V, McCormick W F 1972 Centronuclear myopathy: Disease entity or syndrome? Light- and electromicroscopic study of two cases and review of the literature. Journal of the Neurological Sciences 16:215

Schotland D 1967 Congenital target fibre disease. Transactions of the American Neurological Association 92:107

Schotland D L, DiMauro S, Bonilla E, Scarpa A, Lee C P 1976 Neuromuscular disorder associated with a defect in mitochondrial energy supply. Archives of Neurology 33:475

Schotland D L, Bonilla E, Wakayama Y 1980 Application of the freeze-fracture technique to the study of human neuromuscular disease. Muscle and Nerve 3:21

Schröder M, Adams R D 1968 Ultrastructural morphology of the muscle fibre in myotonic dystrophy. Acta Neuropathologica (Berlin) 10:218

Schutta H S, Kelly A M, Zacks S I 1969 Necrosis and regeneration of muscle in paroxysmal idiopathic myoglobinuria: electron microscopic observations. Brain 92:191

Schwartz G A, Liu C N 1954 Chronic progressive external ophthalmoplegia: clinical and neuropathologic report. Archives of Neurology and Psychiatry 71:31

Schwartz M S, Sargent M, Swash M 1976 Longitudinal fibre splitting in neurogenic muscular disorders: its relation to the pathogenesis of 'myopathic' change. Brain 99:617

Seitelberger F, Wanko T, Gavin M A 1961 The muscle fibre in central core disease. Histochemical and electron microscopic observations. Acta Neuropathologica (Berlin) 1:223

Sengers R C A, ter Haar B G A, Trijbels J M F, Willems J L, Daniels O, Stadhouders A M 1975 Congenital cataract and mitochondrial myopathy of skeletal and heart muscle associated with lactic acidosis after exercise. Journal of Pediatrics 86:873

Shafiq S A, Milhorat A T, Gorycki M S 1967 Fine structure of human muscle in neurogenic atrophy. Neurology (Minneapolis) 17:934

Shapira Y, Cederbaum S D, Cancilla P A, Nielsen D, Lippe B M 1975 Familial poliodystrophy, mitochondrial myopathy and lactic acidemia. Neurology (Minneapolis) 25:614

Sher J H, Rimalovski A B, Athanassiades T J, Aronson S M 1967 Familial myotubular myopathy. Journal of Neuropathology and Experimental Neurology 24:132

Sher J H, Shafiq S A, Schutta H S 1979 Acute myopathy

with selective lysis of myosin filaments. Neurology (Minneapolis) 29:100

Shibasaki H, Santa T, Kuroiwa Y 1973 Late onset mitochondrial myopathy. Journal of the Neurological Sciences 18:301

Shy G M, Magee K R 1956 A new non-progressive myopathy. Brain 79:610

Shy G M, Wanko T, Rowley P T, Engel A G 1961 Studies in familial periodic paralysis. Experimental Neurology 3:53

Shy G M, Engel W K, Somers J E, Wanko T 1963 Nemaline myopathy: A new congenital myopathy. Brain 86:793

Shy G M, Gonatas N K, Perez M 1966 Two childhood myopathies with abnormal mitochondria. I. Megaconial myopathy. II. Pleoconial myopathy. Brain 89:133

Sissons H 1965 Further observations on muscle fibre size. In: Current research in muscular dystrophy. Proceedings of the Third Symposium. Pitman Medical, London, p 107

Skoglund R R 1979 Reversible ataxia, mitochondrial myopathy and lactic acidemia. Neurology (Minneapolis) 29:717

Sloan M F, Franks A J, Exley K A, Davison A M 1978 Acute renal failure due to polymyositis. British Medical Journal 1:6125

Sloper J C, Pegrum G D 1967 Regeneration of crushed mammalian skeletal muscle and effects of steroids. Journal of Pathology and Bacteriology 93:47

Sloper J C, Partridge T A 1980 Skeletal muscle: Regeneration and transplantation studies. British Medical Bulletin 36:153

Speidel C C 1938 Studies on living muscles. I. Growth, injury and repair of striated muscle, as revealed by prolonged observations of individual fibres in living frog tadpoles. American Journal of Anatomy 62:179

Speidel C C 1939 Studies of living muscle. II. Histological changes in single fibres of striated muscle during contraction and clotting. American Journal of Anatomy 65:471

Spiro A J, Shy G M, Gonatas N K 1966 Myotubular myopathy — persistance of fetal muscle in an adolescent boy. Archives of Neurology 14:1

Spiro A J, Prineas J W, Moore C L 1970a A new mitochondrial myopathy in a patient with salt craving. Archives of Neurology 14:1

Spiro A J, Moore C L, Prineas J W, Strasberg P M, Rapin I 1970b A cytochrome-related inherited disorder of the nervous system and muscle. Archives of Neurology 23:103

Sreter F A, Åström K E, Romanul F C A, Young R R, Jones H R Jr 1976 Characteristics of myosin in nemaline myopathy. Journal of the Neurological Sciences 27:99

Stenger R J, Spiro D, Scully R E, Shannon J M 1962 Ultrastructural and physiologic alterations in ischemic skeletal muscle. American Journal of Pathology 40:1

Stout A P 1946 Rhabdomyosarcoma of the skeletal muscles. Annals of Surgery 123:447

Sugie H, Hanson R, Rasmussen G, Verity M A 1982 Congenital neuromuscular disease with type 1 fibre hypotrophy, ophthalmoplegia and myofibril degeneration. Journal of Neurology, Neurosurgery and Psychiatry 45:507

Salaiman W R, Doyle D, Johnson R H, Jennett S 1974 Myopathy with mitochondrial inclusion bodies: histological and metabolic studies. Journal of Neurology, Neurosurgery and Psychiatry 37:1236

Suzuki K, Rapin I 1969 Giant mitochondria in an infant

with microcephaly and seizure disorder. Archives of Neurology 20:62

Swash M, Schwartz M S 1977 Implications of longitudinal muscle fibre splitting in neurogenic and myopathic disorders. Journal of Neurology, Neurosurgery and Psychiatry 40:1152

Swash M, Schwartz M S, Sargeant M K 1978 Pathogenesis of longitudinal splitting of muscle fibres in neurogenic disorders and polymyositis. Neuropathology and Applied Neurobiology 4:99

Szliwowski H B, Drachman P 1975 Ultrastructural aspects of muscle and nerve in Werdnig-Hoffman disease. Acta Neuropathologica (Berlin) 31:281

Tarlow M J, Lake B D, Lloyd J K 1973 Chronic lactic acidosis in association with myopathy. Archives of Disease in Childhood 48:489

Tarui S, Ikuno G, Ikura Y, Tanaka T, Suda M, Nishikawa M 1965 Phosphofructokinase deficiency in skeletal muscle: A new type of glucogenosis. Biochemical and Biophysical Research Communications 19:517

Taylor E W 1915 Progressive vagus — glossopharyngeal paralysis with ptosis: contribution to a group of family diseases. Journal of Nervous and Mental Diseases 42:129

Tomé F M, Fardeau M 1975 Congenital myopathy with 'reducing bodies' in muscle fibres. Acta Neuropathologica (Berlin) 31:207

Tomé F M, Fardeau M, Lenoir G 1977 Ultrastructure of muscle and sensory nerve in Fabry's disease. Acta Neuropathologica (Berlin) 38:187

Tomé F M S, Fardeau M 1980 Nuclear inclusions in oculopharyngeal dystrophy. Acta Neuropathologica (Berlin) 49:85

Tomlinson B E, Walton J N, Rebeiz J J 1969 The effects of aging and of cachexia upon skeletal muscle. A histopathological study. Journal of the Neurological Sciences 9:321

Tsairis P, Engel W K, Kark P 1973 Familial myoclonic epilepsy syndrome associated with skeletal muscle mitochondrial abnormalities. Neurology (Minneapolis) 23:408

Tyler F H 1950 Studies in disorders of muscle. III Pseudohypertrophy of muscle in progressive muscular dystrophy and other neuromuscular disease. Archives of Neurology and Psychiatry 63:425

Tyler F H, Stephens F E, Gunn F D, Perkoff G T 1951 Studies in disorders of muscles. VII Clinical manifestations and inheritance of a type of periodic paralysis without hypopotassemia. Journal of Clinical Investigation 30:492

van Biervliet J P G M, Bruinvis I, Ketting D et al 1977 Hereditary mitochondrial myopathy with lactic acidemia, a de Toni-Fanconi-Debré syndrome and a defective respiratory chain in voluntary striated muscles. Pediatric Research 11:1088

van Wijngaarden G K, Bethlem J, Meijer A E F H, Hülsmann W C, Feltkamp C A 1967 Skeletal muscle disease with abnormal mitochondria. Brain 90:577

Van Unnik A J M 1982 Muscle tumours. In: Mastaglia F L, Walton J (eds) Skeletal muscle pathology. Churchill Livingstone, Edinburgh

Victor M, Hayes R, Adams R D 1962 Oculopharyngeal muscular dystrophy. A familial disease of late life characterized by dysphagia and progressive ptosis of the eyelids. New England Journal of Medicine 267:1267

Walker B E 1963 The origin of myoblasts and the problem of dedifferentiation. Experimental Cell Research 30:80

Wallace S L, Lattes R, Malia J P, Ragen C 1958 Diagnostic significance of the muscle biopsy. American Journal of Medicine 25:600

Walton J N 1957 The limp child. Journal of Neurology, Neurosurgery and Psychiatry 20:144

Walton J N, Adams R D 1958 Polymyositis. Livingstone, Edinburgh

Walton J N, Gardner-Medwin D 1968 Second thoughts on classification of the muscular dystrophies. In: Current research in muscular dystrophy. Proceedings of the Fourth Symposium. Pitman Medical, London

Watkins S C, Cullen M J 1982 Muscle fiber size and shape in Duchenne muscular dystrophy. Neuropathology and Applied Neurobiology 8:11

Whiteley A M, Schwartq M S, Sachs J A, Swash M 1976 Congenital myasthenia gravis: clinical and HLA studies in two brothers. Journal of Neurology, Neurosurgery and Psychiatry 39:1145

Willems J L, Monnens L A M, Trijbels et al 1977 Leigh's encephalomyelopathy in a patient with cytochrome c oxidase deficiency in muscle tissue. Pediatrics 60:850

Wohlfart G 1942 Quantitativ-histologische Studien an der Skelettmuskulatur während der Entwicklung und bei der Atrophie nach Nervendurchschneidung. Zeitschrift für Mikroskopisch-Anatomische Forschung 5:480

Wohlfart G 1949 Muscular atrophy in diseases of the lower motor neuron: contribution to the anatomy of motor units. Archives of Neurology 61: 599–620

Wohlfart G 1951 Dystrophia myotonica and myotonia congenita: Histopathological studies with special reference to changes in muscles. Journal of Neuropathology and Experimental Neurology 10:109

Wohlfart G 1955 Aktuelle Probleme der Muskelpathologie. Deutsche Zeitschrift für Nervenheilkunde 173:426

Worsfold M, Park D C, Pennington R J 1973 Familial 'mitochondrial' myopathy. A myopathy associated with disordered oxidative metabolism in muscle fibres. Part 2. Biochemical findings. Journal of the Neurological Sciences 19:261

Yarom R, Shapira Y 1977 Myosin degeneration in a congenital myopathy. Archives of Neurology 34:114

Yunis E J, Samaha F J 1971 Inclusion body myositis. Laboratory Investigation 25:240

Zelena J 1962 The effect of denervation on muscle development. In: Gutman E (ed) The denervated muscle. Publishing House of Czechoslovak Academy of Sciences, Prague, p 103

Zellweger H, Afifi A, McCormick W F, Mergner W 1967 Severe congenital muscular dystrophy. American Journal of Diseases of Children 114:591

Zellweger H, Ionasescu V 1973 Early onset of myotonic dystrophy in infants. American Journal of Diseases of Children 125:601

The pathological anatomy of the neuromuscular junction

INTRODUCTION

The muscles receive peripheral nerve endings from both alpha and gamma neurones as well as postganglionic fibres of the posterior spinal ganglia and autonomic system. In this chapter we confine ourselves to the pathology of the terminal nerve endings and end-plates of the alpha motor neurones.

Accurate histological diagnosis of neuromuscular disorders requires, in addition to conventional histology and histochemistry on biopsied muscle or nerve, the investigation of intramuscular nerves and nerve endings. Muscle biopsy can be of additional value in neurological diagnosis as it also permits the microscopic investigation of terminal nerve fibres and motor end-plates during life. Because terminal nerves separate from one another after their emergence from the intramuscular nerve bundles, each fibre may be followed in isolation for long distances to the motor end-plates. Visualisation of such terminal nerve fibres and end-plates can be further enhanced by selective stains and by the relatively homogeneous background of the muscle fibres.

Although the anterior horn cell body cannot be included in a muscle biopsy specimen, one may investigate the terminal nerves as well as the motor end-plates and, from these, infer changes in the motor neurone soma. In this regard we are greatly assisted by the concept of 'dying-back' of the neurone (see discussion in Coërs & Woolf 1959, pp. 66–67) first described almost 100 years ago. The 'dying-back' changes represent some of the most characteristic features of the terminal nerve endings and end-plates seen in peripheral nerve or motor neurone disease. As the earliest changes in the anterior horn cell tend to appear in the motor end-plate and in adjacent axonal twigs, the value of the muscle biopsy is greatly enhanced by the simultaneous application of the muscle biopsy to an 'intra-vitam' or enzyme histochemical examination of nerve endings and end-plates.

The standing of muscle biopsy, both as a diagnostic weapon and as a research tool for studying diseased nerve endings and end-plates has been greatly facilitated in the last three decades. The progress in this area has emerged largely as a result of the following contributions: (1) the demonstration of the zonal distribution of the intramuscular nerve endings by motor point biopsies (Coërs 1953a, Coërs & Woolf 1959); (2) the introduction of vital staining of the nerve fibres and endings with methylene blue (Coërs 1952); (3) the application of the modified Koelle's method for simultaneous demonstration of the nerve endings and the end-plate by means of its acetylcholinesterase (AChE) activity (Beermann & Cassend 1976, Pestronk & Drachman 1978a); (4) the discovery of α-bungarotoxin (α-BT) binding to the acetylcholine receptor (AChR) and the subsequent histochemical identification of receptor protein (Lee et al 1967, Fambrough et al 1973); (5) the application of immunoperoxidase techniques for localising AChR with α-BT (Daniels & Vogel 1975), and (6) the use of the electron microscope with or without immunostaining to investigate ultrastructural abnormalities.

ANATOMICAL CONSIDERATIONS

Evolution and histology of the neuromuscular junction

The early belief of Valentin (1836) and Emmert (1836) that the nerve fibres terminated in striated muscle in a branching, arc-like structure which formed networks and sent fibres from the periphery back to the CNS was refuted in a careful study by Wagner (1878), who observed the terminal branching of the axon with loss of its myelin sheath at the junctional site. In vertebrates, three patterns of nerve endings in striated muscle are known (Coërs 1967a): (1) terminal innervation, in which nerve endings are localised at the ends of the myofibres and exemplified in fish; (2) multiple scattered innervation along the length of the myofibres, exemplified in frogs; (3) single, mid-point innervation of each myofibre as seen in many terrestial vertebrates, including man.

Vital staining of the neuromuscular junction

The ability of axons to take up methylene blue was first demonstrated by Ehrlich (1882). Subsequently, Dogiel (1890) and Attias (1912) used this phenomenon to demonstrate nerve endings by immersing the removed tissue to be examined in a methylene blue solution (supravital staining). Weddell (1941a, b) introduced intravital staining by local injection of human cutaneous nerve endings and this was subsequently applied to muscle biopsy in man (Coërs 1952).

Vital staining with methylene blue has the advantage over silver impregnation in that it shows greater detail of the end-plate (Fig. 6.1). Vital staining also allows the demonstration of terminal axoplasmic alterations while they are still in a living or near-living state. Axonal swellings, for example, appear fuller than after fixation and this may be important in correlating electron-microscopic findings.

Histochemistry of the neuromuscular junction

Morphological details and subneural acetylcholinesterase (AChE) activity can be demonstrated by histochemical staining of the end-plate. The ability of cholinesterase staining to characterise morphologically the end-plate in this fashion is apparently due to the high concentration of the enzyme confined to the synaptic folds. The zonal distribution of the motor end-plate at, or near, the centre of each muscle fibre (Fig. 6.2) is best demonstrated by this method (Coërs 1953a).

Two methods have been used to demonstrate subneural cholinesterase activity: the copper thiocholine technique of Koelle (Koelle & Friedenwald 1949, Couteaux 1951, Coërs 1953b) and the indoxyl method of Holt (Holt 1956, Holt & Withers 1956). These methods have been used to describe differences in the light-microscopic morphology of AChE-stained fast and slow-twitch motor end-plates (Nystrom 1968, Dias 1974). The

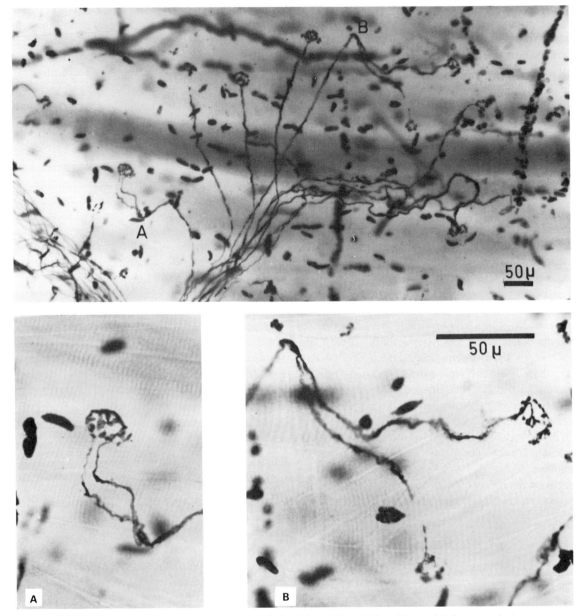

Fig. 6.1 Normal pattern of terminal motor innervation (vital staining with methylene blue, thick frozen section).
A. Ultraterminal ramification subserving two different muscle fibres. B. Distal ramification forming two motor arborisations subserving the same muscle fibre

modified indoxyl staining combined with silver impregnation by Pestronk & Drachman (1978a) can readily be applied to cryosections of 20–30 μm thickness cut from biopsied muscle. The nerve terminals are black-stained (silver) and the end-plates blue (bromoindoxyl) (Fig. 6.3). This method has given consistently good results, allowing a good resolution for evaluating both sprouting and reinnervation processes and may potentially replace the vital staining technique.

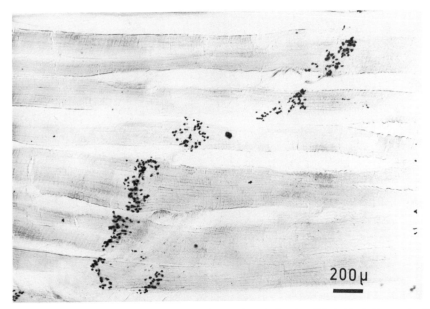

Fig. 6.2 Zone of motor innervation in the palmaris longus of a newborn infant (modified thiocholine method)

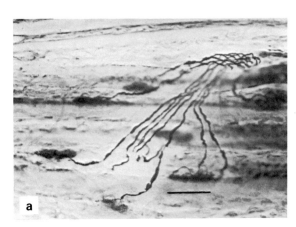

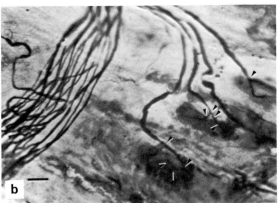

Electron microscopy of the neuromuscular junction

The preferred specimen for electron microscopy (EM) is derived from motor point biopsy and processed by conventional techniques. End-plate regions can be selected prior to plastic embedding by staining a parallel strip fixed in 3% phosphate-buffered glutaraldehyde for AChE. The tissue can then be trimmed for a better yield for EM (de Harven & Coërs 1959, Engel 1970) prior to osmication. The preterminal axon loses its myelin sheath shortly before reaching the myofibre and forming the terminal arborisation. This arborisation can be divided into four layers: (1) Schwann cell; (2) nerve terminal with many synaptic vesicles containing acetylcholine (ACh); (3) junctional folds and cleft; (4) junctional sarcoplasm (Fig. 6.4a). The junctional gap between the nerve terminal and the underlying end-plate region is called the

Fig. 6.3 a. Several motor end-plates stained blue with bromoindoxyl and nerve terminal twigs stained black with silver arising from a preterminal nerve bundle (Pestronk and Drachman method). Scale bar = 30 μm, i.e. approximate length of end-plate ×380. b. Within each of three end-plates a few nerve terminal branch points (arrows) can be seen (Mouse diaphragm). Scale bar = 10 μm; ×550

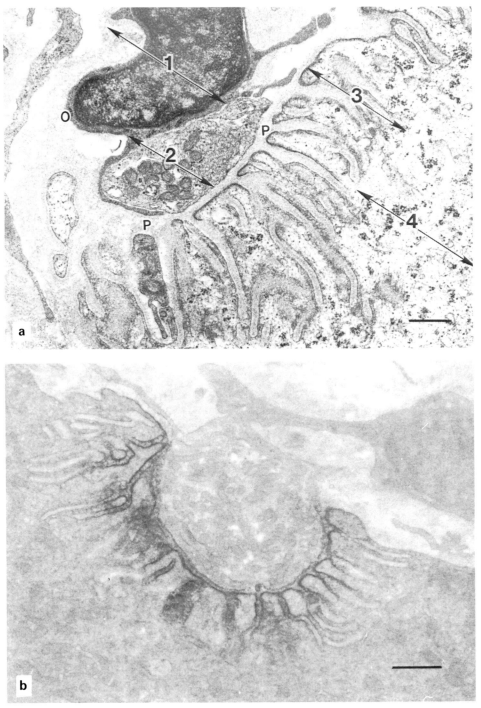

Fig. 6.4 a. Four layers of normal terminal arborisation consisting of: (1) Schwann cell; (2) nerve terminal with many synaptic vesicles and mitochondria, separated by the primary synaptic cleft (P); (3) junctional gap with many secondary synaptic clefts; (4) junctional sarcoplasm. Scale bar = 1 μm ×13 000. b. AChR sites visualised by peroxidase-conjugated α-BT, showing receptor sites distributed mainly at the peaks of secondary synaptic clefts and much less in the deep secondary clefts. Scale bar = 1 μm; ×15 200 (Courtesy of Dr M. Tsujihata, Nagasaki University, Japan)

primary synaptic cleft. When ACh in the synaptic vesicles is discharged through the presynaptic membrane, ACh must travel across the primary synaptic cleft to reach the receptor sites in the postsynaptic membrane at the 'peaks' (Engel et al 1981) of secondary synaptic clefts (Fig. 6.4b). Ultrastructural differences of fast and slow neuromuscular junctions have been reported (Padykula & Gauthier 1970, Duchen 1971). The available ultrastructural data, however, are often too restricted to represent the overall view of the synaptic structures even though attempts have been made to rectify bias in interpretation by morphometric and statistical analysis of given motor end-plates (Engel & Santa 1971, Engel et al 1975). In this regard, the advent of additional qualitative approaches by means of immunocytochemical EM may alleviate certain difficulties in diagnostic interpretation of diseased end-plates. In addition, scanning EM provides a view of both internal and external synaptic surface structures and clefts as well as patterns of nerve terminal branches, rendering with relative ease the identification of two different neuromuscular junctions (Fig. 6.5) and pathological patterns (Fahim et al 1984).

Immunocytochemistry and radiochemistry of the neuromuscular junction

Either immunocytochemical or radiochemical techniques can be applied to the study of the membrane component at the neuromuscular junction, specifically, the acetylcholine receptor (AChR). A neurotoxin, alpha-bungarotoxin (α-BT), irreversibly binds to the AChR and can be labelled with the radioisotope ^{125}I (Fambrough et al 1973) (Fig. 6.6), a fluorescent conjugate (Bursztajn et al 1983) or a peroxidase conjugate (Daniels & Vogel 1975). With these techniques, ultrastructural localisation and turnover rates of AChR-labelled end-plates have been studied in various human neuromuscular diseases (Engel et al 1977, Tsujihata et al 1980, 1984). Similarly, immuno-electron-microscopic studies localising immunoglobulin G (IgG) and complement components (especially C3 and C9) to the endplate have successfully detailed the dynamics and pathogenesis of certain diseases involving the neuromus-

cular junctions (Sahashi et al 1980, Fumagalli et al 1982).

TECHNIQUE OF NEUROMUSCULAR JUNCTION BIOPSY

Selection of muscle

In the selection of muscles for biopsy, a muscle in which the innervation is only partly, although definitely, affected should be chosen because the earliest pathological changes are usually the most characteristic, and the nerve fibres may be diminished or absent in severely affected muscle. For this reason, muscles which show marked weakness should be avoided. A clinically unaffected forearm muscle may be suitable even if the disease process affects all lower motor neurones but produces clinically demonstrable signs only at the distal ends of the longest axons. For example, in generalised peripheral neuropathy the choice of a forearm muscle is justified if there are paraesthesiae in the finger tips. Even in the absence of such symptoms, studying an upper extremity muscle permits exclusion of possible lumbosacral root compression causing obvious lower motor neurone disease in the legs.

An additional advantage in studying a forearm muscle, especially the flexor carpi radialis or palmaris longus, is the relative ease with which the innervation zones (determined by electrical stimulation) can be exposed. Of the two, palmaris longus is the muscle of choice because it has less functional importance and the shortness of its belly facilitates localisation of the nerve endings.

The vastus internus is recommended among the muscles of the quadriceps group, because it has an innervation zone which closely underlies the motor point. The deltoid, on the other hand, has muscle fasciculi running parallel with the surface but they tend to be adherent to the fascia. Biceps brachii can also be used although its motor point does not always correspond to the zone of innervation.

Motor point biopsy

The operative technique for muscle biopsy has been described in detail elsewhere (Coërs &

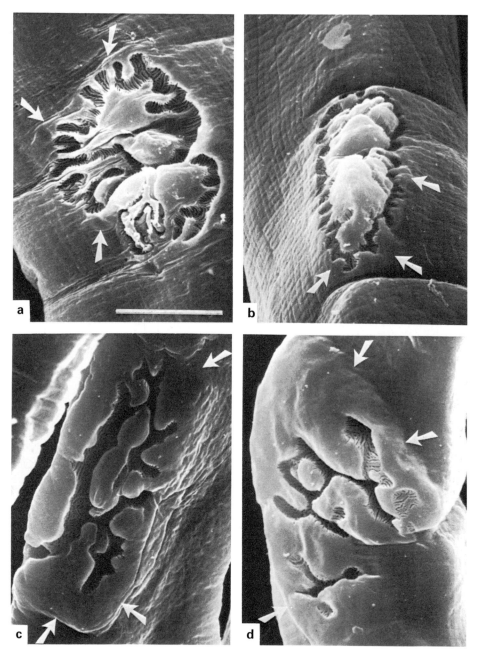

Fig. 6.5 Scanning electron micrographs of fast (EDL) and slow (SOL) twitch muscle end-plates showing the higher and large 'raised area' marked with arrows of SOL end-plates (c & d) with relatively wider primary cleft area than EDL end-plates (a & b). Note part of the nerve terminal still attached to the end-plates (a & b). Scale bar = 10 μm (Reproduced with permission from Fahim et al 1984 and Neuroscience)

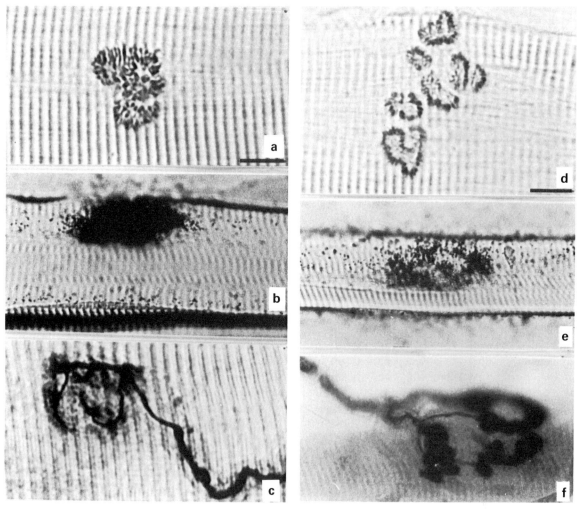

Fig. 6.6 End-plates visualised by AChE staining (a & b) radio-labelled α-BT autoradiography (b & e) and silver staining (c & f) at different ages (a, b, c from a 32-year-old male and d, e, f from a 54-year-old female) showing a propensity of increased number of smaller conglomerates with AChE, of prejunctional AChRs and of preterminal axons entering the end-plates in the older subjects. Scale bar = 20 μm (Reproduced with permission from Oda 1984 and Journal of the Neurological Sciences)

Woolf 1959) and later with certain modifications (Woolf 1962). After local anaesthesia of the subcutaneous tissue, the skin and fascia are incised across the motor point, parallel to the main axis of the muscle fibres for a length of 4–5 cm. Accurate localisation of the terminal innervation area is achieved with electrical stimulation of the exposed muscle. A sterile metallic electrode connected to the cathode of the stimulator delivers currents of 0.1 ms duration at a frequency of 1.0 s. The terminal nerve endings can be localised to the region where a single fasciculus, and not the whole muscle, contracts when stimulated by a current too weak to produce contraction when applied to any other part of that fasciculus. The current should usually be of the order of 0.1–0.5 mA with a stabilised current stimulator and the voltage should be of the order of 1–10 V with a constant-voltage apparatus. The accuracy of the motor point biopsy may be lessened if the innervation zone is enlarged, particularly in muscles with partial denervation, myasthenia gravis or myopathy. On the whole, the yield of the method is about 95% (Harriman 1961).

A strip, not wider than 1 mm, is first removed for electron microscopy with a biopsy forceps applied across the innervation zone. Another strip may be removed from a parallel area for enzyme histochemical, immunocytochemical or radiochemical techniques. For vital staining, the selected fasciculus is injected with a 0.02–0.05% solution of methylene blue in physiological saline, using the finest needle available. The needle is introduced parallel to the direction of the fasciculus and just below its surface, and the solution is gently injected as the needle is being withdrawn. The injection is repeated along a 2–3 cm area, 1–2 mm wide, over 3–5 min using a 10–30 ml of solution. Anaesthetic is not usually necessary but may be used to prevent the rare aching pain which may occur, and does not interfere with the staining. The strips are placed on a gauze moistened with physiological saline, oxygenated for 1 h, and then immersed in a filtered cold aqueous saturated solution of ammonium molybdate at 4°C for 24 h. After washing in three changes of distilled water,the specimens are fixed in 10% formol saline for 24 h. They are then cut as longitudinal frozen sections 50–100 μm thick: thick frozen sections have the advantage of preserving the normal relationship between the subterminal nerve fibres and motor end-plates.

METHODS OF EVALUATION
Terminal innervation ratio (TIR)

When the intramuscular nerves reach the terminal innervation band, they spread into isolated individual fibres which course only a short distance before reaching the muscle fibres and forming their terminal arborisations (Fig. 6.1). These nerve fibres are referred to as terminal axons. On occasion, the terminal axon may branch before reaching the muscle fibres or may branch directly off the motor arborisation. The two arborisations resulting from such a branching usually innervate the same muscle fibre (Fig. 6.1b); less frequently, they innervate two different muscle fibres (Fig. 6.1a). Clinical significance of collateral sprouting has been well reviewed by Wohlfart (1960) and Woolf (1957). This branching can be quantitatively estimated as the Terminal Innervation Ratio (TIR) which is defined as the ratio of the number of myofibres (Nmf) innervated by a given number of subterminal axons (Nnf); [TIR = Nmf/Nnf].

The normal value of TIR, initially based on the findings in 12 individuals who were both clinically and electromyographically normal, was 1.1 ± 0.06 (Coërs 1955). Later studies on 13 neuromuscular biopsies taken from normal volunteer university students showed a mean TIR of 1.12 ± 0.04 (Reske-Nielsen et al 1969). These results were comparable to a group of 43 biopsies taken by us for diagnostic purposes, in which there were no clinical, EMG or histological changes (Coërs et al 1973a); the mean TIR of this group was 1.1 ± 0.05. There was no significant difference between these figures and the values obtained from the volunteer students ($P > 0.2$). The pooled mean TIR from these three groups of biopsies was 1.11, with a standard deviation of 0.05. Values higher than 1.26 (mean + 3 SD) are considered to be abnormal (Coërs et al 1973b).

Excessive branching of intramuscular nerve fibres may occur at various levels, collateral, subterminal or ultraterminal, forming expanded motor endings or several motor arborisations on the same myofibre. This change may be observed either in denervation or myopathy and usually affects hypertrophic muscle fibres (Fig. 6.7). Collateral ramification results in the innervation of different muscle fibres, causing an increase of the functional (true) TIR, i.e. an increase in the number of muscle fibres innervated by a given number of subterminal axons, and represents an expansion of the motor unit by inclusion of muscle fibres from denervated units. The TIR was found to be significantly increased in 87% of patients with denervating disease; in muscular dystrophy, the TIR was within the normal range in 82% of cases, including all cases of Duchenne muscular dystrophy and congenital myopathies (Coërs et al 1973c, 1976). The differential diagnosis of limb-girdle muscular dystrophy and spinal muscular atrophy may therefore be enhanced by studying TIR (Coërs & Telerman-Toppet 1979).

Sprouting index

Instead of using TIR as the index for functional denervation or the amount of sprouting, Pestronk

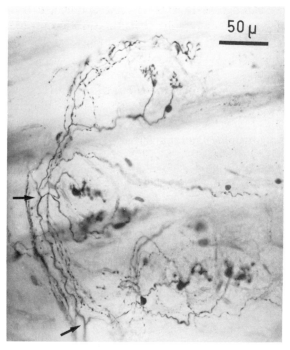

50 μ

Fig. 6.7 Kugelberg–Welander disease. Collateral reinnervation (arrows) and distal branching forming several motor arborisations on hypertrophic muscle fibres. Some axons are abnormally thin and beaded (vital staining with methylene blue)

& Drachman (1978b) introduced another morphometric measurement — the 'sprouting index' — to assess the sprouting response of motor neurones. It is quantitatively evaluated by (1) counting the number of nerve terminal branch points within each end-plate area and (2) measuring the length of each end-plate parallel to the length of the myofibre, as visualised in the combined silver and AChE staining preparation (Fig. 6.3B) (Pestronk & Drachman 1978a). The mean motor end-plate diameter was 32.2 μm $\pm$ 10.5, ranging from 10 to 80 μm (Coërs 1955); the mean value of the motor end-plate area ranged from 177 to 314 μm^2 (Coërs & Hildebrand 1965, Reske-Neilsen et al 1969). The histograms of both the diameters and the surface areas of the motor end-plates corresponded to unimodal-normal or logarithmic-normal distribution curves, indicating a single population of motor nerve endings. Hence, the sprouting index is the mean number of branch points for each muscle multiplied by the

mean end-plate length (μm) for the given muscle. Sprouting activity of terminal axons appears to depend on availability of extrajunctional AChR, as sprouting can be inhibited by blockade of AChR (Pestronk & Drachman 1978b). This contention is well supported by experimental studies of the extent of nerve terminal outgrowth demonstrated by botulinum toxin and α-BT treatment following nerve crush in anti-AChR antibody-treated or AChR-immunised animals (Pestronk & Drachman 1985b). Hence, the sprouting index should reflect the level of available extrajunctional AChR as visualised and measured by isotope- or peroxidase-labelled α-BT.

Ultrastructural morphometric analysis of the neuromuscular junction

Morphometric analysis using planimetry with line and point sampling techniques for the ultrastructure of individual motor end-plates was advocated by Engel & Santa (1971). The parameters included: (1) nerve terminal areas; (2) mitochondrial population; (3) synaptic vesicle concentration; (4) postsynaptic area of clefts and folds; (5) postsynaptic membrane length; (6) postsynaptic membrane profile concentration. Statistical analysis was later applied to correct bias from other variables (Engel et al 1975). By combining the immunoelectron-microscopic technique, such as peroxidase staining for AChR, ultrastructural morphometry becomes more practical and comprehensive. In one study, peroxidase-conjugated α-BT was incubated with thin strips of fresh muscle for several hours and then fixed in 3% glutaraldehyde for several more hours. Following an overnight rinse in the same buffer, small pieces of myofibres with end-plates were dissected and then reacted with diaminobenzidine reagent for 30 min. The specimens were routinely processed for electron microscopy following osmication. Morphometric analysis of the AChR in microphotographs of end-plates included: (1) presynaptic membrane length (PSML) in μm; (2) postsynaptic membrane length with the positive reaction product for AChR in μm (Engel et al 1977). The ratio AChR surface length: PSML is considered to be a useful index for the assessment of functional AChR in the end-plate.

DIAGNOSTIC CONSIDERATIONS

Development and ageing of the neuromuscular junction

During embryonic muscle development, the motor nerve terminals do not make contact with the myotube until the sarcolemmal nuclei attain their peripheral location in the myofibre. Once this occurs, the nerve fibres extend terminal sprouts, together with Schwann cell nuclei, to end at the level of one of these peripheralised muscle nuclei. This close relationship of developing motor end-plates and sarcolemmal nuclear aggregates in human fetuses is well illustrated by Tello (1917). In human muscle up to two years of age, immature end-plates, characterised by simple unbranched and club-like terminations, may be seen in the presence of fully mature end-plates in striated muscle (Coërs & Woolf 1954).

Despite marked variation in size, the structure of the motor nerve endings is fairly constant in normal muscles. However, some abnormal end-plates may also be observed in healthy young mammals (Barker & Ip 1965) and interpreted as indicating an ageing process. Tuffery (1971) reported that the average number of myelinated branches of a single terminal axon increased with age in cats. The effects of ageing on the terminal motor innervation pattern creates a perplexing diagnostic problem. An increase in the number of preterminal axons entering an end-plate and the length of the end-plate correlates with the number of prejunctional AChRs in older subjects (Oda 1984). Oda (1984) also described the propensity of AChRs to form smaller, multiple conglomerates in the older subjects. These findings are in agreement with the scanning-microscopic observations that nerve terminals and the underlying postsynaptic cleft are longer and more branched in aged mice (Fahim et al 1983). Ultrastructural morphometry of end-plates in aged mice reveals pronounced loss of synaptic folds without physiological evidence of denervation or loss of junctional AChR (Fahim & Robbins 1982, Banker et al 1983). These age-related changes in the end-plate architecture are different in functionally diverse muscles (Pestronk et al 1980, Rosenheimer & Smith 1985). A general decline in sprouting is reported in the hind-limb neuromuscular junctions of aged rats whereas the diaphragm is well maintained, suggesting that the direction of age-related changes is somewhat influenced by the functional state of the muscle.

DENERVATION

Amyotrophic lateral sclerosis

In amyotrophic lateral sclerosis (ALS), the terminal motor axons may appear normal or may show thinning or fine beading of the distal axon. The end-plates have an attenuated appearance, with the terminal axonic expansions small, spherical and darkly staining. Although the arborisation may be expanded with an excessive number of terminal expansions, the filaments of the terminal arborisations are usually slender and delicate. This is reflected by the increased mean TIR in 18 cases of ALS of 1.60 ± 0.3 (Telerman-Toppet & Coërs 1978).

Eventually, the attenuation of the end-plates reaches a stage when contact is lost with the muscle fibre and the axon appears to 'die back' from the periphery. Just how long this process takes is not clear, but it is characteristic to find many fine, beaded nerve fibres in the terminal nerve bundles forming plexiform networks on the muscle fibres (Fig. 6.8). These fine, beaded sprouts may be present in the more proximal parts of the motor and spinal nerves and their unstable polarisation may be related to the fasciculations seen in ALS (Woolf 1957, 1962, Coërs & Woolf

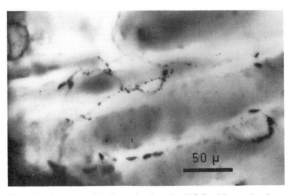

Fig. 6.8 Amyotrophic lateral sclerosis (ALS). Network of fine beaded motor fibres (vital staining with methylene blue)

1959). Bjornskov et al (1975), however, reported increased numbers of segmented and enlarged end-plates in 19 out of 21 ALS patients, although their more recent study of the modified sprouting index failed to demonstrate an increase in axonal sprouting (Bjornskov et al 1984).

The changes seen with the electron microscope in the intramuscular nerve bundles mirror the findings noted with vital staining. Schwann cells may be devoid of axons and there is an increase in collagen covering denuded postsynaptic regions, suggesting a lack of regeneration and reinnervation (Fig. 6.9). The postsynaptic folds, however, are relatively well preserved (Engel et al 1975, Chou 1982). Tsujihata et al (1984) performed a quantitative analysis of AChR in 45 end-plates from 16 ALS patients' biceps muscles by measuring: (1) the postsynaptic area; (2) the AChR surface length, and 3) 'AChR density', arbitrarily calculated by dividing the value of (2) by that of (1). The junctional AChRs were well preserved (Fig. 6.10) in both the highly atrophic myofibres and the denuded postsynaptic folds (Tsujihata et al 1984); in the 139 ALS postsynaptic regions studied, 47 (33.8%) were denuded of nerve terminals while 9.8% of 64 end-plates from five control patients showed denuded postsynaptic regions.

Werdnig–Hoffmann disease

In Werdnig-Hoffmann disease (WHD) the motor axons proximal to the terminal nerve bundles are typically normal, whereas terminal axons form a

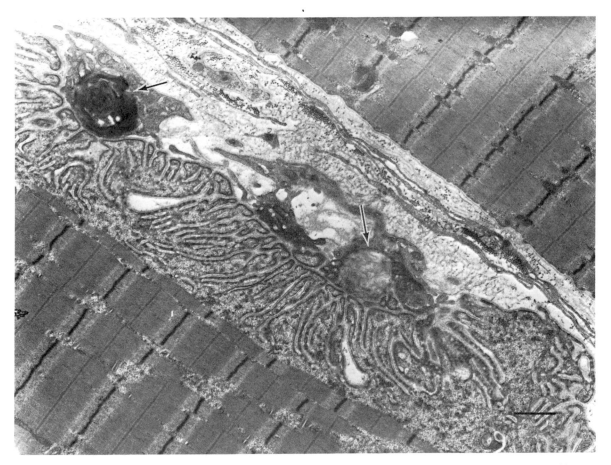

Fig. 6.9 Myeloid figures in degenerating terminal axons (arrows) in biopsied external intercostal muscle from a 47-year-old woman with ALS. Note well-preserved secondary synaptic clefts and sarcomeres near the end-plate. Scale bar = 1 μm

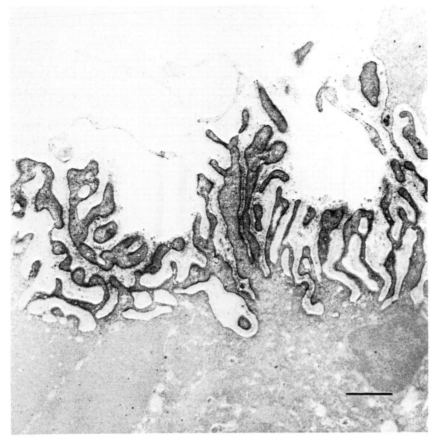

Fig. 6.10 Denuded postsynaptic regions with relatively well-preserved postjunctional folds with abundant junctional AChRs localised mainly along the peak zones of secondary clefts as visualised with peroxidase conjugated α-BT in a 34-year-old male with ALS. Scale bar = 1 μm; ×14 000 (Courtesy of Dr M Tsujihata, Niigata University, Japan)

'tangle' of fine, beaded fibres with scanty branching. From this tangle, the emerging fibres end in a poorly formed end-plate, a finding especially characteristic of slowly progressive disease. This loss of neuromuscular connection makes it impossible to measure the TIR in most biopsies. The tangle is typical of WHD and enables it to be distinguished from other causes of infantile muscular weakness and hypotonia in most cases (Woolf 1960). The beaded fibres may represent immature end-plates and early attempts for motor axons to make contact with a myofibre, as end-plates of varied sizes and shapes are seen with acetylcholine staining (Fig. 6.11). The appearance of the end-plates may vary in WHD depending on the tempo of disease development, as more beaded tangles with little distal sprouting are seen in rapidly fatal cases (Coërs & Woolf

1959). Motor end-plates in two out of six patients with WHD appeared ultrastructurally normal (Szliwowski & Drochmans 1975).

Charcot–Marie–Tooth disease

In Charcot–Marie–Tooth disease (CMT), which has a much slower and milder evolution than ALS, the process of collateral ramification is significantly increased. Consequently, the mean TIR measured in 12 cases of CMT was 2.16 ± 0.56, significantly higher than that of ALS ($P < 0.05$) (Telerman-Toppet & Coërs 1978). This difference indicates that the unaffected motor neurones in CMT have a better capacity to reinnervate adjacent denervated muscle fibres than do their counterparts in ALS. The high value of TIR is also reflected in an increased degree of type

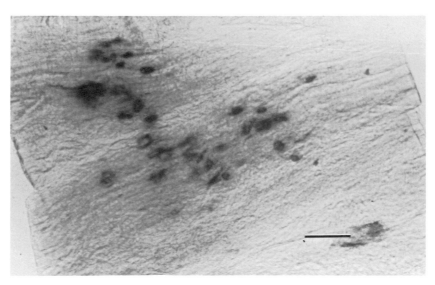

Fig. 6.11 AChE staining of a biopsied muscle from a nine-month-old infant with Werdnig–Hoffmann's disease, showing scattered end-plates of varied sizes and shapes, mostly ring-shaped. Scale bar = 100 μm

grouping and group atrophy in CMT as compared with ALS (Dubowitz & Brooke 1973, Jennekens et al 1974, Telerman-Toppet & Coërs 1978). Electromyographic estimation of fibre density has produced results in agreement with these morphological data (Schwartz et al 1976). Both increased collateral branching and type grouping are an expression of the compensatory increase in the size of residual motor units that occurs in chronic denervation. As in WHD, reticulated axonal networks of very fine beaded nerve fibres wander among myofibres without making visible contact in CMT (Fig. 6.12). An increased TIR is a reliable indication of denervation processes, including both motor neurone diseases and peripheral motor neuropathies, especially in the early stages. Limb immobilisation in experimental animals produces muscle atrophy and denervation-like changes at the neuromuscular junctions especially of type II myofibres and leads to terminal axonal sprouting and ultrastructural remodelling (Pachter & Eberstein 1984).

MYOPATHIES

Duchenne muscular dystrophy

Harriman (1976) studied 42 end-plates from 13 patients with Duchenne muscular dystrophy

(DMD) and concluded that many did not differ from those seen in control specimens, except for some junctions which showed withdrawal of the axon terminals, regenerating neuromuscular junctions and axonal sprouting. The investigation of intramuscular innervation of 19 muscle biopsy specimens did not demonstrate reinnervation through collateral sprouting in DMD. The mean TIR was 1.12 ± 0.06, ranging from 0.01 to 1.23 and not significantly different from the findings in controls ($P > 0.4$) (Coërs & Telerman-Toppet 1977). Although no collateral sprouting secondary to axonal loss occurs, innervation persists in affected muscles. It is easy in methylene blue preparations to follow 'unemployed' nerve fibres traversing connective tissue parallel to the longitudinal axis of the muscle fibres (Fig. 6.13). These nerve fibres are often abnormally thin and beaded, but do not branch excessively. This distorted pattern of motor innervation results in a very marked elongation of the terminal innervation area and a longitudinal scatter of motor end-plates that may reach 10 mm (Fig. 6.14).

This dispersion of motor endings may be explained in two ways. According to Desmedt & Borenstein (1973), focal necrosis can produce a transection of muscle fibres with the consequent formation of denervated segments. 'Unemployed' axons could be accepted by the remaining segment

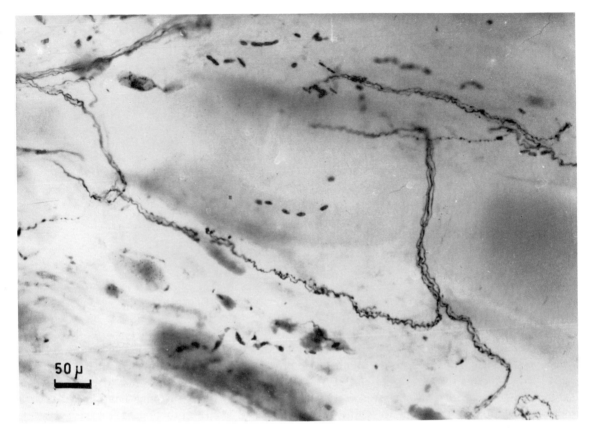

Fig. 6.12 Reticulated motor axons in a case of Charcot–Marie–Tooth disease (vital staining with methylene blue)

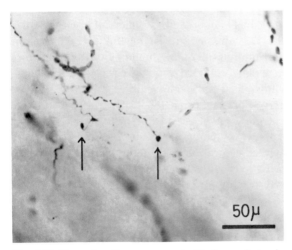

Fig. 6.13 'Unemployed' motor axons in Duchenne dystrophy (vital staining with methylene blue)

of innervated fibres in the vicinity, producing ectopic end-plates. Innervation of regenerated muscle fibres is also known to occur in the early stages of the disease (Desmedt & Borenstein 1976). Another possibility is the dispersion of the motor end-plate secondary to the longitudinal displacement of transected muscle fibres resulting from segmental necrosis or new motor arborisation to myofibres with longitudinal splitting and/or regenerative sprouting.

Morphometric studies of the end-plates by Jerusalem et al (1974) indicate focal atrophy of the postsynaptic regions without abnormalities in the axon terminals. A later study by Engel et al (1975) also revealed focal degeneration of postsynaptic folds and an increased incidence of simplified postsynaptic regions in 47% of end-plate regions studied. Ultrastructural studies on the end-plates of three patients with Becker's muscular dystrophy (BMD) showed markedly

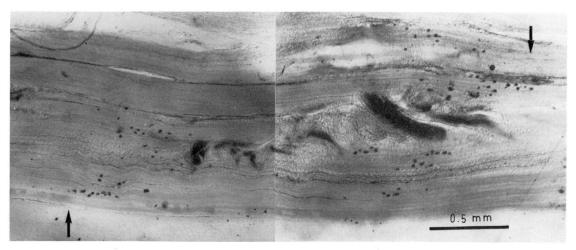

Fig. 6.14 Abnormal dispersion of motor end-plates (arrows) in Duchenne dystrophy (modified Koelle method)

widened sole-plate areas with several terminal axons abutting and forming neuromuscular junctions on the same fibre (Fig. 6.15). The changes appear to be type IA fibre specific and show markedly decreased secondary synaptic clefts both in number and size; a finding which is absent in type II fibres (Fukuhara et al 1985). As most terminal axons show no degenerative changes, the findings suggest that a neurotropic factor may be involved in both DMD and BMD. No reduction in AChR nor extrajunctional spread of AChR was noted in DMD by Sakakibara et al (1977).

Myotonic dystrophy

A very marked distortion of the terminal motor innervation pattern is characteristic of myotonic dystrophy. Subterminal axons are intermingled, often encircling muscle fibres and are difficult to observe individually. The end-plates tend to cover a larger area than normal, while the terminal expansions are larger and more numerous (Coërs & Woolf 1959, Woolf 1962). There is often striking axonal sprouting, leading to the formation of several end-plates on a single muscle fibre, or to the innervation of several muscle fibres, increasing the TIR. More impressive, however, is the tendency for axonal sprouts to wander between muscle fibres, giving off short collateral sprouts terminating in a series of miniature synapses at intervals of 20–50 μm (Coërs & Woolf

1959). Abnormally small, but elongated, end-plates observed in the majority of cases with myotonic dystrophy (MacDermot 1961) may correspond to those miniature synapses or a series of terminal expansions described by Coërs & Woolf (1959). However, electron microscopy of end-plates in 16 biopsy specimens in myotonic dystrophy revealed normal postsynaptic regions in all but one case. Similarly, the ultrastructure of all the motor end-plates except one were normal in four cases of infantile myotonic dystrophy (Karpati et al 1973). Morphometric analysis on 230 nerve terminals from four myotonic dystrophy patients revealed a mild but significant decrease in the presynaptic mitochondrial concentration; no abnormalities were observed in the postsynaptic regions. Hence, the striking findings of terminal expansion and axonal sprouting on light microscopy have not been well correlated with electron-microscopic findings. As in DMD, the postsynaptic membrane length, postsynaptic area of folds and clefts associated with a given nerve terminal, and membrane density (postsynaptic membrane length per unit postsynaptic area) were all decreased in 16 end-plates studied in a case of congenital myotonic dystrophy (Tsujihata et al 1981).

Congenital myopathies

In most of these diseases (central core, nemaline-

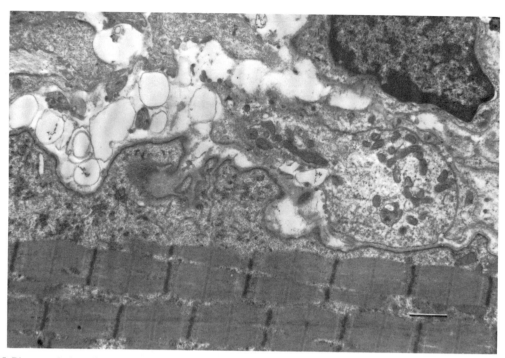

Fig. 6.15 Biceps end-plates from a 14-year-old boy with Becker-type dystrophy since the age of five, showing a marked decrease in the postsynaptic membrane profile concentration and in the synaptic vesicle density in the axon terminal, as well as the denuded zone filled with vacuoles; ×12 000; Scale bar = 1 μm (Courtesy of Dr N. Fukuhara, Kanazawa University, Japan)

rod, centronuclear, multicore diseases and fibre-type disproportion) a neural defect has been suspected and discussed extensively (Chou 1984). Investigation of the intramuscular innervation in these conditions revealed evidence of collateral reinnervation in one case of central core disease (Coërs et al 1976). In all other biopsies, no structural abnormality of motor axons, myelin sheaths or junctional regions suggesting denervation has been well documented. Unusually small and simplified motor endings, suggesting delayed or impaired maturation, have been described in both centronuclear myopathy, familial focal loss of cross striation (Fig. 6.16a) and, to a lesser extent, in nemaline myopathy (Coërs et al 1976, van Wijngaarden 1977). In three siblings with nemaline myopathy, Fukuhara et al (1978) studied 255 neuromuscular junctions from three biopsy specimens and found abundant myelin figures, mitochondria and glycogen in swollen terminal axons. Secondary synaptic clefts were significantly decreased in number and length (Fig. 6.16b), but little evidence of reinnervation was noted.

Distal myopathy

There has been no systematic study of motor nerve terminals or end-plates by light microscopy in distal myopathy. The histopathological features seen in muscle specimens are generally those of myopathic change, although occasional atrophic angular fibres and mild fibre type grouping were described by Markesbery et al (1977). After describing type I fibre atrophy and fibrillation in 13 patients, Edström (1975) advocated a neurogenic factor in this hereditary disease. A large number of denuded postsynaptic regions similar to those noted in amyotrophic lateral sclerosis were found by Engel et al (1975) who examined six end-plates from one patient with distal myopathy. Tsujihata et al (1981) studied 19 end-plates and 25 nerve terminals and concluded that

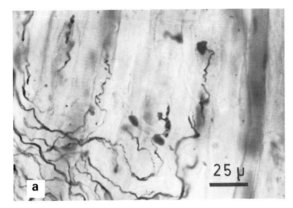

Fig. 6.16 a. Reduced motor endings in familial focal loss of cross-striations (vital staining with methylene blue) b. End-plate from a nine-year-old girl with nemaline myopathy showing paucity of synaptic vesicles but abundant mitochondria, myelin figures, and glycogen in terminal axons. Secondary synaptic clefts were attenuated both in number and length with little sign of reinnervation; ×15 000; Scale bar = 1 μm (Courtesy of Dr. N. Fukuhara, Kanazawa University, Japan)

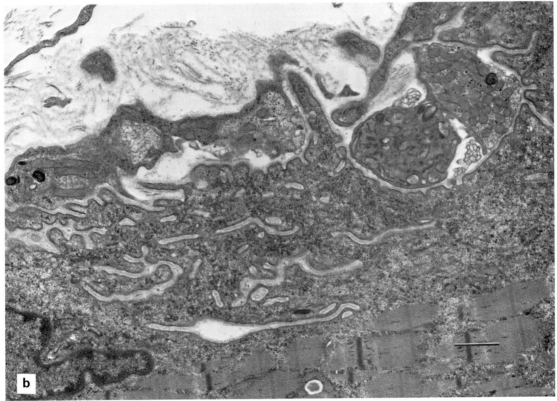

the mean nerve terminal area in μm^2 was increased in distal myopathy (Fig. 6.17); no denuded postsynaptic regions were found.

Polymyositis

In general, the changes in motor innervation observed in 31 cases of various myositides were similar to those seen in other myopathies (Coërs & Carbone 1966, Coërs et al 1973c). The distal parts of the nerve fibres were involved, forming small and irregular motor endings or multiple terminal arborisations through distal branching, resulting in an increased TIR. Usually, the axonal branching occurred in the vicinity of, or within, foci of cellular infiltration where terminal axonal

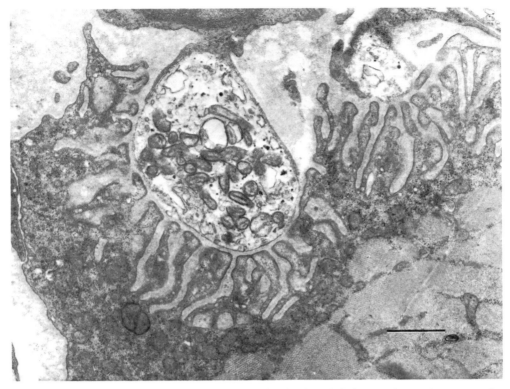

Fig. 6.17 End-plate from a 46-year-old female with distal myopathy showing relatively normal-appearing presynaptic and postsynaptic regions with somewhat swollen nerve terminal; ×19 000; scale bar = 1 μm (Courtesy of Dr M. Tsujihata, Nagasaki University, Japan)

swellings, probably secondary to oedema, could be seen. The mean TIR varied in those 31 myositis cases: it was significantly increased in dermatomyositis (16 cases) and granulomatous (sarcoid) myopathy (six cases), but did not exceed normal in polymyositis (nine cases) (Coërs & Carbone 1966, Coërs 1967b, Coërs et al 1973c). In many of the 19 patients with polymyositis, Pestronk & Drachman (1985a) found reduction of AChRs at neuromuscular junctions as compared with controls, averaging 55% below control values. As in myasthenia gravis, they observed in polymyositis patients the presence of circulating IgG which significantly reduced the number of surface AChRs and increased their rate of degradation in seven out of eight cases. Morphometric analysis on 64 end-plates from five patients with polymyositis revealed several abnormalities of uncertain significance (Engel et al 1975). A small but significant decrease in synaptic vesicle concentration without postsynaptic abnormalities was

described. No morphometric deviation was found in the various parameters of 15 nerve terminals studied by Tsujihata et al (1981), who noted a significant decrease in the postsynaptic membrane length (Fig. 6.18a) and in the membrane density (postsynaptic membrane length per unit postsynaptic area) in 15 postsynaptic regions scanned. However, AChR surface receptors were found to be well preserved (Fig. 6.18b) in 15 end-plates from one patient with polymyositis studied by Tsujihata et al (1980), despite degeneration and simplification of the postsynaptic regions.

MYASTHENIC DISORDERS

Congenital myasthenic syndrome

Four different congenital myasthenic syndromes have been described: (1) end-plate AChE deficiency (Engel et al 1977); (2) a defect in ACh resynthesis or mobilisation (Hart et al 1979); (3)

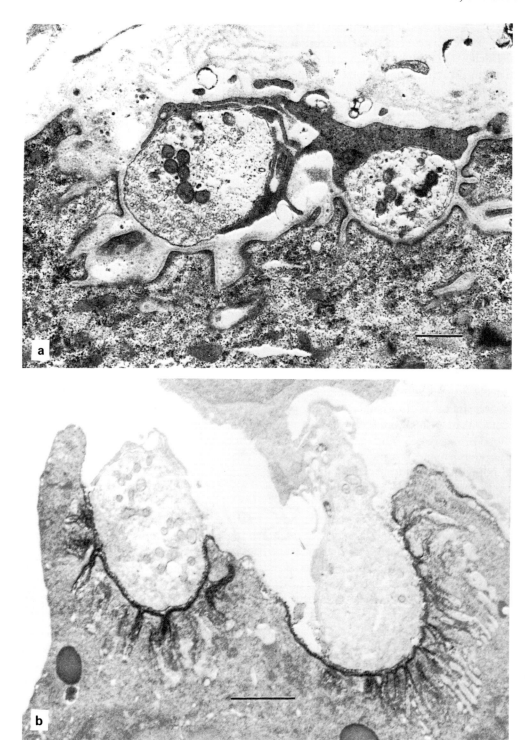

Fig. 6.18 a. End-plate from a 19-year-old female with polymyositis showing a decrease in the postsynaptic membrane length and number with relatively normal-looking nerve terminals; ×15 400; scale bar = 1 μm. b. End-plate from a 34-year-old male with polymyositis showing well-preserved AChRs as visualised with horseradish peroxidase-labelled α-BT; ×20 300, Scale bar = 1 μm (Courtesy of Dr M. Tsujihata, Nagasaki University, Japan)

a defect in the ACh-induced ion changes, or slow-channel syndrome (Engel et al 1982); (4) end-plate AChR deficiency (Vincent et al 1981).

In 1977, Engel et al described a new myasthenic syndrome with end-plate AChE deficiency with characteristic clinical, electrophysiological, ultrastructural and cytochemical features different from those of acquired, autoimmune myasthenia gravis. The patient demonstrated clinical weakness and a decremental response to nerve stimulation. Muscle biopsy revealed a complete absence of AChE from muscle end-plate regions, degenerative postsynaptic changes, but normal AChR and small nerve terminals with a 50% increase in synaptic vesicle density. A defect in the biosynthesis of AChE receptor subunits or their assembly was suspected.

An autosomal recessive congenital myasthenic syndrome caused by a presynaptic defect of ACh resynthesis or mobilisation was reported in 1979 by Hart et al in two siblings with fluctuating ophthalmoparesis, feeding difficulty, easy fatiguability and episodic apnoea; three other siblings died suddenly in infancy. No circulating antibody to AChR was found in any family member and normal amounts of AChR were found in the intercostal muscles. Increased numbers of synaptic vesicles were also found but postsynaptic regions appeared normal in the end-plates. The miniature end-plate potential (mepp) amplitude and the quantum content decreased abnormally after repetitive stimulation over a few minutes. Hence a defect in ACh resynthesis or in the packaging of ACh quanta was suspected.

Six cases (five familial and one sporadic) of a new congenital myasthenic syndrome with onset either in infancy or in late life were described by Engel et al (1982). Selective muscle involvement affected cervical, scapular and finger extensor muscles in addition to ophthalmoparesis. Muscle biopsy specimens revealed predominance of type I fibres, small group atrophy, tubular aggregates and vacuoles near end-plates and abnormal end-plate configuration. AChE activity was abundant at all the end-plates and the activity and kinetic properties of AChE in muscle were normal. Small nerve terminals with an increase in synaptic vesicle density with reduction in the length of the postsynaptic membrane with concomitant loss of

AChRs was also noted. The basic pathogenic mechanism was considered to be a prolonged open time of the AChR ion channel. The ultrastructural changes may correspond to the remarkably elongated and often filamentous motor end-plates with many of the terminal arborisations expanded and spread over a larger area than normal, as described in a case of congenital myasthenia gravis reported by Coërs & Woolf in 1954. No increase in TIR was noted.

End-plate AChR deficiency was demonstrated by reduced α-BT binding in end-plates in three patients reported by Vincent et al (1981). The end-plate AChE was well preserved and end-plate currents were not prolonged. The AChR deficiency was postulated to be secondary to decreased synthesis, reduced resynthesis or accelerated degradation of AChR. The changes were similar to those described in congenital canine myasthenia gravis with deficient junctional AChR: no detectable autoantibodies against AChR, and inherited as an autosomal recessive trait (Oda et al 1984). The four aforementioned types of congenital myasthenic disorders abundantly reflect the complexity of the actual and potential pathological mechanisms involving steps in the sequence of neuromuscular transmission.

Myasthenia gravis

The lesions which cause the profound fatiguability in myasthenia gravis (MG) lie at the neuromuscular junction, as first pointed out by Walker (1934) in a therapeutic trial for MG.

After the initial observation by Woolf et al (1956), Coërs & Telerman-Toppet (1976) studied a series of 45 cases; elongated end-plates were present in 26 biopsies and occurred more frequently in younger patients (Fig. 6.19a). There was no correlation between the incidence of this change and severity of the disease, nor with the histological and histochemical appearances of the muscle fibres. A TIR exceeding the upper limit of normal and suggesting denervation was found in seven biopsies, all from patients over the age of 50.

Denervation in myasthenia gravis has been postulated from the histological and histochemical changes in the muscle fibres (Fenichel & Shy

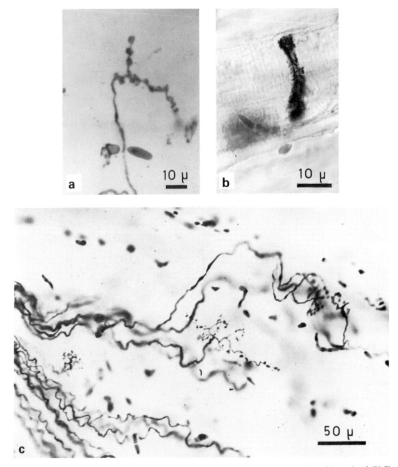

Fig. 6.19 Elongated motor end-plate in myasthenia gravis. a. Vital staining with methylene blue. b. AChE staining with modified Koelle methods. c. Expanded motor endings in myasthenia gravis (vital staining with methylene blue)

1963, Brody & Engel 1964). Distal branching of motor axons forming expanded or multiple motor arborisations may follow to compensate for impaired neuromuscular transmission (Fig. 6.19b, c) similar to the axonal changes obtained by local application of *Clostridium botulinum* toxin (Duchen & Strich 1967).

Quantitative ultrastructural studies involving morphometry of 68 motor end-plates showed the postsynaptic region to be smaller and simpler than normal with widening of the synaptic space (Fig. 6.20) suggesting focal degeneration and regeneration of the junctional folds (Engel & Santa 1971, Santa et al 1972, Gutmann & Chou 1976). The average nerve terminal area was also smaller than normal, but the synaptic vesicle and mitochondrial concentration was normal. The

same changes were induced in animals by prolonged administration of anticholinesterase drugs (Engel et al 1973) and also in experimental autoimmune myasthenia gravis (Engel et al 1976).

Simpson (1960) and Nastuk et al (1960) independently postulated that MG might be an autoimmune disease. In 1973, Patrick & Lindstrom successfully developed a myasthenic syndrome by inoculating eel electric organ AChR in rabbits — a finding confirmed by Sugiyama et al in the same year. Seven to 11 days following immunisation with AChR protein, mononuclear cell infiltration occurred in the end-plate, with degeneration and phagocytosis of the postsynaptic region (Lennon et al 1975). Subsequently, the inflammatory reaction subsided and the intact nerve terminal innervated a simplified postsyn-

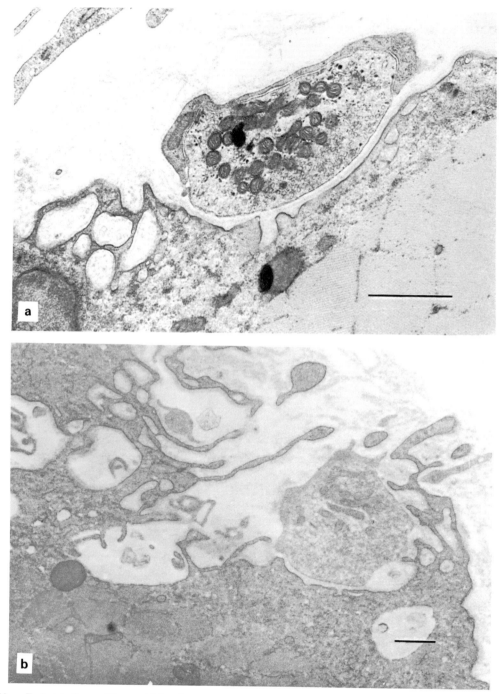

Fig. 6.20 a. End-plate from a 30-year-old female myasthenia gravis patient showing a small, extremely simplified nerve terminal and widened secondary synaptic clefts. Density of the synaptic vesicles and mitochondria appear normal; ×27 000; Scale bar = 1 μm. b. Complete absence of AChR in a motor end-plate from a 25-year-old female myasthenia gravis patient, stained with peroxidase-labelled α-BT. Note also markedly widened and simplified junctional folds; ×13 700; Scale bar = 1 μm (Courtesy of Dr M. Tsujihara, Nagasaki University, Japan)

aptic region. This experimental model of myasthenia gravis suggests that the alterations in the nerve terminals observed in myasthenic patients are secondary to the postsynaptic changes related to autoimmune injury. Elongation and simplification of motor endings could be the earliest consequence of this injury with compensatory distal sprouting occurring at a later stage.

In a study of a large series of individuals including 76 MG patients and 49 control subjects, a highly significant reduction of available AChR at neuromuscular junctions was reported by Pestronk et al (1985). The magnitude of AChR reduction approximately corresponded to the severity of the patient's weakness and the receptor abnormality was widespread even when clinical weakness was restricted. Serum anti-AChR was positive in 88% of 153 electromyographically validated cases of myasthenia gravis and was a highly specific diagnostic test when immunoassayed before treatment by thymectomy or immunosuppressive therapy (Vincent & Newsom-Davis 1985).

Similar ultrastructural abnormalities (Fig. 6.21a) were also described at the end-plates of clinically unaffected limb muscles of patients with ocular myasthenia gravis (Tsujihata et al 1979). The ultrastructural changes were similar to those in denervated and denuded end-plates and the distinction between myasthenic and denervated end-plates has become possible only with the advent of the immunoperoxidase method for localisation of AChR with α-BT. No extrajunctional spread of AChR was observed in myasthenic end-plates (Bender et al 1976) and only faint segmental staining for depleted AChR was seen in the synaptic folds and postsynaptic membranes, especially in simplified end-plates (Fig. 6.21b) (Engel et al 1977). Marked reduction in the morphometric number of AChR was demonstrated in myasthenic end-plates in contrast to normal amounts of AChR in other neuromuscular diseases including limb-girdle dystrophy, polymyositis and amyotrophic lateral sclerosis (Tsujihata et al 1980). In two patients with ocular MG, the amount and distribution of AChR was normal in one (Fig. 6.21b) and decreased in the other. Loss of AChR is attributed to autoimmune attack, but the attachment of the antibody to the receptor

protein does not alone cause myasthenia and activation of the complement cascade appears essential for lysis of the junctional membrane (Rash et al 1976). The severity of the disease was related, not to the amount of IgG bound, but to loss of AChR. Both IgG and the complement system were localised and concentrated around the crests of the postjunctional folds (Engel et al 1977) and within the synaptic spaces on degenerated material in both human and experimental autoimmune MG (Engel et al 1976, 1979, 1981, Lennon et al 1975, Sahashi et al 1978). Activation of the terminal and lytic complement component (C_9) was also demonstrated on the simplified postsynaptic membrane and the degenerated material (Sahashi et al 1980). Autoreactive plasma cells producing anti-AChR autoantibodies were demonstrated in the peripheral blood (Lisak et al 1983) and in lymphoid organs, including the thymus (Scadding et al 1981). Cell lines of autoimmune, AChR-specific T lymphocytes were isolated from several MG patients and the same autologous autoimmune T cells stimulated the production of anti-AChR autoantibodies in vitro (Hohlfeld et al 1986). Thus, several aspects of the disordered immunoregulation in acquired human MG have been steadily clarified and a specific immunotherapy for MG appears imminent in the near future. The end-plate in patients with certain congenital myasthenic syndromes was free from any detectable IgG, C_3 or C_9 (Engel et al 1979) and an antibody-dependent, complement-mediated injury to the postsynaptic membrane was not suggested.

Myasthenic (Lambert–Eaton) syndrome

The myasthenic syndrome, also referred to as the Lambert–Eaton myasthenic syndrome (LEMS), is characterised by proximal muscle weakness and fatiguability which is clinically and electrophysiologically distinct from those seen in MG. The LEMS is often but not invariably associated with carcinoma, especially small-cell carcinoma of the lung (Lambert et al 1956, Eaton & Lambert 1957). Unlike the case in MG, the defect of neuromuscular transmission is improved by repetitive nerve stimulation or by an increase in the external Ca^{2+} concentration. A reduced release of ACh quanta from the nerve terminal by the nerve

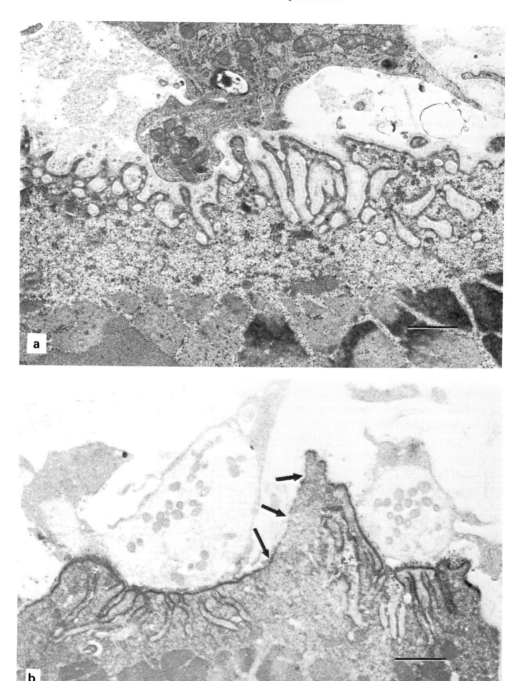

Fig. 6.21 a. End-plate of clinically unaffected limb from a 14-year-old female patient with ocular myasthenia gravis, showing characteristic abnormalities of MG including small nerve terminal, widened and simplified secondary synaptic clefts; ×16 400; scale bar = 1 μm. b. Relatively faint, segmental staining for AChR of postsynaptic folds especially at the simplified secondary clefts (arrows) in the end-plate from the same patient with ocular myasthenia gravis; ×16 200; Scale bar = 1 μm (Courtesy of Dr M. Tsujihata, Nagasaki University, Japan)

action potential is attributed to the failure of neuromuscular transmission. Patients with LEMS show no diminution in the size of mepp amplitude (Lambert & Elmquist 1971) and there is no decrease in the number of AChRs (Engel et al 1977). The LEMS is partly palliated by calcium, guanidine hydrochloride, epinephrine, aminophylline or caffeine (Takamori et al 1973): factors which interfere with the utilisation of calcium have therefore been suspected as the physiological defect. As recently reviewed by Duncan (1982), regulation of intracellular Ca^{2+} is of great importance in governing mepps at the presynaptic terminals. In 1981, Lang et al passively transferred the electrophysiological defect of the LEMS from man to mouse with IgG, providing compelling evidence for an autoimmune pathogenesis of the disease. The target of the pathogenic autoantibodies appeared to be at the presynaptic membrane active zones where a decreased number of active zone particles was demonstrated in freeze-fracture preparations of presynaptic membranes (Fukunaga et al 1982). As the active zones corresponded to sites of synaptic vesicle exocytosis, they may represent the voltage-sensitive calcium channels (Fukunaga et al 1983). However, no laboratory assay is yet available for detecting this IgG autoantibody.

A study by Lambert & Rooke (1965) on 20 muscle biopsy specimens from LEMS patients showed 11 with normal findings; nine had only non-specific alterations in myofibres. Engel & Santa (1971) found no characteristic abnormalities in motor end-plates by light microscopy in five patients. No significant abnormalities were detected by Fukuhara et al (1972) in AChE-stained motor end-plates in four patients with LEMS. Abnormally large and complex end-plates accompanied by increased preterminal axon branching were interpreted as a mild terminal neuropathy in LEMS by Wise & MacDermot (1962). Ultrastructural changes in the neuromuscular junctions in LEMS, however, are striking (Fig. 6.22), in sharp contrast with those in MG, and are characterised by proliferation and enlargement of the secondary synaptic clefts (Engel & Santa 1971, Fukuhara et al 1972). There is a significant increase in the mean area of the secondary postsynaptic clefts and folds and the postsynaptic/presynaptic membrane-length ratio.

Presynaptic terminal axons showed atrophy in 40% of 63 neuromuscular junctions studied by Fukuhara et al (1972). The proliferative and hypertrophic postsynaptic membranes were considered to be secondary to repeated degeneration and regeneration of presynaptic membranes. In a study of 196 end-plates from seven patients with LEMS, Sahashi et al (1978b) concluded that the AChR index was normal and the end-plate changes were clearly distinguishable from those in MG. Recent developments in clinical and basic research into congenital myasthenic syndromes, MG and LEMS have been extensively reviewed by Engel (1984).

CONCLUSION

The study of intramuscular motor nerve terminals and motor end-plates is complementary to conventional muscle histochemistry and may augment the correct diagnosis of neuromuscular diseases. The highly dynamic and complex changes of terminal axons and end-plates which have been described in various neuromuscular diseases reflect the remarkable capability of terminal axons and end-plates for regeneration and remodelling, but are not necessarily disease-specific. However, the basic pathogenetic processes involved in neurogenic and myogenic conditions produce detectable differences in the branching and sprouting patterns of terminal axons and in the end-plates. These differences are partly reflected in the TIR or sprouting index and can be correlated with the functional significance of collateral branching. TIR values have been found to increase significantly in all the chronic neurogenic disorders, whereas they remain normal in most of the myopathies. An increased TIR may also indicate secondary involvement of intramuscular nerves in myositis, myotonic dystrophy and in elderly patients with MG. Rarefaction of intramuscular nerve fibres and a reticular appearance of terminal axons provides additional evidence of denervation. Similarly, the sprouting index is useful in differentiating functional denervation, such as that induced by a presynaptic blocker (botulinum), disuse (tetrodotoxin), or from a postsynaptic blocker (α-BT). As axonal sprouting occurs in

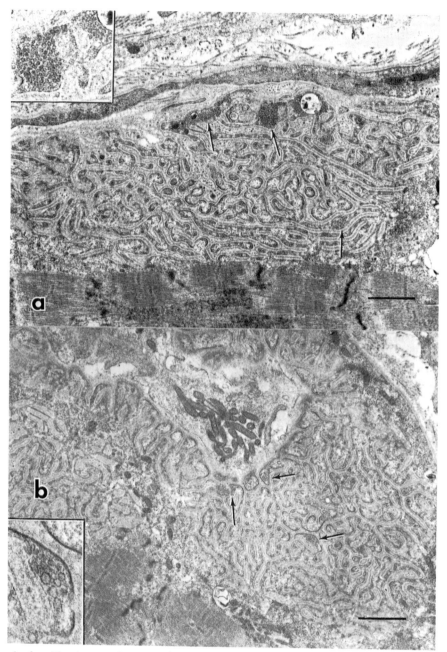

Fig. 6.22 Network of proliferative secondary synaptic clefts in the end-plates from biopsied external intercostal muscle from a patient with the Lambert–Eaton syndrome, showing marked proliferation of caveolae, 30–50 nm in diameter, subjacent to postsynaptic membrane (arrows) in insets. Top inset ×35 200, bottom inset ×66 000; scale bar = 1 μm (Reproduced from Fukuhara et al 1972 with permission from Archives of Neurology, Chicago)

response to diverse physiological states including ageing, immobilisation, hyperactivity, or disuse secondary to muscular dystrophy or impairment of neuromuscular transmission, interpretation of sprouting behaviour must be given with the utmost caution. The extent of sprouting may vary according to the types (type I or II) of myofibres in a given process and modulated by extrajunctional AChR at neuromuscular junctions (Pestronk & Drachman 1985a, b).

In MG, especially in young patients, simplification and elongation of motor arborisation are considered to be characteristic. However, correlation of such a characteristic light-microscopic finding with the ultrastructural finding is not always present. With various sophisticated techniques, including immunoperoxidase staining, freeze-fractured membrane studies and morphometric studies, lesions at either the presynaptic or postsynaptic region can be localised. Among all the neuromuscular diseases, MG provides us with a prime example of a complex disease process in which the concept of pathogenesis has moved from the presynaptic to the postsynaptic region and has become bound up with studies of autoimmune processes and molecular biology. Without various morphological studies on neuromuscular junctions, our current understanding of the pathogenesis of MG or of other myasthenic syndromes would not have been possible. The complexity of the disease processes involved in neuromuscular transmission is also well illustrated in four types of congenital myasthenic syndrome which have no autoimmune basis. The fact that AChR is also affected in the denervation process but not as strikingly as in MG — because only one of two subpopulation AChRs (rapidly reversible AChR) is affected and resynthesised in denervation — attests to the complex metabolic processes involved in neuromuscular transmission (Levitt & Salpeter 1981).

ACKNOWLEDGEMENT

The authors wish to express their gratitude to Dr Janet M Miles for her review as well as discussion of the manuscript and to Mrs Denise Egleton for her efficient clerical assistance.

REFERENCES

Attias G 1912 Die Nerven der Hornhaut des Menschen. Albrecht v. Graefes Archiv für Ophthalmologie 83:207

Banker B Q, Kelly S S, Robbins N 1983 Neuromuscular transmission and correlative morphology in young and old mice. Journal of Physiology 339: 355–375

Barker D, Ip M C 1965 Sprouting and degeneration of mammalian motor axons in normal and de-afferented skeletal muscle. Proceedings of the Royal Society. Series B 163: 538–554

Beermann D H, Cassend R G 1976 Combined silver and acetylcholine esterase method for staining intramuscular innervation. Stain Technology 51: 173–177

Bender A N, Ringel S P, Engel W K 1976 The acetylcholine receptor in normal and pathologic states. Neurology (Minneapolis) 20:477

Bjornskov E K, Dekker N P, Norris F H, Stuart M E 1975 End-plate morphology in amyotrophic lateral sclerosis. Archives of Neurology (Chicago) 32:711

Bjornskov, E K, Norris F H, Mower-Kuby J 1984 Quantitative axon terminal and end-plate morphology in amyotrophic lateral sclerosis. Archives of Neurology 41: 527–530

Brody I A, Engel W K 1964 Denervation of muscle in myasthenia gravis. Archives of Neurology 11: 350–354

Bursztajn S, McManaman J L, Elias S B, Appel S H 1983 Myasthenic globulin enhances the loss of acetylcholine receptor clusters. Science 49: 195–196

Chou S M 1982 Pathology of the neuromuscular junction, Chapter 14. In: Mastaglia F L, Walton J (eds) Skeletal muscle pathology. Churchill Livingstone, p. 427–460

Chou S M 1984 Congenital neuromyopathies, Chapter 7. In: Heffner R R Jr (ed) Contemporary Issues in Surgical Pathology 3: 88–107

Coërs C 1952 The vital staining of muscle biopsies with methylene blue. Journal of Neurology, Neurosurgery and Psychiatry 15:211

Coërs C 1953a Contribution a l'étude de la jonction neuromusculaire II, Topographie zonale de l'innervation, motrice terminale dans les muscles striés. Archives de Biologie 64:49

Coërs C 1953b La detection de la cholinesterase au niveau de la jonction neuromusculaire. Revue belge de pathologie et de médecine expérimentale 22:306

Coërs C 1955 Les variations structurelles normales et pathologiques de la jonction neuromusculaire. Acta Neurologica et Psychiatrica Belgica 55:74

Coërs C 1965 Histology of the myoneural junction in myopathies. In: Paul W M, Daniel E E, Kay C M, Monckton G (eds) Muscle. Pergamon Press, Oxford, p 453

Coërs C 1967a Structure and organization of the myoneural junction. International Review of Cytology 39: 1–16

Coërs C 1967b The histological features of muscle sarcoidosis. Acta Neuropathologica (Berlin) 7: 242–252

Coërs C, Carbone F 1966 La myopathie granulomateuse. Acta Neurologica et Psychiatrica Belgica 66: 353–381

Coërs C, Hildebrand J 1965 Latent neuropathy in diabetes and alcoholism. Neurology (Minneapolis) 15: 19–38

Coërs C, Woolf A L 1954 Etude histologique et histochimique de la jonction neuromusculaire dans la myasthénie. Comptes rendus du Congres des Médecins Alienistes et Neurologistes, Liege, 19–26 July 1954

Coërs C, Woolf A L 1959 The innnervation of muscle. Blackwell, Oxford

Coërs C, Reske-Nielsen E, Harmsen A 1973a The pattern of terminal motor innervation in healthy young adults. Journal of the Neurological Sciences 19:351

Coërs C, Telerman-Toppet N & Gerard J M 1973b Terminal innervation ratio in neuromuscular disease. I Methods and controls. Archives of Neurology 29:210

Coërs C, Telerman-Toppet N, Gerard J M 1973c Terminal innervation ratio in neuromuscular disease. II Disorders of lower motor neuron, peripheral nerve and muscle. Archives of Neurology 29: 215–222

Coërs C, Telerman-Toppet N, Gerard J M, Szliowski H, Bethlem J, Van Wijngaarden G K 1976 Changes in motor innervation and histochemical pattern of muscle fibers in some congenital myopathies. Neurology (Minneapolis) 26: 1046–1053

Coërs C, Telerman-Toppet N 1976 Morphological and histochemical changes of motor units in myasthenia. Annals of the New York Academy of Science 274: 6–19

Coërs C, Telerman-Toppet N 1977 Morphological changes of motor units in Duchenne's muscular dystrophy. Archives of Neurology 34: 396–402

Coërs C, Telerman-Toppet N 1979 Differential diagnosis of limb girdle muscular dystrophy and spinal muscular atrophy. Neurology (Minneapolis) 29: 957–972

Couteaux R 1951 Remarques sur les methodes actuelles de detection histochimique des activités cholinesterasiques. Archives Internationales de Physiologie 59:526

Daniels M P, Vogel Z 1975 Acetylcholine receptor staining: immunoperoxidase visualization of α-bungarotoxin binding sites in muscle endplates. Nature 253:339

de Harven P, Coërs C 1959 Electron microscope study of the human neuromuscular function. Journal of Biophysical and Biochemical Cytology 6: 7–10

Desmedt J E, Borenstein S 1973 Collateral innervation of muscle fibres by motor axons of dystrophic motor units. Nature 264: 500–501

Desmedt J E, Borenstein S 1976 Regeneration in Duchenne dystrophy. Archives of Neurology 33: 642–650

Dias P L R 1974 Surface area of motor end-plates in fast and slow twitch muscles of the rabbit. Journal of Anatomy 117: 453–462

Dogiel A S 1890 Die Nerven der Cornea des Menschen. Anatomischer Anzeiger 5:483

Dubowitz V, Brooke M H 1973 Muscle biopsy: A modern approach. Major Problems in Neurology Vol 2. W. B. Saunders, Eastbourne

Duchen L W 1971 An electron microscopic comparison of motor end-plates of slow and fast skeletal muscle fibres of the mouse. Journal of the Neurological Sciences 14: 37–45

Duchen L W, Strich S J 1967 Changes in the pattern of motor innervation of skeletal muscles in the mouse after local injection of Clostridium botulinum toxin. Journal of Physiology 189: 16–17

Duncan C J 1982 Parallels between spontaneous release of transmitter at the neuromuscular junction and subcellular damage of muscle. Evidence for the underlying common involvement of intracellular Ca^{2+}? Comparative Biochemistry and Physiology 73A: 147–149

Eaton L M, Lambert E H 1957 Electromyography and electric stimulation of nerves in diseases of motor unit: Observations in the myasthenic syndrome associated with malignant tumors. Journal of the American Medical Association 163:1117

Edström L 1975 Histochemical and histopathological changes in skeletal muscle in late-onset hereditary distal myopathy (Welander). Journal of the Neurological Sciences 26:147

Ehrlich P 1882 Zur biologischen Verwertung des Methylenblau. Zentralblatt für die medizinischen Wissenschaften 12:49

Emmert E 1836 Uber di Endigungsweise der Nerven in Den Muskeln, nach Eigenen Untersuchen. C. A. Jenni, Bern p. 1–335

Engel A G 1970 Locating motor end-plates for electron microscopy. Mayo Clinic Proceedings 45: 450–454

Engel A G 1984 Myasthenia gravis and myasthenic syndrome. Annals of Neurology 16: 519–534

Engel A G, Santa T 1971 Histometric analysis of the ultrastructure of the neuromuscular junction in myasthenia gravis and in the myasthenic syndrome. Annals of the New York Academy of Sciences 83: 46–63

Engel A G, Lambert E H, Santa T 1973 Study of long-term anticholinesterase therapy. Effect on neuromuscular transmission and on motor end-plate fine structure. Neurology (Minneapolis) 23:1273

Engel A G, Tsujihata M, Jerusalem 1975 Quantitative assessment of motor endplate ultrastructure in normal and diseased human muscle. In: Dyck P J, Thomas P K, Lambert E H (eds) Peripheral neuropathy, Vol. 2. Saunders, Philadelphia, p 1404

Engel A G, Tsujihata M, Lindstrom J & Lennon V A 1976 The motor end-plate in myasthenia gravis and in experimental autoimmune myasthenia gravis. A quantitative ultrastructural study. Annals of the New York Academy of Sciences 274: 60–79

Engel A G, Lindstrom J M, Lambert E H et al 1977 Ultrastructural localization of the acetylcholine receptor in myasthenia gravis and in its experimental autoimmune model. Neurology (Minneapolis) 27: 307–315

Engel A G, Lambert E H, Mulder D M et al 1979 Investigations of three cases of a newly recognized familial congenital myasthenic syndrome. Annals of Neurology 6:146

Engel A G, Sahashi K, Fumagalli G 1981 The immunopathology of acquired myasthenia gravis. Annals of the New York Academy of Sciences 377:158–174

Engel A G, Lambert E H, Mulder D M et al 1982 A newly recognized myasthenic syndrome attributed to a prolonged open time of the acetylcholine-induced ion channel. Annals of Neurology 11: 553–569

Fahim M A, Robbins N 1982 Ultrastructural studies of young and old mouse neuromuscular junctions. Journal of Neurocytology 11: 641–656

Fahim M A, Holley J A, Robbins N 1983 Scanning and light microscopic study of age changes at a neuromuscular junction in the mouse. Journal of Neurocytology 12: 13–25

Fahim M A, Holley J A, Robbins N 1984 Topographic comparison of neuromuscular junctions in mouse slow and fast twitch muscles. Neuroscience 13: 227–235

Fambrough D M, Drachman D B, Satyamurti S 1973 Neuromuscular junction in myasthenia gravis. Decreased acetylcholine receptors. Science 182: 293–295

Fenichel G M, Shy G M 1963 Muscle biopsy experience in myasthenia gravis. Archives of Neurology 9: 237–243

Fukuhara N, Takamori M, Gutman L, Chou S M 1972 Eaton–Lambert Syndrome: Ultrastructural study of the motor end-plates. Archives of Neurology 27: 67–78

Fukuhara N, Yuasa T, Tsubaki T, Kushiro S, Takasawa N 1978 Nemaline myopathy: histological, histochemical, and ultrastructural studies. Acta Neuropathologica (Berlin) 42:33

Fukuhara N, Suzuki M, Tsubaki T, Kuzhiro S, Takasawa N 1985 Ultrastructural studies on the neuromuscular junction of Becker's muscular dystrophy. Acta Neuropathologica (Berlin) 66: 283–291

Fukunaga H, Engel A G, Osme M, Lambert E H 1982 Paucity and disorganization of presynaptic membrane active zones in the Lambert–Eaton myasthenic syndrome. Muscle and Nerve 5: 686–697

Fukunaga H, Engel A G, Lang B, Newson-Davis J, Vincent A 1983 Passive transfer of Lambert–Eaton myasthenic syndrome with IgG from man to mouse depletes the presynaptic membrane active zones. Proceedings of the National Academy of Sciences 80: 7636–7640

Fumagalli G, Engel A G, Lindstrom J 1982 Ultrastructural aspects of acetylcholine receptor turnover at the normal endplate and in autoimmune myasthenia gravis. Journal of Neuropathology and Experimental Neurology 41: 567–579

Gutmann L, Chou S M 1976 Myasthenia gravis; Current concepts. Archives of Pathology and Laboratory Medicine 100:401

Harriman D 1961 The diagnostic value of motor-point muscle biopsy. In: Garland H G (ed) Scientific aspects of neurology. Livingstone, Edinburgh, p 37

Harriman D G F 1976 A comparison of the fine structure of motor end-plates in Duchenne dystrophy and in human neurogenic diseases. Journal of the Neurological Sciences 28: 233–247

Hart Z, Sahashi K, Lambert E H et al 1979 Congenital, familial, myasthenic syndrome caused by a presynaptic defect of transmitter resynthesis or mobilization. Neurology (NY) 29:556

Hohlfeld R, Kalies I, Kohleisen B et al 1986 Myasthenia gravis: stimulation of antireceptor autoantibodies by autoreactive T cell lines. Neurology (Cleveland) 36: 618–621

Holt S J 1956 The value of fundamental studies of staining reactions in enzyme histochemistry with reference to indoxyl methods of esterases. Journal of Histochemistry and Cytochemistry 4:541

Holt S J, Withers R F J 1956 Cytochemical localization of esterases using indoxyl derivatives. Nature 170:1012

Jennekens F G I, Meijer A E F A, Bethlem J, van Wijugaarden G K 1974 Fibre hybrids in type groups. An investigation of human muscle biopsies. Journal of the Neurological Sciences 23: 337–352

Jerusalem F, Engel A G, Gonez M R 1974 Duchenne dystrophy II, Morphometric study of motor endplate fine structure. Brain 97: 123–130

Karpati G, Carpenter S, Watters G V, Eisen A A, Andermann F 1973 Infantile myotonic dystrophy. Neurology (Minneapolis) 23:1066

Koelle G B, Friedenwald J S 1949 A histochemical method for localizing cholinesterase activity. Proceedings of the Society for Experimental Biology and Medicine 70:617

Lambert E H, Eaton L M, Rooke E D 1956 Defect of neuromuscular conduction associated with malignant neoplasms. American Journal of Physiology 187:612

Lambert E H, Rooke E D 1965 Myasthenic state and lung cancer. In: Brain L, Norris F M (eds) The remote effects of cancer on the nervous system. Grune & Stratton, New York, p 67

Lambert E H, Elmquist D 1971 Quantal component of end-plate potentials in myasthenic syndrome. Annals of the New York Academy of Sciences 183: 183–199

Lang B, Newsom-Davis J, Wray D, Vincent A 1981 Autoimmune etiology for myasthenic (Eaton–Lambert) syndrome. Lancet 2: 224–226

Lee C Y, Tseng L F, Chiu T H 1967 Influence of denervation on localization of neurotoxin from celapid venoms in rat diaphragm. Nature 215:1177

Lennon V, Lindstrom J, Seybold M 1975 Experimental autoimmune myasthenia (EAMG): A model of myasthenia gravis in rats and guinea pigs. Journal of Experimental Medicine 141: 1365–1375

Levitt T A, Salpeter M M 1981 Denervated end-plates have a dual population of junctional acetylcholine receptors. Nature 291: 239–241

Lisak R P, Laramone C, Zweiman B, Moskeovitz A 1983 In vitro synthesis of antibodies to acetylcholine receptors by peripheral blood mononuclear cells of patients with myasthenia gravis. Neurology (Cleveland) 33: 604–608

MacDermot V 1961 The histology of the neuromuscular junction in dystrophia myotonica. Brain 84:75

Markesbery W R, Griggs R C, Herr B 1977 Distal myopathy: electron microscopic and histochemical studies. Neurology (Minneapolis) 27:727

Nastuk W L, Plescia O, Osserman K E 1960 Changes in serum complement activity in patients with myasthenia gravis. Proceedings of the Society for Experimental Biology and Medicine 105:177

Nystrom B 1968 Postnatal development of motor nerve terminals in 'slow-red' and 'fast-white' cat muscles. Acta Neurologica Scandinavica 44: 363–383

Oda K, 1984 Age changes of motor innervating and acetylcholine receptors distribution on human skeletal muscle fibers. Journal of the Neurological Sciences 66: 327–338

Oda K, Lambert E H, Lennon V A, Palmer A C 1984 Congenital canine myasthenia gravis 1. Deficient junctional acetylcholine receptors. Muscle and Nerve 7: 705–716

Pachter B R, Eberstein A 1984 Neuromuscular plasticity following limb immobilization. Journal of Neurocytology 13: 1013–1025

Padykula H A, Gauthier F G 1970 The ultrastructure of neuromuscular junctions of mammalian red, white, and intermediate skeletal muscle fibers. Journal of Cell Biology 46: 27–41

Patrick J, Lindstrom J M 1973 Autoimmune response to acetylcholine receptor. Science 180:871

Pestronk A, Drachman D B 1978a A new stain for quantitative measurement of sprouting at neuromuscular junction. Muscle and Nerve 1: 70–74

Pestronk A, Drachman D B 1978b Motor nerve sprouting and acetylcholine receptors. Science 199: 1223–1225

Pestronk A, Drachman D B, Griffin J W 1980 Effects of aging on nerve sprouting and regeneration. Experimental Neurology 70: 65–82

Pestronk A, Drachman D B 1985a Polymyositis: Reduction of acetylcholine receptions in skeletal muscle. Muscle and Nerve 8: 233–239

Pestronk A, Drachman D B 1985b Motor nerve terminal outgrowth and acetylcholine receptors: Inhibition of terminal growth by α-bungarotoxin and antiacetylcholine receptor antibody. Journal of Neuroscience 5: 751–758

Pestronk A, Dachman D B, Self S G 1985 Measurement of junctional acetylcholine receptors in myasthenia gravis: Clinical correlates. Muscle and Nerve 8: 245–251

Rash J E, Albuquerque E X, Hudson C S 1976 Studies of human myasthenia gravis: Electrophysiological and ultrastructural evidence compatible with antibody attachment to acetylcholine receptor complex. Proceedings of the National Academy of Sciences (USA) 73:4584

Reske-Nielsen E, Coërs C, Harmsen A 1969 Qualitative and quantitative histological study of neuromuscular biopsies from healthy young men. Journal of the Neurological Sciences 10:369

Rosenheimer J L, Smith D 0 1985 Differential changes in the end-plate architecture of functionally diverse muscles during aging. J Neurophysiology 53: 1567–1581

Sahashi K, Engel A G, Lindstrom J M 1978a Ultrastructural localization of immune complex (IgG) and (3) at the endplate in experimental autoimmune myasthenia gravis. Journal of Neuropathology and Experimental Neurology 37:212

Sahashi K, Engel A G, Lambert E M, Sakakibara H 1978b Ultrastructural localization and quantitation of acetylcholine receptor (AChr) in the Lambert–Eaton myasthenic syndrome and and electrophysiological correlation. Journal of Neuropathology and Experimental Neurology 37:684

Sahashi K, Engel A G, Lambert E M, Howard F M Jr 1980 Ultrastructural localization of the terminal and lytic ninth complement component (C9) at the motor endplate in myasthenia gravis. Journal of Neuropathology and Experimental Neurology 30:160

Sakakibara H, Engel A G, Lambert E H 1977 Duchenne dystrophy: Ultrastructural localization of the acetylcholine receptor and intracellular microelectrode studies of neuromuscular transmission. Neurology (Minneapolis) 27: 741–745

Santa T, Engel A G, Lambert E H 1972 Histometric study of neuromuscular junction ultrastructure I. Myasthenia gravis. Neurology (Minneapolis) 22: 71–82

Scadding G K, Vincent A, Newsom-Davis J, Henry K 1981 Acetylcholine receptor antibody synthesis by thymic lymphocytes: correlation with thymic history. Neurology (NY) 31: 935–943

Schwartz M S, Stalberg E, Schiller H H Thiele B 1976 The reinnervated motor unit in man. Journal of the Neurological Sciences 27: 303–312

Simpson J A 1960 Myasthenia gravis: a new hypothesis. Scottish Medical journal 5:419

Sugiyama H, Benda P, Meunier J C, Changeux J P 1973 Immunological characterization of the cholinergic protein from electrophorus electricus, FEBS Letters 35:124

Szliwowski H B, Drochmans P 1975 Ultrastructural aspects of muscle and nerve in Werdnig–Hoffman disease. Acta Neuropathologica (Berlin) 31:281

Takamori M, Ishu N, Mori M 1973 The role of cyclic 3^1, 5^1 adenosine monophosphate in neuromuscular disease. Archives of Neurology 29: 420–424

Telerman-Toppet N, Coërs C 1978 Motor innervation and fiber type pattern in amyotrophic lateral sclerosis and in Charcot–Marie–Tooth disease. Muscle and Nerve 1: 133–139

Tello J F 1917 Genesis de las terminaciones nerviosas motrices y sensitivas. I En el sistema locomotor de los vertebrados superiores. Histogenesis muscular. Trabajos del Instituto Cajal de Investigaciones Biologicas (Madrid) 15: 101–199

Tsujihata M, Hazama R, Ishu N et al 1979 Limb muscle endplates in ocular myasthenia gravis: Quantitative ultrastructural study. Neurology 29: 254–261

Tsujihata M, Hazama R, Ishii N, Yoshihiko I, Takamori M 1980 Ultrastructural localization of acetylcholine receptor at the motor endplate: myasthenia gravis and other neuromuscular diseases. Neurology 30: 1203–1211

Tsujihata M, Hazama R, Yoshimura T, Akira S 1981 The motor end-plate in human neuromuscular disorders: A quantitative study. Journal of Clinical and Electron Microbiology 14: 5–6

Tsujihata M, Hazama R, Yoshimura T, Satoh A, Mori M, Nagataki S 1984 The motor endplate fine structure and ultrastructural localization of acetylcholine receptors in amyotrophic lateral sclerosis. Muscle and Nerve 7: 243–249

Tuffery A R 1971 Growth and degeneration of motor end plates in normal cat hind limb muscles. Journal of Anatomy 110:221

Valentin G 1836 Uber den verlauf und die letzten Enden der Nerven. Nova Acta (Phys Med Acad), Leopoldino-Carolinae, 18: 51–240

Van Wijngaarden G K, Bethlem J, Dingemans K P, Coërs C, Telerman-Toppet N & Gerard J M 1977 Familial focal loss of cross striations. Journal of Neurology 216: 163–172

Vincent A, Cull-Candy S G, Newsom-Davis J et al 1981 Congenital myasthenia: end-plate acetylcholine receptors and electrophysiology in five cases. Muscle and Nerve 4: 306–318

Vincent A, Newsom-Davis J 1985 Acetylcholine receptor antibody as a diagnostic test for myasthenia gravis: results in 153 validated cases and 2967 diagnostic assays. Journal of Neurology, Neurosurgery and Psychiatry 48: 1246–1252

Wagner R 1878 Neue Untersuchungen uber den Bau und die Endigungen der Nerven. (Leipzig) Cited in: Ranvier L Legons sur l'histologie due systeme nerveux. Savy, Paris

Walker M B 1934 Treatment of myasthenia gravis with physostigmine. Lancet 1:1200

Weddell G 1941a The pattern of cutaneous innervation in relation to cutaneous sensibility. Journal of Anatomy 75:346

Weddell G 1941b The multiple innervation of sensory spots in the skin. Journal of Anatomy 75:441

Wise R P, MacDermot V 1962 A myasthenic syndrome associated with bronchial carcinoma. Journal of Neurology, Neurosurgery and Psychiatry 25:31

Wohlfart G 1960 Clinical significance of collateral sprouting of remaining motor nerve fibres in partially denervated muscles. Journal of Experimental Medicine 3: 128–133

Woolf A L 1957 The significance of the sprouting of intramuscular nerves. Nederlands tijdschrift voor geneeskunde 101–102:1506

Woolf A L 1960 Muscle biopsy in the diagnosis of the 'floppy baby': infantile hypotonia. Cerebral Palsy Bulletin 2:19

Woolf A L 1962 Muscle biopsy. In: Williams D (ed) Modern trends in neurology 3rd edn. Butterworth, London

Woolf A L, Bagnall H J, Bauwens P, Bickerstaff, E R 1956 A case of myasthenia gravis with changes in intramuscular nerve endings. Journal of Pathology and Bacteriology 71:173

Histochemical and immunocytochemical studies in neuromuscular diseases

INTRODUCTION

Histochemistry is the combination of morphology and biochemistry. It provides precise localisation of specific chemical moieties and aids the characterisation of a cell. The past few decades have seen an increase in the application of histochemical techniques to many biological problems and they now have an essential diagnostic and research role in the study of neuromuscular disorders.

The main contributions of histochemistry in the study of muscle are: (1) the recognition of fibre types and their response to disease, and to neural, hormonal and other influences; (2) the demonstration of structural defects in muscle fibres; (3) the detection of enzyme deficiencies and the storage of metabolic compounds. Histochemistry has exposed many abnormalities not detected by routine histological stains and the rapidly developing discipline of immunocytochemistry offers similar prospects. Immunocytochemistry has already provided a new insight into the field of neuromuscular disorders and its full potential has yet to be fulfilled.

Histochemistry and immunocytochemistry have had a wide application to both human and animal muscle. As it is not possible to cover all aspects, this review is confined to the histochemical and immunocytochemical aspects of human muscle. The application of these techniques is discussed with regard to normal, diseased and developing muscle.

METHODS

Choice of biopsy material

In humans, as in animals, there may be differences between muscles, particularly with regard to fibre–type proportions (Johnson et al 1973). It is thus desirable to confine studies to the same anatomical groups of muscle so as to become familiar with the normal pattern of that group.

Selection of the muscle for biopsy should be based on clinical assessment of the muscle weakness. It is important not to select a muscle that is so severely involved that the tissue has degenerated to such an extent that no trace of the underlying disease remains; nor, on the other hand, to choose a muscle which is pathologically unaffected. In general, the rectus femoris or vastus lateralis muscles of the quadriceps are easily accessible and suitable for the study of most proximal muscle syndromes. Even within the quadriceps, however, selective involvement of the vasti and relative sparing of the rectus femoris can occur in some diseases (Heckmatt & Dubowitz 1985). In some circumstances the gastrocnemius, deltoid or biceps may also be suitable for biopsy. Ultrasound has proved a useful tool for routine screening to assess the differential involvement of individual muscles and can help to decide which muscle to biopsy.

The choice of biopsy site must also take into account previous invasive techniques, such as electromyography or any form of injection. These sites must be avoided as trauma of this kind can produce pathological changes in muscle (Engel 1967).

Biopsy techniques

All muscle biopsies from both adult and paediatric patients can be performed under local anaesthesia. Premedication of children is often desirable. There is no advantage in the use of general anaesthesia and it may at times be hazardous in patients with neuromuscular disease because of poor respiratory function. To avoid artefacts in the biopsy it is essential that the local anaesthetic infiltrates the skin and subcutaneous tissue only and does not penetrate the muscle itself.

Biopsies can be obtained by an open surgical technique or by using a variety of commercially available needles (Edwards & Maunder 1977). The needle that we favour is that developed by Bergström and it has now been used extensively for the study of adults and children (Edwards et al 1973, 1983, Heckmatt et al 1984). The samples obtained with Bergström-type needles are approximately 3–4 mm in diameter and may contain 1000 or more fibres in transverse section. It is essential that these small pieces are properly orientated under a dissecting microscope before processing. Although this requires some expertise, this is readily acquired by technical staff.

The Bergström needle biopsy technique has the advantage of providing adequate samples by a rapid, simple and less traumatic procedure than open biopsy. In addition, the risk of infection is reduced as the incision is small, no stitches are required and the residual mark is only a few millimetres in length; multiple samples can be made through the same incision; and samples for biochemical studies can be taken rapidly.

Open biopsy procedures provide larger quantities of muscle which may still be necessary for some biochemical techniques not yet adapted to small samples. With open biopsy samples it is also possible to avoid contraction artefacts in the sample by taking the muscle at resting length. This can be achieved either by the use of clamps or by suturing the sample and tying it to a strip of wood before removal. For light microscopy this offers no special advantage as samples are usually transversely orientated and contraction does not adversely affect the appearance. For electron microscopy, contraction may cause distortion and samples stretched before fixation best reveal the sarcomeric regularity. Needle biopsies, however, can provide adequate samples for electron microscopy even though the results may not be quite so aesthetically pleasing as those derived from open biopsies (Sewry 1985).

Specimen preparation

All muscle biopsies must be rapidly frozen. If this is correctly performed, very little ice crystal damage or other artefact is detectable at the light–microscopical level. All histological and histochemical studies can be carried out on cryostat sections and for some enzyme techniques this is essential. Ideally, samples should be frozen as soon as possible after removal but delays of up to 30 minutes have no deleterious effect on the pathological interpretation of biopsies. Some enzymes, e.g. the myosin ATPases, will withstand quite considerable delays in freezing. It is therefore still possible to do meaningful histochemical studies on some post-mortem samples or samples that unavoidably may have to travel from another hospital.

Immunocytochemical studies at both light- and electron-microscopic levels can also be performed on cryostat sections from the same blocks of tissue (Fitzsimons & Sewry 1985, Sewry et al 1985). It is often an advantage to prepare serial sections for both histochemical and immunocytochemical investigations for detailed comparisons. As with histochemical techniques, the localisation of many muscle antigens does not require fixation and in some instances it may have a deleterious effect on antigenicity; some antigens, in contrast, benefit from mild fixation. Most immunocytochemical methods applied to muscle use an indirect technique and utilise a secondary antibody directed against the primary antibody of interest. Amplification of antibody labelling can be obtained using the biotin–avidin technique (Hsu et al 1981). This method, particularly with streptococcal avidin, has the additional benefit of overcoming some problems of non-specific binding to the sarcolemma, connective tissue and necrotic fibres (Fitzsimons & Sewry 1985, Sewry et al 1985). The antibody is visualised by the use of conjugates of enzymes, such as peroxidase, or fluorochromes, such as fluorescein isothiocyanate (FITC), or metals, such as gold. Texas red (Amersham) is a new fluorochrome that we have applied extensively to muscle and found to be brighter and more resistant to fading than other fluorochromes.

Ultrastructural localisation of muscle antigens is usually achieved using electron-dense markers such as ferritin, colloidal gold or enzymes which can be made to produce electron-dense end products (Polak & Varndell 1984).

Histochemical techniques

Histochemical techniques are not performed in isolation and reference is always made to histological preparations. In particular, haematoxylin and eosin, Verhoeff-van Gieson and the modified Gomori trichrome stains (Engel & Cunningham 1963) clearly demonstrate the size and shape of the fibres, the position of nuclei, the presence of interstitial cells, blood vessels, nerves, connective tissue and adipose tissue. In addition, abnormal structures such as rods in nemaline myopathy and abnormal mitochondria can be demonstrated with the trichrome technique (Dubowitz 1985). Other stains are useful in particular circumstances such as Sudan black B or oil red O for lipids, techniques for nucleic acids (DNA and RNA), cresyl fast violet or toluidine blue for metachromatic material and alizarin red for calcium.

Enzyme histochemistry adds an extra dimension to the study of muscle. In the early days a large battery of enzymes was routinely applied to muscle biopsies (Dubowitz & Pearse 1961) but now assessment of diseased muscle can easily be made using a small selection of procedures. Additional methods are of research interest and necessary only in specific circumstances. Details of techniques can be found in manuals such as those by Lojda et al (1979), Bancroft & Stevens (1982), Filipe & Lake (1983) and Pearse (1980, 1985). The following sections will cover the application of the most important enzyme groups and chemical radicals to muscle and will illustrate their pathological value.

Immunocytochemical techniques

Several immunocytochemical studies of human muscle have now been reported and these have provided alternative methods for localising specific enzymes and have expanded our understanding of the precise nature of intracellular and extracellular muscle components. The cellular components and the antibodies localised in human muscle are summarised in Table 7.1.

A variety of lectins have also been applied to human muscle and as similar techniques to those of immunocytochemistry are used to localise them, they are often considered with antibody localisation studies. Lectins are glycoproteins isolated from plants and animals that bind to specific glycoside groups. Lectins have an important role in the characterisation of muscle membranes.

With a variety of techniques, therefore, many

Table 7.1 Immunocytochemical studies of human muscle

Antigen	Localisation
Collagen types I, III, IV, V	Extracellular matrix
Laminin	Extracellular matrix
Fibronectin	Extracellular matrix
HLA ABC class I antigens	Sarcolemma
β_2 microglobulin	Sarcolemma
Neural cell adhesion molecule and antigen 5.1H11	Sarcolemma of fetal and regenerating fibres
Immunoglobulin and complement	Sarcolemma, blood vessels, some fibres
β spectrin-like protein	Subsarcolemmal cytoskeleton
Desmin (skeletin)	Cytoskeleton
Fast, slow and fetal myosins	Myofibrils of specific fibre types
Fast and slow troponin I	Myofibrils of specific fibre types
α actinin	Z line
Myoglobin	Specific fibre types
Cathepsins	Interstitial cells and some fibres
B and T lymphocyte subtypes	Interstitial cells

properties of normal muscle have been established and deviations from the normal pattern can be used as markers for disease and an aid to the diagnosis of neuromuscular disorders.

MUSCLE ENZYMES COMMONLY IDENTIFIED AND STUDIED HISTOCHEMICALLY

Oxidoreductases

The oxidoreductases include a large number of enzymes that catalyse the oxidation of various substrates and provide energy for cell metabolism. They are divided into oxidases, which oxidise by catalysing the reaction between the substrate and oxygen, and the dehydrogenases that oxidise by the transfer of hydrogen from the substrate along a hydrogen acceptor pathway.

Cytochrome-*c* oxidase (EC 1.9.3.1) is a haem–copper enzyme and is part of the succinic oxidase system. It is synonymous with cytochrome a_3 and is entirely intramitochondrial in its localisation. Muscle is rich in cytochrome oxidase and it demonstrates a clear distinction between fibre types because of their varying mitochondrial content. In disease situations cytochrome oxidase

is associated with the tubular aggregates that characterise periodic paralysis syndromes. This led to the suggestion that tubular aggregates originate from mitochondria (Lewis et al 1971) rather than the sarcoplasmic reticulum (Engel et al 1970a). Cytochrome oxidase may be absent in some forms of mitochondrial myopathies.

Peroxidases (EC 1.11.1) are haem–copper oxidases that require peroxide as catalyst. Endogenous peroxidases are present in small amounts in muscle and are found in leucocytes, some erythrocytes and occasionally in some abnormal fibres (Dunn et al 1982). This is of relevance to immunocytochemical studies when peroxidase-labelled antisera are applied and it may then be necessary to remove endogenous peroxidase before proceeding with immunolabelling.

Dehydrogenases. The dehydrogenases oxidise specific substrates anaerobically and the hydrogen removed is usually accepted by the coenzyme nicotinamide adenine dinucleotide (NAD) or nicotinamide adenine dinucleotide phosphate (NADP). Some dehydrogenases do not require a coenzyme and can act as hydrogen acceptors themselves. Succinate and glycerol-3-phosphate dehydrogenases (SDH, EC 1.3.99.1; GPDH, EC 1.1.99.5) are the two enzymes of this type most often demonstrated. The activity of the latter can be increased by vitamin K_3 (menadione) which acts as a hydrogen acceptor (Wattenberg & Leong 1960). This demonstrates the mitochondrial coenzyme-independent GPDH in contrast to the coenzyme-dependent GPDH (glycerol-3-phosphate: NAD^+) (EC 1.1.1.8) which is cytoplasmic.

Oxidation of reduced coenzymes (NADH and NADPH) can be catalysed by flavin enzymes, formerly known as diaphorases. The flavin enzymes can transfer hydrogen to various acceptors, including tetrazolium salts. The flavin enzymes are then called tetrazolium reductases (TR) (NADH-tetrazolium reductase and NADPH-tetrazolium reductase).

Dehydrogenases are demonstrated histochemically using tetrazolium salts. These are soluble, almost colourless, salts which yield a coloured insoluble formazan on reduction. Many dehydrogenases are localised to the mitochondria, exceptions being coenzyme-dependent GPDH and L-lactate dehydrogenase (LDH, EC 1.1.1.27) which are cytoplasmic. Some LDH is firmly bound to mitochondria but most of the enzyme is cytoplasmic. Tetrazolium reductases are firmly bound in mitochondria and the sarcoplasmic reticulum.

The first application of dehydrogenase methods to human muscle was in the investigation of autopsy specimens by Wachstein & Meisel (1955). They found a variation in SDH activity between muscle fibres and observed that the more reactive fibres tended to be smaller in diameter. Dubowitz & Pearse (1960a, 1961) investigated several oxidoreductase enzymes in human muscle biopsies including NAD and NADP tetrazolium reductases, NAD-linked β-hydroxybutyrate (EC 1.1.1.30), isocitrate (EC 1.1.1.41), malate (EC 1.1.1.37), glutamate (EC 1.4.1.2) glycerol-3-phosphate (EC 1.1.1.8), alcohol (EC 1.1.1.1) and L-lactate (EC 1.1.1.27) dehydrogenases, NADP-linked isocitrate (EC 1.1.1.42) and glucose-6-phosphate (EC 1.1.1.49) dehydrogenases and non-coenzyme-linked glycerol-3-phosphate dehydrogenase (EC 1.1.99.5). Positive reactions were obtained with all the enzymes except β-hydroxybutyric dehydrogenase which was negative. The most intense reactions were for NADH-tetrazolium reductase and lactate dehydrogenase and the weakest were glucose-6-phosphate and alcohol dehydrogenases.

Dehydrogenases, in common with oxidases, clearly distinguish between the different fibre types. In normal muscle the NADH-TR and NADPH-TR reactions stain type I fibres more intensely than type II fibres (Fig. 7.1). The fibres showing the least reaction are IIB fibres and those with intermediate activity are IIA fibres. The myofibrils are unstained but the intermyofibrillar network comprising the mitochondria and sarcoplasmic reticulum is well demonstrated. Succinate dehydrogenase (EC 1.3.9.9.1) is entirely mitochondrial and gives similar differentiation of fibre types. In longitudinal section a striated appearance is seen with a series of paired dots located at the A–I junction. Lactate dehydrogenase differentiates fibre types less well with a more uniform intermyofibrillar network, possibly because of the sarcoplasmic LDH. Type I fibres, however, are

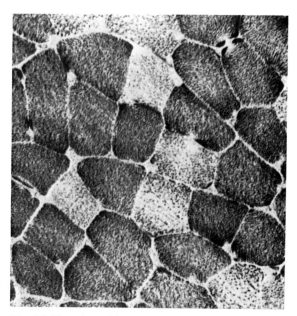

Fig. 7.1 Normal quadriceps muscle showing checkerboard pattern of dark (type I) and light (type II) fibres. NADH-TR ×330

still more intensely stained than type II. Co-enzyme-linked glycerol-3-phosphate dehydrogenase also gives a strong reaction in type I fibres but the coenzyme-independent menadione-linked GPDH is seen predominately in type II fibres. In addition to the differentiation of fibre types, oxidative enzymes often show increased concentration of stain at the periphery of fibres and in areas adjacent to nuclei. If central nuclei are present, areas of increased stain may be seen within the fibre; these probably represent focal aggregates of mitochondria.

In diseased muscle, oxidative enzymes not only reveal alterations in fibre-type proportions and distribution but they also reveal structural changes in the fibre architecture. Many of these are not apparent with routine histological stains. Some changes reflect a specific pathological change and characterise a disorder, whereas others are non-specific and are common pathological features.

Oxidative enzyme staining is the best method to demonstrate the presence of cores. *Cores* are unstained regions of the fibre (Fig. 7.2). The presence of large central cores in most fibres is pathognomonic of central core disease but sporadic cores also occur in other disorders and these fibres

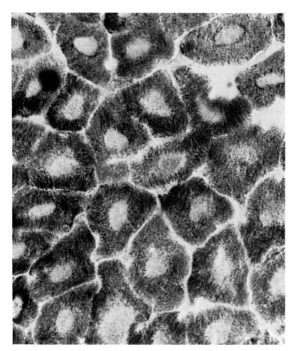

Fig. 7.2 Biopsy from quadriceps of 29-year-old woman showing central cores in most fibres and uniformity of enzyme pattern (type I). NADH-TR ×330

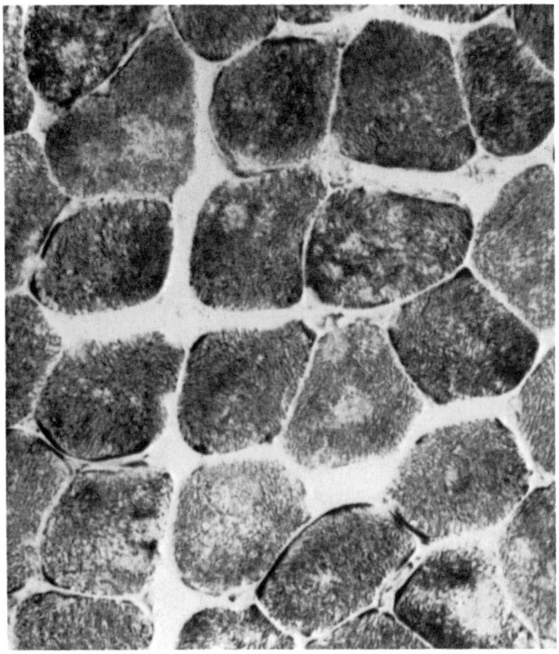

are difficult to distinguish from target fibres associated with denervation (see below). Central cores run most of the length of the fibre. Two types of central core have been identified with myosin adenosine triphosphatase (ATPase) staining: these are structured and unstructured (Neville & Brooke 1973) (see Congenital Myopathies — central core disease pp. 269–270).

Minicores are also easily recognised with oxidative enzymes and are small, focal areas of disruption (Fig. 7.3). The myofibrillar material is disrupted in these regions and they show up as weaker staining areas with the ATPase reactions.

Target fibres resemble central core fibres but are characterised by three distinct zones (Fig. 7.4). The central zone is devoid of enzyme activity and is circumscribed by an intermediate zone with increased oxidative enzyme activity; peripheral to this is a relatively normal zone. Most target fibres are of type I and they are usually associated with denervating disorders.

Common changes, occurring particularly in type I fibres, are disruption and disorientation of the intermyofibrillar network. This may result in patchy staining giving rise to a 'moth-eaten' appearance (Fig. 7.5) or bizarre patterning of the myofibrils in whorled fibres (Fig. 7.6). Oxidative

Fig. 7.3 Deltoid muscle from a 10-year-old child showing minicores (multicores) in many fibres. NADH-TR ×330

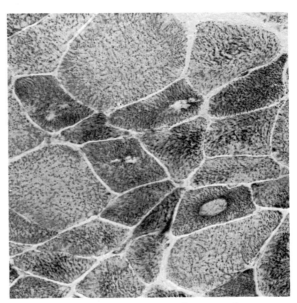

Fig. 7.4 Target fibres with an unreactive core and surrounded by a darker-staining rim or intermediate zone. NADH-TR ×380

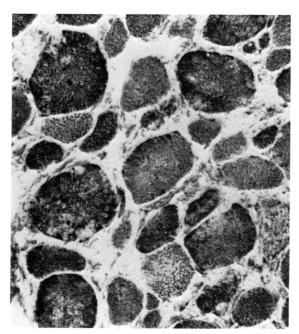

Fig. 7.5 Disruption of intermyofibrillar network in 'moth-eaten' fibres in a nine-year-old boy with congenital muscular dystrophy. NADH-TR ×330

enzyme stains also reveal alterations in the distribution of mitochondria. This is particularly striking in *lobulated fibres*. These have small subsarcolemmal aggregates of stain that project into the fibre (Fig. 7.7). They occur in a variety of disorders but we have not observed them in our extensive studies of paediatric cases (Guerard et al 1985). Suspected structural changes in mitochondria are seen with oxidative enzyme staining as excessively intense regions (Fig. 7.8). They are often granular in appearance and the formazan colour may differ slightly from normal. These regions correspond to the 'ragged red' areas seen with the Gomori trichrome stain. Electron microscopy is needed to confirm the presence of the structural defect.

Transferases

Phosophorylase (EC 2.4.1.1) This cytoplasmic enzyme has an essential role in the utilisation and synthesis of glycogen in muscle. It catalyses a reversible reaction that transfers glucosyl residues from combination with phosphate to a long–chain polysaccharide. A large proportion of phosphorylase in muscle is present in an inactive form,

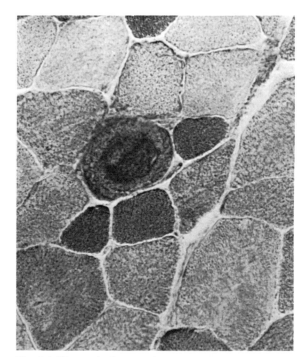

Fig. 7.6 Disorganised pattern in a whorled fibre from a 13-year-old girl with limb girdle dystrophy. NADH-TR ×330

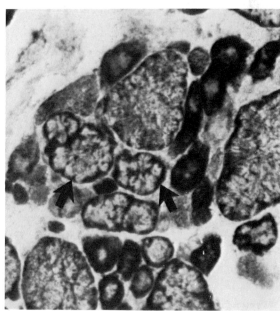

Fig. 7.7 Lobulated fibres (arrows) with marked aggregation of stain at the periphery of the fibre. NADH-TR ×270

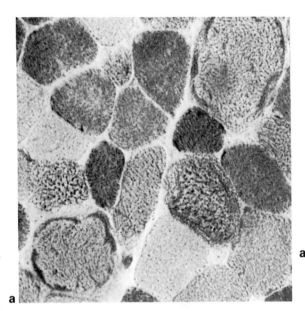

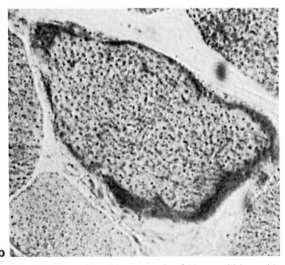

Fig. 7.8 Biopsy from biceps muscle of 11-year-old boy with 'ophthalmoplegia plus' syndrome showing (a) increased oxidative enzyme activity in individual fibres with abnormal mitochondria, NADH-TR ×330; and (b) higher power showing increased activity at the periphery of the fibre, NADH-TR ×830

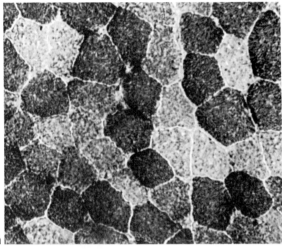

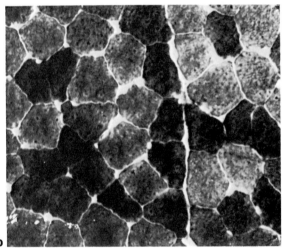

Fig. 7.9 Normal muscle showing reciprocal activity between (a) oxidative enzyme activity and (b) phosphorylase activity in individual fibres. Quadriceps. a. NADH-TR ×330; b. phosphorylase ×330

phosphorylase *b*, and the histochemical demonstration of phosphorylase is dependent on the conversion of this to the active form, phosphorylase *a* (Takeuchi 1956). Enzyme activity is assessed by the resulting glycogen production which is visualised with iodine or the periodic acid-Schiff reaction.

Histochemical staining for phosphorylase shows a variation in activity of individual fibres (Dubowitz & Pearse 1960a,b, 1961). There is a reciprocal relationship between phosphorylase and oxidative enzymes in human muscle (Fig. 7.9). Thus fibres high in phosphorylase are low in oxidative enzymes (type II) and those low in phosphorylase are high in oxidative enzymes (type I). Fibres with staining intensities intermediate between these two extremes are also revealed (Eränkö & Palkama 1961, Godlewski 1963). Changes in the normal fibre-type distributions are demonstrated by the phosphorylase technique but these are more clearly seen with myosin adenosine triphosphatase (ATPase) staining. The main application of the phosphorylase technique is in the study of glycogen storage diseases, in particular type V (McArdle's disease): this is characterised by a total absence of phosphorylase from all fibres.

Deficiencies of 1-phosphofructokinase (EC 2.7.1.56) (Bonilla & Schotland 1970) and the hydrolase myoadenylate deaminase (AMP deaminase, EC 3.5.4.6) (Fishbein et al 1978) can also be revealed histochemically and are useful techniques for the differential diagnosis of the glycogenoses.

Hydrolases

Phosphatases catalyse the hydrolysis of organic esters. They are classified into alkaline or acid phosphatases according to their optimal pH. Most phosphatases catalyse the hydrolysis of a wide range of substrates but some, such as glucose-6-phosphatase (EC 3.1.3.9) and 5′-nucleotidase (EC 3.1.3.5), are substrate-specific. Phosphatases are usually demonstrated either by metal chelation of the released phosphate or by coupling the alcoholic residue to an azo dye. More recently, a method using metachromatic dyes has also been reported (Doriguzzi et al 1983).

Alkaline phosphatase (EC 3.1.3.1) has an optimum pH of 9–10 and is found primarily in cell membranes where active transport occurs, such as endothelium of arteries, endoplasmic reticulum and Golgi apparatus. Normal human muscle fibres appear negative when stained for alkaline phosphatase but arterioles 15–35 μm in diameter are clearly depicted. Large blood vessels and capillaries in human muscle do not stain, unlike those in animal muscle (Engel & Cunningham 1970). In diseased human muscle alkaline phosphatase identifies a particular kind of abnormal fibre (Engel & Cunningham 1970). These fibres are usually small, often contain internal nuclei and most, but not all, have basophilia. Necrotic fibres, however, are negative. Fibres positive for alkaline phosphatase are common in X-linked dystrophies and active myositic conditions. They are also seen in carriers of Duchenne dystrophy and in neurogenic disorders. Occasional positive fibres occur

in other conditions. In dermatomyositis, polymyositis and some acute inflammatory situations there is prominent staining of the endomysial and perimysial connective tissue (Engel 1977). This is considered to be a diagnostic feature of these inflammatory disorders, as it is rarely seen in the dystrophies.

Acid phosphatase (EC 3.1.3.2) has an optimum pH of 4–5 and its main localisation is believed to be in lysosomes. Very little acid phosphatase activity is seen in normal muscle and morphologically identifiable lysosomes are rarely observed ultrastructurally. Using azo dye coupling techniques, acid phosphatase activity is seen associated with muscle spindles and interstitial cells and is present as small discrete subsarcolemmal areas. This activity is often adjacent to nuclei and is probably associated with lipofuscin (Cullen et al 1979). In diseased muscle, acid phosphatase activity is increased. Basophilic fibres show high diffuse activity (Neerunjun & Dubowitz 1977) and such activity is prominent in necrotic areas, both in the fibres and in the associated cellular infiltrate. In type II glycogenosis, acid phosphatase staining is also intense.

Adenosine triphosphatase (ATPase) (EC 3.6.1.3) There are several ATPases in animal tissues that differ in their localisation and biochemical properties in relation to activators and inhibitors. One of the most important histochemically is the calcium-activated myosin-ATPase. This enzyme is responsible for the hydrolysis of ATP which results in the release of energy required for muscle contraction. Histochemical demonstration of myosin ATPase is usually by the metal chelation method at pH 9.4 as applied by Padykula & Hermann (1955). More recently, modifications of their method have been successfully applied to human muscle biopsies (Round et al 1980). The end result of this reaction is the deposition of cobalt sulphide which is seen to be localised to the A band. It gives a clear differentiation into muscle fibre types and distinguishes the lightly stained type I fibres from the heavily stained type II fibres (Fig. 7.10). The ATPase technique forms the basis for the identification of fibre types in diagnostic pathology. In addition to the two main

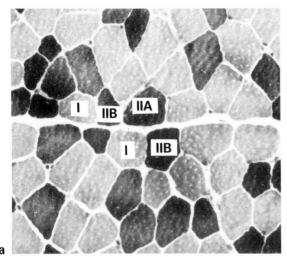

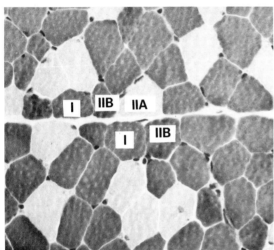

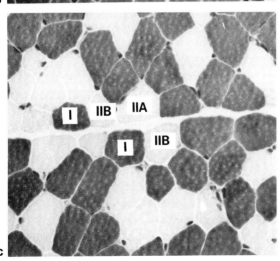

fibre types, Brooke & Kaiser (1970) defined three fibre types in human muscle by utilising a pre-incubation at varying pH (9.4, 4.6 and 4.3). With acid pre-incubation at 4.3 the pattern seen at 9.4 is reversed and type I fibres are heavily stained in contrast to the pale type II fibres. Pre-incubation at pH 4.6 demonstrates three populations of fibres with the type I fibres being heavily stained and the type II fibres subdivided into pale type IIA fibres and darkly stained IIB fibres (Fig. 7.10); in addition, a few fibres, type IIC fibres, stain darkly at pH 9.4 and show some residual staining at pH 4.3 (Fig. 7.11).

In normal muscle, the myosin ATPase reaction reveals a checkerboard pattern of fibre types. The three fibre types I, IIA and IIB, are randomly distributed, present in more or less equal proportions, and show a similar small variation in size. The normal pattern can be influenced by exercise, nerve stimulation, hormones and disease (see Dubowitz 1985). In diseased muscle the changes include selective alteration in size of one fibre type, alterations in the distribution of fibre types (fibre-type grouping) and predominance of one fibre type.

Fig. 7.10 Serial sections from quadriceps muscle showing the three main fibre types (I, IIA, IIB) stained for (a) myosin ATPase, pH 9.4; (b) ATPase after pre-incubation at pH 4.6 and (c) ATPase after pre-incubation at pH 4.3.
Counterstained with haematoxylin and eosin, ×335

HISTOCHEMICAL REACTIONS IN HUMAN MUSCLE

MUSCLE FIBRE TYPE	I	IIA	IIB	IIC
Routine ATP-ase	1+	3+	3+	3+
ATP-ase pre-incubated pH 4.6	3+	0	3+	3+
ATP-ase pre-incubated pH 4.3	3+	0	0	2+
NADH-TR	3+	2+	1+	2+
SDH	3+	2+	1+	2+
α glycerophosphate - menadione linked	0	2+	2+	1+
PAS	1+ + 2+	3+	2+	2+
Phosphorylase	1+ + 0	3+	3+	3+

◯ = 0   ◔ = 1+   ⊗ = 2+   ● = 3+

Fig. 7.11 Histochemical reactions of the different fibre types in human muscle (from Dubowitz & Brooke 1973)

Selective atrophy of type II fibres (Fig. 7.12) is one of the commonest abnormalities associated with muscle pathology. The commonest form of type II atrophy selectively involves type IIB fibres. Although atrophy of type IIA and IIB fibres may occur concomitantly, it is unusual to see selective atrophy of type IIA fibres. Type II atrophy occurs in a wide variety of disorders and in situations where muscle strength is secondarily impaired or when the muscle is not used. It is also a common feature associated with steroid therapy. Although disuse resulting from bedrest is commonly thought to induce type II atrophy, other forms of disuse such as immobilisation following fractures involve type I fibres (Sargeant et al 1977). Selective involvement of type I fibres is less common but may occur in myotonic dystrophy (Engel & Brooke 1966) and some congenital myopathies, such as centronuclear myopathy and nemaline myopathy (see below).

Alterations in the distribution of fibre types are most clearly seen in denervating disorders such as peripheral neuropathies and spinal muscular atrophy. In these situations it is common to find large groups of fibres of one type, in association with groups of atrophic fibres of mixed types (Fig. 7.13). This fibre–type grouping is associated

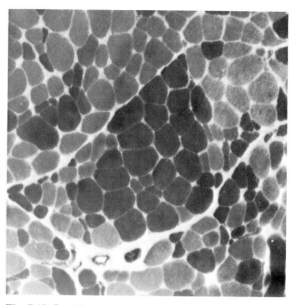

Fig. 7.13 Quadriceps muscle biopsy from a case of peripheral neuropathy showing fibre-type grouping in association with small group atrophy of both fibre types. ATPase 9.4 ×230

with collateral sprouting of terminal axons (Morris & Raybould 1971b) and reinnervation.

Predominance of either fibre type may occur but it is essential that normal limits for the muscle in question are clearly defined. Predominance of type I in the rectus femoris is defined as meaning that more than 55% of the fibres are type I (Dubowitz & Brooke 1973). Type II predominance occurs when more than 80% of the fibres are of type II. Type I predominance tends to be associated with myopathic conditions, particularly the genetically determined dystrophies (Fig. 7.14). Type II predominance is associated with motor neurone diseases.

Esterases. Carboxylic ester hydrolases (EC 3.1.1) hydrolyse carboxylic acids and are classified into three closely related groups — lipases, non-specific esterases and specific esterases. Of particular interest to muscle are the non-specific esterases and the specific cholinesterase, acetyl-cholinesterase (EC 3.1.1.7). Normal muscle fibres show no non-specific esterase staining but the small basophilic fibres, seen in some dystrophies and often referred to as regenerating fibres, show

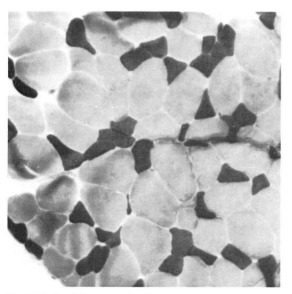

Fig. 7.12 Quadriceps muscle biopsy showing marked type II fibre atrophy. ATPase 9.4 ×160

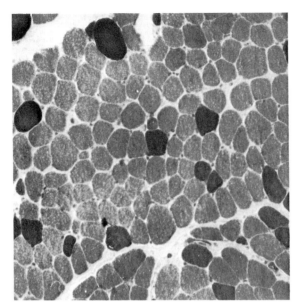

Fig. 7.14 Predominance of type I fibres in a quadriceps biopsy from a boy with Duchenne muscular dystrophy. ATPase 9.4 ×170

a high activity (Engel 1979). The high activity of this and other hydrolytic enzymes in regenerating fibres has led to the term regenerate–degenerate (regen–degen) fibres (Engel 1979).

Acetylcholinesterase in normal fibres is restricted to the motor end-plate. Denervated fibres, basophilic fibres and cultured myotubes, however, show extrajunctional acetylcholine receptors (Engel 1979).

Proteases (peptide hydrolases, EC 3.4) are a group of hydrolytic enzymes classified into endopeptidases and exopeptidases according to the position of the peptide bond they attack (McDonald 1985). Interest in proteases from both classes has risen in recent years because of their involvement in the metabolic turnover of myofibrillar proteins (Bird et al 1978, Kar & Pearson 1978, 1979). In diseased muscle, myofibrillar degradation is increased and is thought to result from increased activities of proteases (Kar & Pearson 1978, Warnes et al 1981). Many of the studies of muscle proteases have been biochemical estimates from homogenates. Recent investigations, however, using fluorescent histochemical methods (Stauber et al 1985), semipermeable techniques (White et al

1985) or immunocytochemical methods (Whitaker et al 1983) have localised a variety of proteolytic enzymes in diseased human muscle. Cathepsins have been demonstrated in muscle fibres in several neuromuscular disorders (Whitaker et al 1983, Stauber et al 1985) and cathepsin D (EC 3.4.23.5) is particularly prominent in basophilic fibres. It is not associated with necrotic fibres and the authors therefore suggested that it may have a role in repair processes (Whitaker et al 1983). Aminopeptidases (L-amino acyl peptide hydrolases, EC. 3.4.11) and dipeptidyl peptide hydrolases (EC 3.4.14) show low activity in muscle fibres from normal and diseased muscle, but higher activity in the interstitial tissue, particularly in relation to mast cells and macrophages (White et al 1985).

Lyases

Adenylate cyclase (AC, EC 4.6.1.1) regulates the synthesis of cyclic adenosine monophosphate (cAMP) from Mg-adenosine triphosphate (MgATP). Its precise localisation in muscle is still uncertain but biochemical studies of the sarcolemma of muscle fibres from dystrophic patients and of cultured myotubes have shown differences in AC activity and its response to inhibitors (Willner et al 1982). Very few histochemical studies of AC have been reported but a technique using an artificial substrate was believed to demonstrate it specifically (Dubrovsky & Engel 1976, Engel 1977). In normal human muscle AC was localised to blood vessels and to the sarcolemma and intermyofibrillar network. Diseased muscle showed high AC activity in basophilic (regenerating) fibres. In Duchenne dystrophy not only were basophilic fibres strongly stained but also several additional fibres that otherwise appeared normal. Denervating disorders showed slight to moderate staining in atrophic fibres.

GLYCOGEN

Glycogen is stored to a varying degree in all muscle fibres. Historically, the periodic acid–Schiff (PAS) stain has been used to demonstrate glycogen but the specificity of the reaction for glycogen has to be checked with α-amylase diges-tion. In normal human muscle the PAS reaction stains type II fibres more intensely than type I (Fig. 7.11). Intermediate fibres are also demon-strated and correspond to IIB fibres. Excessive quantities of glycogen are a characteristic feature of glycogenoses. In some dystrophies, fibres with no detectable PAS staining are often seen.

In addition to demonstrating the presence of glycogen, the PAS stain is also useful for the recognition of ring fibres (Fig. 7.15). These abnormal fibres have a peripheral band of myofi-brils at right angles to the central myofibrils. This gives the appearance of a striated annulet around the fibre. Although these are a non-specific feature, ring fibres frequently occur in myotonic dystrophy and limb girdle dystrophy.

The PAS stain demonstrates not only glycogen but also other polysaccharides, mucopolysacchar-ides and glycoproteins. After α-amylase digestion, PAS is a simple method for revealing the sarco-lemma of the fibres and the position of capillaries. Capillaries can be counted easily using this method (Hermansen & Wachtlova 1971) and numbers can be related to fibre type by comparison with serial ATPase sections (Andersen 1975).

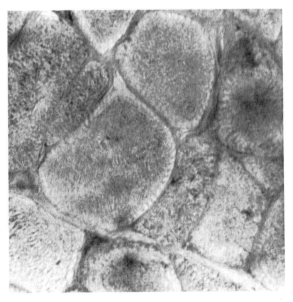

Fig. 7.15 Ring fibres in a quadriceps biopsy from a child with myotonic dystrophy. PAS ×740

LIPID

Neutral lipids in normal muscle fibres appear as small droplets distributed throughout the fibre. The concentration and size of the droplets is related to fibre type. Excessive lipid accumulation in muscle fibres occurs in some disorders affecting lipid metabolism. In other disorders, e.g. poly-myositis, fibres with excess lipid are seen occasionally. The proliferation of adipose tissue that occurs in muscular dystrophies and to some extent in other conditions is clearly demonstrated by lipid stains.

NUCLEIC ACIDS

The demonstration of nucleic acids is sometimes of value, particularly with respect to RNA. The methyl green pyronine reaction and the fluor-escent acridine orange technique differentiate DNA from RNA. Accumulations of RNA are seen in basophilic fibres in diseased muscle and this has led to the dogma that these fibres are regenerating fibres.

QUANTITATION

It is notoriously difficult to judge the size of fibres in a muscle biopsy by simple inspection. A more objective assessment is often necessary for the interpretation of pathological changes and to this end various measurements of fibres have been applied: these include orthogonal diameters, fibre circumference, fibre area and lesser diameter, and fibre-type proportions (Sissons 1965, Adams et al 1968, Edstrom & Nystrom 1969, Reniers et al 1970, Round et al 1982). Measurement of the lesser fibre diameter has had wide acceptance during the past decade as a simple, reproducible measurement of fibre size (Dubowitz & Brooke 1973, Dubowitz 1985). Sections stained for myosin ATPase are usually employed and the data used to construct a histogram showing the vari-ation of each fibre type. In addition, the number of fibres outside the normal range (atrophy and hypertrophy factors) and the degree of variability can be assessed.

Although measurements of fibre diameter can be made easily using an eye-piece micrometer, a variety of computer-assisted systems is now commercially available. These have been applied to several studies of human muscle (see Dubowitz 1985) and demonstrate the importance of quantitation in the objective assessment of biopsies, particularly those with minor pathological changes. In an extensive study of biopsies from carriers of Duchenne muscular dystrophy we have emphasised the need for quantitation (Maunder-Sewry & Dubowitz 1981).

DEVELOPMENT OF MUSCLE

The histochemical development of human fetal muscle can be divided into three distinct phases (Dubowitz 1965, 1968). Until about 18 weeks of gestation there is no easily definable division into fibre types. There may be some variation in enzyme activity but the fibres showing this tend to occur in clusters and do not show a reciprocal reaction between oxidative and phosphorylating enzymes. Between 18 and 28 weeks the fibres can

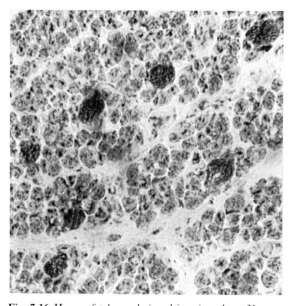

Fig. 7.16 Human fetal muscle (quadriceps) at about 21 weeks' gestation showing a small proportion of darker-staining (type I) fibres. Remaining fibres are uniform in activity and still undifferentiated and correspond to type IIC fibres. NADH-TR ×330

be subdivided into type I and type II in a similar way to adult muscle, but only about 5–10% of the total can be recognised as type I fibres (Fig. 7.16). This corresponds to the distribution of classic Wohlfart B fibres (Wohlfart 1937). Immunocytochemical studies of myosin types suggest that fibre-type differentiation may occur earlier at about 16 weeks gestation (Thornell et al 1984). After 30 weeks gestation the muscle has a checkerboard pattern as in mature muscle. Brooke et al (1971) suggested that the undifferentiated fibres in human fetal muscle are type IIC fibres and that these are the precursors of the type I and type IIA and IIB fibres of mature human muscle. This has been substantiated by the studies of Colling-Saltin (1978).

IMMUNOCYTOCHEMISTRY

The wide variety of antibodies that have been applied to human muscle have already been summarised in Table 7.1 (Fitzsimons & Sewry 1985, Sewry et al 1985).

Extracellular matrix

Immunolocalisation of collagen types has shown that in normal muscle types I and III collagen are localised to the perimysial connective tissue. The endomysium also stains strongly with antibodies to type III collagen but anti-type I staining is relatively weak (Fig. 7.17). Collagen type IV is localised to the basement membrane of muscle fibres, major blood vessels and capillaries (Duance et al 1980, Stephens et al 1982, Dunn et al 1984). In muscle from dystrophic patients, collagen antibodies reflect the increase in connective tissue seen histologically with a marked increase in perimysial and endomysial type III collagen (Fig. 7.17). The distribution of collagen type IV appears to be unaltered but is sometimes intense around small fibres (Fig. 7.18). Fibres that are split or whorled show collagen types I, III and IV, associated with the abnormal membrane features, mentioned above (Fig. 7.19). Neurogenic disorders such as spinal muscular atrophy show an increase in perimysial connective tissue and a concomitant increase in type III collagen.

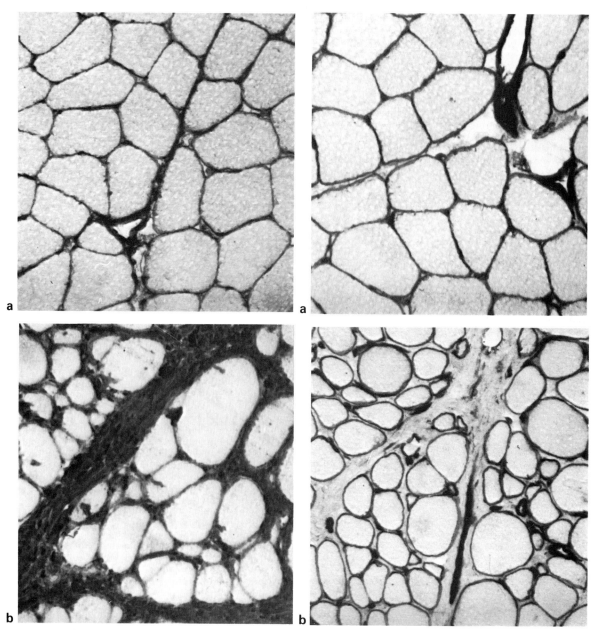

Fig. 7.17 Collagen type III labelled with an avidin-biotin-peroxidase immunotechnique in (a) normal muscle, (b) muscle from a boy with Duchenne muscular dystrophy (DMD). There is a marked increase in staining of the perimysial and endomysial connective tissue in dystrophic muscle. ×230

Fig. 7.18 Collagen type IV labelled with an avidin-biotin-peroxidase immunotechnique in (a) normal muscle, (b) muscle from a boy with Duchenne muscular dystrophy. Staining is confined to the basement membrane of the fibres and blood vessels. ×230

In normal and diseased muscle, staining with antibodies to fibronectin parallels that with collagen type III antibodies whereas antibodies to laminin show a similar distribution to that of type IV collagen (Bertolotto et al 1983, Dunn et al 1984, Sewry et al 1985).

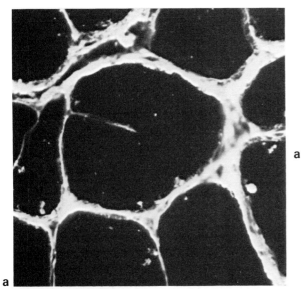

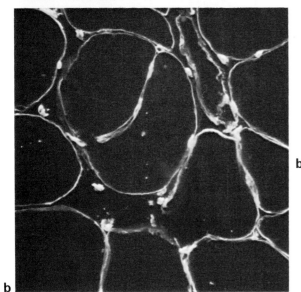

Fig. 7.19 Split fibres in dystrophic muscle stained by an indirect immunofluorescent technique showing (a) type III collagen and (b) type IV collagen associated with the membrane abnormality. ×360

Membrane-associated proteins

Those that have been studied immunocytochemically are HLA A,B,C class I antigens, β2-microglobulin, immunoglobulins and components of the complement pathway, cell adhesion molecules and muscle-specific surface antigens. HLA ABC class I antigens are glycoproteins involved in T-lympho-

cyte reactions to virus and alloantigen–bearing cells. Normal skeletal muscle fibres express minimal or no class I antigens but all fibres in inflammatory myopathies and several fibres in X-linked dystrophies show appreciable labelling with monoclonal antibodies to class I antigens (Appleyard et al 1985) (Fig. 7.20). In addition the class I-associated polypeptide β2-microglobulin is not

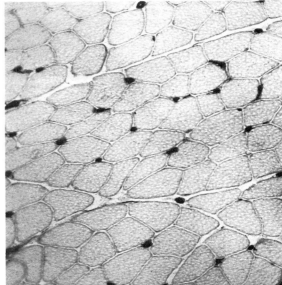

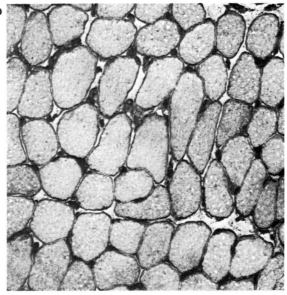

Fig. 7.20 HLA ABC class I antigen localised with an avidin-biotin-peroxidase immunotechnique showing (a) no labelling of the fibres, only the blood vessels in normal muscle but (b) strong labelling of the sarcolemma in muscle from a case of dermatomyositis. ×220

detectable on normal muscle plasma membrane whereas it is in polymyositis.

Immunoglobulin and complement deposition occur in inflammatory disorders, the muscular dystrophies and myasthenia gravis (Engel & Biesecker 1982, Isenberg 1983, Morgan et al 1984). Immunoglobins and complement have been localised to the sarcolemma, blood vessel endothelium and whole muscle fibres. Isenberg (1983) also suggested that immunoglobulin deposition can be used to distinguish myopathic from neuropathic disorders.

The formation of the membrane-attack complex (C5b-9,MAC) on a cell surface is associated with events leading to lysis. Thus antibodies to MAC and to the terminal component C9 are found in necrotic fibres in several diseases (Engel & Biesecker 1982, Cornelio & Dones 1984). Using a monoclonal antibody to C9 we have shown that

MAC is also present as discrete patches on the surface of non-necrotic fibres (Morgan et al 1984) (Fig. 7.21). This suggests a more primary role for complement in muscle necrosis.

Studies of myasthenia gravis have shown immunoglobulin and complement (C3 and C9) at motor end-plates (Engel et al 1977, Sahashi et al 1980). This provides evidence for antibody-dependent complement-mediated injury at the postsynaptic membrane.

Antibodies to the neural cell adhesion molecule (N-CAM) have been localised on the surface of myoblasts and myotubes but not fibroblasts (Moore & Walsh 1985). They have also been identified on human fetal muscle fibres of 10–20 weeks gestation. Normal adult muscle does not express N-CAM but the basophilic fibres in some myopathic conditions are strongly positive. The antibody staining in the basophilic fibres, however, is not confined to the fibre periphery. Similar positively staining fibres have been found in diseased muscle using a monoclonal antibody 5.1H11 directed against human fetal muscle and cultured myogenic cells (Hurko & Walsh 1983).

Cytoskeleton

Human skeletal muscle fibres have been shown to express a β-spectrin-like protein associated with the plasma membrane (Appleyard et al 1984). The periphery of the fibre is clearly delineated (Fig. 7.22) and in neuromuscular disorders there appears to be a slight increase in the intensity of antibody binding in many fibres. Some basophilic fibres, by contrast, show reduced binding and we have identified two types of basophilic fibres according to their β-spectrin binding. One population shows an absence of β-spectrin labelling (Fig. 7.23) whilst the other shows traces (Sewry et al 1986). Necrotic fibres do not label with β-spectrin antibodies. Unlike mature avian muscle (Menold & Repasky 1984) only β-spectrin has been localised in mature and fetal human muscle and α-spectrin antibodies do not bind (Appleyard et al 1984).

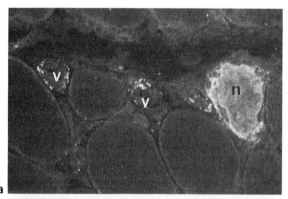
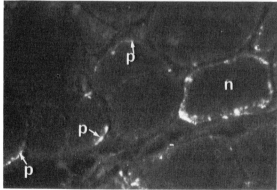

Fig. 7.21 Complement C9 in a case of polymyositis localised with an avidin-biotin-Texas red immunofluorescent technique showing (a) a necrotic fibre (n) with internal staining and two vacuolated fibres (v) with C9 localised to the periphery of the fibres; and (b) a necrotic fibre (n) with a bright peripheral rim and non-necrotic fibres with small localised patches of C9 (p). ×300

Intermediate filaments

Intermediate filaments are a group of immunologically related proteins approximately 10 nm in

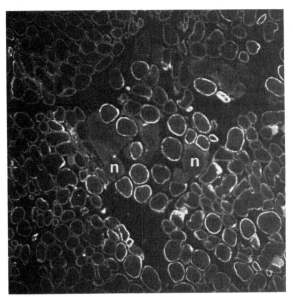

Fig. 7.22 Localisation of β spectrin in a quadriceps biopsy from a case of Duchenne muscular dystrophy using an avidin-biotin-Texas red immunofluorescent technique. All fibres have a brightly stained sarcolemma except the necrotic fibres (n). ×90

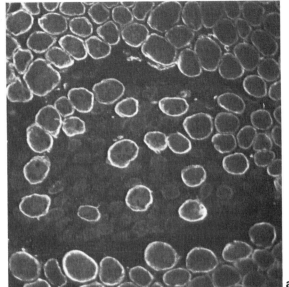

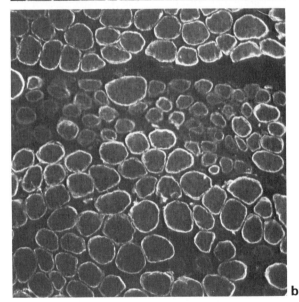

Fig. 7.23 Basophilic fibres in a quadriceps biopsy from a two-year-old boy with Duchenne muscular dystrophy stained for β spectrin with an avidin-biotin-Texas red immunofluorescent technique showing (a) absence of β-spectrin labelling in one group of basophilic fibres and (b) reduced labelling in another group of basophilic fibres in the same biopsy. ×230

diameter that have a characteristic, tissue-associated distribution. Desmin (skeletin) (Thornell et al 1983), vimentin (Lazarides 1980), synemin (Granger & Lazarides 1980) and a neural filament-associated polypeptide (Wang et al 1980) have been identified in muscle fibres and cultured myotubes. Only desmin, however, has been extensively studied in human muscle (Thornell et al 1980, Osborn et al 1982). It is present in small amounts in mature muscle at the periphery of the Z line and links adjacent myofibrils (Lazarides & Hubbard 1976, Thornell et al 1980, 1983). Morphological evidence also suggests a linkage at the M line. The sarcolemma and nuclear membrane may also be associated with desmin, as has been shown in chicken muscle (Tokuyasu et al 1983). In fetal muscle desmin is abundant and it is also prominent in the small basophilic 'regenerating' fibres seen in some dystrophies and myositic conditions (Fig. 7.24). In diseased muscle, changes in desmin distribution accompany the myofibrillar disruption and disorientation seen in cores, mini-cores and ring fibres and with Z line streaming (Thornell et al 1983). Abnormal struc-

tures such as rods and cytoplasmic bodies have also been shown to have desmin associated with them (Jockusch et al 1980, Thornell et al 1980, Osborn & Goebel 1983).

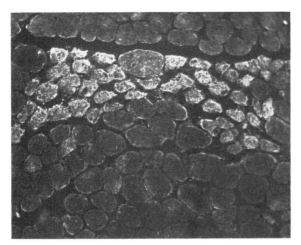

Fig. 7.24 Basophilic fibres in a two-year-old boy with Duchenne muscular dystrophy labelled with anti-desmin monoclonal antibody using an avidin-biotin-Texas red immunofluorescent technique. ×200

Myofibrillar proteins

In addition to the well-established components such as actin and myosin, immunocytochemistry has helped to identify several new proteins associated with the myofibrils (Fitzsimons & Sewry 1985). Several of these recently identified proteins have not yet been studied in human muscle but studies of their distribution in diseased muscle may prove to offer an important contribution to our understanding of the changes that occur.

The contractile proteins that have been studied in man include the myosin and troponin subtypes and α-actinin. Isomyosins can be categorised into two major groups — fast and slow — but there is considerable heterogeneity within these. Both heavy and light chains of myosin are polymorphic; and embryonic, fetal and adult forms of myosin can be identified. Most mature fibres contain only one myosin heavy chain type, slow or fast (Fig. 7.25), corresponding to histochemical fibre types I and II respectively (Billeter et al 1980). A few fibres in dystrophic muscle contain both a slow and a mature form of fast myosin. Some, but not all, of these correspond to type IIC fibres (Fig. 7.26). Other type IIC fibres, however, contain neither slow nor this mature fast myosin. During muscle development there is a transition from embryonic forms of myosin to fetal forms

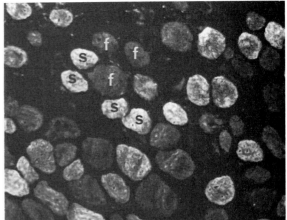

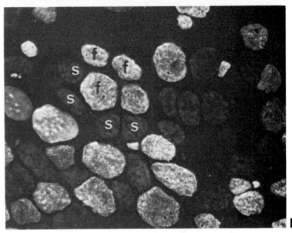

Fig. 7.25 Serial sections from a case of Duchenne muscular dystrophy labelled by an avidin-biotin-Texas red immunofluorescent technique with monoclonal antibodies to (a) slow myosin heavy chain (S) (type I fibres bright) and (b) fast myosin heavy chain (f) (type II fibres bright). ×230 (Antibodies courtesy of Dr R. Fitzsimons, MRC Cambridge)

and finally to the adult forms (Fitzsimons & Hoh 1981). Fetal myotubes have been shown to express adult slow myosin as early as 15–16 weeks' gestation (Thornell et al 1984) but traces of fetal myosin exist up to four weeks of post-natal life (Fitzsimons & Hoh 1981). We have found embryonic myosins in basophilic 'regenerating' fibres in Duchenne muscular dystrophy (Sewry et al 1986) (Fig. 7.27) and in some small fibres in spinal muscular atrophy (R. B. Fitzsimons, personal communication).

Studies of myosin subtypes have been shown to

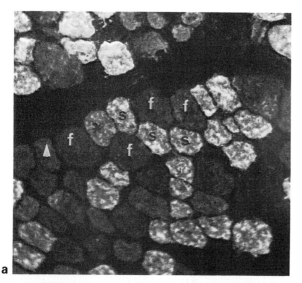

a

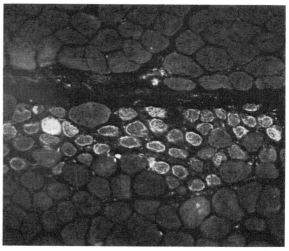

Fig. 7.27 Basophilic fibres from a case of Duchenne muscular dystrophy labelled with monoclonal antibody to embryonic myosin by an avidin-biotin-Texas red immunofluorescent technique. ×220. (Antibody courtesy of Dr R. Fitzsimons, MRC Cambridge)

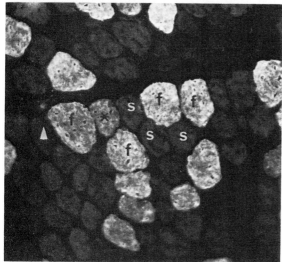

b

Fig. 7.26 Serial sections from a case of Duchenne muscular dystrophy labelled by an avidin-biotin-Texas red immunofluorescent technique with monoclonal antibodies to (a) slow myosin (s), (b) fast myosin (f). Most fibres contain either slow or fast myosin but occasional fibres contain both (★) or contain neither (△). ×300 (Antibodies courtesy of Dr R. Fitzsimons, MRC Cambridge)

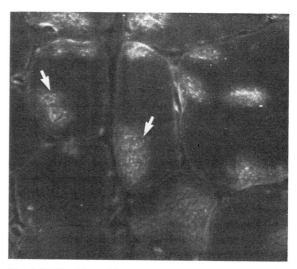

Fig. 7.28 Quadriceps biopsy from a case of nemaline myopathy showing α-actinin antibodies localised to the rods (arrows) using an indirect fluorescent technique. ×400

be of diagnostic value in a case report of a distal myopathy. Histochemical techniques showed uniformity of the fibres but immunostaining with myosin polyclonal antibodies revealed different fibre types (Thornell et al 1984). The investigation of myosin subtypes in diseased human muscle is already producing some interesting data and the expansion of such studies will lead to a better understanding of fibre-type distributions, of fibre-type conversions and of the coexistence of different myosin types within one fibre.

Immunochemically distinct slow and fast forms of troponin I also exist and are segregated into type I and type II fibres. In muscular dystrophies and spinal muscular atrophy, intermediate fibres occur which bind antibodies to fast and to slow troponin I (Dhoot & Pearce 1984a, b).

The major component of the Z line is α-actinin; antibodies to α-actinin have been shown to bind in large quantities to the rod-like structures that characterise nemaline myopathy (Jockusch et al 1980, Jennekens et al 1983) (Fig. 7.28). This supports the origin of rods from the Z line.

Inflammation

Cellular infiltrates are a feature of inflammatory myopathies and other myopathies, including muscular dystrophy. A panel of monoclonal antibodies has been used to characterise the T-cell subsets and B lymphocytes present in the infiltrates and to examine the proportions and distribution of these within biopsies (Arahata & Engel 1984, Engel & Arahata 1984, Giorno et al 1984). It has been found in inflammatory disorders that both suppressor/cytotoxic and helper/inducer phenotypes are present (Fig. 7.29) and the proportion of these varies between perivascular and endomysial areas. Iyer and co-workers (1983) however, have not found a difference in T-cell subpopulations in peripheral blood. Many of the infiltrating T cells in muscle biopsies are positive for HLA-DR and are therefore considered to be activated. In Duchenne muscular dystrophy where

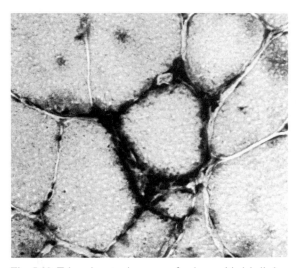

Fig. 7.29 T lymphocytes in a case of polymyositis labelled with an avidin-biotin-peroxidase technique. Counterstained with haematoxylin. ×300

cellular infiltrates are also observed, the suppressor/cytotoxic T-cell phenotype is predominant (Arahata & Engel 1984) suggesting that T-cell-mediated reactions may be involved.

Cathepsin D has also been identified immunochemically in interstitial cells and in invading phagocytes (Whitaker et al 1983).

Necrosis

Muscle fibre necrosis plays an important role in several neuromuscular disorders, in particular the muscular dystrophies and the inflammatory disorders. The cause of necrosis and the events leading to the final destruction of the fibre are, however, not fully understood. Calcium has been implicated as an important factor in necrosis but calcium overload is probably a secondary event (Sewry & Dubowitz 1984).

Necrotic fibres are usually identified by abnormalities in intensity with histological stains such as Gomori's trichrome. These fibres have already reached the terminal stage but little is known about the intermediate steps between the initial damage to the fibre and the 'point of no return'. Immunocytochemistry is revealing new information on the properties of necrotic fibres and may help to elucidate some of the events involved. Necrotic fibres contain C3, C9 (Fig. 7.21) and the membrane-attack complex C5b-9 (Engel & Biesecker 1982, Morgan et al 1984). The same necrotic fibres also contain excess calcium and are penetrated by albumin (Cornelio & Dones 1984). The peroxidase methods used in these studies did not reveal any complement binding to non-necrotic fibres in contrast to our own fluorescent studies with monoclonal antibodies to C9 (Morgan et al 1984) (see section on membranes pp. 256–257).

Necrotic fibres do not bind β-spectrin antibodies but their perimeter is always positive for the basement-membrane proteins lamimin and collagen type IV and they are often positive for HLA A, B, C class I antigens (Sewry et al 1986). Hypercontracted and necrotic fibres do not bind cathepsin D antibodies, suggesting that this lysosomal enzyme is not a marker for necrosis (Whitaker et al 1983).

Immunoglobulin (IgG) is deposited in necrotic

fibres and blood vessels in some muscle disorders (Engel & Biesecker 1982, Isenberg 1983) but caution in interpretation is needed when fluorescein-conjugated secondary antibodies are used, as these may bind non-specifically to necrotic fibres. In addition, IgG is present in the extracellular fluid and immunostaining will reveal binding of IgG to the sarcolemma and to connective tissue (Garlepp & Dawkins 1984). Some IgG may also diffuse from the extracellular fluid into necrotic fluids (Engel & Biesecker 1982).

Lectins

Lectins are proteins or glycoproteins of non-immune origin which bind to specific carbohydrate residues. They can be conjugated to biotin, enzymes or fluorochromes and their binding sites can be localised in tissue sections by similar detection systems as those used for conjugated antibodies (Ponder 1983).

Several lectins with various sugar specificities have been used to stain human muscle at both light-microscopic (Pena et al 1981, Dunn et al 1982, Capaldi et al 1985) and electron-microscopic levels (Bonilla et al 1978, Capaldi et al 1984a, b). Perimysial and endomysial connective tissue is stained by several lectins and parallels the distribution of extracellular matrix antibodies. Split fibres and whorled fibres also bind several lectins (Dunn et al 1982). An increase in staining intensity of the perimysial and endomysial connective tissue in X-linked muscular dystrophies has been reported with peanut agglutinin and wheat-germ agglutinin (Paljarvi et al 1984).

Fibre peripheries are clearly delineated with several lectins (Fig. 7.30) (Capaldi et al 1985). Electron microscopy, however, has revealed an absence of binding of Ricinus communis I agglutinin (RCA I) to the plasma membrane of muscle fibres from cases of Duchenne muscular dystrophy in contrast to its presence in normal muscle (Capaldi 1984a). Blood vessels and capillaries are also positively stained with several lectins. The lectin Bandeiraea simplicifolia agglutinin I (BSA I) is unusual in not staining the capillaries in muscle specimens from patients with blood group O; however, larger blood vessels are positive.

Internal staining of muscle fibres with lectins is

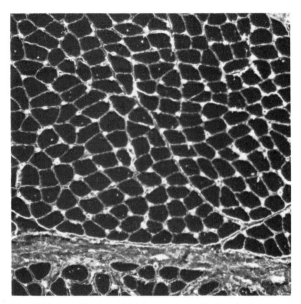

Fig. 7.30 Localisation of Ricinus communis I agglutinin in a quadriceps biopsy from a case of dermatomyositis using an avidin-biotin-Texas red fluorescent technique. The sarcolemma and connective tissue are both heavily labelled. ×150

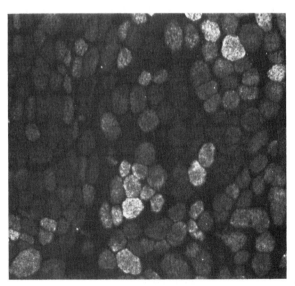

Fig. 7.31 Bandeiraea simplicifolia agglutinin I localisation in a quadriceps biopsy from a case of Duchenne muscular dystrophy using an avidin-biotin fluorescent technique. Several fibres are positively stained. ×120

not observed in normal muscle but in diseased muscle necrotic fibres are often positive. In Duchenne muscular dystrophy some fibres that do not appear to be necrotic stain with BSA I and some of the same fibres also bind C9 antibodies peripherally (Fig. 7.31).

Studies with lectins have shown that, although their binding is not solely governed by monosaccharide specificity, they are useful probes for identifying tissue glycoconjugates and can be used to reveal abnormalities in diseased muscle.

HISTOCHEMICAL CHANGES IN SPECIFIC DISEASES

The muscular dystrophies

Clinical assessment of patients with muscle disorders is often insufficient for accurate diagnosis. Histochemical techniques have an essential role in the differential diagnosis of neuromuscular disorders and they are now extensively applied to the study of the muscular dystrophies, diseases of the lower motor neurone, congenital myopathies and the glycogenoses as well as other, unclassified disorders.

Many of the histochemical abnormalities already referred to are non-specific and may occur in more than one clinical condition but experience has shown that consistent patterns of change can be attributed to certain diseases.

X-linked muscular dystrophies

Duchenne muscular dystrophy. This is the commonest and most severe form of muscular dystrophy. Histology and histochemistry reveal a diffuse pattern of pathology characterised by degeneration, loss of fibres with replacement by adipose and connective tissue, variation in fibre size and increased cellularity.

Both major fibre types show an abnormally wide variation in fibre size with hypertrophy of some and atrophy of others (Fig. 7.32). Some of the variation observed in cross-section is also due to branching of several fibres (Schmalbruch 1984). Mean diameter values, however, are not markedly altered. In an early histochemical study (Dubowitz & Pearse 1961) it was noticed that in advanced cases the abnormally large fibres were type II whereas the atrophic ones were of type I. Subsequent investigations have shown that this is not a consistent feature.

Alterations in fibre-type proportions occur and

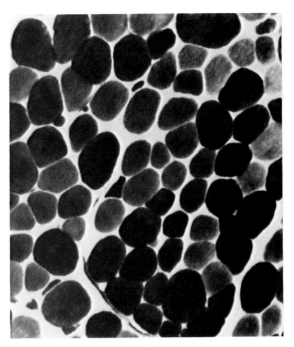

Fig. 7.32 Duchenne muscular dystrophy showing variability in fibre size with hypertrophy and atrophy of both fibre types. ATPase pH 9.4 ×200

a predominance of type I fibres is common (Fig. 7.33). The differentiation into type I and type II fibres with the routine pH 9.4 ATPase, however, is not always clear. Type IIC fibres, which are rare in normal muscle, frequently occur (Johnson & Kucukyalcin 1978, Nonaka et al 1981) and type IIB deficiency is also common.

Architectural changes in the intermyofibrillar network are relatively uncommon compared with other forms of dystrophy. Slight granularity or patchiness of stain are seen on occasion but motheaten and whorled fibres are less common than in other dystrophies (Fig. 7.33).

Degeneration, necrosis and phagocytosis are marked in Duchenne dystrophy. Necrotic fibres frequently occur in groups and they appear pale with the routine histological stains. Their histochemical fibre-type properties, however, are often retained.

Basophilic fibres also commonly occur in small groups and characterise biopsies of early cases. Basophilic fibres are considered to be regenerating fibres because of their high RNA content and the presence of a prominent nucleolus in the nucleus.

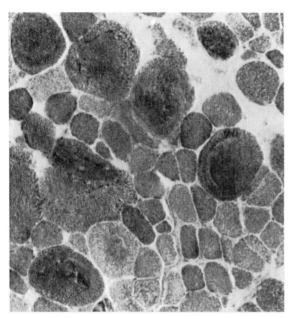

Fig. 7.33 Duchenne muscular dystrophy showing variation in fibre size, predominance of strongly reacting (type I fibres) fibres and presence of whorled fibres. NADH-TR ×200

The nucleus is often centrally placed. Basophilic fibres also contain increased activity of acid and alkaline phosphatases, cathepsin D, non-specific esterases and acetyl cholinesterase. Histochemically, they often correspond to the fetal IIC fibres and immunocytochemically they contain prominent amounts of desmin and embryonic myosin (Figs 7.24, 7.27). We have recently demonstrated, however, that β-spectrin antibodies do not always bind to these basophilic fibres (Fig. 7.23) and that some have complement associated with them. In addition, they all express HLA ABC class I antigens in contrast to normal mature fibres. This raises the question of whether the attempts at regeneration are abnormal or abortive, and whether the regeneration is still active at the stages examined.

Becker muscular dystrophy. This form of X-linked dystrophy is similar in clinical distribution to the Duchenne type but milder in severity (Becker & Kiener 1955). Recent studies with DNA probes have shown that the locus for the Becker type dystrophy is very close to that of Duchenne, suggesting that they may be allelic forms (Dorkins et al 1985).

Muscle biopsies show similar changes to those of Duchenne dystrophy in many cases (Ringel et al 1977, Dubowitz 1985) with a wide variation in the size of both fibre types. Type IIB fibres, however, are not deficient in contrast to Duchenne dystrophy. Some workers (Bradley et al 1978, ten Houten & De Visser 1984) have reported neurogenic changes in Becker dystrophy based on the presence of angular atrophic fibres, small groups of atrophic fibres, slight fibre-type grouping and clumps of pyknotic nuclei. There is no evidence, however, of any direct involvement of the nervous system.

Emery–Dreifuss muscular dystrophy. This is clinically distinct from both other X-linked dystrophies (Emery & Dreifuss 1966). Muscle biopsies usually show only mild changes with variation in fibre size, an increase in internal nuclei, occasional necrotic fibres and focal proliferation of connective tissue. Whorled, split and moth-eaten fibres may also occur (Figs. 7.34, 7.35). Recent studies with DNA probes have shown that the gene is separate from that of Duchenne or Becker dystrophy and is probably located near the end of the long arm of the X-chromosome.

Carriers of X-linked dystrophies. Muscle biopsies from known carriers of Duchenne and Becker muscular dystrophy may show changes (Dubowitz 1963ab, Emery 1963, Pearson et al 1963, Pearce et al 1966, Smith et al 1966, Roy & Dubowitz 1970, Morris & Raybould 1971a). Changes may occur when creatine kinase activity is normal but not all carriers have pathologically abnormal biopsies. The abnormalities are mild and include variation in fibre size, increase in internal nuclei and patchiness or moth-eaten fibres with oxidative enzyme techniques. Some biopsies from carriers are unequivocally abnormal but in others the significance of minor deviations is difficult to assess. We have shown, however, that quantitative assessment provides a good basis for evaluating the changes (Maunder-Sewry & Dubowitz 1981, Dubowitz 1985).

Other dystrophies. A number of histochemical and structural changes appear to be more characteristic of other dystrophic syndromes. The

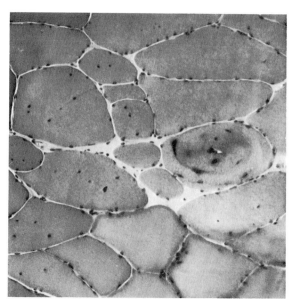

Fig. 7.34 Emery–Dreifuss dystrophy showing variation in fibre size, an increase in internal nuclei, a split fibre and a whorled fibre. Haematoxylin and eosin ×140

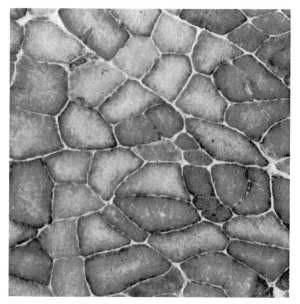

Fig. 7.35 Emery–Dreifuss dystrophy showing a normal fibre type distribution and only minor disruptions of the intermyofibrillar network. NADH-TR ×90

following are some of the more distinctive changes that occur in addition to the 'myopathic' changes in the biopsies.

Limb girdle muscular dystrophy. In contrast to Duchenne muscular dystrophy the standard pH 9.4 ATPase reaction shows good fibre-type differentiation. Oxidative enzyme techniques may show abundant moth-eaten and whorled fibres. Fibre-size variation is often very great with many extremely large fibres. Fibre splitting is common and the number of internal nuclei is often increased. Ring fibres also occur in several cases and are easily seen with the PAS stain or oxidative enzyme stains.

Facioscapulohumeral dystrophy. This slowly progressive form of dystrophy shows variable degrees of pathological change. Some biopsies show good retention of architecture and are characterised by scattered, very atrophic fibres and several hypertrophied fibres. Others are overtly dystrophic and moth-eaten and whorled fibres also occur. An inflammatory response may be a predominant feature in some biopsies.

Congenital muscular dystrophy. The pathological picture in this disorder is often very striking and may be disproportionate to the relatively static or slowly progressive nature of the disease; neither severity nor prognosis can therefore be assessed from the biopsy. There is usually marked proliferation of connective tissue and replacement of muscle by adipose tissue (Fig. 7.36). The residual fibres show some variation in fibre size but degenerative changes are mild. Type I fibres are often predominant and there is a high incidence of moth-eaten fibres.

Myotonic dystrophy. The distinctive features of this condition are selective atrophy of type I fibres and hypertrophy of type II fibres, particularly in the early stages of the disease (Fig. 7.37). Excessive numbers of internal nuclei occur and structural changes such as moth-eaten fibres, ring fibres and sarcoplasmic masses are common (Harper 1979).

Inflammatory myopathies

In dermatomyositis and polymyositis the classic feature is the marked inflammatory response. This, however, may be absent, particularly in

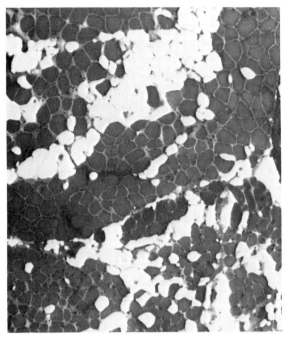

Fig. 7.36 Congenital muscular dystrophy showing replacement of large areas of muscle by adipose tissue and marked variation in fibre size. Haematoxylin and eosin ×75

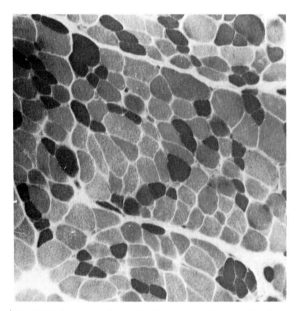

Fig. 7.37 Myotonic dystrophy in a boy aged seven showing atrophy of type 1 fibres (darkly stained) and hypertrophy of type II fibres (pale). ATPase pH 4.3 ×200

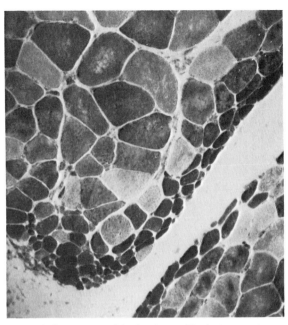

Fig. 7.38 Dermatomyositis showing perifascicular atrophy and the presence of 'moth-eaten' fibres. NADH-TR ×330

acute childhood dermatomyositis. Atrophy of both fibre types occurs and in dermatomyositis this has a characteristic perifascicular distribution (Fig. 7.38). Hypertrophy of fibres does not occur and can be used as a distinguishing feature. Oxidative enzyme staining may show dark-centred fibres, in addition to moth-eaten fibres (Whitaker 1982, Mastaglia & Ojeda 1985a,b, Dubowitz 1985). Vacuolar degeneration is frequently seen and in inclusion body myositis the vacuoles have a basophilic rim and contain basophilic inclusions (Carpenter et al 1978). In dermatomyositis the connective tissue is reactive for alkaline phosphatase (Engel 1977).

Metabolic myopathies

Glycogenoses. The inborn errors of glycogen metabolism have been categorised into seven types (Cori 1958); four of these affect muscle and a fifth (type IV) may also do so. Type II glycogenosis (acid maltase deficiency) — the severest form (Pompe's disease) — affects infants and is usually fatal but there is also a milder myopathy of late onset presenting as a mild proximal weakness. Biopsies characteristically show vacuolation and

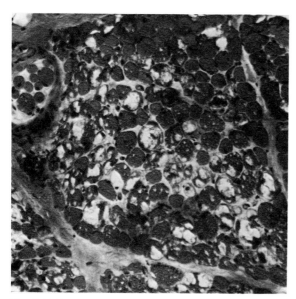

Fig. 7.39 Type II glycogenosis (Pompe's disease) showing marked vacuolation. Haematoxylin and eosin ×390

excess glycogen (Fig. 7.39). The vacuolated fibres also show high activity of acid phosphatase. Vacuolation can also be demonstrated in lymphocytes (Trend et al 1985). Type III glycogenosis (debranching enzyme deficiency) is characterised by an abnormal form of glycogen in cardiac and skeletal muscle and the liver (Illingworth & Cori 1952, Forbes 1953, Krivit et al 1953) due to the absence of amylo-1,6-glucosidase. Changes in biopsies are not marked and the overall architecture is retained. The PAS stain shows a moderately strong reaction but differentiation of fibre types is retained.

Type V glycogenosis (myophosphorylase deficiency). In 1951 McArdle described a myopathy due to a defect in the breakdown of muscle glycogen. It was later shown that this was due to an absence of myophosphorylase (Schmid & Mahler 1959). Pathological changes in muscle biopsies are mild in type V glycogenosis although occasional necrotic fibres may be present. The consistent findings are an absence of phosphorylase and excess glycogen on PAS staining. Different isomeric forms of phosphorylase exist in fetal and cultured muscle compared with mature muscle (Sato et al 1977, DiMauro et al 1978). Thus phos-

phorylase activity can be demonstrated histochemically in regenerating muscle fibres and cultured myotubes from patients with type V glycogenosis (Roelofs et al 1972, Mitsumoto 1979). There is also an infantile form of phosphorylase deficiency which presents as a floppy infant syndrome in the neonatal period.

Type VII glycogenosis. The histological changes are similar to those of McArdle's disease and the absence of phosphofructokinase can be demonstrated histochemically (Bonilla & Schotland 1970).

A number of additional glycogenoses affecting muscle have been identified over the past few years, including lactic dehydrogenase deficiency (Kanno et al 1980), phosphoglycerate kinase deficiency (Rosa et al 1982, DiMauro et al 1983) and phosphoglycerate mutase deficiency (DiMauro et al 1981).

Mitochondrial myopathies. The mitochondrial myopathies are a complex, heterogeneous group of neuromuscular disorders in which structurally abnormal mitochondria in the muscle are associated with an identifiable or presumptive metabolic defect. The structural changes in mitochondria are varied and non-specific (Sewry 1985). No specific abnormality has yet been associated with a particular biochemical defect (Morgan-Hughes 1982).

Mitochondrial myopathies may be overlooked on routine histological staining (although they may show some increased granularity of fibres with H and E and Verhoeff–van Gieson stains) but they are usually suspected from the presence of disrupted, red-staining fibres with the Gomori trichome stain ('ragged-red fibres') and from very strongly reactive fibres on oxidative enzyme preparations (Fig. 7.40). They are confirmed on electron microscopy by the presence of an abnormality in number, size and structure of the mitochondria. Ernster et al (1959) and Luft et al (1962) first recorded a case of myopathy associated with abnormal mitochondria and hypermetabolism. Shy et al (1966) described two cases of myopathy with abnormal mitochondria, which they labelled 'megaconial' and 'pleoconial' myopathy respectively; there was no associated hypermetabolism.

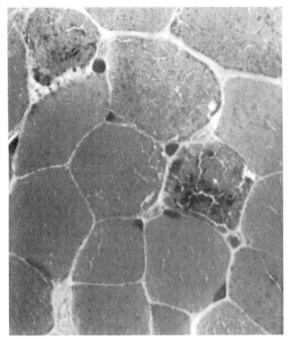

a

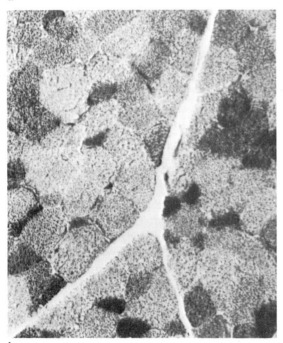

b

Fig. 7.40 Mitochondrial myopathy showing (a) 'ragged red fibres' with the Gomori trichrome stain (×560); and (b) several fibres with intense oxidative activity. NADH-TR ×330

Similar cases were subsequently reported by van Wijngaarden et al (1967) and by Price et al (1967). In all these cases the abnormality could be suspected in the histochemical preparations for oxidative enzymes, which show aggregates of prominent mitochondria, especially in the subsarcolemmal region (Fig. 7.41).

Mitochondrial myopathy is not a single entity, but mitochondrial abnormalities have now been described in a large number of different clinical syndromes of muscle weakness, including the limb girdle and facioscapulohumeral syndromes and cases with distal weakness. Mitochondrial abnormalities are a consistent feature in the so-called oculocraniosomatic syndrome or 'ophthalmoplegia plus' (Kearns & Sayre 1958, Drachmann 1968, Olson et al 1972). In this there is external ophthalmoplegia, pigmentary retinopathy and heart block in association usually with only mild skeletal weakness and with other syndromes affecting the central nervous system.

In floppy infants there is also considerable heterogeneity and at present these mitochondrial myopathies can be categorized into: (1) a fatal mitochondrial myopathy with onset in the neonatal period, associated with renal dysfunction

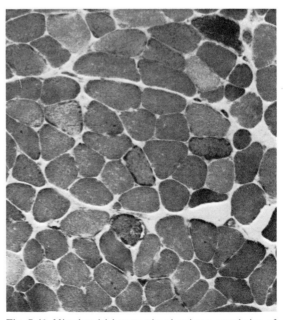

Fig. 7.41 Mitochondrial myopathy showing a population of fibres with intense oxidative activity at the periphery of the fibres. NADH-TR ×120

and a deficiency of cytochrome *c* oxidase; (2) a benign mitochondrial myopathy without renal involvement but associated with cytochrome *c* oxidase deficiency; (3) a benign mitochondrial myopathy without cytochrome *c* deficiency or currently recognisable biochemical deficiency. In addition there is a mitochondrial-lipid-glycogen myopathy without renal involvement or cytochrome oxidase deficiency.

Lipid storage myopathies. In 1970 Engel et al (1970b) reported excess lipid droplets in muscle biopsies from identical twin sisters who had muscle cramps and myoglobinuria some hours after exercise; they postulated a defect in the utilisation of long-chain fatty acids. Bressler (1970) predicted that a deficiency of carnitine or carnitine palmityl transferase (CPT) could account for this lipid storage myopathy. Since then many cases of carnitine or CPT deficiency have been described (Pleasure & Bonilla 1982). In carnitine deficiency lipid accumulation is more striking in type I fibres than type II. Carnitine palmityl transferase deficiency, however, is not usually associated with marked lipid storage in the muscle fibres.

Other metabolic myopathies. Pathological changes can be found in a variety of other metabolic myopathies including malignant hyperpyrexia (Harriman 1982), periodic paralysis (Tomé 1982) and endocrine myopathies (Hudgson & Hall 1982, Dubowitz 1985). Most histochemical features are non-specific and include selective type II atrophy, moth-eaten fibres, core-targetoid fibres and vacuolar changes. In periodic paralysis there is a characteristic vacuolar myopathy, especially during attacks of weakness, and an additional peculiar feature is the presence of tubular aggregates (Engel et al 1970a, Pearse & Johnson 1970, Lewis et al 1971). These are confined to type II fibres and show an intense reaction with oxidative enzymes but lack ATPase staining. With electron microscopy they have a characteristic tubular appearance.

The congenital myopathies

The wider application of histochemical techniques to muscle biopsies in recent decades has helped to delineate a series of conditions with specific structural changes in the muscle. Many of these are not apparent on routine histological preparations. Congenital myopathies usually present in infancy with a floppy infant syndrome, or later with relatively non-progressive muscle weakness.

Central core disease. In 1956 Shy & Magee described a new congenital non-progressive myopathy characterised histologically by amorphous central cores within the fibres. With a trichrome stain the central core stained blue, whereas the periphery was red. The core was strongly positive with the PAS reaction but this was not influenced by diastase treatment. Greenfield et al (1958) subsequently named the condition central core disease. A patient with the same illness was extensively investigated by Engel et al (1961). They found that the core region stained more deeply than the non-core region with a number of acidic as well as basic dyes. With a Gomori trichrome stain, the core regions were purple and the non-core region red; in this case the core did not contain PAS-positive material. Most fibres had a single central core but a second biopsy from the vastus lateralis showed multiple cores in most fibres. Histochemical studies of this biopsy showed that the cores were devoid of enzymes (Dubowitz & Pearse 1960c) and that most of the fibres were high in oxidative enzymes and low in phosphorylase. In longitudinal section the cores ran the length of the fibre. The enzyme pattern in biopsies from both parents was normal and showed the usual division into fibre types and reciprocal relationship of oxidative enzymes and phosphorylase.

Bethlem & Meyjes (1960) described the histological features of a biopsy from the triceps of a Dutch patient with this disease: almost all the fibres had a single central core. There have been several reports of central core disease since the initial cases and the cores have consistently been found to affect type I fibres. In some cases the muscle appears to be undifferentiated and to be composed entirely, or almost entirely, of type I fibres (Dubowitz & Pearse 1960c, Gonatas et al 1965, Dubowitz & Roy 1970). In others, fibre-type differentiation is present and the type I fibres are selectively affected (Dubowitz & Platts

1965, Bethlem et al 1966, Dubowitz & Roy 1970). Occasional cases show involvement of type II fibres (Dubowitz & Brooke 1973, Pongratz et al 1976).

Fibres may have a single central core, a single eccentric core or have multiple cores. There is also an apparent evolution of cores with time (Dubowitz 1985). A four-year-old boy whose mother had centrally placed cores in all type I fibres showed eccentrically placed cores in only 3% of his type I fibres (Fig. 7.42a). A follow-up biopsy 12 years later showed an identical picture to that of his mother with almost every fibre having a single, or occasional multiple, central core (Fig. 7.42b).

The absence of enzyme activity in the cores suggests that they are a non-functional part of the fibre. Histochemical findings are further supported by the electron-microscopic features which show almost complete absence of mitochondria in the core region and varying degrees of myofibrillar disruption (Sewry 1985). Neville & Brooke (1973) suggested that central cores can be divided into 'structured' and 'unstructured' types according to their electron-microscopic appearance. In structured cores the myofibrils are contracted but the striation pattern is retained and ATPase activity remains in the core. Unstructured cores, in contrast, show severe myofibrillar disruption and large amounts of Z line material, while ATPase activity is absent. Cases showing structured and unstructured cores in the same biopsy have been reported (Telermann-Toppet et al 1973, Isaacs et al 1975) but Neville (1979) considers that this is unusual and that it is more common to find only one type of core in a given patient with central core disease.

Engel (1961) observed 'target' fibres in adult patients with long-standing neurogenic atrophies (Fig. 7.4) and in view of their resemblance to central cores suggested that the latter might be due to denervation. Core-like structures have also been observed in experimental animals during reinnervation (Dubowitz 1967) and following tenotomy (Shafiq et al 1969).

Several cases have been reported that show both central cores and rod bodies (nemaline rods) (Afifi et al 1965, Karpati et al 1971, Telermann-Toppet et al 1973, Isaacs et al 1975, Bethlem et al 1978,

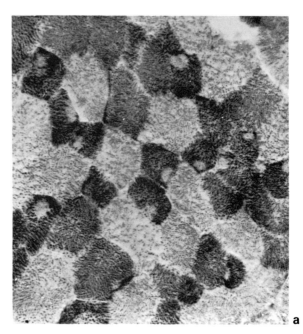

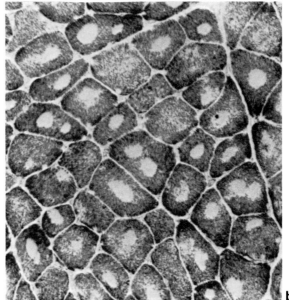

Fig. 7.42 Central core disease. (a) Biopsy from quadriceps of four-year-old boy showing a normal distribution of fibre types and the presence of eccentric cores in several type I fibres. NADH-TR ×330. (b) Biopsy from the same child as in (a) at 16 years of age showing evolution of the disease with uniformity of fibre type and centrally placed cores in almost all fibres. NADH-TR ×200

Dubowitz 1985). This questions the specificity of some morphological entities but in most situations one feature predominates.

Minicore disease (Multicore disease). Ultrastructurally, minicores resemble unstructured cores with marked myofibrillar disruption. They affect varying numbers of sarcomeres but never run the length of the fibre, unlike central cores.

In 1971 Engel et al documented two unrelated children with a benign congenital non-progressive myopathy associated with multifocal areas of degeneration in the muscle fibres. The foci showed a decrease in mitochondrial enzyme activity and also focal myofibrillar degeneration (Fig. 7.3). The condition is probably distinct from central core disease as it appears to have an autosomal recessive inheritance. As in central core disease, there is a tendency for the muscle to show type I fibre predominance and for the minicores to have a predilection for type I fibres (Dubowitz 1978). On routine histological staining the muscle may look essentially normal, apart from some variability in fibre size and the presence of fibres with internal nuclei.

Nemaline myopathy. This is another non-progressive congenital myopathy. The characteristic rod bodies or nemaline rods were first recognised by Conen et al (1963) and Shy et al (1963). The nemaline rods are devoid of enzyme activity and stain red with the Gomori trichrome. They have been shown in electron microscopy to be in continuity with the Z bands (Price et al 1965, Sewry 1985). Recent studies have shown that rods resemble Z lines in several respects. Their lattice structure is similar and both rods and Z lines contain α-actinin and tropomyosin (Schollmeyer et al 1974, Jockusch et al 1980). Desmin is also located at their periphery and they may contain actin (Thornell et al 1980, Yamaguchi et al 1978, 1982).

Nienhuis et al (1967) noted in their cases of nemaline myopathy that all fibres were uniform in enzyme activity and showed no differentiation into fibre types. Other cases may show fibre typing and a tendency towards a bimodal distribution of small and large fibres with the type I fibres being atrophic. In these cases the rods tend to be confined to the atrophic type I fibres (Gonatas et al 1966, Dubowitz 1978) but other cases show involvement of both fibre types (Shafiq et al 1967)

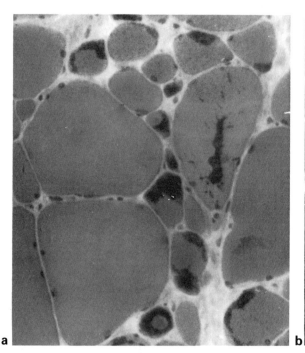
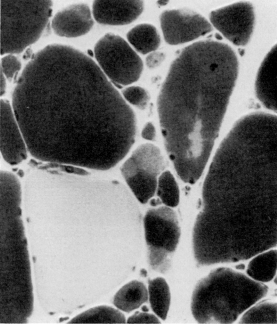

a   b

Fig. 7.43 Nemaline myopathy. Biopsy of gastrocnemius from 12-year-old boy showing (a) variation in fibre size and presence of dark (red) stained rods (Gomori trichrome × 330) and (b) absence of staining in the rods with the ATPase reaction. ATPase, pH 4.3 × 330

or selective involvement of type II fibres (Shy et al 1963) (Fig. 7.43).

Studies of the distribution of rods in several muscles from autopsied cases have shown variation in the proportion of affected fibres between muscles and also in different parts of the same muscle (Shafiq et al 1967). There is no correlation between the number of rods or affected fibres and clinical severity (Nienhuis et al 1967).

Although rods are the characteristic feature of nemaline myopathy, they have been observed in a variety of other conditions and in normal human extraocular muscle (Mukuno 1969) and myotendinous regions.

Centronuclear myopathy (Myotubular myopathy). In the first reported case of this non-progressive (or slowly progressive) myopathy, Spiro et al (1966) suggested the name myotubular myopathy because several fibres had centrally placed prominent nuclei and resembled myotubes of fetal muscle. Sher et al (1967) suggested the term centronuclear myopathy as an alternative name. Their two cases showed normal subdivision into type I and type II fibres, as in mature muscle. Since these early reports a large number of cases have been published. Several differences exist from case to case and subdivisions of centronuclear myopathy are now recognised. These differ clinically, pathologically and genetically (Dubowitz 1980, Fardeau 1982, Heckmatt et al 1985).

The characteristic common to all types is the presence of a population of fibres with central nuclei (Fig. 7.44). The central region also shows a striking aggregation of oxidative enzyme activity, often with a clear halo. Some fibres also show a radial deposition of the intermyofibrillar network. The ATPase reaction shows a consistent absence of activity in the central zones.

Severe X-linked centronuclear myopathy. A severe form of centronuclear myopathy was reported by van Wijngaarden et al (1969) and by Barth et al

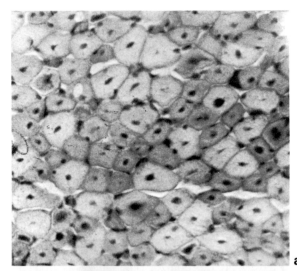
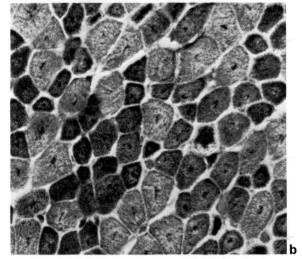
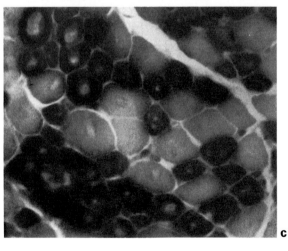

Fig. 7.44 Myotubular myopathy. Biopsy from rectus femoris of 14-year-old boy showing (a) striking internal nuclei (VG ×330). (b) Focal aggregation of oxidative activity at site of nuclei(NADH-TR ×330). (c) 'Holes' in fibres at site of nuclei due to absence of myofibrillar structure. ATPase ×330

(1975) in different families with an apparent X-linked pattern of inheritance and a high mortality. Muscle biopsies show uniform small fibres with few large fibres. Central nuclei are apparent in only a proportion of the fibres in transverse section as they tend to be separated from one another in longitudinal sections and the plane of section may not always pass through the nucleus. The central region shows the characteristic concentration of oxidative enzyme staining and lack of ATPase staining. The female carriers clinically show no signs of the disorder but muscle biopsies may show mild pathological changes with central nuclei in some small fibres (Heckmatt et al 1985).

Centronuclear myopathy with type I fibre hypotrophy. Engel et al (1968) reported an 11-month-old child with severe and progressive weakness, whose muscle had profuse central nuclei, restricted to type I fibres, which were also small in diameter. They suggested that this might represent a maturational arrest, or 'hypotrophy' of the type I fibres rather than an atrophy. Further cases with milder clinical involvement but a similar biopsy picture have been reported by Bethlem et al (1969), Karpati et al (1970) and Dubowitz (1985).

Congenital fibre-type disproportion. In their histographic analysis of muscle biopsies, Brooke & Engel (1969) suggested classifying children's biopsies according to the relative size of type I and type II fibres. Normally the fibre types are of approximately equal diameter. In some cases with a relatively non-progressive weakness, type I fibres were noted to be smaller than type II. Brooke (1973) subsequently delineated a fairly consistent clinical picture, usually presenting with hypotonia at birth or in early infancy and having a benign course. The only abnormality on biopsy is the disproportion in size of the fibre types, with striking and uniform atrophy of the type I fibres and normal-sized or enlarged type II fibres (Fig. 7.45). Type I fibres are frequently predominant.

This condition has to be distinguished from dystrophia myotonica and myotubular myopathy with type I fibre atrophy, which also present with

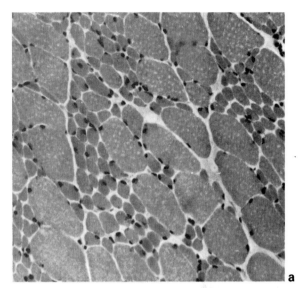

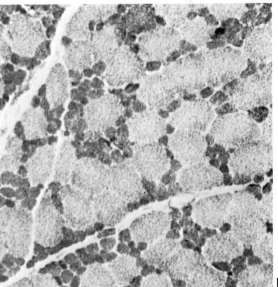

Fig. 7.45 Congenital fibre type disproportion in 4½-year-old floppy weak child, showing (a) presence of two populations of fibres on routine staining (H and E ×200).
(b) Strikingly uniform atrophy (hypotrophy) of type I fibres (dark) in contrast to normal sized or enlarged type II fibres. NADH-TR ×200

hypotonia and weakness in early infancy (Dubowitz & Brooke 1973) and from the early stage of infantile spinal muscular atrophy (Werdnig–Hoffmann disease) (Dubowitz 1980), where all the fibres may be small with type I smaller than type II.

Infantile hypotonia. There are many causes of the floppy infant syndrome and this has been the subject of a separate monograph (Dubowitz 1980). From a practical point of view it is important to separate those cases with weakness and involvement of the lower motor neurone from the floppy infants with hypotonia of 'central' nervous origin or related to more remote disorders. In addition to electrodiagnostic investigations, which offer a useful screening test for identifying a myopathic, neurogenic or normal pattern of muscle activity, muscle biopsy with detailed histochemical study is essential in this group of disorders in order to differentiate between spinal muscular atrophy and congenital muscular dystrophy, or to identify one of the rarer forms of congenital myopathy with specific structural abnormality. In the congenital form of myotonic dystrophy, the muscle may be essentially normal apart from a tendency to atrophy of type I fibres, and the diagnosis is more readily confirmed by clinical and electrodiagnostic assessment of the mother, who invariably has the dominantly inherited condition. In the Prader–Willi syndrome (Prader et al 1956, Prader & Willi 1963) the infant presents with profound hypotonia and associated sucking and swallowing difficulty at birth, but with relatively good muscle power and a gradual resolution of the hypotonia. Muscle biopsy is unlikely to be of diagnostic help as the histological and histochemical patterns are usually normal. The diagnosis then has to rest on the typical clinical features and identifying the deletion in chromosome 15, which is present in about 50% of cases.

Congenital myopathies with abnormal ultra-structural inclusions. The occurrence of some ultrastructural abnormalities has been shown to characterise some congenital myopathies. These include fingerprint body myopathy (Engel et al 1972, Fardeau et al 1976), sarcotubular myopathy (Jerusalem et al 1973), zebra body myopathy (Lake & Wilson 1975), reducing body myopathy (Brooke & Neville 1972, Dubowitz 1985), cytoplasmic body myopathy (Jerusalem et al 1979), and trilaminar muscle fibre disease (Ringel et al 1978). These disorders may show changes in the normal fibre-type-pattern, particularly in relation to fibre size and fibre-type proportions.

Neurogenic atrophies

Many clinical disorders affect the lower motor neurone, some having a proximal distribution of weakness (e.g. the spinal muscular atrophies) and others a distal distribution (e.g. peroneal muscular atrophy). Although the biopsy in all of them will reflect the denervating process, detailed histochemical studies have revealed patterns more or less distinctive for some of these syndromes.

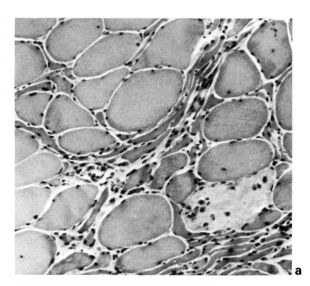

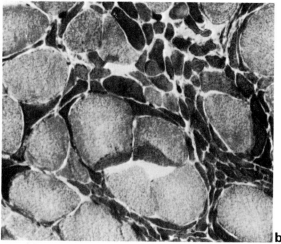

Fig. 7.46 Neurogenic atrophy. Biopsy from quadriceps of 35-year-old man with rapidly progressive motor neurone disease showing (a) large groups of atrophic fibres and also 'myopathic changes' in some large fibres with internal nuclei and presence of necrotic (pale) fibres (H and E ×120). (b) Mixed fibre-type pattern in atrophic fibres and uniformity of enzyme reaction in large fibres. NADH-TR ×120

The characteristic histological change in (long-standing) denervation of muscle is uniform atrophy of groups of muscle fibres, so-called 'large-group atrophy' or 'small-group atrophy', in association with other fibres of normal or enlarged size (Fig. 7.46). Histochemically, the atrophic fibres are of both fibre types, thus helping to distinguish this condition from those with selective atrophy of one fibre type. The large fibres are often uniform in type, suggesting that they are reinnervated rather than normal unaffected fibres, which would have a mixed pattern (Fig. 7.46).

Another pattern characteristic of denervation is fibre type-grouping, where large clusters of the fibre type occur alongside clusters of fibres of the other type (Fig. 7.47). This represents a process of reinnervation of previously denervated fibres, as a result of sprouting of the terminal axons of surviving nerves. It is usually a feature of long-standing and relatively slowly progressive neuropathies and the muscle biopsy may be completely normal apart from the type grouping.

'Target' fibres are also a feature of longstanding denervation (Engel 1961). They resemble central cores in their oxidative enzyme pattern, except for the presence of three zones of activity — the central zone devoid of enzyme activity, the outer normal-staining region of the fibre and an intermediate darkly stained zone (Fig. 7.4) — in contrast to the two zones in central core disease.

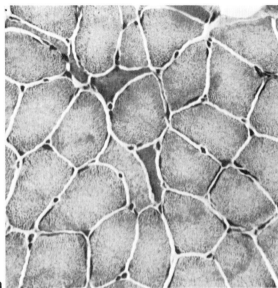

a

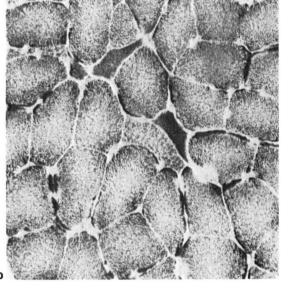

b

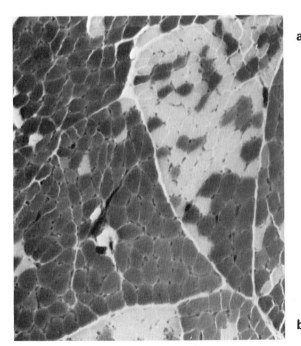

Fig. 7.47 Fibre type-grouping, showing clusters of fibres of uniform fibre type, characteristic of reinnervation. Biopsy of gastrocnemius of five-year-old girl with mild almost non-progressive neurogenic weakness (?spinal muscular atrophy, ?peripheral neuropathy). ATPase ×120

Fig. 7.48 Biopsy from rectus femoris of 12-year-old boy with mild slowly progressive motor neurone disease showing focal angulated atrophic fibres which have intense activity with oxidative enzyme reaction, while remaining fibres are uniform in enzyme activity, suggesting a reinnervation process. (a) VVG ×330; (b) NADH-TR ×330

Another feature suggestive of denervation is the presence of small angulated fibres with a very intense reaction for NADH-tetrazolium reductase (Fig. 7.48). These fibres vary in their ATPase activity, some being strongly reacting (corresponding to type II) and others weakly reacting (corresponding to type I).

Spinal muscular atrophy. One of the common forms of neurogenic atrophy is spinal muscular atrophy, a genetically determined condition (usually autosomal recessive), in which there is degeneration of the anterior horn cells of the cord and at times of cranial nerve nuclei. The condition ranges in severity from the very severe infantile spinal muscular atrophy (Werdnig–Hoffmann disease) at one extreme, to the very mild proximal neurogenic atrophy (Kugelberg–Welander disease) with only limited proximal weakness at the other, and an intermediate group, spanning the two extremes. Overlap in severity may occasionally be observed within a family (Dubowitz 1964).

Biopsies in the severe infantile cases and in cases of intermediate severity look very similar, irrespective of the degree of weakness (Fig. 7.49). They usually show large group atrophy; occasionally a section may show universal atrophy. The atrophic fibres are rounded and of both fibre types. This mixed pattern suggests that, even in the congenital cases, with weakness already present at birth, the process is one of denervation of previously fully mature muscle, already differentiated into fibre types, but a maturational arrest of embryonic fibres has been suggested by some authors in the past (Dubowitz 1966). The large fibres may occur singly or in clusters and tend to be uniform in enzyme activity, suggesting reinnervation of the muscle by sprouting of nerves of one type (Fig. 7.49). They are more often uniformly of type I, but at times type II or even a mixture of the two.

In milder cases there may be less extensive

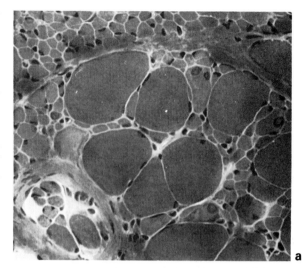

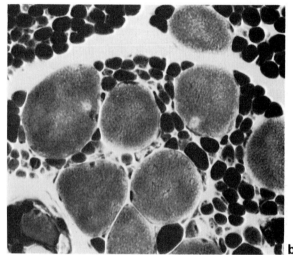

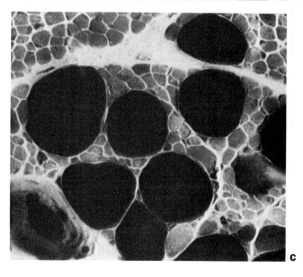

Fig. 7.49 Spinal muscular atrophy of intermediate severity in a 21-month-old child. Rectus femoris shows atrophy of large groups of fibres of mixed fibre type, together with enlarged fibres of uniform enzyme type. Note muscle spindle (bottom left) with intrafusal fibres of size comparable with the atrophic fibres. Serial sections. (a) H and E; (b) ATPase pH 9.4; (c) ATPase pH 4.6 ×330

atrophy and the presence of fibre-type grouping in otherwise normal-looking bundles. However, the extent of the atrophy varies considerably even in cases of equal clinical severity and it is not possible to prognosticate on the basis of the biopsy findings.

In the longstanding Kugelberg–Welander variety, the fibres may in addition show structural changes in the large fibres, such as coil fibres and disruption of the intermyofibrillar network. Some of the large fibres may also have internal nuclei, which are not a feature of the large fibres in the severe forms.

The uniformity of enzyme activity in the large fibres is almost certainly indicative of reinnervation. The influence of innervation on the fibre type has been conclusively demonstrated in recent studies of cross-innervation of slow and fast muscles in animals. Immunocytochemical studies with antibodies to myosin isomers have shown similar patterns of fibre-type grouping and have confirmed that some atrophic fibres contain a fetal form of myosin (R. B. Fitzsimons, personal communication). Further immunocytochemical investigations may reveal the stage at which the denervation occurs.

CONCLUSION

Histochemistry, in particular enzyme histochemistry, has made a considerable contribution to the understanding of normal and diseased muscle. The techniques are essential to the investigation of muscle biopsies and they are now widely accepted as routine procedures. The application of immunocytochemical techniques is providing further insight into the structure and development of normal muscle as well as the changes associated with disease. Immunocytochemistry has opened new avenues of exploration and may yet prove to have the same revolutionary impact on the field of muscle pathology as histochemistry.

ACKNOWLEDGEMENTS

We are grateful to Dr. M. H. Brooke and Baillière Tindall for permission to reproduce Figure 7.11 and to Baillière Tindall for permission to reproduce the following figures: 7.3, 7.4, 7.5, 7.6, 7.7, 7.15, 7.17, 7.18, 7.21b, 7.28, 7.34, 7.35, 7.36, 7.37, 7.39, 7.40, 7.41, 7.42a, 7.42b, 7.43a, 7.43b, 7.44b, 7.44c, 7.45a, 7.45b, 7.48b, 7.49b, 7.49c. We thank Mrs C. Hutson and Mrs C. Lovegrove for technical assistance, Mrs Karen Davidson for photographic assistance and Mrs C. Trand for typing the manuscript.

We also gratefully acknowledge the financial support for the work reported in this chapter from the Muscular Dystrophy Group of Great Britain, the Medical Research Council and the Muscular Dystrophy Association of America.

REFERENCES

Adams R D, Coërs C, Walton J N 1968 Report of a subcommittee on the quantitation of muscle biopsy findings. Journal of the Neurological Sciences 6: 179–188

Afifi A K, Smith J W, Zellweger H 1965 Congenital nonprogressive myopathy. Central core and nemaline myopathy in one family. Neurology 15: 371–381

Andersen P 1975 Capillary density in skeletal muscle of man. Acta Physiologica Scandinavica 95: 203–205

Appleyard S T, Dunn M J, Dubowitz V, Scott M L, Pittman S J, Shotton D M 1984 Monoclonal antibodies detect a spectrin-like protein in normal and dystrophic human skeletal muscle. Proceedings of the National Academy of Sciences (USA) 81: 776–780

Appleyard S T, Dunn M J, Dubowitz V, Rose M L 1985 Increased expression of HLA ABC class I antigens by muscle fibres in Duchenne muscular dystrophy, inflammatory myopathy and other neuromuscular disorders. Lancet i: 361–363

Arahata K, Engel A G 1984 Monoclonal antibody analysis of mononuclear cells in myopathies. I Quantitation of subsets according to diagnosis and sites of accumulation and demonstration and counts of muscle fibers invaded by T cells. Annals of Neurology 16: 193–208

Bancroft J D, Stevens A (eds) 1982 Theory and practice of histological techniques, 2nd edn. Churchill Livingstone, Edinburgh

Barth P G, van Wijngaarden G K, Bethlem J 1975 X-linked myotubular myopathy with fatal neonatal asphyxia. Neurology (Minneapolis) 25: 531–536

Becker P E, Kiener F 1955 Eine neue X-chromosomale Muskeldystrophie. Archiv für Psychiatrie und Nervenkrankenheiten 193:427

Bertolotto A, Palmucci L, Doriguzzi C, Mongini T, Gagnor E, Del Rosso M, Tarone G 1983 Laminin and fibronectin distribution in normal and pathological human muscle. Journal of the Neurological Sciences 60: 377–382

Bethlem J, Meyjes F E P 1960 Congenital, nonprogressive central core disease of Shy and Magee. Psychiatria, Neurologia, Neurochirurgia 63:246

Bethlem J, van Gool J, Hülsmann W C, Meijer A E F H 1966 Familial non-progressive myopathy with muscle cramps after exercise. A new disease associated with cores in the muscle fibres. Brain 89: 569–588

Bethlem J, van Wijngaarden G K, Meijer A E F H, Hülsmann W C 1969 Neuromuscular disease with type 1 fiber atrophy, central nuclei, and myotube-like structures. Neurology 19: 705–710

Bethlem J, Arts W F, Dingermans K P 1978 Common origin of rods, miniature cores and focal loss of cross-striation. Archives of Neurology (Chicago) 35: 555–566

Billeter R, Weber H, Lutz H, Howald H, Eppenberger H M, Jenny E 1980 Myosin types in human skeletal muscle fibers. Histochemistry 65: 249–259

Bird J W C, Spanier A M, Schwartz W N 1978 Cathepsin B and D: proteolytic activity and ultrastructural localisation in skeletal muscle. In: Segal H L, Doyl D J (eds) Protein turnover and lysosome function. Academic Press, New York, p 589–604

Bonilla E, Schotland D L 1970 Histochemical diagnosis of muscle phosphofructokinase deficiency. Archives of Neurology (Chicago) 2: 8–12

Bonilla E, Schotland D L, Wakayama Y 1978 Duchenne dystrophy: focal alterations in the distribution of Concanavalin A binding sites at the muscle cell surface. Annals of Neurology 4: 117–123

Bradley W G, Jones M Z, Mussini J-M, Fawcett P R W 1978 Becker-type muscular dystrophy. Muscle and Nerve 1: 111–132

Bressler R 1970 Carnitine and the twins (editorial). New England Journal of Medicine 282: 745–746

Brooke M H 1973 A neuromuscular disease characterized by fiber type disproportion. In: Kakulas B A (ed) Proceedings of II International Congress on Muscle Disease, ICS No. 237. Excerpta Medica, Amsterdam

Brooke M H, Engel W K 1969 The histographic analysis of human muscle biopsies with regard to fibre types. 4. Children's biopsies. Neurology (Minneapolis) 19: 591–605

Brooke M H, Kaiser K K 1970 Muscle fiber types: how many and what kind? Archives of Neurology 23: 369–379

Brooke M H, Williamson E, Kaiser K K 1971 The behavior of four fiber types in developing and reinnervated muscle. Archives of Neurology 25: 360–366

Brooke M H, Neville H E 1972 Reducing body myopathy. Neurology 22: 829–940

Capaldi M J, Dunn M J, Sewry C A, Dubowitz V 1984a Altered binding of Ricinus communis I lectin by muscle membranes in Duchenne muscular dystrophy. Journal of the Neurological Sciences 63: 129–142

Capaldi M J, Dunn M J, Sewry C A, Dubowitz V 1984b Binding of Ricinus communis I lectin to the muscle cell plasma membrane in diseased muscle. Journal of the Neurological Sciences 64: 315–324

Capaldi M J, Dunn M J, Sewry C A, Dubowitz V 1985 Lectin binding in human skeletal muscle: a comparison of 15 different lectins. Histochemical Journal 17: 81–92

Carpenter S, Karpati G, Heller I, Eisen A 1978 Inclusion body myositis: a distinct variety of idiopathic inflammatory myopathy. Neurology 28: 8–17

Colling-Saltin A 1978 Enzyme histochemistry on skeletal muscle of the human foetus. Journal of the Neurological Sciences 39: 169–185

Conen P E, Murphy E G, Donohue W L 1963 Light and electron microscopic studies of 'myogranules' in a child with hypotonia and muscle weakness. Canadian Medical Association Journal 89: 983–986

Cori G T 1958 Biochemical aspects of glycogen deposition diseases. Modern Problems in Pediatrics 3: 344–358

Cornelio F, Dones I 1984 Muscle fiber degeneration and necrosis in muscular dystrophy and other muscle diseases. Annals of Neurology 6: 694–701

Cullen M J, Appleyard S T, Bindoff L 1979 Morphological aspects of muscle breakdown and lysosomal activation. Annals of the New York Academy of Sciences 317: 440–463

Dhoot G K, Pearce G W 1984a Changes in the distribution of fast and slow forms of troponin I in some neuromuscular disorders. Journal of the Neurological Sciences 65: 1–15

Dhoot G K, Pearce G W 1984b Transformation of fibre types in muscular dystrophies. Journal of the Neurological Sciences 65: 17–28

DiMauro S, Arnold S, Miranda A, Rowland L P 1978 McArdle disease: the mystery of reappearing phosphorylase activity in muscle culture — a fetal isoenzyme. Annals of Neurology 3: 60–66

DiMauro S, Miranda A F, Khan S, Gitlin K, Friedman R 1981 Human muscle phosphoglycerate mutase deficiency: newly discovered metabolic myopathy. Science 212: 1277–1279

DiMauro S, Dalakas M, Miranda A F 1983 Phosphoglycerate kinase deficiency: another cause of recurrent myoglobinuria. Annals of Neurology 13: 11–19

Doriguzzi C, Mongini T, Palmucci L, Schiffer D 1983 A new method for myofibrillar Ca^{++}-ATPase reaction based on the use of metachromatic dyes: its advantages in muscle fibre typing. Histochemistry 79: 289–294

Dorkins H, Junien C, Mandel J L, Wrogemann K, Moison J P, Martinez M et al 1985 Segregation analysis of a marker localised Xp21.2–Xp21.3 in Duchenne and Becker muscular dystrophy families. Human Genetics 71: 103–107

Drachmann D A 1968 Ophthalmoplegia plus, the neurodegenerative disorders associated with progressive external ophthalmoplegia. Archives of Neurology (Chicago) 18: 654–674

Duance V C, Stephens H R, Dunn M J, Bailey A J, Dubowitz V 1980 A role for collagen in the pathogenesis of muscular dystrophy? Nature (London) 284: 470–472

Dubowitz V 1963a Myopathic changes in a muscular dystrophy carrier. Journal of Neurology, Neurosurgery and Psychiatry 26: 322–325

Dubowitz V 1963b Myopathic changes in muscular dystrophy carriers. Proceedings of the Royal Society of Medicine 56: 810–812

Dubowitz V 1964 Infantile muscular atrophy. A prospective study with particular reference to a slowly progressive variety. Brain 87: 707–718

Dubowitz V 1965 Enzyme histochemistry of skeletal muscle. II Developing human muscle. Journal of Neurology, Neurosurgery and Psychiatry 28: 519–524

Dubowitz V 1966 Enzyme histochemistry of skeletal muscle. III Neurogenic muscular atrophies. Journal of Neurology, Neurosurgery and Psychiatry 29: 23–28

Dubowitz V 1967 Pathology of experimentally re-innervated skeletal muscle. Journal of Neurology, Neurosurgery and Psychiatry 30: 99–110

Dubowitz V 1968 Developing and diseased muscle: A histochemical study. Heinemann, London

Dubowitz V 1978 Muscle disorders in childhood. W. B. Saunders, London

Dubowitz V 1980 The floppy infant, 2nd edn. Clinics in Developmental Medicine No. 76. Spastics International Medical Publications. Blackwell, Oxford

Dubowitz V 1985 Muscle biopsy: A practical approach, 2nd edn. Bailliere Tindall, London

Dubowitz V, Pearse A G E 1960a Reciprocal relationship of phosphorylase and oxidative enzymes in skeletal muscle. Nature (London) 185: 701–702

Dubowitz V, Pearse A G E 1960b A comparative histochemical study of oxidative enzyme and phosphorylase activity in skeletal muscle. Histochemie 2: 105–117

Dubowitz V, Pearse A G E 1960c Oxidative enzymes and phosphorylase in central core disease of muscle. Lancet ii: 23–24

Dubowitz V, Pearse A G E 1961 Enzymic activity of normal and diseased human muscle: a histochemical study. Journal of Pathology and Bacteriology 81: 365–378

Dubowitz V, Platts M 1965 Central core disease of muscle with focal wasting. Journal of Neurology, Neurosurgery and Psychiatry 28: 432–437

Dubowitz V, Roy S 1970 Central core disease of muscle: clinical, histochemical and electron microscopic studies of an affected mother and child. Brain 93: 133–146

Dubowitz V, Brooke M H 1973 Muscle biopsy: A modern approach. W. B. Saunders, London

Dubrovsky A L, Engel W K 1976 New histochemical technique for demonstrating adenyl cyclase in nervous tissue and muscle. Archives of Neurology 33:386 (abstract).

Dunn M J, Sewry C A, Dubowitz V 1982 Cytochemical studies of lectin binding by diseased human muscle. Journal of the Neurological Sciences 55: 147–159

Dunn M J, Sewry C A, Statham H E, Dubowitz V 1984 Studies on the extracellular matrix in diseased human muscle. In: Kemp R B, Hinchcliffe J R (eds) Matrices and cell differentiation. Alan R Liss, New York, p 213–231

Edström L, Nyström B 1969 Histochemical types and sizes of fibres in normal human muscles. A biopsy study. Acta Neurologica Scandinavica 45: 257–269

Edwards R H T, Maunder C, Lewis P D, Pearse A G E 1973 Percutaneous needle biopsy in the diagnosis of muscle diseases. Lancet ii: 1070–1071

Edwards R H T, Maunder C A 1977 Muscle biopsy. Hospital Update October: 569–582

Edwards R H T, Round J M, Jones D A 1983 Needle biopsy of skeletal muscle: a review of 10 years' experience. Muscle and Nerve 6: 676–683

Emery A E H 1963 Clinical manifestations in two carriers of Duchenne muscular dystrophy. Lancet i: 1126–1128

Emery A E H, Dreifuss F E 1966 Unusual type of benign X-linked muscular dystrophy. Journal of Neurology, Neurosurgery and Psychiatry 29: 338–342

Engel A G, Gomez M R, Groover R V 1971 Multicore disease. Mayo Clinic Proceedings 10: 666–681

Engel A G, Angelini C, Gomez M R 1972 Fingerprint body myopathy. Mayo Clinic Proceedings 47: 377–388

Engel A G, Lambert E H, Howard F M 1977 Immune complexes (IgG and C3) at the motor end-plate in myasthenia gravis. Ultrastructural and light microscopic localization and electrophysiologic correlations. Mayo Clinic Proceedings 52: 267–296

Engel A G, Biesecker G 1982 Complement activation in muscle fiber necrosis: demonstration of the membrane attack complex of complement in necrotic fibers. Annals of Neurology 12: 289–296

Engel A G, Arahata K 1984 Monoclonal antibody analysis of mononuclear cells in myopathies. II Phenotypes of autoinvasive cells in polymyositis and inclusion body myositis. Annals of Neurology 16: 209–215

Engel W K 1961 Muscle target fibres, a newly recognized sign of denervation. Nature (London) 191: 389–390

Engel W K 1967 Focal myopathic changes produced by electromyographic and hypodermic needles. Archives of Neurology 16: 509–511

Engel W K 1977 Integrative histochemical approach to the defect of Duchenne muscular dystrophy. In: Rowland L P (ed) Pathogenesis of human muscular dystrophies. Excerpta Medica, Amsterdam, p 277–309

Engel W K 1979 Muscle fiber regeneration in human neuromuscular disease. In: Mauro A (ed) Muscle regeneration. Raven Press, New York, p 285–296

Engel W K, Foster J M, Hughes B P, Huxley H E, Mahler R 1961 Central core disease — an investigation of a rare muscle cell abnormality. Brain 84: 167–185

Engel W K, Cunningham G C 1963 Rapid examination of muscle tissue. An improved trichrome method for fresh-frozen biopsy sections. Neurology (Minneapolis), 13: 919–923

Engel W K, Brooke M H 1966 Histochemistry of the myotonic disorders. In: Kuhn E (ed) Progressive Muskeldystrophie, Myotonie, Myasthenie. Springer-Verlag, Stuttgart, p 203

Engel W K, Gold G N, Karpati G 1968 Type I fibre hypotrophy and central nuclei. A rare congenital muscle abnormality with a possible experimental model. Archives of Neurology (Chicago) 18: 435–444

Engel W K, Cunningham G G 1970 Alkaline phosphatase — positive abnormal muscle fibers of humans. Journal of Histochemistry and Cytochemistry 18: 55–57

Engel W K, Bishop D W, Cunningham G G 1970a Tubular aggregates in type II muscle fibers: ultrastructural and histochemical correlation. Journal of Ultrastructural Research 31: 507–525

Engel W K, Vick N A, Glueck C J, Levy R I 1970b A skeletal muscle disorder associated with intermittent symptoms and a possible defect of lipid metabolism. New England Journal of Medicine 282: 697–704

Eränkö O, Palkama A 1961 Improved localization of phosphorylase by the use of polyvinyl pyrrolidine and high substrate concentrations. Journal of Histochemistry and Cytochemistry 9:585

Ernster L, Ikkos D, Luft R 1959 Enzymic activities of human skeletal muscle mitochondria: a tool in clinical metabolic research. Nature 184:1851

Fardeau M 1982 Congenital myopathies. In: Mastaglia F L, Walton J (eds) Skeletal muscle pathology. Churchill Livingstone, Edinburgh, p 161–203

Fardeau M, Tomé F M S, Derambure S 1976 Familial fingerprint body myopathy. Archives of Neurology 33: 724–725

Filipe M I, Lake B D (eds) 1983 Histochemistry in pathology. Churchill Livingstone, Edinburgh

Fishbein W N, Armbrustmacher V W, Griffin J L 1978 Myoadenylate deaminase deficiency — a new disease of muscle. Science 200: 545–548

Fitzsimons R B, Hoh J F Y 1981 Embryonic and foetal

myosins in human skeletal muscle. The presence of foetal myosins in Duchenne muscular dystrophy and infantile spinal muscular astrophy. Journal of the Neurological Sciences 52: 367–384

Fitzsimons R B, Sewry C A 1985 Immunocytochemistry of muscle. In: Dubowitz V Muscle biopsy: A practical approach, 2nd edn. Bailliere Tindall, London, p 184–207

Forbes G B 1953 Glycogen disease. Report of a case with abnormal glycogen storage structure in liver and skeletal muscle. Journal of Pediatrics 42:645

Garlepp M J, Dawkins R L 1984 Immunological aspects. In: Ansell B (ed) Clinics in rheumatic diseases, vol. 10. W B Saunders, London, p 35–51

Giorno R, Barden M T, Kohler P F, Ringel S P 1984 Immunohistochemical characterization of the mononuclear cells infiltrating muscle of patients with inflammatory and non-inflammatory myopathies. Clinical Immunology and Immunopathology 30: 405–412

Godlewski H G 1963 Are active and inactive phosphorylase histochemically distinguishable? Journal of Histochemistry and Cytochemistry 11: 108–112

Gonatas N K, Perez M C, Shy G M, Evangelista I 1965 Central core disease of skeletal muscle. Ultrastructural and cytochemical observations in two cases. American Journal of Pathology 47: 503–524

Gonatas N K, Shy G M, Godfrey E H 1966 Nemaline myopathy. The origin of nemaline structures. New England Journal of Medicine 274: 535–539

Granger B L, Lazarides E 1980 Synemin: a new high molecular weight protein associated with desmin and vimentin filaments in muscle. Cell 22: 727–738

Greenfield J G, Cornman T, Shy G M 1958 The prognostic value of the muscle biopsy in the floppy infant. Brain 81:461

Guerard M J, Sewry C A, Dubowitz V 1985 Lobulated fibres in neuromuscular diseases. Journal of the Neurological Sciences 69: 345–356

Harper P S 1979 Muscle pathology in myotonic dystrophy. In: Harper P S (ed) Myotonic dystrophy. W. B. Saunders, Philadelphia, p 250

Harriman D G F 1982 The pathology of malignant hyperpyrexia. In: Mastaglia F L, Walton J (eds) Skeletal muscle pathology. Churchill Livingstone, Edinburgh, p 575–591

Heckmatt J Z, Moosa A, Hutson C, Maunder-Sewry C A, Dubowitz V 1984 Diagnostic needle muscle biopsy: a practical and reliable alternative to open biopsy. Archives of Disease in Childhood 59: 528–532

Heckmatt J Z, Dubowitz V 1985 Diagnostic advantage of needle biopsy and ultrasound imaging in the detection of focal pathology in a girl with limb girdle dystrophy. Muscle and Nerve 8: 705–709

Heckmatt J Z, Sewry C A, Hodes D, Dubowitz V 1985 Congenital centronuclear (myotubular) myopathy. A clinical, pathological and genetic study in eight children. Brain 108: 941–964

Hermansen L, Wachtlova M 1971 Capillary density of skeletal muscle in well-trained and untrained men. Journal of Applied Physiology 30: 860–863

Hsu S-M, Raine L, Fanger H 1981 Use of avidin-biotin-peroxidase complex (ABC) in immunoperoxidase techniques. Journal of Histochemistry and Cytochemistry 29: 577–580

Hudgson P, Hall R 1982 Endocrine myopathies. In:

Mastaglia F L, Walton J (eds) Skeletal muscle pathology. Churchill Livingstone, Edinburgh, p 393–408

Hurko O, Walsh F S 1983 Human fetal muscle-specific antigen is restricted to regenerating myofibres in diseased adult muscle. Neurology 33: 737–743

Illingworth B, Cori G T 1952 Structure of glycogens and amylopectins. III Normal and abnormal human glycogen. Journal of Biological Chemistry 199: 653

Isaacs H, Heffron J J A, Badenhorst M 1975 Central core disease: a correlated genetic, histochemical, ultrastructural and biochemical study. Journal of Neurology, Neurosurgery and Psychiatry 38: 1177–1186

Isenberg D A 1983 Immunoglobulin deposition in skeletal muscle in primary muscle disease. Quarterly Journal of Medicine 207: 297–310

Iyer V, Lawton A R, Fenichel G M 1983 T-cell subsets in polymyositis. Annals of Neurology 13: 452–453

Jennekens F G I, Roord J J, Veldman H, Willemse J, Jockusch B M 1983 Congenital nemaline myopathy. I Defective organization of α-actinin is restricted to muscle. Muscle and Nerve 6: 61–68

Jerusalem F, Engel A G, Gomez M R 1973 Sarcotubular myopathy; a newly recognized benign, congenital, familial muscle disease. Neurology 23: 897–906

Jerusalem F, Ludin H, Bischoff A, Hartmann G 1979 Cytoplasmic body neuromyopathy presenting as respiratory failure and weight loss. Journal of the Neurological Sciences 41: 1–9

Jockusch B M, Veldman H, Griffiths G W, van Oost B A, Jennekens F G I 1980 Immunofluorescence microscopy of a myopathy. α-Actinin is a major constituent of nemaline rods. Experimental Cell Research 127: 409–420

Johnson M A, Polgar J, Weightman D, Appleton D 1973 Data on the distribution of fibre types in 36 human muscles. An autopsy study. Journal of the Neurological Sciences 18: 111–129

Johnson M A, Kucukyalcin D K 1978 Patterns of abnormal histochemical fibre type differentiation in human muscle biopsies. Journal of the Neurological Sciences 37: 159–178

Kanno T et al 1980 Hereditary deficiency of lactate dehydrogenase M-subunit. Clinica Chimica Acta 108: 267–276

Kar N C, Pearson C M 1978 Muscular dystrophy and activation of proteinases. Muscle and Nerve 1: 308–313

Kar N C, Pearson C M 1979 Activity of some proteolytic enzymes in normal and dystrophic human muscle. Clinical Biochemistry 12: 37–39

Karpati G, Carpenter S, Nelson R F 1970 Type I muscle fibre atrophy and central nuclei. A rare familial neuromuscular disease. Journal of the Neurological Sciences 10: 489–500

Karpati G, Carpenter S, Andermann F 1971 A new concept of childhood nemaline myopathy. Archives of Neurology (Chicago) 24: 291–304

Kearns T P, Sayre G P 1958 Retinitis pigmentosa, external ophthalmoplegia and complete heart block. Archives of Ophthalmology 60: 280–289

Krivit W, Polglase W J, Gunn F D, Tyler F H 1953 Studies in disorders of muscle. IX Glycogen storage disease primarily affecting skeletal muscle and clinically resembling amyotonia congenita. Pediatrics 12: 165–167

Lake B D, Wilson J 1975 Zebra body myopathy: clinical, histochemical and ultrastructural studies. Journal of the Neurological Sciences 24: 437–446

Lazarides E 1980 Intermediate filaments as mechanical integrators of cellular space. Nature (London) 283: 249–256

Lazarides E, Hubbard R D 1976 Immunological characterization of the subunit of the 100 A-filaments from muscle cells. Proceedings of the National Academy of Sciences (USA) 73: 4344–4348

Lewis P D, Pallis C, Pearse A G E 1971 'Myopathy' with tubular aggregates. Journal of the Neurological Sciences 13: 381–388

Lojda Z, Gossrau R, Schiebler T H 1979 Enzyme histochemistry: a laboratory manual. Springer-Verlag, Berlin

Luft R, Ikkos D, Palmieri G, Ernster L, Afzelius B 1962 A case of severe hypermetabolism of nonthyroid origin with a defect in the maintenance of mitochondrial respiratory control: a correlated clinical, biochemical and morphological study. Journal of Clinical Investigation 41: 1776–1801

Mastaglia F L, Ojeda V J 1985a Inflammatory myopathies. Part I. Annals of Neurology 17: 215–227

Mastaglia F L, Ojeda V J 1985b Inflammatory myopathies. Part II. Annals of Neurology 17: 317–323

Maunder-Sewry C A, Dubowitz V 1981 Needle muscle biopsy for carrier detection in Duchenne muscular dystrophy. I Light microscopy — histology, histochemistry and quantitation. Journal of the Neurological Sciences 49: 305–324

McArdle B 1951 Myopathy due to a defect in muscle glycogen breakdown. Clinical Science 10: 13–35

McDonald J K 1985 An overview of protease specificity and catalytic mechanisms: aspects related to nomenclature and classification. Histochemistry Journal 17: 773–785

Menold M M, Repasky E A 1984 Heterogeneity of spectrin distribution among avian muscle fiber types. Muscle and Nerve 7: 408–414

Mitsumoto H 1979 McArdle disease: phosphorylase activity in regenerating muscle fibres. Neurology 29: 258–262

Moore S E, Walsh F S 1985 Specific regulation of N-CAM/D2-CAM cell adhesion molecule during skeletal muscle development. The EMBO Journal 4: 623–630

Morgan B P, Sewry C A, Siddle K, Luzio J P, Campbell A K 1984 Immunolocalization of complement component C9 on necrotic and non-necrotic muscle fibres in myositis using monoclonal antibodies: a primary role of complement in autoimmune cell damage. Immunology 52: 181–188

Morgan-Hughes J A 1982 Mitochondrial myopathies. In: Mastaglia F L, Walton J (eds) Skeletal muscle pathology. Churchill Livingstone, p 309–339

Morris C J, Raybould J A 1971a Histochemically demonstrable fibre abnormalities in normal skeletal muscle and in muscle from carriers of Duchenne muscular dystrophy. Journal of Neurology, Neurosurgery and Psychiatry 34: 348–353

Morris C J, Raybould J A 1971b Fiber type grouping and end-plate diameter in human skeletal muscle. Journal of the Neurological Sciences 13: 181–187

Mukuno K 1969 Electron microscopic studies on human extraocular muscles under pathologic conditions. I. Rod formation in normal and diseased muscles (polymyositis and ocular myasthenia). Japanese Journal of Ophthalmology 13: 35–51

Neerunjun J S, Dubowitz V 1977 Concomitance of basophilia

ribonucleic acid and acid phosphatase activity in regenerating muscle fibres. Journal of the Neurological Sciences 33: 95–109

Neville H E 1979 Ultrastructural changes in diseases of human skeletal muscle. In: Vinken P J, Bruyn G W (eds) Handbook of clinical neurology, vol 40. Diseases of Muscle, Part 1. North-Holland, Amsterdam, p 63–123

Neville H E, Brooke M H 1973 Central core fibers: structured and unstructured. In: Kakulas B (ed) Basic research in myology. Proceedings of International Congress on Muscle Diseases, Part I, ICS No. 294. Excerpta Medica, Amsterdam, p 497–511

Nienhuis A W, Coleman R F, Jann Brown W, Munsat T L, Pearson C M 1967 Nemaline myopathy. A histopathologic and histochemical study. American Journal of Clinical Pathology 48: 1–13

Nonaka I, Takagi A, Sugita H 1981 The significance of type 2C muscle fibres in Duchenne muscular dystrophy. Muscle and Nerve 4: 326–333

Olson W, Engel W K, Walsh G O, Einaugler R 1972 Oculocraniosomatic neuromuscular disease with 'ragged-red' fibers. Archives of Neurology (Chicago) 26: 193–211

Osborn M, Geisler N, Shaw G, Sharp G, Weber K 1982 Intermediate filaments. Cold Spring Harbor Symposia on Quantitative Biology 46: 413–429

Osborn M, Goebel H H 1983 The cytoplasmic bodies in a congenital myopathy can be stained with antibodies to desmin, the muscle-specific intermediate filament protein. Acta Neuropathologica (Berlin) 62: 149–152

Padykula H A, Hermann E 1955 The specificity of the histochemical method for adenosine triphosphate. Journal of Histochemistry and Cytochemistry 3: 170–195

Paljarvi L, Karjalainen K, Kalimo H 1984 Altered muscle saccharide pattern in X-linked muscular dystrophy. Archives of Neurology 41: 39–42

Pearce G W, Pearce J M S, Walton J N 1966 The Duchenne type muscular dystrophy: histopathological studies of the carrier state. Brain 89: 109–120

Pearse A G E 1980 Histochemistry: Theoretical and applied, vol 1, 4th edn. Churchill Livingstone, Edinburgh

Pearse A G E 1985 Histochemistry: Theoretical and applied, vol 2, 4th edn. Churchill Livingstone, Edinburgh

Pearse A G, Johnson M 1970 Histochemistry in the study of normal and diseased muscle with special reference to myopathy with tubular aggregates. In: Walton J N, Canal N, Scarlato G (eds) Muscle diseases, ICS No. 199. Excerpta Medica, Amsterdam, p 25–32

Pearson C M, Fowler W M, Wright S W 1963 X-chromosome mosaicism in females with muscular dystrophy. Proceedings of the National Academy of Sciences (USA) 50: 24–31

Pena S D J, Gordon B B, Karpati G, Carpenter S 1981 Lectin histochemistry of human skeletal muscle. Journal of Histochemistry and Cytochemistry 29: 542–546

Pleasure D, Bonilla E 1982 Skeletal muscle storage diseases: myopathies resulting from errors in carbohydrate and fatty acid metabolism. In: Mastaglia F L, Walton J (eds) Skeletal muscle pathology. Churchill Livingstone, Edinburgh, p 340–359

Polak J M, Varndell I M (eds) 1984 Immunolabelling for electron microscopy. Elsevier, Amsterdam

Ponder B A J 1983 Lectin histochemistry. In: Polak J M, van Noorden S (eds) Immunocytochemistry: Practical applications in pathology and biology. Wright, Bristol, p 129–142

Pongratz D, Heuser M, Koppelwallner C, Hübner G 1976 Central Core Disease mit 'structured cores' in Type-II Fasern. Klinische Wochenschrift 54: 117–122

Prader A, Labhart A, Willi H 1956 Ein Syndrom von Adipositas, Kleinwuchs, Kryptorchismus und Oligophrenie nach myotonieartigem Zustand im Neugeborenenalter. Schweizerische medizinische Wochenschrift 86:1260

Prader A, Willi H 1963 Das Syndrom von Imbezillitat, Adipositas, Muskelhypotonie, Hypogenitalismus, Hypogonadismus, und Diabetes Mellitus mit 'Myatonie'-anamnese. Verh. 2 Int. Kong. Psych. Entw-Stor. Kindes-Alt. Vienna 1961, pt 1, p 353–357

Price H M, Gordon G B, Pearson C M, Munsat T L, Blumberg J M 1965 New evidence for excessive accumulation of Z-band material in nemaline myopathy. Proceedings of the American Academy of Sciences 54: 1398–1406

Price H M, Gordon G B, Munsat T L, Pearson C M 1967 Myopathy with atypical mitochondria in the (type 1) skeletal muscle fibers. Journal of Neuropathology and Experimental Neurology 26: 475–497

Reniers J, Martin L, Joris C 1970 Histochemical and quantitative analysis of muscle biopsies. Journal of the Neurological Sciences 10: 349–367

Ringel S P, Carroll J E, Schold C 1977 The spectrum of mild X-linked recessive muscular dystrophy. Archives of Neurology (Chicago) 34: 408–416

Ringel S P, Neville H E, Duster M C, Carroll J E 1978 A new congenital neuromuscular disease with trilaminar fibers. Neurology 28: 282–289

Roelofs R I, Engel W K, Chauvin P B 1972 Histochemical demonstration of phosphorylase activity in regenerating skeletal muscle fibers from myophosphorylase deficiency patients. Science 177: 795–797

Rosa R, George C, Fardeau M, Calvin M-C, Rapin M, Rosa J 1982 A new case of phosphoglycerate kinase deficiency: PGK creteil associated with rhabdomyolysis and lacking hemolytic anemia. Blood 60: 84–91

Round J M, Matthews Y, Jones D A 1980 A quick simple and reliable method for ATPase in human muscle preparations. Histochemical Journal 12: 707–709

Round J M, Jones D A, Edwards R H T 1982 A flexible microprocessor system for the measurement of cell size. Journal of Clinical Pathology 35: 620–624

Roy S, Dubowitz V 1970 Carrier detection in Duchenne muscular dystrophy. A comparative study of electron microscopy, light microscopy and serum enzymes. Journal of the Neurological Sciences 11: 65–79

Sahashi K, Engel A G, Lambert E H, Howard F M 1980 Ultrastructural localization of the terminal component (C9) at the motor end-plate in myasthenia gravis. Journal of Neuropathology and Experimental Neurology 39: 160–172

Sargeant A S, Davis C T M, Young A, Maunder C A, Edwards R H T 1977 Functional and structural changes after disuse of human muscle. Clinical Science and Molecular Medicine 52: 337–342

Sato K et al 1977 Characterization of glycogen phosphorylase isoenzymes present in cultured skeletal muscle from patients with McArdle's disease. Biochemical and Biophysical Research Communications 78: 663–668

Schmalbruch H 1984 Regenerated muscle fibers in Duchenne muscular dystrophy: A serial section study. Neurology (Cleveland) 34: 60–65

Schmid R, Mahler R 1959 Chronic progressive myopathy with myoglobinuria. Demonstration of a glycogenolytic defect in the muscle. Journal of Clinical Investigation 38:2044

Schollmeyer J V, Goll D, Stromer M H, Dayton W, Singh I, Robson R M 1974 Studies on the composition of the Z disk. Journal of Cell Biology 63:303a

Sewry C A 1985 Ultrastructural changes in diseased muscle. In: Dubowitz V Muscle biopsy: A practical approach, 2nd edn. Bailliere Tindall, London, p 129–183

Sewry C A, Dubowitz V 1984 Calcium and necrosis. In: Serratrice G et al (eds) Neuromuscular diseases. Raven Press, New York, p 131–135

Sewry C A, Appleyard S T, Dunn M J, Capaldi M J 1985 Immunocytochemistry of human skeletal muscle diseases. In: Polak J, van Noorden S (eds) Immunocytochemistry, practical applications in pathology and biology, 2nd edn. Wright, Bristol, p 664–673

Sewry C A, Lovegrove C, Dubowitz V 1986 Immunocytochemistry of basophilic fibres in Duchenne muscular dystrophy. Journal of Neuropathology and Neurobiology 12:429

Shafiq S A, Dubowitz V, Peterson H de C, Milhorat A T 1967 Nemaline myopathy: report of a fatal case with histochemical and electron microscopic studies. Brain 90: 817–828

Shafiq S A, Gorycki M A, Asiedu S A, Milhorat A T 1969 Tenotomy. Effects on the fine structure of the soleus of the rat. Archives of Neurology (Chicago) 20: 625–633

Sher J H, Rimalovski A B, Athanassiades T J, Aronson S M 1967 Familial centronuclear myopathy: a clinical and pathological study. Neurology 17/1: 727–742

Shy G M, Magee K R 1956 A new congenital non-progressive myopathy. Brain 79: 610–621

Shy G M, Engel W K, Somers J E, Wanko T 1963 Nemaline myopathy. A new congenital myopathy. Brain 86: 793–815

Shy G M, Gonatas N K, Perez M 1966 Two childhood myopathies with abnormal mitochondria. Brain 89: 133–158

Sissons H A 1965 Further investigations of muscle fibre size. In: Research in muscular dystrophy. Proceedings of the Third Symposium, Research Committee of the Muscular Dystrophy Group of Great Britain. Pitman Medical, London, p 107

Smith H L, Amick L D, Johnson W W 1966 Detection of subclinical and carrier states in Duchenne muscular dystrophy. Journal of Pediatrics 69: 67–79

Spiro A J, Shy G M, Gonatas N K 1966 Myotubular myopathy. Archives of Neurology (Chicago) 14: 1–14

Stauber W, Fritz V, Dahlmann B, Gauthier F, Kirschke H, Ulrich R 1985 Fluorescence methods for localizing proteinases and proteinase inhibitors in skeletal muscle. Histochemical Journal 17: 787–796

Stephens H R, Duance V C, Dunn M J, Bailey A J, Dubowitz V 1982 Collagen types in neuromuscular diseases. Journal of the Neurological Sciences 53: 45–62

Takeuchi T 1956 Histochemical demonstration of phosphorylase. Journal of Histochemistry and Cytochemistry 4:84

Telerman-Toppet N, Gerard J M, Coërs C 1973 Central core disease; a study of clinically unaffected muscle. Journal of the Neurological Sciences 19: 207–223

ten Houten R, De Visser M 1984 Histopathological findings

in Becker-type muscular dystrophy. Archives of Neurology (Chicago) 41: 729–733

Thornell L-E, Edström L, Eriksson A, Henriksson K-G, Angqvist K A 1980 The distribution of intermediate filament protein (skeletin) in normal and diseased human skeletal muscle. Journal of the Neurological Sciences 47: 153–170

Thornell L-E, Eriksson A, Edström L 1983 Intermediate filaments in human myopathies. In: Dowben R M, Shay J W (eds) Cell and muscle motility, vol. 4. Plenum, New York, p 84–136

Thornell L-E, Billeter R, Butler-Browne G S, Eriksson P O, Ringqvist M, Whalen R G 1984 Development of fiber types in human fetal muscle. An immunocytochemical study. Journal of the Neurological Sciences 66: 107–115

Tokuyasu K T, Dutton A H, Singer S J 1983 Immunoelectron microscopic studies of desmin (skeletin) localization and intermediate filament organization in chicken skeletal muscle. Journal of Cell Biology 96:1727

Tomé F M S 1982 Periodic paralysis and electrolyte disorders. In: Mastaglia F L, Walton J (eds) Skeletal muscle pathology. Churchill Livingstone, London, p 287–308

Trend P St J, Wiles C M, Spencer G T, Morgan-Hughes J A, Lake B D, Patrick A D 1985 Acid maltase deficiency in adults: Diagnosis and management in five cases. Brain 109: 845–860

van Wijngaarden G K, Bethlem J, Meijer A E F H, Hulsmann W Ch, Feltkamp C A 1967 Skeletal muscle disease with abnormal mitochondria. Brain 90: 577–592

van Wijngaarden G K, Fleury P, Bethlem J, Meijer A E F H 1969 Familial 'myotubular' myopathy. Neurology 19: 901–908

Wachstein M, Meisel E 1955 The distribution of demonstrable succinic dehydrogenase and of mitochondria in tongue and skeletal muscle. Journal of Biophysical and Biochemical Cytology 1:483

Wang C, Asai D J, Lazarides E 1980 The 68 000 dalton neurofilaments — associated polypeptide is a component of nonneuronal cells and skeletal myofibrils. Proceedings of the National Academy of Sciences 77: 1541–1545

Warnes D M, Tomaş F M, Ballard J F 1981 Increased rates of myofibrillar protein breakdown in muscle-wasting diseases. Muscle and Nerve 4: 62–66

Wattenberg L W, Leong J L 1960 Effects of coenzyme Q_{10} and menadione on succinic dehydrogenase activity as measured by tetrazolium salt reduction. Journal of Histochemistry and Cytochemistry 8:296

Whitaker J N 1982 Inflammatory myopathy: a review of etiologic and pathogenetic factors. Muscle and Nerve 5: 573–592

Whitaker J N, Bertorini T E, Mendell J R 1983 Immunocytochemical studies of cathepsin D in human skeletal muscle. Annals of Neurology 13: 133–142

White M G, Stoward P J, Christie K N, Anderson J M 1985 Proteases in normal and diseased human skeletal muscle; a preliminary histochemical survey. Histochemical Journal 17: 819–832

Willner J H, Cerri C, Wood D S 1982 Adenylate cyclase in human genetic myopathies. In: Schotland D S (ed) Disorders of the motor unit. Wiley, New York, p 423–440

Wohlfart G 1937 Uber das vorkommen verschiedener Arten von Muskelfasern in der skelett-muskulatur des menschen und einiger saugitere. Acta Psychiatrica et Neurologica, Suppl. 12

Yamaguchi M, Robson R M, Stromer M H, Dahl D S, Oda T 1978 Actin filaments forms the backbone of nemaline myopathy rods. Nature (London) 271: 265–267

Yamaguchi M, Robson R M, Stromer M H, Dahl D S, Oda T 1982 Nemaline myopathy rod bodies: structure and composition. Journal of the Neurological Sciences 56: 35–56

Ultrastructural studies of diseased muscle

INTRODUCTION

Advances in our knowledge of the ultrastructure of diseased muscle have depended upon advances in techniques which disclose previously inaccessible morphological information. Since the fourth edition of this book was published several powerful new procedures have become established and these are referred to in this chapter.

Freeze fracture is a technique which has wide applications in cell biology and which has now been applied to the study of muscle pathology and immunopathology. Freeze fracture permits the electron microscopist an *en face* view of the internal structure of cell membranes and their components and has therefore been employed to study the plasma membrane of dystrophic muscle. It has also been used, e.g., to examine the motor nerve terminals in mice injected with IgG from patients with the Lambert–Eaton syndrome, with dramatic results (see Ch. 9). However it is still clear that there are problems with interpretation of freeze–fracture images because of variability induced by fixation and freezing (Lee et al 1986). This type of work will be further discussed in the section on Duchenne muscular dystrophy (see below).

Another technique, the accuracy of which depends crucially on the preparatory freezing procedures, is X-ray microanalysis which can be used to determine the concentration of individual elements in a section. As the probe size is usually smaller than most organelles, the elemental concentrations from one compartment to another can be compared. Thus Somlyo and her colleagues (Somlyo et al 1981) were able to measure the concentrations of sodium, magnesium, phosphorus, sulphur, chlorine, potassium and calcium in different parts of the sarcotubular system and to examine how these changed during tetanus. Wróblewski's group in Sweden (see below) have applied X-ray microanalysis to human muscle biopsies (Wróblewski et al 1978a,b, 1982) but, thus far, the potential of this very powerful technique has not been fully realised in the examination of diseased muscle.

A third technique which has considerable potential for adding an extra dimension to our understanding of cell ultrastructure is that of electron microscopic (EM) immunocytochemistry. For this a label (peroxidase, ferritin or gold) is conjugated to an antibody against the antigen of interest or, more usually, to a secondary antibody to the primary IgG. By using colloidal gold particles of different sizes, different antigens can be labelled on the same section. An example of dual labelling of tubulin and desmin in skeletal muscle is illustrated in Chapter 2. Examples where peroxidase labelling has been used include the demonstration of the membrane-attack complex of

complement in necrotic muscle fibres (Engel & Biesecker 1982), the localisation of cathepsin D in human skeletal muscle (Whitaker et al 1983) and the detection of a spectrin-like protein in normal and dystrophic human skeletal muscle (Appleyard et al 1984). Ferritin-labelled antibodies have been used for the precise localisation of collagen types III and IV, laminin and fibronectin in Duchenne muscular dystrophy (Dunn et al 1984).

In terms of scientific chronology these three techniques are just emerging from their infancy, yet used singly or in combination with other techniques, such as computer-aided image analysis, they represent advances in approach which are beginning to yield important information in our understanding of muscle disease.

ULTRASTRUCTURAL REACTIONS OF THE MUSCLE FIBRE

During the past 20 years, electron microscopists have become increasingly aware of the fact that

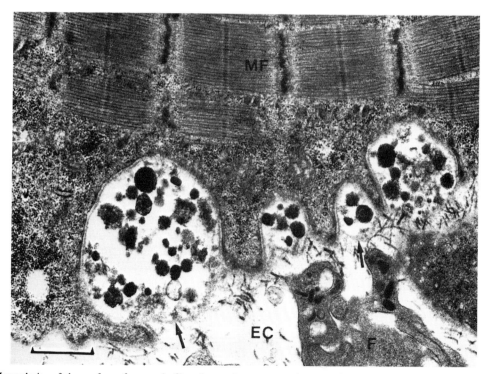

Fig. 8.1 Irregularity of the surface of a muscle fibre due to the presence of exocytotic vacuoles which contain granular and membranous debris enclosed by the basal lamina (arrows). MF = myofibrils; EC = extracellular space; F = fibroblast. Myopathy due to ε-aminocaproic acid. Bar: 1.0 μm

few ultrastructural reactions are specific for particular disease entities. Despite this lack of specificity, certain combinations or sequences of changes (reaction patterns) seen in some disorders are sufficiently distinctive to be of diagnostic value. The more important ultrastructural reactions of the muscle fibre components and the ultrastructural correlates of some of the well-known light microscopic reactions of the muscle fibre are considered below.

Reactions of muscle fibre components

Surface membrane changes. The muscle fibre surface is usually relatively smooth and under normal circumstances the plasma membrane and basal lamina run parallel with each other (Ch. 2). Irregular projections of the surface may be due to the fibre being fixed while contracted but these have also been noted frequently in various neuro-muscular disorders (Neville 1973). Papillary projections from the surface of diseased muscle fibres may be seen in fibres which are undergoing atrophy or in fibres of normal size, and either may be due to loss of fibre bulk or else may be a sequel to extrusion of degradation products from the surface of the fibre (exocytosis) (Fig. 8.1) (Engel & MacDonald 1970). Deep infoldings of the sarcolemma are seen in fibres which are undergoing longitudinal splitting, and are particularly prominent in dystrophia myotonica (Schröder 1970, Casanova & Jerusalem 1979).

In atrophying fibres the basal lamina may separate from the plasma membrane forming redundant folds which may remain even after the rest of the fibre has broken down (Fig. 8.2). Duplication of the basal lamina is a common finding in the muscular dystrophies and other

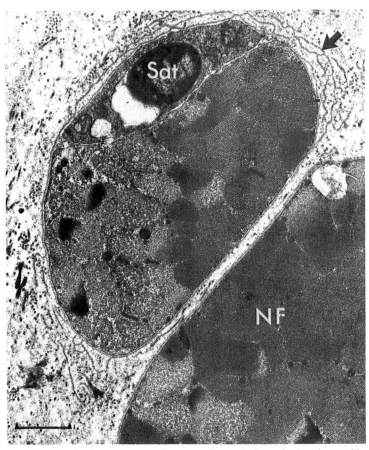

Fig. 8.2 Redundant folds of basal lamina (arrow) surrounding a small muscle fibre. An inactive satellite cell (Sat) is situated internal to the basal lamina. NF = normal muscle fibre. Congenital myotonic dystrophy. Bar: 1.0 μm

necrotising myopathies and is a result of the regenerating fibre producing a new basal lamina while underlying the 'parental' basal lamina. Thickening of the basal lamina is a non-specific finding in a variety of situations (Mastaglia et al 1970).

Focal or more extensive deficits in the plasma membrane are frequently observed in fibres undergoing necrosis. Focal defects have also been described in otherwise normal fibres in carefully prepared material from patients with Duchenne muscular dystrophy (see below). Increased numbers of pinocytotic vesicles associated with the plasma membrane are also found in a variety of situations (Engel & MacDonald 1970).

Nuclear reactions. Changes in the myonuclei are sometimes found in fibres that otherwise appear morphologically normal (Cullen & Mastaglia 1982) but are usually seen in fibres that are atrophic, necrotic or sublethally injured. In a recent review Tomé & Fardeau (1986) have categorised the changes as changes in location, number, shape, size, internal structure or envelope structure. Localisation of all or some of the nuclei in a central or internal position is usually an indication of a chronic myopathic or neurogenic disorder. Central nuclei are particularly prominent in dystrophia myotonica and centronuclear myopathy. Why the nuclei do not move to the periphery, as they do during normal myogenesis, and why some peripheral nuclei should be displaced centrally, is not understood, although changes in the mechanical constraints imposed by the myofibrils are probably involved (Cullen & Mastaglia 1982, Tomé & Fardeau 1986).

Changes in the numbers of nuclei may be caused by the degeneration of individual nuclei prior to fibre necrosis in myopathic conditions. Numbers of myonuclei have been reported to be decreased in children with acquired hypothyroidism (Cheek et al 1971) and in Down's syndrome (Landing & Shankle 1982). In neurogenic atrophy the nuclei tend to aggregate into clumps, where they persist with intact nuclear membranes when most of the other fibre components have been lost. This may give the false impression that numbers have increased.

The myonuclei of diseased muscle fibres often become extremely irregular in shape and deep indentations of the nuclear membrane can give rise to the appearance of 'pseudo-inclusions'. These can be distinguished from real inclusions by being bound by the double nuclear membrane. The indentations of the nucleus can be so extensive that it takes on a spongiform appearance (Fig. 8.3). Irregularly shaped nuclei have been described in polymyositis (Mastaglia & Walton 1971b), distal myopathy (Markesbery et al 1977), inclusion body myositis (Carpenter et al 1978) and dystrophia myotonica (Tomé & Fardeau 1986) and are totally non-specific.

The nuclei of diseased muscle sometimes contain aggregations of filaments of various types. Actin-like 6 nm filaments have been described in polymyositis (Chou 1973, Cullen & Mastaglia 1982). Larger 8.5 nm tubular filaments have been observed in oculopharyngeal muscular dystrophy

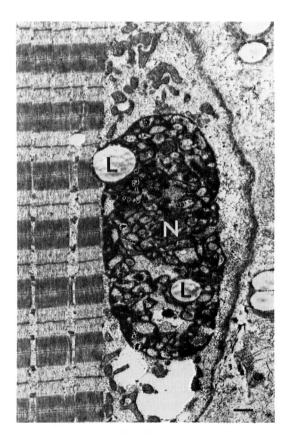

Fig. 8.3 A myonucleus (N) with numerous complex indentations giving 'spongiform' structure. Lipid storage myopathy. L = lipid. Bar: 1 μm

(Tomé & Fardeau 1986), and 16–18 nm tubular filaments in reducing body myopathy (Carpenter et al 1985) and inclusion body myositis (Tomé & Fardeau 1986). In this laboratory we have seen 25 nm filaments in a case of dermatomyositis (Cullen & Mastaglia 1982). The chemical identity of none of these filament types has yet been elucidated, although Carpenter and his colleagues (1985) give a thorough account of the staining properties of the 17 nm filaments found in reducing body myopathy.

Wröblewski and his colleagues (1982) were able to distinguish between two myopathies exhibiting central nuclei on the basis of the elementary spectra produced when subjected to X-ray microanalysis. One of the myopathies (myotubular) exhibited spectra with high sodium and chlorine and low potassium signals which is an indication of immature properties. In the other myopathy the elemental spectra conformed to the adult state. It was concluded that there was an arrest in development in the first but not in the second myopathy.

Reactions of myofibrils. The orderly sarcomere pattern and regular alignment of myofibrils seen in normal muscle may be disorganised in a number of different ways in disease. Focal areas of disruption involving a single or a few adjoining sarcomeres are commonly found in a variety of disorders and their significance is uncertain. In a number of children with a congenital myopathy this was found to be the principal change in the muscle fibres and the terms *multicore* and *minicore*

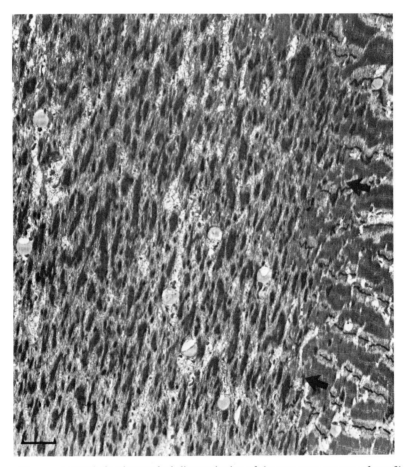

Fig. 8.4 Central core-like area (arrows) showing marked disorganisation of the sarcomere pattern of myofibrils in a muscle fibre. Mitochondrial myopathy. Bar: 2.0 μm

disease were applied (Engel et al 1971). Typically there is Z-line streaming and loss of mitochondria, SR and glycogen within the minicores (Swash & Schwarz 1981, Pagès et al 1985).

More extensive disorganisation of the myofibrils is found in *central cores* and in *target fibres*. Central cores were first described 30 years ago (Shy & Magee 1956). Ultrastructurally they display a variable amount of myofibril disorganisation (Fig. 8.4); Z-line streaming is common (Palmucci et al 1978) and there may be extensive rod formation (Bethlem et al 1978); there is also marked reduction or absence of mitochondria and a lack of intermediate filaments (Thornell et al 1983).

Neville & Brooke (1973) subdivided central cores into structured and unstructured types according to whether the cross-striations and myofibrillar ATPase staining were retained or lost. However both types of core have been reported in the same biopsy (Telerman-Toppet et al 1973, Isaacs et al 1975) although Neville (1979) considers this to be unusual. Sewry (1985) has pointed out that some cores can have both structured and unstructured features.

Target fibres are found in denervating conditions, after reinnervation, and in some myopathies including familial periodic paralysis and polymyositis. Within such fibres, a central zone of marked myofibrillar disorganisation is separated from an outer zone of normal myofibrils by an intermediate zone in which the degree of myofibrillar disarray is relatively mild. Within the

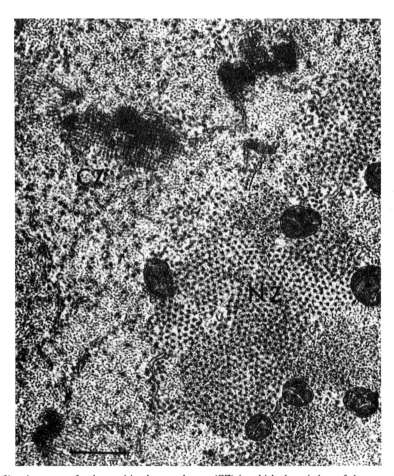

Fig. 8.5 Targetoid fibre in a case of polymyositis. A central zone (CZ) in which there is loss of the normal hexagonal arrangement of thick and thin myofilaments, disorganisation of the sarcoplasmic reticulum and loss of mitochondria borders on a normal portion of the fibre (NZ). Bar: 0.5 μm

central zone there is disruption of the myofibril pattern, spreading of Z-band material, loss of mitochondria and disorganisation of the SR (Fig. 8.5) (Schotland 1969). Autophagic vacuoles and honeycomb structures have also been observed in the target centres with mitochondrial disintegration in the intermediate area (Mrak et al 1982). In so-called *targetoid* fibres, which may be found in both myopathic and neurogenic con-.ditions, the intermediate zone is lacking (Dubowitz & Brooke 1973, Dubowitz 1985).

Z-line streaming is probably the commonest alteration in myofibril structure seen in diseased muscle. It is commonly seen in the areas of disorganisation mentioned above and in a variety of other disorders. At its simplest it appears as an extension of the electron-dense component of the Z line into the adjacent I band. More commonly the density extends throughout the length of the sarcomere and into neighbouring sarcomeres and, at its most severe, zones of Z-line streaming can occupy large areas of a fibre (Fig. 8.6). Z-line streaming should not always be regarded as pathological; a certain amount of Z-line streaming can be detected in normal muscle, especially where there is a 'mismatch' between the Z lines of adjacent myofibrils.

Rod-body formation is the central feature of nemaline myopathy (Shy et al 1963, Hudgson et al 1967) but has now been described in a variety of conditions (Cullen & Mastaglia 1982). The rods are highly electron-dense, usually about the width of a myofibril and up to 7-8 um in length (Fig. 8.7). Biochemical and immunocytochemical evidence indicates that the electron-dense material is α-actinin (Ebashi 1967, Yamaguchi et al 1978a). Longitudinal filaments within the rods may be composed of actin. Desmin is found around the margins of the rods (Jockusch et al 1980, Thornell et al 1980). These observations seem to support suggestions that the rods can be regarded as a lateral polymer of the Z-line subunit (MacDonald & Engel 1971, Stromer et al 1976). Stauber and his colleagues (1986) recently found an apparent absence of dipeptidyl peptidase 1 in two cases of nemaline myopathy and speculate whether this protease might be involved in the post-trans-

lational modification of proteins that are to be assembled into the Z line.

Another structure probably derived from the myofibrils is the *cytoplasmic body* (MacDonald & Engel 1969). These are usually round or oval in profile and have a dense core and a peripheral zone of radially arranged filaments which in some cases connect with adjoining myofibrils (Fig. 8.8). The dense core contains tightly packed randomly arranged filaments. Its biochemical nature is unknown but it is sometimes linked to an adjoining Z line. The radiating filaments resemble actin although a case has been reported in which they contain desmin (Osborn & Goebel 1983). Cytoplasmic bodies have been found in a number of conditions and seem to be non-specific (Cullen & Mastalgia 1982). They have, however, represented a major change in two cases of an unusual form of chronic progressive neuromy-

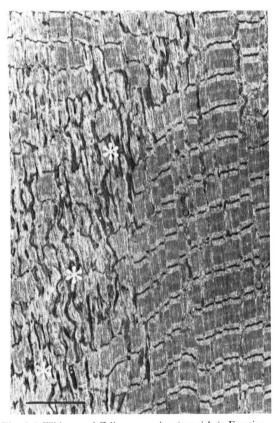

Fig. 8.6 Widespread Z-line streaming (asterisks). Emetine-induced myopathy. Bar: 5 μm (from Bindoff & Cullen 1978 . Journal of the Neurological Sciences 39:1, with permission from Elsevier, North-Holland Biomedical Press)

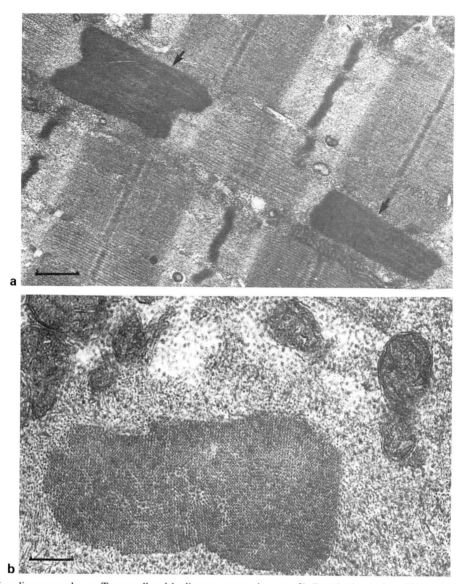

Fig. 8.7 Nemaline myopathy. a. Two small rod bodies are present in a myofibril at the level of the Z lines (arrows). Bar: 0.5 μm. b. Higher magnification of a transversely sectioned rod body showing the characteristic lattice-like appearance. Bar: 0.25 μm

opathy which has been termed 'cytoplasmic body neuromyopathy' (Jerusalem et al 1979).

Filamentous bodies are another class of filamentous structure thought to be derived from the myofibrils. They usually consist of tightly packed masses of 6 nm actin-like filaments and are frequently subsarcolemmal in location (Fig. 8.9). They have been observed in muscular dystrophy

(Hurwitz et al 1967), hypokalaemic periodic paralysis (Odor et al 1967, Macdonald et al 1969) and intermittent claudication (Teräväinen & Makitie 1977). They have also been seen in healthy human muscle (Shafiq et al 1966, Schmalbruch 1968). A similar, but probably unrelated, structure consisting of 10 nm intermediate filaments has been described by Cullen & Mastaglia (1982) and by Thornell and his co-workers (1983).

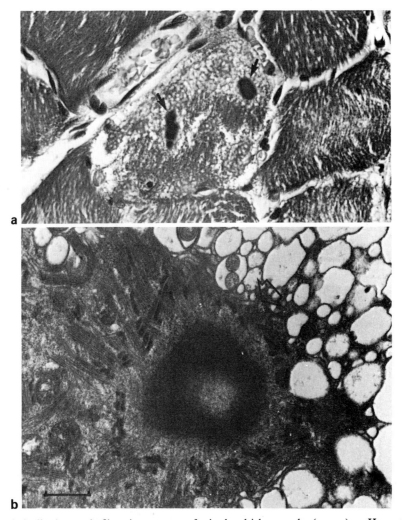

Fig. 8.8 Cytoplasmic bodies in muscle fibres in two cases of mitochondrial myopathy (arrows). a. Haematoxylin and eosin, ×640. b. Electronmicrograph showing electron-dense centre surrounded by radially orientated myofibrils and triads. Bar: 1.0 μm

Ring fibres are fibres in which one or more myofibrils are arranged circumferentially instead of longitudinally (Fig. 8.10). The disorientated myofibrils may be situated in the immediate subsarcolemmal region or, in some instances, are separated from the plasma membrane by an area of sarcoplasm containing disorganised myofilaments, nuclei and other organelles. These peripheral areas are termed sarcoplasmic masses. Ring fibres have been found in a variety of situations including myotonic dystrophy, Becker dystrophy, limb-girdle syndrome and some cases of hypothyroid myopathy (Fardeau 1970).

Reactions of the sarcoplasmic reticulum and T system. The main morphological changes seen in the sarcoplasmic reticulum (SR) in diseased muscle are dilatation and proliferation. Dilatation of the SR appears to be the first ultrastructural change that can be identified in Duchenne muscular dystrophy (Hudgson & Pearce 1969, Cullen & Fulthorpe 1975, Oberc & Engel 1977) (Fig. 8.11). Other conditions in which it has been reported include chronic alcoholism (Rubin et al 1976), distal myopathy (Markesbery et al 1977), myopathy with hyperaldosteronism (Gallai 1977), myotonic dystrophy (Casanova & Jerusalem 1979)

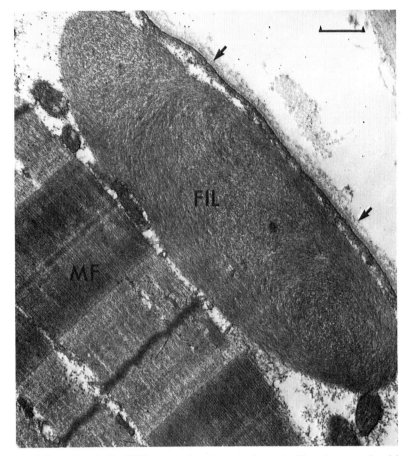

Fig. 8.9 Sub-sarcolemmal filamentous body (FIL) in an otherwise normal muscle fibre. Arrows = basal lamina; MF = myofibrils; Bar: 0.5 μm

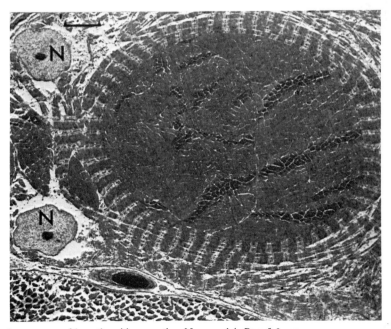

Fig. 8.10 Ring fibre from a case of hypothyroid myopathy. N = nuclei; Bar: 5.0 μm

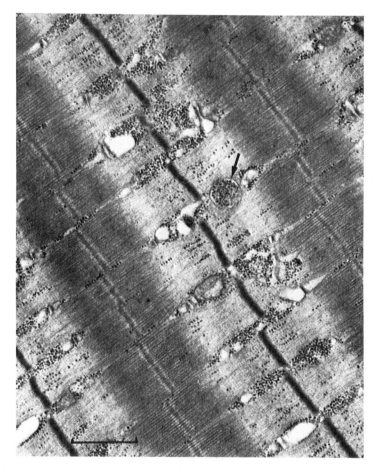

Fig. 8.11 Dilatation of transverse tubules and lateral sacs of the sarcoplasmic reticulum. Arrow = small area of autophagia. Duchenne muscular dystrophy. Bar: 1.0 μm

and perhexiline maleate-induced polyneuropathy (Fardeau et al 1979). Somlyo and her colleagues (1981), using X-ray microanalysis, have shown that dilatation of the SR in frog muscle is associated with calcium overloading, although there is no direct evidence to suggest that this is the case in the human conditions mentioned above.

Proliferation of the SR is frequently seen in atrophic fibres. In denervated muscle the amount of SR appears to increase but this is relative as the sarcotubular reticulum seems to remain longer after the myofibrils and mitochondria have begun to break down (Cullen & Pluskal 1977). After denervation, the SR appears to revert to an immature configuration with frequent duplication or stacking at the triads (Fig. 8.12). This configuration of the sarcotubular system is also seen in

regenerating fibres (Ch. 2). In certain patients localised proliferation of the SR gives rise to tubular aggregates (see below).

Three types of changes to the T tubules are quite commonly seen in diseased muscle: they may become receptacles for cell debris; they may change their orientation, or they may form 'honeycomb' or labyrinthine structures. In healthy muscle the lamina of the tubules usually appear empty but, where the fibres are breaking down, material may be exocytosed into them, resulting in their dilatation. The T tubules open to the outside of the fibres; they may therefore, in effect, be acting as gutters for the disposal of cellular debris (Kelly et al 1986).

In diseased muscle the T tubules often change their orientation from transverse to longitudinal,

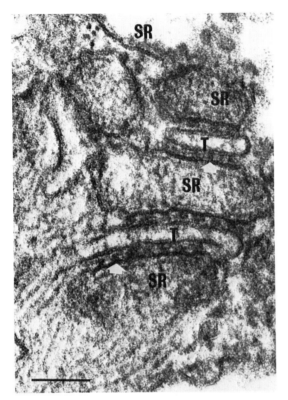

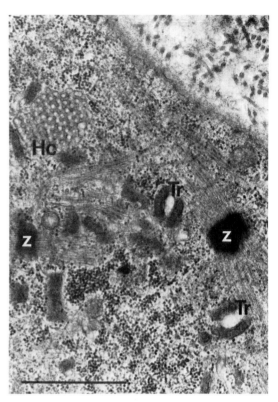

Fig. 8.12 Edge of a small fibre in Werdnig–Hoffman disease. Two T-system elements (T) are sandwiched by three sarcoplasmic reticulum (SR) cisternae. Note the variable appearance of the feet (white arrows) in the junctional gap. Bar: 0.2 μm

Fig. 8.13 Part of an atrophic fibre in a case of Werdnig-Hoffmann disease showing a honeycomb structure (Hc) and prominent misorientated triads (Tr). Z = Z bodies. Bar: 1 μm (from Cullen & Mastaglia 1982)

which is the configuration usually seen in developing and regenerating muscle. This change in orientation is most commonly seen in conditions producing denervation and in other forms of muscle fibre atrophy. At the same time there is often duplication of the tubules and the adherent cisternae of the SR so that complex associations of the T system and SR are formed (Fig. 8.12). 'Honeycomb' structures, first described in denervated rat muscle (Pellegrino & Franzini 1963), take the form of a regular three-dimensional array of interconnecting tubules (Fig. 8.13). They are connected to elements of the T system and their intercommunication with the T tubules has been demonstrated by tracer experiments (Engel & MacDonald 1970, Schotland 1970). They are a non-specific phenomenon and have been described in a large range of unrelated neuromuscular diseases.

Mitochondrial reactions. The number and size of mitochondria in muscle fibres vary considerably. Focal loss of mitochondria is a common accompaniment of myofibrillar disorganisation or breakdown in various myopathies (Engel & MacDonald 1970). Focal increases in mitochondrial numbers have been noted in a variety of myopathies. Peripheral aggregates of morphologically normal mitochondria (Fig. 8.14) have been found to be particularly prominent in corticosteroid myopathy (Engel 1966) and in hypokalaemic periodic paralysis (MacDonald et al 1969). Triangular subsarcolemmal aggregates of normal mitochondria are found in the lobulated fibres which occur in facioscapulohumeral dystrophy and a number of other neuromuscular disorders, and account for the characteristic histochemical appearances of these fibres in oxidative enzyme preparations (Bethlem et al 1973).

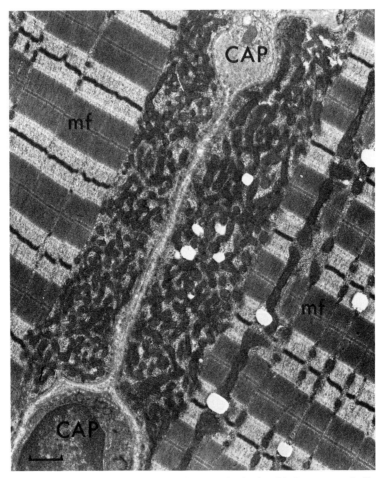

Fig. 8.14 Large sub-sarcolemmal aggregates of morphologically normal mitochondria in two muscle fibres (mf) in a case of mitochondrial myopathy. Two capillaries (CAP) indent the surface of the muscle fibres. Bar: 1.0 μm

Cases in which mitochondria are not only abundant but also show bizarre abnormalities such as increases in size, abnormal cristae and the presence of amorphous, tubular or paracrystalline inclusions are in a separate category (Fig. 8.15). Such changes have been found in various forms of inherited or acquired myopathy but are especially prominent in the group of so-called 'mitochondrial' myopathies in which they represent the most prominent and earliest morphological change seen in muscle fibres (see below, p. 326). The structure of the mitochondrial inclusions has been considered in detail by a number of authors (Chou 1969, Neville 1973, Morgan-Hughes & Landon 1983, Rowland et al 1983, Schmalbruch 1983). Electron-probe X-ray microanalysis of the paracrystalline inclusions has revealed an excess of phosphorus, sulphur, chlorine, potassium and calcium ions over those in control mitochondria (Baruah et al 1983). The relative excess of phosphorus and sulphur suggests that the inclusions are proteinaceous in nature. Electron-dense granules (Fig. 8.16) thought to be calcific, have been noted in a number of situations including glycogen storage disease (Engel & Dale 1968) and hypothyroid myopathy (F. L. Mastaglia, unpublished observations).

Other distinctive changes

Tubular aggregates. These are collections of parallel tubules 60–80 nm in diameter, usually

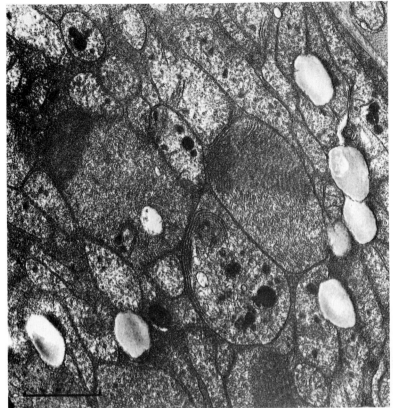

Fig. 8.15a

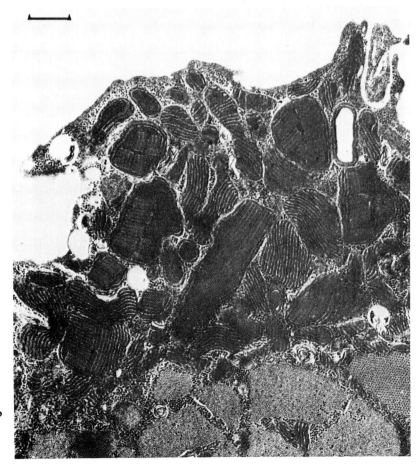

Fig. 8.15b

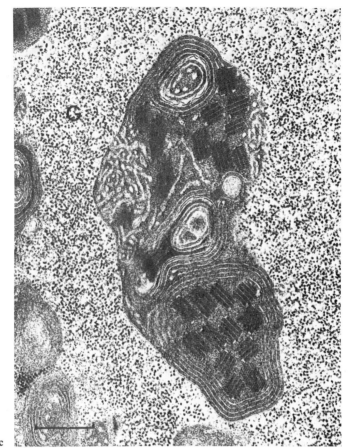

Fig. 8.15c

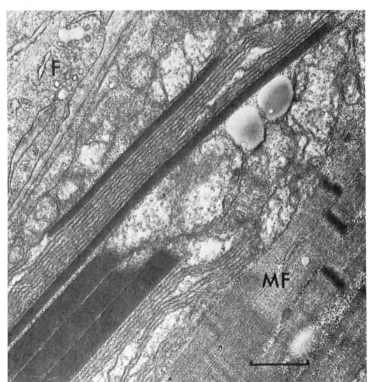

Fig. 8.15d

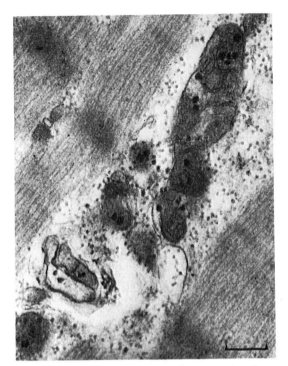

Fig. 8.16 Unduly prominent electron-dense granules of probable calcific nature within mitochondria. Hypothyroid myopathy. Bar: 0.25 μm

found at the edges of Type II fibres in a number of unrelated clinical and experimental conditions, the only definite disease connection apparently being with periodic paralysis (Bradley 1969, Meyers et al 1972, Rosenberg et al 1985, Roullet et al 1985). On morphological criteria there are at least three types of aggregate occurring in the literature: in the first, the commonest, the tubules contain a co-axial non-membranous inner tubule (Fig. 8.17); in the second the tubules have a more densely staining granular core, and in the third the tubules have filaments, approximately 10 nm in diameter, attached around their outer edge. It is clear that the first type, at least, is derived from elements of the sarcoplasmic reticulum (SR).

Concentric laminated bodies. Concentric laminated bodies are hollow cylindrical structures of

characteristic form which occur principally in type II fibres (Payne & Curless 1976). Concentric laminae approximately 7 nm thick, with centre-to-centre spacing of 8.5 nm, make up the walls of the cylinders. The laminae consist of parallel double bands approximately 12 nm wide running circumferentially and projecting about 7 nm at the outside edge with a repeat of 16 nm (Fig. 8.18). There may be up to 25 laminae to each cylinder. Their origin is uncertain. Luft et al (1962) considered that they arise from mitochondria whereas Toga et al (1970) and Payne & Curless (1976) thought that they derive from myofilaments. However they are not membranous and the subunit dimensions do not correspond to those of the thick or thin filaments. They were first described in hypermetabolism of non-thyroid origin (Luft et al 1962) and have since been described in many types of condition, although these do not offer any clue to their origin (Cullen & Mastaglia 1982).

Fingerprint bodies. These consist of short lamellae spaced approximately 30 nm apart and arranged in patterns resembling fingerprints. They are non-specific, having been described in benign congenital myopathy (Engel et al 1972), dystrophia myotonica (Tomé & Fardeau 1973) and oculopharyngeal muscular dystrophy (Julien et al 1974). Their origin is obscure.

Zebra bodies or leptomeres. These are filamentous structures with light bands alternating with thinner darker bands with a repeat of about 150 nm (Fig. 8.19). They are found at normal myotendinous junctions, in normal extraocular muscle and in intrafusal muscle fibres as well as in diseased muscle. They were a frequent finding in a patient with an unusual form of slowly progressive congenital myopathy (Lake & Wilson 1975) and we have observed them in a case of hypothyroid myopathy.

Curvilinear bodies. These structures, which

Fig. 8.15 Mitochondrial myopathy. a. Sub-sarcolemmal collection of pleomorphic mitochondria some of which have electron-dense inclusions and abnormal cristal configurations. Bar: 1.0 μm. b. Peripheral aggregate of mitochondria with paracrystalline inclusions of various types and abnormal cristal patterns. Bar: 0.5 μm. c. Abnormal mitochondrion with rectangular 'parking-lot' inclusions and coiled cristae. G = glycogen granules; Bar: 0.5 μm. d. Electron-dense elongated crystalline mitochondrial inclusions. MF = myofibrils; F = fibroblast; Bar: 0.5 μm

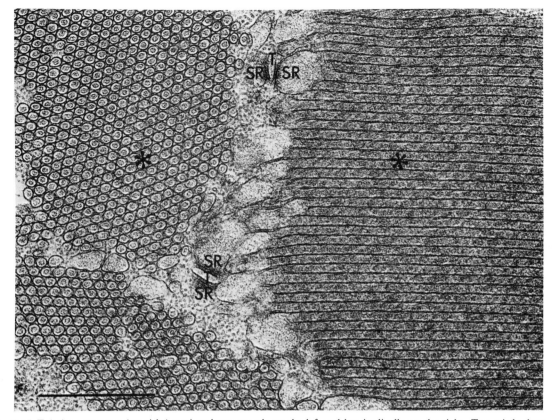

Fig. 8.17 Tubular aggregates (asterisks) sectioned transversely on the left and longitudinally on the right. Two triads show that the sacs from which the tubules are derived are SR. T = T tubule. Bar: 1 μm

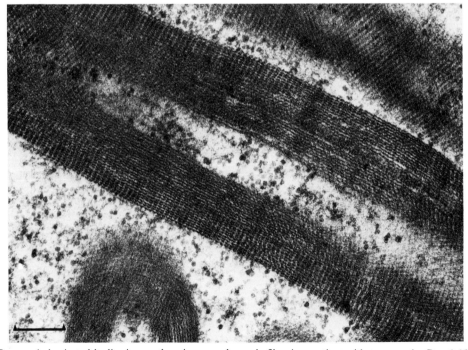

Fig. 8.18 Concentric laminated bodies in an otherwise normal muscle fibre in a patient with acromegaly. Bar: 0.25 μm

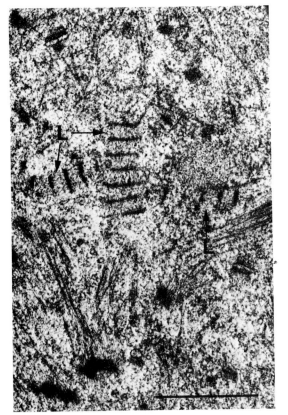

Fig. 8.19 Leptomeres (L) in a disorganised fibre in a patient with hypothyroid myopathy. Bar: 1 μm

appear to be basically membranous in nature, have been observed in association with lipofuscin bodies in chloroquine myopathy (Mastaglia et al 1977, Neville et al 1979) and are identical to the curvilinear bodies described in cerebral glial cells and the neurones in neuronal ceroid-lipofuscinosis (Rapola & Haltia 1973).

Reactions of satellite cells. Several studies have shown that there is a two- to three-fold increase in satellite cell numbers in Duchenne muscular dystrophy (Wakayama & Schotland 1979, Wakayama et al 1979, Cullen & Watkins 1981, Ishimoto et al 1983), distal muscular dystrophy (Nonaka et al 1985), dermatomyositis (Chou & Nonaka 1977) and polymyositis (Ishimoto et al 1983). This holds true whether the numbers are expressed in relation to the number of myonuclei or the numbers of myofibres. Despite the abundance of satellite cells, regeneration eventually fails in dystrophic muscles: it would seem, therefore, that the events causing this failure occur later than the satellite cell or myoblast stage (Watkins & Cullen 1986).

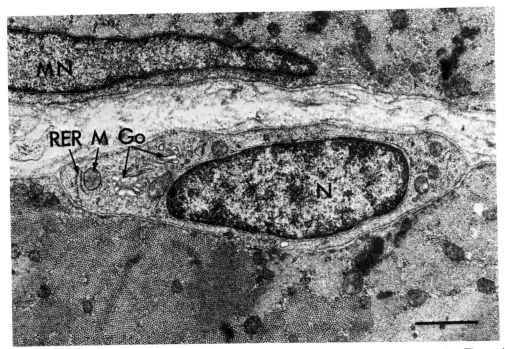

Fig. 8.20 A satellite cell in the quadriceps muscle of a six-year-old boy with Duchenne muscular dystrophy. The section has passed through an area of cytoplasm containing rough endoplasmic reticulum (RER), mitochondria (M) and Golgi apparatus (Go). N = nucleus. Bar: 1 μm (from Watkins & Cullen 1986, with permission from John Wiley)

Satellite cell numbers have also been reported to increase after denervation of experimental animal muscle (Hess & Rossner 1970, Aloisi et al 1973, Ontell 1974, Hanzlikova et al 1975, Schultz 1978, Snow 1983). However, in all these studies the satellite cell numbers were expressed in relation to myonuclear number which can also vary after denervation; the data are therefore difficult to interpret. Normally, growth after re-innervation is by regrowth of existing atrophic myofibres, not by regeneration, *sensu stricto*, of new fibres derived from the progeny of satellite cells. The role, if any, of satellite cells in denervated and reinnervated muscle has not yet been thoroughly examined and remains an interesting area of investigation.

It is widely believed that satellite cells adopt a resting conformation in healthy mature muscle (see Ch. 2, p. 58) and that when they become activated their structure changes as the amount of cytoplasm and the number of cytoplasmic organelles increases. Figure 8.20 shows a profile of such an 'activated' cell in a case of DMD (compare with the resting cell in Fig. 2.21). However, to describe satellite cells as either 'resting' or 'activated' on ultrastructural grounds alone is unjustifiable. In a detailed comparison of satellite cell profiles in DMD, polymyositis and normal controls, Watkins & Cullen (1986) found that the nuclear-to-cytoplasmic area ratios were the same in each sample, i.e. one was as likely to find an 'activated' cell in the control muscle as in the diseased. The cellular constituents were also similar in all three samples; the only detectable difference was that the satellite cells in the DMD sample contained on average more micropinocytotic vesicles or caveolae than those in the normal sample. This was attributed to a generalised cell response to a physiologically altered environment in the dystrophic muscle.

Blood vessel reactions. Ultrastructural observations have been made on the muscle capillaries and other small blood vessels in a variety of neuromuscular disorders. Thickening of the capillary basal lamina is a common finding which is particularly prominent in diabetes (Zacks et al 1962), polymyositis (Vick 1971, Mastaglia & Walton 1971b) and a variety of other disorders. Lamellation of the capillary basal lamina is also

seen in a number of conditions including Duchenne dystrophy, periodic paralysis (Koehler 1977) and polymyositis (Mastaglia & Walton 1971b).

An increase in size of the endothelial cells and increased numbers of pinocytotic vesicles in such cells have been found in polymyositis (Mastaglia & Walton 1971b), Duchenne dystrophy (Jerusalem et al 1974b) and in various other situations and is clearly a non-specific reaction. Degenerative changes in the endothelial cells of small vessels, such as the finding of myelin-like bodies, are also non-specific and have been noted in hypothyroid myopathy and in chloroquine neuromyopathy (Mastaglia et al 1977).

Basic pathological reactions

Atrophy. The most obvious indication of atrophy, whether it results from disuse (Klinkerfuss & Haugh 1970, Mendell & Engel 1971), denervation (Recondo et al 1966, Mastaglia & Walton 1971a) or any other cause, is a reduction in the cross-sectional area of the fibres. This is often accompanied by a change in shape of the fibres: they may become angular in profile and sometimes become heavily indented at the periphery. The main loss of material in the fibres is from the myofibrils which gradually decline in diameter, although this may not become clear until intermyofibrillar spaces develop. The myofibrillar atrophy usually begins at the periphery of the fibres and moves centrally. In longitudinal section there may be clear disorganisation of myofilament and myofibril alignment, although in some situations well-organised myofibrils persist until very late stages of atrophy. Z-line streaming is common in atrophying muscle (Fig. 8.6).

The amount of SR and T system appears to increase in atrophic fibres, although this is probably relative (to the volume of myofibrils) and not a real increase (Stonnington & Engel 1973, Cullen & Pluskal 1977). The T tubules and triads lose their transverse alignment and take up a random or nearly longitudinal orientation. Honeycomb structures are formed in association with the T tubules (Fig. 8.13). The sarcoplasm of atrophic fibres is usually well endowed with Golgi apparatus, rough endoplasmic reticulum and ribosomes (Stonnington & Engel 1973, Cullen et al 1978) suggesting that active synthesis as well as break-down occurs. As the fibres atrophy their edges can become deeply invaginated. The basal lamina follows these invaginations but can also get thrown into redundant empty folds (Fig. 8.2).

The cellular mechanisms controlling myofibre atrophy are still poorly understood. Little is known about how the different myofibrillar proteins are broken down but there is widespread evidence for lysosomal participation (Bird & Roisen 1986). The degradation of purified myofibrillar proteins by cathepsins B and D has been demonstrated using SDS-polyacrylamide-gel electrophoresis (Schwartz & Bird 1977) and immunofluorescence studies have shown an intracellular localisation of cathepsins B and H in developing

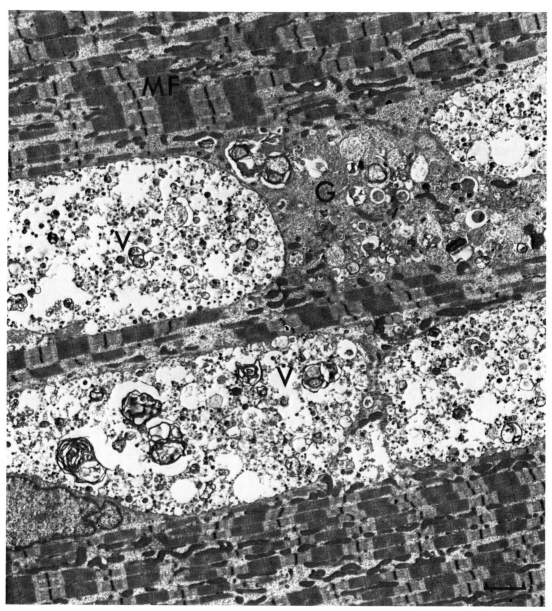

Fig. 8.21 Large autophagic vacuoles (V) containing granular and membranous material. The vacuoles have led to wide separation of the myofibrils (MF). G = glycogen. Vacuolar myopathy of undetermined cause. Bar: 2.0 μm

myoblasts (Bird et al 1982). A major area of uncertainty is the role of non-lysosomal proteinases, such as calpain, which, it has been suggested, may be involved in the release of polypeptides from myofilaments prior to being taken up by lysosomes for digestion (Dayton et al 1976). Recently developed techniques using antibodies against specific enzymes for their ultrastructural localisation should provide information on the intracellular sites of activity of these enzymes and greatly enhance our understanding of the mechanism of protein turnover in muscle.

Hypertrophy. Muscle fibre hypertrophy may occur physiologically as a response to an increased workload in individuals with a high level of physical activity and may also occur in certain disease states. In muscle pathology it is found most markedly in myotonia congenita and in the more slowly progressive muscular dystrophies such as the Becker and limb-girdle varieties. Myofibre hypertrophy is also found in long-standing hypothyroidism and acromegaly where both fibre types are affected (Mastaglia 1973). Muscle fibre hypertrophy, which is presumably of a compensatory nature, is also encountered in states of chronic partial denervation such as the slowly progressive forms of spinal muscle atrophy.

The increased cross-sectional area of the muscle fibres has been shown to be due mainly to an increase in the number of myofibrils (Miledi & Slater 1969). The basic mechanisms involved in the laying down of new myofibrils are still incompletely understood. Longitudinal splitting of myofibrils, once they reach a critical size, may be one of the ways in which they increase their numbers (Goldspink 1972). Hypertrophied fibres contain an increased number of myonuclei, with the new nuclei presumably being incorporated following division of the satellite cells.

Autophagy. Autophagy or self-digestion is a normal cellular activity of living tissues and is a mechanism for the turnover of cytoplasmic components, for the disposal of redundant components and for the use of cell constituents as emergency sources of energy. The process becomes stimulated and especially important when the tissue is exposed to unfavourable conditions

such as starvation, dietary deficiency or inhibition of protein synthesis. When the stress is prolonged, autophagy may be followed by death and necrosis of the cells.

Autophagic vacuoles can be found in small numbers in normal muscle but increase in numbers in both myopathic (Nonaka et al 1985) and neurogenic (Mrak et al 1982) neuromuscular diseases. They are particularly prominent in vincristine and chloroquine myopathies (Rewcastle & Humphrey 1965, Tagerud et al 1986). They contain sarcoplasm, glycogen, mitochondria and other organelles undergoing degradation (Fig. 8.21) but to the authors' knowledge have not been found to contain myofibrillar material. The turnover of myofilaments is thought to occur by non-lysosomal pathways, at least in the early stages (Cullen et al 1978).

Autophagic vacuoles are bounded by single, double or multiple membranes, the source of which is still controversial. For discussion of this question the reader is referred to the article by Cullen & Mastaglia (1982). Some of the conflicting observations could be explained if the initial enveloping membrane were derived from the SR and if the digested debris were, under certain circumstances, exocytosed into the (expanded) T tubules, which thus would act as a gutter to the fibre periphery (Kelly et al 1986). Normally, exocytosis of the cell debris is through the plasma membrane (Fig. 8.1) but, as the T system is continuous with the plasma membrane, it could act as a channel from the interior to the exterior of the muscle fibre.

Necrosis. Although necrosis of a cell may result from a variety of exogenous or endogenous stresses, the immediate cause is the loss by the cell of the ability to maintain physiological homeostasis. The plasma membrane, separating the cell cytoplasm from the extracellular space, ceases to act as an ionic barrier and the cytosol becomes isosmotic with the extracellular fluid. Whereas cell death can usually be recognised without great difficulty in mononuclear cells, it can be much more difficult to distinguish in skeletal muscle because of the multinucleate nature of the myofibres. Part of a fibre may appear healthy, while another part of the same fibre may be clearly necrotic. This segmental necrosis can be observed only in longitudinal sections and has been most commonly observed in Duchenne muscular dystrophy (Adams et al 1962, Schmalbruch 1975, Cullen & Mastaglia 1980). There is often a longitudinal gradient of events from a normal to a necrotic segment of the fibre, but the line of demarcation between the living and the dead part of the fibre can be extremely difficult to identify because conventional electron microscopy can tell us little about the biochemical status of the cell. Thus, one can sometimes be very certain that an area is necrotic (e.g. if phagocytosis is taking place) and can be confident that another area is normal; but the intermediate areas of prenecrosis and early necrosis have to be interpreted with considerable caution. The components of a muscle fibre may appear extremely bizarre without the fibre being necessarily necrotic.

Certain features, however, can be reliable indicators of necrosis. Nuclei can undergo a variety of changes in diseased muscle (see above, p. 287) but in necrotic muscle the changes are terminal: e.g. loss of the membranes of the nuclear envelope (Fig. 8.22) must preclude any normal nuclear function. An intact plasma membrane is also a requisite for normal cell function and a necrotic fibre will usually demonstrate either partial or complete loss of this membrane (Fig. 8.22). In DMD an apparent loss of the plasma membrane may also be a feature of prenecrosis (see below).

The changes to the myofibrils may conveniently be grouped into three main forms. First, there may be severe hypercontraction of the myofibrils. As this can also be caused by mechanical damage to muscle fibres in contact with calcium-containing media (Karpati & Carpenter 1982) it seems likely that it is initiated in vivo by a massive, perhaps rapid, influx of calcium from the extracellular fluid which overwhelms the buffering capacity of the sarcoplasmic reticulum and mitochondria. Secondly, there can be preferential loss of different segments of the myofibrils. Loss of the Z line and I band (Fig. 8.23) has been described in a variety of diseases and conditions (Gonatas et al 1965, Johnson 1969, Afifi 1972, Cullen & Fulthorpe 1982). It is also one of the characteristics of ischaemic (Karpati et al 1974) and postmortem muscle. This suggests that it is caused by

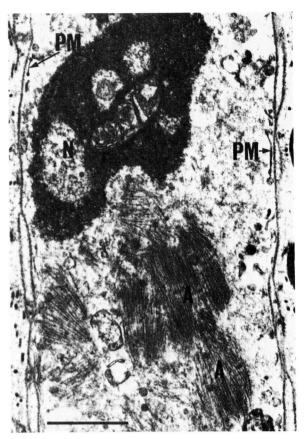

Fig. 8.22 Part of a severely necrotic myofibre in a case of polymyositis showing loss of the nuclear membrane and plasma membrane (PM). A = A band. N = nucleus Bar: 1 μm (from Cullen & Fulthorpe 1982)

a more spatially uniform and gradual rise of cytosol calcium concentrations. The dissolution of the Z line may be mediated by calpain, the calcium-activated neutral protease which is able to extract Z lines, at least in vitro (Busch et al 1972, Dayton et al 1976). A-band loss (Fig. 8.24) is less common than Z-line and I-band loss, but has been described in childhood dermatomyositis, adult dermatomyositis (Carpenter et al 1976), polymyositis (Cullen & Mastaglia 1982) congenital hypotonia (Yarom & Shapira 1977) and a case of polyradiculopathy (Yarom & Reches 1980). The third type of myofibrillar breakdown seen in necrotic fibres involves the reduction of the myofibrils to a homogeneous mixture of filamentous fragments (Fig. 8.25). The mitochondria of necrotic fibres usually round off and the cristae

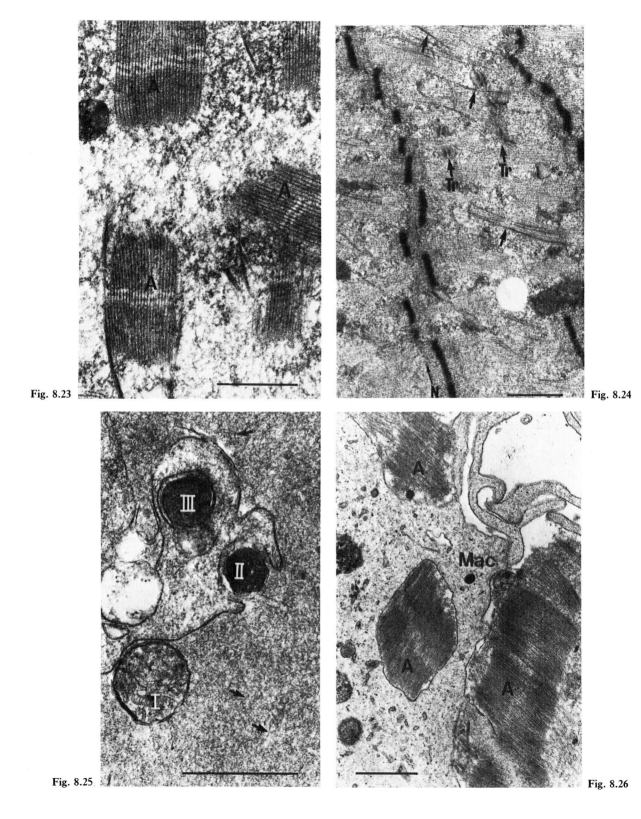

Fig. 8.23

Fig. 8.24

Fig. 8.25

Fig. 8.26

become indistinct or condensed and plate-like. The tubules of the sarcoplasmic reticulum break up into small vesicles which, in hypercontracted fibres, often accumulate between the contraction bands.

Death of the fibres is followed by their phagocytosis by invasive cells which enter through the basal lamina and move through the basal lamina tube. There may be some specialisation by the cells in what they phagocytose and digest. In those fibres in which the Z line and I band are lost it is often possible to see cells which are filled with phagosomes which contain only A bands (Cullen & Fulthorpe 1982). Figure 8.26 shows part of a macrophage ingesting A bands which are nearly intact when they are first taken up; later they become increasingly condensed as they are broken down. Figure 8.25, in contrast, shows part of a macrophage, in a necrotic fibre, which is specialising in ingesting mitochondria.

Regeneration. After mild forms of injury that do not lead to necrosis, degradation and repair of the injured portion occur together and new myofibrils are formed to replace those which have been broken down. The ultrastructural signs of such synthetic activity are the presence of many ribosomes and polyribosomes, and prominent Golgi apparatus and rough endoplasmic reticulum within the sarcoplasm. When necrosis of the muscle fibre occurs, regeneration is brought about by myoblasts which arise internal to the basal lamina of the fibre while its degenerate contents are undergoing phagocytosis (Fig. 8.27). The cytoplasm of these cells contains many ribosomes, polyribosomes and rough endoplasmic reticulum and the nuclei are usually large with prominent nucleoli.

Until quite recently the site of origin of the new myoblasts had been the source of considerable argument. A major impetus to answering this question came with the discovery 25 years ago of the muscle satellite cell (see Ch. 2). A combination of electron-microscopic, tissue-culture (Bischoff 1975, Konigsberg et al 1975) and autoradiographic techniques (Snow 1977, 1978, Hsu et al 1979, Trupin & Hsu 1979) has now shown beyond doubt that the satellite cells are the major, and probably the only, source of new myoblasts in regenerating skeletal muscle. Interestingly, cardiac muscle, which does not possess satellite cells, is unable to regenerate.

The satellite cells undergo mitotic division and generate the population of myoblasts which, in turn, fuse to form multinucleate myotubes. (The normal ratio of myonuclei to satellite cells is approximately 10:1 so the satellite cells need only undergo three or four divisions on average to restore the myonuclear population completely.) Myofilaments and nascent myofibrils appear first in the early myotubes. The first myofibrils usually develop in close conjunction with the plasma membrane, although later they form throughout the body of the myotube. The future positions of the Z lines are marked by ill-defined dense bodies which are linked to narrow bundles of actin filaments (Fig. 8.28). As well as numerous polyribosomes and abundant RER, the developing myotubes contain many microtubules which lie closely parallel with the myofibrils and may be involved in guiding the assembly of the new myofilaments at the myofibril periphery (Antin et al 1981).

Several myotubes may form in parallel in the original basal lamina and normally these will fuse to replace the original myofibre. If, as frequently happens in diseased muscle, the fusion is incomplete, this gives rise to branched fibres which in transverse section can appear as splits (Schmalbruch 1976, 1984, Chou & Nonaka 1977). During

Fig. 8.23 Part of a myofibre in which the Z lines and I bands have been lost. Polymyositis. A = A band. Bar: 1 μm (from Cullen & Mastaglia 1982)

Fig. 8.24 Part of a myofibre in a case of dermatomyositis in which the A bands are absent. There is a small number of individual A filaments (arrows). The triads (Tr) are prominent and are still in their normal position. N = N line. Bar: 1 μm (from Cullen & Mastaglia 1982)

Fig. 8.25 Part of a necrotic fibre on which the myofibrils are reduced to a near-homogeneous pool of filament and fragments of filaments (arrows). The part of the macrophage shown appears to be actively engaged in ingesting muscle mitochondria (Successive steps I, II and III). Duchenne muscular dystrophy. Bar: 1 μm (from Cullen & Mastaglia 1982)

Fig. 8.26 Part of a macrophage (Mac) ingesting A bands (A). Note the near-intact structure of the A band in the early phagosome. Polymyositis. Bar: 1 μm (from Cullen & Fulthorpe 1982)

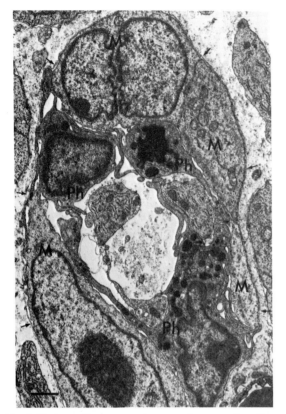

Fig. 8.27 A myofibre at an early stage of regeneration. Four myoblasts (M) or myotubes surround a central area that still contains phagocytic cells (Ph). The boundary of the fibre is delimited by the basal lamina (arrows). X-linked mouse dystrophy. Bar: 1 µm

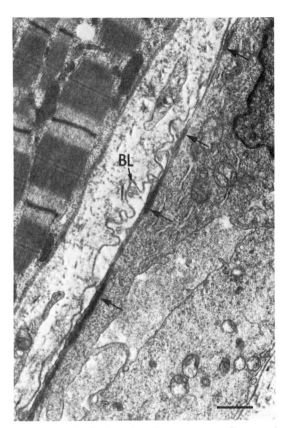

Fig. 8.28 Longitudinal section of a regenerating fibre at about the same stage as that in Fig. 8.27. A nascent myofibril is forming in association with the plasma membrane. The dense bodies (arrows) are Z-line precursors. The young fibre can be distinguished from a capillary by the near absence of pinocytotic vesicles. Duchenne dystrophy. Bar: 1 µm

regeneration the persisting basal lamina of the parent fibre acts as a scaffolding for the developing myotubes. The myotubes later form new basal laminae so a regenerated myofibre usually shows duplication of this outer sheath.

THE MUSCULAR DYSTROPHIES

In the first three editions of this book, this section encompassed the ultrastructural pathology of all the 'classic' muscular dystrophies listed in the World Federation of Neurology classification of neuromuscular disorders (1968, see Appendix to Ch. 13) and defined as progressive, genetically determined, primary degenerative myopathies (Walton 1961). For some years before the publication of the third edition of this book (in 1974)

and certainly since then, clinicopathological and electrophysiological evidence has been adduced to show that some forms of 'dystrophy' do not conform to this definition. In particular, it has become clear that some disorders once thought to be dystrophies are due to degeneration of the anterior horn cell rather than of the skeletal muscle fibre, or at least to changes in the latter which could not be classed as primary necrobiotic degeneration (Bradley 1980). These observations apply particularly to many cases diagnosed in the past as examples of limb-girdle and facioscapulo-humeral dystrophy, both of which should be regarded as syndromes rather than disease entities in their own right. However, we believe that the nosological integrity of Duchenne's disease as a primary necrobiotic myopathy remains unchallenged. Equally, there can be little doubt about the status of myotonic dystrophy on clinical and genetic grounds. Accordingly, this section is restricted to a consideration of the ultrastructural pathology of these two conditions only, without prejudice to any of the current hypotheses about their aetiology and pathogenesis. The ultrastructural abnormalities underlying the facioscapulohumeral and limb-girdle syndromes are discussed in sections concerning spinal muscular atrophy, mitochondrial myopathy etc.

Duchenne muscular dystrophy

Locating the gene. Since the fourth edition of this book was published, there have been very great advances in research aimed at locating and isolating the gene for Duchenne muscular dystrophy (DMD) (Bakker et al 1985, Monaco et al 1985, 1986, Wilcox et al 1985, Kunkel et al 1986). This work has progressed rapidly and investigators working in this field have had regularly to revise or update their conception of the gene. For more specialist accounts of this genetic work the reader is referred to Chapter 26.

One of the immediate benefits of the DNA investigations has been the provision of probes as gene markers that can identify carriers with 98–99% accuracy and can also be used for prenatal diagnosis. This represents a great improvement in the accuracy of counselling for families in whom there is a history of the disease. Although there is a real hope of virtually complete prevention of new cases of the disease in these families, unfortunately there will still be the necessity for the development of a realistic therapy and eventually a cure for the one-third of cases which arise by new mutations. This search for a cure relates directly to the second major objective of the DNA research which is to isolate the entire DMD locus, to clone the gene itself and to identify its product. The hope and expectation is that this will give us some real understanding about the pathogenesis of the disease.

The development of effective therapy when the gene product is known will depend upon an accurate knowledge of the cell biology of the human muscle cell (and in particular, its surface

membrane properties) and of the natural history of the disease. At the moment, it is not even established that muscle tissue is the primary site of the lesion, nor whether the gene is expressed throughout life or at particular developmental stages. Accordingly, in the foreseeable future there will still be an important part to be played by the biochemists, physiologists, morphologists and pathologists who study dystrophic muscle.

Pathophysiology. During the last five years there has been a considerable expansion in the literature on the cell physiology and pathology of dystrophic tissue. In particular, there has been an increase in the number of studies carried out on non-muscle material from Duchenne patients. This work is justified on the assumption that the gene for DMD will be expressed in other tissues besides muscle. In particular, it is often stated that the defect is likely to be expressed in the plasma membrane of the cells being studied (Anand 1983), because widespread credence is given to the hypothesis that there is a systemic or generalised membrane defect in DMD. Thus a large body of work has accumulated which examines the properties of cell membranes in tissues such as erythrocytes, lymphocytes and fibroblasts, where the membranes are more readily available than in muscle. Much of this work was reviewed by Rowland (1980) and by Roses and his co-workers (Roses et al 1980) and another, more recent, assessment would be extremely welcome. Both reviews pointed out that there had been little corroboration of results between laboratories, because of methodological differences and technical variations and limitations. Rowland points out that, e.g. of 27 abnormalities in erythrocytes reported by 1980, there was controversy about all but one of the 18 functions that had been studied in more than one laboratory. The other nine uncontested observations had been reported from only one laboratory. In their conclusions, Roses and his colleagues state that 'It would be prudent to view all reports of abnormalities in the human muscular dystrophies with a healthy degree of scepticism. Experimental corroboration or refutation must be as critically evaluated as the original reports'. This advice is as relevant today as it was in 1980.

The concept of a generalised membrane defect is a development from the membrane hypothesis which itself derives from the 'leaky' membrane theory. The central position of the membrane hypothesis in many workers' thinking justifies a critical assessment of the ultrastructural evidence which supports it.

The membrane hypothesis. At its most fundamental, the membrane hypothesis states that the gene causing DMD exerts its effect by altering one of the components of the plasma membrane. This alteration may be qualitative or quantitative, or perhaps be in the packing of the component. It assumes that all the clinicopathological features of the disease are a consequence of this abnormality.

In his 1980 version of the hypothesis, Rowland confined the effect to an enzyme or structural protein but we prefer to include the membrane phospholipids among the potential components affected. Ultrastructural work on normal muscle (see Ch. 2) has shown that it possesses a membrane skeleton formed by a network of proteins underlying and interacting with the plasma membrane, its major constituent being spectrin. The membrane skeleton is, in turn, linked to the rest of the cytoskeleton. Presumably, any genetic alteration to these sub-membranous components could affect the packing of the membrane constituents, as well as the integrity of the membrane.

The concept of a 'leaky' muscle membrane antedates any ultrastructural evidence of lesions in the membrane by about 15 years, and the development of this concept is well described in Rowland's review (Rowland 1980). Electron-microscopic images of localised loss or perforations in the plasma membrane have been published by several laboratories (Mokri & Engel 1975, Schmalbruch 1975, Carpenter & Karpati 1979, Cullen & Mastaglia 1980) but these images are all difficult to interpret. Figures 8.29 and 8.30 show two typical views taken from two DMD patients. The difficulty in interpretation lies in the fact that loss of the membrane is often observed when the underlying myofibrillar structure is entirely normal (Carpenter & Karpati 1979, Cullen & Mastaglia 1980). If the ionic barrier to the extracellular fluid is lost, it would be expected that the myofibrils would undergo contracture as ionic equilibration with the external environment takes place. In the hyaline fibres, irreversible contracture indeed appears to have occurred (Cullen & Fulthorpe 1975), yet there are many other fibres with perforated membranes in which the myofibrils are relaxed. The question has to be considered, therefore, as to whether the loss of the plasma membrane is an artefact produced by processing for electron microscopy. This seems very unlikely because the membranes are well preserved in other fibres, other cells and even other organelles in the affected fibres, which have all been exposed to the same procedures (Fig. 8.29). It might reasonably be argued that the affected membranes are in some way predisposed to perforation during the processing but this must also mean that the membranes are altered in some way.

The ultrastructural evidence for some kind of alteration in the plasma membrane in DMD is therefore persuasive. However it is not logical to deduce from this that the membrane is the site of the primary lesion in muscular dystrophy: the alteration to the plasma membrane could be secondary to events within the fibre itself. In a study of the changes in pre-necrotic fibres in 15 DMD patients, it was found that the commonest change, and the only one that occurred by itself, was dilatation of the sarcoplasmic reticulum (M. J. Cullen, unpublished observations) (Fig. 8.31). It seems, therefore, that the alterations in the plasma membrane are probably not the first ultrastructural changes occurring in dystrophic muscle (see also Hudgson & Pearce 1969).

The membrane hypothesis is often linked to the concept of calcium overload of the muscle fibres. Normally there is a four orders difference in concentration of calcium ions between the interior ($\sim10^{-7}$M) and the exterior ($\sim10^{-3}$M) of the cell. It is thought that calcium leaks across the defective plasma membrane down the concentration gradient, overwhelming the sequestering capacity of the SR and mitochondria and bringing about either hypercontraction or breakdown of the myofibrils. Cullen & Fulthorpe (1975) speculated on morphological grounds that an abnormally elevated calcium ion level might explain some of

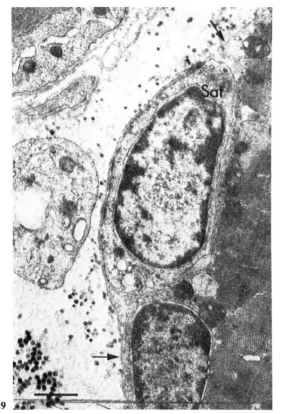

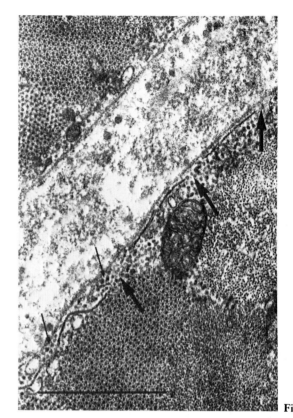

Fig. 8.30

Fig. 8.29 The edge of a fibre in a three-year-old DMD patient showing the absence of plasma membrane beneath the basal lamina (arrows). In contrast the membranes of the myonucleus, mitochondria, satellite cell (Sat) and surrounding cells seem well preserved. Bar: 1 μm

Fig. 8.30 The edge of a fibre in a four-year-old DMD patient showing perforations (large arrows) in the plasma membrane. Glycogen (small arrows) has passed through the perforations. Bar: 1 μm

Fig. 8.31 The edge of a fibre in Duchenne muscular dystrophy in which the only abnormality is dilatation of the sarcoplasmic reticulum (SR). Bar: 1 μm

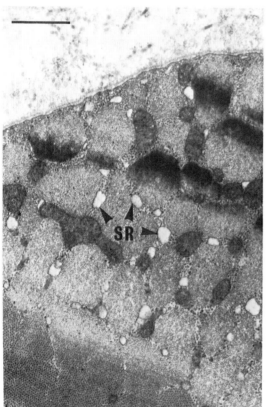

the changes seen in dystrophic muscle. In the same year, Mokri & Engel observed the entry of extracellular fluid containing horseradish peroxidase into fibres with plasma membrane defects and also suggested that intracellular calcium overloading might be an important mechanism of muscle fibre degeneration. Since then there has been a steady accumulation of evidence, both theoretical and material, that there is an association between calcium accumulation and myofibre degeneration in dystrophic muscle (Wrogeman & Pena 1976, Oberc & Engel 1977, Bodensteiner

& Engel 1978, Bertorini et al 1982, Jackson et al 1985).

The remaining question, like that concerning the plasma membrane, is whether the calcium overloading is part of the initial trigger for fibre breakdown. Necrotic tissue normally accumulates calcium: calcium levels therefore should be measured in pre-necrotic fibres. Although the association between a plasma membrane lesion and calcium accumulation is conceptually very attractive, the alternative possibility, that the calcium levels are increased because of an abnormal SR function, should not be overlooked. A technique which might help to answer this question is X-ray microanalysis by which ionic concentrations can be measured with sufficient spatial resolution to allow different compartments of the muscle fibre to be analysed. It is carried out on frozen unfixed material in order to preclude any ionic movement. This has been carried out successfully on normal tissue (Somlyo et al 1981) but, probably because of the difficult techniques of specimen preparation, has not yet been successfully applied to dystrophic tissue.

Freeze-fracture of plasma membranes. Another technique which has advanced rapidly since the fourth edition of this book was published is that of freeze-fracture. This allows an en face view of the internal organisation of membranes (Fig. 8.32). The methodology of the technique and its earlier application to dystrophic muscle is summarised in a review by Shotton (1982). Three main features of the membrane have been examined in normal and dystrophic tissue: intramembranous particles (IMPs), orthogonal arrays and caveolae. Ketelsen (1975) and Yoshioka & Okuda (1977), both examining only one DMD patient, reported an increase in the number of IMPs. In contrast, Schotland's group (who have looked at several series of DMD patients) found a significant diminution in IMPs in both P (protoplasmic) and E (exoplasmic) faces (Schotland et al 1980, 1981, Bonilla et al 1982). They also reported a significant diminution in number of orthogonal arrays from a median of $13.2/\mu m^2$ to almost none and an increase in number of caveolae by 50%. Wakayama and his co-workers (1984) similarly reported a large reduction in the number of orthogonal arrays and also

found that the number of subunit particles per array was reduced from a mean of 21.4 in the controls to 15.2 in the DMD patients (Fig. 8.32). Peluchetti and his colleagues (1985), examining a series of four DMD patients, have similarly found a decrease in orthogonal arrays but, in contrast to the other investigators they found no significant change in the IMPs. All investigators agree that dystrophic muscle plasma membranes have fewer orthogonal arrays and more caveolae than control membranes. The significance of these changes is not understood because the physiological role of both of these components is still unknown. There is still no universal agreement about the changes to the IMPs. These changes may reflect changes in fibre type or maturity in the dystrophic muscle but at the moment it is not possible to examine both histological and freeze-fracture alterations on the same fibre.

Freeze-fracture studies have failed to reveal any lesions which could correspond to the perforations seen in conventional thin-section transmission electron micrographs of DMD muscle (Fig. 8.29, 8.30). This supports the suggestion that the loss of membrane occurs during the tissue processing and that there is some alteration in the membranes of these fibres which predisposes them to this disintegration.

Regeneration in DMD. One of the unexplained features of DMD is that regeneration does not compensate for the wasting that occurs. In contrast to many other conditions and to regeneration following trauma, where there is extensive repair of the muscle, regeneration in DMD fails to keep pace with the breakdown of the muscle fibres. This is crucial because restoration of useful muscle function and strength will be the major aim of therapy when the cause of the disease is discovered.

The inadequacy of the regenerative response is not due simply to a reduced population of satellite cells. Satellite cell numbers are in fact increased two- to three-fold in DMD (Wakayama & Schotland 1979, Cullen & Watkins 1981, Ishimoto et al 1983). The cells are able to undergo mitosis (Fig. 8.33) and the resulting myoblasts are able to fuse as indicated by the presence of multinucleate myotubes in the DMD biopsies

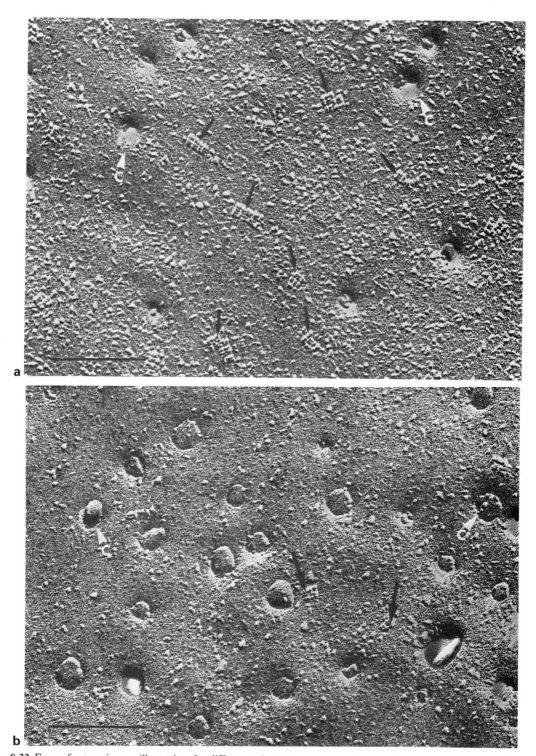

Fig. 8.32 Freeze-fracture images illustrating the differences in orthogonal array (arrows) density and the subunit particle number per array in normal and Duchenne muscle plasma membrane. a. Normal P face. b. Duchenne P face. Note also the increased number of caveolae (c) in the Duchenne. Bar: 1 μm (Electron micrographs kindly provided by Dr Y. Wakayama, Showa University) (from Wakayama et al 1984)

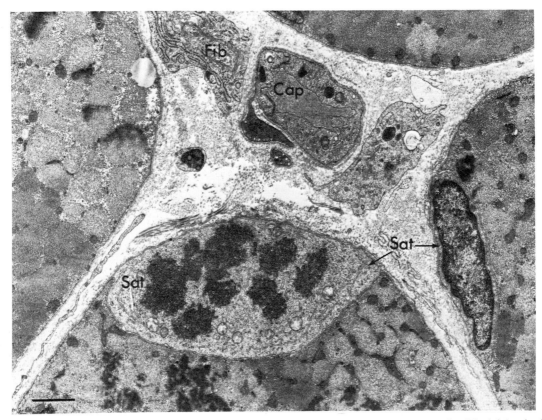

Fig. 8.33 Two satellite cells (Sat) in adjoining fibres in a two-year-old patient with Duchenne dystrophy. The left-hand cell is in mitosis. Fib = fibroblast, Cap = capillary; Bar: 1 μm

(Fig. 8.34). The restriction to regeneration thus appears to operate after myoblast fusion.

Many of the regenerating fibres show ultrastructural abnormalities. The myofibrils are frequently ill-defined and poorly orientated (Fig. 8.35), and the SR and T system are often poorly differentiated and are sometimes dilated. Two more features, perhaps aspects of the same phenomenon, seem particularly relevant to the impaired regeneration. Firstly many of the fibres are extremely small, down to 1–2 μm in diameter (Fig. 8.36) and secondly the edges of the fibres are often indented and fragmented (Fig. 8.37a). At higher magnification it can be seen that in these areas there is an electron-dense 20–40 nm coating to the cytoplasmic face of the plasma membrane (Fig. 8.37b) and fine hook-like bridges extend from the plasma membrane towards the basal lamina. This appearance is exactly like that of the myofibre periphery at a myotendinous junction

(see Ch. 2, Fig. 2.22). It suggests that the growing regenerating fibres react to the proliferating fibrous connective tissue (a striking feature of DMD, see below) by forming pseudo-myotendinous junctions with it. One can thus envisage growth being restricted by the connective tissue and effectively ceasing once the junctions are formed (Watkins & Cullen 1985). In support of this suggestion, Schmalbruch (1984) has reported the formation of myotendinous junctions when branching fibres end blindly in the connective tissue in DMD.

The marked growth in amount of fibrous connective tissue in DMD patients is usually interpreted as a natural secondary response to the wasting of the muscle tissue. The alternative interpretation suggested here is that the wasting of the muscle is partly or wholly caused by the connective tissue having a restricting effect on the regeneration of the myofibres. The interaction

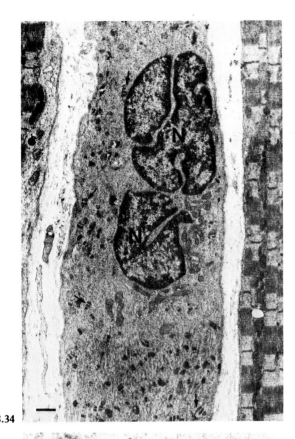

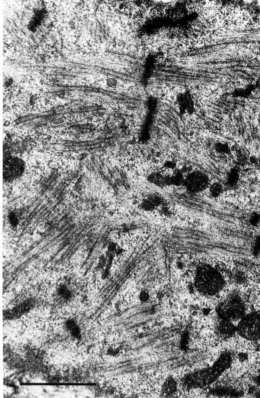

Fig. 8.35

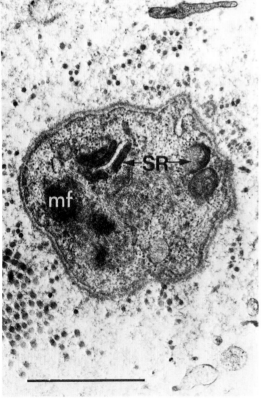

Fig. 8.34 Two nuclei (N) in a regenerating fibre in Duchenne muscular dystrophy. Note the immature triads and pentads (arrows). Bar: 1 μm

Fig. 8.35 Poorly orientated myofibrils in a regenerating fibre in Duchenne muscular dystrophy. Bar: 1 μm

Fig. 8.36 An extremely small myofibre, approximately 1.5 μm in diameter, in a two-year-old patient with Duchenne dystrophy. SR = sarcoplasmic reticulum, mf = myofibril, Bar: 1 μm

between muscle fibres and the surrounding endomysium and perimysium is poorly understood although in DMD it appears to be a very close one (Fig. 8.38). If the considerable amount of work being carried out in different laboratories on DMD fibroblasts (Witkowski 1986) is able to establish a consistent abnormality in their biochemistry or behaviour, the question will then have to be addressed as to how this might bring about the necrosis of the muscle fibres. It might be speculated that this is a muscle surface phenomenon to do with the interface between the plasma membrane and basal lamina (both of muscle origin) on one side and the very closely associated collagen fibrils (of fibroblast origin) on

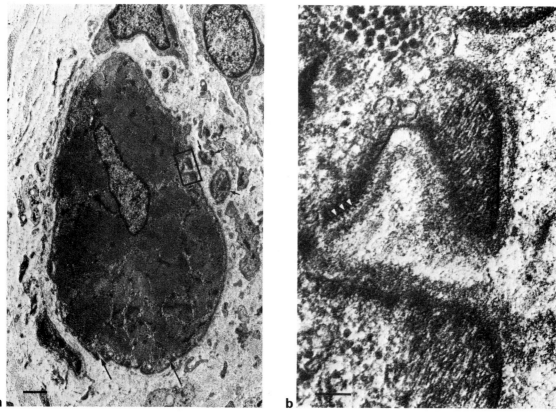

Fig. 8.37 a. A small regenerated fibre in a three-year-old patient with Duchenne muscular dystrophy. The fibre outline is indented (large arrows) and fragmented (small arrows) and there is increased electron density associated with the plasma membrane in these areas. Bar: 1 μm. b. The boxed area of (a) at higher magnification. Electron-dense material lies inside the plasma membrane and bridges (arrows) extend out towards the basal lamina. Bar: 0.1 μm (from Watkins & Cullen 1985, with permission from Blackwell Scientific Publications)

the other. It is difficult to imagine, e.g. that the build-up of collagen around even normal fibres in DMD does not eventually influence their contractility.

Myotonic dystrophy (Steinert's disease)

Myotonic dystrophy is a multisystem disorder in which the numerous clinical manifestations, involving many tissues and organs, may all be attributable to what is (arguably) a common abnormality of excitable membrane function (Roses & Appel 1975). There is no particular reason to believe that the morphological abnormalities in skeletal muscle, as revealed by the light or electron microscope, are likely to help in elucidating the pathogenesis of the condition.

Further to this, the recent demonstration that the gene locus is likely to be situated at or near the apo C locus on autosome 19 (Roses 1986) opens up the possibility of identifying an abnormal gene product. In this case, further pursuit of the morphological minutiae of myotonic dystrophy seems most unlikely to be contributory. Accordingly, this section will be restricted to a brief resumé of the literature in the recent past.

Recent interest has concentrated on the peripheral nervous system in myotonic dystrophy. Pollock & Dyck (1976) failed to find any abnormalities in the population of myelinated fibres in the superficial and deep peroneal nerves of patients with myotonic dystrophy. In a morphometric analysis of the fine structure of those nerves, these authors were unable to find any differences

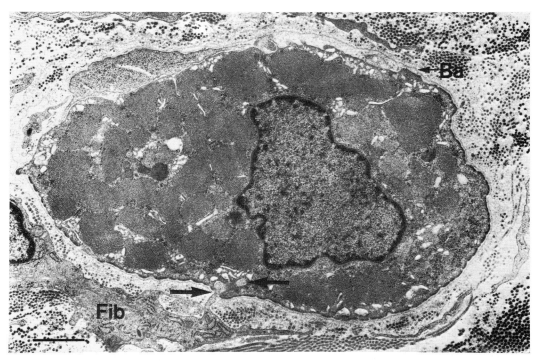

Fig. 8.38 A small regenerated fibre in a four-year-old boy with Duchenne dystrophy. Both the SR and T system are dilated. An adjacent fibroblast-like cell has penetrated the myofibre by extending a cell process (arrows) into a dilated T tubule. Ba = basal lamina. Bar: 1 μm (from Watkins & Cullen 1985, with permission from Blackwell Scientific publications)

between the dystrophic nerves and control material with respect to numbers of myelin lamellae, neurofilaments per unit area and microtubules per unit area of axis cylinder. In contrast, Borenstein et al (1977) reported a case of myotonic dystrophy accompanied by a hypertrophic neuropathy with typical 'onion bulb' formation, extensive endoneurial fibrosis and paracrystalline inclusions in fibroblast processes. Borenstein and colleagues pointed out that any relationship between the nerve and muscle conditions must be conjectural, although there is some physiological evidence for an associated neural defect (McComas et al 1971, Panayiotopoulos & Scarpalezos 1977).

As mentioned in the previous edition, there were a number of accounts in the literature of the ultrastructural pathology of this condition in the late 1960s (Fardeau et al 1965, Klinkerfuss 1967, Samaha et al 1967). None of the ultrastructural changes described in those papers can be regarded as specific although the composite picture they represent may be characteristic (Schröder & Adams 1968). Segmental hyaline degeneration was said to be an infrequent finding in spite of the histopathological evidence of numerous contraction clumps in longitudinal muscle sections, although there was abundant evidence of myofilamentous and myofibrillar disorientation in the muscle fibres. Sarcoplasmic masses, which can be seen either at the periphery or within some muscle fibres with the light microscope, consist of disarrayed myofilaments with associated nuclei, mitochondria and other organelles (Fardeau et al 1965, Schröder & Adams 1968). This type of sub-sarcolemmal change has certain similarities to that seen in some cases of hypothyroid myopathy (Pongratz et al 1979). Circumferentially orientated myofibrils (ring-fibres or ringbinden, Fig. 8.18) may be found either deep to sarcoplasmic masses or beneath the sarcolemma and, in either case, they may represent no more than artefacts of fixation although they can also be seen in rapidly frozen as well as formalin-fixed material. Other changes, such as invagination of nuclear membranes (Johnson & Woolf 1969), the formation of cytoplasmic 'cysts', the accumulation of lipofuscin and myelin-bodies and splitting of muscle fibres (Schröder & Adams 1968) are unlikely to be of primary importance.

POLYMYOSITIS AND DERMATOMYOSITIS

Electron-microscopic studies have provided useful information on the ultrastructural changes in muscle in polymyositis and have contributed significantly to the development of our understanding of the pathogenesis of inflammatory myopathies.

Muscle fibre changes

A variety of degenerative changes has been described in muscle fibres (Shafiq et al 1967c, d, Rose et al 1967, Mintz et al 1968, Chou 1967, 1968, 1969, Mastaglia & Walton 1971b). The most severe of these is the myofibrillar contracture which occurs in entire segments of muscle fibres and which is followed by progressive disruption of the contractile elements and phagocytosis (Fig. 8.26). Less severe changes include areas of focal myofibrillar disorganisation which may take the form of cytoplasmic bodies (Fig. 8.8) or of targetoid areas (Fig. 8.4) and the formation of myelin-like bodies and autophagic vacuoles. The relationship between these latter changes and the segmental necrosis which appears to be the fundamental lesion both at light- and electron-microscopic levels is uncertain. The mechanism of breakdown of the myofibrillar apparatus in degenerating fibres has been discussed in detail by Cullen & Fulthorpe (1982). The regenerative changes in necrotic muscle fibres have been well documented by a number of authors (Shafiq et al 1967b, Engel & MacDonald 1970, Mastaglia & Walton 1971b).

Blood vessel changes

Numerous changes have been described in the small intramuscular blood vessels in polymyositis and dermatomyositis. These include thickening and reduplication of the basement membrane and swelling of endothelial cells which may contain autophagic vacuoles, multivesicular bodies (Shafiq et al 1967c, Gonzalez-Angulo et al 1968, Norton 1970, Mastaglia & Currie 1971) and tuboreticular inclusions within the endoplasmic reticulum (Norton 1970, Hashimoto et al 1971, Nick et al 1971, Jerusalem et al 1974a, Carpenter et al 1976). Such inclusions are found most chacteristically in the childhood form of dermatomyositis (Banker 1975, Carpenter et al 1976, Oshima et al 1979). They have also been described in the endothelium of cutaneous blood vessels (Landry & Winkelmann 1972) and in lymphocytes (Nick et al 1971) in some cases of dermatomyositis; and identical structures are found in the lymphocytes of some normal subjects (White 1972) and in endothelial cells in a variety of other conditions (Györkey et al 1969, Norton 1970, Baringer 1971). The original view that they are viral in nature (Györkey et al 1969, Hashimoto et al 1971) is now regarded as unlikely.

Attention has been drawn to the occurrence of capillary necrosis, particularly in a form of dermatomyositis which occurs in children and young adults (Jerusalem et al 1974a, Carpenter et al 1976), and it has been suggested that the resulting capillary depletion causes progressive ischaemia which is responsible for the muscle fibre damage in this form of dermatomyositis (Carpenter et al 1976). Immune complex deposition has been demonstrated in childhood dermatomyositis by Whitaker & Engel (1972) and by Kissel et al (1986). It has been demonstrated ultrastructurally in the walls of intramuscular blood vessels in a case of polymyositis associated with Waldenström's macroglobulinaemia (Ringel et al 1979).

Inflammatory cells

Electron-microscopic observations on the inflammatory cells in the muscle lesions in polymyositis have provided some support for the view that a cell-mediated immune mechanism is involved in the pathogenesis of the muscle damage. Mastaglia & Currie (1971) found 'activated', 'transformed' and dividing lymphoid cells among the perivascular and interstitial inflammatory cells in two cases of polymyositis. They also found cells resembling lymphoid cells situated internal to the basement membrane of some muscle fibres and in some instances actually lying within the fibre,

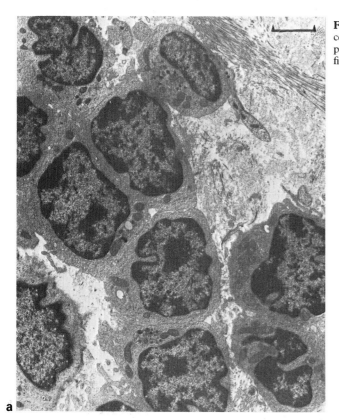

Fig. 8.39 Sub-acute polymyositis. a. Interstitial lymphoid cells. Bar: 2.0 μm. b. Lymphoid cells (LY) which have penetrated the basement membrane (arrowhead) of a muscle fibre (MF). Bar: 1.0 μm

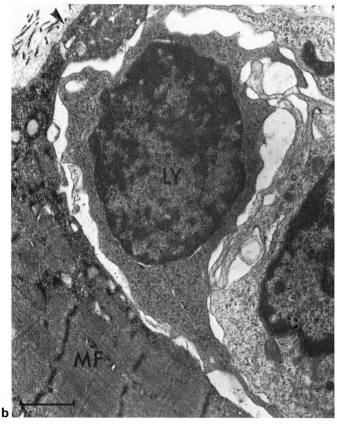

having invaginated the plasma membrane (Fig. 8.39). Similar observations have since been made by Cullen & Fulthorpe (1982). This relationship between lymphoid cells and muscle fibres has also been seen in allogeneic muscle grafts undergoing rejection (Mastaglia et al 1975). An interesting change found in the region of contact between the lymphoid cell and the muscle fibre is the formation of tubular arrays, probably arising from the T system and identical to the honeycomb arrays found within muscle fibres in a variety of conditions. Whether some form of physical contact between activated lymphoid cells and muscle fibres is integral to the mechanism of cell-mediated myotoxicity or whether muscle fibre damage may be effected at a distance by lymphoid cells remains to be determined. Further to this, it seems at least possible that the role of the macrophage in the pathogenesis of myonecrosis in polymyositis has been underestimated. Certainly, macrophages can be seen in the endomysium as well as in necrotic segments in patients who prove refractory to treatment with corticosteroids and other immunosuppressive agents, and they may be the predominant infiltrating cell in some cases, irrespective of their subsequent response to immunosuppression (Emslie-Smith & Hudgson, unpublished work 1987). Further data on the possible pathogenetic role of the large mononuclear cells would be of considerable interest.

'Virus-like' inclusions

Since the original report of myxovirus-like structures in muscle fibres in a case of chronic polymyositis (Chou 1967,1968), virus-like inclusions have been described in at least a further 26 cases. In a number of cases of chronic polymyositis, inclusions consisting of 5–7 nm filaments or of filamentous microtubules of variable diameter (8–25 nm) resembling myxo- or paramyxovirus nucleocapsids have been found (Adams et al 1965, Chou 1967, 1968, Carpenter et al 1970, Hudson et al 1971, Sato et al 1971, Yunis & Samaha 1971, Jerusalem et al 1972, Schochet & McCormick 1973, Hughes & Esiri 1978, Oteruelo 1976, Ketelsen et al 1977, Carpenter et al 1978). In some cases these have been confined to myonuclei or have been present both in nuclei (Fig. 8.40a) and

in the sarcoplasm (Fig. 8.40b) whereas in others inclusions have been found only in the sarcoplasm. Mitochondrial abnormalities and massive accumulations of membranous bodies (myeloid bodies) have also been found consistently in such cases. Many such patients have also had other features in common: a very protracted clinical course; frequent involvement of distal muscle groups, and failure to respond to corticosteroid therapy. The term 'inclusion body myositis' has been applied to such cases and it has been suggested that this represents a distinct form of inflammatory myopathy (Carpenter et al 1978). This is, in fact, unlikely as some cases are clinically very similar to dermatomyositis and may show at least a partial response to treatment with corticosteroids (Lane et al 1985). Indeed, some authorities claim that inclusion bodies of the kind described above occur quite frequently in their material (Banker 1986, Ringel et al 1986) although this has not been our experience.

The nature of the nuclear and sarcoplasmic inclusions in these cases is uncertain. The variable dimensions, sub-structure and distribution within muscle fibres of the filamentous inclusions suggests that they may derive from several different sources. While the possibility remains that, at least in some cases, they are viral in nature, an infective agent has yet to be isolated from any such cases and serological studies have also failed to provide evidence for a myxo- or paramyxovirus infection. On the other hand, if a viral agent is present in muscle in such cases, it may not necessarily be in an infective form, and its isolation may require the use of specialised co–cultivation techniques rather than the conventional tissue culture methods used for the isolation of infective viruses.

A second variety of virus-like inclusions has been described in some cases of acute or sub-acute dermatomyositis. These have been confined to the sarcoplasm and have consisted of paracrystalline arrays of 1.5–3 nm particles resembling viruses of the picorna group (Chou & Gutmann 1970, Mastaglia & Walton 1970, Ben-Basset & Machtey 1972, Sato & Nakamura 1975, Tang et al 1975, De Reuck et al 1977a, Fukuyama et al 1977, Györkey et al 1978), or in one case, of noncrystalline aggregates of 16–24 nm particles resem-

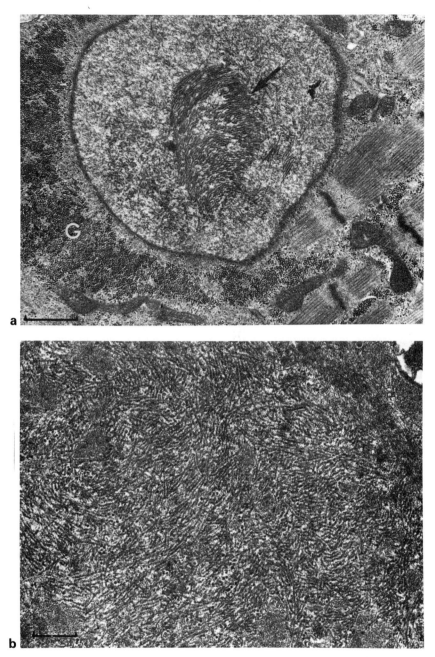

Fig. 8.40 Inclusion body myositis. Intranuclear (arrow) (a) and cytoplasmic (b) aggregates of virus-like filamentous tubules. G = glycogen granules; Bar: (a) 1.0 μm; (b) 0.5 μm

bling viral ribonucleoprotein (Mastaglia & Walton 1970). Attempts at viral isolation from muscle have been successful in only one of these cases in which Coxsackie A9 virus was grown (Tang et al 1975). The finding of identical structures, often without accompanying pathological changes, in malignant hyperpyrexia (Schiller & Mair 1974), Reye's syndrome (Alvira & Mendoza 1975, Hanson & Urizar 1975), idiopathic scoliosis (Webb & Gillespie 1976) and various other situations (Schmalbruch 1967, Caulfield et al 1968) raises the possibility that these structures may not be viral in nature. It has been suggested that paracrystalline arrays of this type may represent one of the forms in which glycogen may be present in muscle fibres. However, Fukuhara (1979), using the cis-platinum (II) technique, has shown that they contain nucleic acids and has concluded that they may, after all, represent an RNA virus.

Cytoplasmic aggregates of larger (87 nm) spherical particles of possible viral origin have also been described in muscle fibres in a young woman with rapidly progressive fatal polymyositis (Martinez et al 1974). Attempts at virus isolation from muscle in this case were also unsuccessful.

The evidence for a viral aetiology in polymyositis and dermatomyositis remains in doubt. Further studies using techniques for the identification of viral genome within cells (Jones et al 1979) and for the isolation of defective or latent virus from tissues, as well as conventional virological technology, are required to clarify the role of viruses in the pathogenesis of these disorders.

METABOLIC MYOPATHIES

An increasing number of genetically determined or acquired systemic metabolic diseases, in which myopathy forms a major part of the clinical syndrome, have been recognised. These include the periodic paralyses and other electrolyte disturbances, the glycogen storage disorders and a number of endocrine disturbances, the most important of which are thyrotoxicosis, hypothyroidism, disturbances of adrenal cortical function and acromegaly. In addition to these disorders, we have included in this section those myopathies in which there is a primary abnormality of mitochondrial structure and function or of lipid metabolism in muscle.

Periodic paralysis syndromes

These rare disorders, which are usually familial, are associated with abrupt rises or falls in the serum potassium level. Hypokalaemic periodic paralysis is also a well-recognised but uncommon

feature of thyrotoxicosis, particularly among Cantonese, Chinese and Thais, and may be the presenting manifestation of the disorder.

Electron-microscopic studies of muscle have been carried out in the hypokalaemic (Shy et al 1961, Pearce 1964, MacDonald et al 1969), the hyperkalaemic (adynamia episodica hereditaria) and so-called normokalaemic forms (Bradley 1969), and in the thyrotoxic form of periodic paralysis (Engel 1966, Norris et al 1968, Takagi et al 1973). The most characteristic ultrastructural change found in muscle fibres in each of these disorders has been a marked dilatation of the sarcotubular system which leads to the formation of the vacuoles (Fig. 8.41) which are seen with the light microscope during paralytic attacks (Pearson 1964). This dilatation is thought to arise in the terminal cisternae of the SR (Bradley 1969) and comparable observations have been made in experimental studies of the effects of chronic hypokalaemia in the rat (Kao & Gordon 1977, De Coster 1979). It is known from light-microscopic observations (Pearson 1964) that the vacuolation of muscle fibres is most striking during attacks of paralysis and that little, if any, abnormality may be seen in biopsies obtained in the interval between attacks. In contrast, dilatation of the SR and other ultrastructural changes may be found even between attacks, although these changes are more marked during an attack, or when weakness becomes established in the later stages of the disease. In one particular study of the hypokalaemic form of periodic paralysis, it was found that the numbers and sizes of vacuoles did not appear to vary appreciably during or between attacks (Gordon et al 1970). That the function of the SR is significantly disturbed during attacks of paralysis is shown by the finding of impaired Ca^{2+}-binding and Mg^{2+}-ATPase activity in SR membranes from cases of thyrotoxic periodic paralysis (Takagi et al 1973).

Several other ultrastructural changes have been prominent in cases of periodic paralysis. These include tubular aggregates (see p. 296), which have been found in cases of hypo- and hyperkalaemic periodic paralysis (Grüner 1966, Odor et al 1967, Engel & MacDonald 1970) and in thyrotoxic periodic paralysis (Bergman et al 1970). As mentioned previously, these structures appear to

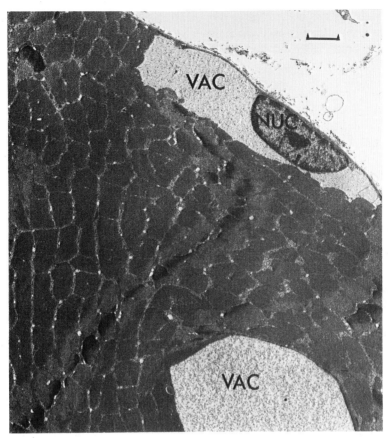

Fig. 8.41 Vacuoles (VAC) containing finely granular material in a muscle fibre in a case of hypokalaemic periodic paralysis. NUC = nucleus; Bar: 2.0 μm

be derived from the SR (Schiaffino et al 1977). Other types of tubular proliferation that probably are also derived from the SR have been described in cases of hypokalaemic periodic paralysis (MacDonald et al 1969). The presence of apparently increased quantities of glycogen lying free in the sarcoplasmic reticulum in the subsarcolemmal region and between myofibrils has been noted in the hypokalaemic (Howes et al 1966, Odor et al 1967), the hyperkalaemic and normokalaemic forms (Bradley 1969) and in thyrotoxic periodic paralysis (Takagi et al 1973) and is in accord with the finding of granular PAS-positive material in the sub-sarcolemmal region in some cases (Engel et al 1967, Brody & Dudley 1969). In some cases this observation was supported by the finding of an increased content of glycogen measured quantitatively (Takagi et al 1973), whereas in others the glycogen content has been found to be within the normal range (Engel et al 1967).

Weller & McArdle (1971) have drawn attention to the finding of a characteristic type of basophilic granular degeneration in muscle fibres in various types of periodic paralysis, which they consider to be caused by the deposition of calcium salts (in a form resembling hydroxyapatite crystals) in association with acid mucopolysaccharide. They postulate that this intracellular deposition of calcium salts occurs initially in the SR, but have also found evidence of calcium deposition in the extracellular space.

Glycogen storage disease

Children with skeletal muscle glycogenosis usually present with infantile hypotonia; adult patients with glycogen storage disease presenting exclusively or predominantly with myopathy are rare. In the relatively few cases of this kind reported to date, a number of different deficiencies of enzymes of the glycolytic pathway have been reported. These have included muscle phosphorylase (Engel et al 1963), acid maltase (α-1, 4-glucosidase) (Courtecuisse et al 1965, Zellweger et al 1965, Cardiff 1966, Smith et al 1966, Isch et al 1966, Hudgson et al 1968, Engel 1970, Martin et al 1973, 1976, Hudgson & Fulthorpe 1975, Schlenska et al 1976, Karpati et al 1977), amylo-1,6-glucosidase (Oliner et al 1961, Murase et al 1973) and possibly phosphoglucomutase (Thomson et al 1963). In addition, a number of familial cases have been reported in which the disorder presented with symptoms indistinguishable from those due to muscle phosphorylase deficiency and in which there were no demonstrable clinical abnormalities at rest. In two families the symptoms were shown to be due to phosphofructokinase deficiency (Tarui et al 1965, Layzer et al 1967) and in one to a possible disturbance of hexosephosphate isomerase activity (Satoyoshi & Kowa 1967).

The light-microscopic changes found in muscle obtained at biopsy in these patients have been essentially similar: a vacuolar myopathy of greater or lesser severity, with accumulation of glycogen granules within the vacuoles, particularly in those lying immediately under the sarcolemma. Electron-microscopic studies have been performed in a number of these conditions. In the case of acid maltase deficiency, Hudgson et al (1968) and Engel (1970) emphasised the sequestration of glycogen within vacuoles lined by a unit membrane, believing this to be a hallmark of a lysosomal storage disorder (Fig. 8.42a, b). They also described vacuoles containing osmiophilic material and complex lipid structures, regarding these as autophagic vacuoles or secondary lysosomes, their contents being the degradation products of phospholipid membranes within the muscle cell. Engel (1970) classified the deposits of glycogen within the muscle according to the abnormal spaces in which they were stored, calling these types 1–4 on the basis of their ultrastructural appearance.

Type 1 spaces. These are sarcoplasmic intermyofibrillar deposits of glycogen which displace other subcellular organelles and which appear to occupy whole segments of affected fibres in some areas. The facile explanation for these deposits has been the rupture of overdistended 'lysosomes' and Hudgson & Fulthorpe (1975) adduced some ultrastructural evidence in support of this (see below). However, it has to be conceded that most of the glycogen appears to be sarcoplasmic in location in both the infantile and late-onset forms of acid maltase deficiency and this has led Cardiff (1966) to question its status as a single-enzyme-defect disease.

Type 2 spaces. Engel (1970) defined these as smooth-contoured sacs lined by continuous unit or double membranes and containing only glycogen (Fig. 8.42a,b). Many of these were quite small (<0.5 μm in diameter) and, in some instances, appeared to be the only abnormality in the muscle cell. Hudgson & Fulthorpe (1975) were able to demonstrate these structures within a satellite cell.

Type 3 spaces. Engel (1970) and Hudgson & Fulthorpe (1975) all described numerous autophagic vacuoles in material from infantile and adult cases (Type 3 spaces). These contained a variety of structures including small dense osmiophilic bodies, lipid droplets and complex membranous structures (Fig. 8.42c). Using Barka's technique (Barka 1964), Engel was able to demonstrate acid phosphatase activity within these spaces in material from three of his cases, supporting the concept that these structures were lysosomal in nature. In contrast, he found no evidence of acid phosphatase activity within the Type 2 spaces or on their membranes, concluding that they may have been abnormal lysosomes deficient in acid hydrolases.

Type 4 spaces. Engel defined these as transitional regions in which admixtures of two or more of the other categories could be seen.

Essentially similar abnormalities to those described above have been reported in a series of subsequent reports on cases of acid maltase de-

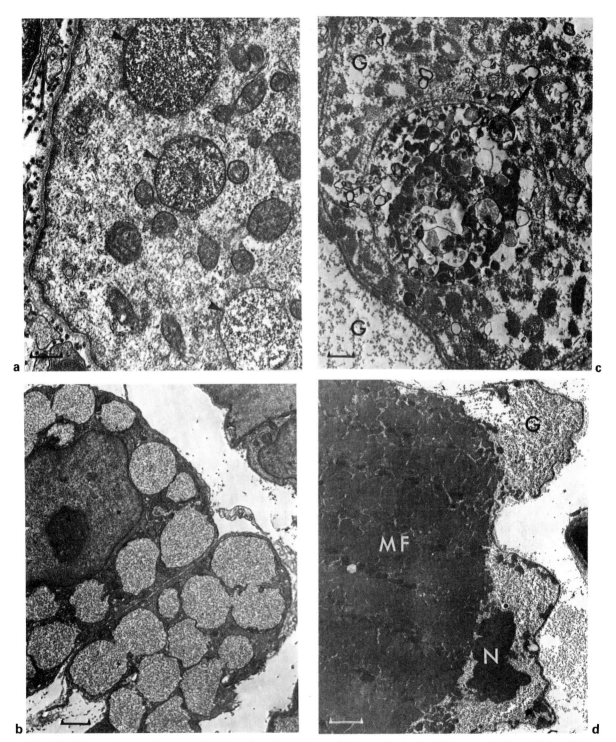

Fig. 8.42 Glycogen storage disease. a. Membrane-bound aggregates of glycogen (arrowheads) in a muscle fibre. Adult acid-maltase deficiency. Bar: 0.5 μm. b. Large membrane-bound collections of glycogen in two interstitial cells. Infantile acid-maltase deficiency (Pompe's disease). Bar: 1.0 μm. c. Autophagic vacuole (arrow) containing sequestered glycogen and other granular and membranous debris in a muscle fibre in which there is also excessive accumulation of free glycogen (G) in the sarcoplasm (some of which has been lost during preparation of the section) leading to separation of the myofibrils. Adult acid-maltase deficiency. Bar: 1.0 μm. d. Sub-sarcolemmal and perinuclear accumulation of glycogen (G) in a case of McArdle's disease. N = nucleus; MF = myofibrils; Bar: 2.0 μm

ficiency by Martin et al (1973, 1976), Schlenska et al (1976) and Karpati et al (1977). In addition, Martin et al (1973) adduced histological and ultra-structural evidence of glycogen storage within the central and peripheral nervous systems in their infantile case, and Karpati et al (1977) found elec-trophysiological and histochemical abnormalities suggesting denervation in material from their case, an adult male. Interestingly, Askanas et al (1976) were able to demonstrate identical changes in muscle grown in tissue cultures established from the biopsy.

In McArdle's disease, glycogen accumulates mainly in the sub-sarcolemmal region (Fig. 8.42d) (Korenyi-Both et al 1977) and in debrancher enzyme deficiency in the intermyofibrillar spaces (Murase et al 1973, DiMauro et al 1979).

In addition to these 'cardinal' ultrastructural features, Engel & Dale (1968), Hudgson et al (1968), Engel (1970) and Hudgson & Fulthorpe (1975) all reported increased numbers of lipid droplets within the muscle fibres of their patients with adult acid maltase deficiency. Hudgson & Fulthorpe were impressed particu-larly by the number of lipid droplets in the ma-terial from their infantile cases and speculated that this may have been due to increased mobilisation of fat stores because of impaired glycogen break-down. Certainly, hyperlipidaemia is well recog-nised in other forms of glycogenosis (Types I, III and VI), possibly because of the chronic hypo-glycaemia associated with these conditions (Jakovics et al 1966) and this mechanism was suggested as a causal factor for the lipid storage myopathy developing in Type I glycogenosis (von Gierke's disease) (Yamaguchi et al 1978b). In this context it is also of interest that mixed glycogen and lipid storage in the presence of structurally abnormal mitochondria has been reported in a child with an improving congenital myopathy (Jerusalem et al 1973a), and in glycogen storage disease associated with structurally and functionally abnormal mito-chondria in a patient with progressive external ophthalmoplegia (DiMauro et al 1973).

Engel & Dale (1968) described a coiled in-clusion in one muscle fibre in their case of late onset adult muscular dystrophy and Engel (1970) found giant mitochondria with crystalloid inclusions in one of his four cases. Hudgson & Fulthorpe

(1975) and Korenyi-Both et al (1977) described concentrically laminated inclusions in material from patients with the adult form of acid maltase deficiency and McArdle's disease respectively. The former authors likened these to the inclusions in the muscle fibres of patients with abnormal carbohydrate tolerance, described by Fisher et al (1972), and of a patient with mucopolysaccharid-osis (Afifi et al 1974a).

Myopathies associated with abnormalities of oxidative metabolism

The history of the mitochondrial myopathies or cytopathies is so well known that it scarcely bears repetition. The reader is referred to the previous edition (Mastaglia & Hudgson 1981), to the comprehensive review by Morgan-Hughes (1982) and to Chapter 25, for detailed references to earlier reports in this area. However it is worth recording that it was an electron-microscopic study (Shy et al 1966) which first established the concept of mitochondrial muscle disease.

Although some early papers questioned the specificity of mitochondrial abnormalities (Shafiq et al 1967d, Fardeau 1970), there is no reasonable doubt that the stereotyped and quite spectacular abnormalities observed histologically, histochemi-cally (Ch. 2, 25) and ultrastructurally are virtually pathognomonic of mitochondrial myopathy (Fig. 2.12). It has to be conceded, however, that it is impossible to predict the clinical presentation of the affected patient on the one hand and the probable metabolic error on the other on the basis of the morphological abnormalities described. The clinical syndromes associated with these abnor-malities and their related metabolic errors (mainly involving the respiratory chain) are discussed in Chapter 25.

Disorders of lipid metabolism

In the last decade it has become clear that there is a group of 'storage' disorders affecting muscle in which neutral lipid accumulates within the muscle fibre, in most cases as a result of defective transport of free fatty acids (FFA) across the mitochondrial membrane to participate in β-oxidation. There appear to be two modes of presentation, one with a relapsing and remitting myopathy and the second with exercise-induced muscle cramps, sometimes accompanied by myoglobinuria (cf. disorders of glycolytic metabolism in muscle). In the first instance, the patients usually present in early adult life with clinical features not unlike those of polymyositis (Bradley et al 1969, Engel & Siekert 1972) and they may even show a partial response to treatment with corticosteroids (Engel & Siekert 1972, Johnson et al 1973). Engel & Angelini (1973) demonstrated deficiency of carnitine, a base with which FFAs combine before crossing the mitochondrial membrane, in one of their cases and this observation has been confirmed in a number of other cases with similar presentations. It has been suggested in the past that carnitine deficiency may be restricted to the skeletal muscle cell in some cases and generalised in others (Engel 1981). However, it has become clear that this distinction is apparent rather than real (Angelini et al 1986); furthermore, recent biochemical studies have shown that carnitine deficiency is likely to be epiphenomenal in many cases, the fundamental metabolic error being acyl coA dehydrogenase deficiencies with fatty aciduria (Turnbull et al 1984). In addition, the sub-sarcolemmal mitochondrial aggregates are usually larger than normal and the individual organelles may contain inclusions. In general terms, however, their appearance is less bizarre than in the 'mitochondrial' myopathies.

Deficiency of the transferase enzyme systems, notably CPT, responsible for transporting the

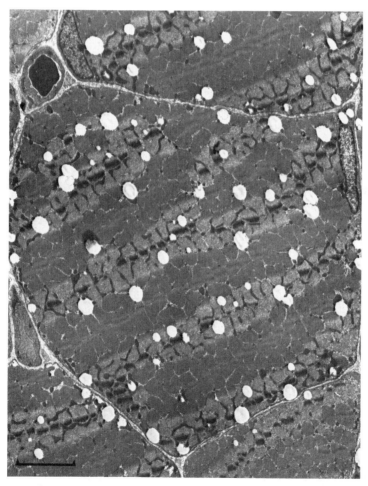

Fig. 8.43 Increased numbers of lipid droplets in muscle fibres in a case of CPT deficiency. Bar: 0.5 μm

acyl-carnitine complex across the mitochondrial membrane, may also lead to lipid accumulation within the muscle fibre (Fig. 8.43) and causes recurrent episodes of exertional muscle pain, cramps and myoglobinuria. In these patients, lipid storage may be demonstrable only while the patient has symptoms, the abnormal accumulations disappearing after a period of rest (Cumming et al 1976).

Myopathies associated with hyperthyroidism and hypothyroidism

Hyperthyroidism. The few electron-microscopic studies of muscle from patients with thyrotoxicosis have shown only relatively minor changes and have not contributed significantly to our understanding of the mechanism of muscle dysfunction in such patients. In a study of biopsy material from two cases of thyrotoxic myopathy, Engel (1966) found prominent papillary projections from the sarcolemma of muscle fibres, large sub-sarcolemmal accumulations of glycogen in some fibres, focal dilatations of transverse tubules and degenerative changes in mitochondria, but no abnormality of the contractile elements. He suggested that the last two changes may have been relevant to the pathogenesis of thyrotoxic myopathy, the mitochondrial abnormalities suggesting the possibility of a disturbance of oxidative metabolism, and the T-tubule changes a possible disturbance of electrical excitation of muscle fibres. Similar changes were found by Gruener et al (1975) who also noted atrophy of both type I and type II fibres.

In thyrotoxic periodic paralysis, glycogen accumulation and distension of the lateral sacs of the SR have been described both during and between attacks of paralysis (Engel 1966, Bergman et al 1970, Takagi et al 1973).

Hypothyroidism. There have been few ultrastructural studies of muscle in patients with hypothyroid myopathy. In general, the changes found have been more striking than those in thyrotoxic myopathy. Norris & Panner (1966) found focal areas of mitochondrial disorganisation, paracrystalline and other types of mitochondrial inclusion, and excessive amounts of glycogen in an adult with a hypertrophic myopathy associated with severe myxoedema. They also noted occasional necrotic fibres but commented that the majority of muscle fibres showed no ultrastructural abnormality. The electron-microscopic findings in the hypertrophic form of myopathy associated with congenital hypothyroidism (Kocher–Debré–Semelaigne syndrome) have been described in a number of cases (Spiro et al 1970, Afifi et al 1974b). Spiro et al (1970) found focal accumulations of glycogen, distension of the SR, and sub-sarcolemmal areas devoid of myofibrils and other organelles in one patient. Afifi et al (1974a), in a study of 10 such children, found very variable ultrastructural changes and commented upon dilatation of the SR, sub-sarcolemmal crescents which in some cases were very large, focal areas of myofibrillar disruption, ring fibres, and the presence of honeycomb-like tubular arrays which were striking in some cases. In a study of a patient with an atrophic form of hypothyroid myopathy, Godet-Guillain & Fardeau (1970) also commented upon the frequency of inclusions and other structural changes in mitochondria, the presence of focal areas of myofibrillar damage which were at times associated with autophagic vacuole formation, dilatation and proliferation of the SR, and abnormal sub-sarcolemmal areas filled with disorganised filaments (sarcoplasmic masses) and often associated with annular myofibrils. They commented upon the similarity of these changes to those found in myotonic dystrophy.

We have confirmed the above observations in a study of four cases of hypothyroid myopathy (unpublished observations). Degenerative changes in mitochondria, and the presence of small myeloid bodies in muscle fibres and in endothelial cells, were the most frequent findings. In addition, in two cases core-like areas of variable size, which were devoid of enzyme activity in histochemical preparations, were prominent and were found to contain finely granular material which bore a superficial resemblance to glycogen but showed unusual staining properties (Fig. 8.44). Mitochondria contained unduly prominent calcific granules (Fig. 8.16) and, in some instances, paracrystalline inclusions.

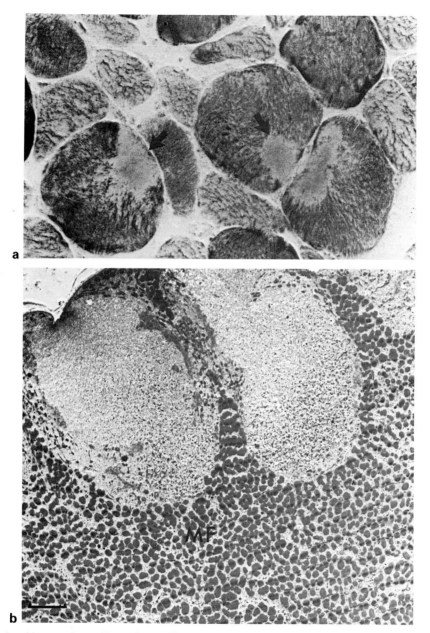

Fig. 8.44 Hypothyroid myopathy. a. Eccentric core-like areas (arrows) are present in three muscle fibres. Succinic dehydrogenase preparation. ×400. b. Electron micrograph of core-like areas showing that they consist of finely granular material with varying staining properties. Similar material separates the myofibrils (MF). Bar: 5.0 μm

The ultrastructural findings therefore suggest that the principal effects of prolonged hypothyroidism are on mitochondria and on carbohydrate metabolism, with the accumulation of glycogen and possibly of some abnormal form of polysaccharide. These findings are in accord with experimental studies which have shown defective oxidative phosphorylation, with changes in mitochondrial morphology and numbers, in thyroidectomised animals (Meijer 1972), and with the impairment of glycogenolysis which has been reported in patients with hypothyroid myopathy (Hurwitz et al 1970, McDaniel et al 1977).

Myopathies associated with disturbances of ACTH and adrenal corticosteroid metabolism

Proximal muscle weakness is commonly found in cases both of Cushing's syndrome and of Addison's disease and is a relatively common finding in patients on long-term corticosteroid therapy, particularly with the fluorinated steroids (see Ch. 29). There have been few studies of the ultrastructural changes in muscle in such cases (Pearce 1964, Engel 1966, Afifi et al 1968). These have not shown any specific changes and have not contributed materially to our understanding of the pathogenesis of the muscle dysfunction. Focal accumulations of mitochondria, and vacuolation and degeneration of these organelles, have been noted in some cases (Pearce 1964, Engel 1966) but it is not clear to what extent these changes were artefactual. Enlargement of muscle mitochondria and similar changes to those found in some of the human cases have also been found in experimental steroid myopathy in the rat and in the rabbit (D'Agostino & Chiga 1966, Ritter 1967, Afifi & Bergman 1969, Freund-Mölbert et al 1973).

Other changes which have been described in the human and experimental myopathy include an increase in intermyofibrillar sarcoplasm, an apparent increase in glycogen (Pearce 1964, D'Agostino & Chiga 1966, Ritter 1967), and neutral lipid droplets (D'Agostino & Chiga 1966, Harriman & Reed 1972, Freund-Mölbert et al 1973) and thickening of the basement membrane of muscle fibres (Afifi et al 1968, Mastaglia et al 1970). The accumulation of glycogen is in accord with the finding of increased glycogen synthetase activity in muscle in experimental steroid myopathy (Shoji et al 1974). Necrosis and calcification of muscle fibres has been found in some of the short-term high-dose experimental animal studies (Afifi & Bergman 1969, Freund-Molbert et al 1973). An acute necrotising myopathy has been reported in human subjects treated with high doses of hydrocortisone for status asthmaticus (MacFarlane & Rosenthal 1977, Van Marle & Woods 1980, Knox et al 1986). Presumably this is analogous to the experimental models referred to above, although no ultrastructural studies have been carried out on the human material, as far as the authors are aware.

The question of the differential involvement of the type II (glycolytic) fibres in human steroid myopathy and of fast-twitch (white) muscles in animals has not been adequately explored in ultrastructural studies.

It is also appropriate to include in this section a reference to the myopathy which develops in patients who have undergone bilateral adrenalectomy for Cushing's syndrome (Prineas et al 1968). A proportion of such patients develop very high serum ACTH levels with generalised skin pigmentation (Nelson's syndrome) and, subsequently, proximal limb muscle weakness. The presence of myopathy was confirmed in these patients electromyographically and Prineas and his colleagues showed histochemically and electron-microscopically that the type I fibres contained excessive amounts of neutral lipid droplets, which were almost exclusively situated beneath the sarcolemma, usually in association with sentinel mitochondria.

CONGENITAL MYOPATHIES

The difficulties encountered in the clinical classification of this heterogeneous group of disorders are discussed in detail in Ch. 20. Unfortunately, the ultrastructural study of biopsy material from 'floppy' infants and other patients with congenital myopathies has not contributed as much as was expected to the clarification of their nosology. However electron-microscopic studies have provided the morphological substrate for the provisional designation of a number of pathological entities since the mid-1950s, although some of their supposedly 'characteristic' structural abnormalities are not entirely specific. Nevertheless, some of these have stood the test of time and are discussed in detail below. In addition, brief accounts are given of the numerous descriptions of single cases of families in which infantile hypotonia or congenital myopathy has been associated with unusual ultrastructural findings in muscle. These disorders

will be discussed under the following headings:
(1) Abnormalities of the contractile apparatus;
(2) Abnormalities of other sarcoplasmic organelles;
(3) Myopathies with intracellular inclusions of various types.

Abnormalities of the contractile apparatus

The first account of a congenital myopathy with a 'specific' pathological basis was given by Shy & Magee (1956) in their description of central core disease, a benign condition usually presenting with infantile hypotonia and with a family history suggesting autosomal dominant inheritance. In this disorder, the type I muscle fibres in particular contain cores in which there are variable degrees of disruption of the normal myofibrillar architecture, the cores being termed 'structured' or 'unstructured', depending upon the degree of abnormality (Neville 1973). In the most severely affected fibres, the cores contain no normal cytoplasmic organelles such as SR or mitochondria. Absence of the latter is reflected in the failure of the appropriate histochemical stains to demonstrate any evidence of oxidative enzyme activity within the cores (Dubowitz & Pearce 1960, Engel et al 1961). Since then a number of variations on the original description have been reported. Afifi et al (1965) described two members of a family in which central cores were demonstrated in biopsy specimens, but in which foci of Z-band degeneration resembling that seen in nemaline myopathy were also found. Engel & MacDonald (1970) described congenital myopathies characterised by the presence of multiple and/or miniature cores (multi- and mini-core disease respectively). In addition Radu et al (1977) described two cases in which the muscle fibres contained structured, unstructured and 'reversed' cores, the latter containing central agglomerations of mitochondria.

Loss of the normal ultrastructure of the contractile elements and reduction in the mitochondrial population occurs also in target and targetoid fibres (Fig. 8.5). These are seen most often in denervated muscle, and focal lesions of a similar nature have been described in patients with progressive congenital muscle weakness (Van Wijngaarden et al 1977, Yarom & Shapira 1977). This curious abnormality is accompanied by type

I fibre predominance, the individual fibres being significantly reduced in diameter. The pathogenetic basis for this condition is unknown, although Van Wijngaarden and colleagues suggested that delayed development of motor nerves may have been involved on the basis of abnormalities demonstrated by supravital staining of the motor end-plates. Van Wijngaarden and colleagues (1977), in a comprehensive review of the literature, considered that several other reported cases were either identical or very similar to their own.

The next disease 'entity' to be described was nemaline myopathy, first reported by Conen et al (1963) under the name 'myogranular' myopathy. Subsequently, sporadic cases, or families with members suffering from the disease, were described by Shy et al (1963), Engel et al (1964), Spiro & Kennedy (1964), Price et al (1965), Gonatas (1966), Gonatas et al (1966), Engel & Gomez (1967), Hudgson et al (1967) and Shafiq et al (1967a). Autopsy confirmation of the widespread distribution of nemaline rods in a patient with adult-onset symptoms diagnosed on biopsy in life has recently been provided by Brownell et al (1978). Bender & Willner (1978), in a histochemical study of a biopsy specimen of muscle obtained from the mother of a patient with myopathy who had been diagnosed on ultrastructural grounds as having nemaline myopathy, found abnormalities closely resembling those seen in the child's biopsy, although the mother's muscle contained no rod bodies. They suggested that this established her status as the gene carrier.

Nemaline myopathy is characterised pathologically by the presence of tiny rod-like bodies (up to 5 μm in length and 1.5 μm in diameter) which lie within the muscle fibre; most of these bodies are concentrated in aggregates at the poles of the muscle nuclei. At the light-microscopic level these 'rod' bodies are usually brilliantly refractile with phase-contrast and interference illumination (Gonatas 1966, Hudgson et al 1967) and stain intensely with the modified Gomori trichrome, picro-Mallory and PTAH stains. Ultrastructurally the rod bodies are electron-dense and the larger ones correspond roughly in size to those seen in light-microscopic sections. These larger bodies may occupy a space in the affected fibres up to two sarcomeres in length and, as in the light-microscopic sections, appear to be concentrated near the poles of the muscle nuclei. Moving away from the nuclei, the bodies steadily decrease in number and it becomes increasingly obvious that they are intimately related to the Z bands (Fig. 8.7a). The smallest ones, in fact, appear to be mere bulbous expansions of the Z bands (Fig. 8.7).

In many illustrations, the rods appear to be 'cross-hatched' due to the presence of transverse and axial striae (Fig. 8.7b). In various reports the transverse striae have had a periodicity of approximately 14.5 nm and the axial ones a periodicity ranging from 12 to 18 nm. The measurements quoted by Price et al (1965) differed significantly from those in most other descriptions of the disease, and led them to propose that the rod bodies might be composed of an altered form of tropomyosin B. Engel & Gomez (1967) found that the periodicity of the striae in the rod bodies in their material did not correspond with that of the crystal lattice of the Z bands. On the basis of experiments involving glycerination of the biopsy and extraction of the filaments with Guba-Straub-ATP solution, followed by treatment of the residue with Szent-Gyorgyi's actin-extracting solution, they suggested that the rods might contain actin, tropomyosin B, a combination of the two, or another protein with solubility properties common to both. However, the most recent evidence available suggests that the rods are composed of α-actinin on a skeleton of actin (Ebashi 1967, Yamaguchi et al 1978a).

As we have pointed out in other sections of this chapter, many so-called specific ultrastructural anomalies, previously identified with discrete clinical syndromes, can occur in a variety of naturally occurring and experimental myopathies. This is certainly the case with nemaline-like degeneration in the Z bands, which can be produced by experimental denervation or tenotomy in animals (Engel et al 1966). Fardeau (1970) has described a similar change in myotonic dystrophy; Cape et al (1970) found rod bodies in material from a patient with polymyositis and we have seen them in various other disorders including muscular dystrophy, mitochondrial myopathy, the myopathy associated with chronic renal failure and in spinal muscular atrophy and glycogen storage disease (Hudgson & Fulthorpe 1975). However, we believe that rod-body formation is still the most important single structural abnormality in some congenital myopathies, particularly those associated with dysmorphogenetic states such as Marfan's syndrome (Hudgson et al 1967).

The last entity to be considered in this section is the 'new' congenital neuromuscular disease with trilaminar fibres described by Ringel et al (1978). In what was clearly an unusual clinical situation, the authors described an infant who was born with a marked increase in muscle tone, paucity of spontaneous movements and increased serum creatine kinase (CK) activity. Biopsy of muscle at the age of seven weeks demonstrated numerous 'trilaminar' fibres containing three concentric zones (see their figures 2 & 3). Electron microscopy revealed that the central zone contained densely packed mitochondria, glycogen, electron-dense material and single myofilaments; the middle zone consisted of deranged myofibrils showing Z-band streaming, and the outer zone resembled a sarcoplasmic mass (see their figures 4–7). Appropriate cytochemical techniques demonstrated extrajunctional AChR between the middle and outer zones in the trilaminar fibres. The authors considered that this finding, together with the child's rigidity, was in keeping with abnormal neural influences of some kind. It is, however, a little difficult to reconcile this with the grossly elevated serum CK activities (2240 i.u./l at birth and 2290 at 14 days) and the gross disruption of the cyto-architecture of the muscle fibres.

Abnormalities of other sarcoplasmic organelles

The first condition to be described under this heading was myotubular myopathy (Spiro et al 1966), now better known as centronuclear myopathy (Sher et al 1967). There are now approximately 50 cases recorded in the literature, although Palmucci et al (1978) have questioned the validity of some of these cases, pointing out that the mere presence of internal nuclei in fibres otherwise resembling myotubes is not sufficient to justify the diagnosis. Nevertheless, there does appear to be a substantial measure of agreement about the histochemical and ultrastructural characteristics of the disease.

In this condition, which appears to be genetically determined (with variable mode of inheritance) and slowly progressive, the majority of the muscle fibres (up to 85% in the cases described by Spiro and colleagues) resemble fetal muscle fibres, being of small diameter and containing central nuclei. Histochemical studies (Sher et al 1967, Kinoshita & Cadman 1968) have shown that oxidative enzyme activity may be either increased or decreased in the central region of the fibres, and that myofibrillar adenosine triphosphatase activity is usually absent centrally (Sher et al 1967). Electron-microscopic studies (Spiro et al 1966, Sher et al 1967, Kinoshita & Cadman 1968) have demonstrated that, in addition to the presence of central nuclei, the central region of the fibres is usually devoid of myofibrils. Sher and her co-workers also found a small number (less than 1%) of centrally situated mitochondria which were vacuolated and contained myelin whorls. In contrast, Campbell et al (1969) found large numbers of similarly placed mitochondria in material from a case of myotubular myopathy studied in this department.

The aetiology and pathogenesis of this condition is unknown, although Spiro and associates (1966) suggested that it may develop as a result of 'maturation arrest' because of the structural resemblances between the myopathic fibres and those seen in fetal skeletal muscle. Bethlem and co-workers (1969) suggested a neurogenic basis for the condition in their discussion of the fourth reported case and Serratrice et al (1978) supported this suggestion. They considered that their histochemical evidence particularly favoured a neurogenic aetiology, their material showing a type I fibre preponderance and atrophy. The authors likened the latter feature to the appearance of type I fibre hypotrophy with internal nuclei (Engel et al 1968) in which a neurogenic basis has also been suggested. In this context, it may also be relevant that De Reuck et al (1977b) described type I fibre atrophy, particularly in respiratory muscle, in a child with severe neonatal respiratory distress. They considered that a neurogenic basis for the

muscle disorder was the most attractive of the possible hypotheses. However, Palmucci et al (1978) claimed that centronuclear myopathy is likely to be a histopathological syndrome produced by several unrelated disease entities, a suggestion mooted previously by Bradley et al (1970).

In 1973, Jerusalem and co-workers described a new, benign congenital disorder in two brothers born of a consanguineous marriage. They called this condition sarcotubular myopathy and reported that it was characterised histopathologically by microvacuolar degeneration affecting the type II more than the type I fibres (see their figures 3 & 4), and which was segmental in distribution in longitudinal sections. Electron micrographs of the affected fibres showed that they contained rows of membrane-bound spaces, some of which were coalescing and some of which were in close relationship to tubular profiles (see their figure 7). Appropriate electron-cytochemical techniques showed that the vacuoles probably originated from the SR rather than the T system. The authors concluded that segmental vacuolation of the SR with selective affection of type II fibres was the characteristic morphological abnormality and they differentiated this from the non-specific dilatation of the SR which occurs in many necrobiotic myopathies and in the periodic paralyses.

Myopathies with intracellular inclusions

The presence of inclusion bodies of various kinds within mitochondria in patients with mitochondrial myopathy and other conditions has already been discussed. In this section, we propose to consider a number of congenital myopathies with inclusions in other compartments of the muscle cell.

Jenis et al (1969) described a fatal congenital myopathy in which they were able to demonstrate eosinophilic crystalline inclusions within the myonuclei, with similar smaller bodies within the sarcoplasm and arising from the Z bands of the muscle fibres. Multiple passage of material from this case through suckling mice and rhesus monkey and human embryonal kidney in tissue culture failed to adduce any evidence of viral infection, but electron microscopy of the intranuclear and sarcoplasmic inclusions indicated that they possessed a crystal lattice not unlike that of nemaline rods (see, in particular, their figure 7). The authors were unable to reach any definite conclusions about the fundamental nature of this condition and particularly about its relationship to other congenital myopathies including nemaline disease. As far as we are aware, no similar case has been described subsequently.

Brooke & Neville (1972) reported two unrelated cases of a progressive congenital myopathy which also had a fatal termination. In each case, light microscopy of muscle biopsies revealed scattered sub-sarcolemmal inclusions which were eosinophilic with haematoxylin and eosin, and red in the modified trichrome preparation. Further histochemical studies demonstrated that the bodies contained both RNA and sulphydryl groups in high concentration, the latter observation prompting the authors to call them 'reducing bodies'. Electron microscopy showed that these bodies were densely osmiophilic, porous structures up to about 10 μm in length. They were not membrane-bound, contained beaded fibrillar material in places and the pores often contained glycogen (see their figures 10 & 13). Speculating on the possible origin of these structures, the authors considered the possibility that they were derived from an RNA virus. They noted, in addition, that the presence of sulphydryl groups in high concentration in skeletal muscle is most unusual, although the sulphydryl-containing amino acid, homocysteine, is produced during the transmethylation of guanidoacetate to creatine.

As far as we know, no other cases of this kind have been reported, although Sahgal & Sahgal (1977) described a non-progressive congenital myopathy characterised by the presence of sub-sarcolemmal inclusions reacting strongly for sulphydryl groups, particularly in type I fibres. However, these inclusions contained granular and filamentous material only at the ultrastructural level and did not resemble the 'reducing bodies' of Brooke & Neville (1972) in any other respect.

At about the same time as the description of reducing-body myopathy appeared, Engel et al (1972) described another curious inclusion in a child with non-progressive weakness since infancy.

These inclusions were observed first by phase-contrast microscopy of semithin Epon sections, and were described as being oval or irregularly circular in shape, invariably subsarcolemmal in situation, often near the muscle nuclei and from 7–10 μm in length. Ultrastructurally they were composed of complex convoluted lamellae arranged in 'fingerprint' patterns (see their figure 5). In each inclusion the lamellae were spaced 30 nm apart and were studded with sawtooth-like projections 6.5 nm wide and 16 nm high, with a period varying from 14.5–16 nm. Predigestion of the muscle with RNase and amylase, disruption of the membranous components of the muscle fibres by glycerination and selective extraction of the myosin and actin filaments, M bands and Z bands, did not alter the appearance of these structures. 'Finger-print' inclusions have been reported in several other cases of congenital myopathy (Fardeau et al 1976), dystrophia myotonica (Tomé & Fardeau 1973) and oculopharyngeal dystrophy (Julien et al 1974). In addition, we have seen a similar structure in material from a patient with uraemic myopathy.

Fardeau's group (Fardeau et al 1978) reported a family with a genetically determined myopathy (autosomal dominant inheritance) with affection of skeletal, pharyngeal and respiratory musculature, cardiomyopathy and lens opacities. The biopsies from affected members of the family revealed what the authors described as 'rubbing out' of the intermyofibrillar network in the type I fibres, electron microscopy showing that this was associated with the deposition of electron-dense granular and filamentous material in the sarcoplasm of the fibres. In some areas, this material was arranged in a meshwork around the myofibrils, although it did not appear to have any structural relationship with the Z band or indeed with any of the other components of the contractile apparatus.

The final condition cited in this section is the recently reported myofibrillar inclusion-body myopathy or cytoplasmic-body neuromyopathy presenting with respiratory insufficiency and weight loss (Clark et al 1978, Jerusalem et al 1979). In this condition the type I fibres contain numerous typical cytoplasmic bodies (Jerusalem et al 1979, see their figure 4). The nature of this condition remains obscure, although some cases are familial with an autosomal dominant form of inheritance.

CONCLUSIONS

The role of electron microscopy in the investigation of diseased muscle has changed since the first edition of this book was published nearly two decades ago. Then, the electron microscope was used principally to acquire basic morphological information about the many different neuromuscular disorders. This cataloguing role is now relatively less important because it has been realised that conventional electron microscopy by itself is unlikely to reveal the basic defect in any one disease. Accordingly, it is being used increasingly in combination with other techniques and the EM specimen itself is being manipulated, probed, fractured and labelled in a variety of ways, some referred to in this chapter. Ultrastructural studies have therefore become less descriptive and more analytical. Increasingly they are being used to pinpoint the location in the specimen of chemical elements (by electron-probe microanalysis), enzymes (by EM cytochemistry) and other proteins (by EM immunolabelling). One might predict that the last-mentioned technique, in particular, is going to transform our view of muscle over the next five years and thereby to provide new insights into the pathogenesis of those muscular disorders which continue to confound medical science.

ACKNOWLEDGEMENTS

The work discussed in this chapter was carried out with the aid of grants from the Medical Research Council and the Muscular Dystrophy Group of Great Britain. We wish to acknowledge the invaluable technical assistance of Mr John Walsh and Mr John Fulthorpe.

The manuscript was typed by Miss Carol Atkinson whose efficient services are greatly appreciated.

REFERENCES

Adams R D, Denny-Brown D, Pearson C M 1962 Diseases of muscle: A study in pathology, 2nd edn. Hoeber, New York

Adams R D, Kakulas B A, Samaha F J 1965 A myopathy with intracellular inclusions. Transactions of the American Neurological Association 90:213

Afifi A K 1972 The myopathology of the prune belly syndrome. Journal of the Neurological Sciences 15:153

Afifi A K, Smith J W, Zellweger H 1965 Congenital non-progressive myopathy. Central core disease and nemaline myopathy in one family. Neurology (Minneapolis) 15:371

Afifi A K, Bergman R A, Harvey J C 1968 Steroid myopathy. Clinical, histologic and cytologic observation. Johns Hopkins Medical Journal 123:158

Afifi A K, Bergman R A 1969 Steroid myopathy. A study of the evolution of the muscle lesion in rabbits. Johns Hopkins Medical Journal 124:66

Afifi A K, der Kaloustian V M, Bahuth W B, Mire-Salman J 1974a Concentrically-laminated membranous inclusions in myofibres of Dyggve-Melchior-Clausen syndrome. Journal of the Neurological Sciences 21:335

Afifi A K, Najjar S S, Mire-Salman J, Bergman R A 1974b The myopathology of the Kocher-Debré-Semelaigne syndrome. Journal of the Neurological Sciences 22:445

Aloisi M, Mussini I, Schiaffino S 1973 Activation of nuclei in denervation and hypertrophy. In: Kakulas B A (ed) Basic research in myology. Excerpta Medica, Amsterdam, p 338

Alvira M M, Mendoza M 1975 Reye's syndrome: A viral myopathy? New England Journal of Medicine 292:1297

Anand R 1983 Cellular membranes in Duchenne muscular dystrohy. European Journal of Biochemistry 15:1211

Angelini C, Trevisan C, Vergani L 1986 Disorders of lipid metabolism. Muscle & Nerve 9:6 (53/Suppl)

Antin P B, Forry-Schandies S, Friedman T M, Tapscott S J, Holtzer H 1981 Taxol induces postmitotic myoblasts to assemble interdigitating microtubule-myosin arrays that exclude actin filaments. Journal of Cell Biology 90:300

Appleyard S T, Dunn M J, Dubowitz V, Scott M L, Pittman S J, Shotton D M 1984 Monoclonal antibodies detect a spectrin-like protein in normal and dystrophic human skeletal muscle. Proceedings of the National Academy of Science 81:767

Askanas V, Engel W K, Di Mauro S, Brooks B R, Mehler M 1976 Adult onset acid maltase deficiency. New England Journal of Medicine 294:573

Bakker E and 15 co-authors 1985 Prenatal diagnosis and carrier detection of Duchenne muscular dystrophy with closely linked RFLPs. Lancet i:654

Banker B Q 1975 Dermatomyositis of childhood. Ultrastructural observations of muscle and intramuscular blood vessels. Journal of Neuropathology and Experimental Neurology 34:46

Banker B Q 1986 The ultrastructural features of dermatomyositis. Muscle and Nerve 9:34 (59/Suppl)

Baringer J R 1971 Tubular aggregates in endoplasmic

reticulum in herpes-simplex encephalitis. New England Journal of Medicine 285:943

Barka T 1964 Electron histochemical localization of acid phosphatase activity in the small intestine of mouse. Journal of Histochemistry and Cytochemistry 12:229

Baruah J K, Sulaiman A R, Kinder D, Murtha T 1983 Electron probe, X-ray microanalysis of mitochondrial paracrystalline inclusions. In: Scarlatto G, Cerri C (eds) Mitochondrial pathology in muscle disease. Piccin, Padua, p 159

Ben-Bassat M, Machtey I 1972 Picornavirus-like structures in acute dermatomyositis. American Journal of Clinical Pathology 58:245

Bender A N, Willner J P 1978 Nemaline (rod) myopathy: the need for histochemical evaluation of affected families. Annals of Neurology 4:37

Bergman R A, Afifi A K, Dunke L M, Johns R T 1970 Muscle pathology in hypokalaemic periodic paralysis with hyperthyroidism. Annals of the New York Academy of Sciences 126:100

Bertorini T E, Bhattacharya S K, Palmieri G M A, Chesney C M, Pifer D, Baker B 1982 Muscle calcium and magnesium content in Duchenne muscular dystrophy. Neurology (New York) 32:1088

Bethlem J, Van Wijngaarden G K, Meijer AEFH, Hülsmann W C 1969 Neuromuscular disease with type I fiber atrophy, central nuclei and myotube-like structures. Neurology (Minneapolis) 19:705

Bethlem J, Van Wijngaarden G K, De Jong J 1973 The incidence of lobulated fibres in the FSH type of muscular dystrophy and the limb-girdle syndrome. Journal of the Neurological Sciences 18:351

Bethlem J, Arts W F, Dingemans K F 1978 Common origin of rods, cores, miniature cores and focal loss of cross-striations. Archives of Neurology 35:555

Bird J W C, Kirschke H, Wood L 1982 Proteolytic enzyme activities in differentiating muscle cells. Federation Proceedings 41: 507–520

Bird J W C, Roisen F J 1986 Lysosomes in muscle: developmental aspects, enzyme activities, and role in protein turnover. In: Engel A G, Banker B Q (eds) Myology. McGraw-Hill, New York, p 745

Bischoff R 1975 Regeneration of single skeletal muscle fibers in vitro. Anatomical Record 182:215

Bodensteiner J B, Engel A G 1978 Intracellular calcium accumulation in Duchenne dystrophy and other myopathies: A study of 567 000 muscle fibers in 114 biopsies. Neurology (Minneapolis) 28:439

Bonilla E, Schotland D L, Wakayama Y 1982 Freeze-fracture studies in human muscular dystrophy. In: Schotland D L (ed) Disorders of the motor unit. John Wiley, New York, p 475

Borenstein S, Noël P, Jacquy J, Flament-Durand J (1977) Myotonic dystrophy with nerve hypertrophy. Journal of the Neurological Sciences 34:87

Bradley W G 1969 Ultrastructural changes in adynamia episodica hereditaria and normokalaemic familial periodic paralysis. Brain 92:379

Bradley W G 1980 Ultrastructural changes in adynamia episodica hereditaria and normokalaemic familial periodic paralysis. Brain 92:379

Bradley W G, Hudgson P, Gardner-Medwin D, Walton J N 1969 Myopathy with abnormal lipid metabolism in skeletal muscle. Lancet 1:495

Bradley W G, Price D L, Watanabe C K 1970 Familial

centronuclear myopathy. Journal of Neurology, Neurosurgery and Psychiatry 33:687

Brody I A, Dudley A W 1969 Thyrotoxic hypokalemic periodic paralysis. Muscle morphology and functional assay of sarcoplasmic reticulum. Archives of Neurology 21:1

Brownell A K W, Gillbert J J, Shaw D T, Garcia B, Wenkeback G F, Lam A K ́S 1978 Adult onset nemaline myopathy. Neurology (Minneapolis) 28:1306

Brooke M H, Neville H E 1972 Reducing body myopathy. Neurology (Minneapolis) 22:829

Busch W A, Stromer M H, Goll D E, Suzuki A 1972 Ca^{2+}-specific removal of Z lines from rabbit skeletal muscle. Journal of Cell Biology 52:367

Campbell M, Rebeiz J J, Walton J N 1969 Myotubular, centronuclear or pericentrinuclear myopathy. Journal of the Neurological Sciences 8:425

Cape C A, Johnson W M, Pitner S E 1970 Nemaline structures in polymyositis. Neurology (Minneapolis) 20:494

Cardiff D R 1966 A histochemical and electron microscopic study of skeletal muscle in a case of Pompe's disease (glycogenosis II). Pediatrics 37:249

Carpenter S, Karpati G, Wolfe L 1970 Virus-like filaments and phospholipid accumulation in skeletal muscle. Neurology (Minneapolis) 20: 889

Carpenter S, Karpati G, Rothman S, Watters G 1976 The childhood type of dermatomyositis. Neurology (Minneapolis) 26:952

Carpenter S, Karpati G, Heller I, Eisen A 1978 Inclusion body myositis: a distinct variety of idiopathic inflammatory myopathy. Neurology (Minneapolis) 28:78

Carpenter S, Karpati G 1979 Duchenne muscular dystrophy. Plasma membrane loss initiates muscle cell necrosis unless it is repaired. Brain 102:147

Carpenter S, Karpati G, Holland P 1985 New observations in reducing body myopathy. Neurology (Cleveland) 35:818

Casanova G, Jerusalem F 1979 Myopathology of myotonic dystrophy. Acta Neuropathologica (Berlin) 45:231

Caulfield J B, Rebeiz J J, Adams R D 1968 Viral involvement of human muscle. Journal of Pathology and Bacteriology 96:232

Cheek D B, Holt A B, Hill D E, Talbert J L 1971 Skeletal muscle cell mass and growth: the concept of the deoxyribonuclei acid unit. Paediatric Research 5:312

Chou S M 1967 Myxovirus-like structures in a case of human chronic polymyositis. Science 158:1453

Chou S M 1968 Myxovirus-like structures and accompanying nuclear changes in chronic polymyositis. Archives of Pathology 86:649

Chou S M 1969 'Megaconial' mitochondria in a case of chronic polymyositis. Acta Neuropathologica (Berlin) 12:68

Chou S M 1973 Prospects of viral etiology in polymyositis. In: Kakulas B A (ed), Clinical studies in myology, Part 2. p 17

Chou S M, Gutmann L 1970 Picornavirus-like crystals in subacute polymyositis. Neurology (Minneapolis) 20:205

Chou S M, Nonaka I 1977 Satellite cells and muscle regeneration in diseased human skeletal muscles. Journal of the Neurological Sciences 34:131

Clark J R, D'Agostino A N, Wilson J, Brooks R R, Cole G C 1978 Autosomal dominant myofibrillar inclusion body myopathy–clinical, histologic histochemical and ultrastructural characteristics. Neurology (Minneapolis) 28:399

Conen P E, Murphy E G, Donohue W L 1963 Light and electron microscopic studies of 'myogranules' in a child with hypotonia and weakness. Canadian Medical Association Journal 89:983

Courtecuisse V, Royer P, Habib R, Monnier C, Demos J 1965 Glycogenose musculaire per deficit d'alpha-1,4-glucosidase simulant une dystrophie musculaire progressive. Archives françaises de pédiatrie 22:1153

Cullen M J, Fulthorpe J J 1975 Stages in fibre breakdown in Duchenne muscular dystrophy. Journal of the Neurological Sciences 24:179

Cullen M J, Pluskal M J 1977 Early changes in the ultrastructure of denervated rat skeletal muscle. Experimental Neurology 56:115

Cullen M J, Appleyard S T. Bindoff L 1978 Morphologic aspects of muscle breakdown and lysosomal activation. Annals of the New York Academy of Sciences 317:440

Cullen M J, Mastaglia F L 1980 Morphological changes in dystrophic muscle. British Medical Bulletin 36:143

Cullen M J, Watkins S C 1981 The role of satellite cells in regeneration in diseased muscle. Advances in the Physiological Sciences 24:341

Cullen M J, Fulthorpe J J 1982 Phagocytosis of the A band following Z line and I band loss. Its significance in skeletal muscle breakdown. Journal of Pathology 138:129

Cullen M J, Mastaglia F L 1982 Pathological reactions of skeletal muscle. In: Mastaglia F L, Walton J N (eds) Skeletal muscle pathology. Churchill Livingstone, Edinburgh, p 88

Cumming W J K, Hardy M, Hudgson P, Walls J 1976 Carnitine palmityl transferase deficiency. Journal of the Neurological Sciences 30:347

D'Agostino A N, Chiga M 1966 Corticosteroid myopathy in rabbits: A light and electron microscopic study. Neurology (Minneapolis) 16:257

Dayton W R, Reville W J, Goll D E, Stromer M H 1976 A Ca^{2+}-activated protease possibly involved in myofibrillar protein turnover. Partial characterization of the purified enzyme. Biochemistry 15:2159

De Coster W J P 1979 Experimental hypokalaemia: ultrastructural changes in rat gastrocnemius muscle. Archives of Neurology 45:79

De Reuck J, De Coster W, Inderadjaja N 1977a Acute viral polymyositis with predominant diaphragm involvement. Journal of the Neurological Sciences 33:453

De Reuck J, Hooft C, De Coster W, Van den Bossche H, Cuvelier C 1977b A progressive congenital myopathy. European Neurology 15:217

DiMauro S, Schotland D L, Bonilla E, Lee C-P, Gambetti P, Rowland L P 1973 Progressive ophthalmoplegia, glycogen storage and abnormal mitochondria. Archives of Neurology 29:170

DiMauro S, Hartwig G B, Hays A et al 1979 Debrancher deficiency: neuromuscular disorder in 5 adults. Annals of Neurology 5:422

Dubowitz V 1985 Muscle biopsy. A practical approach. Bailliere Tindall, London

Dubowitz V, Pearse A G E 1960 Oxidative enzymes and phosphorylase in central core disease of muscle. Lancet 2:23

Dubowitz V, Brooke M H 1973 Muscle biopsy: a modern approach. W B Saunders, London

Dunn M J, Sewry C A, Statham H E, Dubowitz V 1984 Studies on the extracellular matrix in diseased human muscle. In: Demp R B, Hinchcliffe J R, Matrices and cell differentiation. Alan Liss, New York, p 213

Ebashi S 1967 Quoted by C M Pearson. In: Skeletal muscle.

Basic and clinical aspects and illustrative new diseases. Annals of Internal Medicine 67:614

Engel A G 1966 Thyrotoxic and corticosteroid-induced myopathies. Mayo Clinic Proceedings 41:785

Engel A G 1970 Acid maltase deficiency in adult life. Brain 93:599

Engel A G 1981 Metabolic and endocrine myopathies. In: Walton J N (ed) Disorders of Voluntary Muscle 4th edn. Churchill Livingstone, Edinburgh, p 664

Engel A G, Gomez M R 1967 Nemaline (Z disc) myopathy: Observations of the origin, structure and solubility properties of the nemaline structures. Journal of Neuropathology and Experimental Neurology 26:601

Engel A G, Potter C S, Rosevear J W 1967 Studies on carbohydrate metabolism and mitochondrial respiratory activities in primary hypokalemic periodic paralysis. Neurology (Minneapolis) 17:329

Engel A G, Dale A J D 1968 Autophagic glycogenosis of late onset with mitochondrial abnormalities; light and electron microscopic observations. Mayo Clinic Proceedings 43:233

Engel A G, MacDonald R D 1970 Ultrastructural reactions in muscle disease and their light-microscopic correlates. In: Walton J N, Canal N, Scarlato G (eds) Muscle diseases. Excerpta Medica, Amsterdam

Engel A G, Gomez M R, Groover R V 1971 Multicore disease: a recently recognized congenital myopathy associated with multifocal degeneration of muscle fibres. Mayo Clinic Proceedings 46:666

Engel A G, Siekert R G 1972 Lipid storage myopathy responsive to prednisone. Archives of Neurology 27:174

Engel A G, Angelini C, Gomez M R 1972 Fingerprint body myopathy. Mayo Clinic Proceedings 47:377

Engel A G, Angelini C 1973 Carnitine deficiency of human skeletal muscle with associated lipid storage. Science 179:899

Engel A G, Biesecker G 1982 Complement activation in muscle fiber necrosis: demonstration of the membrane attack complex of complement in necrotic fibers. Annals of Neurology 12:289

Engel W K, Foster J B, Hughes B P, Huxley H E, Mahler R 1961 Central core disease: An investigation of a rare muscle cell abnormality. Brain 84:167

Engel W K, Eyerman E L, Williams H E 1963 Late onset type of skeletal muscle phosphorylase deficiency: A new familial variety with completely and partly affected subjects. New England Journal of Medicine 268:135

Engel W K, Wanko T, Fenichel G M 1964 Nemaline myopathy: A second case. Archives of Neurology 11:22

Engel W K, Brooke M H, Nelson P G 1966 Histochemical studies of denervated or tenotomized muscle. Annals of the New York Academy of Sciences 138:160

Engel W K, Gold N, Karpati G 1968 Type I fiber hypotrophy and central nuclei. Archives of Neurology 18:435

Fardeau M 1970 Ultrastructural lesions in progressive muscular dystrophies. A critical study of their specificity. In: Muscle diseases. Proceedings of an International Congress. Excerpta Medica, Amsterdam

Fardeau M, Lapresle J, Milhaud E 1965 Contribution a l'étude des lesions elementaires du muscle squélettique: Ultrastructure des masses sarcoplasmiques laterales (observées dans un cas de dystrophie myotonique). Comptes rendus des seances de la Société de biologie et des filiales 159:15

Fardeau M, Tomé FMS, Derambure S 1976 Familial fingerprint body myopathy. Archives of Neurology 33:724

Fardeau M, Godet-Guillain J, Tomé FMS, Collin H, Gaudeau S, Boffety Cl L, Vernant P 1978 Une nouvelle affection musculaire. Revue Neurologique 131:411

Fardeau M, Tomé FMS, Simon P 1979 Muscle and nerve changes induced by perhexiline maleate in man and mice. Muscle and Nerve 2:24

Fisher E R, Gonzalez A R, Khurana R C , Danowski T S 1972 Unique, concentrically laminated, membranous, inclusions in myofibers. American Journal of Clinical Pathology 48:239

Freund-Mölbert E, Ketelsen U-P, Beckmann R 1973 Ultrastructural study of experimental steroid myopathy. In: Kakulas B A (ed), Basic research in myology. Excerpta Medica, Amsterdam, p 595

Fukuhara N 1979 Electron microscopical demonstration of nucleic acids in virus-like particles in the skeletal muscle of a traffic accident victim. Acta Neuropathologica (Berlin) 47:55

Fukuyama Y, Ando J T, Yokota J 1977 Acute fulminant myoglobinuric polymyositis with picornavirus-like crystals. Journal of Neurology, Neurosurgery and Psychiatry 40:755

Gallai M 1977 Myopathy with hyperaldosteronism — An electron microscopic study. Journal of the Neurological Sciences 32:337

Godet-Guillain J, Fardeau M 1970 Hypothyroid myopathy. Histological and ultrastructural study of an atrophic form. In: J N Walton, N Canal, G. Scarlato (eds) Muscle disease. Excerpta Medica, Amsterdam, p 512

Goldspink D 1972 Postembryonic growth and differentiation of striated muscle. In: Bourne G H, Function of muscle. Academic Press, New York, vol 1 p 179

Gonatas N K 1966 The fine structure of the rod-like bodies in nemaline myopathy and their relation to the Z discs. Journal of Neuropathology and Experimental Neurology 25:409

Gonatas N K, Perez M C, Shy G M, Evangelista I 1965 Central 'core' disease of skeletal muscle. Ultrastructural and cytochemical observations in two cases. American Journal of Pathology 47:503

Gonatas N K, Shy G M, Godfrey E H 1966 The origin of nemaline structures. New England Journal of Medicine 274:535

Gonzalez-Angulo A, Fraga A, Mintz G, Zavala B 1968 Submicroscopic alterations in capillaries of skeletal muscle in polymyositis. American Journal of Medicine 45:873

Gordon A M, Green J R, Lagunoff D 1970 Studies on a patient with hypokalaemic familial periodic paralysis. American Journal of Medicine 48:185

Gruener R, Stern L Z, Payne C, Hannapel L 1975 Hyperthyroid myopathy. Journal of the Neurological Sciences 24:339

Grüner J E 1966 Anomalies du reticulum sarcoplasmique et prolifération des tubules dans le muscle d'une paralysie périodique familiale. Comptes rendus des seances de la Societé de biologie et des filiales 26:555

Györkey F, Min F-W, Sinkovics J G, Györkey P 1969 Systemic lupus erythematosus and myxovirus. New England Journal of Medicine 280:333

Györkey F, Labral G A, Györkey P, Uribe-Botero G, Dressman G-R, Melnick J L 1978 Coxsackie virus aggregates in muscle cells of a polymyositis patient. Intervirology 10:69

Hanson P A, Urizar R E 1975 Reye's syndrome–virus or artifact in muscle. New England Journal of Medicine 293:505

Hanzlikova V, Makova E V, Hnik P 1975 Satellite cells of rat soleus in the process of compensatory hypertrophy combined with denervation. Cell and Tissue Research 160:411

Harriman D G F, Reed R 1972 The incidence of lipid droplets in human skeletal muscle in neuromuscular disorders. Journal of Pathology 106:1

Hashimoto K, Robinson L, Velayos E, Niizuma K 1971 Dermatomyositis. Electron microscopic, immunological, and tissue culture studies of paramyxovirus-like inclusions. Archives of Dermatology 103:120

Hess A, Rosner S 1970 The satellite cell bud and myoblast in denervated mammalian muscle. American Journal of Anatomy 129:21

Howes E L, Price H M, Pearson C M, Blumberg J M 1966 Hypokalemic periodic paralysis: electron microscopic changes in the sarcoplasm. Neurology (Minneapolis) 16:242

Hudgson P, Fulthorpe J J 1975 The pathology of type II skeletal muscle glycogenosis. A light and electronmicroscopic study. Journal of Pathology 116:139

Hudgson P, Gardner-Medwin D, Fulthorpe J J, Walton J N 1967 Nemaline myopathy. Neurology (Minneapolis) 17:1125

Hudgson P, Gardner-Medwin D, Worsfold M, Pennington R J T, Walton J N 1968 Adult myopathy from glycogen storage disease due to acid maltase deficiency. Brain 91:435

Hudgson P, Pearce G W 1969 Ultramicroscopic studies of diseased muscle. In: Walton J N (ed) Disorders of voluntary muscle. 1st edn. Churchill, London, p 277

Hudson A J, Oteruelo F T, Haust M D 1971 Unusual generalised myopathy of late onset. Clinical and morphological study. In: Serratrice G, Roux H (eds) Actualités de pathologie neuromusculaire. L' Expansion Scientifique Française, Paris, p 140

Hughes J T, Esiri M M 1978 Ultrastructural studies in human polymyositis. Journal of the Neurological Sciences 25:347

Hurwitz L J, Carson N A, Allen I V, Fannin T F, Lyttle J A, Neill D W 1967 Clinical, biochemical and histopathological findings in a family with muscular dystrophy. Brain 90:799

Hurwitz L, McCormick D, Allen V I 1970 Reduced muscle α-glucosidase (acid maltase) activity in hypothyroid myopathy. Lancet 1:67

Hsu L, Trupin G L, Roisen F J 1979 The role of satellite cells and myonuclei during myogenesis in vitro. In: Mauro A (ed) Muscle regeneration. Raven Press, New York, p 115

Isaacs H, Heffron J J A, Badenhorst M 1975 Central core disease: a correlated genetic, histochemical, ultramicroscopic and biochemical study. Journal of Neurology, Neurosurgery and Psychiatry 38:1177

Isch F, Juif J-G, Sacrez R, Thiebaut F 1966 Glycogénose musculaire; forme myopathique par déficit en maltase acide. Pédiatrie 21:71

Ishimoto S, Goto I, Ohta M, Kuroiwa Y 1983 A quantitative study of the muscle satellite cells in various neuromuscular disorders. Journal of the Neurological Sciences 62:303

Jackson M J, Jones D A, Edwards R H T 1985

Measurements of calcium and other elements in muscle biopsy samples from patients with Duchenne muscular dystrophy. Clinica Chimica Acta 147:215

Jakovics S, Khachadurian A K, Tsia D Y Y 1966 The hyperlipidemia in glycogen storage disease. Journal of Clinical Laboratory Medicine 68:769

Jenis E H, Lindquist R R, Lister R C 1969 New congenital myopathy with crystalline intramuscular inclusions. Archives of Neurology 20:281

Jerusalem F, Baumgartner G, Wyler R 1972 Virus-ahnliche Einschlusse bei chronischen neuro-muskularen Prozessen. Electronenmikroskopische Biopsiebefunde von 2 Fallen. Archiv für Psychiatrie und Nerven-Krankheiten 215:418

Jerusalem F, Angelini C, Engel A G, Groover R V 1973a Mitochondria-lipid-glycogen (MLG) disease of muscle. Archives of Neurology 29:162

Jerusalem F, Engel A G, Gomez M R 1973b Sarcotubular myopathy. Neurology (Minneapolis) 23:897

Jerusalem F, Engel A G, Gomez M R 1974a Duchenne dystrophy. I. Morphometric study of the muscle microvasculature. Brain 97:115

Jerusalem F, Engel A G, Gomez M R 1974b Duchenne dystrophy. II Morphological study of motor end-plate fine structure. Brain 97:123

Jerusalem F, Ludin H, Bischoff A, Hartmann G 1979 Cytoplasmic body neuromyopathy presenting as respiratory failure and weight loss. Journal of the Neurological Sciences 41:1

Jockusch B M, Veldman H, Griffiths G W, van Oot B A, Jennekens FGT 1980 Immunofluorescence microscopy of a myopathy. α-Actinin is a major constituent of nemaline rods. Experimental Cellular Research 127:409

Johnson A G 1969 Alterations of the Z-lines and I-band myofilaments in human skeletal muscle. Acta Neuropathologica 12:218

Johnson A G, Woolf A L 1969 Abnormal sarcolemmal nuclei encountered in several cases of dystrophia myotonica. Acta Neuropathologica (Berlin) 12:183

Johnson M A, Fulthorpe J J, Hudson P 1973 Lipid storage myopathy. A clinicopathologically recognizable entity. Acta Neuropathologica (Berlin) 24:97

Jones K W, Kinross J, Maitland N, Norval M 1979 Normal human tissues contain RNA and antigens related to infectious adenovirus Type 2. Nature 277:274

Julien J, Vital C L, Vallat J-M, Vallat M, Le Blanc M 1974 Oculopharyngeal muscular dystrophy — a case with abnormal mitochondria and 'fingerprint' inclusions. Journal of the Neurological Sciences 21:165

Kao I, Gordon A M 1977 Alteration of skeletal muscle cellular structures by potassium depletion. Neurology (Minneapolis) 27:855

Karpati G, Carpenter S, Eisen A, Aube M, DiMauro S 1977 The adult form of acid maltase (-1,4-glucosidase) deficiency. Annals of Neurology 1:276

Karpati G, Carpenter S, Melmed C, Eisen A A 1974 Experimental ischaemic myopathy. Journal of the Neurological Sciences 23:129

Karpati G, Carpenter S 1982 Micropuncture lesions of skeletal muscle cells: a new experimental model for the study of muscle cell damage, repair and regeneration. In: Schotland D L (ed) Disorders of the motor unit. John Wiley, New York, p 517

Kelly F J, McGrath J A, Goldspink D F, Cullen M J 1986 A morphological/biochemical study of the actions of

corticosteroids on rat skeletal muscle. Muscle and Nerve 9: 1–10

Ketelsen U P 1975 The plasma membrane of human skeletal muscle cells in the pathological state. Freeze etch studies. In: Bradley W G, Gardner-Medwin D, Walton J N (eds), Recent advances in myology. Excerpta Medica, Amsterdam, p 446

Ketelsen U P, Beckmann R, Zimmerman H, Sauer M 1977 Inclusion body myositis. A 'slow virus' infection of skeletal musculature? Klinische Wochenschrift 55:1063

Kinoshita M, Cadman T E 1968 Myotubular myopathy. Archives of Neurology 18:265

Kissel J T, Mendell J R, Rammohan K W 1986 Microvascular deposition of complement membrane attack complex in dermatomyositis. New England Journal of Medicine 314:329

Klinkerfuss G H 1967 An electron microscopic study of myotonic dystrohy. Archives of Neurology 16:181

Klinkerfuss G H, Haugh M J 1970 Disuse atrophy of muscle. Archives of Neurology 22:309

Knox A J, Mascie-Taylor B H, Muers M F 1986 Acute hydrocortisone myopathy in acute severe asthma. Thorax 41:411

Koehler J 1977 Blood vessel structure in Duchenne muscular dystrophy. 1. Light and electron microscopic observations in resting muscle. Neurology (Minneapolis) 27:861

Konigsberg U R, Lipton B H, Konigsberg I R 1975 The regenerative response of single mature muscle fibres isolated in vitro. Developmental Biology 45:260

Korenyi-Both A, Smith B H, Baruah J K 1977 McArdle's syndrome. Fine structural changes in muscle. Acta Neuropathologica 40:11

Kunkel L M et al (75 Signatories) 1986 Analysis of deletions in DNA from patients with Becker and Duchenne muscular dystrophy. Nature 322:73

Lake B D, Wilson J 1975 Zebra body myopthy. Clinical, histochemical and ultrastructural studies. Journal of the Neurological Sciences 24:437

Landing B H, Shankle W R 1982 Reduced number of skeletal muscle fiber nuclei in Down's syndrome: speculation on a 'shut off' of chromosome 21 in control of DNA and nuclear replication rates, possibly via determination of cell surface area per nucleus. Birth Defects 18:81

Landry M, Winkelmann R K 1972 Tubular cytoplasmic inclusion in dermatomyositis. Mayo Clinic Proceedings 47:479

Lane R J M, Fulthorpe J J, Hudson P 1985 Inclusion body myositis: a case with associated collagen vascular disease responding to treatment. Journal of Neurology, Neurosurgery and Psychiatry 48:270

Layzer R B, Rowland L P, Ranney H M 1967 Muscle phosphofructokinase deficiency. Archives of Neurology 17:512

Lee R E, Poulos A C, Mayer R F, Rash J E 1986 Caveolae preservation in the characterization of human neuromuscular disease. Muscle and Nerve 9:127

Luft R, Ikkos D, Palmieri G, Ernster L, Afzelius B 1962 A case of severe hypermetabolism of non-thyroid origin with a defect in the maintenance of mitochondrial respiratory control: a correlated clinical, biochemical and morphological study. Journal of Clinical Investigation 41:1776

McComas A J, Campbell M J, Sica REP 1971

Electrophysiological study of dystrophia myotonica. Journal of Neurology, Neurosurgery and Psychiatry 34:132

McDaniel H G, Pitman C S, Oh S J, DiMauro S 1977 Carbohydrate metabolism in hypothyroid myopathy. Metabolism 26:867

MacDonald R D, Engel A G 1969 The cytoplasmic body: another structural anomaly of the Z discs. Acta Neuropathologica (Berlin) 14:99

MacDonald R D, Rewcastle N B, Humphrey J G 1969 Myopathy of hypokalaemic periodic paralysis. Archives of Neurology 20:565

MacDonald R D, Engel A G 1971 Observations on organization of Z-disk components and on rod-bodies of Z-disk origin. Journal of Cell Biology 48:431

MacFarlane I A, Rosenthal F D 1977 Severe myopathy after status asthmaticus. Lancet 2:615

Markesbery W R, Griggs R C, Herr B 1977 Distal myopathy: electron microscopic and histochemical studies. Neurology 27:727

Martin J J, De Barsy Th, Van Hoof F, Palladini G 1973 Pompe's disease: An inborn lysosomal disorder with storage of glycogen. Acta Neuropathologica (Berlin) 23:229

Martin J J, De Barsy Th, De Schrijver F, Leroy J G, Palladini G 1976 Acid maltase deficiency (Type II glycogenosis). Journal of the Neurological Sciences 30:155

Martinez A J, Hooshmand H, Indolos Mendoza G, Winston Y E 1974 Fatal polymyositis: Morphogenesis and ultrastructural features. Acta Neuropathologica (Berlin) 29:251

Mastaglia F L 1973 Pathological changes in skeletal muscle in acromegaly. Acta Neuropathologica (Berlin) 24:273

Mastaglia F L, Walton J N 1970 Coxsackie virus-like particles in skeletal muscle from a case of polymyositis. Journal of the Neurological Sciences 11:593

Mastaglia F L, McCollum J P K, Larson P F, Hudgson P 1970 Steroid myopathy complicating McArdle's disease. Journal of Neurology, Neurosurgery and Psychiatry 33:111

Mastaglia F L, Currie S 1971 Immunological and ultrastructural observations on the role of lymphoid cells in the pathogenesis of polymyositis. Acta Neuropathologica (Berlin) 18:1

Mastaglia F L, Walton J N 1971a An electron microscopic study of skeletal muscle from cases of the Kugelberg–Welander syndrome. Acta Neuropathologica (Berlin) 17:201

Mastaglia F L, Walton J N 1971b An ultrastructural study of skeletal muscle in polymyositis. Journal of the Neurological Sciences 12:473

Mastaglia F L, Papadimitriou J M, Dawkins R L 1975 Mechanisms of cell-mediated myotoxicity. Morphological observations in muscle grafts and in muscle exposed to sensitized spleen cells in vivo. Journal of the Neurological Sciences 25:26

Mastaglia F L, Papadimitriou J M, Dawkins R L, Beveridge B 1977 Vacuolar myopathy associated with chloroquine, lupus erythematosus and thymoma. Journal of the Neurological Sciences 34:315

Mastaglia F L, Hudgson P 1981 Ultrastructure of diseased muscle In: Walton J N (ed) Disorders of voluntary muscle 4th edn. Churchill Livingstone, Edinburgh, Ch 9, p 327

Meijer A E F H 1972 Mitochondria with defective respiratory control of oxidative phosphorylation isolated from muscle tissues of thyroidectomised rabbits. Journal of the Neurological Sciences 16:445

Mendell J R, Engel W K 1971 The fine structure of type II muscle fibre atrophy. Neurology (Minneapolis) 21:358

Meyers K R, Gilden D H, Rinaldi C F 1972 Periodic muscle weakness, normokalemia and tubular aggregates. Neurology 22:269

Miledi R, Slater C R 1969 Electron microscopic structure of denervated skeletal muscle. Proceedings of the Royal Society of London, Series B 174:253

Mintz G, Gonzalez-Angulo A, Graga A, Zavala B 1968 Ultrastructure of muscle in polymyositis. American Journal of Medicine 44:216

Mokri B, Engel A G 1975 Duchenne dystrophy: Electron microscopic findings pointing to a basic or early abnormality in the plasma membrane as the muscle fibre. Neurology (Minneapolis) 25:1111

Monaco A P, Neve R L, Colletti-Feener C, Bertelson C J, Kurnit D M, Kunkel L M 1986 Isolation of candidate cDNAs for portion of the Duchenne muscular dystrophy gene. Nature 323:646

Monaco A P, Bertelson C J, Middlesworth W et al 1985 Detection of deletions spanning the Duchenne muscular dystrophy locus using a tightly linked DNA segment. Nature 316:842

Morgan-Hughes J A 1982 Defects of the energy pathways of skeletal muscle. In: Matthews W B, Glaser G H (eds) Recent advances in clinical neurology 3. Churchill Livingstone, Edinburgh, ch 7, p 1

Morgan-Hughes J A, Landon D N 1983 Mitochondrial respiratory chain deficiencies in man. Some histochemical and fine-structure observations. In: Scarlato G, Cerri C (eds) Mitochondrial pathology in muscle diseases. Piccin, Padua p 19

Mrak R E, Saito A, Evans O B, Fleischer S 1982 Autophagic degradation in human skeletal muscle target fibers. Muscle and Nerve 5:745

Murase T, Ikeda H, Muro T, Nakao K, Sugita H 1973 Myopathy associated with Type III glycogenosis. Journal of the Neurological Sciences 20:287

Neville H E 1973 Ultrastructural changes in muscle disease. In: Dubowitz V, Brooke M (eds) Muscle biopsy. Saunders, London, p 383

Neville H E 1979 Ultrastructural changes in diseases of human skeletal muscle. In: Vinken P J, Bruyn G W (eds) Handbook of Clinical Neurology. North Holland, Amsterdam, vol 40, p 63

Neville H E, Brooke M H 1973 Central core fibres: structured and unstructured. In: Kakulas B (ed), Basic research in myology. Excerpta Medica, Amsterdam, p 497

Neville H E, Maunder-Sewry C A, McDougall J, Sewell J R, Dubowitz V 1979 Chloroquine-induced cytosomes with curvilinear profiles in muscle. Muscle and Nerve 2:376

Nick J, Prunieras M, Bakouche P, Reignier A, Nicolle M-H 1971 Inclusions dans les cellules endothéliales et les lymphocytes au cours d'un cas de dermatomyosite. Revue Neurologique 125:22

Nonaka I, Sunohara N, Satoyoshi E, Teerasawa K, Yonemoto K 1985 Autosomal recessive distal muscular dystrophy: a comparative study with distal myopathy with rimmed vacuole formation. Annals of Neurology 17:51

Norris F H, Panner B J 1966 Hypothyroid myopathy: Clinical, electromyographical and ultrastructural observtions. Archives of Neurology 14:574

Norris F H, Panner B J, Stormont J M 1968 Thyrotoxic periodic paralysis. Metabolic and ultrastructural studies. Archives of Neurology 19:88

Norton W L 1970 Comparison of the microangiopathy of systemic lupus erythematosus, dermatomyositis, scleroderma and diabetes mellitus. Laboratory Investigation 22:301

Oberc M A, Engel W K 1977 Ultrastructural localisation of calcium in normal and abnormal skeletal muscle. Laboratory Investigation 36:566

Odor D L, Patel A N, Pearce L A 1967 Familial hypokalemic periodic paralysis with permanent myopathy. Journal of Neuropathy and Experimental Neurology 26:98

Oliner L, Schulman X, Larner J 1961 Myopathy associated with glycogen deposition resulting from generalised lack of amylo -1,6-glucosidase. Clinical Research 243

Ontell M 1974 Muscle satellite cells: a validated technique for light microscopic identification and a quantitative study of changes in their population following denervation. The Anatomical Record 178:211

Osborn M, Goebel H H 1983 The cytoplasmic bodies in a congenital myopathy can be stained with antibodies to desmin, the muscle-specific intermediate filament protein. Acta Neuropathologica (Berlin) 62:149

Oshima Y, Becker L E, Armstrong D L 1979 An electron microscopic study of childhood dermatomyositis. Acta Neuropathologica (Berlin) 47:189

Oteruelo F T 1976 Intranuclear inclusions in a myopathy of late onset. Virchows Archiv Abteilung B. Zeupathologie 20:319

Pagès M, Echenne B, Pages A-M, Dimeglio A, Sires A 1985 Multicore disease and Marfan's syndrome: a case report. European Neurology 24:170

Palmucci L, Bertolotto A, Monga G, Ardizzone G, Schiffer D 1978 Histochemical and ultrastructural findings in a case of centronuclear myopathy. European Neurology 17:327

Panayiotopoulos C P, Scarpalezos S 1977 Dystrophia myotonica. A model of combined neural and myopathic muscle atrophy. Journal of the Neurological Sciences 31:261

Payne C M, Curless R G 1976 Concentric laminated bodies-ultrastructural demonstration of fibre type specificity. Journal of the Neurological Sciences 29:311

Pearce G W 1964 Tissue culture and electron microscopy in muscle disease. In: Walton J N (ed), Disorders of voluntary muscle. 1st edn. Churchill, London

Pearson C M 1964 The periodic paralyses: Differential features and pathological observations in permanent myopathic weakness. Brain 87:341

Pellegrino C, Franzini C 1963 An electron microscopic study of denervation atrophy in red and white skeletal muscle fibers. Journal of Cell Biology 17:327

Peluchetti D, Mora M, Protti A, Cornelio F 1985 Freeze-fracture analysis of the muscle plasma membrane in Duchenne dystrophy. Neurology (Clevelend) 35:928

Pollock M, Dyck P J 1976 Peripheral nerve morphometry in myotonic dystrophy. Archives of Neurology 33:33

Pongratz D, Schultz D, Koppenwallner C H, Hübner G 1979 Wertigkeit der muskelbiopsie in der diagnostia der dystrophia myotonica (Curschmann-Steinert). Klinische Wochenschrift 57:215

Price H M, Gordon G B, Pearson C M, Munsat T L, Blumbert J M 1965 New evidence for accumulation of excessive Z band material in nemaline myopathy. Proceedings of the National Academy of Sciences USA 64:1398

Prineas J W, Hall R, Barwick D D, Watson A J 1968 Myopathy associated with pigmentation following adrenalectomy for Cushing's syndrome. Quarterly Journal of Medicine 37:63

Radu H, Rosu-Serbu A M, Ionescu V, Radu A 1977 Focal abnormalities in mitochondrial distribution in muscle. Acta Neuropathologica (Berlin) 39:25

Rapola J, Haltia M 1973 Cytoplasmic inclusions in the vermiform appendix and skeletal muscle in two types of so-called neuronal ceroid-lipofuscinosis. Brain 96:833

Recondo J de, Fardeau M, Lapresle J 1966 Étude au microscope electronique des lesions musculaires d'atrophie neurogène par atteinte de la corne anterieure (observées dans huit cas de sclerose lateral amyotrophique). Revue Neurologique 114:169

Rewcastle N B, Humphrey J G 1965 Vacuolar myopathy: clinical, histochemical and microscopic study. Archives of Neurology (Chicago) 12:570

Ringel S P, Kenny C, Neville H, Gilden D 1986 Spectrum of inclusion body myositis. Muscle and Nerve 9:218

Ringel S P Neville H E, Duster M C, Carroll J E 1978 A new congenital neuromuscular disease with trilaminar muscle fibers. Neurology (Minneapolis) 28:282

Ringel S P, Thorne E G, Phanuphak P, Lava N S, Kohler P S 1979 Immune complex vasculitis, polymyositis and hyperglobulinaemic purpura. Neurology (Minneapolis) 29:682

Ritter R A 1967 The effect of cortisone on the structure and strength of skeletal muscle. Archives of Neurology 17:493

Rose A L, Walton J N, Pearce G W 1967 Polymyositis: An ultramicroscopic study of muscle biopsy material. Journal of the Neurological Sciences 5:457

Rosenberg N L, Neville H E, Ringel S P 1985 Tubular aggregates. Their association with neuromuscular diseases, including the syndrome of myalgias/cramps. Archives of Neurology 42:973

Roses A D 1986 Genetic linkage of myotonic dystrophy. Muscle and Nerve 9:51

Roses A D, Appel S H 1975 Phosphorylation of component a in the human erythrocyte membrane in myotonic muscular dystrophy. Journal of Membrane Biology 20:51

Roses A D, Hartwig G B, Mabry M, Nagano Y, Miller S E 1980 Red blood cell and fibroblast membranes in Duchenne and myotonic muscular dystrophy. Muscle and Nerve 3:36

Roullet E, Fardeau M, Collin H, Martean R 1985 Myopathie avec agrégates tubulaires. Étude clinique biologique et histologique de deux cas. Revue Neurologique 141:655

Rowland L P 1980 Biochemistry of muscle membranes in Duchenne muscular dystrophy. Muscle and Nerve 3:3

Rowland L P, Hays A P, DiMauro S, De Vivo D C, Behrens M 1983 Diverse clinical disorders associated with morphological abnormalities of mitochondria. In: Scarlato G, Cerri C (eds), Mitochondrial pathology in muscle diseases. Piccin, Padua, p 141

Rubin E, Katz A M, Lieber C S, Stein E, Purzkin S 1976 Muscle damage caused by chronic alcohol consumption. American Journal of Pathology 83:499

Sahgal V, Sahgal S 1977 A new congenital myopathy. Acta Neuropathologica (Berlin) 37:225

Samaha F J, Schröder J M, Rebeiz J, Adams R D 1967 Studies on myotonia. Biochemical and electron microscopic studies on myotonia congenita and myotonia dystrophica. Archives of Neurology 17:22

Sato T, Nakamura N 1975 Myositis and virus. Naika (Tokyo) 35:239

Satoyoshi E, Kowa H 1967 A myopathy due to a glycolytic abnormality. Archives of Neurology 17:248

Schiaffino S, Severin E, Cautini M, Sartore S 1977 Tubular aggregates induced by anoxia in isolated rat skeletal muscle. Laboratory Investigation 37:228

Schiller H H, Mair W G P 1974 Ultrastructural changes of muscle in malignant hyperthermia. Journal of the Neurological Sciences 21:93

Schlenska G K, Heene R, Spalke G, Seiler D 1976 The symptomatology, morphology and biochemistry of glycogenosis type II (Pompe) in the adult. Journal of Neurology 212:237

Schmalbruch H 1967 Kristalloide in menschlichen skelett-muskelfasern. Naturwissenschaften 54:519

Schmalbruch H 1968 Lyse und regeneration von fibrillen in der normalen menschlichen skelettmuskulatur. Virchows Archiv für pathologische Anatomie unde physiologie und für Klinische Medizin 344:159

Schmalbruch H 1975 Segmental fibre breakdown and defects of the plasmalemma in diseased human muscle. Acta Neuropathologica (Berlin) 33:129

Schmalbruch H 1976 Muscle fibre splitting and regeneration in diseased human muscle. Neuropathology and Applied Neurobiology 2:3

Schmalbruch H 1983 The fine structure of mitochondrial abnormalities in muscle diseases. In: Scarlatto G, Cerri C (eds) Mitochondrial pathology in muscle diseases, Piccin, Padua, p 39

Schmalbruch H 1984 Regenerated muscle fibres in Duchenne muscular dystrophy: a serial section study. Neurology (Cleveland) 34:60

Schochet S S, McCormick F 1973 Polymyositis with intra-muscular inclusions. Archives of Neurology 28:280

Schotland D L 1969 An electron microscopic study of target fibers, target-like fibers and related abnormalities in human muscle. Journal of Neuropathology and Experimental Neurology 28:214

Schotland D L 1970 An electron microscopic investigation of myotonic dystrophy. Journal of Neuropathology and Experimental Neurology 29:241

Schotland D L, Bonilla E, Wakayama Y 1981 Application of freeze-fracture technique to the study of human neuromuscular disease. Muscle and Nerve 3:21

Schotland D L, Bonila E, Wakayama Y 1981 Freeze-fracture studies of muscle plasma membrane in human muscular dystrophy. Acta Neuropathologica 54:189

Schröder J M 1970 Sarcolemmal indentations resembling junctional folds in myotonic dystrophy. In: Walton J N, Canal N, Scarlato G (eds) Muscle diseases. Excerpta Medica, Amsterdam, p 109

Schröder J M, Adams R D 1968 The ultrastructural morphology of the muscle fibre in myotonic dystrophy. Acta Neuropathologica (Berlin) 10:218

Schultz E 1978 Changes in the satellite cells of growing muscle following denervation. Anatomical Record 190:299

Schwartz W N, Bird J W C 1977 Degradation of myofibrillar proteins by cathepsins B and D. Biochemical Journal 167:811

Serratrice G, Pellissier J F, Faugère M C, Gastaut J L 1978 Centronuclear myopathy: Possible central nervous system origin. Muscle and Nerve 1:62

Sewry C A 1985 Ultrastructural changes in diseased muscle. In: Dubowitz V Muscle biopsy. A practical approach. Bailliere Tindall, London, p 129

Shafiq S A, Gorycki M, Goldstone L, Milhorat A T 1966 Fine structure of fiber types in normal human muscle. Anatomical Record 156:283

Shafiq S A, Dubowitz V, Peterson H de C, Milhorat A T 1967a Nemaline myopathy: Report of a fatal case with histochemical and electronmicroscopic studies. Brain 90:817

Shafiq S A, Gorycki M A, Milhorat A T 1967b An electron microscopic study of regeneration and satellite cells in human muscle. Neurology (Minneapolis) 17:507

Shafiq S A, Milhorat A T, Gorycki M A 1967c An electron microscopic study of muscle degeneration and changes in blood vessels in polymyositis. Journal of Pathology and Bacteriology 94:139

Shafiq S A, Milhorat A T, Gorycki M A 1967d Giant mitochondria in human muscle with inclusions. Archives of Neurology 17:666

Sher J H, Rimalovski A B, Athanassiades T J, Aronson S M 1967 Familial centronuclear myopathy. Neurology (Minneapolis) 17:721

Shoji S, Takagi A, Sugita H, Toyokura Y 1974 Muscle glycogen metabolism in steroid-induced myopathy in rabbits. Experimental Neurology 45:1

Shotton D M 1982 Quantitative freeze-fracture electon microscopy of dystrophic muscle membranes. Journal of the Neurological Sciences 57:161

Shy G M, Magee K R 1956 A new non-progressive myopathy. Brain 79:610

Shy G M, Wanko T, Rowley P T, Engel A G 1961 Studies in familial periodic paralysis. Experimental Neurology 3:53

Shy G M, Engel W K, Somers J E, Wanko T 1963 Nemaline myopathy: A new congenital myopathy. Brain 86:739

Shy G M, Gonatas N K, Perez M 1966 Two childhood myopathies with abnormal mitochondria. I. Megaconial myopathy. II. Pleoconial myopathy. Brain 89:133

Smith H L, Amick L D, Sidbury J B 1966 Type II glycogenosis: report of a case with 4 year survival and absence of acid maltase associated with an abnormal glycogen. American Journal of Diseases of Children 111:475

Snow M H 1977 Myogenic cell formation in regenerating rat skeletal muscle injured by mincing. II An autoradiographic Study. Anatomical Record 188:201

Snow M H 1978 An autoradiographic study of satellite cell differentiation into regenerating myotubes following transplantation of muscle in young rats. Cell Tissue Research 186:537

Snow M H 1983 A quantitative ultrastructural analysis of satellite cells in denervated fast and slow muscles of the mouse. Anatomical Record 207:593

Somlyo A V, Gonzalez-Serratos H, Shuman H, McClellan G, Somlyo A P 1981 Calcium release and ionic changes in the sarcoplasmic reticulum of tetanized muscle — an electron-probe study. Journal of Cell Biology 90:577

Spiro A J, Kennedy C 1964 Hereditary occurrence of nemaline myopathy. Transactions of the American Neurological Association 89:62

Spiro A J, Shy G M, Gonatas N K 1966 Myotubular myopathy. Archives of Neurology 14:1

Spiro A J, Hirano R L, Beilin R L, Finkelstein J W 1970 Cretinism with muscular hypertrophy (Kocher-Debré-Semelaigne syndrome). Archives of Neurology 23:340

Stauber W T, Riggs J E, Schochet S S, Gutmann L, Crosby T W 1986 Nemaline myopathy. Evidence of dipeptidyl peptidase 1 deficiency. Archives of Neurology 43:39

Stonnington H H, Engel A G 1973 Normal and denervated muscle. Neurology (Minneapolis) 23:714

Stromer M H, Tabatabai L B, Robson R M, Goll D E, Zeece M G 1976 Nemaline myopathy, an integrated study: selective extraction. Experimental Neurology 50:402

Swash M, Schwartz M S 1981 Familial multicore disease with focal loss of cross-striations and ophthalmoplegia. Journal of the Neurological Sciences 52:1

Tagerud S, Jirmanova I, Libelius R 1986 Biochemical and ultrastructural effects of chloroquine on horseradish peroxidase uptake and lysosomal enzyme activities in innervated and denervated mouse skeletal muscle. Journal of the Neurological Sciences 75:159

Takagi A, Schotland D L, Di Mauro S, Rowland L P 1973 Thyrotoxic periodic paralysis. Function of sarcoplasmic reticulum and muscle glycogen. Neurology (Minneapolis) 23:1008

Tang T T, Sedmak G V, Siegesmund K A, McCreadie S R 1975 Chronic myopathy associated with Coxsackie virus type A9. A combined electron microscopical and viral isolation study. New England Journal of Medicine 292:608

Tarui S, Okuno G, Ikura Y, Suda M 1965 Phosphofructokinase deficiency in skeletal muscle: A new type of glycogenosis. Biochemical and Biophysical Research Communications 19:517

Telerman-Toppet N, Gerrard J M, Cöers C 1973 Central core disease: a study of clinically unaffected muscle. Journal of the Neurological Sciences 19:207

Teräväinen H, Mäkitie J 1977 Striated muscle ultrastructure in intermittent claudication. Archives of Pathological Laboratory Medicine 101:230

Thomson W H S, Maclaurin J C, Prineas J W 1963 Skeletal muscle glycogenosis: An investigation of two dissimilar cases. Journal of Neurology, Neurosurgery and Psychiatry 26:60

Thornell L-E, Edström L, Eriksson A, Henriksson K-G, Ängqvist K-A 1980 The distribution of intermediate filament protein (skeletin) in normal and diseased human skeletal muscle: an immunohistochemical and electron-microscopic study. Journal of the Neurological Sciences 47:153

Thornell L-E, Eriksson A, Edström L 1983 Intermediate filaments in human myopathies. In: Dowben R M, Shay J W (eds) Cell and muscle motility. Plenum, New York, vol. 4, p 85

Toga M, Berard-Badier M, Gambarelli D, Pinsard N 1970 Ultrastructure des lesions neuromusculaires dans un cas de dystrophie neuroaxonale infantile ou maladie de Seitelberger. Communication to II Journées Internationales de Pathologie Neuromusculaire, Marseille

Tomé F M S, Fardeau M 1973 'Fingerprint inclusions' in muscle fibres in dystrophia myotonica. Acta Neuropathologica (Berlin) 24:62

Tomé F M S, Fardeau M 1986 Nuclear changes in muscle disorders. Methods and Achievements in Experimental Pathology 12:261

Trupin G L, Hsu L 1979 The identification of myogenic cells in regenerating skeletal muscle. Developmental Biology 68:72

Turnbull D M, Bartlett K, Steven D L, Alberti K G M M, Gibson G J, Johnson M A, McCulloch A J, Sherratt H S A 1984 Lipid storage myopathy and secondary carnite

deficiency due to short acyl-CoA dehydrogenase deficiency. New England Journal of Medicine 311:1232

Van Marle W, Woods K L 1980 Acute hydrocortisone myopathy. British Medical Journal 3:271

Van Wijngaarden G K, Bethlem J, Dingemans K P, Cöers C, Telerman-Toppet N, Gerard J M 1977 Familial focal loss of striations. Journal of Neurology 216:163

Vick N A 1971 Skeletal muscle capillary basement membranes in humans. Acta Neuropathologica (Berlin) 17:1

Wakayama Y, Schotland D L 1979 Muscle satellite cell populations in Duchenne dystrophy. In: Mauro A (ed) Muscle regeneration. Raven Press, New York, p 212

Wakayama Y, Schotland D L, Bonilla E, Orecchio E 1979 Quantitative ultrastructural study of muscle satellite cells in Duchenne dystrophy. Neurology (Minneapolis) 29:401

Wakayama Y, Okayasu H, Shibuya S, Kumagai T 1984 Duchenne dystrophy: reduced density of orthogonal array sub-unit particles in muscle plasma membrane. Neurology (Cleveland) 34:1313

Watkins S C, Cullen M J 1985 Histochemical fibre typing and ultrastructure of the small fibres in Duchenne muscular dystrophy. Neuropathology and Applied Neurobiology 11:447

Watkins S C, Cullen M J 1986 A quantitative comparison of satellite cell ultrastructure in Duchenne muscular dystrophy, polymyositis and normal controls. Muscle and Nerve 9:724

Webb J N, Gillespie W J 1976 Virus-like particles in paraspinal muscle in scoliosis. British Medical Journal 4:912

Weller R O, McArdle B 1971 Calcification within muscle fibres in the periodic paralyses. Brain 94:263

Whitaker J N, Engel W K 1972 Vascular deposits of immunoglobulin and complement in idiopathic inflammatory myopathy. New England Journal of Medicine 286:333

Whitaker J N, Bertorini T E, Mendell J R 1983 Immunocytochemical studies of cathepsin D in human skeletal muscle. Annals of Neurology 13:133

White J G 1972 Lymphocyte inclusion. Annals of Internal Medicine 76:1042

Wilcox D E, Affara N A, Yates J R W, Ferguson-Smith M A, Pearson P L 1985 Multipoint linkage analysis of the short arm of the human X chromosome in families with X-linked muscular dystrophy. Human Genetics 70:365

Witkowski J A 1986 Tissue culture studies of muscle disorders. Part 1. Techniques, cell growth, morphology cell surface. Muscle and Nerve 9:191

Wróblewski R, Gremski W, Nordemar R, Edström L 1978a Electron probe X-ray microanalysis of human skeletal muscles involved in rheumatoid arthritis. Histochemistry 57: 1–8

Wróblewski R, Roomans G, Jansson E, Edström L 1978b Electron probe X-ray microanalysis of human biopsies. Histochemistry 55: 281–292

Wróblewski R, Edström L, Mair W G P 1982 Five different types of centrally nucleated muscle fibres in man: elemental composition and morphological criteria. Journal of Submicroscopic Cytology 14:377

Wrogemann K, Pena S D J 1976 Mitochondrial calcium overload: a general mechanism for cell necrosis in muscle diseases. Lancet i:672

Yamaguchi M, Robson R M, Stromer M H, Dahl D S, Oda T 1978a Actin filaments form the backbone of nemaline myopathy rods. Nature (London) 271:265

Yamaguchi K, Santa T, Inove K, Omae T 1978b Lipid storage in Von Gierke's disease. Journal of the Neurological Sciences 38:195

Yarom R, Shapira Y 1977 Myosin degeneration in a congenital myopathy. Archives of Neurology 34:114

Yarom R, Reches A 1980 Thick filament degeneration in a case of acute quadriplegia. Journal of the Neurological Sciences 45:13

Yoshioka M, Okuda R 1977 Human skeletal muscle fibers in normal and pathological states: freeze-etch observations. Journal of Electronmicroscopy (Tokyo) 26:103

Yunis E J, Samaha F J 1971 Inclusion body myositis. Laboratory Investigation 25:240

Zacks S I, Pegues J J, Elliott F A 1962 Interstitial muscle capillaries in patients with diabetes mellitus: A light and electron microscope study. Metabolism II:381

Zellweger H, Brown B I, McCormick W F, Tu J-B 1965 A mild form of muscular glycogenosis in two brothers with alpha-1,4-glucosidase deficiency. Annals of Paediatrics 205:413

The immunology of neuromuscular disease

INTRODUCTION

Several neuromuscular diseases and syndromes are thought to be immunopathologically mediated. With the exception of acquired myasthenia gravis, the Lambert–Eaton myasthenic syndrome and most probably the chronic demyelinating neuropathy associated with benign IgM paraproteinaemia with antibody activity to a carbohydrate determinant on myelin-associated glycoprotein, the other disorders have not been proved to be immunopathologically mediated and/or autoimmune in aetiology. In order to understand better the data bearing on the role of the immune system in the pathogenesis of these neuromuscular diseases, it is useful to review several important aspects of the immune system.

ORGANISATION OF THE IMMUNE SYSTEM

Studies carried out over the last 10–20 years have demonstrated that the immune system is comprised of many cells and subsets of cells that at one time were thought to represent two or three end-stage cell types. It is now clear that there are many subsets of lymphocytes with different functions. In addition, cells of the same lineage at different stages of maturation may have different functional capacities. Moreover, products of cells of the immune system as well as many other endogenous and exogenous substances are able to alter and/or modify the function of subsets of immune system cells. Indeed, only the nervous system exceeds the immune system in its complexity of cell types and cellular interactions which affect system activity. It is not surprising, therefore, that it has been difficult to provide simple explanations as to the role of the immune system in the aetiology and pathogenesis of many putative immunopathologically mediated disorders.

Lymphocytes were at first divided into T-cells (thymic-dependent), B-cells (thymic-independent and bursal-equivalent) and null cells, based originally on the presence or absence of particular cell-surface characteristics (antigens or receptors). It is clear that the T-cells can be further classified by functional characteristics such as helper-inducer, cytotoxic and suppressor types. These cells may exert their function in a non-specific fashion upon stimulation by non-antigen-specific polyclonal stimulators or in response to specific antigen (Cantor 1984). The interaction with a specific antigen for each T lymphocyte is controlled by a specific receptor for that antigen (Acuto & Reinherz 1985). It is also clear that much of the interaction of T-cells with other T-cells and other cells of the organism is mediated by products of these cells, called lymphokines (Smith 1984).

Each B-cell also reacts with a specific antigen by the nature of the specific immunoglobulin (Ig) on its surface. For B-cells to respond by secreting appropriately the specific immunoglobulin (antibody) interaction with products of T-cells is generally necessary (Fauci 1982, Howard & Paul 1983, Smith 1984). It is, therefore, clear that normal antibody responses depend not only on B-cells but on regulatory T-cells and their products.

Recently we have learned a great deal about those non-T, non-B lymphocytes previously called null cells. Many of these cells mediate cytotoxic effects against tumour cells (in vitro) although little is known about the mechanisms of cell recognition or killing: these cells are called natural killer (NK) cells (Heberman 1982). Cells of this lineage are also able to participate in specific killing of immune targets. Although these cells themselves do not specifically recognise antigens, they interact with the Fc portion (crystallisable fragment of proteolytic digest of Ig) of immunoglobulins (antibodies) that have bound to the specific antigen (The binding to the antigen is mediated by the specific antibody (idiotype) portion

of the molecule contained in the Fab fragment.) (Ziegler & Henney 1977).

The monocyte (circulating phase)-macrophages and related accessory cells of the immune system (dendritic cells and Langerhans cells of the skin) are extremely important in the normal function of the immune system. These cells are involved in the afferent phase (antigen processing and induction of specific sensitised cells), being important in the processing of antigen activation of T-cells and presentation of antigen to the specific lymphocyte. They are also highly important in the efferent phase. (Sensitised cells and products interact with non-specific factors to mediate the functions of the immune system.) They may be activated by lymphokines, attracted to inflammatory sites by chemotactic factors and interact with antigen–antibody reactions by nature of the presence of receptors for the Fc portion of IgG and components of the complement system (Shevach 1984). In addition to participating in immune phagocytosis, macrophages also participate in non-immune phagocytosis. Products of macrophages, such as prostaglandins, may have regulatory as well as direct effector actions (Dore-Duffy et al 1985).

IMMUNOPATHOLOGICAL REACTIONS

The immune system is capable of many complex and interrelated immunological reactions which are necessary for the maintenance of the health of the organism. When these reactions or immune mechanisms are excessive, prolonged, misdirected or inappropriate, they are capable of causing damage to the host and are termed immunopathological reactions. There were originally thought to be four types of reactions (Coombs & Gell 1968) but it has become clear that many more exist, or at least that there are several subtypes. There has been considerable progress in determining the reactants and mediators of these reactions and in determining which of them are likely to be important in several human diseases (Table 9.1). One can also consider diseases associated with autoantibodies to receptors on cell surfaces as an entirely separate immunopathological group of disorders; these antibodies may have inhibitory or

Table 9.1 Immunological effector mechanisms and immunopathological reactions in man and experimental animals

Immunological Mechanism	Reactants	Mediators	Normal Function	Diseases
Reaginic	IgE mast cell or basophil and antigen	vasoactive amines (histamine) arachidonic acid metabolites (leukotrienes, prostaglandins, platelet activating factor), inflammatory cells (neutrophils, eosinophils, mononuclear leucocytes)	parasite killing	allergic respiratory diseases, anaphylaxis
Antibody to self-antigens Direct cytotoxic	IgG or IgM & antigen	complement; inflammatory cells	infections	experimental autoimmune myasthenia gravis, myasthenia gravis, certain haemolytic anaemias
Alteration of membranes & surface receptors (a) sequestration via cell surface activation		immune complex between antigen on circulating cell & antibody; reacts with Fc receptor on reticuloendo-thelial cell	infections	certain haemolytic anaemias, idiopathic thrombocytopenic purpura
(b) block of ligand binding				myasthenia gravis, experimental autoimmune myasthenia gravis, diabetes & acanthocytosis secondary to antibodies to insulin receptor
(c) receptor down-regulation				myasthenia gravis, experimental autoimmune myasthenia gravis
(d) receptor stimulation				autoimmune hyperthyroidism, anti-insulin receptor antibodies
Immune complex deposition	IgG or IgM + antigen (complement)	complement; inflammatory cells	antigen clearance	serum sickness, vasculitides, lupus nephritis, rare haemolytic anaemias & thrombocytopenias (drug-related)
Cell-mediated reactions T-cell mediated (a) delayed hypersensitivity	T-cells (helper-inducer) & antigen, Type II MHC dependent	lymphocytes & lymphokines, monocyte-macrophages	infections with obligate intracellular organisms	experimental allergic encephalomyelitis, experimental allergic neuritis, acute disseminated encephalomyelitis (?), allograft rejection
(b) T-cell cytotoxic	T-cells (cytotoxic) & antigen, Type I MHC dependent	lymphocytes & products, secondary phagocytosis	? tumour necrosis, infection (with obligate intracellular organisms)	certain forms of hepatitis, allograft rejection, graft versus host reaction
ADCC (see p. 352)	K-cells (lymphocytes) & macrophages, Fc & receptor	K-cell & macrophages	? infections, tumour destruction	allograft rejection
NK-cell reactions	NK lymphoctes	NK lymphocytes	? tumour destruction & infections	?

stimulatory effects. These diseases include myasthenia gravis, type B insulin-resistant diabetes mellitus with acanthocytosis, Graves' disease and perhaps some forms of hay fever (asthma). In the discussion to follow of different neuromuscular diseases of man and experimental animals of immunopathological origin, an attempt is made to review the evidence for the possible role of such reactions in these disorders.

TOLERANCE

The immune system normally does not react to self (autoantigens) but, in true autoimmune diseases, the reaction by sensitised cells or antibody to a component of self represents a failure of maintenance of the normal state of self-tolerance. There are several mechanisms that have been proposed by which the immune system prevents the attack on self antigens. These include: (a) clonal deletion (or abortion); (b) suppressor T-cells (antigen-specific or non-specific cells); (c) sequestration of self antigens; (d) idiotype networks; and (e) antigen-specific antigen-induced tolerance (Nossal 1983). There is evidence for and against each of these theories. It is possible that each of these mechanisms may be important but none can completely explain the maintenance of tolerance (Cohen & Lisak 1987).

Burnet (1959) had proposed that exposure to self-antigens during ontogeny renders the immune system unable to react to that antigen and that this tolerance results from deletion of clones of lymphoid cells that recognise that antigen. The presence of both antibodies and T-cells reactive to autoantigens in normal experimental animals and man makes this hypothesis unlikely to be the major explanation for tolerance to self.

In the second scenario, suppressor cells, principally a subset of T lymphocytes, suppress the immune response of other T-cells and B-cells. Failure of these T-cells or a subset of these cells to suppress the activity of other cells that recognise self-antigens would result in the emergence of an autoimmune reaction (Miller & Schwartz 1982).

There is increasing interest in the possibility that the immune system is partly controlled by so-called idiotypic reactions (Jerne 1974). In this system every antibody molecule itself is an antigen which elicits a response by another immunoglobulin molecule: the reaction of the second antibody is to the portion of the first antibody that reacts with the antigen. That antigen-binding site is the idiotype and the antibody elicited by the first antibody is called the anti-idiotype. This second antibody (the anti-idiotype) can also elicit an antibody response called an anti-anti-idiotype. This network is called the idiotypic network. It is not clear if this system extends to antigen-specific cells. Ordinarily this network keeps the immune response in balance; a failure in the network allows the autoimmune antibody to emerge (Zanetti 1985). While there is considerable evidence for elements of this network in experimental animals and, to a lesser degree, in man, there is also considerable evidence that the hypothesis originally offered cannot be correct in its entirety. It is likely that under normal conditions at times of activation of immunoglobulin-producing cells the network becomes operative (Bona & Pernis 1984).

Another mechanism promoting tolerance is sequestration of antigen from the immune system during development. Nervous system antigens which are hidden behind the blood–brain or blood–nerve barrier are examples of such antigens. T-cells recognise antigen in the context of products of the major histocompatibility complex (MHC) expressed on the cell surface (Zinkernagel & Dougherty 1974). The normal nervous system is poor in MHC products (antigens). This MHC-dependent restriction may provide additional protection from the emergence of self-reactive clones (Cowing 1985). The later exposure of an immunologically appropriate cell, genetically programmed with the potential to react to that antigen in the context of MHC antigens, to that self antigen or an exogenous antigen that shares the epitope (molecular mimicry) would then result in an autoimmune response (Fujinami & Oldstone 1985). Normals have been shown to have T-cells which react to self-antigens that are components of organ systems which are relatively sequestered from the immune system and are components of organs that are relatively deficient in MHC-associated antigens, including the central and peripheral nervous systems and the eye (Burns et al 1983). Therefore, some other factors would be required to suppress these autoreactive T-cells.

A final mechanism is antigen-induced tolerance of autoantigen reactive clones. In this system the exposure of antigen-specific cells to that antigen, perhaps in the absence of MHC antigens (Cohn & Epstein 1978), causes suppression of the antigen-specific clones already present in the organism (Feldmann et al 1985).

IMMUNOGENETICS

The immunological response of any particular organism is strongly influenced by the genetic make-up of that individual. Several allelic systems have been identified which determine the response of both humoral (antibody) and cellular elements of the immune response. These genes, therefore, in large part determine whether the host makes a response to a stimulus, be that response appropriate (protective) or inappropriate (failure to respond or an autoreactive response).

The structure of both the heavy and light chains of immunoglobulin molecules is controlled by many genetic elements which create a single gene that determines the structure of both variable and constant regions of the immunoglobulin molecule (Leder 1983, Tonegawa 1983). These regions respectively determine the antigenic specificity and biological properties of each immunoglobulin molecule. These genetic elements are not part of the MHC. In man, the haplotype in the Gm allotype system determines the allotypic nature of an individual's IgG (heavy chains). Similar allotypes have been identified for IgA heavy chains as well as kappa light chains. The genes of this system do not, of course, identify the fine specificity of the control exercised by the variable idiotype region of the heavy or light chains which determines the antigenic specificity of an antibody (immunoglobulin) molecule.

The MHC consists of several types of genes identified by gene products (these can be identified immunologically and are, therefore, themselves antigens) that are of great importance in the genetic control of the immune response. The ability of lymphocytes to react to an antigen requires co-recognition of that antigen with MHC type I (HLA, A, B and C molecules [antigens] in

man for cytotoxic T-cells) or type II (HLA-DR and DQ (DC) also called Ia in man) molecules for helper-inducer T-cells (Zinkernagel & Dougherty 1974, Winchester & Kunkel 1979, Hurley et al 1983, Acuto & Reinherz 1985). The MHC antigens control the response to transplantation (hence their name) and by a high degree of polymorphism and requirement for co-recognition with antigens, influence the capacity for a response of an individual organism to an antigen, be it exogenous or endogenous. It should be noted that the antigens identified to date do not seem to identify the entire repertoire of immune response genes. This need for co-recognition is true for soluble proteins as well as cell surface antigens. Moreover, genes that control other important components of the immune response include the second (C2) and fourth (C4) components of the complement system; and factor B (a component of the alternative complement pathway) (Alper 1981), maps to the MHC.

As noted, the genes have been shown to influence the immunological response of experimental animals, including the ability to develop several immunologically-mediated diseases (McDevitt & Bodmer 1974). For these reasons, there have been many studies to see if there is an increased incidence of different MHC and haplotypes and Gm allotypes in diseases believed to be of immunopathological origin. Among those diseases studied are several neuromuscular disorders (Table 9.2). These MHC antigens may not themselves be the susceptibility determining gene products, but map near the appropriate gene, since these antigens appear in normals. It is also possible that patients may differ from normals who have the same serologically defined DR or DQ type in the pattern of the genes (DNA) that determine the different peptide chains controlling the fine specificity of the gene products (polymorphism) of the MHC II alleles. Alternatively, the MHC antigens might be the important gene product but other environmental factors determine whether a disease develops and which disease.

IDIOPATHIC INFLAMMATORY MYOSITIS

The term 'inflammatory myopathy' encompasses a large number of disorders. A group of these, of

Table 9.2 Immunogenetic markers and neuromuscular disease associations

Disease	HLA Associations	References
Polymyositis	B8; B8, DR3 (Caucasoids); B7, Dw6 (blacks)	Reviewed in Behan & Behan 1985 and Mastaglia & Ojeda 1985b
Dermatomyositis	B8, B14	Reviewed in Behan & Behan 1985 and Mastaglia & Ojeda 1985b
Juvenile dermatomyositis Myasthenia gravis	B6 or none	Reviewed in Behan & Behan 1985 and Mastaglia & Ojeda 1985b
No thymoma, <40 y.o. onset, females, probably males as well	A1, B8, DRw3 (B12 Japan); A1, B8, DR5 (blacks & other non-Caucasoids)	Compston et al 1980, Reviewed in Behan & Shields 1982, Christiansen et al 1984, Engel 1984
No thymoma,>40 y.o. onset, males	A3, B7, DRw2 (B10 Japan)	
thymoma, older onset	? A2, ? A3	
Lambert–Eaton myasthenic syndrome	B8 — idiopathic > carcinomatous	Willcox et al 1985
Guillain–Barré syndrome	None	Adams et al 1977, Stewart et al 1978, Kaslow et al 1984
Chronic demyelinating inflammatory neuropathy	A1, B8, DRw3	Stewart et al 1978, Adams et al 1979
Amyotrophic lateral sclerosis	A3 (classic) or none; B12 (slow progressive) BW35 (rapid progressive guamanian)	Reviewed in Cashman et al 1985
	Gm Allotypes	
Myasthenia gravis	Gm[1,2,21] (Japan); none (Finland)	Nakao et al 1980, Smith et al 1984
Lambert–Eaton	G1m[(2)]	Willcox et al 1985
Amyotrophic lateral sclerosis	None	Reviewed in Cashman et al 1985

unknown aetiology, with certain clinical features in common, are generally referred to as idiopathic inflammatory myopathy or polymyositis and dermatomyositis (Whitaker 1982, Behan & Behan 1985, Mastaglia & Ojeda 1985a, b). It should be noted from the outset that many consider polymyositis and dermatomyositis to be the same disorder, differing only in the occurrence of a characteristic spectrum of skin lesions. While this may eventually be proved to be true, 'lumping' these disorders may obscure differences in immunopathogenesis between polymyositis and dermatomyositis. Indeed, there is immunological and histopathological evidence to support the hypothesis that there are several sub-types of disease embraced by the terms polymyositis and dermatomyositis and that different immunopathological abnormalities and different aetiological factors may be important in these different syndromes (Whitaker 1982, Behan & Behan 1985).

Experimental autoimmune myositis (EAM) and other models

There have been many attempts over the years to develop an experimental laboratory model for polymyositis similar to experimental allergic encephalomyelitis (EAE), experimental allergic neuritis (EAN) and, more recently, experimental autoimmune myasthenia gravis (EAMG). Although some investigators have reported successful production of myositis, this has been a histological finding, while others have been unable to demonstrate reproducibly even histological myositis (Dawkins 1975, Smith et al 1979, Whitaker 1982, Behan & Behan 1985). Recently, SJL mice have been shown consistently to develop histological EAM (Rosenberg et al 1985). The relative roles of cell-mediated and humoral (antibody) effector mechanisms in EAM are not clear. It has not been possible to produce a disorder similar to childhood dermatomyositis by inducing the vascular lesions (Hathaway et al 1970). Polymyositis and both sporadic and familial canine dermatomyositis have been reported (Kornegay et al 1980, Hargis et al 1985).

Immunopathological mechanisms

There are no reported studies to suggest that the serum of patients with polymyositis or dermatomyositis contains IgE class antibodies to muscle. Basophils and mast cells are not prominent in muscle in idiopathic inflammatory myopathies. Eosinophils, which are important cells in reaginic immunity, are seen in eosinophilic polymyositis, a disorder that is part of the hypereosinophilic syndrome — a condition of unknown aetiology in which vasculitis (presumptive immune complex deposition) is frequently observed (Layzer et al 1977).

The possibility that the serum of patients with idiopathic inflammatory myopathies contains antibodies to one or more muscle antigens that are involved in Type II immunopathological reactions has been investigated. There have been reports of deposition of immunoglobulin and complement components at the site of muscle fibre necrosis (Heffner et al 1976, Engel & Biesecker 1982, Isenberg 1983, Morgan et al 1984), a finding that is certainly compatible with the hypothesis that antibodies to muscle are involved in the pathogenesis of these disorders. While the presence of components of the complement system seems to be reproducible, it should be noted that this is not proof that antimuscle antibodies are responsible for this deposition, activation and subsequent fibre necrosis. Immune complex deposition (see below) could also be responsible for complement activation and the alternate pathway of complement can be activated through non-antibody-related mechanisms. The demonstration of immunoglobulin deposition has suggested, to some, non-specific in vitro staining or in vivo deposition (Mastaglia & Ojeda 1985) as a result of changes in the vasculature. Studies of serum of patients with polymyositis and dermatomyositis have not revealed disease-specific increases in antibodies to muscle, muscle extracts or purified muscle antigens such as myoglobin, actin or myosin

(Whitaker 1982, reviewed in Behan & Behan 1985, Mastaglia & Ojeda 1985b). One would expect that pathogenic antibodies would be directed at a surface component rather than at a component of the cytoplasm or nucleus. As noted later, an antibody-dependent cell-mediated cytotoxic reaction could be involved in disease pathogenesis.

The serum of patients with polymyositis frequently contains antibodies to nuclear and/or cytoplasmic antigens and it has been suggested that some of these are relatively specific for clinical subsets of the idiopathic inflammatory myopathies (Table 9.3). It is unlikely that these antibodies are responsible for muscle damage but they may be useful in defining subsets of these disorders and, more importantly, in helping to delineate the cause of some of these syndromes. For example, the Jo antigen is the enzyme that catalyses the charging of histidine to its transfer RNA. Picornaviruses have been shown to interact with the transfer RNA synthetase enzymes (Matthews & Bernstein 1983).

There is considerable evidence to support the possibility that deposition of circulating immune complexes in vessels within muscle is important in the pathogenesis of certain idiopathic inflammatory myopathies. Frank vasculitis is found in the muscle and in other tissues, especially in patients with juvenile dermatomyositis (Banker 1975). Milder changes are also observed, including changes in capillary endothelial cells and basement membrane (Behan & Behan 1985). It should be noted that changes can be noted in vessels at the site of clear-cut cell-mediated non-antibody reactions. Deposition of immunoglobulin and complement in the vessels were described by Whitaker & Engel (1972), but the incidence was highest among patients with juvenile dermatomyositis. Indeed, in studies which did not include a significant number of patients of this subtype, immunoglobulin and complement deposition was seldom, if ever, observed in vessel walls. Recently, evidence of complement activation was found in vessels of patients with dermatomyositis (Kissel et al 1986). Thus, it is possible that immune complex deposition is important in the pathogenesis of some but not all idiopathic inflammatory myopathies. The presence of elevated levels of immune

Table 9.3 Antinuclear and related antibodies in polymyositis/dermatomyositis

Antibody	Disease subset	Antigen	Reference
PM-1	60–70% PM; some childhood DM	unknown	Wolfe et al 1977, Pachman & Cooke 1980
Jo-1	30–40% of PM; 60–70% with pulmonary fibrosis	Histidyl-tRNA synthetase	Arnett et al 1981, Matthews & Bernstein 1983
Mi	exclusively seen with dermatomyositis	Cathodic non-histone protein	Nishikai & Reichlin 1980, Targoff & Reichlin 1985
Ku	PM with scleroderma features	Acidic protein	Mimori et al 1981
PM-Scl	PM with scleroderma features	Nucleus/nucleolar	Reichlin et al 1984
PL-7	Polymyositis	Threonyl-tRNA synthetase	Matthews et al 1984
RNP	Mixed connective tissue disease; some SLE	Ribonucleoprotein	Sharp et al 1972, 1976
Sm	SLE	Non-histone devoid of nucleic acids	
DS-DNA	SLE-active	Native DNA	Zweiman & Lisak 1984, Behan & Behan 1985
Ro	Sjögren's syndrome; some SLE, polymyositis, mothers of infants with congenital heart block	Cytoplasmic antigen	

complexes in the serum of patients with both polymyositis and dermatomyositis has been reported (Behan et al 1982). The nature of antigen in these complexes is not known.

There is long-standing interest in the possibility that some cases of polymyositis may be caused by cell-mediated reactivity to muscle antigens or conceivably to viral antigens in latently infected muscle fibres. Myositis has been described recently in patients with the acquired immune deficiency syndrome (AIDS) (Levy et al 1985). With the exception of one study (Johnson et al 1972), in vitro experiments assessing cell-mediated cytotoxicity have not used HLA-matched human muscle as the target (Currie et al 1971, Dawkins & Mastaglia 1973, Haas & Arnason 1974, Haas 1980). As T-cell cytotoxic reactions apparently do not occur across histocompatibility barriers, the reported cytotoxic reactions may not represent in vitro evidence of T-cell cytotoxicity. These experiments could represent: (a) antibody-dependent cell-mediated cytotoxic (ADCC) reactions; (b) reactions of the blood cells to allogenic histocompatibility antigens on the muscle; or (c) increases in NK cell activity. It should be noted that only one of the studies examined the cytotoxic effect of patients' cells on non-muscle tissue so that

muscle-specific cytotoxicity has not been demonstrated absolutely conclusively. In addition, there are no studies employing purified T-cells or cytotoxic (T8+) T-cells in in vitro cytotoxicity assays. Disease-specific in vitro reactivity to muscle using proliferation of lymphocytes has not been demonstrated (Behan et al 1975, Lisak & Zweiman 1975).

There is, however, some indirect evidence for a role for cell-mediated immunity in polymyositis and dermatomyositis. Graft versus host disease, both clinical and experimental, not infrequently includes an inflammatory myopathy (Anderson et al 1982). Experimental allergic (autoimmune) myositis, a somewhat controversial model of autoimmunity, would seem to be a cell-mediated reaction (see earlier discussion). The strongest evidence of a primary role for a cell-mediated reaction in the idiopathic inflammatory myopathies is the recent work of several groups demonstrating that T-cells, including T8+ cytotoxic-suppressor cells and T4+ helper-delayed type sensitivity cells are the predominant cells in the muscles of these patients. Engel and co-workers have elegantly demonstrated T8+ cells invading muscle fibres, apparently initiating muscle fibre necrosis (Fig. 9.1 and 9.2). The T-cells seem to

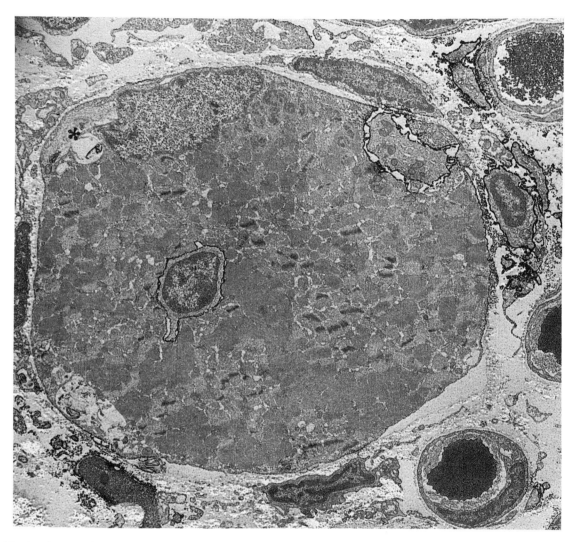

Fig. 9.1 A muscle fibre with surrounding and superficial and deeply placed T8$^+$ invading cells. Small cavities in the fibre (asterisk) probably contained invading cells that retracted during fixation or dehydration, or indicate focal myofibrillar loss near invading cells. The plasma membrane of the fibre facing the invading cells, highlighted by diffusion artefact, shows no deletions. ×6000 (From Arahata & Engel 1986)

be activated (Ia or DR$^+$). In addition, some B-cells and macrophages are also seen but K-cells and NK-cells, at least as defined by monoclonal antibodies, and plasma cells are rarely encountered (Engel & Arahata 1984, Arahata & Engel 1984, 1986). Studies by others support the predominance of T-cells in the inflammatory exudate in muscle (Rowe et al 1981, Behan & Behan 1985, Olsson et al 1985) although there are some differences with regard to T-cell subset analysis.

Thus, there is evidence for both cell-mediated and immune-complex-mediated immunopathologi-cal mechanisms being involved in the pathogenesis of these disorders; there is less evidence for a pathogenic role for anti-muscle antibodies. It may be that more than one mechanism may be important and perhaps different mechanisms predominate in different sub-types of these disorders. It must be emphasised that the evidence is indirect and controversial.

Immunoregulation

If a disorder is immunopathogenic in origin or is

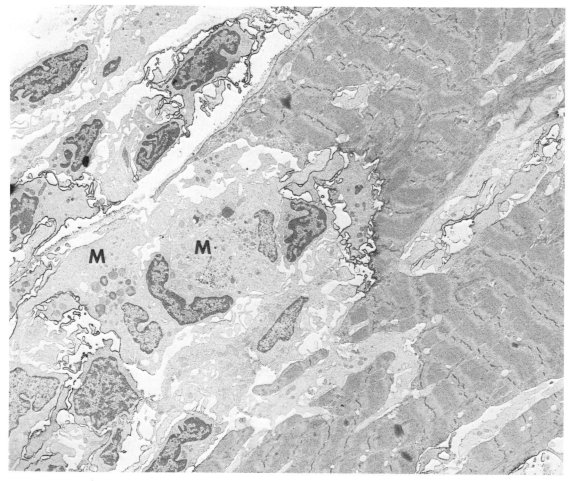

Fig. 9.2 More advanced fibre invasion. The T8 antigen is localised. The muscle fibre is honeycombed by cavities containing both T8$^+$ and T8-negative invading cells and their spike-like extensions. Large invading cells with pale cytoplasm and multiple lysosomal structures are macrophages (M). The muscle fibre is depleted of mitochondria and shows focal myofibrillar degeneration beginning at the Z disk. ×4400 (From Arahata & Engel 1986)

the result of a persistent infection with a common virus, it is important to determine whether there is a defect in the normal regulatory mechanisms which would be permissive for such an abnormal state to develop and persist. Indeed, it has recently been noted that primates with an acquired immune deficiency (AIDS-like) illness have polymyositis-like lesions (Dalakas et al 1986) and similar lesions have recently been described in patients with AIDS (Levy et al 1985).

There have been several studies of the peripheral blood of patients with polymyositis and dermatomyositis which have assessed quantitatively the numbers of various lymphocyte subsets.

Some (Behan et al 1983, Behan & Behan 1985) but not all (Iyer et al 1983) groups of investigators have found a reduction in the number of suppressor T-cells in the blood of such patients. Functional studies have also been performed to assess the immunoregulatory capacity of blood cells. A decrease in some but not other suppressor T-cell activities has been reported (Mastaglia & Ojeda 1985b) and an increase in B-cell activity, manifested by increased serum immunoglobulin levels, which could be a consequence of decrease in suppressor activity, is also seen (Lisak & Zweiman 1976). The relationship between decreased T-cell suppressor activity and number and a reported decrease in the proliferative response of blood cells of patients with polymyositis to phytohaemagglutinin (Behan & Behan 1985) is not clear. One usually associates decreased proliferation of cells to this T-cell mitogen with defects in the number or function of helper rather than in suppressor T-cell defects.

MYASTHENIA GRAVIS

Myasthenia gravis has emerged as the prototypic autoimmune disease. Although its aetiology is unknown, in the past 15 years we have learned much about immunopathological mechanisms important at the end-plate, the nature of important antigenic sites of the acetylcholine (ACh) receptor (AChR), and a good deal about defects in normal immunological control which may have a role in the loss of tolerance and emergence of pathogenic autoantibodies.

Experimental autoimmune myasthenia gravis (EAMG) and other models

Sensitisation of experimental animals with material rich in AChR with the production of weakness and neuromuscular block responsive to acetylcholinesterase inhibitors, was a major development in our understanding of the immunopathogenesis of myasthenia gravis (Patrick & Lindstrom 1973, reviewed in Ashizawa & Appel 1985). It became clear that while T-cells and macrophages were important in the production of antibodies to AChR, the antibodies were responsible for the actual reduction of available AChR at the postsynaptic membrane (Sahashi et al 1978). The EAMG model has continued to be of use in investigation of pathogenic mechanisms by which the antibodies actually cause a decrease in available receptor, as well as in the study of interactions of cells of their immune system that bring about disease induction and, potentially, suppression of the autoimmune response (Christados et al 1981, Pachner & Cantor 1984, Lennon et al 1985). More recently, experimental myasthenia and anti-AChR antibodies have been induced by immunising animals either with antibodies to an agonist of AChR (Wasserman et

al 1982) or with the agonist (Bis Q) itself (Cleveland et al 1983) via the idiotype network.

Monoclonal antibodies produced in rodents against AChR have also provided insight into the events at the end-plate. Because of the exquisite specificity of these immunoglobulins against defined epitopes (antigenic sites) it is possible to employ these monoclonal antibodies in in vitro and in vivo experiments to determine which epitopes serve as potentially pathogenic reactants and to investigate which immunopathological mechanisms involving anti-AChR antibodies are important (see below). Analysis with this degree of specificity is not possible in passive transfer experiments employing heteroantisera or human immunoglobulins (Toyka et al 1975).

Acquired autoimmune myasthenia gravis occurs in several breeds of dogs, as does congenital myasthenia gravis which is not immunologically mediated (Lennon et al 1978).

Immunopathological events at the end-plate

It has become clear that there are several mechanisms by which anti-AChR antibodies cause a reduction in AChR at the muscle end-plate (Lisak & Barchi 1982, Ashizawa & Appel 1985). The original demonstration of serum anti-AChR antibodies employed an assay that detected antibodies directed against the α-bungarotoxin binding site which is close to or perhaps identical to the ligand (ACh) binding site (Almon et al 1974). For some time it was felt that this was not an important mechanism for pathological manifestation in vivo principally because the majority of patients do not have detectable antibodies to this site and the proportion of antibodies blocking α-bungarotoxin binding is small in patients with such antibodies (Whiting et al 1983). However, it is possible that in some patients antibodies which block or alter the confirmation of the ligand binding site may be important in certain stages of the disease. This is supported by the finding that monoclonal antibodies to the α-bungarotoxin binding site cause a rapidly evolving neuromuscular block when passively transferred to avian recipients (Gomez & Richman 1983).

A second mechanism is complement-mediated destruction of the end-plate. It is clear that some end-plates show evidence of necrosis with the presence of both the third and ninth components of the complement cascade (Fig. 9.3) (Engel et al 1977, Sahashi et al 1980). In vitro studies and passive transfer protocols with experimental antibodies and IgG from patients with myasthenia confirm the importance of antibody-determined complement-mediated membrane destruction.

The other important mechanism is antigen-specific antibody-mediated degradation, down-regulation of AChR. AChR, like other membrane constituents, is constantly degraded, resynthesised and inserted into the membrane. It has been demonstrated that an antibody molecule can bind to antigenic sites on adjacent molecules of AChR by virtue of its two antigen-binding sites (bivalent). This results in a cross-linking of adjacent molecules which in turn causes a rearrangement of receptor molecules (Bursztajn et al 1983) and an increased rate of AChR degradation (Appel et al 1977, Kao & Drachman 1977, Drachman et al 1978, Stanley & Drachman 1978). While eventually there is an increase in synthesis, it does not occur acutely and at any rate is insufficient to maintain a normal density of receptor in the membrane. If the immunoglobulin (antibody) binds to two sites in the same molecule, such as on each of the α-chains, there is no increase in receptor-specific degradation (Conti-Tronconi et al 1982).

Although cells can be found at the end-plate in acute stages of EAMG in some species, either in response to complement activation or as an antibody-dependent cell-mediated cytotoxic reaction (ADCC), there is little evidence for such mechanisms being of primary importance in man. It should be noted, however, that there are few, if any, studies of the human end-plate at an equivalent stage of the disease.

Several groups have reported increased in vitro reactivity to AChR by blood and thymic lymphocytes in patients with myasthenia gravis (Abramsky et al 1975, Richman et al 1976, McQuillen et al 1983). This reactivity, while significantly greater than that observed in controls, is quite modest and does not approach the levels of reactivity observed in sensitised animals with EAMG. When one considers passive transfer studies in animals and the pathology of the end-plate in experimental models and in man, one is forced to conclude that a local delayed hypersensitivity reaction or cytotoxic T-cell reaction is not an important pathogenic mechanism in human myasthenia gravis (Lisak et al 1985a).

Antigenic determinants (epitopes)

Anti-AChR antibodies in the serum of patients with MG are not all directed against the same antigenic determinant on the molecule. Antibodies

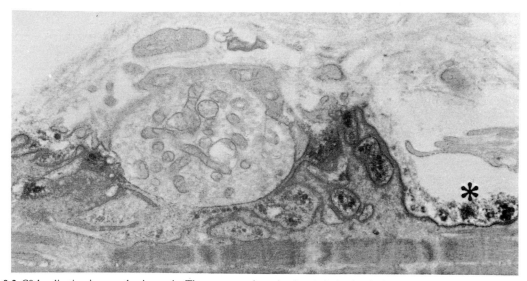

Fig. 9.3 C9 localisation in myasthenia gravis. The postsynaptic region is relatively simple. Reaction for C9 appears on debris in synaptic space, overshort segments of the junctional folds and on material to the right of the folds, and on the surface of the muscle fibre and positioned between layers of basal lamina (asterisk). ×15 300 (From Sahashi et al 1980)

have been detected against all four subunits (α, β, γ, δ) of the protein although the majority seem to be directed to a single region of the α subunits. Two different peptide sequences are believed to be the antigenic determinants (epitopes) that comprise the main immunogenic region (MIR), although this is not certain. A significant role of the MIR as the important epitope for the production of clinically important effector mechanisms in a majority of patients is not proven although rodent monoclonal antibodies to the MIR transfer typical EAMG in passive transfer experiments and are active in muscle tissue culture systems (reviewed in Ashizawa & Appel 1985).

Abnormalities of immunoregulation

As described earlier in this chapter, the emergence of significant levels of pathogenic antibodies to a self-antigen implies one or more abnormalities of normal immunological control and regulatory mechanisms (loss of tolerance). In addition, the occurrence of many autoantibodies in patients with myasthenia, which do not seem to be the result of cross-reactive epitopes in the different tissues and antigens (Gilhus et al 1984), suggests that in some patients there is a broad-based defect in immunoregulation. Indeed, there is evidence for abnormalities of broad-based and AChR-specific immune responses by both blood and thymic cells (Lisak & Barchi 1982, Levinson et al 1985, Lisak et al 1985a).

There have been quantitative analyses of levels of lymphocytes and lymphocyte subsets in the blood of patients with myasthenia gravis, most recently employing monoclonal antibodies that react with subsets with different functional characteristics. While there is no complete agreement, most have found significant, albeit modest, increases in the ratio of helper/suppressor cells, generally reflecting a decrease in suppressor cells (Bahir et al 1981, Skolnik et al 1982). Haynes et al (1983) found a decrease in helper cell numbers in a small number of patients with later onset of disease which was reversed after thymectomy. In vitro evidence for a decrease in T-cell suppressor function has been reported (Mishak & Dau 1981), as has evidence for an increase in vivo B-cell activity (Levinson et al 1981). Thus, there is reason to believe that patients with myasthenia

gravis have a mild decrease in some immunoregulatory capacity not limited to control of the response to AChR.

It is also clear that patients with myasthenia gravis differ from controls with regard to regulation of synthesis of antibodies to acetylcholine receptor. Culture of blood cells of patients with myasthenia in vitro results in detectable synthesis of anti-AChR antibodies in 50–60% of patients without any additional stimulation. The addition of pokeweed mitogen, a T-cell- and monocyte-dependent polyclonal stimulant of B-cell growth and differentiation, results in a dramatic increase in the amount of antibody synthesised, and detectable synthesis of antibody in 70–80% of patients. The amount of antibody correlates with the serum titres of anti-AChR antibodies. The peripheral blood cells of normal individuals rarely synthesise detectable levels of anti-AChR and even then at minimal amounts (Lisak et al 1983b, 1984b). Removal of T8 suppressor lymphocytes from cultures of blood cells from normals does not result in an increase in detectable anti-AChR synthesis. Thus, the lack of anti-AChR synthesis by normals cannot be attributed simply to normal T8 suppressor cell function (Lisak et al 1984b). The most likely explanation is the lack of sufficient numbers of the autoimmune B-cells to respond to non-specific T-cell helper factors. In contrast, the removal of T8 positive cells from cultures of blood from myasthenics does result in an increase in both anti-AChR and total IgG synthesis (Lisak et al 1986a). Therefore, anti-AChR synthesis by abnormal B-cells and helper T-cells, including the AChR-specific helper T-cells reported to be present in the blood of myasthenics (Hohlfeld et al 1984), is subject to some normal immunoregulatory influences. Since we do not know what triggers anti-AChR synthesis in vivo, it is possible that increased numbers of antigen-specific helper T-cells may be important in the loss of immunological tolerance in myasthenics.

It has also been found that the thymus, which is histologically abnormal in the majority of patients with myasthenia, is the site of abnormal immune responses. This is of special interest because of the central role of the thymus in the development of the immune response, the presence of myoid cells in the thymus and the reports of a beneficial effect of thymectomy.

The distribution of T-cell subsets in the thymus seems to be either normal or near-normal in number and in distribution in immunohistological studies (Thomas et al 1982, Kornstein et al 1984). B-cells are probably increased in number in cases of germinal centre hyperplasia although in studies of cells in suspension there seems to be little evidence of an increase in B-cells as assessed by the criteria of surface IgM (Lisak et al 1983c). This dichotomy probably represents dilution of the B-cells by the overwhelming number of T-cells. It may eventually be found that there are differences in the maturational stages of B-cells in the thymus of patients with myasthenia when compared with controls.

Little is known about potential abnormalities in accessory cells in the myasthenic thymus including epithelial cells and dendritic cells. There seems to be an increase in the percentage of DR-positive lymphoid cells in suspensions obtained from thymuses of myasthenic subjects. Whether these are dendritic cells or B-cells that do not bear the other usual B-cell phenotypic markers is not known (Lisak et al 1983c).

Functional studies of thymic lymphocytes have also provided evidence of immunological abnormalities. Despite the fact that relatively few B-cells bear surface IgM, cell suspensions from myasthenic thymuses demonstrate increased spontaneous levels of immunoglobulin-secreting cells, an indicator of enhanced in vivo B-cell activity (Levinson et al 1984). This activity is frequently greater than that of autologous blood cells. It is not clear whether this activity is inherent in the B-cells or represents an abnormal milieu because of abnormal T-cell or accessory-cell function, or because of the presence of AChR itself in the thymus, perhaps in an immunogenetically susceptible subject. The potential for B-cell activation is probably present in the normal thymus, as mitogen stimulation of thymic lymphocytes in vitro results in an equivalent immunoglobulin-secreting cell response, often greater than that of blood cells in control and myasthenic thymic cell suspensions.

It has been shown that thymic lymphocytes secrete anti-AChR in vitro (Vincent et al 1978, McLachlan et al 1981, Newsom-Davis et al 1981, Fujii et al 1986, Lisak et al 1986b) although there is controversy over the response to mitogenic stimulation in vitro and the relative production of thymic and blood cell production of these antibodies. It seems unlikely that the thymus is the major site of in vivo anti-AChR production: normal thymus cells do not synthesise detectable anti-AChR with or without mitogen stimulation; cells from patients with myasthenia and thymoma either do not make anti-AChR or make less than those from patients with germinal centre hyperplasia (Vincent et al 1978, Fujii et al 1984). It is also clear that while much of the IgG synthesised by thymic lymphocytes may be anti-AChR (Fujii et al 1986), other antibodies are synthesised by these cells in vitro (Newsom-Davis et al 1981, Lisak et al 1986b).

It has been reported that thymic cells provide specific help to blood cells of patients with myasthenia gravis, in increasing the in vitro synthesis of anti-AChR but not of other antibodies by the blood cells (Newsom-Davis et al 1981). The exact nature of this help or of the thymic cells involved is not known.

It has been suggested that the thymus may be the site of origin of the autoimmune response in myasthenia gravis (Lisak et al 1976, Werkele & Ketelsen 1977). The roles of accessory antigen-presenting cells and epithelial cells, and the possibility that AChR, perhaps in an altered form, might initiate some cases of myasthenia, requires further investigation. It has been postulated that a viral infection could trigger the autoimmune response (Datta & Schwartz 1974) but evidence for a viral trigger is lacking (Aoki et al 1985, Klavinskis et al 1985). However, it has recently been reported that monoclonal antibodies to AChR react with several Gram-negative bacteria, raising the possibility of stimulation of anti-AChR antibodies in susceptible subjects via molecular mimicry (Stephansson et al 1984).

Anti-idiotype control

There is interest in naturally occurring anti-idiotype antibodies to anti-AChR as possible immunoregulatory modulators in patients with myasthenia gravis and Dwyer et al (1983) have described activity that they feel is compatible with such a possibility; others have failed to detect such activity (Heininger et al 1983). However, if this were important in patients, one would have expected an inverse relation with titre and/or clinical disease. If anti-idiotypic antibodies were important in preventing MG in normals, one might also have expected such activity in serum from normal individuals.

There is also interest in the production of anti-idiotype antibodies as potential therapeutic agents in patients with MG. To date, such antibodies raised to anti-AChR of one individual have not shown extensive cross-reactivity in other patients (Lefvert 1981, Lang et al 1985), a finding not limited to anti-AChR (Kahn 1985). Thus, if such reagents were used, they would have to be produced for individual patients. In addition, anti-idiotype antibodies have not been unequivocally useful in modifying clinical manifestations of disease in animals with EAMG (Fuchs et al 1981, Agius et al 1985), especially once the disease is clinically manifest.

Heterogeneity of myasthenia gravis

Most patients with acquired myasthenia gravis can be shown to have antibodies to AChR, as determined by assays that measure total binding to AChR and/or certain biological effects of such antibodies, such as modulation of AChR, complement-mediated lysis or ligand blocking (Howard et al, in press). It has been suggested that, in others, the autoimmune response is directed at another as yet uncharacterised postsynaptic neuromuscular component (Newsom-Davis et al 1987). One can also find a heterogeneity among patients with myasthenia with serum anti-AChR antibodies. Such heterogeneity may represent different defects in immunological control and different aetiologies leading to similar or identical anti-AChR antibodies with a final common step of neuromuscular block. Such heterogeneity may be represented by differences in age of onset, HLA associations, thymic pathology (hyperplasia vs thymoma vs atrophy) and response to thymectomy (Lisak et al 1985a, Newsom-Davis et al 1987). These factors may not be totally independent variables (Compston et al 1980). In addition, the development of myasthenia gravis as a result of therapy with penicillamine and after bone marrow transplantation in the absence of graft versus host disease (Smith et al 1983, 1987, Cain et al 1986) may represent two other mechanisms allowing for the emergence of the pathogenic anti-AChR antibodies.

LAMBERT–EATON MYASTHENIC SYNDROME

The Eaton–Lambert (or Lambert–Eaton) myasthenic syndrome, a neuromuscular disease in which the muscular symptoms are due to a presynaptic deficit in the release of ACh, now seems to be established as an immunopathologically determined disorder (Newsom-Davis 1985). The syndrome is associated with carcinoma, almost always small (oat)-cell carcinoma of the lung, in approximately 50% of cases. In idiopathic cases there is an increased incidence of other putative immunopathological diseases and of elevated serum titres of several autoantibodies directed at antigens not present in muscle or nerve (Lennon et al 1982). The presynaptic membrane has reduced active zones (Fukunaga et al 1983). It has been shown that serum IgG of patients with both idiopathic and oat-cell carcinoma-associated Lambert–Eaton myasthenic syndrome can passively transfer the characteristic electrophysiological and pathological deficit to immunosuppressed mice (Lang et al 1981, Fukunaga et al 1983, Kim 1985, Newsom-Davis 1985). Indirect supportive evidence for an autoimmune-immunopathological pathogenesis comes from the clinical observation that plasma exchange and immunosuppressive therapy (corticosteroids and cytotoxic agents) have a beneficial effect in many of these patients. The nature of the presynaptic autoantigen is not known but evidence from electrophysiological experiments suggests that it may be in some way related to calcium channels (Newsom-Davis 1985, Prior et al 1985).

The mechanisms responsible for this autoimmune disease are not clear. It has been suggested that the patients with the idiopathic disorder develop antibodies to a presynaptic antigen as part of a more generalised defect in immunoregulatory mechanisms, similar to the multiple autoantibodies frequently seen in patients with myasthenia gravis (Lennon et al 1982). Once the antigen has been identified we may indeed find that some patients with other immunopathologically determined disoders have an increased incidence of antibodies to the Lambert–Eaton antigen without necessarily having the clinical Lambert–Eaton syndrome.

The explanation for the association with oat-cell carcinoma is also uncertain. Patients with neoplasia frequently have abnormal immune function and it has recently been reported that patients with the Lambert–Eaton syndrome associated with oat-cell carcinoma, although not idiopathic cases, have depressed levels of T8 (suppressor/cytotoxic) cells in their blood (Robb et al 1985). Given the theoretical explanation for the emergence of autoimmunity in the idiopathic disorder, the lack of abnormalities in that group is rather surprising. As patients with many types of neoplasia have abnormal immune function we still need an explanation for the very high association with oat-cell carcinoma, which is not a very common tumour. Oat-cell tumours may be associated with other neurological and non-neurological disorders and have been reported to secrete various peptides. However, the increased association of oat-cell carcinoma with the Lambert–Eaton syndrome, and perhaps with other nervous system paraneoplastic syndromes, may lie in possible shared antigens between the nervous system and the Kulchitsky cell in the lung, which is thought to derive from neural crest (Tischler et al 1977, Newsom-Davis 1985). Indeed, patients with the Lambert–Eaton syndrome have prominent autonomic dysfunction, raising the possibility that the target antigen is not limited to the presynaptic region of peripheral motor neurones. Whether a patient develops a remote effect of an oat-cell tumour and, if so, which remote effect may be under immunogenetic control (Willcox et al 1985), is still not known.

ACQUIRED DEMYELINATING NEUROPATHIES

There are several disorders of the PNS which are thought to be immunopathologically-mediated. The evidence is best in the acute and chronic acquired demyelinating neuropathies, although some data suggest a role for the immune system in the pathogenesis of a small number of primarily axonal diseases.

Guillain–Barré syndrome

The Guillain–Barré syndrome (post-infectious, post-immunisation or idiopathic radiculopolyneuritis) is an acquired inflammatory segmental demyelinating disease which develops acutely or subacutely. In approximately two-thirds of patients a preceding associated event (trigger) can be identified. These include infections (often short-lived and banal, involving the respiratory or gastrointestinal tracts or exanthems), immunisations, surgery, or other diseases (lymphomas, systemic lupus erythematosus and acquired immune deficiency syndrome [AIDS] or AIDS-related complex). The relationship between these events and the Guillain–Barré syndrome is not clear and may be different for different triggering events. The disease is generally self-limiting with varying degrees of recovery (often excellent) with remyelination. The presence of inflammatory cells in the nerves and nerve roots which resemble those seen in certain immunopathological experimental and naturally occurring animal diseases, and the association with immunological preceding events in many patients, have naturally led to the view that immunological factors are important in the aetiology and pathogenesis of the Guillain–Barré syndrome (Asbury et al 1969, Steiner & Abramsky 1985).

Experimental and animal models

Experimental models. Experimental allergic neuritis (EAN) is the most widely accepted experimental model of the Guillain–Barré syndrome. It was originally produced by sensitisation of rodents with PNS tissue in adjuvant (Waksman & Adams 1955) and is characterised by perivascular infiltration by mononuclear inflammatory cells, stripping of myelin by monocyte-macrophages, and segmental demyelination (Waksman & Adams 1955, Asbury et al 1969, Steiner & Abramsky 1985); sensitisation with myelin produces the same disorder. More recently it has been possible to produce

EAN by sensitisation with a cathodic PNS myelin protein called P2 (Kadlubowski & Hughes 1979) although it is not clear that P2-induced EAN reproduces all the clinical, electrophysiological, pathological and immunological features of whole-myelin-induced EAN; nevertheless, in general there seems to be little difference in all but serum abnormalities (Rostami et al 1984). It has also been possible to induce a demyelinating, relatively acellular neuropathy by sensitisation of animals with galactocerebroside, a major glycolipid component of myelin (T Saida et al 1979).

The relative roles of cell-mediated and antibody-mediated immune reactions and the number of antigens that serve as the target for these immune reactions in EAN is not certain. Serum from animals with disease induced by whole nerve, myelin or galactocerebroside have high levels of circulating antibodies to galactocerebroside and presumably to other myelin antigens. These sera are capable of mediating complement-mediated demyelination and cytotoxic reactions to Schwann cells in vitro (Armati-Gulson et al 1983) and in vivo (T Saida et al 1978, K Saida et al 1979). It has been possible to transfer EAN, with both inflammation and some degree of demyelination, with lines of helper T-cells specific for reactivity with P2 (Linnington et al 1984, Rostami et al 1985). Whether such lines mediate the entire picture of EAN actively induced with myelin or even with P2 is not as yet known. Thus, in whole-myelin-induced EAN, both cell-mediated and several antibody-mediated reactions to more than one antigen may be involved in the immunopathogenesis of the disorder. When one studies patients with the Guillain–Barré syndrome, this complicated picture must be kept in mind.

Naturally occurring models of the Guillain–Barré syndrome. Several diseases of animals also have features in common with the Guillain–Barré syndrome. These include racoon hound paralysis (Cummings & Haas 1967), acute canine poly-neuropathy (Northington & Brown 1982), cauda equina syndrome of horses (Kadlubowski & Ingram 1981) and Marek's disease of chickens (Stevens et al 1981; see also Ch. 28). Little is known about the immunopathogenesis or aetiology of these disorders. Serum from animals with

acute canine polyneuropathy causes demyelination in vivo after endoneurial injection into rat sciatic nerve, although it is not known if this is mediated by antibodies (Brown et al 1985). The aetiological agent of Marek's disease is a herpes virus and affected chickens go on to develop lymphomas. Serum from these birds contains antibodies to myelin but it is not known if this is a cause or effect of the inflammatory polyneuropathy (Stevens et al 1981). Horses with the cauda equina syndrome have serum antibodies to P2 (Kadlubowski & Ingram 1981), but rats with P2-induced EAN have similar antibodies that seem not to be primarily pathogenic.

Immunopathogenic mechanisms in the Guillain–Barré syndrome. Although there has been a report of elevated serum IgE levels in patients with the Guillain–Barré syndrome, there are no studies showing that this IgE binds to PNS myelin. In addition, the pathology of the Guillain–Barré syndrome does not resemble a reaginic reaction although normal peripheral nerve does contain mast cells.

Much immunological investigation in the Guillain–Barré syndrome has centred on the possibility that antibodies to one or more components of PNS myelin/Schwann cells cause the disease. The evidence that such antibodies exist and are specific to patients with the Guillain–Barré syndrome (or the possibly related chronic or relapsing acquired demyelinating polyneuritis) is very controversial (Cook & Dowling 1981, Lisak et al 1983a, Steiner & Abramsky 1985). Although serum of patients with the Guillain–Barré syndrome has been reported to cause in vitro demyelination (Arnason 1971) and Schwann cell cytotoxicity (Lisak et al 1984a) as well as in vivo demyelination and cellular infiltration (Saida et al 1982, Sumner et al 1982, Feasby et al 1983), it is not clear that this effect is mediated by antibodies (immunoglobulins). In addition, there is little evidence that serum from these patients contains disease-specific antibodies to the three known autoantigens of PNS, P1, P2 and galactocerebroside or to myelin-associated glycoprotein (MAG). Even if antibodies to a myelin component were to be demonstrated, such an antibody might represent either an epiphenomenon (resulting from release of that substance from a nerve injured via another mechanism) or might represent evidence of a heightened immune response to that antigen but one in which another component of the response (cell-mediated immunity) is the primary or only effector mechanism. In addition, non-Ig acute phase reactants in the serum could contribute to demyelination initiated by other mechanisms (Tonnessen et al 1982).

Several groups have reported the presence of circulating immune complexes in the serum of patients with the Guillain–Barré syndrome (Tachovsky et al 1976, Goust et al 1978, Cook & Dowling 1981). Such complexes may be deposited in the glomeruli and be responsible for the proteinuria and rare instances of clinical glomerulonephritis and nephrotic syndrome seen in association with the Guillain–Barré syndrome. (Some have suggested that the Ig deposits represent shared antigens between the nerve and glomerular basement membrane.) There is, however, no evidence that the peripheral nerve is the site of deposition of such immune complexes. Although there are reports of IgG, IgM and complement components in nerves of patients with the Guillain–Barré syndrome, these are not clearly specific and could well represent antibodies to components of the PNS. There is no evidence of vasculitis in the PNS. It is conceivable that if the blood–nerve barrier was made more permeable by another immune process, complexes could then breach the barrier and contribute to the pathological process. Alternatively, it is conceivable that the complexes are responsible for opening the barrier, thus allowing other immune mechanisms to exert their effector role (Reik 1980). It is not clear whether immune complex deposition is involved in the pathogenesis of the Guillain–Barré syndrome (or chronic demyelinating polyneuritis) in patients with systemic lupus erythematosus. As the Guillain–Barré syndrome frequently occurs after other immunological stimuli, the complexes may simply represent part of that immune reaction. It is not known, e.g. whether the antigen in the complexes consists of antigens of the virus that was the triggering event. The persistence of such immune complexes for a longer period than is usually seen with viral infections may represent defects in immunoregulation seen in some patients with the Guillain–Barré syndrome.

On the basis of the similarity in appearance between lesions of EAN and of the Guillain–Barré syndrome, and the clear-cut importance of cell-mediated immunity in EAN, many investigators feel that the Guillain–Barré syndrome is primarily the result of a T-cell mediated immunopathological mechanism directed against some component of myelin and/or Schwann cells (Arnason 1971, Steiner & Abramsky 1985). Even the presence in the blood of antigen-specific T-cells of the helper and/or cytotoxic phenotype would not prove a direct causal relationship; specific demonstration of antigen-specific cells in an increased frequency in nerve and/or blood would be highly supportive, however. Macrophages are prominent in many EAN and Guillain–Barré lesions. Macrophages are important cells in immune phagocytosis because of the presence on their surface of receptors for the Fc portion of IgG and for certain components of complement. Thus, these cells could represent: (a) mediators of an ADCC reaction; (b) cells present in response to the release of lymphokines by antigen-specific T-cells (cell-mediated reaction); and/or, (c) cells phagocytosing myelin injured by other mechanisms.

Immunoregulation. As noted earlier, the development of a disease due to immunopathological mechanisms suggests a failure of normal regulation of the immune response. There have been few systematic studies examining immune regulatory function in patients with the Guillain–Barré syndrome. There have been reports of a decrease in the number and function of suppressor T-cells in some patients as well as a decrease in the numbers of helper T-cells in others (Hughes et al 1983, Lisak et al 1985b). A typical Guillain–Barré syndrome has been reported in patients with immune deficiency in association with transplantation (Drachman et al 1970), Hodgkin's disease (Lisak et al 1977) and with AIDS and the AIDS-related complex (Levy et al 1985, Cornblath et al 1987). It is possible that different defects in immune regulation and loss of tolerance may lead to the same immunopathological mechanism and clinical syndrome. Alternatively, different abnormalities could lead to a different pathogenic mechanism, such as autoimmunity, or perhaps direct involvement of the PNS by a virus (Pepose 1982), in different patients.

Chronic inflammatory demyelinating polyneuropapthy (CIDP)

Patients develop an acquired demyelinating neuropathy in either a chronic progressive pattern, a relapsing pattern, or a relapsing pattern superimposed on a chronic progressive pattern. In addition, a small number of patients with the Guillain–Barré syndrome experience one or, less commonly, more than one recurrence. As noted in Chapter 24, there are striking similarities, in acquired demyelinating neuropathies, to the pathological and physical findings seen in patients with the Guillain–Barré syndrome. There is considerable indirect evidence to support the view that these more chronic and recurrent demyelinating neuropathies result from an imunopathological reaction to PNS myelin and/or Schwann cells.

Much of the evidence for an immunopathogenic cause of the chronic demyelinating neuropathies is based on analogies to the Guillain–Barré syndrome and to acute and chronic forms of EAN (Wisniewski et al 1974, Pollard et al 1975). In addition, there are studies of serum of patients with CIDP suggesting that these patients have antibodies to myelin and/or Schwann cells which could serve in them as the effector mechanism (Nyland & Aarli 1978, Latov et al 1981). Unfortunately, as in the Guillain–Barré syndrome, the evidence is controversial as far as specificity is concerned. Moreover, evidence for an in vitro or systemic or local passive transfer in vivo demyelinating effect is not as strong as in the Guillain–Barré syndrome. With the exception of a sub-group of patients with a monoclonal gammopathy (see below), no clear-cut target antigen has as yet been identified.

There is little known about the possible role of immune complexes in the pathogenesis of CIDP (Dalakas & Engel 1980). The presence of inflammatory cells, including lymphocytes and monocyte-macrophages, in the nerves of patients with CIDP has also raised the possibility that cell-mediated immune processes, such as T-cell-specific delayed-type hypersensitivity or cytotoxicity or an ADCC reaction, are important in the pathogenesis of CIDP. Again, the evidence is indirect and controversial and a probable target antigen has not been clearly identified (Steiner & Abramsky 1985).

There are no systematic studies of immune regulation in CIDP. The occurrence of this syndrome in patients with other disorders associated with abnormalities of immunoregulatory mechanisms such as collagen-vascular diseases (Rechthand et al 1984, Steiner & Abramsky 1985), AIDS and the AIDS-related complex (Snider et al 1983, Cornblath et al 1987) — although other patterns of neuropathy are seen with HLTV III infection (Lipkin et al 1985) — lends credence to the hypothesis that, as in other putative and proven immunopathological disorders, abnormal immunoregulation is involved in the aetiology and pathogenesis of CIDP.

Chronic demyelinating neuropathy associated with paraproteinaemia

Patients with malignant disorders of B-cell lineage associated with monoclonal gammopathy such as multiple myeloma and Waldenstrom's macroglobulinaemia not infrequently develop associated peripheral neuropathies, usually axonal. A syndrome which includes a demyelinating neuropathy in association with osteoblastic myeloma or plasmacytoma has been reported. There is some evidence (not very strong) that myeloma-associated neuropathy may be immunologically mediated (Besinger et al 1981).

A syndrome of chronic progressive demyelinating sensorimotor neuropathy, associated with an IgM (usually kappa light chain) serum paraproteinaemia without evidence of malignancy, also occurs. Several groups have demonstrated that the IgM is an antibody to the myelin-associated glycoprotein, a minor component of both the peripheral and central nervous systems (Braun et al 1982, Steck et al 1983, Steck & Murray 1985). Peripheral nerve biopsies have shown a demyelinating neuropathy with widening of the myelin lamellae but, in all but one case, no inflammation such as is seen in the Guillain–Barré syndrome and CIDP. In situ binding of the IgM paraprotein is demonstrable in biopsy specimens. Recent studies have demonstrated that the IgM binds to a carbohydrate determinant that is part of both myelin-associated glycoprotein and of glycolipids of the peripheral nervous system (Ilyas et al 1984, Quarles 1984). The carbohydrate determinant is also found on the surface of a subpopulation of lymphocytes which have NK function. It has been suggested, but not agreed upon by all investigators, that suppression of NK-cell activity by this autoantibody might be important in the development of this autoimmune neuropathy (Steck & Murray 1985).

Glycolipids have also been identified as antigens for non-MAG-binding IgM paraproteins in some patients with neuropathy (Ilyas et al 1985) and chondroitin sulphate C in patients with axonal neuropathy and epidermolysis (Sherman et al 1983).

MOTOR NEURONE DISEASE (MND) (AMYOTROPHIC LATERAL SCLEROSIS (ALS))

Although motor neurone disease is not generally considered to be a neuromuscular disease likely to have an immunopathological pathogenesis, there has been recent interest in possible involvement of the immune system in this neuromuscular disorder (Cashman et al 1985).

There are several animal models of this disease and several involve viruses which show a relative specificity for anterior horn cells. When this is considered in relation to those human viruses that seem to have relatively high specificity for anterior horn cells (e.g. poliomyelitis), it is not unreasonable to speculate that some cases of MND might be related to viral infection. This would then raise the possibility that loss of anterior horn cells might arise either from direct effects of such a virus on the cell, with or without a resultant inflammatory response, or by immune reaction to the virus or a viral-induced neoantigen. In this scenario, the cell would be an 'innocent bystander'. The strongest argument against this latter possibility is the paucity of reports of inflammation in the spinal cord of patients with MND, even in autopsies performed on cases with rapid progression. There have been no confirmed isolations of virus or proof of a specific viral genome obtained from the nervous system of such patients. Moreover, attempts to demonstrate either decreased or increased in vitro responses to antigens specific for putative aetiological viruses have not yielded consistent results.

A second area of recent study is the question of a possible role of the deposition of immune complexes in pathogenesis. Some (Oldstone et al 1976), but not all groups (Tachovsky 1976, Bartfeld et al 1982, Cashman et al 1985) of investigators have reported an increased incidence of elevated concentrations of immune complexes in the serum of patients with MND, as well as the presence of Ig in a 'lumpy-bumpy' pattern in the renal glomeruli of some patients. However, the few studies of the CNS do not reveal Ig in the CNS except in astrocytes (by immunofluorescence) and this pattern is neither suggestive of immune complex deposition nor is it specific for MND.

For several years there has been interest in a factor in the serum of patients with MND which is toxic to neurones in vitro (Wolfgram & Myers 1973, Roisen et al 1982). Some investigators have not been able to confirm the presence of such a factor (Liveson et al 1975, Lerich & Couture 1978). As the factor has not been characterised, it is impossible to know whether it would also be toxic to other neural and non-neural cell types. It should be remembered that serum from patients with ALS causes in vitro demyelination of CNS organotypic cultures (Bornstein & Appel 1965). It should be pointed out that there is no proof that such toxic circulating factors are immunoglobulins.

There have been several reports of serum monoclonal gammopathy in patients with MND, with the hypothesis that these may represent autoantibodies similar to those described in certain patients with acquired chronic demyelinating neuropathies (Latov 1982, Patten 1984). While such cases occur and, in some instances, the monoclonal Ig may well represent more than the chance occurrence of classic MND and a benign monoclonal gammopathy, to date these cases would seem to be exceptional. It is, of course, possible that other MND patients have potentially pathogenic antibodies not present in sufficient quantity to be detected as a monoclonal spike on electrophoresis.

The most recent interest in a possible immunopathological mechanism in MND has centred on antibodies to a factor produced by muscle that supports terminal neuronal sprouting (Guerney et al 1984). There are problems in accepting this antibody as being important in the pathogenesis of MND. These include: (a) the lack of these antibodies in most MND serum; (b) the nature of the control patients; (c) the lack, as yet, of confirmation by other investigators; (d) how an antibody that inhibits sprouting, a reparative mechanism, rather than being toxic to neurones could be the primary pathological factor in MND. Of some interest, therefore, is the report that an experimental monoclonal antibody to this protein inhibits chicken neurone survival in vitro (Apatoff et al 1984).

There have been few studies of possible defects in immunoregulatory mechanisms in patients with MND. In those published studies there is no hard evidence of a defect in immune regulation in MND patients (Bartfeld et al 1982, Cashman et al 1985).

REFERENCES

Abramsky O, Aharonov A, Webb C, Fuchs S 1975 Cellular immune response to acetylcholine receptor-rich fraction in patients with myasthenia gravis. Clinical and Experimental Immunology 9: 11–16

Acuto O, Reinherz E L 1985 The human T-cell receptor. New England Journal of Medicine 297: 1207–1211

Adams D, Gibson J D, Thomas P K, Batchelor J R, Hughes R A C, Kennedy L, Festenstein H, Sachs J 1977 HLA antigens in Guillain-Barré syndrome. Lancet 2: 504–505

Adams D, Festenstein H, Gibson J P, Hughes R A C, Jaraquemada J, Papasteriadis C, Sachs J, Thomas P K 1979 HLA antigens in chronic relapsing idiopathic inflammatory polyneuropathy. Journal of Neurology, Neurosurgery and Psychiatry 42: 184–186

Agius M A, Geannopoulos C G, Richman D P 1985 Anti-idiotypic modification of the immune response in experimental autoimmune myasthenia gravis. Society for Neuroscience 11:139

Almon R R, Andrew C G, Appel S H 1974 Serum globulin in myasthenia gravis: inhibition of α-bungarotoxin binding to acetylcholine receptors. Science 186: 55–57

Alper C A 1981 Complement and the M H C. In: Dorf M E (ed) The role of the major histocompatibility complex in immunobiology. Garland Press, New York, p 173–122

Anderson B P, Young V, Kean W F, Ludwin S K, Galbraith P R, Anastassiades T P 1982 Polymyositis in chronic graft-versus-host disease. Archives of Neurology 39: 188–190

Aoki T, Drachman D M, Asher D M, Gibbs C J Jr, Bahmanyar S, Wolinsky J 1985 Attempts to implicate viruses in myasthenia gravis. Neurology 35: 185–192

Apatoff B, Antel J P, Gurney M 1984 Autoantibodies in amyotrophic lateral sclerosis. Annals of Neurology 16:109

Appel S H, Anivyl R, McAdams M W, Elias S B 1977 Accelerated degradation of acetylcholine receptor of cultured rat myotubes with myasthenia gravis sera and globulins. Proceedings of the National Academy of Sciences USA 74: 2130–2134

Arahata K, Engel A G 1984 Monoclonal antibody analysis of mononuclear cells in myopathies. I. Quantitation of subsets according to diagnosis and sites of accumulation and demonstrations and counts of muscle fibers invaded by T-cells. Annals of Neurology 16: 198–203

Arahata K, Engel A G 1986 Monoclonal antibody analysis of mononuclear cells in myopathies. III. Immunoelectron microscopic aspects of cell-mediated muscle fiber injury. Annals of Neurology 19: 112–125

Armati-Gulson P, Lisak R P, Kuchmy D, Pollard J 1983 ^{51}Cr release cytoxicity radioimmunoassay to detect immune cytotoxic reactions to rat Schwann cells in vitro. Neuroscience Letters 35: 321–326

Arnason B G W 1971 Idiopathic polyneuritis (Landry-Guillain-Barré-Stohl syndrome) and experimental allergic neuritis: A comparison. Research Publications of the Association for Research in Nervous and Mental Disorders. 49: 156–175

Arnett F C, Hirsch T J, Bias W B, Nishikai M, Reichlin M 1981 The Jo-1 antibody system in myositis: relationships to clinical features and HLA. Journal of Rheumatology 8: 925–930

Asbury A K, Arnason B G W, Adams R D 1969 The inflammatory lesion in idiopathic polyneuritis. Its role in pathogenesis. Medicine 48: 173–215

Ashizawa T, Appel S H 1985 Immunopathologic events at the endplate in myasthenia gravis. In: Steck A J, Lisak R P (guest eds) Immunoneurology (II) Springer Seminars in Immunopathology 8: 177–196

Bahir S, Gaud C, Bach M-A, LeBrigand H, Binet J P, Bach J F 1981 Evaluation of T-cell subsets in myasthenia gravis using anti-T-cell monoclonal antibodies. Clinical and Experimental Immunology 45:1–8

Banker B Q 1975 Dermatomyositis in childhood: Ultrastructural alterations in muscle and intramuscular blood vessels. Journal of Neuropathology and Experimental Neurology 34: 46–75

Bartfeld H, Dham C, Donnenfeld H, Jashnani L, Carp R, Kascsak R, Vilcek J, Rapport M, Wallenstein S 1982 Immunological profile of amyotrophic lateral sclerosis patients and their cell-mediated responses to viral and CNS antigens. Clinical and Experimental Immunology 48: 137–147

Behan P O, Shields J 1982 Genetics. In: Lisak R P, Barchi R L Myasthenia gravis. W B Saunders, Philadelphia, p 37–50

Behan W M H, Behan P O, Simpson J A 1975 Absence of cellular hypersensitivity to muscle and thymic antigens in myasthenia gravis. Journal of Neurology, Neurosurgery and Psychiatry 38: 1039–1047

Behan W M H, Barkas T, Behan P O 1982 Detection of immune complexes in polymyositis. Acta Neurologica Scandinavia 65: 320–334

Behan W M H, Behan P O, Micklem H S, Durward W F 1983 Lymphocyte subset abnormalities in polymyositis. British Medical Journal 287: 181–182

Behan W M H, Behan P O 1985 Immunological features of polymyositis/dermatomyositis. In: Steck A J, Lisak R P (guest eds) Immunoneurology (II). Springer Seminars in Immunopathology 8: 267–294

Besinger U A, Toyka K V, Anzel A P, Neumeier D, Rauscher R, Heininger K 1981 Myeloma neuropathy: Passive transfer from man to mouse. Science 213: 1027–1030

Bona C A, Pernis B 1984 Idiotypic networks. In: Paul W E (ed) Fundamental immunology. Raven Press, New York, p 577–594

Bornstein M B, Appel S H 1965 Tissue culture studies of demyelination. Annals of the New York Academy of Sciences 122: 280–286

Braun P E, Frail D E, Latov N 1982 Myelin-associated glycoprotein is the antigen for a monoclonal IgM in polyneuropathy. Journal of Neurochemistry 39: 1261–1265

Brown M J, Northington J W, Rosen J L, Lisak R P 1985 Acute canine idiopathic polyneuropathy (ACIP) serum demyelinates peripheral nerve in vivo. Journal of Neuroimmunology 7: 239–248

Burnet F M 1959 The clonal selection theory of acquired immunity. Cambridge University Press, New York

Burns J B, Rosenzweig A, Zweiman B, Lisak R P 1983 Isolation of myelin basic protein-reactive T-cell lines from normal human blood. Cellular Immunology 81: 435–440

Bursztajn S, McMassaman J L, Elias S B, Appel S H 1983 Myasthenia globulin enhances the loss of acetylcholine receptor cultures. Science 219: 195–196

Cain G R, Cardinet G H, Cuddon P A, Gale R P, Champlin R 1986 Myasthenia gravis and polymyositis in a dog following fetal hematopoetic cell transplantation. Transplantation 41: 21–25

Cantor H 1984 T lymphocytes. In: Paul W E (ed) Fundamental immunology. Raven Press, New York, p 57–69

Cashman N R, Gurney M E, Antel J P 1985 Immunology of amyotrophic lateral sclerosis. In: Steck A J, Lisak R P (guest eds) Immunoneurology (I). Springer Seminars in Immunopathology 8: 141–152

Christados P, Lennon V A, Kroc C J, Lambert E H, David C S 1981 Genetic control of autoimmunity to acetylcholine receptors: Role of the Ia molecules. Annals of the New York Academy of Sciences 377: 258–277

Christiansen F T, Pollack M S, Garlepp M J, Dawkins R L 1984 Myasthenia gravis and H L A antigens in American blacks and other races. Journal of Neuroimmunology 7: 121–129

Cleveland W L, Wasserman N H, Sarangarajan R, Penn A S, Erlanger B F 1983 Monoclonal antibodies to the acetylcholine receptor by a normally functioning auto-anti-idiotypic mechanism. Nature 305: 56–57

Cohen J A, Lisak R P 1987 Acute disseminated encephalomyelitis. In: Behan P O, Aarli J (eds) Neuroimmunology for clinicians (in press)

Cohen M, Epstein R 1978 T-cell inhibition of humoral responsiveness. II. Theory on the role of restrictive recognition in immune regulation. Cellular Immunology 39: 125–153

Compston D A S, Vincent A, Newsom-Davis J, Batchelor J R 1980 Clinical, pathological, HLA antigen and immunological evidence for disease heterogeneity in myasthenia gravis. Brain 103: 579–601

Conti-Tronconi B M, Gotti C M, Hunkapeller M W, Rafferty M A 1982 Mammalian muscle acetylcholine receptor: a supramolecular structure formed by four related proteins. Science 218: 1227–1229

Cook S D, Dowling P C 1981 The role of autoantibody and immune complexes in the pathogenesis of Guillain–Barré syndrome. Annals of Neurology 9 (Supplement): 70–79

Coombs R R A, Gell P G H 1968 Classification of allergic reactions responsible for clinical hypersensitivity and disease. In: Gell P G H, Coombs R R A (eds) Clinical aspects of immunity. F A Davis, Philadelphia, p 575–596

Cornblath D R, McArthur J C, Kennedy P G E, White A S, Griffin J W 1987 Inflammatory demyelinating peripheral neuropathies associated with human T-cell lymphotropic virus type III infection. Annals of Neurology 21: 32–40

Cowing C 1985 Does T-cell restriction to Ia limit the need for self-tolerance? Immunology Today 6: 72–74

Cummings J F, Haas D C 1967 Coonhound paralysis — an acute idiopathic polyneuritia in dogs resembling Landry-Guillain-Barré syndrome. Journal of the Neurological Sciences 4: 51–81

Currie S, Saunders M, Knowles M, Brown A E 1971 Immunologic aspects of polymyositis. The in vitro activity of lymphocytes on incubation with muscle antigen and with mouse cultures. Quarterly Journal of Medicine 60: 63–84

Dalakas M C, Engel W K 1980 Immunoglobulin and complement deposits in nerves of patients with chronic relapsing polyneuropathy. Archives of Neurology 37: 637–640

Dalakas M C, London W T, Gravell M, Sever J L 1986 Polymyositis in an immunodeficiency disease in monkeys induced by type D retrovirus. Neurology 36: 569–572

Data S K, Schwartz R S 1974 Infectious (?) myasthenia. New England Journal of Medicine 291: 1304–1305

Dawkins R L 1975 Experimental autoallergic polymyositis, polymyositis and myasthenia gravis. Clinical and Experimental Immunology 21: 185–201

Dawkins R L, Mastaglia F L 1973 Cell-mediated cytotoxicity to muscle in polymyositis. Effect of immunosuppression. New England Journal of Medicine 288: 434–438

Dore-Duffy P, Ho S-Y, Longo M 1985 The role of prostaglandins in altered leukocyte function in multiple sclerosis. In: Steck A J, Lisak R P (guest eds) Immunoneurology (II). Springer Seminars in Immunopathology 8: 305–319

Drachman D A, Paterson P Y, Berlin B S, Roguska J 1970 Immunosuppression and the Guillain-Barré syndrome. Archives of Neurology 23: 385–393

Drachman D B, Angus C W, Adams R N, Michelson J D, Hoffman G J 1978 Myasthenic antibodies cross-link acetylcholine receptors to accelerate degradation. New England Journal of Medicine 298: 1116–1121

Dwyer D S, Bradley R J, Urquhart C K, Kearney J F 1983 Naturally occurring anti-idiotypic antibodies in myasthenia gravis patients. Nature 301: 611–614

Engel A G 1984 Myasthenia gravis and myasthenic syndromes. Annals of Neurology 16: 519–534

Engel A G, Lambert E H, Howard F M 1977 Immune complexes (IgG and C3) at the motor end-plate in myasthenia gravis: Ultrastructural and light microscopic localization and electrophysiologic correlations. Mayo Clinic Proceedings 52: 267–280

Engel A G, Biesicker G 1982 Complement activation in muscle fiber necrosis: Demonstration of the membrane attack complex of complement in necrotic fibers. Annals of Neurology 12: 289–296

Engel A G, Arahata K 1984 Monoclonal antibody analysis of

mononuclear cells in myopathies. II. Phenotypes of autoinvasive cells in polymyositis and inclusion body myositis. Annals of Neurology 16: 209–215

Fauci A S 1982 Human B lymphocyte function: cell triggering and immunoregulation. Journal of Infectious Diseases 145: 602–642

Feasby T E, Hahn A F, Gilbert J J 1983 Passive transfer of demyelinating activity in Guillain-Barré polyneuropathy. Neurology 32: 1159–1167

Feldmann M, Zanders E D, Lamb J R 1985 Tolerance in T-cell clones. Immunology Today 6: 58–62

Fuchs S, Bartfeld D, Mochly-Rosen D, Souroujon M, Feingold R 1981 Acetylcholine receptor: molecular dissection and monoclonal antibodies in the study of myasthenia. Annals of the New York Academy of Sciences 377: 110–122

Fujii Y, Manden Y, Nakahara K, Hashimoto J, Kawashima Y 1984 Antibody to acetylcholine receptor in myasthenia gravis: Production by lymphocytes from thymus or thymoma. Neurology 34: 1182–1186

Fujii Y, Hashimoto J, Monden Y, Ito T, Nakahara K, Kawashima Y 1986 Specific activation of lymphocytes against acetylcholine receptor in the thymus in myasthenia gravis. Journal of Immunology 136: 887–891

Fujinami R S, Oldstone M B A 1985 Virus-induced autoimmunity through molecular mimicry. Federation Proceedings 44:1291

Fukunaga H, Engel A G, Osame M, Lambert E H 1982 Paucity and disorganization of presynaptic membrane active zones in the Lambert-Eaton myasthenic syndrome. Muscle and Nerve 5: 686–697

Fukunaga H, Engel A G, Lang B, Newsom-Davis J, Vincent A 1983 Passive transfer of Lambert-Eaton myasthenic syndrome with IgG from man to mouse depletes the presynaptic membrane active zones. Proceedings of the National Academy of Sciences USA 80: 7636–7640

Gilhus N E, Aarli J A, Matre R 1984 Myasthenia gravis: difference between thymoma-associated antibodies and cross-striational skeletal muscle antibodies. Neurology 34: 246–249

Gomez C, Richman D P 1983 Anti-acetylcholine receptor antibodies directed against α-bungarotoxin binding site induce a unique form of experimental myasthenia. Proceedings of the National Academy of Sciences USA 80: 4089–4093

Goust J-M, Chenais F, Carnes J E, Hames C G, Fudenberg H H, Hogan E L 1978 Abnormal T-cell subpopulations and circulating immune complexes in the Guillain-Barré syndrome and multiple sclerosis. Neurology 28: 421–425

Guerney M E, Belton A C, Cashman N, Antel J P 1984 Inhibition of terminal axonal sprouting by serum from patients with amyotrophic lateral sclerosis. New England Journal of Medicine 311: 933–939

Haas D C 1980 Absence of cell-mediated cytotoxicity to muscle cultures in polymyositis. Journal of Rheumatology 7: 671–676

Haas D C, Arnason B G W 1974 Cell-mediated immunity in polymyositis: creatinine phosphokinase release from muscle cultures. Archives of Neurology 31: 192–196

Hargis A M, Haupt K S, Prieur D J, Moore M P 1985 Animal model of human disease. Dermatomyositis: familial canine dermatomyositis. American Journal of Pathology 120: 323–325

Hathaway P W M, Engel W K, Zellweger H 1970 Experimental myopathy after microarterial embolization. Comparison with childhood X-linked pseudohypertrophic muscular dystrophy. Archives of Neurology 22: 365–378

Haynes B F, Harden E A, Olanow C W. Eisenborth G S, Wechsler A S, Hensley L L, Roses A D 1983 Effect of thymectomy on peripheral lymphocyte subsets in myasthenia gravis: Selective effect on T-cells in patients with thymic atrophy. Journal of Immunology 131: 773–777

Heberman R E (ed) 1982 N K cells and other natural effector cells. Academic Press, New York

Heffner R R, Barron S A, Jenis F H, Valeski J C 1976 Skeletal muscle in polymyositis. Immunohistochemical study. Archives of Pathology and Laboratory Medicine 103:310

Heininger K, Hendricks M, Toyka K V, Kalb H 1983 Myasthenia gravis remission not induced by blocking anti-idiotype antibodies. Muscle and Nerve 6: 386–387

Hohlfeld R, Toyka K V, Heininger K, Grosse-Wilde H, Kalis I 1984 Autoimmune human T lymphocytes specific for acetylcholine receptor. Nature 310: 244–246

Howard F, Lennon V, Matsumato J, Finley J 1986 Clinical correlations of antibodies that bind, block and/or modulate human AChRs in myasthenia gravis. Annals of the New York Academy of Sciences (in press)

Howard M, Paul W E 1983 Regulation of B-cell growth and differentiation by soluble factors. Annual Review of Immunology 1: 307–333

Hughes R A C, Aslan S, Gray I A 1983 Lymphocyte subpopulations and suppressor cell activity in acute polyradiculoneuritis (Guillain-Barré syndrome). Clinical and Experimental Immunology 51: 448–454

Hurley C K, Giles R C, Capra J D 1983 The human MHC: evidence for multiple HLA-D-region genes. Immunology Today 4: 219–226

Ilyas A A, Quarles R H, MacIntosh T D, Dobersen M J, Trapp B D, Dalakas M C, Brady R O 1984 IgM in a human neuropathy related to paraproteinemia binds to a carbohydrate determinant in the myelin-associated glycoprotein and to a ganglioside. Proceedings of the National Academy of Sciences USA 81: 1225–1229

Ilyas A A, Quarles R H, Dalakas M C, Brady R O 1985 Polyneuropathy with monoclonal gammopathy: Glycolipids are frequently antigens for IgM paraproteins. Proceedings of the National Academy of Sciences USA 82: 6697–6700

Isenberg D A 1983 Immunoglobulin deposition in skeletal muscle disease. Quarterly Journal of Medicine 52: 297–310

Iyer V, Lawton A R, Finichel G M 1983 T-cell subsets in polymyositis. Annals of Neurology 13: 452–453

Jerne N K 1974 Towards a network theory of the immune system. Annals of the Immunologic Institute Pasteur (Paris) 125: 373–389

Johnson R L, Fink C W, Ziff M 1972 Lymphotoxin formation by lymphocytes and muscle in polymyositis. Journal of Clinical Investigation 51: 2435–2449

Kadlubowski M, Hughes R A C 1979 Identification of the neuritogen for experimental allergic neuritis. Nature 277: 140–141

Kadlubowski M, Ingram P L 1981 Circulating antibodies to the neuritogenic myelin protein P_2 in neuritis of the cauda equina of the horse. Nature 293: 299–306

Kahn S 1985 Human monoclonal IgM autoantibodies with restricted antigenic specificity for myelin express unrelated idiotypes. Journal of the Neurological Sciences 69: 161–170

Kao I, Drachman D B 1977 Myasthenic immunoglobulin accelerates acetylcholine receptor degradation. Science 196: 527–529

Kaslow R A, Sullivan-Bolgai J Z, Hafken B et al 1984 HLA antigens in Guillain-Barré syndrome. Neurology 94: 240–242

Kim G I 1985 Passive transfer of the Lambert-Eaton myasthenic syndrome: neuromuscular transmission in mice injected with plasma. Muscle and Nerve 8: 162–172

Kissel J T, Mendell J R, Rammohan K W 1986 Microvascular deposition of complement membrane attack complex in dermatomyositis. New England Journal of Medicine 314: 329–332

Klavinskis L S, Willcox N, Oxford J S, Newsom-Davis J 1985 Antivirus antibodies in myasthenia gravis. Neurology 35: 1381–1384

Kornegay J N, Gorgacz E J, Dawe D L, Bowen J M, White N A, DeBuysscher E V 1980 Polymyositis in dogs. Journal of the American Veterinary Medical Association 176: 431–438

Kornstein M J, Brooks J J, Anderson A O, Levinson A I, Lisak R P, Zweiman B 1984 The immunohistology of the thymus in myasthenia gravis. American Journal of Pathology 117: 184–194

Lang B, Newsom-Davis J, Wray D, Vincent A, Murray N 1981 Autoimmune aetiology for myasthenic (Eaton-Lambert) syndrome. Lancet ii: 224–226

Lang B, Roberts A J, Vincent A, Newsom-Davis J 1985 Anti-acetylcholine receptor idiotypes in myasthenia gravis analyzed by rabbit antisera. Clinical and Experimental Immunology 60: 637–644

Latov N 1982 Plasma cell dyscrasias and motor neuron disease. In: Rowland L P (ed) Human motor neuron diseases. Raven Press, New York, p 273–279

Latov N, Gross R B, Kostelon J et al 1981 Complement-fixing anti-peripheral nerve myelin antibodies in patients with inflammatory polyneuritis and with polyneuropathy and paraproteinemia. Neurology 31: 1530–1534

Layzer R B, Shearn M A, Satya-Murti S 1977 Eosinophilic polymyositis. Annals of Neurology 1: 65–78

Leder P 1983 Genetics of immunoglobulin production. In: Dixon F J, Fisher D W (eds) The Biology of immunologic disease. Sinauer Associates, p 3–12

Lefvert A K 1981 Anti-idiotypic antibodies against the receptor antibodies in myasthenia gravis. Scandinavian Journal of Immunology 13: 493–497

Lennon V A, Palmer A C, Pflugfelder C, Indrieri R J 1978 Myasthenia gravis in dogs: acetylcholine receptor deficiency with and without autoantibodies. In: Rose N L, Bigzaai P E, Warner N L (eds) Genetic control of autoimmune disease. Elsevier North Holland, Amsterdam, p 295–306

Lennon V A, Lambert E H, Whittingham S, Fairbanks V 1982 Autoimmunity in the Lambert-Eaton myasthenic syndrome. Muscle and Nerve 5: 521–525

Lennon V A, McCormick D J, Lambert E H, Guesmann G E 1985 Region of peptide of acetylcholine receptor α subunit is exposed at neuromuscular junction and induces experimental autoimmune myasthenia gravis, T-cell immunity and modulating autoantibodies. Proceedings of the National Academy of Sciences USA 82: 8805–8809

Lerich J R, Couture J 1978 Amyotrophic lateral sclerosis sera are not cytotoxic to neuroblastoma cells in tissue culture. Annals of Neurology 41: 384–385

Levinson A I, Dziarski A, Lisak R P, Zweiman B,

Moskovitz A R, Brenner T, Abramsky O 1981 Comparative immunoglobulin synthesis by blood lymphocytes in myasthenics and normals. Annals of the New York Academy of Sciences 377: 385–392

Levinson A I, Zweiman B, Lisak R P, Dziarski A I, Moskovitz A R 1984 Thymic lymphocyte activation in myasthenia gravis. Neurology 34: 462–468

Levinson A I, Lisak R P, Zweiman B, Kornstein M J 1985 Phenotypic and functional analysis of lymphocytes in myasthenia gravis. In: Steck A J, Lisak R P (guest eds) Immunoneurology (II). Springer Seminars in Neuropathology 8: 209–234

Levy R M, Bredsen D E, Rosenblum M L 1985 Neurological manifestations of the acquired immunodeficiency syndrome (AIDS): Experience at UCSF and review of the literature. Journal of Neurosurgery 62: 475–495

Linnington C, Izumo S, Suzuki M, Uyemura K, Meyermann R, Wekerle H 1984 A permanent rat T-cell line that mediates experimental allergic neuritis in the Lewis rat in vivo. Journal of Immunology 133: 1946–1950

Lipkin I W, Parry G, Kiprov D, Abrams D 1985 Inflammatory neuropathy in homosexual men with lymphadenopathy. Neurology 35: 1479–1483

Lisak R P, Zweiman B 1975 Mitogen and muscle extract induced in vitro proliferative responses in myasthenia gravis, dermatomyositis and polymyositis. Journal of Neurology, Neurosurgery and Psychiatry 38: 521–524

Lisak R P, Zweiman B 1976 Serum immunoglobulin levels in myasthenia gravis, polymyositis and dermatomyositis. Journal of Neurology, Neurosurgery and Psychiatry 39: 34–37

Lisak R P, Abdou N I, Zweiman B, Zmijewski C, Penn A S 1976 Aspects of lymphocyte function in myasthenia gravis. Annals of the New York Academy of Science 274: 402–410

Lisak R P, Mitchell M, Zweiman B, Orrechio E, Asbury A K 1977 Guillain–Barré syndrome and Hodgkin's disease: Three cases with immunological studies. Annals of Neurology 1: 72–78

Lisak R P, Barchi R L 1982 Myasthenia gravis. W B Saunders, Philadelphia

Lisak R P, Brown M J, Sumner A J 1983a Abnormal serum factors in Guillain–Barré syndrome. Italian Journal of Neurological Sciences 3: 265-272

Lisak R P, Laramore C, Levinson A I, Zweiman B, Moskovitz A R 1983b In vitro synthesis of antibodies to acetylcholine receptor by peripheral blood mononuclear cells of patients with myasthenia gravis. Neurology 33: 604–608

Lisak R P, Zweiman B, Skolnik P, Levinson A I, Moskovitz A R, Guerrero F 1983c Thymic lymphocyte subpopulations in myasthenia gravis. Neurology 33: 868–872

Lisak R P, Kuchmy D, Armati-Gulson P, Brown M. J, Sumner A J 1984a Serum-mediated Schwann cell cytotoxicity in the Guillain–Barré syndrome. Neurology 34: 1240–1243

Lisak R P, Laramore C, Levinson A I, Zweiman B, Moskovitz A R, Witte A 1984b In vitro synthesis of antibodies to acetylcholine receptor by peripheral blood cells: role of suppressor T-cells in normal subjects. Neurology 34: 802–805

Lisak R P, Levinson A I, Zweiman B 1985a Autoimmune aspects of myasthenia gravis. In: Cruse J M, Lewis R E Jr (eds) Concepts in Immunopathology, vol 2. Karger, Basel p 65–101

Lisak R P, Zweiman B, Guerrero F, Moskovitz A R 1985b Circulating T-cell subsets in Guillain–Barré syndrome. Journal of Neuroimmunology 8: 93–101

Lisak R P, Laramore C, Levinson A I, Zweiman B, Moskovitz A R 1986a Suppressor T-cells in myasthenia gravis and antibodies to acetylcholine receptor. Annals of Neurology 19: 87–89

Lisak R P, Levinson A I, Zweiman B, Kornstein M J 1986b Antibodies to acetylcholine receptor and tetanus toxoid: in vitro synthesis by thymic lymphocytes. Journal of Immunology 137: 1221–1225

Liveson J, Fray H, Bornstein M B 1975 The effect of serum from A L S patients on organotypic nerve and muscle tissue cultures. Acta Neuropathologica (Berlin) 32: 127–131

McDevitt H O, Bodmer W F 1974 HL-A, immune response genes and disease. Lancet 2: 1269–1275

McLachlan S M, Nicholson L V B, Venables G et al 1981 Acetylcholine receptor antibody synthesis in lymphocyte cultures. Journal of Clinical and Laboratory Immunology 5: 137–142

McQuillen D P, Koethe S M, McQuillen M P 1983 Cellular response to human acetylcholine receptor in patients with myasthenia gravis. Journal of Neuroimmunology 5: 59–65

Mastaglia F L, Ojeda V J 1985a Inflammatory myopathies: Part 1. Annals of Neurology 17: 215–229

Mastaglia F L, Ojeda V J 1985b Inflammatory myopathies: Part 2. Annals of Neurology 17: 317–323

Matthews M B, Bernstein R M 1983 Myositis autoantibody inhibits histidyl tRNA synthetase: a model for autoimmunity. Nature 304: 177–179

Matthews M B, Reichlin M, Hughes G R V, Bernstein R M 1984 Anti-threonyl-tRNA synthetase, a second myositis-related autoantibody. Journal of Experimental Medicine 160: 420–434

Miller K B, Schwartz R S 1982 Autoimmunity and suppressor T lymphocytes. Advances in Internal Medicine 27: 281–313

Mimori T, Akizu K, Yamagata H, Inada S, Yoshida S, Homma M 1981 Characterization of a high molecular weight acidic nuclear protein recognized by autoantibodies in sera from patients with polymyositis-scleroderma overlap. Journal of Clinical Investigation 68: 611–620

Mishak R P, Dau P C 1981 Lymphocyte binding antibodies and suppressor cell activity in myasthenia gravis. Annals of the New York Academy of Sciences 377: 436–446

Morgan B P, Sewry C A, Siddle K, Luzio J P, Campbell A K 1984 Immunolocalization of complement component C9 on necrotic and non-necrotic muscle fibers in myositis using monoclonal antibodies: A primary role for complement in autoimmune cell damage. Immunology 52: 181–188

Nakao Y, Matsumoto H, Miyazski T, et al 1980 Gm allotypes in myasthenia gravis. Lancet 1: 677–680

Newsom-Davis J 1985 Lambert–Eaton myasthenic syndrome. In: Steck A J, Lisak R P (guest eds) Immunoneurology (I). Springer Seminars in Immunopathology 8: 129–140

Newsom-Davis J, Wilcox N, Calder L 1981 Thymus cells in myasthenia gravis selectively enhance production of anti-acetylcholine receptor antibody by autologous blood lymphocytes. New England Journal of Medicine 305: 1313–1318

Newsom-Davis J, Wilcox N, Schluep M et al 1987 Immunological heterogeneity and cellular mechanisms in myasthenia gravis. Annals of the New York Academy of Sciences (in press)

Nishikai M, Reichlin M 1980 Purification and characterization of a nuclear non-histone basic protein (Mi-1) which reacts with anti-immunoglobulin sera and the sera of patients with dermatomyositis. Molecular Immunology 17: 1129–1141

Nossal G J V 1983 Cellular mechanisms of immunologic tolerance. In: Paul W E, Fathman C G, Metzger H (eds) Annual Review of Immunology. Annual Reviews, Palo Alto, p 33–62

Northington J W, Brown M J 1982 Acute canine idiopathic polyneuropathy: A Guillain–Barré-like syndrome in dogs. Journal of the Neurological Sciences 56: 259–273

Nyland H, Aarli J A 1978 Guillain–Barré syndrome: demonstration of antibodies to peripheral nerve tissue. Acta Neurologica Scandinavica 58: 35–43

Oldstone M B A, Wilson C B, Perrin L H, Norris F H 1976 Evidence for immune complex formation in patients with amyotrophic lateral sclerosis. Lancet 2: 168–172

Olsson T, Henriksson K G, Klareskog L, Farsum U 1985 HLA-DR expression, T lymphocyte phenotypes ILM1 and OKT9 reactive cells in inflammatory myopathy. Muscle and Nerve 8: 419–425

Pachman L M, Cooke N 1980 Juvenile dermatomyositis: a clinical and immunologic study. Journal of Pediatrics 97: 226–234

Pachner A R, Kantor F S 1984 In vitro and in vivo actions of acetylcholine receptor educated T-cell lines in murine experimental autoimmune myasthenia gravis. Clinical and Experimental Immunology 56: 659–668

Patrick J, Lindstrom J 1973 Autoimmune response to acetylcholine receptor. Science 180: 871–872

Patten B M 1984 Neuropathy and motor neuron syndromes associated with plasma cell disease. Acta Neurologica Scandinavica 69: 47–61

Pepose J S 1982 A theory of virus-induced demyelination in the Landry-Guillain–Barré syndrome. Journal of Neurology 227: 93–97

Pollard J D, King R H, Thomas P K 1975 Recurrent experimental allergic neuritis. An electron microscopic study. Journal of Neurological Sciences 24: 365–383

Prior C, Lang B, Wray D, Newsom-Davis J 1985 Action of Lambert-Eaton myasthenic syndrome IgG at mouse motor nerve terminals. Annals of Neurology 17: 587–592

Quarles R H 1984 Myelin-associated glycoprotein in development and disease. Developmental Neuroscience 6: 285–303

Rechthand E, Cornblath D R, Stern B J, Meyerhoff J O 1984 Chronic demyelinating polyneuropathy in systemic lupus erythematosus. Neurology 34: 1375–1377

Reichlin M, Madison P J, Targoff I et al 1984 Antibodies to a nuclear/nucleolar antigen in patients with polymyositis overlap syndromes. Journal of Clinical Immunology 4: 40–44

Reik L Jr 1980 Disseminated vasculomyelinopathy: an immune complex disease. Annals of Neurology 7: 191–196

Richman D P, Patrick J, Arnason B G W 1976 Cellular immunity in myasthenia gravis. New England Journal of Medicine 294: 694–698

Richman D P, Antel J P, Burns J B, Arnason B G W 1981 Nicotinic acetylcholine receptor on human lymphocytes. Annals of the New York Academy of Sciences 377: 427–434

Robb S A, Bowley T J, Willcox H N A, Newsom-Davis J 1985 Circulating T-cell subsets in the Lambert-Eaton myasthenic syndrome. Journal of Neurology, Neurosurgery and Psychiatry 48: 501–505

Roisen F J, Bartfeld H, Donnenfeld H, Baxter J 1982 Neuron specific cytotoxicity of sera from patients with amyotrophic lateral sclerosis. Muscle and Nerve 5: 48–53

Rosenberg N L, Ringel S P, Katzin B L 1985 Experimental autoimmune myositis in SJL/J mice. Annals of Neurology 18:161

Rostami A, Brown M J, Lisak R P, Sumner A J, Zweiman B, Pleasure D E 1984 The role of myelin P_2 protein in the production of experimental allergic neuritis. Annals of Neurology 16: 680–685

Rostami A, Burns J B, Brown M J et al 1985 Transfer of experimental allergic neuritis with P_2-reactive T-cell lines. Cellular Immunology 91: 354–361

Rowe D J, Isenberg D A, McDougall J, Beverly P C L 1981 Characterization of polymyositis infiltrates using monoclonal antibodies to human leukocyte antigen. Clinical and Experimental Immunology 45: 290–298

Sahashi K, Engel A G, Lambert E H, Lennon V 1978 Ultrastructural localization of immune complexes (IgG and C3) at the endplate in experimental autoimmune myasthenia gravis. Journal of Neuropathology and Experimental Neurology 37: 212–223

Sahashi K, Engel A G, Lambert E H, Howard F M Jr 1980 Ultrastructural localization of the terminal and lytic ninth complement component (C9) at the motor endplate in myasthenia gravis. Journal of Neuropathology and Experimental Neurology 39: 160–172

Saida K, Saida T, Brown M J, Silberberg D H, Asbury A K 1979 In vivo demyelination induced by intraneural injection of antigalactocerebroside serum. A morphologic study. American Journal of Pathology 95: 99–116

Saida T, Saida K, Silberberg D H, Brown M J 1978 Transfer of demyelination with experimental neuritis serum. Nature 272: 639–641

Saida T, Saida K, Dorfman S H et al 1979 Experimental allergic neuritis induced by sensitization with galactocerebroside. Science 204: 1103–1106

Saida T, Saida K, Lisak R P, Brown M J, Silberberg D H, Asbury A K 1982 In vivo demyelinating activity of sera from patients with Guillain–Barré syndrome. Annals of Neurology 11: 69–75

Sharp G C, Irvin W S, Tan E M, Gould R C, Holman H R 1972 Mixed connective tissue disease — an apparently distinct rheumatic disease syndrome associated with specific antibody to an extractable nuclear antigen. American Journal of Medicine 52: 148–159

Sharp G C, Irvin W S, May C M et al 1976 Association of antibodies to ribonucleic protein and Sm antigens with mixed connective tissue disease, systemic lupus erythematosus and other rheumatic diseases. New England Journal of Medicine 295: 1149–1154

Sherman W H, Latov N, Hays A P 1983 Monoclonal IgM antibody precipitating with chondroitin sulfate C from patients with axonal polyneuropathy and epidermolysis. Neurology 33: 192–201

Shevach E M 1984 Macrophages and other accessory cells. In: Paul W E (ed) Fundamental immunology. Raven Press, New York, p 71–107

Skolnik P R, Lisak R P, Zweiman B 1982 Monoclonal antibody analysis of blood T-cell subsets in myasthenia gravis. Annals of Neurology 11: 170–176

Smith C I E, Aarli J A, Biberfeld P et al 1983 Myasthenia gravis after bone-marrow transplantation. Evidence for a donor origin. New England Journal of Medicine 309: 1565–1568

Smith C I E, Grubb R, Hammarstrom L, Perskanen R 1984 Gm allotypes in Finnish myasthenia gravis patients. Neurology 34: 1604–1605

Smith C I E, Hammarstrom L, Matell G, Perskanen R, Rabbitts T H 1987 Immunogenetics of myasthenia gravis. Annals of the New York Academy of Sciences (in press)

Smith K A 1984 Lymphokine regulation of T-cell and B-cell function. In: Paul W E (ed) Fundamental immunology. Raven Press, New York, p 559–576

Smith P D, Butler R C, Partridge T S, Sloper J C 1979 Current progress in the study of allergic polymyositis in the guinea pig and man. In: Rose F C (ed) Clinical neuroimmunology. Blackwell, Oxford, p 146–152

Snider W D, Simpson D M, Nielsen S, Gold J W M, Metraka C E, Posner J B 1983 Neurological complications of acquired immune deficiency syndrome: analysis of 50 patients. Annals of Neurology 14: 403–418

Stanley E, Drachman D B 1978 Effect of myasthenic immunoglobulin on acetylcholine receptors of intact mammalian neuromuscular junctions. Science 200: 1285–1287

Steck A J, Murray N, Meier C, Page N, Perruisseau G 1983 Demyelinating neuropathy and monoclonal IgM antibody to myelin-associated glycoprotein. Neurology 33: 19–23

Steck A J, Murray N 1985 Monoclonal antibodies to myelin-associated glycoprotein reveal antigenic structures and suggest pathogenic mechanisms. In: Steck A J, Lisak R P (guest eds) Immunoneurology (1). Springer Seminars in Immunopathology 8: 29–44

Steiner I, Abramsky O 1985 Immunology of Guillain–Barré syndrome. In: Steck A J, Lisak R P (guest eds) Immunoneurology (II) Springer Seminars in Immunopathology 8: 165–176

Stephansson K, Dieperink M E, Richman D P, Gomez C M, Marlton L S 1984 Sharing of antigenic determinants between the nicotinic acetylcholine receptor and proteins in Esherichia coli, Proteus vulgaris, and Klebsiella pneumoniae. New England Journal of Medicine 312: 221–225

Stevens J G, Pepose J S, Cook M L 1981 Marek's disease: A natural model for the Landry–Guillain–Barré syndrome. Annals of Neurology 9(Supplement): 102–106

Stewart G J, Pollard J D, McLeon J G, Wolnizer C M 1978 HLA antigens in the Landry–Guillain–Barré syndrome and chronic relapsing polyneuritis. Annals of Neurology 4: 285–289

Sumner A J, Said G, Idy I, Metral S 1982 Syndrome de Guillain–Barré: Effects electrophysiologiques et morphologiques du serum humain introduit dans l'espace endoneural du nerf sciatique au rat: résultats preliminaires. Revue Neurologique (Paris) 138: 17–24

Tachovsky T, Lisak R P, Koprowski H, Theofilopopoulos A N, Dixon F J 1976 Circulating immune complexes in multiple sclerosis and other neurological diseases. Lancet 2: 997–999

Targoff I N, Reichlin M 1985 The association between Mi-2 antibodies and dermatomyositis. Arthritis and Rheumatism 28: 796–803

Thomas J A, Wilcox H N A, Newsom-Davis J 1982 Immunohistological studies of the thymus in myasthenia gravis: Correlation with clinical state and thymocyte culture responses. Journal of Neuroimmunology 3: 319–355

Tischler A S, Dichter M, Beales B 1977 Electrical excitability of oat cell carcinoma. Journal of Pathology 122: 153–156

Tonegawa S 1983 Somatic generation of antibody diversity. Nature 302: 575–581

Tonnessen T I, Nyland H, Aarli J A 1982 Complement factors and acute phase reactants in the Guillain–Barré syndrome. European Neurology 21: 124–128

Toyka K V, Drachman D B, Pestronk A, Kao I 1975 Myasthenia gravis: passive transfer from man to mouse. Science 190: 397–399

Vincent A, Scadding G K, Thomas H C, Newsom-Davis J 1978 In vitro synthesis of antiacetylcholine receptor antibody by thymic lymphocytes in myasthenia gravis. Lancet 1: 305–307

Waksman B H, Adams R D 1955 Allergic neuritis: Experimental disease of rabbits induced by peripheral nervous tissue and adjuvants. Journal of Experimental Medicine 102: 213–236

Wasserman N H, Penn A S, Freimuth P I et al 1982 Anti-idiotypic route to anti-acetylcholine receptor antibodies and experimental myasthenia gravis. Proceedings of the National Academy of Sciences USA 79: 4810–4814

Werkele H, Ketelsen U-P 1977 Intrathymic pathogenesis and dual genetic control of myasthenia gravis. Lancet 1: 678–680

Whitaker J N 1982 Inflammatory myopathy: a review of etiologic and pathogenetic factors. Muscle and Nerve 5: 573–592

Whitaker J N, Engel W K 1972 Vascular deposits of immunoglobulin and complement in idiopathic inflammatory myopathy. New England Journal of Medicine 286: 333–338

Whiting P J, Vincent A, Newsom-Davis J 1983 Acetylcholine receptor antibody characteristics in myasthenia gravis. Fractionation of alpha-bungarotoxin binding site antibodies and their relationship to IgG subclass. Journal of Neuroimmunology 5: 1–9

Willcox N A, Demaine A G, Newsom-Davis J, Welsh K I, Robb S A, Spiro S G 1985 Increased frequency of IgG heavy chain marker G1m(2) and of HLA-B8 in Lambert–Eaton myasthenic syndrome with and without associated lung carcinoma. Human Immunology 14: 29–36

Winchester R J, Kunkel H G 1979 The human Ia system. Advances in Immunology 28: 221–292

Wisniewski H M, Brostoff S W, Carter H, Eylar E H 1974 Recurrent experimental allergic polyganglioradiculoneuritis. Multiple demyelinating episodes in the rhesus monkey sensitized with rabbit sciatic nerve myelin. Archives of Neurology 30: 347–358

Wolfe J F, Adelstein E, Sharp G C 1977 Antinuclear antibody with distinct specificity for polymyositis. Journal of Clinical Investigation 59: 176–178

Wolfgram F, Myers L 1973 Amyotrophic lateral sclerosis: Effect of serum on anterior horn cells in tissue culture. Science 179: 579–580

Zanetti M 1985 The idiotype network in autoimmune processes. Immunology Today 6: 299–301

Ziegler H K, Henney C S 1977 Studies on the cytotoxic activity of human lymphocytes. II. Interactions between IgG and Fc receptors leading to inhibition of K-cell function. Journal of Immunology 119: 1010–1017

Zinkernagel R M, Dougherty P C 1974 Restriction of in vitro T-cell mediated cytotoxicity in lymphocytic choriomeningitis within a syngeneic or semi-allogeneic system. Nature 248: 701–702

Zweiman B, Lisak R P 1984 Autoantibodies: autoimmunity and immune complexes. In: Henry J (ed) Clinical diagnosis and management by laboratory methods. W B Saunders, Philadelphia, p 924–954

The pathophysiology of excitation in skeletal muscle

INTRODUCTION

Although the generation of force in skeletal muscle ultimately reflects the chemical interaction of actin and myosin, useful muscular activity can occur only when this chemical interaction is faithfully coupled to the electrical activity of a motor neurone. This coupling is provided by the propagation of regenerative spikes or action potentials along the muscle sarcolemma; these impulses originate in the region of the end-plate and subsequently spread across the entire muscle surface, eventually penetrating into the fibre interior along the elements of the T-tubular network. At membrane specialisations known as triads, the T-tubular elements interact closely with the terminal cisternae of the sarcoplasmic reticulum (SR); depolarisation here, in some as yet undefined manner, results in the release of calcium from the SR in a process known as excitation–contraction coupling (for review, see Franzini-Armstrong & Peachey 1981).

If the surface membrane of a muscle fibre fails to generate an action potential in response to end-plate depolarisation, contraction will not take place in spite of normal functioning at the neuromuscular junction and normal properties for all the contractile proteins themselves; inexcitable surface membranes result in muscle paralysis. Conversely, if the surface membrane generates multiple, uncontrolled action potentials in response to a normal stimulus at the neuromuscular junction, sustained contractions can result where only a brief twitch was intended; hyperexcitable surface membranes are one cause of delayed relaxation in neuromuscular disease.

This chapter deals with the processes that

control the action potential in normal skeletal muscle, and with membrane defects that can produce hypo- and hyperexcitable states of the sarcolemma. We then trace the relationship between these factors and the pathogenesis of the myotonic disorders and of the periodic paralyses.

NORMAL MEMBRANE EXCITATION IN SKELETAL MUSCLE

The resting membrane potential

A microelectrode inserted into a normal skeletal muscle fibre will record a potential of 70–90 mV with the inside of the cell negative relative to the extracellular space. This potential is developed across the thin barrier (50–75Å) of the surface membrane. This membrane also marks the boundary across which concentration gradients are established for monovalent and divalent anions and cations between the cytoplasm and the external environment. It is the interrelationship between these concentration gradients and the selective permeability of the surface membrane to these ions that controls the sign and the magnitude of the membrane potential. This potential can be altered either through modification of the concentration gradients themselves or through the modulation of the membrane's ionic conductances.

The interaction between membrane potential, ionic concentration gradients and membrane conductances can best be understood by considering first the simple case of a semipermeable membrane separating two chambers that contain different concentrations of a simple salt solution. Suppose such a membrane (Fig. 10.1), separating a 100 mM solution of KCl on the left-hand side from one of 5 mM on the right, is suddenly made selectively permeable to potassium only. Potassium ions (K^+) will move down their concentration gradient from the side with the highest concentration (the left) to the side with the lowest (the right). However, as the membrane is not permeable to the counterion chloride (Cl^-), any movement of K^+ will produce an imbalance of charge, with more positive ions on the right side of the membrane and more negative ions on the left. This charge imbalance creates a membrane potential whose electrical field will retard the

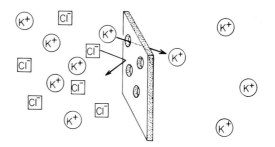

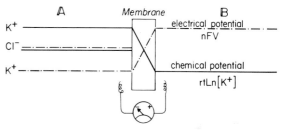

Fig. 10.1 A transmembrane potential develops when a semipermeable membrane separates two solutions with differing concentrations of a permeant ion. In this illustration, the membrane is permeable only to K^+ ions. The electrical potential that results when K^+ ions attempt to move down their concentration gradient will exactly balance the chemical potential produced by that concentration gradient, and the net force acting on a single K^+ ion moving through the membrane will be zero. The membrane potential under these conditions, given by the Nernst equation, will vary as a function of the potassium concentration gradient. Reproduced from Barchi (1980) with permission

further movements of K^+ ions along their chemical gradient. Eventually an equilibrium will be reached where the driving force on a K^+ ion due to the electrical field exactly balances the opposing drive of the concentration gradient and no further net movement of ions occurs. This potential, known as the Nernst potential after the nineteenth-century physiologist who first described it, is given by the simple equation:

$$Vm = \frac{RT}{nF} \ln \left\{ \frac{[K_1^+]}{[K_2^+]} \right\} \qquad (1)$$

where Vm is the membrane potential, $[K_1^+]$ is the concentration of potassium ions on side one, n is the charge on each ion (in this case, $+1$) and R, T, and F are physical constants. The equation predicts that increasing the concentration gradient increases the potential while decreasing the concentration gradient has the opposite effect.

Unfortunately, things are not as simple as this in the case of the muscle membrane. While the sarcolemma is very permeable to K+, and the response of the membrane potential to changes in K+ concentration does approximate to that predicted by the potassium Nernst potential, the membrane is in fact measurably permeable to other ions as well, especially to Na+ and to Cl−. In normal muscle both the concentration gradients and the relative membrane permeabilities for each of these ions have a role in determining the actual membrane potential across the sarcolemma. Although the derivation of the equation describing this situation is complicated, the final result resembles in its general form the simple Nernst relationship:

$$Vm = \frac{RT}{nF} \ln \left\{ \frac{P_K[K_1^+] + P_{Na}[Na_1^+] + P_{Cl}[Cl_2^-]}{P_K[K_2^+] + P_{Na}[Na_2^+] + P_{Cl}[Cl_1^-]} \right\} \quad (2)$$

A new term, P, is now introduced that indicates the membrane's relative permeability to each ionic species. This equation, known as the Goldman–Hodgkin–Katz (GHK) relationship, predicts that the membrane potential will reflect both the concentration gradients for each of the permeant ion species and the relative permeability (P) of the membrane to each of those species. The dependence on relative permeabilities introduced by this equation is extremely important since it predicts that the membrane potential can be altered by modulating membrane permeability alone without any change in the concentration gradients themselves. With the typical concentration gradients for Na+, K+ and Cl− found in mammalian skeletal muscle, the membrane potential can range between −90 mV or so when the permeability to K+ predominates, and +50 mV when the membrane is made selectively permeable to Na+. It is this relationship between permeability and potential that forms the basis for the generation of an action potential.

There is another fundamental difference between the situation described by the Nernst relationship and that quantitated by the GHK equation. With a perfectly selective membrane, the potential predicted by the Nernst equation will persist indefinitely; that is, the equation describes an equilibrium. This is not the case for a membrane permeable to multiple ions as described by the GHK equation. Here, for example, movement of K+ in one direction can be electrically balanced by the movement of Na+ ions along their concentration gradient in the opposite direction. Eventually these gradients will dissipate and the potential itself will disappear. In order for the membrane potential described by equation (2) to persist, there must be a mechanism for maintaining the underlying concentration gradients. Ideally, each ion that crosses the membrane passively must be pumped actively back across the membrane. If this is done, a *steady state* will result; the potential and the concentration gradients remain constant, but at the necessary cost of energy in the form of the ATP needed to run the pump.

In skeletal muscle the major membrane transport protein is the Na+-K+-ATPase. This protein actively transports Na+ against its concentration gradient from the inside of the cell to the extracellular space while simultaneously moving K+ ions in the opposite direction (for a review, see Jorgenson 1982). The coupling of Na+ and K+ in this energy-dependent pumping process is not 1 : 1, however; about three Na+ ions move outwards for each two K+ ions that are transported inwards. If negative counterions cannot keep up with the movement of their positive partners, this asymmetrical pumping will produce a small membrane potential of its own. In normal muscle, the activity of the Na+-K+-ATPase can generate 3–10 mV of hyperpolarisation depending on the level of activity of the enzyme.

Active membrane properties

In muscle, small depolarising current pulses introduced through an intracellular microelectrode produce proportionate changes in the membrane potential as expected for a passive R-C circuit as long as the magnitude of the depolarisation does not exceed 10–15 mV. Larger depolarisations, however, trigger a unique all-or-none regenerative potential change which reflects highly non-linear changes in the underlying properties of the membrane itself. This regenerative spike or action potential is stereotyped in its form, and at its peak produces an internal potential that is actually positive with respect to the extracellular space.

Some insight into the mechanism by which the action potential arises can be gained by studying the relationship between the membrane potential at the peak of the spike and the external concentration of various cations. While the resting potential in muscle is sensitive to changes in external [K⁺] but not to external [Na⁺], the peak of the action potential demonstrates the reverse relationship; it is altered little by variations in [K⁺] but varies with [Na⁺] in a manner resembling a membrane that is permeable only to Na⁺ ions.

Membrane currents during an action potential. The details of the conductance changes that underly the action potential in skeletal muscle have been defined mainly through the use of voltage clamp techniques. After its seminal application to the squid giant axon by Hodgkin & Huxley (1952), this technique was modified for single muscle fibres by Adrian and his colleagues (Adrian et al 1970). Their early findings confirmed that the basic mechanisms involved in producing action potentials in nerve and muscle were the same. The initial rising phase of the action potential is produced by a large, voltage-dependent increase in membrane conductance to sodium ions. The greater the depolarisation, the larger and more rapid is the conductance change; thus, once initiated, the action potential becomes its own stimulus. This increase in sodium conductance is transient, however, and reverts to its resting level within a period of a few milliseconds. This conductance inactivation, in conjunction with a secondary delayed increase in membrane conductance to potassium ions, results in the return of the membrane potential to its normal resting value.

With the use of a voltage clamp, relationships between conductance, voltage, and time have been detailed in muscle for both the sodium and the potassium systems (Adrian et al 1970, Adrian & Marshall 1977). Over the years, a number of points have become clear. First, the membrane proteins controlling these conductances represent two discrete populations of ion channels, each providing a separate time- and voltage-dependent aqueous pathway through the membrane for its selected cation. Secondly, the basic properties of these two channels differ little from comparable sodium and potassium channels involved in the production of action potentials in the nerves and muscles of virtually all multicellular organisms. Thirdly, the action potential is mainly the result of changes in *conductance* of the membrane to these cations; relatively little actual net movement of cations occurs and there is no significant change in the cation concentration gradients across the membrane during a single action potential.

Sodium channel inactivation. The kinetics of current flow through the sodium and potassium channels differ in a very fundamental way. When potassium channels are opened with depolarisation, they tend to stay in the opened state and potassium currents flow throughout the period of depolarisation, terminating only when the membrane repolarises. Sodium channels, on the other hand, open transiently in response to depolarisation and then revert to a non-conducting or inactivated state in spite of persistent depolarisation (for a review, see French & Horn 1983). The process of inactivation in the sodium channel is an extremely important one, and channel inactivation has a central role in the control of membrane excitability. This aspect of sodium channel function requires some additional comment.

The voltage-dependent sodium channel can exist in at least three states. In the normally closed state which predominates at the resting potential, the channel does not allow the movement of cations, but is available to be activated by depolarisation. With rapid depolarisation, a second, opened, state is seen in which sodium ions move freely through the channel pore. With continued depolarisation, the channel enters a third conformation known as the inactivated state; in this state the pore is closed but the channel is no longer able to be activated by depolarisation (Fig. 10.2). All three states appear to be interconvertible, and the inactivated state can be restored to the closed but activatable state simply by repolarising the membrane to its resting level.

In a population of sodium channels, the fraction that will be found in the inactivated state increases with depolarisation. The relationship between steady-state inactivation and membrane potential

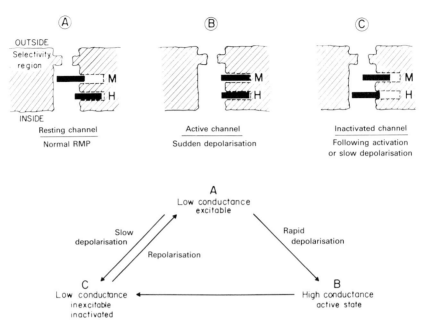

Fig. 10.2 Muscle action potentials are produced largely by transient changes in membrane conductance to sodium ions. Membrane sodium conductance is controlled by a voltage-sensitive sodium channel which provides a water-filled pathway across the muscle surface membrane. In the channel, ion movement is controlled by several 'gates' that switch open or closed as a function of membrane potential and time. At the normal membrane resting potential the channel is closed. Rapid depolarisation results in transient channel opening; during this interval, a Na^+ ion current can flow. Prolonged depolarisation causes a separate 'inactivation' gate to close; the channel no longer conducts Na^+ ions and cannot be opened again by further depolarisation. Repolarisation of the membrane restores the channel to its original closed but activatable state

is sigmoidal, with the midpoint in skeletal muscle at about -50 mV. Prolonged depolarisation can thus paradoxically lead to inactivation of sodium channels and loss of membrane excitability rather than the increased excitability often expected.

Although the actual kinetic inter-relationships between the various conformations of the sodium channel are in fact much more complex, this simple scheme is sufficient to explain many of the basic properties of channel behaviour.

Single channel properties

Our view of the behaviour of sodium and potassium channels as continuously modulated conductance pathways that open and close in a smooth, graded fashion in response to triggering stimuli was based on voltage clamp measurements recording the response of large areas of surface membrane containing many thousands of channel molecules. This view has changed dramatically in recent years with the introduction of a technique known as patch clamping (Neher & Sakmann 1976) (Fig. 10.3a). In this method, very small patches of membrane (less than 1 μm^2 in area) can be isolated at the tip of a fire-polished microelectrode and subjected to the same sort of analysis used with the traditional macroscopic voltage clamp. These patches are so small that they contain only one or two sodium or potassium channels each.

The response of these very small membrane patches to abrupt depolarisation is quite different from that of whole fibres or squid axons. Instead of smoothly modulated changes in membrane current with depolarisation, sharp step-like transitions between discrete current levels are seen at a given driving voltage (Fig. 10.3b). The amplitude of these current steps is constant and the actual change in current occurs so rapidly that

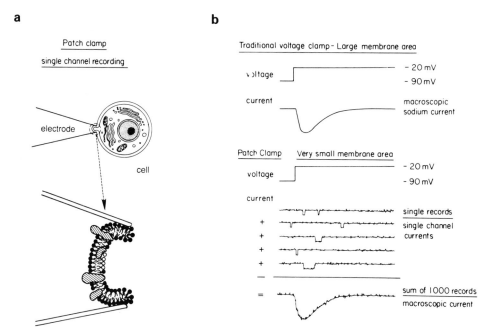

a

Patch clamp

single channel recording

electrode

cell

b

Traditional voltage clamp - Large membrane area

voltage — — −20 mV
— −90 mV

current — macroscopic sodium current

Patch Clamp   Very small membrane area

voltage — −20 mV
— −90 mV

current

+ — single records
+ — single channel currents
+
+
−

= — sum of 1000 records macroscopic current

Fig. 10.3 a. With the technique of patch clamping, a small area of membrane can be sealed so tightly to the tip of a blunt glass microelectrode that it can be removed intact from the cell. The high resistance of the membrane-to-glass seal (usually tens of gigaohms) allows the investigator to resolve the tiny currents flowing through single ion channels in the membrane patch.   b. Classic macroscopic techniques for measuring membrane currents, such as voltage clamp, record the response of thousands of ion channels at a time. The current records often suggest a smoothly graded opening and closing of these channels with time, as shown in this record of membrane sodium currents flowing through the voltage-sensitive sodium channel. Using the patch clamp, the behaviour of single ion channels can be resolved. At this level, sodium channels are seen to open and close abruptly, moving rapidly between a zero conductance state and a characteristic open-channel conductance state. The smooth currents seen with macroscopic techniques really represent the statistical average of the stochastic behaviour of individual channels whose probabilities of opening and closing vary with voltage and time

usually it cannot be accurately resolved (Horn & Patlack 1980). If the same depolarising step is repeated over and over again in the same patch, the characteristics of these current steps remain constant; only their duration and the time of their occurrence during the pulse vary, each in a statistically definable manner. If recordings of these current steps from thousands of such records are averaged, the smooth current increase and self-terminating inactivation characteristic of a traditional voltage clamp record are reproduced.

These small current pulses represent the opening and closing of individual ion channels. Each channel opens very rapidly to a characteristic conductance level, remains opened for a period of time, and then closes again. The interval between the initiation of membrane depolarisation and channel opening varies in a statistical manner for a single channel on multiple trials. Following an

abrupt depolarisation, the probability that a given single channel will be opened increases dramatically for a few milliseconds and then decreases again with time, reflecting the time-dependent onset of inactivation. For skeletal muscle, single sodium channels have a conductance of about 20 pS, resulting in a current flow of several thousand ions through each channel during an average opened interval of 1 ms.

The response of the muscle membrane to depolarisation can no longer be considered as a smooth graded process; the currents recorded with macroscopic techniques such as the traditional voltage clamp actually represent the statistical average of the responses of many thousands of individual channels, each behaving in a stochastic manner in switching between its closed and opened state. The relationship between parameters such as the probability of channel opening and the duration of each channel opening, on the one hand, and the membrane potential and time after depolarisation, on the other, define the response characteristics of the channel in the membrane in a manner analogous to the time- and voltage-dependent rate constants of the classic Hodgkin–Huxley formulation.

Molecular characterisation of muscle sodium channels

Together with an appreciation of single sodium channel events at the biophysical level has come an increasing understanding of the molecular properties of the voltage-sensitive sodium channel protein itself. The sodium channel has now been isolated from rat and rabbit skeletal muscle and partially purified from human muscle (for review, see Barchi 1986); similar sodium channels have been characterised from rat brain and eel electroplax (Agnew 1984). In each case, the isolated proteins look remarkably similar.

The purified sodium channel proteins from each of these sources contain as their sole or predominant component one very large subunit of ~260 kDa (Fig. 10.4). This subunit is a glycoprotein, containing about 23% by weight carbohydrate. In the mammalian skeletal muscle and brain channels, there appear to be one or two additional small subunits of ~38 kDa, which are also heavily glycosylated (Barchi et al 1986).

The purified sodium channels from rat and rabbit muscle have been reconstituted into artificial membranes (Weigele & Barchi 1982, Kraner et al 1985). These purified proteins are capable of voltage-dependent gating of cation currents. Their single-channel properties and cation selectivity characteristics are the same as those of the native sodium channel in vivo, and the channel's behaviour is modified by the same neurotoxins that are effective in intact muscle (Tanaka et al 1983, Kraner et al 1985, Furman et al 1986).

The complete amino-acid sequence for the 260 kDa component of the eel sodium channel has been determined by cloning and sequencing of its messenger RNA using the powerful tools of recombinant DNA technology (Noda et al 1984). Similar sequencing is now complete for the rat brain channel (Noda et al 1986) and partially avail-

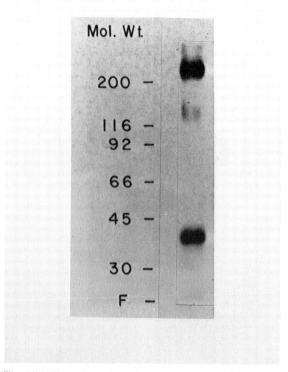

Fig. 10.4 The voltage-dependent sodium channel from mammalian skeletal muscle contains two subunits: one is a very large glycoprotein, the molecular weight of which is ⁻260 000; the molecular weight of the smaller subunit, also a glycoprotein, is 38 000. The channel preparation shown is from rabbit skeletal muscle. Reproduced from Kraner et al (1985) with permission

able for the channel from rat muscle. On the basis of these sequences, several interesting conclusions can now be drawn:

1. These channels are highly homologous, with more than 60% sequence identity between the eel and the rat channels. Not only are the functional aspects of the channel preserved through evolution, but also the same precise amino-acid sequence in many parts of the molecule is retained (Noda et al 1986).

2. The large 260 kDa subunit that contains more than 1800 amino acids is actually made up of four homologous internal segments, almost as if four related subunits had been joined together in a single long chain rather than being synthesised as separate polypeptide seg-

ments. These internal domains must have arisen through a process of gene duplication; the probability that their homology could have occurred by chance alone is certainly less than one part in 10^9 (Noda et al 1984, Guy & Seetharamulu 1986).

3. Detailed analysis of the amino-acid sequence in each of the four homologous domains of the sodium channel large subunit reveals the presence of a number of regions whose local sequence have a high probability of assuming an alpha-helical conformation within the membrane. These regions probably represent membrane-spanning segments and are the most highly conserved regions both between internal domains and between different species (Guy & Seetharamulu 1986). In addition, there is one, and probably two, amphipathic helical segments within each domain ideally suited to participate in the formation of the ion channel itself; the polar faces of these helices may form the lining of the channel's aqueous pore while their remaining hydrophobic surfaces could interact with the other non-polar intramembrane helical segments.

Techniques are now available which allow the investigator to modify single specific amino acids within the primary sequence of huge proteins like the sodium channel. This is done by altering the base sequence in the message encoding for the protein. The altered message can then be amplified, and the message expressed by direct injection into a cell that does not usually produce the channel of interest. Surprisingly, this foreign message is usually translated and processed accurately, and the function of the resultant channel protein can be studied directly in the cell membrane. With this and related approaches borrowed from genetic engineering, the details of the relationship between structure and function in these complex proteins can now be probed.

MEMBRANES AND MUSCLE WEAKNESS IN PERIODIC PARALYSIS

The periodic paralyses are disorders of skeletal muscle characterised by transient episodes of muscle weakness or paralysis. During these episodes there are often profound shifts in the serum potassium concentration. These disorders usually occur as familial syndromes with autosomal dominant inheritance, although clinically indistinguishable sporadic cases do occur (see Ch. 25). The periodic paralyses have traditionally been classified according to the characteristic changes in serum potassium associated with the attacks of weakness, and hypokalaemic, normokalaemic and hyperkalaemic varieties are recognised. This classification is probably simplistic; e.g., it now appears that at least four different types of hyperkalaemic periodic paralysis can be identified (Rudel & Ricker 1985). The details of the clinical presentation of the various forms of periodic paralysis are considered in Chapter 25. We will discuss here some of the common aspects of the membrane events which lead to the development of muscle weakness.

Membrane potential and membrane excitability

Between attacks of paralysis, the resting membrane potential in skeletal muscle of patients with periodic paralysis is usually normal or slightly lower than normal, but excitation–contraction coupling proceeds without difficulty (Shy et al 1961, Creutzfeldt et al 1963, Rieker & Bolte 1966, McComas et al 1968). During the onset of an attack of weakness, muscle strength declines in direct proportion to the loss of muscle membrane excitability, as evidenced by the amplitude of the compound muscle action potential that can be elicited by either direct or indirect stimulation (Gordon et al 1970). At the peak of paralysis, individual muscle fibres exhibit abnormally low resting membrane potentials (Creutzfeldt et al 1963, Hofmann & Smith 1970) and cannot be stimulated to produce an action potential by the usual depolarising current stimuli. Hyperpolarisation of the membrane, on the other hand, will often produce an action potential when the stimulus is terminated — an 'anode break' potential. At the same time, motor nerve action potentials appear normal, processes at the end-plate are intact, and the underlying contractile apparatus responds normally to the direct application of calcium (Engel & Lambert 1969).

Although the details of this scenario vary from

one type of periodic paralysis to another, the basic storyline is the same. Muscle paralysis is associated with failure of action potential generation in the fibre sarcolemma, and this in turn is correlated with a persistent depolarisation of the membrane resting potential. How can these facts be reconciled with our understanding of the molecular basis for action potential generation? We have seen above that prolonged depolarisation will shift the membrane voltage-sensitive sodium channels into an inactivated state. The percentage of the sodium channels in the membrane available for activation varies steeply with voltage near the resting potential (Fig. 10.5). As an action potential can be generated only when the net inward sodium current through these channels exceeds the total outward current carried through all other channels in the membrane, the number of sodium channels available to be opened is critical for normal excitability.

At normal muscle resting potentials, about 70% of the membrane sodium channels are available for activation. With this number of channels, the inward sodium current needed for initiation of the action potential is easily achieved. A persistent depolarisation of only 10–20 mV, however, will increase the fraction of inactivated channels to nearly 50%, and the remaining channels are barely

able to generate the needed inward current density for an action potential. A further small depolarisation renders the membrane totally incapable of generating an action potential even though the sodium channels themselves may be normal in number and in their molecular properties.

If the membrane is once again repolarised to its normal resting level, the equilibrium between closed but activatable channels and inactivated channels shifts back, the fraction of channels available for activation increases, and normal excitability is restored. When action potentials once again couple depolarisation of the neuromuscular junction to calcium release from the sarcoplasmic reticulum, normal muscle function and strength return.

Pathophysiology of membrane depolarisation

This sequence of events appears to be shared by most, if not all, of the periodic paralyses during episodes of muscle weakness. The triggering factors which lead to the underlying membrane depolarisation, however, may be quite different in the various forms of this disease. If we recall the GHK equation (equation 2) describing the origin of the muscle membrane potential, we can appreciate that persistent depolarisation can be produced by a variety of factors. These include an increase in external K^+ concentration, a decrease in external Na^+ concentration, or an increase in membrane permeability to Na^+ relative to that for K^+. Decreasing the contribution to the membrane potential from the electrogenic activity of the Na^+-K^+-ATPase will also depolarise the membrane.

In most of the familial periodic paralyses, membrane depolarisation seems to be due mainly to an increase in the membrane permeability to Na^+ (see Rudel & Ricker 1985, for review). In the toxic paralysis produced by barium ingestion or by experimental potassium deficiency in animals, on the other hand, depolarisation may be the result of a primary decrease in K^+ conductance, again with the ultimate effect of shifting the balance of membrane conductance to favour Na^+ (Kao & Gordon 1975, Gallant 1983). External factors, such as cooling, that lead to a further transient increase in Na^+ conductance or a decrease in electrogenic pump activity will tip the delicately

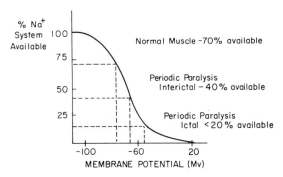

Fig. 10.5 The fraction of the voltage-sensitive sodium channel population that is available for activation varies as a function of the resting membrane potential. Under normal resting conditions in skeletal muscle, about 70% of the channels are ready to be activated. Prolonged depolarisation of the membrane causes inactivation of progressively larger numbers of sodium channels; at resting potentials below about −50 mV, the percentage of channels available falls below the level needed to generate an action potential, and the muscle fibre will fail to contract in response to a signal at the neuromuscular junction

balanced membrane into a more depolarised state, resulting in further inactivation of the voltage-sensitive sodium channel, failure of excitation, and paralysis.

In hypokalaemic periodic paralysis, the increased resting membrane sodium conductance does not involve the voltage-dependent sodium channel, but rather another sodium pathway which may be coupled in some way to the membrane actions of insulin (Rudel et al 1984). In adynamia episodica hereditaria and paramyotonia congenita, the increased sodium conductance is mediated by the sodium channel itself, and can be prevented or reversed by the specific sodium-channel blocker tetrodotoxin (Lehmann-Horn et al 1981, 1983). Of particular interest is the defect in paramyotonia, where the the sodium channel undergoes a temperature-dependent change, functioning normally at 37 °C but becoming persistently opened when cooled to 27 °C (Lehmann-Horn et al 1981). This could be an example of an unstable conformational state produced by the alteration of a single amino-acid code in the channel gene.

Serum K$^+$, membrane potential, and paralysis

The details of the interplay between serum potass-ium, membrane potential and paralysis in the individual disorders remain to be clarified, but shifts in serum K$^+$ probably reflect coupling to sodium movements through the Na$^+$-K$^+$-ATPase system rather than primary events directly respon-sible for paralysis. This coupling can result clini-cally in either hypokalaemia or hyperkalaemia, depending upon the functional state of the Na$^+$-K$^+$-ATPase itself. For example, the increased inward Na$^+$ movement that would be associated with an abnormally large membrane Na$^+$ conduc-tance will be a potent stimulus for pump activity. A sudden increase in Na$^+$ conductance from any specific triggering event will further stimulate this pump. As the Na$^+$-K$^+$-ATPase exchanges extra-cellular K$^+$ for intracellular Na$^+$, pumping activity can rapidly reduce the K$^+$ concentration in the small volume of the extracellular space and produce hypokalaemia. This sort of coupling accounts for the net K$^+$ movement into the cells of normal individuals that follows the adminis-tration of glucose and insulin.

In another setting, the Na$^+$-K$^+$-ATPase may not be able to increase its activity sufficiently to keep pace with an increased Na$^+$ leakage. In this case, progressive depolarisation will result, with inward Na$^+$ movement coupled electrically to outward movement of K$^+$ ions, leading to secondary hyperkalaemia. It is important to realise that either hyperkalaemia or hypokalaemia can result from the same fundamental defect in membrane sodium conductance depending on the magnitude of the conductance change and capacity of the Na$^+$-K$^+$-ATPase to respond to the additional sodium load.

The Na$^+$K$^+$-ATPase may have a pivotal role in the onset of depolarisation as well. A muscle membrane in delicate balance as the result of an increased inward Na$^+$ leak just compensated by a maximally activated pump could be thrown out of balance by the selective slowing of pump activity. This can easily occur with cooling, as the change in activity of energy-dependent pumping with temperature is nearly threefold greater than that for ion movement through an aqueous membrane channel.

HYPEREXCITABLE STATES OF THE MUSCLE MEMBRANE — MYOTONIA

The myotonic syndromes are easily identified among the disorders of the neuromuscular system by their characteristic mechanical and electrical features. Myotonia is expressed clinically as the delayed relaxation of skeletal muscle after a voluntary contraction or a contraction induced by an electrical or mechanical stimulus. This delayed relaxation is a cardinal finding in a number of diseases that vary widely in their inheritance, pathology and prognosis (see Ch. 16); these include myotonia congenita, myotonic dystrophy, paramyotonia congenita, chondrodystrophic myotonia and even some forms of hyperkalaemic periodic paralysis. Myotonia indistinguishable from that found in these natural disorders is also seen as a reaction to several classes of drugs and chemicals and can be reproduced in laboratory animals (Table 10.1).

Patients with myotonia often report painless muscular stiffness that is worst at the beginning

Table 10.1 Neuromuscular disorders associated with myotonia

Inherited disorders	
Man	*Other mammals*
myotonia congenita	congenital myotonia:
dominant and recessive forms	goat
myotonic dystrophy	horse
adynamica episodica	dog
paramyotonia congenita	cattle
chondrodystrophic myotonia	

Acquired disorders

Drug-induced
  Aromatic carboxylic acids
    2,4-D, anthracene-9-carboxylic acid, diuretics
  Inhibitors of sterol synthesis
    20,25-diazacholesterol
    hypocholesterolaemic drugs
      Atromid-S, clofibrate, triparinol
  Steroid administration in dogs

Others
  Iodine intoxication in birds

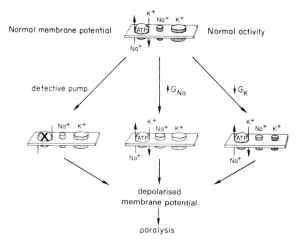

Fig. 10.6 Periodic paralysis is associated with depolarisation of the muscle fibre surface membrane. This depolarisation could result from an increase in membrane Na^+ conductance, a decrease in membrane K^+ conductance, or a reduction in the pumping activity of the membrane Na^+-K^+-ATPase. In the inherited periodic paralyses, an increase in membrane Na^+ conductance appears to be the primary mechanism underlying membrane depolarisation. Adapted with permission from Furman & Barchi (1986)

of movement and that slowly resolves with exercise. Brief muscular contractions are often not impaired, but forceful contractions can cause the muscles to lock in a contracted state, leading to functional disability and falls. Other factors that can aggravate myotonia include muscle cooling, fasting, menstruation, potassium ingestion and sudden emotional arousal.

When examined by electromyography, patients with myotonia exhibit a common picture of increased insertional activity and prolonged, repetitive discharges of motor unit potentials that wax and wane in frequency and amplitude (Fig. 10.6). This prolonged electrical activity correlates with the delay in muscular relaxation and in most of the myotonias is directly responsible for the abnormality of contraction. The waxing and waning frequency of these discharges produce crescendo–decrescendo sound patterns on the audio monitor that early investigators referred to as 'dive bomber potentials'.

The remarkable similarity of the clinical and electrical appearance of myotonia in different muscle diseases initially suggested that a common underlying pathogenetic mechanism might explain this phenomenon at the membrane level in all diseases. Unfortunately, research over the past 20 years has shown that this is not the case (Rudel & Lehmann-Horn 1985). Although one major group of myotonic disorders does share a common

molecular mechanism, clinical myotonia is probably a common expression of a number of otherwise unrelated defects affecting the behaviour of membrane ion channels (Barchi 1982). In the following sections, some of the common themes relating to the appearance of repetitive electrical discharges in the various myotonic disorders will be discussed. The clinical aspects of these diseases are considered in Chapter 16.

Myotonia due to abnormal chloride conductance

Studies in animal models. Much of our knowledge of the pathophysiology of myotonia is based on the detailed electrophysiological and biophysical studies of a naturally occurring congenital myotonia in goats, carried out by Bryant and his colleagues (for a review, see Bryant 1979). This hereditary syndrome is very similar in its appearance to myotonia congenita in humans.

Classic experiments with nerve section and neuromuscular blockade localised the origin of the abnormal electrical activity to the muscle membrane itself (Brown & Harvey 1939). Subsequent measurements on single isolated intercostal muscle fibres demonstrated at the cellular level the correlate of the persistent electrical activity recorded by EMG (Adrian & Bryant 1974). When the surface membrane of a myotonic fibre is depolarised by a constant current, a repetitive series of driven action potentials is seen that is followed by a long, depolarising after-potential (Fig. 10.7). The amplitude of this depolarising after-potential is proportional to the number of action potentials produced during the current pulse. When the after-potential becomes large enough, long trains of self-sustaining, spontaneous action potentials are triggered. These events are not seen in normal fibres where depolarisation generates only a few driven potentials, much smaller after-depolarisations and no spontaneous activity.

Measurement of membrane conductance in these myotonic fibres reveals a remarkable increase in membrane resistance that is caused by the nearly complete absence of the normal membrane conductance to chloride ions (Bryant & Morales-Aguilera 1971). In myotonic goats, this is due to a reduced density of chloride channels rather than a normal number of channels having modified conductance properties, and probably

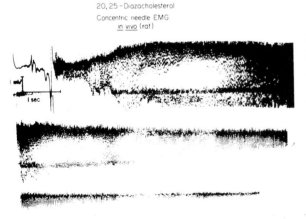

20, 25 – Diazacholesterol
Concentric needle EMG
in vivo (rat)

Fig. 10.7 Sustained membrane electrical activity that follows muscle activation or irritation is the electrical correlate of the delayed relaxation seen in myotonic skeletal muscle. In this example, a myotonic discharge was recorded in response to electrode movement from a rat treated with 20,25-diazacholesterol, an agent that produces a toxic myotonic syndrome. Reproduced from Furman & Barchi (1981) with permission

represents the primary defect in this disorder (Bryant & Owenburg 1980).

The delayed relaxation of myotonic muscle fibres is believed to be the consequence of abnormal repetitive membrane firing that triggers a normal contractile activation process. Unfortunately, there have been few direct measurements of excitation–contraction coupling in myotonic goats. In one study, changes in voltage-dependent contractile activation were interpreted as indicating enhanced calcium re-uptake by the sarcoplasmic reticulum (Bryant 1979), and other findings on purified sarcoplasmic reticulum fragments also suggested an excitation–contraction abnormality (Swift et al 1979). A thorough study of SR function in chemically skinned single fibres from myotonic goats, however, found caffeine-induced contractions and other release and re-uptake parameters to be normal (Wood et al 1980).

Voltage-clamp techniques have been used to study the kinetics of sodium and potassium channel gating in myotonic goat intercostal fibres (Bryant & DeCoursey 1980). Although small changes were seen in the behaviour of both channels in myotonic muscle, these are not in themselves of sufficient magnitude to produce repetitive activity. They may play a part in the modulation of myotonic activity, however.

Human myotonia congenita. Myotonia congenita is an inherited disorder in humans that closely resembles the hereditary myotonia of goats. Myotonia congenita can occur in either an autosomal dominant or a recessive form (Ch. 16). Generalised myotonia is usually noted in childhood at the onset of walking, but the severity of the symptoms does not increase with maturation. Membrane studies in human myotonia congenita indicate that here, too, the primary pathophysiological defect is a drastic reduction in muscle membrane chloride conductance. A specific reduction in sarcolemmal chloride conductance has been found in intercostal muscle biopsies from these patients, through direct measurements using intracellular microelectrodes (Lipicky et al 1971, Lipicky & Bryant 1973).

Toxic myotonic syndromes. A number of

acquired myotonias are also directly due to reduced Cl⁻ conductance in the sarcolemma. For example, carboxylic acids have long been known to induce myotonia. In 1946, the herbicide, 2,4-dichlorophenoxyacetic acid (2,4-D), was reported to produce a myotonic syndrome in man after accidental ingestion (Bucher 1946). Subsequently a group of 33 related hydrocarbon- and halogen-substituted benzoic acids were shown to induce similar symptoms after intraperitoneal injection in animals (Tang et al 1968).

These carboxylic acids produce myotonia by specific block of Cl⁻ conductance pathways. In one study using rat muscle, 19 substituted benzoic acid derivatives reduced membrane Cl⁻ conductance in vitro in a dose-dependent manner, and the inhibitory constant for chloride channel block correlated closely with each compound's ability to produce myotonia both in vivo and in vitro (Palade & Barchi 1977b, Furman & Barchi 1978). At the single-cell level, the electrophysiological features of this myotonia are indistinguishable from those recorded in hereditary myotonia (Bryant 1982).

The physiological basis of myotonia with reduced chloride conductance

The origin of repetitive electrical activity. The repetitive electrical discharges seen in each of the above myotonic disorders can be explained on the basis of the marked reduction in membrane Cl⁻ conductance that they share. At the resting potential, muscle membranes are three to five times more permeable to Cl⁻ than to K⁺, while Na⁺ permeability accounts for less than 1% of the total membrane permeability (Hutter & Noble 1960, Palade & Barchi 1977a). As discussed above, the Na⁺ and K⁺ permeabilities undergo time- and voltage-dependent changes (in response to a depolarising stimulus) that result in the generation of an action potential, while Cl⁻ permeability remains relatively constant during the action potential and Cl⁻ fluxes passively follow cation movements.

During normal muscle activity, action potentials are propagated both longitudinally along the surface sarcolemma and radially into the fibre interior along elements of the T-tubular system.

With each action potential, small amounts of K⁺ move out of the cell while small amounts of Na⁺ and Cl⁻ move inwards. The K⁺ released into the large volume of the extracellular space has little effect on the overall K⁺ concentration, but the situation is different in the limited 'extracellular' volume of the T-tubular system. Measurements indicate that the efflux of K⁺ associated with a single action potential can increase its luminal concentration by 0.3 mM; this change could depolarise the T-tubular membrane by as much as 1.7 mV if the major conductance in the T-tubule were to K⁺ (Adrian & Bryant 1974). With multiple action potentials, the cumulative effect of this intraluminal K⁺ accumulation could be a membrane depolarisation of 10 mV or more.

Under normal conditions, this depolarisation is not reflected in the surface membrane potential because of the large stabilising Cl⁻ conductance that is present in the sarcolemma. In the absence of this Cl⁻ shunt, however, the K⁺ accumulation in the T-tubular lumen produced by a series of action potentials can locally depolarise the surface membrane sufficiently to initiate self-sustaining action potentials (Fig. 10.8). The observed increase in the after-potential of 1 mV per impulse seen in myotonic fibres is compatible with this mechanism (Adrian & Bryant 1974). A study showing that potassium diffuses from the T-tubule with a time constant of 0.4 s (Almers 1972) compares favourably with the after-potential decay time of 0.5 s observed in intact muscle fibres.

The behaviour of myotonic fibres can be reproduced in normal skeletal muscle fibres by blocking Cl⁻ conductance through substitution of an impermeant anion for Cl⁻ (Rudel & Senges 1972) or by specific Cl⁻ channel-blocking compounds (Furman & Barchi 1978). Disconnecting the T-tubular system from the surface membrane by glycerol shock abolishes the long-lasting, depolarising after-potential and sustained spontaneous activity produced by these compounds (Adrian & Bryant 1974), underscoring the importance of the T-tubular system in the generation of this repetitive activity. Figure 10.9 summarises several mechanisms that might lead to the reduced Cl⁻ conductance observed in the membranes of the above myotonic diseases.

The sequence of events in the low chloride-

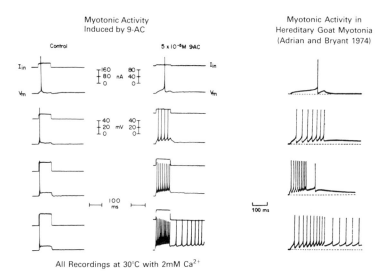

Myotonic Activity
Induced by 9-AC

Myotonic Activity in
Hereditary Goat Myotonia
(Adrian and Bryant 1974)

All Recordings at 30°C with 2mM Ca²⁺

Fig. 10.8 Inherited and acquired myotonic syndromes associated with a reduction in membrane chloride conductance appear very similar at the single cell level. In normal muscle fibres, an intracellular microelectrode will record one or a small number of rapidly accomodating action potentials in response to a depolarising current pulse. In hereditary goat myotonia, or experimental myotonia produced with inhibitors of membrane chloride conductance, depolarisation produces multiple driven action potentials and a prolonged after-depolarisation. If this after-depolarisation exceeds a critical level, continuous self-sustaining action potentials will continue after the depolarising pulse is stopped; this represents myotonia at the single-cell level. Reproduced with permission from Furman & Barchi (1986)

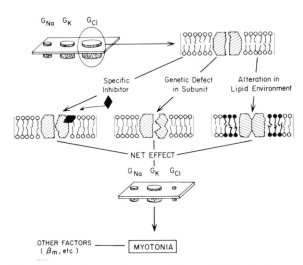

Fig. 10.9 The best-studied group of myotonic disorders is characterised by a pathological reduction in membrane chloride conductance (see Table 10.1). Even within this group, however, there are multiple mechanisms that can ultimately lead to the same membrane abnormality. Chloride channels may be genetically abnormal, or may be specifically blocked by some exogenous or endogenous agent. Alternatively, normal channels might be induced to behave abnormally by an alteration in the membrane-lipid environment in which they reside. In each case the end result is membrane hyperexcitability and clinical myotonia. Reproduced with permission from Furman & Barchi (1986)

conductance myotonias appears to be as follows. Voluntary contraction of a skeletal muscle produces multiple action potentials which originate at the end-plate, propagate along the muscle fibre, and invade the T-tubular system. Each of these action potentials results in a small increase in the T-tubular K^+ concentration. Because of the markedly reduced Cl^- conductance, the effect of this increase in extracellular K^+ is a slight depolarisation. This depolarisation is not large enough to force sodium channels into an inactivated state; rather, as they recover from the normal inactivation that occurs during the depolarisation of the action potential itself, some channels will begin to reopen as a result of this slight depolarisation. Because the sum of opposing currents is much reduced by the lack of a significant Cl^- conductance, the resultant small inward Na^+ current can again initiate depolarisation and recruitment of additional channels so that another action potential develops. The net result of this process is that each action potential creates a transient after-depolarisation that in turn acts as a stimulus for the triggering of the next action potential in the sequence. As long as no channel kinetic parameters are altered, this repetitive chain of potentials can continue indefinitely.

Termination of the myotonic discharge. Results of computer modelling with skeletal muscles confirm the plausibility of this Cl^- hypothesis and indicate that repetitive activity can occur when the membrane Cl^- conductance is reduced to about 15% of normal, a value near the residual conductance found in these myotonic syndromes (Bretag 1973, Barchi 1975, Adrian & Marshall 1976). This modelling has been useful in demonstrating the sensitivity of the repetitive activity to minor changes in sodium channel kinetic parameters; e.g. a slight reduction in the rate recovery from inactivation can completely abolish myotonic activity in spite of a very low Cl^- conductance. In addition, since the magnitude of the actual depolarisation which occurs depends on the K^+ equilibrium potential, small changes in the concentration of K^+ bathing the sarcolemma itself can prevent the appearance of repetitive activity. For example, a slight reduction in external K^+, of a magnitude expected with the activation of the Na^+-K^+-ATPase, will block repetitive firing, as well as the slight hyperpolarisation produced by the electrogenic activity of this pump.

Although the precise factors that alter the frequency of a myotonic discharge and ultimately cause it to stop in a given fibre are unknown, it is easy to speculate on how one or more of these factors could be involved. Continued muscular activity will certainly result in the influx of sufficient Na^+ to activate the Na^+-K^+-ATPase. This activation will have a hyperpolarising electrogenic component, and could as well result in the transient decline in local K^+ concentration outside the sarcolemma. Both factors will slow down the frequency of, or stop, the myotonic discharge. Furthermore, the kinetic parameters of normal sodium channels vary over a considerable range and are probably modulated by cellular processes such as phosphorylation that remain to be completely elucidated. This sort of modulation could also play an important role in modifying myotonic activity.

Hyperactivity vs. paralysis. Why does the depolarisation following an action potential in a myotonic discharge produce hyperexcitability while the depolarisation associated with periodic paralysis results in the loss of all electrical excitability? Part of the answer lies in the magnitude of the depolarisation. In myotonia, the depolarisations are small; they are sufficient to cause some channel activation, yet not large enough to cause a significant increase in steady-state inactivation. A second component is the time-scale on which the depolarisation takes place. The process of channel activation occurs much more rapidly than inactivation; if this were not so, sodium channels would never open during depolarisation, and an action potential could not be produced. With brief depolarisations, activation tends to predominate. Longer depolarisations will eventually lead to inactivation. In myotonia, these depolarising afterpotentials last only for tens of milliseconds. In the periodic paralyses, the magnitude of depolarisation is greater and the duration is essentially indefinite. Here the steady-state effects predominate, and the influence of channel inactivation is the controlling factor. At the onset of membrane depolarisation in periodic paralysis, one might expect transient hyperexcitability if the critical criteria of rapidity and extent are satisfied. Indeed, in at least one form of hyperkalaemic periodic paralysis, hyperirritability and myotonic symptoms immediately precede the development of paralysis. In several other of the periodic paralyses, symptoms of myotonia can be seen in the interictal stages.

Other mechanisms producing membrane hyperexcitability

Low membrane chloride conductance is a common factor that ties together a number of the myotonic disorders, but it certainly does not explain all of them. In myotonic dystrophy, the most common of the human muscle diseases in which myotonia is a major feature, membrane chloride conductance is normal or only slightly reduced (Lipicky 1977). In myotonia produced by 20,25-diazacholesterol, an inhibitor of cholesterol biosynthesis, repetitive electrical activity is again found, although the chloride conductance is reduced only slightly (Furman & Barchi 1981).

Although the exact defect that produces the

myotonic activity in these disorders remains to be elucidated, it is clear that other factors in addition to alterations in Cl⁻ conductance can induce repetitive activity in skeletal muscle. One prominent mechanism by which repetitive activity can be produced is an alteration in the kinetics of channel inactivation. A number of polypeptide neurotoxins that kill by interacting with the sodium channel do so by reducing or eliminating channel inactivation. These toxins characteristically produce repetitive action potentials in excitable membranes that are exposed to them. Similar repetitive activity follows the application of alkaloid toxins such as veratridine or batrachotoxin to muscle; again, the principal effect of these compounds is on sodium channel inactivation.

Any factor that delays the rate or extent of channel inactivation is a potential candidate for the production of repetitive electrical activity. With the failure of sodium inactivation, the repolarisation produced by the activation of potassium channels is incomplete, closed sodium channels are immediately available for activation, and opened, non-inactivated channels can contribute directly to the initiation of a new depolarisation phase. These factors could be exogenous, as with the neurotoxins, or could represent endogenous defects in the channel structure or its environment. It is the latter consideration which has made the concept of a generalised defect in the membrane lipid environment so attractive a hypothesis in myotonic muscular dystrophy.

Factors involving channels other than the sodium or chloride channel may also be implicated in the generation of repetitive electrical activity. For example, a common mechanism for periodic bursting activity in neurones and for rhythmical electrical discharges in cardiac pacemaking cells involves the modulation of calcium-dependent K^+ conductances. However, none of these potential mechanisms has yet been implicated in the production of human myotonic activity. Working out the mechanism of myotonia in myotonic dystrophy remains an elusive yet fertile area for future research.

THE FUTURE

It is clear that a number of neuromuscular diseases involve either primary or secondary defects in membrane ion channels. In the past these channels were difficult to study, especially in human skeletal muscle. Most observations were indirect, and restricted to the electrophysiological measurements of the transmembrane currents that the channels control.

That situation is rapidly changing. Biochemical approaches to the isolation and characterisation of a number of these channels have already been devised, and immunochemical techniques that allow channel isolation from small quantities of tissue are a reality. Details of channel structure can be derived through analysis of channel primary sequences, as deduced from the cloning of messenger RNA or analysis of the genomic DNA; again, such techniques are now applicable to small amounts of tissue and will be invaluable for probing the structure of defective ion channels. Patch clamp methods allow individual ion channels to be studied directly in the muscle membrane, and reconstitution techniques make it possible to measure the single-channel electrophysiological properties of ion channels after purification.

The stage is now set for rapid advances in the study of these disorders characterised by hyperexcitability or hypoexcitability of the muscle membrane and for direct analysis of the relationships between abnormal structure and function in the channel proteins themselves.

REFERENCES

Adrian R H, Chandler W K, Hodgkin A L 1970 Voltage clamp experiments in striated muscle fibers. Journal of Physiology 208: 607–644

Adrian R H, Bryant S H 1974 On the repetitive discharge in myotonic muscle fibres. Journal of Physiology (London) 240: 505–515

Adrian R H, Marshall M W 1976 Action potentials reconstructed in normal and myotonic muscle fibers. Journal of Physiology (London) 258: 125–143

Adrian R H, Marshall M W 1977 Sodium currents in mammalian muscle. Journal of Physiology (London) 268: 233–250

Agnew W 1984 Voltage-regulated sodium channel molecules. Annual Review of Physiology 46: 517–530

Almers W 1972 Potassium conductance changes in skeletal muscle and the potassium concentration in the transverse tubules. Journal of Physiology (London) 225: 33–56

Barchi R L 1975 Myotonia: An evaluation of the chloride hypothesis. Archives of Neurology 32: 175–180

Barchi R L 1980 Excitation and conduction in nerve. In: Sumner A J (ed) The physiology of peripheral nerve disease. W B Saunders, Philadelphia p 1–40

Barchi R L 1982 A mechanistic approach to the myotonic syndromes. Muscle and Nerve 5 Suppl 9: s60–s63

Barchi R L 1986 The biochemistry of sodium channels from mammalian muscle. Annals of the New York Academy of Sciences 479: 179–185

Barchi R L, Casadei J, Gordon R D, Roberts R H 1986 Voltage-sensitive sodium channels; an evolving molecular view. In: Hille, Fambrough (eds) Proteins in excitable membranes. John Wiley, New York

Bretag A H 1973 Mathematical modelling of the myotonic action potential. In: Desmedt J E (ed) New developments in electromyography and clinical neurophysiology vol. 1. Karger, Basel

Brown G L, Harvey A M 1939 Congenital myotonia in the goat. Brain 62: 341–363

Bryant S H 1979 Myotonia in the goat. Annals of the New York Academy of Sciences 317: 314–324

Bryant S H 1982 Abnormal repetitive impulse production in myotonic muscle. In: Culp, Ochoa (eds) Abnormal nerves and muscles as impulse generators. Oxford University Press, New York p 702–725

Bryant S H, Morales-Aguilera A 1971 Chloride conductance in normal and myotonic muscle fibres and the action of monocarboxylic aromatic acids. Journal of Physiology (London) 219: 367–383

Bryant S H, DeCoursey T E 1980 Sodium currents in cut skeletal muscle fibres from normal and myotonic goats. (abstract). Journal of Physiology (London) 307: 31p–32p

Bryant S H, Owenburg K 1980 Characteristics of the chloride channel in skeletal-muscle fibers from myotonic and normal goats. Federation Proceedings 39: 579–579

Bucher N L 1946 Effects of 2,4-dichlorophenoxyacetic acid on experimental animals. Proceedings of the Society for Experimental Biology and Medicine 63: 204–205

Creutzfeldt O D, Abbott B C, Fowler W M, Pearson C M 1963 Muscle membrane potentials in episodic adynamia. Electroencephalography and Clinical Neurophysiology 15: 508–519

Engel A G, Lambert E H 1969 Calcium activation of electrically inexcitable muscle fibers in primary hypokalemic periodic paralysis. Neurology 19: 851–858

Franzini-Armstrong C, Peachey L D 1981 Striated muscle — contractile and control mechanisms. Journal of Cell Biology 91: 166S–186S

French R J, Horn R 1983 Sodium channel gating: models, mimics and modifiers. Annual Review of Biophysics and Bioengineering 12: 319–356

Furman R E, Barchi R L 1978 The pathophysiology of myotonia produced by aromatic carboxylic acids. Annals of Neurology 4: 357–365

Furman R E, Barchi R L 1981 20,25-diazacholesterol myotonia: An electrophysiological study. Annals of Neurology 10: 251–260

Furman R E, Barchi R L 1986 Hyperexcitable and hypoexcitable states in muscle: Myotonia and periodic paralysis. In: Asbury, McKhann, McDonald, (eds) Diseases of the nervous system. W B Saunders, Philadelphia

Furman R E, Tanaka J C, Meuller P, Barchi R L 1986 Voltage-dependent activation in purified reconstituted sodium channels from rabbit T-tubular membranes. Proceedings of the National Academy of Sciences USA 83: 448–492

Gallant E M 1983 Barium-treated mammalian skeletal muscle: similarities to hypokalaemic periodic paralysis. Journal of Physiology (London) 335: 577–590

Gordon A M, Green J R, Lagunoff D 1970 Studies on a patient with hypokalaemic familial periodic paralysis. American Journal of Medicine 48: 185–195

Guy H R, Seetharamulu P 1986 Molecular model of the action potential sodium channel. Proceedings of the National Academy of Sciences USA 83: 508–512

Hodgkin A L, Huxley A F 1952 A quantitative description of membrane current and its application to conduction and excitation in nerve. Journal of Physiology (London) 117: 500–544

Hofmann W W, Smith R A 1970 Hypokalemic periodic paralysis studied in vitro. Brain 93: 445–474

Horn R, Patlack J 1980 Single channel currents from excised patches of muscle membrane. Proceedings of the National Academy of Sciences USA 11: 6930–6934

Hutter O F, Noble D 1960 The chloride conductance of frog skeletal muscle. Journal of Physiology (London) 151: 89–102

Jorgensen P L 1982 Mechanism of the Na^+K^+ pump. Protein structure and conformations of the pure Na^+K^+ATPase. Biochimica et Biophysica Acta 694: 27–68

Kao I, Gordon A M 1975 Mechanism of insulin-produced paralysis of muscle from potassium-depleted rats. Science 188: 740–741

Kraner S D, Tanaka J C, Barchi R L 1985 Purification and functional reconstitution of the voltage-sensitive sodium channel from rabbit T-tubular membranes. Journal of Biological Chemistry 260: 6341–6347

Lehmann-Horn F, Rudel R, Dengler R, Lorkovic H, Hass A, Ricker K 1981 Membrane defects in paramyotonia congenita with and without myotonia in a warm environment. Muscle and Nerve 4: 396–406

Lehmann-Horn F, Rudel R, Ricker K, Lorkovic H, Dengler R, Hopf H C 1983 Two cases of adynamia episodica hereditaria: in vitro investigation of muscle cell membrane and contraction parameters. Muscle and Nerve 6: 113–121

Lipicky R J 1977 Studies in human myotonic dystrophy. In: Rowland L P (ed) Pathogenesis of human muscular dystrophies. Excerpta Medica, Amsterdam

Lipicky R J, Bryant S H, Salmon J H 1971 Cable parameters, sodium, potassium, chloride and water content, and potassium efflux in isolated external intercostal muscles of normal volunteers and patients with myotonia congenita. Journal of Clinical Investigation 50: 2091–2103

Lipicky R J, Bryant S H 1973 A biophysical study of human myotonias. In: Desmedt J E (ed) New developments in electromyography and clinical neurophysiology vol 1. Karger, Basel

McComas A J, Mrozek K, Bradley W G 1968 The nature of the electrophysiological disorder in adynamia episodica. Journal of Neurology, Neurosurgery and Psychiatry 31: 448–452

Neher E, Sakmann B 1976 Single channel currents recorded

from the membrane of denervated frog muscle fibers. Nature (London) 260: 799–802

Noda M, Shimizu S, Tanabe T et al 1984 Primary structure of the Electrophorus electricus sodium channel deduced from cDNA sequence. New Biology and Nature 312: 121–127

Palade P T, Barchi R L 1977a Characteristics of the chloride conductance in muscle fibers of the rat diaphragm. Journal of General Physiology 69: 325–342

Palade P T, Barchi R L 1977b On the inhibition of muscle membrane chloride conductances by aromatic carboxylic acids. Journal of General Physiology 69: 875–896

Riecker G, Bolte H D 1966 Membranpotentiale einzelner Skeletmuskelzellen bei hypokalamischer periodischer Muskelparalyse. Klinische Wochenschrift 44: 804–807

Rudel R, Senges J 1972 Experimental myotonia in mammalian skeletal muscle. Changes in membrane properties. Pfluegers Archiv 331: 324–334

Rudel R, Lehmann-Horn F, Ricker K, Kuther G 1984 Hypokalemic periodic paralysis: in vitro investigation of muscle fiber membrane parameters. Muscle and Nerve 7: 110–120

Rudel R, Lehmann-Horn F 1985 Membrane changes in cells from myotonia patients. Physiological Review 65: 310–346

Rudel R, Ricker K 1985 The primary periodic paralyses. TINS, Nov, p 467–470

Shy G M, Wanko T, Rowley P T, Engel A G 1961 Studies in familial periodic paralysis. Experimental Neorology 3: 53–121

Swift L L, Atkinson J B, Lequire V S 1979 Composition and calcium-transport activity of the sarcoplasmic-reticulum from goats with and without heritable myotonia. Laboratory Investigation 40: 384–390

Tanaka J C, Eccleston J F, Barchi R L 1983 Cation selectivity characteristics of the reconstituted sodium channel from rat skeletal muscle sarcolemma. Journal of Biological Chemistry 258: 7519–7526

Tang A H, Schroeder L A, Keasling H H 1968 U-23,223 (3-chloro-2,5,6-trimethylbenzoic acid), a veratrinic agent selective for the skeletal muscles. Archives Internationales de Pharmacodynamie et de Therapie 175: 319–329

Weigele J B, Barchi R L 1982 Functional reconstitution of the purified sodium channel protein from rat sarcolemma. Proceedings of the National Academy of Sciences USA 79: 3651–3655

Wood D S, Lipicky R J, Bryant S H 1980 Myotonic dystrophy: In vitro physiologic analysis of intact and skinned fibers. Neurology 30: 423–432

Cell biology in relation to neuromuscular disease

INTRODUCTION

Diseased cells in the body are exposed to complex influences which make it difficult to decide whether abnormalities detected are primary lesions. This problem is overcome by isolating and culturing cells in vitro where absence of differences between cultures of diseased and normal cells would suggest that either the disorder is not a primary lesion of that tissue, or that factors present in or absent from the culture environment have prevented full expression of the pathological process. Continued expression of abnormality in cultured cells would suggest, however, that the lesion is intrinsic to the cells.

The first section of this chapter considers those tissue-culture investigations which have increased basic understanding of the process of differentiation of normal muscle cells and especially of the intrinsic and extrinsic factors which affect muscle cell gene expression. In many cases resolution of the molecular events underlying differentiation has been made possible only by the technical advantages of the tissue culture system. The second section deals with tissue culture investigations of specific muscle diseases.

DIFFERENTIATION OF THE NORMAL MUSCLE CELL IN TISSUE CULTURE

Mononucleated cells migrating from the cut surface of vertebrate muscle fragments or released from muscle tissue by enzyme digestion will, under appropriate tissue culture conditions, divide, fuse and differentiate to form syncytial myotubes which contain muscle-specific proteins and may contract spontaneously. In mixed cultures of muscle and nerve cells, functional neuromuscular junctions may be formed.

There are a number of advantages in investigating myogenesis in tissue culture:

1. The cells differentiate more rapidly and with a greater degree of synchrony than in vivo.
2. The living cells are obtained in thin layers, usually only one cell thick and extended in one plane of focus upon a transparent surface and are therefore most suitable for microscopic examination and electrophysiological experiments when alive, or histochemical, immunochemical and autoradiographic experiments when fixed.
3. The closed in vitro system provided by tissue culture makes it particularly easy to control environmental conditions. The closed system is also particularly suitable for the administration of radioactive precursors, testing of drugs, growth and differentiation factors.
4. Methods for obtaining cultures of pure myogenic cells (by cloning or establishment of cell lines) make it possible to investigate myogenesis in the absence of other cells which are usually closely associated with muscle cells in vivo and which may influence events.

Two techniques have been widely used for setting up cultures of muscle cells:

1. The explant technique, in which fragments of muscle, sometimes embedded in a thin layer of clotted plasma, are immersed in tissue culture medium (Carrel 1924) so that mononucleate myogenic cells (myoblasts) emigrate from the cut surface of the fragment (explant). Until relatively recently this was the only successful method for culturing fully differentiated muscle. It was therefore useful in the investigation of those myopathies in which abnormalities are manifested only in late development (Bishop et al 1971, Witkowski et al 1976).
2. The disaggregation technique, in which proteolytic enzymes are used to digest away the intercellular material, reducing the muscle to a suspension of single cells which are seeded out in tissue culture (Moscona & Moscona 1952, Rinaldini 1959, Bischoff 1974, Yasin et al 1976).

From the point where mononucleate cells are obtained in a monolayer on the surface of the tissue culture dishes the process of myogenesis is similar, following either method of establishing

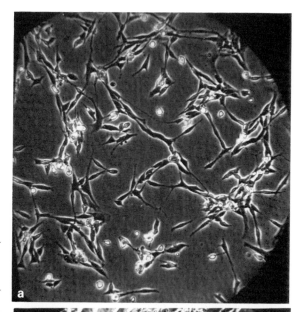

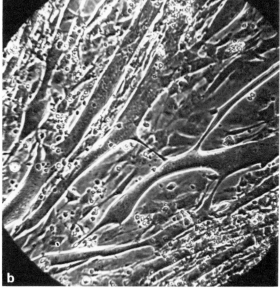

Fig. 11.1 a. Rat myoblasts on the point of fusing. Cells were disaggregated from neo-natal rat muscle by trypsinisation. After two days of proliferation in culture, the cells were detached from the dishes by trypsinisation and the fibroblasts removed from suspension by the 'differential adhesion' method (Yaffe 1968). The myoblasts were then allowed to attach to gelatin-coated culture dishes and grown for a further one day. b. Rat myotubes, differentiated after a further three days

the culture. After a period of cell division, the cells align (Fig. 11.1a) and then undergo fusion to form multinucleate syncytia which further differentiate into myotubes (Fig. 11.1b).

For details of methods the reader is referred to monographs on tissue culture technique by Paul (1970) and Freshney (1983). Techniques for treatment of muscle tissue to obtain myogenic cultures, culture media and methods for preparing pure cultures of muscle cells were reviewed by Witkowski (1977).

Origin of myoblasts

The myoblasts that grow in tissue culture originate either from embryonic or from adult muscle. In rapidly growing embryonic muscle in vivo there are large numbers of dividing myoblasts of recent mesenchymal origin. Hauschka (1974a,b) carried out cell-cloning experiments to estimate proportions of myoblasts present in human fetal limbs of different ages. Muscle cells were prepared by enzymatic disaggregation and plated at cloning densities. The percentage of clones containing myotubes rose from 12% at 31 days' gestation to 90% at 172 days and the plating efficiency rose from 1% to 24% at 88 days' gestation.

Until relatively recently the source of the myogenic cells which grow in tissue culture from adult muscle was not certain. Mauro (1961), in the course of an electron-microscopic study of frog muscle, discovered separate cellular elements in muscle fibres lying within the sarcolemmal membrane but separated from the muscle syncytium by their own membranes, which he named 'satellite cells'. Evidence has now accumulated from studies of muscle regeneration in vivo to suggest that these satellite cells are the main source from which myoblasts in regenerating muscle are derived (see Ch. 1, Ch. 2).

Evidence from tissue-culture experiments also supports the role of the satellite cells in muscle regeneration. Segments of individual differentiated fibres have been dissected and cultured from muscle of quail (Konigsberg et al 1975), rat (Bischoff 1975) and human (Witkowski 1977, p 458). During the first few hours in tissue culture, the fibre showed degenerative changes including the formation of myofibrillar contraction clots and pyknosis of most nuclei. The endomysial tube (basement lamina) remained intact along the entire length of the fibre. Those nuclei which survived were found to be contained within separate mononucleated cells closely applied to and within the endomysial tube. An examination of the fine structure of the mononucleate cells that survived degeneration showed them to be separate, mononucleated cells contained within the basement lamina of the degenerating fibre. These cells were identical (on the basis of their ultrastructure as well as their location) to satellite cells associated with muscle fibres in the source tissue (Konigsberg et al 1975). Regeneration activity seemed to be of two types: quail fibre mononucleate cells divided and cells migrated out from the endomysial tube to form a colony of cells which could undergo myotube formation (Konigsberg et al 1975); rat mononucleate cells divided and remained within the endomysial tube and the satellite-cell progeny began to fuse to form myotubes within the endomysial tube of the original fibre (Bischoff 1975). The myotubes displayed spontaneous contractile activity and extended throughout the length of the endomysial tube.

Trupin et al (1982) investigated the relative contribution of satellite cells and myotubes from neonatal rat muscle during myogenesis in vitro and confirmed results of in vivo autoradiographic studies indicating that satellite cells are the only significant source of regenerating myoblasts in muscle tissue.

Identification of mononucleate cells

Much attention has been given to distinguishing between different mononucleate cells in the stages of culture before the fusion of myoblasts to form myotubes.

Konigsberg (1963) attempted to distinguish myoblasts from fibroblasts of embryonic chick using the method of 'clonal analysis', by which the cells were first separated individually by trypsinisation and then separately plated out at very low density in a culture medium. Many of these cells were then observed to undergo a succession of mitoses to form 'clones' or individual colonies of cells each derived from a single separated cell. These colonies were found to be of two types:

1. Colonies of rather flattened cells that stayed separate from one another and exhibited extensive 'ruffled membranes' at their borders, which were designated 'fibroblasts' (see Fig. 11.2a).
2. Colonies of cells that were most usually fusiform or spindle-shaped with very small regions of 'ruffled membrane' confined to their ends, and which, after ceasing to divide, began fusing with each other to form syncytia in a manner characteristic of the normal pattern of myogenesis. These were designated 'myoblasts' (see Fig. 11.2b).

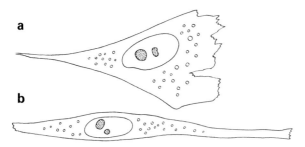

Fig. 11.2 Typical shapes assumed by fibroblasts and by myoblasts in cultures of cells from chick embryo muscle explants, as determined by Konigsberg's cloning techniques: a. typical spread-out fibroblast, b. typical spindle-shaped myoblast

Konigsberg (1963) recorded that in most cases the final character of a colony could be predicted by the morphological appearance of the parent cell of the clone before it began to divide. The results show that, of the 1313 colonies that grew successfully from single cells, 96.5% of the elongated fusiform-shaped cells (Fig. 11.2b) produced colonies of fusing myoblasts, and 85% of the more flattened irregular-shaped cells (Fig. 11.2a) produced colonies of non-fusing cells thereby defined as fibroblasts. Thus, one in 35 of the 'myoblast-like' cells might be expected to be a fibroblast and one in six of the 'fibroblast-like' cells could, conversely, be expected to be a myoblast, which shows that a high degree of correct designation of chick cells is possible on the basis of cell morphology.

A different approach has been used to identify cells by Goyle et al (1973). The morphology of the cells growing from explanted muscle biopsies was compared with that of lipocytes growing from subcutaneous fat explants and of fibroblasts growing from fascia. The lipocytes in young cultures were elongated narrow highly refractile uni- or multinucleated cells with round or oval nuclei. As these cells aged their cytoplasm tended to retract towards the nucleus and they appeared rounded. The young fibroblasts were broader cells with central spherical nuclei and occasionally binucleate cells were seen. The fibroblasts tended to retain their shape as the culture advanced in age. These morphological criteria were used to identify cells migrating from muscle explants.

Morphological criteria are evidently not an entirely dependable means for identifying individual cells in a mixed culture because a cell may sometimes assume uncharacteristic shapes and therefore at any given time a proportion of the cells in a culture will be liable to misclassification. Human myoblasts are flatter than those of rats, mice and birds and for these the only time to distinguish with certainty even clonal colonies of myoblasts is when they have actually shown some differentiation into myotubes. Binucleate cells can arise in cultures of fibroblasts and a cell should possess at least three morphologically normal nuclei before being classified as a myotube. Richler & Yaffe (1970) have commented on the variability of the phenotype even in cloned myogenic cells (i.e. derived from a single cell).

Inheritance of the epigenetic state

One of the remarkable things about the differentiation of cells is that, in many cases, once a cell has been induced to take up a differentiated state it can divide repeatedly and still apparently 'remember' its particular state of differentiation. The fact that, e.g. a muscle cell can reproduce itself under relatively non-specific culture conditions without converting to some other cell type, suggests that muscle cells in vivo are not being continuously induced by humoral influences to maintain their particular state of differentiation. In some way the differentiated state is self-replicating.

An interesting approach to understanding how the state of differentiation is 'remembered' (inheritance of the epigenetic state) has been made in experiments in which muscle cells are induced to fuse with non-muscle cells. Two techniques have been used. In the first, cells were fused by treatment with inactivated Sendai virus (Harris et al 1966) or polyethylene glycol (Konieczny et al 1983) to form heterokaryons in which nuclei from the two donor cells are present in a common cytoplasm derived from both cells. More recently it was shown that intact cells can be reconstituted by fusion of nuclei (mini cells, which make a minimal contribution of cytoplasm) from enucleated cells and cytoplasm from enucleated cells (Ringertz et al 1978).

Carlsson et al (1974a) found that the dormant nucleus of a chick erythrocyte was reactivated when the erythrocyte was fused with a rat myoblast. Activation of both RNA and DNA synthesis was observed. Rat antigens characteristic of nucleoplasm and nucleoli migrated into chick erythrocyte nuclei in rat myoblast x chick erythrocyte heterokaryons. It was postulated that these antigens might represent a class of molecules instrumental in activating chick genes and that, furthermore, the erythrocyte nuclei might possibly be reprogrammed to express the same genes as the rat nuclei which specified the migrating molecules. However, chick myosin could not be detected in the heterokaryons by immunological methods (Carlsson et al 1974b) suggesting that signals controlling the muscle-specific genes present in rat muscle cells were not received and acted upon by chicken erythrocyte nuclei. This lack of response might have been because the nuclei were from cells (erythrocytes) that had undergone terminal differentiation. Linder et al (1979) therefore tested the nuclei of multipotent stem cells to see whether they would respond to gene-regulatory signals present in the foreign cytoplasm. The gene-expression pattern of a mouse embryonal carcinoma cell nucleus was not detectably altered by exposure to myoblast cytoplasm.

Heterokaryons formed by fusing myoblasts at different stages of differentiation have been investigated (Konieczny et al 1983). The results suggest that, when present in a common cytoplasm, the regulatory factors that maintain myoblasts in a proliferating undifferentiated state are dominant over those that govern expression of differentiated gene products.

Myogenic functions are suppressed in heterokaryons formed by fusing differentiated chick myocytes and rat fibroblasts (Wright & Aranoff 1983). This is apparently not due to the influence of the fibroblast cytoplasm. When intact cells were reconstructed by fusion of nuclei from enucleated rat myoblasts with cytoplasm from enucleated mouse fibroblasts, clones derived from the reconstructed cells formed myotubes which produced myosin and developed the cross-striated pattern typical of skeletal muscle. The myogenic programme of the rat myoblast persisted through the enucleation and reconstitution procedures, and was not obviously altered by a period of exposure to mouse fibroblast cytoplasm (Ringertz et al 1978).

There are a few reports that the myogenic cell can forget its commitment to muscle differentiation and can transdifferentiate into another cell type. Schubert & Lacorbiere (1976) reported that the nicotinamide analogue 6-aminonicotinamide and cAMP inhibit myogenesis in a clonal rat cell line from skeletal muscle. Both reagents produced a similar morphological response and stimulated collagen and glycosaminoglycan synthesis, suggesting they had induced a phenotypic transformation of myogenic cells to cells that shared many characteristics with chondrocytes.

Critical final mitosis

Terminal differentiation of myogenic cultures is characterised by cell fusion to form multinucleated myotubes, cessation of DNA synthesis with irreversible withdrawal from the cell cycle and production of muscle-specific proteins.

There are two lines of evidence which demonstrate that, when myoblasts fuse into syncytia, the nuclei do not again divide. Firstly, nuclei within multinucleated myotubes do not incorporate tritiated thymidine into DNA nor are mitotic figures ever observed (Stockdale & Holtzer 1961). Secondly, microspectrophotometric measurements of DNA content per nucleus reveal that all the nuclei within multinucleated myotubes contain only the diploid (2n) complement of DNA (Strehler et al 1963).

Holtzer and his co-workers (Bischoff & Holtzer 1969, Holtzer et al 1972, Dienstmann & Holtzer

1977) have postulated that the transition of a myogenic cell from an actively dividing undifferentiated cell to a post-mitotic cell capable of fusion and biochemical differentiation follows a special mitosis ('quantal' mitosis) during which genes involved in cell proliferation are repressed and the genes needed for differentiation are switched on. The decision to differentiate is made during the phase of DNA synthesis (S) before the 'quantal' mitosis, and sets in motion the metabolic steps required for the subsequent fusion and biochemical differentiation which start during the G_1 phase after 'quantal' division. The major rearrangement of chromatin that occurs during S may make it a particularly suitable time for extensive changes in the genetic programme needed for differentiation. Gurdon & Woodland (1968) have also proposed that a critical mitosis may precede differentiation. They argued that, only during mitosis, when the nuclear membrane disappears transiently, can proteins easily leave the nucleus and new proteins responsible for reprogramming the genes can move from the cytoplasm and bind to the decondensing chromosomes.

Holtzer and his co-workers postulated that the dividing undifferentiated myogenic cell cannot transform into the post-mitotic myoblast without undergoing the critical 'quantal' mitosis. After the 'quantal' mitosis, one or both of the daughter cells is a post-mitotic myoblast. The theory predicts that myogenic cells have only one pathway open to them — either to divide or to differentiate — but not both.

The fact that the tissue-culture environment can be manipulated so that cultured cells will either multiply or differentiate makes it possible to test the quantal mitosis theory. Some investigators (O'Neill & Stockdale 1972, Buckley & Konigsberg 1974) found that chick myogenic cultures which had ceased proliferating and in which differentiation was imminent, and which would presumably have undergone 'quantal' mitosis, could be stimulated to more DNA synthesis and cell division if they were given fresh medium. Inhibition of DNA synthesis did not prevent cell fusion (Doehring & Fischman 1974). More recently, Nadal-Ginard (1978) found that DNA synthesis was not required to switch from growth to differentiation and that, after cell division, rat myogenic

cell line myoblasts had the option either to fuse or to proliferate without intervening DNA synthesis. Furthermore, commitment to differentiation occurred in the G_1 before fusion. In contrast, Dienstmann & Holtzer (1977) found that daily feeding did not prevent fusion and inhibition of DNA synthesis in cells that normally would have multiplied in vitro did not prompt these cells to fuse.

Buckley & Konigsberg (1977) have presented data suggesting that, in vivo, myogenic cells do not withdraw from the cell cycle before fusion, but as a consequence of fusion. According to these investigators, the probability that a cell will fuse is directly correlated to the length of time it spends in G_1 (Buckley & Konigsberg 1974, Konigsberg et al 1978).

Signals for cell fusion

Little is known about the signals which may induce dividing myoblasts to begin fusing.

Zalin & Montague (1974) observed a 10–15-fold spontaneous but transient increase in intracellular cyclic AMP 5–6 h before the onset of fusion in primary chick myoblasts. This correlated with an increase in the activity of adenylate cyclase, the enzyme responsible for the synthesis of cAMP. Adenylate cyclase is embedded in the outer cell membrane in close association with the receptor sites of different kinds of regulatory molecules such as hormones and prostaglandins. Physiological concentrations of prostaglandin E, added to cultures, produced a similar intracellular increase in cAMP, 4 h earlier than that occurring normally, and brought forward the fusion process by a corresponding 4 h. These results suggested that cAMP is acting as a signal for muscle-cell fusion. Two inhibitors of prostaglandin synthesis produced a marked inhibition of cell fusion which it was possible to reverse by the further addition of prostaglandin E_1 (Zalin 1977). These findings provided evidence of prostaglandin synthesis in cultures and suggested that prostaglandin E_1 is required for the generation of a transient increase in intracellular cyclic AMP, which brings about the cellular changes necessary for fusion to occur.

Cyclic AMP is known to exert control by activating an enzyme called protein kinase which transfers a phosphate group to other enzymes (phosphorylation), thus activating them. Scott & Dousa (1978) have shown that some cAMP-dependent protein phosphorylation enzymes are tightly bound to the plasma membrane in myoblasts of the L_6 cell line.

Myoblast fusion

In vivo the cytoplasmic fusion of a large number of mononucleate myoblasts produces a bipolar syncytium several thousand microns long. Myogenic cell fusion in tissue culture has been investigated at the morphological and biochemical levels.

Scanning electron microscope studies of chick myoblasts (Huang et al 1978) showed that spindle-shaped myogenic cells extend microprocesses (150 μm long) which contact and adhere to microprocesses from adjacent cells. Thickening of fused processes occurred as the cells became closer to one another and finally coalesced. Indirect immunofluorescence assay with actin-specific antibody indicated that actin was a major component of the myoblast microprocesses. The occurrence of microvilli or blebs in mammalian myoblasts seems to be more variable (Dupont et al 1979).

Kalderon & Gilula (1979) observed by freeze-fracture scanning electron microscopy and transmission electron microscopy that formation of particle-free domains in the plasma membrane may originate from the fusion of the plasma membrane with submembraneous vesicles. Apposition of these particle-free regions on adjacent interacting cells could then result in cell fusion.

When muscle cells fused to form a multinucleated myotube, their skeletal framework (composed of internal structural fibres, microtrabeculae and the surface lamina) reorganised extensively (Fulton et al 1981). When myoblasts prepared to fuse, the previously continuous surface lamina developed numerous lacunae. The retention of iodinated surface proteins suggested that the lacunae were not formed by the extraction of lamina proteins. The lacunae were probably regions of lipid bilayer devoid of glycoproteins which appeared to be related to fusion and disappeared rapidly after the multinucleate myotube was formed. When muscle cells fused, their internal structural networks interconnected to

form the framework of the myotube. Transmission electron microscopy of skeletal framework whole mounts showed that proliferating myoblasts have a well developed and highly interconnected internal network. Immediately before fusion, these networks were extensively reorganised and destabilised. After fusion, a stable, extensively cross-linked internal structure was reformed, but with a morphology characteristic of the myotube. Muscle cells therefore undergo extensive reorganisation both on the surface and internally at the time of fusion.

Earlier analyses of the cell membrane composition of muscle cells at different stages of differentiation in culture did not reveal major changes in lipid composition (Kent et al 1974) or the activities of phosphatidic acid phosphatase and phospholipase A (Kent & Vagelos 1976). In contrast, the ganglioside content showed changes during differentiation. Cloned cells of a myoblast line showed the presence of GM_3, GM_2, GM_1, and GD_{1a} gangliosides (Whatley et al 1976). The amount of GM_3, GM_2 and GM_1 gangliosides did not vary significantly during the differentiation of myoblasts to myotubes. However, the concentration of GD_{1a} transiently increased almost three-fold just before the fusion of myoblasts, and returned to the basal levels in the myotubes. Mutant myoblasts, selected for 5-azacytidine resistance and unable to fuse, produced only GM_3 and traces of GM_2. It was concluded that GD_{1a} probably participates in the fusion process.

Cell-surface antigens that are specific to various stages of myogenesis have been reported (Friedlander & Fischman 1979, Lee & Kaufman 1981). Use of monoclonal antibodies has shown that some antigenic determinants are highly specific for myoblasts (Grove & Stockdale 1979, Walsh & Ritter 1981, Horowitz et al 1982). The recognition of myoblasts preceding fusion may be mediated by such muscle-specific components (Kaufman 1982).

The possible role of cell-surface glycoproteins and carbohydrates in the cell recognition of myoblasts which precedes fusion is controversial. There have been reports that plant lectins (Den et al 1975, Sandra et al 1977) and β-galactosides (Gartner & Podleski 1975), which bind specifically to carbohydrate moieties, inhibit cell fusion. Other investigators have failed to observe the inhibition of differentiation by β-galactosides (Den et al 1976, Kaufman & Lawless 1980). Myoblasts defective in either the binding or internalisation of several lectins have been isolated (Gilfix & Sanwal 1982). One of these mutants of L6 rat myoblasts lacked both cell surface sialic acid and galactose residues, yet it could fuse, raising the question whether these moieties have any significant role in fusion. These results apparently conflict with the earlier report that neuraminidase strongly inhibits fusion (Schudt & Pette 1976).

Myotube cultures synthesised a fucosyl-glycopeptide not found in dividing myoblast cultures (Marino et al 1980). This was sensitive to neuraminidase, suggesting that it contained sialic acid residues. Its location on the outer myotube plasma membrane was suggested by the observation that it was found in the glycopeptide fraction released by mild trypsin treatment of intact cells in culture. However, differentiated postmitotic myoblasts, the fusion of which had been inhibited by low Ca^{2+} concentration, synthesised the glycopeptide.

Neff et al (1982) have described a monoclonal antibody directed against a complex of three integral membrane glycoproteins (cell stratum attachment (CSAT) antigen) involved in the cell matrix adhesion of myoblasts and fibroblasts (Decker et al 1984). In prefusion myoblasts, which are rapidly detached by CSAT monoclonal antibody, CSAT antigen is distributed diffusely (Damsky et al 1985). After fusion, myotubes become more difficult to detach with CSAT monoclonal antibody. The CSAT antigen is organised in a much more discrete pattern on the myotube surface, becoming enriched at microfilament bundle termini and in lateral lamellae which appear to attach myotubes to the substratum. The results suggest that the organisation of CSAT antigen-adhesive complexes on the surface of myogenic cells can affect the stability of their adhesive contacts. In fibroblasts, CSAT antigen co-distributes with fibronectin, consistent with the suggestion that it participates in the mechanism by which fibroblasts (and probably myogenic cells) attach to fibronectin. The role of fibronectin in the attachment of myogenic cells to the collagen substratum is described in the section, 'The influence of neighbouring fibroblasts on muscle cell differentiation of myogenic cells' (p. 399).

The association of membrane components with the underlying cytoskeleton might regulate the turnover, aggregation and mobility of cell-surface components (Fernandez & Herman 1982, Prives et al 1982). Membrane–cytoskeletal interactions, modulated by contact between neighbouring myoblasts, could alter the topography of the myoblast surface. The altered mobility, aggregation, or loss of membrane components might result in relatively particle-free, highly fluid domains of lipid bilayer and lead to myoblast fusion (Kaufman 1982).

Selective proteolysis may have an important role in myoblast fusion. Strittmatter et al (1982) have shown that inhibition of a carboxypeptidase and a zinc-dependent endoprotease inhibits calcium-induced myoblast fusion. Limited proteolysis during cell fusion may eliminate steric or charge restraints to membrane apposition imposed by large charged-surface glycoprotein molecules, or may permit movement of membrane-bound protein to create particle-free zones of membrane, or again it may generate a polypeptide fragment that mediates fusion.

Membrane union is mediated by the fusion of lipid bilayers in which it is likely that two particular phospholipid classes, phosphatidyl-serine and phosphatidylethanolamine, have a major role. Horowitz et al (1982) found that myoblast plasma membranes possess a distribution of aminophospholipids between cytoplasmic and outer-membrane faces that differ from that described for other animal cells. The eccentric distribution of aminophospholipids is consistent with their participation in fusion.

In recent years, improved methods have been developed for synchronising and/or arresting myogenic cell fusion in monolayer cultures to determine the importance of fusion in triggering the expression of muscle-specific genes. Synchronisation can be achieved by changing the composition of the culture medium, particularly the concentration and type of serum and embryo extract (Yaffe 1971, Emerson & Beckner 1975). Fusion can be arrested by manipulation of the Ca^{2+} concentration of the culture medium using chelating agents such as EGTA (Paterson & Strohman 1972) or Chelex (Vertel & Fischman 1976, Moss & Strohman 1976). Removal of the chelating agent can lead to a very rapid burst of fusion. There is now considerable evidence that, when fusion is blocked, muscle-specific mRNA and proteins can still be synthesised. However, under normal circumstances it does seem that fusion is accompanied by a massive increase in synthesis of muscle-specific proteins.

The influence of neighbouring myogenic cells on muscle cell differentiation

Even before fusion the differentiation of a myogenic cell is almost certainly influenced by neighbouring myogenic cells.

One condition which precedes fusion in culture is the progressive increase in the muscle-cell population density. Konigsberg (1961) has suggested that population density might affect the initiation of fusion by either of two mechanisms. At the higher cell densities, cell-to-cell contacts might occur more frequently, thus increasing the probability of encounters between two cells competent to fuse. Alternatively, increased cell density would accelerate any alterations of the medium generated by the metabolic activities of the cells. In this way, high cell density might facilitate the establishment of a microenvironment, in some way more favourable for the initiation of fusion.

Earlier investigations to discriminate between these two possibilities led to the observation that medium withdrawn from confluent mass cultures supported the development of high proportions of well-differentiated muscle clones (Konigsberg 1963). Later studies (Hauschka & Konigsberg 1966) indicated that depositing a layer of collagen on the surface of the tissue culture dish could substitute for the use of 'conditional medium'. However, Konigsberg (1970) subsequently observed that, when single quail myoblasts were cloned in the absence of collagen, the daughter cells tended to remain in close proximity. Under these conditions of high cell density, fusion occurred earlier than when a collagen substratum was present, and resulted in the formation of a minute clone in which most of the nuclei were in syncytial association.

Further studies (Konigsberg 1971) of quail-cell microcultures of uniform diameter positioned on collagen-treated dishes indicated a diffusion-mediated, cell density-dependent control over the time of initiation of fusion. The onset of fusion was delayed either by decreasing the inoculum size or by increasing the volume of the medium. Furthermore, initiation of fusion was also delayed by continuous circulation of the medium. This delay could be circumvented by increasing the initial cell density or by using media withdrawn from cultures of fusing myoblasts. These results suggested a transmission of the effect of cell density via the medium. Whenever fusion was experimentally delayed, proliferation continued, at an undiminished rate, for longer, generating a larger cell population. This indicated that, although close proximity was a necessary condition for fusion, it was not alone a sufficient condition. Fusion may be promoted by the accumulation of cell products or by the depletion of media constituents. The fusion-promoting activity in the medium did not pass through a dialysis membrane nor a Diaflo® XM 300 membrane during ultrafiltration, indicating that the molecule or molecules involved were larger than a spherical molecule with a molecular weight of 300 000. The activity was not generated by fibroblasts, cardiac muscle or liver cells.

The results of Hauschka & White (1972) also indicated a cell-density effect distinct from the collagen requirement. In these studies, a conditioned medium factor increased that percentage of clones from early embryonic muscle which could express their myogenic potential. Activity was also measured in the presence of a collagen substratum and seemed to reside in a non-dialysable, high molecular weight fraction.

Using a method for both collection and assay of 'conditioning' factors in a defined medium devoid of both serum and embryo extract, Doehring & Fischman (1977) demonstrated that conditioned medium activity is the result both of nutrient depletion and of the addition of macromolecules, probably protein in nature, with a molecular weight greater than 10 000. The active component was not released by other cell types in tissue culture, but was secreted by muscle cells, both pre- and post-fusion.

In contrast, Yeoh & Holtzer (1977) found no evidence that increased cell density induced precocious fusion in myogenic cells. The results of testing conditioned medium prepared by the method of Doehring & Fischman (1977) were less clear. During the early stages of primary cultures in conditioned medium there was more extensive myotube formation, but these cultures degenerated after day 4 in culture.

In order to compare the same population of cells, Quinn & Nameroff (1983) initiated clones in fresh medium and then switched to either new fresh medium or to conditioned medium. Clones were fixed at 12-hour intervals up to 76 hours and then were assayed for the presence of post-mitotic myoblasts by immunoperoxidase staining for muscle myosin heavy chain or muscle-specific creatine kinase. In both media, myogenic cells occurred predominantly in homogeneous positive clones which contained cells in multiples of two. At 76 hours, the percentages of one-, two- and four-cell positive clones were the same in both media. However, the percentages of eight-and 16-cell positive clones were significantly decreased in conditioned medium, and the percentages of small negative clones were concomitantly increased. It was concluded that conditioned medium affects myogenesis by slowing progression through a predetermined series of cell divisions rather than by changing the number of divisions an individual cell will undergo before differentiating terminally.

In tissue culture, myoblasts divide several times; subsequently, some fuse and produce cell-specific proteins while others (possibly analogous to the satellite cells in vivo) remain as mononucleate cells. When the cells from advanced cultures are transferred to new culture dishes it is presumably these mononucleate cells that resume myogenic activity, because whole syncytial myotubes will not normally stick down afresh. Some clue as to the mechanism which underlies this difference in myoblast behaviour has been provided by Nameroff & Holtzer (1969). Embryonic myogenic cells were readily induced to mimic the behaviour of satellite cells by seeding them on a variety of cellular substrates (e.g. five-day cultures of muscle, cartilage or liver). On such substrates presumptive myoblasts did not migrate, fuse, replicate, or synthesise contractile proteins. However, when removed from the inactivating influence of these cellular substrates and subcultured, they migrated, multiplied and fused to

form typical myotubes. Nameroff & Holtzer postulated that the extra-cellular polysaccharide matrix of the cellular substrates is responsible for the observed behaviour.

The influence of neighbouring fibroblasts on muscle cell differentiation

Fibroblasts are responsible for laying down the muscle connective tissue system which involves synthesis of large amounts of collagen which may have an important influence acting as a substratum for muscle cells. In vivo, muscle cells come to lie in bundles enclosed by layers of connective membranes: the endomysium or basement lamina surrounding each individual myotube, the perimysium enclosing a bundle of myotubes, and the epimysium which surrounds a whole series of bundles of myotubes making up the anatomical muscle. It is now established that there are different types of collagen, and it has been shown (Duance et al 1977, Bailey et al 1979) that different connective tissue membranes of muscle contain predominantly one of the collagen types: endomysium contains type V ab; perimysium contains type III; epimysium contains type I.

Hauschka & Konigsberg (1966) demonstrated that, when the culture dish surface was coated with rat tail type I collagen, muscle cell growth and differentiation was promoted. Ketley et al (1976) found that the four different polymorphic forms of collagen (Types I, II, III and IV) were equally effective as substrates for chick myogenesis. In contrast, John & Lawson (1980) found that on a chicken muscle type V collagen, substrate chick myotubes were rounded with nuclei bunched together, whereas on type I collagen the myotubes were aligned in parallel.

Experimental evidence suggests there is a molecular basis for cell–collagen interaction. The initial studies of Hauschka & White (1972) indicated that certain cyanogen bromide peptides of rat skin type I collagen (α1 CB7 and α1 CB8) were particularly active in promoting attachment of cells and clonal differentiation of chick embryo myoblasts. Furthermore, they found that the horse serum in tissue culture medium was critical for enhanced attachment to collagen. More recently it has been established that fibronectin, a cell-surface glycoprotein, promotes cell adhesion to denatured collagen substrata (Pearlstein 1976). Moreover, cold-insoluble globulin, the serum form of fibronectin, must be absorbed on the substratum surface to obtain spreading of a variety of cell types on denatured collagen substrates (Klebe 1974, Kleinmann et al 1976). The sites on type I collagen which bind to fibronectin and are therefore active in cell attachment have been identified as α1 CB7 and α1 CB8 (Kleinmann et al 1976, Dessau et al 1978) which correlates well with the earlier findings of Hauschka & White (1972).

Specific, distinct functional domains have been identified on peptide fragments of fibronectin; one fragment binds to the myoblast, whereas another peptide binds to the collagen matrix (Wagner & Hynes 1980, Ehrismann et al 1981). Precoating of dishes with fibronectin allows parallel alignment of myotubes (Chiquet et al 1981).

Investigations using indirect immunofluorescence techniques have shown changes in the pattern and a decrease in fibrillar fibronectin upon myotube formation (Chen 1977, Frucht et al 1978). In pre-fusion myoblasts, fibronectin was distributed over the cells as a diffuse network. In post-fusion myotubes the fibrillar network of fibronectin disappeared completely. The very small amount of surface fibronectin detectable on some myotubes existed as small discrete patches.

It has been suggested that the ordered deposition of fibronectin may dictate the orientation of cells and guide the formation of unbranched myotubes (Chiquet et al 1981). It seems more likely that this is only one component of the alignment process. If type I collagen were laid down so that molecules or fibrils were aligned in parallel in certain directions by, e.g. fibroblasts, it would require only the transient appearance of fibronectin with its collagen-binding sites at the cell surface to cause all myoblasts to align in parallel prior to fusion.

Humoral influences on myogenesis

In vivo, muscle cells are exposed to complex humoral influences. In culture, myogenic cells usually grow and differentiate in a defined medium, supplemented with serum and chick embryo extract. These supplements may contain nutrients, hormones, growth factors and other factors which have a role in regulating muscle differentiation in vivo.

Serum. The type of serum used in tissue culture can affect both growth and differentiation. Fetal calf serum is considered to favour division of myogenic cells in culture, while horse serum promotes differentiation (Yaffe 1971, Morris & Cole 1972).

It is not usually necessary to use homologous serum for myogenic cells in culture. However, it is interesting that Morgan & Cohen (1974) found that it was necessary to use human serum to obtain extensive development of cross-striations in human myotubes. In addition, Hauschka (1974a) found that human serum alone could replace a mixture of horse serum and chick embryo extract for human fetal myogenic cultures.

There have been numerous attempts to identify the serum components which influence cell proliferation and cell differentiation. De La Haba et al (1966) reported that fusion of chick myoblasts to form myotubes in culture was almost completely inhibited in the absence of horse serum but was restored by addition of high concentrations of insulin to the culture medium although not to the extent obtained if serum was present. When somatotropin and insulin were both added to replace serum, an even greater degree of myotube formation took place, but somatotropin could not replace the effect of insulin. Powers & Florini (1975) found that physiological levels of testosterone stimulated division of rat muscle cells. The effect of testosterone on isolated muscle cells indicates that the effect of male sex hormones results from a direct interaction with muscle rather than from a primary interaction with some other tissue.

Ozawa & Kohama (1978) tested the ability of hormones or extracts from adult chicken tissues to replace or influence the activity of the serum factor. Pituitary gland extracts did not replace the serum factor in a range equivalent to normal serum concentrations of somatotropin, although high concentrations of such an extract showed a significant ability to mimic the serum. Insulin, triiodothyronine, testosterone, dihydrotestosterone and oestradiol did not show any ability to mimic trophic-factor activity. Both pituitary extract and insulin showed a potentiating effect on the trophic factor when added to the medium; however, the concentrations necessary for this effect were too high to be considered physiological. Triiodothyronine, testosterone, dihydrotestosterone and oestradiol did not potentiate the trophic factor; at higher concentrations, these hormones suppressed the activity of the trophic factor.

Since Kohama & Ozawa (1978a) considered that chick embryo extract contained the same active factor as serum they proposed that the results obtained by De La Haba et al (1966) and Powers & Florini (1975) might be due to the hormones having a potentiating effect on this chick embryo extract factor activity. However, testosterone did not potentiate the serum factor when tested in tissue culture (Ozawa & Kohama 1978). Nevertheless, when testosterone was injected into chickens, the activity of the serum then recovered was increased, suggesting that testosterone may have a physiological role in regulating the level of serum factor (Kohama & Ozawa 1978b).

Fibroblast growth factor isolated from bovine pituitary and brain stimulated cell division and delayed myoblast fusion (Gospodarowicz et al 1976). More recently it has been shown that pituitary- and brain-derived fibroblast growth factor can repress the expression of a muscle-specific protein, creatine kinase, in fully differentiated cultures without inducing mitogenic activity (Lathrop et al 1985). However, another factor was isolated from bovine pituitary and brain which promoted differentiation of bovine myoblasts so that 90% of clones contained myotubes (Gospodarowicz et al 1975).

Specific plasma proteins have an important role in myogenesis. The active components of serum have been identified as orosomucoid (an α_1-acid glycoprotein) and α_2-macroglobin (see Paul 1970). Both disappear from the medium during cultivation of cells. Each, alone, has a small effect in stimulating growth; together, they have a marked effect and can replace serum. The macroglobulin can be replaced by non-protein molecules but the acid glycoprotein cannot be replaced. These findings suggest that glycoproteins associated with

Cohn's fraction V are the important components in serum.

Ozawa and his colleagues identified the myotrophic factor in serum and embryo extract as the liver-synthesised iron-binding glycoprotein transferrin (It et al 1982). The myotrophic activities of chicken serum and chick embryo extract were completely lost on removal of transferrin by immunoprecipitation. The activity of transferrin depended not only on its concentration but also on its level of iron saturation: only the iron-bound form of transferrin is effective. The concentration and level of iron saturation of serum transferrin varied during the course of chick development and paralleled the myotrophic activity of the serum. Three main transferrin species (Tf-0, Tf-1 and Tf-2 which have 0, 1 and 2 sialic acid residues per molecule, respectively) were resolved by polyacrylamide-gel isoelectric focusing. As development proceeded, a relative increase occurred in the most acidic species (Tf-2) with decreases in the less acidic one (Tf-0 and Tf-1).

Chicken transferrins isolated from four tissue sources (eggs, embryo extract, serum, nerves) were able to promote myogenesis of chick cells in vitro but mammalian transferrins did not (Beach et al 1985). Comparison of the peptide fragments obtained after chemical or limited proteolytic cleavage demonstrates that the four chicken transferrins were indistinguishable, but they differed considerably from the mammalian transferrins. The structural differences between chicken and mammalian transferrins probably account for the inability of mammalian transferrins to act as mitogens for, and to support myogenesis of, primary chicken muscle cells.

Embryo extract. Chick embryo extract (CEE) has been frequently used to supplement medium in myogenic cultures (reviewed by Witkowski 1977). De La Haba et al (1975) separated CEE into two fractions: a non-filterable fraction (including molecules of molecular weight greater than 10 000) which promoted both the fusion of myoblasts to form syncytia and the further differentiation of these syncytia into myotubes, and a filterable fraction which stimulated myoblast fusion to form syncytia only. The filterable fraction promoted myotube formation if the cells were grown on a collagen substratum. The non-filterable fraction already contained a collagen-like molecule.

It seems likely that there may be active components found in CEE which are also present in serum used as a medium supplement. Kohama & Ozawa (1978a) reported that both CEE and chicken serum stimulated proliferation of chick muscle cultures to about the same degree.

The investigations of Ozawa and his colleagues showed that transferrin was an indispensable component in CEE for avian myogenic cell growth (It et al 1982). However, the growth-promoting activity of CEE was superior to that of transferrin alone. The myotrophic activity of transferrin was potentiated by CEE from which transferrin had been removed by immunoprecipitation (It et al 1982), suggesting the presence in CEE of other factors which promote myogenic cell growth. Analysis of the growth-promoting activity of CEE in the presence of a saturation amount of transferrin (It et al 1985) showed the importance of hypoxanthine-related compounds including RNA present in CEE for promoting avian myoblast proliferation in culture. When added to a basal culture medium, hypoxanthine or adenine markedly promoted quail myoblast proliferation. The concentration of hypoxanthine in CEE was very high (274 μM) and increased twofold during incubation at 37 °C, while that in horse serum was very low (3 μM). The nucleosides and nucleotides of hypoxanthine and adenine were effective, but the deoxynucleosides strongly inhibited the proliferation of avian myoblasts. Furthermore, RNA was also effective but DNA was not. The findings suggested that a supply of raw materials for RNA synthesis is important for optimal proliferation of myoblasts.

Florini & Roberts (1979) have developed a serum- and CEE-free medium for the growth of muscle cells in culture. Rates of cell proliferation essentially equal to those in 10% serum were obtained when rate L6 myoblasts were incubated in Ham's F-12 (defined) medium containing 10^{-5} M fetuin, 10^{-6} M insulin and 10^{-7} M dexamethasone. Addition of other growth factors and hormones in various combinations did not increase myoblast proliferation. Neither fetuin nor insulin could be replaced by other growth factors.

All glucocorticoids tested (but no other steroid hormones) were active. The active material in fetuin was heat-labile and non-dialysable. Primary rat myoblasts proliferated more rapidly than fibroblasts in the medium.

The influence of nerve cells on muscle cell differentiation

Of all tissues, the nervous system exerts the most extended and continuous influence on muscle development and maintenance. The fact that nerve cells and muscle cells can be grown together in tissue culture makes the in vitro system ideal for investigating various aspects of nerve–muscle interaction in a controlled environment.

Excitability of muscle cells in the absence of nerve cells. The cell membrane of the muscle cell differentiating in the absence of nerve cells begins to acquire excitability judged by an increasing response to depolarising stimuli (either a negative electrical pulse to a stimulating electrode or iontophoretically applied acetylcholine). Fambrough & Rash (1971) found that mononucleate myoblasts from chick rat embryo were not sensitive, but multinucleate myotubes were depolarised by acetylcholine (ACh). Mononucleate cells which constructed myofibrils without cell fusion were also ACh-sensitive, suggesting that the appearance of myofibrils and ACh sensitivity are closely linked. The ability of the cell membrane to respond to a depolarising stimulus by generating an action potential is related to an increase in the resting potential caused by the changes in membrane permeability (Fambrough & Rash 1971).

Resting membrane potentials increased from −8 to −55 mV in both rat and chick myoblasts differentiated into large multinucleate myotubes (Ritchie & Fambrough 1975). A progressive increase in the passive permeability of the membrane to K^+ relative to Na^+ ions was observed, which could account for the changes in resting membrane potential with development.

Mononucleated cells of a mouse clonal myogenic cell line had resting potentials of −22.5 mV and responded passively to current stimuli, indicating that they were non-excitable (Amagai et al 1983). On the other hand, multinucleated myotubes had resting membrane potentials ranging from -25 to -79 mV, depending on their stage of development. Newly fused myotubes had relatively less negative resting membrane potentials and showed no response, whereas myotubes later in development showed delayed rectification against depolarising current pulses, proving the development of a voltage-sensitive outward current system. Furthermore, mature myotubes had resting membrane potentials of -58.5 mV and generated fast action potentials having a maximum rate of rise of 315 V/s and a duration of 3.0 ms (measured at half-height). These action potentials were identified as tetrodotoxin-insensitive Na^+ spikes. These results indicate that the membrane excitability of the myogenic cell line develops well after the formation of myotubes, with an increase in membrane resting potential as maturation proceeds.

Human myotubes with well-developed striations had stable resting potentials (-50 mV) and generated all-or-none action potentials (92 mv amplitude) when stimulated (Merickel et al 1981a). The resting permeability of the myotubes was found to be primarily dependent on K^+ and to a lesser extent on Na^+. Changes in external Cl^- did not affect the resting potential or resting conductance indicating that the Cl^- permeability was low compared with the permeabilities of K^+ and Na^+. A small but significant electrogenic Na–K pump component to the resting potential was identified at low K^+ concentrations.

Detection and localisation of acetylcholine receptors and synapse-specific proteins in muscle cells in the absence of nerve cells. The location of acetylcholine receptors (AChR) in cultured muscle cells has been determined using iontophoretically applied ACh or the binding of radioactively labelled or fluorescein-labelled α-bungarotoxin (an AChR-binding neurotoxin prepared from the venom of the Indian cobra). α-Bungarotoxin binding to chick myotubes in culture correlated well with the level of ACh sensitivity (Hartzell & Fambrough 1973). Teng & Fiszman (1976) suggested that receptors were incorporated into the surface membrane from a presynthesised set of receptors. In prefusion myoblasts most AChR may be located in the interior of the myoblasts and appear only at the external cell surface of myotubes. The AChR of myotubes cultured in the absence of nerve were thought to resemble extrajunctional receptors found in vivo, in being sparsely distributed (~300 sites/μm^2) (Land et al 1977) and metabolically unstable (Merlie et al 1976).

However, there have been numerous reports of muscle cells cultured in the absence of nerve cells having several clusters of AChR (Vogel et al 1972, Fischbach & Cohen 1973). Land et al (1977) reported that the α-bungarotoxin site density, after subtracting myoblast background, varied from 54 to 900 sites/μm^2 on primary rat myotubes, with occasional hot spots of 3000 to 4000 sites/μm^2.

Increased external Ca^{2+} concentration caused a marked elevation of AChR levels (Birnbaum et al 1980). Agents known to increase intracellular Ca^{2+} concentration such as ionophore A23187, sodium dantrolene or high external Mg^{2+} concentration enhanced α-bungarotoxin binding. Electrical stimulation or caffeine, both effectors of sarcoplasmic reticulum Ca^{2+} release, brought about a decrease in AChR concentration probably by suppressing its synthesis. Intermediate AChR levels obtained following simultaneous treatments with opposing effects, e.g. electrical stimulation in the presence of high external Ca^{2+} concentration or sodium dantrolene, suggest contradictory effects on a common mediator. These observations indicated a strong correlation between sarcoplasmic reticulum Ca^{2+} levels and AChR concentration on myotubes. Whereas Ca^{2+} accumulation in the sarcoplasmic reticulum was followed by increased AChR synthesis, Ca^{2+} release was accompanied by suppression of receptor synthesis.

The molecular control of the distribution and motion of acetylcholine receptors in the plasma membrane of differentiating rat myotubes was investigated by fluorescein techniques (Axelrod et al 1978). AChRs were tagged with tetramethylrhodamine-labelled α-bungarotoxin and lateral molecular motion in the membrane was measured by the fluorescence photo bleaching recovery technique. AChR lateral motion was inhibited by concanavalin A plant lectin and by anti α-bungarotoxin antibody. AChR cluster and diffuse areas motion were independent of direct metabolic energy requirements and were sensitive to electrical excitation of myotubes. Lipid molecules moved laterally in both AChR cluster and diffuse areas. The AChR lateral motion in diffuse areas and immobility in clusters were not altered by agents which affect extrinsic cell surface proteins, or cytoplasmic microfilaments and microtubules.

A significant population of the AChR tagged with radioactive or fluorescent α-bungarotoxin is retained on the cytoskeletal framework remaining after extraction with the detergent Triton® X-100 using conditions that preserve internal structure (Prives et al 1982a,b). The proportion of non-extracted AChR increased as the myotube differentiated. AChR in patches were retained on the cytoskeleton while diffuse AChR were partially extracted by detergent.

The muscle cell is capable of synthesising other junction-specific proteins in the absence of nerve cells. Hall et al (1982) showed that myotubes of a mouse muscle cell line synthesised in culture the synaptic form of acetylcholinesterase (AChE) and each of three immunologically defined components of the synaptic basal lamina. The 16S AChE had the properties expected of AChE forms with a collagen-like tail and was found in patches on the external cell surface where it appeared to be associated with the extracellular matrix by ionic interactions. Surface patches of one of the synaptic antigens often occurred in close association with AChR clusters, whereas the other antigens and the AChE patches were rarely coincident with AChR clusters. The authors concluded that the muscle cells, in the absence of nerves, synthesised and accumulated on their surface several components that are known to be concentrated in the basal lamina at adult synapses but these were not assembled into a coherent whole as in the adult.

In cultured myotubes the build up of extracellular matrix components was most apparent in plaques overlying AChR clusters (Anderson & Fambrough 1983, Bayne et al 1984). Monoclonal antibodies showed that the ECM components heparan sulphate proteoglycan, laminin and fibronectin were found at 100%, 70–90% and 20% of AChR clusters respectively. The congruence between AChR clusters and heparan sulphate proteoglycan suggests some sort of linkage between the two molecules.

AChE activity has been demonstrated biochemically and cytochemically in cultured muscle cells even before cell fusion (Fluck & Strohman 1973). Uninnervated chick myotubes in culture may contain the 6.5 S, 11 S and 20 S forms of AChE (Kato et al 1980) or the 6.5 S and 11 S only (Cisson et al 1981). The molecular forms of AChE expressed in culture chick myotubes are dependent on the types expressed in the donor muscle (Toutant et al 1983).

The influence of nerve cells on the localisation of acetylcholine receptors. The observation that muscle cells cultured in the absence of nerve cells have clusters of AChR (Vogel et al 1972, Fischbach & Cohen 1973) led to the proposal that the receptor clusters might serve as recognition sites for cholinergic nerves innervating muscle. The clusters might act as pre-formed postsynaptic sites and a cholinergic nerve encountering such a site would form a synapse there. However, evidence suggests that nerve–muscle synapses do not form at pre-existing receptor clusters. Cohen and his colleagues used fluorescein-labelled α-bungarotoxin to follow the distribution of receptors during synapse formation on myocytes cultured from *Xenopus* larvae (Anderson & Cohen 1977, Anderson et al 1977). The fluorescent patches under nerve processes, presumably at synapses, were different in shape from those on myocytes not contacted by nerve cells. In a few cases, the distribution of receptors was followed on a single myocyte while it was contacted by a neurite. Receptor molecules already labelled with fluorescent toxin coalesced under the neurite and adjacent pre-existing fluorescent patches often disappeared. Neural clusters were thus formed by recruitment of surrounding unclustered receptors and perhaps by receptors from dispersed pre-existing clusters as well.

The migration of AChRs to the nerve contact region does not result in a significant decrease in the non-junctional density judged by ACh sensitivity (Gruener & Kidokoro 1982) or α-bungarotoxin binding (Kidokoro & Gruener 1982). Muscle activity caused by spontaneous synaptic potentials does not lead to decreasing AChR density in the non-junctional region (Kidokoro & Gruener 1982).

The relative contribution to neurite-associated receptor patches of AChRs present in the membrane before and after contact was assessed using two fluorescent receptor probes (Role et al 1985). Rhodamine-conjugated α-bungarotoxin was used to label either old or new receptors and a monoclonal antireceptor antibody visualised with a fluorescein second antibody was used to label all receptors. Clusters contained both new and old receptors but within 24 hours of coculture the majority (60–80%) were new. Cholinergic neurites increased the rate of receptor insertion five fold during the first eight hours of neurite-associated cluster formation. The contribution of new receptors to clusters declined with time.

The effect of various types of neurones on AChR clustering in cultured myotubes has been investigated. Spinal cord motor neurones were identified in culture after labelling them in vivo with Lucifer Yellow — wheat-germ agglutinin conjugates (Role et al 1985). All their processes induced receptor clusters on contacted myotubes. Neurones dissociated from ciliary ganglia induced patches to the same extent as motor neurones. In contrast, neurite-associated receptor patches were rarely associated with spinal cord interneurones. Kidokoro and Yeh (1981b) had found that only cholinergic neurones appeared effective in causing receptor localisation.

How nerves induce receptor clustering is unknown. Recently there have been several reports of the effect of soluble factors from nerve tissue on the distribution and site density of AChRs of muscle developing in vitro. Central nervous system extracts caused not only a major increase in AChR site density but also the formation of high-density AChR clusters in cultured cloned rat muscle cells (Podleski et al 1978) and chick cells (Christian et al 1978, Jessel et al 1979, Bauer et al 1981). Saltpeter & Podelski (1982) showed that a soluble brain extract produces AChR clusters with junctional site densities. The extract-induced receptor clustering did not require a decrease in turnover rate, could be produced by a redistribution of existing receptors and resembled the nerve-induced clustering previously described (Anderson & Cohen 1977).

Saline extracts prepared from the electric lobe, the electromotor nerves, and the electric organ of *Torpedo* increased the ACh sensitivity of uninnervated myotubes in culture by increasing the number of AChR and causing clustering (Connolly et al 1982). The active substance was heat-sensitive but not trypsin-sensitive and had a molecular weight of less than 5000.

Tissue culture experiments indicate that nerve cell or glial cell-derived diffusible factors may operate over appreciable distances. Acetylcholinesterase activity in chick muscle cultures was increased by the presence of innervating spinal cord explants (Oh et al 1972). The increased activity could still be obtained if the muscle cells were on one side of a coverslip immersed in medium and the nerve cells on the other, indicating that a functional synapse was not necessary. Furthermore, soluble protein extracts of the spinal cord could induce the same effect, suggesting that nerve cells could produce a diffusible factor. There is evidence that proteins synthesised in the spinal cord can flow distally along the peripheral nerves in vivo (Komiya & Austin 1974). Oh (1976) found that a soluble extract of adult chicken sciatic nerve enhanced the rate and degree of morphological differentiation and maturation, DNA and protein synthesis, and AChE activity of muscle cultures. The active factor (sciatin) had a native molecular weight of 25 000 (Markelonis & Oh 1978). Stimulation of protein synthesis by sciatin did not appear to be mediated by cyclic nucleotides because neither theophylline (an inhibitor of phosphodiesterase) nor imidazole (an inhibitor of adenyl cyclase) affected its action (Markelonis et al 1980). Increased sensitivity to ACh (Kidokoro & Gruener 1982) and an increased relative proportion of long-open-time AChR channels (Brehm et al 1982) was also found in the muscle cells grown in conditioned medium which was prepared by growing muscle cells with neural cells.

The insoluble extracellular matrix (ECM) may be important in interactions between nerve cells and muscle cells. The basal lamina fraction from the electric organ of *Torpedo* contained a proteinaceous factor or factors that organised myotube AChRs into distinct clusters (Wallace et al 1982). Nerve-induced formation of AChR clusters and adjacent plaques of ECM proteoglycan were closely coupled throughout early stages of synapse formation (Anderson et al 1984). Developing junctional accumulations of AChR and proteoglycan appeared and grew progressively throughout a perineural zone that extended along the muscle surface on either side of the nerve process. Junctional proteoglycan deposits appeared to correspond to discrete ultrastructural plaques of basal lamina, which were initially separated by broad expanses of lamina-free muscle surface. The extent of this basal lamina, and a corresponding thickening of the postsynaptic membrane, also increased during the accumulation of AChR and proteoglycan along the path of nerve contact. Presynaptic differentiation of synaptic vesicle clusters became detectable at the developing neuromuscular junction only after the formation of postsynaptic plaques containing both AChR and proteoglycan.

The formation of AChR clusters is inhibited if cocultures of rat myotubes and spinal cord explants are treated with *cis*-hydroxyproline which is a specific inhibitor of collagen production (Kalcheim et al 1982).

The postsynaptic membrane from *Torpedo* electric organ contains, in addition to AChR, a major peripheral membrane protein (molecular weight 43 000) which may be involved in anchoring receptors to the postsynaptic membrane (Peng & Froehner 1985). Clusters of AChR that occurred spontaneously on those cells were stained with a monoclonal antibody to the 43K protein. Newly formed receptor clusters which were induced with positive polypeptide-coated latex beads in a similar fashion to nerve contact were also stained with the monoclonal antibody, suggesting that the 43K protein becomes associated with AChR clusters during a period of active postsynaptic membrane differentiation.

A cell surface glycoprotein, called neural cell adhesion molecule (N-CAM) was found to be essential for the in vitro establishment of physical associations between nerve and muscle, suggesting that binding involving this molecule may be an important early step in synaptogenesis (Rutishauser et al 1983). Anti-(N-CAM) Fab fragments in cultures of spinal cord with skeletal muscle cells specifically block adhesion of spinal cord neurites

and cells to myotubes. However, similar experiments suggested that antibodies to N-CAM L1 did not inhibit synapse formation and synaptic activity in mouse nerve–muscle cocultures (Mehrke et al 1984).

Morphology of the neuromuscular junction in tissue culture. Earlier investigations indicated that the architecture of nerve–muscle contacts in initially dissociated cell cultures, as revealed by silver impregnation and electron microscopy, is rather primitive in comparison with those between explants of spinal cord and attached explants of muscle, which are nearly identical to adult neuromuscular junctions. In short-term cultures, fine neurites terminated over muscle cells in a few simple swellings or boutons, and were not covered by Schwann cells; there were no postsynaptic gutters or folds or membrane thickenings and the muscle fibres were not covered by a basal lamina (Shimada et al 1969a). Rather simple *en plaque* endings and non-muscle nuclei, possibly Schwann cells, were observed in older cultures (Shimada et al 1969b).

More recently the development of synaptic ultrastructure at neuromuscular contacts has been investigated in cultures of dissociated myotomal muscle and spinal cord derived from the embryos of *Xenopus laevis* (Weldon & Cohen 1979). Within one day in culture a few of the neuromuscular contacts already displayed several synaptic specialisations. including 50 nm vesicles clustered against the axolemma, increased axolemmal densities, basal lamina in the cleft and increased sarcolemmal density and subsarcolemmal filamentous material. The myotomal neuromuscular synapse differentiates in culture in much the same way as it does in vivo.

The functioning of the neuromuscular junction in tissue culture. Robbins & Yonezawa (1971) proposed that the neurotransmitter in early junctions in rat cell culture was probably ACh because, in a few cases tested, D-tubocurarine (an antagonist of ACh) completely eliminated excitatory junction potentials. Fischbach (1972) found that the synapses formed between dissociated neurones from chick spinal cord and dissociated myoblasts were cholinergic and that transmitter release (which even in the youngest cultures was quantal) was regulated by Ca^{2+} and Mg^{2+}.

Robbins & Yonezawa (1971) observed nerve–muscle contacts in cultures of rat embryonic spinal cord with either explants of muscle or dissociated myoblasts, with some of the ultrastructural features of neuromuscular junctions. Excitatory junction potentials were obtained by stimulating the spinal cord fragment or nerve fibre and recording with an intracellular electrode in the muscle cell. Excitatory junctional potentials were never found in cells devoid of nerve contacts and were more readily obtained in nerve-contacted myotubes with a large number of nuclei than from myotubes consisting of only a few cells.

The early appearance and functional significance of synaptic AChE were examined in chick spinal cord muscle cocultures (Rubin et al 1979). Synapses were identified by focal extracellular recording and divided into three categories based on their mean time constant of synaptic current decay: fast, intermediate and slow. Patches of AChE were evident at identified synapses within 24 hours of coculture. After four days, 74% of the fast synapses stained for AChE, whereas none of the slow synapses were stained. Thus it is likely that AChE serves to limit the duration of ACh action at newly formed nerve–muscle synapses, just as it does at the adult neuromuscular junction. This conclusion was supported by the fact that methanesulphonyl fluoride, an AChE inhibitor, prolonged synaptic currents at fast, but not at slow, synapses. Furthermore, the mean channel open time of activated AChR estimated by fluctuation analysis was the same at fast and slow synapses.

When the embryonic *Xenopus* muscle cell was contacted by cholinergic neurones, functional synaptic transmission was detected within 10 minutes following the initial contact (Kidokoro & Yeh 1981). Brehm et al (1982) measured the mean channel open time of the AChR channel by extracellularly recorded acetylcholine-induced noise. Muscle cells cultured alone, as well as those cocultured with neural tube cells had two types of AChR channels with either a short open time (0.7 ms) or a long open time (3.0 ms). The relative proportion of the channel type with a long open time increased following coculture with neural tube cells. Prolongation of the mean open time resulted in a greater charge transfer during the activation of AChRs and as a consequence, activation of an equivalent number of AChRs led to a larger depolarisation. An increased ACh sensitivity in muscle cells cocultured with neural tube cells therefore resulted without any increase in AChR density. The prolonging of mean channel open time in the presence of neural tube cells is the opposite of the situation found in vivo where channel open time shortens in the presence of nerve.

Kidokoro (1984) reported that during development in *Xenopus* nerve–muscle cultures miniature end-plate potentials appear at first as subminiature end-plate potentials and subsequently classic miniature end-plate potentials appear.

It is now established that the type of innervation affects gene expression during the differentiation of muscle cells. Experiments in which fast and slow muscle were cross-reinnervated suggested that patterns of impulses may be important, and this was confirmed by direct electrical stimulation of muscle via nerve in vivo (Salmons & Sreter 1976).

Intermittent electrical stimulation of myotube cultures in the total absence of nerves leads to loss of sensitivity to iontophoretically applied acetylcholine and less binding of ^{125}I-labelled α-bungarotoxin in comparison with inactive fibres (Cohen & Fischbach 1973), decreased synthesis of AChR (Shainberg & Burstein 1976) and reduced AChE activity (Walker & Wilson 1975). Repetitive stimulation increased protein synthesis and particularly myosin synthesis (Brevet et al 1976). These investigators did not detect the appearance of proteins characteristic of either fast or slow muscle.

Proteins characteristic of the differentiated myotube in culture

Protein synthesis in the dividing myoblast is geared to cell proliferation while, in the postmitotic myoblast and myotube, synthesis of muscle-specific proteins predominates. With the introduction of two-dimensional gel electrophoresis, gene cloning and monoclonal antibody techniques it has become apparent that many of the myofibrillar proteins and other enzymes occur in different polymorphic forms and are the products of multigene families (Fischman 1982, Buckingham & Minty 1983). Only some of the different polymorphic forms of the proteins are muscle-specific: some may be expressed at different times in muscle development and some are particularly abundant in muscles specialised to carry out a certain physiological function.

Myofibrillar proteins

The predominant protein structures in the differentiated fibre or myotube in vivo are the myofibrils, which comprise about 60% of the cellular protein (Perry 1971). Myotubes in culture can develop cross-striated myofibrils which show spontaneous contractions. Important questions are: To what extent do these myofibrils resemble those in vivo? Does the process of myofibrillogenesis in tissue culture myotubes illuminate the underlying controlling mechanisms?

Morphological investigations. Electron-microscopic investigations have shown that thin and thick filaments organised into myofibrils occur in myotubes and in fusion-blocked mononucleate myoblasts in culture (Holtzer et al 1975, Emerson & Beckner 1975, Moss & Strohmann 1976, Vertel & Fischman 1976).

Non-striated bundles of 6–8 nm microfilaments, running the whole length of the cell and inserted into the cell cortex, appeared before nascent myofibrils in cultured *Xenopus* muscle cells (Peng et al 1981). A number of observations suggested that bundles of microfilaments were precursors to myofibrils: first, nascent myofibrils were anchored to the cell cortex via filaments similar to microfilament bundles; secondly, these filaments in newly formed sarcomeres were often continuous through the middle of the A band — later they broke to form the H zone; thirdly, the filaments appeared to be continuous through the developing Z band, later interacting with the filaments in the Z band to form the staggered appearance. The transition from the regions with incomplete A bands and Z bands to regions of better-defined cross-striation was seen on single

nascent myofibrils. New sarcomeres were added to the distal ends of existing ones.

The effect of taxol, a microtubule-stabilising agent, on chick myogenesis has been investigated (Holtzer et al 1982). Ultrastructurally, taxol-treated post-mitotic myoblasts display microtubule-myosin thick filament arrays from which actin thin filaments were absent. Such arrays appear striated, having normal M and H bands, but they have I bands consisting largely of microtubules. Treatment with 12-O-tetradecanoyl-phorbal-13-acetate followed by taxol revealed more perfectly aligned microtubule-myosin arrays, with normal M and H bands but no Z-band material, sarcoplasmic reticulum (SR), or T-system elements. Apparently, striations can be organised despite the absence of thin filaments and Z-band material.

The way that embryonic myoblasts differentiate in tissue culture in the absence of nerve may be correlated with the future physiological role of the donor muscle (Fremont et al 1983). Slow anterior latissimus dorsi (ALD) and fast posterior latissimus dorsi (PLD) muscles of nine-day-old quail embryos were cultured without neurones for 1–12 weeks. ALD-derived myotubes exhibited wide Z lines, numerous mitochondria and a poorly developed sarcotubular system while PLD-derived myotubes exhibited narrow Z lines, few mitochondria and an abundant sarcotubular system.

Histochemical investigations. Enzymes or substrates can be localised within individual mononucleate cells or myotubes in culture by histochemical techniques.

Gallup et al (1972) found that, during myogenesis in tissue culture, normal human undifferentiated mononucleate myoblasts have strongly glycolytic metabolism (high phosphorylase, high glycogen). In contrast the myotubes have a strongly oxidative metabolism (high NADH-TR) and high myofibrillar ATPase. It is therefore of crucial importance to ensure that cultures being compared are at the same stage of differentiation.

Earlier investigations were unable to detect differentiation of physiologically different muscle fibres in tissue culture (Askanas et al 1972, Askanas & Engel 1975). More recently Fremont et al (1983) found that staining for myofibrillar

ATPase revealed that all well-differentiated ALD-derived myotubes were of the β' type whereas PLD-derived myotubes were of β and βR types.

Immunological investigations. Immunological techniques have been used to investigate the synthesis of myosin during myogenesis in tissue culture using antibodies raised against the native protein (Coleman & Coleman 1968) and against light meromyosin, which is a fragment of the tail region of the myosin heavy chain subunit (Chi et al 1975b). The early work, reporting that antibodies raised to contractile proteins from adult muscle will react with embryonic or cultured muscle, suggested that the proteins were very similar (Holtzer & Sanger 1972). Fluorescein-labelled antibodies against skeletal light meromyosin were bound along the lateral edges of emerging and definitive thick filaments in cultured myotubes (Chi et al 1975a,b).

Masaki (1974) established that the heavy chains of myosins from chicken 'fast white', 'slow red', and cardiac muscles were immunologically distinguishable. The heavy chain of each myosin reacted with its antibody in the presence of SDS, suggesting that differences in primary sequence are involved. Investigations of muscle development in vivo using these highly specific antibodies labelled with fluorescein, indicated that individual myotubes and individual myofibrils at an early stage of development contain all three myosins — fast, slow and cardiac (Masaki & Yoshizaki 1974). Individual cultured myotubes also contained fast and cardiac myosin (Masaki 1973).

Individual human myotubes in culture also displayed multiple reactivity to antimyosin antibodies specific for isomyosins from fast and slow skeletal muscle (Schiaffino et al 1982). When cultured muscle was innervated by the ventral part of fetal rat spinal cord there was a greater degree of differentiation with a large number of cross-striated myotubes but the antibody staining did not differ from that in the non-innervated control cultures.

Indirect immunofluorescence with affinity-purified tropomyosin antibodies demonstrated the presence of filaments containing α and β forms of tropomyosin throughout chick myogenesis in culture (Moss & Schwartz 1981). The fine struc-tural distribution of troponin on thin filaments in developing myofibrils was investigated using immunoelectron microscopy (Obinata et al 1979). Cultured embryonic chick skeletal muscle cells were treated with antibodies against each of the troponin components (troponin T, I and C) from adult chicken muscles. Each antibody was distributed along the thin filaments with a period of 38 nm. It was concluded that these newly synthesised regulatory proteins were assembled at their characteristic positions from the initial phases of myofibrillogenesis.

The occurrence and distribution of M-protein (myomesin), a tightly bound component of the M-line region of myofibrils, was investigated during chick muscle cell differentiation in culture by the indirect immunofluorescence technique (Eppen-berger et al 1981). The protein was first detected in post-mitotic, non-proliferating myoblasts in a regular pattern of fluorescent cross-striations. In electron micrographs of sections through young myotubes it was present within forming H zones of nascent myofibrils. In large myotubes the typical striation pattern in the M-line region of the myofibrils was observed. Myomesin may be a highly specific marker for cross-striated muscle cell differentiation and may have an important role in myofibrillar assembly.

Biochemical investigations

Myosin. The myosin of mammalian myogenic cells in culture differs from that found in differentiated adult muscle. John & Jones (1975) found that radioactively labelled myosin from rat myotubes in culture contained only two light chains which co-electrophoresed with the LC_1 and LC_2 light chains of adult rat fast myosin. There was a high proportion of label in the heavy chain compared with the light chains (13:1). The adult rat myosin preparation had a heavy chain to light chain (LC_1 and LC_2) ratio of 4:1 determined by densitometry suggesting that in myotube myosin either the overall proportion of light chains is less, or the timing of synthesis or turnover differs from that of the heavy chain. Direct analysis of myosin extracted from a large number of cells confirmed that there was a reduced proportion of light chains. The specific Ca^{2+} ATPase of myotube myosin was very low (0.011 μmol ADP/mg myosin/min) compared with that for adult rat myosin (0.38 μmol ADP/mg/min). No labelled myosin could be detected in dividing cultures.

Whalen and his colleagues investigated the nature of the myosin heavy chain present at early stages of muscle development in the rat (Whalen et al 1979). Myosins from cultured myotubes of the myogenic cell line L6 and of primary cultures and from fetal muscle tissue were analysed by polypeptide mapping. The heavy chains of these three myosins had maps different from those of the various adult myosins examined (fast, slow and cardiac). The maps of the heavy chain from the two cultured-cell myosins were very similar. Fetal myosin gave a map in which most of the polypeptides corresponded to those found in the cultured myosin. Developing muscle, either in vivo or in vitro, apparently contains a myosin heavy chain different from the adult type. Similarly, it was shown that cultured myotubes of rat L6 cell line contained an embryonic form of the myosin light chain LC_1 called LC_{1emb} (Whalen et al 1978). Both fetal LC_{1emb} and adult LC_{1F} were synthesised in early fusing primary cultures of rat and calf myoblasts (Whalen et al 1979, Daubas et al 1981). Electrophoresis of myosin in non-denaturing conditions showed that native myosin from L6 cells had a single band corresponding to the embryonic form of myosin which was different from the bands of adult fast and slow myosins (Whalen et al 1981). In organotypic cultures of muscle with spinal cord the adult fast isozyme of myosin was present (Ecob et al 1983).

Investigations of myosin in avian muscle cell cultures are more controversial. Holtzer and his co-workers (Chi et al 1975a,b) used scaled-down biochemical procedures to extract myosin and actomyosin from chick cultures and found that there were different isoenzymatic forms present at different stages of differentiation. The ratio of myosin to actin and the type of myosin light chain in replicating mononucleate cells (myoblasts and fibroblasts) was different from that in fusion-blocked myoblasts and myotubes. The authors suggested that one set of structural genes for the myosin light and heavy chains was active in dividing cells and another set in fusion-blocked myoblasts and myotubes. Chi et al (1975a,b)

reported that the molar ratios of the myosin light chains of myotube myosin and the specific Ca^{2+} ATPase were similar to those of adult fast myosin (see also Sreter et al 1972). Rubinstein & Holtzer (1979) found that only fast myosin light chains were found in myotube cultures derived from myoblasts from either fast or slow muscle regions. In contrast, others have reported that cultured chick myoblasts synthesise the myosin light chains of both fast and slow myosin (Cantini et al 1980).

To obviate the problem of deciding which cells in primary culture synthesise myosin, some investigators have used drugs such as FUdR (Coleman & Coleman 1968) and cytosine arabinoside (Chi et al 1975a,b) to kill proliferating cells leaving cultures of pure myotubes. Others have used a cell cloning technique. Cultures of cloned myoblasts from slow or fast avian skeletal muscles expressed both fast and slow isoforms of myosin light chains (Keller & Emerson 1981, Stockdale et al 1981).

The thin filament proteins: actin, tropomyosin and troponin. The technique of isoelectric focusing enabled Whalen et al (1976) to discover that actin exists in three forms (α, β, and γ) possessing similar biochemical properties and identical molecular weights but having slightly different isoelectric points. Two of the forms (β and γ) were found in prefusion dividing cells and also in cultured non-myogenic cells. The third form (α) was the only one found in fetal muscle tissue and is predominant in myotube cultures. Montarras et al (1982) showed that β-tropomyosin is the predominant isoform in cultured chick myotubes. Cultures of chick myoblasts from slow or fast skeletal muscle expressed both fast and slow isoforms of α-tropomyosin (Montarras & Fiszmann 1983). Similarly, myoblasts from slow or fast quail skeletal muscles express both adult fast and slow isoforms of troponin C (Hastings & Emerson 1982).

The observation that cloned myoblasts from slow or fast avian skeletal muscles express both adult fast and slow isoforms of myosin light chains, and tropomyosin and troponin C, suggests that genes for fast- and slow-muscle isoforms may be co-activated, and a specific subset later repressed during development of distinct muscle types.

The differentiated myofibril in vivo contains myofibrillar proteins in a molar ratio (actin : myosin : tropomyosin : troponin) of 7:1:1:1 (Potter 1974). This suggests a requirement for qualitative and quantitative co-ordination of myofibrillar protein synthesis. Devlin & Emerson (1978) measured the synthesis of specific proteins by autoradiography and fluorography of two-dimensional gels using a scanning densitometer. Contractile proteins synthesised by quail muscle-cell cultures were identified by co-electrophoresis with purified contractile proteins. The results showed that synthesis of myosin heavy chain, myosin light chains LC_1 and LC_2, troponin C and α and β tropomyosin was first detected at the time of myoblast fusion and then increased at least 500-fold to maximum rates which remain constant in myotubes. Both the kinetics of activation and the molar rates of synthesis of these contractile proteins were virtually identical. Muscle-specific actin (α) synthesis also increased at the time of myoblast fusion but this actin was synthesised at three times the rate of the other contractile proteins. The synthesis rate of 30 other muscle cell proteins was measured, and most of these were shown to follow different patterns of regulation. The authors concluded that the synthesis of the contractile proteins is regulated in a co-ordinated manner during myoblast differentiation. The stoichiometry seems to be mainly determined by the respective concentration of the contractile protein mRNAs (Devlin & Emerson 1979).

Shani et al (1981) reported that α-actin synthesis starts a few hours before that of myosin heavy chain and light chains in rat L8 cultures. In the more slowly fusing calf myoblast cultures, different kinetics of accumulation were seen for different contractile proteins (Daubas et al 1981).

Experiments using recombinant DNA probes for measuring levels of contractile protein mRNAs during myoblast fusion have shown a close correlation between mRNA levels and synthesis of the corresponding protein (Buckingham & Minty 1983).

Muscle-specific isoenzymes. The characteristic isoenzyme transitions known to occur in developing muscle in vivo in which an ubiquitous enzyme is replaced by a muscle-specific isoenzy-matic form has also been demonstrated during differentiation of muscle cells in culture in the case of creatine kinase (Delain et al 1974, Turner et al 1976, Morris et al 1976), phosphorylase (Delain et al 1974), phosphofructokinase (Delain et al 1974) and pyruvate kinase (Guguen-Guillouzo et al 1977).

The technique of cellulose polyacetate electrophoresis followed by specific staining has been used to show that the replacement of embryonic brain BB CPK in dividing cultures by muscle MM-CPK in myotube cultures begins in fusion-blocked cells (Turner et al 1976). However, Morris et al (1976), using a combination of electrophoresis and a fluorimetric technique which allowed measurement of low levels of CPK isoenzymes, showed that the early increase in CPK activity during early stages of fusion is of the embryonic BB type and only later does the adult muscle form make a major contribution to the total increase in enzyme activity. A further investigation (Morris & Cole 1977) of increased CPK activity after incubation of cells with radioactive amino acids indicated that while increases in MM-CPK during differentiation involve de novo enzyme synthesis, the early increases in BB-CPK do not but presumably reflect activation of existing enzyme.

Specialised membrane proteins. During the differentiation of the muscle cell the sarcoplasmic reticulum and transverse tubules elaborate the triad structures. One of the components of the sarcoplasmic reticulum is the Ca^{2+}-Mg^{2+}-dependent adenosine triphosphatase (ATPase) and this has been investigated during muscle differentiation in tissue culture. Holland & MacLennan (1976) estimated rates of synthesis at various stages of differentiation from the incorporation of ^3H-leucine into the ATPase which was isolated by antibody precipitation and the enzyme separated by electrophoresis. Synthesis of the sarcoplasmic reticulm ATPase was greatly accelerated as rat myoblasts fuse and differentiate into myotubes, but synthesis did occur in fusion-blocked cells. The concentration of the Ca^{2+}-Mg^{2+}-ATPase measured by selective labelling of the enzyme with ^{32}P ATP also began to increase during fusion of chick myogenic cells (Martonosi et al 1977).

Immunofluorescent staining techniques were used to study the distribution of the Ca^{2+}-Mg^{2+}-dependent ATPase and also calsequestrin, a protein capable of binding Ca^{2+} (Jorgensen et al 1977). These studies at the cellular level confirmed biochemical findings that calsequestrin was synthesised some hours before the ATPase. Immunofluorescent staining of myoblasts showed that calsequestrin first appears in a well-defined region of the cell near one end of the nucleus. Later, the staining occupied progressively larger regions adjacent to the nucleus and took on a fibrous appearance. These observations suggested that calsequestrin first accumulates in the Golgi region and then gradually spreads throughout the cell. In contrast, the ATPase appeared to be concentrated in many small patches or foci throughout the cytoplasm and was never confined to one particular region. In myotubes alternating dark and fluorescent strands parallel to the longitudinal axis of the cells were evident.

Sarcolemmal protein profiles from cultured myotubes and myoblasts have been reported by Hirsch et al 1981.

TISSUE CULTURE INVESTIGATIONS OF NEUROMUSCULAR DISEASES

Duchenne muscular dystrophy (DMD)

DMD myogenic cells

Morphological investigations. The explant technique has been widely used to culture muscle obtained from patients with Duchenne muscular dystrophy. Earlier studies reported differences in morphology and cell migration between normal and DMD cells. Geiger & Garvin (1957) found that DMD myotubes did not differentiate properly and cross-striations did not develop. Other investigators found more extensive growth of cells from DMD biopsies than from normal, and DMD mononucleate cells were smaller than normal (Goyle et al 1967, 1968, Kakulas et al 1968).

Other studies using the explant technique have suggested that there is no significant difference between normal and DMD muscle cells in culture. Morphologically similar cell features in cultures from normal and DMD muscle have been reported by Hermann et al (1960), Askanas & Engel (1975) and Ionasescu et al (1976). Skeate et al (1969) found differentiated myotubes with cross-striations in both normal and DMD muscle cultures. Statistical analysis by Bishop et al (1971) showed no significant differences between normal and diseased muscle in the length, breadth or number of myotubes. Witkowski et al (1976) found that the mononucleate cells, growth rate and degree of differentiation were similar.

In tissue culture of muscle explants from normal fetuses and male fetuses at risk for DMD no differences were found with regard to the ease with which cultures could be established and maintained, or in gross morphology or rate of growth and differentiation in culture (Emery & McGregor 1977); nevertheless, before culture, muscle histology was clearly abnormal in at least one of the at-risk fetuses. The mean area of myotube nuclei in cultures of DMD muscle was found to be significantly larger than that of the myotube nuclei in cultures of normal muscle when measurements were made on fixed and stained preparations (Vassilipoulos et al 1977).

A method for preparing mononucleate cells by enzymatic digestion of human adult skeletal muscle using a mixture of collagenase and trypsin has been described by Yasin et al (1976). An abnormality in cellular behaviour was found in cells prepared from DMD muscle (Thompson et al 1977). The first sign of abnormality was detected four days after plating the cells and consisted of areas where the cells were clustered together in close proximity rather than being more uniformly distributed in a monolayer. The nuclei and the perinuclear cytoplasm of some of the cells in the clusters seemed to be increased in size. There were, however, a proportion of myoblasts which fused to form myotubes in apparently normal fashion. With further differentiation there were a certain number of refractile myotubes but their distribution was again abnormal in that they spanned the gap between the cell clusters. Time-lapse cinematography showed that the clusters enlarged primarily by cell division and, to a lesser extent, by the acquisition of neighbouring cells (Yasin et al 1979); furthermore, none of the single cells surrounding the clusters exhibited contact inhibition of movement. The behaviour was indicative of an abnormality in the cell surface or cell-locomotor machinery of dystrophic cells, as the behaviour was not observed in normal control cultures. In contrast, Ecob-Johnston & Brown (1981) found that multilayered clusters of cells were present in normal muscle-cell cultures and cultures of muscle cells from other neuromuscular diseases but not in the two DMD muscle cell cultures examined.

It is worth while to consider possible explanations for the conflicting observations in investigations using the explant and disaggregation technique. The muscle biopsy used to establish a culture probably contains several cell types including fully differentiated myotubes, myoblasts, satellite cells, fibroblasts and fat cells. Biopsies from pathological muscle may contain higher proportions of some cell types compared with normal muscle biopsies, e.g. muscle tissue is replaced by adipose tissue in advanced cases of DMD and by fibroblastic cells and connective tissue in facioscapulohumeral muscular dystrophy. The differing proportions of cells may influence the appearance of the culture and its growth patterns and this would be particularly dependent on the technique for establishing the culture. When cells are disaggregated by enzyme, all cells that survive the treatment have an equal opportunity to settle on the culture dish surface and establish the monolayer. When an explant culture is set up, only those cells which are capable of migrating from the fragment will appear in the cell monolayer. It is possible that the cells that initiate cluster formation in disaggregation cultures of DMD cells (Thompson et al 1977) are of a cell type that is relatively immobile, would not migrate from explants and would not therefore be seen in cultures set up by the explant technique.

Alternatively, if myogenic cells in a biopsy of DMD muscle were affected by the disease to different degrees there might be selection of the less severely affected cells in the culture environment. Migration out of an explant may be beyond the capability of more severely affected cells, but when disaggregated from the tissue these may remain viable and manifest pathological conditions in the monolayer.

It may take as long for pathological changes to develop in dystrophic myotubes in tissue culture as in vivo. It cannot be ruled out that some techniques of culture, e.g. the disaggregation technique, may bring the cells to the stage of showing pathological changes more rapidly.

To obviate some of these problems the technique of clonal analysis of DMD myogenic cells has been used. A dramatic decrease in the proliferative capacity of cloned DMD myoblasts before they senesce, as compared with control cultures, was reported (Blau et al 1983, Yasin et al 1983). Blau et al (1983) found that, of the DMD myoblast clones obtained, a large proportion contained a morphological class of flat distended cells that had an increased generation time and ceased to proliferate beyond 100–1000 cells but could be induced to fuse and form myotubes. This type of cell was found more frequently in cultures derived from biopsies taken from older DMD boys. It was proposed that the limited capacity of DMD myoblasts to grow is directly related to the progressive muscle degeneration characteristic of the disease.

Yasin et al (1983) found ultrastructural differences between two DMD myogenic clones examined. The cells of one clone had less well-developed myofibrils and a mass of interwoven 7–9 nm filaments.

Freeze fracture electron-microscopic analysis of plasma membranes of cultured DMD muscle cells were not significantly different from controls (Osame et al 1981) suggesting that the morphological abnormalities reported in vivo do not occur at an early stage of differentiation in culture.

Peterson & Crain (1979) have investigated the maturation of human muscle after innervation by fetal mouse spinal cord in long-term cultures. DMD myotubes developed cross-striations and contractions, but some of the striations were off-register and appeared to form swirling patterns within the myotube.

Histochemical, immunochemical and biochemical investigations. Gallup et al (1972) found that DMD myotubes in culture were enzymatically normal (strongly oxidative metabolism (high NADH-TR) and high myofibrillar ATPase) and concluded that the underlying pathological process does not affect enzymatic differentiation. In contrast, Goyle et al (1973) reported differences in succinic dehydrogenase, glucose-6-phosphate dehydrogenase and triglyceride content in cultures from patients with Duchenne muscular dystrophy but the data does not make it clear whether the cells examined were at the mononucleate or myotube stage.

Ionasescu et al (1976) found that total protein synthesis showed a significant decrease in DMD muscle cultures but it was not clear what the proportions of myotubes and fibroblasts were in these cultures. Addition of calcium chloride alone or ionophore A23184 was claimed to normalise the defect in protein synthesis, but synthesis in cultures of DMD cells was still only 60% of that of untreated normal cultures. The membrane-stabilising agents diphenylhydantoin and orgotein also increased total protein synthesis in DMD myogenic cells (Ionasescu et al 1979).

Analysis of ^{3}H-proline incorporation into collagen demonstrated a fourfold increase in ^{3}H-hydroxyproline released into the medium by DMD myogenic clones, while intracellular ^{3}H-hydroxyproline levels showed normal values (Ionasescu & Ionasescu 1982). The collagen turnover of DMD clones was normal. The authors suggested that the increased synthesis of collagen may be a primary defect of the muscle cell.

Walsh and his colleagues (Walsh 1984) were unable to find consistent protein differences between DMD muscle cells and controls (cloned and uncloned) compared using the double-label 2D gel analysis method.

Because of the reported morphological abnormalities of the DMD myotube plasma membrane in vivo there have been several investigations of the plasma membrane of cells in tissue culture. In an electrophysiological investigation Rothman & Bischoff (1983) found that the plasma membrane of DMD myotubes did not have active electrical properties (resting membrane potentials, amplitude or rate of rise of action potentials) that differed from those in controls. The distribution of acetylcholine receptors (detected by ^{125}I-bungarotoxin) was similar in DMD and control cultured myotubes (Franklin et al 1980a).

Ultrastructural examination of concanavalin A-binding sites in cultured DMD myotubes revealed no abnormalities at the cell surface when compared with normal cultured myotubes (Heiman-Patterson et al 1982). Reaction product at the cell surface appeared regular and continuous in both normal and DMD myotubes. These findings indicate that abnormalities of concanavalin surface binding found in biopsied DMD muscle are not present in cultured cells.

No difference was found in the qualitative profile of expression of two X-chromosome linked antigens (12E7 and R1) in a comparison of normal and DMD cultures (Walsh 1984).

Creatine kinase (CK) activities were significantly lower and the amounts of brain-type isoenzyme were significantly higher in DMD muscle cultures compared with controls (Ionasescu et al 1981, Franklin et al 1980b). However there was no difference in the CK levels in the culture medium bathing control and DMD muscle cells (Ionasescu et al 1981). Elevated levels of serum CK resulting from leakage from muscle cells are found in vivo (Ebashi et al 1959).

DMD fibroblasts. DMD skin fibroblasts have been widely investigated because biopsy samples are relatively easy to obtain and culture.

Abnormal growth kinetics of cultured DMD skin fibroblasts and matched normal controls have been reported (Liechti-Gallati et al 1981). DMD fibroblasts showed increased doubling time and a tendency to produce more voluminous cells, thus resembling prematurely ageing cells.

In investigations of purine metabolism, DMD fibroblasts were not significantly different in adenine or adenosine monophosphate uptake and conversion to nucleotides (Willers et al 1982). Activity values of hypoxanthine phosphoribosyl transferase and adenine phosphoribosyl transferase were also similar. However, membrane-bound 5'-nucleotidase activity was reported to be either elevated (Liechti-Gallati et al 1981) or not significantly different (Willers et al 1982).

Polysomes extracted from cultured DMD fibroblasts exhibited a threefold decrease in the rate of protein synthesis in a wheat germ extract system (Boule et al 1979). More recently a poly(U)-directed polyphenylalanine synthesis system was used to test 80 S ribosomes from DMD fibroblasts and normal controls as well as hybrid 80 S couples of subunits from DMD cells and control cells (Poche & Schultz 1985). The activity of ribosomes extracted from the patients was lower than that of normal controls. Of the 80 S hybrid ribosomes, only those consisting of 40 S subunits from DMD cells and 60 S subunits from the control cells showed a similar decrease in activity, suggesting that the defect is based exclusively on an alteration in the small ribosomal subunit.

Comparative investigations of the total protein of normal and DMD fibroblasts have not shown reproducible differences. Analysis of a doubly labelled fibroblast mixture using one-dimensional gel electrophoresis did not detect any consistent anomaly in the major proteins (Pena et al 1978). In contrast Burghes et al (1981) found that there was increased iodination of a 230 000 molecular weight protein which was associated with the outer surface of DMD skin fibroblasts and which was tentatively identified as fibronectin.

Comparison of fibroblast protein composition by two-dimensional gel electrophoresis (Rosenmann et al 1982) indicated that a protein of molecular weight 56 000, isoelectric point 6.4, was missing from DMD cells. It transpired that the normal cells used in this comparison were from preputial skin whereas the DMD fibroblasts were from non-genital skin biopsies. In a further investigation it was found that the protein of interest was also absent in normal fibroblasts if they were from non-genital skin biopsies (Thompson et al 1983).

Intracellular collagen synthesis was significantly decreased and extracellular collagen synthesis increased in rapidly dividing DMD fibroblasts (Ionasescu et al 1977). Prolyl hydroxylase activity was stimulated in fibroblasts exposed in culture to extracts from DMD muscle biopsies characterised by fibrosis compared with extracts from control muscle biopsies (Ulreich et al 1982). As prolyl hydroxylase activity is indicative of the capacity of fibroblasts to manufacture collagen structural macromolecules, it was concluded that the biopsies of dystrophic patients contain one or more factors which promoted this activity.

DMD skin fibroblasts are less adhesive than normal cells (Jones & Witkowski 1979). Their collision efficiencies determined using the couette viscometer were significantly lower than those of normal cells. Quantitative freeze-fracture studies indicated no significant differences in either intramembrane particle density or distribution in DMD fibroblast plasma membranes (Jones et al

1983). Activity of adenylate cyclase in DMD fibroblasts was not different from that in normal controls (Cerri et al 1982) in contrast to DMD myotubes in which the activity was increased (Matawari et al 1976). DMD fibroblasts stain normally with concanavalin A (Newman 1982). When DMD fibroblasts were treated with phospholipase C to degrade plasma membrane phosphatidylcholine, phosphatidylcholine synthesis was at normal control levels suggesting that one membrane repair mechanism was functioning (Wright et al 1984).

Several lysosomal enzymes have been assayed in DMD and age- and sex-matched control fibroblasts (Gelman et al 1980). The activity of 4-glycosidases, cathepsin B and total autoproteolysis at pH 4.0 were unchanged between the groups. However, dipeptidyl aminopeptidase I (cathepsin C) activity was decreased in DMD fibroblasts probably because there were fewer enzyme molecules present in the DMD cells. Disruption of crude lysosomal pellets with nonionic detergents indicated that DMD lysosomes showed less structure-linked latent activity of the enzyme (Davis et al 1982). In intact lysosomes from DMD fibroblasts the apparent K_a for Cl^- of this chloride-requiring enzyme was found to be lower. The apparent increase in entry of Cl^- was closely related with the decreased amount of the enzyme latency. High concentration of extralysosomal Cl^- corrected the abnormality. Electron-microscopic examination of these cells revealed the presence of abundant lamellar bodies, a morphological abnormality commonly associated with impaired lysosomal function (Gelman et al 1981).

Myotonic dystrophy

No morphological abnormalities were observed when myotonic dystrophy muscle cells were cultured by the explant technique (Bishop et al 1971, Witkowski et al 1976) or disaggregation technique (Yasin et al 1977).

Reports describing increased alcianophilia and metachromasia in myotonic fibroblasts have not been confirmed (Hartwig et al 1982). Furthermore, no differences were observed with phase-contrast microscopy or scanning and transmission electron microscopy, in histochemical studies, in growth characteristics, or in ^{35}S-sulphate incorporation studies.

Whether there are electrophysiological abnormalities is open to debate. Merickel et al (1981b) found that control myotubes demonstrated a hyperpolarisation after-potential whereas myotonic myotubes possessed depolarising after-potentials and repetitive bursts. Raising the extracellular or the intracellular calcium concentration in control myotubes caused their hyperpolarising after-potentials to become depolarising, but raising extracellular calcium in myotonic myotubes caused their depolarising after-potentials to become hyperpolarising. Increasing extracellular calcium depressed the slow outward current in myotonic myotubes.

In contrast Talmoush et al (1983) found no evidence that cultured myotonic muscle cells were electrically different from control cells. There was no significant difference in resting membrane potential. When the cells were hyperpolarised to -80 mV, there was no significant difference in effective membrane resistance, effective membrane capacitance, normalised membrane conductance, membrane threshold, action potential amplitude or maximum rate of rise of the action potential. Repetitive discharges were elicited by anodal-break excitation in a few cells from each group.

Myasthenia gravis

The effect of serum from myasthenic patients in which antibodies directed against the patient's own acetylcholine receptors (AChRs) are present has been tested on muscle cells in culture. Human myotubes exposed to sera have a lowered sensitivity to acetylcholine (Bevan et al 1977). Myotubes were incubated with 10% myasthenic serum for 90 min at 37°C before electrophysiological examination in a serum-free recording solution at 23°C. In such conditions, the test serum reduced myotube acetylcholine sensitivity by about 95%.

Antibodies in myasthenic serum reduced α-bungarotoxin binding to AChRs of myotubes of a mouse myogenic cell line by 50% (Gu et al 1985). The number of high-affinity tubocurarine sites was reduced without affecting those of low affinity. More than 80% of the AChR-mediated carbomylcholine-induced ^{22}Na influx was blocked (Maricq et al 1985). In more than 30% of the patches from antibody-treated cells, no channel activity in response to acetylcholine was seen; in contrast, every patch from control cells showed activity. The channels that were seen after antibody treatment were indistinguishable from those seen in normal cells, both in their single-channel conductance and in the kinetic constants used to describe channel opening and closing. Maricq et al (1985) concluded that the antibodies in myasthenic serum inhibit the functional response of AChRs in mouse myotubes to acetylcholine by inactivating individual receptors.

Post-junctional sensitivity of organ-cultured normal muscle fibres and those affected by myasthenia gravis was assessed by comparing miniature end-plate current amplitudes (Cull-Candy et al 1982). No evidence was found for a change in post synaptic sensitivity which ruled out reversible block of receptors by antireceptor antibody as having an important role in myasthenia gravis.

Patients improved clinically after thymectomy but their serum showed no significant difference in ability to decrease residual extrajunctional AChR in myotubes in culture (Hudgson et al 1982).

Other neuromuscular diseases where serum factors may be involved

The possible involvement of serum factors in other neuromuscular diseases in addition to myasthenia has been investigated in tissue culture.

Sera from Guillain–Barré syndrome patients have been observed to demyelinate organotypic cultures of peripheral nerve innervating muscle cells in culture (Dubois-Dalq et al 1971, Hirano et al 1971).

The effect of sera from motor neurone disease patients is more controversial. Originally Wolfgram & Myers (1973) reported that the serum killed anterior horn cells in cultures of embryonic mouse spinal cord but this was not confirmed by Horowich et al (1974). Serum from patients did not have a specific effect on organotypic nerve and muscle cultures (Liveson et al 1975).

The serum of a patient with multiple myeloma and diffuse muscle hypertrophy containing free kappa light chains, tested in human muscle cell cultures, displayed trophic properties (Delaporte et al 1985). Myoblast proliferation was not affected but fusion led to larger and more highly branched myotubes with increased protein synthesis compared with cultures in control serum. An identical trophic effect was also found with the kappa light chains purified from the patient's serum but only in the presence of normal human serum. In vivo, muscle fibres were surrounded by kappa chain deposits.

Metabolic myopathies

The metabolic myopathies can be classified into two groups.

(A) Enzyme deficiency myopathies whose myotubes, when grown in culture, show reappearance of enzyme activity, but which is due to a fetal isoenzyme. So far the following diseases fall into this category:
   1. Myophosphorylase deficiency (McArdle's disease, Glycogenosis V) (Sato et al 1977, DiMauro et al 1978)
   2. Phosphofructokinase deficiency (Davidson et al 1983)
   3. Phosphoglyceromutase deficiency (DiMauro et al 1981, 1982)
   4. Adenylate deaminase deficiency (DiMauro et al 1980)
(B) Enzyme deficiency myopathies in which the myotubes, when grown in culture, do not show reappearance of the enzyme. These involve enzymes that appear to exist in a single molecular form found in most tissues at all stages of development:
   1. Acid maltase deficiency (Glycogenosis II, Pompe's disease) (Askanas et al 1976)
   2. Glycogen debrancher deficiency (Miranda et al 1981)
   3. Carnitine palmitoyltransferase deficiency (Miranda et al 1982)

Other neuromuscular diseases which continue to express abnormalities in tissue culture

Muscle carnitine deficiency. Addition of of L-carnitine increased oxidation of palmitate by carnitine-depleted cultivated human skin fibroblasts from normal subjects and from two patients with muscle carnitine deficiency (Avignan et al 1983). Carnitine reduced incorporation of palmitate into glycerides in normal fibroblasts, suggesting that it may thereby counteract cellular accumulation of glycerides in cells. Fibroblasts from patients with muscle carnitine deficiency took up labelled carnitine at a normal rate. Dexamethasone increased palmitate oxidation by normal human fibroblasts and muscle cells of normal and muscle carnitine-deficient humans. The results parallel the reported effectiveness of carnitine, glucocorticoids, or medium-chain triglycerides in treatment of these patients.

Non-carnitine-deficient familial lipid neuropathy. Electron microscopy of non-innervated cultured muscle from a patient with this disease showed poorly matured muscle fibres containing large 'mushy' mitochondria, lipid droplets, abundant multilaminated inclusions and dense-core dark osmiophilic bodies (Askanas et al 1984). Parallel innervated muscle fibres (cocultured with normal rat motor neurones for two to three weeks) were well cross-striated, had well-developed T tubules and sarcoplasmic reticulum and none of the abnormalities of aneural muscle cultures. Cultured Schwann cells showed ultrastructurally abnormal mitochondria, lipid droplets, dark osmiophilic granular inclusions and numerous 'foamy' vacuoles. The reproduction of abnormalities in culture suggested that there was an intrinsic defect of both muscle and Schwann cells in this disease.

Adrenomyelo-neuropathy. Cultured muscle fibres from biopsies of a patient with a clinically and genetically distinct variant of adrenoleukodystrophy showed amorphous osmiophilic inclusions and multilaminated bodies in the cytoplasm (Askanas et al 1979a). The cytoplasm of cultured Schwann cells contained multilaminated dark inclusions. Cultures of both muscle and Schwann cells contained increased amounts of very-long-chain fatty acids compared with control cultures.

X-linked recessive congenital muscle fibre hypotrophy with central nuclei. At the ultrastructural level cultured fibres from two children with muscle fibres of decreased size and central nuclei in vivo appeared immature, showing increased numbers of ribosomes, unstriated myofibrils, and unusual accumulations of glycogen (Askanas et al 1979b). A decreased level of adenylate cyclase may be responsible for impaired control mechanisms resulting in the other abnormalities observed.

REFERENCES

Amagai Y, Iijima M, Kasai S 1983 Development of excitability during the in vitro differentiation of a newly established myogenic cell line. Japanese Journal of Physiology 33: 547–557

Anderson M J, Cohen M W 1977 Nerve-induced and spontaneous redistribution of acetylcholine receptors on cultured muscle cells. Journal of Physiology 268: 757–773

Anderson M J, Cohen M W, Zorychta E 1977 Effect of innervation on the distribution of acetylcholine receptors on cultured muscle cells. Journal of Physiology 268: 731–736

Anderson M J, Fambrough D M 1983 Aggregates of acetylcholine receptors are associated with plaques of a basal lamina heparan sulfate proteoglycan on the surface of skeletal muscle fibers. Journal of Cell Biology 97: 1396–1411

Anderson M J, Kleier F G, Tanguay K E 1984 Acetylcholine receptor aggregation parallels the deposition of a basal lamina proteoglycan during development of the neuromuscular junction. Journal of Cell Biology 99: 1769–1784

Askanas V, Shafiq S A, Milhorat A T 1972 Histochemistry of cultured aneural chick muscle: morphological maturation without differentiation of fibre types. Experimental Neurology 37: 218–265

Askanas, V, Engel W K, 1975 A new program for investigating adult human skeletal muscle grown aneurally in tissue culture. Neurology (Minneapolis) 25: 58–67

Askanas, V, Engel W K, Di Mauro S, Brooks B R, Mehler M 1976 Adult-onset and maltase deficiency: morphologic and biochemical abnormalities reproduced in cultured muscle. New England Journal of Medicine 294: 573–578

Askanas V, McLaughlin J, Engel W K, Adornato B T 1979a Abnormalities in cultured muscle and peripheral nerve of a patient with adrenomyeloneuropathy. New England Journal of Medicine 301: 588–590

Askanas, V, Engel W K, Reddy N B, et al 1979b X-linked recessive congenital muscle fibre hypertrophy with central nuclei. Abnormalities of growth and adenylate cyclase in muscle tissue cultures. Archives of Neurology (Chicago) 36: 604–609

Askanas, V, Engel W K, Kwan H H, Lawrence J V 1984 Abnormality of cultured muscle and Schwann's cells in familial neuromyopathy. Muscle corrected by neural influence. Archives of Neurology 41: 932–934

Avignan, J, Askanas, V, Engel W K, 1983 Muscle carnitine deficiency: fatty acid metabolism in cultured fibroblasts and muscle cells. Neurology 33: 1021–1026

Axelrod D, Ravdin P M, Podleski T R 1978 Control of acetylcholine receptor mobility and distribution in cultured muscle membranes. A fluorescence study. Biochimica et Biophysica Acta 511: 23–38

Bailey A J, Shellswell G B, Duance V C 1979 Identification and change of collagen types in differentiating myoblasts and developing chick muscle. Nature 278: 67–69

Bauer H C, Daniels M P, Pudimat P A, Jacques L, Sugiyama H, Christian C N 1981 Characterization and partial purification of a neuronal factor which increases acetylcholine receptor aggregation of cultured muscle cells. Brain Research 209: 395–404

Bayne E K, Anderson M J, Fambrough D M 1984 Extracellular matrix organization in developing muscle: correlation with acetylcholine receptor aggregates. Journal of Cell Biology 99: 1486–1501

Beach R L, Popiela M, Festoff B W 1985 Specificity of chicken and mammalian transferrins in myogenesis. Cell Differentiation 16: 93–100

Bevan S, Kullberg R W, Heinemann S F 1977 Human myasthenia sera induce acetylcholine sensitivity of human muscle cells in tissue culture. Nature 267: 263–265

Birnbaum M, Reis M A, Shainberg A 1980 Role of calcium in the regulation of acetylcholine receptor synthesis in cultured muscle cells. Pflugers Archiv. European Journal of Physiology 385: 37–43

Bischoff R 1974 Enzymatic liberation of myogenic cells from adult rat muscle. Anatomical Record 180: 645–662

Bischoff R 1975 Regeneration of single skeletal muscle fibres in vitro. Anatomical Record 182: 215–236

Bischoff R, Holtzer H 1969 Mitosis and the process of differentiation of myogenic cells in vitro. Journal of Cell Biology 41: 188

Bishop A, Gallup B, Skeate Y, Dubovitz V 1971 Morphological studies on normal human muscle in culture. Journal of the Neurological Sciences 13: 333–350

Blau H M, Webster C, Pavlath G K 1983 Defective myoblasts identified in Duchenne muscular dystrophy. Proceedings of the National Academy of Sciences USA 80: 4856–4860

Boule M, Vanasse M, Brakier-Gingras L 1979 Decrease in the rate of protein synthesis by polysomes from cultured fibroblasts of patients and carriers with Duchenne muscular dystrophy. Canadian Journal of Neurological Sciences 6: 355–358

Brehm P, Steinbach J H, Kidikoro Y, 1982 Channel open time of acetylcholine receptor on Xenopus muscle cells in dissociated cell culture. Developmental Biology 91: 31–102

Brevet A, Pinto E, Peacock J, Stockdale F E 1976 Myosin synthesis increased by electrical stimulation of skeletal muscle cell cultures. Science 193: 1152–1158

Buckingham M E, Minty A J 1983 Contractile protein genes. In: McClean N, Gregory A, Flavell, R A (eds) Eukaryotic genes: their structure, activity and regulation. Butterworth, London, p 55–120

Buckley P A, Konigsberg I R 1974 Myogenic fusion and the duration of the post-mitotic gap (G$_1$). Developmental Biology 37: 193–212

Buckley, P A, Konigsberg I R 1977 Do myoblasts in vivo withdraw from the cell cycle? A re-examination. Proceedings of the National Academy of Sciences USA 74: 2031–2035

Burghes A H M, Dunn M J, Statham H E, Dubowitz, V 1981 Analysis of cultured skin fibroblasts from patients with Duchenne muscular dystrophy using electrophoretic techniques. Electrophoresis 1: 295–308

Cantini M, Sartore S, Schiaffino S 1980 Myosin types in cultured muscle cells. Journal of Cell Biology 85: 903–909

Carlsson S-A, Ringertz N R, Savage R E 1974a Intracellular antigen migration in intraspecific myoblast heterokaryons. Experimental Cell Research 84: 255–266

Carlsson S-A, Luger O, Ringertz N R, Savage R E 1974b Phenotypic expression in chick erythrocyte x rat myoblast hybrids and in chick myoblast x rat myoblast hybrids. Experimental Cell Research 84: 47–55

Carrel A 1924 Tissue culture and cell physiology. Physiological Reviews 4: 1–20

Cerri C G, Willner J H, Miranda A F 1982 Adenylate cyclase in Duchenne fibroblasts. Journal of the Neurological Sciences 53: 181–185

Chen L B 1977 Alteration in cell surface LETS protein during myogenesis. Cell 10: 393–400

Chi J C, Fellini S A, Holtzer H 1975a Differences among myosins synthesized in non-myogenic cells, presumptive myoblasts and myoblasts. Proceedings of the National Academy of Sciences USA 72: 4999–5003

Chi J C H, Rubinstein N, Strahs K, Holtzer H 1975b Synthesis of myosin heavy and light chains in muscle cultures. Journal of Cell Biology 67: 523–537

Chiquet M, Eppenberger H M, Turner D C, 1981 Muscle morphogenesis: evidence for an organizing function of exogenous fibronectin. Developmental Biology 88: 220–235

Christian C N, Daniels M P, Sugiyama H, Vogel Z, Jacques L, Nelson P G 1978 A factor from neurones increases the number of acetylcholine receptor aggregates on cultured muscle cells. Proceedings of the National Academy of Sciences USA 75: 4011–4015

Cisson C M, McQuarrie C H, Sketely J, McNamee M G, Wilson B W 1981 Molecular forms of acetylcholinesterase in chick embryonic fast muscle: developmental changes and effects of DFP treatment. Developmental Neuroscience 4: 157–164

Cohen S A, Fischbach G D 1977 Regulation of muscle acetylcholine sensitivity by muscle activity in cell culture. Science 181: 74–78

Coleman J R, Coleman A W 1968 Muscle differentiation and macromolecular synthesis. Journal of Cellular Physiology 72: Suppl 1 19–30

Connolly J A, St.John P A, Fischbach G D 1982 Extracts of electric lobe and electric organ from Torpedo californica increase the total number as well as the number of aggregates of chick myotube acetylcholine receptors. Journal of Neuroscience 2: 1207–1213

Cull-Candy S G, Miledi R, Uchitel O D 1982 Properties of junctional and extrajunctional acetylcholine-receptor channels in organ cultured human muscle fibres. Journal of Physiology 333: 251–267

Damsky C H, Knudsen K A, Bradley D, Buck C A, Horowitz A F 1985 Distribution of the cell substratum attachment (CSAT) antigen on myogenic and fibroblastic cells in culture. Journal of Cell Biology 100: 1528–1539

Daubas P, Caput D, Buckingham M, Gros F 1981 A comparison between the synthesis of contractile proteins and the accumulation of their translatable mRNAs during calf myoblast differentiation. Developmental Biology 84: 133–143

Davidson M, Miranda A F, Bender A N, DiMauro S, Vora S 1983 Muscle phosphofructokinase deficiency. Biochemical and immunological studies of phosphofructokinase isozymes in muscle culture. Journal of Clinical Investigation 72: 545–550

Davis M H, Gelman B B, Gruenstein E 1982 Decreased structure-linked latency of lysosomal dipeptidyl aminopeptidase-I activity in Duchenne muscular dystrophy fibroblasts. Neurology 32: 486–491

Decker C, Greggs R, Duggan K, Stubbs J, Horowitz A 1984 Adhesive multiplicity in the interaction of embryonic fibroblasts and myoblasts with extracellular matrices. Journal of Cell Biology 99: 1398–1404

Delain D, Dreyfus J C, Meienhofer M C, Proux D. Schapira F, Wahrmann J P 1974 Studies on myogenesis in vitro I. Changes of creatine kinase, phosphorylase and phosphofructokinase isozymes. Recent Advances in Myology. Excerpta Medica, Amsterdam, p 344–350

De La Haba G, Cooper E W, Etling V 1966 Hormonal requirements for myogenesis of striated muscle in vitro: insulin and somatotropin. Proceedings of the National Academy of Sciences USA 56: 1719–1723

De La Haba G, Kamali H M, Tiede D M 1975 Myogenesis of avian striated muscle in vitro: role of collagen in myofibre formation. Proceedings of the National Academy of Sciences USA 72: 2729–2732

Delaport C, Drouin F, Ract A R, Varet B, Fardeau M 1985 Effect of a serum from a patient with multiple myeloma and diffuse muscle hypertrophy on the growth of human muscle cells in vitro. Revue Neurologique (Paris) 141: 109–119

Den H, Malinzak D, Keating H J, Rosenberg A 1975 Influence of concanavalin A, wheat germ agglutinin, and soybean agglutinin on the fusion of myoblasts in vitro. Journal of Cell Biology 67: 826–834

Den H, Malinzak D, Rosenberg A 1976 Lack of evidence for the involvement of a β-D-galactosyl-specific lectin in the fusion of chick myoblasts. Biochemical and Biophysical Research Communications 69: 621–627

Dessan W, Adelman B C, Timpl R, Martin G R 1978 Identification of the sites in collagen α chains that bind serum antigelatin factor (c-1g). Biochemical Journal 169: 55–59

Devlin R B, Emerson C P 1978 Co-ordinate regulation of contractile protein synthesis during myoblast differentiation. Cell 13: 599–611

Devlin R B, Emerson C P 1979 Co-ordinate accumulation of contractile protein mRNA during myoblast differentiation. Developmental Biology 69: 202–216

Dienstmann S R, Holtzer H 1977 Skeletal myogenesis. Control of proliferation in a normal cell line lineage. Experimental Cell Research 107: 355–364

DiMauro S, Arnold S, Miranda A, Rowland L P 1978 McArdle disease: the mystery of reappearing phosphorylase activity in muscle culture. Annals of Neurology 3: 60–66

DiMauro S, Miranda A, F, Hays A P, Franck W A, Hoffman G S, Schoenfeldt R S, Singh N 1980 Myodenylate deaminase deficiency — muscle biopsy and muscle culture in a patient with gout. Journal of the Neurological Sciences 47: 191–202

DiMauro S, Miranda A F, Kahn S, Gitlin K 1981 Human muscle phosphoglycerate mutase deficiency: Newly discovered metabolic myopathy. Science 212: 1277–1279

DiMauro S, Miranda A F, Olarte M, Friedman R, Hays A P H 1982 Muscle phosphoglycerate mutase deficiency. Neurology 32: 584–591

Doehring J L, Fischman D A 1974 The in vitro cell fusion of embryonic chick muscle without DNA synthesis. Developmental Biology 36: 225–235

Doehring J L, Fischman D A 1977 A fusion-promoting macromolecular factor in muscle conditioned medium. Experimental Cell Research 105: 437–443

Duance V. C, Restall D J, Beard H, Bourne F J, Bailey A J 1977 The location of three collagen types in skeletal muscle. FEBS Letters 79: 248–252

Dubois-Dalcq N, Buyse M, Buyse G, Gorce F 1971 The action of Gullain-Barré syndrome serum on myelin — a tissue culture and electronmicroscope analysis. Journal of the Neurological Sciences 13: 67–83

Dupont L, Buckingham M E, Gros F 1979 Scanning electron microscopy of mammalian muscle cells during differentiation in tissue culture. Biologie Cellulaire 35: 1–7

Ebashi S, Toyokura Y, Momoi H, Sugita M 1959 High creatine phosphokinase activity of sera of progressive muscular dystrophy patients. Journal of Biochemistry (Tokyo) 46: 103–110

Ecob-Johnston M S, Brown A E 1981 Cluster formation in monolayer cultures of normal and diseased human muscle. Experimental Neurology 71: 390–397

Ecob M S, Butler-Browne G S, Whalen R G 1983 The adult fast isozyme of myosin is present in nerve-muscle tissue culture system. Differentiation 25: 84–87

Ehrismann R, Chiquet M, Turner D C 1981 Mode of action of fibronectin in promoting chicken myoblast attachment. Journal of Biological Chemistry 256: 4056–4062

Emerson C P, Beckner S K 1975 Activation of myosin synthesis in fusing and mononucleated myoblasts. Journal of Molecular Biology 93: 431–447.

Emery A E H, McGregor L 1977 The foetus in Duchenne muscular dystrophy: muscle growth in tissue culture. Clinical Genetics 12: 183–187

Eppenberger H M, Perriard J-C, Rosenberg U B, Strehler E E 1981 The M 165000 m-protein myomesin: a specific protein of cross-striated muscle cells. Journal of Cell Biology 89: 185–193

Fambrough D, Rash J E 1971 Development of acetylcholine sensitivity during myogenesis. Developmental Biology 26: 55–64

Fernandez S A, Herman B A 1982 Topography and mobility of concanavain A receptors during myoblast fusion. In: Pearson M L, Epstein H F (eds) Muscle development. Molecular and cellular control. Cold Spring Harbor Laboratory 319–327

Fischbach G D 1972 Synapse formation between dissociated nerve and muscle cells in low density cell cultures. Developmental Biology 28: 407–429

Fischbach G D, Cohen S A 1973 The distribution of acetylcholine sensitivity over uninnervated and innervated muscle fibres grown in cell culture. Developmental Biology 31: 147–162

Fischman D A 1982 Myofibrillar assembly. In: Pearson M L, Epstein H F (eds) Muscle development. Molecular and cellular control. Cold Spring Harbor Laboratory 397–404

Florini J R, Roberts S B 1979 A serum-free medium for the growth of muscle cells in culture. In Vitro 15: 983–992

Fluck R A, Strohman R C 1973 Acetylcholinesterase activity in developing skeletal muscle cells in vitro. Developmental Biology 33: 417–428

Franklin G I, Yasin R, Hughes B P, Thomson E J 1980a Acetylcholine receptors in cultured human muscle cells. Journal of the Neurological Sciences 47: 317–327

Franklin G I, Cavanagh N P C, Hughes B P, Yasin R, Thompson E J 1980b Creatine kinase isoenzymes in cultured human muscle cells I. Comparison of Duchenne muscular dystrophy with other myopathic and neurogenic diseases. Clinica Chimica Acta 115: 179–189

Fremont P H, Fournier le Ray C, Le Douarin G H 1983 In vitro differentiation in the absence of nerve of avian myoblasts derived from slow and fast muscle rudiments. Cell Differentiation 13: 325–339

Freshney R I 1983 Culture of animal cells: a manual of basic technique. Alan R Liss, New York

Friedlander M, Fischman D A 1979 Immunological studies of the embryonic muscle surface. Journal of Cell Biology 81: 193–214

Frucht L T, Mosher D F, Wendelschafter-Crabb G 1978 Immunocytochemical localization of fibronectin (LETS protein) on the surface of L_6 myoblasts. Cell 13: 263–271

Fulton A B, Prives J, Farmer S R, Penman S 1981 Developmental reorganization of the skeletal framework and its surface lamina in fusing muscle cells. Journal of Cell Biology 91: 103–113

Gallup B, Bishop A, Dubovitz V 1972 Autoradiographic studies of RNA and DNA synthesis during myogenesis in cultures of human, chick and rat muscle. Journal of the Neurological Sciences 17: 127–140

Gartner T K, Podleski T R 1975 Evidence that a membrane bound lectin mediates fusion of L_6 myoblasts. Biochemical and Biophysical Research Communications 67: 972–978

Geiger R S, Garvin J S 1957 Pattern of regeneration of muscle from progressive muscular dystrophy patients cultivated in vitro as compared to normal human skeletal muscle. Journal of Neuropathology and Experimental Neurology 16: 532–543

Gelman B B, Papa L, Davis M H, Gruenstein E 1980 Decreased lysosomal dipeptidyl aminopeptidase I Activity in cultured human skin fibroblasts in Duchenne's muscular dystrophy. Clinical Investigation 65: 1398–1406

Gelman B B, Davis M H, Morris R E, Gruenstein E 1981 Structural changes in lysosomes from cultured human fibroblasts in Duchenne's muscular dystrophy. Journal of Cell Biology 88: 329–337

Gilfix, B M, Sanwal B D 1982 Lectin-resistant myoblasts. In: Pearson M L, Epstein H F (eds) Muscle development. Molecular and cellular control. Cold Spring Harbor Laboratory 329–336

Gospodarowicz D, Weseman J, Moran J 1975 Presence in brain of mitogenic agent promoting proliferation in low density culture. Nature 256: 216–219

Gospodarowicz D, Weseman J, Moran J, Lindstrom J 1976 Effect of fibroblast growth factor on the division and fusion of bovine myoblasts. Journal of Cell Biology 70: 395–405

Goyle S, Kalra S L, Singh B 1967 The growth of normal and dystrophic human skeletal muscle in tissue culture. Neurology (India) 15: 149–151

Goyle S, Kalra S L, Singh B 1968 Further studies on normal and dystrophic human skeletal muscle in tissue culture. Neurology (India) 16: 87–88

Goyle S, Virmani V, Singh B 1973 Cytochemical studies on cells grown in vitro from explants of normal and dystrophic human skeletal muscle, subcutaneous fat and fascia. In: Kakulas B A (ed) Basic research in myology. Excerpta Medica, Amsterdam, p 582–592

Grove B K, Stockdale F E 1979 Monoclonal antibodies to

cell surfaces of differentiating skeletal muscle. Journal of Cell Biology 83: 28a

Gruener R, Kidokoro Y 1982 Acetylcholine sensitivity of innervated and noninnervated Xenopus muscle cells in culture. Developmental Biology 91: 86–92

Gu Y, Silberstein L, Hall Z W 1985 The effects of a myasthenic serum on the acetylcholine receptors of C2 myotubes I Immunological distinction between the two toxin-binding sites of the receptor. Journal of the Neurosciences 5: 1907–1916

Guguen-Guillouzo C, Szajnert M-F, Marie J, Delain D, Schapira F 1977 Differentiation in vivo and in vitro of pyruvate kinase isoenzymes in rat muscle. Biochimie 59: 65–71

Gurdon J B, Woodland H R 1968 The cytoplasmic control of nuclear activity in animal development. Biological Reviews 43: 233

Hall Z W, Silberstein L, Inestrosa N C 1982 Synaptic basal lamina components made by a muscle cell line. In: Pearson M L, Epstein H F (eds) Muscle development. Molecular and cellular control. Cold Spring Harbor Laboratory 459–467

Harris H, Watkins J F, Ford C E, Schoefl G I 1966 Artificial heterokaryons of animal cells from different species. Journal of Cell Science 1: 1–30

Hartwig G B, Miller S E, Frost A P, Roses A D 1982 Myotonic muscular dystrophy: morphology, histochemistry and growth characteristics of cultured skin fibroblasts. Muscle and Nerve 5: 125–130

Hartzell H C, Fambrough D M 1973 Acetylcholine receptor production and incorporation into membranes of developing muscle fibre. Developmental Biology 30: 153–165

Hastings K E M, Emerson C P 1982 cDNA clone analysis of six coregulated mRNAs encoding skeletal muscle contractile proteins. Proceedings of the National Academy of Sciences USA 79: 1553–1557

Hauschka S D 1974a Clonal analysis of vertebrate morphogenesis. II Environmental influences upon human muscle differentiation. Developmental Biology 37: 329–344

Hauschka S D 1974b Clonal analysis of vertebrate morphogenesis. III Developmental changes in the muscle-colony-forming cells of the human foetal limb. Developmental Biology 37: 345–346

Hauschka S D, Konigsberg I R 1966 The influence of collagen on the development of muscle clones. Proceedings of the National Academy of Sciences USA 55: 119–126

Hauschka S D, White N K 1972 Studies of myogenesis in vitro. In: Banker B Q, Przbylski R J, van der Meulen J, Victor M (eds) Research in muscle development and the muscle spindle. Excepta Medica, Amsterdam, p 53–71

Heiman-Patterson T D, Bonilla E, Schotland D L 1982 Concanavalin A binding of the cell surface of Duchenne muscle in vitro. Annals of Neurology 12: 305–307

Hermann H, Konigsberg U R, Robinson G 1960 Observations on culture in vitro of normal and dystrophic muscle tissue. Proceedings of the Society for Experimental Biology and Medicine 105: 217–221

Hirano A, Cook S D, Whitaker J N, Dowling P C, Murray M R 1971 Fine structural aspects of demyelination in vitro — the effect of Guillain-Barré-serum. Journal of Neuropathology and Experimental Neurology 30: 249–265

Hirsch H E, Parks M E, Pardridge W M, Casanello-Ertl D 1981 Sarcolemmal protein profiles from cultured myotubes and myoblasts. Experimental Neurology 73: 837–841

Holland P C, MacLennan D H 1976 Assembly of the sarcoplasmic reticulum. Biosynthesis of the adenosine triphosphatase in rat skeletal muscle cell culture. Journal of Biological Sciences 251: 2030–2036

Holtzer H, Sanger J W 1972 Myogenesis: old views rethought. In: Barnier B, Research in muscle development and the muscle spindle. Excerpta Medica, Amsterdam, p 222–229

Holtzer H, Sanger J W, Ishikawa H, Strahs K 1972 Selected topics in myogenesis. In: The mechanism of muscle contraction. Cold Spring Harbor Symposia on Quantitative Biology 37: 549–566

Holtzer H, Croop J, Dienstman S, Ishikawa H, Somlyo A P 1975 Effects of cytochalasin B and colcemid on myogenic cultures. Proceedings of the National Academy of Sciences USA 72: 513–517

Holtzer H, Forry-Schaudies S, Antin P, Toyama Y, Goldstein M A, Murphy D L 1982 Effects of taxol, a microtubule-stabilizing agent on myogenic cultures. In: Pearson M L, Epstein H F (eds) Muscle development. Molecular and cellular control. Cold Spring Harbor Laboratory, p 383–394

Horowich M S, Engel W K, Chauvin P B 1974 Amyotrophic lateral sclerosis sera applied to cultured motor neurons. Archives of Neurology 30: 332–333

Horowitz A, Neff N, Sessions A, Decker C 1982 Cellular interactions in myogenesis. In: Pearson M L, Epstein H F (eds) Muscle development. Molecular and cellular control. Cold Spring Harbor Laboratory 291–300

Huang H L, Singer R H, Lazarides E 1978 Actin-containing microprocesses in the fusion of cultured chick myoblasts. Muscle and Nerve 1: 219–229

Hudgson P, McAdams M W, Pericak-Vance M A, Edwards A M, Roses A D 1982 Effect of sera from myasthenia gravis patients on acetylcholine receptors in myotube cultures. Journal of the Neurological Sciences 59: 37–45

Ionasescu V, Zellweger H, Ionasescu R, Lara-Brand C, Cancilla P A 1976 Protein synthesis in muscle cultures from patients with Duchenne muscular dystrophy. Acta Neurologica Scandinavica 54: 241–247

Ionasescu V, Lara-Brand C, Zellweger M, Ionasescu R Burmeister L 1977 Fibroblast cultures in Duchenne muscular dystrophy: alterations in synthesis and secretion of collagen and noncollagen proteins. Acta Neurologica Scandinavica 55: 407–417

Ionasescu V, Stern L Z, Ionasescu R, Rubenstein P 1979 Stimulatory effects of drugs for protein synthesis on muscle cell cultures in Duchenne dystrophy. Annals of Neurology 5: 107–110

Ionasescu V, Ionasescu R, Feld R, Witte D, Cancilla P, Kaeding L, Stern L Z 1981 Alterations in creatine kinase in fresh muscle and cell cultures in Duchenne dystrophy. Annals of Neurology 9: 394–399

Ionasescu V, Ionasescu R 1982 Increased collagen synthesis by Duchenne myogenic clones. Journal of the Neurological Sciences 54: 79–87

It I, Kimura I, Ozawa E 1982 A myotrophic protein from chick embryo extract: its purification, identity to transferrin, an indispensibility for avian myogenesis. Developmental Biology 94: 366–377

It I, Kimura I, Ozawa E 1985 Promotion of myoblast proliferation by hypoxanthine and RNA in chick embryo extract. Development, Growth and Differentiation 27: 101–110

Jessel T M, Siegel R E, Fischbach G D 1979 Induction of

acetylcholine receptors on cultured skeletal muscle by a factor extracted from brain and spinal cord. Proceedings of the National Academy of Sciences 76: 5397–5401

John H A, Jones K W 1975 Tissue culture investigations of the effect of nerve on myosin structure and function. In: Bradley W G, Gardner-Medwin D, Walton J N (eds) Recent advances in myology. Excerpta Medica, Amsterdam, p 358–363

John H A, Lawson H 1980 The effect of different collagen types used as substrata on myogenesis in tissue culture. Cell Biology International Reports 4: 841–850

Jones G E, Witkowski J A 1979 Reduced adhesiveness between skin fibroblasts from patients with Duchenne muscular dystrophy. Journal of the Neurological Sciences 43: 465–470

Jones G E, Severs N J, Witkowski J A 1983 Freeze fracture analysis of plasma membranes in Duchenne muscular dystrophy. A study using cultured skin fibroblasts. Journal of the Neurological Sciences 58: 185–193

Jorgensen A O, Kalnins V I, Zubrzycka E, MacLennan D H 1977 Assembly of the sarcoplasmic reticulum: localization by immunofluorescence of sarcoplasmic reticulum proteins in differentiating rat skeletal muscle cell cultures. Journal of Cell Biology 74: 287–298

Kakulas B A, Papadimitriou J M, Knight J D, Mastaglia F L 1968 Normal and abnormal human muscle in tissue culture. Proceedings of the Australian Association of Neurology 5: 79–85

Kalcheim C, Duksin D, Vogel Z 1982 Aggregation of acetylcholine receptors in nerve-muscle cocultures is decreased by inhibitors of collagen production. Neuroscience Letters 31: 265–270

Kalderon N, Gilula N B, 1979 Membrane events involved in myoblast fusion. Journal of Cell Biology 81: 411–425

Kato A C, Vrachliotis A, Fulpius B, Dunant Y 1980 Molecular forms of acetylcholinesterase in chick muscle and ciliary ganglion: embryonic tissues and cultured cells. Developmental Biology 76: 222–228

Kaufman S J 1982 Membrane events during myogenesis. In: Pearson M L, Epstein H F (eds) Muscle development. Molecular and cellular control. Cold Spring Harbor Laboratory 271–280

Kaufman S J, Lawless M L 1980 Thiogalactoside binding lectin and skeletal myogenesis. Differentiation 16: 41–50

Keller L R, Emerson C P 1981 Synthesis of adult myosin light chains by embryonic muscle cultures. Proceedings of the National Academy of Sciences USA 78: 1020–1024

Kent C, Schimmel S O, Vagelos P R 1974 Lipid composition of plasma membranes from developing chick muscle cells in culture. Biochimica et Biophysica Acta 360: 312–321

Kent C, Vagelos P R 1976 Phosphatidic acid phosphatase and phospholipase A activities in plasma membranes from fusing muscle cells. Biochimica et Biophysica Acta 436: 377–386

Ketley J N, Orkin R W, Martin G R 1976 Collagen in developing chick muscle in vivo and in vitro. Experimental Cell Research 99: 261–268

Kidokoro Y 1984 Two types of miniature endplate potentials in Xenopus nerve–muscle cultures. Neuroscience Research 1: 157–170

Kidokoro Y, Yeh E 1981 Synaptic contacts between embryonic Xenopus neurones and myotubes formed from a rat skeletal muscle cell line. Developmental Biology 86: 12–18

Kidokoro Y, Gruener R 1982 Distribution and density of α-bungarotoxin binding sites on innervated and noninnervated Xenopus muscle cells in culture. Developmental Biology 91: 78–85

Klebe R J 1974 Isolation of a collagen-dependent cell attachment factor. Nature 250: 248–251

Kleinmann H K, Goodwin E B, Klebe R J 1976 Localization of the cell attachment region in type I and II collagen. Biochemical and Biophysical Research Communications 72: 426–432

Kohama K, Ozawa E 1978a Muscle trophic factor. II Ontogenic development of activity of a muscle trophic factor in chicken serum. Muscle and Nerve 1: 236–241

Kohama K, Ozawa E 1978b Muscle trophic factor. IV Testosterone-induced increase in muscle trophic factor in chicken serum. Muscle and Nerve 1: 320–321

Komiya Y, Austin L 1974 Axoplasmic flow of protein in the sciatic nerve of normal and dystrophic mice. Experimental Neurology 43: 1–12

Konieczny S F, Lawrence J B, Coleman J R 1983 Analysis of muscle protein expression in polyethylene glycol-induced chicken:rat myoblast heterokaryons. Journal of Cell Biology 97: 1348–1355

Konigsberg I R 1961 Some aspects of myogenesis in vitro. Circulation 24: 447–453

Konigsberg I R 1963 Clonal analysis of myogenesis. Science 140: 1273–1284

Konigsberg I R 1970 The relationship of collagen to the clonal development of embryonic skeletal muscle. In: Balazs E A (ed) Chemistry and molecular biology of intracellular matrix. Academic Press, New York, vol 3

Konigsberg I R 1971 Diffusion-mediated control of myoblast fusion. Developmental Biology 26: 133–152

Konigsberg U R, Lipton B H, Konigsberg I R 1975 The regenerative response of single mature muscle fibres isolated in vitro. Developmental Biology 45: 260–275

Konigsberg I R, Sollmann P A, Mixter L O 1978 The duration of the terminal G of fusing myoblasts. Developmental Biology 63: 11–26

Land B R, Podleski T R, Salpeter E E, Salpeter M M 1977 Acetylcholine receptor distribution on myotubes in culture correlated to acetylcholine sensitivity. Journal of Physiology (London) 269: 155–176

Lathrop B, Olson E, Glaser L 1985 Control by fibroblast growth factor of differentiation in the BC₃H1 muscle cell line. Journal of Cell Biology 100: 1540–1547

Lee H U, Kaufman S J 1981 Use of monoclonal antibodies in the analysis of myoblast development. Developmental Biology 81: 81–95

Liechti-Gallati S, Moser H, Siegrist H P, Wiesmann U, Herschkowitz N N 1981 Abnormal growth kinetics and 5′-nucleotidase activities in cultured skin fibroblasts from patients with Duchenne muscular dystrophy. Pediatric Research 15: 1411–1414

Linder S, Brzeski H, Ringertz N R 1979 Phenotypic expression in cybrids derived from teratocarcinoma cells fused with myoblast cytoplasms. Experimental Cell Research 120: 1–14

Liveson J, Frey H, Bornstein M B 1975 The effect of serum from ALS patients on organotypic nerve and muscle tissue cultures. Acta Neuropathologica (Berlin) 32: 127–131

Maricq A V, Gu Y, Hestrin S, Hall Z 1985 The effects of a myasthenic serum on the acetylcholine receptors of C2 myotubes II. Functional inactivation of the receptor. Journal of the Neurosciences 5: 1917–1924

Marino M, Cossu G, Neri G, Molinaro M 1980 Appearance

of a class of cell-surface fucosyl-glycopeptides in differentiated muscle cells in culture. Developmental Biology 78: 258–267

Markelonis G J, Oh T H 1978 A protein fraction from peripheral nerve having neurotrophic effects on skeletal muscle cells culture. Experimental Neurology 58: 285–295

Markelonis G, Oh T H, Derr D 1980 Stimulation of protein synthesis in cultured skeletal muscle by a trophic protein from sciatic nerve. Experimental Neurology 70: 598–612

Martonosi A, Roufa D, Boland R, Reyes E, Tillack T W 1977 Development of sarcoplasmic reticulum in cultured chicken muscle. Journal of Biochemistry 252: 318–332

Masaki T 1973 Development of myosin in chick embryo. Japanese Journal of Pharmacology 23 (suppl)

Masaki T, Yoshizaki C 1974 Differentiation of myosin in chick embryos. Journal of Biochemistry (Tokyo) 76: 123–133

Matawari S, Miranda A, Rowland L P 1976 Adenyl cyclase abnormality in Duchenne muscular dystrophy muscle cells in culture. Neurology (Minneapolis) 26: 1021–1026

Mauro A 1961 Satellite cells of skeletal muscle fibres. Journal of Biophysical and Biochemical Cytology 9: 493–495

Mehrke G, Jockusch H, Faissner A, Schachner M 1984 Synapse formation and synaptic activity in mammalian nerve-muscle co-culture are not inhibited by antibodies to neural cell adhesion LI. Neuroscience Letters 44: 235–239

Merickel M, Gray R, Chauvin P, Appel S 1981a Electrophysiology of human muscle in culture. Experimental Neurology 72: 281–293

Merickel M, Gray R, Chauvin P, Appel S H 1981b Cultured muscle from myotonic muscular dystrophy patients: altered membrane electrical properties. Proceedings of the National Academy of Sciences USA 78: 648–652

Merlie J P, Changeux J-P, Gros F 1976 Acetylcholine receptor degradation measured by pulse chase labelling. Nature 264: 74–76

Miranda A F, Di Mauro A, Antler A, Stern L Z, Rowland L P 1981 Glycogen debrancher deficiency is reproduced in muscle culture. Annals of Neurology 9: 283–288

Miranda A F, Shanske S, DiMauro S 1982 Developmentally regulated isozyme transitions in normal and diseased human muscle. In: Pearson M L, Epstein H (eds) Muscle development — molecular and cellular control. Cold Spring Harbor Laboratory, p 515–525

Montarras D, Fiszman M Y, Gros F 1982 Changes in tropomyosin during development of chick embryonic skeletal muscles in vivo and during differentiation of chick muscle cells in vitro. Journal of Biological Chemistry 257: 545–548

Montarras D, Fiszman M Y 1983 A new muscle phenotype is expressed by subcultured quail myoblasts from future fast and slow muscle. Journal of Biological Chemistry 258: 3883–3888

Morgan J, Cohen L 1974 Use of papain in the preparation of adult mammalian skeletal muscle for tissue culture. In Vitro 10: 188–195

Morris G E, Cole R J 1972 Cell fusion and differentiation in cultured chick muscle cells. Experimental Cell Research 75: 191–199

Morris G E, Piper M, Cole R J 1976 Differential effects of calcium ion concentration on cell fusion, cell division and creatine kinase activity in muscle cell cultures. Experimental Cell Research 99: 106–114

Morris G E, Cole R J 1977 Biosynthesis of muscle specific creatine kinase during differentiation in vitro. FEBS Letters 79: 183–187

Moscona A, Moscona H 1952 The dissociation and aggregation of cells from organ rudiments of the early chick embryo. Journal of Anatomy 86:287

Moss M, Schwartz R 1981 Regulation of tropomyosin gene expression during myogenesis. Molecular and Cellular Biology 1: 289–301

Moss P S, Strohmann R C 1976 Myosin synthesis by fusion-arrested chick embryo myoblasts in cell culture. Developmental Biology 48: 431–437

Nadal-Ginard B 1978 Commitment, fusion and biochemical differentiation of a myogenic cell line in the absence of DNA synthesis. Cell 15: 855–863

Nameroff M, Holtzer H 1969 Interference with myogenesis. Developmental Biology 19: 380–391

Neff N T, Lowrey C, Decker C, Tovar A, Damsky C, Buck C, Horowitz A F 1982 A monoclonal antibody detaches skeletal muscle from extracellular matrices. Journal of Cell Biology 95: 654–666

Newman G C 1982 Duchenne muscular dystrophy cultured skin fibroblasts stain normally with concanavalin-A. Journal of the Neurological Sciences 54: 353–358

Obinata T, Shimada Y, Matsuda R 1979 Troponin in embryonic chick skeletal muscle cells in vitro. An immunoelectron microscope study. Cellular Biology 81: 59–66

Oh T H 1976 Neurotrophic effects of sciatic nerve extracts on muscle development in culture. Experimental Neurology 50: 376–386

Oh T H, Johnson D D, Kim S V 1972 Neurotrophic effect on isolated chick embryo muscle in culture. Science 178: 1298–1300

O'Neill M C, Stockdale F E 1972 A kinetic analysis of myogenesis in vitro. Journal of Cell Biology 52: 52–65

Osame M, Engel A G, Rebouch C J, Scott R E 1981 Freeze-fracture electronmicroscopic analysis of plasma membranes of cultured muscle cells in Duchenne dystrophy. Neurology 31: 970–979

Ozawa E, Kohama K 1978 Muscle trophic factor III Effect of hormones and tissue extracts on muscle trophic-factor activity. Muscle and Nerve 1: 314–319

Paterson B, Strohman R C 1972 Myosin synthesis in cultures of differentiating chick embryo skeletal muscle. Developmental Biology 29: 113–118

Paul J 1970 Cell and tissue culture. Livingstone, Edinburgh

Pearlstein E 1976 Plasma membrane glycoprotein which mediates cell adhesion of fibroblasts to collagen. Nature 262: 497–500

Pena S D J, Vust A, Tucker D, Hamerton J L, Wrogemann K 1978 Biochemical investigations in cultured skin fibroblasts from patients with Duchenne muscular dystrophy. Clinical Genetics 14: 50–54

Peng H B, Wolosewick J J, Cheng P-C 1981 The development of myofibrils in cultured muscle cells: a whole-mount and thin section electron microscopic study. Developmental Biology 88: 121–136

Peng H B, Froehner S C 1985 Association of the postsynaptic 43K protein with newly formed acetylcholine receptor clusters in cultured muscle cells. Journal of Cell Biology 100: 1698–1705

Perry S V 1971 Development and specialization in muscle and the biochemistry of the dystrophies. Journal of the Neurological Sciences 12: 289–306

Peterson E R, Crain S M 1979 Maturation of human muscle after innervation by foetal mouse spinal cord explants in long term cultures. In: Mauro A (ed) Muscle regeneration. Raven Press, New York, p 305–309

Poche H, Schulze H 1985 Ribosomal protein synthesis in cultured skin fibroblast cells obtained from patients with Duchenne muscular dystrophy. Journal of the Neurological Sciences 70: 295–304

Podelski T R, Axelrod D, Ravdin P, Greenberg I, Johnson M M, Saltpeter M M 1978 Nerve extract induces increase and redistribution of acetylcholine receptors on cloned muscle cells. Proceedings of the National Academy of Sciences USA 75: 2035–2039

Potter J D 1974 The content of troponin, tropomyosin, actin and myosin in rabbit skeletal muscle myofibrils. Archives of Biochemistry and Biophysics 162: 436–441

Powers M L, Florini J R, 1975 A direct effect of testosterone on muscle cells in tissue culture. Endocrinology 97: 1043–1047

Prives J, Hoffman L, Ross A, Serafin N 1982a Interaction of the acetylcholine receptor and acetylcholinesterase of the muscle cell surface with the cytoskeletal framework. In: Pearson M L, Epstein H F (eds) Muscle development. Molecular and cellular control. Cold Spring Harbor Laboratory 301–309

Prives J, Fulton A B, Penman, S, Daniels M P, Christian C N 1982b Interaction of the cytoskeletal framework with acetylcholine receptor on the surface of embryonic muscle cells in culture. Journal of Cell Biology 92: 231–236

Quinn L S, Nameroff M 1983 Analysis of the myogenic lineage in chick embryos IV Effects of conditioned medium. Differentiation 24: 124–130

Richler C, Yaffe D 1970 The in vitro cultivation and differentiation capacities of myogenic cell lines. Developmental Biology 23: 1–12

Rinaldini L M 1959 An improved method for the isolation and quantitative cultivation of embryonic cells. Experimental Cell Research 16: 477–505

Ringertz N R, Krondahl U, Coleman J R 1978 Reconstitution of cells by fusion of cell fragments I Myogenic expression after fusion of minicells from rat myoblasts (L6) with mouse fibroblasts (A9) cytoplasm. Experimental Cell Research 113: 233–246

Ritchie A K, Fambrough D M 1975 Electrophysiological properties of the membrane and acetylcholine receptor in developing rat and chick myotubes. Journal of General Physiology 66: 327–355

Robbins N, Yonezawa T 1971 Developing neuromuscular junctions: first signs of chemical transmission during formation in tissue culture. Science 172: 395–397

Role L W, Matossian V R, O'Brien R J, Fischbach G D 1985 On the mechanism of acetylcholine receptor accumulation at newly formed synapses on chick myotubes. Journal of Neuroscience 5: 2197–2204

Rosenmann E, Kreis C, Thompson R G, Dobbs M, Hamerton J L, Wrogemann K 1982 Analysis of fibroblast proteins from patients with Duchenne muscular dystrophy by two-dimensional gel electrophoresis. Nature 298: 563–565

Rothman S M, Bischoff R 1983 Electrophysiology of Duchenne dystrophy myotubes in tissue culture. Annals of Neurology 13: 176–179

Rubin L L, Schuetze S M, Fischbach G D 1979 Accumulation of acetylcholinesterase at newly formed nerve-muscle synapses. Developmental Biology 69: 46–58

Rubinstein N A, Holtzer H 1979 Fast and slow muscles in tissue culture synthesize only fast myosin. Nature 280: 323–325

Rutishauser U, Grumet M, Edelman G M 1983 Neural cell adhesion molecular mediates initial interactions between spinal cord neurons and muscle cells in culture. Journal of Cell Biology 97: 145–152

Salmons S, Sreter F A 1976 Significance of impulse activity in the transformation of the skeletal muscle type. Nature 263: 30–34

Salpeter M M, Podelski T R 1982 Acetylcholine receptors on primary rat muscle cells redistribute to reach functional site densities after exposure to soluble neuronal extracts. In: Pearson M L, Epstein H F (eds) Muscle development. Molecular and cellular control. Cold Spring Harbor Laboratory 481–495

Sandra A, Leon M A, Przybylski R J 1977 Suppression of myoblast fusion by concanavalin A: Possible involvement of membrane fluidity. Journal of Cell Science 28: 251–263

Sato K, Imai F, Hatayama I, Roelofs R I 1977 Characterization of glycogen phosphorylase isoenzymes present in cultured skeletal muscle from patients with McArdle's disease. Biochemical and Biophysical Research Communications 75: 663–668

Schiaffino S, Askanas V, Engel W K, Vitadello M, Sartore S 1982 Myosin isoenzymes in cultured human muscle. Archives of Neurology 39: 347–349

Schubert D, Lacorbiere M 1976 Phenotypic transformation of clonal myogenic cells to cells resembling chondrocytes. Proceedings of the National Academy of Sciences USA 73: 1989–1993

Schudt C, Pette D 1976 Influence of monosaccharides, medium functions and enzymatic modification on fusion of myoblasts in vitro. Cytobiologie (Stuttgart) 13: 74–84

Scott R E, Dousa T P 1978 Plasma membrane cyclic AMP-dependent protein phosphorylation system in L_6 myoblasts. Biochimica et Biophysica Acta 509: 499–506

Shainberg A, Burstein M 1976 Decrease of acetylcholine receptor synthesis in muscle cultures by electrical stimulation. Nature 264: 368–369

Shani M, Zevin-Sonkin D, Saxel O, Carmon Y, Katcoff D, Nudel U, Yaffe D 1981 The correlation between the synthesis of skeletal muscle actin, myosin heavy chain and myosin light chain and the accumulation of corresponding mRNA sequences during myogenesis. Developmental Biology 86: 483–492

Shimada Y, Fischman D A, Moscona A A 1969a Formation of neuromuscular junctions in embryonic cell cultures. Proceedings of the National Academy of Sciences USA 62: 715–719

Shimada Y, Fischman D A, Moscona A A 1969b The development of nerve-muscle junctions in monolayer cultures of embryonic spinal cord and skeletal muscle cells. Journal of Cell Biology 43: 382–387

Skeate Y, Bishop A, Dubowitz V 1969 Differentiation of diseased human muscle in culture. Cell and Tissue Kinetics 2: 307–310

Sreter F, Holtzer S, Gergley J, Holtzer H 1972 Some properties of embryonic myosin. Journal of Cell Biology 55: 586–594

Stockdale F E, Holtzer H 1961 DNA synthesis and myogenesis. Experimental Cell Research 2: 508–520

Stockdale F E, Saden H, Raman N 1981 Slow muscle myoblasts differentiating in vitro synthesize both slow and fast myosin light chains. Developmental Biology 82: 168–171

Strehler B L, Konigsberg I R, Kelley J E T 1963 Ploidy of myotube nuclei developing in vitro as determined with a recording double-beam micro-spectrophotometer. Experimental Cell Research 32: 232–241

Strittmatter W J, Couch C B, Elias S B 1982 Role of specific proteases in rat myoblast fusion. In: Pearson M L, Epstein H F (eds) Muscle development. Molecular and cellular control. Cold Spring Harbor Laboratory 311–318

Talmoush A J, Askanas V, Nelson P G, Engel W K 1983 Electrophysiologic properties of aneurally cultured muscle from patients with myotonic muscular atrophy. Neurology 33: 311–316

Teng N N H, Fiszman M Y 1976 Appearance of acetylcholine receptors in cultured myoblasts prior to fusion. Journal of Supramolecular Structure 4: 381–387

Thompson E J, Yasin R, van Beers G, Nurse K, Al Ani S 1977 Myogenic defect in human muscular dystrophy. Nature 268: 241–243

Thompson R G, Nickel B, Finlayson A, Meuser R, Hamerton J L, Wrogemann, K 1983 56K Fibroblast protein is not specific for Duchenne muscular dystrophy but for skin biopsy site. Nature 304: 740–741

Toutant J P, Toutant M, Fiszman M Y, Massoulie J M 1983 Expression of the A_{12} form of acetylcholinesterase by developing avian leg muscle cells in vivo and during differentiation in primary cell cultures. Neurochemistry International 5/6: 751–762

Trupin G L, Hse L, Parfett G 1982 An autoradiographic study on the role of satellite cells and myonuclei during myogenesis in vitro. Virchows Archiv B. Cell Pathology 39: 339–349

Turner D C, Gmur R, Siegrist M, Burckhardt E, Eppenberger H M 1976 Differentiation in cultures derived from embryonic chicken muscle I Muscle-specific enzyme changes before fusion in EGTA-synchronised cultures. Developmental Biology 48: 258–283

Ulreich J B, Stern L Z, Chvapil M 1982 Tissue factor influences fibroblast activity in neuromuscular diseases. Experimental Neurology 76: 150–155

Vassilopoulos D, Emery A E H, Gordon N 1977 Nuclear changes in cultured human dystrophic muscle. Experientia 33: 759–760

Vertel B M, Fischman D A 1976 Myosin accumulation in mononucleated cells of chick muscle cultures. Developmental Biology 48: 438–446

Vogel Z, Sytkowski A J, Nirenberg M W 1972 Acetylcholine receptors of muscle grown in vitro. Proceedings of the National Academy of Sciences USA 69: 3180–3184

Wagner D D, Hynes R O 1980 Topological arrangement of the major structural features of fibronectin. Journal of Biological Chemistry 255: 4304–4312

Walker C R, Wilson B W 1975 Control of acetylcholine esterase by contractile activity of cultured muscle cells. Nature 256: 215–216

Wallace B G, Godfrey E W, Nitkin R M, Rubin L L, McMahon U J 1982 An extract of extracellular matrix fraction that organises acetylcholine receptors. In: Pearson M L, Epstein H F (eds) Muscle development, molecular and cellular control. Cold Spring Harbor Laboratory 469–479

Walsh F S 1984 X-chromosome-coded antigens in Duchenne muscular dystrophy. Biochemical Society Transactions 12: 368–371

Walsh F S, Ritter M A 1981 Surface antigen differentiation during human myogenesis in culture. Nature 289: 60–64

Weldon P R, Cohen M W 1979 Development of synaptic ultrastructure at neuromuscular contacts in an amphibian culture system. Journal of Neurocytology 8: 239–259

Whalen R G, Butler-Browne G S, Gros F 1976 Protein synthesis and actin heterogeneity in calf muscle cells in culture. Proceedings of the National Academy of Sciences USA 73: 2018–2022

Whalen R G, Butler-Browne G S, Gros F 1978 Identification of a novel form of myosin light chains present in embryonic muscle tissue and cultured muscle cells. Journal of Molecular Biology 126: 415–431

Whalen R G, Schwartz K, Bouveret P, Sell S M, Gros F 1979 Contractile protein isozymes in muscle development: identification of an embryonic form of myosin heavy chain. Proceedings of the National Academy of Science USA 76: 5197–5201

Whalen R G, Sell S M, Butler-Browne G S, Schwartz K, Bouvert P, Pinset-Harstrom 1 1981 Three myosin heavy-chain isozymes appear sequentially in rat muscle development. Nature 292: 805–809

Whatley R, Ng S K, Rogers J, Murray W C, Sanwal B D 1976 Developmental changes in gangliosides during myogenesis of a rat myoblast cell line and its drug resistant variants. Biochemical and Biophysical Research Communications 70: 180–185

Willers I, Singh S, Goedde H W 1982 Purine metabolism in fibroblasts of patients with Duchenne's muscular dystrophy. Human Heredity 32: 233–239

Witkowski J A 1977 Diseased muscle cells in culture. Biological Reviews 52: 431–476

Witkowski J A, Durbridge M, Dubovitz V 1976 Growth of human muscle in tissue culture. In Vitro 12: 98–106

Wolfgram F, Myers L 1973 Amyotrophic lateral sclerosis-effect of serum on anterior horn cells in tissue culture. Science 179: 579–560

Wright P S, McKinney E, Berry S, Evers A, Kent C 1984 A functional membrane repair system in Duchenne muscular dystrophy fibroblasts. Journal of the Neurological Sciences 64: 259–264

Wright W E, Aranoff J 1983 The suppression of myogenic functions in heterokaryons formed by fusing chick myocytes to diploid rat fibroblasts. Cell Differentiation 12: 299–306

Yaffe D 1968 Retention of differentiation potentialities during prolonged cultivation of myogenic cells. Proceedings of the National Academy of Sciences USA 61: 477–480

Yaffe D 1971 Developmental changes preceding cell fusion during muscle differentiation in vitro. Experimental Cell Research 66: 33–48

Yasin R, van Beers E, Bulien D, Thomson E J 1976 A quantitative procedure for the dissociation of adult mammalian muscle in mononucleated cells. Experimental Cell Research 102: 405–408

Yasin R, van Beers G, Nurse K C E, Al-Ani S, Landon D N, Thompson E J 1977 A quantitative technique for growing human adult skeletal muscle in culture starting from mononucleate cells. Journal of the Neurological Sciences 32: 347–360

Yasin R, van Beers G, Riddle P N, Brown D, Widdowson G, Thompson E J 1979 An abnormality of cell behaviour in human dystrophic muscle cultures: a time-lapse study. Journal of Cell Science 10: 201–310

Yasin R, Walsh F S, Landon D N, Thompson E J 1983 New approaches to the study of human dystrophic muscle cells in culture. Journal of the Neurological Sciences 58: 315–334

Yeoh G C T, Holtzer H 1977 The effect of cell density, conditioned medium and cytosine arabinoside on myogenesis in primary and secondary cultures. Experimental Cell Research 104: 63–78

Zalin R J 1977 Prostaglandins and myoblast fusion. Developmental Biology 59: 241–248

Zalin R J, Montague W 1974 Changes in adenylate cyclase, cyclic AMP and protein kinase levels in chick myoblasts and their relationship to differentiation. Cell 2: 103–107

Experimental muscle diseases

INTRODUCTION

The prime aim of experimental myopathology is to provide insights into the underlying mechanisms involved in the aetiology and pathogenesis of human disorders of voluntary muscle. In this respect there are three distinct avenues of approach. First, there are studies which pertain to the principles of general pathology, e.g. the effects of ischaemia or infection; secondly, there is the experimental investigation of tissue reactions which are more or less specific to muscle, such as denervation; and thirdly, there are the attempts in the laboratory to produce a copy of a natural human or animal myopathy.

In addition to the above there are several research disciplines which, although conforming to the general intent of experimental myopathology, are nevertheless beyond the scope of this review. For instance, there exists a vast body of scientific information concerning many aspects of skeletal muscle obtained experimentally by biologists, biochemists, physiologists and anatomists, much of which is broadly relevant to muscle disease. However, to review such progress is beyond our present intent and only those experimental investigations which are immediately applicable to muscle disease will be considered. Furthermore, although the hereditary muscular dystrophies of animals are sometimes studied experimentally they will not be considered here as a separate chapter is devoted to this topic (Ch. 28).

Much of what is known about the reaction of the muscle fibre in disease is derived from experimental study of the effects of injurious agents when tested in animals. The effects of disuse, denervation, ischaemia, infection and toxins are all well described. Not only is the primary consequence of such noxious influences known, but their continuing effect on the natural history of muscle disease is well understood. As a result of this work it is now possible to 'dissect' a lesion into its histological components, to identify the alterations in each such element and to observe how it contributes towards the overall derangement of architecture. The formulations derived from such experimental analyses are readily applicable to human myopathology, especially in the structural or topographic context.

Considerable progress has also been made in developing laboratory models of human diseases. Examples are the nutritional, toxic and endocrine myopathies, the muscular dystrophies and the immune disorders, such as polymyositis and myasthenia gravis. Experimental myotonia may also be produced in the laboratory by the administration of chemicals. New light has been shed on the histochemical and cytological changes encountered in the human congenital or 'structural' group of myopathies. Examples are the experimental production of 'central cores' and 'rod bodies' and the role of reinnervation in their pathogenesis. Biochemical agents which block oxidative pathways provide models of the so-called 'mitochondrial myopathies', and these might be further studied.

As mentioned above, there is an enormous volume of fundamental information derived from the work of 'basic' scientists. These advances have elucidated the physical qualities of muscle, its biochemistry, histochemistry, physiology, nerve – muscle interactions, trophisms, receptors, the muscle cytoskeleton, the mechanism of muscle contraction and membrane properties, among others. More recent muscle research has concentrated on cell biology and molecular genetics using recombinant DNA technology with 'probes' for the identification of genes governing specific cellular functions.

BASIC MUSCLE REACTIONS

Necrosis and regeneration

Focal or segmental necrosis of the muscle fibre is a frequent and non-specific muscle lesion found in a wide variety of myopathies which together are known as the 'necrobiotic' group. Within the group are the genetic muscular dystrophies, the inflammatory, nutritional, toxic and drug-induced myopathies. Necrosis also occurs as a result of ischaemia or trauma and may even be found in normal muscles following strenuous exercise. For this reason necrosis produced by experiment has been the subject of extensive investigation. Light, phase and electron microscopy, histochemistry, freeze fracture (Wakayama et al 1984) and other methods are utilised in these studies.

As far as can be determined ultrastructurally, the first sign of necrosis is swelling of the mitochondria and dilatation of the sarcoplasmic reticulum (SR). These changes are followed by a loss of definition of other organelles and, often, the 'supercontraction' and homogenation of sarcomeres with dissolution of myofibrils which may also show Z-band streaming. Membranous bodies or 'myelin' figures, lysosomes and autophagic vacuoles appear later. After a short time, zones of complete necrosis may become demarcated from the intact portion of the muscle fibre by a newly formed plasma membrane.

Light microscopy shows removal of debris by macrophages within hours and 'myoblasts' soon appear. Presumably these myoblasts are derived from 'activated satellite cells', although this point is not completely settled. The sequence of regeneration then begins. As debris is being removed the myoblasts multiply and join together, forming myotubes which then gradually increase in size. Regeneration ensues in this manner until complete restoration of the muscle fibre occurs in about four to six weeks, provided that the cause of the original injury is no longer active.

For regeneration to be complete the fibrous endomysial framework of the muscle fibre must remain intact; regeneration of this type is called isomorphic. On the other hand, if the endomysial framework is also destroyed, regenerating myoblasts are unguided and a random mixture of regenerating myotubes and proliferating fibrous tissue results; disorganised regeneration of this type is known as heteromorphic. As well as being akin to a traumatic neuroma, heteromorphic regeneration also bears a resemblance to 'proliferative myositis' and the desmoid tumour.

In the case of complete disruption of the muscle

fibre the regeneration which follows is referred to as being 'discontinuous' (Adams 1975), i.e. interrupted. However, partial injury of the muscle fibre is associated with retention of continuity of the sarcoplasm so that the regeneration which follows is of the 'continuous' type. Injury of this type affects the fibre only internally and thus in a limited manner. On the ultrastructural level, destruction of cytoplasmic organelles is found in the zones of partial injury. Subcellular structures become dense, ill-defined and may undergo lysis. These changes are also associated with increased pinocytosis, membranous bodies, vacuoles and lysosomes. Glycogen tends to accumulate. In 'continuous' regeneration the new sarcomeres and organelles are rapidly re-synthesized by ribosomes in a few days following the removal of necrotic debris by autophagosomes. When viewed with the light microscope in haematoxylin and eosin (H & E) stains, continuous regeneration is amphophilic or basophilic because of large numbers of ribosomes in the area undergoing restoration.

In the vicinity of regeneration, muscle nuclei are swollen, vesicular and contain abundant heteromorphic chromatin. Nucleoli are prominent. Myonuclei may also migrate towards the centre of the muscle fibre in late regeneration, which explains a common non-specific myopathic histological sign.

The effect of trauma. Simple section and crush are popular methods of investigating the reaction to injury of the muscle fibre. In both instances necrosis is soon followed by regeneration so that a model is produced for the histochemical and electron-microscopic evaluation of such reactions.

Following the classic studies of simple crush by Clark (1946) and Clark & Wajda (1947), regeneration after crush was investigated electron-microscopically by Allbrook (1962). These workers confirmed the classic observations of Volkmann (1893). The seminal observations of Clark (1946) were later greatly extended (Reznik 1973). The events which follow localised crush injury to muscle in the first few hours consist of altered morphology with obscured markings. Necrosis, evident as fragmentation and disintegration of sarcoplasm, is followed by phagocytosis of debris, spindle cell proliferation and 'isomorphic' regeneration.

Surprisingly, major trauma to muscle has been little studied experimentally. In this instance there is often associated haemorrhage, and healing is through the formation of granulation tissue. With the destruction of the supporting tissue elements, muscle regeneration is partly obscured by the proliferation of fibroblasts. Later there is collagenous fibrosis. Nevertheless, in such lesions myoblasts and tongue-like myotubes are readily identified, especially in sections stained with phosphotungstic acid haematoxylin (PTAH). The experimental findings are similar to those which occur in accidental massive injury to muscle in man (Anastas & Kakulas 1968). Such lesions may be present clinically as tumorous masses and in this case they are the equivalent in muscle of the 'traumatic' neuroma of peripheral nerve.

Needle myopathy. The effects of needle-induced myopathy have been studied experimentally in the rat. The lesions are characterised initially by haemorrhagic focal destruction followed by cellular infiltration, local necrosis and single fibre degeneration, regeneration and dystrophy-like changes. After several weeks the muscle returns to normal (Mumenthaler & Paakkari 1974).

Muscle transplantation has attracted increasing attention in recent years and numerous reports have appeared (Mauro et al 1970). Factors which affect the success of transplantation of skeletal muscle in the rat were studied by Gutmann & Hanzlikova (1975). The 'morphogenetic effects of cross-transplantation of muscle upon the epimorphic regenerative process' were examined in detail by Carlson (1974). The host reaction of muscle grafts in mice was investigated by Mastaglia et al (1974). Partridge & Sloper (1977) were able to demonstrate a host contribution to the regeneration in muscle heterografts. Proof was obtained by the isolation of two distinct isoenzymic forms of NADP-dependent malate dehydrogenase, as genetic markers in the two strains of mice used (CBA donors and C3H hosts). It was also shown that little, if any, of the newly formed muscle was of donor origin.

Recently, Sola et al (1985) have been successful in the transplantation of skeletal muscle grafted to the heart of dogs.

Experimental ischaemia. The effects of ischaemia differ from those of other metabolic disturbances in that pan-necrosis with loss of the supporting tissues, as well as necrosis of the muscle sarcoplasm, occurs in ischaemia. Therefore, when an end artery is obstructed the zone of necrosis is massive, often haemorrhagic and complete. The regeneration which follows is heteromorphic in type, with muscle buds and 'giant cells' present as well as the haphazard proliferation of fibrous tissue. In the 'end stage' there is little useful regeneration and the formation of a 'mixed' scar occurs in the belly of the muscle.

Scully et al (1961) examined the factors involved in recovery from experimental skeletal muscle ischaemia in dogs. Boehme & Themann (1966) reported structural and ultrastructural changes in striated human muscle caused by chronic ischaemia in amputated human legs. Electron-microscopic observations disclosed fibres in which mitochondria and sarcoplasmic reticulum were well preserved and others in which degeneration of these elements was prominent. Glycogen was actually increased in some fibres. These observations were considered to be relevant to human Volkmann's ischaemic contracture. Ischaemic muscle injury was studied by Adams (1975) and the resulting pan-necrosis described in detail.

The damage resulting from partial ischaemia presents a special circumstance and the studies of Clark (1946) illuminated a number of obscure features of the process. In one series of experiments a small portion of gracilis muscle was completely excised and immediately sutured back: its vascular supply was thus completely disrupted. In another series, the anterior tibial artery was ligated: this produced necrosis in the distal two-thirds of the muscle. Histological examinations were made at several time intervals, with the following results. Oedema was the first pathological reaction, followed by invasion of the area by a large number of polymorphs and macrophages. Phagocytosis of the dead muscle and fibroblastic proliferation soon followed. Clark & Wajda (1947) calculated the growth rate of regenerating fibres to be about 1.5 mm per day. After one to three weeks the average thickness of the fibres was about 30% of normal, and by three months the new muscle fibres were fully restored.

The importance of the endomysial tubes in the regeneration of muscle fibres was demonstrated in Clark's experiments (Clark 1946). The preserved endomysial envelopes ensured that the direction of growth occurred within the original muscle scaffold.

Physical methods

Temperature changes. Experimentally induced temperature changes are known to cause coagulative necrosis (Adams 1975). Gutmann & Guttmann (1942) studied the effect of electrical stimulation upon the prevention of changes secondary to denervation. Nageotte (1937) reported a shredding effect in muscle fibres produced by electrically induced severe contraction in vitro. Muscle changes caused by electrical stimulation have been described by a number of workers (Smith et al 1965). The lesions were produced by AC and DC electrical discharge through the fore and hind limbs of dogs. Skin and subcutaneous tissues were not injured but the skeletal muscle showed subsarcolemmal nuclear proliferation, loss of striations, vacuolisation and ultimately frank necrosis. Changes were indistinguishable, regardless of the type and polarity of the discharge. Ring fibres were not found, although these are reported to be easily produced by tendon-cutting (Bethlem & van Wijngaarden 1963), which also produces target fibres (De Reuck et al 1977). In addition to necrosis caused by burns, supercontraction of myofibrils and nuclear streaming result from electrical injury.

Examination of the ultrastructure of freeze-injured muscle fibres shows dissolution of organelles and rarefaction of myofibrils (Fig. 12.1). Such injuries in partly affected muscle fibres result in the appearance of large numbers of ribosomes as a sign of early repair (see Fig. 12.2).

X-irradiation. Skeletal muscle is relatively resistant to X-irradiation as it is a highly differentiated tissue. The effects of massive experimental X-irradiation were described in the studies of Warren (1943) who considered the vascular changes to be primary. Amino-aciduria resulting from whole-body irradiation was reported (Goyer & Yin 1967). Khan (1974) studied radiation-

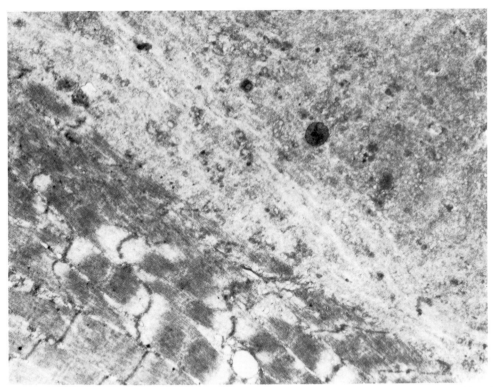

Fig. 12.1 There is total dissolution of organelles in one part of the muscle fibre two days after freeze injury. Uranyl acetate-lead citrate, ×35 000

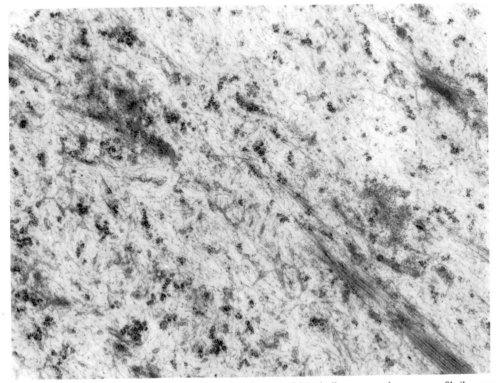

Fig. 12.2 Freeze injury to muscle showing early regenerative changes with polyribosomes and sparse myofibrils seven days after the injury. In this case regeneration is of the 'continuous' type. Uranyl acetate-lead citrate, ×54 600

induced changes in skeletal muscle under the electron microscope.

Nutritional disorders. As already indicated, there are many natural myopathies in animals deserving experimental enquiry, which are also the subject of therapeutic trials. Study of these disorders has provided useful information in relation to the possible aetiology and pathogenesis of human muscle diseases. Many of these animal disorders are genetically determined and are thus true dystrophies; however, the majority result from nutritional deficiencies or are caused by toxic agents. The most common nutritional disorder is vitamin E deficiency which is sometimes associated with selenium deficiency. Otherwise electrolyte disturbances, such as hypokalaemia, are prominent. Other animal myopathies which can be induced by nutritional factors are the thiamine, choline, vitamin D (dogs) and vitamin C (guinea pigs) deficiency disorders (Banker 1960).

Vitamin E deficiency is a very potent cause of muscle fibre necrosis and the resulting myopathic effects are well known (Hadlow 1962). Experimental vitamin E deficiency provides much useful information concerning the pathogenesis of muscle lesions in dystrophic states. In this regard, the Rottnest Island quokka (*Setonix brachyurus*) has proved to be a most useful model (Kakulas & Adams 1966); this is further described below in the context of muscular dystrophy. Howell & Buxton (1975) described α-tocopherol-responsive muscular dystrophy in guinea pigs. Muscle fibre necrosis, regeneration and cellular infiltrates were similar to those which were found in the Rottnest Island quokka with nutritional myopathy. Serum CK levels fell in the guinea pigs, and the animals revived after treatment with α-tocopherol.

Vitamin D deficiency results in defective calcium uptake in the sarcoplasmic reticulum, and protein deficiency will cause pseudomyopathic changes (Francis et al 1974). Ward & Goldspink (1974) studied the response of different muscle fibre types to changes in the activity pattern in protein malnutrition in the mouse.

Rats placed on an iodine-deficient diet by Rosman et al (1978), in order to produce hypothyroidism, unexpectedly developed progressive muscle weakness. The myopathy was due to a deficiency of a number of dietary constituents, only one of which was iodine. Necrosis and atrophy of cells were seen, as well as variability of muscle fibre size and shape.

Human muscle diseases may also result from the ingestion of animal flesh contaminated with animal or plant toxins, e.g. Haff disease and quail myopathy (Kakulas & Adams 1985).

Veterinarians are generally much better informed on these topics than students of human myopathology and much remains to be gained from the simple application of this knowledge to the human subject, especially with regard to the effects of nutritional deficiencies and toxic disorders on muscle.

SPECIAL LESIONS OF MUSCLE

Experimental disuse atrophy

Because reduced mobility is so common in muscle disease, disuse atrophy may be expected to have been the subject of extensive investigation. Myostatic contracture is a phenomenon closely associated with disuse and an understanding of both is essential basic knowledge for those involved in rehabilitation medicine. Joint fixation is rapidly followed by shortening of whole muscle as a result of myostatic contracture. The reduced length is due to the loss of sarcomeres from the muscle fibres, commensurate with the degree of shortening. Experimental studies also demonstrate the reverse effect, i.e. that lengthening of the muscle following a graduated exercise regime is due to the addition of more and more sarcomeres at each end of the muscle fibre.

The usual experimental methods utilised in the study of disuse atrophy are either section of a tendon or muscle or skeletal fixation. Such atrophy is also associated with a reduction in muscle fibre diameter and there is a tendency to darkening of the sarcoplasm by the accumulation of lipofuscin pigment ('brown atrophy' of general pathology).

Following division of the lumbosacral spinal cord segments, Eccles (1941) observed 40% loss of muscle bulk in three weeks as a result of inactivation of the leg muscles. Other workers, such as Ferguson et al (1957), have employed casts.

They also found that tension on a muscle even though it was 'disused' would result in hypertrophy.

The effects of tenotomy have been extensively studied, both by the pioneers (Eccles 1944) and more recently by others. Karpati et al (1972) showed that core-like lesions and nemaline rods were produced in type I fibres of the rat following Achilles tenotomy. They also reported that sciatic neurotomy or thoracic cordotomy prevented the development of the core-like lesions, so that intact innervation was a key factor in their formation.

Engel et al (1966) found that tenotomy in the cat resulted in greater atrophy of the soleus which consists purely of type I fibres. In the gastrocnemius, which is a mixed muscle in the cat, there was greater atrophy of type I fibres and some hypertrophy of type II fibres. Target fibres, rods and sarcoplasmic masses were only observed in the soleus. They also found that tenotomy and denervation resulted in core targetoid fibres in their histochemical studies.

Sarnat and associates (1977) investigated the effects of tenotomy and denervation in the gastro-cnemius muscle of the frog. The normal histochemical pattern persisted after denervation and they found that the small fibres of the gastrocnemius underwent further atrophy while the intermediate and large fibres were essentially unchanged 21–46 days after sciatic neurotomy.

Baker & Hall-Craggs (1980) found that the effects of tenotomy in the rat soleus were maximal one week postoperatively, after which a period of recovery occurred. Core targetoid fibres appeared within a few days of tenotomy and were maximal after one week when examined by electron microscopy. Baker & Hall-Craggs (1980) reported a reduction in sarcomere length following tenotomy. They were also able to demonstrate the appearance of 'unstructured cores' in the tenotomised muscle after one week. Muscle histology returned to normal in six weeks.

In a further study by Baker (1983) it was found that, after tenotomy and within the first few days, the affected fibres of the soleus underwent a complete morphological reorganisation. Initially, necrosis with phagocytosis occurred, especially

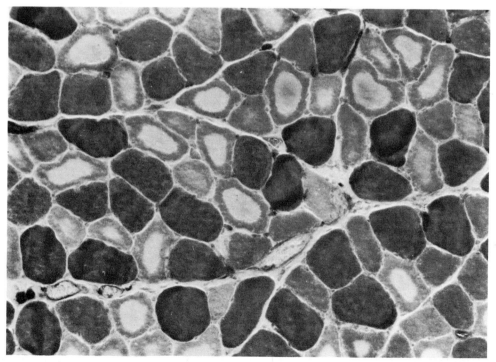

Fig. 12.3 Experimental 'cores' in rat soleus muscle tenotomised seven days previously. The central zones of many muscle fibres fail to stain by the ATPase method at pH 4.6. The muscle fibres with central core-like lesions are probably histochemical type I, ×512

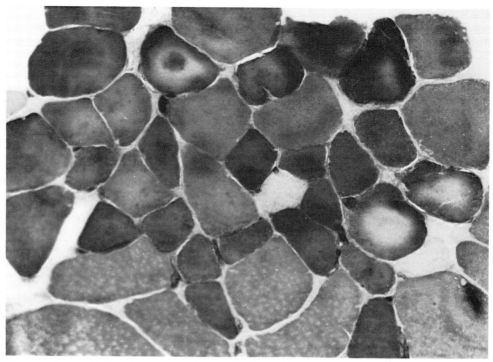

Fig. 12.4 Target and targetoid fibres in gastrocnemius muscle of rat subjected to tenotomy seven days before. ATPase at pH 9.4, ×800

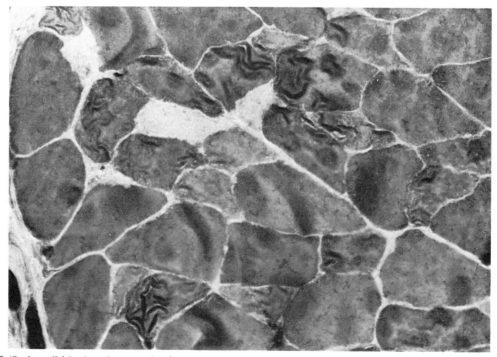

Fig. 12.5 'Snake coils' in the soleus muscle of a rat tenotomised seven days previously. ATPase pH 9.4, ×800

near the tendon. He also found that, by the seventh day, the fibres with central core lessions were associated with regeneration of myofibrils at the periphery of the fibre and this regeneration continued to complete reconstruction. Chou (1984) extensively reviews the topic of the experimental and natural 'core-genic neuro-myopathies' in conjunction with his own experimental observations.

Central cores, targetoid changes, snake coils, Z-band streaming and necrosis, all induced by tenotomy, are illustrated in Figures 12.3–12.7.

Bourne (1973) investigated the effect of zero gravity. In addition to the atrophic changes, he reported circulatory disturbances, redistribution of body fluids and other effects of weightlessness on muscle.

Mendell (1979), in his extensive review of the histochemistry of experimental myopathology, noted that, in general, disuse caused preferential type II fibre atrophy. He also described the histochemistry of increased muscle usage, joint fixation, cordotomy and tenotomy with or without nerve section.

Experimental hypertrophy

Experimental investigation has established that the stimulus for hypertrophy is simply use or work. Controlled exercise of the muscle of laboratory animals shows that hypertrophy occurs only when a muscle contracts with a force greater than that to which it is usually accustomed. For hypertrophy to occur, the contraction should be close

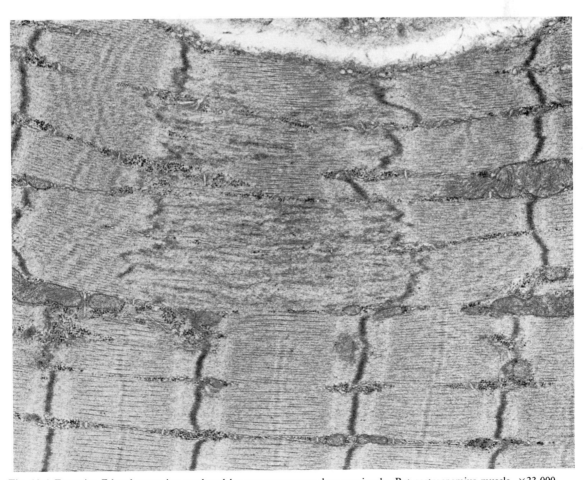

Fig. 12.6 Extensive Z-band streaming produced by tenotomy seven days previously. Rat gastrocnemius muscle, ×23 000

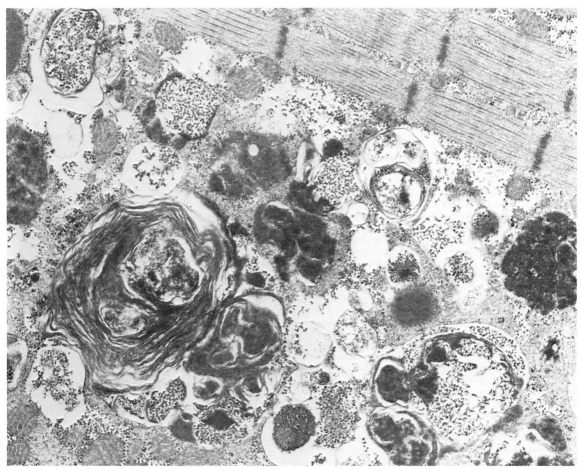

Fig. 12.7 Muscle fibre necrosis in the gastrocnemius muscle of a guinea pig tenotomised 30 days previously. All normal organelles are lost, except for rarified sarcomeres (top right), and are replaced by myelin figures, dense bodies, lysosomes, and abundant glycogen granules. EM, ×25 300

to the maximum power generated. The stimulus is related more to the intensity than to the duration of the effort.

The classic work on exercise hypertrophy is that of Morpurgo (1897) who measured the sartorius muscles of dogs before and after exercising on running wheels for a two-month period. He reported that the number of fibres increased very slightly in each muscle and that hypertrophy of the order of 55% occurred under these conditions. He found that the enlargement was due almost entirely to an increase in the diameter of the individual muscle fibres. He assumed that each enlarged fibre contained a greater number of myofibrils, an observation which was later confirmed by Denny-Brown in 1951.

Endocrine effects on muscle hypertrophy have

been little studied. Papanicolaou & Falk (1938) showed that the temporal muscle of the male guinea pig, which is normally larger than that of the female, remained small if the animal was castrated at puberty. On the other hand, androgenic hormones injected into females caused enlargement of their temporal muscles. Similar effects have been shown for somatotrophin by Bigland & Jehring (1952), who found the number of muscle fibres to be increased in rats treated with somatotrophin.

Experimental denervation atrophy

The close interaction of nerve and muscle has been the subject of investigation and conjecture from the beginning of the serious study of muscle disease. The dependence of muscle on an intact nerve supply, in order to maintain its size, is a long-standing clinical observation. Almost immediately, hypothetical trophic factors were postulated in the last century, as mediators of the phenomenon. The trophic factors which could theoretically exist number more than 15; however, perhaps only one such factor has really been identified, namely acetylcholine, and even this well-known neurotransmitter may not be the actual trophic factor itself (Kakulas & Adams 1985). Trophic factors are postulated for the maintenance of normal fibre size, membrane stability, reinnervation, end-plate production, hypertrophy, splitting, regeneration and histochemical specificity of muscle fibres. It has also been suggested that the human congenital myopathies, many of which show dysmorphic features, may reflect disturbances of a trophic nature (Engel 1979).

Numerous reports of the effects of denervation observed by light microscopy, histochemical studies and electron microscopy are in existence. The first experimental investigation which identified the functional and histochemical specificity of motor units was that of Eccles (1941, 1944). The work of Buller et al (1960) on the physiological relationship between motor nerve and muscle is now well known. Edström & Kugelberg (1968) elegantly confirmed Eccles' observation by histochemical means. It is now well established that the special functional qualities of a motor unit are dictated by the motor neurone to its muscle fibres; this fact is used in routine muscle biopsy diagnosis. The denervation studies of Kugelberg et al (1970) defined the histochemical specificity of muscle fibre types within individual motor units. Peter (1973), in a full review of this subject, concluded that the particular histochemical qualities of a fibre type are governed by the physiological function of the motor unit rather than by anterior horn cell 'trophic' specificity. The histochemical type is thus determined by physiological demand rather than by an 'immutable' motor-unit-specific determinant.

There is considerable interest in the definition of trophic and developmental influences in fetal muscle under experimental conditions, and denervation is employed in such studies (Margreth et al 1974). In the biochemistry of denervated muscle, attention was paid to protein synthesis and oxidation by Gauthier & Schaeffer (1975) and by Kark et al (1975).

Myographic and electroneurographic responses of leg muscles to cross-innervated sciatic nerves are reported to be normal in dystrophic mice united by parabiosis (Douglas 1974). The investigation of neurotrophic influences has extended to the investigation of intramuscular injection of spinal cord homogenate. Such studies demonstrate enhancement of protein synthesis (Crockett & Edgerton 1974).

The histochemistry of regenerating myofibres before and after reinnervation was undertaken to determine the role of 'trophic influences' in creating 'type specificity' of muscle fibres (Reznik 1973, Manolov 1974). It was found that differentiation of regenerated myofibres into several types begins four to five weeks after injury and is related to reinnervation. Unusual checkerboard distributions of type I and type II fibres and heterogeneous myofibres occur in the major part of a muscle which, before injury, contained type II fibres almost exclusively. Additionally, large and small regenerating myofibres had end-plates which were often abnormal. The results suggest that axons sprouting from different motor units proliferate in the same area and innervate new myofibres at random. Such modifications are quite different from the fibre-type grouping described after spontaneous or experimentally induced reinnervation of normal myofibres.

Denervation caused the appearance of central nuclei and muscle-fibre splitting with eventual loss of architecture in the experimental myopathy induced by paroxan and organophosphorus (Wecker & Dettbarn 1977).

The more recent histochemical and electron-microscopic effects of denervation are fully reviewed by Mendell (1979) and details of the observations of the pioneers of experimental denervation may be found in Kakulas & Adams (1985).

Post-denervation hypertrophy. The paradoxical phenomenon of 'denervation hypertrophy' is of considerable experimental interest. Formation of new muscle fibres, i.e. hyperplasia as well as true hypertrophy (of 'intermediate' fibres), is associated with this phenomenon, which is readily produced in the diaphragm of most species and the anterior latissimus dorsi muscle of chickens (Sola et al 1973).

Experimental myotoxicity

Skeletal muscles are prone to injury by drugs and toxins. As a result, numerous toxic chemicals have been investigated for their effects on the muscle fibre. There are also many 'iatrogenic' drug myopathies known clinically and which are the subject of experimental investigation (Kakulas 1982b, Kakulas & Adams 1985, see also Ch. 29).

The effect of metabolic poisons. Powerful metabolic poisons are commonly used in experimental myopathology; e.g. iodoacetate (Lundsgaard 1930) which blocks lactate production by the inhibition of glyceraldehyde-3-phosphate dehydrogenase, causes massive rhabdomyolysis (Fig. 12.8). A metabolic myopathy which may be induced in rabbits by hypoglycaemia following administration of insulin (Tannenberg 1939) is

associated with single-fibre necrosis in both cardiac and skeletal muscle. Another chemical agent investigated experimentally is imidazole, which accelerates the catabolism of cyclic AMP and is associated with myopathic changes in the gastrocnemius muscle of rats (Fenichel & Martin 1974).

Such chemical myopathies usually cause pure sarcoplasmic necrosis and spare the sarcolemmal and endomysial fibrous tissue sheaths. Because of this, in the recovery phase following withdrawal of the agent, connective tissue proliferation is minimal and muscle regeneration is complete. These experimental conditions bear a resemblance to a number of natural and drug-induced metabolic myopathies in man. Again, regeneration is complete when the cause is removed.

Jasmin & Gareau (1961) studied with light microscopy the skeletal muscle lesions produced in rats injected with diphenylenediamine. Swelling and homogenisation were visible in 24 hours, followed by coagulative necrosis. The necrotic muscle

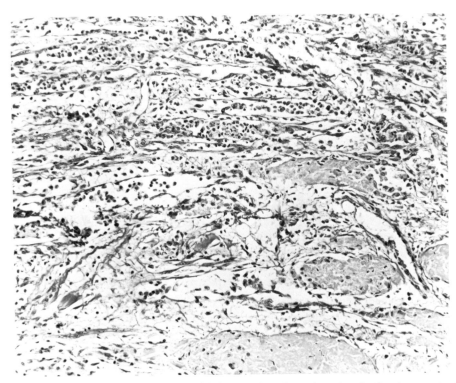

Fig. 12.8 Abdominal wall of rat injected with 0.04 mg of iodoacetate into the peritoneal cavity five days previously. There is widespread muscle destruction. Recent necrosis is present (bottom right) and phagocytosis of debris (above) is in progress. Regenerative changes in the form of elongated spindle cells are conspicuous. H & E ×120

segments acted as foreign bodies and gave rise to a histiocytic reaction with multinucleated giant cells. Regenerative changes occurred parallel to the severity of the lesions with regeneration ad integrum in less than 20 days. Mascres & Jasmin (1975) later used p-phenylenediamine (PPD) to investigate the inflammatory and degenerative patterns of muscle lesions in rats. Fifteen minutes after the injection of PPD, subsarcolemmal oedema was visible in the diaphragm under the electron microscope. Enzymatic changes appeared in the first hour while pathological features were prominent after 24 hours. There was segmental necrosis adjacent to unaltered fibres and several particular types of abnormal fibres such as target, snake coils and core fibres were seen.

Uraemic myopathy may be produced in rats. In this disorder, atrophy of type I fibres occurs but there are no other structural changes (Bundschu et al 1974).

Graham et al (1976) reported that core formation was observed in the muscles of rats intoxicated by triethyltin sulphate (TET). The changes affected only the type I fibres and were observed in the soleus muscle in animals intoxicated with TET for up to 23 days. The development of core-like structures, which occur after tenotomy in association with nemaline body formation and vacuolar degeneration of muscle fibres, may be compared with those structures which are found after emetine intoxication and in which there are large lesions extending throughout the transverse axis of fibres, associated with loss of oxidative enzyme activity. In contrast, alkyltin intoxication differs in that in this case the central nervous system shows intramyelinic vacuolisation.

Biological toxins are powerful myonecrotic agents. Morita (1926) studied the effect of clostridial toxin, such as that from *Clostridium welchii*, which usually destroys connective tissue as well as causing muscle fibre necrosis. The effects of *Clostridium botulinum* were recently studied, with denervation changes being reported by Johnston & Drachman (1974).

Adams (1975) reported fatty degeneration in cardiac muscle after the administration of diphtheria toxin to guinea pigs. However, no consistent changes in skeletal muscle were observed, and he found that direct inoculation of diphtheria organisms into muscle caused lesions which did not differ from those produced by any bacterial necrosis.

Keast (1967), in his studies on the origin of lesions in neonatal mice receiving neomycin sulphate, investigated the effect of *E.coli* endotoxin, and in this way produced widespread muscle fibre necrosis (Fig. 12.9).

Tiger · snake toxin causes skeletal muscle degeneration and subsequent regeneration when injected into the rat (Pluskal et al 1974). The oriental hornet (*Vespa orientalis*) causes a lesion of the muscle transverse-tubular system (Ishay et al 1975). Light-microscopic examination showed that vacuoles appear in the sartorius muscle incubated in hornet venom–Ringer's solution. Under the electron microscope it was observed that these vacuoles were caused by greatly distended T-tubules and terminal cisternae.

Bacteria and viruses. Bacterial myositis has been studied in the laboratory and the subject was reviewed by Banker (1960) and by Adams (1975). As might be expected, pyogenic organisms cause acute abscesses and similar lesions result from injections of turpentine into muscle. Banker (1960) also discussed parasitic infections of muscle.

Many viruses are capable of producing experimental myositis, including mouse encephalomyelitis (GD-VII and FA strains) and the Mitchell strain of lymphocytic choriomeningitis (Rustigan & Pappenheimer 1949). The Coxsackie viruses (Dalldorf 1950) are especially known to cause myositis and Type A (Field 1960) is more active in this regard (Fig. 12.10).

Arboviruses also cause myositis. It has been demonstrated in this connection that myofibrils are severely damaged with accompanying dilatation of T-tubules and of the sarcoplasmic reticulum (SR), with the accumulation of mature arbovirus particles within the cisternae and vacuoles (Sato et al 1974).

Miranda et al (1978) studied influenza virus infection of human skeletal muscle in tissue culture. Using scanning and transmission electron microscopes, they observed cytopathic changes, both in organelles and surface elements. Cell

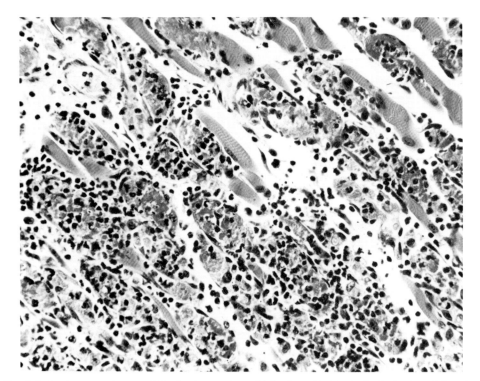

Fig. 12.9 Muscle lesion in neonatal mouse following intraperitoneal injection of 0.01 ml of 10^9 dilution of *E. coli* endotoxin 16 days previously. There is widespread muscle fibre necrosis and macrophage reaction (specimen provided by Mr. D. Keast). H & E ×300

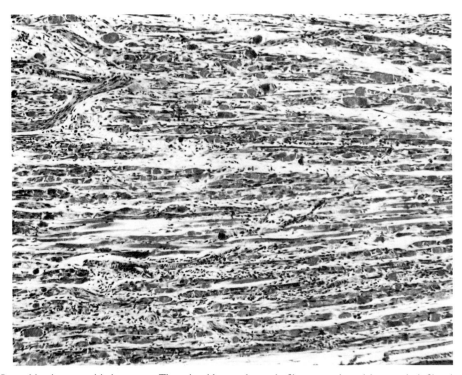

Fig. 12.10 Coxsackie virus myositis in mouse. There is widespread muscle fibre necrosis and leucocytic infiltration (specimen provided by Dr. R. D. Adams). H & E ×80

injury and death appear to be caused by massive accumulation of virus-induced products that alter cellular metabolism in vitro.

Alcohol. The adverse effect of alcohol on muscle has been well studied, both experimentally and in patients with alcoholic myopathy, and poly-focal muscle fibre necrosis is found in both situations. Cessation of exposure to ethanol is associated with rapid reversal of the process: necrosis ceases and regeneration proceeds. Electron–microscopic examination shows that all organelles are affected to some degree, with changes in the mitochondria and dilatations of the SR occurring in the vicinity of the zones of total necrosis.

Extensive biochemical and morphological studies were carried out by Rubin et al (1976) in volunteers in relation to studies of human alcoholic myopathy. Ultrastructural changes consisted of deformation of mitochondria, dilatation of the sarcoplasmic reticulum and increased amounts of fat and glycogen.

Drugs. Emetine, plasmocid and chloroquine are all myotoxic. Myocardial as well as skeletal muscle necrosis occurs in each, while the presence of autophagic lysosomal bodies is a particular feature of chloroquine myopathy. Many of these drug myopathies, while occurring clinically, have also been extensively studied experimentally. Necrosis experimentally induced by plasmocid is shown in Figure 12.11.

Other · drugs, e.g. 20,25-diazocholesterol have been used to study the effects of myotonia. Lithium, phenytoin, quinidine, penicillamine and a number of antibiotics interfere with neuromuscular transmission, producing a type of 'myasthenia' (see Ch. 29).

As may be expected, the cytotoxic and vasoactive drugs are associated with polyfocal muscle fibre necrosis. Pethidine and heroin are also known myotoxic agents and have been investigated experimentally (Kakulas 1982a).

Steroids and other hormones have been subject to experimental study for their effects on muscle (Fig. 12.12). Steroids are associated with type II

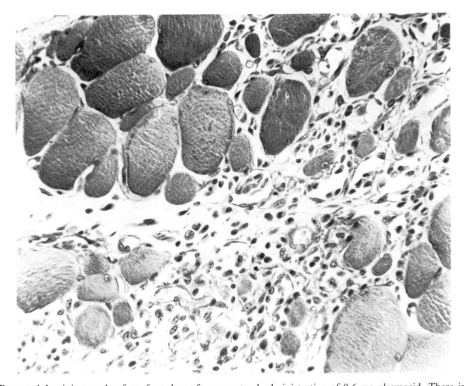

Fig. 12.11 Rectus abdominis muscle of rat four days after parenteral administration of 0.6 mg plasmocid. There is muscle fibre necrosis and macrophage activity (centre, below) and intact fibres (above). Van Gieson stain ×260

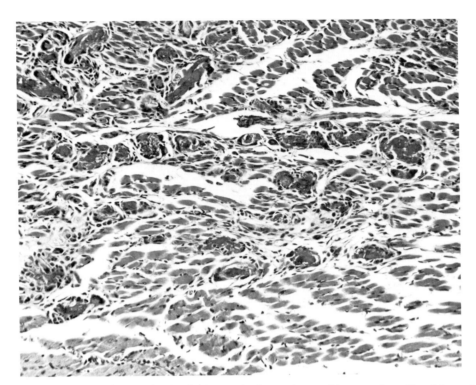

Fig. 12.12 Paravertebral muscles of mouse showing focal necrosis of sarcoplasm and impregnation with calcium salts, injected with 0.1 mg/g body weight hydrocortisone 14 days previously (specimen provided by Mr D. Keast). H & E ×83

atrophy and in some animals will cause muscle fibre necrosis (Ellis 1956).

Other drugs will of course affect muscle by their action on the peripheral nerve. For a review of the drug-induced myopathies see Kakulas (1982b) and Chapter 29.

EXPERIMENTAL MODELS OF HUMAN MYOPATHIES

Most of the work in this area is concerned with three human conditions — progressive muscular dystrophy, myasthenia gravis and polymyositis. The human and animal dystrophies are the subject of intensive enquiry because of their devastating clinical effects. To help achieve an understanding of these conditions the natural dystrophies in animals are carefully investigated and attempts are made to reproduce similar myopathies in the laboratory. Some of this research examines simple chemical or physical injury to muscle, as shown

above. Other methods, such as microembolisation (Engel 1973) and, more particularly, the effects of controlled deprivation of vitamin E (Kakulas & Adams 1966) produce useful models.

Muscular dystrophy occurs in the mouse, chicken, hamster, sheep and other species: myotonia and spinal arthrogryposis occur in goats and spinal muscular atrophy is found in dogs. All are subject to laboratory manipulation and research. These natural animal myopathies are described in Chapter 28.

Muscular dystrophy

Vitamin E. Of the numerous attempts to simulate muscular dystrophy in animals, the myopathy of experimental vitamin E deficiency in the Rottnest Island quokka (*Setonix brachyurus*) more closely resembles the naturally occurring conditions than do some others (Fig. 12.13). In this model there is polyfocal muscle fibre necrosis and reactive cellular changes are concerned with

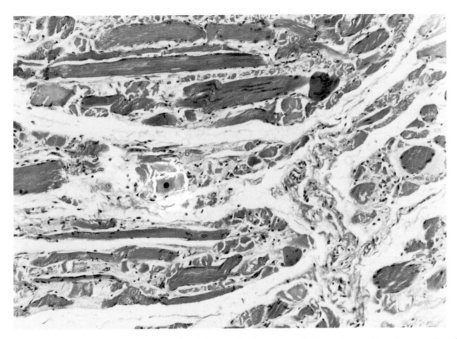

Fig. 12.13 Widespread hyaline and granular necrosis with myophagia of muscle fibres in nutritional myopathy of the Rottnest Island quokka. There is also loss of muscle fibres, fibrous tissue condensation and fat increase. The changes bear a resemblance to those found in human muscular dystrophy, ×142

the removal of debris and regeneration. Using the quokka, it is possible to regulate the deficiency of vitamin E so that the changes which occur in human progressive muscular dystrophy are closely reproduced. These lesions result from chronic continuing necrosis due to marginal deficiency of the vitamin. The proximal distribution of paralysis in the animal also follows the pattern of the human condition.

The early lesions in the vitamin-E-deficient quokka resemble those in the incipient stages of Duchenne muscular dystrophy but they are more acute. There is focal necrosis, attempted regeneration and general disorganisation of muscle architecture. Apart from the lack of the very large round fibres common in the gastrocnemius in Duchenne dystrophy, the muscle changes are very similar in both conditions. At the end of the process, the histopathology consists of a few preserved muscle fibres which are irregular in size and shape while nuclear distribution is disordered. There is also fat and connective tissue increase, which results from collapse of endomysial fibrous tissue.

Numerous laboratory studies continue to take place using dystrophic mice, chickens and hamsters. These include reinnervation experiments after experimental denervation, and studies of the biochemistry of subcellular organelles and of the effects of therapeutic agents (Ashmore & Doerr 1974, Owens et al 1975, Park et al 1975, Wrogemann et al 1975). Jasmin et al (1975) reported that verapamil will prevent hereditary cardiomyopathy in the Syrian hamster.

Microembolisation. Engel (1973) induced focal muscle fibre necrosis in rabbits using microembolisation. The lesions appeared to be grouped, and regeneration ensued. To some extent the lesions resembled those of the naturally occurring human and animal dystrophies. However, this ischaemic myopathy is not now regarded as a useful model of the human disease.

Immunological attempts to produce dystrophic changes are even less successful. In early reports of the use of immunological methods, the changes were considered dystrophic in character by Tal

& Liban (1962). However, the lesions seemed to be more akin to atrophy caused by chronic disuse and poor nutrition.

Myasthenia gravis

Attempts to reproduce MG in the laboratory have a long history. The most popular method is immunisation of the animal using muscle extracts, crude or purified, with or without adjuvant. Many of these experiments have resulted in 'myasthenia', when it is defined simply as excessive fatiguability or increased sensitivity to curare (Goldstein & Whittingham 1966, Whittingham & Mackay 1966). Where reported, histological muscle lesions consist of focal necrosis and inflammation, otherwise the muscles are normal in appearance. Parkes (1966) failed to produce a model for myasthenia gravis by immunological methods in the rat, although muscle fibre necrosis was produced. Nevertheless, Goldstein & Whittingham (1966) considered that they had produced an experimental counterpart to myasthenia gravis. A naturally occurring animal model of myasthenia in the dog is well known (Palmer et al 1974).

Patrick & Lindstrom (1973) discovered that repeated immunisation of rabbits with nicotinic acetylcholine receptor (AChR) purified from the electric organ of *Electrophorus electricus* produced muscular weakness and a decremental electromyographic response on repeated nerve stimulation. The changes were reversible with anticholinesterase drugs. Serum from rabbits immunised with antigens derived from the electrical organs of other eels have serum antibodies to AChR. This antibody is capable of blocking the depolarisation response of the electroplaque to carbamylcholine (Patrick et al 1973).

Later, experimental myasthenia was produced in rabbits injected with isolated nicotinic acetylcholine receptor purified from the electrical organ of *Torpedo marmorata* by affinity chromatography (Heilbronn et al 1975). The rabbits developed flaccid paralysis within three weeks. Experimental myasthenia in monkeys produces ptosis which is reversible with edrophonium (Tarrab-Hazdai et al 1975).

In this manner, investigators have successfully produced experimental myasthenia gravis which closely resembles the human disease and may be passively transferred in breast milk (Sanders et al 1978). Furthermore, Engel et al (1976) have shown morphological and electrophysiological changes at the neuromuscular junction in the rat with experimental autoimmune myasthenia gravis (EAMG). These changes closely resemble the alterations seen at the end-plate in human myasthenia gravis in the chronic phase. In the early phases, mononuclear cells infiltrate the end-plate regions and there is intense degeneration in the postsynaptic area with splitting of abnormal junctional folds from the underlying muscle fibres. Macrophages remove the degenerating folds by phagocytosis and nerve terminals are displaced. Such changes are accompanied by blocked neuromuscular transmission. In the more chronic phase in this experimental model, after day 11 nerve terminals return to the highly simplified postsynaptic regions and the inflammatory reaction subsides. Subsequently postsynaptic folds become reconstituted, but they again degenerate. Immature junctions with poorly differentiated postsynaptic regions and nerve sprouts near end-plates are also observed. Postsynaptic membrane length and miniature end-plate potential (mepp) amplitudes are decreased in all animals in the chronic phase. In another experiment, Lennon et al (1976) demonstrated the passive transfer of EAMG by lymphoid cells.

Toyka et al (1977) reported the passive transfer of myasthenia gravis to mice, with immunoglobulins derived from patients with myasthenia gravis. Typical reductions in mepp occurred and the data suggested that the pathogenesis of myasthenia gravis often involves an antibody-mediated autoimmune attack on the acetylcholine receptors of the neuromuscular junction.

A clear understanding of the pathogenesis of EAMG has emerged from the work of Lindstrom (1978), who first developed the AChR model, and by Engel (1978) who applied a combination of morphological and physiological observations to the problem. The experimental disease has many features in common with naturally occurring MG. The review by Engel (1979) provides full details of these experimental studies. Although the pathogenesis of EAMG is now reasonably well understood, the initiating cause of the autoimmune reaction in human MG still remains to be discovered.

Polymyositis

A variety of experimental methods are used to produce a 'polymyositis-like' disorder in animals. These observations began, indirectly, in 1937 with Kallos & Pagel who observed muscle lesions in rabbits with induced hypersensitivity and bronchial reactions. The suggestion that human polymyositis may be the result of disordered immune function was based on the presence of raised levels of serum globulins in the serum of many patients with the disease, on the sometimes dramatic response to steroid hormones given for therapeutic purposes, and on the known clinical association with disorders of presumed immunological aetiology, e.g. systemic lupus erythematosus (Walton & Adams 1958). An active immunological approach was employed by Pearson in 1956. Although noting that myositis was present, Pearson became more interested in the polyarthritis produced by Freund's adjuvant than in the myositis.

A 'polymyositis-like' condition, subsequently named experimental allergic myositis (EAM), can be produced in rats by immunological methods (Dawkins 1965, Kakulas 1966, 1973). Histological features include focal necrotic and inflammatory changes (Fig. 12.14). Electron microscopy shows that the necrosis affects all ultrastructural elements, but especially the myofibrils, with membranous bodies also prominent.

It has also been shown that in vitro transfer of lymphocytes from animals with EAM produces

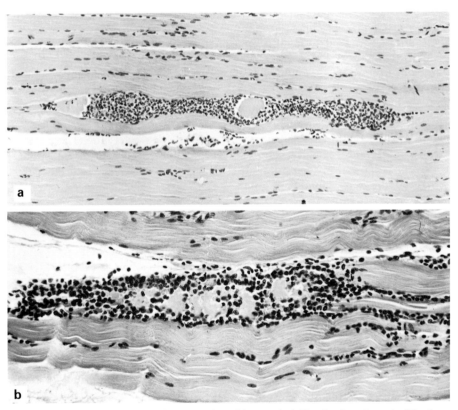

Fig. 12.14 a. Immunologically induced muscle-fibre necrosis and leucocytic infiltration in guinea pig following repeated injections of rabbit muscle and adjuvant. H & E, ×112. b. Focal muscle-fibre necrosis and round-cell collections in rat, produced by similar means. H & E ×208

cytotoxic effects in tissue cultures of fetal rat muscle (Kakulas 1966). Similar experiments with slight variations in technique or animal species give essentially similar results (Webb 1970, Currie et al 1971).

The close relationship of the experimental disease to human polymyositis is demonstrated by the presence of in vitro cytotoxic effects of human lymphocytes from patients with the disease, when these cells are applied to human fetal muscle in culture (Kakulas 1970, 1973). In muscle biopsies of patients with polymyositis, lymphocytes and plasma cells are mainly perivenular and appear to be closely related to necrotic foci (Adams 1973).

Experimental studies of EAM are also directed towards determining the nature of the antigen (Esiri & MacLennan 1975). Myofibrillar antigens appear to be more potent than those of other subcellular components of muscle (Manghani et al 1975). These workers established that lymphocytes from myositic animals are sensitised to the outer surface of muscle cells. The macrophage–migration inhibition test was used to identify the components within the muscle fibres to which lymphocytes are also sensitised. Their studies indicate that there is lymphocyte sensitisation against the myofibrillar fraction and especially against the proteins myosin and tropomyosin. Guinea pigs injected with rabbit myofibrillar fractions and Freund's adjuvant regularly develop myositis. These animals show many more muscle lesions, consisting of areas of round cell infiltration and muscle fibre necrosis, than do those animals given other subcellular fractions

Penn (1977), in reviewing the pathogenesis of myasthenia gravis, polymyositis and dermatomyositis, concludes that the humoral arm of the defence appears to be directly responsible for the lesion in myasthenia gravis, but that cellular mechanisms at the thymic regulatory level are also involved. Cytotoxic T cells seem to produce the lesion of experimental myositis, in which anti-muscle antibodies can be detected, and those of polymyositis and dermatomyositis, in which antibodies have not been convincingly shown. Childhood dermatomyositis is considered to be a probable exception in which antibodies and complement contribute to underlying vasculitis. Immunosuppressive measures can modify or prevent the disease in experimental models and Penn (1977) believes that the evidence indicates a solid rationale for their use in the human diseases, although much more information is required concerning the site of action and appropriate therapeutic planning.

Animal models for polymyositis and dermatomyositis were recently reviewed (Kakulas 1986). In this survey the autoimmune diseases can be viewed as being the result of an excess in the number and ratio of T-4 helper cells compared with T-8 suppressor lymphocytes, whereas the immunodepression syndromes are due to a relative excess of the T-8 suppressor cells. That is to say, autoimmune disease and immunodeficiency syndromes may be regarded as being at opposite ends of a continuous spectrum, or even as mirror images of each other.

Experimental AIDS (acquired immune deficiency syndrome)

Animal models for the experimental study of AIDS are emerging, such as the naturally occurring simian AIDS, which is presumably due to a virus infection (London et al 1983). In simian AIDS, focal necrosis of muscle fibres with inflammatory infiltrates and inclusion bodies are described. However, the changes are possibly due to an opportunistic infection rather than to the simian AIDS virus itself (Kakulas 1986).

Experimental malignant hyperpyrexia (MH)

Malignant hyperthermia may be induced in Pietrain pigs by the administration of halothane and succinylcholine or even by stress. This model allows electrophysiological studies to be undertaken, as well as investigation of the mechanism of heat generation. It is now believed that the cause of MH is excessive leakage of calcium into the cytosol through defects in the terminal cisternae of the T system. Neither of the electrical phenomena — pseudotremor and increase in neuromuscular block — relate to the contracture while steep thermal gradients develop with increasing tissue and skin insulation. Histology and histochemistry show no specific alteration in muscle tissue between attacks (Schiller et al 1974), although necrosis-regeneration is the usual feature of an acute episode.

Tumours

Experimentally induced muscle tumours are also the subject of study. In a biochemical report, muscle acid proteinase, alkaline proteinase arylamidase and cathepsin C were increased and cathepsin E 1 was decreased. Cathepsin A autolytic activity and trypsin inhibitory capacity were unchanged in the extensor digitorum muscle (Holmes et al 1974).

Congenital structural myopathies

It is now well known that the mitochondrial myopathies can be induced experimentally by drugs which block the oxidative pathways. The best-known model is induced by the administration of 2, 4-dinitrophenol: in this case the mitochondria are large, lack the normal cristae and may even contain crystalline inclusions (Fig. 12.15). Mitochondrial abnormalities can also be induced by other agents which block oxidative metabolism (Melmed et al 1975; Sahgal et al 1979) as shown in Figure 12.16. Histochemical preparations for oxidative enzymes (Fig. 12.17) provide an experimental counterpart for the 'ragged red fibres' of the human mitochondrial myopathies.

As mentioned above, tenotomy and disuse may produce core-targetoid changes and rod bodies in type I muscle fibres which closely resemble the

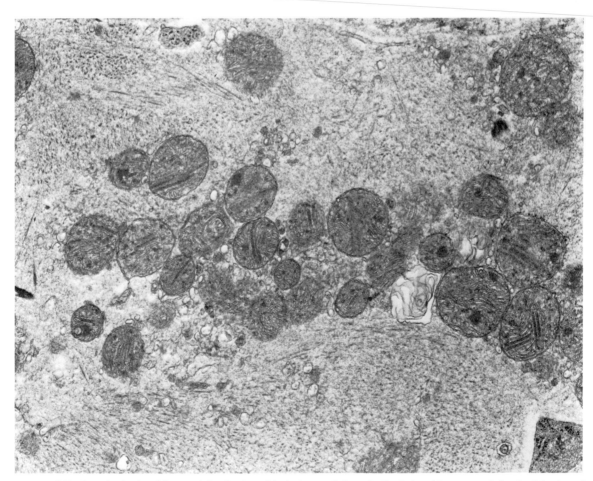

Fig. 12.15 Englarged mitochondria containing laminated inclusions and dense bodies induced in rat muscle by the injection of 2,4-dinitrophenol 24 hours previously. EM, ×25 500

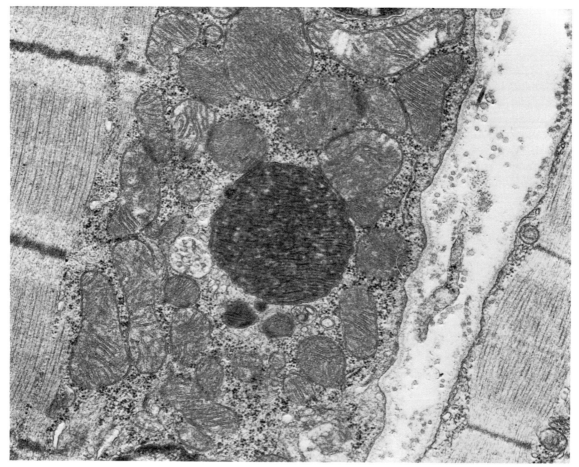

Fig. 12.16 Enlarged mitochondrion showing multi-laminated and dense cristae in rat muscle injected with 2,4-dichlorophenoxyacetate 24 hours previously. EM, ×28 000

human central core and nemaline myopathies (Chou 1984), provided that the nerve supply remains intact.

CONCLUSIONS

The reaction of skeletal muscle to injury of various types is now reasonably well understood as a result of the increasing number of experimental studies and the wider range of techniques applied to the subject in recent years. In this respect, the histochemical and electron-microscopic contributions have been especially relevant.

Nevertheless, it can still be said that the most notable aspect of the pathology of injured muscle is the remarkably stereotyped character of the resulting changes, a fact which is demonstrated by the many diverse agents producing similar results. The elementary lesion in the majority of these conditions is focal necrosis of the muscle fibre with preservation of the endomysial sheath. Focal or segmental necrosis is always followed by a series of reparative changes leading to regeneration which is considered to be an inherent property of skeletal muscle. The sequence of regenerative events is the same regardless of whether the cause is physical, chemical, drug-induced or immunological provided that the duration of action of the noxious influence is finite.

Within the necrobiotic group of myopathies the variability in the microscopic appearance is related more to the severity of noxious influence rather than to its specificity. This fact, together with the

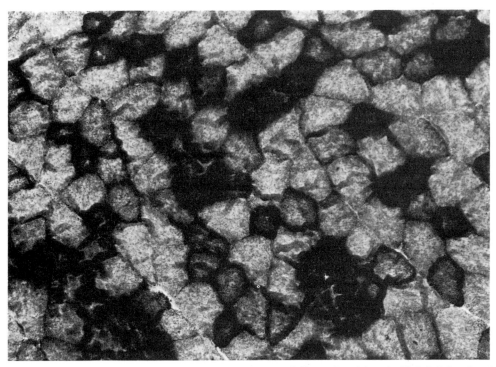

Fig. 12.17 Masses of conglomerated dark staining mitochondria in type I fibres of rat injected with 2,4-dinitrophenol 24 hours previously. The changes are similar to those found in human mitochondrial myopathies. SDH, ×512

topographic distribution of the lesions and the time over which it acts, determines the morphology of the eventual architectural derangement.

However, because the regenerative potential of skeletal muscle is ultimately limited, continuous necrosis will eventually lead to exhaustion of regeneration and outfall of muscle fibres, with fat and fibrous tissue taking up the dead space. This is known as end-stage disease.

If the term 'focal' is used to represent the anatomical aspect of the lesion and if the term 'phasic' refers to the time factor, and the prefixes 'mono' and 'poly' are added, the full spectrum of histopathological changes may be predicted and precisely described (Kakulas 1975). Examples are easily found for each of these possibilities.

The most important of these combinations occurs when the myopathological change is both polyfocal and polyphasic. This common lesion is observed in the muscular dystrophies and is also found in polymyositis and the other necrobiotic myopathies. The changes are therefore similar in the metabolic and nutritional myopathies, both

human and experimental and whenever necrosis continues over a long period.

The characteristic architectural disorganisation of muscle, the common feature of these states, results from the polyfocal and polyphasic necrosis occurring over an extended period. Initially, regenerative changes are prominent but, because the newly formed muscle fibres undergo further necrosis, regeneration is eventually exhausted so that muscle fibres are lost altogether. The non-specific 'myopathic' features of the reduced number of muscle fibres which may remain, such as irregularity in size and shape, central location of nuclei and muscle fibre splitting, are largely due to compensatory hypertrophy and incomplete regeneration.

These principles emphasise that simple morphological similarity of lesions is not an indication of similarity of primary cause. Muscle fibre necrosis is the common denominator in many diverse conditions whether they are infective, toxic, immunological, metabolic, drug-induced, hormonal or genetically determined. The lesions may differ morphologically only because of variability in the severity, anatomical distribution and temporal action of these noxious agents.

It is axiomatic that when the cause of focal muscle fibre necrosis is corrected, removed or neutralised, regeneration will ensue as an inherent biological property of voluntary muscle. This principle applies as much to the (at present) incurable disorders such as muscular dystrophy as it does to the toxic myopathies or polymyositis.

It is evident from the above that experimental myopathology encompasses a very broad field of investigation. A loose definition would include all experimental investigations on skeletal muscle and thus much of laboratory myology. However, because most of these basic data relate only indirectly to disease processes, they are not considered in detail. However, the more disease-orientated aspects of the subject have contributed significantly to the understanding of human myopathies.

The most impressive achievement in the field of pure experiment is probably understanding the experimental model (EAMG) which has contributed to the elucidation of the mechanisms which underlie human myasthenia gravis. Other significant advances are as follows.

Membrane instabilities due to nutritional or chemically induced abnormalities provide avenues for the investigation of muscle diseases characterised by defects of electrolyte transfer such as the periodic paralyses, myotonia congenita and dystrophia myotonica.

The experimental manipulation of hereditary muscular dystrophy in the mouse has also provided useful information concerning the natural history of the lesions in muscular dystrophy (Manda & Kakulas 1986).

The production of rods, target fibres and cores and other histochemical or structural changes similar to those encountered in the congenital group of myopathies is also a useful recent contribution of experimental myopathology. The laboratory production of mitochondrial abnormalities using chemical poisons which act within the oxidative pathways provides useful models for the study of those disorders.

The experimental investigation of the mode of action of myotoxic drugs and toxins in animals gives insights into these unwanted side effects, within this enlarging field of iatrogenic disorders.

Experimental myopathology has shed some light on the basic processes of reaction of the muscle fibre encountered in human diseases and the analytical approach has led to the recognition of the essential elements which comprise the muscle lesions in many of these myopathies. Investigators now await, with some excitement, the application of recombinant DNA technology to these issues.

REFERENCES

Adams R D 1973 In: Kakulas B A (ed) Clinical studies in myology. Excerpta Medica, Amsterdam, p 40

Adams R D 1975 Diseases of muscle. A study in pathology, 3rd edn. Harper & Row, New York

Allbrook D 1962 An electron microscopic study of regenerative skeletal muscle. Journal of Anatomy 96:137

Anastas N C, Kakulas B A 1968 Muscle lesions associated with bony injuries. Proceedings of the Australian Association of Neurologists 5:553

Ashmore C R, Doerr L 1974 Reinnervation of a β-fibered muscle mince by nerve from an α-fibered muscle in normal and dystrophic chicks. In: IIIrd International Congress on Muscle Diseases, International Congress Series No 334, Abstract 130. Excerpta Medica, Amsterdam

Baker J H 1983 Segmental necrosis in tenotomized muscle fibers. Muscle and Nerve 6: 29–39

Baker J H, Hall-Craggs E C G 1980 Recovery from central core degeneration of the tenotomized rat soleus muscle. Muscle and Nerve 3: 151–159

Banker B Q 1960 The experimental myopathies. In: Research Publications. Association for Research in Nervous and Mental Diseases (ch VII) 38:197

Bethlem J, van Wijngaarden G K 1963 The incidence of ringed fibres and sarcoplasmic masses in normal and diseased muscle. Journal of Neurology, Neurosurgery and Psychiatry 26:326

Bigland B, Jehring B 1952 Muscle performance in rats — normal and treated with growth hormone. Journal of Physiology (London) 116: 129–136

Boehme D, Themann H 1966 Structural and ultrastructural changes in striated human muscle caused by chronic ischemia. American Journal of Pathology 49:569

Bourne G H 1973 The effects of weightlessness on muscle. In Kakulas B A (ed) Clinical studies in myology, Part 2. Proceedings of the Second International Congress on Muscle Disease, International Congress Series, No 295, Perth, Western Australia. Excerpta Medica, Amsterdam, p 115–123

Buller A J, Eccles J C, Eccles R M 1960 Interactions between motorneurons and muscles in respect of the characteristic speeds of their response. Journal of Physiology (London) 150: 417–439

Bundschu H D, Pfeilsticker H, Suchenwirth R, Matthews C, Ritz E 1974 Experimental uremic myopathy. In: IIIrd

International Congress on Muscle Diseases, International Congress Series No 334, Abstract 330. Excerpta Medica, Amsterdam

Carlson B M 1974 Morphogenetic effects of cross-transplanted muscles upon an epimorphic regenerative process. In: IIIrd International Congress on Muscle Diseases, International Congress Series No 334, Abstract 273. Excerpta Medica, Amsterdam

Chou S M 1984 Core-genic neuromyopathies. In: Heffner R R Jnr (ed) Muscle pathology. Churchill Livingstone, New York, ch 7, p 83–107

Clark W E Le Gros 1946 An experimental study of the regeneration of mammalian striped muscle. Journal of Anatomy 80:24

Clark W E Le Gros, Wajda H S 1947 The growth and maturation of regenerating striated muscle fibres. Journal of Anatomy 81:56

Crockett J L, Edgerton V R 1974 Enhancement of muscle protein and tetanic tension after intramuscular spinal cord homogenate injections. In: IIIrd International Congress on Muscle Diseases, International Congress Series No 334, Abstract 22. Excerpta Medica, Amsterdam

Currie S, Saunders M, Knowles M, Brown A E 1971 Immunological aspects of polymyositis. The in vitro activity of lymphocytes on incubation with muscle antigen and with muscle cultures. Quarterly Journal of Medicine 40:63

Dalldorf G 1950 The Coxsackie viruses. Bulletin of the New York Academy of Medicine 26:329

Dawkins R L 1965 Experimental myositis associated with hypersensitivity to muscle. Journal of Pathology and Bacteriology 90:619

Denny-Brown D 1951 The influence of tension and innervation on the regeneration of skeletal muscle. Journal of Neuropathology and Experimental Neurology 10: 94–96

De Reuck J, De Coster W, Van der Eecken H 1977 The target phenomenon in rat muscle following tenotomy and neurotomy. Acta Neuropathologica 37:49

Douglas W B 1974 Myographic and electroneurographic responses of leg muscles and cross-innervated sciatic nerves in normal and dystrophic mice (129B6F$_1$ hybrid) united in parabiosis. In: IIIrd International Congress on Muscle Diseases, International Congress Series No 334, Abstract 19. Excerpta Medica, Amsterdam

Eccles J C 1941 Disuse atrophy of skeletal muscle. Medical Journal of Australia 2: 160–164

Eccles J C 1944 Investigations on muscle atrophies arising from disuse and tenotomy. Journal of Physiology (London) 103: 252–266

Edström L, Kugelberg E 1968 Histochemical composition distribution of fibers and fatigability of single motor units. Journal of Neurology, Neurosurgery and Psychiatry 31: 424–433

Ellis J T 1956 Necrosis and regeneration of skeletal muscle in cortisone-treated rabbits. American Journal of Pathology 32: 993–1013

Engel A G 1978 The ultrastructural immunopathology of myasthenia gravis; Abstracts of the International Conference of Plasmapheresis and the Immunobiology of Myasthenia Gravis, June 22–24, 1978. Muscle and Nerve 1:337

Engel A G 1979 Myasthenia gravis. In: Vinken P J, Bruyn G W (eds) Handbook of clinical neurology, vol 41, Diseases of muscle Part II. North Holland, Amsterdam (ch 4), p 92–145

Engel A G, Tsujihata M, Lambert E G, Lindstrom J M, Lennon V A 1976 Experimental autoimmune myasthenia gravis: a sequential and quantitative study of the neuromuscular junction ultrastructure and electrophysiologic correlations. Journal of Neuropathology and Experimental Neurology 35: 569–587

Engel W K 1973 Duchenne muscular dystrophy. A histologically based ischemia hypothesis and comparison with experimental ischemic myopathy. In: Pearson C M, Mostofi F K (eds) The striated muscle. Williams & Wilkins, Baltimore, p 453

Engel W K 1979 Development of the motor unit in vitro vis-a-vis: The pathology of congenital neuromuscular diseases. In: Aguayo A J, Karpati G (eds) Current topics in nerve and muscle research. Selected papers of the Symposia held at the IVth International Congress on Neuromuscular Diseases, Montreal, Canada, September 17–21, 1978. Excerpta Medica, Amsterdam, p 143–153

Engel W K, Brooke M H, Nelson P G 1966 Histochemical studies of denervated or tenotomized cat muscle: Illustrating difficulties in relating experimental animal conditions to human neuromuscular diseases. Annals of the New York Academy of Sciences 138: 160–185

Esiri M M, MacLennan I C M 1975 Some immunological studies of an experimental allergic myositis in rats. In: Bradley W G, Gardner-Medwin D, Walton J N (eds) Recent advances in myology. Excerpta Medica, Amsterdam, p 380–386

Fenichel G M, Martin J T 1974 An experimental myopathy in rats produced with imidazole. In: IIIrd International Congress on Muscle Diseases, International Congress Series No 334, Abstract 331. Excerpta Medica, Amsterdam

Ferguson A B, Vaughan L, Ward L 1957 A study of disuse atrophy of skeletal muscle in the rabbit. Journal of Bone and Joint Surgery (Am) 39A: 583–596

Field E J 1960 Virus infections. In: Bourne G H (ed) The structure and function of muscle. Academic Press, New York, (ch 3) p 85

Francis M J O, Curry O B, Smith R 1974 Vitamin D and muscle: a defect of calcium uptake by sarcoplasmic reticulum in vitamin D deficient rabbits. In: IIIrd International Congress on Muscle Diseases, International Congress Series No 334, Abstract 324. Excerpta Medica, Amsterdam

Gauthier G F, Schaeffer S F 1975 Ultrastructural evidence of early subsarcolemmal protein synthesis in denervated skeletal muscle fibres. In: Bradley W G, Gardner-Medwin G, Walton J N (eds) Recent advances in myology. Excerpta Medica, Amsterdam, p 27–32

Goldstein G, Whittingham S 1966 Experimental autoimmune thymitis. An animal model of human myasthenia gravis. Lancet 2:315

Goyer R A, Yin M W 1967 Taurine and creatine excretion after x-irradiation and plasmocid-induced muscle necrosis in the rat. Radiation Research 30:301

Graham D I, Bonilla E, Gonatas N K, Schotland D L 1976 Core formation in the muscles of rats intoxicated with triethyltin sulfate. Journal of Neuropathology and Experimental Neurology 35:1

Gutmann E, Guttmann L 1942 Effect of electrotherapy on denervated muscles in rabbits. Lancet 1:169

Gutmann E, Hanzlikova V 1975 Factors affecting success of transplantation of skeletal muscle in the rat. In: Bradley W G, Gardner-Medwin D, Walton J N (eds) Recent advances in myology. Excerpta Medica, Amsterdam, p 57–63

Hadlow W J 1962 Diseases of skeletal muscle. In: Innes J R M, Saunders L Z (eds) Comparative neuropathology. Academic Press, New York, p 147–232

Heilbronn E, Mattson C, Stalberg E 1975 Immune response in rabbits to a cholinergic receptor protein: possibly a model for myasthenia gravis. In: Bradley W G, Gardner-Medwin D, Walton J N (eds) Recent advances in myology. Excerpta Medica, Amsterdam, p 486–492

Holmes D, Dickson J A, Pennington R J 1974 Peptide hydrolases in muscle from tumour-bearing rats. In: IIIrd International Congress on Muscle Diseases, International Congress Series No 334, Abstract 326. Excerpta Medica, Amsterdam

Howell J McC, Buxton P H 1975 α-tocopherol responsive muscular dystrophy in guinea pigs. Neuropathology and Applied Neurobiology 1:49

Ishay J, Lass Y, Sandbank U 1975 A lesion of muscle transverse tubular system by oriental hornet (*Vespa orientalis*) venom; electron microscopic and histological study. Toxicon 13:57

Jasmin G, Gareau R 1961 Histopathological study of muscle lesions produced by paraphenylenediamine in rats. British Journal of Experimental Pathology 42:592

Jasmin G, Bajusz E, Solymoss B 1975 Selective prevention by verapamil and other drugs of the hamster hereditary cardiomyopathy. In: Bradley W G, Gardner-Medwin D, Walton J N (eds) Recent advances in myology. Excerpta Medica, Amsterdam, p 413–417

Johnston D M, Drachman D B 1974 Neurotrophic regulation of dynamic properties of skeletal muscle: effects of botulinum toxin and denervation. In: IIIrd International Congress on Muscle Diseases, International Congress Series No 334, Abstract 21. Excerpta Medica, Amsterdam

Kakulas B A 1966 Destruction of differentiated muscle cultures by sensitized lymphoid cells. Journal of Pathology and Bacteriology 91:495

Kakulas B A 1970 The pathogenesis of human muscle disease. In: Walton J N, Canal N, Scarlato G (eds) Muscle diseases. Excerpta Medica, Amsterdam, p 337

Kakulas B A 1973 Observations on the etiology of polymyositis. In: Pearson C M, Mostofi F K (eds) The striated muscle. Williams & Wilkins, Baltimore, p 485–497

Kakulas B A 1975 Experimental muscle diseases. In: Jasmin G, Cantin M (eds) Methods and achievements in experimental pathology, vol 7. Karger, Basel, p 109–131

Kakulas B A 1982a Skeletal muscle. In: Riddell R H (ed) Pathology of drug-induced and toxic diseases. Churchill Livingstone, Edinburgh, (ch 3) p 49–69

Kakulas B A 1982b Toxic and drug-induced myopathies. In: Walton J N, Mastaglia F L (eds) Skeletal muscle pathology. Churchill Livingstone, Edinburgh, (ch 13) p 46–69

Kakulas B A 1987 Animal models of polymyositis/dermatomyositis. In: Dalakas M (ed) Polymyositis and dermatomyositis. Butterworths, Massachusetts (in press)

Kakulas B A, Adams R D 1966 Principles of myopathology as illustrated in the nutritional myopathy of the Rottnest quokka (*Setonix brachyurus*). Annals of the New York Academy of Sciences 138:90

Kakulas B A, Adams R D 1985 Diseases of muscle. Pathological foundations of clinical myology. Harper and Row, Philadelphia

Kallos P, Pagel W 1937 Experimentelle Untersuchungen uber asthma bronchale. Acta Medica Scandinavica 91:292

Kark R A P, Edgerton V R, Whiteman N 1975 Decreased oxidation by muscle after denervation but not disuse atrophy. In: Bradley W G, Gardner-Medwin D, Walton J N (eds) Recent advances in myology. Excerpta Medica, Amsterdam, p 33–41

Karpati G, Carpenter S, Eisen A A 1972 Experimental core-like lesions and nemaline rods: a correlative morphological and physiological study. Archives of Neurology 27: 237–251

Keast D 1967 Personal communication

Khan M Y 1974 Radiation-induced changes in skeletal muscle: an electron microscopic study. Journal of Neuropathology and Experimental Neurology 33:42

Kugelberg E, Edström L, Abbruzzese M 1970 Mapping of motor units in experimentally reinnervated rat muscle. Interpretation of histochemical and atrophic fibre pattern in neurogenic lesions. Journal of Neurology, Neurosurgery and Psychiatry 33:319

Lennon V A, Lindstrom J M, Seybold M E 1976 Experimental autoimmune myasthenia gravis: cellular and humoral immune responses. Annals of the New York Academy of Sciences 274:283

Lindstrom J M 1978 The role of antibodies to the acetylcholine receptor, protein and its component peptides in experimental autoimmune myasthenia gravis in rats. Abstracts of the International Conference on Plasmapheresis and the Immunobiology of Myasthenia Gravis. Muscle and Nerve 1: 335–336

London W T, Sever J L, Madden D L, Gravel M, Dalakas M C, Houff S A et al 1983 Experimental transmission of Simian acquired immunodeficiency syndrome (SAIDS) and kaposi-like skin lesions. Lancet ii: 869–873

Lundsgaard E 1930 Untersuchungen über Muskelkontraktion ohne Milchsäurebildung. Biochem Zeitschrift 217: 162–177

Manda P, Kakulas B 1986 The effect of myotoxic agent iodoacetate on dystrophic mice 129 Re. In: Karoutas G, Logothetis J (eds) Proceedings of the International Society of Hellenic Neuroscientists. Thessalonika, Greece (in press)

Manghani D, Partridge T, Sloper J C, Smith P 1975 Role of myofibrillar antigens in the pathogenesis of experimental myositis, with particular reference to lymphocyte sensitization, the transfer of the disease by lymphocytes, and the preferential attachment of lymphocytes from animals with experimental myositis to cultured muscle cells. In: Bradley W G, Gardner-Medwin D, Walton J N (eds) Recent advances in myology. Excerpta Medica, Amsterdam, p 387–394

Manolov S 1974 Regeneration of rat neuromuscular junctions. In: IIIrd International Congress Series No 334, Abstract 183. Excerpta Medica, Amsterdam

Margreth A, Salviati G, Carraro U 1974 Biochemical characteristics of skeletal muscles in relation to the pattern and rate of activity. In: IIIrd International Congress on Muscle Diseases, International Congress Series No 334, Abstract 10. Excerpta Medica, Amsterdam

Mascres C, Jasmin G 1975 Changes in the muscle fibre induced in the rat by p-phenylenediamine. Pathology and Biology 23:193

Mastaglia F L, Dawkins R L, Papadimitriou J M 1974 A morphological study of muscle grafts in mice. In: IIIrd International Congress on Muscle Diseases, International Congress Series No 334, Abstract 275. Excerpta Medica, Amsterdam

Mauro A, Shafiq S A, Milhorat A T 1970 Regeneration of

striated muscle, and myogenesis. International Congress Series No 218. Excerpta Medica, Amsterdam

Melmed C, Karpati G, Carpenter S 1975 Experimental mitochondrial myopathy produced by in vivo uncoupling of oxidative phosphorylation. Journal of the Neurological Sciences 26: 305–318

Mendell J R 1979 Experimental myopathies: A review of experimental models and their relationship to human neuromuscular diseases. In: Vinken P J, Bruyn G W (eds) Handbook of clinical neurology, vol 30, Part I. North Holland, Amsterdam (ch 4) p 133–182

Miranda A F, Gamboa E T, Armstrong C L, Hsu K C 1978 Susceptibility of human skeletal muscle culture to influenza virus infection, Part 2. Ultrastructural cytopathology. Journal of the Neurological Sciences 36:63

Morita H 1926 An experimental study on the pathology of the black-leg. Journal of the Japanese Society of Veterinary Science 5:1

Morpurgo B 1897 Über activatäts: Hypertrophie der willkürliehen muskeln. Virchow's Archiv für Pathologische Anatomie und Physiologie und fur Klinische Medizin 150: 522–524

Mumenthaler M, Paakkari I 1974 The needle myopathy. An experimental study. In: IIIrd International Congress on Muscle Diseases, International Congress Series No 334, Abstract 341. Excerpta Medica, Amsterdam

Nageotte J 1937 Sur la contraction extreme des muscles squelettiques chez les vertebrés. Zeitschrift für Zellforschung und mikroskopische. Anatomie 26:603

Owens K, Ruth R C, Gottwik M G, McNamara D B, Weglicki W B 1975 Muscular dystrophy of the chicken: distribution of subcellular organelles in zonal gradients. In: Bradley W G, Gardner-Medwin D, Walton J N (eds) Recent advances in myology. Excerpta Medica, Amsterdam, p 395–400

Palmer A C, Harriman D G F, Barker J 1974 Myasthenia in the dog. In: IIIrd International Congress on Muscle Diseases, International Congress Series No 334. Excerpta Medica, Amsterdam

Papanicolaou G N, Falk E A 1938 General muscular hypertrophy induced by androgenic hormone. Science 87: 238–239

Park J H, Chou T H, Hill E J, Pinson R, Bartle E, Connally J et al 1975 Improvement of hereditary avian muscular dystrophy by penicillamine therapy. In: Bradley W G, Gardner-Medwin D, Walton J (eds) Recent advances in myology. Excerpta Medica, Amsterdam, p 401–406

Parkes J D 1966 Attempted production of myasthenia gravis in the rat. British Journal of Experimental Pathology 47:577

Partridge T A, Sloper J C 1977 A host contribution to the regeneration of muscle grafts. Journal of the Neurological Sciences 33:425

Patrick J, Lindstrom J 1973 Autoimmune response to acetylcholine receptor. Science 180:871

Patrick J, Lindstrom J, Culp B, McMillan J 1973 Studies on purified eel acetylcholine receptor and antiacetylcholine receptor antibody. Proceedings of the National Academy of Sciences USA 70:3334

Pearson C M 1956 Development of arthritis, periarthritis and periosteitis in rats given adjuvants. Proceedings of the Society for Experimental Biology and Medicine 91:95

Penn A S 1977 Myasthenia gravis, dermatomyositis, and polymyositis: immunopathological diseases. In: Griggs R C, Moxley R T (eds) Advances in neurology, vol 1. Raven Press, New York, p 41–61

Peter J B 1973 Skeletal muscle: diversity and mutability of its histochemical, electron microscopic, biochemical and physiologic properties. In: Pearson C M, Mostofi F K (eds) The striated muscle. Williams and Wilkins, Baltimore, p 1–18

Pluskal M G, Pennington R J, Johnson M A, Harris J B 1974 Some effects of tiger snake toxin upon skeletal muscle. In: IIIrd International Congress on Muscle Diseases, International Congress Series No 334, Abstract 327. Excerpta Medica, Amsterdam

Reznik M 1973 Current concepts of skeletal muscle regeneration. In: Pearson C M, Mostofi F K (eds) The striated muscle. Williams and Wilkins, Baltimore, p 185–225

Rosman N P, Schapiro M B, Haddow J E 1978 Muscle weakness caused by an iodine-deficient diet: investigation of a nutritional myopathy. Journal of Neuropathology and Experimental Neurology 37:192

Rubin E, Katz A M, Lieber C S, Stein E P, Puszkin S 1976 Muscle damage produced by chronic alcohol consumption. American Journal of Pathology 83:499

Rustigan R, Pappenheimer M 1949 Myositis in mice following intramuscular injection of viruses of the mouse encephalomyelitis group and of certain other neurotropic viruses. Journal of Experimental Medicine 89:69

Sahgal V, Subramani V, Hughes R, Shah A, Singh H 1979 On the pathogenesis of mitochondrial myopathies. An experimental study. Acta Neuropathologica (Berlin) 46:177–183, 1979

Sanders D B, Cobb E E, Winfield J B 1978 Neonatal experimental autoimmune myasthenia gravis. Muscle and Nerve 1:146

Sarnat H B, Portnoy J M, Chi D Y K 1977 Effects of denervation and tenotomy on the gastrocnemius muscle in the frog: A histological and histochemical study. Anatomical Record 187(3): 335–346

Sato T, Sakuragawa N, Tsubaki T 1974 Arbovirus myositis: initiation and multiplication of sindbis virus in mouse skeletal muscles. In: IIIrd International Congress on Muscle Diseases, International Congress Series No 334, Abstract 291. Excerpta Medica, Amsterdam

Schiller H H, Esslen E, Weihe W H, Haldermann G, Teelmann K 1974 Investigations on experimental malignant hyperthermia (MH) in pigs. In: IIIrd International Congress on Muscle Diseases, International Congress Series No 334, Abstract 391. Excerpta Medica, Amsterdam

Scully R E, Shannon J M, Dickersin G R 1961 Factors involved in recovery from experimental muscle ischemia produced in dogs. 1. Histologic and histochemical pattern of ischemic muscle. American Journal of Pathology 39:721

Smith G T, Beeuwkes R, Tomkiewicz Z M, Tadaaki A, Town B 1965 Pathological changes in skin and skeletal muscle following alternating current and capacitor discharge. American Journal of Pathology 47:1

Sola O M, Christensen D L, Martin A W 1973 Hypertrophy and hyperplasia of adult chicken anterior latissimus dorsi muscles following stretch with and without denervation. Experimental Neurology 41:76

Sola O M, Dillard D H, Ivey T D, Haneda K, Itoh T, Thomas R 1985 Autotransplantation of skeletal muscle into myocardium. Circulation 71(2): 341–348

Tal C, Liban E 1962 Experimental production of muscular dystrophy-like lesions in rabbits and guinea pigs by an autoimmune process. British Journal of Experimental Pathology 43:525

Tannenberg J 1939 Pathological changes in the heart, skeletal musculature and liver in rabbits treated with insulin in shock dosage. American Journal of Pathology 15:25

Tarrab-Hazdai R, Aharanov A, Abramsky O, Yaar I, Fuchs S 1975 Passive transfer of experimental autoimmune myasthenia by lymph node cells in inbred guinea pigs. Journal of Experimental Medicine 142:785

Toyka K V, Drachman D B, Griffin D B, Pestronk A, Winkelstein J A, Fischbeck K H et al 1977 Myasthenia gravis; a study of humoral immune mechanisms by passive transfer to mice. New England Journal of Medicine 296:125

Volkmann R 1893 Ueber die Regeneration des quergestreiften Muskelgewebes beim Menschen und Säugethier. Beiträge zue pathologischen Anatomie und zur allgemeinen. Pathologie 12:233

Wakayama Y, Okayasu H, Kumagai T 1984 Quantitative freeze-fracture electron microscopic study of muscle plasma membrane of experimental anoxic myopathy. Journal of the Neurological Sciences 63: 411–421

Walton J N, Adams R D 1958 Polymyositis. Livingstone, Edinburgh

Ward P, Goldspink G 1974 Response of different fibre types to changes in activity pattern and to protein malnutrition. In: IIIrd International Congress on Muscle Diseases, International Congress Series No 334, Abstract 16. Excerpta Medica, Amsterdam

Warren S 1943 Effects of radiation on normal tissues. XIV. Effects on striated muscle. Archives of Pathology 35:347

Webb J N 1970 Experimental immune myositis in guinea pigs. Journal of the Reticulo-endothelial Society 7:305

Wecker L, Dettbarn W D (1977) Effects of denervation on the production of an experimental myopathy. Experimental Neurology 57:94

Whittingham S, Mackay I R 1966 Autoimmune aspects of myasthenia gravis. Proceedings of the Australian Association of Neurologists 4:27

Wrogemann K, Mezon B J, Beockx R L, Thakar J H, Picard S, Blanchaer M C 1975 Defective oxidative phosphorylation: is it responsible for muscle necrosis in muscular dystrophy? In: Bradley W G, Gardner-Medwin D, Walton J N (eds) Recent advances in myology. Excerpta Medica, Amsterdam, p 441–445

Biochemical aspects of muscle disease with particular reference to the muscular dystrophies

INTRODUCTION

In the muscular dystrophies, with which this chapter is primarily concerned, the chemical alterations may initially be limited and subtle but later become widespread and associated with the gradual deterioration of the muscle tissue. Biochemical study of the disease then becomes extremely complicated: the more fundamental changes, those which are presumed to initiate the process of degeneration, are obscured by the numerous secondary disturbances. This is one reason why nothing is yet known of the cause of any type of muscular dystrophy. Moreover, the diagnostic value of many of the secondary changes is limited by the fact that muscle degeneration, whatever the ultimate cause, appears to have many common features.

Since the last edition of this book, numerous papers concerned, directly or indirectly, with the biochemistry of the muscular dystrophies have continued to appear. They report diverse observations, generally with no clear interrelationships and since, at this stage, it is not usually possible to assess their importance vis-a-vis the origin and development of the disease, this survey is made, as in previous editions, on a wide front. In addition, accurate description of the secondary changes associated with the progress of the disease may be valuable in itself, because it may point the way to treating some of these and thus delaying, halting or even reversing degeneration of the muscles.

Some of the reported studies have comprised direct investigation of biochemical changes in biopsied muscle and, increasingly commonly, other tissues from patients. Much work has also been done on laboratory animals with hereditary myopathies, particularly those in the mouse, chicken and hamster, and will be referred to occasionally in this chapter. It is generally recognised that such models are not identical to any of the forms of human muscular dystrophy, but many of the secondary changes in the muscles are similar and it is possible that the underlying defects may be closely related. A useful brief review and discussion of such models has recently been published (Lunt & Marchbanks 1978). More information will be found in Harris (1979). A few biochemical studies have also been carried out on muscle cultured from human patients or affected animals. Although one or two claims have been made that abnormalities can be seen in muscle cultured from patients, not everyone is convinced that the genetic defect will be manifested in the early stages of development of the muscle fibres. Histological abnormalities in dystrophic muscle are not much in evidence at the fetal stage.

As well as the investigation of affected muscle, much relevant research involves studies on normal muscle alone, with special emphasis on those features, such as membrane biochemistry, which it is commonly supposed may be disturbed in dystrophic muscle. Clearly, there is a possibility that the more important alterations in disease may involve facets of muscle biochemistry not yet fully explored in normal tissue. Evidently, it is preferable that, where feasible, such studies should be carried out using human muscle because of possible interspecies differences.

One problem to be faced when reviewing the biochemistry of muscle diseases is the number of potentially important, but unconfirmed, findings in the literature. Unfortunately, in the past, several such promising reports have proved to be unfounded on further investigation, and some caution is necessary in assessing new claims.

Because of the large number of studies which have now been published, it is not practicable to include a fully comprehensive bibliography. Where a choice has to be made, reference will be made to the more recent papers on a particular topic; these usually provide references to the earlier works. Many of the references quoted in the last edition have had to be omitted because of considerations of space. Apologies are offered,

therefore, to those authors whose work is not quoted directly.

The material in this chapter will be of most interest to those concerned directly or indirectly with research into muscle disease, especially muscular dystrophy. Practical clinical applications are restricted to the use of serum enzymes, particularly creatine kinase, in the diagnosis of muscular dystrophy and, most important, in identification of the genetic carriers. This will be discussed fully.

MUSCLE BIOCHEMISTRY

General remarks

It is reasonable to suppose that direct analysis of affected muscle, its chemical composition and enzyme activities, is most likely to lead to understanding of the causes and progression of the muscular dystrophies.

All biochemical studies must take into account the profound histological changes occurring in the affected muscles, notably the proliferation of connective tissue and sometimes of fat, and the structural changes in the fibres. It is evident that marked alterations may occur in the overall chemical and enzymic composition of the muscle tissue merely as a result of these changes. Biochemical research must try to discriminate between these and more fundamental changes. An obvious consideration is the relative decrease in the overall volume of the muscle fibres which is accompanied by the proliferation of connective tissue and increase in fat. Comparison of the concentration of muscle cell constituents in diseased and normal cells expressed in terms of total muscle weight is of little value unless the changes are very large indeed. Some of the early data on changes in composition of diseased muscle were vitiated by lack of a suitable reference base. A simple and reasonably satisfactory way of overcoming this problem is to use as a reference base for comparison the protein of the muscle which will dissolve in dilute alkali at room temperature. This 'non-collagen protein' excludes the alkali-insoluble collagen and elastin and is easily determined — an important requirement of a reference base. Typically it represents over 90% of the total protein of normal muscle but may be less than 50% when the muscle is in an advanced state of degeneration. It is used by most workers and it may be hoped that it will be adopted by all as a reference base. Any criterion which is chosen must be arbitrary to some extent, but the use of such a common procedure will facilitate comparison of results.

Second, where increases in metabolic activities of affected muscle are recorded, it must be asked whether these may be associated with an increase in connective tissue or with invading macrophages; probable instances are mentioned below. Changes will occur also in the relative amounts of vascular and nervous tissue and probably of mast cells. Finally, the presence of regenerating fibres, which have characteristic metabolic profiles, must be considered. Such difficulties as these, which stand in the way of investigations into the more fundamental biochemical defects and the biochemical changes in degenerating fibres, can best be circumvented by study of muscle in which the disease has made only minimal progress. In practice it is normally more difficult to obtain specimens of such muscle for investigation; consequently, there have as yet been relatively few studies of this nature. When volunteered, the availability of muscle biopsies from genetic carriers, particularly from those with high serum creatine kinase activity but minimal histopathological changes, should be valuable. The importance of comparing results with those derived from normal muscle, preferably obtained from individuals of about the same age, must also be emphasised, because many workers have demonstrated that there are age variations in the amounts of enzymes and other proteins in muscle. Furthermore, in view of the recognised quantitative metabolic differences between different muscles, in particular between 'red' and 'white' muscles, it is desirable that the diseased muscle should be compared with the same muscle in the normal subject. In practice the use of the abdominal muscle offers advantages in this respect.

Muscle enzymes — general

Numerous workers have measured the activity of various enzymes in biopsies of diseased muscle, particularly in those obtained from patients with Duchenne muscular dystrophy. However, not more than about 50 enzymes have yet been studied, out of hundreds possible. Nevertheless, many have already been shown to display a changed level of activity in dystrophic muscle. Undoubtedly, many such changes will result merely from the kind of factors mentioned above and can throw little, if any, light on the nature of the disease. Others, however, may represent aspects of fundamental metabolic changes which occur during the progression of the disease.

To assess the significance of observed enzyme changes may often be difficult. Probably, many will be understood only when many other enzymes have been studied at different stages of the disease and meaningful patterns have begun to emerge.

It is a reasonable supposition, by analogy with some other hereditary diseases, that the ultimate defect resulting from the genetic aberration is a complete or partial failure to synthesise a particular enzyme, the activity of which is essential for the maintenance of normal cell structure. It now seems highly probable that the identification of the enzyme or other protein involved in the genetic defect will be achieved in the relatively near future in Duchenne and myotonic dystrophies through the recent dramatic developments in recombinant DNA techniques (see Ch. 26 and Roses et al 1983). Rational therapies may then become possible.

Many of the enzymes which have been measured fall into broad classes, which will now be discussed.

Lysosomal enzymes

A striking feature of many myopathies (human and animal) is an increase, in the diseased muscle, of the activity of many lysosomal enzymes. (The association of such enzymes with lysosomes is based predominantly on investigations with tissues, such as liver, from which lysosomes can be isolated and studied.) These enzymes hydrolyse various cell constituents and have maximum activity in vitro at a low pH, which is assumed to simulate conditions within lysosomes. An extensive series of reports, published by Kar and Pearson from 1972 onwards, on the concentrations of such enzymes in muscle diseases has confirmed earlier findings and added new observations. They have noticed some interesting differences in the degree of elevation of these enzymes in relation to the nature and progression of the disease. An increase in acid cathepsin (probably cathepsin D, EC 3.4.23.5), an enzyme which attacks proteins, was general among the myopathies but was significant in severely affected muscle only (Kar & Pearson 1972a). On the other hand, four other enzymes which degrade proteins or peptides (cathepsin A, EC 3.4.16.1; cathepsin B1, EC 3.4.22.1; and dipeptidyl peptidases I and II, EC 3.4.14.1 and 3.4.14.2) were raised even in the mildly affected muscle in various diseases (Kar & Pearson 1976a, 1977, 1978). It should be noted that, in these studies, cathepsin B1 was measured by the hydrolysis of benzoylarginine 2-naphthylamide; this substrate is split by at least one other peptidase in muscle (Hardy & Pennington 1979). Other lysosomal enzymes, notably acid phosphatase (EC 3.1.3.2), β-acetylglucosaminidase (EC 3.2.1.30), α-fucosidase (EC 3.2.1.51), α-mannosidase (EC 3.2.1.24) and α-glucosidase (EC 3.2.1.20), are increased in advanced cases only (Kar & Pearson 1972b, 1973a). Hooft et al (1966) reported increased aryl sulphatase (EC 3.1.6.1) activity at various stages of progression of Duchenne dystrophy. An increase in acid ribonuclease activity in Duchenne dystrophy was found by Abdullah & Pennington (1968).

It can be assumed that invading macrophages, which are rich in these enzymes, will contribute to these changes. High levels are found also in muscle fibroblasts (Parsons et al 1978). It is difficult to assess the extent of their contribution but, if one assumes that a similar response mechanism operates in various types of muscle damage, there is reason to believe that it does not fully explain the increased activities. Experimentally denervated muscle also shows increased activity of this group of enzymes, but there does not appear to be any appreciable increase in macrophages during the first few days following nerve section. Further evidence that the increase in acid proteinase and cathepsin B1 in denervated muscle is not due to mononuclear cells has been provided by Maskrey et al (1977).

The presence of regenerating muscle fibres may also contribute to the increased concentrations of lysosomal enzymes. Iodice et al (1972) found a decrease in the activity of several cathepsins during maturation of breast muscle in the chicken. However, this again is likely to be only a partial explanation, because regeneration is not seen in denervated muscle.

It would appear likely, therefore, that muscle fibres respond in some way to various damaging influences by an increase in their content of lysosomal enzymes. How this occurs and what may be its biological significance is unknown, as is its contribution to the subsequent degeneration of the fibres. It is, perhaps, of interest to compare the well-studied proliferation of lysosomes which occurs in insect intersegmental muscles when they break down during metamorphosis (Lockshin & Beaulaton 1974). It has, indeed, been postulated by Webb (1974) that muscular dystrophy may be a disturbance of a process of 'cell death' which occurs in normal fetal development. The lysosomal alterations in ischaemic myocardium and their significance, discussed by Wildenthal (1978), may also have some common features.

Nevertheless, it must be stressed that there is still much uncertainty regarding the nature of the function, if any, of acid hydrolases within normal muscle. The activity of these enzymes in muscle homogenates can be increased, under suitable conditions, by the use of detergents; thus they exhibit the 'latency' characteristic of lysosomal enzymes in other tissues. However, the extent to which cells other than the muscle fibres contribute to these activities is not known. Histochemical studies on normal muscle have sometimes failed to show up lysosomal enzymes within the muscle fibres. On the other hand, in muscle affected by disease, such as muscular dystrophy in hamsters (Al-Azzawi & Stoward 1972), denervation (Schiaffino & Hanzlikova 1972), starvation (Bird 1975) or ischaemia (Shannon et al 1974), there is histochemical evidence of the appearance of lysosomes or lysosomal enzymes. Canonico & Bird (1970) fractionated normal rat muscle homogenates by centrifuging on density gradients and obtained evidence for two groups of particle-bound acid hydrolases, one of which they considered to originate from the muscle fibres. Stauber & Ong (1981) localised cathepsin B in discrete granules in rat muscle. Consideration of their results alongside previous work with other lysosomal enzymes led them to the conclusion that muscle fibres contain different populations of lysosomal enzymes.

Enzymes of energy metabolism

Enzymes of glycolysis and related enzymes. Dreyfus et al (1956) showed that the rate of glycolysis of dystrophic muscle was much less than normal; the extent of the decrease paralleled the state of progress of the disease. Assays of individual glycolytic enzymes showed that α-glucan phosphorylase (EC 2.4.1.1), phosphoglucomutase (EC 5.4.2.2) and aldolase (EC 4.1.2.13) had low activity. In contrast, the activity of a number of other enzymes, such as cytochrome oxidase (EC 1.9.3.1), succinate dehydrogenase (EC 1.3.99.1), aconitase (EC 4.2.1.3), fumarase (EC 4.2.1.2) and the aminotransferases (EC 2.6.1.1 and 2.6.1.2), was not significantly different from normal. Other workers, quoted by these authors, had previously carried out similar investigations in experimental neurogenic muscular atrophy; the changes were, in general, similar. They are not, however, an invariable consequence of muscle atrophy because aldolase activity and the rate of glycolysis are largely unimpaired in myopathic mouse muscle. It is of interest, also, that DiMauro et al (1967) reported that, in contrast with other glycolytic enzymes, muscle phosphorylase showed an earlier and more marked loss in progressive muscular dystrophies than in neurogenic diseases. Studies by Vignos & Lefkowitz (1959) showed that the rate of glycolysis is low in the juvenile forms but is essentially normal in the adult forms of muscular dystrophy. The latter workers also found a low activity of creatine kinase (EC 2.7.3.2) in juvenile muscular dystrophy and neurogenic atrophy of muscle, but only marginal changes in adult muscular dystrophy. Many of these findings have been confirmed in extensive investigations by Heyck et al (1963), Hooft et al (1966) and Kleine & Chlond (1967) which have also shown decreases in other enzymes in dystrophic muscle, including adenylate kinase (EC 2.7.4.3) and a number of glycolytic enzymes. The enzyme fructose 1,6-diphosphatase (EC 3.1.3.11), which in muscle may be concerned with

the control of glycolysis is, however, present in normal amounts in various kinds of muscular dystrophy (Kar & Pearson 1972c).

Another enzyme, AMP aminohydrolase (AMP deaminase, EC 3.5.4.6) is markedly decreased in both dystrophic mouse muscle (Pennington 1961) and in muscle from patients with Duchenne dystrophy even at an early stage, while in other muscle diseases a low level is seen only in severely affected muscle (Kar & Pearson 1973b). This enzyme occurs in far greater concentration in skeletal muscle than in other tissues; while its precise role is not yet clear, it may be important in the control of glycolysis in muscle.

This secondary fall in AMP deaminase is, of course, to be distinguished from the inherited deficiency of the muscle isoenzyme of AMP deaminase which has come to light during the last few years (reviewed by Fishbein 1985, and dealt with more fully in Ch. 25 of this volume).

It is of interest that the activity of adenylosuccinase (EC 4.3.2.2) one of the enzymes involved in the resynthesis of AMP from IMP, was unaltered in muscle of patients with muscle diseases (Kar & Pearson 1981a).

Cause of changes. It seems unlikely that the enhanced leakage of these enzymes from diseased muscle, which is described below, is an important cause of their low activities in muscle. Thus there is no increase in serum AMP deaminase in Duchenne dystrophy (R. J. Pennington, unpublished work) while conversely aminotransferases, which are released into the blood, are not decreased in muscle. Moreover it would probably require only a relatively small acceleration in the normal rate of resynthesis to compensate for the leakage.

Work by Dawson & Kaplan (1965), Hooft et al (1966), Kendrick-Jones & Perry (1967) and others, showed that many of the enzymes concerned show a marked increase in activity in the muscles of normal animals during development. Hence, the levels of these enzymes in dystrophic muscle tend to resemble those of normal muscle at an earlier stage of development. A probable partial explanation for the lower enzyme activities in both diseased muscle and fetal muscle is that they are the result, engineered by an adaptive mechanism, of a lower level of physical activity. The increase in certain muscle enzymes during development can be correlated clearly with the use of the muscles (Dawson & Kaplan 1965, Kendrick-Jones & Perry 1967). Moreover, exercise can increase the concentration of muscle enzymes (Kendrick-Jones & Perry 1965) and also of myoglobin (Pattengale & Holloszy 1967). One can only speculate on the possible mechanisms by which muscular activity could influence the concentration of muscle enzymes. Possibly, nerve impulses facilitate the transfer from nerve to muscle of 'trophic' substances which specifically enhance the synthesis of certain muscle enzymes. Alternatively, some product of glycolysis or change in pH or oxygen tension may stimulate the synthesis of these enzymes, thus ensuring that their level would be automatically related to muscle activity. It seems improbable, however, that muscular activity provides a complete explanation for the changes in glycolytic enzymes during development and disease. Mann & Salafsky (1970) reported that the large increases in aldolase and pyruvate kinase (EC 2.7.1.40) observed during the development of the anterior tibial muscle in the kitten were not prevented by immobilising the muscle. Other works (e.g. Riley & Allin 1973), demonstrate that the levels of glycolytic enzymes are influenced by the pattern of nerve impulses.

In so far as these changes directly reflect a delayed development, they accord with other observations as discussed by Vrbová (1983) who has postulated that such immaturity of the muscle makes it unable to withstand the activity imposed by the motor neurone and is thus a primary factor in the aetiology of Duchenne muscular dystrophy.

Isoenzymes. Certain enzymes have also been shown to display in diseased muscle an isoenzyme pattern which is abnormal for adult muscle but resembles that of immature muscle. Isoenzymes are different proteins (or contain varying proportions of the same protein sub-units) with similar enzymic properties; they are usually recognised and differentiated by electrophoresis on gels or other suitable media or by ion-exchange chromatography. Many enzymes display such multiplicity; in many instances, the enzyme pattern varies with the tissue of origin of the enzyme. Wieme & Lauryssens (1962) found differences between normal and diseased human muscle (muscular dystrophy and neurogenic atrophy), in the relative amounts of the five lactate dehydrogenase (EC 1.1.1.27) isoenzymes. The major component of lactate dehydrogenase in most normal muscles is the most slow-moving on electrophoresis (LDH5). They found that, in normal muscle, it represented an average of 31.4% of the total lactate dehydrogenase, but in myopathic muscle only 17.7%. Numerous subsequent investigations have confirmed and extended these findings: it appears that such changes are usually, but not invariably, present in Duchenne dystrophy and many other muscle diseases (Emery 1968, Kowalewski & Rotthauwe 1972). The abnormal isoenzyme pattern in diseased muscle resembles that of normal fetal muscle, a situation parallel to that in the case of total enzyme activities, mentioned above. The abnormal pattern has been observed at a very early stage in Duchenne muscular dystrophy, and Kowalewski & Rotthauwe (1972) could find no correlation between the extent of the change and histological or clinical features. It is possible that, in many instances, the normal mature pattern is never attained. A decreased proportion of LDH5 was reported also in muscle of some female carriers of Duchenne dystrophy (Emery 1964), although Kowaleski & Rotthauwe (1972) could find no abnormalities in their series of carriers.

A similar phenomenon is seen in the case of creatine kinase (Goto et al 1969, Tzvetanova 1971). The 'BB' isoenzyme (found also in brain) is predominant in the early stages of muscle development; at a later stage the 'MB' (hybrid) form is much in evidence. Adult muscle contains largely the 'MM' type, sometimes with a small proportion of 'MB'. In some, but not all, muscles from a variety of muscle disorders, an increased proportion of 'MB' and the presence of 'BB' has been detected by these workers and by Cao et al (1971). Franklin et al (1981) found that cultured muscle cells from primary myopathies but not neurogenic muscle disorders had a greater proportion of 'BB' as well as a reduction in total CK. This was reported also for Duchenne muscular dystrophy by Ionasescu et al (1981). It is not clear how this finding is related to the change in isoenzyme pattern found in the adult muscle.

Adenylate kinase is an enzyme which alters the

level of adenine nucleotides and which, because of this, is considered to have a role in the control of glycolysis. The enzyme in Duchenne muscle is only partly inactivated by Ellman's reagent which, in normal muscle, blocks its activity completely (Schirmer & Thuma 1972). It is not clear whether this is attributable to a change in isoenzyme pattern or to modification of the enzyme protein.

Fat metabolism. Relatively little attention has been paid to fat metabolism in muscular dystrophy, but Lin et al (1972) found that the oxidation of palmitate by skeletal muscle mitochondria was markedly reduced in cases of Duchenne dystrophy where the inheritance of the disease was established but, surprisingly, not in isolated cases. They also found a low activity in female carriers. In a recent paper (Lin et al 1976) these workers have shown that a similar abnormality found in dystrophic mouse muscle is not due to a deficiency of palmityl-CoA synthetase (EC 6.2.1.3). More recently Carrol et al (1985) have reported that the oxidation of [U-^{14}C] palmitic acid but not [1-^{14}C]palmitic acid by muscle homogenates was decreased in Duchenne dystrophy. It was suggested that this is due to a defect in an isoenzyme of one of the enzymes of β-oxidation, acting specifically on shorter-chain acyl-CoAs.

The oxidation of fatty acids in muscle requires carnitine for their transfer across the mitochondrial membrane, and a specific deficiency of this compound is now well recognised (see Ch. 25). In many muscle diseases, in particular Duchenne dystrophy, there appears to be a non-specific lowering of muscle carnitine (Borum et al 1977). Berthillier et al (1982) found that this was particularly marked in the early stages of Duchenne dystrophy; palmitoyl-carnitine transferase (EC 2.3.1.21) activity was increased, however.

Oxidative phosphorylation. Mitochondria isolated from Duchenne muscle appear to have a normal ability to carry out oxidative phosphorylation, unless the disease is far advanced (Olson et al 1968, Peter 1971).

In dystrophic hamsters there is a defect in oxidative phosphorylation which appears to be due to an abnormal accumulation of calcium in the mitochondria (see below).

Pentose phosphate pathway. In human dystrophic muscle there is increased activity of glucose 6-phosphate dehydrogenase (EC 1.1.1.49) and 6-phosphogluconate dehydrogenase (EC 1.1.1.44), the first two enzymes of the pentose phosphate pathway of glucose utilisation. This is, however, a non-specific phenomenon, being seen in various types of experimental muscle damage (reviewed by Wagner et al 1978). Various factors may be responsible for these changes. There is a relatively high level of these enzymes in connective tissue and in macrophages, and Wagner et al (1978) demonstrated a high activity in regenerating muscle fibres. It appears likely that one function of this pathway is the provision of pentoses for nucleic acid synthesis.

Both enzymes transfer electrons between their substrate and NADP, and it is of interest that two other NADP-linked enzymes, isocitrate dehydrogenase (EC 1.1.1.42) and glutathione reductase (EC 1.6.4.2), also increase in dystrophic muscle (McCaman 1960, Heyck et al 1963).

Miscellaneous. Following earlier studies suggesting that there was a deficiency of coenzyme Q in dystrophic muscle, Folkers et al (1974) have reported that treatment with coenzyme Q reduced serum creatine kinase activity in two boys with preclinical Duchenne dystrophy. Coenzyme Q is involved in the electron transport chain in oxidation by mitochondria.

Ellis et al (1973) found that biopsy specimens of Duchenne muscle converted [^{14}C]glucose into fructose to a greater extent than normal muscle. The abnormality was noted also in muscle from genetic carriers of the disease. The same group (West et al 1977) have reported that Duchenne muscle also converted more of the glucose into neutral lipid. Nevertheless, the possible contribution to these results of other cell types, particularly fat cells, must be considered.

Any general inadequacy of the energy supply to the muscles would be expected to be reflected in the levels of high-energy phosphate carriers, ATP and creatine phosphate, in the muscles. Samaha et al (1981) reported that these were normal, when related to myosin as reference base, in Duchenne muscle. Others, e.g. Bertorini et al (1985), have found low levels of adenine nucleotides when related to non-collagen nitrogen. According to

Edwards (1984) a decrease in the phosphocreatine/Pi ratio can be demonstrated by topical magnetic resonance. Because of the lack of an ideal reference base, any changes in the levels of the energy carriers inside the muscle fibres of resting muscle in Duchenne dystrophy remain unknown.

Interference with transfer of energy to specific functions or structures, particularly the cell membranes, can be considered. Feit et al (1983) could find no abnormality in the creatine kinase associated with the M line of the myofibrils in Duchenne muscular dystrophy. This bound enzyme is considered, in the 'phosphocreatine shuttle' hypothesis, to be involved in the transfer of phosphate bond energy to the myofibrils. A similar shuttle may be involved in supplying energy to the sarcolemma. Lane et al (1986) have found that creatine kinase activity is closely associated with human muscle sarcolemma, although this has yet to be studied in dystrophic muscle.

Myotonic dystrophy. It has been recognised for many years that patients with myotonic dystrophy commonly display an excessive pancreatic insulin secretory response to glucose or to other agents. On the other hand, a degree of glucose intolerance has also been widely reported. Poffenbarger et al (1976) obtained evidence against the secretion of a biologically inactive form of insulin in this disease, and their studies showed a balanced secretion of insulin and proinsulin. Karpati (1985) has reviewed the abnormal insulin status in myotonic dystrophy and concludes that there is probably a reduced affinity of insulin receptors, possibly resulting from an abnormality in the physico-chemical microdomain of the plasma membranes.

Protein metabolism

In healthy muscle fibres, as in most animal cells, the proteins, which are the main constituents of the fibres, are in a dynamic state, being continually broken down and resynthesised. The rate at which this occurs has been the subject of a great deal of research using mainly isotopic labelling techniques. Recent studies on man (McKeran et al 1978) gave a myofibril protein catabolic rate of 2.16% or 1.47% per day, depending upon the procedure used. There is good evidence that the individual muscle proteins turn over at different rates. The way in which protein degradation and synthesis are normally integrated to maintain a steady level of protein is still not known. Protein loss in disease could obviously result from either impairment of its synthesis or increased degradation. Meaningful study of protein synthesis in human muscular dystrophy is difficult and the picture is not clear. In a series of reports, Ionasescu and colleagues (see Ionasescu 1975) have studied protein synthesis by ribosomes isolated from muscle affected by various kinds of muscular dystrophy and also from genetic carriers of Duchenne dystrophy. Increased, rather than decreased, activity was generally observed, apparently not always attributable to an increase in the synthesis of collagen. These findings have not been confirmed as yet. Autoradiographic studies by Monckton & Marusyk (1979) showed increased uptake of [3H]leucine apparently associated with regenerating fibres.

More recently, studies on the in vivo incorporation of ^{13}C-labelled leucine into muscle proteins of Duchenne patients have been taken to demonstrate a decrease in protein synthesis in both Duchenne dystrophy (Rennie et al 1982) and myotonic dystrophy (Halliday et al 1985). Such studies, however, must be interpreted with caution in the absence of data on the specific radioactivity of the immediate precursor of protein synthesis, aminoacyl-t-RNA.

Actin in all muscle fibres and myosin in white fibres contain 3-methylhistidine, formed by methylation of histidine residues in the peptide chains. When these proteins are broken down in the cell, the released 3-methylhistidine is not re-utilised but is quantitatively excreted. The urinary ratio of 3-methylhistidine to creatinine (the latter is taken as a measure of total muscle mass) reflects the rate of myofibril protein breakdown. Several workers have reported that this ratio is increased in Duchenne muscular dystrophy. However, the significance of this is debatable when the contribution of urinary 3-methylhistidine from tissues other than muscle, which becomes relatively more important when the muscles are wasted, is taken into account. In neurogenic diseases, however, the computed rate of breakdown was increased, even when this factor was allowed for (Rothig et al 1984). The 3-methylhistidine/creatinine ratio was found to be normal in myotonic dystrophy (Griggs et al 1980).

Some indirect evidence for an accelerated rate of muscle protein breakdown in Duchenne dystrophy was provided by the observation of an increased turnover of alanine relative to muscle mass (Haymond et al 1978).

An in vitro technique for studying protein turnover in pieces of biopsied human muscle was described by Lundholm et al (1976) and was used by them to show a decreased protein synthesis and increased protein breakdown in muscle from cancer patients.

Further work is still required to establish with certainty the relative roles of changes in protein synthesis and breakdown in the various muscle-wasting conditions and possible variation with the phase of the disease. The extent to which such changes may be a result of the presence of regenerating fibres must also be considered.

Human growth hormone was shown by metabolic balance studies to provoke a protein catabolic effect in boys with Duchenne dystrophy, in contrast with its normal anabolic action (Chyatte et al 1973).

Muscle proteinases. The enzymic apparatus for the breakdown of muscle protein, and the factors which control its activity, are still not clear. A number of enzymes (peptide hydrolases) which attack proteins and smaller peptides have been identified in skeletal muscle (see Pennington 1977a), but little is yet known about their participation in protein breakdown in normal and pathological states. The lysosomal cathepsins have already been mentioned, but because of their restricted intracellular distribution and low pH optimum it seems unlikely that these are responsible for the initial attack on muscle proteins, although Schwartz & Bird (1977) have reported that cathepsins B and D are able to degrade myosin and actin. A serine proteinase studied by Katunuma and co-workers shows increased activity in Duchenne muscle (Katunuma et al 1978); it seems likely, however, that this enzyme may be mast cell chymase (EC 3.4.21.39), located in mast cells in the muscle (Park et al 1973). Two

calcium-activated proteinases (EC 3.4.22.17) with different calcium sensitivities, both present in muscle, have been intensively investigated during the past few years (e.g. Penny et al 1985). It was shown by Sugita & Toyokura (1976) that troponin I and troponin C were attacked more readily than troponin T by one of these. They showed also that, in Duchenne muscle, the amounts of troponins I and C decrease more than troponin T, and suggested that the two findings may be related. Kar & Pearson (1976b) have reported that there is increased activity of calcium-activated neutral proteinase in homogenates of muscle from patients with Duchenne and Becker dystrophies, but not in muscle from patients with limb-girdle dystrophy or denervating diseases. A current, widely accepted theory is that calcium-requiring proteinases may become activated in diseased muscle by influx of calcium ions from the extracellular space resulting from a damaged or defective sarcolemma. The enzymes would be expected to have little or no activity in healthy fibres because of their low calcium concentration. Another muscle proteinase with unusually high molecular weight has been discovered recently (Hardy et al 1983).

Increased alkaline proteinase activity in Duchenne muscle was observed by Pennington & Robinson (1968). Another enzyme, dipeptidyl peptidase IV (EC 3.4.14.5), was found to increase sharply in many muscle-wasting conditions (Kar & Pearson 1978): on the other hand, arylamidase and dipeptidyl peptidase III (EC 3.4.14.4), two other peptide hydrolases believed not to be associated with lysosomes, were not significantly altered (Kar & Pearson 1976a, 1978). Proline endopeptidase (EC 3.4.21.26), a proteinase which is particularly abundant in muscle, is also elevated in the muscular dystrophies (Kar & Pearson 1981b).

Animal myopathies. Quite extensive studies have been carried out on muscle protein metabolism in the animal myopathies, especially that seen in the mouse. Although earlier studies pointed to an increased rate of muscle protein synthesis in the dystrophic mouse, Kitchin & Watts (1973) have claimed that there is no difference in the incorporation of labelled amino acid when correction is made for the size of the amino-acid pool; some differences were seen in the case of individual proteins, however. A few studies on protein synthesis with isolated ribosomes have been carried out but have shown no clear picture. There is an increase in alkaline proteinase activity in muscles in the dystrophic mouse (Pennington 1963).

The finding (Stracher et al 1978) that injection of the proteinase inhibitors leupeptin and pepstatin will delay muscle degeneration in dystrophic chickens is of considerable interest. Pepstatin has also been shown to have a beneficial effect in muscular dystrophy in the mouse (Schorr et al 1978). Pepstatin is an inhibitor of cathepsin D, whereas leupeptin inhibits both cathepsin B and the calcium-activated muscle proteinase. The compounds appear to have low toxicity and may be suitable for therapeutic tests in human muscular dystrophy; in addition, they may be used to elucidate the mechanism of protein degradation in diseased muscle.

Contractile proteins

Vignos & Lefkowitz (1959) showed a decrease, relative to non-collagen nitrogen, in the amount of the main contractile protein, myosin, in dystrophic muscle; the change was more marked in adult patients than in the childhood form of muscular dystrophy. Evidence for a change in some of the properties of myosin and associated proteins in Duchenne dystrophy was brought forward by Furukawa & Peter (1971, 1972). Duchenne myosin showed a low ATPase activity and a markedly delayed superprecipitation, presumably related to the low ATPase. The trypsin-sensitive calcium-binding ability of the actomyosin (a property of the troponin component) was less than normal; this was not so in some other muscle diseases studied. On the other hand, Penn et al (1972), using immunodiffusion analysis and agarose electrophoresis, could find no abnormality in myosin in Duchenne or other forms of muscular dystrophy, while Samaha & Thies (1979) have reported that the types and relative proportions of the myosin light chains were unaltered. A number of workers have examined the properties of myosin in animal myopathies but there is as yet no general agreement on how it differs from normal. Smoller & Fineberg (1965) reported that there were extensive differences in composition of myosin from normal and dystrophic mice; however, Oppenheimer et al (1964) found no difference in its behaviour in the ultracentrifuge and it also showed a similar ATPase activity and an ability to combine with actin. Morey et al (1967) were unable to find any difference between myosin from normal and dystrophic chick muscle. It does not seem at all likely, in any event, that the primary defect in human muscular dystrophy is in the contractile system; as is now well recognised, detectable muscle weakness occurs only when the histopathological changes are well established.

Membranes

Sarcolemma. The long-established phenomenon of the leakage of muscle enzymes into the blood in the muscular dystrophies, particularly in Duchenne dystrophy, has commonly been associated with the idea that there is a defect in the structure of the sarcolemma, although opinion varies on whether this is a primary or a secondary change (see Rowland 1976). Biochemical investigation of the sarcolemma is not easy because of the difficulty of isolating it in pure form, as well as the low yield, which necessitates the use of relatively large quantities of muscle. Numerous procedures for preparing sarcolemma from animal muscles have been described.

Peter & Fiehn (1972) found that isolated sarcolemma from patients with myotonic dystrophy had a higher content of unsaturated fatty acids in the phospholipids than normal; a decrease in cholesterol content was also observed. The possible effect of diet upon the fatty acid composition of muscle phospholipids (Alling et al 1974) must be borne in mind, however. Peter et al (1974), on the other hand, reported that there were no significant abnormalities in the proportions of the various sarcolemmal phospholipids in Duchenne or myotonic dystrophy. Fischbeck et al (1983), however, using freeze-fracture study of cholesterol–digitonin complexes, have found increased cholesterol in Duchenne sarcolemma, which they suggest may lead to increased fragility of the membrane. A drastically reduced level of glycerophosphocholine, a derivative of lecithin, in Duchenne muscle has been reported by Chalovich et al (1979). This compound is produced from lysolecithin by lysolecithin phospholipase (EC 3.1.1.5). Further work (Schliselfeld et al 1981) has indicated that there may be a decreased affinity of this enzyme for lysolecithin. These findings accord with a previous report of an increase in lysolecithin, a lytic agent, in Duchenne muscle.

Kunze et al (1980) were unable to detect any differences in the activity of enzymes involved in the synthesis and breakdown of lecithin in Duchenne muscle. Peter et al (1974) found no differences in any of the sarcolemmal ATPase activities; on the other hand, Dhalla et al (1973), using a different procedure for isolation of the sarcolemma, found a lower Na^+,K^+-ATPase (EC 3.6.1.37) and higher Ca^{++}- and Mg^{++}-ATPases in Duchenne dystrophy. It is of particular interest that Niebroj-Dobosz (1981) has reported that the Na^+,K^+-ATPase of Duchenne sarcolemma is stimulated by ouabain, in contrast to the usual inhibition, as this has been found also with erythrocytes (see below).

A careful study by Cerri et al (1981) confirmed earlier observations by a number of workers that the membrane-associated enzyme, adenyl cyclase (EC 4.6.1.1), shows an abnormally low response to catecholamines in Duchenne muscle. This could conceivably be a result of a difference in membrane structure. A similar abnormality had previously been observed also in cultured muscle cells from patients with Duchenne dystrophy (Mawatari et al 1976). The level of cyclic AMP in Duchenne muscle has been reported to be normal (Kito et al 1979).

A specific decrease in cyclic nucleotide phosphodiesterase (EC 3.1.4.16) in Duchenne muscle has been observed by Canal et al (1975). The enzyme 5'-nucleotidase (EC 3.1.3.5) increases in many muscle diseases and the increase can be seen at an early stage in Duchenne dystrophy (Kar & Pearson 1973c). Although earlier histochemical studies pointed to an endomysial location for this enzyme, it has been shown in several studies to be associated with isolated plasma membranes, including the sarcolemma, and appears to be located on the outer surface of the sarcolemma (Woo & Manery 1975).

Evidence for altered membrane properties in muscular dystrophy comes from enzyme leakage studies (see below) and also from a decreased ability to retain injected ^{137}Cs and ^{83}Rb (Lloyd et al 1973); the latter was characteristic of all the muscle diseases studied but was not seen in genetic carriers of Duchenne dystrophy. A decrease in potassium content and an increase in sodium is a well-recognised characteristic of diseased muscle, although recent studies (Edmonds et al 1985) have led to the conclusion that there is little or no substitution of potassium by sodium in the muscle fibres in Duchenne dystrophy. In Duchenne dystrophy, at least, any change is not attributable to increased aldosterone or other causes of renal wastage of potassium, because urinary excretion of sodium, potassium and aldosterone was found not to differ significantly from normal (Garst et al 1977).

Electron-microscopic studies on the sarcolemma in diseased muscle should be mentioned here. Mokri & Engel (1975) and Schmalbruch (1975) demonstrated focal lesions in the plasma membrane of the sarcolemma in Duchenne muscular dystrophy; the latter worker observed similar, although less prominent, changes in other muscle diseases. A more general type of change has been reported by Schotland et al (1977). These workers, using freeze-fracture studies, observed a depletion of particles on both sides of the muscle plasma membrane in Duchenne muscle; such particles are considered to be integral protein components of the membrane. The decrease does not appear preferentially to involve particles of one particular size, thus implying the loss of more than one protein (Fischbeck et al 1984). In myotonic dystrophy, however, an increase in the number of particles was observed (Schotland & Bonilla 1977).

A few studies have been carried out on isolated sarcolemma in animal myopathies. De Kretser & Livett (1977) found changes in its lipid composition in the dystrophic mouse, in particular a fourfold decrease in the relative amount of free cholesterol. However, the sarcolemmal enzymes which they measured were unchanged. Sarcolemma from dystrophic chickens has been reported to show elevated adenylate cyclase (Rodan et al 1974) and increased microviscosity (Sha'afi et al 1975); similar alterations were seen in plasma membranes from liver and erythrocytes.

Recently some groups have undertaken histochemical studies with labelled lectins or antibodies to look for glycoprotein abnormalities on the surface membrane and some differences have been found in diseased muscle (see Ch. 7).

Sarcoplasmic reticulum. An important function of the sarcoplasmic reticulum membrane system in muscle is the re-uptake of calcium following muscle contraction, thus inducing relaxation. Studies showing a decreased ability of Duchenne sarcoplasmic reticulum to take up calcium were reviewed by Peter (1971), who showed also that the affinity for calcium — possibly a more meaningful criterion — was also reduced in Duchenne dystrophy and polymyositis.

Subsequent study of the biochemistry of the sarcoplasmic reticulum in human muscle disease appears to have been sparse until a report by Samaha & Congedo (1977) that, in Duchenne dystrophy, the proteins of the sarcoplasmic reticulum display an abnormal pattern on acrylamide gel electrophoresis. Moreover, the abnormal pattern fell into two types and these workers therefore suggested that Duchenne dystrophy may comprise two biochemically distinct diseases. This study must be interpreted cautiously, however, as the increased proteinase activity in dystrophic muscle may influence the results (Nagy & Samaha 1984).

There appears to be a difference between the effect of muscular dystrophy upon calcium uptake by isolated sarcoplasmic reticulum in the mouse and hamster on the one hand and in the chicken on the other. In the first two animals there is a decrease (Martinosi 1968, Dhalla et al 1975) which is not seen in the chicken (Sylvester & Baskin 1973).

Muscle and calcium

The suggestion that there may be an influx of calcium into diseased muscle from the extracellular space was mentioned earlier, in connection with the calcium-activated proteinase. Bodensteiner & Engel (1978) have supported this possibility by histochemical demonstration of calcium in non-necrotic fibres in diseased muscle; this occurred more frequently in Duchenne dystrophy than in other muscle diseases. Increased numbers of calcium-positive fibres have been reported to occur in a dystrophic fetus (Brambati et al 1980). Wrogemann and his colleagues (see Wrogemann & Nylen 1978) showed that in the muscle of dystrophic hamsters there is an accumulation of calcium in mitochondria at an early stage of the disease. This caused, among other things, a defect in oxidative phosphorylation and could thus contribute to the death of the fibres.

Emery et al (1982) tested the effects of administering verapamil for a year to Duchenne patients and considered the results sufficiently encouraging to undertake trials of other calcium-blocking agents.

A subnormal level of 24, 25-dihydroxyvitamin D in serum in Duchenne patients has recently been reported (Shapira et al 1984) and it was suggested that this might be related to a disturbance in calcium transport in the cells.

Miscellaneous findings

Kar & Pearson, in a long series of studies, have measured the activity (related to non-collagen protein) of several enzymes in muscle biopsy samples obtained from various muscle diseases at different stages. Acyl phosphatase (EC 3.6.1.7), the cellular function of which is not clear, was decreased only in advanced cases of various muscle diseases (Kar & Pearson 1972d). Cholinesterase (EC 3.1.1.7) was increased in Duchenne dystrophy but not in other muscle diseases, whereas β-naphthyl acetate esterase was normal in all cases (Kar & Pearson 1973d). Monoamine oxidase (EC 1.4.3.4) was also normal (Kar & Pearson 1974); thus the reported increase in catecholamines or related compounds in Duchenne muscle (Wright et al 1973) does not appear to be a consequence of reduced activity of this enzyme. Glyoxalase I (EC 4.4.1.5) activity was decreased in Duchenne and limb-girdle dystrophies only, and glyoxalase II (EC 4.4.1.6) was unaltered;

phosphodiesterases I (EC 3.1.4.1) and II showed a non-specific increase which was more marked in advanced cases; lipase (EC 3.1.1.3) was increased in Duchenne dystrophy only (Kar & Pearson 1975a,b,c).

Human muscle contains ribonucleases active at high pH, as well as acid (presumably lysosomal) ribonucleases, and both are markedly increased in Duchenne dystrophy (Abdullah & Pennington 1968).

The similarity in symptoms between the genetic muscular dystrophies and nutritional muscular dystrophy has frequently led to speculation that the former, like the latter, may involve damage by lipid peroxidation. Omaye & Tappel (1974) found increased thiobarbituric acid-reactive products (an index of lipid peroxidation) in muscles of genetically dystrophic mice and chickens. These workers also found increased glutathione peroxidase (EC 1.11.1.9) and glutathione reductase activities, while Bell & Draper (1976) observed an increase in glutathione and glutathione peroxidase in dystrophic mouse muscle; this suggests a possible adaptive increase in the protective mechanism against lipid peroxidation. Increased thiobarbituric acid-reactive products in muscle in the major forms of human muscular dystrophy were found by Kar & Pearson (1979). Increased activity of glutathione reductase and catalase (EC 1.11.1.6.), both of which may exert a protective action, was also found but the enzyme superoxide dismutase, which inhibits lipid peroxidation, was normal. The authors cite the known disruptive effect of lipid peroxidation upon lysosomal membranes as a possible factor in the aetiology of the dystrophies. Superoxide dismutase (EC 1.15.1.1), however, was found to be ineffective in the treatment of Duchenne dystrophy (Stern et al 1982). The postulated effectiveness of penicillamine (a sulphydryl compound) in improving the condition of genetically dystrophic chickens (Chou et al 1975) could result from its protection of lipids or possibly of protein sulphydryl groups.

With regard to muscle constituents other than enzymes, many workers have attempted to characterise the myoglobin in dystrophic muscle. This haem protein functions as an oxygen carrier in muscle. The existence of many genetic variations in haemoglobin popularised the idea that a genetic abnormality in myoglobin might underlie muscular dystrophy. Variable results were obtained, however, in investigations of myoglobin in diseased muscle; these were critically reviewed by Romero-Herrera et al (1973), who discussed possible artefacts in these studies which might account for the reported changes. The latter workers found no abnormalities in tryptic peptides or amino acids in myoglobin from a case of Duchenne muscular dystrophy and one of distal type muscular dystrophy.

The possibility that an abnormality in collagen production may be a causative factor in muscular dystrophy has often been considered. Duance et al (1980) observed that collagen types III and IV could be found within the splits of the muscle fibres in Duchenne and limb-girdle dystrophy and suggest that this may play a part in the dystrophic process. Ionasescu & Ionasescu (1982) have reported that Duchenne myogenic clones show a largely increased extracellular production of collagen, measured by the incorporation of hydroxyproline. As collagen production by fibroblasts also appears to be increased in Duchenne dystrophy (see below) it seems possible that both types of cell contribute to the lesions, if these findings are valid.

Kremzner et al (1978) have noted differences in the concentration of certain polyamines (putrescine, spermidine and spermine) in muscle, in human muscle diseases and in the dystrophic mouse, although the implication of these changes is not clear. The excretion of these compounds is also increased (Russell & Stern 1981).

SERUM ENZYMES

Much attention has been paid to the changes in the activities of certain enzymes in the blood of patients with muscle diseases, and such changes are undoubtedly the most useful contribution to biochemical diagnosis. It would be impossible to catalogue all the individual reports here, but the main findings are outlined.

Creatine kinase

Many of the earlier studies concerned measurement of serum aldolase, but it is now generally acknowledged that increase in the enzyme creatine kinase is the most sensitive index of muscle disease. Furthermore, an increased concentration of this enzyme is rather more specific than that of most enzymes for muscle disease and, in addition, because erythrocytes contain very little creatine kinase, assays in serum are not vitiated by haemolysis of the sample — an important practical point. Creatine kinase transfers a phosphate group from creatine phosphate to ADP forming creatine and ATP. The rate of ATP and creatine formation is usually determined either by colorimetric measurement of creatine or, more commonly, by measuring ATP by means of a coupled enzyme reaction resulting in the reduction of a pyridine nucleotide, which is measured by a change in ultraviolet absorbance. Comparison of the two methods is discussed by Tippett et al (1982). Reagent kits for the coupled enzyme procedure are obtainable from numerous commercial sources, with many variations in detail. Consequently, it is usually necessary for each laboratory to establish its own range of normal serum creatine kinase activities.

It has been found empirically that the logarithms of serum creatine kinase values in healthy subjects show an approximately normal distribution and the confidence limits for the normal range can be determined simply by making use of this. In our laboratory, however, the distribution, even of the logarithms of the normal values, is slightly skewed; we prefer, therefore, to deduce the normal range from a cumulative frequency curve plotted on logarithmic paper. With this procedure, 97.5% of all values for adult women do not exceed 60 units (μmol/min, measured at 37°C) per litre. It is generally accepted (e.g. Munsat et al 1973) that men have a higher mean level than women, presumably because of the relatively greater muscle mass of the men. Factors, other than disease, which may affect serum creatine kinase levels, are discussed below.

The most striking increases in serum creatine kinase concentration occur in Duchenne-type dystrophy; values of up to several hundred times normal are common in early cases. As in the case of aldolase, the levels decline markedly as the disease progresses (Pearce et al 1964a). There is a particularly sharp fall around the age of 10 years, probably because the patient starts to use a wheel-chair at that age (Thomson et al 1974). In adult dystrophies and myotonic dystrophy there is usually an increased level although not as high as is seen in the Duchenne type. Variable results are obtained in polymyositis; occasionally, extremely high values are found and the serum activity of this enzyme is normally raised in untreated cases. Representative data are given by Pearce et al (1964a). Increased values in the overtly neurogenic muscle diseases appear to be more common than was once supposed (Koufen & Consbruch 1970, Williams & Bruford 1970). The author and his colleagues have recorded many raised values in cases of spinal muscular atrophy. Further information is given by Pennington (1977b).

The syndrome of malignant hyperpyrexia occurring under anaesthesia is associated with a myopathy, and some affected individuals and their relatives are known to have raised serum creatine kinase levels. However, there does not appear to be a good correlation between susceptibility to the condition and increased creatine kinase activity (Ellis et al 1975).

An important aspect of the use of serum enzymes in the detection of Duchenne muscular dystrophy is that a substantial rise may occur long before clinical symptoms are evident. The time course of such early changes in several serum enzymes was followed closely by Heyck et al (1966). In the brother of a patient with Duchenne dystrophy they found increased activities directly after birth, peak values at 14–22 months and, subsequently, a slow decline. At 28 months there were still no clinical signs of muscular dystrophy, although the disease had been confirmed by biopsy. Such early detection can be useful in establishing the mother as a genetic carrier, apart from facilitating the study of the disease at an early stage. Population screening by rapid creatine kinase tests on dried blood samples has been initiated at some centres.

The time course of the elevations in fetal serum enzymes in Duchenne dystrophy is not established. Measurement at 16–18 weeks' gestation by a number of groups for possible prenatal diagnosis has shown, at most, only slight rises. The possibility cannot be excluded that a large increase takes place at birth, when the maternal influence is lost.

Genetic carriers. In many hereditary diseases it has long been recognised that clinically normal carriers of the abnormal gene may show, to a minor degree, biochemical abnormalities characteristic of the disease. Many of the mothers who transmit the gene for Duchenne-type dystrophy have some increase in serum enzyme activities. Measurable differences are seen most commonly in the case of serum creatine kinase. Findings at many centres suggest that about two-thirds of all carriers have a serum creatine kinase above the normal range. The difference is often small; thus Pearce et al (1964b) found that about one-half of the raised values were less than twice the upper limit of the normal range. It is, therefore, necessary to take account of factors which influence serum creatine kinase levels in normal individuals, in order to derive the maximum value from the test. Many workers have recorded changes with age, the most recent being Lane & Roses (1981) and Livingstone et al (1982), in which earlier studies are reviewed. It is generally agreed that levels are higher in younger girls. Meltzer (1971) also noted an effect of race; the mean level in Negroes was higher than that in Caucasians. Early pregnancy is associated with a lowering of serum creatine kinase (Blyth & Hughes 1971, King et al 1972). There is, however, some disagreement about the effect of contraceptive pills (Simpson et al 1974). Numerous studies have shown that physical exercise, if sufficiently severe and prolonged, can cause marked increases in serum enzyme activities and should therefore be avoided for at least one day before the test.

There is good evidence (Nicholson et al 1979) that a higher carrier detection rate can be achieved by measuring creatine kinase early in life. Percy et al (1982) also found a seasonal variation in the efficiency of detection, this being highest in November.

A few carriers display very high serum creatine kinase activities, up to about one hundred times the normal upper limit. These differences among carriers have not, so far, been consistently related to any other features such as the degree of histopathological or electrophysiological changes, and the underlying basis of this wide variation is not clear. It is generally considered that the pathological changes in carriers can be explained by the inactivation in each muscle cell nucleus of either the paternal (normal) or maternal (abnormal) X chromosome, according to the Lyon hypothesis. This is complicated by the multinucleate nature of the muscle fibres; it seems reasonable to assume that the degree of abnormality will be related to the proportion of abnormal X chromosomes in the fibre, although the effective range of action of each individual nucleus is unknown.

Other enzymes

Apart from creatine kinase, many other enzymes appear in increased amounts in the blood in muscular dystrophy although, in most cases, the relative rise is less. Aldolase, aspartate and alanine aminotransferases, and lactate dehydrogenase received early study. In addition, glucose phosphate isomerase (EC 5.3.1.9) (Dreyfus et al 1958) phosphoglucomutase (Berni et al 1961), α-hydroxybutyrate dehydrogenase (EC 1.1.1.30) (Cutillo et al 1962) and malate dehydrogenase (EC 1.1.1.37) (Chowdhury et al 1962) increase; a rise in malate dehydrogenase was found only in childhood dystrophy. Carbonic anhydrase III (EC 4.2.1.1), a muscle-specific isoenzyme of carbonic anhydrase, is markedly elevated in Duchenne dystrophy (Carter et al 1983). On the other hand, β-acetylglucosaminidase and arylsulphatase A, both lysosomal enzymes, were raised in some patients with active polymyositis or dermatomyositis and certain other inflammatory diseases, but not in the muscular dystrophies (Kar & Pearson 1972e). Negative results have been reported for cholinesterase, 5′-nucleotidase, adenosine triphosphatase, isocitrate dehydrogenase, acid and alkaline (EC 3.1.3.1) phosphatases and γ-glutamyl transpeptidase (EC 2.3.2.2).

Serum pyruvate kinase is elevated in Duchenne muscular dystrophy and some carriers. Some but not all laboratories (some using discriminant analysis) have found this enzyme to be a useful adjunct to creatine kinase in carrier detection (see Muir et al 1983). Zatz et al (1978) found that pyruvate kinase activities were raised much more frequently than were those of creatine kinase in facioscapulohumeral muscular dystrophy.

This is an appropriate place to mention studies

on serum myoglobin. With the advent of a sensitive radioimmunoassay, several workers have been able to show increased levels of serum myoglobin in patients with muscle disease and in carriers of Duchenne dystrophy. Whereas some (Kagen et al 1980, Nicholson 1981) have found it to be a valuable new tool in carrier detection, others (Edwards et al 1984, Percy et al 1984) have found it to have little or no advantage when used in addition to creatine kinase.

Isoenzymes

Several studies have shown that the increase in serum lactate dehydrogenase activity in muscular dystrophy is due mainly to an increase in the more negatively charged components (LDH 1–3). This reflects the change in the isoenzyme composition of dystrophic muscle, mentioned above (Yasmineh et al 1978). In the last few years more attention has been given to isoenzymes of creatine kinase in the serum. There is general agreement (see Takahashi et al 1977) that, in the majority of cases of Duchenne dystrophy, the MB isoenzyme can be detected; this isoenzyme is rarely seen in normal serum. In other neuromuscular diseases MB is commonly found, but less frequently than in Duchenne dystrophy. Cardiac muscle normally contains the MB isoenzyme, but its presence in serum in Duchenne dystrophy does not appear to be related to cardiac involvement in the disease (Silverman et al 1976) and presumably reflects the changed isoenzyme pattern of the muscle.

Hamada et al (1981) have reported the presence of an unusual isoenzyme of adenylate kinase in Duchenne serum; it may be a fetal type of isoenzyme.

Leakage of enzymes from muscle fibres

There can be little doubt that the increased amounts of the above-mentioned enzymes appearing in the blood originate largely or wholly in the muscle tissue itself, leaking out of the fibres as the latter are affected by the disease. The enzymes concerned are known to be present in high concentration in muscle. Creatine kinase, which shows a particularly sharp rise, is present in higher concentration in skeletal muscle than in

other tissues; in fact, there is relatively little in many tissues including liver and kidney. That the serum aldolase in muscular dystrophy originates in the muscle accords with the observation of the Paris workers (Dreyfus et al 1958) that the serum enzyme has no activity on fructose-1-phosphate; e.g. the liver enzyme has high activity towards this compound as well as towards fructose 1,6-diphosphate. The fact that higher enzyme levels are seen in the earlier stages of the disease is understandable because, in this phase, there will be large numbers of fibres which are involved but still rich in enzymes.

When considering the significance of the enzyme leakage from diseased muscle, we find it useful to have some idea of the rate at which this occurs, in relation to the amount of enzyme in the muscle. A rough estimate may be made, although this involves some uncertainties, especially in the rate of clearance from the blood. Bär & Ohlendorf (1970) estimated the clearance rate from the rate of fall in the concentration of plasma enzymes following their rapid release into the blood after, e.g., a myocardial infarction. In the case of creatine kinase they concluded that about 5% of the plasma enzyme was lost per hour. However, a more recent estimate of the clearance of injected creatine kinase in the dog (Rapaport 1975) gave a rate which was about one order greater than this. As the creatine kinase concentration in human muscle is about 500 IU/g it can be readily deduced, using the former estimate, that even in a patient with very high serum creatine kinase activity (10 000 IU/l) less than 1% of the total creatine kinase in the muscle must leak out per day.

Reasons for enzyme leakage

It is not yet possible to give an adequate explanation for the release of intracellular constituents from diseased muscles. Most of the enzymes detected in increased amounts in the blood in muscle disease are major 'soluble' (sarcoplasmic) enzymes in muscle, although the mitochondrial form of aspartate aminotransferase is also found (Matsuda et al 1978). There are a number of possible factors involved in the release, but their relative importance cannot be stated with certainty.

Clearly, enzymes and other constituents may be lost from necrotic fibres, but this is not generally considered to be the whole explanation, because high serum enzyme activities in very early stages of Duchenne dystrophy and in some genetic carriers of this disease may not be paralleled by a prominent degree of necrosis. The reported focal rupture of the sarcolemma, mentioned above, may be important; its contribution to the leakage process can better be judged when it has been studied in the very early stages of Duchenne dystrophy.

An alternative possibility, that there is a general change in the structure of the sarcolemma at the molecular level, is widely held to account for the leakage. Such a mechanism might be expected to lead to a more selective passage of cell constituents, and it does appear that the leakage is a selective process. Thus, in Duchenne dystrophy the level of serum creatine kinase activity may be of the order of 100 times that of aldolase, whereas the activities of these enzymes in muscle are of the same order, and the blood clearance rates appear to be similar (Bär & Ohlendorf 1970). Two of the major muscle enzymes, phosphofructokinase (EC 2.7.1.11; Rowland et al 1968) and AMP deaminase (R. J. Pennington, unpublished work) could not be detected in serum in Duchenne dystrophy. As would be expected, molecular size appears to play some part in the selectivity. The molecular weight of aldolase (150 000) is greater than that of creatine kinase (81 000), while that of phosphofructokinase is very high (400 000). On the other hand, Husic & Suelter (1980, 1983) have emphasised the importance of the rate of clearance of the enzymes from the blood. They showed that injected AMP deaminase disappeared very rapidly from the blood of normal and dystrophic chickens. This factor, rather than its molecular weight (320 000), could explain the absence of a rise in the plasma in muscular dystrophy. A further factor to be considered is that the so-called 'soluble' enzymes of muscle may bind variably to intracellular structures (see Clarke & Masters 1976).

Origin of increased permeability. As discussed above, the leakage of enzymes from diseased muscle fibres is at present a main pillar of support for the supposition that there is a sarcolemmal defect in muscular dystrophy. This concept has been particularly associated with the Duchenne type, where the leakage is exceptionally high. While the existence of such a disturbance in the membrane seems very probable, its immediate cause is not known and may have to await further advances in our knowledge of the structure and function of membranes. This is, at present, a very active field of research. Some workers have inclined to the belief that an inherited defect in the structure of sarcolemma is the ultimate cause of Duchenne dystrophy. The evidence from this extreme view, however, is not very convincing. As mentioned above, increased serum enzyme levels are found in many human muscle disorders and are seen also in animal myopathies. A similar phenomenon is encountered also in many other diseases; thus, enzyme leakage is a widespread, non-specific consequence of tissue damage. The very early increase in serum creatine kinase activity in Duchenne dystrophy has been thought to have special significance, but even the earliest reported rise, in a 20-week-old fetus (Mahoney et al 1977) was accompanied by characteristic histopathological changes in the muscles. The hypothesis of a primary membrane defect has stimulated many workers to look for abnormalities in the more accessible plasma membranes of blood cells and fibroblasts. Somer (1980), however, found no significant difference between Duchenne patients and controls in the rate of release of lactate dehydrogenase from lymphocytes. Although changes in these cells have been reported (see below), the general picture is not clear and little attention has been given to their aetiology.

Apart from a genetically determined defect in membrane structure, other possibilities are that membranes may be damaged by a circulating factor or may be affected by a disturbance in the metabolism of the fibres. An intérference in energy supply to the membrane is worth considering here, as there is evidence that such interference can increase enzyme efflux; such an effect may eventually be understood in the terms of the modern fluid-mosaic concept of membrane structure. Mendell et al (1972) found that ligature of the aorta in rats markedly increased many plasma enzymes, although there was little muscle necrosis. Other studies along these lines are discussed by Pennington (1977b). Some workers, e.g. Jones et al (1983), have demonstrated increased rates of enzyme efflux from isolated muscles when the energy supply is interfered with. Studies on the influence of corticosteroids and other drugs upon enzyme efflux (Cohen et al 1977, Verrill et al 1977, de Leiris et al 1978) may also help eventually in the understanding of the phenomenon in muscular dystrophy. Calcium has also been implicated in enzyme release from muscle (Anand & Emery 1980).

Marked muscle wasting is not always associated with enzyme leakage. In the protein-deficiency disease kwashiorkor, serum creatine kinase activity is, on average, lower than normal (Reindorp & Whitehead 1971). Rapid muscle atrophy of neurogenic origin may occur without appreciable increase in serum enzyme levels, and experimental nerve section in animals does not usually cause an appreciable rise. Furthermore, steroid myopathy seldom, if ever, produces such an increase. In these conditions, therefore, membrane integrity in this respect seems unimpaired. Nevertheless, Pellegrino & Bibbiani (1964) were able to demonstrate in vitro an increased permeability to aldolase in denervated muscle.

SERUM PROTEINS, INCLUDING GLYCOPROTEINS AND LIPOPROTEINS

Characteristic quantitative disturbances of the normal electrophoretic pattern of serum proteins occur in many diseases. Comprehensive investigations of human and animal myopathies were described by Oppenheimer & Milhorat (1961). An increase in the α_2-globulin fraction appears to be the most consistent alteration in serum proteins in muscle disease. They also showed that there was a high level of sialic acid in the serum of muscular dystrophy cases; the highest proportion of sialic acid in serum occurs in the α_2-globulin fraction. Small and non-specific serum glycoprotein changes were recorded also by these workers.

More recently Jones (1982) found an elevated α_2-macroglobulin concentration in Duchenne serum, and suggested that this may be involved in controlling elevated muscle proteinase activity.

Oppenheimer & Milhorat (1961) found a decrease in albumin in cases of myositis and of scoliosis and an increase in γ-globulin in the latter. Corridori (1960) found no change in the serum electrophoretic pattern in myasthenia gravis. In various myopathies, Ionasescu & Lucal (1960) reported decreased albumin, increased α_1- and β-globulins and normal γ-globulin. Puricelli et al (1961) have found raised β-globulin and lowered α_1- and γ-globulin in dystrophia myotonica.

An increase in the β_1-globulin, haemopexin, in Duchenne patients and carriers has been reported, but not all workers could confirm the rise in carriers (Lane et al 1979).

In general there has been little attempt to investigate in depth the serum protein changes brought out by the analytical data. However, Wochner et al (1966) have shown that there is a reduced amount of immunoglobulin G (IgG) in myotonic dystrophy and that catabolism of IgG is greatly accelerated. Serum concentrations and catabolic rates of IgM and IgA were normal.

Little work has been carried out on plasma lipoproteins in muscle disease, the most recent study being that of Arthur et al (1983) who found that isolated low-density lipoprotein fractions from Duchenne patients had increased electrophoretic mobility.

Turning to investigations on individual lipid components, both Danowski et al (1956a) and Oppenheimer & Milhorat (1961) noted some decrease in serum cholesterol in children with muscular dystrophy. It is perhaps worth mentioning that this finding represents a biochemical difference between human muscular dystrophy and muscular dystrophy caused by vitamin E deficiency in the rabbit; in the latter case, serum cholesterol increases sharply. This, and other biochemical differences, need not necessarily rule out the idea that human muscular dystrophy is a consequence of a genetic defect in the utilisation of vitamin E — a hypothesis to which a few workers have inclined in the past. Inadequate utilisation of vitamin E in one species might not have the same effect as an inadequate supply of the vitamin in another species. However, there is at present no good evidence for any fundamental relationship between nutritional and hereditary muscular dystrophy. Wakamatsu et al (1970) have observed an increase in serum desmosterol, total cholesterol and triglyceride in myotonic dystrophy; these workers suggest a pathogenic role for abnormal lipid metabolism in this disease.

CREATINURIA

The urine of normal adults contains little or no creatine but its anhydride, creatinine, is excreted in considerable and quite constant amounts (1–2 g/day). One of the earliest discovered characteristics of myopathy, reported over 50 years ago, was a marked increase in creatine excretion; extensive investigations by numerous workers have shown this to be true of almost all types of muscle disease. (It may occur also in some other conditions such as fasting and hyperthyroidism.) Typical data are given by Van Pilsum & Wolin (1958) whose analytical techniques were probably more specific than those used in many earlier studies. They found creatinuria in a wide variety of diseases affecting the muscles, although the exception was myasthenia gravis, and creatinuria was slight in myotonic dystrophy. In most cases there was also a decrease in urinary creatinine and an increased blood creatine, both of which findings have been reported frequently, and an increase in urinary guanidoacetic acid, a precursor of creatine in the body. (It is suggested by the authors that the rise in blood creatine may inhibit to some extent the methylation of guanidoacetic acid to form creatine.) Others (e.g. Danowski et al 1956b) have demonstrated a decreased creatine tolerance in muscular dystrophy patients.

It is now generally accepted that creatinuria is a non-specific manifestation of muscle atrophy, and that there is an obvious connection between the two. Creatine is synthesised (its synthesis involving glycine, arginine and methionine) largely in tissues other than muscle; kidney, liver and pancreas are probably the most important, although there is some doubt about their relative contributions. Most of the creatine formed is rapidly taken up by the muscle fibres and is converted reversibly, by the action of creatine kinase, to creatine phosphate. (The latter represents an important reserve of energy for muscular contraction.) Creatinine arises, probably

spontaneously, from the creatine and creatine phosphate. If the amount of muscle is reduced because of wasting, creatine will be removed less rapidly from the blood, the blood level will be higher and more will be excreted by the kidneys. It seems likely that, in myotonic dystrophy, the production of creatine is also diminished, possibly because of endocrine disturbances; consequently creatinuria is low or absent. Myotonic subjects, like normal individuals, show creatinuria after administration of methyltestosterone (Zierler et al 1949). It is of interest that dystrophic mice of the Bar Harbor strain do not show an increase in creatine excretion (Perkoff & Tyler 1958); this disease has been shown to resemble myotonic dystrophy in other respects also.

It appears from the work of Fitch & Sinton (1964) that a contributory cause of the creatinuria of muscular dystrophy may be the inability of the remaining muscle to retain creatine normally. The half-time of the decrease in specific radioactivity of urine creatinine after intravenous injection of creatine labelled with ^{14}C was considerably decreased in patients with Duchenne and facioscapulohumeral muscular dystrophy. On the other hand, patients with amyotrophic lateral sclerosis and a myopathy of late onset showed a normal rate of decrease. The nature of the defect in the dystrophic muscle is not clear; it may represent either an alteration in cell membrane properties or a change in the intracellular binding of creatine. This is discussed by Fitch (1977).

AMINOACIDURIA

Normal individuals regularly excrete small quantities of several amino acids in the urine, although the nature and amounts show considerable variation. Bank et al (1971) determined quantitatively, by column chromatography, the concentration of 33 amino acids in the plasma and urine of patients with muscle disease. In Duchenne dystrophy, plasma amino acids were normal and there was no characteristic pattern of aminoaciduria, although excretion of taurine was frequently increased. No abnormalities were observed in a smaller number of cases of limb-girdle and facioscapulohumeral dystrophy and myotonic dystrophy. Emery &

Burt (1972), however, in a larger study of patients with myotonic dystrophy, have reported significantly increased excretion (related to creatinine) of threonine, glycine, glutamine, serine and ornithine.

The excretion of hydroxyproline is decreased in patients with muscular dystrophy: a quantitative study by Kibrick et al (1964) showed decreased excretion at all stages in Duchenne dystrophy. The results were less clear-cut in the case of other muscle diseases. This amino acid is found only in collagen and elastin and its reduced excretion may be related to the formation of extra connective tissue in muscular dystrophy.

Enhanced urinary excretion of N^G, N^G-dimethylarginine in the muscular dystrophies has been reported by two laboratories (Inoue et al 1979, Lou 1979). This compound is mainly localised in non-histone nuclear proteins in the cell nucleus.

OTHER CHANGES IN BODY FLUIDS

The early thorough studies of Danowski and his co-workers (1956b) on childhood muscular dystrophy demonstrated increases in serum inorganic phosphate and calcium and a decrease in chloride. In each case the effect was small, with considerable overlap of the individual values, but the mean difference was highly significant. There was no indication that the difference from normal was any greater or less in the more advanced cases. No difference was found in serum total carbon dioxide, sodium, potassium, total protein, albumin or globulin or in fasting levels of venous whole-blood non-protein nitrogen and sugar. In a further paper, dealing with endocrine studies (Danowski et al 1956a), these workers reported normal serum corticoids and urinary gonadotrophin and 17-oxosteroid excretion in their patients. On the other hand, the children with muscular dystrophy had serum protein-bound iodine values in the upper half of the normal range or above it; however, they were able to dispose of administered thyroxine at a normal rate. The same group (Fergus et al 1956) also confirmed an earlier observation that the blood sugar response to adrenaline injection is subnormal in dystrophy patients. The accompanying decreases in serum

inorganic phosphate, potassium and total carbon dioxide were also found to be less than normal in Duchenne dystrophy (Murphy et al 1973) and there were no alterations in the urinary excretion of adrenaline, noradrenaline or 5-hydroxyindole-acetic acid (Mendell et al 1972).

Smith et al (1962) investigated serum magnesium levels in muscular dystrophy. They were able to show that, although much less magnesium can be detected (by EDTA titration), in untreated serum, normal values are found if the analyses are carried out after wet-ashing or on serum ultrafiltrates. This finding indicates that, in serum from the patients, magnesium is bound to an unusually high extent by some constituent of large molecular weight, presumably protein.

Some evidence has been put forward (Gross 1977) for a difference in urinary peptides in Duchenne muscular dystrophy, but the nature and origin of this difference is obscure. Frearson et al (1981) reported the presence of two extra protein spots on electropherograms of urine from boys with Duchenne dystrophy; one of the spots was present in other muscle diseases. It was considered that these were a result of the muscle damage.

Kondo et al (1967) reported that about one-third of the patients with Duchenne dystrophy which they studied excreted nicotinamide-adenine dinucleotide (NAD) in the urine; this ribose-containing coenzyme was absent from the urine of normal subjects. An increase in the excretion of a glucose-containing tetrasaccharide has also been noted (Lundblad et al 1979).

In two rare familial muscle disorders an alteration in blood composition appears to be all-important. In hypokalaemic periodic paralysis (see Ch. 25) the attacks are associated with a rapid fall in serum potassium, which may persist for days. This fall is apparently due to a shift of the ion into the cells and probably results in hyperpolarisation of the fibres, with consequent paralysis. The underlying biochemical mechanism remains unknown. The other condition, in which attacks are precipitated by a high serum potassium, is equally obscure.

Myoglobinuria may occur in inflammatory myopathies (Kagen 1977). It is also found in a number of metabolic disorders of muscle (see Ch. 25) as well as in certain rare muscle disorders of unknown aetiology, in which it occurs spasmodically.

In myotonic dystrophy, abnormalities in the composition of bile acids in bile and serum have been recorded (Tanaka et al 1982). It was suggested that this could influence muscle contraction and membrane fluidity.

BIOCHEMICAL STUDIES OF OTHER TISSUES

Erythrocytes

The past decade has seen a remarkable surge of interest in investigations directed at red blood cells from patients with muscle diseases, particularly Duchenne muscular dystrophy. In fact, the majority of papers on the biochemistry of muscular dystrophy appear to have been concerned with such studies. The relatively ready availability of blood samples has doubtless been a contributory factor. Attention has been focused mainly on the plasma membrane of the erythrocyte, motivated by the possibility, discussed earlier, that there may be a general abnormality in plasma membranes in this disease. Some of these reports are contradictory, in some cases apparently because of inadequate planning and control of the studies, but probably also because of the sensitivity of red-cell ghosts to small variations, often not explicit, in the procedures used in their preparation and washing. It is possible that even circadian changes in erythrocytes, reported by a number of workers (e.g. Hartman et al 1976), may have to be taken into account. The literature now contains an extremely large number of reported abnormalities, with, in most cases, no clear relationship between them. The putative defect in membrane structure, which may be responsible for those of the described changes which are valid, is unknown. Usually, only the more recent papers will be quoted; reference to earlier reports can generally be obtained from these.

The earliest and most widely studied feature is the abnormal response of myosin ATPase to the cardiac glycoside, ouabain, which normally inhibits the enzyme. Various groups have reported different results: that in Duchenne and sometimes other forms of muscular dystrophy the enzyme is stimulated by ouabain, shows subnormal inhibition or responds normally (see Mawatari et al 1981). Although there are variations in experimental details between the studies, none of these appear to correlate with the differences in the findings. Interest is, however, heightened by the observation of an abnormal response to ouabain by the sarcolemmal ATPase of the myopathic hamster (Dhalla et al 1975), mouse (de Kretser & Livett 1977), and Duchenne patient (Niebroj-Dobosz 1981).

Most, but not all workers have found an increase in the Ca^{2+}, Mg^+-ATPase of Duchenne red cells although the details (kinetics, etc) have differed (Dunn et al 1982). This calcium-pump enzyme maintains the low intracellular calcium concentration. Luthra et al (1979) could find no evidence for a difference in calmodulin, which activates this enzyme. Some of the other postulated red cell changes could be explained by an alteration in the cell's handling of calcium (Godin et al 1978) but there appear to have been no reliable measurements of erythrocyte calcium levels in Duchenne dystrophy. Contradictory reports have appeared on the relative rates of transport of calcium in both Duchenne and myotonic dystrophy (Johnson et al 1983). An enhancement of the sensitivity of calcium-induced changes to calcium loading of the cells has been reported in one or two instances but others (Szibor et al 1981) have failed to find this.

An increased autophosphorylation of the spectrin component, protein band II, separated on polyacrylamide gels, reported by Roses et al (1976) has been confirmed by one group but not by others. In myotonic dystrophy a different abnormality was found, notably a decrease in phosphorylation of band III. These findings are reviewed by Tsung & Palek (1980). Anand & Emery (1981) could find no difference in two-dimensional peptide mapping of bands I and II in Duchenne dystrophy. Several workers, e.g. Tsuchiya et al (1981), have reported that the extractability of spectrin from red cells is decreased in Duchenne dystrophy.

It is well known that the behaviour of membrane enzymes may be affected by their lipid environment. Several attempts have been made to find abnormalities in the lipid composition of red-cell membranes in muscular dystrophy. A number of such have been reported but disagreements exist; some of the reported abnormalities concern minor lipid components, which are difficult to analyse accurately. Not all workers have taken precautions to prevent autoxidation of polyunsaturated fatty acids which can lead to selective loss of phospholipids. Moreover, in some of the studies the values given for the normals have been atypical. As pointed out by McLaughlin & Engel (1979), who were unable to detect any abnormalities in Duchenne dystrophy or myotonic dystrophy, the red cell lipids can be influenced by diet.

Hunter et al (1983) made the interesting observation that the phosphatidylcholine in Duchenne erythrocytes appeared to be more accessible to added phospholipase, suggesting that a greater proportion is present in the outer lipid layer of the membrane.

The use of electron spin resonance or fluorescence polarisation techniques after incorporating suitable 'probe' molecules into the membrane is widely used in searching for abnormalities in the molecular organisation of membranes. These have been applied by a number of groups to Duchenne dystrophy and, although precise interpretation of the signals is difficult and the techniques and findings have differed in detail, most results have suggested an increased molecular rigidity of the membrane. The opposite has been found in myotonic dystrophy; Butterfield (1981), however, found that this difference was manifested only after storing the washed cells and suggested that metabolic deprivation is necessary before the abnormality is evident. These studies are reviewed in more detail by Jones & Witkowski (1983). Using electron spin resonance, Clark et al (1983) found that the change in response with temperature of Duchenne erythrocytes did not show the break found with normal red cells. This is of particular interest as other groups have noted a similar phenomenon and it has been seen also in the case of the membrane Na^+,K^+-ATPase (Austin et al 1983).

Other reported biochemical abnormalities in erythrocytes in Duchenne dystrophy include an increased rate of potassium efflux (Howland 1974), raised phospholipase A activity (Iyer et al

1976), found also in myotonic dystrophy, and a decrease in glutathione reductase (Hunter & Kunjlata 1983) Physical properties of erythrocytes have also been investigated. A change of shape has been postulated but is controversial (Matheson et al 1976) as are the claims of a reduced deformability (Conlon et al 1983). An increase in osmotic fragility of Duchenne red cells, observed by most workers who have measured this property, appears to be more soundly based. Kim et al (1980) observed this difference in young erythrocytes.

As discussed above, a change in membrane behaviour could possibly arise from interference with energy-supplying mechanisms in the cell; energy in the form of ATP is required to drive the ion pumps and possibly for other membrane functions. However, reports on the ATP content of Duchenne erythrocytes have been contradictory (Kalofoutis & Poulakis 1984).

There appears to be no difference in the age distribution of erythrocytes in Duchenne dystrophy (Campbell et al 1977). The possibility that changes in red-cell membranes in patients with muscle disease may result from alterations in the blood plasma has not been widely examined. This is surprising because there is a ready exchange of lipids between membrane and plasma (see Bruckdorfer & Graham 1976). (It may be important that this occurs also with muscle membranes (Graham & Green 1967)). However, three independent reports (see Lloyd & Emery 1981) have demonstrated that the abnormal response of the ATPase to ouabain in Duchenne muscular dystrophy can be induced in normal red cells by incubation with Duchenne plasma. Austin et al (1983) found that the monophasic response to temperature of the ATPase can also be induced by this means, while Iyer et al (1977) obtained evidence that plasma factors may be involved in the abnormal protein phosphorylation which they observed in myotonic dystrophy.

Differences between normal and Duchenne serum in their effects on the properties of cultured skin fibroblasts have also been claimed (Ulreich et al 1982). Such effects of circulating factors, particularly if reversible, may explain some of the divergencies in the findings on red cell characteristics in muscular dystrophy.

Skin fibroblasts

During the last few years, numerous studies have been carried out on cultured skin fibroblasts from patients with Duchenne muscular dystrophy and other muscle diseases. Once cultures are established they are a continuously available source of cells for those searching for generalised defects in these diseases or exploring the possibility that connective tissue abnormality may be a causative factor. Unfortunately some investigators have procured their cultures from different sources, introducing possibilities of variability, due to the age of the subject and differences in the site of biopsy. In particular, biopsies of young boys are often taken from the foreskin, which has special properties (Thompson et al 1983). These factors must be taken into account when evaluating reported abnormalities. Studies indicating reduced adhesiveness of Duchenne cells (Jones & Witkowski 1983, Kent 1983) have suggested changes in the membrane surface. Workers at Cincinatti have reported in a series of papers that Duchenne fibroblasts have a reduced level and decreased latency of the lysosomal enzyme, dipeptidylpeptidase I, associated with increased chloride permeability of the lysosome (Davis et al 1982). The author's laboratory, however, has failed to confirm the decrease in enzyme activity. Both Ionasescu et al (1977) and Thompson et al (1982) have found an increased production of extracellular collagen (measured by the incorporation of [^{14}C] proline) by Duchenne fibroblasts.

The phospholipid and fatty acid composition of fibroblasts in Duchenne dystrophy was found to be normal by Kohlschutter et al (1976) and [1-^{14}C] acetate incorporation into fibroblast lipids was normal in myotonic dystrophy (Thomas & Harper 1978).

Other tissues

Platelets from patients with Duchenne dystrophy but not from those with other neuromuscular disorders have been reported to show a decreased rate of uptake of serotonin (Murphy et al 1973). Platelet aggregation displayed reduced sensitivity to adrenaline (Yarom et al 1983), in contrast to myotonic dystrophy, where the sensitivity was increased.

Cap formation in lymphocytes, i.e. aggregation of surface immunoglobulin molecules in response to binding of antigen, is decreased in a number of diseases. It is a complex phenomenon influenced by many factors such as membrane fluidity, energy supply and probably calcium. Following a report of a decrease in capping in both patients and carriers of Duchenne dystrophy, many laboratories, e.g. Goldsmith et al (1984), have attempted to confirm this finding. The assessment of capping requires experience and critical judgement and despite much attention to the details of the procedure not all workers have been able to confirm this result and the situation is still to be resolved fully.

In a recent study (Klip et al 1985) using the sensitive calcium indicator, Quin 2, the free cytoplasmic calcium level in Duchenne lymphocytes was found to be normal.

The pattern of plasma enzyme elevations in disease commonly provides clues pinpointing the affected tissues. In Duchenne dystrophy the pattern can be attributed largely to damaged muscles, although Kleine (1970) has concluded that it also implicates other tissues, such as liver and heart. Two characteristic liver enzymes, γ-glutamyltransferase (Rosalki & Thompson 1971) and sorbitol dehydrogenase (EC 1.1.1.14) (Kar & Pearson 1973e), appear to show normal serum levels. Danowski et al (1956a, b) and others have, nevertheless, reported that there are occasional abnormalities in liver function tests. Gammaglutamyltransferase levels, however, have been found to be increased in myotonic dystrophy (Alevizos et al 1976).

Paulson et al (1974) could find no evidence for a circulatory abnormality in Duchenne or limbgirdle dystrophy. They found, using the xenon-133 injection method, that muscle blood flow was normal at rest and during exercise-induced hyperaemia. Capillary diffusion capacity, measured with ^{51}Cr-EDTA, was at least as high as normal. These results, therefore, provided no evidence for the hypothesis that ischaemia may be important in the pathogenesis of Duchenne dystrophy.

Particular interest has been shown in the possibility of chemical alterations in the nervous system in Duchenne muscular dystrophy, in view of the theory (reviewed by Sica & McComas 1978) that the muscle damage has a neural origin. Muscle can atrophy as a result of damage to its motor nerve. Moreover, following the work of Buller et al (1960) on the effect of cross-innervation in reversing the contraction time of fast and slow muscles, it is now recognised that the nervous system may exert a more discriminating control over the metabolism of muscle fibres than was previously realised. Romanul & Van Der Meulen (1966), Dubowitz & Newman (1967) and others have shown by cross-innervation and histochemical techniques that the characteristic enzyme profile of red and white fibres is influenced by their motor nerves. The relative amounts of myoglobin in the two muscle types are also altered by cross-innervation (McPherson & Tokunaga 1967), while Guth & Watson (1967) have shown that this procedure alters the protein electrophoresis pattern of the slow muscle towards that characteristic of a fast muscle. Quantitative enzyme studies by Prewitt & Salafsky (1970) have shown that, after cross-innervation, the activities of the glycolytic enzymes, aldolase and pyruvate kinase, increase in the soleus and decrease in the flexor digitorum longus. It remains to be seen whether these effects result in some way from the different pattern of impulses from the different motor nerves, or whether they are due to passage from the nerves of 'trophic' factors which influence the synthesis of specific proteins in the muscle. The former possibility now seems more likely. The existence of trophic factors has often been suggested but direct evidence is slight. Some workers (e.g. Appeltauer & Korr 1977) maintain that they have demonstrated a transfer of compounds from nerve to muscle; a disturbance in the passage of such 'trophic' factors could be invoked in muscular dystrophy. Confirmation and extension of these studies is required, however. The existence of such a detailed control of muscle metabolism by the nerve, whatever its mechanism, might allow for the possibility that muscle disease could result from changes in the nerve which are more subtle than those occurring in the recognised neurogenic disorders and which have, so far, escaped observation. There is scant biochemical evidence, however, for changes in the nervous system in human muscular dystrophies. Changes in cerebrospinal fluid (CSF) protein in adult muscular dystrophies have been observed by Kjellin & Stibler (1976), but their origin is not clear.

CONCLUSION

In conclusion, an attempt has been made in this chapter to review the main biochemical approaches to the investigation of muscle diseases (particularly the muscular dystrophies) and to comment on the implications of the findings. Research is proceeding at an increasing pace and one can merely draw a line under what has been achieved up to a particular moment. Relatively little has been said about the endocrine and metabolic myopathies, which are discussed fully in Chapter 25 and to which major recent advances such as nuclear magnetic resonance spectrosocopy are of particular relevance. Some practical success has been attained, as in the improved diagnosis of muscular dystrophy and the identification of carriers of the X-linked Duchenne gene. However, in spite of attacks on a number of fronts, biochemical research has not yet achieved a breakthrough leading to the cure of any major muscle disease, because of the complexities of the problems involved. Researchers studying diseased muscle must at present bear in mind the fact that understanding of the disease may involve as yet undiscovered features of the chemistry of normal muscle. Undoubtedly the combined results of research on both the normal and the diseased state will eventually solve these problems.

ACKNOWLEDGEMENTS

I am grateful to the Medical Research Council, the Muscular Dystrophy Group of Great Britain and the Muscular Dystrophy Association of America for financial assistance for some of the work referred to in this chapter.

REFERENCES

Abdullah F, Pennington R J 1968 Ribonucleases in normal and dystrophic human muscle. Clinica Chimica Acta 20:365

Al-Azzawi H T, Stoward P J 1972 Abstracts of Sixth symposium on Current Research in Muscular Dystrophy and Related Diseases, Abstract No 29. Muscular Dystrophy Group of Great Britain

Alevizos B, Spengos M, Vassilpoulos D, Stefanis C 1976 γ-glutamyl transpeptidase — elevated activity in myotonic dystrophy. Journal of the Neurological Sciences 28:225

Alling C, Bruce A, Karlsson I, Svennerholm L, 1974 Effect of different dietary levels of essential fatty acids on the fatty acid composition of lecithin in rat skeletal muscle. Nutrition and Metabolism 16:1

Anand R, Emery A E H 1980 Calcium stimulated enzyme efflux from human skeletal muscle. Research Communications in Clinical Pathology and Pharmacology 28:541

Anand R, Emery A E H 1981 Erythrocyte spectrin in Duchenne muscular dystrophy. Clinica Chimica Acta 117:345

Appeltauer G S L, Korr I M 1977 Further electrophoretic studies on proteins of neuronal origin in skeletal muscle. Experimental Neurology 57:713

Arthur H, de Niese M, Jeffrey P L, Austin L 1983 Plasma lipoproteins in Duchenne muscular dystrophy. Biochemistry International 6:307

Austin L, Katz S, Jeffrey P L, Shield L, Arthur H, Mazzoni M 1983 Thermodynamic behaviour of membrane enzymes in Duchenne muscular dystrophy. Journal of the Neurological Sciences 58:143

Bank W J, Rowland L P, Ipsen J 1971 Amino acids of plasma and urine in diseases of muscle. Archives of Neurology 24:176

Bär U, Ohlendorf S 1970 Studien zur Enzymelimination. I. Halbwertszeiten einiger Zellenzyme beim Menschen. Klinische Wochenschrift 48:776

Bell R R, Draper H H 1976 Glutathione peroxidase activity and glutathione concentration in genetically dystrophic mice. Proceedings of the Society for Experimental Biology and Medicine 152:520

Berni C M, Rea F, Schettini F 1961 Demonstration of the phosphoglucomutase acitvity in the serum of children with progressive muscular dystrophy. Bollettino della Societa Italiana di Biologia Sperimentale 37:845

Berthillier G, Eichenberger D, Carrier H N, Guibaud P, Got R 1982 Carnitine metabolism in early stages of Duchenne muscular dystrophy. Clinica Chimica Acta 122:3

Bertorini T E, Palmieri G M A, Griffin J et al 1985 Chronic allopurinol and adenine therapy in Duchenne muscular dystrophy: effects on muscle function, nucleotide degradation and muscle ATP and ADP content. Neurology 35:61

Bird J W C 1975 Skeletal muscle lysosomes. In: Dingle J T, Dean R T (eds) Lysosomes in biology and pathology. North Holland, Amsterdam p 75

Blyth H, Hughes B P 1971 Pregnancy and serum-CPK levels in potential carriers of 'severe' X- linked muscular dystrophy. Lancet 1:855

Bodensteiner J B, Engel A G 1978 Intracellular calcium accumulation in Duchenne dystrophy and other myopathies: A Study of 567 000 muscle fibres in 114 biopsies. Neurology (Minneapolis) 28:439

Borum P R, Broquist H P, Roelofs R I 1977 Muscle carnitine levels in neuromuscular disease. Journal of the Neurological Sciences 34:279

Brambati B, Cornelio F, Dworzak F, Dones I 1980 Calcium-positive muscle fibres in fetuses at risk for Duchenne muscular dystrophy. Lancet ii:969

Bruckdorfer K R, Graham J M 1976 The exchange of cholesterol and phospholipids between cell membranes and lipoproteins. In: Chapman D, Wallach D F H (eds) Biological membranes, vol. 3. Academic Press, New York, p 103

Buller A J, Eccles J C, Eccles R M 1960 Interactions between motoneurones and muscles in respect of characteristic speeds of their responses. Journal of Physiology (London) 150:417

Butterfield D A 1981 Myotonic muscular dystrophy. Time-dependent alterations in erythrocyte membrane fluidity. Journal of the Neurological Sciences 52:61

Campbell J C W, Suelter C H, Puite R H 1977 5'-AMP aminohydrolase activity in erythrocytes from normal and dystrophic individuals. Clinica Chimica Acta 79:379

Canal N, Frattola L, Smirne S 1975 The metabolism of cyclic-3'-5'-adenosine monophosphate (cAMP) in diseased muscle. Journal of Neurology 208:259

Canonico P G, Bird J W C 1970 Lysosomes in skeletal muscle tissue. Zonal centrifugation evidence for multiple cellular sources. Journal of Cell Biology 45:321

Cao A, de Virgilis S, Lippi C, Coppa G 1971 Serum and muscle creatine kinase isoenzymes and serum aspartate aminotransferase isoenzymes in progressive muscular dystrophy. Enzyme 12:49

Carrol J E, Norris B J, Brooke M H 1985 Defective (U-¹⁴C) palmitic acid oxidation in Duchenne muscular dystrophy. Neurology 35:96

Carter N D, Heath R, Jeffrey S, Jackson M J, Newham D J, Edwards R H T 1983 Carbonic anhydrase III in Duchenne muscular dystrophy. Clinica Chimica Acta 133:201

Cerri C, Willner J H, Rowland L P 1981 Assay of adenylate cyclase in homogenates of control and Duchenne skeletal muscle. Clinica Chemica Acta 11:133

Chalovich J M, Burt C T, Danon M J, Glonek T, Barany M 1979 Phosphodiesters in muscular dystrophies. Annals of the New York Academy of Sciences 317:649

Chou T, Hill E J, Bartle E et al 1975 Beneficial effects of penicillamine treatment of hereditary avian muscular dystrophy. Journal of Clinical Investigation 56:842

Chowdhury S R, Pearson C M, Fowler W W Jr, Griffith W H 1962 Serum enzyme studies in muscular dystrophy. III. Serum malic dehydrogenase 5-nucleotidase and adenosine triphosphatase. Proceedings of the Society of Experimental Biology and Medicine 109:227

Chyatte S B, Rudman D, Patterson J H et al 1973 Human growth hormone and estrogens in boys with Duchenne muscular dystrophy. Archives of Physical Medicine and Rehabilitation 54:248

Clark A D, Nash G B, Patel K J, Wyard S J 1983 Electron spin resonance spin label studies of the erythrocyte membrane in Duchenne muscular dystrophy. American Journal of Medical Genetics 16:153

Clarke F M, Masters C J 1976 Interactions between muscle proteins and glycolytic enzymes. International Journal of Biochemistry 7:359

Cohen L, Morgan J, Bozyk M E 1977 Variable effects of

corticosteroid treatment on serum enzyme activities in Duchenne's muscular dystrophy. Research Communications in Chemical Pathology and Pharmacology 17:529

Conlon T, Lingard P S, Tomkins J K 1983 Deformability and cell membrane properties of erythrocytes in Duchenne muscular dystrophy. Clinica Chimica Acta 130:139

Corridori F 1960 Studies on the electrophoretic picture of the serum proteins and glycoproteins in progressive muscular dystrophy and myotonic dystrophy. Rivista Sperimentale di Freniatria 84:52

Cutillo S, Colletta A, Lupi L, Canani M B 1962 The relationship between lactic and α-hydroxybutyric dehydrogenase of the serum in children with progressive muscular dystrophy. Bollettino della Societa Italiana di Biologia Sperimentale 38:691

Danowski T S, Bastiani R M, McWilliams F D, Mateer F M, Greenman L 1956a Muscular dystrophy. IV. Endocrine studies. American Journal of Diseases of Children 91:356

Danowski T S, Wirth P M, Leinberger M H, Randall L A, Peters J H 1956b Muscular dystrophy. III. Serum blood solutes and other laboratory indices. American Journal of Diseases of Children 91:346

Davis M H, Gelman B B, Gruenstein E 1982 Decreased structure-linked latency of lysosomal depeptidyl aminopeptidase-I activity in Duchenne muscular dystrophy fibroblasts. Neurology 32:486

Dawson D M, Kaplan N O 1965 Factors influencing the concentration of enzymes in various muscles. Journal of Biological Chemistry 240:3215

de Kretser T, Livett B G 1977 Skeletal-muscle sarcolemma from normal and dystrophic mice. Biochemical Journal 168:229

Dhalla N S, McNamara D B, Balasubramanian V, Greenlaw R, Tucker F R 1973 Alterations of adenosine triphosphatase activities in dystrophic muscle sarcolemma. Research Communications in Chemical Pathology and Pharmacology 6:643

Dhalla N S, Singh A, Lee S L, Anand M B, Bernatsky A M, Jasmin G 1975 Defective membrane systems in dystrophic skeletal muscle of the UM-X7.1 strain of genetically myopathic hamster. Clinical Science and Molecular Medicine 49:359

DiMauro S, Angelini G, Catani C 1967 Enzymes of the glycogen cycle and glycolysis in various human neuromuscular disorders. Journal of Neurology, Neurosurgery and Psychiatry 30:411

Dreyfus J C, Schapira G, Schapira F, Demos J 1956 Activités enzymatiques du muscle humain. Recherches sur la biochimie comparée de l'homme normal et myopathique et du rat. Clinica Chimica Acta 1:434

Dreyfus J C, Schapira G, Schapira F 1958 Serum enzymes in the physiopathology of muscle. Annals of the New York Academy of Sciences 75 (I):235

Duance V C, Stephens H R, Dunn M, Bailey A J, Dubowitz V 1980 A role for collagen in the pathogenesis of muscular dystrophy? Nature 284:470

Dubowitz V, Newman D L 1967 Change in enzyme pattern after cross-innervation of fast and slow skeletal muscle. Nature 214:840

Dunn M J, Burghes A H M, Dubowitz V 1982 Erythrocyte-ghost Ca^{2+}-stimulated Mg^{2+}-dependent adenosine triphosphatase in Duchenne muscular dystrophy. Biochemical Journal 201:445

Edmonds C J, Smith T, Griffiths R D, Mackenzie J, Edwards R H T 1985 Total body potassium and water, and exchangeable sodium in muscular dystrophy. Clinical Science 68:379

Edwards R H T 1984 Nuclear magnetic resonance and other new techniques for the study of metabolism in human muscular dystrophy. Italian Journal of Neurological Sciences (Suppl 3) 75

Edwards R J, Rodeck C H, Watts D C 1984 The diagnostic value of plasma myoglobin levels in the adult and fetus at risk for Duchenne muscular dystrophy. Journal of the Neurological Sciences 63:173

Ellis, D A, Strickland J M, Eccleston J F 1973 The direct interconversion of glucose and fructose in human skeletal muscle with special reference to childhood muscular dystrophy. Clinical Science 44:321

Ellis F R, Clarke I M C, Modgill M, Currie S, Harriman D G F 1975 Evaluation of creatinine phosphokinase in screening patients for malignant hyperpyrexia. British Medical Journal 3:511

Emery A E H 1964 Electrophoretic pattern of lactate dehydrogenase in carriers and patients with Duchenne muscular dystrophy. Nature 201:1044

Emery A E H 1968 Muscle lactate dehydrogenase isoenzymes in hereditary myopathies. Journal of the Neurological Sciences 7:137

Emery A E H, Burt D 1972 Amino acid, creatine and creatinine studies in myotonic dystrophy. Clinica Chimica Acta 39:361

Emery A E H, Skinner R, Howden L C, Matthews M B 1982 Verapamil in Duchenne muscular dystrophy. Lancet i:559

Feit H, Fuseler J, Cook J D 1983 Myofibrillar creatine kinase in Duchenne and avian muscular dystrophy. Biochemical Medicine 29:355

Fergus E B, Nichols W R, Horne L M, Danowski T S 1956 Muscular dystrophy. VI. Diminished blood sugar and serum electrolyte response to epinephrine. American Journal of Diseases of Children 91:436

Fischbeck K H, Bonilla E, Schotland D L 1983 Freeze-fracture analysis of plasma membrane cholesterol in Duchenne muscle. Annals of Neurology 5:532

Fischbeck K H, Bonilla E, Schotland D L 1984. Distribution of freeze-fracture particle sizes in Duchenne muscle plasma membrane. Neurology 34:534

Fishbein W N 1985 Myoadenylate deaminase deficiency: inherited and acquired forms. Biochemical Medicine 33:158

Fitch C D 1977 Significance of abnormalities in creatine metabolism. In: Rowland L P (ed) Pathogenesis of human muscular dystrophies. Excerpta Medica, Amsterdam, p 329

Fitch C D, Sinton D W 1964 A study of creatine metabolism in diseases causing muscle wasting. Journal of Clinical Investigation 43:444

Folkers K, Nakamura R, Littarru G P, Zellweger H, Brunkhorst J B, Williams C W, Jr, Langston J H 1974 Effect of coenzyme Q on serum levels of creatine phosphokinase in preclinical muscular dystrophy. Proceedings of the National Academy of Sciences USA 71:2098

Franklin G I, Cavanagh N P C, Hughes B P, Yasin R, Thompson E J 1981 Creatine kinase isoenzymes in cultured human muscle cells. I. Comparison of Duchenne muscular dystrophy with other myopathic and neurogenic disease. Clinica Chimica Acta 115:179

Frearson N, Taylor R D, Perry S V 1981 Proteins in the urine associated with Duchenne muscular dystrophy and other neuromuscular diseases. Clinical Science 61:141

Furukawa T, Peter J B 1971 Superprecipitation and adenosine triphosphatase activity in myosin B in Duchenne muscular dystrophy. Neurology (Minneapolis) 21:290

Furukawa T, Peter J B 1972 Muscular dystrophy and other myopathies. Troponin activity of natural actomyosin from skeletal muscle. Archives of Neurology, 26:385

Garst, J B, Vignos P J Jr, Hadaday M, Matthews D N 1977. Urinary sodium, potassium and aldosterone in Duchenne muscular dystrophy. Journal of Clinical Endocrinology and Metabolism 44:185

Godin D V, Bridges M A, MacLeod P J M 1978 Chemical compositional studies of erythrocyte membranes in Duchenne muscular dystrophy. Research Communications in Chemical Pathology and Pharmacology 20:331

Goldsmith B M, Drachman D B, Gruener H-D, Miller W G, Self S S 1984 Blind evaluation of lymphocyte capping in Duchenne muscular dystrophy. Neurology 34:821

Goto I, Nagamine M, Katsuki S 1969 Creatine phosphokinase isoenzymes in muscles. Human fetus and patients. Archives of Neurology 20:422

Graham J M Green C 1967 The binding of sterols in cellular membranes. Biochemical Journal 103:16c

Griggs, R C, Moxley R T, Forbes G B 1980 3-Methyl-histidine excretion in myotonic dystrophy. Neurology 30:1262

Gross S 1977 Peptides in Duchenne muscular dystrophy. Clinical Chemistry, 23:299

Guth L, Watson P K 1967 The influence of innervation on the soluble proteins of slow and fast muscles of the rat. Experimental Neurology 17:107

Halliday D, Ford G C, Edwards R H T, Rennie M J, Griggs R C 1985 In vivo estimation of muscle protein synthesis in myotonic dystrophy. Annals of Neurology 17:65

Hamada M, Okuda H, Oda K et al 1981 An aberrant adenylate kinase isoenzyme from the serum of patients with Duchenne muscular dystrophy. Biochemica et Biophysica Acta 660:227

Hardy M F, Pennington R J T 1979 Separation of cathepsin B1 and related enzymes from rat skeletal muscle. Biochimica et Biophysica Acta 577: 253

Hardy M F, Mantle D, Pennington R J T 1983 Characteristics of a new muscle proteinase. Biochemical Society Transactions 11:348

Harris J B (ed) 1979 Muscular dystrophy and other inherited diseases of muscle. Annals of the New York Academy of Sciences 317

Hartman H, Ashkenazi I, Epel B L 1976 Circadian changes in membrane properties of human red blood cells in vitro, as measured by a membrane probe. FEBS Letters 67:161

Haymond M W, Strobel K E, deVivo, D C 1978 Muscle wasting and carbohydrate homeostasis in Duchenne muscular dystrophy. Neurology 28:1224

Heyck H, Laudahn G, Luders C-J 1963 Fermentaktivitatsbestimmungen in der gesunden, menschlichen Muskulatur und bei Myopathien. II Mitteilung. Enzymaktivitatsveranderungen im Muskel bei Dystrophia musculorum progressiva. Klinische Wochenschrift 41:500

Heyck H, Laudahn G, Carsten P M 1966 Enzymaktivatatsbestimmungen bei Dystrophia musculorem progressiva. IV. Mitteilung. Die Serumenzymkinetic im praklinischen Stadium des Typus Duchenne wahrend der ersten Lebensjahre. Klinische Wochenschrift 41:695

Hooft C, de Laey P, Lambert Y 1966 Étude comparative de l'activité enzymatique du tissu musculaire de l'enfant normal et d'enfants atteints de dystrophie musculaire progressive aux différents stades de la maladie. Revue Française d'Études Cliniques et Biologiques 11:510

Howland, J L 1974 Abnormal potassium conductance associated with genetic muscular dystrophy. Nature 251:724

Hunter M I S, Kunjlata A 1983 Red cell catalase and glutathione reductase in Duchenne muscular dystrophy. IRCS Medical Science: Biochemistry 11:341

Hunter M I S, Lao M S de Vane P J 1983 Is erythrocyte membrane phospholipid organisation abnormal in Duchenne muscular dystrophy? Clinica Chimica Acta 128:69

Husic H D, Suelter C H 1980 The rapid disappearance of muscle AMP aminohydrolase from blood plasma of normal and dystrophic chickens. Biochemical and Biophysical Research Communications 95:228

Husic H D, Suelter C H 1983 The levels of creatine kinase and adenylate kinase in the plasma of dystrophic chickens reflect the rate of loss of these enzymes from the circulation. Biochemical Medicine 29:318

Iodice A A, Chin J, Perker S, Weinstock I M 1972 Cathepsins A, B, C, D and autolysis during development of breast muscle of normal and dystrophic chickens. Archives of Biochemistry and Biophysics 152:166

Ionasescu V 1975 Distinction between Duchenne and other muscular dystrophies by ribosomal protein synthesis. Journal of Medical Genetics 12:49

Ionasescu V, Lucal N 1960 Changes in the serum electropherogram in myopathies. Review of Neurology, 102:253

Ionasescu V, Lara-Braud C, Zellweger H, Ionasescu R, Burmeister L 1977 Fibroblast cultures in Duchenne muscular dystrophy. Alterations in synthesis and secretion of collagen and non-collagen proteins. Acta Neurologica Scandinavica 55:407

Ionasescu V, Ionasescu R, Feld R, Witte D, Cancilla P, Kaeding L, Stern L Z 1981 Alterations in creatine kinase in fresh muscle and cell cultures in Duchenne dystrophy. Annals of Neurology 9:394

Ionasescu V, Ionasescu R 1982 Increased collagen synthesis by Duchenne myogenic clones. Journal of Neurological Sciences 54:79

Inoue R, Miyake M, Kanawaza A, Sato M, Kakimoto Y 1979 Decrease of 3-methylhistidine and increase of N^G, N^G-dimethylarginine in the urine of patients with muscular dystrophy. Metabolism 28:801

Iyer S L, Katyare S S, Howland J L 1976 Elevated erythrocyte phospholipase A associated with Duchenne and myotonic muscular dystrophy. Neuroscience Letters 2:103

Iyer S L, Hoenig P A, Sherblom A P, Howland J L 1977 Membrane function affected by genetic muscular dystrophy. I. Erythrocyte ghost protein kinase. Biochemical Medicine 18:384

Johnson R, Somer H, Karli P, Saris N E 1983 Erythrocyte flexibility, ATPase activities and Ca efflux in patients with Duchenne muscular dystrophy, myotonic dystrophy and congenital myotonia. Journal of the Neurological Sciences 58:399

Jones D A, Jackson M J, Edwards, R H T 1983 Release of intracellular enzymes from an isolated mammalian skeletal muscle preparation. Clinical Science 65:193

Jones, G E, Witkowski J A 1983 Membrane abnormalities in Duchenne muscular dystrophy. Journal of the Neurological Sciences 58:159

Jones G L 1982 Plasma antiproteases in Duchenne muscular dystrophy. Biochemical Medicine 27:1

Kagen L J 1977 Myoglobinemia in inflammatory myopathies. Journal of the American Medical Association 237:1448

Kagen L J, Moussavi S, Miller S L, Tsairis P 1980 Serum myoglobin in muscular dystrophy. Muscle and Nerve 3:221

Kalofoutis A, Poulakis Z 1984 Phosphate compounds in erythrocytes and plasma in Duchenne muscular dystrophy. Clinical Chemistry 30:1101

Kar N C, Pearson C M 1972a Acid, neutral and alkaline cathepsins in normal and diseased human muscle. Enzyme 13:188

Kar N C, Pearson C M 1972b Acid hydrolases in normal and diseased human muscle. Clinica Chimica Acta 40:341

Kar N C, Pearson C M 1972c Fructose 1, 6-diphosphatase in normal and diseased human muscle. Clinica Chimica Acta 38:252

Kar N C, Pearson C M 1972d Acyl phosphatase in normal and diseased human muscle. Clinica Chimica Acta 40:262

Kar N C, Pearson C M 1972e Serum β-acetylglucos-aminidase and arylsulfatase A in inflammatory disorders of muscle and connective tissue. Proceedings of the Society for Experimental Biology and Medicine 140:1480

Kar N C, Pearson C M 1973a Glycosidases in normal and diseased human muscle. Clinica Chimica Acta 45:269

Kar N C, Pearson C M 1973b Muscle adenylic acid deaminase activity. Selective decrease in early-onset Duchenne muscular dystrophy. Neurology (Minneapolis) 23:478

Kar N C, Pearson C M 1973c 5'-Nucleotidase activity of normal and dystrophic human muscle. Proceedings of the Society for Experimental Biology and Medicine 143:1125

Kar N C, Pearson C M 1973d Cholinesterase and esterase activity in normal and dystrophic human muscle. Biochemical Medicine 7:452

Kar N C, Pearson C M 1973e Sorbitol dehydrogenase in muscle disease. Lancet 1:673

Kar N C, Pearson C M 1974 Monoamine oxidase activity in normal and dystrophic human muscle. Clinica Chimica Acta 50:431

Kar N C, Pearson C M 1975a Glyoxalase enzyme system in human muscular dystrophy. Clinica Chimica Acta 65:153

Kar N C, Pearson C M 1975b Phosphodiesterases in normal and dystrophic human muscle. Proceedings of the Society for Experimental Biology and Medicine 148:1005

Kar N C, Pearson C M 1975c Lipase activity in normal and dystrophic human muscle. Biochemical Medicine 14:135

Kar N C, Pearson C M 1976a Arylamidase and cathepsin A activity of normal and dystrophic human muscle. Proceedings of the Society for Experimental Biology and Medicine 151:583

Kar N C, Pearson C M 1976b A calcium-activated neutral protease in normal and dystrophic human muscle. Clinica Chimica Acta 73:293

Kar·N C, Pearson C M 1977 Early elevation of cathepsin B1 in human muscle disease. Biochemical Medicine 18:126

Kar N C, Pearson C M 1978 Dipeptidyl peptidases in human muscle disease. Clinica Chimica Acta 82:185

Kar N C, Pearson C M 1979 Catalase, superoxide dismutase, glutathione reductase and thiobarbituric acid-reactive products in normal and dystrophic human muscle. Clinica Chimica Acta 94:277

Kar N C, Pearson C M 1981a Adenylosuccinase in human muscular dystrophy. Muscle and Nerve 4:174

Kar N C, Pearson C M 1981b Post-proline-cleaving enzyme in normal and dystrophic human muscle. Clinica Chimica Acta 111:271

Karpati G 1985 Abnormal insulin homeostasis in myotonic dystrophy. Trends in Neurological Sciences 8:141

Katunuma N, Yasogawa N, Kito K, Sanada Y, Kawai H, Miyoshi K 1978 Abnormal expression of a serine protease in human dystrophic muscle. Journal of Biochemistry (Japan) 83:625

Kendrick-Jones J, Perry S V 1965 Enzymatic adaptation to contractile activity in skeletal muscle. Nature 208:1068

Kendrick-Jones J, Perry S V 1967 The enzymes of adenine nucleotide metabolism in developing skeletal muscle. Biochemical Journal 103:207

Kent C 1983 Increased rate of cell-substratum detachment of fibroblasts from patients with Duchenne muscular dystrophy. Proceedings of the National Academy of Sciences USA 80:3086

Kibrick A C, Hashiro C, Walters M, Milhorat A T 1964 Hydroxyproline excretion in urine of patients with muscular dystrophy and other muscle diseases. Proceedings of the Society for Experimental Biology and Medicine 115:662

Kim H D, Luthra M G, Watts R P, Stern L Z 1980 Factors influencing osmotic fragility of red blood cells in Duchenne muscular dystrophy. Neurology 30:726

King B, Spikesman A, Emery A E H 1972 The effect of pregnancy on serum levels of creatine kinase. Clinica Chimica Acta 36:267

Kitchin S E, Watts D C 1973 Comparison of the turnover patterns of total and individual muscle proteins in normal mice and those with hereditary muscular dystrophy. Biochemical Journal 136:1017

Kito S, Yamamoto M, Itoga E, Kishida T 1979 Cyclic nucleotides in progressive muscular dystrophy. European Neurology 18:356

Kjellin K G, Stibler H 1976 Isoelectric focusing and electrophoresis of cerebrospinal fluid proteins in muscular dystrophies and spinal muscular atrophies. Journal of the Neurological Sciences 27:45

Kleine T O 1970 Evidence for the release of enzymes from different organs in Duchenne's muscular dystrophy. Clinica Chimica Acta 29:227

Kleine T O, Chlond H 1967 Enzymmuster gesunder skelett-, herz und glatter Muskelatur des Menschen sowie ihrer pathologischen Veränderungen. mit besonderer Berücksichtigung der progressiven Muskeldystrophie (Erb). Clinica Chimica Acta 15:19

Klip A, Elder B, Ruiz-Funes H P, Buchwald M, Grinstein S 1985 The free cytoplasmic Ca^{2+} levels in Duchenne muscular dystrophy lymphocytes. Muscle and Nerve 8:317

Kohlschütter A, Wiesmann U N, Herschkowitz N, Ferber E 1976 Phospholipid composition of cultivated skin fibroblasts in Duchenne's muscular dystrophy. Clinica Chimica Acta 70:463

Kondo F, Abe E, Ikeda M 1967 Occasional appearance of diphosphopyridine nucleotide in urine of patients with progressive muscular dystrophy. Tohoku Journal of Experimental Medicine 91:191

Koufen H, Consbruch U 1970 Die Serum-Creatin-Phosphokinase-(CPK)-Aktivität bei amyotropher

Lateralsklerose (ALS) und anderen neurogenen Muskelatrophien unter Berücksichtigung differentialdiagnosticher Aspekte. Der Nervenarzt 41:599

Kowalewski S, Rotthauwe H-W 1972 LDH-Isoenzyme in Muskel bei neuromuskulären Erkrankungen und bei Konduktorinnen der recessiv X-chromosomalen Muskeldystrophie (Duchenne). Zeitschrift für Kinderheilkunde 113:55

Kremzner L T, Tennyson V M, Miranda A F 1978 Polyamine metabolism in normal, denervated and dystrophic muscle. Advances in Polyamine Research 2:241

Kunze D, Rüstow B, Olthoff D 1980 Studies of selected enzymes of phospholipid metabolism in the dystrophic human muscle. Clinica Chimica Acta 108:211

Lane R J M, Maskrey P, Nicholson G A et al 1979 An evaluation of some carrier detection techniques in Duchenne muscular dystrophy. Journal of the Neurological Sciences 43:377

Lane R J M, Roses A D 1981 Variation of serum creatine kinase levels with age in normal females: implications for genetic counselling in Duchenne muscular dystrophy. Clinica Chimica Acta 113:75

Lane R J M, Watmough N J, Champaneria S, Pennington R J T 1986 Creatin kinase activity in human skeletal muscle membranes. Biochemical Society Transactions 14:126

Leiris de J, Peyrot M, Feuvray D 1978 Pharmacological reduction of ischaemia-induced enzyme release from isolated rat hearts. Journal of Molecular Medicine 3:11

Lin C H, Hudson A J, Strickland K P 1972 Fatty acid oxidation by skeletal muscle mitochondria in Duchenne muscular dystrophy. Life Sciences (Part II) 11:355

Lin C H, Hudson A J, Strickland K P 1976 Palmityl-CoA synthetase activity in the muscle of dystrophic mice. Life Sciences 18:613

Livingstone I R, Gardner-Medwin D, Pennington R J T, Walton J N 1982 Serum creatine kinase and pyruvate kinase activities in normal adolescent females. Journal of the Neurological Sciences 54:349

Lloyd, R D, Mays C W, McFarland S S, Zundel, W S, Tyler F H 1973 Metabolism of ⁸³Rb and ¹³⁷Cs in persons with muscle disease. Radiation Research 54:463

Lloyd S J, Emery A E H 1981 A possible circulating plasma factor in Duchenne muscular dystrophy. Clinica Chimica Acta 112:85

Lockshin R A, Beaulaton J 1974 Programmed cell death. Cytochemical evidence for lysosomes during the normal breakdown of the intersegmental muscles. Journal of Ultrastructure Research 46:43

Lou M F 1979 Human muscular dystrophy: elevation of urinary dimethylarginines. Science 203:668

Lundblad A, Svensson S, Yamashina I, Ohta M 1979 Increased urinary excretion of a glucose-containing tetrasaccharide in patients with Duchenne muscular dystrophy. FEBS Letters 97:249

Lundholm K, Bylund A, Holm J, Schersten T 1976 Skeletal muscle metabolism in patients with malignant tumour. European Journal of Cancer 12:465

Lunt G G, Marchbanks R M (eds) 1978 The biochemistry of myasthenia gravis and muscular dystrophy. Academic Press, London, p 239

Luthra M G, Stern L Z, Kim H D 1979 (Ca⁺⁺ + Mg⁺⁺)-ATPase of red cells in Duchenne and myotonic dystrophy: effect of soluble cytoplasmic activator. Neurology 29:835

McCaman M W 1960 Dehydrogenase activities in dystrophic mice. Science 132:621

McKeran R O, Halliday D, Purkiss P 1978 Comparison of human myofibrillar protein catabolic rate derived from 3-methylhistidine excretion with synthetic rate from muscle biopsies during L-[α-¹⁵N]lysine infusion. Clinical Science and Molecular Medicine 54:471

McLaughlin J, Engel W K 1979 Lipid composition of erythrocytes. Findings in Duchenne's muscular dystrophy and myogenic atrophy. Archives of Neurology 36:351

McPherson A, Tokunaga J 1967 Effects of cross-innervation on the myoglobin content of tonic and phasic muscles. Journal of Physiology 188:121

Mahoney M J, Haseltine F P, Hobbins, J C, Banker B Q, Caskey C T, Golbus M S 1977 Prenatal diagnosis of Duchenne's muscular dystrophy. New England Journal of Medicine 297:968

Mann W S, Salafsky B 1970 Enzymic and physiological studies on normal and diseased developing fast and slow cat muscles. Journal of Physiology 208:33

Martinosi A 1968 Sarcoplasmic reticulum. VI. Microsomal Ca²⁺ transport in genetic muscular dystrophy of mice. Proceedings of the Society for Experimental Biology and Medicine 127:824

Maskrey P, Pluskal M G, Harris J B, Pennington R J T 1977 Studies on increased acid hydrolase activities in denervated muscle. Journal of Neurochemistry 28:403

Matheson D W, Engel W K, Derrer E C 1976 Erythrocyte shape in Duchenne muscular dystrophy. Neurology (Minneapolis) 26:1182

Matsuda I, Miyoshino S, Miike T et al 1978 Mitochondrial fraction of serum glutamic-oxaloacetic transaminase in Duchenne muscular dystrophy. Clinica Chimica Acta 83:231

Mawatari S, Igisu H, Kuroiwa Y, Myoshino S 1981 Na⁺ + K⁺ATPase of erythrocyte membranes in Duchenne muscular dystrophy. Neurology 31:293

Mawatari S, Miranda A, Rowland L P 1976 Adenyl cyclase abnormality in Duchenne muscular dystrophy: muscle cells in culture. Neurology (Minneapolis) 26:1021

Meltzer H Y 1971 Factors affecting serum creatine phosphokinase levels in the general population. The role of race, activity and age. Clinica Chimica Acta 33:165

Mendell J R, Engel W K, Derrer E C 1972a Increased plasma enzyme concentrations in rats with functional ischaemia of muscle provide a possible model of Duchenne muscular dystrophy. Nature 239:522

Mendell J R, Murphy D, Engel W K, Chase T N, Gordon E 1972b Catecholamines and indoleamines in patients with Duchenne muscular dystrophy. Archives of Neurology 27:518

Mokri B, Engel A G 1975 Duchenne dystrophy: Electron microscopic findings pointing to a basic or early abnormality in the plasma membrane of the muscle fibre. Neurology (Minneapolis) 25:1111

Monckton G, Marusyk H 1979 The incorporation of ³H(G)L-leucine into single muscle fibres in Duchenne dystrophy and Charcot–Marie–Tooth disease. Le Journal Canadien des Sciences Neurologiques 6:53

Morey K S, Tarczy-Hornoch K, Richards E G, Brown W D 1967 Myosin from dystrophic and control chicken muscle. I. Preparation and preliminary characterisation. Archives of Biochemistry 119:491

Muir W A, Knoke J, Martin A, Vignos P, McErlean A 1983 Improved detection of Duchenne muscular dystrophy heterozygotes using discriminant analysis of creatine kinase levels. American Journal of Medical Genetics 14:125

Munsat T L, Baloh R, Pearson C M, Fowler W Jr 1973 Serum enzyme alterations in neuromuscular disorders. Journal of the American Medical Association 226:1536

Murphy D L, Mendell J R, Engel W K 1973 Serotonin and platelet function in Duchenne muscular dystrophy. Archives of Neurology 28:239

Nagy B, Samaha F J 1984 Duchenne dystrophic muscles possess protease activity affecting the calcium-adenosine triphosphatase of sarcoplasmic reticulum. IRCS Medical Science: Biochemistry 12:828

Nicholson G A, Gardner-Medwin D, Pennington R J T, Walton J N 1979 Carrier detection in Duchenne muscular dystrophy: assessment of the effect of age on detection rate with serum-creatine-kinase activity. Lancet (ii):692

Nicholson L V B 1981 Serum myoglobin in muscular dystrophy and carrier detection. Journal of the Neurological Sciences 51:411

Niebroj-Dobosz I 1981 $(Na^+ + K^+) Mg^{2+}$-ATPase of muscle plasma membranes in Duchenne muscular dystrophy. Neurology 31:331

Olson E, Vignos P J Jr, Woodlock J, Perry T 1968 Oxidative phosphorylation of skeletal muscle in human muscular dystrophy. Journal of Laboratory and Clinical Medicine 71:220

Omaye S T, Tappel A L 1974 Glutathione peroxidase, glutathione reductase and thiobarbituric acid-reactive products in muscles of chickens and mice with genetic muscular dystrophy. Life Sciences 15:137

Oppenheimer H, Milhorat A T 1961 Serum proteins, lipoproteins and glycoproteins in muscular dystrophy and related diseases. Annals of the New York Academy of Sciences 94 (I):308

Oppenheimer H, Bárány K, Milhorat A T 1964 Myosin from mice with hereditary muscular dystrophy. Proceedings of the Society for Experimental Biology and Medicine 116:877

Park D C, Parsons M E, Pennington R J T 1973 Evidence for mast cell origin of proteinase in skeletal muscle homogenates. Biochemical Society Transactions 1:730

Parsons M E, Parsons R, Pennington R J T 1978 Peptide hydrolase activities in rat muscle cultures. International Journal of Biochemistry 9:745

Pattengale P K, Holloszy J O 1967 Augmentation of skeletal muscle myoglobin by a program of treadmill running. American Journal of Physiology 213:783

Paulson O B, Engel A G, Gomez M R 1974 Muscle blood flow in Duchenne type muscular dystrophy, limbgirdle dystrophy, polymyositis and in normal controls. Journal of Neurology, Neurosurgery and Psychiatry 37:685

Pearce J M S, Pennington R J T, Walton J N 1964a Serum enzyme studies in muscle disease. Part II: Serum creatine kinase activity in muscular dystrophy and in other myopathic and neuropathic disorders. Journal of Neurology, Neurosurgery and Psychiatry 27:96

Pearce J M S, Pennington R J T, Walton J N 1964b Serum enzyme studies in muscle disease. Part III: Serum creatine kinase activity in relatives of patients with the Duchenne type of muscular dystrophy. Journal of Neurology, Neurosurgery and Psychiatry 27:181

Pellegrino C, Bibbiani C 1964 Increase of muscle permeability to aldolase in several experimental atrophies. Nature 204:483

Penn A S, Cloak R A, Rowland L P 1972 Myosin from

normal and dystrophic human muscle. Immunochemical and electrophoretic studies. Archives of Neurology 27:159

Pennington R J T 1961 5'-Adenylic acid deaminase in dystrophic mouse muscle. Nature 192:884

Pennington R J T 1963 Biochemistry of dystrophic muscle. 2. Some enzyme changes in dystrophic mouse muscle. Biochemical Journal 88:64

Pennington R J T, Robinson J E 1968 Cathepsin activity in normal and dystrophic human muscle. Enzymologia Biologica et Clinica 9:175

Pennington R J T 1977a Proteinases of muscle. In: Barrett A J (ed) Proteinases in mammalian cells and tissues. North Holland, Amsterdam, p 515

Pennington R J T 1977b Serum enzymes. In: Rowland L P (ed) Pathogenesis of human muscular dystrophies. Excerpta Medica, Amsterdam, p 341

Penny I F, Taylor M A J, Harris A G, Etherington D J 1985 Purification and immunological characterization of two calcium-activated neutral proteinases from rabbit skeletal muscle. Biochimica et Biophysica Acta 829:244

Percy M E, Andrews D F, Thompson M W, 1982 Serum creatine kinase in the detection of Duchenne muscular dystrophy carriers: effects of season and multiple testing. Muscle and Nerve 5:58

Percy M E, Pichora A, Chang L S, Manchester K E, Andrews D F 1984 Serum myoglobin in Duchenne muscular dystrophy carrier detection: a comparison with creatine kinase and hemopexin using logistic discrimination. Americal Journal of Medical Genetics 18:279

Perkoff G T, Tyler F H 1958 Creatine metabolism in the Bar Harbor strain dystrophic mouse. Metabolism 7:745

Peter J B 1971 Biochemical approaches to the study of muscle disease. Birth Defects 7:38

Peter J B, Fiehn W 1972 Distinctive lipid abnormalities in sarcolemma from patients with muscular dystrophy. Clinical Research 20:192

Peter J B, Fiehn W, Nagatomo T, Andiman R, Stempel K, Bowman R 1974 Studies of sarcolemma from normal and diseased skeletal muscle. In: Milhorat A T (ed) Exploratory concepts in muscular dystrophy, II. Excerpta Medica, Amsterdam, p 479

Poffenbarger P L, Pozefsky T, Soeldner J S 1976 The direct relationship of proinsulin-insulin hypersecretion to basal serum levels of cholesterol and triglyceride in myotonic dystrophy. Journal of Laboratory and Clinical Medicine 87:384

Prewitt M A, Salafsky B 1970 Enzymic and histochemical changes in fast and slow muscles after cross-innervation. American Journal of Physiology 218:69

Puricelli H A, Cacciatore J, Hermida M E, Toffoli de Matheos M 1961 Electrophoretic investigations of the proteins and lipids of the plasma in Steinert's disease. Acta Neuropsichiatrica Argentina 7:293

Rapaport E 1975 The fractional disappearance rate of the separate isoenzymes of creatine phosphokinase in the dog. Cardiovascular Research 9:473

Reindorp S, Whitehead R G 1971 Changes in serum creatine kinase and other biological measurements associated with musculature in children recovering from kwashiorkor. British Journal of Nutrition 25:273

Rennie M J, Edwards R H T, Millward D J, Wolman S L, Halliday D, Matthews D E 1982 Effects of Duchenne muscular dystrophy on muscle protein synthesis. Nature 296:165

Riley D A, Allin D F 1973 The effects of inactivity, programmed stimulation and denervation on the histochemistry of skeletal muscle fibre types. Experimental Neurology 40:391

Rodan S B, Hintz R L, Sha'afi R I, Rodan G A 1974 The activity of membrane bound enzymes in muscular dystrophic chicks. Nature 252:589

Romanul F C A, Van Der Meulen J P 1966 Reversal of the enzyme profiles of muscle fibres in fast and slow muscles by cross-innervation. Nature 212:1369

Romero-Herrera A E, Lehmann H, Tomlinson B E, Walton J N 1973 Myoglobin in primary muscular disease. I. Duchenne muscular dystrophy and II. Muscular dystrophy of distal type. Journal of Medical Genetics 10:309

Rosalki S B, Thompson W H S 1971 Serum gammaglutamyl transpeptidase in muscle disease. Clinica Chimica Acta 33:264

Roses A D, Herbstreith M, Metcalf B, Appel S H 1976 Increased phosphorylated components of erythrocyte membrane spectrin band II with reference to Duchenne muscular dystrophy. Journal of Neurological Sciences 30:167

Roses, A D, Pericak-Vance M A, Yamaoka L H, Stubblefield E, Stajich J, Vance J M, Roses M J, Carter D B 1983 Recombinant DNA strategies in genetic neurological diseases. Muscle and Nerve 6:339

Rothig H-J, Bernhardt W, Afting E-G 1984 Excretion of total and muscular N-methylhistidine and creatinine in muscle diseases. Muscle and Nerve 7:374

Rowland L P 1976 Pathogenesis of muscular dystrophies. Archives of Neurology 33:315

Rowland L P, Layzer R B, Kagen L J 1968 Lack of some muscle proteins in serum of patients with Duchenne dystrophy. Archives of Neurology 18:272

Russell D H, Stern L Z 1981 Altered polyamine excretion in Duchenne muscular dystrophy. Neurology 31:80

Samaha F J, Congedo C Z 1977 Two biochemical types of Duchenne dystrophy: Sarcoplasmic reticulum membrane proteins. Annals of Neurology 1:125

Samaha F J, Thies W H 1979 Myosin light chains in Duchenne dystrophy and paraplegic muscle. Neurology 29:122

Samaha F J, Davis B, Nagy B 1981 Duchenne muscular dystrophy: adenosine triphosphate and creatine phosphate content in muscle. Neurology 31:916

Schiaffino S, Hanzlikova V 1972 Studies on the effect of denervation in developing muscle. II. The lysosomal system. Journal of Ultrastructure Research 39:1

Schirmer R H, Thuma E 1972 Sensitivity of adenylate kinase isozymes from normal and dystrophic human muscle to sulfhydryl reagents. Biochimica et Biophysica Acta 268:92

Schliselfeld L H, Barany M, Danon M J, Abraham E, Kleps R A 1981 Lysolecithin phospholipase activities of muscles from control and Duchenne muscular dystrophy subjects. Molecular Physiology 1:61

Schmalbruch H 1975 Segmental fibre breakdown and defects of the plasmalemma in diseased human muscle. Acta Neuropathologica 33:129

Schorr E E C, Arnason B G W, Aström K, Darzynkiewicz Z 1978 Treatment of mouse muscular dystrophy with the protease inhibitor pepstatin. Journal of Neuropathology and Experimental Neurology 37:263

Schotland D L, Bonilla E 1977 Myotonic dystrophy: Alteration in the internal molecular architecture of the muscle plasma membrane. Neurology (Minneapolis) 27:379

Schotland D L, Bonilla E, Van Meter M 1977 Duchenne dystrophy: Alteration in muscle plasma membrane structure. Science 196:1005

Schwartz W N, Bird J W C 1977 Degradation of myofibrillar proteins by cathepsins B and D. Biochemical Journal 167:811

Sha'afi R I, Rodan S B, Hintz R L, Fernandez S M, Rodan G A 1975 Abnormalities in membrane microviscosity and ion transport in genetic muscular dystrophy. Nature 254:525

Shannon A D, Adams E P, Courtice F C 1974 The lysosomal enzymes acid phosphatase and β-glucuronidase in muscle following a period of ischaemia. Australian Journal of Experimental Biology and Medical Science 52:157

Shapira Y A, Patz D, Menczel J et al 1984 Low serum 24, 25-dihydroxyvitamin D in Duchenne muscular dystrophy. Neurology 34:1192

Sica R E P, McComas A J 1978 The neural hypothesis of muscular dystrophy. Le Journal Canadien des Sciences Neurologiques 5:189

Silverman L M, Mendell J R, Sahenk Z, Fontana M B 1976 Significance of creatine phosphokinase isoenzymes in Duchenne muscular dystrophy. Neurology (Minneapolis) 26:561

Simpson J, Zellweger H, Burmeister L F, Christee R, Nielsen M K 1974 Effect of oral contraceptive pills on the level of creatine phosphokinase with regard to carrier detection in Duchenne muscular dystrophy. Clinica Chimica Acta 52:219

Smith H L, Fischer R L, Etteldorf J N 1962 Magnesium and calcium in human muscular dystrophy. American Journal of Diseases of Children 103:771

Smoller M, Fineberg R A 1965 Studies of myosin in hereditary muscular dystrophy in mice. Journal of Clinical Investigation 44:615

Somer H 1980 Enzyme release from isolated erythrocytes and lymphocytes in Duchenne muscular dystrophy. Journal of the Neurological Sciences 48:445

Stauber W T, Ong S-H 1981 Fluorescence demonstration of cathepsin B activity in skeletal, cardiac and vascular smooth muscle. Journal of Histochemistry and Cytochemistry 29:866

Stern L Z, Ringel S P, Ziter F A, Menander-Huber K B, Ionasescu V, Pellegrino R J, Snyder R D 1982 Drug trial of superoxide dismutase in Duchenne's muscular dystrophy. Archives of Neurology 39:342

Stracher A, McGowan E B, Shafiq A 1978 Muscular dystrophy: inhibition of degeneration in vivo with protease inhibitors. Science 200:50

Sugita H, Toyokura Y 1976 Alteration of troponin subunits in progressive muscular dystrophy (DMP). II. Mechanism of the alteration of troponin subunits in DMP. Proceedings of the Japan Academy 52:260

Sylvester R, Baskin R J 1973 Kinetics of calcium uptake in normal and dystrophic sarcoplasmic reticulum. Biochemical Medicine 8:213

Szibor R, Till U, Losche W, Steinbicker V 1981 Red cell response to A23187 and valiomycine in Duchenne muscular dystrophy. Acta Biologica et Medica Germanica 40:1187

Takahashi K, Shutta K, Matsuo B, Takai T, Takao H, Imura H 1977 Serum creatine kinase isoenzymes in Duchenne muscular dystrophy. Clinica Chimica Acta 75:435

Tanaka K, Takeshita K, Takita M 1982 Abnormalities of

bile from patients with myotonic muscular dystrophy. Clinical Science 62:627

Thompson R G, Sponder E S, Rosenmann E, Hamerton J L, Wrogemann K 1982 Proline incorporation by cultured skin fibroblasts from patients with Duchenne muscular dystrophy. Journal of the Neurological Sciences 57:41

Thompson R G, Nickel B, Finlayson S, Meuser R, Hamerton J L, Wrogemann K 1983 56K fibroblast protein not specific for Duchenne muscular dystrophy but for skin biopsy site. Nature 304:740

Thomas N S T, Harper P S 1978 Myotonic dystrophy: Studies on the lipid composition and metabolism of erythrocytes and skin fibroblasts. Clinica Chimica Acta 83:13

Thomson W H S, Sweetin J C, Elton R A 1974 The neurogenic and myogenic hypotheses in human (Duchenne) muscular dystrophy. Nature 249:151

Tippett P A, Dennis N R, Machin D, Price C P, Clayton B E 1982 Creatine kinase activity in the detection of carriers of Duchenne muscular dystrophy: comparison of two methods. Clinica Chimica Acta 121:345

Tsuchiya Y, Sugita H, Ishiura S, Imahori K 1981 Spectrin extractability from erythrocytes in Duchenne muscular dystrophies and the effect of proteases on erythrocyte ghosts. Clinica Chimica Acta 109:285

Tsung P, Palek J 1980 Red cell membrane protein phosphorylation in hemolytic anemias and muscular dystrophies. Muscle and Nerve 3:55

Tzvetanova E 1971 Creatine kinase isoenzymes in muscle tissue of patients with neuromuscular diseases amd human fetuses. Enzyme 12:279

Ulreich J B, Stern L Z, Holubec H, Chvapil M 1982 Dystrophic and normal fibroblast activity modulated by sera from patients with Duchenne muscular dystrophy. Abstracts of the 5th International Congress on Neuromuscular Diseases, No. M066

Van Pilsum J F, Wolin E A 1958 Guanidinium compounds in blood and urine of patients suffering from muscle disorders. Journal of Laboratory and Clinical Medicine 51:219

Verrill H L, Pickard N A, Gruemer H D 1977 Mechanisms of cellular enzyme release. I. Alteration in membrane fluidity and permeability. Clinical Chemistry 23:2219

Vignos P J, Lefkowitz M 1959 A biochemical study of certain skeletal muscle constituents in human progressive muscular dystrophy. Journal of Clinical Investigation 38:873

Vrbová G 1983 Hypothesis; Duchenne dystrophy viewed as a disturbance of nerve–muscle interactions. Muscle and Nerve 6:671

Wagner K R, Kauffman F C, Max S R 1978 The pentose phosphate pathway in regenerating skeletal muscle. Biochemical Journal 170:17

Wakamatsu H, Nakamura H, Ito K et al 1970 Serum desmosterol and other lipids in myotonic dystrophy. A possible pathogenesis of myotonic dystrophy. Keio Journal of Medicine 19:145

Webb J N 1974 Muscular dystrophy and muscle cell death in normal and fetal development. Nature 252:233

West D P, Ellis D A, Strickland J M 1977 Incorporation of U-^{14}C glucose into neutral lipids and sn-glycerol-3-phosphate in muscle from Duchenne muscular dystrophy and control patients. Journal of the Neurological Sciences 33:131

Wieme R J, Lauryssens M J 1962 Lactate dehydrogenase multiplicity in normal and diseased human muscle. Lancet 1:433

Wildenthal K 1978 Lysosomal alterations in ischaemic myocardium: Result or cause of myocellular damage? Journal of Molecular and Cellular Cardiology 10:595

Williams E R, Bruford A 1970 Creatine phosphokinase in motor neurone disease. Clinica Chimica Acta 27:53

Wochner R D, Drews G, Strober W, Waldmann T A 1966 Accelerated breakdown of immunoglobulin G (IgG) in myotonic dystrophy: A hereditary error of immunoglobulin catabolism. Journal of Clinical Investigation 45:321

Woo Y, Manery J E 1975 5'-Nucleotidase: an ecto-enzyme of frog muscle. Biochimica et Biophysica Acta 397:144

Wright T L, O'Neill J A, Olson W H 1973 Abnormal intrafibrillar monoamines in sex-linked muscular dystrophy. Neurology (Minneapolis) 23:511

Wrogemann K, Nylen E G 1978 Mitochondrial calcium overloading in cardiomyopathic hamsters. Journal of Molecular and Cellular Cardiology 10:185

Yarom R, Meyer S, More R, Liebergall M, Eldor A 1983 Platelet abnormalities in muscular dystrophy. Thrombosis and Haemostasis 49:168

Yasmineh W G, Ibrahim G A, Abbasnezhad M, Awad E A 1978 Isoenzyme distribution of creatine kinase and lactate dehydrogenase in serum and skeletal muscle in Duchenne muscular dystrophy, collagen disease and other muscular disorders. Clinical Chemistry 24:1985

Zatz M, Schapiro L J, Campion D S, Oda E, Kaback M M 1978 Serum pyruvate-kinase (PK) and creatine phosphokinase (CPK) in progressive muscular dystrophies. Journal of the Neurological Sciences 36:349

Zierler K, Folk B P, Magladery J W, Lilienthal J L Jr 1949 On creatinuria in man. The roles of the renal tubule and of muscle mass. Bulletin of the Johns Hopkins Hospital 85:370

Clinical examination, differential diagnosis and classification

INTRODUCTION

The neuromuscular disorders are those conditions in which the patient's symptoms result from abnormalities in the lower motor neurones (including the motor nuclei of the cranial nerves, the anterior horn cells of the spinal cord, the spinal motor roots, the motor fibres of the peripheral nerves), the neuromuscular junction and the voluntary muscles themselves. Lesions or pathological processes involving the spinal cord, spinal roots or peripheral nerves often involve sensory as well as motor pathways, thus causing pain, paraesthesiae and sensory loss which may vary in character and distribution depending upon the nature and site of the lesion or process concerned. Some such symptoms and their accompanying signs are considered in Chapters 24 and 27. This chapter concentrates upon the clinical manifestations of motor dysfunction resulting from disease of the neuromuscular apparatus.

SYMPTOMS AND SIGNS IN NEUROMUSCULAR DISEASE

Although the neuromuscular disorders are many, the symptoms which they produce are few, pain and weakness being the most frequent; limpness, fatigue, wasting, spontaneous movements, palpable tenderness, local or diffuse swelling of nerves and/or muscles and contractures are the only others of importance. Often a definite diagnosis can and should be reached only after biochemical, electrophysiological and histological investigation. However, this in no way diminishes the importance of the clinical history and examination, which will usually restrict the differential diagnosis to a few conditions and will also be invaluable in indicating the best site for electromyography and muscle biopsy. These all-important investigations can be inconclusive or even misleading if a muscle in too advanced or too early a stage of the disease is chosen.

In the following catalogue of the clinical features of neuromuscular disease, symptoms and signs are often necessarily discussed together but, as far as possible, points arising from the history are mentioned before the findings on examination. Details of methods of eliciting physical signs are generally omitted but useful accounts of these are given in de Jong (1979), Bickerstaff (1980), Asbury & Gilliat (1984), Ross Russell & Wiles (1985) and 'Aids to the examination of the peripheral nervous system' (Medical Research Council 1986). Valuable information on the examination of children will be found in Paine & Oppé (1966), Gordon (1976), Dubowitz (1978), Gamstorp (1984) and Pact et al (1984).

Family history

The familial occurrence of a disorder is of obvious diagnostic help. Sometimes, however, the course of the disease may differ greatly in different family members; this can be particularly striking in infantile and juvenile spinal muscular atrophy and in glycogen-storage disease of muscle, where slowly progressive proximal weakness in one sib may bear little resemblance to the severe and rapidly fatal disease in another. Better-understood examples include the homozygous and heterozygous forms of distal muscular dystrophy, inter-sib variation in the peroneal muscular atrophy syndrome and the subclinical myopathy of female carriers of the Duchenne dystrophy gene.

On the whole it is among the X-linked and autosomal dominant conditions that the family history is most helpful; the early diagnosis of Duchenne, facioscapulohumeral and myotonic muscular dystrophy or of the periodic paralyses is much easier if others in the family have been affected. In obscure myopathies parental consanguinity may, on the other hand, direct attention to the possibility of an autosomal recessive disorder. The patient's statement that there is 'no

family history of muscle disease' should not be accepted without a detailed pedigree enquiry. Especially in myotonic dystrophy, facioscapulohumeral dystrophy, peroneal muscular atrophy and its variants and in the congenital myopathies it is a common experience to find previously unrecognised cases when the whole family is carefully examined.

Muscle pain at rest

Painful muscular contraction is the basis of many common symptoms, including tension headache, low back pain and 'fibrositis'. Fear, often irrational and unconscious (such as that associated with depression and anxiety), and minor trauma may each be responsible. In a particularly sophisticated form these mechanisms may give rise to writer's cramp and other occupational neuroses. (I do not accept the view that these disorders represent focal forms of dystonia.) Painful muscle spasm is also a common accompaniment of joint disease. Furthermore, pain is often referred to muscle from other sites. These banal but important conditions are usually easily recognised if considered.

Cramp is a transient, involuntary and painful localised muscular contraction which may follow unaccustomed exertion, or result from sodium depletion, uraemia, tetany or drugs but is much more often unexplained. In spinal cord lesions, especially multiple sclerosis, *flexor spasms* due to spasticity may be very painful. In *compression of spinal roots or nerves* resulting, say, from intervertebral disc disease or peripheral nerve entrapment, pain often radiates along the cutaneous dermatome innervated by the sensory component of the spinal or peripheral nerve concerned, but sometimes dull aching pain is felt in the muscles innervated by its motor component. Nerve trunks may become tender or painful on palpation or stretching when one or more component roots is so affected, or at or near sites of entrapment. Tapping over a nerve at such a site can give, not only pain, but also paraesthesiae radiating down its cutaneous sensory distribution. *Neuralgic amyotrophy* begins with severe aching pain in the shoulder or arm followed after a few days by wasting and weakness which usually involves the serratus anterior, trapezius, deltoid, biceps or spinati. Often there is a preceding febrile illness. The pain generally clears up after a few weeks and the weakness after a few months but both may persist for several months and weakness is very occasionally permanent. In both *poliomyelitis* and the *Guillain–Barré syndrome* the onset of weakness may be preceded by pain, and in poliomyelitis there is often visible fasciculation at this stage. Other painful *polyneuropathies* are those associated with alcoholism, porphyria, arsenic poisoning and polyarteritis nodosa. In yet others, including those due to deficiency of vitamin B1 or B12, the muscles are tender. In diabetic amyotrophy, usually due to a mononeuropathy of the femoral nerve, less often of the lumbar plexus, there is pain in and atrophy of the quadriceps or rarely of other muscles. Myalgia is common in virus infections and varies in severity from the commonly experienced in influenza, to the more severe pain of benign myalgic encephalomyelitis and the very severe diaphragmatic pain of *Coxsackie B myalgia (Bornholm disease)*. *Polymyalgia rheumatica* affects elderly people who may be severely incapacitated by muscular pains in the arms and legs without weakness or sensory change; the ESR is always raised and the condition responds well to steroid therapy. *Polymyositis* is not often painful but some muscular tenderness is found in acute and severe cases.

Pain on exertion

This is usually attributable to muscle ischaemia, illustrated by the familiar experiment of exercising the forearm muscles with a cuff at above arterial pressure around the arm or by 'intermittent claudication' resulting from atherosclerotic occlusion of the iliac or femoro-popliteal arteries. Occasionally the weakness and paraesthesiae in the leg and foot during walking, which result from intermittent ischaemia of the spinal cord or cauda equina, may cause confusion. In *McArdle's disease* (myophosphorylase deficiency), and related disorders of muscle glycolytic metabolism including phosphofructokinase deficiency, the earliest symptom is usually an aching sensation in the calves during walking, becoming more painful if the patient perseveres; other muscles become similarly

painful, often with temporary contracture, if vigorously exercised. However, many patients with this symptom are investigated enthusiastically with disappointingly negative results, and the cause of benign exertional cramps in otherwise apparently healthy people is poorly understood. Undoubtedly some patients who complain bitterly of diffuse muscular pain brought on or accentuated by exercise are tense, introspective and obsessional and some respond to treatment with antidepressive and/or tranquillising remedies, but there is a small group of individuals presumed to have an as yet unidentified metabolic disorder of muscle in whom exertional muscle pain may be dramatically relieved by calcium antagonist drugs such as verapamil (Walton 1981, Lane et al 1986). Some such patients may prove to have Ca^{2+} ATPase deficiency. Rare causes of exertional muscle pain and cramp, often associated with myoglobinuria, include some of the lipid storage myopathies and especially carnitine palmityl transferase deficiency. Sometimes cramp on exertion is a feature of muscular dystrophy, early motor neurone disease or even early spasticity but it is rarely, if ever, a presenting symptom in the absence of other signs of these disorders.

Weakness as a symptom

The disability to which muscle weakness gives rise depends not only on the muscles involved but upon the patient's way of life. Few people use any of their muscles to full capacity and sometimes quite profound weakness goes unnoticed by apparently intelligent people. It is not, therefore, surprising that difficulty in walking is a common presentation of muscle disease, as this is a form of exertion that few escape. Difficulty in running, in climbing stairs or on to bus platforms and in getting out of low chairs are the usual early symptoms of proximal lower limb weakness; often shoulder-girdle weakness is equally severe but asymptomatic. Those whose occupation involves lifting weights or the arrangement of complex hairstyles may, however, notice upper-limb weakness first. Quadriceps weakness sometimes causes sudden falls because of the resulting instability of the knee, and muscle weakness may not even be considered if the idea of 'drop attacks' enters the examiner's mind. Distal weakness leads to tripping over carpets, kerbs and stairs and to weakness of the hands often first described as clumsiness. Patients who complain of difficulty in walking *down* stairs often turn out to have spasticity of the legs or cerebellar ataxia.

The mode of onset and progression of the weakness are very important in neuromuscular disease. A rapid onset after a minor febrile illness may suggest poliomyelitis or the Guillain–Barré syndrome. It is less well known that spinal muscular atrophy, either Werdnig–Hoffmann disease or its benign variant, may present in this way and may then show further less rapid progression. Benign spinal muscular atrophy is also notable for its tendency to undergo static periods, lasting sometimes for many years, between phases of deterioration. Many of the hereditary myopathies progress steadily at rates which vary widely from one condition to another but tend to be fairly uniform among cases of each disease. The inflammatory myopathies, however, and especially polymyositis, have a wide spectrum of progression from a fulminating course of a few days to an indolent one spanning several decades. The periodic paralyses cause recurrent episodes of weakness which usually give little diagnostic difficulty, especially when there is a family history. In sporadic cases, thyrotoxicosis and hyperaldosteronism must be excluded. A story of remission and relapse over longer periods suggests myasthenia gravis or a relapsing peripheral neuropathy

Weakness — the patient in action

The first stage of the examination in a suspected neuromuscular disorder is to watch the patient in action — his posture and gait especially. The facial appearance can be critical in giving the first clue to the diagnosis — myotonic dystrophy is the supreme example of this among muscle disorders because of the many features which are immediately evident — baldness, apathy, atrophy of temporal and sternomastoid muscles, masseter weakness, ptosis, drooping of the cheeks and lower lip, and sometimes cataract. In facioscapulohumeral dystrophy only the everted position of the lips and the lack of facial lines may be apparent at first. Here the facial weakness must

be demonstrated by movement. The 'snarl' of myasthenia gravis is shown in Chapter 19 (Fig. 19.5). In facioscapulohumeral dystrophy the shoulders have a strikingly sloping posture and a characteristic sign is the remarkable elevation of the scapula which occurs when the arm is abducted (Ch. 15, Fig. 15.6). *Winging of the scapulae at rest* is seen in serratus palsies and in limb-girdle muscular dystrophy but it must generally be brought out by putting serratus anterior into action in the other types of muscular dystrophy and in the many other conditions in which it occurs. *Kyphoscoliosis* is seen early in Friedreich's ataxia and neurofibromatosis. In the muscular dystrophies and in the spinal muscular atrophies it may, if unchecked, become severe, but not until muscular weakness is obvious; thus it is important in management but not in the diagnosis of these conditions. However, contractures of the calf muscles and of the hip flexors can contribute significantly to the lordotic tip-toe position which patients with muscular dystrophy often adopt at a stage when the diagnosis is still in doubt. The posture and appearance of the hands and feet are characteristic and usually easy to recognise in various nerve palsies, tetany, peroneal muscular atrophy and the other hereditary neuropathies, motor neurone disease and syringomyelia.

The *gait* can be invaluable in convincing the examiner that weakness is present, and in indicating its approximate distribution. Not too much more should be expected of it and it is a mistake to suggest that any abnormal gait is 'pathognomonic' of a specific neuromuscular disorder. In general the 'steppage' gait of pure peripheral muscle weakness (e.g. in peroneal muscular atrophy) is noticeably more fluent and confident than the combination of foot-drop with sensory ataxia seen in the sensory or mixed neuropathies and in tabes. In the spastic foot-drop of pyramidal tract disease the foot is dragged rather than lifted. Mild weakness of dorsiflexion is easily detected if patients are asked to walk on their heels, and calf weakness when they walk on their toes. The waddling lordotic gait of proximal lower-limb weakness is even less specific. It is seen most typically in the childhood muscular dystrophies when it is often associated with a tip-toe stance. In benign spinal muscular atrophy and polymyositis a similar gait is common; in the former the waddle may be even more extreme but the lordosis is often less. The gait in disorders of the hip joint, such as the epiphyseal dysplasias, can be deceptively similar and in young children who cannot co-operate in muscle testing, investigations may be pursued to a late stage before a radiograph reveals the true diagnosis. In early and doubtful cases of proximal weakness it is invaluable to watch the patient running and trying to hurry up stairs. Attempts to run may resemble a 'racing walk' and the hands may push on the knees or pull on the banister when climbing stairs. These signs are usually the earliest detectable in Duchenne dystrophy.

Gowers' sign, illustrated in Chapter 15 (Fig. 15.1), is also valuable but, in the very early stages of pelvic girdle weakness, patients may be able to stand up fairly easily with only perhaps a brief push with a hand on one knee. Weakness of the quadriceps muscle is best shown during attempts to climb stairs or to stand up from a low stool without using the arms. Much can be learned by asking a patient to sit up from the lying position; weakness of the anterior neck muscles causes the head to lag instead of being the first part to be lifted from the couch, weakness of either hip flexion or of abdominal muscles can make the manoeuvre impossible, and localised weakness of upper or lower abdominal muscles will cause the umbilicus to shift from the mid position. Early paraspinal weakness can be tested when the patient is prone by asking him to lift the head and shoulders backwards from the couch.

It is also important to consider methods of assessing clinically respiratory insufficiency secondary to involvement of the muscles of the thoracic cage and diaphragm. Such weakness may develop rapidly, e.g. in acute polymyositis or in the acute polyneuropathies such as the Guillain–Barré syndrome. It sometimes develops, as a rule much more insidiously, in the muscular dystrophies and/or spinal muscular atrophies and in motor neurone disease, but much less often in the metabolic myopathies, and may then cause alveolar hypoventilation and CO_2 retention which can be easily overlooked. Breathlessness (as a symptom) and use of the accessory muscles of respiration (as a sign), if overt, imply actual or impending respiratory insufficiency, which can be confirmed, of course, by spirometry and other

appropriate respiratory function tests; but, in the first instance, asking the patient to count aloud as quickly as possible without taking a breath is a simple and useful bedside test: inability to count beyond about 15 implies potentially grave insufficiency, possibly requiring assisted respiration. Diaphragmatic movement can be crudely assessed by observing movement of the abdominal wall during deep inspiration and expiration, intercostal efficiency by observing the movements of the chest wall. Indrawing of the lower ribs at the diaphragmatic attachment during inspiration as a result of intercostal weakness is an important (and common) sign in Werdnig–Hoffman disease; unilateral or bilateral diaphragmatic paralysis develops in some cases of limb-girdle muscular dystrophy, chronic spinal muscular atrophy and motor neurone disease.

For comparative studies and particularly in treatment trials it is useful to record, not only the strength of individual muscles, but also the patient's overall disability. The following scheme, modified from Vignos & Archibald (1960), is suitable for cases of muscular dystrophy but can be adapted for other purposes if, e.g., information about early loss of function in the arms or bulbar muscles is important.

Grade 0 Preclinical. All activities normal.
Grade 1 Walks normally. Unable to run freely.
Grade 2 Detectable defect in posture or gait. Climbs stairs without using the banister.
Grade 3 Climbs stairs only with the banister.
Grade 4 Walks without assistance. Unable to climb stairs.
Grade 5 Walks without assistance. Unable to rise from a chair.
Grade 6 Walks only with calipers or other aids.
Grade 7 Unable to walk. Sits erect in a chair. Able to roll a wheelchair and eat and drink normally.
Grade 8 Sits unsupported in chair. Unable to roll wheelchair or unable to drink from a glass unassisted.
Grade 9 Unable to sit erect without support or unable to eat or drink without assistance.
Grade 10 Confined to bed. Requires help for all activities.

In the early stages further quantitative information can be gained by timing the patient walking over measured distances, climbing standard stairs, standing up from the supine position or from a low chair, or from low stools of graded height. In children especially these functional muscle tests are more valid than measurements of strengths of individual muscles.

Weakness — detailed muscle testing

The examiner of a patient with muscular weakness must determine whether weakness is genuine or spurious, its degree, distribution and symmetry and whether it changes after exercise. The last point is dealt with in the section on fatiguability.

The question of the reality of the weakness is put first, not through cynicism, but because it poses a common problem. Ill patients can develop severe weakness which is easily missed unless careful muscle testing is performed. Compression neuropathies following general anaesthesia, and drug-induced neuropathies developing in the course of illnesses such as tuberculosis or renal failure are obvious examples, but perhaps most notable is the myopathy associated with osteomalacia in renal failure or malabsorption, which is very commonly ignored. In addition, weakness in myasthenia gravis or thyrotoxic myopathy has been attributed to neurasthenia. The obverse problem of spurious or hysterical weakness masquerading as neuromuscular disease is more easily dealt with because the situation invites careful neurological examination. Spasticity and extrapyramidal rigidity or akinesia may give an initial impression of weakness. Pain due to joint disease is a common pitfall in muscle testing and is especially liable to cause confusion at the hips and knees. The position is often made more complex by the genuine weakness and wasting which may develop, e.g. in the quadriceps in rheumatoid disease or osteoarthritis of the knee, or in the small muscles of an arthritic hand. The diagnosis of hysterical weakness or malingering depends chiefly on the discovery of inconsistencies when the clinical signs are considered as a whole, but much can be learned in the course of manual muscle testing. There is often a momentary initial contraction of reasonable strength, followed by a sudden 'give' in the resistance, not found in true weakness except in the presence of pain. An important caveat relates to the curiously intermittent muscular contraction, or rapid fatigue resembling this sign, which are common in so-called benign myalgic encephalomyelitis. Some believe firmly that this syndrome is organic while others are equally adamant that it is often a manifestation of mass hysteria. The other useful sign in malingering and the less sophisticated degrees of hysteria is a display of massive apparent effort to little effect accompanied by simultaneous contraction in agonist and antagonist muscles, with a failure of synergist and stabilising muscles to contract, although they are strong when tested separately. Thus, in testing quadriceps in a case of suspected hysteria, an unobtrusive hand on the hamstrings on the same side may give valuable information.

Much can be learned about the extent and severity of muscle weakness by watching the patient in action, walking, hopping, jumping, climbing stairs, getting up from the floor or from a chair, sitting up from a couch, trying to lift his arms above his head or writing his name. A great deal of time can be saved by these tests and, indeed, some muscles such as those of the abdomen and trunk cannot be satisfactorily tested in any other way. In examining young children this may be the only possible approach. However, detailed information is best acquired by manual testing of each muscle or group in turn. The proper methods for these tests are briefly summarised in Table 14.1 and are more fully described and illustrated in several texts including Bickerstaff (1980), the Medical Research Council memorandum (1986) and Pact et al (1984). A few of the more important tests are illustrated in Figures 14.1–14.5. The precise positioning of the limb and of the examiner's resistance are very important but, with practice, the methods are reliable. Usually isometric resistance is applied to the fully contracted muscle until it gives way (the 'break' test) but in some circumstances it is useful to test a muscle's strength throughout its full range of movement. It is best to palpate the contracting muscle at the same time. The results are usually expressed on the scale used in the Medical Research Council memorandum (1986):

Table 14.1 The nerve and root supply of the principal muscles with methods of testing their actions. Modified from Gray's Anatomy (1967) and M.R.C. memorandum (1986). Where any single root supplying a particular muscle is more important than the others it is printed in bold type.

Nerve	Muscle	Roots	Action tested
Accessory nerve	Trapezius	spinal root	Elevation of shoulders. Adduction of scapulae
	Sternocleidomastoid	spinal root	Tilting of head to same side with rotation to opposite side
Brachial plexus	Pectoralis major		
	Clavicular part	**C5**, C6	Adduction of elevated arm
	Sternocostal part	C6, **C7**, **C8**	Adduction and forward depression of arm
	Serratus anterior	C5, C6, C7	Fixation of the scapula during forward thrusting of the arm
	Rhomboids	C4, C5	Elevation and fixation of scapulae
	Supraspinatus	**C5**, C6	Initiation of abduction of arm
	Infraspinatus	**C5**, C6	External rotation of arm
	Latissimus dorsi	C6, **C7**, C8	Adduction of horizontal, externally rotated arm. Coughing
Axillary nerve	Deltoid	**C5**, C6	Lateral and forward elevation of arm to horizontal
Musculocutaneous nerve	Biceps	**C5**, C6	Flexion of the supinated forearm
	Brachialis		
Radial nerve	Triceps	C6, **C7**, C8	Extension of forearm
	Brachioradialis	C5; **C6**	Flexion of semi-prone forearm
	Extensor carpi radialis longus	**C6**	Extension of wrist to radial side
Posterior interosseus nerve	Supinator	C6, C7	Supination of extended forearm
	Extensor digitorum	**C7**, C8	Extension of proximal phalanges
	Extensor carpi ulnaris	**C7**, C8	Extension of wrist to ulnar side
	Extensor indicis	**C7**, C8	Extension of proximal phalanx of index finger
	Abductor pollicis longus	**C7**, C8	Abduction of first metacarpal in plane at right angle to palm
	Extensor pollicis longus	**C7**, C8	Extension at first interphalangeal joint
	Extensor pollicis brevis	**C7**, C8	Extension at first metacarpophalangeal joint
Median nerve	Pronator teres	C6, C7	Pronation of extended forearm
	Flexor carpi radialis	C6, C7	Flexion of wrist to radial side
	Flexor digitorum superficialis	C7, **C8**, T1	Flexion of middle phalanges
	Abductor pollicis brevis (ulnar nerve rarely)	C8, **T1**	Abduction of first metacarpal in plane at right angle to palm
	Flexor pollicis brevis (more often ulnar nerve)	C8, **T1**	Flexion of proximal phalanx of thumb
	Opponens pollicis (rarely ulnar nerve)	C8, **T1**	Opposition of thumb against fifth finger
	1st and 2nd lumbricals	C8, **T1**	Extension of middle phalanges while proximal phalanges are fixed in extension
Anterior interosseous nerve	Flexor digitorum profundus (lateral part)	**C8**, T1	Flexion of terminal phalanges of index and middle fingers
	Flexor pollicis longus	**C8**, T1	Flexion of distal phalanx of the thumb
Ulnar nerve	Flexor carpi ulnaris	C7, **C8**, T1	Observe tendon during testing abductor digiti minimi
	Flexor digitorum profundus (medial part)	C7, **C8**	Flexion of distal phalanges of ring and little fingers
	Hypothenar muscles	C8, **T1**	Abduction and opposition of little finger
	3rd and 4th lumbricals	C8, **T1**	Extension of middle phalanges while proximal phalanges are fixed in extension
	Adductor policis	C8, **T1**	Adduction of thumb against palmar surface of index finger
	Flexor pollicis brevis (sometimes median nerve)	**C8**, T1	Flexion of proximal phalanx of the thumb
	Interossei	C8, **T1**	Abduction and adduction of the fingers

Table 14.1 — continued

Nerve	Muscle	Roots	Action tested
Femoral nerve	Iliopsoas (and lumbar nerves)	**L1**, **L2**2, L3	Hip flexion from semi-flexed position
	Sartorius	L2, L3	Hip flexion from externally rotated position
	Quadriceps (rectus femoris and the lateral and medial vasti)	L2, **L3**, **L4**	Extension at the knee
Obturator nerve	Adductor longus magnus* brevis	**L2**, **L3**, L4	Adduction of the thigh
Superior gluteal nerve	Gluteus medius	**L4**, **L5**, S1	Abduction of the thigh. Internal rotation of the thigh
	Tensor fasciae latae	L4, L5	
Inferior gluteal nerve	Gluteus maximus	**L5**, **S1**, S2	Extension of the thigh
Sciatic nerve	Biceps femoris	L5, **S1** S2	
	Semitendinosus	L5, **S1**, S2	Flexion at the knee
	Semimembranosus	L5, **S1**, S2	
Peroneal nerve (deep)	Anterior tibial	**L4**, L5	Dorsiflexion of the foot
	Extensor digitorum longus	**L5**, S1	Dorsiflexion of the toes
	Extensor hallucis longus	**L5**, S1	Dorsiflexion of great toe
	Extensor digitorum brevis	L5, S1	Dorsiflexion of the toes
Peroneal nerve (superfic.)	Peroneus longus	L5, S1	Eversion of the foot
	Peroneus brevis		
Tibial nerve	Gastrocnemius	**S1**, S2	Plantar-flexion of the foot
	Soleus	S1, **S2**	
	Tibialis posterior	L4, **L5**	Inversion of plantar-flexed foot
	Flexor digitorum longus	L5, **S1**, **S2**	Flexion of toes (distal phalanges)
	Flexor hallucis longus	L5, **S1**, **S2**	Flexion of great toe (distal phalanx)
	Flexor digitorum brevis	S1, S2	Flexion of toes (middle phalanges)
	Flexor hallucis brevis	S1, S2	Flexion of great toe (proximal phalanx)
Pudendal nerve	Perineal muscles	S2, S3, S4	Tension of anal sphincter

* Adductor magnus is partly supplied by the sciatic nerve.

Grade 0 No contraction.
Grade 1 Flicker or trace of contraction.
Grade 2 Active movement with gravity eliminated.
Grade 3 Active movement against gravity.
Grade 4 Active movement against gravity and resistance.
Grade 5 Normal power.

Grades 4−, 4 and 4+ may be used to indicate movement against slight, moderate and strong resistance respectively. For accurate comparative work there is no substitute for measurement, but here the difficulties of using standard methods and of eliminating gravity and friction are multiplied and skill and experience are required to assess whether the patient is exerting his full strength. Non-extensive strain gauges have theoretical advantages but, in practice, a spring balance held by the examiner is often as good an instrument as any because the 'feel' of the patient's effort can be assessed at the same time. The Hammersmith myometer gives reasonably accurate and reproducible measurements of muscle power in clinical practice (Edwards & McDonnell 1974, Dubowitz 1978).

Broadly speaking, the interpretation of any muscle weakness which is found is often an exercise in applied anatomy when the lesion is in the lower motor neurone and a matter of pattern recognition in the myopathies. The diagnosis of upper motor neurone lesions requires a combination of these approaches and is beyond the scope of this chapter. Localised weakness in a single limb is usually neurogenic although the effects of muscle trauma such as severe ischaemia or tendon rupture sometimes cause confusion. Details of the root and nerve supply of the principal muscles are given in Table 14.1. When localised weakness seems to fit into no anatomical pattern, poliomyel-

Table 14.2 An outline of some of the common patterns of muscular weakness and atrophy in various disorders

Weakness	Generalised	Mainly distal	Mainly proximal	Symmetrical — highly selective	Asymmetrical

With little or no wasting	Polymyositis
	Myasthenia gravis
	Myasthenic-
	  myopathic
	  syndrome
	Periodic paralyses
	Hypothyroidism
	Addison's disease
	Steroid myopathy
		U.M.N. lesions	Polymyositis
			Myasthenia gravis
			Myasthenic-
			  myopathic
			  syndrome
			Myopathy with
			  osteomalacia
			Periodic paralyses
			Steroid myopathy
			Hypothyroidism
			Upper motor
			  neurone lesions
				Periodic paralyses	Periodic paralyses
					Peripheral
					  neuropathy
					U.M.N. lesion

With wasting	Werdnig-
	  Hoffmann
	  disease
	Benign congenital
	  myopathies
	M.N.D.
	(Polymyositis)
		Most peripheral
		  neuropathies
		Peroneal muscular
		  atrophy
		M.N.D.
		Distal myopathy
		Myotonic
		  dystrophy*
		Ocular myopathy
		(U.M.N. lesions)
			Muscular
			  dystrophy†
			Spinal muscular
			  atrophy
			Thyrotoxic
			  myopathy
			Glycogen-storage
			  diseases
			Lipid storage
			  myopathies
			Myasthenic-
			  myopathic
			  syndrome
			Motor neuropathy
			M.N.D.
			Polymyositis
				Muscular
				  dystrophy†
				Spinal muscular
				  atrophy
				Thyrotoxic
				  myopathy
				M.N.D.
				Motor neuropathy
				Ocular myopathy
				Glycogen-storage
				  disease
				(Poliomyelitis)
					M.N.D.
					Poliomyelitis
					Peripheral
					  neuropathy
					Spinal muscular
					  atrophy
					(Limb-girdle
					  muscular
					  dystrophy)

M.N.D. = motor neurone disease. U.M.N. = upper motor neurone.

Unusual presentations are given in brackets. Causes of purely localised weakness have been excluded.
* In myotonic dystrophy the weakness is semi-distal, i.e. involves the forearm and the leg but not small hand muscles at first.
† 'Muscular dystrophy' refers to the X-linked, limb-girdle and facioscapulohumeral types.

itis and early motor neurone disease or localised spinal muscular atrophy should be considered. It is difficult to discuss briefly the patterns of muscular involvement in the various myopathies. Nor is it proper to consider the diagnostic value of these patterns without reference to other important points such as the duration and mode of progression of the disease, the presence of other symptoms, the presence or absence of wasting or reflex change, and so on. However, the information given in Table 14.2 may be helpful as an approximate guide and further details are given in the section on differential diagnosis in Chapter 15. It is of special importance to decide whether proximal muscle weakness involves all the shoulder girdle or pelvic muscles to about the same degree (e.g. as in polymyositis or thyrotoxic and other metabolic myopathies) or certain muscles selectively. A selective, symmetrical pattern of involvement in a chronic progressive myopathy is suggestive of muscular dystrophy, although spinal muscular atrophy and other disorders may imitate this. The exact distribution of this selective involvement may be of great help in distinguishing one form of muscular dystrophy from another, especially in the early stages. An atypical distribution of weakness and wasting in a case of apparent muscular dystrophy should arouse immediate suspicions about the diagnosis and will underline the need for full investigation, including muscle biopsy.

Fatiguability

Muscular weakness which is variable in degree and is made worse by repeated contraction is typical of myasthenia. It must be distinguished from simple fatigue due to slight fixed muscular

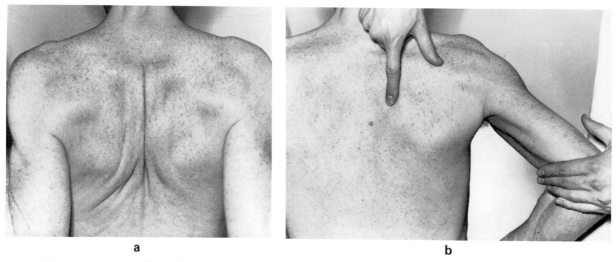

Fig. 14.1 a. The horizontal fibres of trapezius adduct the scapulae when the shoulders are braced backwards (normal subject). b. The rhomboids may be felt when the elbow is pushed backwards against resistance. The overlying trapezius is relaxed (normal subject)

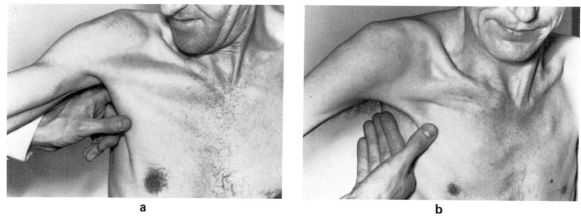

Fig. 14.2 The arm is being adducted and depressed against resistance, the sternocostal fibres of pectoralis major are clearly seen and felt. a. normal subject, b. Becker type of muscular dystrophy

weakness and from stiffness or pain induced by exercise. Clinical demonstration of myasthenia is usually possible if the strength of an affected muscle is compared with its contralateral equivalent before and after repeated contraction. The reverse phenomenon, weakness which improves during the first few contractions following rest may occur in the myasthenic–myopathic or Eaton–Lambert syndrome. The clinical features of these conditions are described in Chapters 19 and 27. Although typical cases are easily recognised,

patients do not always notice the effect of exercise. It is, therefore, wise to try the effect of intravenous edrophonium in every case of obscure muscular weakness; this should be an early investigation whenever muscular weakness is not associated with conspicuous wasting, especially if the tendon reflexes are preserved. Retention of the tendon reflexes is typical of myasthenia gravis while in the Eaton–Lambert syndrome they are lost early. Another point of distinction between these disorders is the tendency for the lower limbs

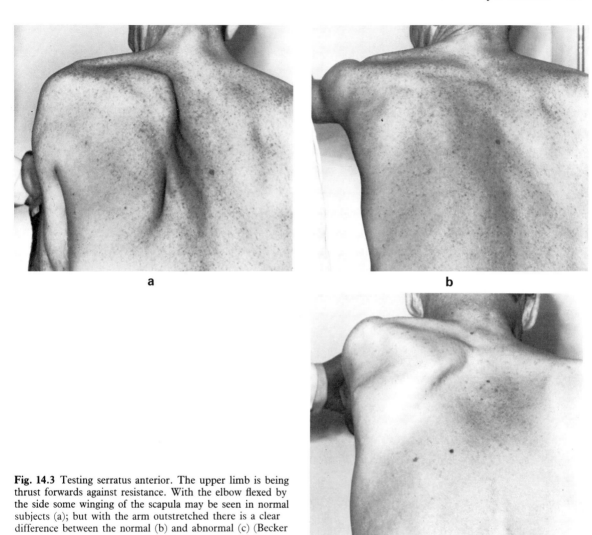

Fig. 14.3 Testing serratus anterior. The upper limb is being thrust forwards against resistance. With the elbow flexed by the side some winging of the scapula may be seen in normal subjects (a); but with the arm outstretched there is a clear difference between the normal (b) and abnormal (c) (Becker dystrophy)

to be affected first in the myasthenic–myopathic syndrome while myasthenia gravis rarely presents in this way.

Atrophy

Atrophy brings patients to the doctor much less often than weakness but may do so in motor neurone disease or syringomyelia, when the small muscles of the hand are affected, and occasionally in other disorders. As a physical sign of muscle disease, however, atrophy is second in importance only to weakness. It is particularly valuable to compare the degrees of atrophy and weakness in affected muscles; this is illustrated in Table 14.2.

In most patients atrophy can be recognised by systematic inspection of the muscles but in some women and in the obese it is difficult to assess. When asymmetry is suspected, limb girth must be measured at points equidistant from well-defined bony landmarks on the two sides. Palpation of the muscles during contraction is often helpful and computed tomography can be very useful (O'Doherty et al 1977). Sometimes confusion is caused by congenital absence of muscles (most often of pectoralis major, Fig. 14.6). Atrophy may

a b

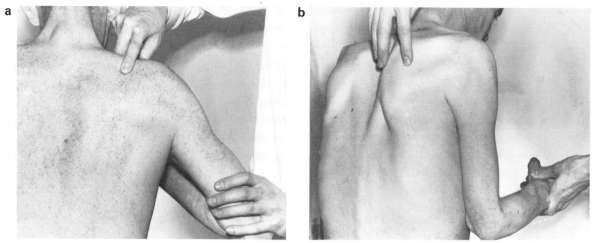

Fig. 14.4 a. Supraspinatus acts as the principal abductor with the elbow close to the trunk. Its contraction can easily be felt (normal subject). b. Infraspinatus is tested during external rotation of the arm against resistance. The wasting of the muscle can be seen and felt (Becker dystrophy)

a b

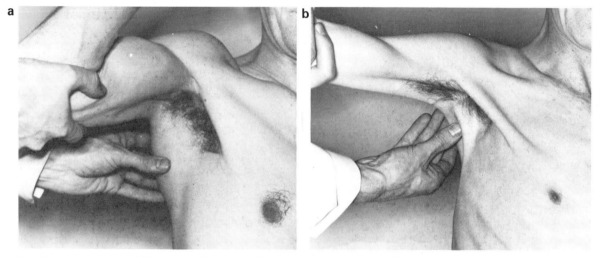

Fig. 14.5 Latissimus dorsi. The elbow of the externally rotated arm is being pushed downwards against resistance, the difference between the normal bulky muscle (a) and the wasted remnant in Becker muscular dystrophy (b) is clear

involve only part of a muscle. This is often seen in limb-girdle dystrophy or spinal muscular atrophy, in which localised dimples are seen when muscles are contracted against resistance; in the late stages the uppermost third of the deltoid muscle is often wasted and fibrotic while the lower two-thirds are soft and much bulkier, even hypertrophic. A similar combination of atrophy and hypertrophy is sometimes found in quadriceps, usually with atrophy of medial, and partial hypertrophy of lateral, vasti. Another important cause

of focal atrophy of part of a muscle is infarction. Focal atrophy may be simulated by the appearances after rupture of a tendon (e.g. long head of biceps brachii) or of the perimysial sheath (giving a muscle hernia).

The significance of patterns of muscle involvement is discussed in the section on weakness. In most lower motor neurone disorders and in many myopathies, muscle wasting and weakness go hand in hand. In motor neurone disease there tends to be proportionately more wasting and in

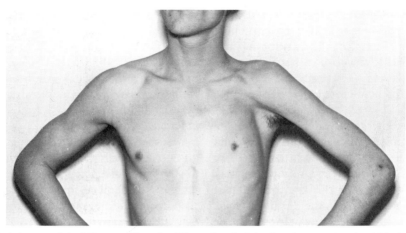

Fig. 14.6 Congenital absence of the left pectoralis major. The patient had developed a secondary brachial plexus lesion and the wasting of the left deltoid can be seen

muscular dystrophy proportionately more weakness, but these points are subtle and often not of much help. However Table 14.2 lists myopathies in which quite severe weakness may be associated with very little atrophy; because several of these are treatable, this finding should be recognised as being of great significance. The most important such conditions are myasthenia gravis, polymyositis, periodic paralysis and the myopathy of osteomalacia; careful investigation to exclude these four conditions (and other metabolic myopathies) is necessary in any case of muscle weakness in which atrophy is not prominent. Such investigations should include an edrophonium test, measurement of evoked muscle action potentials during and after repetitive nerve stimulation, electromyography (including single fibre studies with measurement of 'jitter' and 'blocking'), estimation of the serum creatine kinase activity, calcium, phosphorus, alkaline phosphatase and potassium, assay of circulating antibodies against the acetylcholine receptor (AChR) and muscle biopsy. When the weakness is recent, atrophy may not have had time to develop. Following complete traumatic denervation, clinical atrophy becomes evident after about two weeks and is maximal after about 12 weeks. Another potential pitfall is the atrophy which may develop after many years in myasthenia gravis, polymyositis, periodic paralysis and in McArdle's disease and other metabolic myopathies.

The reverse situation, muscular atrophy with little or no weakness, is common in many wasting diseases such as tuberculosis, malnutrition, carcinomatosis or simple atrophy due to ageing. In fact, muscular atrophy in the elderly, especially in certain lower limb muscles, such as soleus, is associated with histological appearances indistinguishable from those of denervation and seems to be due to a progressive loss of anterior horn cells in the spinal cord consequent upon ageing processes (Jennekens et al 1971). Some cases of thyrotoxic myopathy are masked by the generalised weight loss which occurs in this condition and similarly the myasthenic–myopathic syndrome of Eaton and Lambert sometimes goes unrecognised in the general malaise and weight loss of carcinomatosis.

Muscular hypertrophy and pseudohypertrophy

It is very doubtful whether a general increase in muscle bulk is ever a primary pathological phenomenon. Of all the muscle diseases it is seen most strikingly in myotonia congenita, where the muscle hypertrophy may resemble that of a professional weight-lifter. The strength of the muscles in this condition is consistent with their bulk and work hypertrophy induced by the myotonia seems to be responsible. It may even be that the bulky muscles seen in the 'pseudohypertrophic' forms of muscular dystrophy initially pass through a similar phase. Certainly the enlarged muscles seen in early Duchenne dystrophy are relatively strong (e.g. the calves, deltoids and lateral vastus) and contain a high proportion of hypertrophied fibres. Later in the disease replacement by fat and connective tissue sometimes maintains bulk despite muscle fibre loss. This is the stage of pseudohypertrophy. Failure to distinguish between these two stages is perhaps responsible for contradictory descriptions of the consistency of these muscles as 'rubbery' and 'inelastic' or 'firm' and 'doughy'. In fact they are generally firm while strong and soft when weak but, apart from establishing this fact, palpation of muscle is not of much help in the diagnosis of the muscular dystrophies. Only inspection of the muscles or measurement can make it clear whether they are abnormally bulky or not.

Enlargement of muscles is fairly common in limb-girdle muscular dystrophy and very common in the Becker type as well as in the Duchenne. It is also a fairly common clinical feature in manifesting carriers of the Duchenne gene. It is also seen in the myopathy of hypothyroidism and occasionally in polymyositis or cysticercosis and localised tender swellings in muscle may be a consequence of infarction (in various vasculitides), of pyogenic infection (in tropical myositis) or of localised nodular myositis (Ch. 17). However, it is not pathognomonic of myopathy as it also occurs in spinal muscular atrophy. There now seems to be general agreement that so-called hypertrophia musculorum vera is not a specific disease entity but a syndrome of diffuse muscular hypertrophy of multiple aetiology. In de Lange's syndrome of athetosis and mental defect (1934), muscle hypertrophy may be the result of continuous muscle spasm.

Spontaneous movement

Two closely similar forms of spontaneous movement may signify neuromuscular disease or dysfunction, viz., fasciculation and myokymia. Both are painless contractions of small groups of muscle fibres which may cause visible movement of the overlying skin but not usually of neighbouring joints. These points distinguish them not only from the contraction of single fibres (fibrillation) which is detectable only by electromyography or by examination of the exposed muscle which 'is involved in a confusion of very small twitches' — 'without either apparent rhythm or obvious centre of activity' (Denny-Brown & Pennybacker 1938), but also from tremor, myoclonus, chorea and other more overt movements unrelated to muscular disease. Both fasciculation and myokymia may be felt by the patient.

Fasciculations are brief twitches of groups or bundles of fibres which often involve the same group repetitively over short periods but may be totally irregular. They are best seen where the muscle is superficial, in the hands and especially the tongue and can often be induced by percussing or pinching the muscle. They occur in active degenerative disorders of the anterior horn cell but may be induced in normal individuals by anticholinesterase drugs. Fasciculation is a valuable clue to diagnosis in motor neurone disease and in spinal muscular atrophy and should be sought particularly in the tongue, which should lie relaxed in the floor of the mouth. Absence of fasciculation, however, does not by any means exclude anterior horn cell disease. Spontaneous benign fasciculation is not uncommon in normal subjects, especially in the calf or small hand muscles. It cannot be distinguished with certainty from the pathological type, but fasciculation which is seen *only* after movement or strong contraction, and is not associated with muscle weakness, is usually benign. Rarely, fasciculation occurs in inflammatory or compressive nerve root lesions, but here its character is different, for it usually involves large fasciculi and tends to occur repetitively in the same fasciculus during minimal contraction but not during complete relaxation. It corresponds to the 'giant units' recorded in the electromyogram. While exertional muscle pain and cramps are sometimes associated with benign fasciculation, some patients with this combination of symptoms appear to have a benign polyneuropathy (Hudson et al 1978).

Myokymia is sometimes used, imprecisely, simply to identify coarse, benign fasciculation but, more correctly, it refers to a slower contraction of independent small bands or strips of muscle fibres which give an undulating or rippling appearance to the overlying skin, the movement often being recognisably in the direction of the muscle fibres. The difference between the single twitch of fasciculation and the tetanic contraction of myokymia may be evident only on electromyography in difficult cases. Myokymia is rare; it is seen in some cases of thyrotoxicosis, or more often with cramp, hyperhidrosis, myotonia-like contractions and muscular atrophy in various combinations (Gamstorp & Wohlfart 1959, Gardner-Medwin & Walton 1969, Albers et al 1981). The syndrome is closely related to, if not identical with, the 'syndrome of continuous muscle fibre activity and spasm' described by Isaacs in 1961, later called 'neuromyotonia' by Mertens & Zschocke (1965), but the latter is a misnomer as the phenomenon differs from true myotonia. This activity is abolished by neuromuscular block but not by proximal nerve block, which suggests that it arises in the distal part of the α-motor neurone. It may be associated with mild peripheral neuropathy (Wallis et al 1970) and is sometimes familial (Welch et al 1972, Ashizawa et al 1983, Auger et al 1984). Most cases are sporadic and of unknown aetiology but the onset in two reported cases was related to exposure to dichlorophenoxyacetic acid herbicide (Wallis et al 1970) or an alcoholic debauch (Williamson & Brooke 1972). Rarely, laryngeal muscles are involved, causing hoarseness and exertional dyspnoea (Jackson et al 1979), while reflex myoclonus (Leigh et al 1980) and muscular stiffness and hypertrophy resembling that of the stiff-man syndrome (Valli et al 1983, Zisfein et al 1983, Auger et al 1984) have also been reported. The condition usually responds to treatment with phenytoin or carbamazepine (Zisfein et al 1983).

An interesting episodic variety of myokymia involving one side of the face (facial myokymia) may occur in multiple sclerosis or as an isolated phenomenon (Matthews 1966). The recurrent twitches of the eyelid or of particular parts of muscles, which are commonly experienced by normal people and are often called myokymia, are probably more closely related to benign fasciculations; they have no pathological significance but are often induced by fatigue.

Facial clonic spasm or hemifacial spasm is a recurrent twitch of part, or sometimes the whole, of the musculature supplied by the facial nerve on one side. Rarely it is bilateral. The movement is stereotyped in form but irregular in timing and the former point distinguishes it from chorea and facial dyskinesia. Facial tic or habit spasm is often similar, but less rapidly repeated. Tetany, tetanus and blepharospasm due to ocular irritation, to facial spasticity or to Meige's (Brueghel's) syndrome of blepharospasm-oromandibular-facial dystonia should be considered in differential diagnosis. Hemifacial spasm is an intractable condition usually seen after the fifth decade. It has been attributed to an irritative lesion of the facial nerve in its canal but is more often due to compression of the intracranial trunk of the nerve by an aberrant artery (see Walton 1985). Sometimes it is seen in geniculate herpes or Paget's disease of the skull.

Movement induced by contraction or stimulation

Myotonia is easier to describe than to define because its pathophysiology is still incompletely understood (Ch. 16). Denny-Brown & Nevin (1941) found that it persisted after nerve block or curarisation, and it is associated with a defect of chloride conductance in the muscle fibre membrane (Adrian & Marshall 1976). Clinically it is characterised by failure of the muscle to relax immediately after voluntary contraction has ceased and often a dimple persists for a few seconds after percussion of a muscle. Electromyographically a specific form of high-frequency discharge occurs after voluntary contraction on electrical or mechanical stimulation of the muscle (see Ch. 30). The diseases associated with myotonia and their differentiation are discussed in Chapter 16. In infants with myotonia the face and eyelids may fail to relax for several seconds after a sneeze or cry, the cry itself may sound strangled and the limbs may seem stiff. Later in life, patients complain of stiffness of the limbs, difficulty in walking or inability to relax the grip. Generally myotonia improves after repeated contraction and is worsened by cold. These effects are so striking in paramyotonia that it may be necessary to ask the patient to chill the hands in cold water before any abnormality can be demonstrated. Grip myotonia is shown by failure of relaxation lasting usually for 5–10 s after a tight contraction but occasionally for as long as a minute. Often the fingers and thumb remain flexed at the metacarpophalangeal joints while the other joints are extended. Percussion myotonia in the thenar eminence results not only in a dimple but in slow tonic opposition of the thumb and gradual relaxation lasting altogether 2–10 s. A small tendon hammer may be used to percuss the tongue against a spatula placed over the lower teeth when a persistent dimple is again seen. There is little difficulty in recognising myotonia once the possibility of its presence has occurred to the examiner. However, percussion myotonia may be confused with *myoidema*, an electrically silent ridge (not a depression) induced by percussion of atrophic muscles in such wasting conditions as tuberculosis and malabsorption (Denny-Brown & Pennybacker 1938, Salick & Pearson 1967). Contraction myotonia can really be mistaken only for the very similar but electrically distinct phenomenon which may be associated with myokymia (Gamstorp & Wohlfart 1959) and with the pseudomyotonia of hypothyroidism (Hoffmann's syndrome) (see Ch. 16). Leyburn & Walton (1959) described a method of quantitative assessment of myotonia for use in trials of treatment.

Tetany may be associated with hypocalcaemia, with alkalosis and possibly with hypomagnesaemia. It is heralded by tingling in the extremities or lips and, in the latent phase, spasms may be induced by nerve percussion (Chvostek's sign) or ischaemia (Trousseau's sign). Later, stridor and dyspnoea may occur and intermittent muscle cramp and spasm develop. Although these spasms can occur spontaneously they are increased by mechanical stimulation or contraction of the muscle as the excitability of both nerve and muscle is increased. They affect chiefly the hands, which adopt the 'main d'accoucheur' position, and the feet. More generalised involvement with opisthotonos may develop in severe cases and may be accompanied by colic and fits. Only in this advanced stage is tetany painful.

In *tetanus* the hyperexcitability of the nerves and muscles resembles that of tetany. In addition, however, there is usually an underlying state of continuous muscle spasm which results in the well-known features of trismus, neck retraction and the risus sardonicus. This predilection for the face and neck contrasts with the carpopedal spasm of early tetany although the muscles involved early

in tetanus may also depend on the site of the infection. Indeed the spasm may remain localised in some cases, usually in partly immunised subjects. In the later stages the spasm usually becomes widespread and any movement or external stimulus induces paroxysmal and painful exacerbations. The bite of the American Black Widow spider (*Lactrodectus mactans*) may result in a similar condition of painful muscle spasm. The *stiff-man syndrome* is a poorly understood disorder in which progressive spasms usually begin in the proximal muscles and may become generalised. It is discussed further in Chapter 27.

Cramp contracture is electrically silent shortening of the muscles induced by exertion. It is seen in McArdle's disease, phosphofructokinase deficiency and in other related forms of glycogenstorage disease of muscle (Lehoczky et al 1965, Satayoshi & Kowa 1967, and see Ch. 25). Perkoff et al (1966) showed that a similar reversible metabolic disorder with cramp contracture can occur in chronic alcoholism after heavy drinking bouts. The exercised muscle develops aching or cramping pain and then becomes stiff and weak. Continued gentle exercise allows some patients to enter a 'second wind' stage with lessening of the pain as they continue. More often the pain forces them to halt and if the muscle is then examined it is found to be shortened, tense and tender. Only electromyography can distinguish this from true cramp in doubtful cases. The contracture lasts from a few minutes to several hours, depending on its severity. Very severe pain which passes off rapidly is not due to McArdle's disease.

Muscle tone

In infants hypotonia is an early and important indication of muscle disease. The problem of diagnosis of the 'floppy infant' is dealt with in Chapter 20 and all that needs to be said here is that the cause may lie in the brain (especially the parietal lobes and cerebellum), the anterior horns or posterior columns of the spinal cord, the motor or sensory nerves, the myoneural junctions or the muscle fibres and possibly sometimes in the muscle spindles or ligaments. Hypotonia can also result from malnutrition, malabsorption and metabolic disorders. Part of the diagnostic problem may lie in the failure to define the precise meaning of tone and hypotonia. André-Thomas et al (1960) described methods for testing several different aspects of muscle tone, each of which may be disturbed independently. Thus the *consistency* of a muscle may be tested by wobbling it laterally with a finger, by shaking the limbs and by palpation, its *extensibilité* by slow movement of joints through their full range and its *'passivité'* by, e.g., measuring the amplitude of the flapping movement when the proximal part of a limb is shaken. The *recoil* of a muscle suddenly released from a fully stretched position is another manifestation of tone. The different functions of tonic and phasic reflexes account for some of the apparent inconsistencies when tone is tested in different ways but, in general, the pathological significance of the various manifestations is not properly understood. In muscle disease consistency and *'passivité'* are more often abnormal than *'extensibilité'*. Other useful signs of hypotonia are the hanging posture of the head and limbs when the baby is lifted supine with the hand under his back and the tendency to slip through the hands when he is lifted with hands under the axillae. It is important to recall that tone normally decreases from birth until the second to sixth month and gradually increases again in later childhood.

In *children* beyond the 'floppy infant' stage, hypotonia is a valuable sign before full cooperation in muscle strength tests is possible. An important example is the looseness of the shoulders in early Duchenne dystrophy.

In *adults* most myopathies and disorders of the lower motor neurone produce a moderate reduction in muscle tone. Because of the much more definitive information given by assessing muscle atrophy and power, tone is rarely of much importance in diagnosis, except when apparently out of keeping with other signs. Thus, in cases of combined pyramidal tract and lower motor neurone involvement, as in some hereditary ataxias and motor neurone disease, spasticity in weak, wasted, areflexic muscles may be in the only indication of the upper motor neurone lesion.

Palpation of nerves and muscles

As mentioned above, peripheral nerves may become tender to palpation at sites of entrapment (as with the ulnar nerve behind the medial epicondyle of the humerus) or when their component roots are compressed or irritated (as with the sciatic nerve in sciatica due to lumbar intervertebral disc prolapse). Localised swelling or hypertrophy of peripheral nerves can occur in leprosy or neurofibromatosis, more generalised enlargement, even involving the greater auricular nerve, in cases of hypertrophic neuropathy (as in some cases of peroneal muscular atrophy and related disorders, or in recurrent demyelinating peripheral neuropathy).

The importance of palpation in assessing muscle tone, atrophy, hypertrophy or weakness has already been stressed. In addition, local areas of tenderness may be discovered, an event which often provides more satisfaction for the anxious patient than for the thoughtful physician, as the cause of such local tenderness is only rarely found. Nevertheless in some fairly well-defined syndromes such as 'tennis elbow', attributable to a localised tendonitis at the lateral epicondyle of the humerus or in the region of the neck of the radius resulting from repetitive movement, useful treatment may result. Palpable masses in muscle are generally either areas of local spasm, post-traumatic haematomata or, less commonly, infarcts (in polyarteritis nodosa) or areas of localised nodular myositis. Differentiation between these can be difficult in acute cases. Sometimes the bony swellings of myositis ossificans can be felt and, rarely, a local mass turns out to be a tumour, either primary in muscle (rhabdomyosarcoma), or expanding from deeper structures such as an osteogenic sarcoma. Herniation of muscle fibres through a ruptured perimysial sheath (a muscle hernia) may feel deceptively like a tumour.

Reflex change

Markedly different patterns of reflex change may be found in otherwise similar disorders. In peripheral neuropathy, even without obvious sensory loss, the tendon reflexes are usually abolished early and are often absent in muscles which seem otherwise unaffected. In the muscular dystrophies, loss of reflexes tends to follow closely the degree of weakness and they are absent in any markedly weak muscle. In motor neurone disease, however, substantial wasting and weakness may be found in muscles with brisk reflexes, presumably because of the survival of some motor units with intact peripheral nerve conduction in the presence of corticospinal tract involvement. Poly-myositis, myasthenia gravis and the myopathy of osteomalacia or hyperparathyroidism are other disorders in which the reflexes tend to be preserved in weak muscles. They are valuable in distinguishing between myasthenia gravis (in which they are preserved) and the myasthenic syndrome associated with carcinoma (in which they are abolished early). It is well known that in hypothyroidism, with or without myopathy, the rates of contraction and relaxation in the reflex response are characteristically slow and, less often, excessively rapid responses are found in thyrotoxicosis.

The plantar responses are, of course, generally flexor in neuromuscular disorders. Generally speaking, the discovery of extensor plantar responses in cases of proximal muscle weakness should arouse suspicions of motor neurone disease or of those rare instances of spinal muscular atrophy in which there is evidence of pyramidal tract dysfunction (Gardner-Medwin et al 1967).

Contracture

Contracture is a state of shortening of a muscle not caused by active contraction. It may be acute and spontaneously reversible, as in McArdle's disease, but far more often it is the result of the rearrange-ment of collagen fibrils within the muscle over a longer period. At this stage it is fully reversible by repeated stretching. Later, actual fibrosis may make it increasingly difficult to treat. Contracture often follows failure of a muscle to grow in length or progressive shortening when its action is not opposed by a sufficiently powerful antagonist or one which is becoming steadily weaker. Palpation of the muscle during attempts at passive move-ment at the affected joint will rapidly distinguish contracture from joint ankylosis in one case and active contraction in another although, occasionally, examination under general anaesthesia may be necessary when both are present. When the relevant muscles are inaccessible, e.g. at the hip joint or in the 'frozen shoulder' syndrome, these distinctions may be difficult and, indeed, in the latter condition, muscles may pass through all

three stages of spasm, contracture and atrophy due to ankylosis. Demonstration of contractures is usually easy, but they may be missed at the shoulder if the scapula is not fixed, and at the hips if the lumbar lordosis is not first eliminated by flexing the opposite hip so that the thigh touches the abdomen.

Contractures develop in many chronic muscle diseases, whether neurogenic or myopathic, and are especially prominent in the syndrome of arthrogryposis multiplex congenita, in muscular dystrophy of the Duchenne type, and in polio-myelitis and the spinal muscular atrophies. In muscular dystrophy they are an important source of early difficulty in walking (see Ch. 15). In acute polymyositis they occasionally develop rapidly within a few weeks, even in muscles with surpris-ingly little weakness. In progressive myosclerosis (another syndrome of multiple aetiology), contrac-ture may be the major cause of disability; here, no weakness may be detectable, but the muscles have a woody or fibrotic consistency.

The muscles supplied by the cranial nerves

The examination of the *external ocular muscles* is a complex art which is described by Cogan (1978) and Leigh & Zee (1983). Only a few points of special relevance to muscle disease are mentioned here. Pareses which do not conform to the pattern of single or multiple nerve palsies suggest a local muscular disorder, but this may be caused by expanding orbital lesions as well as by inflamma-tory, metabolic or degenerative myopathies. Thus, in polymyositis the ocular muscles are occasionally involved, as they are in the rare orbital myositis and the closely related condition of orbital pseudo-tumour, which is often unilateral but sometimes bilateral, giving proptosis as well as impaired ocular movement and usually a raised erythrocyte sedimentation rate. In the ocular, oculopharyngeal and myotonic muscular dystrophies, ptosis in-variably occurs before ocular pareses, and diplopia is only rarely an early symptom. Later, ocular myopathy may progress to complete external ophthalmoplegia. An isolated superior rectus palsy is often the earliest feature of ophthalmic Graves' disease. If proptosis is not obvious in such cases it should be sought using an exophthalmometer;

in most cases, conjunctival oedema is also present. Myasthenia gravis is a great imitator of ocular palsies and should be considered wherever diagnosis is uncertain. Maintaining upward gaze for a full minute will usually induce some ptosis in such cases but, even if it does not, an edrophonium test should always be tried. Electronystagmographic recording of optokinetic nystagmus or tonometry performed before and after edrophonium has proved helpful in diagnosis but measurement of serum AChR antibodies is more reliable. In children, bilateral facial weakness apparently associated with bilateral sixth nerve palsies suggests Möbius' syndrome, which can be a purely myopathic disorder (sometimes being one manifestation of myotubular myopathy) in some cases although it is certainly the result of nuclear agenesis in others. Another imitator of abducens palsy is Duane's syndrome, in which impaired abduction of the affected eye is associated with ptosis and enophthalmos during adduction. It is due to fibrosis of the external rectus muscle and may be bilateral. This anomaly is sometimes dominantly inherited.

The *muscles of mastication* may be affected late in the course of many disorders but are often involved in early myasthenia gravis, in which the hand supporting the lower jaw is a useful clue to diagnosis, in tetanus (trismus) and in myotonic dystrophy, in which wasting of the temporal and masseter muscles and a drooping jaw contribute to the typical facial appearance. The rare branchial myopathy can give bilateral masseter hypertrophy. Trismus may also be of emotional origin or can occur transiently in patients receiving phenothiazines.

The facial muscles are commonly involved in myopathies and rather uncommonly in motor neurone disease. A brisk jaw jerk will usually distinguish the latter. Bilateral lower motor neurone weakness, e.g. in the Guillain-Barré syndrome, sarcoidosis, acute leukaemia in childhood, poliomyelitis and pontine lesions may sometimes be confirmed by loss of taste, but may closely resemble myopathic weakness. A useful distinguishing point is inability to close the eyes in facial nerve lesions; this is less often seen in myopathy except in advanced facioscapulohumeral dystrophy. In young children, gross facial myopathy is usually due to Möbius' syndrome or myotonic dystrophy. In facioscapulohumeral dystrophy the involvement may be severe or slight and is best shown by asking the patient to shut his eyes tightly, or to hold air in his mouth under pressure. In the middle and late stages of Duchenne dystrophy, facial weakness is rarely absent, though usually slight. Failure to retract the corners of the mouth and to blow out the cheeks are the most useful signs.

Dysarthria and dysphagia are both common in myasthenia gravis and polymyositis. In the myotonic and oculopharyngeal muscular dystrophies dysphagia alone is more frequent. Bulbar involvement in poliomyelitis, motor neurone disease and acute polyneuritis are also well known.

The *sternomastoid* muscles are severely wasted and weak in dystrophia myotonica and often in such neurogenic disorders as motor neurone disease, poliomyelitis and craniovertebral anomalies involving the accessory nerve. Of the other myopathies, myasthenia gravis and polymyositis are two in which weakness of neck flexion or extension may be particularly prominent. Selective trapezius weakness may occur in the limb-girdle type of muscular dystrophy and in accessory nerve lesions.

The *tongue* is important in diagnosis because of the ease with which it shows fasciculation, especially in motor neurone disease and other spinal muscular atrophies, as discussed above. Few myopathies affect the tongue. In dystrophia myotonica, lingual dysarthria is more often a sign of myotonia than of weakness. In Duchenne dystrophy the speech is often indistinct and sometimes the tongue is enlarged. Tongue hypertrophy is also a rare manifestation of late-onset glycogen-storage disease due to acid maltase deficiency. A curiously selective form of atrophy of the tongue in myasthenia gravis is illustrated in Chapter 19 (Fig. 19.3).

Important non-muscular symptoms and signs

In polymyositis these are particularly important and Raynaud's phenomenon, dysphagia and, above all, skin changes may help in diagnosis. The rash in dermatomyositis may involve the face, trunk or limbs, but in difficult cases the eyelids and nail beds should be examined with particular care. In other obscure myopathies uveitis, erythema nodosum, or dyspnoea with pulmonary infiltration may suggest sarcoidosis; anaemia, proteinuria, rashes, arthropathy, pleurisy or splenomegaly, the collagen diseases; tight shiny skin over the face or fingers, systemic sclerosis; and diarrhoea or steatorrhoea, uraemia, bony tenderness or radiological abnormalities in the bones, osteomalacia or hyperparathyroidism. In all these cases the myopathy may be the presenting feature before the more usual symptoms are obvious. Rarely, this also occurs in thyrotoxic myopathy in which, however, thyroid function tests will be abnormal. The same is true of the myopathy of hypothyroidism (Wilson & Walton 1959) but in Cushing's syndrome, Addison's disease and acromegaly or hypopituitarism, the myopathy usually amounts to no more than an incidental part of the disease. Severe fatiguability with increased skin pigmentation after bilateral adrenalectomy for Cushing's disease should arouse suspicion of very high levels of circulating ACTH (Nelson's Syndrome) (Prineas et al 1968). Myoglobinuria is associated not only with 'idiopathic' paroxysmal rhabdomyolysis but sometimes also with severe necrotising myopathy in polymyositis, acute alcoholism and other intoxications, and after exercise in the anterior tibial syndrome, McArdle's disease and carnitine palmityl transferase deficiency (see Ch. 25). The inherited myopathies may be associated with other congenital abnormalities; these are especially prominent in the myotonic and ocular dystrophies (see Ch. 15), in nemaline myopathy (a high-arched palate, long face, protruding jaw and dental malocclusion), in a-β-lipoproteinaemia (steatorrhoea, retinal degeneration, ataxia and acanthocytosis), in ataxia telangiectasia (ataxia, conjunctival telangiectasia and recurrent infections); and in Types II and III glycogen-storage disease in which hepatic involvement and (in Type II) cardiac, cerebral and spinal cord involvement occur.

APPENDIX

The following classification of neuromuscular disorders was originally prepared for the Research Group on Neuromuscular Diseases of the World Federation of Neurology (1968) and is reprinted here with many changes and additions. Abbreviated references are given to some conditions not described in extenso in the relevant chapters in this book.

The term 'amyotrophy' is used repeatedly, not in the literal sense of 'muscular atrophy' but with the more restricted meaning of neurogenic muscular atrophy as distinct from myopathy or primary disease of muscle. As this is a classification of neuromuscular disorders, those diseases of roots and peripheral nerves which give rise solely to sensory, as distinct from motor, dysfunction are omitted. Questionable entites of doubtful nosology are preceded by a question mark.

I. SPINAL MUSCULAR ATROPHIES AND OTHER DYSFUNCTIONS OF ANTERIOR HORN CELLS

A. *Genetically determined*

1. Infantile and juvenile spinal muscular atrophy
    (*a*) acute infantile spinal muscular atrophy (Werdnig–Hoffmann disease) (autosomal recessive)
    (*b*) arthrogryposis multiplex due to anterior horn cell disease (see British Medical Journal 1981 283: 2)
    (*c*) pseudomyopathic familial spinal muscular atrophy — autosomal recessive (Kugelberg & Welander) — X-linked (Tsukagoshi et al 1970 Neurology (Minneapolis) 20:1188, Harding et al 1982 Journal of Neurology, Neurosurgery and Psychiatry 45:1012, Schanen et al 1984 Revue Neurologique (Paris) 140:720); with testicular failure (Arbizu et al 1983 Journal of the Neurological Sciences 59:371), dominant (Zellweger et al 1972 Neurology (Minneapolis) 22:957, Pearn 1978 Journal of the Neurological Sciences 38:263)
    (*d*) scapuloperoneal form of spinal muscular atrophy — (recessive or dominant) (Kaeser 1965 Brain 88: 407); dominant, with secondary myopathic and inflammatory changes and cardiopathy (Jennekens et al 1975 Brain 98:709); X-linked with cardiopathy (Mawatari et al 1973 Archives of Neurology 28:55)
    (*e*) distal spinal muscular atrophy (Dyck & Lambert 1968 Archives of Neurology 18:619, Pearn & Hudgson 1979 Journal of the Neurological Sciences 43:183, Harding & Thomas 1980 Journal of the Neurological Sciences 45:337); with optic atrophy and nerve deafness, (Iwashita et al 1970 Archives of Neurology 22:357); with vocal cord paralysis (Young & Harper 1980 Journal of Neurology, Neurosurgery and Psychiatry 43:413); predominantly involving the upper limbs (Serratrice 1984 Revue Neurologique (Paris) 140:368, van Gent et al 1985 Journal of Neurology, Neurosurgery and Psychiatry 48:266)
    (*f*) markedly asymmetrical or restricted spinal muscular atrophy, perhaps restricted to one upper extremity (Hashimoto et al 1976 Journal of Neurology 211:105, Sobue et al 1978 Annals of Neurology 3:429, Harding et al 1983 Journal of the Neurological Sciences 59:69)
    (*g*) spinal muscular atrophy with cystinuria and leucinuria (Radu et al 1974 Journal of Neurology 207:73)
    (*h*) spinal muscular atrophy with pallidonigral degeneration (Serratrice et al 1983 Neurology (Cleveland) 33:306)
2. Guam motor neurone disease*
3. Familial motor neurone disease (other than the Guam type) (Horton et al 1976 Neurology (Minneapolis) 26:460)
4. Familial bulbar palsy
    (*a*) progressive spinal muscular atrophy with bulbar palsy

---

* There is now considerable evidence to suggest that Guam motor neurone disease is due to environmental factors and not genetically determined, but this is not yet proven.

(Dobkin & Verity 1976 Neurology (Minneapolis) 26:754, Ringel et al 1978 Muscle and Nerve 1:297)
- (b) infantile and juvenile progressive bulbar palsy (Gomez et al 1962 Archives of Neurology 6:317, Markand & Daly 1971 Neurology (Minneapolis) 21:753)
- (c) recessive X-linked bulbar palsy (Tsukagoshi et al 1965 Archives of Neurology 12:597, Kennedy et al 1968 Neurology (Minneapolis) 18:671)

5. Amyotrophy in the parkinsonism-dementia complex and the juvenile amyotrophic lateral sclerosis-dementia complex (Staal & Went 1968 Neurology (Minneapolis) 18:800)
6. Amyotrophy in heredofamilial ataxias
   - (a) in Friedreich's ataxia
   - (b) in hereditary spastic paraplegia
   - (c) in autosomal dominant cerebellar ataxia
   - (d) in X-linked recessive spinocerebellar ataxia
   - (e) in dyssynergia cerebellaris myoclonica (Ramsay Hunt)
   - (f) in ataxia telangiectasia
   - (g) in the Kjellin syndrome (see Harding 1984 The hereditary ataxias. Churchill Livingstone)
7. Amyotrophy in Huntington's chorea
8. Amyotrophy in Marinesco-Sjögren syndrome (Alter & Kennedy 1968 Minnesota Medicine 51:901)
9. Amyotrophy in infantile neuroaxonal dystrophy (Huttenlocher & Gilles 1967 Neurology (Minneapolis) 17:1174)

B *Congenital (developmental abnormalities)*
1. Möbius' syndrome (agenesis of cranial nerve nuclei). Möbius' syndrome with peripheral neuropathy and hypogonadism (Abid et al 1978 Journal of the Neurological Sciences 35:309). Möbius' syndrome with absence of pectoral muscle
2. Congenital absence of muscles (pectorals, abdominals, etc.) (? possibly better classified under disorders of muscle but it is not known whether the appropriate anterior horn cells are absent)
   - (a) congenital absence of pectoral muscle with syndactyly (David 1972 New England Journal of Medicine 287:487)
3. Hydromyelia with amyotrophy
4. Spinal dysraphism with amyotrophy
5. Meningomyelocele with amyotrophy
6. Aplasia of spinal cord (amyelia)
7. Syringomyelia or syringobulbia with amyotrophy (note close relationship with Chiari malformation)
8. Anterior horn cell disease with pontocerebellar hypoplasia (Goutières et al 1977 Journal of Neurology, Neurosurgery and Psychiatry 40:370)
9. Arthrogryposis multiplex congenita of non-neural and non-myopathic origin

C. *Traumatic*
C-I. *Physical* (Amyotrophy due to destruction or compression of anterior horn cells)
1. Birth injury to spinal cord
2. Spinal tumours
3. Haematomyelia
4. Infective masses, e.g.
   - (a) tuberculoma
   - (b) gumma
   - (c) parasitic cyst
5. Other causes of spinal cord compression
6. Ischaemic
   - (a) occlusion or stenosis of anterior spinal artery
   - (b) progressive vascular myelopathy (Jellinger & Neumayer 1962 Acta Neurologica et Psychiatrica Belgica 62:944)
7. Amyotrophy in multiple sclerosis and neuromyelitis optica

8. Amyotrophy in transverse myelitis
9. Amyotrophy following electrical injury (Farrell & Starr 1968 Neurology (Minneapolis) 18:601, Holbrook et al 1970 British Medical Journal 4:659)

C-II. *Toxic (Toxins acting on the motor neurone)*
1. Tetanus toxin
2. Strychnine
3. Botulinum toxin (adult botulism and infantile botulism) (Clay et al 1977 Archives of Neurology 34:236, Arnon 1980 Annual Review of Medicine 31:541)
4. Lead (Campbell et al 1970 Journal of Neurology, Neurosurgery and Psychiatry 33:877, Boothby et al 1974 Archives of Neurology 3:18)
5. Saxitoxin and related toxins

D. *Infective amyotrophy*
1. Paralytic acute anterior poliomyelitis
   - (a) due to poliomyelitis virus
   - (b) due to other enteroviruses (including Coxsackie viruses)
2. Russian spring-summer encephalitis with amyotrophy
3. Herpes zoster (including Ramsay Hunt syndrome — so-called geniculate herpes) (Thomas & Howard 1972 Neurology (Minneapolis) 22:715)

E. *Amyotrophy of unknown aetiology*
1. Motor neurone disease
   - (a) progressive bulbar palsy
   - (b) progressive muscular atrophy
   - (c) amyotrophic lateral sclerosis
2. Juvenile motor neurone disease (van Bogaert 1925 Revue Neurologique 1:180, Nelson & Prensky 1972 Archives of Neurology 27:300)
3. ? Progressive amyotrophy following old poliomyelitis (Mulder et al 1972 Mayo Clinic Proceedings 47:756, Wiechers & Hubbell 1981 Muscle and Nerve 4:524)
4. Progressive amyotrophy following encephalitis lethargica (Greenfield & Matthews 1954 Journal of Neurology, Neurosurgery and Psychiatry 17:50)
5. Amyotrophy in orthostatic hypotension (the Shy-Drager syndrome of progressive multisystem degeneration)
6. Amyotrophy in Pick's disease (Minauf & Jellinger 1969 Archives Psychiatry Nervenkeilhunde 212:279)
7. Amyotrophy in ataxia telangiectasia (Goodman et al 1969 Bulletin of the Los Angeles Neurology Society 34:1)
8. Chronic neurogenic quadriceps amyotrophy (Furukawa et al 1977 Annals of Neurology 2:528)

F. *Amyotrophy in malignant disease*
1. ? Carcinomatous motor neurone disease (Brain et al 1965 Brain 88:479). This association is now thought unlikely to be of significance
2. Spinal muscular atrophy in Waldenstrom's macroglobulinaemia (Peters & Chatanoff 1968 Neurology (Minneapolis) 18: 101)

G. *Dysfunction of the motor neurone in metabolic disorders*
1. Tetany in
   - (a) hypocalcaemia
   - (b) magnesium deficiency
   - (c) alkalosis
2. ? Hypoglycaemia (organic hyperinsulinism) with amyotrophy (Tom & Richardson 1951 Journal of Neuropathology and Experimental Neurology 10:57, Harrison 1976 Journal of Neurology, Neurosurgery and Psychiatry 39:465)

H. *Myokymia, cramps, benign fasciculation**

* It is by no means certain that the origin of these disorders lies in dysfunction of the anterior horn cells.

II. DISORDERS OF MOTOR NERVE ROOTS

A. *Congenital*

1. Associated with meningomyelocele and other anomalies
2. Arthrogryposis multiplex congenita (radicular type) (Peta et al 1968 Neurology (Minneapolis) 18:926)

B. *Traumatic*

B-I. *Physical*

1. Laceration, contusion, distraction or avulsion of roots
2. Compression of roots by:
   (*a*) vertebral osteoarthritis
   (*b*) prolapsed intervetebral disc
   (*c*) Paget's disease
   (*d*) tumour in the spinal canal or intervertebral foramina
   (*e*) vertebral collapse
3. Ischaemia
4. Radiation

B-II. *Toxic*

1. Toxic agents (injected local anaesthetics, phenol, etc.)

C. *Inflammatory*

C-I. *Infective*

1. Radiculopathy in meningitis
2. Syphilis
3. Granulomatous arachnoiditis of other causes (including spinal tuberculosis and sarcoidosis)
4. Bilharziasis

C-II. *Post-infective, allergic or immunologically mediated*

1. Acute inflammatory (post-infective) polyradiculoneuropathy (Guillain–Barré syndrome)
2. Polyradiculoneuropathy following inoculation
3. Serum neuropathy

D. *Neoplastic*

1. Neurofibroma
2. Meningioma
3. Metastases
4. Reticulosis
5. Vascular malformations

III. DISORDERS OF PERIPHERAL NERVES*

A. *Genetically determined*

1. Hereditary motor and sensory neuropathy. The hereditary motor and sensory neuropathies (HMSN) have been classified by Dyck into several different types (see Dyck et al (eds) 1983 Peripheral neuropathies, 2nd edn. Saunders p 1600–1655. Types I and II are commonly known as peroneal muscular atrophy or Charcot–Marie–Tooth disease (Harding & Thomas 1980 Brain 103:255)

   (*a*)HMSN I (hypertrophic type) } usually autosomal dominant; sometimes
   Roussy–Lévy syndrome is a variant } autosomal recessive inheritance
   (*b*) HMSN II (neuronal type) }

   (*c*) HMSN III (Dejerine Sottas disease). Autosomal recessive inheritance. Cases of congenital hypomyelination neuropathy (Guzetta et al 1982 Brain 105:395, Kennedy et al 1977 Archives of Neurology 34:337) are probably variants
   (*d*) HMSN IV (heredopathia atactica polyneuritiformis; Refsum's syndrome). Autosomal recessive inheritance
   (*e*) Marinesco–Sjögren syndrome (Serratrice et al 1973 Revue Neurologique (Paris) 128:432)
2. Hereditary neuropathies associated with specific defects

---

* Only disorders involving motor or mixed nerves are included and those confined to sensory or autonomic nerves have not been included in this classification.

(*a*) amyloidosis
   (i) type I — Portuguese type (Andrade 1952 Brain 75:408)
   (ii) type II — Indiana type (Rukavina et al 1956 Medicine (Baltimore) 35:239)
   (iii) type III — Iowa type (Van Allen et al 1969 Neurology (Minneapolis) 19:10)
   (iv) type IV — Finnish type (Meretoja & Teppo 1971 Acta Pathologica Microbiologica Scandinavica 79:432, Boysen et al 1979 Journal of Neurology, Neurosurgery and Psychiatry 42:1020)
(*b*) porphyria; usually acute intermittent variety, but also variegate and hereditary coproporphyria
(*c*) a- alpha-lipoproteinaemia (Tangier disease) (Pollock et al 1983 Brain 106:911)
(*d*) a-beta-lipoproteinaemia (Bassen–Kornzweig syndrome) Neuropathy probably due to vitamin E deficiency
(*e*) metachromatic leukodystrophy (sulphatide lipidosis); late infantile, juvenile, adult onset and other variants are recognised
(*f*) globoid cell leukodystrophy (Krabbe's disease)
(*g*) Cockayne's syndrome (Moosa & Dubowitz 1970 Archives of Disease in Childhood 45:474)
(*h*) adrenoleukodystrophy and adrenomyeloneuropathy (Griffin et al 1977 Neurology (Minneapolis) 12:1107)
(*i*) Fabry's disease (alpha-galactoside A deficiency; glycosphingolipid lipidosis (Bischoff et al 1968 Klinische Wochenschrift 46:666)
(*j*) Refsum's syndrome (phytanic acid storage disease) — see A1(*d*)
(*k*) glycogenoses
   (i) type II (Pompe's disease) (Smith et al 1967 Neurology (Minneapolis) 17:537)
   (ii) type III (Cori's disease) (Ugawa et al 1986 Annals of Neurology 19:294)
(*l*) primary hyperoxaluria (Hall et al 1976 Journal of the Neurological Sciences 29:343)

3. Miscellaneous hereditary neuropathies
   (*a*) hereditary liability to pressure palsies; includes 'tomaculous' neuropathies (Madrid & Bradley 1975 Journal of the Neurological Sciences 25:45) and 'globular' neuropathy (Dayan et al 1968 Journal of Neurology, Neurosurgery and Psychiatry 31:552)
   (*b*) familial recurrent brachial plexus neuropathy (Taylor 1960 Brain 83:113); probably a variant of 3 (*a*)
   (*c*) giant axonal neuropathy; some cases probable autosomal recessive inheritance
   (*d*) ataxia telangiectasia (Dunn 1973 Developmental Medicine and Child Neurology 15:324)
   (*e*) mitochondrial myopathies (Yiannikas & McLeod 1968 Annals of Neurology 20:249)
   (*f*) Riley–Day syndrome (familial dysautonomia) (Aguayo et al 1971 Archives of Neurology 24:105)
   (*g*) neurofibromatosis (von Recklinghausen's disease)
   (*h*) hereditary hypertrophic neuropathy with paraproteinaemia (Gibberd & Gavrilescu 1966 Neurology (Minneapolis) 16:130)
   (*i*) hereditary polyneuropathy with oligophrenia, premature menopause and acromicria (Lundberg 1971 European Neurology 5:84) — ? mitochondrial
   (*j*) neuropathy in the neuroectodermal syndrome with dominant inheritance (Flynn & Aird 1965 Journal of the Neurological Sciences 2:161)
   (*k*) subacute necrotising encephalomyelopathy (Leigh's disease) (Goebel et al 1986 Muscle and Nerve 9:1657)

(*l*) peripheral neuropathy associated with xeroderma pigmentosum (Mimaki et al 1986 Annals of Neurology 20:70

B. *Congenital*
Congenital neuropathy with arthrogryposis multiplex congenita (Hooshmand et al 1971 Archives of Neurology 24:561)

C. *Traumatic*
C-I. *Physical*
1. Laceration, contusion, compression or distraction of nerves or plexuses
2. Birth trauma to brachial plexus
   (*a*) Erb's paralysis
   (*b*) Klumpke's paralysis
3. Entrapment neuropathies
   (*a*) of cranial nerves
      (i) facial nerve compression in the stylomastoid foramen (Bell's palsy)
      (ii) clonic facial spasm (hemifacial spasm)
      (iii) recurrent familial facial palsy (Melkersson's syndrome)
   (*b*) of the upper extremity
      (i) thoracic inlet and cervico-axillary canal, including cervical rib
      (ii) median nerve in the forearm (pronator syndrome)
      (iii) median nerve at the wrist (carpal tunnel syndrome)
      (iv) ulnar nerve at the elbow (cubital tunnel syndrome)
      (v) ulnar nerve at the wrist or its deep branch in the palm
      (vi) radial nerve in the spiral groove
      (vii) radial nerve in the forearm
      (viii) posterior interosseous nerve in the forearm
      (ix) anterior interosseous nerve
      (x) suprascapular nerve at the shoulder
      (xi) long thoracic nerve at the shoulder
      (xii) axillary nerve at the shoulder
      (xiii) musculocutaneous nerve in the upper arm
   (*c*) of the lower extremity
      (i) sciatic nerve at the pelvic exit
      (ii) obturator nerve in the obturator canal
      (iii) ilioinguinal nerve at the groin
      (iv) femoral nerve in the groin or upper thigh
      (v) common peroneal nerve around the fibular neck
      (vi) deep peroneal nerve (Gutmann 1970 Journal of Neurology, Neurosurgery and Psychiatry 33:450)
      (vii) tibial nerve
      (viii) posterior tibial nerve in the tarsal tunnel
   (*d*) of the trunk
      (i) intercostal neuropathy
   (*e*) multiple entrapments in mucopolysaccharidosis (Karpati et al 1974 Archives of Neurology 31:418)
4. Electric shock (Farrell & Starr 1968 Neurology (Minneapolis) 18:601)
5. Burns
6. Radiation injury (Stoll & Andrews 1966 British Medical Journal 1:834)
7. Ischaemic neuropathy*
   (*a*) giant cell arteritis
   (*b*) mononeuropathy in polyarteritis nodosa

* Peripheral nerve lesions occurring in these disorders are believed to be ischaemic but other pathological processes may well be involved.

(*c*) neuropathy in disseminated lupus erythematosus
(*d*) diabetes mellitus (some cases)
(*e*) post-irradiation neuropathy
(*f*) neuropathy in peripheral vascular disease
(*g*) dysproteinaemic neuropathy
(*h*) neuropathy in subacute bacterial endocarditis (Jones & Siekert 1968 Archives of Neurology 19:535)
(*i*) mononeuropathy in necrotizing angiitis due to amphetamine or other drugs (Stafford et al 1975 Neurology (Minneapolis) 25:570)
(*j*) neuropathy in rheumatoid arthritis (Pallis 8 Scott 1965 British Medical Journal 1: 1141, Dyck et al 1972 Mayo Clinic Proceedings 47:462)
(*k*) neuropathy in sarcoidosis — sometimes associated with angiitis (Nemni et al 1981 Neurology (Minneapolis) 31:1217)
(*l*) Churg–Strauss syndrome
(*m*) Wegener's granulomatosis

C-II. *Toxic*
1. Drugs
   amiodarone — carbamazepine — chloral — chloroquine — clioquinol (subacute myelo-opticoneuropathy) — cytotoxic agents (especially nitrogen mustard and vincristine) — dapsone — diphenylhydantoin — disulfiram (Bradley & Hewer 1966 British Medical Journal 2:449) — emetine — ethionamide — glutethimide — hydrallazine — indomethacin — iproniazid — isoniazid — lithium — metronidazole (Coxon & Pallis 1976 Journal of Neurology, Neurosurgery and Psychiatry 39:403) — methaqualone — metronidazole — misonidazole — nitrofurantoin — perhexiline — phenytoin — sodium cyanate — stilbamidine — streptomycin — sulphanilamide — taxol — thalidomide — trichloroethylene — vinca alkaloids etc.
2. Inorganic substances
   (*a*) heavy metals
      antimony — arsenic — bismuth — copper — gold — lead — mercury (Pink disease, Minimata disease) — thallium
   (*b*) other inorganic substances
      phosphorus
3. Organic substances (N.B. some of these cause giant axonal neuropathy) (see Carpenter et al 1974 Archives of Neurology 31:312) acrylamide — alcohol — aniline — bush tea — carbon disulphide — carbon monoxide* — carbon tetrachloride — dinitrobenzol — dinitrophenol — ethylene oxide hexachlorophene — n-hexane (Herskowitz et al 1971 New England Journal of Medicine 285:82) — methyl butyl ketone — pentachlorophenol and DDT — polychlorinated biphenyl (in cooking oil) (Chia & Chu 1985 Journal of Neurology, Neurosurgery and Psychiatry 48:894) — tetrachlorethane — trichlorethylene — other organic chlorine derivatives — triorthocresylphosphate
4. Toxins derived from bacteria
   (*a*) botulism
   (*b*) diphtheria
   (*c*) dysentery
   (*d*) tetanus
5. Toxins derived from other organisms: saxitoxin–cigatuera
6. Buckthorn neuropathy (Mitchell et al 1978 Neuropathology and Experimental Neurology 4:85)

C-III. *Of uncertain aetiology (? toxic, ? nutritional)*
1. Neuropathy and amyotrophy in
   (*a*) Jamaican and other tropical neuropathy
   (*b*) South Indian paraplegia
   (*c*) neuropathy in tropical ataxia (Nigeria) (Williams &

Osuntokun 1969 Archives of Neurology 21:475) (probably due to cyanide in cassava root) and tropical spastic paraparesis

2. Neuropathy in the Spanish toxic oil syndrome (Cruz Martinez et al 1984 Muscle and Nerve 7: 12)

D. *Inflammatory*

D-I. *Infective*

1. Direct infection of nerves
   (*a*) leprosy
   (*b*) syphilis
   (*c*) brucellosis
   (*d*) leptospirosis
   (*e*) herpes simplex
   (*f*)) herpes zoster
   (*g*) HTLV III infection (AIDS)
   (*h*) trypanosomiasis

2. Neuropathies occurring in other infections
   (*a*) gonorrhoea
   (*b*) malaria
   (*c*) meningitis
   (*d*) mumps
   (*e*) paratyphoid
   (*f*) puerperal sepsis
   (*g*) septicaemia
   (*h*) smallpox
   (*i*) tuberculosis
   (*j*) typhoid
   (*k*) typhus
   (*l*) subacute bacterial endocarditis
   (*m*) Legionnaire's disease

D-II. *Post-infective (allergic)*

1. Post-infective neuropathies (? allergic)
   (*a*) chicken pox
   (*b*) infectious hepatitis
   (*c*) measles
   (*d*) upper respiratory tract infection
   (*e*) infectious mononucleosis
   (*f*) influenza
   (*g*) vaccinia

2. Post-infective polyneuropathy (probably immunologically mediated)
   (*a*) acute post-infective polyradiculoneuropathy (Guillain–Barré syndrome)
   (*b*) chronic progressive polyneuropathy
   (*c*) recurrent polyneuropathy (Austin 1958 Brain 81:157)
   (*d*) the Miller Fisher syndrome (Meinenberg & Ryffel 1983 Archives of Neurology 40:402)

3. Neuropathy in connective tissue disorders see *C I-7*
   (*a*) systemic lupus erythematosus
   (*b*) polyarteritis nodosa
   (*c*) rheumatoid arthritis
   (*d*) scleroderma (systemic sclerosis)
   (*e*) thrombotic thrombocytopenic purpura (thrombotic microangiopathy)
   (*f*) giant-cell arteritis
   (*g*) mixed connective tissue disease
   (*h*) Churg–Strauss syndrome
   (*i*) Sjögren's (sicca) syndrome

4. Neuropathy in sarcoidosis

5. Serum neuropathy

E. *Metabolic neuropathy*

1. Nutritional
   (*a*) specific deficiencies
       (i) cyanocobalamin deficiency
       (ii) folic acid deficiency
       (iii) vitamin E deficiency
   (*b*) of uncertain aetiology (probably B_1, B_2 and B_6 vitamin deficiency)
       (i) in chronic alcoholism
       (ii) beri-beri
       (iii) burning feet syndrome
       (iv) famine oedema and kwashiorkor
       (v) in hyperemesis gravidarum
       (vi) in pregnancy
       (vii) pellagra
       (viii) in gluten-sensitive enteropathy (Cooke & Smith 1966 Brain 89:683)

2. Neuropathies associated with endocrine disorders
   (*a*) diabetes mellitus
       (i) polyneuropathy
       (ii) mononeuropathy (including diabetic amyotrophy)
       (iii) thoracic radiculopathy (Kikta et al 1982 Annals of Neurology 11:80)
       (iv) autonomic neuropathy
   (*b*) thyroid disorders
       (i) hyperthyroidism (Feibel & Campa 1976 Journal of Neurology, Neurosurgery and Psychiatry 39:491)
       (ii) primary hypothyroidism (Dyck & Lambert 1970 Journal of Neuropathology and Experimental Neurology 29:631)
       (iii) hypothyroidism secondary to thyrotropin deficiency (Grabow & Chou 1968 Archives of Neurology 19:284)
   (*c*) neuropathy in organic hyperinsulinism (Mulder et al 1956 Neurology (Minneapolis) 6:627)
   (*d*) in acromegaly (Steward 1966 Archives of Neurology 14:107)

3. Neuropathy in blood dyscrasias
   (*a*) polycythaemia vera
   (*b*) leukaemia
   (*c*) bleeding disorders — haemorrhage into nerves
   (*d*) in sickle-cell disease
   (*e*) myelofibrosis

4. Neuropathy in renal failure
   (*a*) uraemic polyneuropathy (Asbury et al 1963 Archives of Neurology 8:413)
   (*b*) mononeuritis multiplex following dialysis (Meyrier et al 1972 British Medical Journal 2:252)

5. Neuropathy in liver disease including primary biliary cirrhosis (Dayan & Williams 1967 Lancet ii:133, Thomas & Walker 1965 Brain 88:1079)

6. Neuropathy in porphyria
   (*a*) genetically determined
       (i) acute intermittent porphyria (Swedish type)
       (ii) variegated porphyria (South African type)
       (iii) porphyria cutanea tarda
   (*b*) acquired
       (i) hexachlorobenzene poisoning

7. Dysglobulinaemic neuropathy
   (*a*) macroglobulinaemia
   (*b*) cryoglobulinaemia
   (*c*) with benign IgG paraproteinaemia (Read et al 1978 Journal of Neurology, Neurosurgery and Psychiatry 41:215)
   (*d*) in multiple myeloma (Vallat et al 1980 Annals of Neurology 8:179)
   (*e*) in macroglobulinaemia with IgM plasma-cell dyscrasia (Rowland et al 1982 Annals of Neurology 11:532)

F. *Neuropathy in malignant disease*

1. Carcinomatous neuropathy
2. Neuropathy in reticulosis
3. Neuropathy in myelomatosis (see also dysglobulinaemic neuropathy above)
G. *Miscellaneous neuropathies*
1. Neuropathy in:
    (a) chronic obstructive pulmonary disease (Appenzeller et al 1968 American Journal of Medicine 44:873)
    (b) total lipodystrophy (Tuck & McLeod 1983 Australian Medical Journal 13:65)
    (c) acrodermatitis chronica atrophicans (Hopf 1975 Journal of Neurology, Neurosurgery and Psychiatry 38:452)
    (d) neuropathy in critical illness (Bolton et al 1987 Brain in press)
2. Chronic sensorimotor neuropathy of undetermined cause
3. Chronic idiopathic ataxic neuropathy (Dalakas 1986 Annals of Neurology 19:545)
H. *Tumours of nerves*
1. Arising from supporting structures and/or axons
    (a) plexiform neuroma
    (b) traumatic neuroma
    (c) myelinic neuroma
2. Arising from supporting structures
    (a) Schwannoma (neurinoma, neurofibroma), including acoustic neuroma
    (b) fibroma
    (c) neurogenic sarcoma
    (d) haemangioma
    (e) lipoma
    (f) neuroepithelioma
I. *Functional disorders of peripheral nerves**
1. Stiff-man syndrome (Moersch & Woltman 1956 Mayo Clinic Proceedings 31:421)
2. Myokymia — hyperhidrosis — impaired muscle relaxation (Gamst orp & Wohlfart 1959 Acta Psychiatrica Scandinavica 34:181)
3. ? Recurrent muscle spasms of central origin (Satayoshi & Yamada 1967 Archives of Neurology 16:254)
4. ? 'Painful legs and moving toes' (Spillane et al 1971 Brain 94:541)
5. ? Ekbom's syndrome ('restless legs') (Harriman et al 1970 Brain 93:393)
IV. DISORDERS OF NEUROMUSCULAR TRANSMISSION
A. *Genetically determined*
1. Hereditary myasthenia
    (a) congenital and juvenile (Bowman 1948 Pediatrics 1:472, see Bundey 1972 Journal of Neurology, Neurosurgery and Psychiatry 35:41, Honeybourne et al 1982 45:854)
    (b) myasthenia with myopathy (McQuillen 1966 Brain 89:121)
2. Pseudocholinesterase deficiency (suxamethonium paralysis)
B. *Congenital or developmental myasthenia*
1. Putative defect in ACh synthesis or packaging
2. Congenital end-plate acetylcholinesterase deficiency
3. Slow-channel syndrome
4. Congenital end-plate AChR deficiency (see Engel A G 1984 Annals of Neurology 16:519, and Ch. 25)
5. Decrease of MEPP amplitude without AChR deficiency
C. *Toxic*
1. Botulism
2. Tick paralysis
3. Puff-fish paralysis (tetrodotoxin)

* The cause of these disorders is uncertain; they may be due to spinal cord or central neuronal dysfunction.

4. Magnesium intoxication
5. Kanamycin and other antibiotics (McQuillen et al 1968 Archives of Neurology 18:402)
6. Penicillamine-induced myasthenia (Garlepp et al 1983 British Medical Journal 1:338)
7. Other drugs (see Ch. 29)
D. *Autoimmune*
1. Myasthenia gravis and its variants
    (a) transient neonatal myasthenia (Namba et al 1970 Pediatrics 45:488)
    (b) ocular myasthenia
        (i) with peripheral neuropathy and spastic paraparesis (Brust et al 1974 Neurology (Minneapolis) 24:755)
    (c) generalised myasthenia
        (i) severe, especially in young women, correlated with HL-A8 antigen
        (ii) in older patients, often with thymoma and with HL-A2 or A3 antigen
    (d) myasthenia with thyrotoxicosis
    (e) myasthenia with hypothyroidism (Takamori et al 1972 Archives of Neurology 26:326)
    (f) myasthenia with other autoimmune diseases
    (g) myasthenia with features of the myasthenic-myopathic syndrome (Schwartz & Stalberg 1975 Neurology (Minneapolis) 25:80)
    (h) myasthenia with the Satoyoshi syndrome (muscle cramps, alopecia and diarrhoea, Satoh et al 1983, Neurology (Cleveland) 33:1209)
E. *Other myasthenic syndromes*
1. Myasthenic–myopathic syndrome (Eaton–Lambert)
    (a) with malignant disease
    (b) without malignant disease
2. Symptomatic myasthenia
    (a) in polymyositis and systemic lupus
    (b) in motor neurone disease
    (c) in chronic polyneuropathy
F. *Cholinergic paralysis*
1. Poisoning with anticholinesterase compounds (e.g. nerve gases)
2. Depolarising drugs
3. Black Widow spider venom
V. DISORDERS OF MUSCLE
A. *Genetically determined myopathies*
1. The muscular dystrophies
    (a) X-linked types
        (i) X-linked recessive (severe) (Duchenne)
        (ii) X-linked Duchenne dystrophy due to chromosomal translocation in females or to Turner's syndrome (Gomez et al 1977 Neurology (Minneapolis) 27:537; Zatz et al 1981 Journal of Medical Genetics 18:442)
        (iii) X-linked recessive (mild) (Becker)
        (iv) X-linked recessive (mild) with contractures and cardiomyopathy (Emery-Dreifuss) (Rowland et al 1979 Annals of Neurology 5:111, Hopkins et al 1981 Annals of Neurology 10:230)
        (v) X-linked recessive myopathy (mild) with acanthocytosis (Swash et al 1983 Brain 106:717)
        (vi) myopathy in manifesting Duchenne carriers
        (vii) X-linked myopathy with glycerol kinase deficiency (Guggenheim et al 1980 Annals of Neurology 7:441)
        (viii) X-linked recessive congenital muscle hypotrophy with central nuclei (Askanas et al 1979 Archives of Neurology 36:604)

(b) facioscapulohumeral (Landouzy & Dejerine)
  (i) autosomal dominant involving face, scapulohumeral and anterior tibial muscles
  (ii) with inflammatory changes in muscle (Munsat et al 1972 Neurology (Minneapolis) 22:335)
  (iii) with Möbius' syndrome (Hanson & Rowland 1971 Archives of Neurology 24:31)
  (iv) with sensorineural deafness and Coats' disease of the retina (Taylor et al 1982 Annals of Neurology 12:395, Korf et al 1985 Annals of Neurology 17:513)
(c) scapuloperoneal muscular dystrophy
  (i) autosomal dominant (Thomas et al 1975 Journal of Neurology, Neurosurgery and Psychiatry 38:1008)
  (ii) X-linked (Thomas et al 1972 Journal of Neurology, Neurosurgery and Psychiatry 35:208)
  (iii) with inflammatory changes and cardiopathy (Jennekens et al 1975 Brain 98:709)
(d) limb-girdle muscular dystrophy
  (i) autosomal recessive or sporadic (Erb; Leyden & Möbius)
  (ii) myopathy limited to quadriceps (Swash & Heathfield 1983 Journal of Neurology, Neurosurgery and Psychiatry 46:355)
  (iii) autosomal dominant, of late onset (Coster et al 1974 European Neurology 12:159, Bethlem and van Wijngaarden 1976 Brain 99:91)
(e) autosomal recessive dystrophy of childhood, resembling Duchenne, but more benign and affecting both sexes (especially frequent in Tunisia and other parts of the Middle East) (Ben Hamida et al 1983 Muscle and Nerve 6:469)
(f) distal muscular dystrophy
  (i) autosomal dominant variety of late onset (Welander)
  (ii) autosomal dominant variety with infantile onset (Bautista et al 1978 Journal of the Neurological Sciences 37:149)
  (iii) autosomal recessive variety (Scoppetta et al 1984 Muscle and Nerve 7:478); with rimmed vacuole formation and lamellar (myeloid) bodies (Nonaka et al 1985 Annals of Neurology 17:51)
  (iv) hereditary distal myopathy with characteristic sarcoplasmic bodies and intermediate (skeletin) filaments (Edström et al 1980 Journal of the Neurological Sciences 47:171)
  (v) autosomal recessive with high serum CK activity (Myoshi et al 1986 Brain 109:31)
(g) autosomal dominant dystrophy with humeropelvic distribution and cardiomyopathy (Fenichel et al 1982 Neurology (Minneapolis) 32:1399)
(h) autosomal dominant Emery-Dreifuss dystrophy (Miller et al 1985 Neurology (Cleveland) 35:1230)
(i) ocular myopathy (progressive external ophthalmoplegia)★
  (i) isolated (dominant)
  (ii) with pigmentary retinal degeneration (dominant or sporadic)
  (iii) with retinal degeneration, short stature, heart block, ataxia, etc. (Kearns & Sayre, Berenberg et al 1977 Annals of Neurology 1:37)
(j) oculopharyngeal muscular dystrophy (Little & Perl 1982 Journal of the Neurological Sciences 53:145)

(k) oculopharyngeal myopathy with distal myopathy and cardiomyopathy (Goto et al 1977 Journal of Neurology, Neurosurgery and Psychiatry 40:600)
(l) familial multicore disease (see below) with ophthalmoplegia (Swash & Schwartz 1981 Journal of the Neurological Sciences 52:1)
(m) congenital ophthalmoplegia in the Goldenhar-Gorlin syndrome (Aleksic et al 1976 Neurology (Minneapolis) 26:638)
(n) neonatal ophthalmoplegia with microfibres (Hanson et al 1977 Neurology (Minneapolis) 27:974)
(o) nemaline myopathy with ophthalmoplegia and mitochondrial abnormalities (Fukunaga et al 1980 Journal of the Neurological Sciences 46:169)
2. Obscure congenital myopathies of unknown aetiology
(a) congenital muscular dystrophy (including some cases of arthrogryposis multiplex congenita): some cases with severe mental retardation (Fukuyama et al 1981 Brain Development 3:1)
(b) benign congenital myopathy without specific features (Turner 1940 Brain 63:163)
(c) ? congenital universal muscular hypoplasia★ (Krabbe 1947 Nordisk Medicin 35:1756)
(d) benign congenital or infantile hypotonia (Walton), amyotonia congenita (Oppenheim)†
(e) central core disease
(f) nemaline, or rod-body, myopathy
(g) myotubular or centronuclear myopathy
  (i) (Spiro et al 1966 Archives of Neurology 14:1, Elder et al 1983 Journal of the Neurological Sciences 60:79)
  (ii) X-linked variety (Wijngaarden et al 1969 Neurology (Minneapolis) 19:901)
  (iii) with type I fibre atrophy (Bethlem et al 1970 Archives of Neurology 23:70)
(h) familial myosclerosis (myodysplasia fibrosa multiplex) myopathy in Marfan's syndrome (Goebel et al 1973
(i) Neurology (Minneapolis) 23:1257)
  (i) centronuclear myopathy with type I fibre hypotrophy and 'fingerprint' inclusions with Marfan's syndrome (Jadro-Santel et al 1980 Journal of the Neurological Sciences 45:43)
(j) familial congenital myopathy with cataract and gonadal dysgenesis (Bassöe 1956 Journal of Clinical Endocrinology 16:1614)
(k) myopathies with characteristic histochemical abnormalities
  (i) type I fibre hypotrophy (Engel W K et al 1968 Archives of Neurology 18:435; Bender and Bender 1977 Neurology (Minneapolis) 27:206)
  (ii) congenital fibre type disproportion (Curless & Nelson 1977 Annals of Neurology 2:455: Sulaiman et al 1983 Journal of Neurology, Neurosurgery and Psychiatry 46:175)
  (iii) congenital myopathy with uniform fibre type (type I) (Oh & Danon 1983 Archives of Neurology 40:147)
  (iv) congenital fibre type disproportion in Krabbe's

★ The primary myopathic nature of some of these cases is unproven.

★ It is now clear that this disorder is not a specific entity as some cases previously so described have been found, on further investigation, to be suffering from nemaline myopathy.
† This is not a single entity and many such cases are probably not myopathic in origin.

disease (Dehkharghani et al 1981 Archives of Neurology 38:585)

    (v) reducing body myopathy (Brooke & Neville 1971 Neurology (Minneapolis) 21:412)

    (vi) congenital neuromuscular disease with trilaminar muscle fibres (Ringel et al 1978 Neurology 28:282)

    (vii) congenital myopathy with multifocal degeneration of muscle fibres (Engel A G et al 1971 Mayo Clinic Proceedings 46:666)

(l) the rigid spine myopathy (probably of multiple aetiology but in certain cases undoubtedly of myopathic origin) (Poewe et al 1985 Journal of Neurology, Neurosurgery and Psychiatry 48:887)

(m) myopathy with features of both centronuclear myopathy and multicores (Lee & Yip 1981 Journal of the Neurological Sciences 50:277, Fitzsimons & McLeod 1982 Journal of the Neurological Sciences 57:395)

(n) myopathies with cytoplasmic inclusions

    (i) (Nakashima et al 1970 Archives of Neurology 22:270)

    (ii) with 'fingerprint' inclusions (Engel A G et al 1972 Mayo Clinic Proceedings 47:377)

(o) 'multicore disease' (Engel A G & Groover 1971 Neurology (Minneapolis) 21:413, Vanneste & Stam 1982 Journal of Neurology, Neurosurgery and Psychiatry 45:360)

(p) sarcotubular myopathy (Jerusalem et al 1973 Neurology (Minneapolis) 23:897)

(q) myopathy with tubular aggregates (Morgan-Hughes et al 1970 Brain 93:873) — (see also D-II)

(r) familial neuromuscular disease with type I fibre hypoplasia, tubular aggregates, cardiomyopathy, and myasthenic features (Dobkin & Verity 1978 Neurology (Minneapolis) 28:1135)

(s) myopathy with crystalline intranuclear inclusions (Jenis et al 1969 Archives of Neurology 20:281)

(t) autosomal dominant 'spheroid body' myopathy (Goebel et al 1978 Muscle and Nerve 1: 14)

(u) hypertrophic branchial myopathy (Mancall et al 1974 Neurology (Minneapolis) 24:1166)

(v) monomelic hypertrophic myopathy (Celesia et al 1967 Archives of Neurology 17:69)

(w) cytoplasmic body neuromyopathy with respiratory failure and weight loss (Jerusalem et al 1979 Journal of the Neurological Sciences 41:1)

(x) zebra body myopathy (Lake & Wilson 1975 Journal of the Neurological Sciences 24:437)

3. Myotonic disorders

(a) dystrophia myotonica (myotonia atrophica)
    (i) adult form
    (ii) infantile hypotonic form

(b) myotonia congenita (autosomal dominant form, Thomsen)

(c) myotonia congenita (autosomal recessive form)

(d) myotonia, dwarfism, diffuse bone disease and unusual eye and face abnormality (chondrodystrophic myotonia — the Schwartz–Jampel syndrome)

(e) paramyotonia congenita (Eulenburg)

(f) paramyotonia without paralysis on exposure to cold (de Jong)

(g) familial granulovacuolar lobular myopathy with electrical myotonia (Juguilon et al 1982 Journal of the Neurological Sciences 56:133)

B. Trauma to muscle by external agents

B-I. Physical

1. Crush syndrome

2. Ischaemic infarction or atrophy

    (a) in peripheral vascular disease (Engel & Hawley 1977 Journal of Neurology 215:161)

    (b) in polyarteritis nodosa and other vasculitides

    (c) in diabetes mellitus (Banker & Chester 1973 Neurology (Minneapolis), 23:667)

3. Volkmann's contracture

4. Anterior tibial syndrome

5. Posterior compartment (tibial) syndrome (British Medical Journal 1975 3:193)

6. Congenital or idiopathic torticollis (Sarnat & Morrissy 1981 Muscle and Nerve 4:374)

B-II. Toxic

1. Haff disease

2. Snake-bite by *Enhydrina schistosa* (Malayan sea snake)

3. Saxitoxin poisoning

4. Rhabdomyolysis caused by hornet venom (Shilkin et al 1972 British Medical Journal 1:156)

B-III. Drugs

1. Steroid myopathy

2. Chloroquine myopathy

3. ? Bretylium tosylate myopathy (Campbell & Montuschi 1960 Lancet ii:789)

4. Emetine

5. Vincristine

6. Diazocholesterol (myotonia)

7. Clofibrate

8. Carbenoxolone (Mohamed et al 1966 British Medical Journal 1:1581)

9. Amphotericin B (K^+ depletion)

10. Anodiaquine

11. Colchicine

12. Meperidine (Aberfeld et al 1968 Archives of Neurology 19:384)

13. Pethidine (Mastaglia et al 1971 British Medical Journal 4:532)

14. Pentazocine (Steiner et al 1973 Archives of Neurology 28:408)

15. Polymyxin E (Vanhaeverbeck et al 1974 Journal of Neurology, Neurosurgery and Psychiatry 37:1343)

16. Triorthocresylphosphate (Prineas 1969 Archives of Neurology 21:150)

17. Imidazole (Martin et al 1977 Neurology (Minneapolis) 27:484)

18. Epsilon aminocaproic acid (EACA) (Lane et al 1979 Postgraduate Medical Journal 55:282, Kennard et al 1980 Muscle and Nerve 3:202)

19. Cimetidine (Feest & Read 1980 British Medical Journal 281: 1284)

20. Enfluorane anaesthesia (Caccia et al 1978 Journal of the Neurological Sciences 39:61)

21. Iron overload during haemodialysis (Bregman et al 1980 Lancet ii:876)

22. Gasoline sniffing-myopathy with myoglobinuria (Kovanen et al 1983 Neurology (Cleveland) 33: 629)

C. Inflammatory

C-I. Infections of muscle

1. Viral myositis (see Mastaglia & Ojeda 1985 Annals of Neurology 17: 215)

    (a) benign acute myositis due to:
        influenza A and B
        parainfluenza
        adenovirus 2

    (b) acute rhabdomyolysis due to:
        influenza A and B

Coxsackie B5
Echo 9
adenovirus 21
herpes simplex
Epstein-Barr
(c) epidemic pleurodynia due to:
Coxsackie B5 (also Bl, 3 and 4)
(d) postviral fatigue syndrome or benign postinfection myositis (Schwartz et al 1978 British Medical Journal 2:1256)

2. Bacterial
(a) gas gangrene (*Cl. welchii*)
(b) tetanus (*Cl. tetani*)
(c) staphylococci and other pyogenic agents (septic myositis)
(d) leprous myositis
(e) tropical myositis (usually pyogenic)

3. Fungal myositis (e.g. disseminated candidiasis)

4. Protozoal myositis
(a) toxoplasmosis (Rowland & Greer 1961 Neurology (Minneapolis) 11:367; Behan et al 1983 Acta Neuropathologica (Berlin) 61:246)
(b) sarcosporidiosis
(c) trypanosomiasis cruzi (Chagas disease)
(d) amoebiasis
(e) sarcocystis

5. Cestode myositis
(a) cysticercosis
(b) coenurosis
(c) hydatidosis
(d) sparganosis

6. Nematode myositis
(a) trichinosis
(b) toxocariasis
(c) cutaneous larva migrans (Ancylostoma)

C-II. Other inflammatory disorders of muscle

1. Polymyositis (Group I of Walton & Adams) (possibly an organ-specific autoimmune disease)
(a) acute polymyositis with myoglobinuria
(b) subacute polymyositis
(c) chronic polymyositis (including chronic myositis fibrosa)

2. Dermatomyositis

3. Polymyositis (Group II of Walton & Adams) when occurring as one feature of a non-organspecific autoimmune disease
(a) polymyositis in mixed connective tissue disease
(b) polymyositis in disseminated lupus erythematosus
(c) polymyositis in rheumatic fever
(d) polymyositis in rheumatoid arthritis
(e) polymyositis in scleroderma and/or systemic sclerosis
(f) scleroderma (morphoea) with myopathy
(g) ocular myositis (pseudotumour of the orbit)
(h) muscle infarction and/or polymyositis in polyarteritis nodosa
(i) polymyopathy in Sjögren's disease (Denka & Old 1969 American Journal of Clinical Pathology 151:631, Ringel et al 1982 Archives of Neurology 39:157)
(j) ? polymyopathy in Werner's disease (see Epstein et al 1966 Medicine (Baltimore) 45:177) — nature of muscle atrophy uncertain
(k) localised nodular myositis (see Ch. 17)
(l) myositis of chronic graft versus host disease (Reyes et al 1983 Neurology (Cleveland) 33:1222)
(m) benign acute childhood myositis (Antony et al 1979 Neurology (Minneapolis) 29:1068)

(n) acne fulminans with inflammatory myopathy (Noseworthy et al 1980 Annals of Neurology 8:67)

4. Polymyositis or dermatomyositis (Group IV of Walton & Adams) occurring possibly as a conditioned autoimmune response in malignant disease

5. Polymyositis with associated virus particles (Chou 1967 Science 158:1453, Carpenter et al 1970 Neurology (Minneapolis) 20:889)

6. Acute fulminant myoglobinuric polymyositis with picornavirus-like particles (Fukuyama et al 1977 Journal of Neurology, Neurosurgery and Psychiatry 40:775)

7. Eosinophilic polymyositis (Layzer et al 1977 Annals of Neurology 1:65); with hyperimmunoglobulin E (Symmans et al 1986 Annals of Internal Medicine 104:26)

8. Inclusion body myositis (Carpenter et al 1978 Neurology (Minneapolis) 28:8, Julien et al 1982 Journal of the Neurological Sciences 55:15)

C-III. Inflammatory disorders of muscle of unknown aetiology

1. Sarcoidosis with myopathy

2. Granulomatous polymyositis (Lynch & Bansal 1973 Journal of the Neurological Sciences 18:1) and giant cell myositis (Namba et al 1974 Archives of Neurology 31:27)

3. Polymyalgia rheumatica

4. Localised myositis ossificans

5. Fibrositis and nodular fasciitis

6. ? Myopathy in relapsing panniculitis (Weber–Christian syndrome)

7. Myositis with necrotising fasciitis (Carruthers et al 1975 British Medical Journal 3:355)

8. ? Myopathy in psoriasis (Mormum et al 1970 Dermatologia (Basel) 140:214)

9. Myopathy in Reye's syndrome (Hanson & Urizar 1977 Annals of Neurology 1:431)

10. Myositis ossificans (generalised)

D. Metabolic myopathies

D-I. Muscle disorder associated with endocrine disease

1. Thyrotoxicosis
(a) myopathy
(b) myasthenia gravis
(c) periodic paralysis

2. Myxoedema
(a) girdle myopathy
(b) Debré-Semelaigne syndrome (cretins) (Debré & Semelaigne 1935 American Journal of Diseases of Children 50:1351)
(c) Hoffmann syndrome (adults) (Hoffmann 1897 Deutsche Zeitschrift für Nervenheilkunde 9: 278)
(d) pseudomyotonia
(e) ? neuromyopathy following ^{131}I therapy

3. Hypopituitarism with myopathy

4. Acromegaly with muscle hypertrophy (and/or muscular atrophy) (Mastaglia et al 1970 Lancet ii: 907)

5. Exophthalmic ophthalmoplegia (infiltrative ophthalmopathy or ophthalmic Graves' disease)

6. Cushing's disease myopathy (and corticosteroid myopathy)

7. ACTH myopathy in Nelson's syndrome (Prineas et al 1968 Quarterly Journal of Medicine 37:63)

8. Addison's disease with myopathy

9. Primary aldosteronism (with hypokalaemic periodic paralysis)

10. Hyperparathyroidism with myopathy (Cholod et al 1970 American Journal of Medicine 48:700)

11. Hypoparathyroidism with myopathy (Shane et al 1980 Neurology 30:192)

12. Myopathy in other forms of metabolic bone disease
(a) osteomalacia

(i) idiopathic steatorrhoea

(ii) malabsorption after partial gastrectomy (Ekbom et al 1964 Acta Medica Scandinavica 176:493)

(iii) renal acidosis

(iv) hypophosphataemia (Schott & Wills 1975 Journal of Neurology, Neurosurgery and Psychiatry 38:297)

(v) due to anticonvulsants (Marsden et al 1973 British Medical Journal 4:526)

13. Myopathy with calcitonin-secreting medullary carcinoma of the thyroid (Cunliffe et al 1970 American Journal of Medicine 48:120)

D-II. Genetically-determined metabolic myopathies

1. Glycogen storage disease involving muscle

(a) glycogenosis type I due to glucose-6-phosphatase deficiency (von Gierke's disease) (gives hypotonia without direct muscular involvement)

(b) glycogenosis type II (Pompe's disease) due to amylo-1,4 glucosidase deficiency

(i) acute infantile form

(ii) adult or late onset variety (see Loonen et al 1981 Neurology (Minneapolis) 31:1209)

(c) glycogenosis type III (Cori–Forbes disease) due to debrancher enzyme (amylo-1,6 glucosidase) deficiency (DiMauro et al 1979 Annals of Neurology 5:422)

(d) glycogenosis type IV (Andersen's disease) due to brancher enzyme (1,4 glucan: 1,4 glucan-6-glycosyl transferase) deficiency (Ferguson et al 1983 Journal of the Neurological Sciences 60:337)

(e) glycogenosis type V (McArdle's disease) due to phosphorylase deficiency

(i) usual form with onset in childhood

(ii) fatal infantile form (DiMauro & Hartlage 1978 Neurology (Minneapolis) 28:1124)

(iii) late-onset myophosphorylase deficiency (Kost & Verity 1980 Muscle and Nerve 3:195)

(f) glycogenosis type VII (Tarui's disease) due to phosphofructokinase deficiency (Hays et al 1981 Neurology (Minneapolis) 31:1077)

(g) phosphoglycerate kinase deficiency (Bresolin et al 1984 Muscle and Nerve 7:542)

(h) phosphoglycerate mutase deficiency

(i) lactate dehydrogenase deficiency (for (h) and (i) see DiMauro et al 1982 Neurology (Minneapolis) 32:584)

(j) lysosomal glycogen storage disease without acid maltase deficiency (Danon et al 1981 Neurology (New York) 31:51, Riggs et al 1983 Neurology (Cleveland) 33:873)

(k) mixed enzyme deficiencies (e.g. phosphofructokinase and phosphorylase b kinase) (Danon et al 1981 Neurology (New York) 31:1303)

2. Other inherited disorders of carbohydrate metabolism

(a) glycerol kinase deficiency in X-linked myopathy (Guggenheim et al 1980 Annals of Neurology 7:441)

(b) muscle fructose 1,6-diphosphatase deficiency with atypical central core disease (Kar et al 1980 Journal of the Neurological Sciences 48:243)

(c) myoadenylate deaminase deficiency (with cramps and exertional myalgia) (DiMauro et al 1980 Journal of the Neurological Sciences 47:191, Kelemen et al 1982 Neurology (New York) 32:857)

3. Familial periodic paralysis and related syndromes

(a) hypokalaemic periodic paralysis

(b) hyperkalaemic periodic paralysis (adynamia episodica hereditaria)

(c) normokalaemic periodic paralysis (probably a variant of (b)) (Poskanzer & Kerr 1961 American Journal of Medicine 31:328)

(d) myotonic periodic paralysis (paramyotonia congenita) (possibly a variant of (b))

(e) thyrotoxic periodic paralysis

4. Mitochondrial and lipid storage myopathies (modified from Morgan-Hughes et al 1982 Brain 105:553)

(a) monocarboxylase translocase deficiency

(b) deficiencies involving the carnitine acyl-carnitine carrier system

(i) muscle carnitine deficiency

(ii) systemic carnitine deficiency

(iii) partial muscle carnitine deficiencies

(iv) carnitine palmityl transferase (CPT) deficiency (including heterogeneous forms (Donato et al 1981 Journal of the Neurological Sciences 50: 207), CPT II deficiency with normal CPT I (Scholte et al 1979 Journal of the Neurological Sciences 40:39; Trevisan et al 1984 Neurology (Cleveland) 34:353), CPT deficiency with myoglobinuria and respiratory failure (Bertorini et al 1980 Neurology (Minneapolis) 30:263) and with cold-induced rhabdomyolysis (Brownell et al 1979 Canadian Journal of Medical Science 6:367)

(v) combined carnitine and CPT deficiencies

(vi) autosomal dominant lipid storage neuromyopathy with normal carnitine and CPT (Askanas et al 1985 Neurology (Cleveland) 35:66)

(c) lipid storage myopathies of uncertain origin (see Ch. 25)

(d) defects of mitochondrial substrate utilisation

(i) pyruvate decarboxylase deficiency

(ii) dihydrolipoyl transacetylase deficiency

(iii) dihydrolipoyl dehydrogenase deficiency

(iv) pyruvate dehydrogenase phosphatase deficiency

(v) pyruvate carboxylase deficiency

(vi) carnitine acetyltransferase deficiency

N.B. Many disorders in this group cause myopathy but the clinical picture is often dominated by progressive encephalopathy, hypotonia, lactic acidosis and respiratory insufficiency

(e) defects of the respiratory chain

(i) defects of NADH oxidation

(ii) cytochrome b deficiency

(iii) cytochrome c oxidase (aa₃) deficiency

(iv) combined cytochrome deficiencies (aa₃ +b)

(v) encephalomyopathy with decreased succinate-cytochrome c reductase deficiency (Riggs et al 1984 Neurology (Cleveland) 34:48)

(f) defects of energy conservation and transduction

(i) hypermetabolic mitochondrial myopathy (Luft's disease)

(ii) other mitochondrial myopathies with 'loose coupling'

(iii) mitochondrial ATPase deficiency

N.B. The mitochondrial and lipid storage myopathies give a bewildering variety of symptoms including ophthalmoplegia, severe hypotonia, cramps and myoglobinuria, exercise-induced muscle pain and muscular weakness of variable severity occurring at many different stages of life. The mitochondrial encephalomyopathies also embrace a very wide variety of syndromes (see Kuriyama et al 1984 Neurology (Cleveland) 34:72 and Ch. 25); lactic acidosis and multiple cerebral infarcts are among the commoner manifestations of cerebral involvement (Pavlakis et al 1984 Annals of Neurology 16:481).

5. Malignant hyperpyrexia, induced by halothane, suxamethonium, ketamine, psychotropic agents and many other anaesthetic agents and drugs (see Lane & Mastaglia 1978 Lancet ii: 562 and Ch. 25)
6. Progressive myositis ossificans (see Pitt & Hamilton 1984 Journal of the Royal Society of Medicine 77:68)
7. Progressive muscle spasm, alopecia, diarrhoea and malabsorption (Satoyoshi's disease) (Satoyoshi 1978 Neurology (Minneapolis) 28:458)
8. Myopathy in lysine-cystinuria (Clara & Lowenthal 1966 Journal of the Neurological Sciences 3:433)
9. Myopathy in xanthinuria (Chalmers et al 1969 Quarterly Journal of Medicine 38:493)
10. Myopathy in Lafora disease (Coleman et al 1974 Archives of Neurology 31:396)
11. Myopathy with tubular aggregates, often associated with myalgia (Brumback et al 1981 Journal of Neurology, Neurosurgery and Psychiatry 44:250, Rohkamm et al 1983 Neurology (Cleveland) 33:331, Niakan et al 1985 Journal of Neurology, Neurosurgery and Psychiatry 48:882)
12. Cytoplasmic body myopathy (Patel et al 1983 Journal of the Neurological Sciences 60:281)
13. Benign reducing body myopathy (Oh et al 1983 Muscle and Nerve 6:278)
14. Myopathy due to a deficiency of relaxing factor (Brody's disease); now believed to be due to a deficiency of Ca^{2+}-adenosine-triphosphatase in sarcoplasmic reticulum (Brody 1969 New England Journal of Medicine 281:187, Karpati et al 1986 Annals of Neurology 20:38)

D-III. Other metabolic myopathies
1. Alcoholic myopathy
   (a) acute, with rhabdomyolysis and myoglobinuria
   (b) subacute or chronic proximal (Hudgson 1984 British Medical Journal 1:585)
   (c) hypokalaemic (Rubinstein & Wainapel 1977 Archives of Neurology 34:553)
2. Nutritional myopathy
   (a) protein deficiency; malnutrition due to anorexia nervosa or malabsorption
   (b) human myopathy due to vitamin E deficiency (Neville et al 1983 Neurology (Cleveland) 33:483)
   (c) chronic myopathy with hypercalcaemia and hypophosphataemia
3. Myopathy in chronic renal failure (Floyd et al 1974 Quarterly Journal of Medicine 43:509)
4. Acute polymyopathy during total parenteral nutrition (Stewart & Hensley 1981 British Medical Journal 2:1578)
5. Potassium depletion myopathy (Comi et al 1985 Muscle and Nerve 8:17)
6. Carnitine deficiency induced during haemodialysis (Battistella et al 1978 Lancet i:939)
7. Riboflavin-responsive lipid myopathy with carnitine deficiency (Carroll et al 1981 Neurology (New York) 31:1557)
8. Myoglobinuria (other than that due to glycogen storage disease, mitochondrial or lipid storage myopathies and CPT deficiency) (see Rowland 1984 Canadian Journal of Neurological Sciences 11:1)
   (a) exertion (including military training, running, skiing, anterior tibial syndrome, status epilepticus, electric shock, myoclonus, severe dystonia)
   (b) crush or ischaemic injury to muscle (see above)
   (c) metabolic depression or distortion (including CO or drug intoxication, diabetic ketoacidosis, hyperosmolar states, renal tubular acidosis, hyper- and hyponatraemia, hypokalaemia and hypophosphataemia)

(d) due to drugs and toxins (see above), including the ingestion of quail (Bateman 1977 US Office of Naval Research)
(e) abnormalities of body temperature (including hypothermia due to cold or hypothyroidism, or fever due to toxins, vaccines, heat stroke, malignant hyperpyrexia or the malignant neuroleptic syndrome)
(f) infections (including viral, bacterial and mycoplasma infections and the toxic shock syndrome)
(g) autoimmune muscle disease (polymyositis and dermatomyositis)
(h) idiopathic recurrent or paroxysmal rhabdomyolysis with myoglobinuria, sometimes leading to myopathy with persistent weakness (Korein et al 1959 Neurology (Minneapolis) 9:767, Favara et al 1967 American Journal of Medicine 42:196, Bermils et al 1983 Neurology (Cleveland) 33:1613)
(i) chronic myopathy due to drugs (chloroquine, emetine, steroids, penicillin, vincristine, colchicine; repeated intramuscular injections of meperidine or pentazocine)

E. Myopathy associated with malignant disease
1. Carcinomatous myopathy (other than polymyositis)
2. Myasthenic–myopathic syndrome
3. Carcinomatous embolic myopathy (Heffner 1971 Neurology (Minneapolis) 21:841)
4. Proximal myopathy due to discrete carcinomatous metastases in muscle (Doshi & Fowler 1983 Journal of Neurology, Neurosurgery and Psychiatry 46:358)
5. Myopathy in the carcinoid syndrome (Swash et al 1975 Archives of Neurology 32:572)

F. Myopathy associated with myasthenia gravis

G. Myopathy in thalassaemia (Logothetis et al 1972 Neurology (Minneapolis) 22:294)

H. Other disorders of muscle of unknown or uncertain aetiology
1. Acute muscle necrosis
   (a) of unknown cause
   (b) in chronic alcoholism
   (c) in carcinoma (Urich & Wilkinson 1970 Journal of Neurology, Neurosurgery and Psychiatry 33:398)
2. Amyloid myopathy
   (a) primary familial
   (b) primary sporadic (sometimes causing pseudohypertrophy of muscle) (Ringel & Claman 1982 Archives of Neurology 39:413)
   (c) in myelomatosis
   (d) with angiopathy (Bruni et al 1977 Canadian Journal of Neurological Sciences 2:77)
3. Disuse atrophy
4. Muscle cachexia (in wasting diseases and in the elderly)
5. Muscle wasting in contralateral cerebral lesions (particularly of parietal lobe)

I. Tumours of muscle
1. Rhabdomyoma
2. Rhabdomyosarcoma
   (a) adult pleomorphic type
   (b) embryonal botryoid type
   (c) embryonal alveolar type
3. Desmoid fibroma
4. Alveolar sarcoma
5. Angioma
6. Other connective tissue tumours occasionally occurring in muscle

VI. SOME DISORDERS OF SUPRASPINAL TONAL REGULATION WHICH MAY MIMIC NEUROMUSCULAR DISORDERS
1. Muscular hypertrophy, extrapyramidal disorders and

mental deficiency (de Lange 1934 American Journal of Diseases of Children 48:243)
2. Prader–Willi syndrome
3. Hypotonia in mental defect
4. Hypotonia in metabolic disorders
5. Hypotonia in cerebral palsy (atonic diplegia)
6. Hypotonia in cerebellar diplegia and other cerebellar ataxias
7. Hypotonia in rheumatic chorea
8. Hypotonia in acrodynia (Pink disease)
9. Hypotonia in the cerebrohepatorenal syndrome (Bowen et al 1964 Johns Hopkins Medical Journal 114:402)

REFERENCES

Adrian R H, Marshall M W 1976 Action potentials reconstructed in normal and myotonic muscle fibres. Journal of Physiology 258:125

Albers J W, Allen A A, Bastron J A, Daube J R 1981 Limb myokymia. Muscle and Nerve 4:494

André-Thomas A, Chesni Y, Dargassies S S-A 1960 The neurological examination of the infant. National Spastics Society, London

Asbury A K, Gilliatt R W 1984 Peripheral nerve disorders — a practical approach. Butterworth, London

Ashizawa T, Butler I J, Harati Y, Roongta S M 1983 A dominantly inherited syndrome with continuous motor neuron discharges. Annals of Neurology 13:285

Auger R G, Daube J R, Gomez M R, Lambert E H 1984 Hereditary form of sustained muscle activity of peripheral nerve origin causing generalized myokymia and muscle stiffness. Annals of Neurology 15:13

Bickerstaff E R 1980 Neurological examination in clinical practice, 14th edn. Blackwell, Oxford

Cogan D G 1978 Neurology of the ocular muscles, 3rd edn. Thomas, Springfield, Illinois

de Jong R N 1979 The neurologic examination, 4th edn. Harper and Row, New York

de Lange C 1934 Congenital hypertrophy of muscles, extrapyramidal motor disturbances and mental deficiency. American Journal of Diseases of Childhood 48:243

Denny-Brown D, Pennybacker J B 1938 Fibrillation and fasciculation in voluntary muscle. Brain 61:311

Denny-Brown D, Nevin S 1941 The phenomenon of myotonia. Brain 64:1

Dubowitz V 1978 Muscle disorders in childhood. Saunders, London

Edwards R H T, McDonnell M 1974 Hand-held dynamometer for evaluating voluntary muscle function. Lancet ii:757

Gamstorp I 1984 Pediatric neurology, 2nd edn. Appleton-Century-Crofts, New York

Gamstorp I, Wohlfart G 1959 A syndrome characterised by myokymia, myotonia, muscular wasting and increased perspiration. Acta Psychiatrica Scandinavica 34:181

Gardner-Medwin D, Hudson P, Walton J N 1967 Benign spinal muscular atrophy arising in childhood and adolescence. Journal of the Neurological Sciences 5:121

Gardner-Medwin D, Walton J N 1969 Myokymia with impaired muscular relaxation. Lancet i:127

Gordon N S 1976 Paediatric neurology for the clinician. Spastics International Medical Publications, Heinemann, London

Gray's Anatomy 1967 34th edn. Davies D V, Coupland R E (eds) Longmans, London

Hudson A J, Brown W F, Gilbert J J 1978 The muscular pain-fasciculation syndrome. Neurology (Minneapolis) 28:1105

Isaacs H 1961 A syndrome of continuous muscle fibre activity. Journal of Neurology, Neurosurgery and Psychiatry 24:319

Jackson D L, Satya-Murti S, Davis L, Drachman D B 1979 Isaacs syndrome with laryngeal involvement: an unusual presentation of myokymia. Neurology (Minneapolis) 29:1612

Jennekens F G I, Tomlinson B E, Walton J N 1971 Histochemical aspects of five limb muscles in old age: an autopsy study. Journal of the Neurological Sciences 14:259

Lane R J M, Turnbull D M, Welch J, Walton J N 1986 A double-blind, placebo-controlled, crossover study of verapamil in exertional muscle pain.

Lehoczky T, Halasy M, Simon G, Harmos G 1965 Glycogenic myopathy: a case of skeletal muscle-glycogenosis in twins. Journal of the Neurological Sciences 2:366

Leigh P N, Rothwell J C, Traub M, Marsden C D 1980 A patient with reflex myoclonus and muscle rigidity: 'jerking stiff-man syndrome'. Journal of Neurology, Neurosurgery and Psychiatry 43:1125

Leigh R J, Zee D S 1983 The neurology of eye movements. F A Davis, Philadelphia

Leyburn P, Walton J N 1959 The treatment of myotonia: a controlled trial. Brain 82:81

Matthews W B 1966 Facial myokymia. Journal of Neurology, Neurosurgery and Psychiatry 29:35

Medical Research Council 1986 Aids to the examination of the peripheral nervous system, Memorandum no. 45, 3rd edn. Baillière Tindall, Eastbourne

Mertens H-G, Zschocke S 1965 Neuromyotonie. Klinische Wochenschrift 43:917

O'Doherty D S, Schellinger D, Raptopoulos V 1977 Computed tomographic patterns of pseudohypertrophic muscular dystrophy: preliminary results. Journal of Computer Assisted Tomography 1:482

Pact V, Sirotkin-Roses M, Beatus J 1984 The muscle testing handbook. Little Brown, Boston, Toronto

Paine R S, Oppé T E 1966 Neurological examination of children. National Spastics Society and Heinemann, London

Perkoff G T, Hardy P, Velez-Garcia E 1966 Reversible acute muscular syndrome in chronic alcoholism. New England Journal of Medicine 274:1277

Prineas J, Hall R, Barwick D D, Watson A J 1968 Myopathy associated with pigmentation following adrenalectomy for Cushing's syndrome. Quarterly Journal of Medicine 37:63

Ross Russell R W, Wiles C M 1985 Neurology. Integrated Clinical Science Series. Heinemann, London

Salick A I, Pearson C M 1967 Electrical silence of myoidema. Neurology (Minneapolis) 17:899

Satayoshi E, Kowa H 1967 A myopathy due to glycolytic abnormality. Archives of Neurology 17:248

Valli G, Barbieri S, Cappa S, Pellegrini G, Scarlato G 1983 Syndromes of abnormal muscular activity: overlap between continuous muscle fibre activity and the stiff man syndrome. Journal of Neurology, Neurosurgery and Psychiatry 46:241

Vignos P J, Archibald K C 1960 Maintenance of ambulation in childhood muscular dystrophy. Journal of Chronic Diseases 12:273

Wallis W E, Poznak A V, Plum F 1970 Generalized muscular stiffness, fasciculation, and myokymia of peripheral nerve origin. Archives of Neurology 22:430

Walton J N 1981 Diffuse exercise-induced muscle pain of undetermined cause relieved by verapamil. Lancet i:993.

Walton J N 1985 Brain's Diseases of the Nervous System, 9th edn. Oxford University Press, Oxford, p 116

Welch L K, Appenzeller O, Bicknell J M 1972 Peripheral neuropathy with myokymia, sustained muscular contraction, and continuous motor unit activity. Neurology (Minneapolis) 22:161

Williamson E, Brooke M H 1972 Myokymia and the motor unit: a histochemical study. Archives of Neurology 26:11

Wilson J, Walton J N 1959 Some muscular manifestations of hypothyroidism. Journal of Neurology, Neurosurgery and Psychiatry 22:320

World Federation of Neurology: Research Group on Neuromuscular Diseases 1968 Classification of the neuromuscular disorders. Journal of the Neurological Sciences 6:165

Zisfein J, Sivak M, Aron A M, Bender A N 1983 Isaacs' syndrome with muscle hypertrophy reversed by phenytoin therapy. Archives of Neurology 40:241

The muscular dystrophies

INTRODUCTION

The study of the progressive degenerative disorders of muscle began in the mid-nineteenth century, especially in France and Germany. Aran (1850) and Wachsmuth (1855) reviewed the subject with little attempt at classification of disease states or the distinction of neurogenic from myopathic disease. Meryon (1852) gave the first clear account of progressive muscular paralysis in young boys and demonstrated that it was due to 'granular degeneration' of the muscles without changes in the anterior horns of the spinal cord or in the motor roots. Later, Duchenne (1868) gave a vivid description of this disorder, now given his name, and Gowers' (1879) was the first comprehensive account in English and is still one of the finest. Both Duchenne and Gowers emphasised the 'pseudohypertrophic' enlargement of certain muscles. Leyden (1876) and Möbius (1879) described a familial form of degeneration affecting the muscles of the pelvic girdle. In 1884 Erb described a juvenile or scapulohumeral form, and stressed that this disease was due to a primary degeneration of the muscles which he later (Erb 1891) named muscular dystrophy. The classic description of the facioscapulohumeral form was published by Landouzy & Dejerine (1884) although cases had earlier been recorded and photographed by Duchenne (1862). 'Muscular dystrophy' in the external ocular muscles was reported by Hutchinson (1879) and Fuchs (1890); the discovery in recent years that mitochondrial disorders are responsible for many such cases has made the title of muscular dystrophy inappropriate. Howard (1908) and Batten (1909) suggested that some cases of amyotonia congenita (Oppenheim 1900) were the result of a simple atrophic variety of congenital muscular dystrophy. In 1930 Ullrich reported a distinct 'atonic-sclerotic' type of congenital muscular dystrophy and later another variant associated with cerebral anomalies was reported from Japan by Fukuyama et al (1960). Gowers (1902) described a distal form of the disease. There is now some doubt about the true nature of his cases, but Welander (1951) gave a full account of a distal muscular dystrophy occurring in Sweden and later two other forms of distal muscular dystrophy were distinguished. The benign form of X–linked muscular dystrophy was distinguished from the Duchenne type by Becker & Keiner (1955). Victor et al (1962) delineated oculopharyngeal muscular dystrophy, separating it from the other ocular myopathies. A scapuloperoneal distribution of muscular weakness is seen in certain cases of spinal muscular atrophy, of which it seems to form a distinct subtype. In some kindreds a similar disorder of myopathic origin constitutes, in effect, another form of muscular dystrophy (Seitz 1957). It is now apparent that both X-linked and autosomal dominant varieties of scapuloperoneal myopathy exist, the former having been characterised first by Emery & Dreifuss (1966).

Apart from the delineation and description of the disorders which fall within the definition of the muscular dystrophies, the principal recent advances in the field have been in our understanding of the X-linked muscular dystrophies. The use of genetic theory and of serum creatine kinase (CK) assays to assess the probability that female relatives were carriers of the gene was developed during the 1960s and 1970s; in addition to its direct contribution to the prevention of Duchenne dystrophy, this work maintained a high level of research interest in the genetics of the X-linked dystrophies. The discovery that a few females with otherwise typical Duchenne muscular dystrophy had translocations involving the Xp21 site on the short arm of one of their X-chromosomes provided the first direct evidence of the site of the gene for Duchenne dystrophy; this rapidly led to the realisation that the Becker and Duchenne genes were probably allelic and not sited at opposite ends of the chromosome as had previously been believed. More importantly, it led

to the application of recombinant DNA studies to this part of the X-chromosome and to the discovery of a number of increasingly closely linked restriction fragment length polymorphisms (RFLPs) which can now be used in many families to estimate the probability of the carrier status in females and the probability that a male fetus is affected. The discovery of further polymorphisms and the application of the technique to a higher proportion of families at risk have become the dominant factor in the current clinical and research approach to muscular dystrophy★.

Before the clinical aspects of these disorders are described, the dual problem of the definition of muscular dystrophy and the proper classification of the diseases which have been given this name must be discussed.

The problem of definition

In the nineteenth century, while the clinical syndromes were being delineated, much attention was paid to the distinction between muscular atrophy resulting from pathological changes in the nervous system and those disorders, or 'myopathies', in which the primary pathological change was in muscle. The myopathies are now known to include not only genetic disorders but also many which are inflammatory, metabolic or endocrine in nature. The muscle pathology, at first identifiable only at autopsy, was correlated gradually with clinical syndromes. Duchenne defined characteristic responses of muscle to electrical stimulation and Erb, among others, defined typical histological appearances of muscle which could later be used to characterise myopathies in living patients. In particular Erb (1891) described the characteristic histological appearances by which he defined 'muscular dystrophy' (see Ch. 5). The investigative techniques of clinical enzymology and electromyography have improved our ability to diagnose muscular dystrophy, but as an operational definition for use in the diagnosis of individual cases we are still dependent upon: (1) the recognition of a specific clinical syndrome; and (2) the recognition of the specific, or at least

---

★ The Duchenne gene has now been identified and partially characterised (see Ch. 26).

compatible, histological features in muscle biopsy material. Yet a wider conceptual definition is plainly needed and Walton (1961) suggested that the term 'muscular dystrophy' should be reserved for cases of progressive, genetically determined, primary degenerative myopathy.

As our understanding of the essential lesions underlying each type of muscular dystrophy advances, this definition may become difficult to sustain and will be replaced by more accurate ones, e.g. the congenital muscular dystrophies are by no means always progressive. Furthermore, the concept of primary degenerative disorders in general is being eroded by the discovery of underlying specific metabolic disorders in many conditions. Some examples of the ocular and oculopharyngeal 'muscular dystrophies' and of the facioscapulohumeral syndrome are now recognised to be mitochondrial disorders. Some of the 'congenital myopathies', such as nemaline myopathy, are often slowly progressive, thus falling within our definition, yet because of their different and characteristic histology they are not called muscular dystrophies.

Interest in the relationship between muscular dystrophy and neurogenic atrophy was re-awakened by Kugelberg & Welander (1956) who described 12 patients with spinal muscular atrophy closely resembling muscular dystrophy. This disorder proved to be a common cause of confusion and its existence necessitated careful clinical, electromyographic and histological examination in every patient to avoid errors in diagnosis. Then followed the discovery that, not only in spinal muscular atrophy but also in other chronic denervating disorders, 'secondary myopathic changes' may occur in muscle (Tyrer & Sutherland 1961, Drachman et al 1967) so that, in advanced cases, anterior horn cell disease and primary myopathy may be indistinguishable by any criteria short of autopsy. This has made it necessary to reconsider the pathogenesis of many of the rarer chronic 'myopathies', including the less well-established muscular dystrophies, and this reassessment is still incomplete.

Electrophysiological studies favouring an apparent disorder of anterior horn cell function even in Duchenne muscular dystrophy (McComas et al 1971) led to a 'neurogenic theory' of the aetiology of the disease which, after a period of popularity in the early 1970s, fell out of favour because of lack of confirmatory evidence. However, those muscular dystrophies which are more difficult to define by strict criteria than the Duchenne type provide a continual source of confusion: cases of 'limb-girdle', scapuloperoneal and facioscapulohumeral 'syndromes' in which investigation indicates myopathic or neurogenic features, or both, are commonplace in the literature and in clinical practice. It is clear that at this stage no more adequate general definition of muscular dystrophy is possible.

The problem of classification

The hereditary nature of the muscular dystrophies was recognised early, but attempts to apply the principles of genetics to certain categories led to much confusion. Thus, in studying the traditional pseudohypertrophic, pelvic girdle atrophic, facio-scapulohumeral and juvenile scapulohumeral forms, Bell (1943) and others found examples of autosomal recessive, dominant and X-linked recessive inheritance in each of the clinical varieties of the disease.

This confusion led to many attempts to produce a revised classification, taking into account both clinical and genetic criteria. Notable contributions were made by Tyler & Wintrobe (1950), Levison (1951), Stevenson (1953), Becker (1953, 1964), Lamy & de Grouchy (1954), Walton & Nattrass (1954), Morton & Chung (1959) and Emery & Walton (1967). Several of these revised classifications were reviewed in previous editions of this book.

In the absence of any absolute definition of muscular dystrophy or of a known biochemical basis for any of the types, classification consists of listing those disorders which conform to the operational definition and which seem to be separate entities on genetic, clinical and pathological grounds. The sporadic case, in which no genetic evidence is available, presents particular difficulties in diagnosis and classification. In the present state of knowledge, the X-linked and dominant disorders are therefore often better characterised than those of autosomal recessive inheritance. These nosological difficulties are discussed in relation to individual disorders in the sections which follow, but it is important to point out here that we have now virtually abandoned the term 'limb-girdle muscular dystrophy', used in the past to encompass a variety of different disorders, in favour of the more specific terms used in the classification below.

The myotonic disorders are discussed in a separate chapter, and myotonic dystrophy (which differs in so many ways from the 'pure' muscular dystrophies) is therefore excluded from the following working classification. Some of the less well-established clinical types are qualified with question marks.

The muscular dystrophies

(a) X-linked muscular dystrophies
   Duchenne
   Becker
   Emery–Dreifuss
   ? Hereditary myopathy confined to females
(b) Autosomal recessive muscular dystrophies
   Scapulohumeral
   Autosomal recessive in childhood
   ? Late onset proximal (lower limbs)
   ? Quadriceps myopathy
   Distal
   Congenital
   Ullrich
   Fukuyama
(c) Autosomal dominant muscular dystrophies
   Facioscapulohumeral
   Scapuloperoneal
   Late-onset proximal
   Distal (adult-onset)
   Distal (juvenile)
   ? Ocular
   Oculopharyngeal

General principles of diagnosis

An unqualified diagnosis of 'muscular dystrophy' is never justifiable. Every case must be allotted firmly to one of the categories listed above; any which seem not to be typical of any specific type should be regarded with suspicion and should be thoroughly investigated, a point of great importance because several of the other myopathic disorders are treatable. In the early stages, or in any doubtful case, a firm diagnosis should be made only after investigation including estimation of serum enzymes, especially of CK activity, electromyography (EMG) and muscle biopsy. Nevertheless, the clinical diagnosis of advanced cases of the well-established types is rarely difficult, especially in the Duchenne and facioscapulohumeral types. It is based upon a clear history of the onset and progression of the symptoms, the pattern of inheritance and a detailed examination of the muscles, which will reveal the pattern of selective muscular wasting and weakness that is characteristic of each type of muscular dystrophy.

Differential diagnosis from other disorders. This matter is considered in detail in Chapter 14, but for completeness an outline is given here.

When a waddling gait is caused by *disease of the hip joints* there will be no wasting, weakness, hypotonia or reflex change and, in this situation, the hips should always be X-rayed even if passive movements of the joints are full.

Spinal muscular atrophy is an important imitator of muscular dystrophy in childhood and early adult life (Kugelberg & Welander 1956). There may have been a previously affected sib in the family, sometimes with a more severe infantile form. The weakness may have developed gradually or may apparently have been precipitated by an acute infection, an injury or a prophylactic immunisation. Often the course is variable with periods of improvement. The muscle weakness is chiefly proximal and often selective with corresponding atrophy, and hypertrophy may occur, all points which cause confusion with muscular dystrophy. Unfortunately, the selective muscular weakness in spinal muscular atrophy, unlike that of the muscular dystrophies, has no consistent or recognisable pattern: indeed, the recognition that the pattern is slightly 'wrong' for any muscular dystrophy is often the first clue to diagnosis. Another helpful but inconstant clue is fasciculation of the tongue, which should be sought in all such cases; less often there is fasciculation elsewhere. Such features as tremor, talipes, distal, asymmetrical or even focal muscle weakness and the loss of tendon reflexes in relatively well-preserved muscles are not constant characteristics of spinal muscular atrophy, but they occur frequently and are helpful clues to the diagnosis when they are found. The serum CK activity may be normal but it is often raised. Electromyography and muscle biopsy are the only reliable ways of distinguishing this disorder.

In a small proportion of cases of motor neurone disease the weakness is chiefly proximal, but fasciculation and signs of corticospinal tract involvement in the form of brisk reflexes or extensor plantar responses are almost invariable, and clearly distinguish the disorder from muscular dystrophy.

In *polymyositis* the progression of the disease is usually more rapid than in muscular dystrophy, and spontaneous remissions may occur. The generalised proximal (and sometimes also distal) weakness contrasts with the selective weakness in muscular dystrophy and, in particular, often affects both the anterior and posterior neck muscles. Dysphagia is common in polymyositis and rare in dystrophy. Except in very chronic cases, muscular atrophy in polymyositis is less severe than that in dystrophic muscles with an equal degree of weakness; muscle hypertrophy is rare. The tendon reflexes tend to be spared in polymyositis, except in advanced cases, whereas they are lost as soon as there is significant weakness of the relevant muscle in muscular dystrophy. In dermatomyositis the skin changes are often diagnostic.

When all these points are considered, there is rarely doubt as to whether a child has polymyositis or muscular dystrophy. Nevertheless, diagnosis is so important that a muscle biopsy should always be performed. The same criteria apply to adult cases, but some indolent cases of polymyositis in middle age may be mistaken for 'limb-girdle dystrophies' of late onset. Here the diagnosis is essentially a pathological one, but controversy may persist even after autopsy.

The various *congenital myopathies* often present with hypotonia in infancy, but may also cause gait disturbances in later childhood. In occasional cases, clinical diagnosis is possible, e.g. when a child has the skeletal dysmorphism of nemaline myopathy; however, the diagnosis in this group is essentially pathological: this further underlines the importance of full investigation, including histochemical and electron-microscopic studies of muscle biopsies, in all cases of unusual muscle disease.

The presence of bone pain should raise the possibility of a *myopathy associated with metabolic bone disease*. The absence of muscle wasting and the brisk tendon reflexes are useful clinical points in such cases (Smith & Stern 1967).

The myopathy sometimes associated with *thyrotoxicosis* can imitate muscular dystrophy, especially when the hyperthyroidism is not clinically obvious. The condition should be excluded by laboratory tests whenever there is proximal weakness and wasting, especially in the upper limbs, with a rather short history or with an unusual pattern of selective muscle involvement.

Diagnosis of the type of muscular dystrophy. The differentiation of the many varieties of muscular dystrophy should be made, ideally, on both clinical and genetic grounds. Unfortunately this is rarely possible; many patients have no family history of the disease and, furthermore, the different genetic varieties of the disease cannot always be distinguished clinically. This problem is most acute in cases of the Duchenne, autosomal recessive childhood and Becker types. Nevertheless, the differentiation of the X-linked disorders from the similar autosomal recessive type is of great importance for genetic counselling. For example, the daughters of a man with Becker dystrophy are all obligate carriers and may transmit the disease to their sons, whereas the daughters of a man with an autosomal recessive muscular dystrophy carry a very small risk of having affected children. On the other hand, the Duchenne, scapuloperoneal and facioscapulohumeral types, for example, can generally be differentiated from each other, even in their early stages, on the basis of the age of onset, the rate of progression and the pattern of selective muscle involvement. The technique of CT scanning of muscle is potentially a valuable aid to the analysis of selective muscle involvement and may prove helpful in subtle problems of differential diagnosis in the future (Bulcke et al 1981, Jones et al 1983,

Stern et al 1984). Ultrasound imaging, although non-invasive, is much less revealing (Heckmatt et al 1982). Further points in differential diagnosis are discussed in relation to the individual types of muscular dystrophy.

The general principles of management

(1) The first stage of management is diagnosis. Precision in diagnosis is important, not only to exclude treatable disorders but to provide an accurate basis for prognosis and genetic counselling. Furthermore, diagnosis in any disabled patient involves not only identification of the nature of the disease, but also assessment of the degree of handicap, so that appropriate remedial therapy and services can be provided.

(2) Telling the patient, or the parents, the diagnosis and prognosis is a vital stage in management, which will often determine their whole subsequent attitude and approach to the disease. It must be done with sensitivity by a physician who knows the patient personally and has a sound understanding of the disease and its implications. We believe that, in general, adult patients or the parents of affected children should be given a full and accurate account in order to allow them to make constructive plans for the future. It is valuable to balance the bad news with an offer of a programme of management and of continuing practical help and support. Most patients also find some comfort in knowing about the extensive world-wide research into the pathogenesis and potential treatment of the muscular dystrophies.

(3) Genetic advice must be offered at the earliest opportunity, not only to the immediate family but, in the X-linked and dominant disorders, to other relatives at risk of having affected children.

(4) Useful mobility should be maintained as a major priority. Exercise promotes physical fitness and muscle strength, and we believe that regular exercise should become a lifelong habit for all patients. Obesity should be avoided. Contractures can be at least partly controlled by regular stretching. Surgery should be undertaken only with great circumspection, should be as simple and brief as possible and must, above all, be done only in conjunction with well-organised programmes for rapid postoperative mobilisation (see Ch. 22).

In general, surgical procedures should be done only when they are likely to provide an important functional benefit which can be obtained in no other way. Anaesthesia should be avoided, or undertaken only with special precautions to avoid respiratory or cardiac complications. Regular breathing exercises and, where appropriate, postural drainage help to delay the onset of respiratory failure.

(5) A bewildering variety of practical aids and equipment for the disabled has beome available in recent years. Many are invaluable, but careful assessment and trial may be necessary to solve specific problems for individual patients. Wheelchairs and lifting equipment, in particular, must be selected with professional skill. Occasional but regular consultation with an occupational therapist, sometimes linked with visits to one of the many 'Aids Centres' now established in Britain and other countries, may greatly reduce the disabling effects of the disease. It is of the greatest psychological importance that patients and their families should know in advance of such solutions to problems, so that they may live expecting to remain reasonably independent and successful. Professional help should also be provided in planning for ideal access and convenience in the home, school or place of work.

(6) Innumerable practical and emotional problems, large and small, occur during the lives of severely handicapped people, and these commonly affect other members of the family. It is an important part of the management to make sure that an appropriate professional person is available on a continuing basis to suggest solutions and to provide support. A medical social worker with experience of the disease can often fill this role and may be able to foresee and prevent many difficulties. She can also advise on the many grants and special services available for these patients. We have found that psychiatric help is very rarely needed when emotional support and practical help are provided in this way.

(7) Employment, marriage and child-bearing are feasible, and often very successful, in patients with muscular dystrophy in whom the onset is in adolescence or later. Employment and marriage are very rare in the Duchenne type, although sheltered employment is possible for a short period in

some cases. It is an important responsibility of the doctor at the time of diagnosis of the late-onset muscular dystrophies to advise about the aspects of the prognosis affecting employment, so that appropriate training and careers may be planned in advance.

Additional points in the management of specific types of muscular dystrophy are discussed in subsequent sections of this chapter and the principles of management of neuromuscular disease are described in detail in Chapter 21.

THE TYPES OF MUSCULAR DYSTROPHY

Severe X-linked (Duchenne) muscular dystrophy

This, the commonest muscular dystrophy, is an X-linked recessive trait and thus, in its typical form, affects only males. Very rarely, females with Turner's syndrome or with a translocation involving part of one X-chromosome at the Xp21 site are affected. Minor or abortive forms occur in occasional female carriers (manifesting carriers) of the gene, but never in males. It is characterised by: (a) onset of symptoms usually before the fourth year, rarely as late as the seventh; (b) symmetrical and at first selective involvement of the muscles of the pelvic and pectoral girdles; (c) hypertrophy of the calves and certain other muscles at some stage of the disease in almost every case; (d) relentlessly progressive weakness in every case, leading to inability to walk within 10 years of the onset and later to contractures and thoracic deformity; (e) invariable cardiac involvement; (f) frequent, but not invariable, intellectual impairment; (g) death by the second or third decade caused by respiratory or, less frequently, cardiac failure, often associated with inanition and respiratory infection; (h) very high activity of certain muscle enzymes, notably CK in serum in the early stages of the disease; and (i) certain characteristic histological features in muscle.

Incidence. The most reliable estimates of the incidence of Duchenne muscular dystrophy range from 18 to 30 per 100 000 liveborn males, and of its prevalence in the population as a whole from 1.9 to 4.8 per 100 000. One-third of cases are new mutants, one-third have a previous family history and one-third are born to unwitting and often mutant carriers. The mutation rate is about $7–10 \times 10^{-5}$ per gene per generation (Moser et al 1964, Gardner-Medwin 1970, 1982a, Brooks & Emery 1977, Danieli et al 1977, Davie & Emery 1978, Cowan et al 1980, Monckton et al 1982, Nigro et al 1983, Williams et al 1983, Moser 1984).

Occurrence in girls. Most young girls with a severe progressive muscular dystrophy have the autosomal recessive form (see p. 545).

Theoretically, a girl homozygous for the Duchenne gene might result from the union of a female carrier with an affected man or one in whom a gonadal mutation of the gene had occurred, but this has never been reported.

Cases of true Duchenne dystrophy in girls with Turner's syndrome (XO genotype) have been reported, but are very rare (Walton 1956a, Ferrier et al 1965, Jalbert et al 1966).

In 1977 a girl with Duchenne muscular dystrophy and a reciprocal translocation of parts of the short arms of chromosomes X and 21 was described by Verellen et al (1977). Subsequently, a number of affected girls with translocations based at the Xp21 site of one of their X-chromosomes have been reported (Greenstein et al 1977, Canki et al 1979, Lindenbaum et al 1979, Jacobs et al 1981, Zatz et al 1981, Emanuel et al 1983, Verellen-Dumoulin et al 1984, Nevin et al 1986). Their clinical features appear to conform closely to those of affected boys and their importance lies in their being the origin of the discovery of the site of the Duchenne gene and hence of all recent attempts to identify the gene itself by recombinant DNA technology. It appears that damage to only one of the pair of genes gives rise to the disease, not because these girls are all carriers of the mutant gene on their other X-chromosome, but because the damage prevents the random inactivation of the abnormal X-chromosome so that only the normal X is inactivated in all the relevant cells.

A few remarkable pairs of identical twin girls have now been reported, in which one twin has progressive muscular dystrophy while the other is entirely unaffected (Gomez et al 1977, Burn et al 1986): the dystrophy in such cases appears to be typical of the Duchenne type; no chromosome deletions have been found. Burn has suggested, and has provided some supporting evidence, that in such cases early random inactivation of the normal X-chromosome in some cells and of the other X, containing the mutant Duchenne gene, in other cells might contribute to the causation of the twinning process in the early carrier zygote. The resultant twins, both actually heterozygous for the Duchenne gene, might as a result have quite different phenotypes, one normal and the other typical of Duchenne muscular dystrophy. If this explanation is correct, one might expect early fetal loss of one twin to result occasionally in apparently isolated heterozygotes of each type (totally non-manifesting carriers, and fully affected girls with a normal karyotype).

More mildly affected 'manifesting heterozygotes' are more frequently seen and may inadvertently be diagnosed as cases of 'limb-girdle dystrophy' (see p. 540).

Symptoms. The earliest symptom is usually clumsiness in walking, with a tendency to fall. In many cases, the first attempts to walk are delayed and are awkward from the beginning. About half are still unable to walk at the age of 18 months. General developmental delay, especially involving speech, is not uncommon and may divert the clinician's attention from the neuromuscular problem. In other cases, progress may be apparently normal until the third year and very occasionally parents do not report anything abnormal until the sixth or seventh year. Then the child's walking begins to lack briskness and freedom of movement; often this is erroneously attributed to 'laziness' or flat feet, or some other comparatively trivial complaint. It is common to find that parents who have had a dystrophic child can detect the earliest signs of the disease in a second son, at a time when no abnormal signs can be identified by an experienced clinician. Inability to run, to hop and especially to jump over a small object with both feet together are often useful early guides. Soon the boy has increasing difficulty in climbing stairs and in rising from the floor (Fig. 15.1). The method of rolling from supine to prone and then climbing up the legs to reach a standing position is characteristic (Gowers 1879).

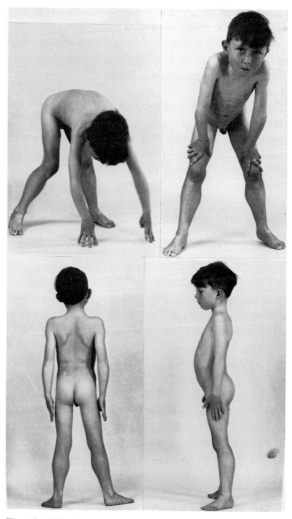

Fig. 15.1 The Duchenne type of muscular dystrophy: note the hypertrophy of the calves and the characteristic method of rising from the floor (Walton 1962)

He walks with a waddle and protrudes his abdomen, later rising on to his toes with feet wide apart and shoulders and chin drawn back. A detailed study of the pathomechanics of the typical gait was made by Sutherland et al (1981). Weakness of the upper limbs is often not reported until up to five years after the onset, but it can be found on examination long before this.

Course. At the age of four or five years the boy's growth may outstrip the progress of the disease, giving a false impression of improvement; otherwise deterioration is continuous and most patients become unable to walk between the ages of seven and 12 years. The mean age is about 9.5 years (Gardner-Medwin 1982a). Despite the apparently intermittent rapid progression of the disease as critical milestones of disability are reached (such as inability to rise from the floor, to climb stairs or to walk) Ziter et al (1977) showed that the decline in measured muscle strength is continuous and linear. More recently, efforts to improve the standards of therapeutic trials have resulted in a number of studies of the rate of natural progression of the disease. Particularly useful data are given by Allsop & Ziter (1981), Scott et al (1982) and Brooke et al (1983).

A rapid increase in weakness may follow bed rest for minor illness, fractures or surgery, but the childhood exanthems rarely affect the condition if the child is kept active. Surgical procedures designed to lengthen Achilles tendons are particularly dangerous in this respect. Archibald & Vignos (1959) stressed the importance of early contractures of the hip flexors in accentuating postural difficulties and leading to early confinement to a wheelchair. Once the wheelchair stage is reached, other contractures develop rapidly, especially in the hamstrings and biceps, and weakness of spinal muscles almost invariably leads to increasing scoliosis. Eventually the deformity may make even a wheelchair existence impossible and the patient is confined to bed, able to speak, swallow and breathe, but otherwise retaining feeble power only in the movements of the face, in the grip and in plantar-flexion of the feet and toes. Only a quarter of cases survive beyond the age of 21 years and survival beyond 25 years is rare (Gardner-Medwin 1982a, Johnston et al 1985). Death usually results from chest infection with respiratory and sometimes cardiac failure.

Suggestions that more than one genetic entity may be concealed within what we now reognise as Duchenne dystrophy (Emery et al 1979) have received little support and there is some contrary evidence (O'Brien et al 1983). A few puzzling instances are recorded in which great variation in severity occurs within a family (Furukawa & Peter 1977, Gardner-Medwin 1982b) but in general the course of the disease is fairly uniform.

In one striking exception a very atypical benign course of the disease in one of 10 affected males in a family was reported by Zatz et al (1981). The mildly affected boy also had growth hormone deficiency, a fact of possible pathogenetic importance.

Physical examination. Weakness and wasting usually begin in the iliopsoas, quadriceps and gluteus muscles and soon spread to involve the anterior tibial group. In the upper limbs, the costal origin of pectoralis major, the latissimus dorsi, the biceps, triceps and brachioradialis muscles are the first involved. Scapular winging occurs, but is not prominent in the early stages. Hypotonia at the shoulders when the child is lifted is a useful early sign. Later, power is better retained in the wrist flexors than extensors, in the hamstrings than in quadriceps, in the invertors of the foot than in the evertors and in neck extension than in flexion. The calf muscles may remain remarkably strong for several years. Slight facial weakness, especially of movements of the mouth, is usual in the later stages. Progressive deterioration of respiratory function occurs and is discussed in a later paragraph.

Muscular hypertrophy, later followed by the pseudohypertrophic phase of fatty replacement of muscle, is commonly seen in the calves (Fig. 15.1) and muscles of mastication, less often in the deltoids, wrist extensors and quadriceps and occasionally in other muscles. Denervation of muscle (as in poliomyelitis) may abolish it, and it usually disappears spontaneously as the disease progresses. It is rare for cases of otherwise typical Duchenne muscular dystrophy to show no muscular enlargement at any stage of the disease. Macroglossia is not uncommon.

The tendon reflexes are diminished in the upper limbs early in the disease and the knee jerks also disappear soon. The ankle jerks, however, remain brisk until a comparatively late stage. Contractures generally develop first in the calf muscles and hip flexors and abductors and give rise to progressive plantar-flexion and inversion of the feet, and to hip contractures with compensatory lumbar lordosis; they are seen later in the hamstrings, biceps brachii and flexors of the wrists and fingers.

Some of the children become generally wasted as the disease progresses, but many become very obese, presumably because of a combination of excessive feeding and immobility. Studies of endocrine function have failed to reveal why some are thin and others obese. Sexual development is usually normal, but puberty may be delayed.

Intellectual changes. Intellectual retardation is common (Allen & Rodgin 1960, Worden & Vignos 1962): indeed, it occurred in Duchenne's earliest case and led him to believe at first that the disorder was of cerebral origin. About one-third of cases have an intelligence quotient (IQ) below 75 and a significant minority are below 50; about one tenth are above 100. Mean IQ levels in different series vary between about 70 and 85 (Dubowitz 1965, Zellweger & Hanson 1967a, Cohen et al 1968, Prosser et al 1969, Kozicka et al 1971, Marsh & Munsat 1974, Kohno 1978, Leibowitz & Dubowitz 1981); however, the most thorough population surveys (Cohen et al 1968, Kohno 1978) gave the highest figures for mean IQ. Verbal ability is usually most severely affected. Karagan et al (1980) attempted to analyse this verbal deficit in seven selected boys and concluded that verbal expression and memory for patterns, numbers and verbal labels were more severely impaired than some other verbal skills. In addition to the intellectual deficit, Leibowitz & Dubowitz (1981) identified behaviour problems in more than one-third of their cases. There is no evidence of progressive intellectual deterioration, however, and, except in the series described by Rosman (1970), the severity of the muscular and intellectual involvements are not correlated. The intelligence levels of affected sibs are often similar, but no abnormality has been found in carriers, and the sons of known carriers are no more severely affected than are sporadic cases (Prosser et al 1969). Kozicka et al (1971) found that the electroencephalogram (EEG) was abnormal more often in retarded cases, but the study by Barwick et al (1965) revealed no consistent EEG abnormality. Rosman & Kakulas (1966) found cerebral-neuronal heterotopias at autopsy in three retarded boys with Duchenne dystrophy, but not in four patients with normal intelligence. Their cases were somewhat atypical, however, and Dubowitz & Crome (1969) found no significant abnormality in the brain in 21 autopsied patients, in five of whom the IQ had been below 60.

Skeletal changes. The pattern of skeletal deformity occurring in patients with Duchenne muscular dystrophy was reviewed by Walton & Warrick (1954). The changes, which are secondary to disuse, include narrowing of the shafts and rarefaction of the ends of the long bones (Fig. 15.2), impaired development of flat bones and coxa valga. At a later stage there is almost invariably severe spinal curvature, widespread decalcification and eventually gross distortion and disorganisation of the skeletal system. These changes render the affected bones liable to fracture as a result of minimal trauma, and a child may fracture a femur on falling from a wheelchair. A few patients develop a long thoracolumbar lordosis instead of the more usual kyphoscoliosis (Wilkins & Gibson 1976).

Cardiac involvement. This is probably invariable in the true Duchenne form of the disease,

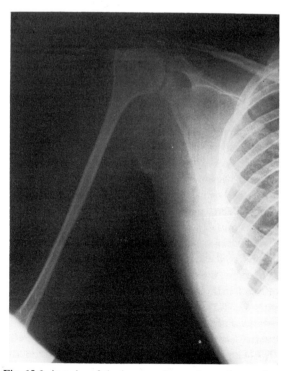

Fig. 15.2 Atrophy of the humerus in an advanced case of Duchenne muscular dystrophy (Walton 1962)

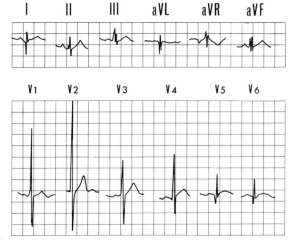

Fig. 15.3 Typical ECG recorded from a boy of 14 with Duchenne muscular dystrophy. There are narrow but deep Q waves in leads I, aVL, V_5 and V_6, and RSR_1 pattern in aVR and dominant R waves in V_1 and V_2

although it may not be detectable in the early stages (Zatuchni et al 1951, Walton & Nattrass 1954, Manning & Cropp 1958, Perloff et al 1966, Slucka 1968). Persistent tachycardia is common and sudden death from myocardial failure may occur (Berenbaum & Horowitz 1956) but chronic cardiac failure is rare. Of particular importance is the characteristic electrocardiogram (ECG) which shows tall R waves in the right precordial leads and deep Q waves in the limb leads and the left precordial leads (Fig. 15.3). Schott et al (1955), Skyring & McKusick (1961), Perloff et al (1966) and Emery (1972) have claimed that this ECG pattern is of diagnostic value in distinguishing between the juvenile forms of muscular dystrophy. Perloff et al (1967) have shown that the pathological basis for this distinctive ECG in two cases was interstitial and replacement fibrosis of the basal part of the left ventricular free wall. Echocardiography has indicated relatively good preservation of myocardial function in Duchenne dystrophy, despite the ECG changes. There is, however, some reduction in the rate of diastolic relaxation (Kovick et al 1975, Ahmad et al 1978) and more recent studies have shown impairment of left ventricular contraction and relaxation and, in boys with thoracic distortion, an abnormally high incidence of mitral valve prolapse (Danilowicz et al

1980, Goldberg et al 1980, Reeves et al 1980, Hunsaker et al 1982). Hunsaker et al (1982) documented a decline in function over 10 years.

Hunter (1980) points out that the impairment of physical fitness which results from enforced immobility may contribute to the abnormalities that are found. Despite its usual association with thoracic distortion, mitral valve prolapse seems to result from involvement of the papillary muscle by the cardiomyopathy (Sanyal et al 1980).

A variety of disturbances of rhythm, including labile tachycardia, may be demonstrated by careful investigation (Sanyal and Johnson 1982) but they are relatively uncommon as clinical problems. Disease of the nodal arteries may account for some of these (James 1962, Perloff et al 1967).

Respiratory muscle involvement. The respiratory muscles are always affected in Duchenne dystrophy and when scoliosis and thoracic distortion occur they further diminish the efficiency of respiration. Respiratory failure compounded by infection is the major cause of death.

The vital capacity begins to fall below normal as early as the seventh year, by the age of 14 is on average only 50% of normal and at 21 only 20% (Rideau 1978, Rideau et al 1981). The expiratory reserve volume component of the vital capacity is affected earlier than the inspiratory component. The tidal volume is relatively preserved but the maximum ventilatory capacity is progressively impaired. The maximum expiratory and inspiratory pressures that can be exerted begin to decline at about the same stage (Inkley et al 1974). The loss of expiratory force is particularly important because it makes attempts to cough ineffective and contributes further to the risk of acquiring and succumbing to infections.

Rideau et al (1981) were able to correlate the age at which the vital capacity reached its plateau with the duration of ultimate survival. Kurz et al (1983) studied the relationship of thoracic spinal curvature to vital capacity and concluded that, in addition to the effect of age on the latter, each additional 10 degrees of curvature diminished the vital capacity by 4%.

Only in the last stages of the disease is quiet respiration affected. Because the accessory muscles of respiration are themselves extremely weak, their visible use, often a slight heaving movement of the shoulders, is a very significant bad prognostic sign. The tidal volume, though not reduced, cannot be increased to meet demands and so the respiratory rate increases instead. The central respiratory responses to oxygen and CO_2 are normal (Begin et al 1980). Carbon dioxide retention is also a late feature, usually apparent as morning drowsiness but occasionally causing headache and even papilloedema in extreme cases (Burke et al 1971). Fear of falling asleep is a common and disturbing feature for the patient and the whole family as the respiratory reserve fails.

Pathogenesis. This is unknown. Hypotheses in the recent past have suggested a defect in muscle fibre regeneration which interfered with the repair of the normal wear and tear of muscle (Hudgson et al 1967); the occurrence of multiple microscopic infarcts of muscle due to a hypothetical vascular lesion in intramuscular arterioles (Mendell et al 1971) and a functional defect in spinal anterior horn cells in some way induces a trophic degenerative lesion in muscle (McComas et al 1971). None of these hypotheses has stood up to critical investigation, although each was supported by some items of experimental evidence. At present a hypothesis, rather more promising than the previous ones, postulates a defect in the sarcolemmal membrane which allows a substance or substances, as yet unknown but which could possibly be calcium, to enter the muscle fibre too freely, and there to activate neutral proteases which, in turn, maintain an excessive degree of muscle catabolism and lead to muscle fibre necrosis (Mokri & Engel 1975, Rowland 1976, Ebashi & Sugita 1978, Wakayama et al 1983, see also Ch. 13).

The genetic defect. The gene for Duchenne dystrophy was found to be located near the Xp21 site on the short arm of the X-chromosome when translocations resulting from breaks at that site were found in a small number of affected females (Verellen et al 1977 and others reviewed by Verellen-Dumoulin et al 1984). This led in due course to the discovery of the first of several cloned DNA sequences closely linked to the Duchenne gene (Murray et al 1982). Some closely linked genes which have recognised clinical effects include that for ornithine transcarbamylase deficiency (Lindgren et al 1984); presumably also those for a number of associated disorders found in a boy with a minor Xp21 deletion — chronic granulomatous disease (cytochrome b-245 deficiency), a form of retinitis pigmentosa and the McLeod red cell phenotype (Francke et al 1985 and genes for congenital adrenal hypoplasia and glycerol kinase deficiency (Guggenheim et al 1980, Renier et al 1983, Dunger et al 1986). The Duchenne gene is also close to a block of ribosomal RNA genes (Worton et al 1984). For recent information on the identification of the Duchenne gene, see Ch. 26.

Diagnosis. The typical distribution of muscular weakness, wasting and hypertrophy, the characteristic gait, best seen when the child attempts to run or to climb stairs, the characteristic very high levels of serum CK activity and the rather typical histological appearances in muscle biopsy sections (see below) all make the diagnosis, once suspected, relatively easy to confirm.

The conditions which may superficially resemble Duchenne muscular dystrophy in clinical practice are spinal muscular atrophy, polymyositis, the myopathy associated with osteomalacia or renal failure, and certain congenital and metabolic myopathies including central core disease, juvenile acid maltase deficiency and carnitine deficiency. Detailed clinical examination and investigation including serum CK estimation and muscle biopsy will rarely leave the matter in doubt. The more difficult differential diagnoses from autosomal recessive muscular dystrophy in a young boy and from Becker dystrophy are discussed in the sections on those disorders.

Between the ages of one and five years, serum CK activity in Duchenne muscular dystrophy is 100–300 times the upper limit of the normal range and other muscle enzymes (aldolase, SGOT, pyruvate kinase, lactic dehydrogenase and others) are also grossly elevated (see Ch. 13). The only other comparable gradually progressive myopathies which may give such high serum enzyme levels are the Becker and autosomal recessive types of childhood muscular dystrophy (see below). The diagnosis may be made at birth (Heyck et al 1966). In the neonatal period the normal range of serum CK activity is higher than in older infants (Gilboa & Swanson 1976) but in a large-scale screening survey the activities in newborn infants with Duchenne muscular dystrophy were at least 2.5 times the highest normal figures and 20–50 times the normal mean (Dellamonica 1978). After birth CK activity rises over the first year or so and then falls gradually from the age of two or three years so that, in very advanced cases, it is only one to five times the upper normal limit.

The muscle biopsy in the first few weeks of life may show only a small excess of endomysial connective tissue and the presence of many large hyaline muscle fibres. As the activity of the disease reaches its peak, the muscle fascicles become 'fossilised' by a mesh of perimysial and endomysial connective tissue, the scattered hyaline fibres remain prominent, and active muscle necrosis, phagocytosis and regeneration are conspicuous. Gradually the muscle fibres, which are rounded, often showing splitting and central nuclei, and which vary greatly in size, are replaced by increasing quantities of fat. In the late stages of the disease so little muscle may be left in the mass of fat and fibrous tissue that the biopsy is no longer diagnostic. It is our view that the diagnosis of a new case of muscular dystrophy is so important to the patient and his family that muscle biopsy should always be performed to confirm it.

For clinical trials of treatment rigid diagnostic criteria are required. Like many simple concepts, Duchenne muscular dystrophy has proved difficult to define in unequivocal terms which are not unwieldy. The lengthy criteria of Brooke et al (1981) can be recommended to those planning trials on a large scale: however, they do not rigorously exclude severe cases of Becker dystrophy or boys with autosomal recessive childhood dystrophy (see below) and in small scale trials such individuals might by chance bias the results.

In practice the confirmation of the diagnosis of Duchenne muscular dystrophy is usually easy: The difficulty lies in early clinical recognition of the disease. The mean age at diagnosis in the UK is about 5.8 years (Gardner-Medwin et al 1978). This delay may result in the conception of further preventable cases in the family. The development of a micro-method of CK analysis which can be performed on a dried blood spot (Zellweger & Antonik 1975) has enabled large-scale neonatal screening projects to be set up in several parts of the world (Zellweger & Antonik 1975, Beckmann and Scheuerbrandt 1976, Dellamonica 1978, Dellamonica et al 1978, Drummond 1979, Scheuerbrandt et al 1986). Altogether more than 250 000 newborn males have been screened and the incidence of Duchenne muscular dystrophy among them has been 1 in 4 000 males (1 in 3 700 of the 176 000 males screened by Scheuerbrandt et al 1986). At best, neonatal screening can theoretically prevent 12–15% of cases and its effect upon the parents' relationship with their newborn son is unpredictable and potentially psychologically hazardous. The alternative strategy of screening boys with psychomotor developmental delay at the age of about 18 months would be less effective but would still be valuable and would probably have less harmful emotional consequences (Gardner-Medwin et al 1978, Gardner-Medwin 1979a, Crisp et al 1982).

The possibility of prenatal diagnosis of Duchenne muscular dystrophy was considered following the development of micro-methods of CK estimation and the technique of fetal (placental) blood sampling under direct endoscopic control. Golbus et al (1979), who had earlier reported successful prenatal diagnosis by this technique in one case, found it unreliable in a series of 24 fetuses at risk. R J Edwards et al (1984) similarly found the method inadequate for ruling out the disease in high-risk fetuses. A prenatal test would be valuable only if it were capable of distinguishing affected from normal male fetuses with a high degree of reliability. The use of DNA probes for prenatal diagnosis, first reported by Bakker et al (1985), is being applied with increasing success in carefully selected families who have been shown to carry appropriately informative marker genes, and is likely to become more widely applicable as new probes are discovered. It is important to recognise that this, like all other techniques of prenatal diagnosis, is essentially a method for permitting couples at risk to have normal children instead of remaining childless. They contribute little to *prevention* of the disease.

Prevention and carrier detection. About one-third of cases of Duchenne muscular dystrophy in a population not subjected to genetic counselling are theoretically preventable. The contribution which early diagnosis can make to prevention has already been discussed. Considerably more cases could be prevented by the active tracing, investigation and counselling of potential female carriers. The clinician who makes the diagnosis of Duchenne muscular dystrophy thereby acquires the responsibility of making genetic advice available to his patient's female relatives.

The most important achievements of recent muscular dystrophy research have been in carrier detection. For a woman known to be a carrier of the gene for one of the X-linked dystrophies there is a 1 in 4 chance that any pregnancy will result in an affected son. Genetic counselling may be considered in three stages: pedigree analysis, tests for the carrier state and the tracing through the family of markers closely linked to the Duchenne gene by the use of recombinant DNA techniques.

Pedigree analysis. When a woman at risk seeks genetic advice, examination of the family history will allow her to be assigned to one of the following categories (Pearce et al 1964, Thompson et al 1967). Definite carriers are those mothers of an affected son who have also an affected brother, maternal uncle, sister's son or other male relative in the female line of inheritance; also mothers of affected sons by different, non-consanguineous fathers. Probable carriers are the mothers of two or more affected sons, who have no other affected relatives; in practice they should be counselled as known carriers. Possible carriers are the mothers of isolated cases and the sisters and other female relatives of affected males. The possible carriers may have a high risk of heterozygosity (as in the daughter of a definite carrier where the risk is 1 in 2), or a low risk (as in a distant female cousin with many unaffected males in intervening generations). In all of them, the probability may be calculated after examination of the pedigree (Weismann et al 1965, Emery & Morton 1968).

Tests for the carrier state. The next stage in carrier identification depends upon the fact that many, and perhaps all, true carriers have a slight degree of myopathy which can usually be detected by investigation: óccasionally it gives rise to definite muscular hypertrophy (Emery 1963) or weakness (Chung et al 1960, Moser et al 1964) but in the great majority it is subclinical. The most successful method of detecting the myopathy is by estimating certain serum enzyme levels, of which CK is the most valuable. The experience of a number of investigators was reviewed in previous editions of this chapter and in Gardner-Medwin et al (1971). Major series were reported by Hughes (1963), Sugita & Tyler (1963), Milhorat & Goldstone (1965), Wilson et al (1965), Dreyfus et al (1966), Emery & Walton (1967), Thompson et al (1967), Hausmanowa-Petrusewicz et al (1968) and Griggs et al (1985). About 70–75% of definite carriers can be 'detected' in this way. However, in some of these series the normal range of CK activity was rather strictly interpreted and the proportion of carriers with activity above the 97% confidence limits of the normal range was considerably less than 70% (see especially Griggs et al 1985). It is therefore important in interpreting the significance of serum CK activity in potential carriers to know the relative probability of a given CK level being found in a carrier compared with a normal person. This relative probability may then be combined with the prior probability obtained from the pedigree, on Bayesian principles, to obtain the overall risk for the individual (Emery & Morton 1968, Dennis et al 1976).

In fact, women at risk are seeking evidence that they are normal, not that they are carriers. No study of carriers has expressed the results in terms of the detection of normal individuals among groups of possible carriers, but superficial examination of the available data indicates that this more critical 'detection rate' is much lower than the carrier detection rate.

Spurious elevation of serum CK activity may occur after exercise in normal subjects, and possibly more so in carriers (see Gardner-Medwin et al 1971, Gaines et al 1982, Herrmann et al 1982) but discrimination of normal and carrier subjects is not much improved. Falsely low levels have been reported in early pregnancy (Blyth & Hughes 1971, Emery & King 1971). Serum activity of another enzyme, pyruvate kinase, is also increased in many carriers and may be less affected by pregnancy (Zatz et al 1983). Recent reports have also stressed the potential effect of age upon CK levels in carriers and in normal females, in both of whom a decline has been reported in the second and third decades. There is some evidence that carriers may be more readily identified in childhood, but more comparisons with series of normal children are needed before early diagnosis of carriers can be relied upon (Nicholson et al 1979).

Other methods of carrier detection are now of more theoretical than practical importance because none is capable of detecting all carriers (or any individual as unequivocally normal) and the contribution they can make to calculations of probabilities is small in comparison with the value of CK estimation: therefore, only a brief review is given here.

Electromyography may detect some carriers. The most useful methods have been EMG sampling of multiple muscles as a preliminary to muscle biopsy (Smith et al 1966), measurement of the absolute refractory period of muscle fibres (Caruso & Buchthal 1965), measurement of the duration and number of phases of the motor unit action potentials (van den Bosch 1963, Hausmanowa-Petrusewicz et al 1968, Gardner-Medwin 1968) and analysis of the interference pattern by the use of an automatic spike counter and computer (Willison 1967, Moosa et al 1972, Toulouse et al 1985). Only 50–70% of definite carriers can be identified. The most careful comparison with normal control subjects is essential.

The histology of muscle biopsy material is abnormal in some carriers (Dubowitz 1963, Emery 1965, Milhorat et al 1966, Pearce et al 1966, Roy & Dubowitz 1970) but negative or uncertain results are frequent. Other methods which give some positive results are ultrasound or CT scan imaging (Rott et al 1984), muscle electron microscopy (Afifi et al 1973), studies of the isoenzyme pattern of lactate dehydrogenase in muscle biopsy specimens (Emery 1964, 1965) and possibly in the serum of some carriers (Hooshmand et al 1969), measurement of serum activity of pyruvate kinase (Sage et al 1979, Zatz & Otto 1980, Griggs et al 1985), electrocardiography (Mann et al 1968, Emery 1969, Lane et al 1980), the measurement in vitro of protein synthesis by polyribosomes in biopsied muscle (Ionasescu et al 1976), the detection of myoglobinaemia (Adornato et al 1978, Nicholson 1981) and the frequency of the 'capping' phenomenon in lymphocytes (Pickard et al 1978). The highest detection rates have so far been obtained by the use of a combination of several methods in each potential carrier (Hausmanowa-Petrusewicz et al 1968, Radu et al 1968, Gardner-Medwin et al 1971, Nicholson 1981, Percy et al 1982, 1984). However, great caution must be used in interpreting minor deviations from normal in one or more items in a battery of tests, because the confidence limits for the normal range for the battery as a whole are not usually available.

Definitely abnormal results from any of these investigations make it highly probable that a woman is indeed a carrier. When the results are all normal or borderline, advice is given in terms of the probability that she is a carrier, estimated from the precise level of her serum CK within the normal range, together with the application of Bayes' theorem to her pedigree (Emery & Morton 1968, Emery & Holloway 1977).

Risk estimation using DNA probes. The use of recombinant DNA technology in genetic counselling is discussed fully in Chapter 26. The field is a rapidly changing one and only a few brief observations are appropriate here. Two of the vital initial contributions were made by Murray et al (1982) and Monaco et al (1985). Useful recent genetic studies include those of Pembrey et al (1984) and Williams et al (1986).

The technique can be used directly to 'detect' carriers only when there is actually a deletion of closely linked flanking genes at the Xp21 site in the affected members of the family which can be shown to occur also in the females in question, and even this is liable to occasional errors. Deletions appear to occur in fewer than 10% of affected males (Monaco et al 1985). Carriers can otherwise be traced only by the use of linkage studies.

The use of DNA probes is essentially a matter of identifying, by the use of restriction enzymes and gene probes, specific fragments of the X-chromosome which are very close to the site of the Duchenne gene and then following these through the family to see whether a female at risk is likely or unlikely to have inherited the same fragment as is found on the X-chromosome of her affected male relative(s). Where possible, flanking probes on either side of, and within, the very extensive site of the Duchenne gene are used to diminish the likelihood of crossing over. The technique may be of no value in families where there is no surviving affected individual or where certain other critical family members are not available for testing, or when identical polymorphisms on both sides of the family obscure the source of the fragments identified. Furthermore, the Duchenne gene appears to be at an unstable site so that mutations, chromosome breaks, deletions, and crossing over (separating the Duchenne gene from its closely neighbouring genes between one generation and the next) are all more frequent than they are elsewhere on the chromosome. Nevertheless, when conditions are favourable, the technique is a powerful one. It has the advantages over all previous methods of carrier detection that: (1) it is independent of the presence or absence of minimal myopathy in carriers; and (2) it can often be used in conjunction with chorion biopsy for prenatal diagnosis (Bakker et al 1985), sometimes even in situations where the carrier status of the mother is uncertain, although caution is required in the interpretation of the results (Williams et al 1986).

The use of DNA probes is now an established and very valuable technique for predicting the genetic risk in an increasing proportion of Duchenne families. Indeed it has become the most important method but, for the present, it is vital to realise that it is not infallible and has not rendered obsolete the methods based on classic pedigree analysis and serum CK testing: all of these methods should be used in combination until specific identification of the Duchenne gene itself is achieved and the subsequent use of gene-specific probes becomes established as a reliable technique.

The effectiveness of systematic carrier tracing and counselling has been demonstrated in Ontario, Western Australia, Northern England and Brazil (Hutton & Thompson 1976, Kakulas & Hurse 1978, Gardner-Medwin 1978, Zatz 1983) and a valuable comprehensive review of the prevention of Duchenne muscular dystrophy was published by Moser (1984).

Management. No treatment is at present known which has any definite influence upon muscular dystrophy. The drugs which have been tried in the past, and the use of therapeutic trials are discussed in Chapter 21.

The absence of specific treatment for muscular dystrophy makes it all the more important to prevent its physical, emotional, social and educational complications and to provide active support for the family throughout the course of the disease. The clinician's first responsibility is to provide an unequivocal diagnosis and enough information and constructive suggestions to enable the family to formulate practical plans for the future. These must be given in relaxed sessions after the initial shock has passed (Firth 1983). Females potentially at risk of being carriers should be actively traced and offered genetic advice at this time. In the early stages, the most useful activities for the parents to encourage are regular physical exercise, appropriate eating habits to prevent obesity, and social activities, sporting and cultural interests, hobbies and education to provide a basis for interests in the later stages of the disease.

Vignos & Watkins (1966) showed that organised programmes of maximum resistance exercise may increase muscular strength in the adult forms. Such programmes are more difficult in childhood and there is still no really satisfactory published trial of the effect of active exercise in Duchenne muscular dystrophy; however, it is the common experience that Duchenne boys benefit from exercise and, conversely, that rest is detrimental. Bed rest for minor illness or trauma should be avoided whenever possible and regular walking, swimming and games, a little more than the boy really wants to do, should be encouraged. Older boys can do more formal and deliberate exercises and, in the late stages, these should be continued with emphasis on the upper limbs and on breathing exercises. Wheelchair sports provide both exercise and a boost for morale.

Unlike the muscular weakness, contractures are to some extent preventable and reversible. Hip flexion and equinus contractures may significantly alter the stance and interfere with walking at a stage when the muscular weakness alone is not severe enough to prevent ambulation; passive stretching of the hip flexors and iliotibial bands and of soleus and gastrocnemius may therefore be an important part of management. Prone lying to prevent hip flexion contracture is useful. Vignos et al (1963) recommended passive stretching for at least 5 s repeated 10 times, twice a day. Others suggest more prolonged continuous stretching (Kottke et al 1966) but, in the face of relatively weak antagonist muscles, no intermittent regime of stretching will be entirely successful. Splinting at night may be successful at the ankle but is not feasible at other joints. The dangers of anaesthesia and the increased weakness which follows immobility demand that minor surgery be undertaken only if immediate postoperative mobilisation is prepared for in advance. However, surgical management of equinus deformity can be successful in the hands of surgeons with special experience of the postoperative management in muscular dystrophy (Williams et al 1984).

Spencer & Vignos (1962) and Vignos et al (1963) pioneered the active management of the combined weakness and contractures in Duchenne muscular dystrophy, recommending a combination of subcutaneous tenotomy (with brief anaesthesia) and subsequent vigorous physiotherapy and bracing; they enabled some of their patients to walk for two or more years longer than usual. Siegel et al (1968), Roy & Gibson (1970), Miller & Dunn (1982) and Heckmatt et al (1985) recommended similar measures. In recent years Vignos and his colleagues have developed stricter criteria for the application of this technique based on the residual strength and bulk of muscle, the rate of loss of muscle, vital capacity and motivation of the patient (Vignos et al 1983). If tenotomies are to be performed, rapid mobilisation and the maintenance of the corrected position with light alloy calipers are essential. From our own experience we can confirm that it is feasible to prolong ambulation in this way; however, one must set against the advantages of this, the sense of relief which patients often feel on accepting a wheelchair existence after a period of exhaustingly difficult walking with frequent falls, and also the time taken up by physiotherapy and the application of complex braces, often at the expense of schooling, and often for the sake of less useful mobility than is possible in a wheelchair (Gardner-Medwin 1977, 1979b). None the less, all families should have the chance to discuss bracing before the need for it arises. When the boy and his parents are both enthusiastic, it can be very successful in preserving a useful range of activities and in maintaining morale; there is increasing evidence that it also delays the onset of kyphoscoliosis.

When a wheelchair is required it should at first be hand-propelled to provide exercise, but should be replaced with an electrically propelled chair as soon as it no longer provides independent mobility. It is essential not only to select the right chair for the individual's needs, but to adapt the house and, if necessary, the school, to provide full access for the wheelchair. We often recommend subcutaneous Achilles tenotomy in the early wheelchair stage with subsequent use of below-knee cosmetic splints to prevent the unsightly equinovarus contractures which otherwise occur, simply to allow these boys to wear normal footwear. If cosmetic splints are worn consistently from the moment that the ability to walk is lost, the need for tenotomy can sometimes be avoided, especially if splints are also worn at night. Contractures at the hips, knees, elbows and wrists occur in the late stages in almost all cases, but these require surgical management only in rare instances where they are persistently painful. Elbow and wrist contractures respond, at least partly, to regular stretching.

Progressive scoliosis usually begins soon after patients become unable to walk (Robin & Brief 1971) and the prevention of scoliosis is one practical reason for the artificial maintenance of ambulation in appropriate cases. Once it has become established and fixed, it is very difficult to correct or even control and it may go on to cause severe thoracic distortion, respiratory impairment and a major threat to life.

Attempts at early prevention of scoliosis are usually concentrated on achieving a good posture in the wheelchair but Rideau (1978) has suggested that the position in sleep may also be relevant. Proper support of the feet and a firm, comfortable seat position can encourage a symmetrical upright posture. Discouragement of a single habitual sleeping posture may possibly prevent asymmetrical hip flexion and hip abduction contractures, but the origin of these can often be traced back to asymmetry of stance before the wheelchair stage. Once a curvature appears, some form of spinal support is urgently required, but the *prophylactic* use of spinal orthoses is more controversial (Vignos et al 1963, Young et al 1984). Often they are not well accepted by the boys; the more effectively they support the spine the more they limit activity, so there is some risk that they may actually hasten loss of strength in the muscles of the trunk while also impairing the quality of life. Moulded wheelchair inserts, designed to lock the intervertebral facet joints, and thus to prevent rotation of the spine by inducing an artificial lumbar lordosis, were an important innovation (Wilkins & Gibson 1976) but they depend for their effect on limiting freedom of movement. Low-set lumbar/thoracic lightweight cosmetic orthoses can induce a lordosis while allowing more movement and not restricting respiration and undoubtedly they can help to limit the development of scoliosis, but a cycle of incomplete control of curvature, discomfort, disuse and further curvature is easily set up and failure is frequent (Seeger et al 1984).

Robin & Brief (1971), Robin (1977) and Gibson et al (1978) introduced spinal fusion with insertion of a Harrington rod as an alternative to bracing when scoliosis was uncontrolled. Increasing experience with the methods of anaesthesia and postoperative care required, and the proper assessment of respiratory function, allowed important advances in the management of scoliosis to be made using this technique (Milne & Rosales 1982, Swank et al 1982, Weimann et al 1983). The more recent introduction of the Luque type of segmental instrumentation allows more rapid postoperative

mobilisation and has widened the potential scope of surgery (Taddonio 1982, Siegel 1982, Rideau et al 1984, Sussman 1984, 1985). It has even been suggested that spinal orthoses should no longer be used because they serve only to delay the development of spinal curvature until respiratory function has deteriorated too far for surgery to be possible (Rideau et al 1984, Sussman 1984). This presupposes the availability of a skilled surgical team which can operate without delay at the critical moment. It may also leave boys, who for any reason become unsuitable for surgery, with an irreversible curvature. It is widely agreed that orthoses rarely control scolioses which start early and quickly reach a Cobb angle of more than 25 degrees, that surgery is often unsuccessful if the curve is greater than 50 degrees and that the hazards of operation become unacceptable if the vital capacity is less than about 40% of the predicted normal value. Policies in many units are currently in a state of flux: our own at present is to provide spinal orthoses as soon as the patient is unable to walk, to examine the spine every three months and to offer surgery by the Luque procedure if the curve exceeds 20 degrees at a stage when the vital capacity is still sufficient for safe anaesthesia. In deciding the ultimate 'correct' policy, it will be important to consider not only the effect upon the curvature itself but on the comfort and functional ability of the boys: e.g. some have found the use of their arms restricted after the operation.

Many aids such as hoists, bath aids and specially adapted clothing are available; these and adaptations to homes and schools can be provided, after their effectiveness and acceptability for each family have been assessed. An occupational therapist may play a leading part in management when these measures are required. The practical help, advice and emotional support of a social worker are also important. The long inexorable deterioration of the disease is punctuated by crises occurring at the time of diagnosis, of inability to walk, of changing or leaving school and of illness. Fears of fatal illness, of another child being affected, or pregnancies either in the mother or in her carrier daughters, may be added to the frequent misguided sense of marital guilt on the part of carriers and to the prolonged maintenance of family facades to avoid sharing knowledge, fears and often myths about the disorder. Social isolation is common. Boys may become overprotected, frightened, petulant, resentful, aggressive and lonely. Reactive depression is far commoner in parents than in boys. A survey of parents' attitudes to their predicaments was reported by Firth et al (1983). Many of these problems can be prevented or alleviated by a medical social worker familiar with both the disease and the family.

The combined physical and intellectual handicap presents formidable educational problems. Psychological assessment of aptitudes as well as limitations can assist in planning both education and hobbies. Many boys with poor verbal skills show special competence in design and modelling. The social isolation of home education should be avoided whenever possible and education should be dovetailed with the limited opportunities that are likely to be available when the boy leaves school.

Complications include obesity in the wheelchair stage; this is easier to prevent than to treat. The calorie requirements of some immobile boys are very low and expert dietary advice may be required to maintain a balanced diet. In a valuable study, R H T Edwards et al (1984) showed that strict dieting for weight reduction has no deleterious effect on muscle bulk or function in Duchenne boys. Fractures, especially of the lower end of the femur, often occur in the more adventurous wheelchair users. The atrophic bones mend remarkably well and only very limited splinting is needed, especially in the lower limbs. No attempt should be made to correct contractures at the same time. Boys who fracture a femur while still ambulant can often be mobilised in a cast and thus avoid the very grave risk of being unable to walk after a prolonged period of standard immobilisation (Hsu & Garcia-Ariz 1981). Dependent oedema and bedsores are surprisingly rare complications in Duchenne dystrophy.

Anaesthesia may be hazardous (Cobham & Davis 1964, Boba 1970, Genever 1971, Yamashita et al 1976) and should be administered by an experienced anaesthetist in hospital, even for minor dental and other procedures. With care, general anaesthesia for muscle biopsy or incidental surgery in young patients with Duchenne muscular dystrophy is usually uneventful. However, there are now several case reports of cardiac arrest

or rhabdomyolysis induced by anaesthesia (Genever 1971, Watters et al 1977, Miller et al 1978, Seay et al 1978, Bolthauser et al 1980, Lintner et al 1982) and in very occasional cases the full syndrome of malignant hyperpyrexia occurs, confirmed by in vitro tests of muscle sensitivity to halothane or caffeine (Oka et al 1982, Brownell et al 1983, Kelfer et al 1983, Rosenberg & Heiman-Patterson 1983). It is probably wise to avoid using halothane or suxamethonium whenever possible in cases of known or suspected Duchenne muscular dystrophy; certainly, dantrolene should be available for immediate use. However, it would be wrong to deny Duchenne patients surgical treatment on the basis of the small number of reported problems and, in fact, in many of the recorded cases the muscular dystrophy was recognised only after the anaesthetic problem had occurred.

Respiratory insufficiency often gives rise to no symptoms until sudden decompensation occurs during respiratory infections or other sudden stresses. Death may then occur very suddenly in acute respiratory failure, occasionally with terminal heart failure. Cardiac arrhythmias, although often postulated as a cause of sudden death, are rarely observed and delaying respiratory failure seems to be the only useful approach to prophylaxis. Regular breathing exercises and the prevention of scoliosis are important and all parents should be taught to use postural drainage during respiratory infections, together with appropriate antibiotic therapy. Artificial ventilation during such infections may be appropriate (and effective) in some circumstances, but tracheostomy or long-term ventilation, even on an intermittent nocturnal basis, are rarely justifiable. Sudden fluctuations in serum potassium, perhaps related to the limited total body (muscle) potassium pool, may cause difficulties in the management of acute illness or in postoperative care.

Useful reviews of the management of Duchenne muscular dystrophy include those of Siegel (1977, 1978), Robin & Falewski de Leon (1977), Dubowitz (1978) and Bossingham et al (1979).

Benign X-linked (Becker) muscular dystrophy

The existence of a distinct benign X-linked recessive form of muscular dystrophy was first recognised by Becker & Keiner (1955) who described a family and quoted earlier reports of similar pedigrees. In a family later recognised as being affected with Becker (or possibly, in retrospect the Emery–Dreifuss variety) rather than with Duchenne dystrophy, linkage with colour blindness was noted (Philip et al 1956). Subsequent reports by Becker (1957, 1962), Moser et al (1964), Mabry et al (1965), Rotthauwe & Kowalewski (1965a), Markand et al (1969), Emery & Skinner (1976), Ringel et al (1977), Bradley et al (1978b) and others, made it clear that the benign cases are distinct and are not simply part of a spectrum of severity. Indeed, the Becker type of muscular dystrophy is now more clearly characterised than some of the traditional categories. Families are occasionally found in which cases of the Becker and Duchenne types seem to coexist (Furukawa & Peter 1977, Fischbeck & Schotland 1983), but these probably just reflect the extremes of variation in severity of the two disorders. Genetic linkage data at first suggested that the Duchenne and Becker genes occupied widely separated loci on the X-chromosome (Skinner et al 1974, Zatz et al 1974), but these studies were statistically inconclusive and there is now firm evidence, based on linkage to cloned DNA sequences, that the Becker and Duchenne genes are both located at the Xp21 site on the short arm of the X-chromosome, and they are probably allelic (Kingston et al 1983, 1984).

Incidence. Perhaps because of the difficulty of identifying sporadic cases, few reliable figures for incidence or prevalence are available. It is our impression that the incidence is of the order of one-tenth to one-fifth and the prevalence of the order of one-third to one-half that of the Duchenne type (Gardner-Medwin 1970). Emery & Skinner (1976) found the fertility of affected males to be 67% that of their unaffected brothers. These figures imply an incidence of about 3–6 per 100 000 male births, a prevalence of about 1 per 100 000 of the whole population and a mutation rate of about 0.3–0.6×10^{-5} per gene per generation, but these figures are very tentative. Among 420 000 male births in Alberta in 1950–74 the incidence was 1.67 per 100 000 and the prevalence amongst 989 000 males was 1.72 per 100 000 (Monckton et al 1982). Four cases were identified

in three neonatal screening programmes (Drummond 1979, Planchu et al 1980, Scheuerbrandt et al 1986) but in an overlapping screening period the French group found two or three possible Becker cases (Guibaud et al 1981) so the identified incidence among 242 000 males was 1.67–2.9 per 100 000. The serum CK activity in the Becker cases at birth was significantly lower than in the Duchenne cases and neonatal screening cannot yet be regarded as reliable in this condition.

Clinical features. The selective muscle involvement is virtually identical to that in Duchenne muscular dystrophy. Symptoms are noticed in the lower limbs 5–10 years before the upper limbs, but examination will usually reveal the typically affected shoulder muscles in any patient with symptoms. There is selective bilateral and symmetrical wasting and weakness of the costal origin of pectoralis major, latissimus dorsi, brachioradialis, hip flexors and extensors and medial vastus of quadriceps. Later the supinator, biceps, triceps, serratus anterior and neck flexors become weak, and the adductors and abductors of the thigh and anterior tibial muscles are involved. Deltoids, the flexors and extensors of the wrists and fingers, small hand muscles, hamstrings and calf muscles are relatively preserved. Computed tomography scans are a valuable new means of analysing the selective muscle involvement (de Visser & Verbeeten 1985b). The face is virtually completely spared, even in the late stages. The tendon reflexes are impaired and later absent in affected muscles. Hypertrophy of the calves is a prominent and almost constant feature, and the deltoids, extensor muscles in the forearm, lateral vasti of the quadriceps and anterior tibial muscles are commonly hypertrophic at some stage of the disease. The calf enlargement affects both the gastrocnemii and soleus muscles and may precede all other symptoms by several years. Muscle cramp in the early stages is more frequent than in any other type of muscular dystrophy except myotonic dystrophy. Occasionally this is so severe that decompressive fasciotomy has been suggested (Henry & Neville 1984). The first symptoms otherwise are usually difficulty in running or in hurrying up stairs and, later, in doing heavy work with the arms. The lordotic standing posture and waddling gait are very similar to those seen in Duchenne muscular dystrophy. Contractures are not a feature in typical Becker dystrophy until the patient is confined to a wheelchair, but pes cavus is reported in between 15% (Bradley et al 1978b) and 70% (Ringel et al 1977) of cases. Scoliosis, although emphasised by Ringel et al 1977 is usually not severe and thoracic distortion is very uncommon. Respiratory failure seems to be rare (Rideau et al 1981).

Early cardiac involvement is not a feature in typical Becker dystrophy. In the late stages a few patients have significant ECG abnormalities including, in different individuals, bundle-branch block, Q waves, increased R/S ratios and T-wave changes. A few develop clinical cardiac failure and this is sometimes the cause of death (Mabry et al 1965, Markand et al 1969, Emery & Skinner 1976, Bradley et al 1978b). Myocardial involvement seems to be more prominent in a few families (Wadia et al 1976).

Although most patients with Becker muscular dystrophy are of normal intelligence, and some are of superior intelligence, there does seem to be a significant minority with mental retardation (Zellweger & Hanson 1967b, Emery & Skinner 1976, Ringel et al 1977, Bradley et al 1978b, Karagan & Sorensen 1981). The last-named authors found the mean full scale IQ (WAIS or WISC) in 16 cases to be 94, verbal 90, performance 99. As in patients with Duchenne dystrophy, this retardation appears to be non-progressive and, in our experience, may rarely be the presenting problem with later recognition of muscle weakness.

Hallen (1970) reported a high incidence of hypogonadism in 'pelvic-girdle' types of muscular dystrophy including the Becker type. We have not encountered this or any other systemic manifestation of this disease, and the fertility of cases reported by Emery & Skinner (1976) and mentioned above is not consistent with hypogonadism.

Course of the disease. This is the principal point of distinction from the Duchenne type. In Becker cases, symptoms may begin as early as one and as late as 45 years of age, but in the great majority the onset is between the ages of five and 15 years. It seems likely that, in cases reporting a very late onset, clinical examination would have revealed signs of involvement earlier. Few patients are able to run after the second decade. Emery & Skinner (1976) reported the following mean ages and ranges for the 'milestones' of the disease: onset 11.1 years (range 2.5–21); inability to walk 27.1 years (range 12–38) (some patients continued to walk up to the age of 63); death 42.2 years (range 23–63). Shaw & Dreifuss (1969) and Bradley et al (1978b) reported very similar figures, but in the experience of Becker (1964) the age at onset extends from five to 30 years and only 10% become unable to walk before the age of 40 years. Emery & Skinner (1976) gave figures for Duchenne cases for comparison as follows: onset 2.8 years (range 0–6); inability to walk 8.5 years (range 6–12); death 16.0 years (range 8–22). They found that in 90% of Becker cases the onset was after 4.7 years and that in 90% of Duchenne cases it was before this age; that 97% of patients became unable to walk after and before 11.2 years respectively, and that 94% died after and before the age of 20.3 years respectively. These figures are of great value in the differential diagnosis. Our own figures also suggest that the age at which independent walking is lost is the best distinguishing criterion, 93% of each group lying on either side of the borderline at 12 years (Gardner-Medwin 1982b). There is no evidence that the course in Becker dystrophy is intermittently progressive or that the disease arrests at any stage, although progression may be almost imperceptibly slow for long periods.

Diagnosis. The Becker type of muscular dystrophy is distinguished from the Duchenne type by its severity and rate of progression, and from the scapuloperoneal and autosomal recessive forms by the selective muscle involvement. Detailed muscle examination will usually distinguish cases of spinal muscular atrophy (SMA), but cases of the latter with similar selective weakness, muscle hypertrophy and X-linked inheritance have been described (Pearn & Hudgson 1978, Bouwsma & van Wijngaarden 1980). Unlike most cases of SMA, all of these males with calf hypertrophy have raised serum CK activities, although not always in the Becker range. They raise doubts about the distinction of neuropathic and myopathic muscle disorders. De Visser & Verbeeten (1985b) showed quite different CT scan appearances of muscle in Becker dystrophy and typical SMA, but this has not been applied yet to X-linked SMA.

Investigation will usually leave little doubt about the diagnosis. The serum CK activity is extremely high in the preclinical and early stages of the disease and falls steeply with age (Rotthauwe & Kowalewski 1965a, Emery & Skinner 1976, Bradley et al 1978b). In the first 10 years of life the serum CK levels are comparable with those seen in Duchenne cases at the same age (25–200 times normal). After the age of 20 the serum CK levels are lower, 1–10 times normal in the Emery & Skinner (1976) series and usually 2–60 times normal in the Newcastle series (Bradley et al 1978b). It seems likely, but is not yet certain, that the disease can be ruled out by a normal serum CK activity in the preclinical age group.

The EMG usually demonstrates a pattern of short-duration low-amplitude polyphasic potentials with some fibrillation potentials and positive waves (Zellweger & Hanson 1967b, Markand et al 1969, Bradley et al 1978b). Bradley et al reported that the findings in some cases suggested neurogenic atrophy, but giant motor units and grossly reduced interference patterns are not seen in Becker muscular dystrophy. As in Duchenne muscular dystrophy, high-frequency and myotonic discharges are occasionally seen.

The histological findings in Becker muscular dystrophy have been reviewed by Dubowitz & Brooke (1973), Ringel et al (1977) and Bradley et al (1978b). Random variation in fibre size (both atrophy and hypertrophy), fibre splitting, central nuclei and fibrosis are the major features. Active necrosis and regeneration are more prominent in young patients. Bradley et al (1978b) discuss the difficulty of differentiating the findings from those of neurogenic atrophy in some cases.

Carrier detection and prevention. Carrier detection in Becker muscular dystrophy is less satisfactory than in the Duchenne type. Carriers only occasionally have detectable muscle weakness (Aguilar et al 1978). Rotthauwe & Kowalewski (1965b), Wilson et al (1965) and Zatz et al (1980) showed that some carriers can be identified by serum CK estimation and a few have abnormal EMGs (Gardner-Medwin 1968). The largest study was that of Skinner et al (1975) who found that about 60% of definite carriers have serum CK activities above their normal 95% confidence limits (and about 40% above the 99% limit). They found a distinct fall in CK levels with age throughout the first to eighth decades, indicating the great importance of early testing for genetic counselling in this disease. Accurate estimates of the risks for potential Becker carriers can be made only in laboratories with extensive experience of the disease. The calculations involved are discussed by Baraitser (1982) and Grimm (1984).

The principles of counselling in Becker and Duchenne families are the same. All the daughters of affected males are, however, definite carriers of the gene.

Manifesting female carriers of X-linked muscular dystrophies

The occasional occurrence of severe Duchenne dystrophy in girls and the problems of identifying non-manifesting potential carriers at risk were discussed above. Here we are concerned with the fact that female carriers of the Duchenne and Becker genes may have an overt myopathy sufficient to lead to a diagnosis of 'limb-girdle muscular dystrophy' (Fig. 15.4).

Gowers (1879), in his study of Duchenne muscular dystrophy, described one family with evident X-linked inheritance in which a female was severely affected. Moser & Emery (1974) reviewed more than 20 manifesting carriers reported in the previous 40 years adding 22 personal cases and others have been studied since then (Bulcke et al 1981, Yoshioka 1981, Olson & Fenichel 1982, de Visser & Verbeeten 1985a). The equivalent situation in Becker dystrophy carriers was reported by Aguilar et al (1978). Overt myopathy appears to lie at one end of the spectrum of the degree of Lyonisation of the X-linked genes and, not surprisingly, the severity of manifestation varies considerably from barely detectable weakness, or isolated calf hypertrophy, to progressive disabling weakness. The special case of discordant manifestation in identical twin

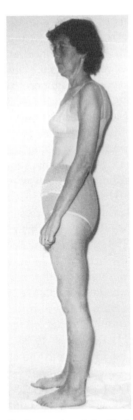

Fig. 15.4 A manifesting carrier of the Duchenne gene, aged 35 with a three-year history of progressive proximal muscle weakness, diagnosed as 'limb-girdle muscular dystrophy', serum CK activity 11× normal. Three years later her son, aged five, was found to have Duchenne muscular dystrophy

Manifesting carriers usually have very high serum CK activities, except in the late stage of the disorder. The ECG is sometimes abnormal with tall R waves in the right precordial leads, but more often the changes are mild and within the normal range (Emery 1972, Moser & Emery 1974).

Muscle biopsy in manifesting carriers often shows isolated hyaline or necrotic fibres or small foci of necrosis and is sometimes severely dystrophic (Dubowitz 1963, Emery 1965, Pearce et al 1966, Yoshioka 1981, de Visser & Verbeeten 1985a). The use of computed tomography to identify selective muscle involvement in these patients (Bulcke et al 1981, de Visser and Verbetten 1985a) may prove valuable in the differential diagnosis from other 'limb girdle syndromes'.

Moser & Emery (1974) revealingly estimated the prevalence of manifesting carriers in the female population to be 22.4×10^{-6} and pointed out that this was comparable to the incidence of 'limb-girdle dystrophy', and that many females presenting with limb-girdle weakness could be accounted for in this way.

At present it seems justifiable to regard the Duchenne carrier state as being the likeliest diagnosis when a female with a normal karyotype presents with progressive proximal myopathy in 'Duchenne' distribution, calf hypertrophy, a very high serum CK activity and randomly scattered necrotic fibres in the muscle biopsy. Additional evidence in favour would be similar symptoms or a raised serum CK level in her mother or other females in the maternal line, asymmetry of the calf hypertrophy or an ECG showing tall R waves over the right precordium. Such patients should be offered appropriate genetic counselling. The differential diagnosis from autosomal recessive childhood muscular dystrophy is discussed below (p. 545).

girls is discussed on page 525. Moser & Emery (1974) showed that the manifesting carrier state often occurs in several members of a family.

The age at the onset of symptoms varies from early childhood to the fourth decade and the course is often progressive. We personally know of three cases in which the ability to walk was lost in the fifth to sixth decades. Moser & Emery (1974) reported progression in 12 of 22 cases: all but four had calf muscle hypertrophy and one of these had presented in childhood, 50 years earlier, with swollen calves; she became unable to walk at the age of 53. The weakness and calf hypertrophy are sometimes asymmetrical. The literature is disappointingly silent on the subject of the precise distribution of muscle wasting and weakness but such information as there is suggests that this is the same as in Duchenne cases.

Hereditary myopathy limited to females

Two reports suggest that X-linked dominant inheritance may occur in a form of muscular dystrophy. The lack of investigation of the muscle disorder in the large pedigree reported by Hertrich (1957) precludes accurate diagnosis. Henson et al (1967) recorded eight cases, all

female, in two generations: they had a high incidence of miscarriages; symptoms of a proximal
myopathy began in the first or second decade and
progressed to severe disability by the age of 30.
They had a waddling gait, lumbar lordosis and
weakness of the truncal and proximal muscles of
the limbs, especially glutei and hamstrings. The
deltoids and medial gastrocnemii were wasted; the
facial muscles were spared. Serum CK activity was
9–15 times normal in adults but normal in two
affected children. Muscle biopsy showed a necrotising myopathy.

This may be a separate form of X-linked
muscular dystrophy, lethal in affected males
before birth.

Emery–Dreifuss muscular dystrophy (X-linked scapuloperoneal myopathy)

A family of eight affected males in three generations with clear evidence of X-linked inheritance
was recorded on three occasions by Dreifuss &
Hogan (1961), Emery & Dreifuss (1966) and
McKusick (1971). The disorder was quite distinct
from Becker dystrophy. The symptoms began at
four to five years and weakness progressed slowly.
It was described as affecting only the proximal
muscles in the upper and lower limbs but it now
appears that the distal muscles of the lower limbs
were also affected in the earliest stages (A.E.H.
Emery, personal communication). Muscle hypertrophy was absent except in one case. Contractures of the biceps and calf muscles were a striking
and early feature. Every patient over the age of 25
had cardiac involvement, either atrial fibrillation
or atrio-ventricular block. The serum CK activities were 6–7 times normal in the second decade
and fell subsequently. Some female carriers had
raised serum CK levels. For some years this
family was regarded as having an unique
'Emery–Dreifuss' type of muscular dystrophy. A
female with an identical clinical picture was
reported by Takamoto et al (1984); no explanation
is yet apparent.

Meanwhile, cases of a progressive scapuloperoneal syndrome of myopathic origin and with X-
linked inheritance were described by Rotthauwe
et al (1972), Thomas et al (1972), Hassan et al

(1979), Hopkins et al (1981), Dickey et al (1984)
and Dubowitz (1985). The symptoms began in
early childhood and progressed over four to six
decades. There was wasting and weakness in
scapuloperoneal or humeroperoneal distribution
with or without mild facial weakness. Muscle
hypertrophy was absent. Contractures at the
elbows and of the posterior neck muscles and calf
muscles were prominent and in some cases there
was pes cavus. Many cases required Achilles
tenotomies. Cardiomyopathy was present in three
of the cases of Thomas et al (1972) and atrioventricular block in some cases described by
Rotthauwe et al (1972), Hopkins et al (1981) and
Dickey et al (1984). Heart disease was the usual
cause of death. Several cases required cardiac
pacemakers. In some families the symptoms of
heart block were the dominant problem, causing
a major threat to life in the third or fourth decade
and evidence of the skeletal myopathy was relatively trivial (Hassan et al 1979); this contrasts
with the opposite situation in the original kindred
described by Emery & Dreifuss (1966). The
serum CK activity was raised two- to twentyfold
in the first 25–35 years of life but was normal in
older cases. Female carriers had normal serum CK
levels, but Dickey et al found two carriers with
ECG evidence of premature atrial beats and one
with chronic bradycardia and cardiomegaly: the
EMG suggested myopathy. Occasional necrosis
and phagocytosis, central nuclei, type I fibre
atrophy, type II predominance and proliferation
of connective tissue were the main features of
muscle biopsies, but in young children only scattered fibre atrophy and type 11 fibre predominance may be seen. In the family described by
Thomas et al (1972) the disorder was closely
linked with deutan colour blindness.

Rowland et al (1979) described a single case in
which muscle weakness was humeroperoneal in
distribution. They used the term 'Emery–Dreifuss
muscular dystrophy' for their own and the many
other scapulo-humero-peroneal cases in the literature, defining the cardinal features as X-linked
inheritance of myopathy or neuromyopathy associated with early elbow contractures and subsequent heart block. Their lead was followed by
Hopkins et al (1981) and Dickey et al (1984) and

it is now widely agreed that, despite the apparent differences in the distribution of the muscle involvement in the lower limbs, the Emery–Dreifuss and scapuloperoneal syndromes are, in fact, identical. There is now evidence that the gene responsible for the Emery–Dreifuss variety of X-linked dystrophy lies close to the tip of the long arm of the X-chromosome (See Ch. 26).

Scapuloperoneal syndromes are much more frequently neurogenic than myopathic in origin (Kaeser 1965, Emery et al 1968, see also Ch. 23). Those cases in which autosomal dominant inheritance is recorded and which are neither neurogenic in origin, nor abortive or incompletely expressed examples of facioscapulohumeral muscular dystrophy (Ricker & Mertens 1968, Kazakov et al 1976), are discussed below. The remarkably similar X-linked scapuloperoneal spinal muscular atrophy described by Mawatari & Katayama (1973) closely resembled the Emery–Dreifuss type of muscular dystrophy; indeed the cases of Waters et al (1975), in which both myopathic and neurogenic features occurred, were the same individuals as those later reported as cases of Emery–Dreifuss dystrophy by Hopkins et al (1981). This raises the question of whether the scapuloperoneal syndrome may be a neuromyopathy in which the neural and muscular features predominate in different individuals. It is unfortunate that in the only autopsied case (Thomas et al 1972) the spinal cord was not examined.

'Limb-girdle muscular dystrophy', an obsolete term

In previous editions of this book the term 'limb-girdle muscular dystrophy' was retained, though with an increasingly restricted application. In this edition we abandon it virtually completely.

Stevenson (1953) in a genetic population study contrasted the X-linked and the dominant facioscapulohumeral dystrophies with a separate operational category which he called 'autosomal limb-girdle muscular dystrophy'. The term 'limb-girdle muscular dystrophy' was used by Walton & Nattrass (1954) to describe cases of both sexes, usually autosomal recessive in inheritance, in which the facial muscles were not involved, and the symptoms of proximal muscle weakness began in the second or third decade and progressed slowly to a stage of severe disability about 20 years after the onset, with some shortening of life expectancy. This definition encompassed the classic pelvic girdle atrophic (Leyden–Möbius) and juvenile scapulohumeral (Erb) forms, but because of the variability and overlap of the clinical features the overall inclusive term seemed preferable. Since that time, the Becker type of muscular dystrophy, the Kugelberg–Welander 'pseudo-myopathic' type of spinal muscular atrophy, the scapuloperoneal syndromes, a variety of 'congenital myopathies' which may sometimes cause symptoms only in the second and third decades, and many acquired metabolic and other myopathies have been described and characterised. Manifesting female carriers of the Duchenne gene have also been recognised. Many cases diagnosed as limb-girdle muscular dystrophy in the past have, in fact, suffered from one or other of these disorders. The 'limb-girdle type of muscular dystrophy' has not shared as an entity in the rapid increase in research and medical writing about the muscular dystrophies in the last 30 years. A high proportion of cases has always been found to be sporadic (Morton & Chung 1959), which has added to the difficulty of delineating familial entities. Consequently the term has too often been applied indiscriminately to any non-Duchenne proximal type of muscular dystrophy and has too automatically been equated with autosomal recessive inheritance.

We recognise that some cases of progressive proximal muscle weakness present serious difficulties in diagnosis and that some such temporary label as 'limb-girdle syndrome' may be required following inconclusive investigations in the hope that follow-up may lead to a definitive diagnosis. But we now regard it as totally unsatisfactory to use the term 'limb-girdle muscular dystrophy' for this purpose and urge that all cases bearing such a label should be reassessed. In most cases it will be found possible to make a positive diagnosis of one of the following disorders. Where this is not possible, and where good clinical and pathological evidence identifying distinctive features are present, the cases should be recorded in detail in the literature so that our understanding of this difficult group can advance.

The disorders usually overlooked under the title of limb girdle dystrophy are:

(1) *Scapulohumeral muscular dystrophy.*
(2) *The autosomal recessive childhood form of muscular dystrophy.*
(3) *The dominant late onset form of proximal muscular dystrophy.*
(4) *Becker muscular dystrophy.* A very important group. Many clinicians are reluctant to diagnose Becker dystrophy in the absence of evidence of X-linked inheritance. This may have serious genetic consequences. The clinical and pathological features of this disorder are sufficiently characteristic for a presumptive diagnosis to be made even in isolated cases. Isolated males presenting in the first three decades of life with pelvifemoral muscular dystrophy associated with muscle hypertrophy are almost all of the Becker type. They should be examined in detail to ascertain whether the precise distribution of muscle weakness conforms to the Becker pattern and, if it does and the investigations are compatible, genetic advice should be given on the basis of X-linked inheritance.
(5) *Emery–Dreifuss muscular dystrophy.*
(6) *Manifesting carriers of the gene for Duchenne (or Becker) dystrophy.* The very variable degree of severity amongst manifesting carriers makes this category particularly difficult to diagnose in isolated cases (Fig. 15.4) (see p. 540).
(7) *'Myopathy confined to the quadriceps'* (see p. 548).
(8) *The autosomal dominant form of scapuloperoneal muscular dystrophy.*
(9) *The Kugelberg–Welander form of spinal muscular atrophy* (often with 'secondary myopathic change' as a cause of confusion).
(10) *Central core disease* or one of several other congenital myopathies with 'late onset' variants including nemaline, centronuclear and various mitochondrial myopathies.
(11) *Metabolic myopathies* including glycogen storage and lipid storage myopathies.
(12) *Various non-genetic myopathies* including polymyositis, sarcoidosis, thyrotoxicosis, hypothyroidism etc.

Scapulohumeral muscular dystrophy (Erb 1884)

This is a decidedly uncommon muscular dystrophy which first becomes apparent in early adult life and predominantly affects the upper limb girdle (Fig. 15.5). Becker (1964) did not include any such cases in his comprehensive review of myopathies in Baden. The weakness is at first most prominent in the biceps, triceps, trapezius, rhomboid and serratus anterior muscles, and scapular winging is a major feature. The deltoid is relatively preserved. The proximal muscles of the lower limbs are affected later, especially the hip flexors and quadriceps with relative preservation of the hamstrings and muscles below the knees. The facial, forearm and hand muscles are also strikingly preserved until the later stages. The condition is usually very slowly but continuously progressive. Ten or even 20 years may elapse before the weakness spreads from the upper to the lower limbs. Moser et al (1966) reported 15 cases of this type from Switzerland where it appears to be relatively common. The sexes were equally affected. The age at onset in their cases varied from nine to 31 years but was usually 14–23 years. Hypertrophy of muscles was absent except in one doubtful case, and appears to be rare in this disorder. The serum CK activity was 22 times the normal in the youngest case (aged 14) and normal or only slightly raised (1–5 times normal) in cases over 20 years of age. Our experience of a few cases is similar.

Contractures often develop in relation to joints in which the active range of movement is limited, but such contractures are not an early feature. The heart is not involved, and intelligence is normal.

The differential diagnosis of this clinical syndrome includes the Emery–Dreifuss and facioscapulohumeral types of muscular dystrophy and, above all, spinal muscular atrophy. Any patient showing intermittent progression or asymmetry of muscle weakness is particularly likely to have the latter disorder. Nemaline myopathy and thyrotoxic myopathy may present similar features. Diagnosis depends on the clinical and biochemical findings, on the EMG which shows myopathic changes without specific features, and on muscle biopsy to exclude features of the congenital myopathies or denervation. The myopathic features in biopsies of these cases are not well

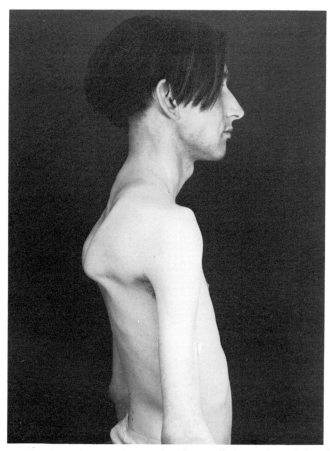

Fig. 15.5 Scapulohumeral muscular dystrophy: note the atrophy of upper limb muscles and the winged scapulae

characterised but appear to be relatively indolent. One of the few cases reported under this title with modern published pathological findings seems to be an atypical example with dominant inheritance (Dubowitz 1978, p. 50).

One of the major disabilities in these patients is in raising the arms. The deltoids may be quite strong, but scapular fixation is very poor. Fixing the scapulae by bracing is not easy and contracture at the shoulder joint may limit the benefit of attempting this. Surgical fixation in carefully selected cases may be valuable (Copeland & Howard 1978), but the contractures must be overcome first.

Childhood muscular dystrophy with autosomal recessive inheritance

This has been one of the most difficult categories of muscular dystrophy to delineate. Proof of auto-somal recessive inheritance in any given family is rarely possible and therefore the arguments for the existence of this disorder have depended upon the occasional occurrence of muscular dystrophy in girls and in a few families in which consanguinity of the parents has made autosomal recessive inheritance likely. Gull (1862) gave a very early account of two sisters with 'granular and fatty degeneration' of the muscles. Stevenson (1953) reviewed the early case reports of muscular dystrophy in girls. Lamy & de Grouchy (1954) in their genetic assessment of 102 families with muscular dystrophy with a 'pelvifemoral onset' concluded that in about 90% the inheritance was X-linked and, in about 10%, autosomal recessive. However, in these reports the paucity of clinical information and in particular the lack of EMG or histological evidence make it impossible to be sure that many of the cases described were not, in fact, examples of benign spinal muscular atrophy

(Kugelberg & Welander 1956). The same reservations must be advanced in the assessment of more recent case reports (Stevenson 1955 (Case D58), Blyth & Pugh 1959, Johnston 1964) although many of these cases must surely have been examples of muscular dystrophy. Cases which can be fairly confidently accepted as examples of autosomal recessive childhood dystrophy were those of Kloepfer & Talley (1958, Pedigree 1), Jackson & Carey (1961), Jackson & Strehler (1968), Stern (1972), Ionasescu & Zellweger (1974), Kakulas et al (1975), Shokeir & Kobrinsky (1976) and Dubowitz (1978). Hazama et al (1979) reported six girls including two sisters who were severely mentally retarded, a feature unique to them. Moser et al (1966), in their review of 'limb-girdle dystrophy' in Switzerland, included 14 cases without facial involvement in which the lower limb muscles were first affected: in nine, the symptoms began between three and nine years of age and in the rest at 15–27 years. It is interesting that the cases of Jackson & Carey (1961) and Shokeir & Kobrinsky (1976) were of Swiss descent. The latter cases had some involvement of facial muscles, and Moser et al (1966) also distinguished a separate autosomal recessive group of seven cases, with onset from the age of three to 17 years, in which the facial muscles were affected. Whether these represent yet another entity within the autosomal recessive muscular dystrophies is not clear. In our experience, slight facial involvement does seem to be a feature in a minority of cases with autosomal recessive inheritance. The pure lower limb-girdle group of Moser et al (1966) showed no calf enlargement and their serum CK activities were normal or raised up to tenfold. The experience of Becker (1964) was different: in south Germany he found that autosomal recessive pelvifemoral dystrophy closely resembled his benign X-linked cases, often showing calf hypertrophy. His recessive cases showed high rates of parental consanguinity and tended to come from small country villages. Penn et al (1970) reviewed this subject very thoroughly and concluded that, at that date, no convincing case of true Duchenne dystrophy had been recorded in a female of normal karyotype and that girls with muscular dystrophy had a separate

disorder, generally distinguishable on clinical grounds.

Recent studies from North Africa (Ben Hamida et al 1983, Salih et al 1983), have characterised a severe autosomal recessive muscular dystrophy seen in large consanguineous kindreds there. Many features were closely similar to those of Duchenne muscular dystrophy including steadily progressive weakness in a broadly similar distribution, hypertrophy of the calf muscles, in Ben Hamida's cases a very high serum CK activity in the early stages (50–200 × the normal limit), and a destructive necrotising biopsy picture. In Salih's cases the serum CK was only up to 15 × normal. The age at onset varied greatly, even within each family, from three to 12 years, and the inability to walk from 10 to 30 years (usually 15–20 years in Ben Hamida's cases and 11–14 years in Salih's). Deaths, recorded only in Salih's cases, usually occurred at between 15 and 20 years. ECGs were often abnormal (Salih et al 1983) but showed ST-depression and T wave changes and not the deep Q waves seen in Duchenne cases. Impaired respiratory function appeared to be a major cause of death (Salih et al 1984).

In a study of 12 affected girls (and two affected brothers) ascertained in a national survey in the UK, Gardner-Medwin & Johnston (1984) concluded that most if not all had an autosomal recessive form of muscular dystrophy. All had early-onset progressive dystrophy with very high CK activity. Points which appeared to help in the distinction from Duchenne muscular dystrophy were: (1) toe walking as a prominent early feature (aged 1–5 years) before the onset of *difficulty* in walking; (2) ability to walk retained to 11–15 years or later; (3) relatively more severe weakness of the deltoid muscles compared with biceps and triceps but otherwise weakness, atrophy and hypertrophy of muscles consistent with the Duchenne pattern; (4) normal ECG; (5) normal intelligence; (6) relatively less severe destruction of muscle in biopsies before the age of 10 years, preservation of the histochemical fibre types and a focal pattern of pathology, typically with foci of tens to hundreds of necrotic, atrophic or regenerating fibres seen against a background of relatively preserved fibres. In retrospect a similar biopsy pattern may be discerned in some cases described earlier, e.g. those of Kakulas et al (1975), Dubowitz (1978, Fig. 2–40), Salih et al (1983) and Ben Hamida et al (1983). Several authors have found type I fibre predominance in muscle biopsies from these cases.

In summary, therefore, it seems that this form of the disease is similar to the Duchenne type but rather more benign. Variation in severity occurs even within families. The incidence is unknown but, except in North Africa, where it may be more frequent than Duchenne dystrophy, it is probably 15–30 times less frequent. The onset may be in the second year or as late as the fourteenth, but is most usual in the second half of the first decade. Early toe walking is a common characteristic. Progression is comparatively slow and patients usually become unable to walk in their early twenties, sometimes as early as 12 years or as late as 44 years, and many survive to the fifth decade or later (Jackson & Strehler 1968). The weakness is chiefly proximal and has not been differentiated clearly in its distribution from that of Duchenne dystrophy, although in some families the facial muscles are spared and in others are much more severely affected. Relatively weak deltoids may be a helpful diagnostic feature. Muscle hypertrophy is present in some affected families. Intelligence is normal. ECGs are normal in most cases but this is not a reliable guide because several of the cases described by Jackson & Carey (1961) had QRS changes resembling the typical Duchenne pattern. The serum CK activity may be only moderately raised (up to 10 times the normal limit) but in many cases is in the Duchenne range and, in Jackson and Strehler's cases, high levels were found in the preclinical stages. A strikingly multifocal pattern of necrosis may be a distinctive feature of the pathology.

Dubowitz (1978) described some cases of a 'limb-girdle myopathy' associated with cramps and myoglobinuria, in which glycogen- and lipid-storage diseases had been ruled out. Their significance is not clear.

The principles of management of autosomal recessive childhood muscular dystrophy are the same as for the Duchenne type, taking into account the better prognosis.

Autosomal recessive muscular dystrophy of proximal lower limb distribution and late onset

It is very doubtful whether any entity of this type remains after elimination of the disorders listed on page 544, that is whether any quintessential 'limb-girdle muscular dystrophy' exists. The review of proximal muscular dystrophies in Switzerland (Moser et al 1966) included five cases affecting the lower limbs with an onset after the age of 15 years. Dubowitz & Brooke (1973) mention reviewing 18 cases of 'limb-girdle dystrophy' and illustrate three of them with a relatively late onset varying from 14 to 33 years; in the second edition (Dubowitz 1985) only one of the three remains. In this case and the four sporadic cases reported by Bethlem et al (1973) (of whom two had a suspiciously early onset) lobulated and whorled fibres were prominent but not specific features. The myopathy was relatively slowly progressive. Serum CK activities varied from 86 to 850 iu/l. Two patients had electrophysiological and histological features of denervation as well as of myopathy, a dilemma very commonly posed by cases of the 'limb-girdle syndrome'. Bethlem et al (1973) described similar pathology in two additional sibs with a probably dominant mode of inheritance and it is difficult to know whether rare sporadic cases of this type might be new mutant dominants or are truly examples of a rare autosomal recessive disorder. Similar uncertainties were encountered in the study of Bradley (1979) who found a 2:1 male predominance (suggesting contamination of the series by X-linked disorders) and only 33% of cases with no features of a denervating component to the pathology.

We repeat that most sporadic cases which present themselves in the guise of a 'limb-girdle dystrophy' may well be, if male, isolated cases of Becker dystrophy and, if female, manifesting carriers of the Duchenne gene.

Clearly, this group of cases demands yet further study.

Sporadic (?autosomal recessive) distal muscular dystrophy

An autosomal dominant form of distal muscular dystrophy has been recognised for many years (see

p. 554). Recently some cases have been described with probable autosomal recessive inheritance and a rather rapidly progressive course from the onset in the second or third decade to the stage of being unable to walk within about 10 years (Markesbery et al 1974, Miller et al 1979, de Visser 1983, Nonaka et al 1985, Miyoshi et al 1986). Nonaka et al and Miyoshi et al reviewed some earlier reports, mainly from the Japanese literature, and reported a total of 22 additional cases. One of the cases of Miyoshi et al was examined at autopsy. Nonaka et al contrasted the dystrophic pathology with that seen in a very similar clinical disorder in which muscle biopsy shows rimmed vacuoles in the muscle fibres with the serum CK activity only slightly raised. Another less severe autosomal recessive distal myopathy, with filamentous inclusions in muscle fibres, was reported by Matsubara & Tanabe (1982).

The earliest feature is usually atrophy of the calf muscles and of the small muscles of the hands. The patients find it more difficult to stand on their toes than on their heels. Proximal muscles are more mildly affected. Serum CK activities are 40–100 times normal in the early stages and the muscle biopsy shows evidence of active fibre necrosis and regeneration. The muscle pathology was reviewed by Markesbery et al (1977).

Although most cases have been sporadic, Miyoshi et al (1986) provided strong evidence favouring autosomal recessive inheritance in their cases.

Quadriceps myopathy

'Myopathy confined to the quadriceps' (Bramwell 1922) should be discussed here. The muscle weakness, of adult onset (20–25 years), rarely remains confined to the quadriceps if cases are re-examined after many years (Walton 1956b, Turner & Heathfield 1961). Van Wijngaarden et al (1968) described two brothers with widespread myopathic changes in the EMG although the clinical involvement was limited to the quadriceps. The cases of Espir & Matthews (1973) suggested dominant inheritance. All other cases have been sporadic. Recent reviews suggest that the condition is heterogeneous, some cases having neurogenic

atrophy with secondary myopathic change (Boddie & Stewart-Wynne 1974, and possibly the cases of Espir & Matthews 1973), and others a very indolent limb-girdle myopathy (Swash & Heathfield 1983). Some may be sporadic cases of the dominant late-onset limb-girdle dystrophy of Bacon & Smith (1971), described in a later section. The serum CK activity may be raised by up to tenfold.

Congenital muscular dystrophy

The congenital muscular dystrophies can be defined as genetically determined necrotising myopathies with muscle weakness evident from the time of birth. They tend to be relatively non-progressive. There appear to be several different types, in addition to congenital myotonic dystrophy which is discussed in Chapter 16, but much remains to be learned about the nosology of these disorders and some similar cases may even represent non-genetic disorders acquired in utero. The term was first used by Howard (1908) and several cases were recorded over the following 50 years which are difficult now to classify. Since the 1950s numerous *congenital myopathies* with more or less specific histological features have been defined (see Ch. 20), and a clearer picture of the dystrophies has emerged.

Banker et al (1957), Greenfield et al (1958), O'Brien (1962), Pearson & Fowler (1963), Gubbay et al (1966) and Zellweger et al (1967) described cases with congenital hypotonia and severe but relatively non-progressive muscular weakness, in which the muscle histology was typical of muscular dystrophy. In several children there was associated arthrogryposis multiplex.

These cases formed the basis of our current concepts of the usual form of congenital muscular dystrophy seen in Europe and the USA which is further described below. The hypotonic-sclerotic type of Ullrich and the Fukuyama type, both most commonly seen in Japan, are treated separately.

In addition there are a few closely related conditions which need to be distinguished. Two of these may represent rare separate forms of congenital dystrophy, each represented by a large consanguineous pedigree. The large kindred with autosomal recessive inheritance described by

Lebenthal et al (1970) is atypical in having a high incidence of associated congenital heart disease. Five cases, four of them related in a manner suggesting autosomal recessive inheritance, were described by Goebel et al (1980). They had congenital weakness, possibly slightly progressive, with progressive scoliosis. In three cases, progressive right ventricular cardiac dilatation, of which the pathology was not established, developed after the age of nine years and was fatal in two of them. The muscle pathology was compatible with a congenital dystrophy; the serum CK activities were normal or slightly raised.

Another distinct type of congenital muscular dystrophy, associated with severe mental retardation, mild hydrocephalus, congenital glaucoma, cataracts, other eye anomalies and renal anomalies, occurs in Finland (Santavuori et al 1977). The serum CK activity is very high in early childhood but in cases that survive into adult life it falls to normal. Towfighi et al (1984) described seven rather similar cases from the USA, mostly surviving for less than a year, with detailed neuropathological findings.

Early concepts of congenital muscular dystrophy were also confused by the inclusion of milder and more severe cases which are now thought to be distinct. Thus the benign congenital myopathy classically described by Batten (1903, 1909), Turner (1940) and Turner & Lees (1962) differs from the muscular dystrophies in its non-progressive course and in the absence of specific histological features.

A few cases of a 'rapidly-progressive type of congenital muscular dystrophy' have been reported (de Lange 1937, Lewis & Besant 1962, Short, 1963, Wharton 1965): of these, only Wharton's two cases survived beyond the age of six months. The clinical features in these cases varied considerably and the pathological evidence was in general inconclusive. The cases of Short (1963) bear a close resemblance to the X-linked type of centronuclear myopathy (see Ch. 20). Futher evidence is needed before the existence of a rapidly progressive form of congenital muscular dystrophy can be accepted.

We may now discuss the typical congenital muscular dystrophies of Western countries. In a series of cases from Finland, described by Donner et al (1975), the symptoms progressed slightly in the first few years of life and thereafter remained static. A similar clinical picture was found in the cases reported by Vasella et al (1967), Lazaro et al (1979) and McMenamin et al (1982b). Serratrice et al (1980) reviewed 92 cases from the literature.

The essential features of this disorder are severe hypotonia present from birth, associated with static or very slowly progressive muscular wasting and weakness. Fetal movements are often impaired. Contractures at birth are common but not invariable, and they may develop later. Some children have difficulty in sucking and breathing in the neonatal period. There is often facial weakness and Donner et al (1975) emphasised severe head lag. The diagnosis can be made with confidence only by examination of the muscle histology. The 'dystrophic' appearances are often severe to a degree that seems out of proportion with the clinical disability, although in some mild cases there are simply myopathic changes without specific features. Afifi et al (1969) and Fidzianska et al (1982) emphasised the excessive collagen proliferation and paucity of muscle fibre regeneration. In late childhood the serum aldolase and CK activities are often normal or only a little raised. However Donner et al (1975) reported figures up to 30 times normal in the first three years, falling to 1–5 times normal by the age of five years. Sibs are often affected, but rigorous evidence of autosomal recessive inheritance is lacking.

It is uncommon, but not unknown, for cases of Duchenne dystrophy to be hypotonic at birth and some patients with 'autosomal recessive childhood dystrophy' have been noted to show this sign. In cases where the distinction is difficult, the serum CK activity would be expected to persist at much higher levels in these dystrophies than in congenital dystrophy at the age of two to three years, and usually diagnosis should also be possible on histological grounds.

Most children with congenital muscular dystrophy learn to walk at between 18 months and eight years, although strenuous efforts to overcome contractures, and the use of supporting calipers, may be needed (Jones et al 1979). The mortality in early childhood is high despite the non-progressive course.

Intelligence is usually normal. A few cases are found to have a disorder of cerebral white matter showing as low attenuation on CT scans; this has been described in the presence of normal intelligence (Nogen 1980) or mild non-progressive mental retardation and epilepsy (Echenne et al 1984), or epilepsy and rapidly progressive dementia in the second decade (Egger et al 1983). Among Egger's cases were two affected sibs. Delayed myelination giving a similar CT scan appearance is a frequent feature of Fukuyama muscular dystrophy (see below) and may reflect a non-progressive and possibly temporary delay in myelination (Ishikawa 1982, Peters et al 1984). Occasionally more extensive cerebral malformation is associated with congenital muscular dystrophy (Fowler & Manson 1973).

Hypotonic-sclerotic muscular dystrophy (Ullrich)

Ullrich described this form of congenital muscular dystrophy in 1930 and descriptions appeared only in the German literature until 1977, since when there have been a few reports in English, all originating from Japan (Furukawa & Toyokura 1977, Nihei et al 1979, Nonaka et al 1981). These authors described 10 cases, and Nihei et al (1979) reviewed 15 cases from the literature.

The features are non-progressive congenital myopathy with slender muscles, contractures of the proximal muscles but hypotonic, hyperextensible distal muscles, relative sparing of the facial muscles, prominence of the calcaneus, high arched palate, hyperhidrosis and normal intelligence. Some cases have preserved tendon reflexes. Secondary scoliosis and torticollis are frequent. Nonaka et al (1981) suggest that some cases may be slowly progressive. The serum CK is normal or nearly so, EMG studies have shown non-specific myopathic features and muscle biopsies show variation in fibre size, poor histochemical fibre differentiation often with Type 1 predominance, fatty and connective tissue replacement and relatively little evidence of muscle fibre degeneration.

Sibs of both sexes may be affected and there is an increased rate of consanguinity, suggesting autosomal recessive inheritance.

Fukuyama muscular dystrophy

This distinctive type of congenital muscular dystrophy, first described by Fukuyama et al (1960), is now one of the most clearly documented muscular dystrophies (Kamoshita et al 1976, Fukuyama et al 1981). In Japan it is approximately half as frequent as Duchenne dystrophy; elsewhere, only a few reports have appeared (Krijgsman et al 1980, McMenamin et al 1982a, Goebel et al 1983, Peters et al 1984).

The principal features are progressive muscular dystrophy of early onset, severe mental retardation and epilepsy. The onset is before eight months but only a few cases have impairment of fetal movements. Congenital arthrogryposis is not a feature. The peak of motor development is at two to five years after which slow deterioration occurs. Many patients learn to crawl but very few to walk. The muscle weakness is generalised with progressive contractures; the facial muscles are affected; calf hypertrophy is frequent. Mental retardation is severe, the IQ 30–50 in most cases. About half have some intelligible speech. Mild microcephaly is frequent. Febrile and non-febrile convulsions occur in more than half of all cases, usually with focal paroxysmal discharges in the EEG (Segawa et al 1979). CT brain scans commonly show low-density white matter (Yoshioka et al 1980, Fukuyama et al 1981) in addition to slight cerebral atrophy. Optic atrophy is rare.

The serum CK activities are comparable to those in Duchenne dystrophy, being 10–50 times the normal limit between six months and six years, later falling towards the normal range. Muscle biopsy (Fukuyama et al 1981, Nonaka et al 1982) reveals extensive connective tissue infiltration, destruction of the fascicular architecture, a lesser degree of fatty infiltration, muscle fibre atrophy without hypertrophy and type 1 fibre predominance. Necrosis, phagocytosis and regeneration are less severe than in Duchenne dystrophy but otherwise the appearances are similar.

Mild myocardial abnormalities may be found at autopsy but ECGs during life have been normal.

The cerebral pathology has been described in 24 cases by Fukuyama et al (1981) and in more detail in five cases by Takada et al (1984). Multifocal cerebral and cerebellar cortical dysplasia, micropolygyria, aberrant fascicles of myelinated nerve fibres and a degree of myelin pallor and gliosis in white matter were the main features. The possible relationship of these findings to a prenatal infection has been discussed but there is no firm evidence for this. The neuropathology suggests a lesion dating from, at the latest, the fifth month of gestation.

A detailed genetic study provides strong evidence of autosomal recessive inheritance (Fukuyama & Ohsawa 1984).

There is little information in the available literature on the management of these cases or on survival. Of the 24 autopsied cases reviewed by Fukuyama et al (1981), four were under two years, four aged two to nine years, 11 aged 10–19 years, four aged 20–22 years and in one the age was unknown.

Facioscapulohumeral (FSH) muscular dystrophy

This variety of muscular dystrophy is characterised by: (1) expression in either sex; (2) transmission usually as an autosomal dominant trait; (3) onset at any age from childhood until adult life; (4) the frequent occurrence of abortive or mildly affected cases; (5) initial involvement of the face and shoulder-girdle muscles with subsequent spread to the muscles of the lower limbs; (6) the rarity of muscular hypertrophy; (7) the infrequent occurrence of muscular contractures and skeletal deformity; (8) insidious progress of the disease with prolonged periods of apparent arrest. Although cases occur in which the disease progresses unusually rapidly, most patients survive and remain active to a normal age.

This type of muscular dystrophy is one of the more clearly defined forms but some cases may cause confusion. Apparently isolated or recessive cases of facioscapulohumeral muscular dystrophy may occur (Moser et al 1966). There is little published evidence as to whether the pattern of muscle involvement is precisely the same in dominant and recessive cases. Cases with minimal facial involvement must be distinguished from examples of the 'scapuloperoneal syndrome' (see p. 542 & 554). Cases of spinal muscular atrophy may closely resemble facioscapulohumeral muscular dystrophy, even showing dominant inheritance (Fenichel et al 1967) but they are more often sporadic. A review of cases with muscular atrophy in facioscapulohumeral distribution undertaken in Newcastle (W. G. Bradley, unpublished work) revealed almost equal numbers with 'myopathic' and 'neurogenic' histological findings on muscle biopsy, and a single family with a mitochondrial myopathy (Hudgson et al 1972, Bradley et al 1978a). A further diagnostic difficulty was first reported by Munsat & Piper (1971) who found inflammatory changes resembling polymyositis in muscle in the early stages of the disease in two families, while true polymyositis with full resolution after therapy may show a similar clinical picture (Rothstein et al 1971). Kazakov et al (1974) in a study of 200 cases, divided faciosca-pulohumeral muscular dystrophy into two groups: in the larger, the late lower-limb involvement primarily affected the anterior tibial and peroneal muscles while, in a smaller number, the proximal pelvic girdle muscles were more severely affected; these groups of patients appeared to be genetically distinct. The investigations did not rigorously exclude neurogenic atrophy, so considerable doubts remain about the atypical 'proximal' group.

One of the most striking features of this variety, as previously described by Tyler & Wintrobe (1950) and Walton (1955, 1956a), is the occurrence of partly affected or abortive cases. Many of these patients are unaware that they are suffering from the disease in a mild form and it is therefore very important that, in any study of inheritance, all available family members should be examined. In these abortive cases the disease may remain confined to one or two muscle groups indefinitely.

Cases in which facial weakness is present at birth or in early infancy present special problems (Hanson & Rowland 1971, Brooke 1977, Carroll & Brooke 1979). Not only may the symptoms be severe, but many patients have been reported as having bilateral sensorineural deafness (Carroll & Brooke 1979, Taylor et al 1982, Wulff et al 1982,

Meyerson et al 1984, Korf et al 1985). Some, but not all, of these cases (Taylor et al 1982, Wulff et al 1982) also had Coats' disease of the retina, an association previously noted in four sibs with FSH dystrophy and deafness who were also mentally retarded (Small 1968). Some of these cases have been sporadic but in others FSH dystrophy both with and without deafness was seen in affected parents in whom the onset was not in infancy. Coats' disease has sometimes involved affected sibs but not their dystrophic parents. The association between these three features has not been elucidated, and at present it would be premature to suggest that the combination represents a distinct genetic disorder.

Incidence. This is quoted as 0.4–5.0 per 100 000 (Morton & Chung 1959, Becker 1964). Morton and Chung quoted a *prevalence* of 0.2 per 100 000 and Monckton et al (1982), 1.52 per 100 000. Evidently the frequency of this type of muscular dystrophy varies considerably in different populations.

Symptoms. The first symptoms of this form of muscular dystrophy usually appear in the second decade, or less often in the first, while occasionally the onset is apparently delayed until much later in life. Rarely, facial weakness is present at birth or in early infancy. The symptomatology is virtually identical to that of scapulohumeral muscular dystrophy in that the weakness usually begins in the same shoulder-girdle muscles. The pelvic girdle muscles are affected much later, but early involvement of the anterior tibial and peroneal muscles is typical. The additional feature which characterises this form is the facial weakness. Many patients are aware of the progressive change in their facial appearance and realise that they are unable to close their eyes properly and that they cannot whistle. When weakness is advanced they cannot pronounce labials and speech becomes characteristically indistinct. Scoliosis may occur, but much more often an extensive and severe lumbar lordosis develops. The consequent pelvic tilt, combined with foot-drop and, in some cases, hyperextension of the knees, gives a characteristic gait disturbance, different from that seen in the other muscular

dystrophies. When sensorineural deafness is present it is usually found at the age or four to six years because of speech delay. It has not been documented at birth, and in one case was absent at two years and present at six years (Korf et al 1985). Coats' disease has developed at various ages between six months and 13 years.

Course of the disease. This form of muscular dystrophy is very benign in many cases, and there are some who have had the disease since adolescence and who remain active, although with increasing disability, in late life. Even within the same family there may, however, be considerable variation in severity between individuals. There are some in whom the rate of progression is rapid, and walking becomes impossible in middle life, or even in the second or third decade, but this is unusual and in many there are long periods, often of several years, when there is no apparent progression.

The life expectancy in most patients with this form of disease is therefore normal, but in the more rapidly progressive cases, death from respiratory infection can occur in middle life. Rarely, the infantile form is severe enough to be fatal in childhood (McGarry et al 1983).

Physical examination. Muscular hypertrophy is rare in this form, but occasionally occurs in the calves and deltoid muscles.

The facial appearance is characteristic: the face is unlined and wrinkles are often missing from the forehead and around the eyes. There is a typical pouting appearance of the lips and a transverse smile. Affected individuals usually cannot close their eyes or bury their eye-lashes on command, while few can retain air under pressure within the mouth. Occasionally, the facial weakness is so slight as to be difficult to elicit.

The pattern of muscular involvement in the upper and lower limbs is similar to that described above in scapulohumeral dystrophy, but elevation of the scapulae on abduction of the arms (Fig. 15.6) is rather characteristic of the faciosca-pulohumeral disorder. The neck flexors, serrati, pectorals, biceps, triceps and extensors of the wrists are selectively involved, with relative

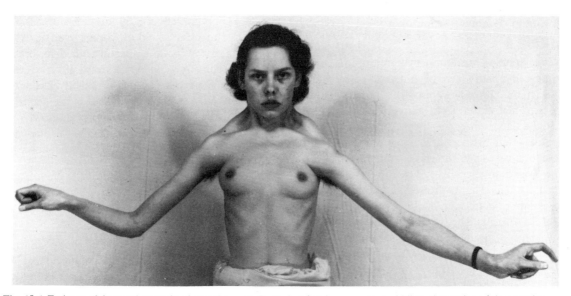

Fig. 15.6 Facioscapulohumeral muscular dystrophy: note the typical facial appearance and bilateral elevation of the scapulae (Walton 1962)

sparing of the deltoids and wrist flexors. Some asymmetry of the muscular weakness and wasting is seen in a proportion of cases. One helpful distinction is involvement of the anterior tibial muscles, which is often found in the facioscapulohumeral type but is rare in the early stages of scapulohumeral dystrophy. Muscular contractures and skeletal distortion occur late, if at all; cardiac involvement is rare and the range of intelligence is normal.

Diagnosis and management. Myotonic dystrophy, myotubular, nemaline and mitochondrial myopathies, the Möbius syndrome and myasthenia gravis may all present with various combinations of facial and limb muscle weakness. None of these conforms to the precise pattern of muscle involvement seen in FSH muscular dystrophy but, once myasthenia and myotonia have been excluded, muscle biopsy is usually essential to make an accurate diagnosis. The FSH form of spinal muscular atrophy may be suspected because of slightly atypical or asymmetrical muscle weakness or the rapid development of weakness in certain muscles. The EMG and biopsy are diagnostic. In FSH muscular dystrophy, as in spinal muscular atrophy, the serum CK activity is often normal or only slightly raised (up to five times normal, rarely more). The muscle biopsy often shows only minimal myopathic changes. Fibre hypertrophy, scattered very atrophic fibres and occasional 'moth-eaten' fibres are seen (Dubowitz 1985). Preclinical cases do not have raised serum enzyme levels and there is no reliable method of preclinical diagnosis. In few, if any, patients aged over 25 years are there no signs at all of the disease, but very careful examination may be required to detect signs in slightly affected individuals, even in their fifties and sixties.

The inflammatory changes frequently seen in muscle biopsies are often unassociated with symptoms and then require no treatment, but significant muscular aching does occur quite often in this disease and sometimes responds to a short course of steroids. There is no indication for prolonged steroid therapy, nor is any other effective treatment known. A few patients require operations for scapular fixation or spinal fusion (Copeland & Howard 1978) but for most, regular active muscle exercise is the only physical treatment necessary.

Early diagnosis of deafness or retinal disease is important. Early treatment of the latter may prevent or delay the complication of retinal detachment.

Autosomal dominant scapuloperoneal myopathy

Cases of sporadic or dominantly inherited scapuloperoneal myopathy have been described by Ricker & Mertens (1968), Thomas et al (1975) and others. They differ from the X-linked cases in having a later onset in the second to the fifth decade, often with initial foot-drop. The progression is very slow and most patients continue to walk thoughout their lives. The serum CK activity is usually only slightly raised but occasionally is very high (Thomas et al 1975). The condition must be distinguished from the more frequent neurogenic scapuloperoneal syndrome, but this may be difficult in the presence of secondary myopathic change in the latter (Feigenbaum & Munsat 1970): indeed, proof, from examination of the spinal cord at autopsy, of the existence of an autosomal myopathic form has not yet been reported. The possibility that some recorded cases have· 'incomplete' or abortive forms of facioscapulohumeral muscular dystrophy is suggested by the large kindred reported by Kazakov et al (1976) in which facial weakness was a late and mild feature in many cases.

Recently Chakrabarti & Pearce (1981) have reported three sibs and their father with a scapuloperoneal myopathy and a pattern of early contractures and later severe heart block closely resembling that of the X-linked form (see p. 542). The onset of muscle symptoms occurred in the first two years of life. This appears to be yet another distinct variant in this complex group of disorders.

Proximal myopathies of late onset and dominant inheritance

Sporadic cases of 'menopausal' myopathy have been described for many years (Nevin 1936, Walton & Adams 1958, Corsi et al 1965). They may well be heterogeneous and their genetic status is obscure. Large pedigrees with autosomal dominant inheritance have been described by Schneiderman et al (1969), Bacon & Smith (1971) and de Coster et al (1974). Proximal lower-limb weakness predominated but affected the quadriceps particularly in the cases of Bacon & Smith

(1971) and relatively mildly in those of Schneiderman et al (1969). The myopathic changes on muscle biopsy were non-specific and deteriorated with increasing age (Bacon & Smith 1971). Serum enzyme activities were normal or slightly increased. The onset of symptoms was in the late teens or in the third decade and weakness progressed very slowly, walking being maintained until after the seventh decade in some cases. Early diagnosis for genetic counselling appears to depend wholly on careful clinical examination. In the kindred described by Schneiderman et al (1969) there was close genetic linkage with the Pelger–Huet anomaly of polymorphonuclear leucocyte nuclei. The 'Barnes type of muscular dystrophy' (Barnes 1932), a dominantly inherited condition of late onset with initial striking muscle hypertrophy, has recently been shown to be of neurogenic origin (D. Riddoch, personal communication 1974).

A type of muscular dystrophy with dominant inheritance, childhood onset, calf hypertrophy and a curious histological picture with capillary proliferation *within* muscle fibres was described by Hastings et al (1980) in a single family.

Distal myopathies with dominant inheritance

Distal myopathy was first described by Gowers in 1902; however, many observers now feel that the patient he described may have been suffering from myotonic dystrophy. In 1907 Spiller pointed out the distinction from 'Charcot–Marie–Tooth disease' or hereditary sensorimotor neuropathies (HSMN) in which confusion may still arise because secondary changes suggestive of myopathy may be seen in muscle biopsy specimens (Greenfield et al 1957, Tyrer & Sutherland 1961).

Initial involvement of peripheral limb muscles serves to distinguish these conditions from the scapulohumeral and scapuloperoneal muscular dystrophies, which they otherwise resemble; in the early stages the appearances in the limb are similar to those of HSMN type 1 but in the latter condition there is usually impairment of vibration sense in the extremities, and impaired nerve conduction. Some cases of mitochondrial myopathy with distal muscle weakness may resemble the juvenile form (Salmon et al 1971, Lapresle et al 1972) and electron microscopy of muscle may be required to distinguish them (Bautista et al 1978). The difficulty in distinguishing distal myopathy from distal chronic spinal muscular atrophy should not be underestimated (Summer et al 1971).

Adult form. Welander (1951, 1957) has had a wide experience of the distal form of muscular dystrophy, which in Sweden is inherited as a dominant character, begins usually between the age of 40 and 60 years, and affects both sexes, although it is commoner in men than in women. It usually begins in the small muscles of the hands and slowly spreads proximally; in the legs the anterior tibial muscles and the calves are affected first. The condition is comparatively benign, but proximal weakness occurs in a few more severe cases which are probably homozygous for the dominant gene (Welander 1957).

Welander's experience of over 250 cases is unique. In Great Britain and in the USA this form of the disease is rare; in Newcastle upon Tyne most of the few cases we have observed appeared to be sporadic and have probably had the newly described autosomal recessive form (see p. 547). In these patients the rate of progress of the disease was somewhat more rapid than in the Swedish cases, and most of them were severely disabled within 10–15 years of the onset, but the pattern of muscular involvement was similar to that described by Welander. The serum CK activity is as high as 20–100 times normal in sporadic cases but is normal or only slightly raised in cases where the onset is much later. Tomlinson et al (1974) described a non-Scandinavian dominantly inherited case with autopsy findings and Markesbery et al (1977) described the muscle pathology in one such patient.

We conclude that the firmly established Swedish form of dominantly inherited distal myopathy in which onset is in adult life is occasionally found in non-Swedish patients, but that most cases seen elsewhere are probably of the recessive or juvenile forms. Another relatively severe distal myopathy with dominant inheritance described by Edström et al (1980) differs clinically in the greater involvement of flexor than extensor muscles in the upper limbs and in being complicated by cardiomyopathy, and histologically in the

occurrence of sarcoplasmic bodies, intermediate-sized filaments and leptomeric fibrils in the muscle fibres.

Juvenile form. Biemond (1955) described a juvenile form of distal 'myopathy' which was subsequently found to be neurogenic in origin. Others (Ciani & Gherardi 1963, Magee & de Jong 1965, van der Does de Willebois et al 1968, Bautista et al 1978) have described similar families where the disease seemed more clearly myopathic, although some doubts remain. Like the late form, these early-onset cases are dominant in inheritance. Symptoms begin by the age of two years and progress slowly with eventual arrest. The serum CK activity is up to 20 times normal in some early cases but is normal in later life. Van der Does de Willebois et al (1968) published histochemical studies in which atrophy of the type I muscle fibres appeared to be a prominent feature.

Ocular myopathy or progressive external ophthalmoplegia

Involvement of the external ocular muscles is extremely unusual in any of the preceding types of muscular dystrophy, but may occur in myotonic dystrophy. Patients who developed ptosis followed by progressive limitation of ocular movements without significant diplopia were described by Hutchinson (1879) and Fuchs (1890) and were reviewed by Kiloh & Nevin (1951). Fuchs (1890), Sandifer (1946) and Kiloh & Nevin (1951) obtained eyelid muscle during corrective operations and interpreted the histology as showing myopathy. Kiloh & Nevin reviewed the literature on autopsied cases and were unconvinced by descriptions of mild changes in the oculomotor nuclei: they therefore concluded that progressive external ophthalmoplegia is a form of muscular dystrophy. Authors writing more recently agree that it is impossible to make a firm diagnosis of primary myopathy on the basis of external ocular muscle histology alone. Full autopsies showing normal brain stem nuclei and 'dystrophic' changes in ocular and limb muscles were reported by Schwartz & Liu (1954), Cogan et al (1962) and Ross (1963). Dominant inheritance has been described in a number of families. Ross (1963, 1964) found that some such patients were peculiarly sensitive to curare but did not improve with anticholinesterase drugs. Surgical correction of ptosis often relieves the only symptom.

The situation was for a long time confused until the delineation of the syndrome of progressive external ophthalmoplegia associated with clinical features of central nervous system involvement and retinal pigmentation (Erdbrink 1957, Walsh 1957, Kearns & Sayre 1958, Drachman 1968, Rosenberg et al 1968). This relationship between myopathic and central nervous system pathology in the 'Kearns–Sayre syndrome' was clarified by the discovery of widespread mitochondrial pathology in these cases (Olson et al 1972, Schneck et al 1973). Later, a partial deficiency of cytochrome oxidase function was identified in many cases of the Kearns–Sayre syndrome but the precise mitochondrial defect remains uncertain. This, and other mitochondrial disorders of the muscle and brain, are discussed further in Chapter 25.

It is now clear that a mitochondrial myopathy is also responsible for some, but not all, cases of uncomplicated progressive external ophthalmoplegia (Morgan-Hughes & Mair 1973, Danta et al 1975). Some other cases have associated spinal muscular atrophy (Rosenberg et al 1968, Aberfeld & Namba 1969) or peripheral neuropathy (Stephens et al 1958, Drachman 1968). The term 'ocular muscular dystrophy' is becoming increasingly unfashionable, but it remains the most accurate available description for some otherwise unexplained hereditary ocular myopathies.

Oculopharyngeal muscular dystrophy

Victor et al (1962) separated cases of ocular myopathy with dysphagia as a group to which they gave the name oculopharyngeal myopathy. Bray et al (1965) supported this subdivision and defined the other distinguishing features, of which the most valuable was the age of onset (mean 23 years for the ocular cases and 40 for the oculopharyngeal). Many of the reported cases have been of French-Canadian stock (Taylor 1915, Hayes et al 1963, Peterman et al 1964, Barbeau 1966, Murphy & Drachman 1968) but occasional cases, often sporadic, have occurred elsewhere. The inheritance in familial cases is dominant. Rebeiz et al (1969), Little & Perl (1982) and several other authors confirmed the primary myopathic nature of cases at autopsy but in the case studied by Schmitt & Krause (1981) there was also evidence of a peripheral neuropathy, possibly incidental. In this type of muscular dystrophy, as in ocular myopathy, muscle biopsy may reveal evidence of a mitochondrial myopathy (Morgan-Hughes & Mair 1973, Julien et al 1974) but more frequently the myopathic findings are less specific, including moth-eaten and whorled fibres, rimmed vacuoles and occasional atypical ragged-red fibres. A transient inflammatory response is sometimes seen (Bosch et al 1979).

Typically, the disorder starts with ptosis in the fourth to sixth decade and dysphagia a decade or so later: both progress slowly. The external ophthalmoplegia is evident on examination by the age of about 40–50 years but rarely causes symptoms. Mild weakness of the face, neck muscles and proximal limb muscles is commonly seen.

This disorder bears some resemblance to myotonic dystrophy, not only in some of the clinical and genetic features, but in the probable involvement of smooth muscle (Lewis 1966) and reports of gonadal atrophy (Lundberg 1962) and abnormalities of immunoglobulins (Russe et al 1967) in some families.

A closely similar syndrome with autosomal recessive inheritance and an earlier onset has been described by Fried et al (1975).

REFERENCES

Aberfeld D C, Namba T 1969 Progressive ophthalmoplegia in Kugelberg-Welander disease: report of a case. Archives of Neurology 20:253

Adornato B T, Kagen L J, Engel W K 1978 Myoglobinemia in Duchenne muscular dystrophy patients and carriers: a new adjunct to carrier detection. Lancet 2:499

Afifi A K, Zellweger H, McCormick W F, Mergner W 1969 Congenital muscular dystrophy: light and electron microscopic observations. Journal of Neurology, Neurosurgery and Psychiatry 32:273

Afifi A K, Bergman R A, Zellweger H 1973 A possible role for electron microscopy in detection of carriers of

Duchenne type muscular dystrophy. Journal of Neurology, Neurosurgery and Psychiatry 36:643

Aguilar L, Lisker R, Ramos G G 1978 Unusual inheritance of Becker type muscular dystrophy. Journal of Medical Genetics 15:116

Ahmad M, Sanderson J E, Dubowitz V, Hallidie-Smith K A 1978 Echocardiograph assessment of left ventricular function in Duchenne's muscular dystrophy. British Heart Journal 40:734

Allen J E , Rodgin D W 1960 Mental retardation in association with progressive muscular dystrophy. American Journal of Diseases of Childhood 100:208

Allsop K G , Ziter F A 1981 Loss of strength and functional decline in Duchenne's dystrophy. Archives of Neurology 38: 406–411

Aran F A 1850 Recherches sur une maladie non encore décrite du systeme musculaire (atrophie musculaire progressive). Archives générales de médecine 24:5

Archibald K C, Vignos P J 1959 A study of contractures in muscular dystrophy. Archives of Physical Medicine 40:150

Bacon P A, Smith B 1971 Familial muscular dystrophy of late onset. Journal of Neurology, Neurosurgery and Psychiatry 34:93

Bakker E, Goor N, Wrogemann K et al 1985 Prenatal diagnosis and carrier detection of Duchenne muscular dystrophy with closely linked RFLPs. Lancet 1: 655–658

Banker B Q, Victor M, Adams R D 1957 Arthrogryposis multiplex due to congenital muscular dystrophy. Brain 80:319

Baraitser M 1982 The genetics of neurological disorders. Oxford University Press, Oxford

Barbeau A 1966 The syndrome of hereditary late onset ptosis and dysphagia in French Canada. In: Kuhn E (ed) Progressive Muskeldystrophie, Myotonie, Myasthenie. Springer-Verlag, New York

Barnes S 1932 Report of a myopathic family with hypertrophic, pseudohypertrophic, atrophic and terminal (distal in the upper extremities) stages. Brain 55:1

Barwick D D, Osselton J W, Walton J N 1965 Electroencephalographic studies in hereditary myopathy. Journal of Neurology, Neurosurgery and Psychiatry 28:109

Batten F E 1903 Three cases of myopathy, infantile type. Brain 26:147

Batten F E 1909 The myopathies or muscular dystrophies; critical review. Quarterly Journal of Medicine 3:313

Bautista J, Rafel E, Castilla J M, Alberca R 1978 Hereditary distal myopathy with onset in early infancy. Journal of the Neurological Sciences 37:149

Becker P E 1953 Dystrophia Musculorum Progressiva. George Thieme, Stuttgart

Becker P E 1957 Neue Ergebnisse der Genetik der Muskeldystrophien. Acta Geneticae Medicae et Gemellologiae (Roma) 7:303

Becker P E 1962 Two new families of benign sex-linked recessive muscular dystrophy. Revue Canadienne de Biologie 21:551

Becker P E 1964 Myopathien. In: Becker P E (ed) Humangenetik: Ein kurzes Handbuch in funf Banden, Band 111/1. George Thieme, Stuttgart, p 411

Becker P E, Keiner F 1955 Eine neue X-chromosomale Muskeldystrophie. Archiv für Psychiatrie und Nervenkrankheiten 193:427

Beckmann R, Scheuerbrandt G 1976 Screening auf erhohte CK-Aktivitaten. Kinderarzt 7:1267

Begin R, Bureau M-A, Lupien L, Lemieux B 1980 Control of breathing in Duchenne's muscular dystrophy. American Journal of Medicine 69; 227–234

Bell J 1943 On pseudohypertrophic and allied types of progressive muscular dystrophy. In: Treasury of human inheritance, vol. IV, part IV. Cambridge University Press, London

Ben Hamida M, Fardeau M, Attia N 1983 Severe childhood muscular dystrophy affecting both sexes and frequent in Tunisia. Muscle and Nerve 6: 469–480

Berenbaum A A, Horowitz W 1956 Heart involvement in progressive muscular dystrophy. Report of a case with sudden death. American Heart Journal 51:622

Bethlem J, van Wijngaarden G K, de Jong J 1973 The incidence of lobulated fibres in the facioscapulohumeral type of muscular dystrophy and the limb-girdle syndrome. Journal of the Neurological Sciences 18: 351–358

Biemond A 1955 Myopathia distalis juvenilis hereditaria. Acta Psychiatrica et Neurologica Scandinavica 30:25

Blyth H, Pugh R J 1959 Muscular dystrophy in childhood. The genetic aspect. A field study in the Leeds region of clinical types and their inheritance. Annals of Human Genetics 33:127

Blyth H, Hughes B P 1971 Pregnancy and serum-C.P.K. levels in potential carriers of 'severe' X-linked muscular dystrophy. Lancet 1:855

Boba A 1970 Fatal postanesthetic complications in two muscular dystrophic patients. Journal of Pediatric Surgery 5:71

Boddie H G, Stewart-Wynne E G 1974 Quadriceps myopathy — entity or syndrome? Archives of Neurology 31:60

Bolthauser E, Steinmann B, Meyer A, Jerusalem F 1980 Anaesthesia-induced rhabdomyolysis in Duchenne muscular dystrophy. British Journal of Anaesthesia 52:559

Bosch E P, Gowans J D C, Munsat T 1979 Inflammatory myopathy in oculopharyngeal dystrophy. Muscle and Nerve 2: 73–77

Bossingham D H, Williams E, Nichols P J R 1979 Severe childhood neuromuscular disease: The management of Duchenne muscular dystrophy and spinal muscular atrophy. Muscular Dystrophy Group of Great Britain, London

Bouwsma G, van Wijngaarden G K 1980 Spinal muscular atrophy and hypertrophy of the calves. Journal of the Neurological Sciences 44: 275–279

Bradley W G 1979 The limb-girdle syndromes. In: Vinken P J, Bruyn G W (eds) Handbook of clinical neurology, vol 40. North Holland, Amsterdam, Ch 11

Bradley W G, Tomlinson B E, Hardy M 1978a Further studies of mitochondrial and lipid storage myopathies. Journal of the Neurological Sciences 35:201

Bradley W G, Jones M Z, Mussini J-M, Fawcett P R W 1978b Becker-type muscular dystrophy. Muscle and Nerve 1:111

Bramwell E 1922 Observations on myopathy. Proceedings of the Royal Society of Medicine 16:1

Bray G M, Kaarsoo M, Ross R T 1965 Ocular myopathy with dysphagia. Neurology (Minneapolis) 15:678

Brooke M H 1977 A clinician's view of neuromuscular diseases. Williams and Wilkins, Baltimore

Brooke M H, Griggs R C, Mendell J R, Fenichel G M, Shumate J B, Pellegrino R J 1981 Clinical trial in Duchenne dystrophy. 1. The design of the protocol. Muscle and Nerve 4: 186–197

Brooke M H, Fenichel G M, Griggs R C, Mendell J R,

Moxley R, Miller J P, Province M A and the CIDD Group 1983 Clinical investigation in Duchenne dystrophy: 2. Determination of the 'power' of therapeutic trials based on the natural history. Muscle and Nerve 6: 91–103

Brooks A P, Emery A E H 1977 The incidence of Duchenne muscular dystrophy in the south east of Scotland. Clinical Genetics 11:290

Brownell A K W, Paasuke R T, Elash A, Fowlow S B, Seagram C G F, Diewold R J, Friesen C 1983 Malignant hyperthermia in Duchenne muscular dystrophy. Anesthesiology 58: 180–182

Bulcke J A, Crolla D, Termote J-L, Baert A, Palmers Y, van den Bergh R 1981 Computed tomography of muscle. Muscle and Nerve 4: 67–72

Burke S S, Grove N M, Houser C R, Johnson D M 1971 Respiratory aspects of pseudohypertrophic muscular dystrophy. American Journal of Diseases of Childhood 121:230

Burn J, Povey S, Boyd Y, Munro E A, West L, Harper K, Thomas D 1986 Duchenne muscular dystrophy in one of monozygotic twin girls. Journal of Medical Genetics 23: 494–500

Canki N, Dutrillaux B, Tivadar I (1979) Dystrophie musculaire de Duchenne chez une petite fille porteuse d'une translocation t(X;3)(p21; q13) de novo. Annales de Génétique (Paris) 22: 35–39

Carroll J E, Brooke M H 1979 Infantile facioscapulohumeral dystrophy. In: Serratrice G, Roux H (eds) Peroneal atrophies and related disorders. Masson, New York

Caruso G, Buchthal F 1965 Refractory period of muscle and electromyographic findings in relatives of patients with muscular dystrophy. Brain 88:29

Chakrabarti A, Pearce J M S 1981 Scapuloperoneal syndrome with cardiomyopathy: report of a family with autosomal dominant inheritance. Journal of Neurology, Neurosurgery and Psychiatry 44: 1146–1152

Chung C S, Morton N E, Peters H A 1960 Serum enzymes and genetic carriers in muscular dystrophy. American Journal of Human Genetics 12:52

Ciani N, Gherardi F 1963 Due casi di myopathia distalis juvenilis hereditaria. Rivista di Neurologia 33:731

Cobham I G, Davis H S 1964 Anesthesia for muscular dystrophy patients. Anesthesia and Analgesia — Current Researches 43:22

Cogan D G, Kuwabara T, Richardson E P 1962 Pathology of abiotrophic ophthalmoplegia externa. Bulletin of the Johns Hopkins Hospital 111:42

Cohen H J, Molnar G E, Taft L T 1968 The genetic relationship of progressive muscular dystrophy (Duchenne type) and mental retardation. Developmental Medicine and Child Neurology 10:754

Copeland S A, Howard R C 1978 Thoracoscapular fusion for facioscapulohumeral dystrophy. Journal of Bone and Joint Surgery 60B:547

Corsi A, Gentili C, Todesco C V 1965 The relationship of menopausal muscular dystrophy to other diseases of muscle. A study of 17 cases. Journal of the Neurological Sciences 2:397

Cowan J, Macdessi J, Stark A, Morgan G 1980 Incidence of Duchenne muscular dystrophy in New South Wales and the Australian Capital Territory. Journal of Medical Genetics 17: 245–249

Crisp D E, Ziter F A, Bray P F 1982 Diagnostic delay in Duchenne's mucular dystrophy. Journal of the American Medical Association 247: 478–480

Danieli G A, Mostacciuolo M L, Bonfante A, Angelini C 1977 Duchenne muscular dystrophy: a population study. Human Genetics 35:225

Danilowicz D, Rutkowski M, Myung D, Schively D 1980 Echocardiography in Duchenne muscular dystrophy. Muscle and Nerve 3: 298–303

Danta G, Hilton R C, Lynch P G 1975 Chronic progressive ophthalmoplegia. Brain 98:473

Davie A M, Emery A E H 1978 Estimation of proportion of mutants among cases of Duchenne muscular dystrophy. Journal of Medical Genetics 15: 339–345

de Coster W, de Reuck J, Thiery E 1974 A late autosomal dominant form of limb-girdle muscular dystrophy: a clinical, genetic and morphological study. European Neurology 12: 159–172

de Lange C 1937 Studien uber angeborene Lahmugen bzw. angeborene Hypotonie. Acta Paediatrica 20, (Suppl III): 33

de Visser M 1983 Computed tomographic findings of the skeletal musculature in sporadic distal myopathy with early adult onset. Journal of the Neurological Sciences 59: 331–339

de Visser M, Verbeeten B 1985a Computed tomographic findings in manifesting carriers of Duchenne muscular dystrophy. Clinical Genetics 27: 269–275

de Visser M, Verbeeten B 1985b Computed tomography of the skeletal musculature in Becker-type muscular dystrophy and benign infantile spinal muscular atrophy. Muscle and Nerve 8: 435–444

Dellamonica C 1978 Etude de la réaction couplée, créatine-kinase/luciferase. Application au depistage systematique neonatal de la myopathie de Duchenne de Boulogne. Thesis for the Université Claude Bernard, Lyon

Dellamonica C, Robert J M, Cotte J, Collombel C, Dorche C 1978 Systematic neonatal screening for Duchenne muscular dystrophy. Lancet 2: 1100 (letter)

Dennis N R, Evans K, Clayton B, Carter C O 1976 Use of creatine kinase for detecting severe X-linked muscular dystrophy carriers. British Medical Journal 2:577

Dickey R P, Ziter F A, Smith R A 1984 Emery-Dreifuss muscular dystrophy. Journal of Pediatrics 104: 555–559

Donner M, Rapola J, Somer H 1975 Congenital muscular dystrophy: a clinicopathological and follow-up study of 15 patients. Neuropadiatrie 6:239

Drachman D A 1968 Ophthalmoplegia plus; the neurodegenerative disorders associated with progressive external ophthalmoplegia. Archives of Neurology 18:654

Drachman D B, Murphy S R, Nigam M P, Hills J R 1967 'Myopathic' changes in chronically denervated muscle. Archives of Neurology 16:14

Dreifuss F E, Hogan G R 1961 Survival in x-chromosomal muscular dystrophy. Neurology (Minneapolis) 11:734

Dreyfus J C, Schapira F, Demos J, Rosa R, Schapira G 1966 The value of serum enzyme determinations in the identification of dystrophic carriers. Annals of the New York Academy of Sciences 138:304

Drummond L M 1979 Creatine phosphokinase levels in the newborn and their use in screening for Duchenne muscular dystrophy. Archives of Disease in Childhood 54: 362–366

Dubowitz V 1963 Myopathic changes in muscular dystrophy carrier. Journal of Neurology, Neurosurgery and Psychiatry 26:322

Dubowitz V 1965 Intellectual impairment in muscular dystrophy. Archives of Disease in Childhood 40; 296

Dubowitz V 1978 Muscle disorders in childhood. Saunders, London

Dubowitz V 1985 Muscle biopsy: A practical approach, 2nd edn. Bailliere Tindall, London

Dubowitz V, Crome L 1969 The central nervous system in Duchenne muscular dystrophy. Brain 92:805

Dubowitz V, Brooke M H 1973 Muscle biopsy: A modern approach. Saunders, London

Duchenne G B 1862 Album de photographies pathologiques: complémentaire du livre intitulé D'Electrisation Localisée. Bailliere, Paris

Duchenne G B 1868 Recherches sur la paralysie musculaire pseudo-hypertrophique ou paralysie myosclerosique. Archives générales de médecine 11:5,178,305,421,552

Dunger D B, Pembrey M, Pearson P et al 1986 Deletion on the X chromosome detected by direct DNA analysis in one of two unrelated boys with glycerol kinase deficiency, adrenal hypoplasia, and Duchenne muscular dystrophy. Lancet 1: 585–587

Ebashi S, Sugita H 1978 The role of calcium in physiological and pathological processes of skeletal muscle. In: Abstracts of the IVth International Congress on Neuromuscular Diseases, Montreal

Echenne B, Pages M, Marty-Double C 1984 Congenital muscular dystrophy with cerebral white matter spongiosis. Brain and Development 6: 491–495

Edström L, Thornell L-E, Eriksson A 1980 A new type of hereditary distal myopathy with characteristic sarcoplasmic bodies and intermediate (skeletin) filaments. Journal of the Neurological Sciences 47: 171–190

Edwards R H T, Round J M, Jackson M J, Griffiths R D, Lilburn M F 1984 Weight reduction in boys with muscular dystrophy. Developmental Medicine and Child Neurology 26: 384–390

Edwards R J, Watts D C, Watts R L, Rodeck C H 1984 Creatine kinase estimation in pure fetal blood samples for the prenatal diagnosis of Duchenne muscular dystrophy. Prenatal Diagnosis 4: 267–277

Egger J, Kendall B E, Erdohazi M, Lake B D, Wilson J, Brett E M 1983 Involvement of the central nervous system in congenital muscular dystrophies. Developmental Medicine and Child Neurology 25: 32–42

Emanuel B S, Zackai E H, Tucker S H 1983 Further evidence for Xp21 location of Duchenne muscular dystrophy (DMD) locus: X; 9 translocation in a female with DMD. Journal of Medical Genetics 20: 461–463

Emery A E H 1963 Clinical manifestations in two carriers of Duchenne muscular dystrophy. Lancet 1:1126

Emery A E H 1964 Electrophoretic pattern of lactic dehydrogenase in carriers and patients with Duchenne muscular dystrophy. Nature 201:1044

Emery A E H 1965 Muscle histology in carriers of Duchenne muscular dystrophy. Journal of Medical Genetics 2:1

Emery A E H 1969 Abnormalities of the electrocardiogram in female carriers of Duchenne muscular dystrophy. British Medical Journal 2: 418

Emery A E H 1972 Abnormalities of the electrocardiogram in hereditary myopathies. Journal of Medical Genetics 9: 8–12

Emery A E H, Dreifuss F E 1966 Unusual type of benign X-linked muscular dystrophy. Journal of Neurology, Neurosurgery and Psychiatry 29:338

Emery A E H, Walton J N 1967 The genetics of muscular dystrophy. In: Steinberg A G, Bearn A G, (eds) Progress in medical genetics, Vol. V. Grune and Stratton, New York

Emery A E H, Morton R 1968 Genetic counselling in lethal X-linked disorders. Genetica et Statistica Medica (Basel) 18:534

Emery A E H, King B 1971 Pregnancy and serum-creatine-kinase levels in potential carriers of Duchenne X-linked muscular dystrophy. Lancet 1:1013

Emery A E H, Skinner R 1976 Clinical studies in benign (Becker type) X-linked muscular dystrophy. Clinical Genetics 10:189

Emery A E H, Holloway S 1977 Use of normal daughters' and sisters' creatine kinase levels in estimating heterozygosity in Duchenne muscular dystrophy. Human Heredity 27:118

Emery A E H, Skinner R, Holloway S 1979 A study of possible heterogeneity in Duchenne muscular dystrophy. Clinical Genetics 15: 444–449

Emery E S, Fenichel G M, Eng G 1968 A spinal muscular atrophy with scapuloperoneal distribution. Archives of Neurology 18:129

Erb W H 1884 Uber die 'juvenile form' der progressiven Muskelatrophie ihre beziehungen zur sogennanten Pseudohypertrophie der Muskeln. Deutsches Archiv für klinische Medizin 34:467

Erb W H 1891 Dystrophia muscularis progressiva: Klinische und pathologischanatomische Studien. Deutsche Zeitschrift für Nervenheilkunde 1:13

Erdbrink W L 1957 Ocular myopathy associated with retinitis pigmentosa. Archives of Ophthalmology 57:335

Espir M L E, Matthews W B 1973 Hereditary quadriceps myopathy. Journal of Neurology, Neurosurgery and Psychiatry 36: 1041

Feigenbaum J A, Munsat T L 1970 A neuromuscular syndrome of scapuloperoneal distribution. Bulletin of the Los Angeles Neurological Societies 35:47

Fenichel G M, Emery E S, Hunt P 1967 Neurogenic atrophy simulating facioscapulohumeral dystrophy: a dominant form. Archives of Neurology 17:257

Ferrier P, Bamatter F, Klein D 1965 Muscular dystrophy (Duchenne) in a girl with Turner's syndrome. Journal of Medical Genetics 2: 38

Fidzianska A, Goebel H H, Lenard H G, Heckmann C 1982 Congenital muscular dystrophy (CMD) — A collagen formative disease? Journal of the Neurological Sciences 55: 79–90

Firth M A 1983 Diagnosis of Duchenne muscular dystrophy: experiences of parents of sufferers. British Medical Journal 286: 700–701

Firth M A, Gardner-Medwin D, Hosking G, Wilkinson E 1983 Interviews with parents of boys suffering from Duchenne muscular dystrophy. Developmental Medicine and Child Neurology 25: 466–471

Fischbeck K H, Schotland D L 1983 Variability of X-linked muscular dystrophy. Annals of Neurology 13:217

Fowler M, Manson J I 1973 Congenital muscular dystrophy with malformation of the nervous system. In: Kakulas B A (ed) Clinical studies in myology. International Congress Series no. 295. Excerpta Medica, Amsterdam, p 192–197

Francke U, Ochs H D, de Martinville B et al 1985 Minor Xp21 chromosome deletion in a male associated with expression of Duchenne muscular dystrophy, chronic granulomatous disease, retinitis pigmentosa and McLeod syndrome. American Journal of Human Genetics 37: 250–267

Fried K, Arlozorov A, Spira R 1975 Autosomal recessive

oculopharyngeal muscular dystrophy. Journal of Medical Genetics 12:416

Fuchs E 1890 Ueber isolieren doppelseitige Ptosia. Archiv für Ophthalmologie 36:234

Fukuyama Y, Kawazura M, Haruna H 1960 A peculiar form of congenital progressive muscular dystrophy: report of fifteen cases. Paediatria Universitatis, Tokyo 4: 5–8

Fukuyama Y, Osawa M, Suzuki H 1981 Congenital progressive muscular dystrophy of the Fukuyama type: clinical, genetic and pathological considerations. Brain & Development 6: 373–390

Furukawa T, Peter J B 1977 X-linked muscular dystrophy. Fukuyama type congenital muscular dystrophy. Brain and development 6: 373–390

Furukawa T, Peter J B 1977 X-linked muscular dystrophy. Annals of Neurology 2: 414–416

Furukawa T, Toyokura Y 1977 Congenital hypotonic-sclerotic muscular dystrophy. Journal of Medical Genetics 14: 426–429

Gaines R F, Pueschel S M, Sassaman E A, Driscoll J L 1982 Effect of exercise on serum creatine kinase in carriers of Duchenne muscular dystrophy. Journal of Medical Genetics 19: 4–7

Gardner-Medwin D 1968 Studies of the carrier state in the Duchenne type of muscular dystrophy. 2. Quantitative electromyography as a method of carrier detection. Journal of Neurology, Neurosurgery and Psychiatry 31:124

Gardner-Medwin D 1970 Mutation rate in Duchenne type of muscular dystrophy. Journal of Medical Genetics 7:334

Gardner-Medwin D 1977 Objectives in the management of Duchenne muscular dystrophy. Israel Journal of Medical Sciences 13:229

Gardner-Medwin D 1978 Strategie per la prevenzione della distrofia muscolare di Duchenne. In: Distrofia Muscolare: alla ricerca di nuove frontiere. The Mario Negri Institute for Pharmacological Research and the Carlo Besta Neurological Institute, Milan, p 4–9

Gardner-Medwin D 1979a Controversies about Duchenne muscular dystrophy; (1) Neonatal screening. Developmental Medicine and Child Neurology 21:390

Gardner-Medwin D 1979b Controversies about Duchenne muscular dystrophy. (2) Bracing for ambulation. Developmental Medicine and Child Neurology 21: 659–662

Gardner-Medwin D 1982a The natural history of Duchenne muscular dystrophy. In: Wise G B, Blaw M E, Procopis P G (eds) Topics in child neurology, vol 2. SP Medical and Scientific Books, New York

Gardner-Medwin D 1982b Uncertainties in the diagnosis of Duchenne muscular dystrophy. Cardiomyology (Naples) 1: 15–20

Gardner-Medwin D, Pennington R J, Walton J N 1971 The detection of carriers of X-linked muscular dystrophy genes: A review of some methods studied in Newcastle upon Tyne. Journal of the Neurological Sciences 13:459

Gardner-Medwin D, Bundey S, Green S 1978 Early diagnosis of Duchenne muscular dystrophy. Lancet 1:1102 (letter)

Gardner-Medwin D, Johnston H M 1984 Severe muscular dystrophy in girls. Journal of the Neurological Sciences 64: 79–87

Genever E E 1971 Suxamethonium-induced cardiac arrest in unsuspected pseudohypertrophic muscular dystrophy. British Journal of Anaesthesia 43:984

Gibson D A, Koreska J, Robertson D, Kahn A, Albisser A M 1978 The management of spinal deformity in

Duchenne's muscular dystrophy. Orthopedic Clinics of North America 9: 437–450

Gilboa N, Swanson J R 1976 Serum creatine phosphokinase in normal newborns. Archives of Disease in Childhood 51:283

Goebel H H, Lennard H-G, Lagenbeck U, Mehl B 1980 A form of congenital muscular dystrophy, Brain and Development 2: 387–400

Goebel H H, Fidzianska S, Lennard H-G, Osse G, Hori A 1983 A morphological study of non-Japanese congenital muscular dystrophy associated with cerebral lesions. Brain and Development 5: 292–301

Golbus M S, Stephens J D, Mahoney M J, Hobbins J C, Haseltine F P, Caskey C T, Banker B Q 1979 Failure of fetal creatine phosphokinase as a diagnostic indicator of Duchenne muscular dystrophy. New England Journal of Medicine 300: 860–861

Goldberg S J, Feldman L, Reinecke C, Stern L Z, Sahn D J, Allen H D 1980 Echocardiographic determination of contraction and relaxation measurements of the left ventricular wall in normal subjects and muscular dystrophy. Circulation 62: 1061–1069

Gomez M R, Engel A G, Dewald G, Peterson H A 1977 Failure of inactivation of Duchenne dystrophy X-chromosome in one of female identical twins. Neurology (Minneapolis) 27:537

Gowers W R 1879 Pseudohypertrophic muscular paralysis. Churchill, London

Gowers W R 1902 A lecture on myopathy and a distal form. British Medical Journal 2:89

Greenfield J G, Shy G M, Alvord E C, Berg L 1957 An atlas of muscle pathology in neuromuscular diseases. Livingstone, Edinburgh

Greenfield J G, Cornman T, Shy G M 1958 The prognostic value of the muscle biopsy in the 'floppy infant'. Brain 81:461

Greenstein R M, Reardon M P, Chan T S 1977 An X/autosome translocation in a girl with Duchenne muscular dystrophy (DMD). Evidence for DMD gene localisation. Pediatric Research 11:457

Griggs R C, Mendell J R, Brooke M H et al, the CIDD group 1985 Clinical investigation in Duchenne dystrophy: V. Use of creatine kinase and pyruvate kinase in carrier detection. Muscle and Nerve 8: 60–67

Grimm T 1984 Genetic counselling in Becker type X-linked muscular dystrophy. II: practical considerations. American Journal of Medical Genetics 18:719–713

Gubbay S S, Walton J N, Pearce G W 1966 Clinical and pathological study of a case of congenital muscular dystrophy. Journal of Neurology, Neurosurgery and Psychiatry 29:500

Guggenheim M A, McCabe E R B, Roig M, Goodman S I, Lum G M, Bullen W W, Ringel S P 1980 Glycerol kinase deficiency with neuromuscular, skeletal, and adrenal abnormalities. Annals of Neurology 7: 441–449

Guibaud P, Carrier H N, Planchu H, Lauras B, Jolivet M J, Robert J M 1981 Manifestations musculaires précoces, cliniques et histopathologiques, chez 14 garçons présentant dans la première année une activité sérique élevée de creatine-phosphokinase. Journale de Génétique Humaine 29: 71–84

Gull W W 1862 Case of progressive atrophy of the muscles of the hands. Guy's Hospital Reports 8: 244–250

Hallen O 1970 Zur Frage der Kombination endokriner Symptome und Syndrome mit der Dystrophia musculorum progressiva. Deutsche Zeitschrift für Nervenheilkunde 197:101

Hanson P A, Rowland L P 1971 Möbius syndrome and facioscapulohumeral muscular dystrophy. Archives of Neurology 24:31

Hassan Z ul, Fastabend C P, Mohanty P K, Isaacs E R 1979 Atrioventricular block and supraventricular arrythmias with X-linked muscular dystrophy. Circulation 60: 1365–1369

Hastings B A, Groothuis D R, Vick N A 1980 Dominantly inherited pseudohypertrophic muscular dystrophy with internalized capillaries. Archives of Neurology 37: 709–714

Hausmanowa-Petrusewicz I, Prot J, Niebroj-Dobosz I et al 1968 Studies of healthy relatives of patients with Duchenne muscular dystrophy. Journal of the Neurological Sciences 7:645

Hayes R, London W, Seidman J, Embree L 1963 Oculopharyngeal muscular dystrophy. New England Journal of Medicine 268:163

Hazama R, Tsujihata M, Mori M, Mori K 1979 Muscular dystrophy in six young girls. Neurology 29: 1486–1491

Heckmatt J Z, Leeman S, Dubowitz V 1982 Ultrasound imaging in the diagnosis of muscle disease. Journal of Pediatrics 101: 656–660

Heckmatt J Z, Dubowitz V, Hyde S A, Florence J, Gabain A C, Thompson N 1985 Prolongation of walking in Duchenne muscular dystrophy with lightweight orthoses: review of 57 cases. Developmental Medicine and Child Neurology 27: 149–154

Henry A N, Neville B G R 1984 Gastrocnemius fasciotomy in Becker muscular dystrophy. Lancet 1: 1350–1351 (letter)

Henson T E, Muller J, De Myer W E 1967 Hereditary myopathy limited to females. Archives of Neurology 17:238

Herrmann F H, Spiegler A, Wiedemann G 1982 Muscle provocation test. A sensitive method for discrimination between carriers and noncarriers of Duchenne muscular dystrophy. Human Genetics 61: 102–103

Hertrich O 1957 Kasuistiche Mitteilung uber eine Sippe mit dominant vererblicher, wahrscheinlich weiblich geschlechtsbebundener progressiver Muskeldystrophie des Schultergurteltyps. Nervenarzt 28:325

Heyck H, Laudahn G, Carsten P M 1966 Enzymaktivitatsbestimmungen bei Dystrophia musculorum progressiva. IV Mitteilung. Klinische Wochenschrift 44:695

Hooshmand H, Dove J, Suter C 1969 The use of serum lactate dehydrogenase isoenzymes in the diagnosis of muscle diseases. Neurology (Minneapolis) 19:26

Hopkins L C, Jackson J A, Elsas L J 1981 Emery-Dreifuss humeroperoneal muscular dystrophy: An X-linked myopathy with unusual contractures and bradycardia. Annals of Neurology 10: 230–237

Howard R 1908 A case of congenital defect of the muscular system (dystrophia muscularis congenita) and its association with congenital talipes equinovarus. Proceedings of the Royal Society of Medicine (Pathological Section) 1: 157–166

Hsu J D, Garcia-Ariz M 1981 Fracture of the femur in the Duchenne muscular dystrophy patient. Journal of Pediatric Orthopedics 1: 203–207

Hudgson P, Pearce G W, Walton J N 1967 Preclinical muscular dystrophy: histopathological changes observed on muscle biopsy. Brain 90:565

Hudgson P, Bradley W G, Jenkison M 1972 Familial 'mitochondrial' myopathy: a myopathy associated with disordered oxidative metabolism in muscle fibres. Part 1. Clinical, electrophysiological and pathological findings. Journal of the Neurological Sciences 16:343

Hughes B P 1963 Serum enzyme studies with special reference to the Duchenne type dystrophy. In: Research in muscular dystrophy. Proceedings of the 2nd Symposium on Current Research in Muscular Dystrophy. Pitman, London, p 167

Hunsaker R H, Fulkerson P K, Barry F J, Lewis R P, Leier C V, Unverferth D V 1982 Cardiac function in Duchenne's muscular dystrophy: results of 10-year follow-up study and non-invasive tests. The American Journal of Medicine 73: 235–238

Hunter S 1980 The heart in muscular dystrophy. British Medical Bulletin 36: 133–134

Hutchinson J 1879 An ophthalmoplegia externa or symmetrical immobility (partial) of the eye with ptosis. Transactions of the Medico-Chirurgical Society of Edinburgh 62:307

Hutton E M, Thompson M W 1976 Carrier detection and genetic counselling in Duchenne muscular dystrophy: a follow-up study. Journal of the Canadian Medical Association 115:749

Inkley S R, Oldenburg F C, Vignos P J 1974 Pulmonary function in Duchenne muscular dystrophy related to stage of disease. The American Journal of Medicine 56:297

Ionasescu V, Zellweger H 1974 Duchenne muscular dystrophy in young girls? Acta Neurologica Scandinavica 50:619

Ionasescu V, Zellweger H, Burmeister L 1976 Detection of carriers and genetic counseling in Duchenne muscular dystrophy by ribosomal protein synthesis. Acta Neurologica Scandinavica 54:442

Ishikawa A 1982 Fukuyama-type congenital muscular dystrophy. Archives of Neurology 39:671

Jackson C E, Carey J H 1961 Progressive muscular dystrophy: autosomal recessive type. Pediatrics 28:77

Jackson C E, Strehler D A 1968 Limb girdle muscular dystrophy: clinical manifestations and detection of preclinical disease. Pediatrics 41:495

Jacobs P A, Hunt P A, Mayer M, Bart R D 1981 Duchenne muscular dystrophy (DMD) in a female with an X/autosome translocation: further evidence that the DMD locus is at Xp21. American Journal of Human Genetics 33: 513–518

Jalbert P, Mouriquand C, Beaudoing A, Jaillard M 1966 Myopathie progressive de type Duchenne et mosaique XO/XX/XXX: Considerations sur la génèse de la fibre musculaire striée. Annales de Génétique 9:104

James T N 1962 Observations on the cardiovascular involvement, including the cardiac conduction system, in progressive muscular dystrophy. American Heart Journal 63:48

Johnston E W, Reynolds T, Stauch D 1985 Duchenne muscular dystrophy: a case with prolonged survival. Archives of Physical Medicine and Rehabilitation 66: 260–261

Johnston H A 1964 Severe muscular dystrophy in girls. Journal of Medical Genetics 1:79

Jones D A, Round J M, Edwards R H T, Grindwood S R, Tofts P S 1983 Size and composition of the calf and quadriceps muscles in Duchenne muscular dystrophy: A tomographic and histochemical study. Journal of the Neurological Sciences 60: 307–322

Jones R, Khan R, Hughes S, Dubowitz V 1979 Congenital muscular dystrophy: the importance of early diagnosis and orthopaedic management in the long term prognosis. Journal of Bone and Joint Surgery 61B: 13–17

Julien J, Vital C, Vallat J M, le Blanc M 1974 Oculopharyngeal muscular dystrophy: A case with abnormal mitochondria and 'fingerprint' inclusions. Journal of the Neurological Sciences 21:165

Kaeser H E 1965 Scapuloperoneal muscular atrophy. Brain 88:407

Kakulas B A, Cullity P E, Maguire P 1975 Muscular dystrophy in young girls. Proceedings of the Australian Association of Neurologists 12:75

Kakulas B A, Hurse P V 1978 Twelve years of genetic counselling in muscular dystrophy in Western Australia. In Abstracts of the IVth International Congress of Neuromuscular Diseases, Montreal

Kamoshita S, Konishi Y, Segawa M, Fukuyama Y 1976 Congenital muscular dystrophy as a disease of the central nervous system. Archives of Neurology 33:513

Karagan N J, Richman L C, Sorensen J P 1980 Analysis of verbal disability in Duchenne muscular dystrophy. Journal of Nervous and Mental Diseases 168: 419–423

Karagan N J, Sorensen J P 1981 Intellectual functioning in non-Duchenne muscular dystrophy. Neurology (New York) 31: 448–452

Kazakov V M, Bogorodinsky D K, Znoyko Z V, Skorometz A A 1974 The facio-scapulo-limb (or the facioscapulohumeral) type of muscular dystrophy: clinical and genetic study of 200 cases. European Neurology 11:236

Kazakov V M, Bogorodinsky D K, Skorometz A A 1976 The myogenic scapuloperoneal syndrome. Muscular dystrophy in the K kindred: Clinical study and genetics. Clinical Genetics 10:41

Kearns T P, Sayre G P 1958 Retinitis pigmentosa, external ophthalmoplegia and complete heart block. Archives of Ophthalmology 60:280

Kelfer H M, Singer W D, Reynolds R N 1983 Malignant hyperthermia in a child with muscular dystrophy. Pediatrics 71: 118–119

Kiloh L G, Nevin S 1951 Progressive dystrophy of external ocular muscles (ocular myopathy). Brain 74:115

Kingston H M, Thomas N S T, Pearson P L, Sarfarazi M, Harper P S 1983 Genetic linkage between Becker muscular dystrophy and a polymorphic DNA sequence on the short arm of the X-chromosome. Journal of Medical Genetics 20: 255–258

Kingston H M, Sarfarazi M, Thomas N S T, Harper P S 1984 Localisation of the Becker muscular dystrophy gene on the short arm of the X chromosome by linkage to cloned DNA sequences. Human Genetics 67: 6–17

Kloepfer H W, Talley 1958 Autosomal recessive inheritance of Duchenne type muscular dystrophy. Annals of Human Genetics 22:138

Kohno K 1978 Mental retardation in Duchenne muscular dystrophy. In: Abstracts of the IVth International Congress on Neuromuscular Diseases, Montreal

Korf B R, Bresnan M J, Schapiro F, Sotrel A, Abroms I F 1985 Facioscapulohumeral dystrophy presenting in infancy with facial diplegia and sensorineural deafness. Annals of Neurology 17: 513–516

Kottke F J, Pauley D L, Ptak R A 1966 The rationale for prolonged stretching for correction of shortening of connective tissue. Archives of Physical Medicine 47:345

Kovick R B, Fogelman A M, Abbasi A S, Peter J P, Pearce M L 1975 Echocardiographic evaluation of posterior left ventricular wall motion in muscular dystrophy. Circulation. 52:447

Kozicka A, Prot J, Wasilewski R 1971 Mental retardation in patients with Duchenne progressive muscular dystrophy. Journal of the Neurological Sciences 14:209

Krijgsman J B, Barth P G, Stam F C, Slooff J L, Jaspar H H J 1980 Congenital muscular dystrophy and cerebral dysgenesis in a Dutch family. Neuropadiatrie 11: 108–120

Kugelberg E, Welander L 1956 Heredofamilial juvenile muscular atrophy simulating muscular dystrophy. Archives of Neurology and Psychiatry 75:500

Kurz L T, Mubarak S J, Schultz P, Park S M, Leach J 1983 Correlation of scoliosis and pulmonary function in Duchenne muscular dystrophy. Journal of Pediatric Orthopedics 3: 347–353

Lamy M, de Grouchy J 1954 L'hérédité de la myopathie (formes basses). Journal de Génétique Humaine 3:219

Landouzy L, Dejerine J 1884 De la myopathie atrophique progressive (myopathie héréditaire), débutant, dans l'enfance, par le face, sans alteration du système nerveux. Comptes Rendus Hebdomadaires des Séances de l'Academie des Sciences 98:53

Lane R J M, Gardner-Medwin D, Roses A D 1980 Electrocardiographic abnormalities in carriers of Duchenne muscular dystrophy. Neurology (Minneapolis) 30:497

Lapresle J M, Fardeau M, Godet-Guillain J 1972 Myopathie distale congénitale avec hypertrophie des mollets — Présence d'anomalies mitochondriales à la biopsie musculaire. Journal of the Neurological Sciences 17:87

Lazaro R P, Fenichel G M, Kilroy A W 1979 Congenital muscular dystrophy: case reports and reappraisal. Muscle and Nerve 2: 349–355

Lebenthal E, Shochet S B, Adam A et al 1970 Arthrogryposis multiplex congenita: Twenty-three cases in an Arab kindred. Pediatrics 46: 891–899

Leibowitz D, Dubowitz V 1981 Intellect and behaviour in Duchenne muscular dystrophy. Developmental Medicine and Child Neurology 23: 577–590

Levison H 1951 Dystrophia musculorum progressiva. Ejnar Munksgaards Forlag, Copenhagen

Lewis A J, Besant D F 1962 Muscular dystrophy in infancy: Report of 2 cases in siblings with diaphragmatic weakness. Journal of Pediatrics 60:376

Lewis I 1966 Late-onset muscular dystrophy: oculopharyngoesophageal variety. Canadian Medical Association Journal 95:146

Leyden E 1876 Klinik der Ruckenmarks-Krankheiten, vol. 2. Hirchwald, Berlin, p. 531

Lindenbaum R H, Clark G, Patel C, Moncrieff M, Hughes J T 1979 Muscular dystrophy in an X;1 translocation female suggests that Duchenne locus is on X chromosome short arm. Journal of Medical Genetics 16: 389–392

Lindgren V, de Martinville B, Horwich A L, Rosenberg L E, Francke U 1984 Human ornithine transcarbamylase locus mapped to band Xp21.1 near the Duchenne muscular dystrophy locus. Science 226:698–700

Lintner S P K, Thomas P R, Withington P S, Hall M G 1982 Suxamethonium associated hypertonicity and cardiac arrest in unsuspected pseudohypertrophic muscular dystrophy. British Journal of Anaesthesia 54: 1331–1332

Little B W, Perl D P 1982 Oculopharyngeal muscular dystrophy: An autopsied case from the French-Canadian kindred. Journal of the Neurological Sciences 53: 145–158

Lundberg P O 1962 Ocular myopathy with hypogonadism. Acta Neurologica Scandinavica 38:142

Mabry C C, Roeckel I E, Munich R L, Robertson D 1965 X-linked pseudohypertrophic muscular dystrophy with a late onset and slow progression. New England Journal of Medicine 273:1062

Magee K R, de Jong R N 1965 Hereditary distal myopathy with onset in infancy. Archives of Neurology 13:387

Mann O, de Leon A C, Perloff J K, Simanis J, Horrigan F D 1968 Duchenne's muscular dystrophy: the electrocardiogram in female relatives. American Journal of Medical Science 255:376

Manning G W, Cropp G J 1958 The electrocardiogram in progressive muscular dystrophy. British Heart Journal 20:410

Markand D N, North R R, D'Agostino A N, Daly D D 1969 Benign sex-linked muscular dystrophy. Clinical and pathological features. Neurology (Minneapolis) 19:612

Markesbery W R, Griggs R C, Leach R P, Lapham L W 1974 Late onset hereditary distal myopathy. Neurology (Minneapolis) 23:127

Markesbery W R, Griggs R C, Herr B 1977 Distal myopathy: electron microscopic and histochemical studies. Neurology (Minneapolis) 27: 727–735

Marsh G G, Munsat T L 1974 Evidence for early impairment of verbal intelligence in Duchenne muscular dystrophy. Archives of Disease in Childhood 49:118

Matsubara S, Tanabe H 1982 Hereditary distal myopathy with filamentous inclusions. Acta Neurologica Scandinavica 65: 363–368

Mawatari S, Katayama K 1973 Scapulohumeral muscular atrophy with cardiomyopathy: an X-linked recessive trait. Archives of Neurology 28:55

McComas A J, Sica R E P, Currie S 1971 An electrophysiological study of Duchenne dystrophy. Journal of Neurology, Neurosurgery and Psychiatry 34:461

McGarry J, Garg B, Silbert S 1983 Death in childhood due to facio-scapulo-humeral dystrophy. Acta Neurologica Scandinavica 68: 61–63

McKusick V A 1971 X-linked muscular dystrophy, benign form with contractures. Birth Defects VII, 2: 113–115

McMenamin J B, Becker L E, Murphy E G 1982a Fukuyama-type congenital muscular dystrophy. Journal of Pediatrics 101: 580–582

McMenamin J B, Becker L E, Murphy, E G 1982b Congenital muscular dystrophy: a clinicopathologic report of 24 cases. Journal of Pediatrics 100: 692–697

Mendell J R, Engel W K, Derrer E C 1971 Duchenne muscular dystrophy: functional ischemia reproduces its characteristic lesions. Science 172: 1143–1145

Meryon E 1852 On granular and fatty degeneration of the voluntary muscles. Medico-Chirurgical Transactions (London) 35:73

Meyerson M D, Lewis E, Ill K 1984 Facioscapulohumeral muscular dystrophy and accompanying hearing loss. Archives of Otolaryngology 110: 261–266

Milhorat A T, Goldstone L 1965 The carrier state in muscular dystrophy of the Duchenne type: identification by serum creatine kinase level. Journal of the American Medical Association 194:130

Milhorat A T, Shafiq S A & Goldstone L 1966 Changes in muscle structure in dystrophic patients, carriers and normal siblings seen by electron microscopy, correlation with levels of serum creatine phosphokinase (CPK). Annals of the New York Academy of Sciences 138:246

Miller E D, Sanders D B, Rowlingson J C, Berry F A, Sussman M D, Epstein R M 1978 Anesthesia-induced rhabdomyolysis in a patient with Duchenne's muscular dystrophy. Anesthesiology 48: 146–148

Miller G, Dunn N 1982 An outline of the management and prognosis of Duchenne muscular dystrophy in Western Australia. Australian Paediatric Journal 18: 277–282

Miller R G, Blank N K, Layzer R B 1979 Sporadic distal myopathy with early adult onset. Annals of Neurology 5: 220–227

Milne B, Rosales J K 1982 Anaesthetic considerations in patients with muscular dystrophy undergoing spinal fusion and Harrington rod insertion. Canadian Anaesthetic Society Journal 29: 250–253

Miyoshi K, Kawai H, Iwasa M, Kusaka K, Nishino H 1986 Autosomal recessive distal muscular dystrophy as a new type of progressive muscular dystrophy: Seventeen cases in eight families including an autopsied case. Brain 109: 31–54

Möbius P J 1879 Ueber die hereditaren nervenkrankheiten. Sammlung klinischer Vortage 171:1505

Mokri B, Engel A G 1975 Duchenne dystrophy: electron microscopic findings pointing to a basic or early abnormality in the plasma membrane of the muscle fibre. Neurology (Minneapolis) 25:1111

Monaco A P, Bertelson C J, Middlesworth W et al 1985 Detection of deletions spanning the Duchenne muscular dystrophy locus using a tightly linked DNA segment. Nature 316: 842–845

Monckton G, Hoskin V, Warren S 1982 Prevalence and incidence of muscular dystrophy in Alberta, Canada. Clinical Genetics 21: 19–24

Moosa A, Brown B H, Dubowitz V 1972 Quantitative electromyography: carrier detection in Duchenne type muscular dystrophy using a new automatic technique. Journal of Neurology, Neurosurgery and Psychiatry 35:841

Morgan-Hughes J A, Mair W G P 1973 Atypical muscle mitochondria in oculoskeletal myopathy. Brain 96:215

Morton N E, Chung C S 1959 Formal genetics of muscular dystrophy. American Journal of Human Genetics 11:360

Moser H 1984 Duchenne muscular dystrophy: pathogenetic aspects and genetic prevention. Human Genetics 66: 17–40

Moser H, Emery A E H 1974 The manifesting carrier in Duchenne muscular dystrophy. Clinical Genetics 5:271

Moser von H, Weismann U, Richterich R, Rossi E 1964 Progressive Muskeldystrophie. VI Haufigkeit, Klinik und Genetik der Duchenne form. Schweizerische Medizinische Wochenschrift 94: 1610–1621

Moser von H, Wiesmann U, Richterich R, Rossi E 1966 Progressive Muskeldystrophie. VIII Haufigkeit, Klinik und Genetik der Typen I und III. Schweizerische Medizinische Wochenschrift 96:169

Munsat T L, Piper D 1971 Genetically determined inflammatory myopathy with facioscapulohumeral distribution. Neurology (Minneapolis) 21:440

Murphy S F, Drachman D B 1968 The oculopharyngeal syndrome. Journal of the American Medical Association 203:1003

Murray J M, Davies K E, Harper P S, Meredith L, Mueller C R, Williamson R 1982 Linkage relationship of a cloned DNA sequence on the short arm of the X chromosome to Duchenne muscular dystrophy. Nature 300: 69–71

Nevin N C, Hughes A E, Calwell M, Lim J H K 1986 Duchenne muscular dystrophy in a female with a translocation involving Xp21. Journal of Medical Genetics 23: 171–187

Nevin S 1936 Two cases of muscular degeneration occurring in late adult life, with a review of the recorded cases of late progressive muscular dystrophy (late progressive myopathy). Quarterly Journal of Medicine 5:51

Nicholson G A, Gardner-Medwin D, Pennington R J T, Walton J N 1979 Carrier detection in Duchenne muscular dystrophy: assessment of the effect of age on detection-rate with serum-creatine-kinase-activity. Lancet 1:692

Nicholson L V B 1981 Serum myoglobin in muscular dystrophy and carrier detection. Journal of the Neurological Sciences 51: 411–426

Nigro G, Comi L I, Limongelli F M et al 1983 Prospective study of X-linked progressive muscular dystrophy in Campania. Muscle and Nerve 6: 253–262

Nihei K, Kamoshita S, Atsumi T 1979 A case of Ullrich's disease. Brain and Development 1: 61–67

Nogen A G 1980 Congenital muscle disease and abnormal findings on computerised tomography. Developmental Medicine and Child Neurology 22: 658–663

Nonaka I, Une Y, Ishihara T, Miyoshino S, Nakashima T, Sugita H 1981 A clinical and histological study of Ullrich's disease (congenital atonic-sclerotic muscular dystrophy). Neuropediatrics 12: 197–208

Nonaka I, Sugita H, Takada K, Kumagai K 1982 Muscle histochemistry in congenital muscular dystrophy with central nervous system involvement. Muscle and Nerve 5: 102–106

Nonaka I, Sunohara N, Satayoshi E, Terasawa K, Yonemoto K 1985 Autosomal recessive distal muscular dystrophy: a comparative study with distal myopathy with rimmed vacuole fomation. Annals of Neurology 17: 51–59

O'Brien M D 1962 An infantile muscular dystrophy: report of a case with autopsy findings. Guy's Hospital Reports 111:98

O'Brien T, Harper P S, Davies K E, Murray J M, Sarfarazi M, Williamson R 1983 Absence of genetic heterogeneity in Duchenne muscular dystrophy shown by a linkage study using two cloned DNA sequences. Journal of Medical Genetics 20: 249–251

Oka S, Igarashi Y, Takagi A, Nishida M, Sato K, Nakada K, Ikeda K 1982 Malignant hyperpyrexia and Duchenne muscular dystrophy: a case report. Canadian Anaesthetists' Society Journal 29: 627–629

Olson B J, Fenichel G M 1982 Progressive muscle disease in a young woman with family history of Duchenne's muscular dystrophy. Archives of Neurology 39: 378–380

Olson W, Engel W K, Walsh G O, Einaugler R 1972 Oculocraniosomatic neuromuscular disease with 'ragged-red' fibres: histochemical and ultrastructural changes in limb muscles of a group of patients with idiopathic progressive external ophthalmoplegia. Archives of Neurology 26:193

Oppenheim H 1900 Ueber allgemeine und localisierte atonie der muskulatur (myatonie) im fruhen kindesalter. Monatsschrift für Psychiatrie und Neurologie 8:232

Pearce G W, Pearce J M S, Walton J N 1966 The Duchenne type muscular dystrophy: histopathological studies of the carrier state. Brain 89:109

Pearce J M S, Pennington R J T, Walton J N 1964 Serum enzyme studies in muscle disease. III. Serum creatine kinase activity in relatives of patients with the Duchenne type of muscular dystrophy. Journal of Neurology, Neurosurgery and Psychiatry 27:181

Pearn J H, Hudgson P 1978 A new syndrome — spinal muscular atrophy with adolescent onset and hypertrophied calves, simulating Becker dystrophy. Lancet 1:1059

Pearson C M, Fowler W G 1963 Hereditary non-progressive muscular dystrophy inducing arthrogryposis syndrome. Brain 86:75

Pembrey M E, Davies K E, Winter R M, Elles R G, Williamson R, Fazzone T A, Walker C 1984 Clinical use of DNA markers linked to the gene for Duchenne muscular dystrophy. Archives of Disease in Childhood 59: 208–216

Penn A S, Lisak R P, Rowland L P 1970 Muscular dystrophy in young girls. Neurology (Minneapolis) 20:147

Percy M E, Andrews D F, Thompson M W 1982 Duchenne muscular dystrophy carrier detection using logistic discrimination: serum creatine kinase, hemopexin, pyruvate kinase, and lactate dehydrogenase in combination. American Journal of Medical Genetics 13: 27–38

Percy M E, Pichora G A, Chang L S, Manchester K E, Andrews D F 1984 Serum myoglobin in Duchenne muscular dystrophy carrier detection: A comparison with creatine kinase and hemopexin using logistic discrimination, American Journal of Medical Genetics 18: 279–287

Perloff J K, de Leon A C, O'Doherty D 1966 The cardiomyopathy of progressive muscular dystrophy. Circulation 33:625

Perloff J K, Roberts W C, de Leon A C, O'Doherty D 1967 The distinctive electrocardiogram of Duchenne's progressive muscular dystrophy. American Journal of Medicine 42:179

Peterman A F, Lillington G A, Jamplis R W 1964 Progressive muscular dystrophy with ptosis and dysphagia. Archives of Neurology 10:38

Peters A C B, Bots G T A M, Roos R A C, van Gelderen H H 1984 Fukuyama type congenital muscular dystrophy: two Dutch siblings. Brain and Development 6: 406–416

Philip U, Walton J N, Smith C A B 1956 Colour-blindness and the Duchenne-type muscular dystrophy. Annals of Human Genetics 21:155

Pickard N A, Gruemer H-D, Verrill H L et al 1978 Systemic membrane defect in the proximal muscular dystrophies. New England Journal of Medicine 299:841

Planchu H, Dellamonica C, Cotte J, Robert J M 1980 Duchenne muscular dystrophy: systematic neonatal screening and earlier detection of carriers. Journal de Génétique Humaine 28: 65–82

Prosser E J, Murphy E J, Thompson M W 1969 Intelligence and the gene for Duchenne muscular dystrophy. Archives of Disease in Childhood 44:221

Radu H, Migea S, Torok Z, Bordeianu L, Radu A 1968 Carrier detection in X-linked Duchenne type muscular dystrophy: a pluridimensional investigation. Journal of the Neurological Sciences 6:289

Rebeiz J J, Caulfield J B, Adams R D 1969 Oculopharyngeal dystrophy — a presenescent myopathy: a clinico-pathologic study. In: Progress in neuro-ophthalmology (International Congress Series No. 176). Excerpta Medica, Amsterdam, p 12

Reeves W C, Griggs R, Nanda N C, Thompson K, Gramiak R 1980 Echocardiographic evaluation of cardiac abnormalities in Duchenne's dystrophy and myotonic muscular dystrophy. Archives of Neurology 37: 273–277

Renier W O, Nabben F A E, Hustinx T W J et al 1983

Congenital adrenal hypoplasia, progressive muscular dystrophy, and severe mental retardation, in association with glycerol kinase deficiency, in male sibs. Clinical Genetics 24: 243–251

Ricker K, Mertens H-G 1968 The differential diagnosis of the myogenic (facio)-scapulo-peroneal syndrome. European Neurology 1:275

Ricker K, Mertens H-G, Schimrigk K 1968 The neurogenic scapuloperoneal syndrome. European Neurology 1:257

Rideau Y 1978 Outlines of Muscular Dystrophy. SREREM, Poitiers, France

Rideau Y, Jankowski L W, Grellet J 1981 Respiratory function in the muscular dystrophies. Muscle and Nerve 4: 155–164

Rideau Y, Glorion B, Delaubier A, Tarle O, Bach J 1984 The treatment of scoliosis in Duchenne muscular dystrophy. Muscle and Nerve 7: 281–286

Ringel S P, Carroll J E, Schold C 1977 The spectrum of mild X-linked recessive muscular dystrophy. Archives of Neurology 34:408

Robin G C 1977 Scoliosis in Duchenne muscular dystrophy. Israel Journal of Medical Sciences 13: 203–206

Robin G C, Brief L P 1971 Scoliosis in childhood muscular dystrophy. Journal of Bone and Joint Surgery 53A:466

Robin G C, Falewski de Leon G 1977 (eds) Symposium on Muscular Dystrophy. Israel Journal of Medical Sciences 13: 85–236

Rosenberg H, Heiman-Patterson T 1983 Duchenne's muscular dystrophy and malignant hyperthermia: Another warning. Anesthesiology 59:362

Rosenberg R N, Schotland D L, Lovelace R E, Rowland L P 1968 Progressive ophthalmoplegia: report of cases. Archives of Neurology 19:362

Rosman N P 1970 The cerebral defect and myopathy in Duchenne muscular dystrophy: a comparative clinico-pathological study. Neurology (Minneapolis) 20:329

Rosman N P, Kakulas B A 1966 Mental deficiency associated with muscular dystrophy. A neuropathological study. Brain 89:769

Ross R T 1963 Ocular myopathy sensitive to curare. Brain 86:67

Ross R T 1964 The effect of decamethonium on curare sensitive ocular myopathy. Neurology (Minneapolis) 14:684

Rothstein T L, Carlson C B , Sumi S M 1971 Polymyositis with facioscapulohumeral distribution. Archives of Neurology 25:313

Rott H-D, Rodl W, Santellani M, Nebel G 1984 Duchenne's muscular dystrophy: carrier detection by imaging techniques. Journal de Génétique Humaine 32: 287–290

Rotthauwe H-W, Kowalewski S 1965a Klinische und biochemische Untersuchungen bei Myopathien. 111. Mitteilung. Recessive x-chromosomale Muskeldystrophie mit relativ gutartigem Verlauf. Klinische Wochenschrift 43:158

Rotthauwe H-W, Kowalewski S 1965b Klinische und biochemische Untersuchungen bei Myopathien. 11 Mitteilung. Die Bedeutung der Serum-Kreatin-Phosphokinase und der Serum-Aldolase fur die Idendifizierung von Heterozygoten der recessive X-chromosomalen Formen der progressiven Muskel-dystrophie (Typ 111a und b). Klinische Wochenschrift 43: 150–158

Rotthauwe H-W, Mortier W, Beyer H 1972 Neuer Typ einer recessive X-chromosomal verebten

Muskeldystrophie: Scapulo-humero-distale Muskeldystrophie mit fruhzeitigen Kontrakturen und Herzrhythmusstorungen. Humangenetik 16:181

Rowland L P 1976 Pathogenesis of muscular dystrophies. Archives of Neurology 33:315

Rowland L P, Fetell M, Olarte M, Hays A, Singh N, Wanat F E 1979 Emery-Dreifuss muscular dystrophy. Annals of Neurology 5: 111–117

Roy L, Gibson D A 1970 Pseudohypertrophic muscular dystrophy and its surgical management: review of 30 patients. Canadian Journal of Surgery 13:13

Roy S, Dubowitz V 1970 Carrier detection in Duchenne muscular dystrophy: a comparative study of electron microscopy, light microscopy and serum enzymes. Journal of the Neurological Sciences 11:65

Russe H, Busey H, Barbeau A 1967 Immunoglobulin changes in oculopharyngeal muscular dystrophy. Proceedings of the 2nd International Congress ·of Neurogenetics, Montreal

Sage J, Inati Y, Samaha F 1979 The importance of serum pyruvate kinase in neuromuscular diseases and carrier states. Muscle and Nerve 2: 390–393

Salih M A M, Omer M I A, Bayoumi R A, Karrar O, Johnson M 1983 Severe autosomal recessive muscular dystrophy in an extended Sudanese kindred. Developmental Medicine and Child Neurology 25:43–52

Salih M A M, Ekmejian A, Omer M I A 1984 Respiratory insufficiency in a severe autosomal recessive form of muscular dystrophy. Annals of Tropical Paediatrics 4: 45–48

Salmon M A, Esiri M M, Ruderman N B 1971 Myopathic disorder associated with mitochondrial abnormalities, hyperglycaemia and hyperketonaemia. Lancet 2:290

Sandifer P H 1946 Chronic progressive ophthalmoplegia of myopathic origin. Journal of Neurology, Neurosurgery and Psychiatry 9:81

Santavuori P, Leisti J, Kruus S 1977 Muscle, eye and brain disease: a new syndrome. Neuropadiatrie 8 (suppl):553

Sanyal S K, Johnson W W, Dische M R, Pitner S E, Beard C 1980 Dystrophic degeneration of papillary muscle and ventricular myocardium: a basis for mitral valve prolapse in Duchenne's muscular dystrophy. Circulation 62: 430–438

Sanyal S K, Johnson W W 1982 Cardiac conduction abnormalities in children with Duchenne's muscular dystrophy. Circulation 66: 853–863

Scheuerbrandt G, Lundin A, Lovgren T, Mortier W 1986 Screening for Duchenne muscular dystrophy: an improved screening test for creatine kinase and its application in an infant screening program. Muscle and Nerve 9: 11–23

Schmitt H P, Krause K-H 1981 An autopsy study of a familial oculopharyngeal muscular dystrophy with distal spread and neurogenic involvement. Muscle and Nerve 4: 296–305

Schneck L, Adachi M, Briet P, Wolintz A, Volk B W 1973 Ophthalmoplegia plus with morphological and chemical studies of cerebellar and muscle tissue. Journal of the Neurological Sciences 19:37

Schneiderman L J, Sampson W I, Schoene W C, Haydon G B 1969 Genetic studies of a family with two unusual autosomal dominant conditions: muscular dystrophy and Pelger-Huet anomaly. American Journal of Medicine 46:380

Schott J, Jacobi M, Wald M A 1955 Electrocardiographic patterns in the differential diagnosis of progressive muscular dystrophy. American Jounal of Medical Science 229:517

Schwartz G A, Liu C-N 1954 Chronic progressive external ophthalmoplegia: a clinical and neuropathologic report. Archives of Neurology and Psychiatry 71:31

Scott O M, Hyde S A, Goddard C, Dubowitz V 1982 Quantitation of muscle function in children: a prospective study in Duchenne muscular dystrophy, Muscle and Nerve 5: 291–301

Seay A R, Ziter F A, Thompson J A 1978 Cardiac arrest during induction of anesthesia in Duchenne muscular dystrophy. Journal of Pediatrics 93: 88–90

Seeger B R, Sutherland A D'A, Clark M S 1984 Orthotic management of scoliosis in Duchenne muscular dystrophy. Archives of Physical Medicine and Rehabilitation 65: 83–86

Segawa M, Nomura Y, Hachimori K, Shinoyama N, Hosaka A, Mizuno Y 1979 Fukuyama type congenital muscular dystrophy as a natural model of childhood epilepsy. Brain and Development 2: 113–119

Seitz D 1957 Zur nosologischen Stellung des sogenannten scapulo-peronealen Syndroms. Deutsche Zeitschrift für Nervenheilkunde 175:547

Serratrice G, Cros D, Pellissier J-F, Gastaut J-L, Pouget J 1980 Dystrophie musculaire congénitale. Revue Neurologique (Paris) 136: 445–472

Shaw R F, Dreifuss F E 1969 Mild and severe forms of X-linked muscular dystrophy. Archives of Neurology 20:451

Shokeir M H K, Kobrinsky N L 1976 Autosomal recessive muscular dystrophy in Manitoba Hutterites. Clinical Genetics 9:197

Short J K 1963 Congenital muscular dystrophy: a case report with autopsy findings. Neurology (Minneapolis) 13:526

Siegel I M 1977 The clinical management of muscle disease. Heinemann, London

Siegel I M 1978 The management of muscular dystrophy: a clinical review. Muscle and Nerve 1: 453–460

Siegel I M 1982 Spinal stabilization in Duchenne muscular dystrophy: rationale and method. Muscle and Nerve 54: 417–418

Siegel I M, Miller J E, Ray R D 1968 Subcutaneous lower limb tenotomy in the treatment of pseudohypertrophic muscular dystrophy. Journal of Bone and Joint Surgery 50A:1437

Skinner R, Smith C, Emery A E H 1974 Linkage between the loci for benign (Becker type) X-borne muscular dystrophy and deutan colour blindness. Journal of Medical Genetics 11:317

Skinner R, Emery A E H, Anderson, A J B, Foxall C 1975 The detection of carriers of benign (Becker-type) X-linked muscular dystrophy. Journal of Medical Genetics 12:131

Skyring A, McKusick V A 1961 Clinical, genetic and electrocardiographic studies in childhood muscular dystrophy. American Journal of Medical Science 242:534

Slucka C 1968 The electrocardiogram in Duchenne progressive muscular dystrophy. Circulation 38:933

Small R G 1968 Coat's disease and muscular dystrophy. Transaction of the American Academy of Ophthalmology and Otolaryngology 72: 225–231

Smith H L, Amick L D, Johnson W W 1966 Detection of subclinical and carrier states in Duchenne muscular dystrophy. Journal of Pediatrics 69:676

Smith R, Stern G 1967 Myopathy, osteomalacia and hyperparathyroidism. Brain 90:593

Spencer G E, Vignos P J 1962 Bracing for ambulation in childhood progressive muscular dystrophy. Journal of Bone and Joint Surgery 44A:234

Spiller W G 1907 Myopathy of the distal type and its relation to the neural form of muscular atrophy (Charcot-Marie-Tooth type). Journal of Nervous and Mental Disease 34:14

Stephens J, Hoover M L, Denst J 1958 On familial ataxia, neural amyotrophy, and their association with progressive external ophthalmoplegia. Brain 81: 556–566

Stern L M 1972 Four cases of Duchenne-type muscular dystrophy in girls. Medical Journal of Australia 2: 1066–1069

Stern L M, Caudrey D J, Perrett L V, Boldt D W 1984 Progression of muscular dystrophy assessed by computed tomography. Developmental Medicine and Child Neurology 26: 569–573

Stevenson A C 1953 Muscular dystrophy in Northern Ireland. Annals of Eugenics 18:50

Stevenson A C 1955 Muscular dystrophy in Northern Ireland. An account of nine additional families. Annals of Human Genetics 19:159

Sugita H, Tyler F H 1963 Pathogenesis of muscular dystrophy. Transactions of the Association of American Physicians 76:231

Sumner D, Crawfurd M d'A, Harriman D G F 1971 Distal muscular dystrophy in an English family. Brain 94:51

Sussman M D 1984 Advantage of early spinal stabilization and fusion in patients with Duchenne muscular dystrophy. Journal of Pediatric Orthopedics 4: 532–537

Sussman M D 1985 Treatment of scoliosis in Duchenne muscular dystrophy. Developmental Medicine and Child Neurology 27: 522–524

Sutherland D H, Olshen R, Cooper L, Wyatt M, Leach J, Mubarak S, Schultz P 1981 Pathomechanics of gait in Duchenne muscular dystrophy. Developmental Medicine and Child Neurology 23: 3–22

Swank S M, Brown J C, Perry R E 1982 Spinal fusion in Duchenne's muscular dystrophy. Spine 7: 484–491

Swash M, Heathfield K W G 1983 Quadriceps myopathy: a variant of the limb-girdle syndrome. Journal of Neurology, Neurosurgery and Psychiatry 46: 355–357

Taddonio R F 1982 Segmental spinal instrumentation in the management of neuromuscular spinal deformity. Spine 7: 305–311

Takada K, Nakamura H, Tanaka J 1984 Cortical dysplasia in congenital muscular dystrophy with central nervous system involvement (Fukuyama type). Journal of Neuropathology and Experimental Neurology 43: 395–407

Takamoto K, Hirose K, Uono M, Nonaka I 1984 A genetic variant of Emery-Dreifuss disease. Archives of Neurology 41: 1292–1293

Taylor D A, Carroll J E, Smith M E, Johnson M O, Johnston G P, Brooke M H 1982 Facioscapulohumeral dystrophy associated with hearing loss and Coats syndrome. Annals of Neurology 12: 395–398

Taylor E W 1915 Progressive vagus-glossopharyngeal paralysis with ptosis. A contribution to the group of family diseases. Journal of Nervous and Mental Disease 42:129

Thomas P K, Calne D B, Elliott C F 1972 X-linked scapuloperoneal syndrome. Journal of Neurology, Neurosurgery and Psychiatry 35:208

Thomas P K, Schott G D, Morgan-Hughes J A 1975 Adult onset scapuloperoneal myopathy. Journal of Neurology, Neurosurgery and Psychiatry 38:1008

Thompson M W, Murphy E G, McAlpine P J 1967 An assessment of the creatine kinase test in the detection of carriers of Duchenne muscular dystrophy. Journal of Pediatrics 71:82

Tomlinson B E, Walton J N, Irving D 1974 Spinal cord limb motor neurones in muscular dystrophy. Journal of the Neurological Sciences 22: 305–327

Toulouse P, Coatrieux J L, LeMarec B 1985 An attempt to differentiate female relatives of Duchenne type dystrophy from healthy subjects using automatic EMG analysis. Journal of the Neurological Sciences 67: 45–55

Towfighi J, Sassani J W, Suzuki K, Ladda R L 1984 Cerebro-ocular dysplasia-muscular dystrophy (COD-MD) syndrome. Acta Neuropathologica (Berlin) 65: 110–123

Turner J W A 1940 The relationship between amyotonia congenita and congenital myopathy. Brain 63:163

Turner J W A, Heathfield K W G 1961 Quadriceps myopathy occurring in middle age. Journal of Neurology, Neurosurgery and Psychiatry 24:18

Turner J W A, Lees F 1962 Congenital myopathy — a fifty year follow up. Brain 85:733

Tyler F H, Wintrobe M M 1950 Studies in disorders of muscle. 1. The problem of progressive muscular dystrophy. Annals of Internal Medicine 32:72

Tyrer J H, Sutherland J M 1961 The primary spino-cerebellar atrophies and their associated defects, with a study of the foot deformity. Brain 84:289

Ullrich O 1930 Kongenitale, atonisch-sklerotische Muskeldystrophie. Mschr. Kinderheilk 47: 502–510

van den Bosch J 1963 Investigations of the carrier state in the Duchenne type dystrophy. Proceedings of the 2nd Symposium on Research in Muscular Dystrophy. Pitman, London, p 23

van der Does de Willebois A E M, Bethlem J, Meijer A E F H, Simons A J R 1968 Distal myopathy with onset in early infancy. Neurology (Minneapolis) 18:383

van Wijngaarden G K, Hagen C J, Bethlem J, Meijer A E F H 1968 Myopathy of the quadriceps muscles. Journal of the Neurological Sciences 7:201

Vasella F, Mumenthaler M, Rossi E, Moser H, Weismann U 1967 Die kongenitale Muskeldystrophie. Deutsch Z. Nervenheilk 190: 349–374

Verrellen C, Freund M, De Meyer R, Laterre C, Scholberg B, Frederic J 1977 Progressive muscular dystrophy of the Duchenne type in a young girl associated with an aberration of chromosome X. In: Littlefield J W (ed) 5th International Congress of Birth Defects, Montreal. Excerpta Medica, Amsterdam, p 42

Verellen-Dumoulin C, Freund M, De Meyer R et al 1984 Expression of an X-linked muscular dystrophy in a female due to translocation involving Xp21 and non-random inactivation of the normal X-chromosome. Human Genetics 67: 115–119

Victor M, Hayes R, Adams R D 1962 Oculopharyngeal muscular dystrophy. A familial disease of late life characterised by dysphagia and progressive ptosis of the eyelids. New England Journal of Medicine 267:1267

Vignos P J, Spencer G E, Archibald K C 1963 Management of progressive muscular dystrophy of childhood. Journal of the American Medical Association 184:89

Vignos P J, Watkins M P 1966 The effect of exercise in muscular dystrophy. Journal of the American Medical Association 197:843

Vignos P J, Wagner M B, Kaplan J S, Spencer G E 1983 Predicting the success of reambulation in patients with Duchenne muscular dystrophy. Journal of Bone and Joint Surgery 65A: 719–728

Wachsmuth A 1855 Ueber progressive Muskelatrophie. Zeitschrift für rationell Medizin 7:1

Wadia R S, Wadgaonkar S U, Amin R B, Sardesai H V 1976 An unusual family of benign 'X' linked muscular dystrophy with cardiac involvement. Journal of Medical Genetics 13:352

Wakayama Y, Bonilla E, Schotland D L 1983 Plasma membrane abnormalities in infants with Duchenne muscular dystrophy. Neurology (Cleveland) 33: 1368–1370

Walsh F B 1957 Clinical neuro-ophthalmology, 2nd edn. Balliere, Tindall and Cox, London

Walton J N 1955 On the inheritance of muscular dystrophy. Annals of Human Genetics 20:1

Walton J N 1956a The inheritance of muscular dystrophy: further observations. Annals of Human Genetics 21:40

Walton J N 1956b Two cases of myopathy limited to the quadriceps. Journal of Neurology and Psychiatry 19:160

Walton J N 1961 Muscular dystrophy and its relation to the other myopathies. Research Publications of the Association of Nervous and Mental Diseases 38:378

Walton J N 1962 Clinical aspects of human muscular dystrophy. In: Bourne G H, Golarz N (eds) Muscular dystrophy in man and animals. Karger, Basel

Walton J N, Nattrass F J 1954 On the classification, natural history and treatment of the myopathies. Brain 77:169

Walton J N, Warrick C K 1954 Osseous changes in myopathy. British Journal of Radiology 27:1

Walton J N, Adams R D 1958 Polymyositis. Livingstone,

Walton J N 1962 In: Bourne G H, Golarz N (eds) Muscular dystrophy in man and animals. Karger, Basel

Waters D D, Nutter D O, Hopkins L C, Dorney E R 1975 Cardiac features of an unusual X-linked humeroperoneal neuromuscular disease. New England Journal of Medicine 293:1017

Watters G, Karpati G, Kaplan B 1977 Post-anesthetic augmentation of muscle damage as a presenting sign in three patients with Duchenne muscular dystrophy. Canadian Journal of Neurological Sciences 4:228

Weimann R L, Gibson D A, Moseley C F, Jones D C 1983 Surgical stabilization of the spine in Duchenne muscular dystrophy. Spine 8: 776–780

Welander L 1951 Myopathia distalis tarda hereditaria. Acta Medica Scandinavica 264 (Suppl. 1)

Welander L 1957 Homozygous appearance of distal myopathy. Acta Geneticae Medicae et Gemellologiae 7:321

Wharton B A 1965 an unusual variety of muscular dystrophy. Lancet 1:603

Wiesmann U, Moser H, Richterich R, Rossi E 1965 Progressive Muskeldystrophie. VII. Die Erfassung von Heterozygoten der Duchenne-Muskeldystrophie durch Messung der Serum-Kreatin-Kinase unter lokalisierter Arbeitsbelastung in Anoxie. Klinische Wochenschrift 43:1015

Wilkins K E, Gibson D A 1976 The patterns of spinal deformity in Duchenne muscular dystrophy. Journal of Bone and Joint Surgery 58A:24

Williams E A, Read L, Ellis A, Morris P, Galasko C S B 1984 The management of equinus deformity in Duchenne muscular dystrophy. Journal of Bone and Joint Surgery 66B: 546–550

Williams H, Sarfarazi M, Brown C, Thomas N, Harper P S 1986 The use of flanking markers in prediction for

Duchenne muscular dystrophy. Archives of Disease in Childhood 61: 218–222

Williams W R, Thompson M W, Morton N E 1983 Complex segregation analysis and computer-assisted genetic risk assessment for Duchenne muscular dystrophy. American Journal of Medical Genetics 14: 315–333

Willison R G 1967 Quantitative electromyography: the detection of carriers of Duchenne dystrophy. Proceedings of the 2nd International Congress of Neurogenetics, Montreal

Wilson K M, Evans K A, Carter C O 1965 Creatine kinase levels in women who carry genes for three types of muscular dystrophy. British Medical Journal 1:750

Worden D K, Vignos P J 1962 Intellectual function in childhood progressive muscular dystrophy. Pediatrics 29:968

Worton R G, Duff C, Sylvester J E, Schmickel R D, Willard H F 1984 Duchenne muscular dystrophy involving translocation of the dmd gene next to ribosomal RNA genes. Science 224: 1447–1449

Wulff J D, Lin J T, Kepes J J 1982 Inflammatory facioscapulohumeral muscular dystrophy and Coats syndrome. Annals of Neurology 12: 398–401

Yamashita M, Matsuki A, Oyama T 1976 General anaesthesia for a patient with progressive muscular dystrophy. Anaesthetist 25:76

Yoshioka M 1981 Clinically manifesting carriers in Duchenne muscular dystrophy. Clinical Genetics 20: 6–12

Yoshioka M, Okuno T, Honda Y, Nakano Y 1980 Central nervous system involvement in progressive muscular dystrophy. Archives of Disease in Childhood 55: 589–594

Young A, Johnson D, O'Gorman E, McMillan T, Chase A P 1984 A new spinal brace for use in Duchenne muscular dystrophy. Developmental Medicine and Child Neurology 26: 808–813

Zatuchni J, Aegerter E E, Molthan L, Schuman C R 1951 The heart in progressive muscular dystrophy. Circulation 3:846

Zatz M 1983 Effects of genetic counselling on Duchenne muscular dystrophy families in Brazil. American Journal of Medical Genetics 15: 483–490

Zatz M, Itskan S B, Sanger R, Frota-Pessoa O, Saldanha P H 1974 New linkage data for the X-linked types of muscular dystrophy and G6PD variants, colour blindness and Xg blood groups. Journal of Medical Genetics 11:321

Zatz M, Otto P A 1980 The use of concomitant serum pyruvate-kinase and creatine-phosphokinase for carrier detection in Duchenne's muscular dystrophy through discriminant analysis. Journal of the Neurological Sciences 47: 411–417

Zatz M, Shapiro L J, Campion D S, Kaback M M, Otto P A 1980 Serum pyruvate-kinase and creatine-phosphokinase in female relatives and patients with X-linked muscular dystrophies (Duchenne and Becker). Journal of the Neurological Sciences 46: 267–279

Zatz M, Vianna-Morgante A M, Campos P, Diament A J 1981 Translocation (X;6) in a female with Duchenne muscular dystrophy: implications for the localisation of the DMD locus. Journal of Medical Genetics 18: 442–447

Zatz M, Passos M R, Bortolini E R 1983 Serum pyruvate-kinase activity during pregnancy in potential carriers for Duchenne muscular dystrophy. American Journal of Medical Genetics 15: 149–151

Zellweger H, Antonik A 1975 Newborn screening for Duchenne muscular dystrophy. Pediatrics 55:30

Zellweger H, Hanson J W 1967a Psychometric studies in muscular dystrophy type IIIa (Duchenne). Developmental Medicine and Child Neurology 9:576

Zellweger H, Hanson J W (1967b) Slowly progressive X-linked recessive muscular dystrophy (type IIIb). Archives of Internal Medicine 120:525

Zellweger H, Afifi A, McCormick W F, Mergner W 1967 Severe congenital muscular dystrophy. American Journal of Diseases of Childhood 114:591

Ziter F A, Allsop K G, Tyler F H 1977 Assessment of muscle strength in Duchenne muscular dystrophy. Neurology 27: 981–984

The myotonic disorders

INTRODUCTION

The myotonic disorders form a group of distinct genetic conditions, the unifying feature of which is myotonia. They vary considerably in their additional features and in the extent to which myotonia is the principal cause of symptoms; all follow clear Mendelian inheritance, but are likely to be determined by separate specific genes. At present we do not understand the primary defect in any of the group, nor can we always explain the aetiology of the myotonia in precise physiological terms. None the less, there is a considerable body of clinical, electrophysiological, biochemical and genetic information about the disorders and about the nature of myotonia as judged from experimental models, which should soon become integrated to give a fuller understanding of the various mechanisms of pathogenesis. This chapter will cncentrate on the clinical and genetic aspects; electrophysiology and histological studies are referred to briefly, but are discussed more fully in Chapters 5, 7, 8, 10 and 30.

MYOTONIA

Before describing the individual myotonic disorders, it is necessary to clarify what is meant by the term myotonia. At a clinical level it refers to the state of delayed relaxation of a muscle or group of muscles seen after voluntary contraction, or following a stimulus such as percussion. Symptomatically this state is usually perceived as 'stiffness', although an element of weakness may be noted. The muscle group involved will largely determine the nature of the complaint; stiffness of grip is the most frequent, while involvement of tongue and pharynx may produce speech disturbance.

As a physical sign, myotonia may be observed in response to a specific action (e.g. delay in relaxation after a firm grip) or in response to direct percussion of a muscle (e.g. the thenar eminence or the tongue). It should be noted that percussion should be firm and that the muscle itself, not a tendon, must be percussed.

At the electrophysiological level the characteristic feature of myotonia is the occurrence of repetitive action potentials after a stimulus, often in sequences of diminishing amplitude and sometimes of diminishing frequency which, when reproduced on a loudspeaker, give the so-called 'dive-bomber' effect. These potentials are absent when the muscle is at complete rest, in contrast to states of increased presynaptic activity; they are unaffected by curarisation, again demonstrating that myotonia is intrinsic to the muscle (Bryant 1973). Further details of experimental work on the nature of myotonia are given at the end of this chapter.

Myotonia has several other general features that help to distinguish it from other states of impaired relaxation. The first of these is 'warm-up', a term that refers to the diminution seen with continued exercise of the muscle group over a period of 5–30 min. This feature is often well recognised by patients, who use it to overcome disability produced by initial myotonia. In occasional patients with myotonia, and notably in the disorder paramyotonia, a paradoxical response is seen (Haynes & Thrush 1972), with myotonia aggravated by exercise.

Most patients with myotonia find their symptoms aggravated by cold, even though electrophysiological studies mostly show no change or even improvement. Again, paramyotonia shows a specific relationship to cold. A final aspect of myotonia often not fully appreciated is the weakness that may accompany the delayed relaxation; this can be assessed quantitatively (Rudel & Lehmann-Horn 1985) after the element of stiffness has been blocked by specific drugs and it may exist in the absence of any dystrophic changes in the muscles.

From the above outline it can be seen that the diagnosis of myotonia requires a specific electrophysiological state as well as specific clinical features. A number of other causes of muscle stiffness or impaired relaxation exist, some of which are listed in Table 16.1, and which require careful distinction from true myotonia because their aetiology is entirely different. Familial cramping syndromes are generally painful, while the contractures are electrically silent, as are those due to such metabolic causes as McArdle's disease. The reflex relaxation delay of hypothyroidism is distinguishable by absence of direct percussion myotonia, although occasional hypothyroid patients may also show true myotonia. Presynaptic disorders characteristically show persistent electrical activity when the muscle is resting, while the repetitive potentials sometimes seen in polymyositis and motor neurone disease are not associated with clinical features of myotonia.

MYOTONIC DYSTROPHY (DYSTROPHIA MYOTONIA; STEINERT'S DISEASE)

This is by far the commonest of the myotonic disorders with a prevalence of about 5 per 100 000 (Harper 1979, p. 228), at least ten times that of myotonia congenita; this high frequency, together with its remarkable variability, make it the most likely diagnosis whenever myotonia is encountered, even though the features may not appear typical. It is a disorder that frequently presents to clinicians other than the neurologist and the uncomplaining, even evasive attitude of some patients makes it important to have myotonic dystrophy in mind in a wide variety of clinical situations. For fuller accounts of this much-studied condition readers are referred to the monographs of Caughey & Myrianthopoulos (1963) and Harper (1979).

Table 16.1 Muscle stiffness mimicking myotonia

Metabolic contractures (e.g. McArdle syndrome)
Tetany
Familial cramp syndromes (various types)
Delayed reflex relaxation (e.g. hypothyroidism)
Presynaptic disorders (e.g. stiff man syndrome; myokymia)
Other disorders associated with atypical repetitive discharges (e.g. polymyositis; motor neurone disease)

Clinical features

Fig. 16.1 shows the relative frequency of the various presenting symptoms in the author's personal series of cases; Table 16.2 lists the principal neuromuscular features, which are often characteristic when sought, but which may not always be complained of, or even mentioned by the patient. *Myotonia* is usually not as severe as in the non-progressive myotonias such as myotonia congenita. It is often accepted as a nuisance rather than regarded as a symptom of illness; patients presenting in adult life may give a clear history of myotonia extending back for decades, even into childhood. The hands are most affected, although examination will usually show percussion myotonia elsewhere, in particular in the tongue. Generalised severe myotonia affecting gait, speech and eyelids is uncommon but may occur. Such patients can be extremely difficult to distinguish from those with myotonia congenita, but observation over a prolonged period, or study of relatives, usually clarifies matters.

Muscle weakness is the commonest symptom causing referral to the neurologist, but is extremely variable in both extent and in rate of progression. The complaint is often of general weakness and fatigue, but the distribution of weakness on examination is more specific. Both upper and lower limbs show predominantly distal weakness, in contrast to the proximal involvement seen in most other muscular dystrophies, while the anterior neck muscles, notably sternomastoids,

Table 16.2 Myotonic dystrophy — distribution of muscle involvement

Usual
 Ptosis
 Facial muscles
 Sternomastoids
 Foot dorsiflexors
 Distal forearm muscles

Frequent
 Small hand muscles
 Palate and pharynx
 Quadriceps
 Diaphragm and intercostals
 Tongue

show a selective involvement that may be extreme. Facial weakness is often marked (Fig. 16.2) and ptosis may be visible as a longstanding feature in photographs. Facial and jaw weakness together may produce dysarthria.

Onset and progression of muscle symptoms are highly variable, even if the congenital form of the disorder, considered below, is omitted. The typical 'adult' form of the disorder may develop at any age from late childhood onwards; usually progression is very slow, with marked loss of function recorded over decades rather than years; occasional patients, however, show a rapid deterioration and may become wheel-chair-bound. Since remissions are not a feature of myotonic dystrophy, the best guide to prognosis is the course over the preceding 5–10 years.

Patients with advanced disease may show additional neuromuscular problems. Diaphrag-

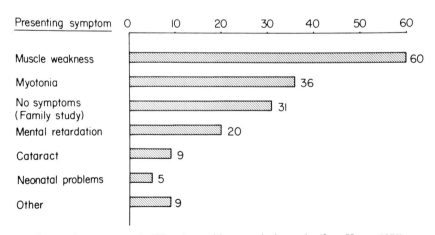

Fig. 16.1 Frequency of presenting symptoms in 170 patients with myotonic dystrophy (from Harper 1979)

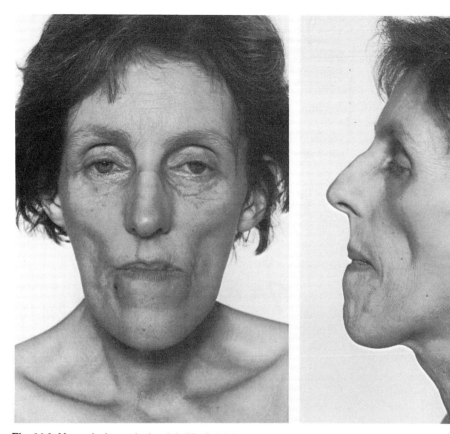

Fig. 16.2 Myotonic dystrophy in adult life: facial features, showing wasting of facial, jaw and sternomastoid muscles

matic involvement may lead to frequent chest infections, to hypoventilation (Benaim & Worster-Drought 1954, Coccagna et al 1975, Carroll et al 1977) and to aspiration of food or gastric contents. Foot drop may be conspicuous and can be helped by toe-springs or light splints. Neck weakness may become extreme and be associated with neck pain and headache, due to cervical osteoarthritis in some cases. Myotonia may diminish rather than increase in such severe cases.

Smooth and cardiac muscle involvement

Table 16.3 lists some of the problems that may result from this. Oesophageal function is frequently abnormal, as seen by barium studies and manometry (Bosma & Brodie 1969, Goldberg & Sheft 1972), but dysphagia is not a prominent symptom. Colonic problems are seen principally in childhood cases (Lenard et al 1977), where constipation,

'spastic colon' symptoms and even faecal soiling can be severe and refractory to treatment. Uterine involvement can lead to maternal complications at delivery (Shore 1975, Sarnat et al 1976), and should be anticipated in any patient who is pregnant or likely to become so.

Cardiac problems have been recognised for many years since the early studies of Evans (1944)

Table 16.3 Smooth muscle involvement in myotonic dystrophy

Pharynx and oesophagus	Delayed relaxation, dysphagia, aspiration
Gallbladder	Delayed emptying; frequent calculi
Colon	'Spastic colon' symptoms, megacolon
Uterus	Incoordinate contraction in labour
Ciliary body	Low intraocular pressure

and Church (1967). Conduction defects vary from asymptomatic first degree heart block to complex A–V dissociation, while tachyarrhythmias, of which atrial flutter is the commonest, may result in a cardiac referral at a time when the neuromuscular features are unrecognised (Cannon 1962, Holt & Lambert 1964). Most instances of sudden death in myotonic dystrophy are likely to occur in patients with at least some evidence of conduction problems (Harper 1979, p. 93); there is no increase in atheromatous heart disease (Orndahl et al 1964). The neurologist has a special responsibility to ensure that all patients have regular cardiac evaluation including electrocardiography (ECG), since this aspect of the disorder is both more lethal and more treatable than are the neuromuscular features.

The dangers associated with anaesthesia and surgery may appropriately be mentioned at this point, as most disasters are cardio-respiratory in nature. There appears to be a real sensitivity to anaesthetics and muscle relaxants in the sense that conventional doses produce prolonged apnoea and drowsiness (Kaufman 1960). Abdominal surgery, such as cholecystectomy and hysterectomy (Hook et al 1975) is more hazardous than such procedures as cataract extraction and orthopaedic measures. It should particularly be noted that it is not only patients with severe muscle disease who are at risk, but those with minimal symptoms, who may not mention their disorder to surgeon or anaesthetist. Again, the neurologist has a special responsibility to his patients and colleagues to ensure that the hazards are both recognised by the patient and noted prominently in the medical record.

Other clinical features (Table 16.4)

The most striking feature of many (but by no means all) myotonic dystrophy patients is a marked degree of apathy and inertia, resulting in much less symptomatic complaint than would seem reasonable for a given degree of weakness and myotonia, but also in a much less adequate level of function. This aspect is most commonly commented on by spouses and other relatives, and may be the deciding factor in determining whether a patient can continue work. Somnolence can be

Table 16.4 Myotonic dystrophy — extramuscular features

CNS	Lethargy, somnolence; mental retardation (children)
Peripheral nerve	Abnormalities in terminal arborisation (usually insignificant clinically)
Ophthalmic	Cataract, retinopathy, blepharitis
Endocrine	Testicular atrophy; complications of pregnancy and labour; diabetes; early balding

prominent, even in those with little involvement of respiratory muscles. All these features, along with the occurrence of mental retardation in the congenital form, indicate a degree of central nervous system involvement in the disorder, though the objective radiological and neuropathological changes are not striking. A thorough neuropsychiatric study has recently been carried out. Involvement of peripheral nerve is insignificant at a clinical level, but has been documented pathologically (Panayiotopoulos & Scarpalezos 1976); most of the changes involve the terminal arborisations (Coërs & Woolf 1959) and may be secondary to the myotonia; the same is probably true of the changes seen in muscle spindles (Swash 1972, Swash & Fox 1975).

Cataract has been recognised to be an integral part of myotonic dystrophy since the earliest descriptions (Fleischer 1918) and the disorder should be considered in any case of cataract in early adult life. In the older patients cataract may be the only symptomatic clinical problem, with only minimal myotonia to indicate the diagnosis. Such patients commonly remain undiagnosed until more typical myotonic dystrophy is recognised in another relative, and their prognosis for retaining normal muscle function is excellent. The results of cataract surgery are good, but some patients have an associated retinopathy that must be considered if visual acuity remains poor (Burian & Burns 1967). In its early stages the cataract of myotonic dystrophy is highly specific, with multi-coloured, refractile opacities visible in the anterior and posterior subcapsular regions when examined with a slit lamp (Vogt 1921, Junge 1966). The presence of such opacities is a valuable confirmatory sign in the doubtful case, as well as a useful predictive test in those at risk (Bundey et al 1970, Polgar et al 1972, Harper 1973). Full ophthalmic assessment, including slit lamp examination, is an essential part of the evaluation of all patients.

Endocrine abnormalities are frequent, but do not usually cause serious symptoms. Testicular atrophy is seen in most post-pubertal males (Marshall 1959); the atrophy affects the tubular structure more than the interstitial cells (Harper et al 1972a), and does not cause loss of secondary sexual function. Fertility is moderately reduced in both sexes, but there is a high fetal wastage in females (O'Brien & Harper 1984). Alterations in the pituitary fossa and occasional pituitary tumours may result from persistently increased gonadotrophin secretion (Banna et al 1973). Clinical diabetes is infrequent (Harper 1979, p. 126) but most patients show a consistent hyperinsulinism and insulin resistance, even at an early stage of their illness (Huff et al 1967, Barbosa et al 1974, Walsh et al 1970), a finding that has led to suggestions of a defect in insulin metabolism as a primary cause of the disease (see below).

Clinical investigations

Most cases of myotonic dystrophy can be diagnosed without the need for complex investigations; Table 16.5 shows those that are generally most helpful.

Serum creatine kinase activity is usually moderately elevated, but a normal level by no means excludes the presence of the disorder.

Electromyography should always be performed where there is doubt as to the diagnosis or where clinical myotonia is equivocal. Most patients will show typical myotonic discharges and increased insertion activity, together with a reduced size of

Table 16.5 Clinical investigations in myotonic dystrophy

Electromyography

Muscle biopsy

Ophthalmic assessment (cataract, retinopathy)

Electrocardiogram (conduction defects)

Serum creatine kinase activity

Glucose tolerance test

the action potential and polyphasic potentials, indicating an active dystrophic process. Absence of the latter may favour the diagnosis of a nonprogressive myotonia, but does not prove it. Nerve conduction velocities are normal. Muscle biopsy should be done whenever the diagnosis is not entirely certain. The changes, discussed more fully in Chapter 5, are often characteristic (Brooke & Engel 1969, Casanova & Jerusalem 1979), with increased central nuclei in chains, ringed fibres, sarcoplasmic masses and a type I fibre predominance, while on electron microscopy Z-band and I-line degeneration with abnormally shaped mitochondria are the most conspicuous features (Aleu & Afifi 1964, Schotland 1970).

Ophthalmic assessment for lens opacities has already been mentioned; blood glucose and glucose tolerance tests should be done to exclude incipient diabetes. The ECG will detect most conduction defects; fuller cardiac assessment is needed only if this is abnormal or if episodes of arrhythmia have occurred. Other investigations needed will depend on the presence of specific problems. Finally, a careful family study and documented pedigree should be regarded as an essential investigation: most apparently isolated cases prove not to be so on closer investigation, and it is the undiagnosed family members who may be most at risk, either of unexpected complications, or of having a severely affected child.

Congenital myotonic dystrophy (Vanier 1960, Dodge et al 1966, Dyken & Harper 1973, Harper 1975a, b)

Although the onset of typical myotonic dystrophy can frequently be traced back to childhood, the congenital form of the disorder is a clinically (and probably aetiologically) distinctive form that until recently has been considerably underdiagnosed; even now it is not recognised by many adult neurologists and general paediatricians, though with modern techniques such as neonatal intensive care and ventilation it is becoming recognised as one of the major neuromuscular causes of respiratory failure.

Some of the prominent features are listed in Table 16.6 and it will be noticed that many of these are quite unlike those normally seen in

Table 16.6 Congenital myotonic dystrophy — principal clinical features

Intrauterine
    Hydramnios
    Poor fetal movement

Neonatal
    Hypotonia (no significant myotonia)
    Respiratory failure
    Feeding problems
    Talipes (sometimes more general contractures)
    Disproportionate face and jaw weakness
    Thin ribs, elevated diaphragm on X-ray

Later
    Facial diplegia
    Jaw weakness
    Mental retardation

myotonic dystrophy of later life; conversely, myotonia is not seen as a clinical feature. Most of the symptoms can be traced back into intrauterine life: indeed, in a pregnancy at risk the disorder can often be predicted by the poor fetal movements and polyhydramnios. The hypotonia and immobility of the affected newborn infant may be profound; the lungs are hypoplastic (Silver et al 1984). Inadequate ventilation previously resulted in death for many without a specific diagnosis, but most now survive following resuscitation to allow the recognition that a generalised neuromuscular disorder is present.

Unless a family history of myotonic dystrophy has been recognised, it may be difficult to distinguish congenital myotonic dystrophy from other congenital myopathies or allied disorders. Helpful features include a disproportionate weakness of face and jaw (Fig. 16.3), the occurrence of a greatly raised and hypoplastic diaphragm on chest X-ray and at autopsy (Bossen et al 1974). (Thin ribs on X-ray result from hypoplastic intercostal muscles.) Talipes is frequent, but more general contractures sometimes occur. In most cases confirmation is obtained by the recognition of features of myotonic dystrophy in the mother, which are often mild and relatively symptomless. Careful electromyography may show a few myotonic potentials (Swift et al 1975), but this becomes conspicuous only after infancy. Muscle biopsy is helpful, not only in allowing other specific causes to be recognised, but also in showing unusual features of immature fibres

(Sarnat & Silbert 1976, Silver et al 1984), with central nuclei, abundant satellite cells and, on histochemical examination, a peripheral region lacking oxidative enzymes (Karpati et al 1973, Farkas et al 1974).

The outlook for severely affected congenital cases is poor with regard to both physical and mental function, and mental retardation is present in almost all survivors, even when anoxia has not been a major problem. Thus the undertaking of major measures of resuscitation or of corrective surgery in an infant recognised as being affected in the newborn period deserves careful consideration and discussion with the parents. Death is unusual once neonatal complications are overcome and once an active course is embarked on it is not easy to abandon.

The factors producing congenital myotonic dystrophy remain an enigma. The immediate cause is clearly a widespread and severe hypoplasia of muscle; the histology suggests that this results from immaturity rather than from degeneration (Sarnat & Silbert 1976). The exclusively maternal transmission of truly congenital cases suggests a maternal factor impeding muscle maturation (Harper & Dyken 1972), but it has not been identified. Suggestions of an abnormality in bile salts (Tanaka et al 1982) in mothers of affected infants or of hyperinsulinism as a causative factor have not been confirmed, nor has any clear immunological defect, such as that involved in congenital myasthenia gravis, been found. The fact that congenitally affected infants commonly improve in childhood, but later develop more typical 'adult' features, suggests that they possess the ordinary gene for the disorder as well as being exposed to the unknown maternal effect; this is confirmed by the finding that approximately half the sibs are unaffected (Harper 1975b), follow-up after a ten-year interval confirming that almost all such sibs are indeed free from the disorder (O'Brien et al 1983).

Genetic problems in myotonic dystrophy

The inheritance of myotonic dystrophy has been studied extensively in many surveys, yet a number of controversial features remain (Harper 1985). Recently the localisation of the gene has provided

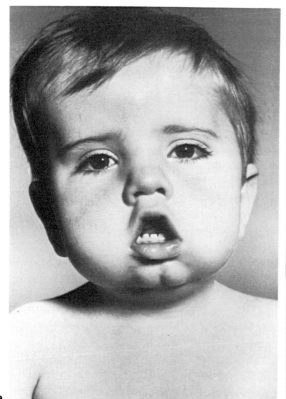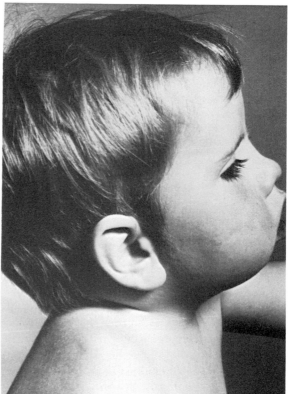

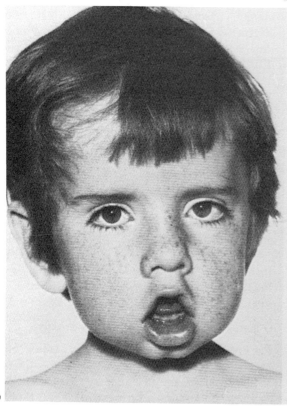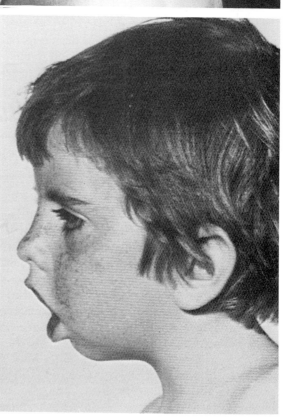

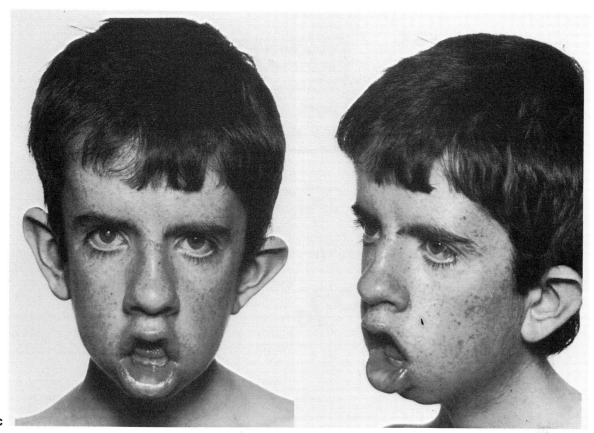

c

Fig. 16.3 Congenital myotonic dystrophy, showing the facial diplegia and the evolution of the facial appearance in the same patient.   a. age 2 years;   b. age 6 years;   c. age 15 years

an example of the power of modern molecular genetic techniques and is leading to practical applications in prediction (Harper et al 1985). It is quite possible that myotonic dystrophy will prove an example of the value of what has come to be known as 'reverse genetics' in which the key to understanding disordered function will come from isolation of the gene, rather than the converse (Weatherall 1985).

Table 16.7 summarises some of the most

Table 16.7 Myotonic dystrophy — genetic aspects

Autosomal dominant

Located on chromosome 19

Extreme variability within a family

Congenital cases maternally transmitted

New mutation extremely rare

important genetic features of myotonic dystrophy, the application of which should be integral to clinical practice. Inheritance is invariably autosomal dominant, so the offspring of an affected person of either sex have a 50% risk of inheriting the gene. Furthermore, almost all those with the gene manifest the disease to some extent (i.e. complete penetrance) although severity varies greatly. Very few cases result from new mutations, making careful testing of sibs (and often more distant relatives) essential, even if the case is apparently isolated. Finally, the occurrence of severe congenital myotonic dystrophy in the children of affected women makes it particularly important that all affected women in the reproductive age group should be fully aware of the risks.

Exclusion of the myotonic dystrophy gene is still less certain than is a positive diagnosis (Polgar et al 1972, Harper 1972, 1973). In the great majority of adult relatives who are normal on careful clinical examination, electromyography and slit-lamp examination of the cases prove to be unaffected, but occasionally individuals who appear to be entirely normal as judged by the results of all studies may show abnormalities on repeat investigation. Many ancillary tests have been advocated to detect such individuals, including insulin studies (Walsh et al 1970), altered immunoglobulins (Grove et al 1973), electroretinography (Burian & Burns 1967) and red blood cell membrane abnormalities (Roses & Appel 1973), but all are unreliable as predictive tests. Similarly, there is no evidence that muscle biopsy will detect gene carriers that are normal by other tests. The need for a test that is reliable at all ages and is independent of any variation in expression of the disorder has emphasised the importance of detection of the gene itself. The current situation (one that is changing rapidly) is outlined below.

Gene markers and myotonic dystrophy

The search for genetic markers in myotonic dystrophy is nothing new. Indeed the first major study of genetic linkage in man by Mohr (1954) showed a suggestion of linkage with the Lutheran blood group, in addition to firm linkage between this marker and the secretor locus. This suggestion was confirmed by later studies (Renwick et al 1971, Harper et al 1972b), and other markers were shown to be linked, including the Lewis blood group and the third component of complement (C_3). The demonstration that the fetus could be secretor typed using amniotic fluid raised the possibility of prenatal prediction (Harper et al 1971), but really useful clinical application was precluded by the relatively high error rate resulting from recombination, as well as by the occurrence of informative marker types in only a minority of those requiring prediction.

Until 1981 the chromosomal location of myotonic dystrophy was entirely unknown, but late in that year chromosome 19 was identified as the site by the localisation of C_3 to the chromosome (Whitehead et al 1982). Confirmation was provided by testing another known chromosome 19 marker, the enzyme peptidase D, in myotonic dystrophy families and finding it to be closely linked (O'Brien et al 1983b). Unfortunately, this marker is only rarely polymorphic and so can be used only in exceptional families.

Localising the disorder to a specific chromosome has allowed the techniques of recombinant DNA analysis (discussed more generally in Chapter 26) to be applied to myotonic dystrophy, with the result that a considerable number of DNA sequences have been localised to chromosome 19, some of which are proving to be useful markers for myotonic dystrophy (Harper et al 1985, Shaw et al 1986). Some of these are the DNA sequences for specific genes, such as those for apolipoproteins C_2 and E, the low-density-lipoprotein receptor and the receptors for insulin and poliovirus; others are DNA sequences of no known function, but showing inherited polymorphisms, which have been isolated from DNA sources enriched for chromosome 19. Table 16.8 shows some of these markers, while Fig. 16.4 shows an approximate gene map of chromosome 19.

Before these markers can be used clinically in the prediction of myotonic dystrophy, their closeness must be estimated by extensive family studies; one important finding of these has been that all except the closest show a much greater error rate from recombination when the female is the affected parent than for the male (Sherman et al 1985). This substantial difference is especially unfortunate because it is for the offspring of

Table 16.8 Genetic markers on chromosome 19 linked to myotonic dystrophy

Protein markers
    Lutheran blood group
    Lewis blood group
    Secretor locus
⋆ Peptidase D

Specific genes
⋆ Apolipoprotein C_2
    Complement C_3
    Low-density-lipoprotein receptor

Other cloned DNA sequences
    lJ2
    17–1
    Cos 1–13
    4–1

⋆Sufficiently close to allow clinical application

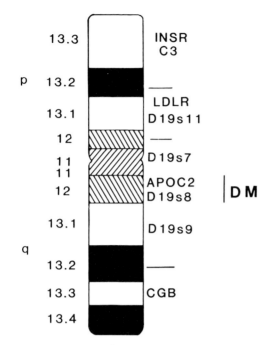

Fig. 16.4 Genetic map of chromosome 19, showing the provisional localisation of the myotonic dystrophy gene and linked markers (From Shaw et al 1986)

affected women, with the danger of severe congenital disease, that prenatal prediction is especially needed. At present the closest and most useful marker appears to be the ApoC2 gene probe (Shaw et al 1985), which on combined data seems to be at least 95% accurate in both sexes. Prenatal prediction is feasible in the first trimester of pregnancy using chorion villus biopsy; Fig. 16.5 shows this marker and examples of its use in carrier detection and prenatal diagnosis (Meredith et al 1986). Recently Roses et al (1986) have reported a further closely linked probe (LDR 152) that has so far shown no recombination with myotonic dystrophy and which may be closer than ApoC2; although not highly polymorphic, this should be a useful aid in diagnostic prediction.

Rapid increase in the number and accuracy of gene markers in myotonic dystrophy is now to be expected, so that a combination of closely linked DNA markers should soon provide reliable prediction and prenatal diagnosis for the disorder. This puts even greater responsibility on to those clinicians caring for patients to ensure that family members receive accurate genetic counselling and

are aware of the new developments and, in particular, that prenatal testing needs to be done in the first trimester. Equally important is that a sample of blood (or other tissue) should be taken for DNA isolation, especially in advanced cases or in severely and congenitally affected patients in whom death is imminent, because knowledge of the genotype of such cases may be critical in allowing prediction in relatives. There is currently no test that is specific for the disease and that can be used without also typing other family members.

Experimental studies in myotonic dystrophy

The literature on experimental work is considerable but so far largely inconclusive. Early work concentrated largely on abnormalities in skeletal muscle and on endocrine defects; subsequently lipid metabolism and disturbances in cell membrane structure and function were studied. As these studies have all given variable or negative results, or have reflected secondary changes, and have been fully reviewed previously (Caughey & Myrianthopoulos 1963, Harper 1979), they are not discussed here. The defect in insulin response has received much study (Moxley et al 1984); skeletal muscle shows a reduced response to insulin, but no decrease in insulin receptor numbers. Halliday et al (1985) also demonstrated reduced muscle protein anabolism, suggesting that the impaired insulin response may also be involved in muscle wasting. Further findings, both requiring independent confirmation, are those of increased calcium accumulation and efflux in both muscle and red blood cells (Plishker et al 1978), and the occurrence of receptor sites for the bee venom apomin, in myotonic dystrophy muscle (Renaud et al 1986). Despite the absence of a specific defect, abnormality of a protein component of the sarcolemmal muscle membrane and membranes of other cells still seems the most reasonable working hypothesis, and this is supported by the work on myotonia itself, discussed at the end of this chapter.

Currently, the most likely route to the elucidation of a specific defect lies through the genetic studies already outlined above. The localisation of the gene to a restricted area of chromosome 19 is

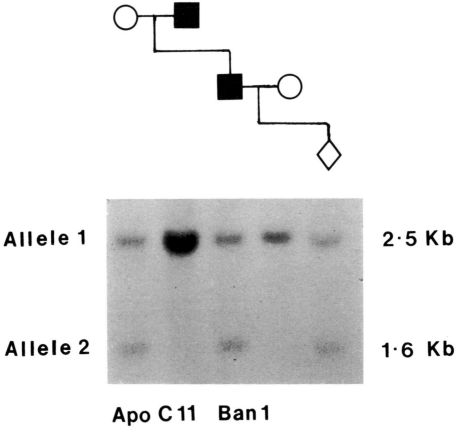

Fig. 16.5 The use of the ApoC2 gene probe in prenatal prediction. The fetus has inherited from the affected parent that marker allele received from the healthy grandparent and is predicted as normal in the absence of recombination (From Lunt et al 1986)

in itself a major advance, because one can immediately discard a gene or gene product not on this chromosome as being unrelated to the primary defect. Correspondingly, specific genes that are on chromosome 19 become of especial interest as 'candidate genes', and can be tested in detail. Thus the recognition that the insulin receptor is on chromosome 19 (Yang-Feng et al 1985), together with the known insulin abnormalities in myotonic dystrophy, made this an obvious possibility to test. It was rapidly ruled out by the finding that it was on a different part of the chromosome and that it showed recombination with myotonic dystrophy in family studies (Shaw et al 1986).

Now that close markers for the myotonic dystrophy gene exist, these can themselves be used to isolate the actual gene. New techniques such as pulsed-field electrophoresis, which allows separation of large, intact DNA sequences (Schwartz & Cantor 1984, Shaw 1986), should allow a detailed analysis of relevant sequences and provides an excellent chance of identifying the gene. A convergence of the DNA and protein approaches should soon be seen, and a detailed molecular analysis of the defect is likely to yield exciting results, perhaps comparable to those already emerging for the X-linked muscular dystrophies (Monaco et al 1985, 1986).

Management

A number of drugs can help to relieve myotonia, but none can alter the natural history of myotonic dystrophy or significantly alter its associated symptoms. Among the anti-myotonic drugs phenytoin is the best first choice, except for women considering pregnancy, in whom its teratogenic potential must be considered. A relatively low dose, such as 100 mg three times daily, is usually satisfactory. Other useful drugs include procainamide and quinine, but both have effects on cardiac conduction and should be avoided in those patients with clinical or ECG evidence of conduction disorder. Most physicians find that only a few of their patients, usually those with minimal weakness, continue to take drug therapy for their myotonia; in view of the chronicity of the disorder and the potential for iatrogenic drug effects they may be wiser than we think.

Until a drug of real value is found, the clinician should concentrate on educating his patients, and those other doctors whom they may encounter, about the disease, its potential implications, and the importance of avoiding complications from cardiac arrhythmias, anaesthesia and surgery — in other words, how to live with a disorder that is normally relatively benign and how to keep out of trouble. Such advice may seem obvious, but it is surprising how often it is not given, or not followed, even when the patient has been assessed in a specialist unit. Most clear indications for surgery, such as cataract extraction, or in children, correction of talipes, can be undertaken with care, but the patient should beware of minor surgery for trivial reasons or laparotomy for non-specific abdominal problems.

On the positive side, benefit can result from simple measures such as provision of head supports in the car or on a chair, with a cervical collar if headache of cervical origin is a problem. A thorough home assessment by a skilled occupational therapist will soon pinpoint which problems are actually hampering the patients' optimal function; a wheelchair commonly helps outdoor mobility, even though few patients become wheelchair-bound. Dietary advice can help those patients with dysphagia or with recurrent chest infection from aspiration. For the present these relatively simple measures, accompanied by the encouragement and support that all families with a chronically disabling disorder need, are the best we can offer, and are much better than the lack of long-term interest that they so often receive.

THE NON-PROGRESSIVE MYOTONIAS

This group of rare disorders, even when taken as a whole, is much less common than myotonic dystrophy; there is considerable heterogeneity within this group, recognised largely as a result of the work of Becker (1971, 1977); it is probable also that a significant number of cases remain unrecognised.

Myotonia congenita, dominant type
(Thomsen's disease)

This was the first of the myotonic disorders to be documented, the occurrence in his own family being recorded by Dr Julius Thomsen in 1876. Although it is extremely rare, its benign nature and dominant inheritance have resulted in a number of large kindreds being recognised, allowing a clear separation of the condition to be made from myotonic dystrophy, although some early cases of the latter without affected relatives can be difficult to distinguish. Myotonia is the principal feature; in contrast to myotonic dystrophy it is actively complained of and widespread, usually aggravated by cold and reduced by exercise. Eyelid myotonia is prominent; speech may be affected by tongue and jaw stiffness; on examination, myotonia is readily elicited by percussion of most muscle groups. Some patients show a generalised myotonic reaction to a sudden shock, with sudden rigidity resulting in falling, an occurrence that can be mistakenly attributed to a central nervous system cause.

Onset is commonly in mid-childhood; there is essentially a static course after puberty, although most patients adapt to their symptoms. Men are usually more severely affected than women. No significant or progressive weakness or wasting occurs: indeed, muscle hypertrophy is common, although less marked than in the recessive form discussed below. Lifespan is normal and there are no associated cardiac and extra-muscular problems. Histological changes in muscle are usually minimal (Fisher et al 1975), although absence of Group IIB fibres on staining for the myosin ATPase reaction has been noted (Crews et al 1976).

Myotonia congenita, recessive type

This disorder was recognised as distinct from Thomsen's disease only after Becker's study (1971, 1977), and was first reported in the English literature only 15 years ago (Harper & Johnston 1972). It is probably twice as common as the dominant form, but its recessive mode of inheritance means that it is seen usually only in sibs or isolated cases. Consanguinity of the healthy parents is frequent. Myotonia is more severe than in Thomsen's disease and may be disabling; some degree of progressive weakness may occur, while muscle hypertrophy can be striking. On muscle biopsy, degenerative changes can be found which might in isolation suggest early myotonic dystrophy, but the clinical features are too distinctive for confusion to occur. Myotonia in an infant is likely to be due to one of the forms of myotonia congenita, not to congenital myotonic dystrophy. Other distinct forms of myotonia may also exist, the best documented being that seen in several families in which myotonia congenita is associated with painful and electrically silent cramps (Sanders 1976).

Therapy for myotonia is effective and appreciated by the patient in both forms of myotonia congenita, in contrast with myotonic dystrophy, where few patients persist with it (Griggs 1977). The agents discussed for myotonic dystrophy are those also suitable for myotonia congenita, with phenytoin as first choice, except when there is a possibility of pregnancy.

Paramyotonia congenita (Becker 1970)

The distinguishing feature of this exceedingly rare condition, first described by Eulenberg in 1886, is the occurrence of prolonged cold-induced contracture of muscle, which may last for several minutes and may be followed by flaccid weakness in the affected area lasting for hours. More typical myotonic stiffness is also seen, but again differs from that in myotonia congenita in being exacerbated rather than relieved by exercise. Electromyography shows typical myotonic potentials but the prolonged cold-induced reaction is electrically silent (Haynes & Thrush 1972). Inheritance is autosomal dominant, the course is static, and there are no extramuscular features. Muscle biopsy shows variation in fibre diameter, lack of histochemical differentiation into type I and II fibres and some increase in central nuclei, but the extent of the changes seen has varied according to different reports (Thrush et al 1972).

The drug tocainide has been found to be effective and specific in blocking the cold-induced response of paramyotonia (Ricker et al 1980), but there have been recent reports of toxicity which suggest caution in its use, particularly as treatment would need to be life-long. The myotonia reponds to phenytoin or procainamide, but these drugs do not' block the cold-induced response. Efficient central heating and avoidance of outdoor occupations in cold climates are as helpful as drug treatment.

Myotonic periodic paralysis (Adynamia episodica (Gamstorp's disease)

Myotonia in this dominantly inherited disorder (Gamstorp 1956, Danowski et al 1975) is generally mild and often recorded only on electromyography. The feature that distinguishes it from other myotonic disorders is the occurrence of episodic flaccid weakness in attacks lasting up to several days, usually generalised and sometimes severe, but always sparing the respiratory, bulbar and ocular muscles. The weakness is not cold-induced or localised as in paramyotonia, nor are the episodes sudden as in the generalised myotonic reaction of myotonia congenita. Electrolyte changes are absent or inconsistent, distinguishing the otherwise similar hypokalaemic periodic paralysis. The disorder is essentially non-progressive, but patients with severe, repeated attacks may show some permanent weakness. The principal change seen on muscle biopsy is dilatation of the sarcoplasmic reticulum.

The most effective therapeutic agent is acetazolamide (Griggs 1977), which diminishes both the severity and the duration of the episodes of weakness, and is more effective than chlorothiazide and other diuretics.

Chondrodystrophic myotonia (Schwartz–Jampel syndrome)

This unusual disorder, which is recessively inherited, is characterised by the onset in infancy of severe muscle stiffness, giving blepharospasm, painful generalised muscle spasms and feeding difficulty (Schwartz & Jampel 1962, Fitch et al 1971). With increasing age the facial appearance becomes pinched and the voice weak, while muscle hypertrophy may occur. The skeletal features consist of delayed bone growth, particularly involving vertebrae, together with joint contractures; the X-ray appearances of the spine are similar to those seen in Morquio's syndrome.

Electromyography shows both characteristic myotonia and also continuous electrical activity of presynaptic origin (Fowler et al 1974). The latter persists during anaesthesia and may be related to the diffuse distribution of acetylcholinesterase over the muscle fibres, which is seen on histochemical investigation (Fowler et al 1974). There are few other histological changes in muscle. Treatment with benzodiazepam and related drugs is more effective than with anti-myotonic agents.

Other causes of myotonia

Apart from the effects of the experimental agents discussed below (some originally used in therapy), myotonia is uncommon as a complication of drug treatment. Propranolol has been recorded as unmasking myotonia in early myotonic dystrophy (Blessing & Walsh 1977), but the extent of use of beta-blocking drugs makes it unlikely that this is a significant problem. Hypothyroidism may cause generalised muscle stiffness associated with delayed muscle relaxation and with repetitive potentials on electromyography, but the discharges differ in nature from those of typical myotonia. Similarly, while myotonia has been recorded in association with a bronchial neoplasm, this is exceptional and may also reflect presynaptic effects. Most of the causes of muscle stiffness likely to cause clinical confusion with the myotonic disorders can be distinguished electrophysiologically, as indicated by Table 16.1 earlier in this chapter.

EXPERIMENTAL APPROACHES TO MYOTONIA

Quite apart from investigations of the various individual myotonic disorders, there is a large body of experimental work on the nature of myotonia itself and its relationship to the disease states. Detailed accounts of the earlier work are given by Bryant (1973, 1977), while more recent evidence is discussed by Rudel & Lehmann-Horn (1985) and Rudel (1986). The broad conclusion to emerge from this work so far is that myotonia may be associated with more than one form of electrophysiological defect, that the type of defect may vary between the different myotonic disorders, and that a number of different molecular defects will eventually be found to be responsible, key functions of the muscle membrane being the most likely sites for these defects.

A focus of many studies has been the animal model provided by the myotonic goat (Bryant 1973), which shows an inherited disorder closely resembling the dominant (Thomsen) form of human myotonia congenita. The muscle fibre membrane shows an increased resistance due to decreased chloride ion conduction, the resting membrane potential being normal (Bryant 1969). Exactly the same findings are seen in isolated muscle fibres in human myotonia congenita (Lipicky & Bryant 1971). Possible causes for the abnormality include a decreased number of chloride channels, alteration in their properties or blockage by some substance (Bryant 1982). The first of these suggestions currently seems most likely, but should be testable when the structure of the molecules involved has been elucidated.

A separate line of evidence bearing on the mechanisms of myotonia comes from chemical agents inducing myotonia. The two principal groups are the aromatic monocarboxylic acids (Bryant & Morales-Aguilera 1971) such as (2, 4-dichlorophenoxy) acetic acid (2, 4-D) and the hypocholesterolaemic agents such as 20, 25-diazacholesterol (Winer et al 1965). Both groups produce a reduced chloride conductance comparable to that of the myotonic goat or Thomsen's disease, but their mechanisms differ. The first group appears closer in action to the natural disorders, with a similar 'warm up' phenomenon, patterns of action potentials and antagonism by drugs such as tocainide (Dengler & Rudel 1979). The second group acts by gradual replacement of cholesterol by desmosterol in the sarcolemma (Peter & Campion 1977) so that the abnormality cannot be rapidly reversed. The occurrence of cataract with some hypocholesterolaemic drugs and an initial report of raised desmosterol levels in myotonic dystrophy (Wakamatsu et al 1972) suggested a possible causal relationship with this disorder, but other workers have found no desmosterol increase, while the enzyme involved in cholesterol–desmosterol conversion is on a different chromosome from that for myotonic dystrophy (Croce et al 1973).

The nature of the myotonia in myotonic dystrophy appears, in fact, to differ from that in myotonia congenita (both dominant and recessive), as well as from that in the myotonic goat and in drug-induced myotonia; there has also been much less consistency in the results of different studies. Most work has shown a reduced resting membrane potential with increased sodium conductance (Gruener 1977, Hofmann & DeNardo 1968), but other studies have shown contrary findings (Lipicky 1977, Lipicky & Bryant 1973). Changes in chloride conductance have been inconsistent. One reason for this variability could be the damage to fibres by the dystrophic process; at present the precise primary defect producing the myotonia is no clearer than the overall primary defect in the disorder.

Two further points currently under study that could bear on the nature of the myotonia in myotonic dystrophy are the increased insulin sensitivity seen in skeletal muscle and the demonstration of reduced protein synthesis in the muscle of affected patients, both mentioned earlier.

The use of cultured muscle cells provides one means of investigating some of these discrepancies, but again results in myotonic dystrophy are contradictory, with one study finding a reduced resting potential (Merickel et al 1981), and the other obtaining normal results (Tahmoush et al 1983). Similarly, studies of membrane ATPases have been highly variable and are probably normal, while the various studies on red blood cell and muscle membrane structural proteins (Roses & Appel 1973) have again not produced any generally accepted or consistent abnormality. Clearer results have emerged from biochemical studies of sarcolemmal membrane in myotonia congenita, where a markedly abnormal pattern of fatty acids has been found in the dominant form, but not in the recessive, suggesting a structural defect of the membrane in the former (Kühn & Seiler (1970). In paramyotonia a different, but equally striking, abnormality of fatty acid distribution was found (Fiehn et al 1974), but few patients have been studied so far.

From this brief account of our current knowledge of myotonia and its relationship to the various myotonic disorders, it is clear that our knowledge remains fragmentary. The fact that all the major disorders are Mendelian in nature, however, and that in the case of myotonic dystrophy we are close to identifying the abnormal gene, gives good reason to hope that hypotheses based on clinical, electrophysiological and biochemical studies will soon become testable at the molecular level, in terms both of specific components of the muscle membrane and of specific DNA sequences from the appropriate regions. Only when such a convergence becomes a reality is it likely that we will develop a complete understanding of the myotonic disorders.

REFERENCES

Aleu F P, Afifi A K 1964 Ultrastructure of muscle in myotonic dystrophy. Preliminary observations. American Journal of Pathology 45: 221–223

Banna M, Bradley W G, Pearce G W 1973 Massive pituitary adenoma in a patient with dystrophia myotonica. Journal of the Neurological Sciences 20: 1–6

Barbosa J, Nuttall F Q, Kennedy W, Geotz F 1974 Plasma insulin in patients with myotonic dystrophy and their relatives. Medicine 53: 307–323

Becker P E 1970 Paramyotonia congenita (Eulenberg). Thieme, Stuttgart

Becker P E 1971 Genetic approaches to the nosology of muscle disease. Myotonias and similar disorders. In: Birth defects, original article series 7: 52–62

Becker P E 1977 Myotonia congenita and syndromes associated with myotonia. Thieme, Stuttgart

Benaim S, Worster-Drought C 1954 Dystrophia myotonica with myotonia of the diaphragm causing pulmonary hypoventilation with anoxaemia and secondary polycythaemia. Medicine Illustrated 8: 221–226

Blessing W, Walsh J C 1977 Myotonia precipitated by propranolol therapy. Lancet 1: 73–74

Bosma J F, Brodie D R 1969 Cineradiographic demonstration of pharyngeal area myotonia in myotonic dystrophy patients. Radiology 92: 104–109

Bossen E H, Sehlburne J D, Verkauf B S 1974 Respiratory muscle involvement in infantile myotonic dystrophy. Archives of Pathology 97: 250–252

Brooke M H, Engel W K 1969 The histographic analysis of human muscle biopsies with regard to fiber types. 3. Myotonias, myasthenia gravis and hypokalemic periodic paralysis. Neurology 19: 469–477

Bryant S H 1969 Cable properties of external intercostal muscle fibres from myotonic and nonmyotonic goats. Journal of Physiology (London) 204: 539–550

Bryant S H 1973 The electrophysiology of myotonia, with a review of congenital myotonia of goat. In: Desmedt J E (ed) New developments in electromyography and clinical neurophysiology, vol. 1. Karger, Basel, p 420–450

Bryant S H 1977 The physiological basis of myotonia. In: Rowland L P (ed) Pathogenesis of human muscular dystrophies. Excerpta Medica, Amsterdam, p 715–728

Bryant S H 1982 Physical basis of myotonia. In: Schotland D L (ed), Disorders of the motor unit. Wiley, New York, p 381–389

Bryant S H, Morales-Aguilera A 1971 Chloride conductance in normal and myotonic muscle fibres and the action of monocarboxylic aromatic acids. Journal of Physiology (London) 219: 361–383

Bundy S, Carter C O, Soothill J F 1970 Early recognition of heterozygotes for the gene for dystrophia myotonica. Journal of Neurology, Neurosurgery and Psychiatry 33: 279–293

Burian H M, Burns C A 1967 Ocular changes in myotonic dystrophy. American Journal of Ophthalmology 63: 22–34

Cannon P J 1962 The heart and lungs in myotonic dystrophy. American Journal of Medicine 32: 765–755

Carroll J E, Zwillich C W, Weil J V 1977 Ventilatory response in myotonic dystrophy. Neurology 27: 1125–1128

Casanova G, Jerusalem F 1979 Myopathology of myotonic dystrophy. A morphometric study. Acta Neuropathologica (Berlin) 45: 231–240

Caughey J E, Myrianthopoulos N C 1963 Dystrophia myotonica and related disorders. C Thomas, Springfield

Church S C 1967 The heart in myotonica atrophica. Archives of Internal Medicine 119: 176–181

Coccagna G, Mantouant M, Parch C, Miron F, Lugares E 1975 Alveolar hypoventilation and hypersomnia in myotonic dystrophy. Journal of Neurology, Neurosurgery and Psychiatry 38: 977–984

Coërs C, Woolf A L 1959 The innervation of muscle. Oxford

Crews J, Kaiser K K, Brooke M H 1976 Muscle pathology of myotonia congenita. Journal of the Neurological Sciences 28: 449–457

Croce C M, Kieba I, Kropowski H, Molion M, Rothblat G M 1973 Restoration of the conversion of desmosterol to cholesterol in L-cells after hybridization with human fibroblasts. Proceedings of the National Academy of Sciences USA 71: 110–113

Danowski T S, Fisher E R, Vidalon C, Vester J W, Thompson R, Nolans S T, Sunder J H 1975 Clinical and ultrastructural observations in a kindred with normal hyperkalaemic periodic paralysis. Journal of Medical Genetics 12 20–28

Dengler R, Rudel R 1979 Effects of tocainide on normal and myotonic mammalian skeletal muscle. Drug Research 29: 270–273

Dodge P R, Gamstorp I, Byers R K, Russell P 1966 Myotonic dystrophy in infancy and childhood. Paediatrics 35: 3–19

Dyken P R, Harper P S 1973 Congenital dystrophia myotonica. Neurology (Minneapolis) 23: 465–473

Eulenburg A 1886 Uber eine familiare, durch 6 generationen

verfolgbare form congenitaler paramyotonie. Neurol. Centralbl. 5:265

Evans W 1944 The heart in myotonia atrophica. British Heart Journal 4: 41–47

Farkas E, Tomé F M S, Fardeau M, Arsenionunes M L, Dreyfuss P, Doebler M F 1974 Histochemical and ultrastructual study of muscle biopsy in three cases of dystrophia myotonica in the newborn child. Journal of the Neurological Sciences 21: 273–288

Fiehn W, Peter J B, Seiler D, Kuhn E 1974 Abnormalities of the sarcolemma in myopathies. In: Hausmanowa-Petrusewicz I, H Jedrejowska (eds). Structure and function of normal and diseased muscle and peripheral nerve. Polish Medicine, Warsaw, p 205–209

Fisher E R, Danowski T S, Ahmad U et al 1975 Electron microscopical study of a family with myotonia congenita. Archives of Neurology 99: 607–610

Fitch N, Karpati G, Pinsky L 1971 Congenital blepharophimosis, joint contractures and muscular hypotonia. Neurology (Minneapolis) 21: 1214–1220

Fleischer B 1918 Uber myotonischer dystrophie mit katarakt. Albrecht von Graefes' Archives of Ophthalmology 96: 91–133

Fowler W M, Layzer R B, Taylor R G et al 1974 The Schwartz–Jampel syndrome. Its clinical, physiological and histological expression. Journal of the Neurological Sciences 22: 127–146

Gamstorp I 1956 Adynamia episodica hereditaria. Acta Pediatrica (Uppsala) 45 (Suppl 108): 1–126

Goldberg H I, Sheft D J 1972 Oesophageal and colon changes in myotonia dystrophica. Gastroenterology 63: 134–139

Griggs R C 1977 The myotonic disorders and the periodic paralyses. In: Griggs R C, Moxley R T (eds) Advances in neurology, vol. 17. Raven Press, New York, p 143–159

Grove D I, O'Callaghan S J, Burston T O, Forbes I J 1973 Immunological function in dystrophia myotonica. British Medical Journal 3: 81–83

Gruener R 1977 In vitro membrane excitability of diseases of human muscle In: Rowland L P (ed) Pathogenesis of human muscular dystrophy. Excerpta Medica, Amsterdam, p 242–258

Halliday D, Ford G C, Edwards R H T, Rennie M J, Griggs R C 1985 In vivo estimation of muscle protein synthesis in myotonic dystrophy. Annals of Neurology 17: 65–69

Harper P S 1972 Genetic studies in myotonic dystrophy. Thesis for degree of D. M., University of Oxford

Harper P S 1973 Presymptomatic detection and genetic counselling in myotonic dystrophy. Clinical Genetics 4: 134–140

Harper P S 1975a Congenital myotonic dystrophy in Britain. I. Clinical aspects. Archives of Disease in Childhood 50: 505–513

Harper P S 1975b Congenital myotonic dystrophy in Britain. II. Genetic basis. Archives of Disease in Childhood 50:514

Harper P S 1979 Myotonic dystrophy 2nd edn. W. B. Saunders, Philadelphia (in press)

Harper P S 1985 Myotonic dystrophy and related disorders. In: Emery A E H, Rimoin D (eds) Principles and practice of medical genetics. Churchill Livingstone, Edinburgh

Harper P S, Bias W B, Hutchinson J R, McKusick V A 1971 ABH secretor status of the foetus: a genetic marker identifiable by amniocentesis. Journal of Medical Genetics 8: 438–440

Harper P S, Dyken P R 1972 Early onset dystrophia

myotonia — evidence supporting a maternal environmental factor. Lancet 2: 53–55

Harper P S, Johnston D M 1972 Recessively inherited myotonia congenita. Journal of Medical Genetics 9: 213–215

Harper P S, Penny R, Foley T Jr, Migeon C J, Blizzard R M 1972a Gonadal function in males with myotonic dystrophy. Journal of Clinical Endocrinology and Metabolism 35: 852–856

Harper P S, Rivas M L, Bias W B M, Hutchinson J R, Dyken P R, McKusick V A 1972b Genetic linkage confirmed between the loci for myotonic dystrophy, ABH secretion and Lutheran blood group. American Journal of Human Genetics

Harper P S, Shaw D, Meredith L, Sarfarazi M, Brook D, Huson S 1985 Gene mapping and myotonic dystrophy. In: Berg K (ed) Medical genetics: past, present, future. Alan R. Liss, p. 61–76

Haynes J, Thrush D C 1972 Paramyotonia congenita: an electrophysiological study. Brain 95: 553–558

Hofmann W W, DeNardo G L 1968 Sodium flux in myotonic muscular dystrophy. American Journal of Physiology 214: 330–336

Holt J M, Lambert E H 1964 Heart disease as the presenting feature in myotonia atrophica. British Heart Journal 26: 433–436

Hook R, Anderson E F, Noto P 1975 Anaesthetic management of a patient with myotonia dystrophia. Anaesthesiology 43: 689–692

Huff T A, Horton E S, Lebovitz H E 1967 Abnormal insulin secretion in myotonic dystrophy. New England Journal of Medicine 277: 837–841

Junge J 1966 Ocular changes in dystrophia myotonica, paramyotonia and myotonia congenita. Documenta Ophthalmologica 21: 1–115

Karpati G, Carpenter S, Watters G V, Eisen A E, Andermann F 1973 Infantile myotonic dystrophy. Histochemical and electron microscopic features in skeletal muscle. Neurology 23: 1066–1077

Kaufman L 1960 Anaesthesia in dystrophia myotonica. A review of the hazards of anaesthesia. Proceedings of the Royal Society of London 53: 183–188

Kühn E, Seiler D 1970 Biochemische Besonderheiten und Unterschiede der autosomal dominant und autosomal recessiv vererbten Myotonia Congenita. Klinische Wochenschrift 48: 1134–1136

Lenard H G, Goebel H H, Weigel W 1977 Smooth muscle involvement in congenital myotonic dystrophy. Neuropediatrie 8: 42–52

Lipicky R J 1977 Studies in human myotonic dystrophy. In: Pathogenesis of human muscular dystrophy. Rowland L P (ed) Excerpta Medica, Amsterdam, 729–738

Lipicky R J, Bryant S H 1971 Ion content, potassium flux and cable properties of myotonic, human, external intercostal muscle. Transactions of the American Neurological Association 96: 34–38

Lipicky R J, Bryant S H 1973 A biophysical study of the human myotonias. In: Desmedt J E(ed) New Developments in electromyography and clinical neurophysiology. Karger, Basel, p 451–463

Lunt P W, Meredith A L, Harper P S 1986 First trimester prediction in fetus at risk for myotonic dystrophy. Lancet 2: 350–351

Marshall J 1959 Observations on endocrine function in dystrophia myotonica. Brain 82: 221–231

Meredith A L, Huson S M, Lunt P W et al 1986 Application of a closly linked polymorphism of restriction fragment length to counselling and prenatal testing in families with myotonic dystrophy. British Medical Journal 293: 1353–1356

Merickel M, Gray R, Chauvin, Appel S 1981 Cultured muscle from myotonic muscular dystrophy patients: altered membrane electrical properties. Proceedings of the National Academy of Sciences USA 78: 648–652

Mohr J 1954 A study of linkage in man. Munksgaard, Copenhagen

Monaco A P, Bertelson C J, Middlesworth W et al 1985 Detection of deletions spanning the Duchenne muscular dystrophy locus using a tightly linked DNA segment. Nature 316: 842–845

Moxley R T, Corbett A J, Minaker K L, Rowe J W 1984 Whole body insulin resistance in myotonic dystrophy. Annals of Neurology 15: 157–163

O'Brien T, Newcombe R G, Harper P S 1983a Outlook for a clinically normal child in a sibship with congenital myotonic dystrophy. Journal of Pediatrics 103: 762–763

O'Brien T, Ball S, Sarfarazi M, Harper P S, Robson E B 1983b Genetic linkage between the loci for myotonic dystrophy and peptidase D. Annals of Human Genetics 47: 117–121

O'Brien T, Harper P S 1984 Reproductive problems and neonatal loss in women with myotonic dystrophy. British Journal of Obstetrics and Gynaecology 4: 170–173

Orndahl G, Thulesius O, Enestrom S, Dehlin O 1964 The heart in myotonic disease. Acta Medica Scandinavica 176: 479–491

Panayiotopoulos C P, Scarpalezos S 1976 Dystrophica myotonica. Peripheral nerve involvement and pathogenetic implications. Journal of the Neurological Sciences 27: 1–16

Peter J B, Campion D S 1977 Animal models of myotonia. In: Rowland L P (ed) Pathogenesis of human muscular dystrophies. Excerpta Medica, Amsterdam, p 739–746

Plishker G A, Gitelman H J, Appel S H 1978 Myotonic muscular dystrophy: Altered calcium transport in erythrocytes. Science 200: 323–325

Polgar J G, Bradley W G, Upton A R M et al 1972 The early detection of dystrophia myotonica. Brain 95: 761–776

Renaud J-F, Desnuelle C, Schmid-Antomarchi H, Hugues M, Serratrice G, Lazdunski M 1986 Expression of apamin receptor in muscles of patients with myotonic muscular dystrophy. Nature 319: 678–680

Renwick J H, Bundey S E, Ferguson-Smith M A, Izatt M M 1971 Confirmation of the linkage of the loci for myotonic dystrophy and the ABH secretor. Journal of Medical Genetics 8: 407–416

Ricker K, Haass A, Rudel R, Bohlen R, Mertens 1980 Successful treatment of paramyotonia congenita (Eulenberg): Muscle stiffness and weakness prevented by tocainide. Journal of Neurology, Neurosurgery and Psychiatry 42: 818–826

Roses A D, Appel S H 1973 Protein kinase activity in erythrocyte ghosts of patients with myotonic muscular dystrophy. Proceedings of the National Academy of Sciences USA 70: 1855–1859

Roses A D, Pericak-Vance M A, Ross D A, Yamaoka L, Bartlett R J 1986 RFLPs at the D19S19 locus of human chromosome 19 linked to myotonic dystrophy. Nucleic Acids Research 14:5569

Rudel R 1986 The pathophysiological basis of the myotonias

and of the periodic paralyses. In: Engel A, Banker B Q (eds) Myology. McGraw-Hill, New York, Ch 41

Rudel R, Lehmann-Horn F 1985 Membrane changes in cells from myotonia patients. Physiological Reviews 65: 310–356

Sanders D B 1976 Myotonia congenita with painful muscle contractions. Archives of Neurology 33: 580–582

Sarnat H B, Silbert S W 1976 Maturational arrest of fetal muscle in neonatal myotonic dystrophy. Archives of Neurology 33: 466–474

Sarnat H B, O'Connor T, Byrne P A 1976 Clinical effects of myotonic dystrophy on pregnancy and the neonate. Archives of Neurology 33: 459–465

Schotland D L 1970 An electron-microscopic investigation of myotonic dystrophy. Journal of Neuropathology and Experimental Neurology 29: 241–253

Schwartz D C, Cantor C R 1984 Separation of yeast chromosome-sized DNAs by pulsed field gradient gel electrophoresis. Cell 37: 67–75

Schwartz O, Jampel R S 1962 Congenital blepharophimosis associated with a unique generalised myopathy. Archives of Ophthalmology 68:52

Shaw D J 1986 A new strategy for mapping the human genome. Journal of Medical Genetics 23: 421–424

Shaw D J, Meredith A L, Sarfarazi M, Huson S M, Brook J D, Myklebost O, Harper P S 1985 The apolipoprotein CII gene: subchromosomal localisation and linkage to the myotonic dystrophy locus. Human Genetics 70: 271–273

Shaw D J, Brook J D, Meredith A L, Harley H G, Sarfarazi M, Harper P S 1986 Gene mapping and chromosome 19. Journal of Medical Genetics 23: 2N–10

Sherman S L, Ball S P, Robson E B 1985 A genetic map of chromosome 19 based on family linkage date. Annals of Human Genetics 49: 181–187

Shore R N 1975 Myotonic dystrophy: hazards of pregnancy and infancy. Developmental Medicine and Child Neurology 17: 356–361

Silver M M, Vilos G A, Silver M D, Shaheed W S, Turner K L 1984 Morphologic and morphometric analyses of muscle in the neonatal myotonic dystrophy syndrome. Human Pathology 15: 1171–1182

Swash M 1972 The morphology and innervation of the muscle spindle in dystrophia myotonica. Brain 95: 357–368

Swash M, Fox K P 1975 Abnormal intrafusal muscle fibres in myotonic dystrophy: a study using serial sections.

Journal of Neurology, Neurosurgery and Psychiatry 38: 91–99

Swift T R, Ignacio O J, Dyken P R 1975 Neonatal dystrophia myotonica: Electrophysiologic studies. American Journal of Disease in Childhood 129: 734–737

Tahmoush A J, Askansas V, Nels P G, Engel W K 1983 Electrophysiological properties of aneurally cultured muscle from patients with myotonic muscular atrophy. Neurology 33: 311–316

Tanaka K, Takeshita K, Takita M 1982 Abnormalities of bile acids in serum and bile from patients with myotonic muscular dystrophy. Clinical Science 62: 627–642

Thomsen J 1876 Tonische Krämpfe in willkurlich beweglichen Muskeln in folge von erebter psychisher Disposition (ataxia muscularis). Archiv für psychiatr und Nervenkrank-heiten vereinigt mit Zeitschrift für die gesamte Neurologie und Psychiatrie 6: 702–718

Thrush D C, Morris C J, Salmon M V 1972 Paramyotonia congenita: a clinical, histochemical and pathological study. Brain 95: 537–552

Vanier T M 1960 Dystrophia myotonica in childhood. British Medical Journal 2: 1284–1288

Vogt A 1921 Die Cataract bei myotonische Dystrophie. Schweiz. Med. Wochenschrift 29: 669–674

Wakamatsu H, Nakamura H, Ho K, Okajima S, Goto Y, Anazawa W 1972 Concentration and fatty acid composition of serum lipids in myotonia dystrophica, with special reference to pathogenesis. Hormone and Metabolism Research 4: 458–462

Walsh J C, Turtle J R, Miller S, McLeod J G 1970 Abnormalities of insulin secretion in dystrophia myotonica. Brain 93: 731–742

Weatherall D J 1985 The new genetics and clinical practice. Oxford University Press

Whitehead A S, Solomon E, Chambers S, Bodmer W F, Povey S, Fey G 1982 Assignment of the structural gene for the third component of human complement to chromosome 19. Proceedings of the National Academy of Sciences USA 79: 5021–5025

Winer N, Mart J M, Somers J E, Wolcott L, Dale H E 1965 Induced myotonia in man and goat. Journal of Laboratory and Clinical Medicine 66: 758–769

Yang-Feng T L, Francke U, Ullrich A 1985 Gene for human insulin receptor: localisation to site on chromosome 19 involved in pre-B-cell leukemia. Science 288: 728–731

The inflammatory myopathies

INTRODUCTION

The term myositis is appropriate when inflammation affects muscle, either one or many muscles. Table 17.1 lists the inflammatory myopathies. The main divisions are idiopathic myositis, including polymyositis and granulomatous myositis, and infective (viral, bacterial and protozoal).

POLYMYOSITIS

Definition

Polymyositis is an acquired myopathy in which muscle undergoes degeneration with inflammation. Proximal myopathy occurs and sometimes dysphagia and weakness of neck muscles. In one-third of cases there are the skin changes of dermatomyositis; in a similar number of cases, arthralgia occurs. The abbreviations PM for polymyositis and DM for dermatomyositis are used in this chapter even though generally not acceptable, given the possibility of confusion with diabetes mellitus (Pachman & Maryjowski 1984). Precipitants and associated conditions include viral infections, drugs, connective-tissue disorders and malignancy. Important investigations are muscle biopsy, electromyography (EMG) and serum creatine kinase (CK) estimation. Histological changes comprise segmental muscle fibre necrosis, regeneration and perifascicular atrophy accompanied by lymphocytic infiltration, interstitial and perivascular. The EMG shows spontaneous activity, myopathic units on volition and high-frequency discharges. The aetiology is obscure; an immunopathogenesis is suggested by both clinical features and experimental work.

Table 17.1 The inflammatory myopathies

Idiopathic
    Polymyositis–Dermatomyositis (PM–DM)
        Simple PM
        DM
        PM-DM with malignancy
        Childhood DM
        PM with connective-tissue disorders (CTD)
    (Myasthenia gravis)
    Granulomatous myositis
    Inclusion body myositis
    Eosinophilic myositis
    Localised myositis
        Focal nodular myositis
        Localised nodular myositis
        Proliferative myositis
        Orbital myositis
Infective
    Viral
        Acute
            Benign myositis
            Rhabdomyolysis
            Pleurodynia
        Chronic 'DM-like'
            Degenerative
    Fungal
    Bacterial
        Pyomyositis: 'tropical' myositis
        Clostridial
    Parasitic (see Ch. 18)
        Toxoplasmosis
        Cysticercosis
        Trichinosis

Table 17.2 PM–DM: Clinical features

Symptom	Incidence
Muscular	
Weakness	
Proximal	>75%
Distal	30%
Neck flexors	65%
Dysphagia	50%
Myalgia	65%
Atrophy	50%
Contractures	15%
Skin Changes	
Classic DM	30%
Minor atypical	25%
Other	
Raynaud's phenomenon	25%
Arthralgia	50%

rash is usually noticed before muscle weakness. Muscular pain is an early symptom in acute cases, typically in the shoulder muscles. Joint pains are an uncommon presentation.

Clinical pattern. The disorder evolves in weeks to months. In DM the onset is often rapid, with limb weakness and dysphagia developing in two weeks (Bohan & Peter 1975). At the other extreme, PM can result in weakness progressing slowly enough for dystrophy to be mimicked. In Table 17.2 clinical features are listed with an indication of their frequency.

Muscular symptoms. Weakness occurs during the course of every case. That affecting pelvic girdle muscles causes difficulty in climbing stairs and in standing up from beds and low chairs. Shoulder muscle weakness impairs elevation of the arms (Fig. 17.1); this affects tasks such as hanging out clothes, using high shelves and even brushing the hair if weakness is marked. Neck weakness affects raising the head from the pillow in bed. Dysphagia results from pharyngeal muscle weakness. Respiratory muscle involvement is unusual.

Atypical distribution can include facial (Bates et al 1973), distal (Hollinrake 1969) and crural weakness confined to the legs (Bharucha & Morgan Hughes 1981) or even just one muscle as in quadriceps myositis (Mohr & Knowlson 1977); only investigation will clarify. Recurrent painful nodules in muscles are characteristic of localised

Clinical features

Precipitants. These are evident only in a minority but have some aetiological significance.

The use of D-penicillamine in rheumatoid arthritis can induce PM (Doyle et al 1983, Swartz & Silver 1984). It can also precipitate other autoimmune disorders such as polyneuritis and myasthenia gravis. Genetic factors may be important in determining which disorders occur (Garlepp & Dawkins 1984). The myopathy is self-limiting although steroid therapy may be necessary.

Infections such as rubella (Landry & Winkelmann 1972) and toxoplasmosis (Kagen et al 1974) have been reported as triggering factors. In these instances the diagnosis of PM must remain uncertain when the same infective agents can cause myopathy directly.

Presentation. Muscle weakness is the initial feature in the majority of cases. In DM, the skin

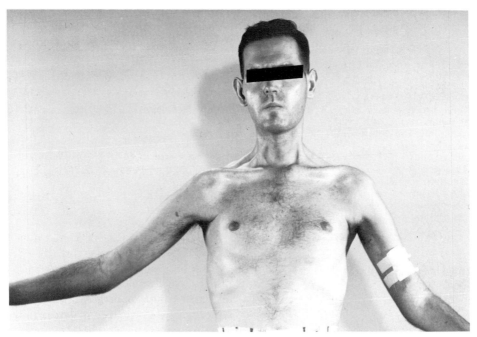

Fig. 17.1 Polymyositis with proximal muscle wasting and weakness and sclerotic skin changes (courtesy of Dr. C M Pearson)

nodular myositis (Cumming et al 1977). Unusual features in PM include fatiguability (Johns et al 1971) which may be responsive to anticholinesterase drugs (Vasilescu et al 1978). Fibrosing myositis results in early contractures (Bradley et al 1973); otherwise in PM these are a late and uncommon feature. Atrophy is slight compared with that in dystrophy.

Skin changes. In DM an erythematous rash affects the face and arms; in the face it is most marked on the cheeks and round the eyes; it spreads to the neck and upper chest (Fig. 17.2). The arms are involved proximally and distally. Sometimes the upper eyelids show a distinctive violet suffusion. Thicker patches of dermatitis occur on the extensor surfaces of the limbs, with induration and scaling. They are found over the elbows, fingers and sometimes the knees and ankles. There is hyperaemia at the base of the finger nails with red, atrophic skin at the ends of the fingers. In many, although not all, cases the dermatitis fluctuates with the myositis, getting worse when it does. In acute myositis there may be subcutaneous oedema proximally in the limbs, without superficial dermatitis (Venables et al

1982). In some patients there are skin changes which are insufficient to warrant the term 'DM'. Besides digital 'acrosclerosis', they include transient erythematous and eczematous rashes, also telangiectasia and disturbances in pigmentation affecting face and chest.

Joint symptoms. Joint pains occur during the course of the myopathy in half of all patients. Occasionally joint involvement is as overt as in rheumatoid arthritis. PM complicating connective-tissue disorders is considered later in this chapter.

Peripheral nerve involvement. This is exceptional and the term 'neuromyositis' can rarely be invoked. It depends on clinical findings such as areflexia and sensory loss and on slowing of nerve conduction and changes on nerve and motor point biopsy (Harriman & Currie 1974). The reflexes in PM are normal or minimally depressed. Henriksson & Stålberg (1978) felt that most denervation with reinnervation was secondary to muscle fibre damage.

Visceral involvement. Cardiac involvement in PM is indicated by the high incidence of abnormality

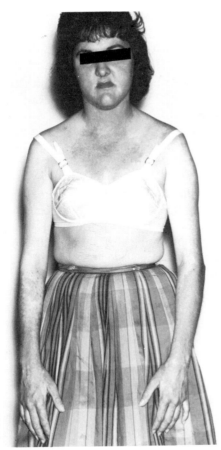

Fig. 17.2 Dermatomyositis with erythematous rash on face, neck and lower arms (courtesy of Dr. C M Pearson)

on electrocardiography and echocardiography (Gottdiener et al 1978) and of raised serum CK-MB isoenzyme levels (Strongwater et al 1983). Occasionally it leads to heart failure and arrhythmia; myocardial myositis can be shown at autopsy (Bohan et al 1977, Haupt & Hutchins 1982). Typically, the cardiac problem becomes apparent during the course of the skeletal muscle disorder but it may antedate it (Rechavia et al 1985); in such a case, histological confirmation might require transvenous endomyocardial biopsy.

Pulmonary involvement takes the form of fibrosing alveolitis (Fergusson et al 1983); it occurs in about 5% of cases (Frazier & Miller 1974). Pulmonary hypertension can result from vasculitis (Bunch et al 1981).

Gastrointestinal involvement includes reduced motility of oesophageal smooth muscle (Jacob et al 1983). This and small bowel dysfunction are most likely with PM in the context of mixed connective-tissue disorder. In childhood DM, vasculitis occasionally leads to ulceration with gastrointestinal haemorrhage (Banker & Victor 1966).

Renal failure due to myoglobinuria is a rare event in acute PM or DM (Sloan et al 1978).

Epidemiology

Incidence. The annual incidence of two to five cases per million is world wide, giving no support to the possibility of environmental factors. In North America an age-adjusted incidence of five per million per year was given by Medsger et al (1970). The rate was higher for black women than for white. That in the UK was similar (Rose & Walton 1966). The incidence in Israel was less than half this, about two per million per year (Benbassat et al 1980). In Japan the prevalence rate has been given as five per 10^5 population (Araki et al 1983).

Age. The condition shows a bimodal age distribution, being commonest in childhood and late middle-age. The peak range is 40 to 70 years but the condition can occur at any age.

Sex. Twice as many women as men are affected. This ratio also holds for the childhood disorder.

Genetic aspects
Familial. Familial PM-DM is rare. Childhood DM has been reported in twins (Cook et al 1963, Harati et al 1984), in first cousins (Lambie & Duff 1963) and in father and daughter (Lewkonia & Buxton 1973). Denman (1984) reported sisters with multiple autoimmune disorders including PM.

Histocompatibility studies. These have not shown clear-cut genetic predisposition to PM-DM. An increased incidence of HLA-B8 has been reported in juvenile DM (Pachman & Cooke 1980) and adult PM (Behan et al 1978) but the findings have not been universal (Walker et al 1982). There is also a weak association between HLA-DR3 and PM (Hirsch et al 1981). Genetic factors may determine the patterns of auto-antibodies such as anti-Jo-1 (Arnett et al 1981).

Hereditary X-linked agammaglobulinaemia. This has been reported in association with childhood DM and cerebral vasculitis (Gotoff et al 1972, Rosen 1974). Familial hypogammaglobulinaemia was associated with DM and viral encephalitis in the case of Webster et al (1978). The nosological position of the myopathy in these cases is considered in the section on viral myositis.

Hereditary complement deficiency has been reported in a case of DM (Leddy et al 1975), the C2 component being absent.

Associated disorders

Connective tissue disorders (CTD). PM is usually grouped with these. One of them is present as an associated disorder in 20% of patients with PM (Bohan et al 1977). PM occurring with other CTD is more refractory to treatment and carries a worse prognosis than the condition in general. However, this does not hold true for the benign PM which complicates mixed CTD (Sharp et al 1972). PM and other types of myopathy in CTD are considered later in this chapter. True PM with symptomatic weakness and the typical changes on biopsy occurs in only a small percentage of cases of systemic lupus erythematosus (SLE), rheumatoid arthritis and progressive systemic sclerosis (PSS). In SLE, the figure is under 10% (Tsokos et al 1981, Foote et al 1982, Isenberg 1984). The incidence in PSS is comparable (West et al 1981). In rheumatoid arthritis and Sjögren's syndrome, PM is uncommon. It may be overlooked when movement is restricted by the arthritis.

Neoplasia. PM-DM is relatively uncommon and its concurrence with neoplasia means that it represents one of the paraneoplastic or non-metastatic neurological syndromes of malignancy. In the series of Callen (1984) the myopathy occurred before the appearance of the neoplasm, concurrently with it or following it, in equal proportions. DM was a marker of malignancy in roughly 24%. The incidence of malignancy overall in PM-DM was about 10%. Callen's figures suggested that for pure PM the association was not a strong one. Bohan et al (1977) gave comparable figures to those of Callen: thus over 20% of older men with DM had underlying malignancy. Even so, in less than 10% of cases did DM present simultaneously and follow a parallel course to that of the neoplasm. No specific tumour type is associated with DM: the malignancies are assorted, with the common ones, bronchial and genital carcinoma, occurring as in the general population. In the rare cases of juvenile DM with neoplasia, the latter may be unusual, such as ovarian dysgerminoma (Solomon & Maurer 1983). Callen (1984) stressed the need to separate the skin changes of DM from those of CTD with PM: in one there is the possibility of malignancy whereas in the other there is not. Exceptionally, the dermatosis is specific for neoplasm, affecting the usual sites for DM but showing the pathognomonic red suffusion of 'malignant erythema'. The failure of PM-DM to respond to therapy is not a pointer to underlying malignancy, according to Callen (1984). He is a convincing advocate of a limited search for malignancy in cases of adult DM. This is corroborated by Manchul et al (1985); although they found a similar figure for the incidence of malignancy in myositis to those of Bohan et al (1977) and Callen (1984), the neoplasms usually presented concurrently with the myositis. There was no increased incidence of neoplasm developing during the course of PM-DM, making late or repeated screening unnecessary. Their series also differed in that the association with neoplasm went for PM as well as for DM and for women as well as for men.

Classification

The PM-DM complex is heterogeneous; subdividing it is of value only if this aids diagnosis and management and gives a guide to prognosis and aetiology. Table 17.3 represents a simple classification. Acute PM can be myolytic enough to produce symptomatic myoglobinuria. This is a

Table 17.3 PM–DM: Classification

Polymyositis
    Isolated ('pure' or 'simple')
    (Acute myolytic)

Dermatomyositis
    Juvenile vasculitic DM

PM with CTD

Drug-induced PM–DM

Paraneoplastic PM–DM

Table 17.4 PM–DM: Clinical investigations

Major
    Serum creatine kinase (CK) estimation
    Electromyography (EMG)
    Muscle biopsy
Minor
    Erythrocyte sedimentation rate
    Blood count
    Other serum enzymes
    Serum myoglobin
        Urinary myoglobin
    Tests for CTD
    Limited malignancy screen

rare and unimportant subdivision even though in the individual case it must be recognised and treated appropriately. DM is clearly separable because of the skin lesions; in addition, the myopathy shows subtle differences from that of isolated or pure PM. Indeed, juvenile DM may be part of such a widespread vascular disorder that it is distinguishable as a form of primary vasculitis. When PM is associated with CTD it may be more refractory to treatment and thus carry a worse prognosis. The severity and ubiquity of the vasculitis in juvenile DM correlates with such a worse prognosis (Crowe et al 1982). Vasculitis is common to DM and to PM with CTD but the conditions are distinctive. There is little justification in placing in a separate group PM-DM when it occurs with malignancy; muscle fibre necrosis may outweigh inflammation in 'paraneoplastic' PM-DM, but not consistently (Bohan et al 1977).

Clinical investigations

The triad of key investigations comprises serum creatine kinase (CK) estimation, EMG and muscle biopsy. These and other investigations are listed in Table 17.4.

Serum creatine kinase (CK) estimation. This gives a sensitive and specific indication of muscle cell necrosis. High CK activity is found in acute disease, falling with remission. Changes in concentrations may antedate those in clinical status. In chronic PM-DM the levels may be normal throughout the course (Schwarz et al 1980).

Electromyography (EMG). The characteristic findings are: first, spontaneous activity, with fibrillation and increased insertional activity; secondly polyphasic potentials of small amplitude and short duration; and thirdly high-frequency discharges on mechanical stimulation of the muscle. Multiple sampling of several muscles is desirable; even with this, no abnormality is found in 10% (Bohan et al 1977). The picture is that of a mixture of myopathy and denervation, the latter increasing with the duration of the disorder (Mechler 1974).

The EMG gives an indication of which muscle to sample, although biopsy at the site of needling itself must be avoided. Biopsy can be of the corresponding muscle on the opposite side or of vastus internus after sampling of vastus externus.

Muscle biopsy. Early biopsy is desirable to establish the diagnosis and to allow therapy to begin. The site is usually quadriceps or deltoid. Needle as opposed to open biopsy allows multiple sampling but can mean that changes in architecture, such as perifascicular atrophy, are missed. Conchotome biopsy (Henriksson 1979) is half-way to open biopsy.

Muscle: light-microscopy changes. The pathology of PM-DM is considered with that of other myopathies in Chapter 5 and is only summarised here (Table 17.5). Degenerative-necrobiotic changes comprise segmental necrosis and degeneration (Fig. 17.3); they are indistinguishable for PM and DM, juvenile and adult, according to Glynn (1984). Perifascicular areas are the most liable to damage (Fig. 17.4). Regenerating fibres are also seen. Additional myopathic changes may appear non-specific, such as the centralisation of nuclei;

Table 17.5 PM–DM Pathology: Light microscopy

Muscle fibre
  Segmental necrosis
  Degeneration
  Regeneration

Inflammatory cell infiltration
  Epimysial
  Interstitial
  Perivascular

Vascular endothelial changes
  Perifascicular atrophy

nevertheless, they give a guide to severity and thus there is an inverse correlation between the percentage of fibres with central nuclei and the response to steroid therapy (Schwartz et al 1980). Inflammatory changes are seen in 75% (Bohan et al 1977) with foci of lymphocytes, perivascular and endomysial in location. In juvenile DM, vasculitis is prominent with infiltration and endothelial necrosis; perifascicular atrophy may be marked

and micro-infarcts are seen (Carpenter et al 1976, Carpenter & Karpati 1981). Vascular changes can occur in adult DM but not PM. Motor end-plate abnormalities are frequent, although evidence of denervation is rare.

Skin: Light microscopy changes. There is atrophy with or without inflammation. The poikiloderma is distinctive.

Muscle: Ultramicroscopy. This is considered in Chapter 8. Degenerative and regenerative changes are common to other myopathies. Inflammatory cells can be seen traversing vessel walls and infiltrating muscle fibres. Endothelial reduplication is found in juvenile DM. Particles resembling both Coxsackie virus and myxovirus have been reported.

Other clinical investigations
Erythrocyte sedimentation rate. This is raised in

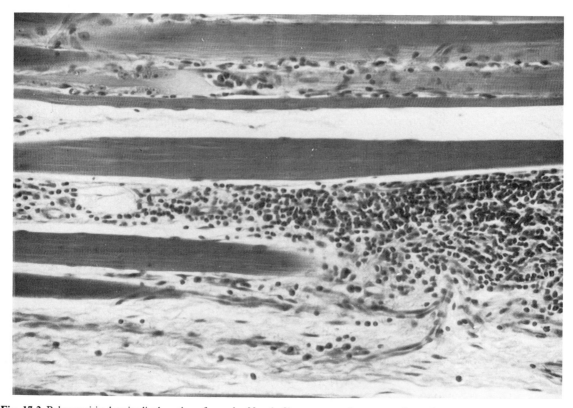

Fig. 17.3 Polymyositis: longitudinal section of muscle. Muscle fibre near top shows necrosis on the right, regeneration on the left. Interstitial lymphocytic infiltration fills the lower field on the right. H & E, ×53 (courtesy of Dr. D G F Harriman)

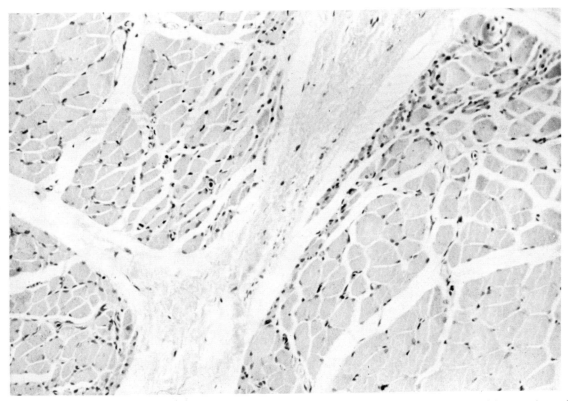

Fig. 17.4 Dermatomyositis: transverse section of muscle. Perifascicular fibre atrophy is seen on either side of the central strand of perimysial connective tissue. H & E, ×22.5 (courtesy of Dr. D G F Harriman)

most acute cases, particularly when there is systemic upset.

Serum enzymes. Aldolase and glutamic oxalo-acetic transaminase are released into the serum by muscle cell necrosis. In practice their estimation is of less value than is that of serum CK.

Serum myoglobin estimation. Myoglobin is raised in blood and urine in the acute forms (Kagen 1977, Nishikai & Reichlin 1977). Serum CK estimation at present remains the better guide to activity.

Tests for antinuclear antibodies. Antinuclear factor is found in about 10% of cases of PM with CTD (Bohan et al 1977). The antinuclear antibody termed anti-Jo-l is frequently but not exclusively associated with PM (Mathews & Bernstein 1983, Yoshida et al 1983). It is associated with PM-DM in which there is interstitial lung disease and overlap features such as Raynaud's, arthritis and the sicca (Sjögren's) syndrome (Bernstein et al 1984). Reichlin & Arnett (1984) found that 89% of PM-DM cases had positive serological results with demonstrable auto-antibody. The autoimmune responses showed great heterogeneity but there were clear relationships between certain specific immune responses and certain clinical syndromes, e.g. anti-Jo-l with isolated pure PM. They felt that genetic factors might determine these relationships.

Special investigations

The above serological findings lead us into the realm of special investigations which are less to do with the diagnosis of PM-DM than with its aetiology. Most are immunological and are considered fully in Chapter 9. They are listed here in Table 17.6.

Table 17.6 PM–DM: Special investigations of pathogenetic significance

Serological tests
  Antinuclear antibodies
    Anti-Jo-l etc.
  Complement levels
  Immunoglobulins
    IgG levels

In vitro lymphocyte studies
  Transformation
  Macrophage migration
  In-vitro cytotoxicity

Whole-body scanning of muscle
Scintigraphy of muscle

Immunochemistry of muscle
  Immunoglobulin deposition
  Complement deposition
  Monoclonal antibody markers for lymphoid cells

Serum protein estimations. Alterations in serum immunoglobulin levels are found inconstantly. In isolated cases there is selective deficiency, such as IgA deficiency (Carroll et al 1976). Serum complement levels vary, with conflicting evidence as to whether activation occurs. Immunofluorescence studies of muscle have shown deposits of immunoproteins in vessel walls. Monoclonal gammopathy can be associated with cases of PM and, in these, may be a factor in the damage to muscle cells. Kiprov & Miller (1984) found monoclonal paraprotein (IgG K light chain) in serum as well as deposited on sarcolemmal basement membrane. Immunosuppressive therapy removed both serum and muscle antibodies, as well as resulting in clinical remission.

In vitro lymphocyte studies. Increased transformation of peripheral blood lymphocytes on culture with muscle extracts may be an epiphenomenon. Macrophage migration studies are a further method by which lymphocytes sensitised to muscle have been demonstrated. Cytotoxicity of such lymphocytes for muscle cells in vitro may parallel in vivo damage to muscle fibres by T cells. This technique has been made more specific by the use of human fetal muscle cells which have been marked with tritium-labelled carnitine (Cambridge & Stern 1981).

Whole-body scanning of muscle. This can confirm active disease (Brown et al 1976) although it does not indicate which individual muscles are affected. Equally, muscle scintigraphy with 99 m technetium-labelled phosphate complexes has not proved a guide to muscles appropriate for biopsy, nor is increased uptake specific to inflammatory myopathies (Messina et al 1982).

Immunocytochemistry of muscle. Immunoglobulin and complement deposition occurs in vessel walls, the more so with the vasculitis of juvenile DM (Whitaker & Engel 1972, Isenberg 1983). Vascular permeability is increased in PM (Isenberg & McKeran 1982). Necrotic muscle fibres contain complement components which may cause cell damage (Engel & Biesecker 1982). The use of monoclonal antibody markers shows that the lymphocytes in infiltrates are mostly T cells (Rowe et al 1981). Subset studies show suppressor-cytotoxic cells invading muscle fibres (Arahata & Engel 1984, Giorno et al 1984).

Diagnostic criteria

The clinical picture and investigatory triad of biopsy, serum enzymes and EMG amount to four main criteria for the diagnosis of PM-DM (Bohan & Peter 1975, Hudgson & Peter 1984). These are given below in summary.
(1) Proximal muscle weakness with or without myalgia, developing over weeks to months, with or without dermatosis.
(2) Pathological changes of muscle fibre necrosis and cellular infiltration, with or without perifascicular atrophy.
(3) Raised serum CK activity (and/or aldolase and myoglobin levels).
(4) EMG changes of myopathy (short-duration, polyphasic potentials) with spontaneous fibrillation and increased insertional activity.

The first criterion, that of the clinical picture, is indispensable. The others are dependent on such factors as the activity and chronicity of the disorder and the vagaries of sampling. Use of the criteria may allow definition of the subgroups of PM-DM, as well as giving a degree of probability in the individual case.

Differential diagnosis

The diagnosis of PM usually comes to mind when a patient has painful weak muscles. The common

Table 17.7 PM–DM: Differential diagnosis

Connective tissue disorders
  Mixed CTD
  RA
  SLE
  PSS
  Polymyalgia rheumatica

Myasthenia gravis

Granulomatous myopathy

Infective myopathy
  Toxoplasmosis
  Trichinosis
  Viral

Hereditary myopathy
  Muscular dystrophy
    Facioscapulohumeral
  Metabolic myopathy
    McArdle's disease
    Other glycogen storage diseases
    Carnitine myopathy

Endocrine myopathy
  Steroid myopathy
  Thyrotoxic myopathy

Neurogenic atrophy
  Chronic spinal muscular atrophy
  Motor neurone disease

Drug-induced and other toxic myopathies

Paraneoplastic myopathies besides PM–DM

Rhabdomyolysis from other causes

alternative is a rheumatic condition, e.g. affecting the shoulder joints. Rheumatoid arthritis can be complicated both by a myositis and by drug-induced myopathy. Acute PM can mimic other CTD. It also must be distinguished from myositis due to infection, either viral or parasitic. Chronic PM must be separated from congenital or hereditary myopathy as it is treatable whereas the latter is not. DM may be mistaken for a dermatosis affecting solely the skin. The main conditions entering the differential diagnosis are listed in Table 17.7.

Rheumatic conditions. The possibility of PM is often invoked when pain on active movement against resistance gives the impression of proximal weakness. Careful testing will usually separate real from apparent weakness. Polymyalgia rheumatica causes early morning stiffness as well as pain around the shoulders. The patients are elderly. The ESR is usually very high. Electromyography in this and other CTD should give negative results for myopathy. There will be cases in which biopsy is necessary for the correct diagnosis.

Infective myopathies. Acute viral involvement of muscle may have a peculiar distribution, affecting the thoracic cage in the pleurodynia of Bornholm, or the lower legs in the acute myositis of childhood. Benign myalgic encephalomyelitis is a nebulous entity. The occasional case of chronic myopathy appears to be directly due to virus; thus, Coxsackie virus was implicated by Tang et al (1975). Biopsy may separate viral myopathy from true PM. Inclusion body myositis is characterised by painless weakness affecting distal as well as proximal muscles and by distinctive light-microscopic changes (Carpenter et al 1978). Tropical or suppurative myositis is focal, involving one or more muscles, and should be separable from PM. Toxoplasmic myositis can simulate PM, requiring serological tests for identification (Rowland & Greer 1961, Kagen 1984).

Congenital myopathies. In general, the proximal weakness of PM-DM lacks the selectivity of involvement seen in muscular dystrophy and benign spinal muscular atrophy, such as biceps and brachioradialis involvement with sparing of the deltoids. Limb-girdle dystrophy and chronic PM may be hard to distinguish from each other even with biopsy. Facioscapulohumeral dystrophy has a distinctive distribution; rarely, this is mimicked in PM (Bates et al 1973). In addition, this form of dystrophy can apparently have a myositic phase, transiently responsive to steroid therapy. Similarly, in benign chronic spinal muscular atrophy, secondary myopathic change can result in high levels of serum CK. Metabolic myopathies, such as McArdle's disease, glycogen storage disease and carnitine myopathy, can be painful or improve with steroid therapy. In these myopathies, the tendon reflexes may be preserved even in affected muscles; this is a feature held in common with PM-DM.

Other disorders. Isolated rhabdomyolysis is rarely due to PM. The necrotising myopathy of neoplasia is a separate entity and exceptionally rare. Thyrotoxic myopathy should be recognisable. Steroid-induced lipid myopathy must be considered in the appropriate circumstances. Myasthenia gravis usually has oculo-faciopharyngeal as well as shoulder girdle involvement, with fatiguability; it co-exists with PM, but rarely. The progressive muscular atrophy form of MND occasionally produces a picture which only biopsy will clarify. It should be noted that weakness of the neck extensor muscles can occur in all three disorders, viz. PM, myasthenia gravis and MND.

Aetiology

The idiopathic myositis of the PM-DM complex is probably due to autoimmune responses (see Ch. 9) initiated by viruses in many cases. Many viruses attack muscles, producing short-lived clinical syndromes. Such viruses localised to muscle cells could provoke a self-perpetuating immunopathological reaction in susceptible patients. The viruses would be latent, hence their being so hard to recover from muscle tissue. Such latent virus could be reactivated by the immunosuppression of malignancy, thus explaining the link between this and PM-DM. Similar mechanisms to that involving viruses could obtain with rarer precipitants, such as BCG with its adjuvant effect on the immune system and penicillamine indirectly stimulating this, usually in the context of RA. The antinuclear antibodies seen especially in the overlap syndromes with PM constitute sound evidence for autoimmunity. Their presence is influenced by genetic factors. Production of an antibody such as anti-Jo-1 is unlikely to be part of the prime initiating event. Vascular endothelial cells trap antigenic material, viral and otherwise: the increase in vascular permeability in PM and the prominent vasculitis of juvenile DM indicate that damage to vessels is one of the earliest changes.

Therapy

Steroid therapy. The use of this in PM-DM is well established. Early, adequate initial therapy is important. The dose of prednisolone is 60–80 mg per day in divided doses; in an acute case this can go up to 1.5 mg per kg body weight per day. In severe juvenile DM with vasculitis, 2 mg per kg is advisable (Pachman & Maryjowski 1984) and may be given parenterally four times a day to

ensure even dosage. Pulsed therapy with methyl-prednisolone is a different method of giving steroids rapidly; high dosage is maintained for at least a month then tapered gradually according to clinical status and serial CK levels in acute cases. The schedule for reduction comprises a 5 mg reduction weekly to 30 mg a day then further reduction at a slower rate (Mastaglia & Ojeda 1985). The maintenance dosage of between 5 and 15 mg per day is usually reached by six months. It is needed indefinitely in most cases although in older patients with milder disease almost half can have their steroids discontinued or substantially reduced within three years of diagnosis (Hoffman et al 1983, Baron & Small 1985). Alternate-day use is another schedule for maintenance therapy. Countertherapy with diuretics, calcium and potassium supplements and ranitidine are appropriate in some patients. Steroid-induced myopathy can be distinguished by EMG, normal CK and, if necessary, needle biopsy.

Immunosuppressive therapy. Cytotoxic immunosuppressive therapy can be brought in if the condition is refractory or relapsing despite 5–10 weeks of high-dose steroid therapy. Some advocate the simultaneous use of steroid therapy with another immunosuppressive drug from the outset. Exceptional cases require two simultaneously administered agents in addition to steroids such as chlorambucil and methotrexate (Wallace et al 1985). This combination of an alkylating agent and an antimetabolite constitutes aggressive therapy but the short- and long-term risks can be minimised by monitoring and by gradual decrease in dosage. Methotrexate is a rapidly acting drug and can therefore be used as an alternative or a supplement to steroid therapy. It is given as a weekly intravenous injection of 25–50 mg (Fisher et al 1979, Niakan et al 1980). Azathioprine in doses of 2–2.5 mg/kg body weight/day is another drug for initiating treatment, although it is perhaps more appropriate as maintenance therapy (Bunch et al 1981). Cyclophosphamide has also been advocated (Niakan et al 1980).

Plasmapheresis. This can be used in patients whose disorder is not responding to drug therapy (Dau 1981) although Wallace et al (1985) consider that combination immunosuppressive drug therapy is superior.

Irradiation. Total-body low-dose irradiation (150 rads over five weeks) is a possibility in the acute case which is refractory to all other forms of therapy (Engel et al 1981, Hubbard et al 1982) and in the chronic case which does not respond on relapse (Morgan et al 1985). The therapy is immunosuppressive, inducing lymphopenia; it is not without risk of severe bone-marrow suppression.

Therapy for calcification. Soft-tissue calcification at pressure points is a major problem in one-third of cases of juvenile DM. Warfarin may reduce the deposits (Berger & Hadler 1983), possibly by reducing the formation of calcium-binding gamma-carboxyglutamic acid (Lian et al 1982).

Prognosis

Steroid therapy has improved the prognosis: prolonged remission is achieved in more than 50%; relapses occur in less than one-quarter of patients, usually within two years of onset. The outlook in childhood PM is good, in general, although that in juvenile DM is less so. The prognosis for the myositis may be worse when it is associated with CTD. This is not the experience of all observers (Bohan et al 1977); in particular, myositis with mixed CTD is relatively benign. In young adults, there remains the possibility that other CTD may develop later in the course of PM. When PM-DM is associated with malignancy, the latter is responsible for the poorer outlook although in occasional cases the myopathy itself has been refractory to therapy (Callen 1984). Benbassat et al (1985) found three features. viz. failure to remit with therapy, persistent leucocytosis, and age, to be poor prognostic factors but not overlap syndromes or cardiac complications, as in some other series. The causes of death in their series were not directly related to the myopathy; these comprised neoplasm, ischaemic heart disease and non-specific pulmonary disorders. In general, it is not yet clear if the use of other forms of therapy besides steroids has increased the remission rate.

MYOPATHY IN CONNECTIVE-TISSUE DISORDERS (CTD)

The connective-tissue disorders (CTD) include the ill-defined vasculitides. PM in CTD has been considered on page 592. The term 'overlap myositis' is used when a case satisfies criteria for both PM and another CTD. There are further cases in which the CTD is not clear-cut. As well as PM, changes in muscle which may be found in CTD include those of denervation, focal nodular myositis, non-specific myopathy and drug-induced myopathy.

Myopathy in rheumatoid arthritis (RA)

Wasting of muscles is common in RA; only partly can it be ascribed to disuse. Histologically, it is mainly type IIB muscle fibre atrophy.

Inflammatory cell infiltration in muscles occurs not only as part of PM in RA but also in focal nodular myositis and in some forms of arteritis (Kim & Collins 1980). The PM in RA is not distinctive (Haslock et al 1970). Focal nodular myositis (Fig. 17.5) is classically associated with long-standing RA (Yates 1976). Arteritis affects small vessels, with infiltration and fibrinoid necrosis.

Apart from non-specific atrophy, the changes of denervation are sometimes present, with scattered atrophic fibres rather than marked group atrophy (Kim & Collins 1980).

Drug-induced myopathy in RA includes steroid myopathy (Askari et al 1977); this is becoming less common with the decline in use of long-term steroid therapy. Penicillamine-induced myositis can also occur.

Myopathy in systemic lupus erythematosus (SLE)

Muscular symptoms occur in as many as 50% of patients with SLE (Isenberg & Snaith 1981): they comprise muscle pains, tenderness and weakness. Joint symptoms, including arthralgia, are commoner in patients with muscle symptoms. It appears that pain in joints frequently simulates muscle involvement. Actual PM occurs in between 5% (Isenberg 1984) and 8% (Tsokos et al 1981) of patients.

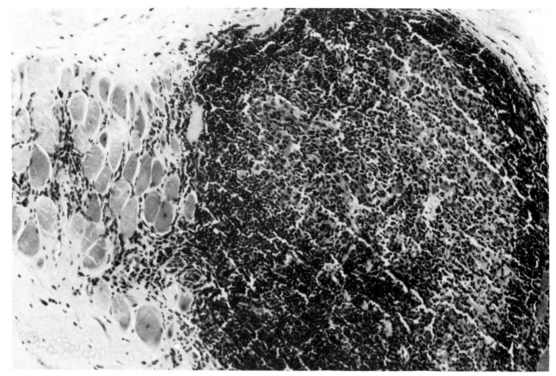

Fig. 17.5 'Focal nodular myositis' in rheumatoid arthritis. A lymphoid follicle with minor myopathic changes in adjacent muscle fibres, thus central nuclei. H & E, ×36 (courtesy of Dr. D G F Harriman)

Vacuolar myopathy is sometimes seen (Sibrans & Holley 1967), the histological changes comprising central vacuolation of muscle fibre segments. There is an association between vacuolar change and a clinical picture in which generalised myalgia is more prominent than muscle weakness.

Myopathy in progressive systemic sclerosis (PSS)

When muscle weakness with wasting occurs in PSS, it is usually the result of disuse atrophy (Rodnan 1979). However, 10% of cases show clinical and laboratory evidence of 'overlap myositis' (Clements et al 1978). This is a proximal myopathy with a distribution similar to that of isolated PM, involving deltoid and pectoral muscles, although sometimes the anterior tibial muscles and diaphragm are involved. The myopathy is usually chronic and relatively mild, without elevation of serum enzymes. The histological counterpart of this consists of atrophy and fibrosis outweighing necrosis and infiltration.

Clements et al (1978) separate a polymyopathy which lacks the features of myositis. On EMG the potentials are polyphasic but of normal amplitude and duration. There is interstitial fibrosis and variation in fibre size on biopsy. The condition rarely responds to steroid therapy.

Myopathy in other CTD

Sjögren's syndrome. Overt myositis was found in 9% of cases in one recent series (Pavlides et al 1982). In some cases there are histological findings which are uncommon in primary PM; thus, small and medium-sized blood vessels may show marked inflammatory changes (Ringel et al 1982); sometimes plasma cells predominate in the perivascular and interstitial infiltrates.

Vasculitis

Polyarteritis nodosa. This CTD is the one which is most commonly associated with muscle symptoms. Myalgia occurs in 75% of cases; however, biopsies are abnormal in only 30%. The changes usually comprise vasculitis; only rarely does this result in damage to muscle fibres.

Nodular myositis. This has been reported, progressing to systemic vasculitis (Allen et al 1980).

Polymyalgia rheumatica. Like polyarteritis nodosa, this disorder produces myalgia without myopathy, clinically or on investigation. It is more important in the differential diagnosis of PM.

Wegener's disease. This is considered under 'granulomatous myositis'; although panarteritis occurs in this condition.

GRANULOMATOUS MYOSITIS

Granulomatous muscle disorders occur either as part of sarcoidosis or separately (Kagen 1984). In

Table 17.8 Granulomatous myositis

Sarcoidosis
    Asymptomatic microscopic granulomata
    Palpable muscle nodules
    Acute generalised myositis
    Chronic myopathy

Isolated myositis without systemic involvement

Granulomatous or giant-cell myositis with thymoma

Myositis with other primary disorder

addition, there are isolated reports of an association with other disorders (Table 17.8).

Sarcoid myositis

Symptomatic myopathy is rare, occurring in less than 1% of patients with sarcoidosis (Kagen 1984). Palpable nodules in muscle are also exceptional; they may be accompanied by subcutaneous nodules. Conversely, asymptomatic granulomata may be found on muscle biopsy (Fig. 17.6) in up

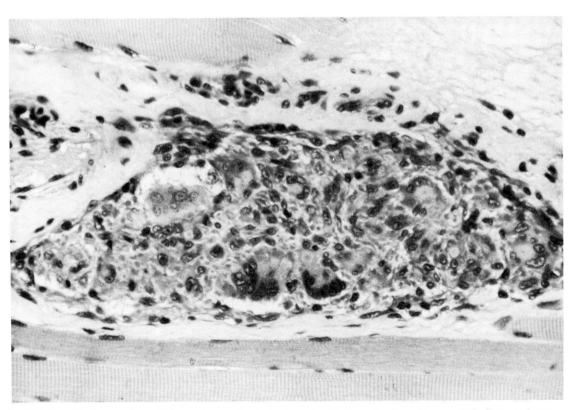

Fig. 17.6 Sarcoidosis: large interstitial granuloma with giant cells and epitheliod cells. The adjacent muscle fibres are intact. H & E, ×19 (courtesy of Dr. D G F Harriman)

to 50% of cases if multiple sections are studied. The clinical syndrome of sarcoid myositis is usually chronic. When acute myopathy does occur, it resembles PM; even the rash of DM may be mimicked (Itoh et al 1980). Such acute myositis is steroid-responsive whereas the more typical chronic, atrophic myopathy is not. Asymptomatic muscle involvement does not warrant treatment.

Isolated granulomatous myositis

This rare entity comprises a chronic proximal myopathy. Other muscles can be involved and there may be dysphagia. Typically, it affects middle-aged women. Like chronic sarcoid myositis, it does not respond to steroid therapy. The pathology is that of granulomata in muscle (Hewlett & Brownell 1975). There is no inflammatory cell infiltration except as part of the granulomata; exceptionally, there is widespread muscle fibre degeneration and regeneration as in one case described by Hewlett & Brownell. The diagnosis of isolated granulomatous myositis is tenable only if there are no granulomata in other tissues.

Granulomatous myositis with thymoma

This is a rare and distinctive variant of granulomatous myositis in which the myopathy is associated with thymoma and myasthenia gravis (Namba et al 1974). Cardiac muscle is involved, as well as skeletal. Auto-allergic thyroiditis is a further association. Once again, the disorder affects middle-aged women. The myopathy is severe, with raised serum CK levels indicating muscle cell necrosis. Granulomatous or 'giant-cell' myocarditis produces arrhythmia and congestive heart failure. The thymoma is a benign lymphocytic neoplasm, the same type as that underlying isolated myasthenia gravis in 10% of cases. Occasionally it is epithelial or mixed cell in origin; rarely it is locally malignant. It may precede the myopathy by months to years. Abnormalities of thyroid function are common and biopsy shows thyroiditis with lymphocytic infiltration. Further disturbance of immune function is shown by proneness to fungal and viral infections.

Granulomatous myositis with other disorders

Wegener's disease. Rarely, skeletal muscle is involved in this systemic disorder, the pathology of which comprises granulomata, inflammatory-cell infiltrates and a necrotising panarteritis similar to that of polyarteritis nodosa. The unique case described by Judge et al (1977) comprised chronic myopathy with no inflammation in a biopsy specimen but IgG staining of muscle fibres on immunofluorescence studies. The patient developed glomerulonephritis and pulmonary vasculitis.

Crohn's disease. A case of Crohn's disease has been described in which there was granulomatous myopathy in addition to the usual inflammatory bowel disease (Menard et al 1976).

EOSINOPHILIC MYOSITIS

Eosinophilic syndromes can include infiltration of muscle as well as of other tissues. Occasionally there is symptomatic myopathy, presenting as muscle pain and tenderness with proximal weakness. Localised myopathy may occur, affecting only thigh or calf. Exceptionally, the myopathy predominates (Layzer et al 1977, Stark 1979). The condition is acute, with raised serum CK levels. Electromyography confirms myopathy. On muscle biopsy there is muscle-cell necrosis and regeneration. Eosinophils are prominent among the inflammatory cells which form perivascular and interstitial collections.

The systemic effects in the eosinophilic syndromes include peripheral blood eosinophilia, pulmonary and cardiac involvement and the prognosis is poor. Steroid therapy is sometimes of benefit, in the disorder at large and in the myopathy, but the response is variable.

There appear to be several different syndromes. One with a more chronic, relapsing course has muscle pain and weakness as prominent features, with partial responsiveness to steroids (Serratrice et al 1980). As muscle infiltration with eosinophils may occur, the term 'eosinophilic myositis' has been used for this condition (Yonker & Panush 1985). Another variant is not a myopathy at all but rather a fasciitis affecting the skin, without evidence of muscle involvement (Simon et al 1982). As has been stated, genuine myopathy deserving the label 'eosinophilic PM' (Layzer et al 1977) is exceptionally rare.

FOCAL MYOSITIS

Nodular myositis

Focal nodular myositis is found in muscles of patients with CTD; it is asymptomatic and not a clinical entity. 'Localised nodular myositis' is characterised by recurrent painful nodules in muscles with circumscribed areas of myositis on biopsy. It may proceed to generalised PM (Cumming et al 1977), of which it is a variant.

Isolated focal myositis

A non-infective myositis affecting a single muscle has been described (Heffner et al 1977) with an indolent onset compared with that of pyomyositis ('tropical myositis'). It is also known as pseudotumour and can be mistaken for sarcoma of muscle. The histology comprises necrosis and infiltration. The condition does not recur after excision nor is it followed by generalised PM.

Proliferative myositis

This is a further entity in which abnormality is confined to one muscle or limb (Enzinger & Dulcey 1967). In some instances it appears to result in pseudotumour through repeated trauma provoking fibrous proliferation combined with excessive muscle fibre regeneration.

Orbital myositis

This can occur in isolation (Bullen & Younge 1982, Spoor & Hartel 1983) and with CTD (Grimson & Simons 1983). It consists of painful ophthalmoplegia, typically in young adults. It is usually confined to a single muscle, swelling of which can be shown by CT-scanning. It is steroid-responsive but may be relapsing (Ludwig & Tomsak 1983). The differential diagnosis of the condition is from conditions such as thyrotoxic ophthalmoplegia (Graves' ophthalmopathy), orbital lymphoid pseudotumour and infection.

INCLUSION BODY MYOSITIS

This disorder is a chronic myopathy which presents clinically as slowly progressive weakness with wasting, and pathologically is distinguished by the presence of inclusion bodies in both the nuclei and cytoplasm of skeletal muscle cells (Carpenter et al 1978, Danon et al 1982, Julien et al 1982).

Clinical features

Typically, the disorder affects elderly men; however, there is a suggestion from the case reports accumulating that there may be a bimodal age–sex distribution, with young women affected as well as old men. The usual absence of features such as muscle and joint pains and skin rashes means that, among the variants of PM, only chronic isolated PM resembles it. The distribution of weakness is that of a myopathy with the proximal muscles involved, but the pelvic girdle musculature is usually more affected than the shoulder girdle. There may be distal weakness in addition, occasionally marked, and facial weakness may occur, as well as dysphagia. The condition has no firm associations although it has been described with disorders in which there is disturbed immunity, such as Sjögren's syndrome (Chad et al 1982, Gutmann et al 1985), thrombocytopenia (Riggs et al 1984) and sarcoidosis.

Investigations

The serum CK is usually normal, as in indolent myositis in general. The findings on EMG can mimic those of PM in that there is a mixture of myopathic and neuropathic changes (Danon et al 1982, Eisen et al 1983); sometimes the EMG picture is entirely myopathic. Motor nerve conduction velocities may be reduced and sensory latencies prolonged (Gutmann et al 1985).

Pathological findings

Histological studies show muscle cell necrosis, vacuolation and regeneration with infiltration by lymphocytic inflammatory cells. The vacuoles are membrane-lined and may be single or multiple. They occur in 5–10% of the fibres; the vacuoles contain basophilic masses. Grouped atrophy is a further indication of denervation.

Electron microscopy is the surest way of showing the inclusion bodies, although they may

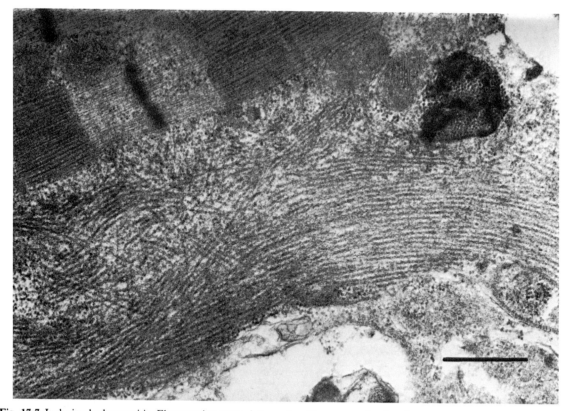

Fig. 17.7 Inclusion body myositis. Electronmicroscopy: intranuclear filaments randomly orientated, 20 nm in diameter (Courtesy of Dr P. Hudgson). Bar = 1.0 μm

be seen as eosinophilic bodies on light microscopy. The cytoplasmic bodies vary in shape and in staining; intranuclear inclusions tend to be acidophilic. Electron microscopy reveals that they are aggregates of microtubular filaments 10–25 nm in diameter and about 2 μm in length (Fig. 17.7). These may be viral in origin, either adenovirus (Mikol et al 1982) or myxovirus. The basophilic masses in the vacuoles are shown to be whorls.

Treatment

The condition is not responsive to steroid therapy; nevertheless, it is relatively benign. In one patient, progression appeared to be halted by total-body irradiation (Kelly et al 1984). Arahata & Engel (1984) found evidence of T cell-mediated injury to muscle fibres which were invaded by suppressor-cytotoxic cells, autoinvasive T cells and macrophages. The case described by Lane et al (1985) responded well to combination therapy with azathioprine and steroids. This patient had

Raynaud's phenomenon, the skin rash of DM and interstitial pulmonary fibrosis. The case therefore called into question the status of inclusion body myositis as a separate nosological entity.

VIRAL MYOSITIS

Viral infections of muscle represent the commonest acquired myopathy, even if the syndromes are almost all benign and short-lived. A number of DNA and RNA viruses can cause an acute myopathy (Table 17.9). The acute syndromes comprise benign acute myositis, acute rhabdomyolysis and epidemic pleurodynia.

Acute childhood myositis

Post-influenzal. This can be epidemic (Farrell et al 1980, Ruff & Secrist 1982) or sporadic. Epidemics are confined to children, sparing adults. The condition has occurred during both A

Table 17.9 Viral myositis

Clinical syndrome	Virus
Acute	
Benign myositis	Influenza A & B
	Parainfluenza
	Adenovirus 2
Rhabdomyolysis	Influenza A & B
	Coxsackie B5
	Echo 9
	Adenovirus 21
	Herpes simplex
	Epstein–Barr
	(Mycoplasma
	pneumoniae)
Epidemic pleurodynia	Coxsackie B5
	(Bl, 3 & 4)
Chronic myopathy	
'DM-like' syndrome of	
agammaglobulinaemia	Echo
Degenerative myopathy	
(Tang)	Coxsackie A9

and B influenza epidemics. Sporadic cases have followed influenza A and B and also parainfluenza (McKinlay & Mitchell 1976).

The myopathic syndrome follows the initial syndrome of influenza by a few days. Thus, there is recovery from the influenza but then severe muscle pain with tenderness and sometimes swelling occurs, developing during two to four days. Typically, both calves are affected; the thighs also may be involved. The condition is usually localised to these but other muscles can be affected. The children refuse to walk and keep their feet plantar-flexed to reduce the pain. The myopathy lasts five to seven days and the whole course is always less than a month (Mejlszenkier et al 1973).

Investigations. The serum CK activity is usually raised in the acute phase. On EMG there are myopathic changes, which are generalised even if slight (Ruff & Secrist 1982). Biopsy shows myositis with necrosis and regeneration. There are foci of inflammatory cells, both mononuclear cells and polymorphs (Antony et al 1979, Ruff & Secrist 1982). The inflammatory changes may be scanty. In general, biopsy is, of course, unjustified.

Aetiology. It is not known whether particular strains of virus can cause myositis following systemic disorder or whether there is individual susceptibility on the part of the host. Virus is usually not isolatable although influenza virus has been found in acute necrotising myopathy. Greco et al (1977) showed budding myxovirus in muscle cells on electron-microscopy. The condition appears to be self limiting, only rarely leading on to chronic myopathy (Schwartz et al 1978). Features which need explaining include the narrow age group, the focal involvement, the small numbers affected in an epidemic and the lack of recurrence in individuals (Mastaglia & Ojeda 1985).

Acute rhabdomyolysis

This sporadic disorder usually affects adults. It is severe, sometimes fatal, and results in profound weakness and myoglobinuria. It has been described in association with infection with a number of different viruses, including Echo (Jehn & Fink 1980, Josselson et al 1980) and adenovirus (Wright et al 1979). Only exceptionally have viruses been isolated and the role of viruses is uncertain. There is the possibility of a metabolic effect on mitochondria, involving fatty acid oxidation as in Reye's syndrome (DeVivo 1978).

Epidemic pleurodynia

Coxsackie B5 virus infection is notably associated with this acute syndrome of painful trunk muscles, those of chest, back, abdomen and sometimes the shoulders. It occurs in outbreaks, affecting children rather than adults. There is headache and fever accompanied by axial muscle pains.

Other viral myositides

More chronic syndromes include the DM-like syndrome occurring with echovirus infection in patients with agammaglobulinaemia (Webster et al 1978, Lederman & Winkelstein 1983) and in hepatitis B infection (Pittsley et al 1978). In the case described by Mease et al (1981) meningoencephalitis and myositis-fasciitis due to Echovirus 11 occurred in a patient with X-linked agammaglobulinaemia. Both conditions responded to regular injections of modified intravenous immunoglobulin. If the frequency of injections was reduced, the disorders reappeared, implying persistence of virus with relapse when host immunity dropped (Mease et al 1985). The syndrome appears to be a multisystem disorder affecting central nervous system as well as muscle, with Echovirus persisting in the CSF, sometimes for years (Webster 1984). The onset of myopathy is insidious while the erythematous rash is usually transient, so the condition differs from idiopathic or isolated DM. There may be little muscle weakness; rather, there is stiffness due to contractures around joints. The encephalitis is a late and serious development. It is probably correct to regard the syndrome as a DM-like one, rather than identical to isolated DM. Nevertheless, it does raise questions both of nosology and aetiology. Coxsackie virus is one more commonly associated with PM-DM, with raised titres (Travers et al 1977, Schiraldi & Iandolo 1978) and complement-fixing antibody to Coxsackie B in a high percentage of cases of juvenile DM (Christensen et al 1983).

The post-viral fatigue syndrome 'benign myalgic encephalomyelitis' forms an uncertain entity. There is a reduction in isometric muscle strength and minor EMG and histological changes. There may be a derangement of metabolism, as shown by early acidosis on exercise (Arnold et al 1984).

FUNGAL MYOSITIS

This is rare. It occurs as part of a generalised infection in the immunocompromised, e.g. in patients with candidiasis. Affected muscles are painful and the overlying skin may be involved, with papules. Biopsy of muscle or of skin shows the infection (Kressell et al 1978).

TROPICAL (BACTERIAL) MYOSITIS OR PYOMYOSITIS

Tropical myositis consists of the formation of one or more abscesses in muscle, the term 'pyomyositis' being an alternative. It is common in tropical regions (Chiedozi 1979); when it does occur in a temperate zone, the subject may recently have returned from the tropics. It may be precipitated by parasitic (filarial) and viral infections (Schlech et al 1981, Kallen et al 1982). Otherwise, infection of an individual muscle occurs only from local causes. An example of this is percutaneous nephrostomy resulting in the clostridial psoas myositis, with air shown by CT-scan, described by Wells et al (1985). However, the commonest precipitating factor is minor local trauma. There is a history of antecedent trauma in 50% of North American cases. In 60% of these the abscesses are multiple (Gibson et al 1984). Normally, skeletal muscle is resistant to metastatic infections. It seems likely that more than one specific factor can remove that imperviousness (Gibson et al 1984). The organism is *Staphylococcus aureus* in 90%, with *Streptococcus* in a small number of cases. The spread is haematogenous except in those cases in which there is direct extension, as from osteomyelitis. The muscles commonly affected are large ones, the glutei and quadriceps, also shoulder and axial muscles; the abscess forms deep inside such muscles. The condition evolves in three stages over as many weeks: initially there is local pain and swelling with pyrexia for a week; there is a leucocytosis, sometimes with eosinophilia, and a raised ESR. On examination the swelling is tender and the overlying skin is indurated. In some cases signs of inflammation in surrounding tissues may be absent because the affected muscle is so deep. At the suppurative stage, the abscess can be demonstrated by CT-scanning and ultrasonography; CT-scanning not only aids in localising but also in differentiating from other causes of swelling such as haematoma and tumour. If treatment is delayed, generalised sepsis with metastatic seeding may occur. Management comprises surgical drainage covered by full doses of a beta-lactamase-resistant penicillin. The affected muscle recovers quickly, its imperviousness to bacterial invasion returning.

REFERENCES

Allen I, Mullally B, Mawhinney H, Sawhney B, McKee P 1980 The nodular form of polymyositis — a possible manifestation of vasculitis. Journal of Pathology 131: 183–191

Antony J H, Procopis P G, Ouvrier R A 1979 Benign acute childhood myositis. Neurology 29: 1068–1071

Arahata K, Engel A G 1984 Monoclonal antibodies: analysis of mononuclear cells in myopathies. 1: Quantitation of subsets according to diagnosis and sites of accumulation and demonstration and counts of muscle fibres invaded by T cells. Annals of Neurology 16: 193–208

Araki S, Uchino M, Yoshida O 1983 Epidemiologic study of multiple sclerosis, myasthenia gravis, and polymyositis in the city of Kumamoto, Japan. Clinical Neurology 23: 838–841

Arnett F C, Hirsch T J, Bias W B et al 1981 The Jo-l antibody system in myositis: relationships to clinical features and HLA. Journal of Rheumatology 8: 925–930

Arnold D L, Bore P J, Radda G K, Styles P, Taylor D J 1984 Excessive intracellular acidosis of skeletal muscle on exercise in a patient with a post-viral exhaustion fatigue syndrome. Lancet 1: 1367–1369

Askari A, Vignos P J, Moskowitz R W 1977 Steroid myopathy in connective tissue disease. American Journal of Medicine 61: 485–492

Banker B Q, Victor M 1966 Dermatomyositis (systemic angiopathy) of childhood. Medicine 45: 261–289

Baron M, Small P 1985 Polymyositis/Dermatomyositis: clinical features and outcome in 22 patients. Journal of Rheumatology 12: 283–286

Bates D, Stevens J C, Hudgson P 1973 'Polymyositis' with involvement of facial and distal musculature. Journal of the Neurological Sciences 19: 105–108

Behan W M H, Behan P O, Dick H 1978 HLA-B8 in polymyositis. New England Journal of Medicine 298: 1260–1261

Benbassat J, Geffel D, Zlotnick A 1980 Epidemiology of polymyositis-dermatomyositis in Israel, 1960–76. Israel Journal of Medical Sciences 16: 197–200

Benbassat J, Geffel D, Larholt K, Sukenik S, Morgenstern V, Zlotnick A 1985 Prognostic factors in polymyositis/dermatomyositis. Arthritis and Rheumatism 28: 249–255

Berger R G, Hadler N M 1983 Treatment of calcinosis universalis secondary to dermatomyositis or scleroderma with low dose warfarin (Abstract). Arthritis and Rheumatism 26: 511

Bernstein R M, Morgan S H, Chapman J 1984 Anti-Jo-l antibody: a marker for myositis with interstitial lung disease. British Medical Journal 289: 151–152

Bharucha N E, Morgan-Hughes J A 1981 Chronic focal polymyositis in the adult. Journal of Neurology, Neurosurgery and Psychiatry 44: 419–425

Bohan A, Peter J B 1975 Polymyositis and dermatomyositis. New England Journal of Medicine 292: 344–347, 403–407

Bohan A, Peter J B, Bowman R L, Pearson C M 1977 A computer-assisted analysis of 153 patients with polymyositis and dermatomyositis. Medicine (Baltimore) 56: 255–286

Bradley W G, Hudgson P, Gardner-Medwin D, Walton J N 1973 The syndrome of myosclerosis. Journal of Neurology, Neurosurgery and Psychiatry 36: 651–660

Brown M, Swift T R, Spies S M 1976 Radioisotope scanning in inflammatory muscle disease. Neurology (Minneapolis) 26: 517–520

Bullen C L, Younge B R 1982 Chronic orbital myositis. Archives of Ophthalmology 100: 1749–1751

Bunch T W, Tancredi R G, Lie J T 1981 Pulmonary hypertension in polymyositis. Chest 79: 105–107

Callen J P 1984 Myositis and malignancy. Clinics in Rheumatic Diseases 10: 117–130

Cambridge G, Stern C M M 1981 The uptake of tritium-labelled carnitine by monolayer cultures of human fetal muscle and its potential as a label in cytotoxicity studies. Clinical and Experimental Immunology 44: 211–219

Carpenter S, Karpati G, Rothman S, Watters G 1976 The childhood type of dermatomyositis. Neurology 26: 952–962

Carpenter S, Karpati G, Heller I, Eisen A 1978 Inclusion body myositis: a distinct variety of idiopathic inflammatory myopathy. Neurology 28: 8–17

Carpenter S, Karpati G 1981 The major inflammatory myopathies of unknown cause. Pathology Annual 16: 205–237

Carroll J E, Silverman A, Isobe Y, Brown W R, Kelts K A, Brooke M H 1976 Inflammatory myopathy, IgA deficiency and intestinal malabsorption. Journal of Pediatrics 89:216

Chad D, Good P, Adelman L, Bradley W G, Mills J 1982 Inclusion body myositis associated with Sjögren's syndrome. Archives of Neurology 39: 186–188

Chiedozi L C 1979 Pyomyositis. Review of 205 cases in 112 patients. American Journal of Surgery 137: 255–259

Christensen M L, Pachman L M, Maryjowski M C, Friedman J M 1983 Antibody to Coxsackie-B virus: increased incidence in sera from children with recently diagnosed juvenile dermatomyositis. (Abstract) Arthritis and Rheumatism 26: S24

Clements P J, First D E, Campion D S et al 1978 Muscle disease in progressive systemic sclerosis. Diagnostic and therapeutic considerations. Arthritis and Rheumatism 21: 62–71

Cook C D, Rosen F S, Banker B Q 1963 Dermatomyositis and focal scleroderma. Pediatric Clinics of North America 10: 979–1016

Crowe W E, Bove K E, Levinson J E, Hilton P K 1982 Clinical and pathogenic implications of histopathology in childhood polydermatomyositis. Arthritis and Rheumatism 25: 126–139

Cumming W J K, Weiser R, Teoh R, Hudgson P, Walton J N 1977 Localised nodular myositis: a clinical and pathological variant of polymyositis. Quarterly Journal of Medicine 46: 531–546

Danon M J, Reyes M G, Perurena O H, Masdeu J C, Manaligod J R 1982 Inclusion body myositis. Archives of Neurology 39; 760–764

Dau P C 1981 Plasmapheresis in idiopathic inflammatory myopathies. Archives of Neurology 38: 544–552

Denman A M 1984 Aetiology. Clinics in Rheumatic Diseases 10: 9–33

DeVivo D C 1978 Reye syndrome: a metabolic response to an acute mitochondrial insult. Neurology (NY) 28: 105–107

Doyle D R, McCurley T L, Sergent J S 1983 Fatal polymyositis in D-penicillamine-treated rheumatoid arthritis. Annals of Internal Medicine 98: 327–330

Eisen A Berry K, Gibson G 1983 Inclusion body myositis (IBM): myopathy or neuropathy? Neurology (Cleveland) 33: 1109–1114

Engel A G, Biesecker G 1982 Complement activation in muscle fibre necrosis: demonstration of the membrane attack complex of complement in necrotic fibres. Annals of Neurology 12: 289–296

Engel W K, Lighter A S, Galdi A P 1981 Polymyositis: remarkable response to total body irradiation (letter). Lancet 1: 658

Enzinger F M, Dulcey F P 1967 Proliferative myositis. Report of 33 cases. Cancer 20: 2213–2223

Farrell M K, Partin J C, Bove K E 1980 Epidemic influenza myopathy in Cincinnati in 1977. Journal of Pediatrics 96: 545–551

Fergusson R J, Davidson N M, Nuki G, Crompton G K 1983 Dermatomyositis and rapidly progressive fibrosing alveolitis. Thorax 38: 71–72

Fisher T J, Rachelefsky G S, Klein R B et al 1979 Childhood dermatomyositis and polymyositis. Treatment with methotrexate and prednisone. American Journal of Diseases of Childhood. 133: 386–389

Foote R A, Kimbrough S M, Stevens J C 1982 Lupus myositis. Muscle and Nerve 5: 65–68

Frazier A R, Miller R D 1974 Interstitial pneumonitis in association with polymyositis and dermatomyositis. Chest 65: 403–407

Garlepp W J, Dawkins R L 1984 Immunological aspects. Clinics in Rheumatic Diseases 10: 35–51

Gibson R K, Rosenthal S J, Lukert B P 1984 Pyomyositis. Increasing recognition in temperate climates. American Journal of Medicine 77: 768–772

Giorno R, Barden M T, Kohler P F, Ringel S P 1984 Immunohistochemical characterization of the mononuclear cell infiltrating muscle of patients with inflammatory and non-inflammatory myopathies. Clinical Immunology and Immunopathology 30: 405–412

Glynn L E 1984 Histopathology. Clinics in Rheumatic Diseases 10: 53–73

Gotoff S P, Smith R D, Sugar O 1972 Dermatomyositis with cerebral vasculitis in a patient with agammaglobulinaemia. American Journal of Diseases of Children 123: 53–56

Gottdiener J S, Sherber H S, Hawley R J et al 1978 Cardiac manifestations in polymyositis. American Journal of Cardiology 41: 1141–1149

Greco T P, Askanase P W, Kashgarian M 1977 Postviral myositis: myxovirus-like structures in affected muscle. Annals of Internal Medicine 86: 193–194

Grimson B S, Simons K B 1983 Orbital inflammation, myositis and systemic lupus erythematosus. Archives of Ophthalmology 101: 736–738

Gutmann L, Govindan S, Riggs J E, Schochet S S 1985 Inclusion body myositis and Sjögren's syndrome. Archives of Neurology 42: 1021–1022

Harati Y, Bergman E W, Niakan E 1984 Postviral childhood dermatomyositis in monozygotic twins. Neurology 34 (suppl 1): 289

Harriman D G F, Currie S 1974 A propos des neuromyosites. In: Serratrice G, Roux H, Recordier A M (eds) Troisièmes Journées Internationales de Pathologie Neuromusculaire. Masson, Paris, p 138–140

Haslock D I, Wright V, Harriman D G F 1970 Neuromuscular disorders in rheumatoid arthritis. A motor point muscle biopsy study. Quarterly Journal of Medicine 39: 335–358

Haupt H M, Hutchins G M 1982 The heart and conduction system in polymyositis-dermatomyositis: a clinicopathological study of 16 autopsied patients. American Journal of Cardiology 50: 998–1006

Heffner R R, Armbrustmacher V W, Earle K M 1977 Focal myositis. Cancer 40: 301–306

Henriksson K G 1979 'Semi-open' muscle biopsy technique. A simple outpatient procedure. Acta Neurologica Scandinavica 59: 317–323

Henriksson K G, Stålberg E 1978 The terminal innervation pattern in polymyositis: a histochemical and SFEMG study. Muscle and Nerve 1 (1): 3–13

Hewlett R H, Brownell B 1975 Granulomatous myopathy: Its relationship to sarcoidosis and polymyositis. Journal of Neurology, Neurosurgery and Psychiatry 30: 1090–1099

Hirsch T J, Enlow R W, Bias W B, Arnett F C 1981 HLA-D related (DR) antigens in various forms of myositis. Human Immunology 3: 181–186

Hoffman G S, Franck W A, Raddatz D A 1983 Presentation, treatment and prognosis of idiopathic inflammatory muscle disease in a rural hospital. American Journal of Medicine 75: 433–438

Hollinrake K 1969 Polymyositis presenting as distal muscle weakness. A case report. Journal of the Neurological Sciences 8: 479–484

Hubbard W N, Walport M J, Halnan K E, Beaney R P, Hughes G R V 1982 Remission from polymyositis after total body irradiation. British Medical Journal 284: 1915–1916

Hudson P, Peter J B 1984 Classification. Clinics in Rheumatic Diseases 10: 3–8

Isenberg D A 1983 Immunoglobulin deposition in skeletal muscle in primary muscle disease. Quarterly Journal of Medicine 52: 297–310

Isenberg D 1984 Myositis in other connective tissue disorders. Clinics in Rheumatic Diseases 10: 151–174

Isenberg D A, Snaith M L 1981 Muscle disease in systemic lupus erythematosus: a study of its nature, frequency and cause. Journal of Rheumatology 8: 917–924

Isenberg D A, McKeran R O 1982 A study of vascular permeability in normal skeletal muscle and inflammatory myopathies using a fluorescent dye technique with percutaneous needle biopsy. Journal of the Neurological Sciences 53: 423–431

Itoh J, Akiguchi I, Midorikawa R, Kameyama M 1980 Sarcoid myopathy with typical rash of dermatomyositis. Neurology (NY) 30: 1118–1121

Jacob H, Berkowitz D, McDonald E, Bernstein L H, Beneventano T 1983 The esophageal motility disorder of polymyositis. A prospective study. Archives of Internal Medicine 143: 2262–2264

Jehn U W, Fink M K 1980 Myositis, myoglobinemia, and myoglobinuria associated with entero-virus echo 9 infection. Archives of Neurology 37: 457–458

Johns T R, Crowley W J, Miller J Q, Campa J F 1971 The syndrome of myasthenia and polymyositis with comments on therapy. Annals of the New York Academy of Sciences 183: 64–71

Josselson J, Pula T, Sadler J H 1980 Acute rhabdomyolysis associated with an echovirus 9 infection. Archives of Internal Medicine 140: 1671–1672

Judge D M, McGlynn T J, Abt A B, Luderer J R, Ward S P 1977 Immunologic myopathy: Linear IgG deposition and fulminant terminal episode. Archives of Pathology 101: 362

Julien J, Vital C I, Vallat J M et al 1982 Inclusion body myositis. Journal of the Neurological Sciences 55: 15–24

Kagen L J 1977 Myoglobinemia in inflammatory myopathies. Journal of the American Medical Association 237: 1448–1452

Kagen L J 1984 Less common causes of myositis. Clinics in Rheumatic Diseases 10: 175–187

Kagen L J, Kimball A C, Christian C L 1974 Serologic evidence of toxoplasmosis among patients with polymyositis. American Journal of Medicine 56: 186–191

Kallen P, Nies K M, Louie J S et al 1982 Tropical pyomyositis. Arthritis and Rheumatism 25: 107–110

Kelly J J, Madoc-Jones H, Adelman L R, Munsat T L 1984 Treatment of refractory polymyositis with total body irradiation (abstract). Neurology (Cleveland) 34 (suppl 1): 80

Kim R C, Collins G H 1980 The neuropathology of rheumatoid disease. Human Pathology 12: 5–15

Kiprov D D, Miller R G 1984 Polymyositis associated with monoclonal gammopathy. Lancet 2: 1183–1186

Kressell B, Szewczyk C, Tuazon C 1978 Early clinical recognition of disseminated candidiasis by muscle and skin biopsy. Archives of Internal Medicine 138: 429–433

Lambie J A, Duff I F 1963 Familial occurrence of dermatomyositis. Case reports and a family survey. Annals of Internal Medicine 59: 839

Landry M, Winkelmann R K 1972 Tubular cytoplasmic inclusion in dermatomyositis. Mayo Clinic Proceedings 47: 479–492

Lane R J M, Fulthorpe J J, Hudgson P 1985 Inclusion body myositis: a case with associated collagen vascular disease responding to treatment. Journal of Neurology, Neurosurgery and Psychiatry 48: 270–273

Layzer R B, Shearn M A, Satya-Murti S 1977 Eosinophilic polymyositis. Annals of Neurology 1: 65–71

Leddy J P, Griggs R C, Klemperer M R, Franks M M 1975 Hereditary complement (C₂) deficiency with dermatomyositis. American Journal of Medicine 58: 83–91

Lederman H M, Winkelstein J A 1983 Congenital agammaglobulinemia (Cay): the clinical course of 88 patients (Abstract). Pediatric Research 17: 25YA

Lewkonia R M, Buxton P H 1973 Myositis in father and daughter. Journal of Neurology, Neurosurgery and Psychiatry 36: 820

Lian J B, Pachman L M, Gundberg C M, Maryjowski M C 1982 Gammacarboxyglutamate excretion and calcinosis in juvenile dermatomyositis. Arthritis and Rheumatism 25: 1094–1100

Ludwig I, Tomsak R L 1983 Acute recurrent orbital myositis. Journal of Clinical Neuroophthalmology 3: 41–47

McKinlay I A, Mitchell I 1976 Transient acute myositis in childhood. Archives of Disease in Childhood 51: 135–137

Manchul L A, Jin A, Pritchard K I et al 1985 The frequency of malignant neoplasms in patients with polymyositis-dermatomyositis. Archives of Internal Medicine 145: 1835–1839

Mastaglia F L, Ojeda V J 1985 Inflammatory myopathies. Annals of Neurology 17: 215–277, 317–323

Mathews M B, Bernstein R M 1983 Myositis autoantibody inhibits histidyl-tRNA synthetase: a model for autoimmunity. Nature 304: 177–179

Mease P J, Ochs H D, Wedgwood R J 1981 Successful treatment of echo virus meningoencephalitis and myositis-fasciitis with intravenous immune globulin therapy in a patient with X-linked agammaglobulinemia. New England Journal of Medicine 304: 1278–1281

Mease P J, Ochs H D, Corey L, Dragavon J, Wedgwood R J 1985 Echovirus encephalitis/myositis in X-linked agammaglobulinemia. New England Journal of Medicine 313: 758

Mechler F 1974 Changing electromyographic findings during chronic course of polymyositis. Journal of the Neurological Sciences 23: 237–242

Medsger T A, Dawson W N, Masi A T 1970 The epidemiology of polymyositis. American Journal of Medicine 48: 715–723

Mejlszenkier J D, Safran A E, Healy J J 1973 The myositis of influenza. Archives of Neurology 29: 441–443

Ménard D B, Haddad H, Blain et al 1976 Granulomatous myositis and myopathy associated with Crohn's disease. New England Journal of Medicine 295: 818–819

Messina C, Bonnano N, Baldari S, Vita G 1982 Muscle uptake of 99 m technetium pyrophosphate in patients with neuromuscular disorders. A quantitative study. Journal of the Neurological Sciences 53: 1–7

Mikol J, Felten-Papaiconomou A, Ferchal F et al 1982 Inclusion body myositis: clinicopathological studies and isolation of an adenovirus type 2 from muscle biopsy specimen. Annals of Neurology 11: 576–581

Mohr P D, Knowlson T G 1977 Quadriceps myositis: an appraisal of the diagnostic criteria of quadriceps myopathy. Postgraduate Medical Journal 53: 757–760

Morgan S H, Bernstein R M, Hughes G R V 1985 Intractable polymyositis: prolonged remission induced by total body irradiation. Journal of the Royal Society of Medicine 78: 496–497

Namba T, Brunner N G, Grob D 1974 Idiopathic giant cell polymyositis. Archives of Neurology 31: 27–30

Niakan E, Pitner S E, Whitaker J N, Bertorini T E 1980 Immunosuppressive agents in corticosteroid-refractory childhood dermatomyositis. Neurology (NY) 30: 286–291

Nishikai M, Reichlin M 1977 Radioimmunoassay of serum myoglobin in polymyositis and other conditions. Arthritis and Rheumatism 20: 1514–1518

Pachman L M, Cooke N 1980 Juvenile dermatomyositis: a clinical and immunologic study. Journal of Pediatrics 96: 226–234

Pachman L M, Maryjowski M C 1984 Juvenile dermatomyositis and polymyositis. Clinics in Rheumatic Diseases 10: 95–115

Pavlides N A, Karsh J, Moutsopoulos H M 1982 The clinical picture of primary Sjögren's syndrome: a retrospective study. Journal of Rheumatology 9: 685–690

Pittsley R A, Shearn M A, Kaufman L 1978 Acute hepatitis B simulating dermatomyositis. Journal of the American Medical Association 239:959

Rechavia E, Rotenberg Z, Fuchs J, Strasberg B 1985 Polymyositis heart disease. Chest 88: 309–311

Reichlin M, Arnett F C 1984 Multiplicity of antibodies in myositis sera. Arthritis and Rheumatism 27: 1150–1156

Riggs J E, Schochet S S, Gutman L et al 1984 Inclusion body myositis and chronic immune thrombocytopenia. Archives of Neurology 41: 93–95

Ringel S P, Forstot J Z, Tan E M et al 1982 Sjögren's syndrome and polymyositis or dermatomyositis. Archives of Neurology 39: 157–173

Rodnan G P 1979 Progressive systemic sclerosis. In: McCarty D J (ed) Arthritis and allied conditions, 9th edn. Lea & Febiger, Philadelphia, p 770–771

Rose A L, Walton J N 1966 Polymyositis: A survey of 89 cases with particular reference to treatment and prognosis. Brain 89: 747–768

Rosen F S 1974 The primary immunodeficiency. Pediatric Clinics of North America 21: 533–549

Rowe D J, Isenberg D A, McDougall J, Beverley P C L 1981 Characterization of polymyositis infiltrates using monoclonal antibodies to human leucocyte antigens. Clinical and Experimental Immunology 45: 290–298

Rowland L P, Greer M 1961 Toxoplasmic polymyositis. Neurology (Minneapolis) 11: 367

Ruff R L, Secrist D 1982 Viral studies in benign acute childhood myositis. Archives of Neurology 39: 261–263

Schiraldi E, Iandolo E 1978 Polymyositis accompanying Coxsackie Virus B2 infection. Infection 6: 32–34

Schlech W F III, Moulton P, Kaiser A B 1981 Pyomyositis:

tropical disease in a temperate climate. American Journal of Medicine 71: 900–902

Schwartz H A, Slavin G, Ward P, Ansell B M 1980 Muscle biopsy in polymyositis and dermatomyositis: clinicopathological study. Annals in Rheumatic Disease 39: 500–507

Schwartz M S, Swash M, Gross M 1978 Benign postinfection polymyositis. British Medical Journal ii: 1256–1257

Serratrice G, Pellissier J F, Cros D et al 1980 Relapsing eosinophilic perimyositis. Journal of Rheumatology 7: 199–205

Sharp G C, Irvin W S, Tan E M et al 1972 Mixed connective tissue disease — apparently distinct rheumatic disease syndrome associated with a specific antibody to an extractable nuclear antigen (ENA). American Journal of Medicine 52: 148–159.

Sibrans D F, Holley H L 1967 Vacuolar myopathy in a patient with a positive LE cell preparation. Arthritis and Rheumatism 10: 141–146

Simon D B, Ringel S P, Sufit R L 1982 Clinical spectrum of fascial inflammation. Muscle and Nerve 5: 525–537

Sloan M F, Franks A J, Exley K E, Davison A M 1978 Acute renal failure due to polymyositis. British Medical Journal 1: 1457

Solomon S D, Maurer K H 1983 Association of dermatomyositis and dysgerminoma in a 16-year-old patient. Arthritis and Rheumatism 26: 572–573

Spoor T C, Hartel W C 1983 Orbital myositis. Journal of Clinical Neuroophthalmology 3: 67–74

Stark R J 1979 Eosinophilic polymyositis. Archives of Neurology 36: 721–722

Strongwater S L, Annesley T, Schnitzer T J 1983 Myocardial involvement in polymyositis. Journal of Rheumatology 10: 459–463

Swartz M O, Silver R M 1984 D-Penicillamine induced polymyositis in juvenile chronic arthritis. Report of a case. Journal of Rheumatology 11: 251

Tang T T, Sedmak G V, Siegesmund K A, McCreadie S R 1975 Chronic myopathy associated with Coxsackie virus Type A9. A combined electron microscopical and viral isolation study. New England Journal of Medicine 292: 608–611

Travers R L, Hughes G R V, Cambridge G, Sewell J R 1977 Coxsackie B neutralization titres in polymyositis/dermatomyositis. Lancet i: 1268

Tsokos G C, Moutsopoulos H M, Steinberg A 1981 Muscle involvement in systemic lupus erythematosus. Journal of the American Medical Association 246: 766–768

Vasilescu C, Bucur G, Petrovici A, Florescu A 1978 Myasthenia in patients with dermatomyositis. Clinical, electrophysiological and ultrastructural studies. Journal of the Neurological Sciences 38: 129–144

Venables G S, Bates D, Cartlidge N E F, Hudgson P 1982 Acute polymyositis with subcutaneous oedema. Journal of the Neurological Sciences 55: 161–164

Walker G L, Mastaglia F L, Roberts D F 1982 A search for genetic influence in idiopathic inflammatory myopathy. Acta Neurologica Scandinavica 66: 432–443

Wallace D J, Metzger A L, White K K 1985 Combination immunosuppressive treatment of steroid-resistant dermatomyositis/polymyositis. Arthritis and Rheumatism 28: 590–592

Webster A D B 1984 Echovirus disease in hypogammaglobulinaemic patients. Clinics in Rheumatic Diseases 10: 189–203

Webster A D B, Tripp J H, Hayward A R et al 1978 Echovirus encephalitis and myositis in primary immunoglobulin deficiency. Archives of Disease in Childhood 53: 33

Wells A D, Fletcher M S, Teare E L, Walters H L, Yates-Bell A J 1985 Clostridial myositis of the psoas complicating nephrostomy. British Journal of Surgery 72: 582

West S G, Killian P J, Lawless O J 1981 Association of myositis and myocarditis in progressive systemic sclerosis. Arthritis and Rheumatism 24: 662–667

Whitaker J N, Engel W K 1972 Vascular deposits of immunoglobulin and complement in idiopathic inflammatory myopathy. New England Journal of Medicine 286: 333–338

Wright J, Conchonnai G, Hodges G R 1979 Adenovirus type 21 infection: concurrence with pneumonia, rhabdomyolysis and myoglobinuria in an adult. Journal of the American Medical Association 242: 2120–2121

Yates D A H 1976 Myositis as a complication of rheumatoid disease. In: Eberl R, Rosenthal M (eds) Organic manifestations and complications in rheumatoid arthritis. F K Schattauer, Stuttgart

Yonker R A, Panush R S 1985 Idiopathic eosinophilic myositis with pre-existing fibromyalgia. Journal of Rheumatology 12: 165–167

Yoshida A, Akizuki M, Mimori T et al 1983 The precipitating antibody to an acidic nuclear protein antigen, the Jo-l, in connective tissue diseases. A marker for a subset of polymyositis with interstitial pulmonary fibrosis. Arthritis and Rheumatism 26: 604–611

Involvement of human muscle by parasites

INTRODUCTION

A large body of data concerning parasitic involvement of human muscle is available to workers in tropical medicine and related fields. In this review we have attempted to summarise this information, emphasising features — both clinical and pathological — of relevance to neurological practice.

Muscle lesions (of varying severity and clinical relevance) are encountered in at least four protozoal diseases of man (toxoplasmosis, sarcosporidiosis, African and American trypanosomiasis). The larval stages of the life cycle of at least five cestodes (tapeworms) may develop in human muscle and result in conditions known as cysticercosis, coenurosis, unilocular and alveolar hydatidosis, and sparganosis. Finally the larvae of various nematodes may be found in muscle, causing diseases such as trichinosis and toxocariasis. In the following short accounts of these conditions parasitological and epidemiological data are kept to a minimum, and the clinical accounts emphasise muscle involvement. The parasitic disorders which may affect muscle are summarised in Table 18.1.

PROTOZOAL DISORDERS

Sarcosporidiosis and toxoplasmosis

Protozoal parasites of the class Sporozoasida may be found in the striated muscle of many mammals and some birds. They have occasionally been reported in man. They are given the generic name *Sarcocystis*. The muscle lesions are known as sarcocysts. *Sarcocystis* and certain species of *Isos-*

Table 18.1 Some clinical and pathological features of parasitic involvement of human muscle[1]

Parasite	Refs.	[2]Disease	Weakness	Wasting	Pain	Tenderness	Nodules	Local mass	Diffuse enlargement	Cardiac muscle involvement	Systemic illness	Calcification in muscle	Parasites in muscle fibres	Parasites between fibres	Diffuse inflammatory change	Abscesses	Inflammatory cell aggregates without parasites	'Tracks' in muscle	Involvement of central nervous system	Comments
1. Protozoa																				
Toxoplasma gondii	1–5	Toxoplasmosis	o	o	o	o	o	o	o	+	+	o	+	o	+	o	+	o	+	Possible relation to polymyositis
Sarcocystis lindemanni	6–11	Sarcosporidiosis	[±]	[±]	[±]	[±]	+	o	o	+	o	o	+	o	+	o	+	o	o	Sarcocysts. Possible relation to polymyositis
Trypanosoma gambiense	12–16	African trypanosomiasis	+	+	o	o	o	o	o	+	+	o	o	o	+	o	+	o	+	Not known in what proportions terminal weakness and wasting are 'myopathic', 'neuropathic' or 'cachectic'
Trypanosoma cruzi	17–18	American trypanosomiasis (Chagas' disease)	o	o	o	o	o	o	o	+	+	o	+	o	+	o	+	o	+	Leishmanial phase in muscle 'pseudocysts'
2. Cestodes																				
Taenia solium	19–25	Cysticercosis	[±]	[±]	[±]	[±]	+	o	[++]	+	[±]	+	o	+	[±]	o	[±]	o	+	Occasional weakness, pain and tenderness (in pseudohypertrophic type only)
Multiceps brauni	26–30	Coenurosis of muscle	o	o	o	o	o	+	o	o	o	o	o	+	[±]	o	[+]	o	o	Cerebral coenurosis is due to a different species (*M. multiceps*)
Echinococcus granulosus	31–37	Unilocular hydatidosis	o	o	[+]	o	o	+	o	+	+	+	+	+	o	o	[+]	o	+	Rupture may cause severe pain and oedema

																Comments
Echinococcus multilocularis	38–40	Alveolar hydatidosis	o	o	[+]	[+]	o	[+]	o	–	[+]	[+]	–	o	+	No capsule. Locally invasive. May metastasise
Spirometra mansonoides	41–46	Sparganosis	o	o	+	+	o	o	o	o	+	+	+	o		Local mass may be mobile
3. Nematodes *Trichinella spiralis*	47–55	Trichinosis	[++]	o	[+]	+	++	++	o	+	[+]	++	o	+		Profuse fibrillation (intracellular parasite 'denervates' part of muscle fibre). Calcification, visible microscopically, *not visible radiologically*
Toxocara canis *Toxocara cati*	56–58	Toxocariasis (visceral larva migrans)	o	o	[±]	[+]	o	o	o	o	+	+	+	+		Possible relation to 'eosinophilic myositis'
Ascaris lumbricoides, A. sui, A. devosi, A. columnaris, Neoascaris vitulorum, Parascaris equorum, Toxascaris leonina, T. transfuga	59–60	? Visceral larva migrans	o	o	o	o	o	o	o	+	o	+	[+]	o		Doubtful involvement of nervous system (? coincidental toxocariasis)

[1]Decreasing degrees of severity are indicated on a scale ranging from ++ to ±. Absence of a feature is shown by o. Parentheses indicate that a particular feature has occasionally been reported. The absence of a symbol implies that information was not available to us.

[2]*References* (Key references are italicised).
[1]Faust et al 1975. [2]Frenkel 1973. [3]**Kagan et al 1974.** [4]**Rabinowicz 1971.** [5]Samuels & Rietschel 1976. [6]Dastur & Iyer 1955. [7]Kean & Breslau 1964. [8]*Jeffery 1974.* [9]Liu & Roberts 1965. [10]Markus et al 1974. [11]McGill & Goodbody 1957. [12]Goodwin 1970. [13]Janssen et al 1956. [14]Koten & de Raadt 1969. [15]Losos & Idede 1972. [16]*Poltera et al 1977.* [17]Faust et al 1970. [18]*Köberle 1968.* [19]Dixon & Lipscomb 1961. [20]Jacob & Mathew 1968. [21]Jolly & Pallis 1971. [22]*MacArthur 1950.* [23]McGill 1948. [24]Sawhney et al 1976. [25]Slais 1970. [26]Fain 1956. [27]Orihel et al 1970. [28]Raper & Dockeray 1956. [29]*Templeton 1968.* [30]Wilson et al 1972. [31]Arana-Iñiguez 1978. [32]Blanco et al 1949. [33]*Dew 1951.* [34]*Dévé 1949.* [35]*Dew 1951.* [36]Lorenzetti 1962. [37]Pearson & Rose 1960. [38]*Abuladze 1964.* [39]Hunter et al 1976. [40]Schimrigk & Emser 1978. [41]Ali-Khan et al 1973. [42]Cho & Patel 1978. [43]*Mueller et al 1963.* [44]Muller 1975. [45]*Wirth & Farrow 1961.* [46]Brashear et al 1971. [47]Brashear et al 1971. [48]Davis et al 1976. [49]Despommier et al 1975. [50]Drachman & Tuncbay 1965. [51]Gould 1954. [52]*Gould 1970.* [53]Gross & Ochoa 1979. [54]Marcus &Miller 1955. [55]Stoll 1947. [56]Beaver et al 1952. [57]*Dent et al 1956.* [58]Woodruff 1970. [59]Nichols 1956. [60]Sprent 1965.

pora are probably different stages in the life cycle of the same parasite.

Carnivorism is important in the transmission of this infection. It is believed that the life cycle involves two vertebrate hosts: a 'prey' (ungulates, rodents, birds, etc.) and a 'predator' (dog, cat, cheetah, etc.). The prey is infected by eating sporocysts passed in the faeces of the predator. Asexual multiplication takes place in the lymphoid cells of the prey. When predator eats prey, sexual reproduction of the parasite takes place in the intestinal submucosa of the predator and free sporocysts are discharged into the lumen of the gut. There is thus a biologically intriguing alternation of generations in two different vertebrate hosts. Man's fate is sometimes to act as an *Isospora*-passing predator, sometimes as a sarcocyst-ridden prey. The sporocysts most

readily available to modern man for ingestion are probably those in his own faeces.

Sarcocysts are cylindrical bodies, usually 400–1000 μm in length and about 100 μm in diameter. They are sometimes much longer and may then be visible to the naked eye as minute white threads. *Sarcocystis lindemanii* (the species found in man) may produce cysts 5 cm long. These cylindrical structures (sometimes referred to as Miescher's tubes) have a hyaline, radially striated limiting membrane, from which septa arise (Fig. 18.1). These divide the tube into compartments containing round, oval or sickle-shaped bodies, 12–16 μm long and 4–10 μm wide, called sporozoites or 'Rainey's corpuscles'. Microscopic calcification may occur (Greve 1985), but this is never radiologically evident.

The only other parasite forming morphologi-

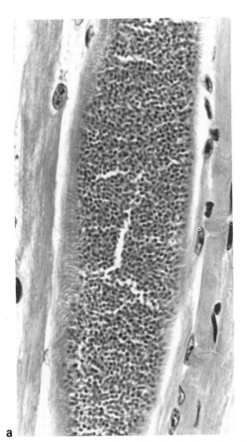 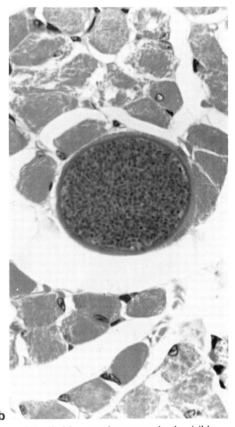

Fig. 18.1 Sarcocysts in muscle. a. Longitudinal section. Radial striations of the limiting membrane are clearly visible. b. Transverse section. H & E ×600

cally similar structures in human muscle is *Toxoplasma gondii*. Differentiation is based on the length and diameter of the cysts (smaller in toxoplasmosis), on the thickness and striations of the capsule, on the division of the cyst by septa, and on the size of the sporozoites (more than twice as large in sarcosporidiosis).

Patients have occasionally presented with features conceivably related to the presence of parasites in muscle. Thus Liu & Roberts (1965) described a patient with a chronic, painful, indurated area of the chest wall. This was excised and showed sarcocysts, surrounded by areas of lymphocytic and eosinophilic cellular infiltration, giant cells and interstitial fibrosis. Jeffery (1974) reviewed the whole subject of human sarcosporidiosis in some detail. His report included the description of a 21-year-old Gurkha soldier presenting with a painful lump in the thigh. Necrotic muscle tissue was evacuated and sarcocysts were found in an area of relatively unaffected muscle taken from the periphery of the lesion.

Rarely sarcosporidiosis is found in association with other disease (see e.g. McGill & Goodbody 1957, Agarwal & Srivastava 1983). However the weight of evidence suggests coincidence rather than any causal relationship, and that human sarcosporidiosis is generally an asymptomatic disorder.

African trypanosomiasis

African trypanosomiasis is transmitted by the 'bite' of tsetse flies of the genus *Glossina*. These act as biological vectors: part of the life cycle of the parasite takes place in their tissues.

The trypanosomes (*T. rhodesiense* and *T. gambiense*) multiply in the gut of the fly, but do not involve cells. Crithidial forms metamorphose into metacyclic (infective) trypanosomes. It is this form which is 'injected' when man is 'bitten'.

Myositis is a feature of trypanosomal infections in rats (Losos & Idede 1972). Patients with African trypanosomiasis may show gross muscle wasting, but it remains uncertain to what extent this is 'cachectic' in origin (many patients dying of this disease have concomitant illnesses such as tuberculosis). It is possible, however, that the wasting may be due, at times, to primary changes in muscle (perhaps immunologically induced). Occasionally it may be of neurogenic origin. Examination of skeletal muscle has very seldom been carried out. Lesions of the spinal roots have been reported (Janssen et al 1956, Poltera et al 1977). In the otherwise very detailed study by the last-named group of workers, systematic investigation of skeletal muscle was undertaken in only one instance, samples being obtained from the upper and lower limbs, the recti abdominis and the diaphragm. The striated muscles showed atrophic fibres, sometimes accompanied by a patchy chronic cellular infiltration. There were eosinophilic degenerative changes of variable severity. The changes were most marked in the diaphragm. The illustrated appearance was not that of neural atrophy. Further studies are needed in this field.

American trypanosomiasis

American trypanosomiasis (caused by *Trypanosoma cruzi*) is transmitted through the infected faeces, deposited on human skin, of several species of reduviid or triatomine bugs which 'bite' and defaecate after feeding. Opossums, armadillos, wood and water rats and raccoons act as natural reservoirs. The spread of the disease to man is related to the adaptation of the vector bugs to living and breeding in and around primitive rural habitations. Man himself then becomes an important reservoir host.

Many infections are clinically silent. Swelling is an early local response to the inoculation of infective material and may characteristically involve one eye and one side of the face. There may be generalised lymphadenopathy, fever and malaise. Trypanosomal forms of the parasite are present in the blood during this stage.

The parasites show a predilection for cells of neuroectodermal or mesenchymal origin (cardiac and skeletal muscle, and lymphoid cells). There may be early myocarditis or meningoencephalitis. In infected cells the organism goes into a leishmanial phase (unlike what happens in African trypanosomiasis). The *Leishmania* multiply by binary fission, distend the cell, and produce a leishmanial pseudocyst. Cyst rupture releases crithidial and further trypanosomal forms which re-enter the circulation causing febrile relapses. Death of intracellular *Leishmania* produces an inflammatory reaction, which may be severe in non-immune individuals.

Skeletal muscle involvement may be florid although it is usually asymptomatic. Chronic myocarditis is common. Chronic Chagas' disease is a late complication of American trypanosomiasis. It is characterised by megacolon and megaoesophagus, brought about by lesions of the intrinsic autonomic innervation of the gastrointestinal tract. Pathogenetic mechanisms are still poorly understood.

CESTODES

Cysticercosis

Man is the only definitive host of the cestodes *Taenia solium* and *Taenia saginata*. Ripe proglottids are shed in human faeces. The released ova are consumed by an intermediate host. The pig (occasionally sheep, bears, cats, dogs and monkeys) has this role in the *T. solium* cycle. Various bovidae are involved in the life cycle of *T. saginata*.

The embryos, freed in the gut of the intermediate host, burrow through the intestinal mucosa and are widely distributed through mesenteric venules and lymphatic channels, to skeletal and cardiac muscle, the nervous system and other tissues where, within two to three months, they develop into infective bladder worms or cysticerci. The larval forms of *T. solium* and *T. saginata* are known respectively as *Cysticercus cellulosae* and *Cysticercus bovis*. These forms were recognised and named before their relationship to their parent worms was recognised. The pseudo-generic names have no taxonomic significance.

When parasitised undercooked pork or beef is eaten by man, the scolex (head) of the cysticercus evaginates like the finger of a glove and becomes attached to the gut wall. The human host then develops an adult tapeworm, *not* cysticercosis. The point needs emphasising as it is still widely misunderstood.

Probably the only way in which man can contract *cysticercosis* is by doing what the pig normally does, i.e. by eating *T. solium* ova (his own or someone else's — usually the latter). It should be noted, that, for reasons that are poorly understood, the ingestion by man of the ova of *T. saginata* hardly ever produces cysticercosis.

T. solium taeniasis has virtually disappeared from Europe. The same has happened in many other places. In the Middle East, Muslim Africa, and Indonesia it was always a very rare or non-existent condition because of religious practices which forbid the consumption of pork. Human cysticercosis continues to occur, however, in India, Mongolia, Korea, China, Central and South America and South Africa (Slais 1970).

Muscle involvement. Involvement of the central nervous system in cysticercosis is very common and will not be further discussed. Involvement of skeletal muscle has been known since the condition was first recognised. In early accounts it was thought to be rare, but it is now known to be common. There was positive evidence of such invasion in 429 of the 450 cases of cysticercosis surveyed by Dixon & Lipscomb (1961). The morbid anatomy of the condition is well described in standard textbooks and articles (MacArthur 1950, Trelles & Trelles 1978 and notably by Slais 1970).

Pseudohypertrophic myopathy. Although it had been described earlier, pseudohypertrophic myopathy in cysticercosis was first drawn to the attention of neurologists by Jacob & Mathew in 1968. In 1971 Jolly & Pallis reviewed seven of the previously reported cases and described two of their own. Since then, further cases have been reported, and it is now possible to describe the clinical and pathological features of this interesting condition in more detail.

All but one of the 16 cases of muscular pseudohypertrophy shown by biopsy to be due to cysticercosis have been reported from India. The main features are summarised in Table 18.2. Eleven males and five females have been affected, their ages ranging from 10 to 45 years.

The thighs, calves, glutei and shoulder girdles are, as a rule, massively enlarged, the patients

Table 18.2 Summary of clinical and laboratory findings in reported cases of pseudohypertrophic myopathy due to cysticercosis

Authors	Year	Cases reported	Sex	Age	Identifiable initial illness	Weakness	Pain	Tenderness	Subcutaneous nodules	Tongue involvement	Eye involvement	Heart involvement	CNS involvement	Calcified muscle cysts	Ova in stool or history of taeniasis	EMG	CPK	Eosinophila
Priest	1926	1	M	24	+	+	+I	+	+	0	+	+	+	NI	0	0	0	+
McRobert	1944	1	M	25	0	0	0	0	+	0	0	NI	+	0	0	0	0	+
McGill	1947,	2	M	25	0	++	0	0	+	+	0	NI	+	0	0	0	0	+
	1948*		M	20	+	++ (calves)	I	0	+	+	0	NI	0	? scolices only	0	0	0	0
Singh & Jolly	1957	1	F	22	0	0	0	±	+	0	papillitis	NI	+	0	0	0	0	+
Prakash & Kumar	1965	1	M	14	0	0	0	+	+	+	0	Abnormal ECG	+	? scolices only	+	0	0	+
Jacob & Mathew	1968	1	M	30	0	±	0	±	+	+	+	0	+	0	0	NI	NI	+
Armbrust-Figueiredo et al	1970	1	F	35	+	+	I	0	0	0	0	Cardiac failure	+	0	+	NI	NI	0
Jolly & Pallis	1971	2**	M	22	0	0	0	0	0	+	+	Abnormal ECG	+	0	0	0	0	NI
Rao et al	1972	1	M	25	0	0	0	0	+	+	0	0	+	0	0	0	0	NI
Salgoakar & Watcha	1974	1	M	10	+	0	0	0	+	+	0	0	0	0	0	NI	NI	0
			M	11	+	±	0	0	+	+	proptosis; swollen disc	0	+	0	0	N	N	+
Vigg & Rai	1975	2	F	45	0	+	++	++	+	+	0	0	+	0	0	0	0	+
			F	35	+	±	±	NI	+	0	0	0	+	0	0	0	0	+
Sawhney et al	1976	1	F	24	0	+	+	0	+	0	+	Non-specific T wave changes	+	NI	NI	Abnormal	N	+
Vijayan et al	1977	1	M	17	0	+	0	0	+	+	+	NI	+	0	0	0	0	NI

* Same cases described in two communications
** Cases 3 and 4

I = Initial muscle pain
NI = No information

often being described as having developed a 'Herculean' appearance (Fig. 18.2). The nuchal musculature, erector spinae, masseters and forearm muscles may be notably involved. The pseudohypertrophy is invariably bilateral and symmetrical.

The enlarged muscles are usually firm. There may be slight overlying oedema. No individual nodules can usually be felt, probably because the muscles are so tightly packed with cysticerci. The nodules may occasionally be felt on contraction.

In six instances there was no detectable weakness in the enlarged muscles. In seven cases there was mild to moderate, predominantly proximal paresis, and in one case paresis seems to have been confined to the calf musculature. Two patients

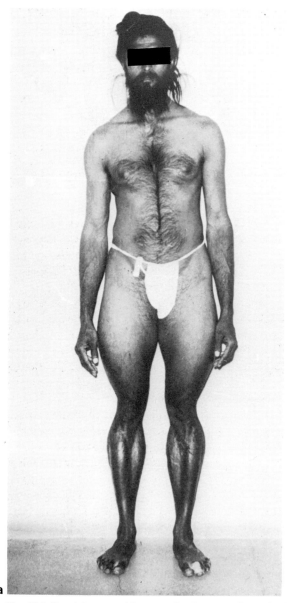
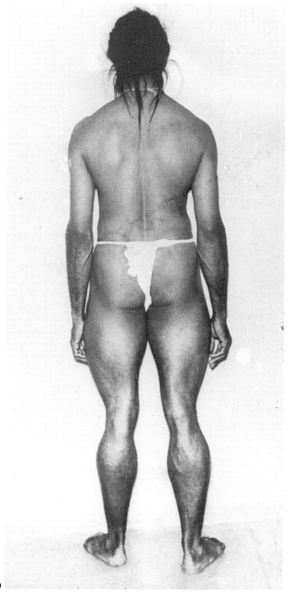

a

b

Fig. 18.2 Pseudohypertrophic myopathy due to cysticercosis (Reproduced from Jolly & Pallis (1971) with kind permission of the authors, editor and publisher)

were described as very weak. In no case was power increased in a manner commensurate with muscle bulk.

Muscle pain was experienced before the onset of the pseudohypertrophy in several instances, but at the time of presentation was seldom a prominent feature. In most patients the muscular enlargement had been entirely painless throughout the whole of its course. Definite muscle tenderness was elicited in two of the 16 cases and in a further two slight tenderness may have been present.

The muscle enlargement had come on insidiously in all cases, over a period varying from a few weeks to 18 months or more. In six instances an initial illness could be identified, often consisting of fever, pain in the limbs and occasionally urticaria or pruritus. In some cases muscular enlargement had been noted within two or three weeks of such an illness.

In 14 of the 16 patients, muscular enlargement had occurred in a context of palpable subcutaneous nodules, i.e. of clinically obvious cysticercosis. Lingual cysticerci were seen in no fewer than 10 instances and ocular cysticerci in two. Two patients had evidence of cardiac failure and a further three had abnormal electrocardiograms. There was evidence of involvement of the nervous system in 14 instances (usually epilepsy, but occasionally mental change or a focal neurological deficit). Calcification of the parasites in muscle was encountered only twice and seemed to be early (i.e. confined to the scolices).

Muscle biopsy will reveal numerous tense cysts, 1 cm or more in length (Fig. 18.3). The muscle fibres are not hypertrophied. Regions in the immediate vicinity of the cysticerci occasionally show variable cellular infiltration with polymorphs, lymphocytes, plasma cells and/or eosinophils, and occasional degenerative changes and areas of focal fibrosis. Sawhney et al (1976), however, illustrated changes 'not in continuity with the inflammatory reaction seen around the cysts'. These consisted of swollen muscle fibres with loss of cross-striation and central migration of nuclei. Their finding implied, they thought, 'an affection of the muscle fibres per se in the disease process'. They did not report, however, on the appearances of sections of muscle from above and below the affected areas. We believe that as likely

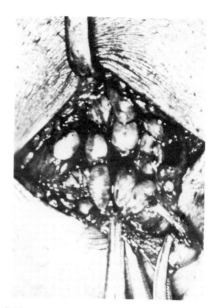

Fig. 18.3 Numerous tense cysticerci, presenting at the biopsy site in gastrocnemius muscle (case of Prakash & Kumar 1965 reproduced with kind permission of the authors, editor and publisher)

an explanation for their observations is the phenomenon reported by Drachman & Tuncbay (1965) — in cases of obvious trichinosis — to account for 'extensive myositis without trichinae'.

Electromyography was used in such cases by Salgaokar & Watcha (1974) who reported normal findings in the proximal muscle groups of their patient. Sawhney et al (1976) reported motor units 'averaging' 300–800 μV and 4–8 ms in duration, 10–15% of which were polyphasic. They interpreted these findings as indicative of myopathy.

We believe muscle enlargement in cysticercosis to be related to larval death, not to the initial dissemination. The cysts found in such cases are invariably very tense and never contain viable parasites. Very little is known of the natural history of the disorder but there is evidence to suggest that it may be a spontaneously reversible condition.

Treatment. Intestinal taeniasis, if present, should be treated. Drug-induced larval death, and the subsequent appearance of further tense cysts, may for a while aggravate the pseudohypertrophy.

The new pyrazino-isoquinoline anthelminthic

praziquantel is clinically effective against a wide spectrum of cestode and trematode infections in animals and humans (Andrews et al 1983, Pearson & Guerrant 1983). At low concentrations the drug paralyses adult worms, causing them to loosen their attachment to host tissues. At higher concentrations it produces vesiculation of the tegument of susceptible parasites (including the larval form of *T. solium*) and release of the contents of the parasite with activation of host defence mechanisms and eventual destruction of the worms. Massive cysticercosis of muscle should be treated cautiously, for the abrupt destruction of large numbers of larvae and the associated oedema may have deleterious effects, particularly if the nervous system is also massively involved. The use of biphasic courses of dexamethasone and praziquantel has been described by de Ghetaldi et al (1983). The dose of praziquantel used was 50 mg/kg/day (given in three divided doses) for 14 days. The use of prolonged high-dose praziquantel therapy for human cysticercosis is still under investigation (Sotelo et al 1984).

Coenurosis

The word coenurus refers to the polycephalous larval form of certain taeniid worms of the genus *Multiceps*, the adults of which inhabit the intestine of dogs and other canidae. The term is descriptive and has no taxonomic significance.

On farm or field, herbivorous mammals may swallow the ova passed by dogs infected by *Multiceps multiceps*. The embryos burrow through the intestinal mucosa and disseminate widely. Affected sheep may develop a neurological disorder known as 'staggers'. Other possible intermediate hosts include rabbits, wild rodents, certain monkeys and — occasionally — man, in whom cerebral symptoms may also be prominent. The cycle is completed when dogs gain access to infected sheep tissue.

In parts of tropical Africa where *M. multiceps* seems to be very rare the taeniid *M. brauni* is found in the gut of the domestic dog, fox and jackal, the usual intermediate hosts being wild rodents or porcupines. Cases of human coenurosis reported from such areas all seem to have shown predominant subcutaneous or muscle involvement.

Coenuri are glistening, globular or ovoid unilocular cysts, each containing several scolices which seem to bud from the inner surface of the cyst wall. The cysts vary in size from that of an almond to that of an apricot. They are usually filled with a milky, gelatinous fluid. They contain neither brood capsules nor daughter cysts. They are surrounded by an adventitious capsule derived from the host, composed of dense collagenous fibrous tissue infiltrated with plasma cells, lymphocytes and occasional histiocytes and eosinophils.

A coenurus is one of the causes of a palpable, occasionally slightly tender, 'tumour' in muscle. The 'tumour' is usually solitary and — in muscle — almost invariably unilocular. The vast majority occur on the trunk. The intercostal and anterior abdominal muscles are favourite sites (Templeton 1971). Coenuri may also be found in the neck, in relation to the sternomastoid or trapezius muscles.

The preoperative diagnosis is usually fibroma or lipoma. When the excised 'tumour' is cut across, and the multiple scolices are revealed in the cyst, macroscopic diagnosis should be obvious.

Hydatidosis

The two canid tapeworms (*Echinococcus granulosus* and *Echinococcus multilocularis*) may cause hydatid disease in man. Muscle involvement has been reported with both types of infection.

Ova of *E. granulosus*, discharged in dogs' faeces, are ingested by the intermediate host (usually sheep but occasionally goats, cattle, pigs, wild herbivores or man). After hatching, the embryos penetrate the venules of the intestinal wall and become established in the liver. If they can get beyond the hepatic circulation they lodge in the lungs. A small proportion may reach other tissues such as muscle or bone. The natural cycle is completed when dogs eat ovine offal. In echinococcosis due to *E. multilocularis*, the natural reservoir is in foxes, although dogs and cats may also harbour the parent tapeworm. The usual intermediate hosts are wild rodents. Man may become infected by consuming fruit and vegetables contaminated by the excreta of foxes.

The classic morphological appearance of hydatid cysts due to *E. granulosus* is well described in standard textbooks and will not be recapitulated. Unlike the large single cysts produced by this tapeworm the larval stage of *E. multilocularis* consists of a honeycomb-like aggregate in innumerable small cysts. There is no proper limiting capsule. The lesion may look like the cut surface of a slice of bread. It may have a necrotic centre, resembling an abscess. It behaves locally like an invasive tumour and true metastases may occur.

In sheep-rearing countries, where hydatidosis is common, hydatid disease of muscle is not rare. Muscle is in fact the third most frequent site (after liver and lung) in which cysts may be found. Over 5% of cases of human hydatid disease may show lesions of muscle (Dévé 1949, Dew 1951). Goinard & Salasc (1931) reported a personal series of 33 cases.

The initial lesion probably occurs within an individual muscle fibre (Dévé 1936). Only about one-third of muscle hydatids contain viable scolices. They are most commonly encountered in the paravertebral gutters and in the limb-girdle musculature, particularly in the thigh. They are rare distally.

In many parts of the world a hydatid is the commonest cause of a benign muscle tumour. Physical examination will reveal a deep, slowly growing, poorly mobile, spherical or lobulated mass, of variable size and firm consistency. The exact shape of the tumour will often be influenced by adjacent bone and limiting fascia. Pain is rare, although patients may complain of a dull ache in the relevant muscle after use. A hydatid 'thrill' can seldom be elicited. The lesion may occasionally calcify. Secondary infection of hydatids is not uncommon. The condition may then present as an abscess.

Hydatids in muscle cause neither weakness nor tenderness. The occurrence of myotonia in three out of five members of a family with evidence of muscle involvement due to *E. multilocularis* (Schimrigk & Emser 1978) was probably fortuitous. The family was thought to be suffering from myotonia congenita.

Sparganosis

The term sparganosis refers to the extra-intestinal infection of vertebrate hosts by the plerocercoid larvae (or spargana) of pseudophyllidean (diphyllobothriid) tapeworms of the genus *Spirometra*. These tapeworms are related to *D. latum* (well known to haematologists and neurologists as an occasional cause of vitamin B_{12} deficiency) but differ in that they cannot complete their life cycle and develop their adult form in man. Two intermediate hosts are needed: the first a copepod crustacean, the second a vertebrate.

The adult worms live in the gut of carnivores. In the Far East '*Spirometra mansoni*' is a common intestinal parasite of dogs and cats. In the United States *Spirometra mansonoides* has been found in bobcats, occasionally in domestic cats and — more rarely — in dogs.

Infected carnivores pass mature proglottids. The ova hatch in ponds or streams, liberating a ciliated coracidium. The coracidia are swallowed by water-fleas of the genus *Cyclops* in whose haemocoele they mature, becoming procercoid larvae. When such larvae are then eaten by frogs, lizards, snakes, birds or small mammals the procercoid larva is liberated in the gut of the vertebrate host, penetrates the intestinal wall and is distributed to the tissues, where it matures to a migrating, plerocercoid larva.

In the USA, natural paratenic (carrier) hosts include mice, rhesus monkeys, water snakes and the pig, raccoon and opossum. In Korea various species of snake have been incriminated. Unlike *Diphyllobothrium*, the plerocercoids are not found in fish. It is only when the paratenic host is consumed by the definitive (carnivore) host that the life cycle is completed and that an adult tapeworm can again develop.

Man can become infected in one of four ways:
(1) by the accidental ingestion of procercoid-infected copepods (as in drinking unboiled, unfiltered, infected water). The procercoid will then penetrate the human gut and become a plerocercoid;
(2) by eating the infected, uncooked, plerocercoid-containing flesh of frogs, snakes or certain fish, for purposes of nutrition or — more often in parts of South East Asia — as a 'tonic'. The plerocercoid is then transmitted from one paratenic (carrier) host to another. It remains a plerocercoid however, for the adult worm cannot develop in man;
(3) through eating uncooked pork (Becklund 1962, Corkum 1966). Spargana are known to develop in pigs allowed to forage in woodland areas, where they may become infected through

the ingestion of snakes, frogs or small mammals infected with plerocercoids — or through drinking water from ponds containing infected copepods;

(4) by using the raw flesh of plerocercoid-infected 'split frogs' or snakes as poultices. The practice, long prevalent in Thailand and Vietnam, of dressing ulcers, wounds or infected eyes with such poultices doubtless accounted for many cases of ocular sparganosis.

Clinical features. In ocular sparganosis there is often an intense inflammatory reaction with periorbital oedema. Retrobulbar lesions produce lagophthalmos and the threat of corneal ulceration. The early phases of infection by the gastro-intestinal route are usually asymptomatic. In soft tissues the clinical features vary. The usual presentation is as a slightly fluctuant subcutaneous or superficial intramuscular lump, about 5 cm in diameter, often suspected of being a lipoma. Occasionally the lump presents with signs of inflammation. A characteristic although uncommon feature is the tendency of the lumps to move slowly downwards, over several weeks or months — as correctly observed by many patients and repeatedly doubted at first interview by many doctors.

Involved muscles have included the rectus abdominis, thigh muscles, pectoralis major and calf muscles. In many cases, other parts of the body will have been involved, although from the descriptions it is not always clear whether the lesions were entirely subcutaneous or could have extended deeper. In a given lesion there is usually a single, viable larva.

A case in which a live sparganum was extracted from the biceps muscle was reported by Ali-Khan et al (1973). Cho & Patel (1978) report a case in which the parasite, deep in the right thigh, was surrounded by granulomatous tissue showing a striking histological similarity to the nodules of rheumatoid arthritis. The length of the excised parasite may lead to misdiagnosis of guinea-worm (dracunculiasis).

NEMATODES

Trichinosis

The larvae of *Trichinella spiralis* may be found in the muscles of many facultative or obligatory carnivores. Natural infection is readily transmitted between species — or by cannibalism within a given species.

Trichinosis, among carnivores, is world-wide, its distribution independent of climate. It is encountered from equatorial to arctic regions. The prevalence of human trichinosis, on the other hand, is patchy and deeply influenced by cultural factors.

Human infection takes place through eating parasitised ('measly') pork in the form of raw or undercooked sausage, smoked ham or pickled trotters — or more exotic foods such as boar or bear meat. (Pigs are infected by eating infected rats, or by being fed uncooked swill containing, inter alia, the offal of other pigs.)

After ingestion of infected meat, viable larvae are released and pass into the duodenum and jejunum where, after moulting, they very rapidly develop into adult worms. The male dies after copulation but the viviparous female (which may reach a size of 4 mm) burrows into the intestinal mucosa and starts producing larvae within a week of ingestion. During the next two or three weeks each female may produce over a thousand 'second-generation larvae' which enter the systemic circulation (via the lymphatics and the right side of the heart) and seed into many tissues.

In striated muscle the larvae penetrate the sarcolemma and grow until after 16 days they reach a length of 800–1000 μm and a width of 30 μm. They show no preference for any particular fibre type (Ochoa & Pallis 1980) (Fig. 18.4). Three weeks after penetration they have increased their length tenfold, becoming coiled in the process (Fig. 18.5). An ellipsoidal collagenous capsule about 500 μm long and 250 μm wide is formed by the muscle cell around the coiled-up larvae. It takes about three months for this capsule to develop fully. Although widely distributed, the larvae seem to encyst in this manner in striated muscle only. Encysted larvae may remain viable for many years. Calcification may begin within 6–9 months. Following death of the trichinae some cysts may be completely resorbed. The penetration of a striated muscle fibre by a larva results in the destruction both of the penetrated fibre and of some adjacent ones.

The extraocular muscles, masseters, diaphragm, muscles of the tongue, larynx and neck, intercos-

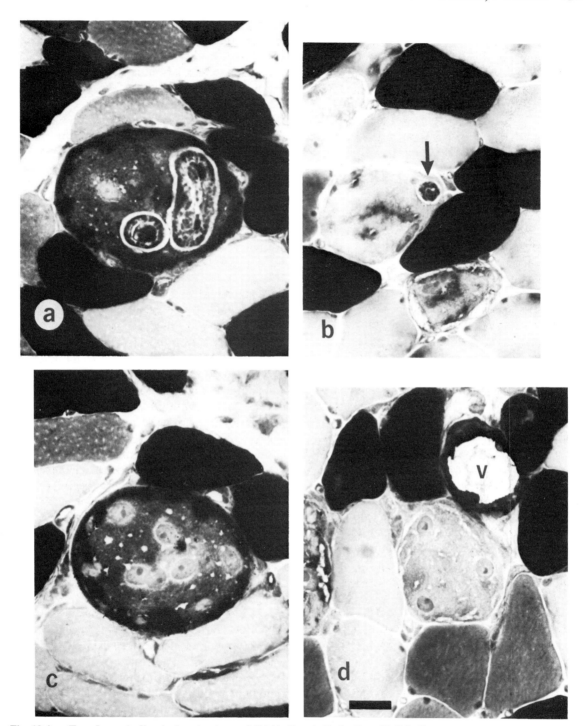

Fig. 18.4 a. Type I muscle fibre harbouring larva of *Trichinella spiralis*. b. Type II (A?) fibre cut across parasite (arrowed). c. Distended type I fibre with reactive nuclei, probably cut close to a parasite. d. Type II (A?) fibre showing similar changes to those in the fibre in (c)

ATPase pH 4.6: Black = Type I   Common Bar = 25 μm
               White = Type IIA   V = blood vessel
               Intermediate = Type IIB

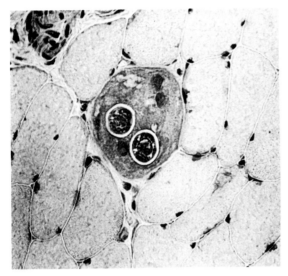

Fig. 18.5 Muscle fibre containing slightly coiled larva of *Trichinella spiralis*, cut across twice

tals and deltoid are most heavily involved. In some epidemics parasitisation predominated in diaphragm, calves and forearm muscles. Sites of attachment to tendons are particularly prone to be affected.

Many infections are asymptomatic, with diaphragm counts of less than 10 larvae per gram. Muscular symptoms probably arise when the larval count reaches 100 per gram. One patient (Davis et al 1976) survived a deltoid concentration of 4000 larvae per gram. Fatal cases, according to Gould (1970) may carry up to 100 million larvae to the grave with them. A worm's eye view of the human connection could only be depressing, for this massive parasitisation of man is clearly a demographic dead-end.

Clinical features. The first diagnostically helpful sign is often periorbital oedema. The whole face may be grotesquely bloated. Patients may be misdiagnosed as suffering from angio-neurotic oedema or even from renal disease. There may be chemosis, a widespread facial erythema and subconjunctival haemorrhages. Patients may present to ophthalmologists with complaints of conjunctivitis or of pain in one or both eyeballs often related to eye movement. The combination of severe photophobia, fever and headache may lead to misdiagnoses of meningitis. Diagnosis may

be very difficult as there may be neck stiffness, probably from myositis of the nuchal musculature. A macular rash, more persistent than that of typhoid, is seen in 10% of cases. Subungual 'splinters' and retinal haemorrhages are not uncommon.

Myalgia is an early and common complaint, although often preceded by fever and by periorbital oedema. Involvement of the ocular muscles, masseters and tongue leaves its imprint on the symptomatology. Masticatory difficulties or even trismus may occur. Oedema of the tongue and pharyngeal muscles may cause dysphagia. The calves and forearms are usually painful. Lumbar pains may be excruciating. Myalgia reaches its height during the third week of the illness, seldom extending into the fourth or fifth weeks.

The involved muscles may be patchily tender but the most striking feature is undoubtedly their weakness. In part, this is a genuine paresis. But there is also a considerable reluctance to move, any movement tending to produce 'tension pain' in both agonists and antagonists. Occasionally, the limb muscles may be grossly swollen. An 'oedematous' patient with puffy face, swollen legs and very tender muscles will almost certainly prove to have trichinosis.

The weakness may be extreme, patients rapidly becoming tetraplegic from muscle involvement. There is probably no other disorder of muscle, except periodic paralysis, in which such severe weakness develops in so short a time. The tendon reflexes may be impaired.

Calf pain may result in an early reluctance to stand, of a degree that would not be warranted by paresis or general prostration. Patients may attempt to remain ambulant by walking on their toes. When they take to bed, they tend to remain immobile. Early contractures may ensue.

Involvement of the central nervous system is well documented in the more massive infections. Its manifestations are protean and include stupor, frank meningitis, brain-stem involvement and various combinations of upper motor neurone and radicular signs. These are of variable pathogenesis (haemorrhage, vasculitis, oedema, granulomatous nodules). Larval embolisation into capillaries is encountered but is much less common than vasculitis. The marked response of neurological signs to steroid medication is probably related to these manifestations of hypersensitivity. Confusing symptoms may be encountered. Diplopia is more often than not of myopathic origin. Dyspnoea may be due to asthma, the pain of deep breathing, cardiac failure or ventilatory insufficiency of myopathic type. Misdiagnoses of poliomyelitis, polyneuritis and even myasthenia have been reported.

In severe cases the illness reaches its height in from two to four weeks. Paresis and asthenia may be protracted and convalescence delayed. In various epidemics of human trichinosis, 2–10% of recognised cases have proved fatal. Death usually results from non-specific myocarditis, pneumonia or encephalitis.

Electromyography. Marcus & Miller (1955) described a patient with widespread, severe trichinosis who exhibited 'the most profuse fibrillation of denervation the examiner had ever seen'. There was gross weakness and some wasting. Although the authors attributed the fibrillation, wasting and weakness to 'lower motor neurone changes' we believe a more likely mechanism is the one suggested to account for 'profuse spontaneous fibrillation in all muscles sampled' in the case described by Gross & Ochoa (1979). These authors incriminated 'disconnection of fragments of muscle fibres from their end-plate regions due to focal muscle necrosis'. The implications of such a mechanism are considerable. They might help in the electromyographic differentiation of those parasitic myopathies in which the parasites lie *within* muscle fibres from those in which the parasites lie *between* muscle fibres.

Treatment. The antihelminthic thiabendazole (2-(thiazolyl)-benzimidazole) was introduced into the therapy of human trichinosis in 1964. It also has a profound effect on larvae already in muscle, damaging or killing substantial numbers of them. The suggested intake is 50 mg/kg/day, taken in divided doses. Medication should be continued until symptoms subside or incapacitating side effects appear, but should not be continued for more than a week. Side effects include anorexia and various gastrointestinal upsets, slight dizziness, and occasionally, drowsiness.

Treatment of trichinosis with thiabendazole alone may result in a Herxheimer-like reaction. This is probably due to massive dissolution of larvae with abrupt release of protein-breakdown products into the circulation. Corticosteroids are therefore usually prescribed concurrently with — or even a little earlier than — thiabendazole. Such a regime would seem to associate the larvicidal effect of one drug, the immunosuppressive effect of the other and the combined anti-inflammatory effects of both.

Toxocariasis

Toxocara canis is a widely distributed ascarid of dogs, in which species its life cycle resembles that of *Ascaris lumbricoides* in man. Its ova are infective to man. *Toxocara cati* (a common feline ascarid) may also cause human toxocariasis.

Human toxocariasis occurs when ova, present in dog or cat faeces, get into the mouths of children, playing in yards or gardens. The ova hatch in the child's jejunum and the liberated larvae enter mesenteric venules or lymphatics. They are then carried to extraintestinal sites, usually the liver but sometimes to the lungs and even beyond: to brain, eye or muscle. The larvae may remain alive and actively motile in such tissues, boring their way in various directions.

Granulomatous lesions caused by larvae may be few or many, depending on the number of ingested eggs, and on the degree of sensitisation of the invaded host. In the liver they appear as subcapsular white nodules or plaques, 5–10 mm in diameter and easily visible to the naked eye. Lesions in human muscle are less numerous but may nevertheless be detected by the use of a hand lens (Dent et al 1956). Using a pepsin technique these workers recovered a mean of 5 larvae per gram of skeletal muscle in a child with toxocariasis who had died from a post-transfusion hepatitis. They suggested that the recovery of *Toxocara* larvae by this technique might be applied to muscle and liver biopsy specimens, as a diagnostic procedure in suspected cases. As far as we know, muscle biopsy has seldom been used for this purpose.

Florid disease is rare, the most usual presentation being a chronically ill child with an enlarged liver, pneumonitis and sustained eosinophilia. Muscle pain may occasionally be a feature (Hunter et al 1976).

Diagnostic procedures are reviewed by Woodruff (1970). The morphological differentiation of various larvae capable of causing visceral larva migrans is discussed in detail by Nichols (1956).

REFERENCES

Abuladze K I 1964 Alveococci as parasites in man. In: Taeniata of animals and man and diseases caused by them. Iztadel'stvo 'Nauka', Moscow (English version: Israel Program for Scientific translations, 1970, Jerusalem) p 379–383

Agarwal P K, Srivastava A N 1983 Sarcocystis in man: a report of two cases. Histopathology 7: 783–787

Ali-Khan Z, Irving R T, Wignall N, Bowmer E J 1973 Imported sparganosis in Canada. Canadian Medical Association Journal 108: 590–593

Andrews P, Thomas H, Pohlke R, Seubert J 1983 Praziquantel. Medical Research Review 3: 147–200

Arana-Iñiguez R 1978 Echinococcus. In: Vinken P J, Bruyn G W (eds) Handbook of clinical neurology Vol 35. North-Holland, Amsterdam, p 175–208

Armbrust-Figueiredo J, Speciali J G, Lison M P 1970 Forma miopatica da cisticercose. Arquivos de Neuropsiquiatria 28: 385–390

Beaver P C, Snyder C H, Carrera G M, Dent J H, Lafferty J W 1952 Chronic eosinophilia due to visceral larva migrans. Pediatrics 9: 7–19

Becklund W W 1962 Occurrence of a larval trematode (Diplostomatidae) in a larval cestode (Diphyllobothriidae) from Sus scrofa in Florida. Journal of Parasitology 48:286

Blanco A E, Mozador J L, Minetti R 1949 Los quistes hidatidicos musculares. Archivos internacionales de la Hidatidosis 9: 221–253

Brashear R E, Martin R R, Glover J L 1971 Trichinosis and respiratory failure. American Review of Respiratory Diseases 104: 245–249

Cho C, Patel S P 1978 Human sparganosis in Northern United States. New York State Journal of Medicine 78: 1456–1458

Corkum K C 1966 Sparganosis in some vertebrates in Louisiana and observations of a human infection. Journal of Parasitology 55: 444–448

Dastur D K, Iyer C G S 1955 Sarcocystis of human muscle. Bulletin of the Neurological Society of India 2: 25–27

Davis M J, Cilo M, Plaitakis A, Yahr M D 1976 Trichinosis: a severe myopathic involvement with recovery. Neurology (Minneapolis) 26: 37–40

De Ghetaldi L D, Norman R M, Douville A W 1983 Cerebral cysticercosis treated biphasically with dexamethasone and praziquantel. Annals of Internal Medicine 99: 170–181

Dent J H, Nichols R L, Beaver P C, Carrera G M, Staggers R J 1956 Visceral larva migrans with a case report. American Journal of Pathology 32: 777–803

Despommier D, Aron L, Turgeon L 1975 Trichinella spiralis: Growth of the intracellular (muscle) larva. Experimental Parasitology 37: 108–116

Dévé F 1936 Sur le siège initial des kystes hydatiques musculaires. Comptes rendus de la Société de Biologie 123: 764–765

Dévé F 1949 L'échinococcose primitive. Masson, Paris, p 79

Dew R H 1951 Hydatid disease. In: Lord Horder (ed)

British encyclopaedia of medical practice 2nd edn. Vol 4. Butterworth, London, p 587–614

Dixon H B F, Lipscomb F M 1961 Cysticercosis: an analysis and follow-up of 450 cases. In: Special report series. Medical Research Council, London

Drachman D A, Tuncbay T O 1965 The remote myopathy of trichinosis. Neurology (Minneapolis) 15: 1127–1135

Fain A 1956 Coenurus of Taenia brauni Setti parasitic in man and animals from the Belgian Congo and Ruanda-Urundi. Nature 178:1353

Faust E C, Russell P F, Jung R C 1970 Craig and Faust's clinical parasitology 8th edn. Lea and Febiger, Philadelphia

Faust E C, Beaver P C, Jung R C 1975 Animal agents and vectors of human disease 4th edn. Lea and Febiger, Philadelphia, p 92–96

Frenkel J K 1973 Toxoplasmosis: Parasite life cycle, pathology and immunology of toxoplasmosis. In: Hammond D M, Long P (eds) The Coccidia: Eimeria, Toxoplasma, Isospora and related genera. University Park Press, Baltimore, p 343–410

Goinard P, Salasc J 1931 Sur les kystes hydatiques des muscles voluntaires. Journal de Chirurgie 54: 320–331

Goodwin L G 1970 The pathology of African trypanosomiasis. Transactions of the Royal Society of Tropical Medicine and Hygiene 64: 797–812

Gould S E 1954 Eye and orbit in trichinosis. Bulletin of the New York Academy of Medicine 30: 726–729

Gould S E 1970 Trichinosis in man and animals. Thomas Springfield, Illinois, p 147–189

Greve E 1985 Sarcosporidiosis — an overlooked zoonosis. Danish Medical Bulletin 32: 228–230

Gross B, Ochoa J 1979 Trichinosis: A clinical report and histochemistry of muscle. Muscle and Nerve 2: 394–398

Hunter G W, Swatzwelder J C, Clyde D E 1976 Tropical Medicine 5th edn. Saunders, Philadelphia

Jacob J C, Mathew N T 1968 Pseudohypertrophic myopathy in cysticercosis. Neurology (Minneapolis) 18: 767–771

Janssen P, van Bogaert L, Haymaker W 1956 Pathology of the peripheral nervous system in African trypanosomiasis. Study of 7 cases. Journal of Neuropathology and Experimental Neurology 15: 269–287

Jeffery H C 1974 Sarcosporidiosis in man. Transactions of the Royal Society of Tropical Medicine and Hygiene 68: 17–29

Jolly S S, Pallis C 1971 Muscular pseudohypertrophy due to cysticercosis. Journal of the Neurological Sciences 12: 155–162

Kagan L J, Kimball A C, Christian C L 1974 Serologic evidence of toxoplasmosis among patients with polymyositis. American Journal of Medicine 56: 186–191

Kean B H, Breslau R C 1964 Cardiac sarcosporidiosis. In: Parasites of the human heart. Grune and Stratton, New York, p 74–83

Köberle F 1968 Chagas' disease and Chagas' syndromes: the

pathology of American trypanosomiasis. Advances in Parasitology 6: 63–116

Koten J W, de Raadt 1969 Myocarditis in Trypanosoma rhodesiense infections. Transactions of the Royal Society of Tropical Medicine and Hygiene 63: 485–489

Liu C T, Roberts L M 1965 Sarcosporidiosis in a Bantu woman. American Journal of Clinical Pathology 44: 639: 641

Lorenzetti L 1962 Contributo alla conoscenza dell'echinococcosi primitiva dei muscoli. Gazzetta internazionale di medicine e chirurgia 67: 2775–2795

Losos G J, Idede B O 1972 Review of pathology of diseases in domestic and laboratory animals caused by Trypanosoma congolense, T. vivax, T. brucei, T. rhodesiense and T. gambiense. Veterinary Pathology (Suppl) 9: 1–56

MacArthur W P 1950 In: Lord Horder (ed) British encyclopaedia of medical practice, Vol 4, 2nd edn. Butterworth, London, p 111

McGill R J 1947 Cysticercosis resembling a myopathy. Indian Journal of Medical Sciences 1: 109–114

McGill R J 1948 Cysticercosis resembling myopathy. Lancet 2: 728–730

McGill R J, Goodbody R A 1957 Sarcosporidiosis in man with periarteritis nodosa. British Medical Journal 2: 333–334

McRobert G R 1944 Somatic taeniasis (solium cysticercosis). Indian Medical Gazette 79: 399–400

Marcus S, Miller R V 1955 An atypical case of trichinosis with report of electromyographic findings. Annals of Internal Medicine 43: 615–622

Markus M B, Killick-Kendrick R, Garnham P C 1974 The coccidial nature and life-cycle of Sarcocystis. Journal of Tropical Medicine and Hygiene 77: 248–259

Mueller J F 1938 Studies on Sparganum mansonoides and Sparganum proliferum. American Journal of Tropical Medicine 18: 303–328

Mueller J F, Hart E P, Walsh W P 1963 Human sparganosis in the United States. Journal of Parasitology 48: 294–296

Muller R 1975 Worms and disease. Heinemann, London

Nichols R L 1956 The etiology of visceral larva migrans. II. Comparative larval morphology of Ascaris lumbricoides, Necator americanus, Strongyloides stercoralis and Ancylostoma caninum. Journal of Parasitology 42: 363–399

Ochoa, J, Pallis C 1980 Trichinella thrives in both oxidative and glycolytic human muscle fibres. Journal of Neurology, Neurosurgery and Psychiatry 43: 281–282

Orihel T C, Gonzales F, Beaver P C 1970 Coenurus from neck of Texas woman. American Journal of Tropical Medicine and Hygiene 19: 255–257

Pearson C M, Rose A S 1960 The inflammatory disorders of muscle. In: Adams R D, Eaton L M, Shy G M (eds) Neuromuscular disorders (the motor unit and its disorders), Vol 38. Williams and Wilkins, Baltimore, p 433

Pearson R D, Guerrant R L 1983 Praziquantel: Major advance in anthelminthic therapy. Annals of Internal Medicine 99: 195–198

Poltera A A, Owor R, Cox J N 1977 Pathological aspects of human African trypanosomiasis (HAT) in Uganda. A post-mortem study of 14 cases. Virchows Archiv A. Pathological Anatomy and Histology 373: 249–265

Prakash C, Kumar A 1965 Cysticercosis with taeniasis in a vegetarian. Journal of Tropical Medicine and Hygiene 68: 100–103

Priest R 1926 A case of extensive somatic dissemination of cysticercus cellulosae in man. British Medical Journal 2: 471–472

Rabinowicz J 1971 A case of acquired toxoplasmosis in the adult. In: Hentsch D (ed) Toxoplasmosis. Huber, Berne, p 197–219

Rao C M, Sattar S A, Gopal P S, Reddy C C M, Sadasivudu B 1972 Cysticercosis resembling myopathy. Report of a case. Indian Journal of Medical Sciences 26: 841–843

Raper A B, Dockeray G D 1956 Coenurus cysts in man: five cases from East Africa. Annals of Tropical Medicine and Parasitology 50: 121–128

Salgaokar S V, Watcha M F 1974 Muscular hypertrophy in cysticercosis: a case report. Journal of Postgraduate Medicine 20: 148–152

Samuels B S, Rietschel R L 1976 Polymyositis and toxoplasmosis. Journal of the American Medical Association 235: 60–61

Sawhney B B, Chopra J S, Banerji A K, Wahi P L 1976 Pseudohypertrophic myopathy in cysticercosis. Neurology (Minneapolis) 26: 270–272

Schimrigk K, Emser W 1978 Parasitic myositis caused by Echinococcus alveolaris. European Neurology 17: 1–7

Singh A, Jolly S S 1957 Cysticercosis: case report. Indian Journal of Medical Sciences 11: 98–100

Slais J 1970 The morphology and pathogenicity of bladder worms: Cysticercus cellulosae and Cysticercus bovis. Academia, Prague

Sotelo J, Escobedo F, Rodriguez-Carbajal, Torres B, Rubio-Donnadieu F 1984 Therapy of parenchymal brain cysticercosis with praziquantel. New England Journal of Medicine 310: 1001–1007

Sprent J F A 1965 Ascaridoid larva migrans: differentiation of larvae in tissues. Transactions of the Royal Society of Tropical Medicine and Hygiene 59: 365–366

Stoll N R 1947 This wormy world. Journal of Parasitology 33: 1–18

Templeton A C 1968 Human coenurus infection. A report of 14 cases from Uganda. Transactions of the Royal Society of Tropical Medicine and Hygiene 62: 251–255

Templeton A C 1971 Anatomical and geographical location of human coenurus infection. Tropical and Geographical Medicine 23: 105–108

Trelles J O, Trelles L 1978 In: Vinken P J, Bruyn G W (eds) Handbook of clinical neurology, Vol 35. North Holland, Amsterdam, p 291–320

Vigg B, Rai V 1975 Muscular involvement in cysticercosis with pseudo-hypertrophy of muscles. Journal of the Association of Physicians of India 23: 593–595

Vijayan G P, Venkataraman S, Suri M L, Seth H M, Hoon R S 1977 Neurological and related manifestations of cysticercosis. Tropical and Geographical Medicine 29: 271–278

Wilson C V L C, Wayte D M, Addae R O 1972 Human coenurosis: the first reported case from Ghana. Transactions of the Royal Society of Tropical Medicine and Hygiene 66: 611–623

Wirth W A, Farrow C C 1961 Human sparganosis. Case report and review of the subject. Journal of the American Medical Association 177: 6–9

Woodruff A W 1970 Toxocariasis. British Medical Journal 3: 663–669

Myasthenia gravis and related syndromes

HISTORICAL INTRODUCTION

Myasthenia gravis is a specific muscular disease characterised by the development of an abnormal amount of weakness in voluntary muscles following repetitive activation or prolonged tension, with a marked tendency to recovery of motor power after a period of inactivity or lessened muscular tension. Some authorities consider that a positive response to anticholinesterase drugs should also be included in the definition. It is important to agree on a definition because the literature contains many reports of cases of doubtful provenance. In particular, the term myasthenia has a less restricted meaning in the French language.

A case described by Thomas Willis (1672) is generally accepted as the first description of the disease. Later landmarks are the papers by Erb, Goldflam and Jolly in the nineteenth century (see Simpson 1983). The clinical picture was established by the review of Campbell & Bramwell (1900). Laquer & Weigert (1901) first noted a relationship with the thymus gland. Attention was concentrated on the concept of neuromuscular block by the demonstration by Walker (1934) of the beneficial effect of physostigmine. Twenty-five years of electrical and pharmacological studies ignored the pathogenesis until Simpson (1960) suggested that the link between thymus and muscle was immunological, with production of antibody against acetylcholine receptors (AChR) at the end-plates. The chance finding of Patrick & Lindstrom (1973) that animals used to raise antibody against acetylcholine receptor protein, purified from the electroplaques of the electric eel, became weak with an illness like myasthenia gravis, confirmed the feasibility of the mechanism. Since then this autoimmune hypothesis has been accepted and has become the rationale for modern treatment.

The molecular biology of nicotinic AChRs and of their ion channels is being disclosed, with clarification of the congenital myasthenias (Ch. 20). For a good review, see Engel (1984). Apart from showing that polyclonal antibodies are myasthenogenic only when they involve the main immunogenic region of the macromolecule (five subunits), detailed description has too little relevance to acquired myasthenia gravis to justify a full description here.

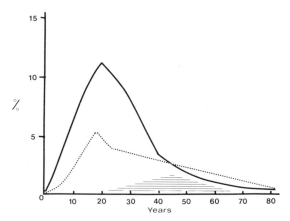

Fig. 19.1 Distribution of age at first myasthenic symptom: female, no thymoma ——————
male, no thymoma ················
thymoma, both sexes

NATURAL HISTORY

Myasthenia gravis affects all races. Estimates of prevalence range from 1 in 50 000 to 1 in 10 000 of the population. Females are affected twice as often as males, the disproportion being 4.5:1 in the first decade, but reversing in later life (Fig. 19.1). The modal age of onset is about 20 years for each sex but because of the different distribution curves the mean age is a little lower for women (26 years) than men (31 years) (Simpson 1958, 1960). These ages refer to patients without a thymoma. A thymic tumour (Fig. 19.2) is found in 10–15% of cases, about 60% of whom are male (Schwab & Leland 1953, Simpson 1958). Myasthenia associated with thymic tumour (benign or malignant) tends to appear at a later age and is rare under the age of 30 years. Muscular weakness is usually severe and difficult to control with any form of treatment, including thymectomy.

If the thymus is not removed the prognosis is worse for women, according to Simpson (1958). The opposite findings, noted by Grob (1958) may have been due to the higher incidence, in females, of the ocular type of myasthenia in his series.

Onset of symptoms is usually insidious but may be sudden, apparently precipitated by an emotional upset or a febrile illness and less commonly by physical exertion. Symptoms may first appear during pregnancy or the puerperium. If myasthenia is already present before pregnancy it tends to remit at the end of the first trimester

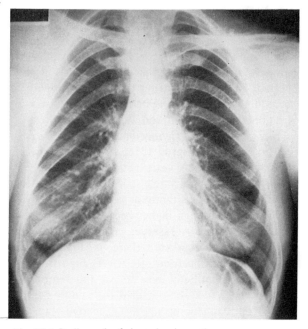

Fig. 19.2 Radiograph of chest showing a thymoma

and to relapse soon after childbirth, but this is not invariable. An abnormal response to a relaxant drug used during anaesthesia may be the first indication of myasthenia gravis or of one of the symptomatic myasthenias.

The initial symptom, especially if it is ptosis or diplopia, may subside for months or years, and later remissions may follow relapses. Remissions of more than a month occur in fewer than half of the cases, and usually only in the early years of the illness in patients treated without thymectomy or steroids, becoming less frequent and prolonged as time goes on. More than one long remission is uncommon, and if myasthenic symptoms return after an absence of a year or more and if muscles other than the extraocular are involved, the disease is usually progressive. Relapses are precipitated by the same factors as initial attacks, but additional causes are menstruation, extremes of cold or heat (especially a hot bath or a stuffy atmosphere), inoculation or vaccination and, occasionally, allergy. Bright sunlight may precipitate ptosis and blurred vision, and a few patients declare that it causes generalised weakness.

It is useful to divide the clinical course into three stages (Simpson 1969a). The clinical state is most labile during the first five to seven years (Stage 1). Although the most significant remissions occur in Stage 1, most of the deaths directly attributable to the disease occur in this period, particularly during the first year, with a second danger period at four to seven years, in progressive cases (Simpson 1958).

To be effective, thymectomy must be carried out in Stage 1 (Simpson 1958, 1960, Papatestas et al 1976). After 10 years (Stage 2) death from myasthenia per se rarely occurs, although the patient may be constantly at risk of asphyxiation from inhaled foreign bodies because of the diminished respiratory reserve. Although further progression is unlikely, there is little or no response to thymectomy. Relatively high titres of antireceptor antibody may persist and temporary improvement may be obtained from immunosuppressive treatment or plasma exchange, but the role of the thymus appears to be diminished. After 15 years or more, some cases enter Stage 3, with persisting weakness, a higher incidence of muscular atrophy, and a reduced response to anticholinesterase drugs. Steroids may still be beneficial in this 'burned out' stage, but thymectomy is of no value and other immunosuppressive regimes have not been assessed. Presumably, permanent morphological changes have occurred at the neuromuscular junctions.

Clinical staging, based on analysis of many cases, is of some value in selecting treatment but it remains difficult to prognosticate for the individual. Grading by 'severity' is less useful. The classification most commonly used (Osserman 1958) is as follows:

I Ocular myasthenia.

IIA Mild generalised myasthenia with slow progression; no crises; drug-responsive.

IIB Moderate generalised myasthenia; severe skeletal and bulbar involvement, but no crises; drug response is less satisfactory.

III Acute fulminating myasthenia; rapid progression of severe symptoms with respiratory crises and poor drug response; high incidence of thymoma; high mortality.

IV Late severe myasthenia; same as III, but takes two years to progress from Classes I or II; crises; high mortality.

These grades, reputed to be a progressive series from I, with good prognosis, to III and IV with poor prognosis, do not represent either discrete types or stages in a progression. It is a tautology to say that purely ocular myasthenia is 'safe' whereas weakness of respiratory muscles in a rapidly deteriorating disorder is dangerous to life. The future course cannot be predicted, although it is widely accepted that it is likely to be benign if signs remain confined to the extraocular muscles for two years. Grob (1953) and Ferguson et al (1955) report this type of history in 20–30% of cases, but it has been rare in my experience, except in males. Conversely, the prognosis is worse (with early death) if a thymoma is present, despite initial benefit from thymectomy.

SYMPTOMS AND SIGNS

The characteristic feature of myasthenia gravis is variability in the strength of affected muscles, rather than a generalised tiredness. It varies from day to day and even from hour to hour, classically increasing towards evening. Surprisingly, few patients comment on this until asked about it. It is not invariable: many patients are weakest on rising. Short-term weakness is often due to physical exertion but the emotional state is an important determinant. Affected muscles lose

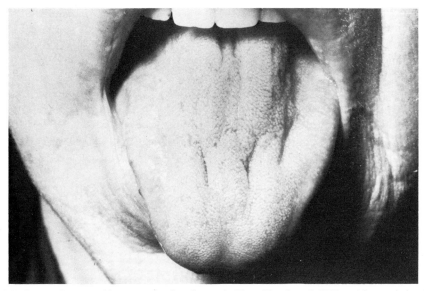

Fig. 19.3 The triple furrowed tongue (there may be four furrows). From Engel et al 1977a, with permission from the publishers

further strength if contraction is maintained or repeated (so-called 'pathological fatiguability'). The contracting muscle may lengthen gradually if it is supporting a load, or a coarse tremor develops with increasing 'rest periods' until the attempt to sustain the contraction ceases. In the eye muscles this may cause a pseudonystagmus. Gradual 'fatigue' is not always seen and failure of contraction may be sudden, suggesting neurotic weakness to the inexperienced. Recovery after rest is often incomplete, even with optimal anticholinesterase dosage, especially in Stage 2. In Stage 3, there may be weakness which cannot be reversed with these drugs, and muscular atrophy is not uncommon, especially in males (Simpson 1958). The most commonly affected muscles are the extraocular muscles, triceps brachii, quadriceps femoris, and the tongue. Atrophy of the tongue is curiously selective, often giving triple longitudinal furrowing (Fig. 19.3) which, though rare, is very characteristic of myasthenia gravis (Wilson 1954). It seems to have been first described by Buzzard in 1905.

The symptoms associated with weakness of ocular, facial, and other muscles are readily appreciated. The distribution of clinically weak muscles in a large series of cases is shown in Figure 19.4, which also shows that the probability

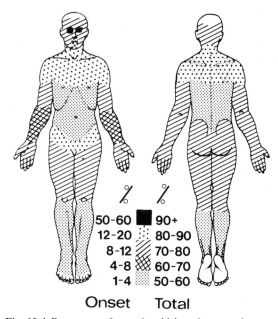

Fig. 19.4 Percentage of cases in which various muscle groups are affected at the onset (left of key) and at some time during the illness (right of key)

of weakness starting in a muscle group matches its overall probability of being involved. Without going into all possible variations, attention is drawn to the early and frequent involvement of the extraocular muscles and levatores palpebrarum (more than 90% of cases), usually associated with weakness of orbiculares oculorum, an almost diagnostic combination. The facies is characteristic (Fig. 19.5). Speech and chewing weakness, difficulty in holding up the head, and proximal limb weakness (more in the upper than the lower limbs) are typical. Fortunately, the chest muscles and diaphragm are not involved until later. Nevertheless, any muscle or part of a muscle may be affected and the distribution is commonly asymmetrical. When the history or physical examination suggests the possibility of myasthenia gravis, the most commonly affected muscles should be subjected to a fatigue test and the response to edrophonium assessed. Some appropriate tests for use in doubtful cases are described below, but usually an appropriate performance test is readily improvised during the consultation.

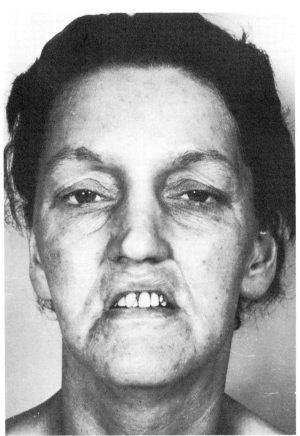

Fig. 19.5 The myasthenic 'snarl' and ptosis (from Engel et al 1977a with permission)

Tendon reflexes are surprisingly brisk and clonus may be present (but with a flexor plantar response). If a reflex is elicited repetitively, the jerk may decrease progressively until it disappears. Persistent absence of many tendon reflexes should suggest that weakness is due to carcinomatous myasthenia rather than to myasthenia gravis, but localised absence may be due to muscular atrophy. Differential diagnosis from the carcinomatous syndrome may be difficult because, in Stage 3, responsiveness to anticholinesterases is lost and some patients (usually men) find that muscle power is increased by exercise. Their muscles may show an incrementing response to tetanisation (Simpson 1966a, Schwartz & Stålberg 1975a, b).

Abnormalities of sensation

Normal sensation is the rule, although cases of myasthenia gravis have been reported with unexplained sensory loss, especially transitory trigeminal anaesthesia. Paraesthesiae of hands, thighs or face (Harvey 1948, Simpson 1960) and the common sensation of 'stiffness' probably have a mechanical explanation. Patients may complain of pain in weak muscles, especially in the neck, the back, and around the eyes. This is normally attributable to the extra effort required to maintain posture, but sometimes there appears to be a true myositis. Sudden substernal ache at the onset of the disease is an occasional and unexplained symptom.

Disorders of other organs

Disorders of the thyroid gland (including subclinical disease indicated by serum antibody studies) are more frequent in a myasthenic population but only a minority have abnormal thyroid function tests, and these patients are as commonly hypothyroid as hyperthyroid (Simpson 1966b, 1968). Millikan & Haines (1953) found that the incidence of hyperthyroidism before, during, or after detectable myasthenia gravis was about 5%. If all thyroid disorders are added, the incidence may be as high as 9% in males and 18% in females (Simpson 1958, Downes et al 1966). Many of these patients have thyrotoxic symptoms or signs for only a few months and these may precede myasthenic symptoms by many years. Thyrotoxic symptoms may be subsiding when myasthenia appears and vice versa. In a limited period of observation this may lead to the conclusion that the disorders have a 'see-saw' relationship to each other (McEachern & Parnell 1948).

It was clearly shown by Engel (1961) that myasthenia could not be caused by hyperthyroidism. The linkage between them is probably genetic and immunological rather than hormonal, and involves all non-tumour diseases of the thyroid including non-toxic goitre (Rowland et al 1956, Simpson, 1958, 1968, Bundey et al 1972), spontaneous myxoedema (Feinberg et al 1957, Sahay et al 1965), and Hashimoto's disease (Simpson 1960, 1964, 1966c, Becker et al 1964). Many myasthenics resemble thyrotoxic patients in other ways. Slight exophthalmos and thickening of the upper eyelids are common (Simpson 1960). The 'lid twitch sign' (transient upward overshoot of the upper eyelid on abruptly looking upwards, followed by a slower return to ptosis) described by Cogan (1965) is readily distinguished from thyrotoxic lid-lag. Many patients complain of excessive sweating, even without taking anticholinesterase drugs (Simpson 1960, Pirskanen 1976). There may also be a genetic as well as an immunological linkage between myasthenia gravis and other diseases. Primary adrenal insufficiency of autoimmune type is rare (Bosch et al 1978). An arthropathy resembling rheumatoid arthritis or ankylosing spondylitis is not uncommon in myasthenics or their relatives (Simpson 1960, 1966c, Oosterhuis 1964, Namba & Grob 1970).

Aplastic anaemia associated with thymic tumour is rare in myasthenic patients (Green 1958, Simpson 1960). A more common association is pernicious anaemia (Simpson 1960, 1964, 1966c) which has a genetic linkage to myasthenia gravis (Simpson 1976). Other immunological disorders occasionally associated (individually and familially) with myasthenia are systemic lupus erythematosus (Harvey et al 1954, Simpson 1960, Alarcón-Segovia et al 1963, Wolf & Barrows 1966), vitiligo (Simpson 1964), pemphigus vulgaris (Wolf et al 1966, Beutner et al 1968, Hausmanowa-Petrusewicz et al 1969, Vetters et al 1973), ulcerative colitis (Osserman 1958, Alarcón-Segovia

et al 1963), sarcoidosis (Simpson 1960, Downes et al 1966), Sjögren's disease (Downes et al 1966, Simpson 1966c, Wolf et al 1966), and hepatitis (Simpson 1960, Whittingham et al 1970).

Associated disorders which probably have an immunological basis or cause immunodeficiency are acrocyanosis, haemolytic anaemia, nephritis (Simpson 1960, Oosterhuis 1964), reticuloses (Alter & Osnato 1930, Symmers 1932, Simpson 1960, Cohen & Waxman 1967), diabetes mellitus (Simpson 1960), and herpes zoster (J A Simpson unpublished work).

Associated disorders which are relatively more common in myasthenics than those listed above, but in which no immunological pathology has yet been identified, are epilepsy (Hoefer et al 1958, Simpson 1960) and psychosis (Hayman 1941, Simpson 1960, Storm-Mathisen 1961). Emotional disturbances are common (Brolley & Hollender 1955, Meyer 1966).

Neonatal myasthenia

About one in seven live-born children of myastenic mothers shows evidence of myasthenia at birth and, if the affected child survives, there is complete recovery in 1–12 weeks (mean 18 days) without later relapse. The literature was reviewed by Namba et al (1970). There is no correlation between the severity of the infant's symptoms and the duration of the mother's illness or the severity of the mother's myasthenia during pregnancy. It is extremely rare for a myasthenic mother to have more than one affected child. Previous thymectomy does not abolish the possibility that the baby will be myasthenic, but the transient nature of neonatal myasthenia suggests that the child is affected by a factor transmitted from the mother. Maternal anti-ACh receptor antibody is transferred to the infant (Lindstrom et al 1976b), but it is becoming evident that this probably occurs in all pregnancies, although only one in seven (Simpson 1960) results in clinical neonatal myasthenia. It does not depend on a high maternal titre of antibody or on non-specific inhibition by α-fetoprotein (Brenner et al 1980). Reactions of anti-idiotypic antibody with anti-AChR antibodies of mother and child suggest that the clinically affected infant synthesises its own antibody, possibly due to transplacental transfer of a cell clone from the mother (Lefvert & Osterman 1983). A myasthenic syndrome may be apparent in the new-born child of a mother without myasthenia, and may then persist throughout life. This congenital myasthenia is not autoimmune in type and is not related to myasthenia gravis (Ch. 20) although some children with congenital myasthenia have low blood levels of IgA (Bundey et al 1972, Behan et al 1976a).

GENETIC FACTORS

There is now clear evidence for a genetic factor in myasthenia gravis. Although a study by Jacob et al (1968) showed no secondary cases of myasthenia gravis in 448 relatives of 70 myasthenic patients, and Herrmann (1971) was unable to establish a definite genetic mechanism in his study of families containing more than one case, Simpson (1960, 1968) suggested that a genetic factor could have variable expression, accounting for the familial linkage with thyroid disease, arthropathy, pernicious anaemia and diabetes mellitus (p. 632). Jacob et al (1968) found no association between myasthenia gravis and the ABO rhesus blood groups or with secretor status or the ability to taste phenylthiocarbamide (PTC). Bundey (1972) recognised an early-onset form of childhood myasthenia with autosomal recessive inheritance of the trait. Her study gave limited support to the concept of alternative gene expression.

Linkage with human histocompatibility antigens, reported in earlier editions of this book, has been confirmed in many countries (Pirskanen et al 1972, Behan et al 1973, Fritze et al 1973, Dick et al 1974, Feltkamp et al 1974, Pirskanen 1976). There is a frequent association with HLA-A1-B8-DW3 haplotypes, but it is clear that the association is not a direct one and not obligatory (Dick et al 1974, Pirskanen 1976). Compston et al (1980) related these haplotypes to non-thymoma myasthenia of women with onset under age 40. They found an increased association with HLA-A3, B7, DRw2 antigens in the later onset, predominantly male group. An increased frequency of HLA-A2 or -A3 in patients with thymoma, reported by

Feltkamp et al (1974) and Fritze et al (1974) was not noted by Dick et al (1974), by Pirskanen (1976) or by Compston et al (1980). Another histocompatibility antigen system, such as the LD antigens (Kaakinen et al 1975) situated near the SD loci bearing HL-A genes, may exhibit a stronger association with myasthenia gravis and with autoimmune disorders; both the SD and LD gene loci are close to some loci controlling immunological responsiveness (Ir genes). With respect to immunoglobulin (Gm) phenotypes, Garlepp et al (1984) found no significant linkage disequilibrium associated with anti-AChR antibodies, but the phenotype Gm (3;5) was associated with the development of antistriational antibody in males and older females. Genetic factors probably constitute risk factors for autoimmune diseases. (Adams (1977) suggests V genes.) The relative scarcity of familial cases of myasthenia gravis (3.4%, Namba et al 1971a; 7.2% in Finland, Pirskanen 1977) and involvement of only one of monozygotic twins (Simpson 1960, 1965, Namba et al 1971b) indicate that many aetiological factors may be involved. Twin studies are reviewed by Behan & Shields (1982).

CLINICAL CHEMISTRY

There are no consistent changes in blood chemistry in myasthenia gravis. Abnormalities of glucose tolerance (Cohen & King 1932, Simpson 1960, 1966b, Frenkel 1963), adrenocortical hypofunction (Simpson 1966b, Bosch et al 1978) and hyper- and hypothyroid function in the absence of clinical endocrinopathies (Simpson 1966b, 1968) are likely to be due to genetic and/or autoimmune linkage. Diminished pregnanediol excretion (Schrire 1959) has not been confirmed (Simpson 1966b).

Hypergammaglobulinaemia occurs in cases associated with other autoimmune diseases (Simpson 1960, 1966b) or with thymoma (Oosterhuis et al 1964) and some, but relatively few, of these patients have a raised erythrocyte sedimentation rate (ESR). Isolated instances of monoclonal gammopathy have been described (Rowland et al 1969). Hypogammaglobulinaemia sometimes occurs (Thévenard & Mende 1955, Simpson 1966b) and may be associated with a thymoma (Te Velde et al 1966, Cohen & Waxman 1967).

Depressed levels of IgA were found in juvenile-onset myasthenia by Bundey et al (1972); Simpson et al (1976) found a selective decrease in IgA in 10 of 50 myasthenic patients, and this was not influenced by thymectomy. The lowest levels were in three patients with congenital myasthenia who had undergone thymectomy. Bramis et al (1976) confirmed that serum IgA concentration may be subnormal. In their series the lowest concentrations were associated with thymomas or other neoplasms. Decreased IgA concentrations tended to be associated with many or prominent germinal centres in the thymus and levels increased slowly after thymectomy. There were no congenital cases in the series of Lisak & Zweiman (1975) who found normal IgA levels in 19 myasthenic patients. These workers reported a slight but significant depression of the mean IgM level (raised in some subjects, especially with a thymoma). Serum IgG tended to be above normal. There was no consistent pattern and the immunoglobulin levels did not correlate with the clinical state.

Nastuk et al (1960) measured serum complement levels serially in myasthenic patients and stated that they were lower during active disease, rising to normal or super-normal levels in remission. Plescia et al (1966) found reduced levels of C2 and C4 and inhibitors to these components. Simpson et al (1976) found no abnormality of Cl_q, C3, C4, C7 and C3 proactivator. They also measured C3 conversion products with C3 activator levels, and CH50 units. All were normal although examined in active and remittent cases. Behan & Behan (1979) re-examined this material when Engel (1977a) demonstrated localisation of IgG and C3 at motor end-plates. Depression of C4 component was found in 34% of myasthenic patients and 29% had circulating immune complexes. The greatest immunological abnormalities were found in patients with mild disease.

Elevated globulin levels in the cerebrospinal fluid (CSF) of 10 patients were recorded by Simpson (1960, 1966b), who reviewed previous isolated reports and concluded that there was associated disease which may be of immunological type. Reports that anti-ACh receptor antibody may be present in the CSF (Lefvert & Pirskanen 1977) have not been confirmed.

IMMUNOLOGICAL STUDIES

The hypothesis by Simpson (1960) that a thymus-controlled lymphocyte-derived antibody against ACh receptor could be the proximate cause of myasthenia gravis could not be confirmed by immunofluorescence techniques then available (McFarlin et al 1966): however, using high-resolution electron microscopy, Rash et al (1976) found material ('fuzzy coats'), resembling IgG in its configuration and dimensions, in the region of the receptors in the neuromuscular junction. The presence of IgG and of the C3 component of complement at the postsynaptic membranes of human myasthenic neuromuscular junctions was convincingly demonstrated by Engel et al (1977a, b) by an immunoperoxidase method. These authors proposed that subsequent sequential activation of C5–C9 would complete the attack phase of the complement reaction sequence and set the stage for lytic destruction of the postsynaptic membrane. It remains possible that antibody or immune complex may block receptors competitively. The rapid beneficial effect of plasma exchange (p. 649) might support this concept but not necessarily so, because the regeneration of receptors is probably very rapid (Devreotes & Fambrough 1975) and there is usually a time lag of two days or more before muscle power is restored (Newsom-Davis et al 1978). Passive transfer of myasthenic immune complexes would help to differentiate between the three main possibilities: (1) lysis of postsynaptic membrane; (2) immunopharmacological blockade, and (3) IgG-induced modulation of AChR. Passive transfer of myasthenia from man to mouse by human myasthenic serum was demonstrated by Toyka et al (1975). It may be necessary to have previous reduction of the transmission safety factor in order to demonstrate the passive transfer (Stahlberg et al 1978) or to use animals of specific H2 haplotype (Fuchs et al 1976). Tissue culture experiments suggest that receptor blockade (Drachman et al 1977) and accelerated degradation of ACh receptors (Anwyl et al 1977, Kao & Drachman 1977b) may both be involved. Synthesis of AChR appears not to be affected by immunoglobulin from myasthenic patients (Drachman 1978).

Serum antibody acting directly on acetylcholine receptor sites has not been identified by standard immunological techniques, but its existence is strongly indicated by a number of methods demonstrating the presence in myasthenic serum of an IgG which will prevent access of α-bungarotoxins (α-Bgtx) to nicotinic receptors, indicating high affinity of the immunoglobulin for receptor or closely adjacent material. Early assays, based on measuring the inhibition of binding of α-Bgtx to extrajunctional receptors of denervated rat muscle (Almon et al 1974), or to junctional receptors of human muscle (Bender et al 1975), were of low sensitivity. Indirect evidence of an antibody in myasthenic serum which cross-reacts with AChR from electrogenic tissue of *Torpedo californica* is provided by complement fixation (Aharonov et al 1975a).

More sensitive assays are based on the binding of antibody to AChR linked to isotope-labelled α-Bgtx. The antibody-AChR-α-Bgtx complexes are then precipitated, together with carrier immunoglobulin, by adding anti-immunoglobulin and the radioactivity of the resulting pellet is measured (Appel et al 1975, Lindstrom 1977). The globulin detected by this method blocks the access of α-Bgtx to the AChR site by binding the receptor complex at a site different from, but in close proximity to, the acetylcholine site which, apparently, is not usually the target for the antibody. Most of the monoclonal antibodies isolated by recent studies bind to the main immunogenic region of the alpha subunits of the receptor macromolecule (Tzartos et al 1983). Lefvert (1982) reports antibody reaction outside the toxin-binding site of myasthenic and denervated muscle in higher titre than against normal muscle (suggesting presentation of unusual epitopes on extra-junctional and myasthenic end-plate receptors). It is increasingly clear that the anti-AChR antibody response is polyclonal, but not all antibodies are pathogenic — only those to the exposed area of the receptor macromolecule, but α-Bgtx binding may be inhibited by antibodies not directed against the toxin-binding sites (Barkas et al 1982). In some reports (Lindstrom et al 1976b) the titre of antibody measured by this radioimmunoassay correlates reasonably well with the severity of the disease, but only if AChR from human muscle is used. In other reports (Lefvert et al 1978, Newsom-Davis et al 1978) the correlation is rather low. No significant titre of antibody is found in serum from congenital myasthenia (Newsom-Davis et al 1978). Antibody has been detected in sera from infants with neonatal myasthenia, as well as from their mothers (Lindstrom et al 1976b, Keesey et al 1977, Lefvert et al 1978), but some infants with receptor antibodies have no detectable weakness, possibly because of receptor antigenic difference between mother and child (Simpson 1960, Keesey et al 1977). Lefvert et al (1978) have suggested that IgG antibody detected by radioimmunoassay may not be a primary cause of the disease, because it is sometimes preceded by IgM antibodies in the early stages of myasthenia. Anti-AChR antibodies are predominantly of the IgG1 and IgG2 subclasses, rich in k-light-chain. IgG3 antibodies, even richer in k-light-chains, and reacting better with receptors from ocular muscles than limb muscles, have been significantly more prominent in sera from patients with ocular myasthenia.

The titre of IgG antibody against AChR is higher in myasthenia gravis associated with thymoma and falls with all the procedures listed later as immunosuppressive (p. 647).

Antimyosin antibodies are found in sera from some myasthenics, the titre being highest in those with a thymoma (Strauss et al 1960, Beutner et al 1962, van der Geld et al 1964, Djanian et al 1964). Using an immunofluorescence technique, binding of antibody to A bands of skeletal muscle is seen only with myasthenic sera and is highly correlated with the presence of a thymoma (Vetters 1965). The A-band antibody also reacts with myoid cells in the thymus (Feltkamp-Vroom 1966). Antibodies to other antigens of skeletal and cardiac muscle occur in myasthenic sera and are usually associated with a thymoma. Aarli has studied an acid-extractable antigen (CA antigen) which is considered to be specific for thymoma-associated myasthenia (Aarli & Thunold 1981, Gilhus et al 1984). It is probably a membrane antigen unrelated to the cross-striational pattern of the muscle fibre. Antisera to the CA extract react strongly with neoplastic epithelial cells of the human thymoma. Other antibodies commonly found in sera from myasthenic patients are antinuclear factor, antithyroid and antigastric substances. Rheumatoid factor may also be present in the blood. It does not usually correlate closely with a history of arthritis (Simpson 1964, 1966b), but may do so (Aarli et al 1975). Patients with pemphigus vulgaris have antiepithelial antibody (Noguchi & Nishitani 1976). Specific antineuronal and antispermatogonia nuclear antibodies in sera of patients with myasthenia gravis have been reported by Martin et al (1974). Clearly, there is a wide spectrum of autoantibodies (Simpson 1983) and they are also more frequent in sera from relatives of myasthenics (Feltkamp et al 1974), supporting the suggestion of genetic predisposition to autoimmune diseases which may include myasthenia gravis when the anti-AChR antibody titre is raised.

It is premature to attribute a pathogenetic role to the 'receptor antibody', although changes in titre closely follow the clinical severity of myasthenia and the passive transfer studies described above are impressive. Protection may be provided by development of anti-idiotype antibodies. They occur in myasthenia gravis (Dwyer et al 1983) but their biological role is uncertain. Experimentally raised anti-idiotypic antibodies against anti-AChR globulin are unique to the individual (Barkas & Simpson 1982, Waldor et al 1983).

There is also uncertainty about the role of cell-mediated immunity (CMI). There are now many reports of minor abnormalities of T-cell subsets (too numerous to list, see reviews by Behan et al 1975, Vincent 1980, Clementi & Conti-Tronconi 1983). Many indicate a deficit of T-suppressor cells, often antigen-dependent and it is probable that abnormality of regulatory T cells precedes the production of anti-self antibodies. The term CMI is now restricted to immunological reactions involving autoaggressive lymphocytes and macrophages without antibody or complement dependence, as in delayed-type hypersensitivity. This type of immune response is minimal in human myasthenia gravis and in the animal model.

Experimental autoimmune myasthenia gravis

Animal models of myasthenia evoked by inoculation of nicotinic receptors and termed experimental autoimmune myasthenia gravis (EAMG) are described in Chapters 9 and 12.

The successful production of EAMG depends on there being some interspecies cross-reactivity of AChR: at first, the sera of animals immunised with electroplaque AChR have antibodies recognising the electric organ in much higher concentration than that of antibodies recognising the AChR of the animal's muscle. At a later stage of the immune response the absolute amount of antibody against recipient AChR is high (Lindstrom et al 1976a) suggesting true autoimmunity. Passive transfer of EAMG by lymph node cells in the guinea pig (Tarrab-Hazdai et al 1975a) and rat (Lennon et al 1976), and by γ-globulin in the rat (Lindstrom et al 1976b) supports the theory that the proximate mechanism of myasthenia is autoimmune. But the human disease does not result from inoculation of foreign AChR and there is evidence that syngeneic AChR released from damaged muscle does not evoke an antibody response in the human or rat (Lindstrom et al 1976b). It has been suggested that a source of antibody-stimulating AChR may be the myoid cells of the thymus. Myoid cells have long been known to cross-react with antimyosin antibody (van der Geld & Strauss 1966) and have been shown by Kao & Drachman (1977a) to have surface ACh receptors which may be separate but immunologically related target organs in myasthenia gravis (Aharanov et al 1975b). It is unlikely that myoid cells provide a triggering antigen stimulus for the autoimmune reaction. Goldstein & Whittingham (1966) reported a myasthenic syndrome in guinea pigs inoculated with calf thymus, muscle, or lymph node and attributed this to 'autoimmune thymitis' with liberation from the thymus of a neuromuscular blocking substance. Other workers did not confirm their findings (e.g. Vetters et al 1969). The conflicting experimental results and conclusions were critically reviewed by Simpson

(1978). The Goldstein hypothesis would make it difficult to account for myasthenia originating after thymectomy, or would require ad hoc explanations for associated autoimmune disorders if the primary source of autoantigen were the thymic myoid cell.

THYMUS GLAND

There are pathological changes in 70–80% of patients with myasthenia gravis. The most consistent finding is lymphoid hyperplasia of cortex and medulla with T lymphocytes in both parts, not mainly in the cortex as in normal subjects (Aarli et al 1979). It is commonly associated with numerous germinal centres in the medulla (Castleman & Norris 1949) (Fig. 19.6). (The term 'hyperplasia' is criticised by Levine 1979.) The normal gland is not involuted, as suggested by earlier observers. Germinal centres are characteristic of several autoimmune disorders

and are not unique to myasthenia gravis. Their significance is uncertain because the prevalence of germinal centres in the thymus bears no clear relationship to the duration or severity of the disease, or to the clinical response to thymectomy (Vetters & Simpson 1974). Levine (1979) points out that germinal centres are separated by basal lamina from the true thymic parenchyma. These extra-parenchymal centres have venules with high endothelium, like lymph nodes. Bofill et al (1985) agree that germinal centres are reactive and stress the importance of hyperplasia of medullary epithelium. Preponderance of B cells in thymic germinal centres (Abdou et al 1974) has been interpreted as an expression of antibody formation against inappropriate T-cell clones, or excess antibody production attributable to lack of suppressor cells. Some thymic lymphocytes synthesise anti-AChR in culture, but usually from thymuses of patients with long duration of disease (Scadding et al 1981). Intrathymic production of antibody is unlikely to be a major mechanism. Thymic cells

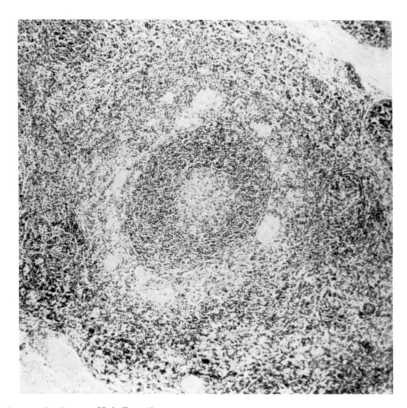

Fig. 19.6 Germinal centre in thymus, H & E, ×42

increase production of anti-AChR antibody by autologous peripheral blood lymphocytes (Newsom-Davis et al 1981). This is not T-cell dependent and may result from rare antigen-presenting cells in germinal centres (Willcox et al 1984). Papatestas et al (1976) found lower counts of peripheral blood lymphocytes in patients with many germinal centres and suggested that the latter may indicate a state of immunosuppression. A. L. Goldstein et al (1976) suggested that a thymic hormone, thymosin, influences precursor T cells, possibly via an adenylate cyclase-dependent process, and that genetic factors and/or viral infection may lead to a deficiency of suppressor or regulatory T cells which in turn removes the mechanisms controlling B-cell function (including formation of autoantibodies). The source of thymosin is unknown; it would be premature to identify it with the granules described in the thymus by Vetters & MacAdam (1972, 1973). Immunoreactivity for thymosin α_1 is localised on thymic epithelial cells at the periphery of Hassall's corpuscles and on some circulating T cells (Dalakas et al 1981). The concept of the role of the thymus in autoimmune disease is more plausible than the alternative that the thymus is itself a target for immunological attack ('thymitis') with consequent release of a neuromuscular blocking substance, as in the theories of Strauss et al (1966) and G. Goldstein (Goldstein & Whittingham 1966). (The 'thymin' of G. Goldstein must not be confused with the 'thymosin' of A. L. Goldstein.)

Wekerle et al (1981) propose that B cells in the thymus and peripheral lymph nodes are instructed by anti-AChR helper T-cell lines whose antigen-reactivity critically depends on presentation of antigen (AChR on myoid cells) and that this interaction is restricted by the HLA phenotype of the presenting cells which are probably epithelial. Their hypothesis would isolate myasthenia gravis from the other autoimmune diseases with which it is associated clinically and genetically. An alternative hypothesis, which I prefer, is aberrant expression of HLA-DR antigens on the antigen-presenting thymic epithelial cells. An idiotype mimicry model, as in the original Simpson (1960) hypothesis, remains possible (Cleveland et al 1983).

Whatever the mechanism, there is general agreement that anti-AChR and antimyosin antibody titres are higher in the presence of a thymoma and that this correlates with clinical severity. A thymoma is usually encapsulated and may be cystic and calcified, but it is sometimes malignant. Invasiveness is limited, spread being usually confined to the thorax and occasionally to the lymph nodes of the neck. An account of the histological types described has been given by Iverson (1956). The thymoma which occurs in myasthenia gravis shows a predominance of lymphocytes and epithelial cells which may have an acinar structure. The spindle-celled thymoma has no special association with myasthenia gravis. Indeed, the benign neoplasm may be an associated disorder, the important tissue being the adjacent non-tumour thymus which commonly contains germinal centres (Castleman 1955, Alpert et al 1971).

MUSCLE AND NERVE

Despite frequent statements in the past that myasthenia gravis is a disease without morbid anatomy, the lymphocyte infiltrations of muscle described by Weigert (1901) and termed lymphorrhages (Fig.19.7) by Buzzard (1905) are found repeatedly in such cases, but not invariably. According to Oosterhuis & Bethlem (1973) they are seen particularly in patients with a thymoma. On rare occasions they occur at the end-plates (Wiesendanger & D'Alessandsi 1963). Buzzard (1905) also reported degenerative changes of muscle fibres which were re-investigated and classified by Russell (1953). These changes were regarded as non-specific. Simpson (1960) suggested that they may indicate cell-mediated immunological damage, a concept supported by Rule & Kornfeld (1971).

In some muscles of some patients, denervation atrophy has been reported, the criteria being groups of small muscle fibres with angular cross-sectional contours, and 'target' fibres (Fenichel & Shy 1963, Brody & Engel 1964, Oosterhuis & Bethlem 1973 and others). The histochemical pattern is usually normal but type II fibre atrophy is not uncommon (Brooke & Engel 1969). These changes are not uniquely associated with denervation due to presynaptic pathology: Coërs &

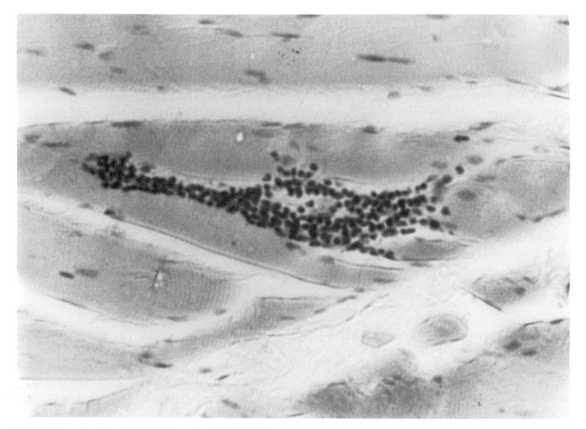

Fig. 19.7 Lymphorrhage in skeletal muscle, H & E ×189

Telerman-Toppet (1976) rarely found the increased terminal innervation ratio which they regard as a sensitive index of denervation with reinnervation.

The peripheral nerve trunks are histologically normal in human myasthenia gravis (Oosterhuis & Bethlem 1973) and in EAMG (Hill et al 1977). Collateral sprouting, a hallmark of conventional denervation, is rare in myasthenia and occurs mainly in older patients (Coërs et al 1973). By intravital staining with methylene blue, Coërs & Desmedt (1959) demonstrated two types of abnormality of the terminal arborisation of motor nerves (Fig. 19.8): a 'dystrophic' type, considered to be a reaction to muscle fibre degeneration, and a 'dysplastic' type highly characteristic of myasthenia gravis. In the latter there are few terminal knobs and these are arranged serially along a scanty number of terminal branches ending in a remarkably elongated end-plate region, especially in young patients (Coërs & Telerman-Toppet 1976). Bickerstaff & Woolf (1960) and MacDermot (1960) confirmed these findings and also described prolific ultraterminal sprouting, important evidence of vigorous but aberrant regeneration.

Ultramicroscopic studies of the end-plate region show poor development of junctional folds and of secondary clefts (Zacks et al 1962, Woolf 1966, Engel & Santa 1971, Fardeau et al 1974). These changes are accompanied by abnormal reduction of the subneural apparatus (Engel & Santa 1971) (Fig. 19.9). Bergman et al (1971) also noted abnormalities of muscle and nerve fibres, damage to Schwann cells, and grossly thickened basement membrane of capillaries but these findings are inconsistent, as are minor changes described in nerve terminals such as dense bodies, myelin figures, mitochondrial abnormalities, and decreased numbers of synaptic vesicles (see review by Engel

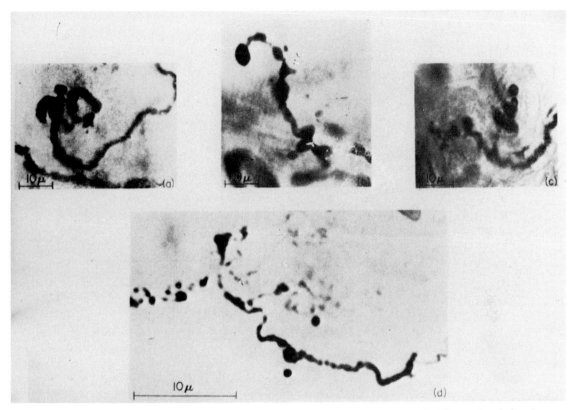

Fig. 19.8 Methylene blue preparations of human motor nerve terminals. a. Normal end-plate. b. Elongated end-plate from a case of myasthenia gravis. c. Motor end-plate with shrunken terminal expansions from a case of myasthenia gravis resistant to neostigmine. d. Axonal sprout with diminutive ending in a case of myasthenia gravis with prominent lymphorrhages — myositic response, previously termed 'dystrophic' (Simpson 1969b, with permission from the publishers and by courtesy of the late Dr A. L. Woolf)

& Santa 1971). Fardeau et al (1974) reported that synaptic vesicles had a normal diameter (about 60 nm) but that the vesicular stacks (at the presumed release sites of ACh) were rarely visible. Nevertheless, they agreed with Engel & Santa (1971) that the changes predominate in the subneural apparatus, which is grossly elongated although the mean nerve terminal area is reduced (measured into the folds). It is generally agreed that the postsynaptic membrane disorganisation is not caused by anticholinesterase medication and that it is of functional significance, because the use of labelled α-Bgtx to identify receptor sites has shown reduced amounts of AChR to a degree which correlates linearly with the decreased miniature end-plate potential amplitude (Engel et al 1977b). Localisation of the IgG and C3 compo-nent of complement to receptors of end-plates obtained only from myasthenic patients was identified by Engel et al (1977a) (Fig. 19.10). From morphometric analysis of electron micro-graphs, these authors found that immune complexes are more abundant in the less severely affected patients than in those with more severe myasthenia (who have less AChR remaining in their end-plates). They interpret this as evidence for a destructive autoimmune reaction involving the postsynaptic membrane. There is functional evidence that anti-AChR antibody increases the degradation and internalisation of junctional (and extrajunctional) receptors of muscle (Reiness & Weinberg 1978) and induces modulation of AChR (Heinemann et al 1978) without involving complement. Fambrough et al (1973) demon-

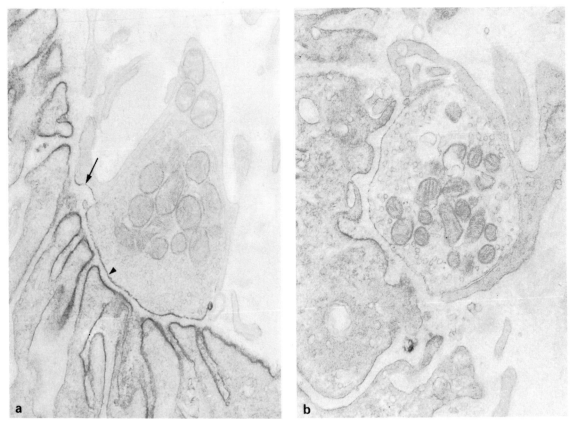

Fig. 19.9 End-plate regions of external intercostal muscles. Acetylcholine receptor sites are stained by α-Bgtx conjugated to horseradish perioxidase, × 22 300. In (a), from a normal subject, AChR is associated with terminal expansions and deeper surfaces of the postsynaptic folds; the presynaptic membrane (arrrowhead) stained by leaching, and Schwann cell membrane (arrow) facing crest of folds are lightly stained. In (b), from a case of moderately severe myasthenia gravis, the postsynaptic regions are simplified, only segments of it react for AChR (Engel et al 1977b)

strated that the number of ACh receptors is decreased by 70–90%, assuming absence of a population of receptors inaccessible to α-Bgtx (Fambrough 1979). Immunopharmacological blockade, as suggested by Simpson (1960), remains a possibility which is supported by the prompt relapse of myasthenic symptoms noted after retransfusion of homologous cell-free lymph (Matell et al 1976), and by the indication that serum from myasthenic patients reduces the mepp amplitude of rat end-plates, an effect which can be reversed by washing with a control solution (Shibuya et al 1978). The relative importance in the human disease of modulation and internalisation, complement-mediated lysis and blockade of receptors is discussed by Engel (1984) and may vary from case to case.

CAUSATION OF MYASTHENIA GRAVIS

The clinical, pathological, and immunological data now available, with the model provided by EAMG, provide strong support for the Simpson hypothesis of myasthenia gravis as a genetically predisposed autoimmune disorder, the proximate mechanism being destruction of end-plate ACh receptors by a complement-fixing antibody reaction. It is probable, although not proved, that cell-mediated immunity and immunopharmacological blockade of receptors are also important. It is still not known what starts the immunological reaction, although a viral attack on thymus or muscle is an attractive hypothesis. This would account for the occasional finding of IgM antibodies, supplanted by the IgG type in early myasthenia (Lefvert et

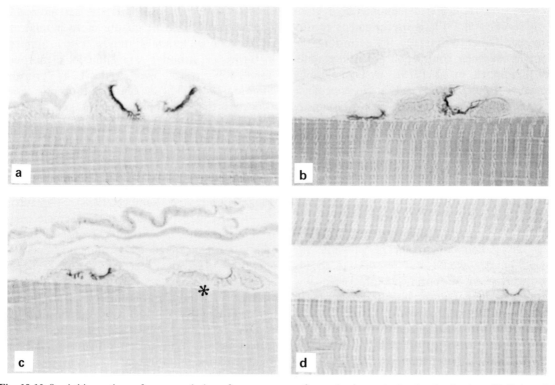

Fig. 19.10 Semi-thin sections of motor end-plates from two cases of myasthenia gravis showing localisation of IgG (a and c) and C3 component of complement (b and d). Reaction at the end-plates is more intense in the case of mild myasthenia gravis (a and b) than in the more severe case (c and d). One of two end-plate regions in c (*) displays only a trace of IgG. Background staining is absent. Unstained sections photographed with a green filter, ×1425 (Engel et al 1977a)

al 1978). Tindall et al (1978) report elevated titres of complement-fixing antibody to cytomegalovirus (CMV) in myasthenics not treated with thymectomy or steroids. Their suggestion that there is persistent viral antigenic stimulation in the myasthenic thymus, arising from incorporation of viral protein into myoid cell surface membranes with subsequent induction of anti-AChR antibody, would be consistent with the thymitis theory reviewed above; the same criticisms would be valid. Nevertheless, virus-induced breakdown of immune surveillance with lack of recognition of self — a strong possibility in all autoimmune diseases — is more likely to be due to infection of cells of the lymphoid system, as a mutagenic agent, than to infection of target organs. Immunodeficiency is a possible background to myasthenia gravis (Dawkins et al 1975a, Simpson et al 1976) but also to CMV infection. Some important biological aspects of myasthenia gravis are

discussed by Rule & Kornfeld (1971) and Drachman (1981).

DIAGNOSTIC TESTS AND CLINICAL PHYSIOLOGY

Performance tests

The abnormal fatiguability of skeletal muscles shown by bedside tests (p. 495) may be documented in many ways, providing objective data which may be important in the assessment of the pharmacological tests described below, or in evaluating treatment. Diaphragmatic movement, or the ability to swallow a mouthful of barium before and after intramuscular injection of edrophonium, may be observed on the fluoroscope; the objective measurement of diplopia, e.g. with prisms, may be valuable in demonstrating the changing extent of weakness. A recording dynamometer or ergo-gram (Greene et al 1961) is useful and is readily improvised. Other techniques for recording the amount of muscular contraction are ocular tono-metry (Campbell et al 1970), nystagmography (Spector & Daroff 1976) and audio-impedance measurement of the stapedius reflex (Blom & Zakrissor 1974). These tests are all occasionally useful when muscular weakness is confined to the appropriate sites.

Electrophysiology

In 1895, Jolly showed that the pathological fatigu-ability of myasthenia could be reproduced by faradic stimulation of a motor nerve while the 'fatigued' muscle would still respond to locally applied galvanism. Electromyographic recording shows that the loss of power when the motor nerve is supramaximally and repetitively stimulated is accompanied by a decrement of the evoked action potential of the muscle, while the antidromically conducted nerve action potential is unchanged in amplitude. In view of the ultrastructural and immunological data, it is unnecessary to present all the facts of neurophysiological observation relevant to the nature of the functional abnor-mality. For this purpose the reader is referred to reviews by Slomić et al (1968), Simpson (1969b) and Kim (1982). It is now accepted that the essen-tial lesion is degeneration of ACh receptors on the postsynaptic membrane, with or without immu-nopharmacological blockade, but it is clear from these studies and from computer analysis of evoked motor unit potentials (Ballantyne & Hansen 1974) that additional, if less important, prejunctional and muscle fibre lesions may co-exist. The essential electrical features are: (1) subnormal amplitude of spontaneous miniature end-plate potentials (mepps), (2) transmission failure due to lowered safety factor, and (3) intact prejunctional potentiation mechanisms. It has been assumed that a lowered safety factor uncovers a physiological decrement of quantal release following a train of nerve impulses; contemporary studies challenge this. Prejunctional nicotinic receptors may also be involved in the disorder.

Subnormal amplitudes of mepps, identified by Elmqvist and colleagues, were at first attributed to production of small quanta of ACh following a prejunctional lesion (Elmqvist 1965), although on theoretical grounds a postjunctional morphol-ogical abnormality was at least as probable (Simpson 1971). The evidence of a receptor lesion reconciles the electrophysiological and morpho-logical findings. Decreased amplitude of spon-taneous mepps in biopsied intercostal muscle can be used as a diagnostic test because this finding is probably unique to myasthenia gravis, but meticulous technique is necessary for reliable results (Elmqvist & Lambert 1968). Spontaneous negative discharges recorded with macroelectrodes at the end-plate zone (motor point) of human muscle are considered to be miniature end-plate potentials. Lovelace et al (1970) reported reduction in frequency of firing and of burst duration, but the amplitude was only slightly reduced. Grob (1971) found no significant differ-ence between these values and those from normal subjects but he had greater difficulty in locating the negative spontaneous discharges in myasthenic subjects. The value of analysis of spontaneous end-plate activity (not to be confused with 'end-plate noise') has not been proved.

Tests of reduced safety factor for transmission

Electromyographic signs of transmission failure at the neuromuscular junction (Fig. 19.11) are fundamentally: (1) evidence of a decremental muscular response to slow repetitive supramax-imal per-neural stimulation in the presence of a normal antidromically conducted motor nerve potential and normal direct muscular excitability; (2) increased 'jitter' and blockings of single muscle fibre responses to repeated nerve impulses (volun-tary or evoked). Both are due to subnormal end-plate potentials, summed from subnormal minia-ture end-plate potentials. The practical appli-cations of these principles are described in Chapter 30 but some riders must be added. Certain electrophysiological phenomena point to additional presynaptic and muscle fibre abnor-malities. The decrementing response and increased 'jitter' are non-specific indicators of a reduced safety factor for transmission at the neuromuscular junction. Their presence supports a clinical diag-

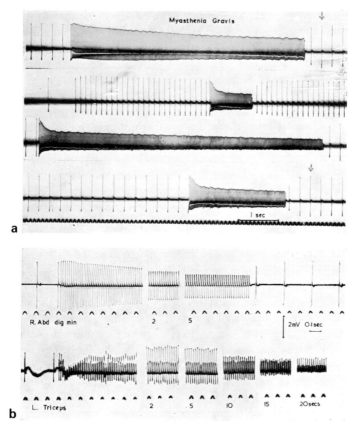

Fig. 19.11 Electromyograms from patients with myasthenia gravis: a. Ulnar nerve at wrist stimulated with supramaximal shock, repeated 4, 8 and 50 times/s. Action potential recorded from abductor digiti minimi muscle by surface electrodes shows decrement ('fatigue') with fast tetanisation only. Note post-tetanic facilitation at arrows. b. The classic response from abductor digiti minimi, but the triceps shows a temporary incremental response

nosis of a myasthenic reaction but does not indicate the type of lesion. Normal findings do not exclude a diagnosis of myasthenia gravis. Their role is to support a tentative clinical diagnosis and they do not strengthen the evidence if 'fatiguable' weakness is demonstrable at the gross level.

Pharmacological tests

The reduced safety factor also increases susceptibility to neuromuscular blocking drugs of competitive type such as D-tubocurarine (Ch. 30) and quinine bisulphate. Agonist-competitors, mainly quaternary ammonium drugs such as decamethonium and suxamethonium, have increased agonist and decreased blocking effect. Their use in diagnosis is of historical interest only but should be known to anaesthetists as the paralysant effect is unpredictable in myasthenics and recovery may be prolonged. The myasthenic end-plate has reduced sensitivity to acetylcholine (Engbaek 1951) because of the loss of receptors in the postsynaptic membrane. Acetylcholine is more effective if its hydrolysis is slowed by inhibiting the acetylcholinesterase at the end-plates. Neostigmine, pyridostigmine and other anticholinesterase drugs given orally or parenterally cause temporary restoration of muscle power but the response is delayed and persists for one to six hours, which is inconvenient. The prolonged action and muscarinic stimulation are unpleasant if the subject does not, in fact, have myasthenia. The short-acting anticholinesterase, edrophonium, is more suitable on both counts although it is necessary to inject the drug intravenously and to adopt a strict protocol.

Edrophonium test. The short antimyasthenic effect of edrophonium chloride (Tensilon®) makes it very suitable for a diagnostic test. A syringe is loaded with 1 ml (10 mg) for intravenous injection. Initially 2 mg should be injected to detect sensitivity but if there is no response the remaining 8 mg is injected after 30 s (Osserman & Kaplan 1953). Within 0.5–1 min there is improvement if weakness is due to myasthenia gravis, but weakness returns in 4–5 min. Some normal subjects experience no obvious effects, while others feel a tight sensation around the eyes and fasciculation may be seen for a few seconds. If weakness is due to cholinergic crisis in a patient under treatment it is transiently increased and fasciculation may occur. Unfortunately, respiratory weakness may be increased to an extent endangering life.

The positive responses described are valuable and reliable when present, but failure to obtain improvement or fasciculation does not indicate either that weakness is not myasthenic or that it is cholinergic. Negative responses are sometimes found, but false positive results are very rare provided that only objective criteria are used. Subjective 'improvement' should never be relied on, especially when the test is used to assess the adequacy of treatment. The test is best performed at the time of greatest activity of the therapeutic drug: where pyridostigmine is being used, it should be performed one hour after a dose.

Because of the differing degree of involvement of different muscles, it is important to test respiratory and bulbar but not ocular muscles when the test is carried out to differentiate between myasthenic and cholinergic weakness. These vital muscles may be overdosed while the ocular muscles are still underdosed, and failure to recognise this may lead to fatal overdosage. An equivocal or 'adequate' response should always be taken to mean that further dosage may be dangerous.

Neostigmine test. Although the latency is greater, a favourable response to injection of neostigmine remains the most convincing evidence of myasthenia gravis because its duration is sufficient to permit repeated testing of all muscles (Viets & Schwab 1935). The duration makes it unsuitable when cholinergic crisis is suspected. Neostigmine methylsulphate is injected intramuscularly (1.5 mg) alone or combined with 0.6 mg of atropine sulphate. Improvement begins in 10–15 min but is most obvious after 30 min. The same preparation may be used intravenously (0.5 mg), when the response is more rapid but the danger of ventricular fibrillation or arrest is greater. The drug should never be given by this route unless accompanied or preceded by atropine. The response to 15 mg of neostigmine bromide orally may be sufficient to make the diagnosis clear. If any of the parenteral tests are equivocal and the diagnosis of myasthenia gravis seems highly probable on clinical grounds, it is worth carrying out a therapeutic trial with oral medication for a week.

The Walker effect

The report by Mary Walker (1938) that exercising a myasthenic limb muscle induced extraocular paresis has not been confirmed by experienced observers (Johns et al 1956) but was supported by Tsukiyama et al (1959). The test is usually conducted with exercise distal to a tourniquet and Patten (1975) postulated that under hypoxic conditions the myasthenic muscle releases lactic acid which adversely affects other muscles when the cuff is released, possibly by lowering the serum calcium levels. I have never witnessed a convincing Walker effect. There is no acceptable evidence of a blocking substance in serum (Nastuk et al 1959). Cell-free lymph re-injected into a myasthenic patient precipitated weakness which had been reduced by thoracic duct drainage (Matellet al 1976) and passive transfer from man to mouse has been described above. These effects are attributed to immunoglobulin. There is no convincing evidence for a role of other 'myasthenic toxins' originating in muscle or thymus.

RADIOLOGY OF THYMUS

The thymus gland is not seen in chest radiographs unless there is a thymoma. Small tumours localised to part of the gland may remain invisible, but those seen at surgery before the gland is sectioned can almost always be detected on straight films of the chest (posteroanterior and lateral) (Fig. 19.2) assisted by tomography if necessary. Pneumo-mediastinography or thymic venography are unnecessary and are not recommended. Isotopic scanning of the mediastinum with selenome-thionine-75 (Cowan et al 1971) or gallium-67 citrate (Swick et al 1976) gives good imaging of thymomas. As the radiopharmaceutical agent accumulates in numerous tissues, false positive studies are reported, but negative studies are considered to be of value in ruling out the presence of a thymoma. Gallium-67 has become the preferred isotope. It may be valuable in detecting recurrences of malignant thymoma after operation. A large thymus is visible on computed tomography and may be wrongly assumed to be a thymoma (Brown et al 1983).

TREATMENT

There are three facets of treatment: (1) immuno-suppression; (2) elevation of the safety factor for neuromuscular transmission; (3) avoidance of factors which lower the safety factor or further embarrass respiration.

Immunosuppressive measures

In principle, the autoimmune disorder may respond to removal or suppression of the thymus, ultrathymic immunosuppression, or removal of antibodies and immuno-aggressive cells.

Thymectomy. For a long time the value of thymectomy was obscured by failure to appreciate that results are different in cases with a thymoma (Keynes 1955). In cases without a thymoma there is a clear benefit in favour of thymectomy, regardless of age or sex of the patient, provided that the disease is still in Stage 1 (Simpson 1958). The contrary view of Papatestas et al (1971) was later reversed (Papatestas et al 1976). Published series since 1960 are too numerous to review but all support these conclusions (Oosterhuis 1984).

There is no clear indication as to which patients are most likely to benefit, apart from those in whom the disease has been of short duration.

Failure of thymectomy to prevent myasthenic death occurs more often in patients requiring a large dose of anticholinesterase drugs, but if they do survive (which is now the rule) the ultimate state is not, apparently, correlated with preoperative severity. Patients with severe bulbar weakness are most likely to die, despite operation. On the other hand, if myasthenia remains confined to the extraocular muscles for two years, the prognosis for life is so good that thymectomy has not been considered justified (Grob 1953, Ferguson et al 1955): nevertheless, I believe that it is unusual for weakness to remain so restricted and the operation is now entirely safe, regardless of the surgical method (Fraser et al 1978). The surgical technique (sternal split or transcervical incision) is a matter of choice by the surgeon. Operative morbidity is less with the transcervical approach, but complete removal of the gland is less certain and this is considered desirable if possible. Prejudice against the sternal splitting operation is due to the belief that respiratory support by endotracheal intubation is usually necessary. It is generally unnecessary if anticholinesterase medication is not discontinued (Fraser et al 1978). Undoubtedly, sites of aberrant thymic tissue are easier to reach with the sternal incision.

Even in Stage 1 (active stage), thymectomy is not a cure: it arrests deterioration, promotes remission and makes the further course more benign; this is increasingly evident with the passage of time (Simpson 1958, Perlo et al 1966, Papatestas et al 1976). It is still controversial whether the pathology of the thymus is important. It is generally agreed that the long-term outlook is much poorer if there is a thymoma, although for five to ten years the results of thymectomy may be excellent. Indeed, there are many records of myasthenia becoming first clinically apparent months or years after removal of a thymoma (Koch et al 1970). There are conflicting reports about the correlation between the presence of germinal centres and the response to surgery: some reported series are too small for analysis; others have assessed the histology subjectively. Not surprisingly, they disagree with each other. Differing conclusions are: (1) there is no relationship between thymic histology and postoperative response (Castleman & Norris 1949, Seybold et al

1971, Reinglass & Brickel 1973); (2) a favourable response correlates with the presence of numerous germinal centres (MacKay et al 1968, Genkins et al 1975, Sambrook et al 1976); (3) a favourable response is more likely after removal of glands with few germinal centres (Alpert et al 1971). Vetters & Simpson (1974) used an accurate morphometric technique and also found a tendency for patients with relatively unreactive thymus glands to obtain a better result from thymectomy, but the difference was not statistically significant and others have considered that there is no relationship at all.

The response to thymectomy is unpredictable. It may be immediate or delayed. The more favourable course in comparison with cases without thymectomy often becomes apparent in the second or third year and is most evident with early thymectomy (Simpson 1958, Genkins et al 1975). A major relapse occurs very rarely: a postulated growth of 'aberrant' or incompletely removed thymic tissue has not been confirmed in most cases although undoubtedly present in some (Joseph & Johns 1973). There is often a temporary improvement during the first few days, which may be so rapid that it is obvious as soon as the patient recovers from the anaesthetic, even though no neostigmine has been injected throughout the operation. A previous ptosis may be replaced by lid retraction. Unfortunately the dose of anticholinesterase drugs may require progressive increase on the third or fourth day but it is extremely important to recognise the extent of the temporary remission as, during this period, a previously ineffective dose of neostigmine may cause a cholinergic crisis. In the past, many postoperative deaths were caused in this way. To avoid this, many experts stop anti-cholinesterase medication before operation and resume two to three days later, meanwhile supporting breathing by artificial ventilation, commonly by tracheostomy. With careful attention to dosage, neither measure is required (Fraser et al 1978).

The delayed response to thymectomy, and the inferior response when operation is postponed beyond stage 1, suggest that T cells controlling antibody formation by B cells continue to be active for some time after thymectomy in some extrathymic site, and that it would be rational to follow thymectomy with immunosuppressive drugs aimed at these cells, and not merely in the most seriously affected patients. It might be argued that adequate chemical immunosuppression would remove the need for thymectomy. This should certainly be investigated but the proof will have to be convincing now that thymectomy carries no operative mortality.

Suppression of the thymus. Alternative means of suppressing the thymus have not been shown to be as effective. Carotid sinus denervation, claimed to cause adrenocortical hypertrophy and thymic atrophy, has been abandoned. Radiotherapy as a method of destroying thymic function is less certain than thymectomy and may cause initial deterioration. Preoperative radiotherapy has been advised before removal of a thymoma (Keynes 1955) and also for non-tumour cases (Schulz & Schwab 1971). The additional benefit has not been proved.

Ultrathymic immunosuppression. Whole-body irradiation reduces the total pool of immune cells and all subsets are equally at risk. Thiopurines and nitrogen mustards depress immune responses by suppression of T-cell-mediated humoral responses, most effectively at the time of antigen presentation and proliferation of antigen-specific T cells. They therefore have the potential of selective suppression of T/B-cell interactions leading to production of IgG class antibodies, but in practice have an appreciable risk of side effects which endanger life. Despite 20 years of clinical trials, cytotoxic drugs have not been established as being superior to thymectomy alone.

Azathioprine. Even in a dosage of 100 mg/day, significant reduction of myasthenia gravis is delayed for 2–24 months, control is inadequate (Hertel et al 1979) and relapse follows withdrawal of treatment after prolonged suppression of symptoms (Hohlfeld et al 1985). When used as a 'steroid sparer' with low-dose prednisolone, the metabolic complications of both drugs are reduced but the risk of uncontrolled infection is not, and the clinical advantage has not been established.

Cyclophosphamide. This alkylating immunosuppressant has greater activity than azathioprine against B cells and other replicating cells. It is more toxic to the gonads. Lymphomas and leukaemias occur more commonly and enhancement of infection is greater. Clinical and neurological remission of myasthenia may be obtained with cumulative dosage of 30 g over a period of one to two years but relapse is common when treatment is stopped (Perez et al 1981).

No cytotoxic immunosuppressive regime has been shown to induce permanent remission, and all are hazardous, but they may have a limited role in treatment of patients who have not been offered thymectomy during clinical stage 1.

Corticosteroids; adrenocorticotrophin. Early reports of 'rebound' remission after initial deterioration of myasthenia treated by ACTH were not followed up because of early fatalities, until the management of crisis situations improved and intensive therapy units became commonplace. It was then possible to use larger doses of ACTH or prednisolone with striking benefit. In the first seven to ten days of treatment there is often clinical deterioration which is associated with a rise of receptor antibody preceding a sustained fall (Lefvert et al 1978), with marked remission of symptoms. As intubation and supported respiration may become necessary, the treatment should be started in hospital. It appears that any corticosteroid or timing regime may be used (Brunner et al 1976) at any clinical stage including the most advanced. Serum concentration of anti-AChR antibody decreases and anticholinesterase dosage may be reduced progressively (but not abruptly withdrawn). A recommended regime is prednisone 100 mg daily or on alternate days for a month or more. Subsequent withdrawal of prednisone must be very gradual, by no more than 10 mg decrements at six to eight week intervals. Pascuzzi et al (1982) reported no satisfactory improvement in 20% of 116 patients. The median time to maximal improvement was five to six months. Only 14% of patients could discontinue steroid treatment and this was not improved by previous thymectomy. Most benefit is experienced by patients over the age of 50 years, but individual responsiveness is not predictable. Results of treatment are impressive, but the side effects and hazards are not negligible (Brunner et al 1976, Mann et al

1976). It is not known how long steroid treatment must be continued. In my opinion it is not a treatment of first choice but should be reserved for patients not responding to thymectomy and anticholinesterases and preferably not until three years or more after operation. Some early reports were certainly over-enthusiastic and not supported by controlled trial (Howard et al 1976). Indeed, it is by no means certain that the benefit from steroids is due to immunosuppression. A direct neuromuscular action is possible, perhaps on regeneration of end-plates or on acetylcholine release (Weir 1982).

Antilymphocyte and antithymocyte sera. It is possible that cytotoxic and steroid immunosuppression may act on immunocompetent cells in division, presumably in the reticuloendothelial system, and so the phase of activity may be critical. This limitation may not apply to these sera. Antilymphocyte serum acts to deplete paracortical lymph node areas where recirculation of antigen-sensitive lymphocytes occurs. An additional action may be to coat the receptor sites of the lymphocytes. Antithymocyte serum has been used in myasthenic patients with varying degrees of clinical improvement, especially when used after thymectomy (Pirofsky et al 1971, Roux et al 1974). Aureggi et al (1970) also used antilymphocyte serum. Although of theoretical importance, these antisera appear to be of limited practical value.

Removal of antibodies and immunoaggressive cells. Drainage of lymph from the thoracic duct, with removal of 0.5–2.0 l daily, to a total of 4–5 l, causes improvement of myasthenic weakness within 48 h. Although the lymph volume increases again in a few days, there is maintained improvement for a year or more (Matell et al 1976). This treatment has been supplanted by plasmapheresis.

Plasma exchange (plasmapheresis) is an effective method for reducing serum anti-AChR antibody. Newsom-Davis et al (1978), who first used the treatment, reported progressive improvement in strength, commonly after two days. We have had good results with six exchanges of 4 litres. Plasmapheresis followed by immunosuppressive therapy may give long remissions. In most cases, however, relapse occurs in one to three weeks.

Some authors recommend repeated courses of plasmapheresis (Newsom-Davis et al 1981).

Unfortunately, relapse at five to six months is sometimes severe. Susceptibility to infection is temporarily increased by antibody depletion, the role of which is still being assessed. There is no direct relationship between the magnitude of fall in antibody titre and improvement. If it merely removed an immunopharmacological block, antibody depletion would be restricted to the management of myasthenic crises or for preoperative preparation, but it may also permit synthesis of new receptors if followed by long-term immunosuppression (Newsom-Davis et al 1978). The rapid changes in the safety factor for neuromuscular transmission require careful adjustment of anticholinesterase dosage. The efficacy of lymph duct drainage and plasmapheresis depends on the fact that the antireceptor antibody regenerates more slowly than the main pool of immunoglobulin. Nevertheless, increased susceptibility to infection is a hazard, and feedback overproduction of auto-antibodies (Bystryn et al 1971) may be dangerous. A method of inhibiting their production selectively would be ideal.

Induction of anti-idiotypic antibodies. A second-best procedure would be selective destruction of autoantibody. Preliminary experimental induction of anti-idiotypic antibodies by immunisation against AChR-educated lymphocytes has been reported (Schwartz et al 1978). If confirmed and extended to the human, this would provide a highly effective treatment for myasthenia gravis, but Barkas & Simpson (1982) found that anti-idiotypic antisera do not cross-react between individuals or species. Favourable response to polyclonal antibody mixtures has been reported (Fatch-Moghadam et al 1984). Meanwhile, although treatment of the immunological basis of myasthenia gravis must be a prime consideration, it is always necessary to raise the safety factor for neuromuscular transmission. Anticholinesterase medication should be continued in an appropriate dosage throughout all immunosuppressive treatment.

Choice of treatment. Protagonists of thymectomy,

immunosuppression and plasmapheresis vigorously support their favoured regime in the literature. I believe that treatment should be based on certain principles: (1) Anticholinesterase drugs must be used with discretion to avoid cholinergic poisoning: there is no evidence that long-term use in therapeutic dosage is harmful in man. (2) Thymectomy is safe and of proven value although rarely curative. (3) Death from myasthenia gravis is rare after the second year if choking is avoided. (4) Immunosuppressant drugs have serious side effects and can rarely be withdrawn without relapse resulting. I therefore recommend that all myasthenics should take pyridostigmine in adequate but not excessive dosage (see below). Anti-immunological therapy is a parallel, not an alternative treatment.

Every patient should be offered thymectomy if there is clinical evidence that myasthenia is not confined to the extraocular muscles and symptoms have not been present for more than seven years. Sex and age do not influence the results if account is taken of the appropriate natural history. If myasthenia is generalised, the severity is not relevant because the future course is not predictable. Late spontaneous remissions are rare. With longer duration before diagnosis, thymectomy is still indicated if there is radiological or serological evidence of thymoma as the tumour is potentially invasive. Late cases failing to respond to pharmacological treatment have less to gain but nothing to lose from thymectomy supervised by an experienced neurologist.

No special preparation is required if the policy of early thymectomy is followed (Fraser et al 1978). It should be delayed until a 'crisis' (see below) is controlled by plasmapheresis or steroids if necessary. Otherwise preoperative steroid therapy is unnecessary. Preparation for operation and treatment of 'crisis' are the only indications for plasmapheresis. Steroids undoubtedly suppress autoimmune reactivity and would be strongly endorsed but for the serious and irreversible side effects. I use them (usually prednisolone) only for patients with life-threatening weakness or where there is a contraindication to surgery. I consider that cytotoxic drugs have little advantage and greater risk. After using them to gain experience

I have abandoned azathioprine and cyclophosphamide. If newer immunoregulatory drugs prove less
toxic, the audit will be different.

Insertion of new receptors. The rate of insertion
of AChR receptors is increased by anti-AChR antibody in EAMG and is highest in denervated
muscle. It appears to be indirectly related to the
concentration of receptors already present in the
postjunctional membrane. Anabolic steroids have
no significant clinical effect (J. A. Simpson,
unpublished work). De Baets (1984) found a
protective effect in rat EAMG but this was related
to lower antibody titres in the hormone-treated
animals.

Elevation of the safety factor for transmission

Anticholinesterase drugs. Inhibitors of end-
plate acetylcholinesterase raise the safety factor for
neuromuscular transmission by preventing hydrolysis of ACh and so prolonging the occupancy of
receptor sites by ACh. Anticholinesterases do not
increase production of ACh and so are effective for
as long as the transmitter is released at motor
nerve endings and the ACh receptors of the end-
plates are intact. In stage 3 myasthenia this may
not be so, at least in some muscles ('neostigmine
resistance'). On the other hand, if inhibition of
cholinesterase is carried to excess, so that ACh
persists at receptor sites, the end-plate remains
depolarised or becomes desensitised ('cholinergic
(blockade') (see p. 653).

Anticholinesterases which have been used
previously include physostigmine (eserine), galan-
thamine, ambenonium, bis-quaternary compounds
such as distigmine bromide, and alkyl phosphates.
They have been abandoned, either because they
cross the blood–brain barrier, with central
actions, or because their prolonged action leads to
cumulative poisoning.

Edrophonium chloride (Tensilon®). This hydroxy-
anilinium salt, administered intravenously
(2–10 mg) has a peak action in 2–3 min, which
rapidly subsides. Although some effect is still
apparent 20–30 min later, this is too brief for
therapeutic purposes. It is used to confirm the
diagnosis of myasthenia or to differentiate between
underdosage and overdosage of anticholinesterases
(p. 653).

Neostigmine bromide (Prostigmin®). The 15 mg
tablet of neostigmine has a cholinergic activity
which evokes a surge of muscular power for
30–60 min, followed by continued activity at a
lower level for 2–6 h. Subsequently, strength is
rapidly lost, making it difficult to adjust the
timing of dosage. Most myasthenics prefer pyridostigmine for this reason. The 'boost' effect of
neostigmine is valuable if taken 30 min before a
meal or a special physical effort.

Pyridostigmine bromide (Mestinon®). Pyridostigmine has less peak effect than neostigmine and its
plateau of activity is very little longer but it wanes
more slowly, allowing a sustained blood level to
be achieved by judiciously timed dosage: this
varies from 2–8 h and the frequency must again
be established by trial. The 60 mg tablet of pyridostigmine is approximately equivalent to the
15 mg tablet of neostigmine. Each of these drugs
should be given by mouth (crushed tablet by
nasogastric tube if necessary) in preference to
parenteral injection, but in some patients absorption is erratic and it is then necessary to rely on
subcutaneous or intramuscular injection of neostigmine methylsulphate (1 mg having an effect
equivalent to 15 mg neostigmine or 60 mg pyridostigmine given orally). It should rarely be given
intravenously as bradycardia may be dangerous.

**Potentiation of ACh release and muscular
responsiveness.** A number of drugs raise the
safety factor for transmission by potentiating
release of ACh presynaptically and/or by sensitisation of ACh receptors or muscle contraction. The
major action is uncertain and they are inferior to
anticholinesterases in treatment of myasthenia
gravis. Guanidine and the aminopyridines are
discussed on p. 657.

Adrenaline; ephedrine etc. Adrenaline and its
amine analogues have exceedingly weak anticholinesterase activity. They are of no practical value
for myasthenia gravis but ephedrine may be

beneficial by combating the bronchoconstriction caused by anticholinesterases (Ringvist & Ringvist 1971). The oral dose is 10–25 mg thrice daily.

Veratrum alkaloids; germine esters. Drugs of this group 'amplify' the muscle response by causing repetitive firing of nerve endings and of the stimulated muscle. Their potential value is insufficient to compensate for important side effects such as hypotension, cardiac arrhythmias and sensory symptoms, although Flacke et al (1966) found these negligible with germine in short-term studies.

Potassium; aldosterone inhibitors. Potassium was once used extensively as an adjuvant in myasthenia gravis. The rationale was obscure and the benefit not documented. It may cause nausea and diarrhoea resembling cholinergic crisis. Spironolactone, given to conserve potassium (Gottleib & Laurent 1961), is of no proven value although it gives a sensation of well-being. Provision of potassium to counteract loss of intracellular potassium during steroid therapy is quite another matter and its use is rational (Critchley et al 1977).

Theophylline; caffeine etc. Phosphodiesterase inhibitors (which increase intracellular cAMP) have been reported to increase the strength of myasthenic patients by increasing Ca^{++} flux at the prejunctional membrane (Dretchen & Standaert 1981). Appel et al (1981) reported stimulation of receptor synthesis of myotubes in culture from calcium and cyclic nucleotides.

Drugs which may lower the safety factor

Enemas may cause sudden death in myasthenics (Keynes 1950). The mechanism is unknown, but may involve stretching of a bowel rendered tonic by anticholinesterases. Corticosteroids, adrenocorticotrophin and thyroxin may cause temporary deterioration. Respiratory depressants, including morphine and sedatives, must be used with care, but diazepam is relatively safe. Myasthenic syndromes are very occasionally caused by penicillamine and β-adrenergic blocking drugs (p. 655), but there is no evidence that these remedies aggravate spontaneous myasthenia gravis. Several drugs

regularly lower the safety factor for transmission at the neuromuscular junction and should be used (with appropriate adjustment of anticholinesterase dosage) only if the indication is clamant (see Ch. 29).

Inhibitors of production or release of ACh. A number of aminoglycoside antibiotics have this action, including streptomycin, dihydrostreptomycin, neomycin, kanamycin, gentamycin, viomycin, bacitracin, polymyxin A and B, and colistin, especially with renal insufficiency (Hokkanen 1964). Low ionised serum calcium may be implicated in a presynaptic action (Wright & McQuillen 1971).

Blockers of ACh receptors or of muscle response. Any neuromuscular blocking drug must be used with caution in myasthenia gravis. Despite the increased sensitivity to curare (p. 645), D-tubocurarine is the best if relaxation for surgery is required, because its mode of action is consistent and is antagonised by neostigmine. The anomalous responses to depolarising drugs (decamethonium, and suxamethonium and others) are dose-dependent and vary in different muscles (Churchill-Davidson & Richardson 1952).

Membrane stabilisers (hydantoinates, quinine, quinidine, procainamide) are, in principle, harmful but rarely cause significant deterioration.

MYASTHENIC CRISIS

There is little justification for this traditional term, which implies sudden spontaneous exacerbation of disease activity. Unquestionably, most cases in the past were examples of unrecognised cholinergic crisis or asphyxia. It is, of course, true that weakness is increased by unusual physical exertion, emotional upset, an infection or childbirth, but it responds to management of the stressful situation. The drugs listed above, which lower the safety factor for transmission or depress respiration, should be used with caution. Myasthenic crisis is rare in well-managed patients.

The absence of cholinergic signs and the presence of a favourable response to the edrophonium test (p. 646) indicate the cause of the severe weakness. If it is necessary to increase the dose of anticholinesterase medication, the only suitable method in emergency is intramuscular injection of neostigmine. Endotracheal intubation is necessary if pulmonary ventilation is failing, or there is severe dysphagia. Thick, glairy bronchial secretion must be aspirated by bronchoscopic suction. Tracheostomy is not required unless the need for passive ventilation continues for more than one week. Once respiration is safeguarded, treatment can proceed methodically without panic measures, the dose of neostigmine or pyridostigmine being regulated by repeated edrophonium titration (Osserman & Kaplan 1953). It is possible that plasma exchange may produce rapid improvement but it cannot be relied on.

CHOLINERGIC CRISIS

Mild muscarinic effects of anticholinesterase medication (colic, diarrhoea, belching, nausea) are not uncommon in myasthenic patients, although less prominent than in normal subjects taking the same dose. More severe muscarinic signs such as vomiting, sweating, hypersalivation, lachrymation, miosis and pallor are less common and indicate that the dose is nearing a dangerous level. The most valuable indication of impending danger is the size of the pupil. It should not be allowed to contract to less than 2 mm diameter in normal room lighting. Bradycardia is very unusual with oral medication, but may be prominent and lead to cardiac arrest with intravenous medication. Hypotension occurs with severe cholinergic poisoning. In the most severe cases, confusion and coma indicate block of cerebral synapses. The use of an antagonist such as atropine sulphate (0.3–0.6 mg) is obligatory with intravenous dosage, but need not be given if the cholinergic drug is administered orally or by subcutaneous injection, unless colic is intolerable. The disadvantage of suppressing the muscarinic symptoms is that more serious nicotonic signs may be overlooked (Schwab 1954). There is, however, no evidence that atropine inhibits the nicotinic signs, the earliest of which is fasciculation of muscles. This need not be a serious sign as it will first appear in muscles unaffected by myasthenia.

Persistent fasciculation in the leg muscles is consistent with excellent clinical control. Conversely, a depolarisation block may be reached without previous fasciculation, or the latter may be transient and therefore overlooked. A muscle may pass from myasthenic weakness to cholinergic block without passing through a stage of normal strength. Poisoning has reached a dangerous level ('cholinergic crisis') when weakness increases because of depolarisation block. This may be difficult to recognise and undoubtedly accounts for most cases of 'neostigmine resistance' not attributable to muscular atrophy. It must be emphasised that different muscles will reflect their degree of myasthenic involvement. Thus, some muscles may suffer cholinergic block while others still require further anticholinesterase medication. As the muscles of respiration are often relatively spared by myasthenia, they may be blocked by a dose of neostigmine which is insufficient for the ocular or limb muscles. It is extremely important to measure the effect of a test dose of edrophonium on the respiratory and bulbar muscles as well as on the more easily tested muscles. Even though short-acting, the additional cholinergic effect of edrophonium may be fatal in cholinergic crisis. In these circumstances atropine should be injected first and there should be facilities for immediate assisted respiration. The test is described on page 646.

Cholinergic paralysis requires urgent treatment. A cuffed endotracheal tube should be passed at once and positive-pressure respiration started. Tracheostomy may be necessary if this has to be prolonged. Atropine sulphate should be injected intravenously (2 mg/h) until signs of atropine toxicity develop. Specific antidotes for anticholinesterase poisoning are not satisfactory in clinical practice. Drugs of the oxime group have some effect on overdosage of quaternary ammonium anticholinesterases (Grob & Johns 1958). Personal experience is limited to pyridine-2-aldoxime (2-PAM) and methane sulphonate (P_2S) but their latency has been found to be too long and their potency and duration of action inadequate for satisfactory treament. Physiological antagonism can be obtained by the use of D-tubocurarine if respiration is artificially controlled. In these circumstances there is little need for an antidote other than atropine to protect the cardiovascular system. Controlled respiration and repeated atropine injection pending the recovery of the neuromuscular response is the most satisfactory form of treatment available at present. Anticholinesterase medication should not be resumed until there is a clear 'myasthenic' type of response to edrophonium on two successive occasions at intervals of 1 h. On resumption, neostigmine should be given by injection and an adequate dose discovered by trial, guided by edrophonium testing. Only when this has been done should oral medication be resumed, at first with neostigmine and then with longer-acting drugs by cautious substitution and prolongation of dose-interval.

DIFFERENTIAL DIAGNOSIS

Myasthenia gravis has to be differentiated from the symptomatic myasthenias described below. More commonly, the problem is to fail to recognise the existence of a myasthenic disorder; once considered, the diagnosis is rarely in doubt. Positive EMG tests (p. 644) are confirmatory but negative tests do not invalidate the diagnosis. A properly conducted edrophonium test, with objective response, is very reliable and a raised titre of anti-AChR antibody in the blood is diagnostic of myasthenia gravis. A normal titre does not, however, exclude the diagnosis.

Myasthenia gravis is commonly mistaken for hysteria because it is so often precipitated by emotional disturbances, and physical signs may be absent if the patient has rested before examination. The intermittent nature of the symptoms and the frequent occurrence of diplopia and dysarthria or other bulbar symptoms may suggest multiple sclerosis. Motor neurone disease, parkinsonism, peripheral neuropathy, and endocrine disorders, particularly thyrotoxicosis, may cause weakness which increases with effort; hypokalaemic states, periodic paralysis, paroxysmal myoglobinuria, botulism, craft palsies and other disorders causing transient paralysis may be confused with myasthenia gravis.

The most difficult disorders to differentiate from myasthenia gravis are the condition termed 'pseudoptosis', mitochondrial myopathy and the congenital syndromes with facial and extraocular palsies including congenital ptosis, ocular myopathy and the Von Graefe–Moebius syndrome. None of these conditions responds favourably to anticholinesterase drugs.

OTHER MYASTHENIC SYNDROMES

The syndrome of progressively decreasing muscular power during continuous or repeated contraction, which is relieved by rest, will result from any disorder which lowers the safety factor for neuromuscular transmission, short of complete block. Many of the types described in the literature are detected only during EMG or pharmacological studies and do not show pathological fatiguability on clinical testing. The lesion may be either pre- or post-junctional. Thus Churchill-Davidson & Wise (1963) examined children under the age of six months and found that successive muscle responses to repetitive stimulation of the motor nerve showed a decrement of amplitude, followed by post-tetanic facilitation. Furthermore, such infants were remarkably resistant to high doses of depolarising drugs such as decamethonium. At birth, human motor end-plates are immature, many consisting of terminal clubs, and a terminal arborisation (if present) is simple. Many immature end-plates are seen in children up to the age of two years (Coërs & Woolf 1959). It is possible that maturation arrest might account for the unusual case of benign congenital myopathy with myasthenic features described by Walton et al (1956) and for the congenital myasthenic syndrome in a 15-year-old boy described by Engel et al (1976a). Neither of these patients had a worthwhile response to neostigmine. In the case described by Engel et al (1976a) there was acetylcholinesterase deficiency in the subneural apparatus of the motor end-plates and no increase in anti-AChR antibody. The congenital myasthenias are described more fully in Chapter 20.

Cholinesterase deficiency

Deficiency of pseudocholinesterase may be genetic or acquired. In normal life there is no muscular weakness, but prolonged apnoea occurs if the affected person is given a depolarising relaxant drug (e.g. suxamethonium) and this disorder must then be distinguished from carcinomatous myasthenia. The genetic variety has a number of phenotypes which may be identified by measuring the inhibitory effect of dibucaine or fluorine (Lehmann & Liddell 1969).

Acquired deficiency of pseudocholinesterase is caused by liver disease, pregnancy, and use of certain drugs, phenelzine (a monoamine oxidase inhibitor) and echothiophate (an organophosphorus compound used as eye drops for glaucoma) (Pantuck & Pantuck 1975). The most important and the only necessary treatment for prolonged response to suxamethonium is adequate pulmonary ventilation, continued for several hours if necessary.

Nutritional, metabolic and toxic myasthenia

A disease named kubisagari in Japan was described in the late nineteenth century. This was an outbreak of paralysis with ptosis and bulbar symptoms. Similar epidemics occurred in prisoner-of-war camps in the Far East. Denny-Brown (1947) reported that parenteral administration of thiamine caused the symptoms to disappear in one week but Japanese authorities now consider that kubisagari was synonymous with myasthenia gravis.

In rare cases of peripheral neuropathy a decrementing response to serial stimulation may be seen, as in diabetic neuropathy, Guillain–Barré syndrome and post-zoster motor neuropathy (Simpson & Lenman 1959, Simpson 1966a). It is also found in other lower motor neurone diseases including poliomyelitis, syringomyelia and motor neurone disease. This statement refers to the electrophysiological findings: clinical myasthenia is exceedingly rare in disorders of the lower motor neurones. One condition in which it has been described is acute idiopathic porphyria, in which the myasthenic weakness is said to respond to neostigmine (Gillhespy & Smith 1954).

Muscular weakness of 'myasthenic' type in chewers of tobacco which had fermented as the result of contamination by *Clostridium perfringens* was described by French authors (Coulonjou & Salaun 1952). This organism usually causes severe myositis (gas gangrene) and it is possible that minimal muscular damage was responsible for the symptoms described, but it is interesting to consider the possibility of an exotoxin such as that produced by *Cl. botulinum*.

Treatment of patients with a number of β-adrenergic-blocking drugs has resulted in a clinical syndrome described as resembling myasthenia gravis by Herishanu & Rosenberg (1975) who attributed it to a neuromuscular-depressant effect described by previous workers. It should be remembered that serious adverse reactions to some β-blockers are immunological in nature (Behan et al 1976b).

A number of patients have developed typical myasthenia gravis while taking D-penicillamine for rheumatoid arthritis or Wilson's disease (Bucknall 1977). Marked falls of serum IgA and other immunoglobulins have been reported with penicillamine treatment for non-immunological diseases (Stephens & Fenton 1977) and a lupus reaction has been induced (Golding & Walshe 1977). It therefore seems likely that myasthenia results directly from the drug (and not from association with rheumatoid arthritis) and that it has an immunological pathogenesis. It clears up when D-penicillamine is withdrawn. Nevertheless, as only two cases of myasthenia have occurred during treatment of Wilson's disease (Dawkins et al 1975b), existing immunological abnormality or genetic constitution may be important predisposing factors. Penicillamine-induced myasthenia gravis has been found to be associated with HLA haplotypes A1, A8 by Bucknall (1977) and Bw, DR1 by Garlepp et al (1983).

Polymyositis and related disorders

A myasthenic type of weakness is commonly present at some stage of polymyositis and dermatomyositis (Walton & Adams 1958). The decrementing neuromuscular response is similar to that of myasthenia gravis and there is usually an initial favourable response to edrophonium or neostigmine. Typically, the 'fatiguability' is transient or the response to anticholinesterase drugs is not maintained after the first few doses. A similar transient myasthenic syndrome occurs in systemic lupus erythematosus but classic myasthenia gravis also occurs in that disease (Harvey et al 1954). As interstitial myositis may occur in myasthenia gravis, and the diagnostic status of anticholinesterase responsiveness is debatable, it is clear that the diagnosis will often give rise to disagreement. The most reasonable interpretation is that all are autoimmune diseases which often show clinical and serological overlap and association with thymic tumours. Dermatomyositis is particularly related to carcinoma. The EMG findings were described by Simpson (1966a) who drew attention to a marked facilitation during rapid stimulation, and occasional slow augmentation of tension and EMG on voluntary contraction (Simpson & Lenman 1959). These authors and Simpson (1966a) described a number of patients in whom the incrementing response was the major reaction. None of their cases had a malignant tumour or developed one subsequently and some had other EMG or histological characteristics of polymyositis. This intermediate group, which constitutes an important link between polymyositis and the carcinomatous myasthenic syndrome, is now classified as an autoimmune form of Lambert–Eaton syndrome.

Lambert–Eaton syndrome

The occasional occurrence of a myasthenic type of muscular weakness associated with malignant tumours was first recognised when Anderson et al (1953) reported prolonged apnoea after administration of succinylcholine to a patient with bronchial neoplasm, and similar patients were reported in the next two years. As the neuromuscular block was reversed by edrophonium, these authors recognised an abnormal end-plate responsiveness resembling that occurring in myasthenia gravis (p. 646). Croft (1958) found abnormal responses to relaxant drugs in patients with carcinomatous neuropathy, not all of whom had symptoms of muscular fatiguability, and drew attention to absence of the tendon jerks. The clinical syndrome was first clearly defined by Lambert et al (1961). They found later that the syndrome is usually related to malignant tumour, either contemporaneously or preceding it by several years, but mainly in men over the age of 40, whereas most women with this syndrome do not develop a recognised neoplasm. The tumour is

usually a small-cell or oat-cell carcinoma of bronchus; Greene et al (1968) drew attention to possible histological differences in the tumour cells, suggesting a secretory function. Less commonly the syndrome has occurred with intrathoracic reticulum cell sarcoma (Rooke et al 1960) and with carcinoma of breast, colon, stomach, prostate and other organs (Adams 1975).

Association of the non-carcinomatous type with autoimmune diseases was noted by Gutman et al (1972) and Lang et al (1981). Patients with both types of Lambert–Eaton syndrome have a linkage disequilibrium for HLA-B8 and DRw3 antigens and the IgG heavy chain marker Glm(2) (Willcox et al 1985).

The principal symptoms are weakness and fatiguability of proximal muscles of the extremities, particularly of the pelvic girdle and thighs. Careful manual testing often reveals a delay in development of strength at the onset of maximal voluntary contraction. Ptosis may be present, but striking differences from myasthenia gravis are that symptoms of involvement of ocular and bulbar muscular weakness either do not occur, or are mild and transient, and that the tendon reflexes are depressed or absent. Common complaints are aching of the lower limbs, peripheral paraesthesiae, dryness of the mouth and loss of potency.

The significance of these symptoms is commonly apparent in retrospect after the patient has had prolonged apnoea following administration of a muscle-relaxant drug during surgical procedures. The diagnosis is then readily confirmed by characteristic EMG responses to repetitive supramaximal motor nerve stimulation. The rested muscle shows a pronounced depression of the response to a single stimulus. Low rates of stimulation evoke further decrement: stimulation rates above 10/s evoke markedly incremental responses (Lambert et al 1965, Lambert 1966). For further details see Chapter 30. Intracellular recordings from the end-plate region of single muscle fibres reveal normal miniature end-plate potentials but subthreshold end-plate potentials which vary greatly, indicating that a very low number of ACh quanta are released from the nerve ending until it is stimulated repetitively (Elmqvist & Lambert 1968). Pharmacological studies on biopsied muscle have shown a reduction in the number of quanta of acetylcholine released from the nerve terminal and also of non-quantal release ('molecular leakage') (Molenaar et al 1982). The transmission characteristics are similar, but not identical, to those of a normal neuromuscular junction exposed to a high Mg^{2+} concentration. The blood level of Mg^{2+} is normal. The quantum content of the end-plate potential is raised by increasing the external calcium ion concentration and with the addition of guanidine.

Pathology. The clinical neurophysiology and pharmacology indicate a prejunctional abnormality of ACh release. In light microscopic specimens, stained intravitally with methylene blue, Wise & MacDermot (1962) noted irregularity of calibre and abnormal swelling of axons of intramuscular nerve fibres, increased preterminal branching, and abnormally large and complex end-plates which they regarded as consistent with a mild peripheral neuropathy. Engel & Santa (1971) found no significant abnormality in the mean area of motor nerve terminals, and a normal number of synaptic vesicles, but there was possibly a decrease in the mean diameter of the vesicles and of the mean area of mitochondria in the nerve terminals. Freeze-fracture studies of the neuromuscular junction showed loss and disorganisation of presynaptic active zone particles, possibly representing distorted calcium channels (Fukunaga et al 1983a). Engel & Santa (1971) also drew attention to an overdevelopment of the post-junctional region, highly complex secondary clefts and folds, and the sacroplasmic folds contained numerous pinocytotic vesicles. At present it is not understood why the post-junctional region is altered in this way or how it contributes to the functional deficit.

There is indirect evidence for antibody-mediated attack on the presynaptic active zone particles (see below). Serum antibody against ACh receptors is not increased (Lindstrom et al 1976a). There is no report on anti-axonal antibody.

Pathogenesis. Speculation about the possible causes of the cancer-related myasthenic syndrome has postulated tumour-derived neurotoxin (Ishikawa et al 1977), polypeptide hormone (Simpson 1982) and immunological disorder (cf previous editions). Immunogenesis is virtually certain, as Newsom-Davis and colleagues have demonstrated that the IgG fraction of plasma from affected patients when injected into mice evokes a similar syndrome (Lang et al 1983, 1984). It is probable that an IgG antibody binds to nerve terminal determinants concerned with release of ACh, causing the distortion of active zones observed by Fukunaga et al (1983a, b). The London and Mayo Clinic groups in collaboration showed that paucity and disorganisation of active zone particles and reduction of quantal content of ACh could be induced in the nerve terminals of mice injected with IgG from patients with the myasthenic syndrome. Late components of complement are not required (Prior et al 1985). Voltage-dependent calcium channels necessary for quantal release of ACh may be damaged. Presumably the postsynaptic changes which are so distinctive morphologically must be secondary. The mechanism of induction of the apparent antibody is unknown. As in most autoimmune disorders, a reduction of circulating suppressor T cells (as marked by the OK T8 monoclonal antibody) has been reported (Robb et al 1985) but, surprisingly, only in the tumour-associated type.

Treatment. Evidence for humoral autoimmunity has encouraged treatment with corticosteroids (previously used empirically), cytotoxic immunosuppressants and plasma exchange as for myasthenia gravis (Newsom-Davis & Murray 1984). The most favourable treatment regime has not yet been established. Pending recovery of nerve terminal function, release of acetylcholine may be potentiated by several drugs. Anticholinesterase drugs (e.g. pyridostigmine) are temporarily beneficial. Guanidine hydrochloride is strikingly effective on prolonged administration. Lambert (1966) recommended 20–30 mg/kg/day in divided dosage: the effect is superior to that of 4-aminopyridine or 3-4-diaminopyridine (Lundh et al 1977, 1983), both of which lower the threshold for seizures. Where tumour has not been identified but may be occult, immunosuppressant treatment may accelerate growth of oat-cell carcinoma and Newsom-Davis & Murray (1984) advise caution in heavy smokers with the Glm(2) heavy chain phenotype.

REFERENCES

Aarli J A, Milde E-J, Thunold S 1975 Arthritis in myasthenia gravis. Journal of Neurology, Neurosurgery and Psychiatry 38:1048

Aarli J A, Heimann P, Matre R, Thunold S, Tonder O 1979 Lymphocyte subpopulations in thymus and blood from patients with myasthenia gravis. Journal of Neurology, Neurosurgery and Psychiatry 42:29

Aarli J A, Thunold S 1981 Serological detection of thymoma in myasthenia gravis. European Neurology 20:380

Abdou N I, Lisak R P, Zweiman B, Abramson I, Penn A S 1974 The thymus in myasthenia gravis. Evidence for altered cell populations. New England Journal of Medicine 291:1271

Adams D D 1977 In: Holborow E J, Reeves W G (eds) Immunology in medicine. Academic Press, London, p 373

Adams R D 1975 Diseases of muscle. A study in pathology, 3rd edn. Harper and Row, Maryland

Aharonov A, Tarrab-Hazdai R, Abramsky O, Fuchs S 1975a Humoral antibodies to acetylcholine receptor in patients with myasthenia gravis. Lancet 2:340

Aharanov A, Tarrab-Hazdai R, Abramsky O, Fuchs S 1975b Immunological relationship between acetylcholine receptor and thymus — a possible significance in myasthenia gravis. Proceedings of the National Academy of Sciences USA 72:1456

Alarcón-Segovia D, Galbraith R F, Maldonado J E, Howard F M 1963 Systemic lupus erythematosus following thymectomy for myasthenia gravis. Lancet 2:662

Almon R R, Andrew C G, Appel S H 1974 Serum globulin in myasthenia gravis: inhibition of α-bungarotoxin binding to acetylcholine receptors. Science 186:55

Alpert L I, Papatestas A, Kark A, Osserman R S, Osserman K 1971 A histologic reappraisal of the thymus in myasthenia gravis. Archives of Pathology 91:55

Alter N M, Osnato M 1930 Myasthenia gravis with status lymphaticus and multiple thymic granulomas. Archives of Neurology and Psychiatry 23:345

Anderson H J, Churchill-Davidson H C, Richardson A T 1953 Bronchial neoplasm with myasthenia. Prolonged apnoea after administration of succinylcholine. Lancet 2:1291

Anwyl R, Appel S H, Narahashi T 1977 Myasthenia gravis serum reduces acetylcholine sensitivity in cultured rat myotubes. Nature 267:262

Appel S H, Almon R R, Levy N 1975 Acetylcholine receptor antibodies in myasthenia gravis. New England Journal of Medicine 293:760

Appel S H, Blosser J C, McManaman O, Ashizawa T, Elias S B 1981 The effects of carbamylcholine, calcium, and cyclic nucleotides on acetylcholine receptor synthesis in cultured myotubes. Annals of the New York Academy of Sciences 377:189

Aureggi A, Cirelli A, Virno F, Nigro G 1970 Prime osservazioni sul trattamento della miastenia grave con immunoglobulina antilinfocite ed antitimocite. Medicina Clinica e Sperimentale 20:1

Ballantyne J P, Hansen S 1974 Computer method for the analysis of evoked motor unit potentials. I. Control subjects and patients with myasthenia gravis. Journal of Neurology, Neurosurgery and Psychiatry 37:1187

Barkas T, Simpson J A 1982 Lack of inter-animal cross-reaction of anti- acetylcholine receptor antibodies at the receptor-binding site as demonstrated by heterologous anti-idiotype antisera: implications for immunotherapy of myasthenia gravis. Clinical and Experimental Immunology 47:119

Barkas T, Gairns J M, Kerr J M, Coggins J R, Simpson J A 1982 Alfa bungarotoxin binding to the nicotinic acetylcholine receptor is inhibited by two distinct subpopulations of anti-receptor antibodies. European Journal of Immunology 12:757

Becker K L, Titus J L, McConahey W M, Woolner L B 1964 Morphologic evidence of thyroiditis in myasthenia gravis. Journal of the American Medical Association 187:994

Behan P O, Simpson J A, Dick H 1973 Immune response genes in myasthenia gravis. Lancet 2:1033, 1220

Behan P O, Simpson J A, Behan W M H 1976a Decreased serum IgA in myasthenia gravis. Lancet 2:593

Behan P O, Behan W M H, Zacharias F J, Nicholls J T 1976b Immunological abnormalities in patients who had the oculomucocutaneous syndrome associated with practolol therapy. Lancet 2:984

Behan P O, Shields J 1982 Genetics. In: Lisak R P, Barchi R L (eds) Myasthenia gravis. Saunders, Philadelphia, p 37

Behan W M H, Behan P O, Simpson J A 1975 Absence of cellular hypersensitivity to muscle and thymic antigens in myasthenia gravis. Journal of Neurology, Neurosurgery and Psychiatry 38:1039

Behan W M H, Behan P O 1979 Immune complexes in myasthenia gravis. Journal of Neurology, Neurosurgery and Psychiatry 42:595

Bender A N, Ringel S P, Engel W K, Daniels M P, Vogel Z 1975 Myasthenia gravis: a serum factor blocking acetylcholine receptors of the human neuromuscular junction. Lancet 1:607

Bergman R A, Johns R J, Afifi A K 1971 Ultra-structural alterations in muscle from patients with myasthenia gravis and Eaton-Lambert syndrome. Annals of the New York Academy of Sciences 183:88

Beutner E H, Witebsky E, Ricken D, Adler R H 1962 Studies on autoantibodies in myasthenia gravis. Journal of the American Medical Association 182:46

Beutner E H, Chorzelski T P, Hale W L, Hausmanowa-Petrusewicz I 1968 Autoimmunity in concurrent myasthenia gravis and pemphigus erythematosus. Journal of the American Medical Association 203:845

Bickerstaff E R, Woolf A L 1960 The intramuscular nerve endings in myasthenia gravis. Brain 83:10

Blom S, Zakrisson J E 1974 The stapedius reflex in the diagnosis of myasthenia gravis. Journal of the Neurological Sciences 21:71

Bosch E P, Reith P E, Granner D K 1978 Myasthenia gravis and Schmidt syndrome. Neurology (Minneapolis) 27:1179

Bofill M, Janossy G, Willcox N, Chilosi M, Trejdosiewicz L K, Newsom- Davis J 1985 Microenvironments in the normal thymus and the thymus in myasthenia gravis. American Journal of Pathology 119:462

Bramis J, Sloane C, Papatestas A E, Genkins G, Aufses A H 1976 Serum IgA in myasthenia gravis. Lancet 1:1243

Brenner T, Beyth Y, Abramsky O 1980 Inhibitory effect of α-fetoprotein on the binding of myasthenia gravis antibody to acetylcholine receptor. Proceedings of the National Academy of Sciences USA 77:3635

Brody I A, Engel W K 1964 Denervation of muscle in myasthenia gravis. Archives of Neurology 11:350

Brolley N, Hollender N H 1955 Psychological problems of patients with myasthenia gravis. Journal of Nervous and Mental Disorders 122:178

Brooke M H, Engel W K 1969 The histographic analysis of human muscle biopsies with regard to fiber types. 3. Myotonias, myasthenia gravis, and hypokalemic periodic paralysis. Neurology (Minneapolis) 19:469

Brown L R, Muhm J R, Sheedy P F, Unni K K, Bernatz P E, Hermann R C 1983 The value of computed tomography in myasthenia gravis. American Journal of Roentgenology 140:31

Brunner N G, Berger C L, Namba T, Grob D 1976 Corticotropin and corticosteroids in generalized myasthenia gravis: comparative studies and role in management. Annals of the New York Academy of Sciences 274:577

Bucknall R C 1977 Myasthenia associated with D-penicillamine therapy in rheumatoid arthritis. Proceedings of the Royal Society of Medicine 70 suppl 3:114

Bundey S 1972 A genetic study of infantile and juvenile myasthenia gravis. Journal of Neurology, Neurosurgery and Psychiatry 35:41

Bundey S, Doniach D, Soothill J T 1972 Immunological studies in patients with juvenile-onset myasthenia gravis and in their relatives. Clinical and Experimental Immunology 11:321

Buzzard E F 1905 The clinical history and post-mortem examination of five cases of myasthenia gravis. Brain 28:438

Bystryn J-C, Schenkein I, Uhr J W 1971 A model for the regulation of antibody synthesis by serum antibody. In: Amos B (ed) Progress in immunology. Academic Press, New York, p 627

Campbell H, Bramwell E 1900 Myasthenia gravis. Brain 23:277

Campbell M J, Simpson E, Crombie A L, Walton J N 1970 Ocular myasthenia: evaluation of Tensilon® tomography and electromyography as diagnostic tests. Journal of Neurology, Neurosurgery and Psychiatry 33:639

Castleman B 1955 Tumors of the thymus gland. In: Atlas of tumor pathology, Section V. Armed Forces Institute of Pathology, Washington, facs 19:7

Castleman B, Norris E H 1949 The pathology of the thymus in myasthenia gravis. A study of 35 cases. Medicine (Baltimore) 28:27

Churchill-Davidson H C, Richardson A T 1952 The action of decamethonium iodide (C.10) in myasthenia gravis. Journal of Neurology, Neurosurgery and Psychiatry 15:129

Churchill-Davidson H C, Wise R P 1963 Neuromuscular transmission in the newborn infant. Anesthesiology 24:271

Clementi F, Conti-Tronconi B M 1983 Cellular immunity in myasthenia gravis. In: Albuquerque E X, Eldefrawi A T Myasthenia gravis. Chapman and Hall, London, p 423

Cleveland W L, Wasserman N H, Sarangarajan R, Penn A S, Erlanger B F 1983 Monoclonal antibodies to the acetylcholine receptor by a normally functioning auto-anti-idiotypic mechanism. Nature (London) 305:56

Coërs C, Desmedt J E 1959 Mise en evidence d'une malformation caractéristique de la jonction neuromusculaire dans la myasthénie: correlations histo- et physiopathologique. Acta Neurologica Belgica 59:539

Coërs C, Woolf A L 1959 The innervation of muscle. A biopsy study. Blackwell, Oxford

Coërs C, Telerman-Toppet N, Gerard J M 1973 Terminal innervation ratio in neuromuscular diseases. 1. Methods and controls. 2. Disorders of lower motor neurone, peripheral nerves and muscles. Archives of Neurology 29:210, 215

Coërs C, Telerman-Toppet N 1976 Morphological and histochemical changes of motor units in myasthenia. Annals of the New York Academy of Sciences 274:6

Cogan D G 1965 Myasthenia gravis: A review of the disease and a description of lid-twitch as a characteristic sign. Archives of Ophthalmology 74:217

Cohen S J, King F H 1932 Relation between myasthenia gravis and exophthalmic goitre. Archives of Neurology and Psychiatry 28:1338

Cohen S M, Waxman S 1967 Myasthenia gravis, chronic lymphocytic leukemia, and autoimmune hemolytic anemia. Archives of Internal Medicine 120:717

Compston D A S, Vincent A, Newsom-Davis J, Batchelor J R 1980 Clinical, pathological, HLA antigen and immunological evidence for disease heterogeneity in myasthenia gravis. Brain 103:579

Coulonjou R, Salaun A 1952 Sur un syndrome myasthénique fréquemment rencontre chez des chiqueurs de tabac. Semaine des Hôpitaux de Paris 28:3968

Cowan R J, Maynard C D, Witcofski R L, Janeway R, Toole J F 1971 Selenomethionine Se 75 thymus scans in myasthenia gravis. Journal of the American Medical Association 215:978

Critchley M, Herman K J, Harrison M, Shields R A, Liversedge L A 1977 Value of exchangeable electrolyte measurement in the treatment of myasthenia gravis. Journal of Neurology, Neurosurgery and Psychiatry 40:250

Croft P B 1958 Abnormal responses to muscle relaxants in carcinomatous neuropathy. British Medical Journal 1:181

Dalakas M C, Engel W K, McLure J F, Goldstein A L, Askanas V 1981 Immunocytochemical localization of thymosin- alpha 1 in thymic epithelial cells of normal and myasthenia gravis patients and in thymic cultures. Journal of the Neurological Sciences 50:239

Dau P C 1981 Response to plasmapheresis and immunosuppressive drug therapy in sixty myasthenia gravis patients. Annals of the New York Academy of Sciences 377:700

Dawkins R L, Robinson J, Wetherall J D 1975a The significance of immunological disturbances in myasthenia gravis: evidence for two subtypes. In: Bradley W G, Gardner-Medwin D, Walton J N (eds) Recent advances in myology. Excerpta Medica, Amsterdam, p 503

Dawkins R L, Zilko P J, Owen E T 1975b Penicillamine therapy, antistriational antibody, and myasthenia gravis. British Medical Journal 4:759

De Baets M H 1984 Autoimmunity to cell surface receptors. Leiter-Nyrels, Maastricht

Denny-Brown D 1947 Neurological conditions resulting from prolonged and severe dietary restriction. Medicine (Baltimore) 26:41

Devreotes P N, Fambrough D M 1975 Acetylcholine receptor turnover in membranes of developing muscle fibers. Journal of Cell Biology 65:335

Dick H M, Behan P O, Simpson J A, Durward W F 1974 The inheritance of HL-A antigens in myasthenia gravis. Journal of Immunogenetics 1:401

Djanian A Y, Beutner E H, Witebsky E 1964 Tanned-cell haemagglutination test for detection of antibodies in sera of patients with myasthenia gravis. Journal of Laboratory and Clinical Medicine 63:60

Downes J M, Greenwood B M, Wray S H 1966 Auto-immune aspects of myasthenia gravis. Quarterly Journal of Medicine 35:85

Drachman D B 1978 Myasthenia gravis. New England Journal of Medicine 298:136

Drachman D B 1981 The biology of myasthenia gravis. Annual Reviews of Neurosciences 4:195

Drachman D B, Kao L, Angus C W, Murphy A 1977 Effect of myasthenic immunoglobulin on acetylcholine receptors of cultured muscle. Annals of Neurology 1:504

Dretchen K L, Standaert F G 1981 Cyclic nucleotides and anti myasthenia drugs. Annals of the New York Academy of Sciences 377:889

Dwyer D S, Bradley R J, Urquhart C K, Kearney J F 1983 Naturally occurring anti-idiotypic antibodies in myasthenia gravis patients. Nature (London) 301:611

Elmqvist D 1965 Neuromuscular transmission with special reference to myasthenia gravis. Acta Physiologica Scandinavica (64 suppl) 249:1

Elmqvist D, Lambert E H 1968 Detailed analysis of neuromuscular transmission in a patient with the myasthenic syndrome sometimes associated with bronchogenic carcinoma. Mayo Clinic Proceedings 43:68

Engbaek L 1951 Acetylcholine sensitivity in diseases of the motor system with special regard to myasthenia gravis. Electroencephalography and Clinical Neurophysiology 3:155

Engel A G 1961 Thyroid function and myasthenia gravis. Archives of Neurology 4:663

Engel A G, Santa T 1971 Histometric analysis of the ultrastructure of the neuromuscular junction in myasthenia gravis and in the myasthenic syndrome. Annals of the New York Academy of Sciences 183:46

Engel A G, Lambert E H, Gomez M R 1976a A new myasthenic syndrome with end-plate acetylcholinesterase (AChE) deficiency, small nerve terminals, and reduced acetylcholine release. Transactions of the American Neurological Association 101:11

Engel A G, Tsujihata M, Lindstrom J M, Lennon V A 1976b The motor end plate in myasthenia gravis and in experimental autoimmune myasthenia gravis. Annals of the New York Academy of Sciences 274:60

Engel A G, Lambert E H, Howard F M 1977a Immune complexes (IgG and C3) at the motor end-plate in myasthenia gravis. Ultrastructural and light microscopic localization and electrophysiologic correlations. Mayo Clinic Proceedings 52:267

Engel A G, Lindstrom J M, Lambert E H, Lennon V A 1977b Ultrastructural localisation of the acetylcholine receptor in myasthenia gravis and in its experimental autoimmune model. Neurology (Minneapolis) 27:307

Engel A G 1984 Myasthenia gravis and myasthenic syndromes. Annals of Neurology 16:519

Fambrough D M 1979 Control of acetylcholine receptor in skeletal muscle. Physiological Reviews 59:165

Fambrough D M, Drachman D B, Satyamurti S 1973 Neuromuscular junction in myasthenia gravis: decreased acetylcholine receptors. Science 182:293

Fardeau M, Godet-Guillain J, Chevallay M 1974 Ultrastructural changes of the motor end-plates in myasthenia gravis and myasthenic syndrome. In: Subirana A, Espadaler J M (eds) Neurology. Proceedings of the X International Congress of Neurology, Barcelona 1973, International Congress Series No 319. Excerpta Medica, Amsterdam, p 427

Fateh-Moghadam A, Wick M, Besinger V and Geursen R G 1984 High-dose intravenous gammaglobulin for myasthenia gravis. Lancet 1:848

Feinberg W D, Underdahl L O, Eaton L M 1957 Myasthenia gravis and myxoedema. Proceedings of the Staff Meetings of the Mayo Clinic 32:299

Feltkamp T E W, van den Berg-Loonen P M, Nijenhuis L E et al 1974 Myasthenia gravis, autoantibodies and HL-A antigens. British Medical Journal 1:131

Feltkamp-Vroom T 1977 Myoid cells in human thymus. Lancet 2:1320

Fenichel G M, Shy G M 1963 Muscle biopsy experience in myasthenia gravis. Archives of Neurology 9:237

Ferguson F R, Hutchinson E C, Liversedge L A 1955 Myasthenia gravis. Results of medical management. Lancet 2:636

Flacke W, Caviness V S, Samaha F G 1966 The action of germine diacetate, a veratrine alkaloid without hypotensive activity, in patients with myasthenia gravis. New England Journal of Medicine 275:1207

Fraser K, Simpson J A, Crawford J 1978 The place of surgery in the treatment of myasthenia gravis. British Journal of Surgery 65:301

Frenkel M 1963 The effect of insulin and potassium in myasthenia gravis. Archives of Neurology 9:447

Fritze D, Herrmann C, Smith G S, Walford R L 1973 HL-A types in myasthenia gravis. Lancet 2:211

Fritze D, Herrmann C, Naeim F, Smith G S, Walford R L 1974 HL-A antigens in myasthenia gravis. Lancet 1:240

Fuchs S, Nevo D, Tarrab-Hazdai R, Yaar I 1976 Strain differences in the autoimmune response of mice to acetylcholine receptors. Nature 263:329

Fukunaga H, Engel A G, Osame M, Lambert E H 1983a Paucity and disorganisation of presynaptic membrane active zones in the Lambert-Eaton myasthenic syndrome. Muscle and Nerve 5:686

Fukunaga H, Engel A G, Lang B, Newsom-Davis J, Vincent A 1983b Passive transfer of Lambert-Eaton myasthenic syndrome with IgG from man to mouse depletes the presynaptic membrane active zones. Proceedings of the National Academy of Sciences USA 80:7636

Garlepp M J H, Dawkins R L, Christiansen F T 1983 HLA antigens and acetylcholine receptor antibodies in penicillamine induced myasthenia gravis. British Medical Journal 286:338

Garlepp M J, Kay P H, Dawkins R L 1984 Immunoglobulin allotype association with autoantibodies in myasthenia gravis. Disease Markers 2:429

Geld H van der, Feltkamp T E W, Oosterhuis H J G H 1964 Reactivity of myasthenia gravis serum γ-globulin with skeletal muscle and thymus demonstrated by immunofluorescence. Proceedings of the Society for Experimental Biology and Medicine 115:782

Geld H van der, Strauss A J L 1966 Myasthenia gravis. Lancet 1:57

Genkins G, Papatestas A E, Horowitz S H, Kornfeld P 1975 Studies on myasthenia gravis: early thymectomy. American Journal of Medicine 58:517

Gilhus N E, Aarli J A, Matre R 1984 Myasthenia gravis: difference between thymoma-associated antibodies and cross-striational skeletal muscle antibodies. Neurology 34:246

Gillhespy R O, Smith S G 1954 Porphyria treated with neostigmine. Lancet 1:908

Golding D N, Walshe J M 1977 Arthropathy of Wilson's

disease. Study of clinical and radiological features in 32 patients. Annals of Rheumatic Diseases 36:99

Goldstein A L, Thurman G B, Cohen G H, Rossio J L 1976 The endocrine thymus: potential role for thymosin in the treatment of autoimmune disease. Annals of the New York Academy of Sciences 274:390

Goldstein G, Whittingham S 1966 Experimental autoimmune thymitis. An animal model of human myasthenia gravis. Lancet 2:315

Gottlieb B, Laurent L P E 1961 Spironolactone in the treatment of myasthenia gravis. Lancet 2:528

Green P 1958 Aplastic anaemia associated with thymoma. Report of two cases. Canadian Medical Association Journal 78:419

Greene J G, Divertie M B, Brown A L, Lambert E H 1968 Small cell carcinoma of lung. Observations on four patients including one with a myasthenic syndrome. Archives of Internal Medicine 122:333

Greene R, Rideout D F, Shaw M L 1961 Ergometry in the diagnosis of myasthenia gravis. Lanc' t 2:281

Grob D 1953 Course and management of myasthenia gravis. Journal of the American Medical Association 153:529

Grob D 1958 Myasthenia gravis. Current status of pathogenesis, clinical manifestations, and management. Journal of Chronic Diseases 8:536

Grob D 1971 Spontaneous end-plate activity in normal subjects and in patients with myasthenia gravis. Annals of the New York Academy of Sciences 183:248

Grob D, Johns R J 1958 Use of oximes in the treatment of intoxication by anticholinesterase compounds in patients with myasthenia gravis. American Journal of Medicine 24:512

Gutman L, Crosby T W, Takamori M, Martin J D 1972 The Eaton-Lambert syndrome and auto-immune disorders. American Journal of Medicine 53:354

Harvey A M 1948 Some preliminary observations on the clinical course of myasthenia gravis before and after thymectomy. Bulletin of the New York Academy of Medicine 24:505

Harvey A M, Shulman L E, Tumulty P A, Cowley C L, Schoenrich E H 1954 Systemic lupus erythematosus. Review of the literature and clinical analysis of 138 cases. Medicine (Baltimore) 33:291

Hausmanowa-Petrusewicz I, Chorzelski T, Strugalska H 1969 Three year observation of a myasthenic syndrome concurrent with other autoimmune syndromes in a patient with thymoma. Journal of the Neurological Sciences 9:273

Hayman M 1941 Myasthenia gravis and psychosis. Report of a case with observations on its psychosomatic implications. Psychosomatic Medicine 3:120

Heinemann S, Merlie J, Lindstrom J 1978 Modulation of acetylcholine receptor in rat diaphragm by anti-receptor sera. Nature 274:65

Herishanu Y, Rosenberg P 1975 β-blockers and myasthenia gravis. Annals of Internal Medicine 83:834

Herrmann C 1971 The familial occurrence of myasthenia gravis. Annals of the New York Academy of Sciences 183:334

Hertel G, Mertens H G, Reuther P, Ricker K 1979 The treatment of myasthenia gravis with azathioprine. In: Dau P C (ed) Plasmapheresis and the immunobiology of myasthenia gravis. Houghton Mifflin, Boston, p 315

Hill P K, Lindstrom J M, Lennon V A, Dyck P J 1977 Experimental autoimmune myasthenia gravis: no morphometric abnormalities of nerve trunks. Neurology (Minneapolis) 27:200

Hoefer P F A, Aranow H, Rowland L P 1958 Myasthenia gravis and epilepsy. Archives of Neurology and Psychiatry 80:10

Hohlfeld R, Toyka K V, Besinger V A, Gerhold B, Heininger K 1985 Myasthenia gravis; reactivation of clinical disease and of autoimmune factors after discontinuation of long-term azathioprine. Annals of Neurology 17:238

Hokkanen E 1964 The aggravating effect of some antibiotics on the neuromuscular blockade in myasthenia gravis. Acta Neurologica Scandinavica 40:346

Howard F M, Duane D D, Lambert E H, Daube J R 1976 Alternate day prednisone. Preliminary report of a double-blind controlled study. Annals of the New York Academy of Sciences 274:596

Ishikawa K, Engelhardt J K, Fujisawa T, Okamoto T, Katjuki H 1977 A neuromuscular transmission block produced by a cancer tissue extract derived from a patient with the myasthenic syndrome. Neurology (Minneapolis) 27:140

Iverson L 1956 Thymoma. A review and reclassification. American Journal of Pathology 32:695

Jacob A, Clack E R, Emery A E H 1968 Genetic study of sample of 70 patients with myasthenia gravis. Journal of Medical Genetics 5:257

Johns R J, Grob D, Harvey A M 1956 Studies in neuromuscular function. 2. Effects of nerve stimulation in normal subjects and in patients with myasthenia gravis. Bulletin of the Johns Hopkins Hospital 99:125

Joseph B S, Johns T R 1973 Recurrence of non-neoplastic thymus after thymectomy for myasthenia gravis. Neurology (Minneapolis) 23:109

Kaakinen A, Pirskanen R, Tiilikainen A 1975 LD antigens associated with HL-A8 and myasthenia gravis. Tissue Antigens 6:175

Kao I, Drachman D B 1977a Thymic muscle cells bear acetylcholine receptors: possible relation to myasthenia gravis. Science 195:74

Kao I, Drachman D B 1977b Myasthenic immunoglobulin accelerates acetylcholine receptor degradation. Science 196:527

Keesey J, Lindstrom J, Cokely H, Herrman C 1977 Anti-acetylcholine receptor antibody in neonatal myasthenia gravis. New England Journal of Medicine 296:1

Keynes G 1950 Thymectomy for myasthenia gravis. In: Maingot R H (ed) Techniques in British surgery. Saunders, Philadelphia, p 126

Keynes G 1955 Investigations into thymic disease and tumour formation. British Journal of Surgery 42:449

Kim Y I 1982 Neuromuscular transmission in myasthenia gravis. Seminars in Neurology 2:199

Koch R, Regli F, Reinle W 1970 Myasthenia gravis nach Thymektomie. Schweizerische medizinische Wochenschrift 100:65

Laquer L, Weigert C 1901 Beitrage zur Lehre von der Erb'schen Krankheit ueber die Erb-sche Krankheit (Myasthenia Gravis). Neurologisches Zentralblatt 20:594

Lambert E H, Rooke E D, Eaton J M, Hodgson C H 1961 Myasthenic syndrome occasionally associated with bronchial neoplasm: neurophysiologic studies. In: Viets H R (ed) Myasthenia gravis. Thomas, Springfield, p 362

Lambert E H, Okihiro M, Rooke E D 1965 Clinical physiology of the neuromuscular junction. In: Paul W M,

Daniel E E, Kay C M, Monckton G (eds) Muscle. Pergamon Press, New York, p 487

Lambert E H 1966 Defects of neuromuscular transmission in syndromes other than myasthenia gravis. Annals of the New York Academy of Sciences 135:367

Lang B, Newsom-Davis J, Wray D, Vincent A 1981 Autoimmune aetiology for myasthenic (Eaton-Lambert) syndrome. Lancet 2:224

Lang B, Newsom-Davis J, Prior C, Wray D 1983 Antibodies to motor nerve terminals: an electrophysiological study of a human myasthenic syndrome transferred to mouse. Journal of Physiology (London) 344:335

Lang B, Molenaar P, Newsom-Davis J, Vincent A 1984 Passive transfer of Lambert-Eaton myasthenic syndrome in mice: decreased rates of resting and evoked release of acetylcholine from skeletal muscle. Journal of Neurochemistry 42:658

Lefvert A K 1982 Differences in the interaction of acetylcholine receptor antibodies with receptor from normal, denervated and myasthenic human muscle. Journal of Neurology, Neurosurgery and Psychiatry 45:70

Lefvert A K, Pirskanen R 1977 Acetylcholine receptor antibodies in cerebrospinal fluid of patients with myasthenia gravis. Lancet 2:351

Lefvert A K, Bergstrom K, Matell G, Osterman P O, Pirskanen R 1978 Determination of acetylcholine receptor antibody in myasthenia gravis: clinical usefulness and pathogenetic implications. Journal of Neurology, Neurosurgery and Psychiatry 41:394

Lefvert A K, Osterman P O 1983 Newborn infants to myasthenic mothers: a clinical study and an investigation of acetylcholine receptor antibody in 17 children. Neurology 33:133

Lehmann H, Liddell J 1969 Human cholinesterase (pseudocholinesterase): genetic variants and their recognition. British Journal of Anaesthesia 41:235

Lennon V A, Lindstrom J M, Seybold M E 1976 Experimental autoimmune myasthenia gravis: cellular and humoral immune responses. Annals of the New York Academy of Sciences 274:283

Levine G D 1979 Pathology of the thymus in myasthenia gravis: current concepts. In: Dau P C (ed) Plasmapheresis and the immunobiology of myasthenia gravis. Houghton Mifflin, Boston, p 113

Lindstrom J 1977 An assay for antibodies to human acetylcholine receptor in serum from patients with myasthenia gravis. Clinical Immunology and Immunopathology 7:36

Lindstrom J M, Engel A G, Seybold M E, Lennon V A, Lambert E H 1976a Pathological mechanisms for experimental autoimmune myasthenia gravis. Journal of Experimental Medicine 144:739

Lindstrom J M, Seybold M E, Lennon V A, Whittingham S, Duane D D 1976b Antibody to acetylcholine receptor in myasthenia gravis. Prevalence, clinical correlates, and diagnostic value. Neurology (Minneapolis) 26:1054

Lisak R P, Zweiman B 1975 Mitogen and muscle extract induced in vitro proliferative responses in myasthenia gravis, dermatomyositis and polymyositis. Journal of Neurology, Neurosurgery and Psychiatry 38:521

Lovelace R E, Stone R, Zablow L 1970 A new test for myasthenia gravis: recording of miniature end-plate potentials in situ. Neurology (Minneapolis) 20:385

Lundh H, Nilsson O, Rosen I 1977 4-Aminopyridine — a new drug tested in the treatment of Eaton-Lambert

syndrome. Journal of Neurology, Neurosurgery and Psychiatry 40:1109

Lundh H, Nilsson O, Rosen I 1983 Novel drug of choice in Eaton-Lambert syndrome. Journal of Neurology, Neurosurgery and Psychiatry 46:684

MacDermot V 1960 The changes in the motor end-plate in myasthenia gravis. Brain 83:24

McEachern D, Parnell J L 1948 The relationship of hyperthyroidism to myasthenia gravis. Journal of Clinical Endocrinology 8:842

McFarlin D E, Engel W K, Strauss A J L 1966 Does myasthenic serum bind to the neuromuscular junction? Annals of the New York Academy of Sciences 135:656

MacKay I R, Whittingham S, Goldstein G, Currie T T, Hare W S C 1968 Myasthenia gravis: clinical, serological and histological studies in relation to thymectomy. Australasian Annals of Medicine 17:1

Mann J D, Johns T R, Campa J F 1976 Long-term administration of corticosteroids in myasthenia gravis. Neurology (Minneapolis) 26:729

Martin L, Herr J C, Wanamaker W, Kornguth S 1974 Demonstration of specific antineuronal nuclear antibodies in sera of patients with myasthenia gravis. Indirect and direct immunofluorescence. Neurology (Minneapolis) 24:680

Matell G, Bergstrom K, Franksson C et al 1976 Effects of some immunosuppressive procedures on myasthenia gravis. Annals of the New York Academy of Sciences 274:659

Meyer E 1966 Psychological disturbances in myasthenia gravis: a predictive study. Annals of the New York Academy of Sciences 135:417

Millikan C, Haines S F 1953 The thyroid gland in relation to neuromuscular disease. In: Metabolic and toxic diseases of the nervous system. Research Publications, Association for Research in Nervous and Mental Disease, 32:61

Molenaar P C, Newsom-Davis J, Polak R L, Vincent A 1982 Eaton-Lambert syndrome: acetylcholine and choline acetyltransferase in skeletal muscle. Neurology 32:1062

Namba T, Grob D 1970 Familial concurrence of myasthenia gravis and rheumatoid arthritis. Archives of Internal Medicine 125:1056

Namba T, Brown S B, Grob D 1970 Neonatal myasthenia gravis: report of two cases and review of the literature. Pediatrics 45:488

Namba T, Brunner N G, Brown S B, Mugurama M, Grob D 1971a Familial myasthenia gravis. Report of 27 patients in 12 families and review of 164 patients in 73 families. Archives of Neurology 25:49

Namba T, Shapiro M S, Brunner N G, Grob D 1971b Myasthenia gravis occurring in twins. Journal of Neurology, Neurosurgery and Psychiatry 34:531

Nastuk W L, Strauss A J L, Osserman K E 1959 Search for a neuromuscular blocking agent in the blood of patients with myasthenia gravis. American Journal of Medicine 26:394

Nastuk W L, Plescia O J, Osserman K E 1960 Changes in serum complement activity in patients with myasthenia gravis. Proceedings of the Society for Experimental Biology and Medicine 105:177

Newsom-Davis J, Pinching A J, Vincent A, Wilson S G 1978 Function of circulating antibody to acetylcholine receptor in myasthenia gravis: investigation by plasma exchange. Neurology (Minneapolis) 28:266

Newsom-Davis J, Willcox N, Scadding G, Calder L, Vincent A 1981 Anti-acetylcholine receptor antibody synthesis by cultured lymphocytes in myasthenia gravis: thymic and peripheral blood cell interactions. Annals of the New York Academy of Sciences 377:393

Newsom-Davis J, Murray N F 1984 Plasma exchange and immunosuppressive drug treatment in the Lambert-Eaton myasthenic syndrome. Neurology 34:480

Noguchi S, Nishitani H 1976 Immunologic studies of a case of myasthenia gravis associated with pemphigus vulgaris after thymectomy. Neurology (Minneapolis) 26:1075

Oosterhuis H J G H 1964 Studies in myasthenia gravis. Part I (a clinical study of 180 patients). Journal of the Neurological Sciences 1:512

Oosterhuis H J G H 1984 Myasthenia gravis. Churchill Livingstone, Edinburgh

Oosterhuis H J G H, van der Geld H, Feltkamp T E W, Peetoom F 1964 Myasthenia gravis with hypergammaglobulinaemia and antibodies. Journal of Neurology, Neurosurgery and Psychiatry 27:345

Oosterhuis H, Bethlem J 1973 Neurogenic muscle involvement in myasthenia gravis. A clinical and histopathological study. Journal of Neurology, Neurosurgery and Psychiatry 36:244

Osserman K E 1958 Myasthenia gravis. Grune and Stratton, New York

Osserman K E, Kaplan L I 1953 Studies in myasthenia gravis: use of edrophonium chloride (Tensilon®) in differentiating myasthenia from cholinergic weakness. Archives of Neurology and Psychiatry (Chicago) 70:385

Pantuck E J, Pantuck C B 1975 Cholinesterases and anticholinesterases. In: Katz R (ed) Muscle relaxants. Excerpta Medica, Amsterdam, p 143

Papatestas A E, Alpert L I, Osserman K E, Osserman R S, Kark A E 1971 Studies in myasthenia gravis: effects of thymectomy. American Journal of Medicine 50:465

Papatestas A E, Genkins G, Horowitz S H, Kornfeld P 1976 Thymectomy in myasthenia gravis: pathologic, clinical and electrophysiologic correlations. Annals of the New York Academy of Sciences 274:555

Pascuzzi R M, Coslett H B, Johns T R 1982 Myasthenia gravis treatment with long-term corticosteroids: a report of 116 cases. Seminars in Neurology 2:250

Patrick J, Lindstrom J 1973 Autoimmune response to acetylcholine receptor. Science 180:871

Patten B M 1975 A hypothesis to account for the Mary Walker phenomenon. Annals of Internal Medicine 82:411

Perez M C, Buot W L, Mercado-Danguilan C, Bagabaldo Z G, Renales L D 1981 Stable remissions in myasthenia gravis. Neurology 31:32

Perlo V P, Poskanzer D C, Schwab R S, Viets H R, Osserman K E, Genkins G 1966 Myasthenia gravis: evaluation of treatment in 1355 patients. Neurology (Minneapolis) 16:431

Pirofsky B, Reid R H, Bardana E J, Bayrakci C 1971 Antithymocyte antisera therapy in non surgical immunologic disease. Transplantation Proceedings 111:769

Pirskanen R 1976 Genetic associations between myasthenia gravis and the HL-A system. Journal of Neurology, Neurosurgery and Psychiatry 39:23

Pirskanen R 1977 Genetic aspects of myasthenia gravis. A family study of 264 Finnish patients. Acta Neurologica Scandinavica 56:365

Pirskanen R, Tiilikainen A, Hokkanen E 1972 Histocompatibility (HL-A) antigens associated with myasthenia gravis. A preliminary report. Annals of Clinical Research 4:304

Plescia O J, Segovia J M, Strampp A 1966 An assessment of changes in the complement level of myasthenic sera. Annals of the New York Academy of Sciences 135:580

Prior C, Lang B, Wray D, Newsom-Davis J 1985 Action of Lambert-Eaton myasthenic syndrome IgG at mouse motor nerve terminals. Annals of Neurology 17:587

Rash J E, Albuquerque E X, Hudson C S, Mayer R S, Setterfield J R 1976 Studies of human myasthenia gravis: electrophysiological and ultrastructural evidence compatible with antibody attachment to acetylcholine receptor complex. Proceedings of the National Academy of Sciences USA 73:4584

Reiness C G, Weinberg C B 1978 Antibody to acetylcholine receptor increases degradation of junctional and extrajunctional receptors in adult muscle. Nature 274:68

Reinglass J L, Brickel A C J 1973 The prognostic significance of thymic germinal center proliferation in myasthenia gravis. Neurology (Minneapolis) 23:69

Ringvist I, Ringvist T 1971 Respiratory mechanics in untreated myasthenia gravis with special reference to the respiratory forces. Acta Medica Scandinavica 190:499

Robb S A, Bowley T J, Willcox H N A, Newsom-Davis J 1985 Circulating T cell subsets in the Lambert-Eaton myasthenic syndrome. Journal of Neurology, Neurosurgery and Psychiatry 48:501

Rooke E D, Eaton L M, Lambert E H, Hodgson C H 1960 Myasthenia and malignant intrathoracic tumor. Medical Clinics of North America 44:977

Roux H, Serratrice G, Pollini S 1974 Antithymic and antilymphocytic globulins in the treatment of some neuromuscular disorders. In: Hausmanowa-Petrusewicz I, Jedrzejowska H (eds) Structure and function of normal and diseased muscle and peripheral nerve. Polish Medical Publishers, Warsaw, p 265

Rowland L P, Hoefer P F A, Aranow H, Merritt H H 1956 Fatalities in myasthenia gravis. Neurology (Minneapolis) 6:307

Rowland L P, Osserman E F, Scharfman W B, Balsam R F, Ball S 1969 Myasthenia gravis with a myeloma-type, gamma-G (IgG) immunoglobulin abnormality. American Journal of Medicine 46:599

Rule A H, Kornfeld P 1971 Studies in myasthenia gravis: biologic aspects. The Mount Sinai Journal of Medicine 38:538

Russell D S 1953 Histological changes in the striped muscles in myasthenia gravis. Journal of Pathology and Bacteriology 65:279

Sahay B M, Blendis L M, Greene R 1965 Relation between myasthenia gravis and thyroid disease. British Medical Journal 1:762

Sambrook M A, Reid H, Mohr P D, Boddie H G 1976 Myasthenia gravis: clinical and histological features in relation to thymectomy. Journal of Neurology, Neurosurgery and Psychiatry 39:38

Scadding G K, Vincent A, Newsom-Davis J, Henry K 1981 Acetylcholine receptor antibody synthesis by thymic lymphocytes: correlation with thymic histology. Neurology 31:935

Schrire I 1959 Progesterone metabolism in myasthenia gravis. Quarterly Journal of Medicine 28:59

Schulz M D, Schwab R S 1971 Results of thymic (mediastinal) irradiation in patients with myasthenia gravis. Annals of the New York Academy of Sciences 183:303

Schwab R S 1954 Belladonna drugs in cholinergic poisoning

during treatment of myasthenia gravis. Journal of the American Medical Association 155:1445

Schwab R S, Leland C C 1953 Sex and age in myasthenia gravis as critical factors in incidence and remissions. Journal of the American Medical Association 153:1270

Schwartz M, Novick D, Givol D, Fuchs S 1978 Induction of anti-idiotypic antibodies by immunisation with syngeneic spleen cells educated with acetylcholine receptor. Nature 273:543

Schwartz M S, Stalberg E 1975a Myasthenia gravis with features of the myasthenic syndrome. An investigation with electrophysiologic methods including single-fiber electromyography. Neurology (Minneapolis) 25:80

Schwartz M S, Stalberg E 1975b Single fibre electromyographic studies in myasthenia gravis with repetitive nerve stimulation. Journal of Neurology, Neurosurgery and Psychiatry 38:678

Seybold M E, Howard F M, Duane D D, Payne W S, Harrison E C 1971 Thymectomy in juvenile myasthenia gravis. Archives of Neurology 25:385

Shibuya N, Mori K, Nakazawa Y 1978 Serum factor blocks neuromuscular transmission in myasthenia gravis: electrophysiologic study with intracellular microelectrodes. Neurology (Minneapolis) 28:804

Simpson J A 1958 An evaluation of thymectomy in myasthenia gravis. Brain 81:112

Simpson J A 1960 Myasthenia gravis: a new hypothesis. Scottish Medical Journal 5:419

Simpson J A 1964 Immunological disturbances in myasthenia gravis: with a report of Hashimoto's disease developing after thymectomy. Journal of Neurology, Neurosurgery and Psychiatry 27:485

Simpson J A 1975 Myasthenia gravis. In: Cumings J N, Kremer M (eds) Biochemical aspects of neurological disorders, second series. Blackwell, Oxford, p 53

Simpson J A 1966a Disorders of neuromuscular transmission. Proceedings of the Royal Society of Medicine 59:993

Simpson J A 1966b The biochemistry of myasthenia gravis. In: Kuhn E (ed) Progressive Muskeldystrophie, Myotonie, Myasthenie. Springer, Berlin, p 339

Simpson J A 1966c Myasthenia gravis as an autoimmune disease. Clinical aspects. Annals of the New York Academy of Sciences 135:506

Simpson J A 1968 The correlations between myasthenia gravis and disorders of the thyroid gland. In: Research in muscular dystrophy. Proceedings of the 4th Symposium. Pitman, London, p 31

Simpson J A 1969a Myasthenia gravis. In: Walton J N, Canal N, Scarlato G (eds) Muscle diseases. Excerpta Medica, Amsterdam, p 14

Simpson J A 1969b The defect in myasthenia gravis. In: Bittar E E, Bittar N (eds) The biological basis of medicine — III. Academic Press, London p 345

Simpson J A 1971 A morphological explanation of the transmission defect in myasthenia gravis. Annals of the New York Academy of Sciences 183:241

Simpson J A 1976 Neurological disorders. In: Israels M C G, Delamore I W (eds) Haematological aspects of systemic disease. Saunders, London, p 440

Simpson J A 1978 Myasthenia gravis: a personal view of pathogenesis and mechanism. Muscle and Nerve 1:45, 151

Simpson J A 1982 The myasthenic (Eaton-Lambert) syndrome associated with carcinoma. Enzyme induction as a possible mechanism of paraneoplastic syndromes. Scottish Medical Journal 27:220

Simpson J A 1983 Current concepts and history of the autoimmune nature of myasthenia gravis. In: Albuquerque E X, Eldefrawi A T (eds) Myasthenia gravis. Chapman and Hall, London, p 3

Simpson J A, Lenman J A R 1959 The effect of frequency of stimulation in neuromuscular diseases. Electroencephalography and Clinical Neurophysiology 11:604

Simpson J A, Behan P O, Dick H 1976 Studies on the nature of autoimmunity in myasthenia gravis. Evidence for an immunodeficiency type. Annals of the New York Academy of Sciences 274:382

Slomić A, Rosenfalck A, Buchthal F 1968 Electrical and mechanical responses of normal and myasthenic muscle, with particular reference to the staircase phenomenon. Brain Research 10:1

Spector R H, Daroff R B 1976 Edrophonium infra red optokinetic nystagmography in the diagnosis of myasthenia gravis. Annals of the New York Academy of Sciences 274:642

Stahlberg E, Mattson C, Uddgard A et al 1978 Increased decremental response in experimental autoimmune myasthenic rabbits following infusion of human myasthenic IgG. In: Lunt G G, Marchbanks R M (eds) The biochemistry of myasthenia gravis and muscular dystrophy. Academic Press, London, p 179

Stephens A D, Fenton J C B 1977 Serum immunoglobulins in D-penicillamine-treated cystinurics. Proceedings of the Royal Society of Medicine 70 (suppl 3):31

Storm-Mathisen A 1961 Myasthenia gravis. Aschehoug/Almquist and Wiksell, Oslo/Stockholm

Strauss A J L, Seegal B C, Hsu K C, Burkholder P M, Nastuk W L, Osserman K E 1960 Immunofluorescence demonstration of a muscle binding, complement-fixing serum globulin fraction in myasthenia gravis. Proceedings of the Society for Experimental Biology and Medicine 105:184

Strauss A J L, Smith C W, Cage G W, van der Geld H W R, McFarlin D E, Barlow M 1966 Further studies on the specificity of presumed immune associations of myasthenia gravis and considerations of possible pathogenic implications. Annals of the New York Academy of Sciences 135:557

Struppler A 1954 Elektromyographische Studien zun Wirkungsmechanismus Endplatten blockierender Stoffe. Aerztliche Forschung 8:564

Swick H M, Preston D F, McQuillen M P 1976 Gallium scans in myasthenia gravis. Annals of the New York Academy of Sciences 274:536

Symmers D 1932 Malignant tumours and tumour-like growths of the thymic region. Annals of Surgery 95:544

Tarrab-Hazdai R, Aharanov A, Abramsky O, Yaar I, Fuchs S 1975 Passive transfer of experimental autoimmune myasthenia by lymph node cells in inbred guinea pigs. Journal of Experimental Medicine 142:785

Te Velde K, Huber J, van der Slikke L B 1966 Primary acquired hypogammaglobulinemia, myasthenia and thymoma. Annals of Internal Medicine 65:554

Thevenard A, Mende D 1955 Etude electrophorétique de proteins sérique par la méthode de Tiselius dans la myasthénie d'Erb-Goldflam. Revue Neurologique (Paris) 92:143

Tindall R S A, Cloud R, Luby J, Rosenberg R N 1978 Serum antibodies to cytomegalovirus in myasthenia gravis:

effects of thymectomy and steroids. Neurology (Minneapolis) 28:273

Toyka K V, Drachman D B, Pestronk A, Kao I 1975 Myasthenia gravis: passive transfer from man to mouse. Science 190:397

Tsukiyama K, Nakai A, Mine R, Kitani T 1959 Studies on a myasthenic substance present in the serum of a patient with myasthenia gravis. Medical Journal of Osaka University 10:159

Tzartos S, Langeberg L, Hochschwender S, Lindstrom J 1983 Demonstration of a main immunogenic region on acetylcholine receptors from human muscle using monoclonal antibodies to human receptor. FEBS Letters 158 (1):116

Vetters J M 1965 Immunofluorescence staining patterns in skeletal muscle using serum of myasthenic patients and normal controls. Immunology 9:93

Vetters J M, MacAdam R F 1972 Hormone production in the human thymus. Lancet 2:1203

Vetters J M, Simpson J A, Folkarde A 1969 Experimental myasthenia gravis. Lancet 2:28

Vetters J M, MacAdam 1973 Fine structural evidence for hormone secretion by the human thymus. Journal of Clinical Pathology 26:194

Vetters J M, Saikia N K, Wood J, Simpson J A 1973 Pemphigus vulgaris and myasthenia gravis. British Journal of Dermatology 88:437

Vetters J M, Simpson J A 1974 Comparison of thymic histology with response to thymectomy in myasthenia gravis. Journal of Neurology, Neurosurgery and Psychiatry 37:1139

Viets H R, Schwab R S 1935 Prostigmin in the diagnosis of myasthenia gravis. New England Journal of Medicine 213:1280

Vincent A 1980 Immunology of acetylcholine receptors in relation to myasthenia gravis. Physiological Reviews 60:775

Vincent A 1983 Humoral immunity in myasthenia gravis and the Eaton-Lambert syndrome In: Albuquerque E X, Eldefrawi A T Myasthenia gravis. Chapman and Hall, London, p 297

Vincent A, Newsom-Davis J 1979 Absence of anti-acetylcholine receptor antibodies in congenital myasthenia gravis. Lancet 1:441

Waldor M C, Sriram S, McDevitt H O, Steinman L 1983 In vivo therapy with monoclonal anti-Ia antibody suppresses immune responses to acetylcholine receptor. Proceedings of the National Academy of Sciences USA 80:2713

Walker M B 1934 Treatment of myasthenia gravis with physostigmine. Lancet 1:1200

Walker M B 1938 Myasthenia gravis: a case in which fatigue of the forearm muscles could induce paralysis of the extra-ocular muscles. Proceedings of the Royal Society of Medicine 31:722

Walton J N, Geschwind N, Simpson J A 1956 Benign congenital myopathy with myasthenic features. Journal of Neurology, Neurosurgery and Psychiatry 19:224

Walton J N, Adams R D 1958 Polymyositis. Livingstone, Edinburgh

Weir A I 1982 The effects of corticosteroid treatment on neuromuscular transmission in rats with experimental auto-immune myasthenia gravis (EAMG). Journal of Physiology 329:43P

Weigert C 1901 Pathologisch-anatomischer Beitrag zur Erbach'en Krankheit (Myasthenia Gravis). Neurologisches Zentralblatt 20:597

Wekerle H, Hohlfeld R, Ketelsen U-P, Kalden J R, Kalies I 1981 Thymic myogenesis, T-lymphocytes and the pathogenesis of myasthenia gravis. Annals of the New York Academy of Sciences 377:455

Whittingham S, Mackay I R, Kiss Z S 1970 An interplay of genetic and environmental factors in familial hepatitis and myasthenia gravis. Gut 11:811

Wiesendanger M, D'Alessandsi A 1963 Myasthenia gravis mit fokaler Infiltration der Endplattenzone. Acta Neuropathologica 2:246

Willcox H N A, Newsom-Davis J, Calder L R 1984 Cell types required for anti-acetylcholine receptor antibody synthesis by cultured thymocytes and blood lymphocytes in myasthenia gravis. Clinical and Experimental Immunology 58:47

Willcox N, Demaine A G, Newsom-Davis J, Welsh K I, Robb S A, Spiro S G 1985 Increased frequency of IgG heavy chain marker Glm (2) and of HLA-B8 in Lambert-Eaton myasthenic syndrome with and without associated lung carcinoma. Human Immunology 14:29

Willis T 1672 De anima brutorum. Oxford, p 404

Wilson S A K 1954 In: Bruce A N (ed) Neurology, 2nd edn. Butterworth, London, p 1730

Wise R P, MacDermot V 1962 A myasthenic syndrome associated with bronchial carcinoma. Journal of Neurology, Neurosurgery and Psychiatry 25:31

Wolf S M, Barrows H S 1966 Myasthenia gravis and systemic lupus erythematosus. Archives of Neurology 14:254

Wolf S M, Rowland L P, Schotland D L, McKinney A S, Hoefer P F A, Aranow N 1966 Myasthenia as an autoimmune disease: clinical aspects. Annals of the New York Academy of Sciences 135:517

Woolf A L 1966 Morphology of the myasthenic neuromuscular junction. Annals of the New York Academy of Sciences 135:35

Wright E A, McQuillen M P 1971 Antibiotic-induced neuromuscular blockade. Annals of the New York Academy of Sciences 183:358

Zacks S I, Bauer W C, Blumberg J M 1962 The fine structure of the myasthenic neuromuscular junction. Journal of Neuropathology 21:335

Neuromuscular disorders in infancy and childhood

INTRODUCTION

This chapter attempts two tasks: to give an account of some disorders, particularly the congenital myopathies and congenital myasthenias, which are not covered elsewhere and then to describe in broader terms the various clinical presentations of the neuromuscular diseases in childhood. Professor Sir Peter Tizard wrote the corresponding chapter in earlier editions and much of the matter, especially in the section on hypotonia, is his and is gratefully acknowledged.

Children present several special problems to the neurologist: they demand special approaches to history-taking and examination; their disorders are superimposed on the shifting ground of continuous development, and they are subject to a very wide variety of disorders, many of them rare, of which a high proportion are unknown in adult life. Most of the serious neuromuscular diseases which affect children are genetically determined and so the need for genetic counselling pervades the strategies of management and may impose a sense of urgency for accurate diagnosis and prognosis even upon clinical situations which might otherwise properly be subjected to the test of time.

Normal muscle activity in young infants is evident mainly in their tone and posture, so hypotonia is the dominant presenting feature of most neuromuscular disorders presenting in the first year or so of life. However, hypotonia is also the earliest sign of many systemic illnesses and disorders of the central nervous system, so a discussion of the hypotonic infant must cover a wide field. Other important presenting features of congenital neuromuscular disorders are contractures (arthrogryposis) and dysfunction of certain critical muscles, especially those of sucking, swallowing and respiration, but also those of eye movement and facial expression.

Later in childhood the disorders causing progressive muscle weakness dominate the scene but the intermittent paralyses, muscle pain and stiffness or myoglobinuria may be the principal problems in various disorders. Each of these will be discussed in turn after an initial account of the congenital myopathies.

More detailed accounts of neuromuscular disease in childhood include those of Dubowitz (1978, 1980, 1985), Brooke (1977), Brook et al (1979), Swaiman & Wright (1979) and (for the spinal muscular atrophies) Hausmanowa-Petrusewicz (1978) and Gamstorp & Sarnat (1984). Quantitative data for muscle power in normal children are given by Hosking et al (1976) and Newman et al (1984). The technique and use of needle muscle biopsy in children will be found in Heckmatt et al (1984) and Dubowitz (1985).

THE CONGENITAL MYOPATHIES

Most of the true myopathies present at birth are genetically determined, and in the rest the cause is usually unknown. On the other hand, many of the genetic disorders customarily described as congenital myopathies may not cause symptoms until later in childhood or even adult life, by which time many acquired myopathies including polymyositis and the endocrine disorders must be considered in the differential diagnosis. It is best, therefore, to consider these myopathies as 'genetic and idiopathic myopathies' and to classify them more or less in diminishing order of our understanding of their nature, as follows. For completeness two final categories of functional disorders of the muscle fibre and disorders of muscle connective tissue are included:

(1) Genetic myopathies with specific biochemical defects
  Glycogen storage diseases
  Lipid storage diseases
  Disorders of the cytochrome system
(2) Genetic myopathies with structurally abnormal mitochondria

(3) Genetic myopathies with periodic 'metabolic' manifestations
  Periodic paralyses
  Malignant hyperpyrexia
  Familial myoglobinuria and idiopathic rhabdomyolysis
(4) Genetic myopathies with specific structural changes in fibres
  Central core disease
  Minicore disease
  Nemaline myopathy
  Centronuclear myopathy
  Finger-print myopathy
  Etc.
(5) Genetic myopathies with changes in the histo-chemical fibre types
(6) Genetic myopathies with progressive degeneration of muscle fibres (the muscular dystrophies)
(7) Genetic myopathies with non-specific changes in fibres
(8) Genetic disorders of neuromuscular transmission
(9) Genetic disorders with abnormal muscle fibre activity
  Myotonic disorders
  Myokymia
  Muscle rigidity
(10) Genetic disorders of muscle connective tissue
  Progressive fibrodysplasia ossificans (myositis ossificans)
  Myosclerosis

Only a few of the categories in this list are discussed below; descriptions of the others can be found in Chapters 15, 19 and 25. This chapter concentrates on clinical aspects of the congenital myopathies because their pathological features are described in Chapters 5, 6, 7 and 8.

Genetic myopathies with specific biochemical defects

These are covered in Chapter 25. Here only a few selected comments are needed. (1) The muscle glycogenoses include not only the classic forms but also atypical variants. Thus Pompe's disease usually presents in the first few weeks of life with progressive muscle weakness and hypotonia, cardiomyopathy, an enlarging liver and mild dementia. However, more slowly progressive variants may present later in infancy or in adolescence, the latter especially resembling a muscular dystrophy (as may debrancher enzyme deficiency). Conversely, muscle phosphorylase deficiency may uncommonly cause its characteristic muscle fatigue and pain on exercise in late childhood but a rare severe variant causes a rapidly progressive and fatal myopathy in the first few weeks of life (DiMauro & Hartlage 1978). Severe variants of phosphorylase kinase deficiency (Ohtani et al 1982) and combined deficiency of phosphofructokinase and phosphorylase b kinase (Danon et al 1981) may present with delayed development and muscle weakness (and also corneal ulceration) in the first or second year. (2) Reye's syndrome with muscle weakness, or recurrent episodes of Reye's syndrome, should alert one to the possibility of systemic carnitine deficiency. Fluctuating muscle weakness or associated liver enlargement or cardiomyopathy are other possible indicators. Carnitine deficiency may present at any period of childhood. Although not all cases found to have low serum (or muscle) carnitine concentrations will respond to oral carnitine therapy, a therapeutic trial is always justified. (3) The discovery of lipid storage myopathy should prompt a search for possible therapeutic measures. Several different forms of lipid storage myopathy are known and a few of these will be found to respond to treatment with propranolol (Martyn et al 1981) or with carnitine, a low-fat diet or other measures. Turnbull et al (1986) have reported the case of a child with a severe myopathy and hepatomegaly, progressing rapidly from the age of five months and associated with intense lipid storage in muscle and the excretion of dicarboxylic acids, glutaric acid and 2- and 3- methyl butyryl glycine in the urine. Treatment with riboflavine, carnitine, glycine and a low-fat diet resulted in a very great improvement (Fig. 20.1).

Genetic myopathies with abnormal muscle mitochondria

Many different types of muscle disease associated with abnormal muscle mitochondria have been described, several of which are accompanied by involvement of the brain and other organs. The early reports inevitably concentrated largely on the abnormalities seen by electron microscopy. The mitochondria may be too large or too numerous, are often distorted and may contain paracrystalline or amorphous inclusions. None of these features corresponds with particular clinical features which are equally variable. Mitochondrial myopathy may be suspected on light microscopy when there is an excess of oxidative enzyme activity in the subsarcolemmal regions of type I fibres, or a 'ragged red' appearance of the same regions of fibres stained by the Gomori trichrome method. Often there is some associated lipid accumulation and in some cases glycogen may accumulate as well (Jerusalem et al 1973b). Great advances have been achieved in recent years in our understanding of the disorders of mitochondrial metabolism (see DiMauro et al 1985 and Ch. 25). There is a defect in cellular respiratory function in many of these disorders to which the visible mitochondrial changes are secondary; in others, no doubt, the defect remains to be discovered, but possibly some may represent primary disorders of mitochondrial structure. Known metabolic abnormalities include deficiencies of carnitine and carnitine palmityl transferase and several disorders of cytochrome function. In this chapter a simple clinical classification seems appropriate.

Hypermetabolic myopathy. Two cases are known, both with fever, heat intolerance, excessive appetite, polydipsia, weight loss and fatigue starting in childhood with negative family histories (Luft et al 1962, Haydar et al 1971). Oxidative phosphorylation was uncoupled and thyroid function was normal (DiMauro et al 1976). Chloramphenicol gave some relief in Haydar's case, presumably by suppressing mitochondrial function.

Progressive muscular weakness and fatigue. Many cases have been described with a slowly progressive myopathy, the symptoms of which usually begin at the age of 5–10 years and in which fatigue is often out of proportion to the degree of muscle weakness but without true myasthenia (Coleman et al 1967). Some cases, including the original case of 'megaconial myopathy' described by Shy et al (1966), have had symptoms from birth. Variations on the theme are reported by van Wijngaarden et al (1967) and by Schotland

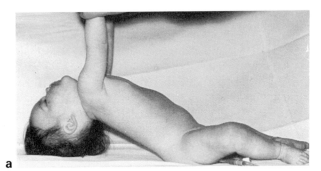

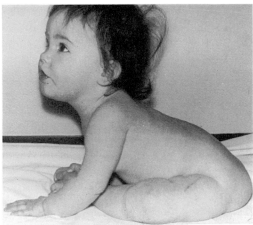

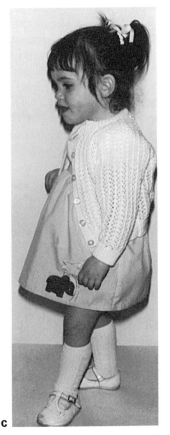

Fig. 20.1 Lipid storage myopathy with type II glutaric aciduria. a. At 6 months of age; severe paresis before treatment; b. After 10 weeks of treatment; c. At 20 months of age

et al (1976) who reported a defect in mitochondrial energy supply in a patient aged 37 years whose symptoms dated from early childhood. Defects have been found in the complex I or complex III components of the cytochrome system in several such patients (Morgan-Hughes et al 1977, Land et al 1981, see DiMauro et al 1985).

Hypotonia with salt-craving and periodic muscular weakness. Shy et al (1966) described the case of a child who was hypotonic from birth and who had episodes of severe muscular weakness lasting 10–14 days, associated with salt craving. His otherwise normal brother also craved salt. The muscle contained very numerous mitochondria ('pleoconial myopathy'). The authors recognised the similarity of the symptoms to those of normo-kalaemic periodic paralysis but showed that the conditions were different. Spiro et al (1970b) reported a similar case without the periodic exacerbations.

Progressive external ophthalmoplegia and the Kearns–Sayre syndrome. The most frequently encountered clinical syndrome of mitochondrial myopathy comprises ptosis and progressive external ophthalmoplegia with or without skeletal muscle weakness. This ocular syndrome has successively been regarded in the last 90 years as an ocular form of muscular dystrophy, and as 'ophthalmoplegia plus' (referring to its association with various disorders of central nervous system function) before the mitochondrial pathology was recognised. There is a wide range of age at onset. The oculopharyngeal type of muscular dystrophy (see Ch. 15) is a separate and well-defined entity.

In the Kearns–Sayre syndrome there is, in addition, a pigmentary degeneration of the retina and heart block, together with various combinations of growth failure, nerve deafness, ataxia, dementia and a raised cerebrospinal fluid (CSF) protein level. The onset is always before the age of 20 years. Recurrent encephalopathy in some cases is associated with patchy low-density lesions seen on CT scanning of the brain and a spongiform degeneration at autopsy; mitochondrial abnormalities have long been recognised to occur in the cerebellum as well as in muscle (Schneck et al 1973).

There is no absolute clinical or histological distinction from other mitochondrial myopathies: e.g. McLeod et al (1975) and Bogousslavsky et al (1982) reported patients with many of the features of the Kearns–Sayre syndrome but with normal eye movements; Spiro et al (1970a) described a father and son with a similar syndrome, but with more prominent dementia and with no retinal degeneration, in whom a defect of the complex III component of the cytochrome system was identified.

Distal myopathy with hyperglycaemia. A girl of five years described by Salmon et al (1971) had a distal myopathy from the first year of life, fasting hyperglycaemia with ketosis and low insulin levels but a normal insulin response to glucose loading. There were mitochondrial abnormalities and lipid accumulation in the muscle. Male relatives in three generations had raised serum CK activity and hyperglycaemia. Lapresle et al (1972) reported a family with apparently dominant inheritance of congenital foot drop with facial and sternomastoid weakness and mitochondrial changes in the muscle biopsy.

Facioscapulohumeral syndrome. Hudgson et al (1972) reported a family with at least eight affected members in four generations in which a mitochondrial myopathy gave rise to a facioscapulohumeral syndrome of muscle weakness. The age at onset varied from six to 50 years. The affected child later developed severe lactic acidosis (Bradley et al 1978) and has since died of a progressive encephalopathy (P. Hudgson, personal communication).

Various non-muscular presentations. It is not unusual for patients to be found to have a mitochondrial myopathy in the course of investigation of other symptoms, e.g. cardiomyopathy and short stature (Rawles & Weller 1974, Sengers et al 1976), progressive ataxia and dementia (Spiro et al 1970a), familial myoclonic epilepsy, myoclonic jerks and ataxia (Tsairis et al 1973, Rosing et al 1985), Leigh's disease (Crosby & Chou 1974, Willems et al 1977, Miyabayashi et al 1984), Alpers' progressive cortical degeneration of infancy (Sandbank & Lerman 1972) and Menkes' trichopoliodystrophy (French et al 1972).

Mitochondrial myopathy and lactic acidosis. Tarlow et al (1973) first drew attention to the association of lassitude and episodic vomiting with lactic and pyruvic acidosis in a child who also had a mitochondrial myopathy, although van Wijngaarden et al (1967) had earlier found lactic acidosis in one of their patients. Since then, many examples have been reported and it seems clear that in many of the syndromes described above, including the Kearns–Sayre syndrome, a critical failure in mitochondrial metabolic function may result in lactic acidosis. In addition, however, to this rather general association between lactic acidosis and mitochondrial disease, a number of more specific syndromes seem to have emerged.

Sengers et al (1975) described a syndrome occurring in seven children from three unrelated families in whom cataracts in infancy and effort intolerance were associated with cardiomyopathy, mitochondrial myopathy and lactic acidosis after exercise. The brothers with lactic acidosis described by Rawles & Weller (1974) also suffered from cardiomyopathy and fatigue but without cataracts.

One of the most sinister of the mitochondrial myopathy syndromes is that first described in two papers relating to the same two sisters (D'Agostino et al 1968, Hackett et al 1973) and later also by Gardner-Medwin et al (1975), Shapira et al (1975), Hart et al (1977) and others reviewed by Pavlakis et al (1984). The cardinal features in the first decade are the onset of growth failure, headaches, vomiting, fatigue and hirsutism at about the age of four years, worsening gradually thereafter. By about 10 years there is marked shortness of stature, the muscles are slim and fatigue easily, but are not very weak, and there is a degree of nerve deafness. Episodes of confusion or even coma may follow exertion. Some cases have seizures. There is no ophthalmoplegia, but ptosis and mild facial weakness may occur. There is lactic acidosis and muscle biopsy reveals a mitochondrial myopathy. During the second decade intermittent subacute episodes of encephalopathy occur, associated in some cases with patchy 'moth-eaten' areas of low density shown by computerised axial tomography of the brain. These occur mainly in white matter but the clinical effect is patchy loss of cortical function with dysphasia, dyspraxia, agnosia, cortical blindness or overt hemiparesis in various combinations. In other cases calcification is seen in the basal ganglia, usually related to hypoparathyroidism. Most patients have died by the age of 16 to 18 years. Autopsies have revealed focal cortical neuronal loss with gliosis and vascular proliferation, and oedema or spongiform change of the adjacent white matter. No electron microscopy of the central nervous system has yet been reported. Although three pairs of affected sibs have been reported, the genetic position is not clear because various other relatives suffered similar, less severe, symptoms.

Finally, there is now an extensive literature on congenital lactic acidosis of which a number of types with different enzyme defects have been described. These tend to cause severe mental retardation with acidosis. In the case described by Brunette et al (1972) a specific enzyme defect was found (pyruvate carboxylase). Fatal infantile lactic acidosis with severe weakness and hypotonia, a mitochondrial myopathy and, in some cases, ophthalmoplegia, renal tubular defects and seizures has been reported in at least 12 patients with a deficiency of cytochrome c oxidase (DiMauro et al 1980, Bresolin et al 1985). The symptoms develop within three weeks after birth. One similar case recovered spontaneously, both biochemically and clinically, to be left with a mild myopathy at the age of 33 months (DiMauro et al 1983). The spontaneously improving mitochondrial–lipid–glycogen disease of Jerusalem et al (1973b), may have been identical (DiMauro et al 1985).

Management of mitochondrial myopathy. The diagnosis can often be suspected if one of the clinical syndromes is recognised. The histochemical findings with or without lipid droplets in the muscle fibres are very suggestive, but the initial diagnosis is generally based on the ultrastructural findings. It is wise to obtain enough muscle at the time of biopsy to rule out carnitine deficiency. Studies of mitochondrial function in vitro require several grams of fresh unfrozen muscle tissue and can be performed only in highly specialised laboratories, so that a more specific diagnosis has rarely been possible in young children and, indeed, has been achieved in very few adult cases.

A few therapeutic manoeuvres may be of limited value. Most important is the recognition of heart block in the Kearns–Sayre syndrome and the provision of a cardiac pacemaker when necessary. Close surveillance is essential because the degree of conduction block can deteriorate rapidly. Treatment with combined vitamins C and K may be valuable in complex III deficiency (see DiMauro et al 1985). Oral carnitine may be helpful in many, but not all, cases of muscle and systemic carnitine deficiency. Steroids also make a contribution in muscle carnitine deficiency, and were of temporary benefit in the case described by Shapira et al (1975). Dubowitz (1978, p. 99, 102) pointed out that respiratory failure may result partly from a failure in central control of ventilation and he was able to maintain a child's breathing with a home ventilator for a time.

Genetic counselling in the mitochondrial disorders is particularly difficult. Clear evidence of Mendelian inheritance is rarely found but sibs, parents and more distant relatives are quite often affected in various syndromes. Direct maternal transmission in the mitochondrial DNA of the ovum is probably responsible for some familial cases (Egger & Wilson 1983, Rosing et al 1985). Further research into the genetics of the mitochondrial myopathies is clearly needed.

Genetic myopathies with specific structural changes in fibres

Central core disease. Although it was the first of this group of myopathies to be described (Shy & Magee 1956), central core disease is uncommon. It can be recognised only by histochemical and ultrastructural examination of the muscle. The cores in the muscle fibres may be single or multiple, central or peripheral but they extend for a considerable distance along the fibre. They are seen almost exclusively in type I fibres and are devoid of mitochondria or oxidative enzymes; the myofibril structure in the core may be disrupted or may be intact and the fibres are otherwise normal. Type I fibre predominance is usual and sometimes type II fibres are virtually absent. Morgan-Hughes et al (1973) reported a mother with central core disease whose two clinically affected children had muscle with type I predominance but no cores.

Three or more clinical syndromes of central core disease seem to exist, but cores have also been described after experimental tenotomy and in association with other types of muscle pathology, so their presence should be interpreted with caution if the clinical situation is unusual.

Most cases present with moderate infantile hypotonia and often with delay in walking until three or four years of age. Thereafter there is no deterioration, but hurried walking and climbing stairs remain difficult. The inheritance is autosomal dominant. Brooke (1977) has pointed out that affected families often recognise and make light of the symptoms and may come under observation only incidentally. The weakness is greater in the legs than in the arms, and muscle wasting is usually slight. The facial muscles are usually, but not always, spared. The tendon reflexes are diminished but present in most cases. A common feature is congenital dislocation of the hips (Armstrong et al 1971) and in some families talipes is prominent either from birth or later in life while others have flat feet. Kyphoscoliosis may occur.

The serum creatine kinase (CK) activity is usually normal. Electromyographic (EMG) abnormalities are often slight and unhelpful. Cruz Martinez et al (1979) reviewed the EMG findings and reported an increase in the density of muscle fibres belonging to individual motor units, a finding presumably related to the predominance of type I fibres. Isaacs et al (1975) reported a reduction in calcium uptake by the sarcoplasmic reticulum in two cases. Although both Cruz Martinez et al and Isaacs et al interpreted their findings as giving evidence of denervation, more direct and definite evidence of a neurogenic basis for central core disease is lacking, its pathogenesis

remains obscure and it is probably best to classify it for the present among the congenital myopathies.

Dubowitz & Platts (1965) reported an affected brother and sister whose unaffected parents were first cousins, making autosomal recessive inheritance likely. These cases were atypical also in both having focal wasting of the muscles of the right arm from childhood and more generalised weakness in the fourth decade.

The family reported by Bethlem et al (1966) was unique in having only minimal weakness and in having suffered since childhood from severe painless stiffness of the muscles induced by running, climbing stairs or walking on tiptoe, and lasting for several minutes.

In addition, various sporadic and atypical cases have been reported, including one with congenital contractures, who had an unaffected identical twin (Cohen et al 1978) and another with late-onset pes cavus with no clinical abnormality of muscle (Telerman-Toppet et al 1973).

Denborough et al (1973) described a patient with central core disease who had an extensive family history of malignant hyperpyrexia and was herself susceptible. Eng et al (1978) and Frank et al (1980) reviewed the association of these two disorders and concluded that it was rare but not coincidental. An atypically elevated serum CK activity in central core disease appears to indicate a risk of susceptibility to malignant hyperpyrexia.

Minicore (multicore) disease. Most authors have followed Engel et al (1971) and Heffner et al (1976) in calling this condition multicore disease. 'Minicore', proposed by Currie et al (1974) distinguishes the typical appearance of the muscle biopsy more precisely from that of central core disease. The minicores extend for only a few sarcomeres, but have the same histochemical and ultrastructural appearance as central cores. Type I fibre predominance is usual but, unlike central cores, minicores occur in both fibre types.

Ten reported cases were reviewed by Taratuto et al (1978); Dubowitz (1985) recorded seven more and several others have been reported. In the typical form of the disease the clinical features have been rather uniform. There is infantile hypotonia, delay in motor development and continuing but non-progressive muscle weakness tending to be proximal in distribution, modest wasting, often some mild asymmetry of involvement, and impairment, rarely absence, of the tendon reflexes. The face is often affected, neck flexion may be weak and typically the ocular muscles are unaffected. The serum CK activity is normal and the EMG usually indicates a myopathic disorder.

One of the cases of Engel et al (1971) had a family history of neuromuscular symptoms in three generations and Vanneste & Stam (1982) found minicores in muscle biopsies from the asymptomatic mother and sister of their patient; otherwise only sibs or sporadic cases have been affected and the inheritance is therefore probably autosomal recessive.

There have been reports of several atypical cases. A child reported by Gadoth et al (1978) had muscle biopsy findings perhaps more akin to minicore than central core disease. The patient's non-progressive myopathy was punctuated by exacerbations of weakness during, and for some time after, febrile illnesses. Koch et al (1985) described a severely affected infant who also had an atrial septal defect and who died after anaesthesia. A late-onset case with proximal weakness progressing from the age of 33 years was reported by Bonnette et al (1974). Chudley et al (1985) reported two affected sibs who also had severe mental retardation, vertical ophthalmoplegia, facial anomalies, short stature, hypogonadism and hypoplasia of the pituitary fossa. Swash & Schwartz (1981) discussed a possibly separate variant of minicore disease in which there is associated ophthalmoplegia and, in addition to minicores, the muscle biopsy shows focal loss of cross-striations.

Nemaline (rod body) myopathy. This condition was first described by Shy et al (1963) and by Conen et al (1963) and has since become the most frequently reported and most intensively studied of the congenital myopathies. It has been reviewed by Kuitonnen et al (1972) and Brooke et al (1979). The pathogenesis is unknown but recently a deficiency of dipeptidyl peptidase 1 has been found in two cases (Stauber et al 1986).

The characteristic tiny rod bodies (they are not really 'nemaline' or thread-like) are derived from the disorganisation of the material from which the Z bands of the sarcomeres are formed. They may reflect a defect in the regulation of the length of actin filaments (Yamaguchi et al 1982). They form clusters or irregular palisades and are often seen near active vesicular nuclei. They may be inconspicuous and are best seen in thick sections stained with toluidine blue or trichrome stains, or under phase contrast when they are usually refractile. Their ultrastructure is also characteristic. As in central core disease, type I fibre predominance is usual and, indeed, rods and cores or minicores may occur together (Afifi et al 1965, Dubowitz 1978 p. 83). Rods are seen in a variety of clinical and experimental myopathies and are, therefore, not in themselves specific; nevertheless, the typical clinical features of the congenital myopathy with which they are usually associated have now been so well defined as to leave no doubt that 'nemaline myopathy' is a specific genetic disorder. In addition, however, nemaline rods may be seen in adults with a late-onset progressive myopathy (Heffernan et al 1968) and it is still not clear whether such cases should be considered to be distinct or part of a spectrum of disease severity; the latter seems more likely. The pathogenesis is unknown and, although various pieces of evidence have indicated a neurogenic lesion in some cases, notably the post-mortem evidence of loss of anterior horn cells in a patient with abundant nemaline rods in the muscle fibres (Dahl & Klutzow 1974), the overall evidence seems still to point to a primary myopathy.

The typical patient is hypotonic in infancy with delayed motor development and with strikingly slender muscles, which are often not as weak as they look. There is usually definite facial weakness (Fig. 20.2a) and often nasal speech due to palatal weakness. The muscle involvement is indeed universal and the cases of Conen et al (1963) and Hopkins et al (1966) were initially diagnosed as having 'Krabbe's universal muscle hypoplasia' (Krabbe 1958), a term no longer in use. The tendon reflexes are reduced or absent. Various skeletal features including a high-arched palate, dental malocclusion, scoliosis and pes cavus, although by no means confined to nemaline myopathy, are common and combine with the facial weakness and muscle hypoplasia to present

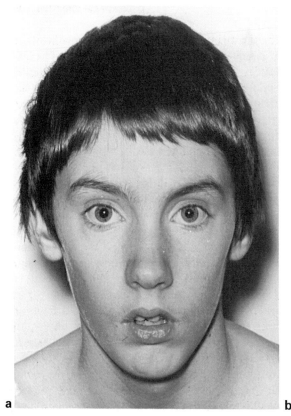

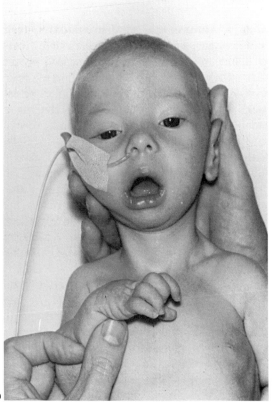

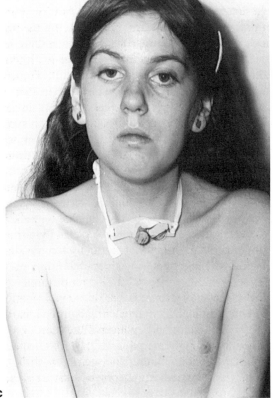

Fig. 20.2 Nemaline myopathy. a. Facies, a boy aged 12 years; b. Severe neonatal form, a boy at 3 weeks old; c. A girl of 13 years, shortly after she had developed severe nocturnal respiratory failure

a striking clinical picture from which the diagnosis may often be suspected. Most cases are moderately severely disabled throughout childhood. In the neonatal period the disease may be severe and cause early death (Shafiq et al 1967, Eeg-Olofsson et al 1983) and there is now evidence that this form of nemaline myopathy is a distinct autosomal recessive entity (Fig. 20.2b). The disorder is usually considered to be non-progressive, but undoubtedly deterioration can occur; e.g. some relatives may be found to have subclinical involvement and it is likely that in some cases they will develop symptoms in adult life (Hopkins et al 1966). Furthermore, progressive respiratory failure is now frequently recognised in the first and second decades (Kuitonnen et al 1972, Dubowitz 1978) and often proves fatal. Serial testing of respiratory function may reveal striking abnormalities months or years before serious respiratory symptoms occur, but excessive fatigue and morning headaches are warning symptoms. One of Dubowitz's cases first presented with acute respiratory failue while hill-walking (Dubowitz 1978). A patient described by us in 1969 (Fulthorpe et al 1969) later developed severe disabling respiratory failure at the age of 13 years (Fig. 20.2c). Regular overnight use of a negative pressure cuirass ventilator at home, together with tracheostomy, has controlled this and she has remained fully ambulant for more than eight years. Loss of central respiratory drive and muscle weakness may both be factors in such cases (Riley et al 1977). Deterioration of nemaline myopathy in the third or fourth decade may also be attributable to cardiomyopathy, either with nemaline rods in the heart muscle (Meier et al 1984) or without (Stoessl et al 1985).

Many families have now been described with affected parents and children, and autosomal dominant inheritance is very likely (Kondo & Yuasa 1980); however, no very extensive pedigrees have been recorded. Sporadic cases with normal biopsies in both parents have been reported but in other families rods have been found in *both* asymptomatic parents, suggesting autosomal recessive inheritance (Arts et al 1978). Even X-linked dominant inheritance has been suggested because of an apparent excess of female patients and the predominance of affected mothers (see Brooke et al 1979) but this is improbable because the disorder may apparently be transmitted by a father to his sons (Gonatas et al 1966).

Centronuclear (myotubular) myopathies. One of the histological characteristics of myopathic disorders in general is the tendency for muscle fibre nuclei to drift away from their normal subsarcolemmal position towards the centre of the fibre. In the centronuclear myopathies, however, central nuclei dominate a histological picture in which abnormal variation in fibre size and often a tendency to type I fibre predominance are the only other major features. Spiro et al (1966), who first drew attention to this disorder, described a boy aged 12 years with congenital but progressive muscle weakness and ophthalmoplegia. His muscle fibres contained central nuclei, often vesicular with prominent nucleoli, which were

surrounded by clear areas devoid of myofibrils and ATPase activity, and sometimes lacking oxidative enzyme activity also, but containing mitochondria. They likened these fibres to the myotubes found in early fetal muscle, postulated that the disorder might represent arrested maturation of muscle fibres and named it 'myotubular myopathy'. Since then many cases have been described and the more non-committal name 'centronuclear myopathy' is now generally preferred because the fibres usually lack the perinuclear clear areas and differ in several other respects from fetal myotubes. Much overlapping clinical, genetic and pathological variation has emerged; for the present purpose a genetic and clinical classification seems to be appropriate.

Early infantile ophthalmoplegic myopathy with probable autosomal recessive inheritance. Patients in this category resemble that described by Spiro et al (1966) and include those reported by Sher et al (1967), Bethlem et al (1968), Coleman et al (1968), Campbell et al (1969), Ortiz de Zarate & Maruffo (1970) and Bill et al (1979). The condition is apparent in the first year of life because of developmental delay, usually without severe hypotonia at first although this may appear later. By the time of diagnosis in the first or second decade there has usually been slight deterioration in gait or some other evidence of gradual progression. Ptosis, strabismus, partial external ophthalmoplegia (for all directions of gaze), facial weakness (not invariable), generalised muscular weakness and wasting, and tendon areflexia are the usual features. Sternomastoid weakness and foot drop are prominent in some cases. Dysarthria is frequent but dysphagia is uncommon. The face may be long and thin and foot deformities and scoliosis may develop. Most patients become unable to walk in the second decade. Intelligence is generally normal but several patients have had convulsions, including the patient described by Spiro et al (1966), whose history was complicated by subdural haematomas; it is not yet certain whether the association with convulsions is coincidental. The serum CK activity is normal or, more often, raised two- or three-fold and the EMG shows myopathic abnormalities. The genetic position is puzzling: both sexes are affected; most cases are sporadic but affected sibs have been recorded (Sher et al 1967, Bradley et al 1970) and in some families subclinical centronuclear myopathy has been found in the mother (Sher et al 1967, Coleman et al 1968). It is, therefore, not yet possible to distinguish autosomal recessive inheritance with manifestation in the heterozygote from autosomal dominant inheritance with variable expressivity. It is possible that the brother and sister reported by Hurwitz et al (1969), with hypotonia and ophthalmoplegia and a family history of aminoaciduria, may have had centronuclear myopathy, as both the clinical and histological features were compatible.

Possibly this category should be defined a little less strictly. In the otherwise typical case described by Kinoshita & Cadman (1968) the symptoms developed at the age of four years and there was ptosis but no ophthalmoplegia. Similarly, the patient of Bethlem et al (1970) had no involvement of the cranial musculature; the symptoms developed at five years and had progressed only slowly at 35 years. A boy with a mild clinical myopathy and with 'hypotrophy' of type I fibres was reported by Inokuchi et al (1975): he had areflexia; the eye movements were not mentioned; sucking had been abnormal in infancy. Ten cases in which the onset was in infancy, the eye movements were normal and the biopsy showed type I fibre atrophy with central nuclei were reviewed by Peyronnard et al (1982); these may represent a separate autosomal recessive entity. The nosological situation overlaps here with that of the 'fibre-type disproportions'. The affected brothers described by Bradley et al (1970) did have ophthalmoplegia but the onset was at eight and 15 years respectively and they deteriorated and died at the age of 34 years. In contrast, the patient of Campbell et al (1969) died at the age of 27 months and in occasional cases there have been life-threatening hypotonia and respiratory difficulties in the neonatal period (Coleman et al 1967, Bender & Bender 1977).

Cases with autosomal dominant inheritance and late onset. The family reported by McLeod et al (1972) is unique in having 16 affected members in five generations. Biopsies were taken from two

members. In most, symptoms began in the third decade but in three (including two of the only three children at risk) the disease began in early childhood (in the second year). The myopathy was usually proximal in emphasis but in some cases showed a scapuloperoneal distribution. The eye muscles were spared, although some had slight facial weakness. While the symptoms were slowly progressive, lifespan was normal. The serum CK activity was normal.

There have been other cases with dominant inheritance, mostly with a relatively late onset (Karpati et al 1970, see Heckmatt et al 1985) and other adult-onset cases have been reported by Vital et al (1970) and Harriman & Haleem (1972).

Severe X-linked centronuclear myopathy. X-linked centronuclear myopathy was first reported in two unrelated Dutch families by van Wijngaarden et al (1969) and Barth et al (1975). The males involved were severely affected, often fatally, with hypotonia and respiratory insufficiency at birth (Fig. 20.3), but the survivors tended to improve and two aged 26 and 33 years were not severely disabled. In the patients of van Wijngaarden et al (1969) the clinical features including ophthalmoplegia and facial weakness, as well as the pathology, were remarkably similar to those of the autosomal recessive cases already described. Further severe X-linked cases were described by Bruyland et al (1984) and Heckmatt et al (1985). They showed that female carriers of the gene may have mild clinical signs of a myopathy, or an excess of central nuclei in the muscle biopsy. Askanas et al (1979) found persistent ultrastructural abnormalities in cultured muscle cells from two affected infants and a deficiency of adenylate cyclase associated with the muscle fibre membrane.

Earlier, Engel et al (1968) had reported a similar severely hypotonic male infant who died aged 18 months. The pathology was reported under the title of 'Type I fibre hypotrophy and central nuclei' which for a time was regarded as a disorder separate from centronuclear myopathy. Then Meyers et al (1974) studied a second affected brother and obtained a family history of recurrent male stillbirths in the mother's generation, suggesting X-linked inheritance. The second child

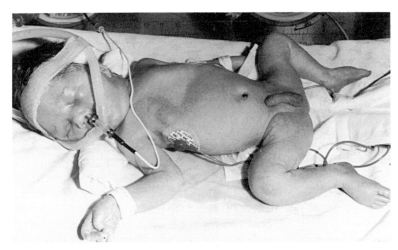

Fig. 20.3 X-linked centronuclear myopathy. A boy born seven weeks pre-term, photographed at 10 days of age. Severe hypotonia and ophthalmoplegia. Needed assisted ventilation for six weeks. Died at five months old

was apnoeic at birth and profoundly hypotonic, and died at seven months. These brothers had no facial weakness, and eye movements were normal. The serum CK activities were normal and the EMGs were inconclusive. These cases are now widely regarded as examples of X-linked centro-nuclear myopathy. A boy with similar clinical and pathological features in infancy who showed striking improvement by the age of six years was reported by Ricoy & Cabello (1985).

Unusual features associated with centronuclear myopathy. The patient of Harriman & Haleem (1972), a woman of 67 years, had marked hyper-trophy of the calves.

The association of cardiomyopathy with centro-nuclear myopathy is recorded by Bethlem et al (1969) in a girl of 16 years, and by Verhiest et al (1976) in two brothers. The boys had early sucking difficulties, delayed motor development and generalised myopathy with ptosis, but the eye movements were not mentioned.

Hawkes & Absolon (1975) reported a man of 29 with typical features of the ophthalmoplegic form but, in addition, cataracts and electromyographic myotonia. His father had cataracts and unilateral congenital ptosis. The cataracts were seen only with a slit lamp. A similar case, but without ptosis or ophthalmoplegia, was reported by Vallat et al (1985). Gil-Peralta et al (1978) described two

affected sibs with clinical myotonia. This condition seems to be distinct both from the typical centronuclear myopathies and from myotonic dystrophy.

Other congenital myopathies with structural abnormalities in muscle fibres

Finger-print inclusion myopathy. Six cases have been reported by Engel et al (1972), Gordon et al (1974), Fardeau et al (1976) and Curless et al (1978a). They include identical twin brothers (Curless et al) half brothers (Fardeau et al) and isolated female cases, in one of which non-progressive congenital myopathy had been present for 54 years before diagnosis (Gordon et al). Subsarcolemmal inclusions resembling finger-prints were associated with a few small areas of focal loss of myofibrillar structure (not unlike minicores) and, in some cases, type I fibre predominance.

All cases were hypotonic in infancy with delayed motor development (walking at between two years and, in Gordon's patient, 12 years) and with no deterioration. The muscles were slim with retained reflexes and mild to moderate weakness. The cranial musculature was normal. Four of the six cases were mildly mentally retarded. Serum CK levels were normal or slightly raised. One patient was thought to show some beneficial response to neostigmine but had no other evidence of myasthenia (Gordon et al 1974). Finger-print inclusions have also been seen in various other disorders including dermatomyositis, myotonic dystrophy and oculopharyngeal dystrophy (see Curless et al 1978a) but the features of the six cases mentioned are sufficiently similar to comprise a clinical entity. The genetic situation is obscure.

Reducing body myopathy. A rather heterogeneous group of isolated cases has been described by Brooke & Neville (1972), and by Dubowitz (1985) (see also Dubowitz 1978, Tomé & Fardeau 1975, Dudley et al 1978, Oh et al 1983, Carpenter et al 1985). The common factor is the presence of sub-sarcolemmal inclusion bodies rich in RNA and sulphydryl groups and capable of reducing nitroblue tetrazolium stain. Their ultrastructure is also diagnostic. Two sibs were reported by Hübner and Pongratz (see Carpenter et al 1985) suggesting a genetic basis. However, in two other cases (Dubowitz 1978, Carpenter et al 1985) there have been high serum antibody titres against Coxsackie virus, the significance of which is not clear.

The patients of Brooke and Neville were hypotonic in infancy. Their weakness progressed and both died, at nine months and two years of age respectively. The older child had facial weakness and contractures and was of normal intelligence. The serum CK activity was normal. Another infant (Dudley et al 1978) died at two and a half months of age after a different type of illness consisting of respiratory paralysis due to progressive board-like rigidity of the muscles of the neck, chest and abdomen, and finally of the limbs; his parents were a father and daughter.

Dubowitz's patient developed a progressive asymmetrical myopathy at the age of four years and died three years later. In addition to reducing bodies, she had histological evidence of a severe degenerative myopathy. Her Coxsackie B virus antibody titre was high and she was treated as having a possible subacute viral polymyositis, responding temporarily to cyclophosphamide but not to steroids. The patients described by Oh et al (1983) and Carpenter et al (1985) developed a slowly progressive proximal myopathy from the age of about one year; the weakness fluctuated in Oh's patient.

The less severely affected patient of Tomé & Fardeau (1975) had a non-progressive proximal myopathy without facial involvement and with normal serum CK activity. In an adult patient with scapuloperoneal myopathy reported by Sahgal & Sahgal (1977) the ultrastructural findings were atypical.

Other congenital myopathies with inclusions. Adams et al (1965) reported a man with lifelong weakness culminating in rapid deterioration for two years. He had a necrotising myopathy and the muscle fibres contained a variety of sarcoplasmic and nuclear inclusions.

Jenis et al (1969) described an infant with severe hypotonia and weakness who died, aged two months, of respiratory failure. There were numerous crystalline inclusions in muscle fibre nuclei and in the cytoplasm.

'Sarcotubular myopathy' was reported by Jerusalem et al (1973a) in two brothers with consanguineous parents. There was mild non-progressive myopathy dating from early infancy. The muscle fibres contained vacuoles derived from the sarcoplasmic reticulum and the T system.

Subsarcolemmal 'tubular aggregates' are found in some patients with muscle cramp on exercise (Lazaro et al 1980) and in a wide variety of other neuromuscular disorders, but they have also been seen in a form of very slowly progressive myopathy, beginning in the second decade, in families with autosomal dominant inheritance (Rohkamm et al 1983, Pierobon-Bormioli et al 1985) and in one of the genetically determined myasthenic syndromes (Engel et al 1982 and see p. 683–85).

'Zebra-body' inclusions were found in the muscle of a boy of 15 years with a vacuolar congenital myopathy (Lake & Wilson 1975). Their specificity is uncertain.

'Cap disease'. Fidzianska et al (1981) reported a single case of a boy with a severe non-progressive congenital myopathy with facial and general muscle weakness and wasting, and a scoliosis. In 70% of the muscle fibres a peripheral ring or a segment ('cap') was deficient in ATPase and myosin and on electron microscopy these zones were shown to contain disorganised myofibrils. The authors postulated a defect in myofilament synthesis or myoblast fusion.

Dense *'cytoplasmic bodies'*, differing from nemaline rods, have been described in a form of non-progressive congenital proximal myopathy with mildly raised serum CK activity, but also in a variety of other myopathies (Goebel et al 1981). Rather similar structures, *'spheroid bodies'*, were found in the muscle fibres of several members of a family who had an autosomal dominant slowly progressive proximal myopathy with the onset of symptoms varying from early childhood to the fourth decade (Goebel et al 1978).

Other 'structural' congenital myopathies. Ringel et al (1978) reported a remarkable child with severe muscular rigidity at birth and very high serum CK activity (45 times normal) who gradually improved over 10 months. The EMG was electrically silent. Muscle biopsy revealed that the fibres had an unusual trilaminar structure.

Brooke (1977, p. 217) described a lace-like structure of the sarcoplasm of type II fibres on oxidative enzyme staining in two members of a large family of 'toe-walkers'. Electron microscopy gave normal results.

Cancilla et al (1971) reported a brother and sister aged two and five years with infantile hypotonia, delayed motor development and mild weakness without areflexia, whose muscle biopsies showed atrophy of type I fibres and apparent lysis of their myofibrils.

Genetic myopathies with changes in the histochemical fibre types

Details of the techniques of histochemical fibre typing and of the patterns found at various stages of the development of normal muscles in man will be found in Chapter 7.

It has already been made clear that in many of the congenital myopathies, notably central core disease, nemaline myopathy and centronuclear myopathy, an abnormal predominance of type I fibres (those concerned with slow oxidative postural activity) is found. Sometimes affected members in families with central core disease may have evidence only of type I fibre predominance on muscle biopsy (Morgan-Hughes et al 1973). It is not unusual, when investigating a hypotonic child, to find no other pathological change and because such cases tend to improve they are ipso facto included in the category 'benign congenital hypotonia'. Indeed, it is not yet clear whether fibre-type predominance is a cause of hypotonia or a result of it. Very similar patterns of fibre-type predominance have been found in muscle biopsies from hypotonic children with primary disorders of the central nervous system (Curless et al 1978b).

However, in addition to inequality of the numbers of type I and II fibres there may be inequality in their size. Usually the small fibres are of type II and this pattern may be found in a wide variety of disorders, especially muscle disuse. Children with small type I fibres have been described as having 'congenital fibre-type disproportion'.

Congenital fibre-type disproportion. Brooke (1973) suggested this name for a group of hypotonic children with no significant pathology other than the small size of their type I fibres. The pattern had emerged from a previous wider analysis of the histochemical patterns found in children's muscle biopsies (Brooke & Engel 1969). Other patients with the same biopsy findings had been found to have cerebellar disease or myotonic dystrophy, but 22 cases seemed to comprise a clinical entity. There was hypotonia, often quite severe, at or soon after birth, which might deteriorate for up to one year but thereafter remained static. Congenital contractures, often with dislocation of the hips, were frequent and high-arched palates, short stature and later kyphoscoliosis were each seen in about half the cases (Fig. 20.4). The tendon reflexes were usually diminished but present, the serum CK activity was normal or slightly increased and the EMG was normal or mildly 'myopathic'. Walking was delayed beyond 18 months in all but one case and in some beyond three years. Brooke emphasised the relatively good prognosis, but later modified this because most of his cases remained significantly disabled (Brooke

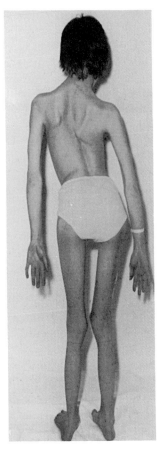

Fig. 20.4 Congenital fibre-type disproportion. A girl of 16 years. Hypotonia since birth; sat at 12 months; walked at 20 months; scoliosis and respiratory insufficiency for three years; stature below 3rd centile. Sister affected

et al 1979). One patient turned out to have facio-scapulohumeral dystrophy. Mild neuromuscular symptoms were present in first-degree or more distant relatives of several cases.

Other cases, subsequently described by Fardeau et al (1975), Lenard and Goebel (1975), Martin et al (1976), Dubowitz (1978), Sulaiman et al (1983) and many others, have on the whole tended to confirm the existence of this disorder as an entity, although some doubts remain. For instance Martin et al (1976) reported that their patient's mother had been alcoholic during her pregnancy and they also found identical biopsy appearances in two cases of globoid cell leucodystrophy and one of Pompe's glycogenosis. Dubowitz pointed out the importance of making the diagnosis only

when the type II muscle fibres were normal or large, in order to avoid confusion with congenital myotonic dystrophy. Lenard & Goebel (1975) reported a child with life-threatening hypotonia and respiratory insufficiency in the neonatal period. The occurrence of an apparently dominant mode of transmission in some families was confirmed by Fardeau et al (1975).

When the clinical and histochemical findings are typical, one is justified in making a provisional diagnosis of congenital fibre-type disproportion, but follow-up assessments for some years are essential. Some cases may be found later to have central hypotonia. Because of the relatively good long-term outlook it is important to prevent and treat spinal deformities enthusiastically to avoid further respiratory insufficiency; the contractures should also be given vigorous attention. There is little doubt that the next few years will bring a clearer understanding of the nature of this disorder and its pathogenesis. Its status as an entity is fragile and as a primary myopathy even more so.

Other abnormalities of size and number of histochemical fibre types. Given two basic fibre types of which either may predominate, or which may be equal in number, and of which either or both may be small or normal (or rarely large) in size, there is wide scope for variation. One may add the presence or absence of central nuclei in the centronuclear myopathies. In practice many of the possible combinations have been reported, and Farkas-Bargeton et al (1978) and Argov et al (1984) suggested that defective neural control of the functional maturation of the muscle fibres might be responsible.

In congenital myotonic dystrophy there may be relatively small type I fibres, but the type II fibres also are often smaller than normal. Relatively small type II fibres are unusual in the context of congenital myopathy. Brooke & Engel (1969) and Matsuoka et al (1974) described children with this finding who had infantile hypotonia, markedly delayed motor development, normal facial and eye movements, preserved reflexes, a non-progressive course and normal intelligence. One of the patients of Argov et al (1984) with type II fibre hypoplasia had impaired central control of vertical gaze. Dubrovsky et al (1978) reported a different clinical pattern associated with type II fibre hypoplasia in a six-year-old child with non-progressive distal muscle weakness and atrophy, bilateral external ophthalmoplegia and cataracts. The EMG suggested neurogenic atrophy.

Extremely small fibres of both types in a very hypotonic baby aged two weeks reverted to normal at 10 months, together with the hypotonia, but severe congenital ophthalmoplegia and slight facial weakness persisted (Hanson et al 1977).

Congenital myopathies with muscle fibre necrosis

The muscular dystrophies are discussed in detail in Chapter 15. It is only necessary to mention here that both 'congenital muscular dystrophy' and congenital myotonic dystrophy (Ch. 16) differ sharply from the other muscular dystrophies in being virtually non-progressive and, indeed, necrosis is not a feature of the muscle pathology in myotonic dystrophy. Nevertheless, both may cause profound and life-threatening hypotonia and muscular paralysis in the first few days and weeks of life. Infants born before term, as they often are, with myotonic dystrophy are particularly at risk. Both may give rise to congenital contractures which are often widespread in congenital muscular dystrophy, but tend to be restricted to the ankles in myotonic dystrophy.

Thompson (1982) reported three cases of a congenital necrotising myopathy with some inflammatory features and an apparent response to steroids, and suggested that they were suffering from an acquired 'infantile myositis', but the evidence distinguishing this from congenital muscular dystrophy was not conclusive.

Genetic myopathies with non-specific changes in fibres — 'Minimal change myopathy'

Everyone who investigates children with neuromuscular disorders is familiar with patients who have undoubted muscular weakness without helpful diagnostic features and whose muscle biopsies show equally non-specific changes. When the symptoms date from infancy and the myopathic features include muscle destruction,

fatty replacement, fibrosis and marked variation in the fibre size the label is often 'congenital muscular dystrophy' (q.v., Ch. 15). When the changes are milder, the term 'benign congenital myopathy', 'minimal change myopathy' (Dubowitz 1985) or some other non-committal term is applied. Such cases are by no means uncommon but are, naturally, reported in the medical literature only when the author is drawing attention to the problems they pose (Fenichel & Bazelon 1966, Lenard & Goebel 1980) or when they have some unusual feature such as an extensive family history (Turner & Lees 1962). Undoubtedly, many of the cases diagnosed in the past would have been classified differently had they undergone full histochemical or ultrastructural investigations; in others, no doubt, ill-luck or ill-judgement in choosing the site for muscle biopsy has led to the failure to reach a more definite conclusion.

In the cases reported by Turner & Lees (1962), six of 13 sibs were affected with hypotonia from birth and had been followed up without evidence of progression of the disorder for 50 years. The pathology was confined to one post-mortem examination of a bedridden patient, but served to confirm the primary myopathic nature of the disorder. Flexion deformities of the fingers occurred in the adult affected members and in an unaffected aunt and a daughter.

Bethlem & van Wijngaarden (1976) described three kindreds in which dominant inheritance of a benign myopathy occurred over four and five generations. Some had congenital torticollis; otherwise the symptoms had started at about five years of age and had progressed extremely slowly. Proximal muscles were mainly affected, but flexion contractures of the fingers were a prominent feature. The muscle biopsy findings were non-specific, but lobulated fibres, of the type seen often in the late-onset types of muscular dystrophy, were prominent. In this situation the distinction between a 'benign familial myopathy' and a very mild muscular dystrophy is semantic.

'Myosclerosis'. Sometimes, non-specific myopathic features in the muscle biopsy may be accompanied by an apparently disproportionate amount of fibrous tissue around and within the fascicles of muscle fibres. The muscles may feel hard and

have striking contractures and the electromyographer may encounter a grating sensation as he inserts his needle. Such cases raise the question of whether such a condition as 'primary myosclerosis' exists. Cases have been reported by Löwenthal (1954) and by Bradley et al (1973) but it must be confessed that considerable doubt remains as to whether they constitute a specific entity. In isolated cases, especially if the pathology is confined to a few muscles, the possibility of fibrosis induced by previous intramuscular drug injection must be considered (see Ch. 25). Chronic and benign spinal muscular atrophy sometimes gives a similar picture.

DISORDERS OF NEUROMUSCULAR TRANSMISSION

Myasthenia

Myasthenia is relatively uncommon in infancy or childhood. Of 447 cases collected by Millichap & Dodge (1960), 16 showed signs of the disease at, or soon after, birth and 35 presented between the ages of one and 16 years. In a series of 217 cases presenting in infancy, childhood or adolescence (Osserman 1958), 34 had symptoms at, or within a few days of birth and eight more within the first two years of life.

For many years it has been recognised that some cases of infantile myasthenia are genetically determined; Bundey (1972) demonstrated that autosomal recessive inheritance made a major contribution in those cases presenting before the age of two years. However, the ability to distinguish autoimmune myasthenia gravis from other myasthenic syndromes by measuring serum antibodies against the acetylcholine receptor (AChR), and the development of in vitro techniques for studying the structure and function of the neuromuscular junction have together led to the recognition of a number of new entities (Engel 1984) and to a clearer understanding of some of the traditional categories (Fenichel 1978, 1983). The current position may be summarised as follows:

Autoimmune myasthenia gravis
(1) Generalised

(2) Ocular
(3) Transient neonatal

Genetically determined myasthenia
(1) Congenital, mainly ocular
   a. End-plate receptor deficiency in some cases
(2) Familial infantile
   a. Defective ACh (re-)synthesis in some cases
(3) Other myasthenic syndromes present from birth
   a. Acetylcholinesterase deficiency in the end-plates
   b. With contractures and defective secondary synaptic clefts
(4) 'Limb-girdle' syndromes resembling myopathies
   a. With tubular aggregates and prolonged ion channel opening
   b. With small quanta of acetylcholine
(5) ? Benign congenital myopathy with myasthenic features

Other disorders of neuromuscular transmission
(1) Botulism
   a. Acute intoxication
   b. Infantile form
(2) Eaton–Lambert syndrome
(3) Other toxic causes

Autoimmune myasthenia in childhood. Children as young as one to two years may develop myasthenia gravis, either generalised or restricted to the external ocular muscles. They never have thymomas. The disorder is essentially identical to that seen in other age groups and is fully described in Chapter 19. The patient of Oberklaid & Hopkins (1976) was six months old at the onset and died at 10 months. Without AChR antibody titres it is impossible to distinguish in this kind of case between extremely early autoimmune myasthenia and a genetic disorder. Similarly, some early descriptions of a fulminatingly acute form, threatening life within 24 hours of the onset, were not backed up by AChR antibody assays but may well be genuine examples of this disorder (see Fenichel 1978).

Fukuyama et al (1973) discussed the outcome in 51 patients aged between nine months and 11 years at the onset, who had apparently not been subjected to thymectomy; very few had remitted within 12 years, although most had 'improved'. Cavanagh (1980) and Bjerre & Hallberg (1983) pointed out the sketchy nature of the published evidence about the role of thymectomy in children. Nevertheless, the usual policy in children with generalised myasthenia and AChR antibodies (as in older people) is to perform a thymectomy as soon as possible, to use steroids if necessary to induce a remission and to rely upon anticholinesterase drugs as sparingly as possible for the control of symptoms. The position regarding purely (or predominantly) ocular autoimmune myasthenia is difficult. Few regard it as justifying thymectomy, yet it tends to be relatively difficult to control by other means.

Transient neonatal myasthenia gravis. In most cases of myasthenia presenting at birth, the mother is affected and the baby's transient weakness is attributed to the placental transfer of maternal antibodies. Nevertheless, very few babies born to myasthenic mothers (10 out of 71 in Osserman's series; Osserman 1958) have symptoms of the condition, and the severity of their symptoms bears no obvious relation to the severity or duration of the mother's illness or to her AChR antibody titre. There is evidence that such babies also produce endogenous AChR antibodies (see Engel 1984).

Early diagnosis is important because, although the myasthenia is transient, lasting for a few days to a few weeks, it is generalised and may be severe or even fatal unless appropriate treatment is given. Signs may be present at birth, or may be delayed for as long as three days, and they often deteriorate over the first few days. The main features are generalised hypotonia, a weak cry, respiratory insufficiency, intermittent cyanosis especially during feeds, and difficulty and fatigue in sucking and swallowing. In a hypotonic baby, reduced mobility of the face, with constantly open eyes and mouth or (less often) ptosis, should suggest the diagnosis.

An intramuscular test dose of 0.05 mg prostigmine or 0.3 mg pyridostigmine bromide, or a subcutaneous dose of 0.1 ml Tensilon® (edrophonium chloride 1 mg) will confirm the diagnosis. Tube feeding and assisted ventilation may be required. Maintenance therapy, when necessary, consists of 1–5 mg of prostigmine or 4–20 mg of pyridostigmine bromide orally with feeds. The size and frequency of the dose will have to be adjusted according to the degree and duration of relief of symptoms and must be reduced as spontaneous recovery takes place.

Genetically determined myasthenia

'Congenital myasthenia'. This name is by convention applied to an autosomal recessive disorder present from birth (but not always noticed until later) in which ptosis and external ophthalmoplegia are the dominant features; there may also be mild involvement of the facial and skeletal muscles. There is a good response to anticholinesterase drugs and a decremental response can be found on electromyography even in clinically normal limb muscles. The condition usually remains relatively mild over many years but does not improve, and some patients develop progressive skeletal muscle weakness (Ford 1966, see Fenichel 1978, 1983) while in others the condition remains localised for many years (Whitley et al 1976). AChR antibodies are assumed to be absent in all cases although the evidence is based on small numbers (Vincent & Newsom-Davis 1979). Thymectomy is contraindicated in this, as in all other non-autoimmune myasthenic disorders.

Vincent et al (1981) studied five patients with myasthenia dating from birth, of whom three had the features of this syndrome. In all these three cases there were findings indicating a defect in the acetylcholine receptors. These patients had a partial response to anticholesterase drugs, possibly enhanced by treatment with 3,4-diaminopyridine (J. Newsom-Davis, personal communication). A fourth child (case 3) with more generalised symptoms in infancy and the later development of ophthalmoplegia (by the age of 13 years) had a different postsynaptic defect.

A single patient (their case 2) conforming to this clinical pattern was investigated by Lecky et al (1986) and the findings also suggested a postsynaptic defect, possibly in the structure of the AChR macromolecule.

Familial infantile myasthenia. Again by convention this term is used for patients with an autosomal recessive disorder causing generalised and often life-threatening myasthenia in the newborn period (Fenichel 1978, 1983). Ocular muscle involvement is absent or at least not a prominent feature. Respiratory failure, recurrent severe apnoeic attacks during crying, and choking and cyanosis during feeding are the dominant symptoms. There is a useful response to anticholinesterase drugs but ventilation and tracheostomy are sometimes required in the early stages. The myasthenia tends to improve over several weeks and it may be possible to withdraw medication but recurrent acute exacerbations pose a threat throughout infancy and early childhood and many of the reported cases have died unexpectedly. In the family reported by Gieron & Korthals (1985) exacerbations continued in adult life. Affected sibs may show a wide variation in the severity of symptoms; the patient of Robertson et al (1980) required continuous anticholinesterase treatment at the age of 14 years but a brother had had only recurrent respiratory depression in infancy with complete remission. The AChR antibody titres are normal (Robertson et al 1980, Gieron & Korthals 1985). Steroid therapy and thymectomy are valueless. In addition to the generally cited reports, some typical cases have escaped notice because of confusion over nomenclature (e.g. McLean et al 1973).

A typical case of this type studied by Hart et al (1979) was found to have evidence of a presynaptic transmission defect of acetylcholine resynthesis or packaging (see also Engel 1984). A decremental response of the muscle action potential could be obtained only after prolonged nerve stimulation.

Other myasthenic syndromes present from birth. A boy with lifelong generalised myasthenia dating from the first week of life and including bulbar and ocular muscle involvement was found by Engel et al (1977) to have a deficiency of acetylcholinesterase in the end-plates. There was no response to anticholinesterase drugs, repetitive stimuli gave a decremental response and single stimuli applied to motor nerves induced repetitive muscle action potentials.

Smit et al (1984, 1987) described a patient born with multiple contractures and severe generalised

myasthenic weakness whose fetal movements had been impaired. In the next two months he had recurrent myasthenic crises but he improved with treatment with pyridostigmine. Study of biopsy samples revealed a structural defect in the secondary synaptic clefts and an altered distribution of the acetylcholine receptors.

Slowly progressive weakness. For many years patients have been described with 'benign congenital myopathy' who survived into adult life with some elements of fluctuation or fatiguability but with a limited response to anticholinesterase drugs (Rowland & Eskanazi 1956, Walton et al 1956).

McQuillen (1966) described a brother and sister who developed a 'limb-girdle' syndrome of proximal and distal weakness in the early teens and who showed a striking response to prostigmine. The ocular and bulbar muscles were not involved. Other similar cases have been described (Fenichel 1978, 1983), some of them with tubular aggregates in the muscle fibres on biopsy, but the pathogenesis of this condition remains obscure.

However, Morgan-Hughes et al (1981) found tubular aggregates in the muscle biopsy and evidence both of reduced numbers of AChRs and of a reduction in their affinity for ACh in a man of 32 years. This patient presented with a 14-month history of myasthenia resembling the autoimmune disease clinically and electrophysiologically, but with absent AChR antibody and no response to anticholinesterase drugs.

Engel et al (1982) described and investigated six patients who all had lifelong muscle weakness and who were shown to have identical postsynaptic neuromuscular transmission defects with a prolonged open-time of the acetylcholine-induced ion channel. The inheritance was autosomal dominant. From early infancy they had weakness of the neck and scapular muscles, the finger extensors, usually (but not always) the external ocular muscles and sometimes other muscles including the face. Periodic exacerbations of the weakness occurred but apparently not typical myasthenic fatigue. Their symptoms progressed gradually and as adults they had muscle wasting but in most cases normal reflexes. The overall picture resembled a congenital muscular dystrophy or myopathy more than myasthenia. AChR antibody titres and serum CK activity were normal. The EMG showed a characteristic repetitive firing response after single nerve stimuli, and a decremental response in affected muscles. Muscle biopsies showed variation in fibre size, fibre splitting, some mild fibrosis, type I fibre predominance and grouping (which could be mistaken for neurogenic atrophy) and tubular aggregates and vacuoles. It is likely that patients with this disorder are usually overlooked. Treatment with anticholinesterase drugs, however, has been disappointing.

A patient of Lecky et al (1986, case 1) had lifelong muscle weakness without diurnal fluctuation which involved the face and proximal limb muscles more than the distal ones. There was ptosis but the eye movements were not recorded. The tendon reflexes were sluggish. There was no response to edrophonium but some improvement with 3,4-diaminopyridine. The serum AChR antibody titre and CK activity were normal. The patient had delayed puberty and an impaired growth hormone response to insulin. EMG showed a limited decremental response and no repetitive firing but there was increased jitter. Muscle biopsy was normal. In vitro studies suggested a reduced amount of ACh per quantum but did not exclude a postsynaptic defect in ACh sensitivity. In one of the patients (case 1) of Vincent et al (1981) there were similar clinical features and findings and on investigation this patient responded to treatment with 4-aminopyridine. He had full external ocular movements. The response to treatment in such patients, who lack obvious clinical evidence of myasthenia, makes it particularly important to use sophisticated electrophysiological studies to identify them.

Other defects of neuromuscular transmission

Infantile botulism. Two infants, aged two and three months, who became hypotonic over a period of a few days and had difficulty in sucking and swallowing, were found to have evidence of neuromuscular blockade on electromyography and both *Clostridium botulinum* organisms and toxin in the faeces. Both made a spontaneous recovery (Pickett et al 1976). Other cases have been described, all with a similar history (Midura &

Arnon 1976, Turner et al 1978). The pupils are fixed and dilated. Constipation seems to be a constant feature, perhaps related to the production of the toxin in the bowel. This disorder is quite distinct from the acute effects of ingestion of *C. botulinum* toxin. It may be mistaken for Werdnig–Hoffmann disease.

The Eaton–Lambert syndrome (see Ch. 19) is exceedingly rare in childhood but has been described in association with leukaemia (Shapira et al 1974) and in a child with no detectable tumour (Chelmicka-Schorr et al 1979).

CLINICAL PROBLEMS IN CHILDREN WITH NEUROMUSCULAR DISORDERS

Hypotonia

Analysis of muscle tone in the assessment of the neurological status of the infant was reviewed by André-Thomas and his colleagues in a book translated from the French by Mac Keith et al (1960). These authors divided tone into two types, tonus passif and tonus actif, the former being subdivided into extensibilité and passivité. Extensibilité is the capacity of the muscle to be lengthened; as it is measured by the amplitude of slow passive movement of a segment of a limb at a joint, it is presumably also a measure of ligamentous laxity. Passivité is the lack of resistance to passive movement, as tested for instance by flapping the hand, and may be regarded as the reciprocal of 'tone' as it is usually understood by British neurologists. Observation of spontaneous posture and active movements, as well as the power of recoil when a limb is rapidly moved by the examiner from its position of rest, are used in the assessment of tonus actif.

In short, 'hypotonia' alone is an inadequate clinical term and its analysis requires assessment of posture, spontaneous movement and reflex responses as well as of the power, extensibility and resistance to rapid passive movements of the muscles.

The differential diagnosis of infantile hypotonia may arise either when a baby is relatively immobile and limp at birth or in the first few days and weeks of life or, more often, because of delay in the development of control of posture at about six months of age and onwards.

The normal infant at birth. The normal infant moves its limbs vigorously for about half an hour after birth and, following a period of quiescence, again at about three to four hours of age (Desmond et al 1963) and thereafter whenever it is awake and crying, periods of quiet wakefulness in newborn babies being few and brief. Moreover, even when a newborn baby is quiet it exhibits marked flexural tone when lying or suspended prone or supine, and it is not possible fully to extend the thighs or legs by passive stretching. Passive movements of the limbs give the impression of hypertonia, which should, of course, be equal bilaterally provided that the head is kept in a central position to eliminate the influence of the asymmetrical tonic neck reflex on the limbs. A beat or two of ankle clonus is normal. Even at birth there is some postural control of the head: on being sat up, the newborn baby will balance its head for a brief period in the upright position before it flops forward; an anencephalic baby will keep its head upright.

The development of postural control in the normal infant. It is important to realise that the muscle tone of the normal infant diminishes during the first month of life to be regained later. The newborn baby can support his head and may take his weight on his legs more firmly than he will do again until the age of six to nine months. Control of body posture develops in stages from head to foot (Illingworth 1972, Touwen 1976) but there is, of course, considerable variability in healthy children. The following is a brief outline of the average age at which each accomplishment is acquired.

Some *control of the head* is evident at birth. By about six weeks of age a baby can extend its head against gravity to the midline when held prone, by three months it can flex against gravity when held supine. By three months it will raise the shoulders and fully extend the head when lying prone; by five to six months a baby lying supine will raise its head in anticipation of being picked up.

By three months a baby lying supine will extend its *arms* towards a preferred object and by five months will reach out and grasp the object with one hand.

Trunk and legs. At six months most babies will sit with support and even for brief periods without support, propping themselves up by the arms placed between the abducted thighs; 50% of normal Newcastle infants are sitting unsupported at 6.4 months, 90% at 8.1 months and 97% at 9.3 months; 50% are walking unaided at 12.8 months, 90% at 15.8 months and 97% at 18.4 months (Neligan & Prudham 1969). The percentile figures for Denver infants are a little different, but the Denver Developmental Screening Test is useful and straightforward to apply (Frankenburg & Dodds 1967, Bryant et al 1979).

The hypotonic infant. The sight of a newborn hypotonic infant lying awake and motionless with outstretched limbs is in striking contrast to the appearance of the normal baby. Typically the hips are fully abducted, the knees flexed and the elbows extended. Hypotonia can be confirmed on handling and lifting the infant, when instead of its curling up, the head, trunk and limbs will flop about under the influence of gravity (Fig. 20.5a). Resistance to passive movement of the limbs and head will be decreased, passivité will be increased and so will extensibilité, as evinced by wrapping each arm round the neck (the 'scarf' sign) or by flexing the thighs on the trunk with the legs fully extended at the knees.

Almost all hypotonic infants move less actively than normal babies. Dubowitz (1978, 1980) emphasises the difference between the paralysed floppy baby with neuromuscular disease and the baby with central hypotonia but without significant weakness who can withdraw from a painful stimulus or support the limbs briefly against gravity (Fig. 20.5b). The distinction is important and useful but by no means always easy to see; some disorders of the central nervous system may give rise to severe paralysis.

Asking the mother about the fetal movements may elicit some evidence about the duration of the hypotonia before birth. Contractures at birth imply fetal immobility, and dislocation of the hips is quite frequent when prenatal hypotonia of the

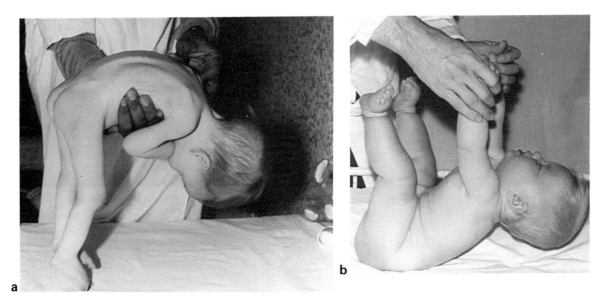

Fig. 20.5 Two infants with severe central hypotonia and no neuromuscular disease. a. Severe mental retardation; a boy 11 months old; b. Prader–Willi syndrome; a boy of 9 months. Abnormal 'passivité' contrasts with active contraction against gravity

muscles of the lower limbs has diminished the normal forces required to form the acetabula properly. Fetal impairment of swallowing is an important cause of polyhydramnios.

Causes of hypotonia. Diminished movement and limpness in the *newborn baby* may be caused by extreme prematurity, by any severe systemic illness, by drugs given to the mother or by lesions of the brain, spinal cord, peripheral nerves, myoneural junction, muscles and ligaments. Severe generalised illness (such as respiratory distress or septicaemia) or cerebral disorders (especially malformation, bleeding, infection or the effects of asphyxia) are by far the commonest causes but, in the absence of obvious illness, and especially when the baby is alert, one must consider the possibility of a number of less common disorders in the differential diagnosis. These include spinal cord injury, spinal muscular atrophy, congenital myotonic dystrophy, myasthenia and various types of congenital myopathy.

There are also numerous causes for *delay in the development of postural control* and many babies who display retarded motor development give the clinical impression of hypotonia. Attempts to measure muscle tone objectively have been made

(Rondot et al 1958) but not applied in a systematic fashion to this problem. It is uncommon for muscular hypotonia and weakness to develop in a previously normal infant so rapidly that they command attention in themselves, or cause actual regression in development. Such an event clearly implies a progressive disorder, whether cerebral, spinal or neuromuscular in origin. Even these more often result in developmental delay before any regression is seen, and so timing the 'onset' of the disease, an important point in differential diagnosis, may be a difficult matter, greatly influenced by the parents' experience, powers of observation and memory (Pearn 1974).

Any chronic debilitating illness in early infancy and many conditions adversely affecting growth (malnutrition, malabsorption syndromes, metabolic diseases, congenital heart malformations, congenital defects of the renal tract, chronic pulmonary diseases, etc) may result in delayed motor control and hypotonia, but can usually be differentiated fairly easily by the history, symptoms and signs. Mental handicap may not be as easily distinguished because the conventional yardsticks of mental development in infancy are so dependent on motor performance; attention must be directed to alertness, awareness, and language development as well as to the specific dysmorphic or other characteristics of the different conditions underlying the mental handicap. It is important not to confuse the absence of facial expression caused by muscle weakness with that of retardation.

It is not uncommon to find delay in postural control and hypotonia, otherwise inexplicable, in infants who have lacked normal care in the early weeks of life (Buda et al 1972). In such cases the cause may be apparent in simple parental neglect, frequent change of foster parent or institutional life, but in other cases the lack of normal mothering is by no means always obvious to the clinician — the mother's anxiety being attributed to the baby's condition, rather than the baby's condition to the mother's endogenous depression and consequent failure to 'identify' with her infant.

When normal variation, chronic disease other than in the nervous system, mental defect and emotional deprivation can be excluded, the causes of hypotonia and delayed development in infancy must lie in disorders of cerebral motor control, of the spinal cord, anterior horn cells, peripheral nerves or myoneural junction, or of muscles, ligaments and tendons.

Paine's follow-up study (Paine 1963) put the differential diagnostic problem into perspective. The following were the final diagnoses in 111 'floppy' infants reviewed at from six months to 20 years of age: various forms of cerebral palsy 48; cerebral degenerative disease 3; brain tumour 1; mental retardation 28; spinal cord injury 1; spinal muscular atrophy 4; myopathy 4; benign congenital hypotonia 18; and disease outside the nervous system 4. In contrast, no fewer than 67 of Walton's series of 109 cases (Walton 1956) were eventually diagnosed as having spinal muscular atrophy, but here the initial diagnosis in each case was 'amyotonia congenita' whereas Paine's series of children simply presented with delay in postural control.

Some non-neuromuscular causes of hypotonia

Acute metabolic disease in the newborn. An inborn error of metabolism — particularly an organic acidaemia, aminoacidaemia or hyper-ammonaemia — should be suspected in a baby who is well at birth but develops profound hypotonia, respiratory failure, poor feeding and drowsiness within the first few days, without evidence of infection or intracranial haemorrhage. Hyperventilation is an important clue to the underlying metabolic acidosis in these disorders. Checking for hypoglycaemia, ketonuria, an unusual odour of the urine and acidosis are important initial stages in their investigation.

These metabolic disorders may, incidentally, present only much later when an acute illness causes a catabolic state and decompensation. They are important because some of them respond to dietary treatment, and some organic acidaemias respond to treatment with biotin or vitamin B_{12} (Barnes et al 1970, Keeton & Moosa 1976, Charles et al 1979). Leigh's disease, which is often associated with lactic acidaemia, also presents with profound hypotonia in a previously normal baby and is often mistaken at first for a neuromuscular disease.

Spinal cord injury, tumours and myelodysplasia. Deformity or injury of the spinal cord at birth may result in the classic picture of the floppy infant, but the arms are often spared. Birth injury to the spinal cord was first accurately described by Crothers (1923). The cord is damaged by stretching or by avulsion of the spinal roots forming the brachial plexus. Most cases follow difficult breech delivery which may be complicated by the rare distal form of brachial plexus palsy (Klumpke) causing paralysis of the small muscles of the hand and the long flexors of the hand and fingers. A minority of spinal cord injuries, namely those complicating difficult vertex delivery, are more usually associated with brachial plexus palsy of the proximal type (Erb) involving mainly the abductors of the upper arm and flexors and supinators of the forearm (Crothers & Putnam 1927).

The initial complete flaccidity and immobility of the lower limbs and trunk in spinal cord injury may result in a mistaken diagnosis of a general neuromuscular disorder, especially if there are also brachial plexus lesions. However, the presence of sphincter and sensory abnormalities will reveal the true diagnosis even if the localised nature of the paralysis is not at first obvious. There is likely to be retention of urine and a patulous anus for several days and pinching the skin of the lower half of the body, although it may later cause reflex withdrawal, will not result in a cry or grimace. After the first few days, however, normal sphincter action may be regained and sensory loss may be difficult to detect. The CSF may contain blood. The subject is reviewed by Towbin (1969) and Byers (1975).

Spinal tumours in infancy are uncommon and are easily overlooked at first if there is extensive paralysis involving the intercostal or abdominal muscles as well as the limbs. Tumours extending over many segments of the cord, whether intramedullary (glioma or ependymoma) or extramedullary such as a neuroblastoma, are fairly characteristic at this age. They provide the same pitfalls in diagnosis as extensive cord injury.

Myelodysplasia is usually obvious at birth in the form of meningomyelocele. In cases where the deformity is hidden, however, there are nearly always overlying skin defects (hair, haemangioma, lipoma or congenital dermal sinus) and X-rays will reveal the spinal deformity.

Cerebral causes of hypotonia at birth. The higher control of muscle tone in the newborn is not well understood. Anencephalic and grossly hydranencephalic newborn infants may exhibit normal muscle tone, but whereas *absence* of cerebral hemispheres may not be associated with hyper- or hypotonicity, *damage* to or disease of the hemispheres may.

Muscular hypotonia is characteristic of 'terminal' asphyxia at birth, in which apnoea is associated with pallor, bradycardia and unresponsiveness to physical stimuli. 'Cerebral depression' in the first few days of life may follow severe asphyxia at birth or a traumatic labour, or may occur unexpectedly in the presence of prenatally determined disease or deformity of the brain. Temporary cerebral depression may follow administration of sedative drugs to the mother in labour and hypotonia is a particularly striking feature when diazepam is used in cases of pre-eclamptic toxaemia. The appearance of a pallid, motionless, hypotonic baby with open eyes and with increasingly frequent periods of apnoea and cyanosis is characteristic of cerebral depression in the newborn. Automatisms, such as the Moro, rooting, nasopalpebral and sucking reflexes are absent. The mortality is high, especially in the first 48 hours of life, and massive intracranial haemorrhage is a common post-mortem finding. Artificial ventilation is increasingly used, and with considerable success, in managing these babies. In those who survive, the hypotonia usually gives place after a day or two either to normal muscle tone and movement or to a clinical state suggesting cerebral irritation, signs of which include hypertonia, hyperactivity, easily elicited automatisms and multifocal fits. The hypotonia caused by a cerebral lesion acquired at birth only infrequently persists after the first few days of life and in these cases lack of alertness or responsiveness, and preservation of the tendon reflexes usually help to differentiate the condition from lower motor neurone or muscular disorders.

Hypotonia as a feature of cerebral palsy. Persistent hypotonia following a perinatal cerebral catastrophe is very rare and its pathological basis is uncertain. It is of interest in this context that Woolf (1960) reported the case of one infant with bilateral cerebral softening secondary to birth asphyxia, accompanied by vacuolar degeneration of anterior horn cells. Flaccidity is, however, often seen in the early months in infants who later prove to be cases of spastic diplegia, athetosis, ataxia or mental defect (as Sigmund Freud realised nearly a century ago). Most infants with more persistent central hypotonia will be found to have a chromosomal disorder, the Prader–Willi syndrome, or other disorders of cerebral or cerebellar development associated with mental defect or persistent congenital ataxia respectively (Lesny 1979). There is thus no evidence to support the widespread concept of a permanent hypotonic category of cerebral palsy. Some infants with cerebral disorders originating before or at birth are found to have delayed maturation of muscle fibres — a fetal or neonatal pattern persisting for longer than usual (Fenichel 1967, Curless et al 1978b), and some cases of 'fibre-type disproportion' seem to fall into this category.

The hypotonic stage of spastic diplegia. Spastic

diplegia is the typical type of cerebral palsy seen in preterm infants, although it is not confined to this group. Ingram (1955) found that 40% of his cases went through a hypotonic stage in early infancy. Within a few weeks after birth physical examination shows hypotonia and diminished tendon reflexes, but automatisms such as the Moro reflex and palmar grasp reflexes are too easily elicited and tonic neck reflexes are conspicuous. Transition to a dystonic stage usually takes place within six months. By then early spasticity is indicated by hyperadduction of the thighs and plantar flexion of the feet on upright suspension, and spread of the knee jerk to the adductors of one or both thighs. Obviously, microcephaly, signs of cerebral sensory defects or intellectual retardation, when present, will suggest a cerebral cause for the hypotonia, usually associated later with an extensive spastic quadriplegia.

The hypotonic stage of athetosis. Hypotonia is characteristic of athetosis and choreoathetosis in infancy, but the tendon reflexes tend to be brisk in contrast to the diminished muscle tone, and tonic neck reflexes are usually easily elicited. Polani (1959) studied the natural history of choreoathetosis. About one-third of his patients displayed marked muscular hypotonia from about the second month and this might still be apparent by one year of age. Usually opisthotonic episodes and athetoid tongue-thrusting begin within the first year.

Ataxic syndromes in infancy. Muscular hypotonia and delay in postural control are often the presenting symptoms of ataxic syndromes of infancy and childhood, whether attributable to prenatal cerebellar hypoplasia, to perinatal events or to degenerative processes. An important minority of these cases results from congenital hypothyroidism. At first, congenital ataxia presents a clinical picture of generalised hypotonia, paucity of spontaneous movement, hyperextensibility of joints, absent automatisms and poor postural control. Intention tremor and incoordination of voluntary movement emerge as the child begins to reach out for objects.

Similarly, degenerative diseases producing ataxia, such as Friedreich's and other hereditary ataxias and ataxia telangiectasia, may present with delay in acquisition of motor control and hypotonia. *Intermittent* ataxia (Blass et al 1971), whether caused by intoxication, benign paroxysmal vertigo, a IVth ventricular tumour, an aminoacidaemia or lactic acidosis, or the syndrome of idiopathic familial intermittent ataxia, may be difficult at first to distinguish from periodic paralysis in very young children.

Mental retardation. Delay in motor development in the first year of life is frequently the presenting symptom of mental retardation and is often accompanied by hypotonia. Later, the child generally proves to have no detectable motor defect while the learning difficulties gradually become apparent. However, there are several conditions, of which Down syndrome and the Prader–Willi syndrome are the best known, in which hypotonia in the early stages is particularly conspicuous.

Down syndrome is usually accompanied by flaccidity from birth until about one year of age and the tendon reflexes may be difficult to obtain. In the neonatal period, hypotonia is more frequently found in patients with trisomy 21 than in those with translocations of the 13/21, 15/21 and 21/21 types. Bazelon et al (1967) claimed that hypotonia is much improved in children with Down sydrome by the oral administration of 5-hydroxytryptophan; this substance is the immediate metabolic precursor of serotonin, the whole-blood level of which is reduced in trisomic Down syndrome (Rosner et al 1965). Unfortunately there is no associated improvement in function.

The Prader–Willi syndrome is an entity characterised by short stature, obesity, mild to moderate mental retardation, cryptorchidism and genital hypoplasia (Prader et al 1956, Laurence 1967, Zellweger & Schneider 1968) and is associated in many cases with a deletion of part of chromosome 15 at or near the q12 site (Fear et al 1985). Most cases have from birth shown marked generalised hypotonia, areflexia, paucity of movement and feeble sucking. Tube feeding is commonly required in the first few weeks of life. After several months the infants become more active and the tendon reflexes are elicitable but moderate hypotonia persists. Excessive appetite and obesity develop in the second or third year. Children with the Prader–Willi syndrome (Fig. 20.6) have recognisably similar faces (Laurence 1967, Dubowitz 1980, Stephenson 1980).

Muscular hypotonia is a feature of *several other chromosomal defects*, but peripheral nerve and muscle have rarely been studied in these conditions. Muscular hypotonia and multiple malformations are prominent in trisomy 13, and in trisomy 18 initial hypotonia is later replaced by hypertonia. Hypotonia is also characteristic of infants with the cri du chat syndrome (partial deletion of the short arm of chromosome 5). Three

chromosomal disorders which may present with hypotonia as the dominant clinical problem are ring chromosome 14 (Fig. 20.7), ring chromosome 22 and possibly translocation of the long arm of chromosome 10; but even in these disorders minor dysmorphic features provide a clue to the diagnosis. One-third of cases of XXXXY karyotype have been noted to be hypotonic (Smith 1982).

The association of mental retardation with hypotonia by no means rules out serious neuromuscular disease. Both in Duchenne muscular dystrophy and in congenital myotonic dystrophy, mental retardation may be severe and may divert attention from the muscular weakness. Boys with unex-

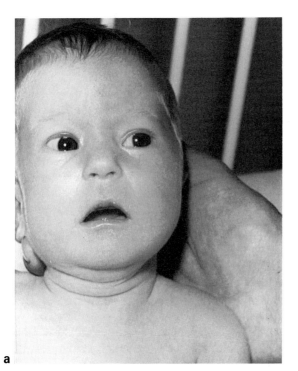

a

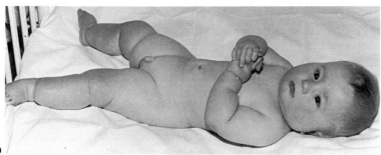

b

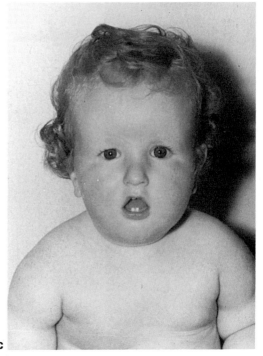

c

Fig. 20.6 Prader–Willi syndrome.
a. Facies, a girl at three weeks old. Severe hypotonia, needed tube-feeding for 10 weeks. At five years her stature was below the 3rd centile, her weight near the 97th; b. Facies, hypotonic posture, hypogenitalism, obesity at nine months of age. Same patient as 20.5(b); c. Facies, a boy aged nine months

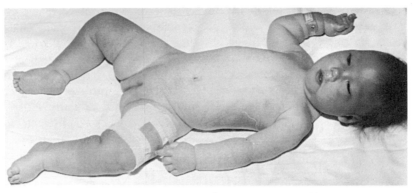

Fig. 20.7 Chromosome anomaly (ring chromosome 14). Hypotonia and weakness were the dominant problems. Mild facial dysmorphism. EMG and needle muscle biopsy normal. Here aged 10 months

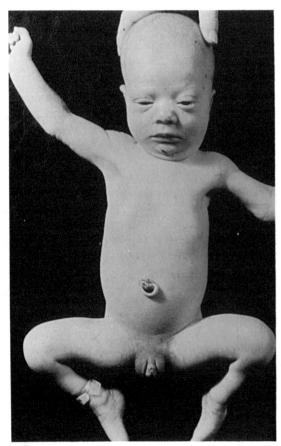

Fig. 20.8 Zellweger (cerebrohepatorenal) syndrome, Profound hypotonia, areflexia and seizures from day 1; liver dysfunction. Here aged two weeks

plained delay in walking or in speech development should be tested for Duchenne muscular dystrophy by estimation of the serum CK activity (see

Ch. 15). Mental retardation is a major feature of Fukuyama muscular dystrophy (Ch. 15), of Lowe syndrome (X-linked hypotonia, myopathy, cataracts and renal aminoaciduria), of a syndrome of retardation, eye anomalies and progressive myopathy (Santavuori et al 1977) and of another with similar features associated with mucolipidosis type IV (Zlotogora et al 1983), of Pompe disease, systemic carnitine deficiency and of certain lipid storage and mitochondrial diseases.

Mental retardation is also found with severe hypotonia, although not with overt myopathy, in Zellweger's cerebrohepatorenal syndrome (Fig. 20.8), neonatal adrenoleucodystrophy (Aubourg et al 1986) and the Smith–Lemli–Opitz syndrome (Smith 1982). In the early stages of certain neurodegenerative diseases (especially Tay–Sachs and Niemann–Pick diseases, generalised gangliosidosis and infantile neuroaxonal dystrophy) the motor disturbance is first evident as hypotonia. In the leucodystrophies and in Tay–Sachs disease, hypotonia of the neck and trunk muscles may co-exist with spasticity of the limbs (Fig. 20.9). In the Krabbe and metachromatic types of leucodystrophy the associated peripheral neuropathy also causes areflexia in the presence of spasticity.

Skeletal, tendinous and ligamentous causes of hypotonia. It may be difficult to make a clinical distinction between ligamentous laxity and muscular hypotonia in early infancy. Later in childhood the hyperextensibility of the joints with otherwise relatively normal muscle tone becomes

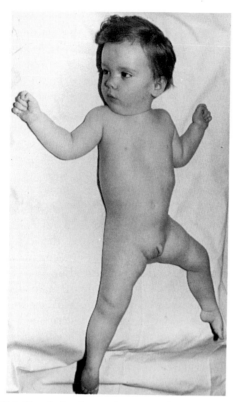

Fig. 20.9 Tay–Sachs disease. Progressive hypotonia, blindness and megalencephaly since seven months. Here aged 21 months. Note the asymmetrical tonic neck reflex

apparent. Certain congenital disorders of connective tissue may be accompanied by delay in postural control and apparent hypotonia due to hyperextensibility of joints.

In Marfan's syndrome and especially in a similar 'marfanoid' syndrome (Walker et al 1969) joint laxity is prominent and in the former some muscular weakness occurs. 'Marfanoid' features have often been mentioned in nemaline myopathy but in fact bear little resemblance to true Marfan's disease. Ehlers–Danlos syndrome must also be considered in the differential diagnosis of the limp child. Eight varieties of this are now recognised of which two (types III and VII) present with joint laxity and recurrent dislocations of joints as the main features while, in the other types, elastic skin, bruising and other features are more prominent (Byers et al 1983). Osteogenesis imperfecta has been reported as presenting with delay in walking and hypotonia (Tizard 1949); the mild autosomal dominant form (type 1) is the relevant one of the four types described and ligamentous laxity and deep blue sclera are striking features (Sillence et al 1979).

Benign congenital hypotonia. This much-maligned term arose from the work of Walton (1956, 1957) who obtained follow-up information on 109 infants diagnosed as having 'amyotonia congenita' during the period 1930–54. Oppenheim's concept of 'myatonia', put forward in 1900 for hypotonic children with a favourable prognosis, had become debased and Walton found that, half a century later, the terms 'myatonia' or 'amyotonia congenita' were sometimes used to encompass all of the infantile hypotonias including Werdnig–Hoffmann disease. Seventeen of his 109 cases had hypotonia of unknown cause, but with recovery which was complete in eight and incomplete in nine cases. The term 'benign congenital hypotonia' was 'used as a descriptive title' for these cases whose 'condition appears to have been due to a widespread congenital muscular hypotonia of undetermined aetiology which eventually recovered completely' (Walton 1956). In the same year, central core disease was first described and, in the period of more than a quarter of a century which has passed since then, many other disorders giving hypotonia with incomplete recovery have been recognised and are now generally classified among the congenital myopathies described earlier in this chapter. The nature of those cases which show complete recovery, and for which Walton now reserves the term 'benign congenital hypotonia', has been less satisfactorily clarified. Brooke & Engel (1969) found that some of them had type I fibre predominance in the muscle biopsy but others have no histological abnormality at all on the evidence of current techniques. No doubt, entities within this group will be identified in the future; meanwhile 'benign congenital hypotonia' remains, at any particular state of the art, a valuable term for those residual cases for whom, after full investigation, no more accurate label exists. It should be reserved for patients: (1) who are hypotonic at or soon after birth, sometimes quite severely; but (2) who retain active limb movements and tendon reflexes; and (3) whose motor development is delayed but shows improvement over a period of months or years; and (4) whose serum enzyme activities, EMGs and biopsies are essentially normal. However, it is quite reasonably argued that muscle biopsy is not justified in an apparently benign situation when it can lead to no effective treatment, unless genetic counselling will be influenced by the result. Certainly, biopsy should be performed in this situation only when full histochemical and electron-microscopic studies will be done, for otherwise it is certain to be inconclusive.

The paediatrician with an interest in the development of the child's motor functions tends to look at hypotonia in a different light. For instance Lundberg (1979) reviewed 78 children who had delayed development of gross motor functions, such as sitting and walking, but had relatively well-developed manipulative functions and no abnormal neurological signs. She found that only three were diagnosed as having neuromuscular disease. Of 65 children whose walking was delayed beyond 27 months, 72% had been significantly hypotonic in infancy, and 28% had a family history of late walking. Half of them were 'bottom shufflers' and 30% had a family history of bottom-shuffling. A common sign among the late walkers in whom no cause for the delay was found was the 'sitting on air' posture of flexion of the hips and extension of the knees while being suspended under the arms.

Whether one thinks of such children as having 'benign congenital hypotonia' or 'dissociated motor development', the essential need in management is to provide the child with the stimulation and equipment and the family with the understanding of the situation and the support that they need, to allow him to develop without the loss of opportunities which may, in the long run, prove more handicapping than the neuromuscular problem itself.

The place of neuromuscular investigations in infantile hypotonia. It will be evident that most hypotonic newborn infants are not suffering from neuromuscular disorders. Most will be found to be ill or mentally retarded or in the early stages of cerebral palsy. On the other hand the baby may become asphyxiated or otherwise ill *because* of neuromuscular problems and when there is apparently disproportionate hypotonia or muscle atrophy, or

unexplained respiratory failure, neuromuscular disease must be suspected. Recognition of a neuromuscular problem is much easier when the baby is fully alert with no signs of central nervous system dysfunction and no dysmorphic features, and especially when there is a history of diminished fetal movement, or if weakness of the cranial muscles or the presence of congenital contractures draw attention to the muscles. Early resort to muscle biopsy has the dual disadvantage that the passage of time may, within a few weeks, reveal evidence for an alternative cause for the hypotonia and that muscle histology and histochemistry in the newborn are more difficult to interpret than in older children. In many of the congenital myopathies and in Werdnig–Hoffmann disease very early biopsy may be misleading.

However it is obviously important to diagnose myasthenia as quickly as possible (see p. 683). Disorders of life-threatening severity and those that are clearly progressive must also be diagnosed as soon as possible, not only to rule out treatable conditions, but for the sake of future genetic counselling.

The serum CK activity is rarely very helpful in neonatal myopathies, but it does provide a valuable clue to the diagnosis of congenital muscular dystrophy if it is very high. Similarly, electromyography may be difficult to interpret in the newborn but in difficult cases is sometimes helpful. Nerve conduction studies are valuable in ruling out peripheral neuropathies. Ultrasonic or CT scanning of muscle are non-specific tests which, however, may provide enough evidence for or against a neuromuscular disorder to help in planning a strategy of early management of the problem.

The following strategy of management may be found helpful in suspected neuromuscular disease of the newborn.
(1) Rule out myasthenia, transplacental drug intoxication and metabolic acidosis. Consider the Prader–Willi syndrome (facies, genitalia, swallowing) and other chromosome anomalies. Consider congenital myotonic dystrophy (examine the mother).
(2) In all uncertain cases check the serum CK level, nerve conduction velocity and if necessary do an ultrasound muscle scan.
(3) In life-threatening cases proceed to EMG and

muscle biopsy. Be prepared to repeat these later if they give an uncertain result.

(4) In less severe cases, after full consultation with the parents, delay further investigation until after a period of follow-up. This may last a few weeks to a few years depending (inversely) on the severity of the residual problem. Repeated clinical examination over a period will usually allow a provisional diagnosis to be made and an appropriate moment for further investigation to be chosen. In cases that improve considerably or remain mild, remember that a biopsy that is 'within normal limits' or 'non-specific' can inspire little confidence if it is performed too early. Above all, muscle biopsy should never be performed unless experienced laboratory services are available for histochemical and electron-microscopic examination.

Arthrogryposis multiplex congenita

The presence of multiple joint contractures at birth is clearly a situation with many causes, and individual appraisal of each patient is essential if one is to avoid overlooking the relatively unusual cases which have a simple genetic basis, an underlying progressive disease or important associated anomalies. The condition in most patients follows a non-progressive course and most are of normal intelligence. Arthrogryposis is seen in about one in 10 000 live births.

To qualify as having arthrogryposis multiplex congenita (AMC) a patient must have joint contractures present at birth in at least two different areas of the body (Fisher et al 1970). The more limited condition of congenital talipes, however, is analogous in having many different causes which include denervation of the lower limbs (as in spina bifida), oligohydramnios (which perhaps acts by restricting movement) and a large group of cases of unknown origin. In a typical case of AMC there is equinovarus deformity of the feet, the hips are abducted and flexed or extended, the knees and elbows incompletely extended, the forearms pronated and the hands flexed with a claw-like apposition of thenar and hypothenar eminences. There may be considerable variation upon this distribution. The muscles acting at the affected joints are typically wasted.

It is currently thought that the condition can result from a number of different pathological processes which cause immobilisation of the limbs during, or shortly after, the embryonic formation of joints (Dodge 1960). In support of this view, Jago (1970) described a typical case of arthrogryposis in an infant born to a mother who had had tetanus at the tenth to twelfth week of pregnancy and was treated with D-tubocurarine for 10 days.

Arthrogryposis, then, may result from immobility imposed on the fetus by external factors, including oligohydramnios, but it also occurs in a number of rare complex syndromes which affect the fetal joints directly or indirectly: Beckerman & Buchino (1978), Hall et al (1982) and Hall (1983) provided extensive lists of these. However, the most frequent causes, and those most relevant to this chapter are disorders of nerve and muscle.

Most cases are found to have a neurogenic basis (Brandt 1947, Drachman & Banker 1963, Besser & Behar 1967). Typically there is asymmetry of the weakness and joint involvement suggesting patchy loss of anterior horn cells and the spinal cord lesion appears to be non-progressive in almost all cases. Although joint contractures may be found at birth in Werdnig–Hoffmann disease, these are uncommon and never severe, and the joint deformity is fully correctable by passive stretching. Clarren & Hall (1983) compared the pathology in the two conditions and found that in Werdnig–Hoffmann disease there was a general loss of the anterior horn cells, whereas in neurogenic arthrogryposis only the alpha motor neurones were lost and the smaller neurones were present in increased numbers. It seems clear, therefore, that neurogenic arthrogryposis is not simply a variant of Werdnig–Hoffmann disease and indeed the two conditions appear to be unrelated entities.

Krugliak et al (1978) described an infant with arthrogryposis in whom post-mortem examination demonstrated apparently total agenesis of the muscle spindles in addition to loss of the anterior horn cells.

A primary myopathy with features of 'congenital muscular dystrophy' (q.v. Ch. 15) is much more rarely the basis of arthrogryposis (Banker et al 1957, Pearson & Fowler 1963). The former authors suggested that the posture induced by the contractures was characteristically different in the myopathic disorders, with flexion of the hips and knees and adduction of the legs, as well as kyphoscoliosis, chest deformity and torticollis. It is unlikely that these criteria are reliable for clinical diagnosis. The 'dystrophic' nature of the muscle pathology in myopathic AMC has been questioned by many authors, notably by Dastur et al (1972) who studied the histological and histochemical features of 26 cases of all types. A primary failure of muscle embryogenesis with secondary fibrosis and disorganisation of muscle architecture seems more likely than a degenerative process in these cases. In the Ullrich type of muscular dystrophy the proximal muscles of both the upper and lower limbs show contractures while the distal joints are hyperextensible (Ch. 15).

Der Kaloustian et al (1972) reported a myopathic form of arthrogryposis in which massive accumulation of glycogen in muscle fibres was found on biopsy.

There is no doubt that both the the EMG and the muscle histology may be difficult to interpret in arthrogryposis, presumably because of the chronicity of the lesion, the associated disuse atrophy and the problems of 'secondary myopathic change in denervated muscle'. Nevertheless, investigation will permit most cases to be assigned to a neurogenic or myopathic category (Bharucha et al 1972, Dastur et al 1972). CT scanning may make a contribution to this assessment (Abbing et al 1985).

Neurogenic AMC may be associated with severe malformation of the brain causing severe retardation, microcephaly and optic atrophy (Fowler 1959, Frischknecht et al 1960) and sometimes with more subtle cerebral atrophy and mild educational subnormality (Ek 1958, Bharucha et al 1972) but most patients, whether of the neurogenic or myopathic type, are intellectually normal (Wynne-Davies & Lloyd-Roberts 1976). Bargeton et al (1961) and Peña et al (1968) described cases of arthrogryposis of autosomal recessive genetic origin, in which the pathology consisted of a peculiar nodular fibrosis of the anterior spinal roots. Congenital familial polyneuropathy may also cause arthrogryposis confined, however, to the lower limbs (Yuill & Lynch 1974). A similar clinical pattern, due probably to anterior horn cell disease, in an extensive family with dominant inheritance was recorded by Fleury & Hageman (1985).

Autosomal recessive inheritance occurs in myopathic AMC (Lebenthal et al 1970). Dominant inheritance was reported in a father and two daughters with relatively mild myopathic features (Daentl et al 1974).

Although the anterior horn cell form of AMC can occur in more than one member of a family (Ek 1958), it has also been reported in only one of pairs of identical twins; hence the genetic position is uncertain, and the condition may well be heterogeneous. In a survey of all the cases of AMC seen in four large centres in Great Britain, Wynne-Davies & Lloyd-Roberts (1976) found none that were familial and concluded that a variety of environmental factors acting in utero were responsible, although these could rarely be identified. Wynne-Davies et al (1981) confirmed these conclusions in a wider study of an epidemic of arthrogryposis which occurred in the 1950s and 1960s in three widely separated parts of the world. They were unable to identify the causative factors involved, but complications early in pregnancy were a frequent concomitant.

Early and vigorous orthopaedic management of the deformities of arthrogryposis is usually successful in correcting them and because the underlying disorder in the great majority of cases is non-progressive the effort is well worth while. The treatment has been reviewed by Friedlander et al (1968) and Lloyd-Roberts & Lettin (1970).

Muscle contractures and spinal deformities later in childhood

Congenital contractures, not amounting to arthrogryposis multiplex, occur in several of the congenital myopathies, notably in central core disease, congenital myotonic dystrophy and fibre-type disproportion, and also in nemaline myopathy, some of the congenital polyneuropathies and in some cases of infantile spinal muscular atrophy (SMA). In SMA fixed contractures at birth suggest a degree of chronicity of the lesion that makes it more likely that the case may fall into the slowly progressive or static type II category rather than into the inevitably progressive type I (Werdnig–Hoffmann disease).

Later in childhood contractures develop especially in the most severe neuromuscular diseases including Duchenne muscular dystrophy and SMA; they may contribute substantially to the child's disability. Regular stretching of the shortened muscles by the parents and the school physiotherapist, while by no means completely successful, makes a major contribution and attention to the sitting posture and sometimes the use of night splints may be valuable. Except at the ankles, where stretching techniques are rarely totally effective, tenotomy is not usually needed when a child has been regularly supervised. The use of tenotomy in the late stages of diseases with a poor prognosis must have a clear purpose, such as improving the child's appearance, posture, or handling, because it will rarely achieve any improvement in function. This is in sharp contrast to its value in arthrogryposis and other congenital contractures with relatively good muscle power. Contractures acquired later, either in the feet or elsewhere, following fractures, immobilisation or neglect, may benefit from the same approach.

Localised contractures in otherwise normal muscles are usually the sequel of earlier intramuscular injections of drugs (Norman et al 1970, Hoefnagel et al 1978).

In some cases of polymyositis in childhood, contractures may develop in a matter of a few days or weeks. Recurrent inflammatory lesions in muscle going on to ossification and contractures are characteristic of fibrodysplasia ossificans progressiva (see Ch. 27).

The management of kyphoscoliosis is discussed in relation to Duchenne muscular dystrophy in Chapter 15. The importance of preventive bracing applies a fortiori to disorders with a potentially better prognosis, such as spinal muscular atrophy and fibre-type disproportion, in which, however, increasing thoracic distortion may pose a major threat to life.

A disorder in which contractures play a major part is the *rigid spine syndrome*, so named by Dubowitz (1973, 1978). Further cases have been described by Goebel et al (1977), Seay et al (1977) and Goto et al (1979). The syndrome has been recorded only in males, although Dubowitz (1978) mentions seeing a female patient. The patients described had noted the cervical contractures by

the age of six or seven years. Some had been normal until that time, others had had earlier muscle weakness and delay in walking. The condition is usually diagnosed late in the second decade, by which time the affected boy has severe contracture of the posterior cervical and paraspinal muscles and slighter elbow and knee contractures. The muscles are generally very thin but only slightly weak. A patient of Professor Sir John Walton's was able to run upstairs but had difficulty in walking down because of severe neck retraction. Neck flexion, however, is very weak and there is no doubt that there is a generalised mild myopathy. Muscle biopsy of the rigid muscles reveals excessive endomysial and perimysial fibrosis, and variation in fibre size. Goebel et al (1977) and Seay et al (1977) found fibre-type disproportion in biceps in their cases. There are no reports of familial cases at present. Somewhat similar contractures and muscle weakness are seen in the Emery–Dreifuss type of muscular dystrophy (see Ch. 15).

Acute muscular weakness in childhood

In the countries which provide immunisation against poliomyelitis it has become a rare event to see a child who has developed severe generalised muscular weakness over a period of hours or a few days.

Poliomyelitis must still be considered, especially in travellers from abroad. ECHO and Coxsackie viruses very occasionally cause an almost indistinguishable illness. The multifocal distribution of the weakness, the relation to a preceding febrile illness and the development of a purely motor deficit over a few days sometimes accompanied by pain and by fasciculation are all characteristic. Poliomyelitis has been reported as an uncommon occurrence in newborn babies (Pugh & Dudgeon 1954, Bates 1955). It seems clear, from the onset of the disease within the first few days of life, that the virus can be transmitted via the placenta. In many cases the mother has had the paralytic form of the disease shortly before or after the birth of the infant. In other cases, infection through faecal contamination from the mother in the birth process or postnatal infection may have taken place. The infant may have little fever and no diarrhoea. The extent of the paralysis is variable, but in many cases has been widespread with a fatal outcome. Focal myocarditis has been a common post-mortem finding in addition to the typical central nervous system changes.

Some patients who later are shown to have chronic spinal muscular atrophy develop symptoms for the first time very suddenly over a few days or even hours in an illness which may resemble poliomyelitis. This often occurs, however, during the course of one of the common childhood fevers or may follow immunisation. Recovery, if any occurs, is very slight after such an episode. Later in the course of the disease, episodes of deterioration are quite often a feature, again with very limited improvement or none at all, so that the disability in these patients tends to deteriorate in a series of steps rather than taking the more continuous downhill course which is seen in the muscular dystrophies and indeed in many other cases of spinal muscular atrophy.

Other causes of rapidly progressive paralysis which must be considered and which are more fully described in other chapters are acute polyneuritis, the periodic paralyses, myasthenia gravis, acute myositis and acute rhabdomyolysis. Botulism causes bulbar weakness, blurred vision and diplopia followed by generalised flaccid paralysis and areflexia. Poisoning with organo-phosphorus compounds, curare or an overdose of an anticholinesterase drug may have to be considered in some cases. In young infants, quite acute weakness and hypotonia may occur in Leigh's disease and the organic acidaemias.

Acute post-infectious polyneuritis (Ch. 24) is uncommon before the age of four years and rare before two years. The presenting symptoms and course of the illness are similar in childhood and adult life. It is not uncommon to be able to diagnose the preceding viral infection serologically and the Epstein–Barr virus is an important one among many causative agents. The disease as it affects children has been reviewed by Peterman et al (1959), Paulson (1970) and Eberle et al (1975).

Acute transient viral myosits (Ch. 17) may cause a rather painful generalised paralysis after a prodromal febrile illness of several days; the serum CK level is 5–50 times normal; recovery occurs in a few days. McKinlay & Mitchell (1976)

described eight patients aged between five and nine years.

Acute weakness may result from fluctuations in serum potassium levels (Ch. 25). Any condition causing considerable hypokalaemia is likely to be associated with muscular weakness, hypotonia and areflexia. Cushing's disease and primary aldosteronism are rare in young children, but gastrointestinal and renal losses of potassium may occur in a number of infantile diseases such as chronic diarrhoea and vomiting, congenital alkalosis of gastrointestinal origin, renal tubular acidosis and galactosaemia, and the hypokalaemia produces muscular weakness, hypotonia and depression of tendon reflexes. The hypokalaemic, hyperkalaemic and normokalaemic forms of periodic paralysis may all be seen in childhood: indeed, the hyperkalaemic form almost always begins in the first decade. In their series of 108 cases, Gamstorp et al (1957) found that 45% had attacks before the age of five years and 90% before the age of 10 years. Their youngest patient was eight months old at the onset. The symptoms last a few minutes at first but become more prolonged in adolescence. The treatment of attacks of hyperkalaemic periodic paralysis with inhaled salbutamol, introduced by Wang & Clausen (1976) has proved useful in children. The hypokalaemic form tends to start later but may do so at as early as three years (Howes et al 1966, Buruma et al 1985). As the attacks continue, a permanent myopathy may develop and this may be seen even in children (Pearson 1964, Dyken et al 1969). The normokalaemic form of periodic paralysis also begins before the age of 10 years (Poskanzer & Kerr 1961) and causes recurrent severe tetraparesis lasting usually for several days or even weeks. A similar clinical pattern of weakness was described by Shy et al (1966) in the 'pleoconial' type of mitochondrial myopathy.

Acute focal muscular weakness of lower motor neurone type may result from birth trauma or other injuries to the brachial plexus or from poliomyelitis. Acute radiculitis or mononeuritis multiplex are two of the many potential neurological complications of the tick-borne *Borrelia* infection known as Lyme disease (Reik et al 1979, Bruhn 1984).

Two other conditions are of special interest in

children. Recurrent attacks of neuralgic amyotrophy (brachial neuritis) occur in some families in which the trait is inherited as an autosomal dominant (Geiger et al 1974, Dunn et al 1978). As in the sporadic adult disease, quite severe local pain precedes acute weakness, usually in certain proximal muscles of the upper limb but sometimes in the forearm. There is profound atrophy; recovery takes many months and may be incomplete. Sometimes there is autonomic involvement. Attacks may occur from the first year of life but do so at long intervals, usually of several years. Rarely there is vocal cord paresis. Several authors have noted hypoteleorism in affected members of the families.

Amyotrophy following asthma ('post-asthmatic pseudo-poliomyelitis') was first described by Hopkins (1974) in a series of 10 cases. Three more were reported by Danta (1975) and Ilett et al (1977). Acute paralysis, preceded in most cases by pain, occurred four to ten days after an acute asthmatic attack. The weakness resolved slowly and very incompletely. In several of Hopkins' patients the leg was affected, a situation which is very rare in neuralgic amyotrophy if, indeed, it ever occurs. In Hopkins' series, CSF pleocytosis was the rule, often with a raised protein level, but in one of the patients of Ilett et al (1977) the CSF was normal. There seemed to be no consistent relationship to any of the drugs given for the asthma, or to any particular virus infection.

Fluctuating and intermittent muscular weakness in childhood

In addition to the periodic paralyses there are several disorders in which muscular weakness varies from time to time.

Repeated episodes of temporary paralysis occur also in mitochondrial myopathy as Shy et al (1966) pointed out over 20 years ago. Recurrent subacute attacks of muscular weakness, especially if they follow physical stress and are associated with nausea or vomiting, should arouse suspicion of carnitine deficiency or mitochondrial myopathy. The discrete episodes of focal neuropathic paralysis in familial brachial neuritis have been mentioned and families have been reported in which recurrent pressure palsies occur against a background of a permanent subclinical generalised peripheral neuropathy. Chronic relapsing polyneuropathy is a sporadic inflammatory disorder in which recurrent episodes of severe demyelinating motor and sensory neuropathy occur and lead to permanent weakness. It is important to recognise this because of the good response to steroids in some cases. The CSF protein is increased. Attacks may start in childhood and the disorder has occurred in early infancy (Pasternak et al 1982). There is an association with certain HLA haplotypes (Thomas 1979).

The fluctuating weakness and fatiguability which occur in myasthenia gravis are rarely mimicked by any other disorder. A degree of fluctuation over a longer time-scale is often seen in the myopathy of carnitine deficiency and has been reported in reducing-body myopathy. A striking sense of fatigue which seems out of proportion to the muscular weakness is a feature of some of the mitochondrial myopathies, but it is not possible to induce true loss of power by repeated muscle contraction in these cases. The degree of weakness in the mitochondrial myopathies may also vary from time to time, but not to a great degree. Rarely one encounters cases of apparent congenital myopathy in which fluctuation in symptoms is a prominent feature and some of these cases may well be unrecognised examples of genetic disorders of neuromuscular transmission (p. 683–85).

Progressive muscular weakness

The rate at which muscular weakness develops and progresses is of vital importance both in diagnosis and prognosis. Table 20.1 gives an indication of the rate of progression of the most important neuromuscular disorders which may be considered in differential diagnosis at various periods of childhood. This approach has its limitations, however, because the rate of progression may vary from case to case, may change during the course of the illness and in any case may be difficult to gauge in the early stages.

Other valuable clues to diagnosis include the degree of muscle atrophy in relation to the weakness, the broad pattern of distribution of the weakness (whether proximal, distal or generalised), whether the weakness within this broad

Table 20.1 Progressive muscular weakness

Apparent rate of progression at time of presentation	Onset			
	First 6 months	First 2 years	2–10 years	Adolescence
Progressive over hours or days	Myasthenia Werdnig–Hoffmann disease Spinal tumour Metabolic acidoses Cytochrome oxidase deficiency Carnitine deficiency (Chronic SMA) (Poliomyelitis) (Rhabdomyolysis) (Botulism)	Poliomyelitis Myasthenia gravis Chronic SMA Hyperkalaemic P.P. Rhabdomyolysis (Guillain–Barré) Organicacidaemia Leigh's disease	Poliomyelitis Guillain–Barré syndrome Hyperkalaemic P.P. Hypokalaemic P.P. Myasthenia gravis Rhabdomyolysis Acute myositis (Pleoconial myopathy)	Poliomyelitis Guillain–Barré syndrome All 3 periodic paralyses Myasthenia gravis Acute myositis
Weeks or months	Werdnig–Hoffmann disease Pompe's disease Congenital MD Mitochondrial myopathy Nemaline myopathy Centronuclear myopathy Leigh's disease Congenital polyneuropathy Metabolic myopathies	Chronic SMA Dermatomyositis Myasthenia Carnitine deficiency Metachromatic leucodystrophy Leigh's disease Metabolic myopathies	Dermatomyositis Chronic SMA Kearns–Sayre syndrome Carnitine deficiency Myasthenia gravis Metabolic myopathies (Refsum's disease)	Myasthenia Polymyositis Carnitine deficiency Metabolic myopathies (MLD neuropathy) (Dermatomyositis) (Refsum's disease)
Years	Chronic SMA Nemaline myopathy Centronuclear myopathy Rarely FSH MD Mitochondrial myopathy HMSN type III Hypothyroidism	Duchenne MD Autosomal recessive MD Rarely polymyositis Chronic SMA Glycogen storage disease Kearns–Sayre syndrome Carnitine deficiency Other mitochondrial myopathies Myasthenic myopathies Distal MD & SMA Fukuyama MD Centronuclear myopathy	Duchenne MD Becker MD Emery–Dreifuss MD Autosomal recessive MD Chronic SMA Scapuloperoneal SMA Kearns–Sayre syndrome Glycogen storage disease Carnitine deficiency Mitochondrial myopathies HMSN I and II (Polymyositis)	Becker MD Emery–Dreifuss MD FSH MD Chronic SMA Glycogen storage disease Carnitine deficiency HMSN I and II Myotonic MD
Static or progressive over decades	Chronic SMA Central core disease Minicore disease Fibre-type disproportion Congenital myotonic MD Duchenne MD Congenital MD Fingerprint myopathy	Duchenne MD Autosomal recessive MD Fingerprint myopathy Central core disease	Duchenne MD Autosomal recessive MD Myotonic MD Becker MD Emery–Dreifuss MD (Central core disease)	Becker MD Myotonic MD FSH MD Manifesting female DMD cariers

pattern is highly selective for particular muscles or not, whether the face and other cranial muscles are involved, the presence or absence of fasciculation, fatiguability, reflex changes or symptoms and signs of involvement of other tissues, the degree of abnormality in serum CK activity and in other enzymes, and the findings in the EMG and muscle biopsy. Many of these points are discussed in Chapter 14, and here we confine discussion of the progressive disorders to a few comments upon some of the most important conditions.

Duchenne muscular dystrophy. The diagnosis is easy to confirm (Ch. 15). The problem is to remember to consider it when a child presents with the early symptoms. It is not uncommonly overlooked until after another affected child has been born in the family. The earliest sign in most cases is delay in walking (50% walk only after the age of 18 months). General psychomotor delay is quite frequent and speech may be immature. At first the gait disturbance is easier to recognise when the patient tries to run or to climb stairs. From an early age, boys with this condition are unable to jump with both feet together and they roll on to their faces before standing up from the floor. The full 'Gowers' manoeuvre' of climbing up the legs is not apparent until the age of four to six years. A few are hypotonic during the first few months of life. Unexplained developmental delay in any young boy warrants an estimation of his serum CK activity. Although the very high serum CK levels, present from birth, indicate that active destruction of muscle occurs from the beginning, clinical evidence of progression may not be apparent until the age of four to seven years.

Spinal muscular atrophy (SMA). After Duchenne muscular dystrophy, SMA is by far the commonest neuromuscular disorder in childhood. The nosology of the spinal muscular atrophies is complex. They vary greatly in age at onset, rate of progression and distribution of weakness, and attempts to classify them on these grounds have often proved to be genetically invalid (see Ch. 23, 26), while purely genetic classifications lead to a state of apparent clinical confusion. The following list of apparent genetic entities, modified from Pearn (1980), in no sense comprises a nosological classification because the criteria for inclusion in the categories are so mixed, but it does provide a basis for a brief discussion of the diagnosis and management in childhood. More detail will be found in Chapter 23.

Autosomal recessive
(1) Progressive infantile spinal muscular atrophy ('Acute Werdnig–Hoffmann disease')
(2) Chronic childhood SMA (proximal or generalised) including the phenotypes 'Arrested Werdnig–Hoffmann disease', 'Intermediate SMA' 'Kugelberg–Welander syndrome'
(3) Infantile SMA with initial diaphragmatic paralysis
(4) Infantile SMA with cerebellar hypoplasia
(5) Adult-onset SMA (proximal)
(6) Distal SMA (infantile onset)
(7) Facioscapulohumeral SMA
(8) Bulbar SMA (Fazio-Londe disease)
(9) SMA in hexosaminidase deficiency

Autosomal dominant
(10) Autosomal dominant scapuloperoneal SMA
(11) Distal SMA (juvenile onset)
(12) Other autosomal dominant SMAs (adult onset)

X-linked
(13) X-linked scapuloperoneal SMA
(14) X-linked bulbar/distal SMA
(15) ? SMA with calf hypertrophy and high serum CK activity (a doubtful entity)

Most cases fall into one of the first two categories. Progressive infantile SMA may present at any time in the first five months of life and is best distinguished from the chronic cases, not by the age at onset which may be evident from diminished fetal movement as early as the thirty-fifth week of gestation in both acute and chronic cases, but by its relentlessly progressive course. It is therefore prudent to wait for clear evidence of deterioration before offering a firm prognosis when the clinical picture of severe paralytic hypotonia, areflexia and fasciculation of the tongue makes the diagnosis of infantile SMA obvious.

Muscle biopsy appears not to be of help in distinguishing progressive from non-progressive cases. Other conditions which may present a very similar clinical picture are congenital peripheral neuropathy of the type reported by Lyon (1969), described below, and perhaps infantile botulism.

Two other distinct genetic forms of acute infantile spinal muscular atrophy have been described. In one the infants present with diaphragmatic paralysis within the first few months of life, and may only later develop limb paralysis (Mellins et al 1974, McWilliam et al 1985, Murphy et al 1985, Schapira & Swash 1985). This situation contrasts with the usual relative preservation of the phrenic motor neurones in Werdnig–Hoffmann disease (Kuzuhara & Chou 1981). In the other distinct form, neuropathological examination reveals hypoplasia of the cerebellum and ventral pons, and sometimes of the thalamus, as well as anterior horn cell degeneration. Some cases have more widespread degenerative change in grey and white matter. During life, both the motor and sensory nerve conduction velocities are very slow. Such children are usually already severely hypotonic at birth and may be less socially responsive than children with typical Werdnig–Hoffmann disease (Norman 1961, Weinberg & Kirkpatrick 1975, Goutières et al 1977, Steiman et al 1980, de Leon et al 1984).

The discovery of apparent vitamin E deficiency in Werdnig–Hoffmann disease has, unfortunately, not been shown to have any aetiological or therapeutic relevance (Shapira et al 1981).

The term *chronic childhood SMA* embraces cases of Kugelberg–Welander syndrome (type III SMA) and of the intermediate or type II variety (Emery 1971). It covers a wide range of cases in which the onset may be as early as fetal life or as late at least as the end of the first decade, and in which the severity may vary equally widely. The fact that such variation may occur within a single family suggests that only one genetic entity is involved but undoubtedly the severely affected infant who never learns to sit unsupported and who survives in a helpless condition with major contractures and spinal deformity for anything from a few months to three or more decades presents a very different problem in clinical management from the previously normal five-year-old who begins to develop a waddling gait. It is also characteristic of chronic SMA that it may progress irregularly, intermittently or not at all, and it is therefore exceptionally difficult to give an accurate prognosis in an individual case, even after a considerable period of observation. A few cases present with the sudden development of weakness over a matter of hours or days, usually in association with an infection or immunisation, and with subsequently a relatively static or chronic course. The Kugelberg–Welander syndrome resembles the muscular dystrophies (and very few other neuromuscular disorders) in causing strikingly selective muscular weakness. It differs in causing no recognisable pattern of selection and in often being asymmetrical. Fasciculation, so helpful in diagnosis when present, may be absent or inconspicuous in as many as 50% of cases. The feet tend to evert rather than adopting the equinovarus position seen in Duchenne muscular dystrophy. The serum CK may be normal or considerably elevated and even the EMG, so valuable in co-operative adult patients, may be confusing or quite often even normal in children if they are unable to maintain a strong volitional contraction of the needled muscle. It is therefore particularly important to select an appropriate and moderately severely affected muscle for biopsy in trying to reach a definitive diagnosis. It is difficult to assess the power of individual muscles in an unco-operative or obese child; careful palpation of the degree of atrophy will often be helpful in diagnosis and in choosing a muscle for biopsy. When the choice is difficult, visualising the muscles by ultrasound or even CT scanning may be helpful.

Investigation of the cause of SMA is almost always disappointing. Recently a few cases of juvenile SMA (onset five to 16 years) have been found to have hexosaminidase A deficiency. Some of them, but not all, had additional features such as dysarthria, ataxia, pyramidal signs, mild dementia or episodic psychosis (Johnson et al 1982, Mitsumoto et al 1985, Parnes et al 1985).

A number of restricted non-progressive forms of congenital anterior horn cell disease exist, probably not of genetic origin and probably akin to neurogenic arthrogryposis multiplex (q.v.). Often only the lower limbs are affected, but cases in which amyotrophy is confined to the upper limbs are also described (Darwish et al 1981). Segmental upper limb *progressive* amyotrophy of the type seen in young adults, especially in the Far East, may also occur in children (Sobue et al 1978, Tan 1985).

Rapidly fatal forms of juvenile anterior horn cell disease include the bulbar (Fazio–Londe) type (q.v.) and juvenile motor neurone disease (Nelson & Prensky 1972), both mercifully rare.

The principles of management of spinal muscular atrophy follow in many respects those laid down for Duchenne muscular dystrophy in Chapters 15, 21 and 22. Active orthopaedic measures to deal with contractures and spinal deformity are, however, even more important because of the possibility of prolonged arrest of progression of the disease and because thoracic distortion due to kyphoscoliosis presents one of the major hazards to life by contributing to respiratory insufficiency. Rigid spinal braces applied to very late and advanced cases of spinal curvature may actually make the respiratory function worse (Noble-Jamieson et al 1986). Active spinal bracing as soon as a hypotonic child begins to sit up is therefore usually the best policy, but spinal fusion during adolescence is often necessary. It must be expertly performed after very careful assessment of respiratory function (Aprin et al 1982, Riddick et al 1982). Active and intensive postoperative care, including active exercise of limb muscles, is a vital component of this type of management. The provision of lightweight walking calipers is useful in some cases and is worth trying in very young children (from two years of age) if they have strong enough trunk muscles.

Other progressive myopathies. The other important conditions to consider in a progressive muscular disorder in childhood include dermatomyositis or, much less commonly, pure polymyositis (see Ch. 17), muscle carnitine deficiency, glycogen storage disease (especially the juvenile forms of acid maltase deficiency and debrancher enzyme deficiency), mitochondrial myopathy, nemaline myopathy, centronuclear myopathy, the Becker, autosomal recessive and facioscapulohumeral types of muscular dystrophy, myotonic dystrophy and the myopathies associated with renal failure, metabolic bone disease, malabsorp-

tion, chronic cholestasis, hypothyroidism, Cushing's syndrome (and steroid therapy), and the various peripheral neuropathies. Some of the myopathies may mimic muscular dystrophy, especially dermatomyositis, muscle carnitine deficiency, acid maltase and debrancher enzyme deficiency and sometimes the myopathy of metabolic bone disease — a point of great importance because several of these disorders are potentially treatable. The myopathy associated with vitamin E deficiency in chronic cholestasis is also treatable with high doses of the vitamin (Guggenheim et al 1982). Vitamin E deficiency is seen also as a consequence of the malabsorption in a-β-lipoproteinaemia, and was reported by Burck et al (1981) in a child with an autosomal recessive neuromyopathy and ataxia. Further discussion of these important disorders of childhood will be found elsewhere in this volume.

Skeletal myopathy and cardiomyopathy. Cardiomyopathy is a constant feature of Pompe's disease and a frequent one of certain types of lipid storage myopathy and particularly of systemic carnitine deficiency in childhood (see ch. 25). Other rare metabolic myopathies with cardiac involvement in childhood include β-galactosidase deficiency (Kohlschutter et al 1982) and a polysaccharide storage disease described by Karpati et al (1969). Heart block is a frequent component of the Kearns–Sayre syndrome, and may be seen in various other mitochondrial myopathies in childhood. It is a rare feature in children with myotonic dystrophy. Cardiac involvement is an important but usually a late feature in Duchenne, Becker and especially Emery–Dreifuss muscular dystrophy (q.v. Ch. 15), and has been described as a late feature in nemaline myopathy (page 675) and centronuclear myopathy (Verhiest et al 1976). All of these possibilities must be considered when a child presents with combined skeletal and cardiac myopathy.

However, it is not unusual to encounter children with this combination of features in whom no satisfactory diagnosis emerges on investigation — or even at post-mortem examination — for such children usually have only moderate skeletal muscle weakness while their cardiomyopathy may progress relentlessly. Only a few such cases appear in the literature (e.g. Fried et al 1979, Dubowitz 1985 p. 632–633) but the author has seen four cases, all with a fatal outcome. The muscles are strikingly hypotonic, muscle biopsy has revealed type II fibre atrophy or no significant abnormality and the cardiac pathology has been a cardiomyopathy with or without associated endocardial fibroelastosis. A boy aged 18 years (case 11) reported by Shafiq et al (1972), who had cardiomyopathy and mild myopathy with type I fibre atrophy, in retrospect seems to have had the clinical features of Emery–Dreifuss muscular dystrophy. Lenard & Goebel (1980) did muscle biopsies in 10 children with cardiomyopathy but with clinically normal skeletal muscle and found type II fibre atrophy in four of them.

Myopathy and bone disorders. A number of genetically determined bone dysplasias may cause a pseudomyopathic waddling gait because of involvement of the hips or spine. In at least one condition, however, progressive diaphyseal dysplasia (Camurato–Engelmann disease), striking muscular atrophy and weakness appears to be an integral feature of the pathology (Sparkes & Graham 1972, Naveh et al 1985) and muscle pain and fatigue are prominent symptoms. X-rays show thickening and hyperostosis of the diaphyses of the long bones; growth is not affected.

In childhood, as in adult life, chronic osteomalacia in nutritional or renal disorders may be associated with a reversible myopathy. Coeliac disease has been described as presenting with a dystrophy-like progressive myopathy (Hardoff et al 1980).

Both bone and muscle may be involved in thalassaemia major. Logothetis et al (1972) found myopathic features in one-fifth of their 138 cases and muscle atrophy in one-third. Those with myopathy tended to be of shorter stature with more bone complications than those without.

Facial, bulbar and external ocular muscle weakness in infancy

Traumatic unilateral *facial weakness* is not uncommon in the newborn and usually disappears in a few days or weeks. Persistent congenital paralysis is much rarer, and may reflect nuclear agenesis.

Bell's palsy occurs in young children and may be associated with acute viral infections or occasionally with arterial hypertension. Recurrent attacks, especially if bilateral, raise the possibility of Melkersson's syndrome or very rarely sarcoidosis (Jasper & Denny 1968). The silent development of facial weakness, first on one side and then on the other, occurs especially in meningeal leukaemia or pontine glioma. Subacute progression of facial and other cranial nerve palsies may occur in the tick-borne infection Lyme disease, which responds to treatment with penicillin.

Bilateral facial weakness in the newborn may result from bilateral nuclear agenesis (Moebius syndrome) when it is usually accompanied by bilateral lateral rectus palsies and sometimes by bulbar paresis and mild amyotrophy of the limbs. A few patients are also mentally handicapped. A rare association of Moebius syndrome with the Poland anomaly (unilateral absence of the pectoralis major muscle) has also been established (Parker et al 1981). In an apparently distinct disorder the features of Moebius syndrome are associated with hypogonadotrophic hypogonadism and a late-onset progressive neuropathy (Abid et al 1978).

Several of the congenital myopathies may produce prominent facial weakness, especially centronuclear myopathy, nemaline myopathy, minicore disease and less often mitochondrial myopathy, carnitine deficiency, central core disease and fibre-type disproportion. Myasthenia gravis must be ruled out. Congenital myotonic dystrophy causes very prominent facial diplegia with a triangular open mouth together with hypotonia and feeding difficulties, and an infantile form of facioscapulohumeral dystrophy exists in which difficulty in closing the mouth to suck or inability to smile or to close the eyes may be a first symptom. In both of these diseases, examination of the parents gives the essential clue to the diagnosis. Infantile SMA (Werdnig–Hoffmann disease) may affect the face, but rarely profoundly. In Fazio–Londe disease (Gomez et al 1962) progressive bulbar paralysis may be accompanied by facial weakness and eventually by paralysis of all the cranial muscles, including those of the eyes. Some cases, but not all, also have signs of limb muscle weakness. Cranial polyneuritis, meningeal lymphoma or leukaemia and pontine glioma must be excluded before this rare disease can justifiably be diagnosed.

Apart from rare congenital or post-infectious lesions, isolated paralyses affecting the *Xth and XIIth cranial nerves* are uncommon. A unilateral XIIth nerve lesion may be seen in the Arnold–Chiari malformation. Bulbar paralysis may occur in meningeal and medullary neoplasm. Bulbar paralysis in the neonate, in association with more generalised hypotonia or paralysis, suggests myasthenia, Werdnig–Hoffmann disease or congenital myotonic dystrophy, but may also occur in nemaline and centronuclear myopathy, in fibre-type disproportion and in the Prader–Willi syndrome. Later in childhood, bulbar paralysis as an important feature of a generalised muscular problem should bring to mind myasthenia, botulism or the Guillain–Barré syndrome or, if the pace is slower, dermatomyositis, myotonic dystrophy, nemaline myopathy or centronuclear myopathy.

External ocular palsies are not uncommon in the newborn period, and must be distinguished from the Duane syndrome and from more extensive external ophthalmoplegia. The congenital neuromuscular disorders most often associated with ophthalmoplegia are myasthenia, centronuclear myopathy and the Moebius syndrome; but it may occur in minicore disease. The later development of ophthalmoplegia may be seen in the same disorders but is also a major feature of the Kearns–Sayre syndrome and very occasionally of other variants of mitochondrial myopathy and of Fazio–Londe disease. None of these should be diagnosed until the possibility of a brain stem lesion or of myasthenia gravis has been considered.

Peripheral motor neuropathy in childhood

The distinction between a predominantly motor neuropathy in a child and the very similar distal form of SMA and, even rarer, the distal type of muscular dystrophy, can really be made only on the basis of electro-physiological and histological investigations. Some cases of mitochondrial myopathy also present with distal weakness and, in the facioscapulohumeral and scapuloperoneal syndromes, the distal lower limb involvement may be sufficiently predominant in the early stages to cause confusion.

No attempt is made here to cover all the peripheral neuropathies of childhood and a systematic account will be found in Chapter 24. Nutritional deficiencies and diphtheria are now rare diseases in developed countries and so is acrodynia (Pink disease), since the elimination of mercury from teething powders. Lead poisoning causes an encephalopathy rather than a polyneuropathy in childhood. Certain insecticides and drugs may produce peripheral neuropathy (Watters & Barlow 1967). This problem is mostly encountered during the treatment of children with malignant tumours with cytotoxic drugs, especially vincristine or cisplatin. Otherwise in clinical practice the Guillain–Barré syndrome and Charcot–Marie–Tooth disease (hereditary motor and sensory neuropathy type I — HMSN I) are seen far more frequently than other types. The former has been mentioned above in relation to acute muscular weakness.

HMSN I. 'Peroneal muscular atrophy' often begins in childhood and in some cases as early as the first year of life. The foot deformity usually causes more disability than the weakness itself at first, and responds well to orthopaedic treatment. Weakness of the hands may become a serious problem during the school years. Diagnosis is straightforward on the basis of profound slowing of nerve conduction. It is a common experience to find subclinical involvement in one of the parents and it is important to seek this by clinical and, if necessary, neurophysiological examination for genetic counselling purposes.

HMSN II. The axonal form of 'peroneal muscular atrophy' is also seen in childhood but much less frequently. Both sporadic cases (possibly recessive) and, more often, families with dominant inheritance occur. The onset is usually a little later than in HMSN I, but the clinical problems are similar.

HMSN III. Dejerine–Sottas disease is a rare

but very disabling disorder, usually producing symptoms in the first two years of life, rarely later. Hypertrophic nerves (also seen in HMSN I), a high CSF protein, and early and severe weakness and deformity are the helpful diagnostic features. Scoliosis is common.

Giant axonal neuropathy. Cases of this rare disorder were first described by Asbury et al (1972) and Carpenter et al (1974). A progressive peripheral motor and sensory neuropathy of axonal type begins at the age of two to three years and progresses to become severe within a few years. Both children in the above reports were intelligent and like all subsequently reported cases they had abnormal tightly curled hair which is often blond. Later case reports have mentioned various additional features including ataxia, learning disorders and sexual precocity, and in some cases the neuropathy has taken a much slower course (Ionasescu et al 1983). Nerve biopsy shows remarkable segmental enlargement of axons, distended with neurofilaments. Abnormal cytoplasmic filaments may possibly also be found in other intraneural cells including fibroblasts and endothelial cells. Affected sibs have been recorded (Takebe et al 1981).

Congenital peripheral neuropathies. Charcot–Marie–Tooth disease (HMSN I) may present at birth in rare instances (Vanasse & Dubowitz 1979). One type of congenital peripheral neuropathy resembles Werdnig–Hoffmann disease in presenting with severe hypotonia and areflexia in early infancy, but with profound slowing of nerve conduction, a raised CSF protein level (usually) and, in the peripheral nerve, virtually total absence of myelin sheaths and hypertrophic reduplication of the basement membrane (Lyon 1969, Anderson et al 1973, Kasman & Bernstein 1974, Karch & Urich 1975, Goebel et al 1976, Kennedy et al 1977, and others reviewed by Harati & Butler 1985). Both parents of one child had slight slowing of nerve conduction (Kennedy et al 1977). Joosten et al (1974) described two sibs aged 12 and 14 years in whom the symptoms had started in the second or third year of life and had progressed much more in one than the other, but whose nerve pathology was

similar to that in the Lyon type. This disorder may be fatal in infancy but most of the cases described have survived at least into their second decade.

A much milder form of congenital peripheral neuropathy was described by Yuill & Lynch (1974) and was inherited as a dominant trait, but there was no information about histology and in only one case were nerve conduction studies performed.

Other genetically determined peripheral neuropathies seen in childhood include Refsum disease, porphyria, and several others in which the clinical features of the neuropathy are largely sensory rather than motor (including Friedreich's ataxia, Fabry disease, Tangier disease, a-β-lipoproteinaemia and the various disorders classified as hereditary sensory neuropathies). A clinically overt peripheral neuropathy may also occur in some of the progressive degenerative disorders of the central nervous system, particularly in metachromatic leucodystrophy, infantile neuroaxonal dystrophy and the Cockayne syndrome, while a subclinical neuropathy, of no significance to the patient but helpful in diagnosis, may be found by nerve conduction studies in Krabbe (globoid cell) leucodystrophy (Moosa 1971) and in Canavan disease.

In the typical infantile form of metachromatic leucodystrophy, deterioration of gait and speech begin at about the age of one year and progress over several months to a state of severe retardation with a spastic tetraparesis, optic atrophy and severe distal muscle wasting. The tendon reflexes are diminished soon after the onset. In some cases the disorder presents later, usually with cerebral symptoms but occasionally with a pure progressive demyelinating peripheral neuropathy (Yudell et al 1967). In all forms of the disease the CSF protein level is raised, metachromatic staining may be seen in the nerve biopsy and the underlying deficiency or abnormality of the enzyme aryl-sulphatase A may be demonstrated in white blood cells.

In infantile neuroaxonal dystrophy, progressive mental retardation and optic atrophy in the first year of life are sometimes associated with severe hypotonia and muscle paralysis resembling that of

SMA (Huttenlocher & Gilles 1967). The diagnosis is difficult without a brain biopsy but can be achieved in at least some cases by the biopsy of peripheral nerve or even by examination of the nerve twigs in a conjunctival biopsy (Arsenio-Nunes & Goutières 1978).

In Cockayne dwarfism, progressive growth failure and dementia starting in the first five years of life are associated with a characteristic light-sensitive rash, deep-set eyes and a peripheral neuropathy (Moosa & Dubowitz 1970). Other features are intracranial calcification and a mild retinal pigmentary degeneration.

Cramps and abnormal muscle contraction

Cramp, although less frequent in childhood than in later life, is no better understood. Limb pains are a common stress symptom in children. Muscle rigidity and weakness in the newborn are an uncommon but long-established manifestation of congenital hypothyroidism (the Debré–Semelaigne syndrome) and acquired hypothyroidism later in childhood may also present with painful muscle cramps after exercise.

Of the overt muscle disorders, patients with the myotonic and, for some reason, the Becker type of muscular dystrophy are chiefly plagued by cramps. Stiffness on exertion, sometimes amounting to cramp, is a feature of the early stages of McArdle disease, phosphofructokinase deficiency, carnitine palmityl transferase deficiency and certain disorders of the cytochrome system. In persistent cases of exertional or post-exertional cramp it is therefore appropriate to do an ischaemic lactate test and to measure the serum CK activity after exercise performed during a fast (see Ch. 13). The urine should also be examined for myoglobin. Similar symptoms, starting in childhood, may occur in muscle adenylate deaminase deficiency (Fishbein et al 1978, Kelemen et al 1982). The serum CK activity is often increased during attacks of pain. Painless stiffness of the muscles after exertion may also occur in a variant of central core disease (Bethlem et al 1966) and in a myopathy with subsarcolemmal tubular aggregates (Lazaro et al 1980). Brody (1969) described a single case in which muscle contracture induced by exercise appeared to result from a defect in

muscle relaxing factor. This condition is now thought to be due to calcium ATPase deficiency.

Dystonia and tetany must be considered as possible causes of persistent cramping of muscle during activity. Rigidity, equal in degree to that seen in tetanus, has already been mentioned as one of the presentations of reducing-body myopathy (Dudley et al 1978) and of a myopathy with trilaminar fibres (Ringel et al 1978).

The myotonic disorders occurring in childhood are discussed in Chapter 16.

Myokymia with impaired muscular relaxation (also called 'neuromyotonia' and 'continuous muscle fibre activity') is a slowly progressive disorder, which usually begins between the ages of 15 and 25 years but may do so earlier, even in infancy, and gives rise to muscular stiffness and cramps (Isaacs 1961, Gardner-Medwin & Walton 1969). The distal muscles of the feet and hands are mainly affected, but disabling laryngeal spasm occurs in some cases; there may be associated hyperhidrosis. Claw-like deformities of the feet are common and close inspection of the muscles, especially the small hand muscles, reveals irregular undulating contractions which have been likened to a 'bag of worms'. Distal muscle atrophy is usual but secondary muscle hypertrophy may occur if the myokymia is very active. The EMG shows continuous motor unit activity at rest and the activity can be blocked by curare but not by peripheral nerve blockade. Some cases show evidence of a mild peripheral neuropathy; it is not certain whether this is a secondary phenomenon. Almost all cases are sporadic but dominant inheritance has been described (McGuire et al 1984). The condition responds to treatment with carbamazepine or, less certainly, phenytoin. Similar activity occurs in chondrodystrophic myotonia (see Ch. 16).

Myoglobinuria in childhood

Children, like adults, may develop myoglobinuria as a result of crush injury or intoxication (see Ch. 13, 25).

Paroxysmal myoglobinuria occurring after exertion is a rare phenomenon in childhood. McArdle's disease, although causing stiffness on exertion in some cases during the first decade of life (Williams & Hosking 1985), does not cause myoglobinuria at such an early stage, but phosphofructokinase deficiency may do so. Several of the reported cases of carnitine palmityl transferase deficiency have first developed the typical post-exertional cramps and myoglobinuria during childhood. A few cases occur in which these clinical symptoms in childhood are associated with no detectable evidence of glycogen- or lipid-storage myopathy and, no doubt, other comparable metabolic disorders remain to be discovered.

Paroxysmal myoglobinuria occurring without exertion is a much more devastating illness because it results from acute necrosis of muscle (rhabdomyolysis). It tends to follow viral infection in childhood and may occur as early as the first few months of life. Acute muscle weakness and respiratory failure may be complicated by renal failure and may be fatal. Coxsackie virus infections seem to be one of the important precipitants and in some cases evidence may be found of a direct fulminating viral myositis (Fukuyama et al 1977). In other cases, attacks may be precipitated by cold (Raifman et al 1978). Recurrent attacks may affect several sibs in a family (Favara et al 1967, Savage et al 1971). Intensive respiratory care and often renal dialysis are vital in the treatment of this dangerous disorder.

Malignant hyperpyrexia, like acute rhabdo-myolysis, may cause sufficient myoglobinuria to induce uraemia in those patients who survive the initial emergency.

Rarely, recurrent myoglobinuria may accompany a progressive myopathy comparable to muscular dystrophy. Meyer–Betz (1910) described this situation in a boy of 13 years and Dubowitz (1978, p. 48) illustrates the case of a boy of seven years with cramps and myoglobinuria associated with a chronic 'dystrophic' myopathy.

Malignant hyperpyrexia. The incidence in children is high, one in 15 000 anaesthetics administered. Apart from the usual dominantly inherited syndrome of susceptibility, an association has been suggested with several conditions in childhood including central core disease (q.v.), Duchenne muscular dystrophy (q.v.), myotonia congenita, a family history of the sudden infant death syndrome (Denborough et al 1982) and a syndrome occurring in males of ptosis, low-set ears, hypoplasia of the mandible, thoracic kyphosis, short stature and cryptorchidism (King et al 1972). The associations with all of these except the first and the last are weak and such patients should not be denied anaesthesia; it is prudent, however, to avoid the use of halothane or suxamethonium.

REFERENCES

Abbing P J R, Hageman G, Willemse J 1985 CT-scanning of skeletal muscle in arthrogryposis multiplex congenita. Brain and Development 7: 484–491

Abid F, Hall R, Hudgson P, Weiser R 1978 Moebius syndrome, peripheral neuropathy and hypogonadotrophic hypogonadism. Journal of the Neurological Sciences 35: 309–315

Adams R D, Kakulas B A, Samaha F A 1965 A myopathy with cellular inclusions. Transactions of the American Neurological Association 90: 213–216

Afifi A K, Smith J W, Zellweger H 1965 Congenital non-progressive myopathy: Central core disease and nemaline myopathy in one family. Neurology (Minneapolis) 15:371

Anderson R M, Dennett X, Hopkins I J, Shield L K 1973 Hypertrophic interstitial polyneuropathy in infancy: Clinical and pathologic features in two cases. Journal of Pediatrics 82: 619–624

Aprin H, Bowen J R, MacEwen G D, Hall J E 1982 Spine fusion in patients with spinal muscular atrophy. Journal of Bone and Joint Surgery 64A: 1179–1187

Argov Z, Gardner-Medwin D, Johnson M A, Mastaglia F L 1984 Patterns of muscle fiber-type disproportion in hypotonic infants. Archives of Neurology 41: 53–57

Armstrong R M, Koenigsberger R, Mellinger J, Lovelace R E 1971 Central core disease with congenital hip dislocation: study of two familes. Neurology (Minneapolis) 21: 369–376

Arsenio-Nunes M L, Goutières F 1978 Diagnosis of infantile neuroaxonal dystrophy by conjunctival biopsy. Journal of Neurology, Neurosurgery and Psychiatry 41: 511–515

Arts W F, Bethlem J, Dingemans K P, Eriksson A W 1978 Investigations on the inheritance of nemaline myopathy. Archives of Neurology 35: 72–77

Asbury A K, Gale M K, Cox S C, Baringer J R, Berg B O 1972 Giant axonal neuropathy — A unique case with segmental neurofilamentous masses. Acta Neuropathologica (Berlin) 20: 237–247

Askanas V, Engel W K, Reddy N B, et al 1979 X-linked recessive congenital muscle fiber hypotrophy with central nuclei: abnormalities of growth and adenylate cyclase in muscle tissue cultures. Archives of Neurology 36: 604–609

Aubourg P, Scotto J, Rocchiccioli F, Feldmann-Pautrat D,

Robain O 1986 Neonatal adrenoleukodystrophy. Journal of Neurology, Neurosurgery and Psychiatry 49: 77–86

Banker B Q, Victor M, Adams R D 1957 Arthrogryposis multiplex due to congenital muscular dystrophy. Brain 80: 319–334

Bargeton E, Nezelof C, Guran P, Job J-C 1961 Étude anatomique d'un cas d'arthrogrypose multiple congénitale et familiale. Revue Neurologique 104: 479–489

Barnes N D, Hull D, Balgobin L, Gompertz D 1970 Biotin-responsive propionicacidaemia. Lancet 2: 244–245

Barth P G, van Wijngaarden G K, Bethlem J 1975 X-linked myotubular myopathy with fatal neonatal asphyxia. Neurology (Minneapolis) 25: 531–536

Bates T 1955 Poliomyelitis in pregnancy, fetus and newborn. American Journal of Diseases of Children 90:189

Bazelon M, Paine R S, Cowie V A, Hunt P, Houck J C, Mahanand D 1967 Reversal of hypotonia in infants with Down's syndrome by administration of 5-hydroxytryptophan. Lancet 1:1130

Beckerman R C, Buchino J J 1978 Arthrogryposis multiplex congenita as part of an inherited symptom complex: two case reports and a review of the literature. Pediatrics 61: 417–422

Bender A N, Bender M B 1977 Muscle fiber hypotrophy with intact neuromuscular junctions: A study of a patient with congenital neuromuscular disease and ophthalmoplegia. Neurology (Minneapolis) 27: 206–212

Besser M, Behar A 1967 Arthrogryposis accompanying congenital spinal-type muscular atrophy. Archives of Disease in Childhood 42:666

Bethlem J, van Gool J, Hulsmann W C, Meijer A E F H 1966 Familial non-progressive myopathy with muscle cramps after exercise. A new disease associated with cores in the muscle fibres. Brain 89:569

Bethlem J, Meijer A E F H, Schellens J P M, Vroom J J 1968 Centronuclear myopathy. European Neurology 1:325

Bethlem J, van Wijngaarden G K, Meijer A E F H, Hulsmann W C 1969 Neuromuscular disease with type 1 fiber atrophy, central nuclei, and myotube-like structures. Neurology (Minneapolis) 19:705

Bethlem J, van Wijngaarden G K, Mumenthaler M, Meijer A E F H 1970 Centronuclear myopathy with Type 1 fiber atrophy and 'myotubes'. Archives of Neurology 23: 70–73

Bethlem J, van Wijngaarden G K 1976 Benign myopathy, with autosomal dominant inheritance: A report on three pedigrees. Brain 99: 91–100

Bharucha E P, Pandya S S, Dastur D K 1972 Arthrogryposis multiplex congenita. Journal of Neurology, Neurosurgery and Psychiatry 35: 425–434

Bill P L A, Cole G, Proctor N S F 1979 Centronuclear myopathy. Journal of Neurology, Neurosurgery and Psychiatry 42: 548–556

Bjerre I, Hallberg A 1983 Myasthenia gravis: immunological studies in a young child treated with thymectomy and immunosuppressive drugs. Neuropediatrics 14: 106–109

Blass J P, Kark R A P, Engel W K 1971 Clinical studies of a patient with pyruvate decarboxylase deficiency. Archives of Neurology 25: 449–460

Bogousslavsky J, Perentes E, Deruaz J P, Regli F 1982 Mitochondrial myopathy and cardiomyopathy with neurodegenerative features and multiple brain infarcts. Journal of the Neurological Sciences 55: 351–357

Bonnette H, Roelofs R, Olson W H 1974 Multicore disease: report of a case with onset in middle age. Neurology (Minneapolis) 24: 1039–1044

Bradley W G, Price D L, Watanabe C K 1970 Familial centronuclear myopathy. Journal of Neurology, Neurosurgery and Psychiatry 33: 687–693

Bradley W G, Hudson P, Gardner-Medwin D, Walton J N 1973 The syndrome of myosclerosis. Journal of Neurology, Neurosurgery and Psychiatry 36: 651–660

Bradley W G, Tomlinson B E, Hardy M 1978 Further studies of mitochondrial and lipid storage myopathies. Journal of the Neurological Sciences 35: 201–210

Brandt S 1947 A case of arthrogryposis multiplex congenita. Acta Paediatrica 34:365

Bresolin N, Zeviani M, Bonilla E, et al 1985 Fatal infantile cytochrome c oxidase deficiency: decrease of immunologically detectable enzyme in muscle. Neurology 35: 802–812

Brody I A 1969 Muscle contracture induced by exercise: A syndrome attributable to decreased relaxing factor. New England Journal of Medicine 281:187

Brooke M H 1973 Congenital fiber type disproportion. In: Kakulas B A (ed) Clinical studies in myology, part 2. Excerpta Medica, Amsterdam, p 147–159

Brooke M H 1977 A clinician's view of neuromuscular disease. Williams and Wilkins, Baltimore

Brooke M H, Engel W K 1969 The histographic analysis of human muscle biopsies with regard to fiber types: 4. Children's biopsies. Neurology (Minneapolis) 19: 591–605

Brooke M H, Neville H E 1972 Reducing body myopathy. Neurology (Minneapolis) 22:829

Brooke M H, Carroll J E, Ringel S P 1979 Congenital hypotonia revisited. Muscle and Nerve 2: 84–100

Bruhn F W 1984 Lyme disease. American Journal of Diseases of Children 138: 467–470

Brunette M G, Delvin E, Hazel B, Scriver C R 1972 Thiamine-responsive lactic acidosis in a patient with deficient low-KM pyruvate carboxylase activity in liver. Pediatrics 50: 702–711

Bruyland M, Liebaers I, Sacre L, Vandeplas Y, De Meirleir L, Martin J J 1984 Neonatal myotubular myopathy with a probable X-linked inheritance: observations on a new family with a review of the literature. Journal of Neurology 231: 220–222

Bryant G M, Davies K J, Newcombe R G 1979 Standardisation of the Denver developmental screening test for Cardiff children. Developmental Medicine and Child Neurology 21: 353–364

Buda F B, Rothney W B, Rabe E F 1972 Hypotonia and the maternal-child relationship. American Journal of Diseases of Children 124: 906

Bundey S 1972 A genetic study of infantile and juvenile myasthenia gravis. Journal of Neurology, Neurosurgery and Psychiatry 35: 41–51

Burck U, Goebel H H, Kuhlendahl H D, Meier C, Goebel K M 1981 Neuromyopathy and vitamin E deficiency in man. Neuropediatrics 12: 267–278

Buruma O J S, Bots G T A M, Went L N 1985 Familial hypokalemic periodic paralysis: 50-year follow-up of a large family. Archives of Neurology 42: 28–31

Byers P H, Holbrook K A, Barsh G S 1983 Ehlers–Danlos syndrome. In: Emery A E H, Rimoin D L (eds) Principles and practice of medical genetics. Churchill Livingstone, Edinburgh, ch 58

Byers R K 1975 Spinal-cord injuries during birth. Developmental Medicine and Child Neurology 17: 103–110

Campbell M J, Rebeiz J J, Walton J N 1969

Myotubular, centronuclear or pericentronuclear myopathy? Journal of the Neurological Sciences 8: 425–443

Cancilla P A, Kalyanaraman K, Verity M A, Munsat T, Pearson C M 1971 Familial myopathy with probable lysis of myofibrils in type 1 fibers. Neurology (Minneapolis) 21: 579–585

Carpenter S, Karpati G, Andermann F, Gold R 1974 Giant axonal neuropathy: A clinically and morphologically distinct neurological disease. Archives of Neurology 31: 312–316

Carpenter S, Karpati G, Holland P 1985 New observations in reducing body myopathy. Neurology 35: 818–827

Cavanagh N P C 1980 The role of thymectomy in childhood myasthenia. Developmental Medicine and Child Neurology 22: 668–674

Charles B M, Hosking G, Green A, Pollitt R, Bartlett K, Taitz L S 1979 Biotin-responsive alopecia and developmental regression. Lancet 2: 118–120

Chelmicka-Schorr E, Bernstein L P, Zurbrugg E B, Huttenlocher P R 1979 Eaton–Lambert syndrome in a 9-year-old girl. Archives of Neurology 36: 572–574

Chudley A E, Rozdilsky B, Houston C S, Becker L E, Knoll J H 1985 Multicore disease in sibs with severe mental retardation, short stature, facial anomalies, hypoplasia of the pituitary fossa, and hypogonadotrophic hypogonadism. American Journal of Medical Genetics 20: 145–158

Clarren S K, Hall J G 1983 Neuropathic findings in the spinal cords of 10 infants with arthrogryposis. Journal of the Neurological Sciences 58: 89–102

Cohen M E, Duffner P K, Heffner R 1978 Central core disease in one of identical twins. Journal of Neurology, Neurosurgery and Psychiatry 41: 659–663

Coleman R F, Nienhuis A W, Brown W J, Munsat T L, Pearson C M 1967 New myopathy with mitochondrial enzyme hyperactivity. Journal of the American Medical Association 199: 624–630

Coleman R F, Thompson L R, Nienhuis A W, Munsat T L, Pearson C M 1968 Histochemical investigation of 'myotubular' myopathy. Archives of Pathology 86: 365–376

Conen P E, Murphy E G, Donohue W L 1963 Light and electron microscopic studies of 'myogranules' in a child with hypotonia and muscle weakness. Canadian Medical Association Journal 89: 983–986

Crosby T W, Chou S M 1974 'Ragged-red' fibers in Leigh's disease. Neurology (Minneapolis) 24: 49–54

Crothers B 1923 Injury of the spinal cord in breech extractions as an important cause of foetal death and paraplegia in childhood. American Journal of Medical Science 165:94

Crothers B, Putnam M C 1927 Obstetrical injuries of the spinal cord. Medicine (Baltimore) 6:41

Cruz Martinez A, Ferrer M T, López-Terradas J M, Pascual-Castroviejo I, Mingo P 1979 Single fibre electromyography in central core disease. Journal of Neurology, Neurosurgery and Psychiatry 42: 662–667

Curless R G, Payne C M, Brinner F M 1978a Fingerprint body myopathy: a report of twins. Developmental Medicine and Child Neurology 20: 793–798

Curless R G, Nelson M B, Brinner F 1978b Histological patterns of muscle in infants with developmental brain abnormalities. Developmental Medicine and Child Neurology 20: 159–166

Currie S, Noronha M, Harriman D 1974 'Minicore' disease.

In: Bradley W G (ed) Abstracts of the IIIrd International Congress on Muscle Diseases. Excerpta Medica, Amsterdam, p 12

Daentl D L, Berg B O, Layzer R B, Epstein C J 1974 A new familial arthrogryposis without weakness. Neurology (Minneapolis) 24: 55–60

D'Agostino A N, Ziter F A, Rallison M L, Bray P F 1968 Familial myopathy with abnormal muscle mitochondria. Archives of Neurology 18: 388–401

Dahl D S, Klutzow F W 1974 Congenital rod disease: Further evidence of innervational abnormalities as the basis for the clinico-pathologic features. Journal of the Neurological Sciences 23: 371–385

Danon M J, Carpenter S, Manaligod J R, Schliselfeld L H 1981 Fatal infantile glycogen storage disease: deficiency of phosphofructokinase and phosphorylase b kinase. Neurology (New York) 31: 1303–1307

Danta G 1975 Electrophysiological study of amyotrophy associated with acute asthma (asthmatic amyotrophy). Journal of Neurology, Neurosurgery and Psychiatry 38: 1016–1021

Darwish H, Sarnat H, Archer C, Brownell K, Kotagal S 1981 Congenital cervical spinal atrophy. Muscle and Nerve 4: 106–110

Dastur D K, Razzak Z A, Bharucha E P 1972 Arthrogryposis multiplex congenita: part 2: Muscle pathology and pathogenesis. Journal of Neurology, Neurosurgery and Psychiatry 35: 435–450

de Leon G A, Grover W D, D'Cruz D A 1984 Amyotrophic cerebellar hypoplasia: a specific form of infantile spinal atrophy. Acta Neuropathologica (Berlin) 63: 282–286

Denborough M A, Dennett X, Anderson R M 1973 Central-core disease and malignant hyperpyrexia. British Medical Journal 1: 272–273

Denborough M A, Galloway G J, Hopkinson K C 1982 Malignant hyperpyrexia and sudden infant death. Lancet 2: 1068–1069

Der Kaloustian V M, Afifi A K, Mire J 1972 The myopathic variety of arthrogryposis multiplex congenita: A disorder with autosomal recessive inheritance. Journal of Pediatrics 81:76

Desmond M M, Franklin R R, Valebona C, Hill R M, Plumb R, Arnold H, Watts J 1963 The clinical behaviour of the newly born. Journal of Pediatrics 62:307

DiMauro S, Bonilla E, Lee C P, Schotland D L, Scarpa A, Conn H, Chance B 1976 Luft's disease; further biochemical and ultrastructural studies of skeletal muscle in the second case. Journal of the Neurological Sciences 27: 217–232

DiMauro S, Hartlage P L 1978 Fatal infantile form of muscle phosphorylase deficiency. Neurology 28: 1124–1129

DiMauro S, Mendell J R, Sahenk Z, Bachman D, Scarpa A, Scofield R M, Reiner C 1980 Fatal infantile mitochondrial myopathy and renal dysfunction due to cytochrome-c-oxidase deficiency. Neurology 30: 795–804

DiMauro S, Nicholson J F, Hays A P, Eastwood A B, Papadimitiou A, Koenigsberger R, DeVivo D C 1983 Benign infantile mitochondrial myopathy due to reversible cytochrome c oxidase deficiency. Annals of Neurology 14: 226–234

DiMauro S, Bonilla E, Zeviani M, Nakagawa M, DeVivo D C 1985 Mitochondrial myopathies. Annals of Neurology 17: 521–538

Dodge P R 1960 Neuromuscular disorders. Research

Publications of the Association for Research into Nervous and Mental Disease 38:497

Drachman D B, Banker B Q 1963 Arthrogryposis multiplex congenita: Case due to disease of the anterior horn cells. Archives of Neurology 8: 77–93

Dubowitz V 1973 Rigid spine syndrome: A muscle syndrome in search of a name. Proceedings of the Royal Society of Medicine 66: 219–220

Dubowitz V 1978 Muscle disorders in childhood. Saunders, London

Dubowitz V 1980 The floppy infant, 2nd edn. Spastics International Medical Publications, London

Dubowitz V 1985 Muscle biopsy: A practical approach, 2nd edn. Baillière Tindall, London

Dubowitz V, Platts M 1965 Central core disease of muscle with focal wasting. Journal of Neurology, Neurosurgery and Psychiatry 28: 432–437

Dubrovsky A L, Taratuto A L, Martino R 1978 Type II hypotrophy and ophthalmoplegia: Another congenital neuromuscular disease? In: Abstracts of the IVth International Congress of Neuromuscular Diseases (Montreal)

Dudley A W, Dudley M A, Varakis J M, Blackburn W R 1978 Progressive tetany and reducing bodies in a neonate: A new myopathy. In: Abstracts of the IVth International Congress of Neuromuscular Diseases (Montreal)

Dunn H G, Daube J R, Gomez M R 1978 Heredofamilial brachial plexus neuropathy (hereditary neuralgic amyotrophy with brachial predilection) in childhood. Developmental Medicine and Child Neurology 20: 28–46

Dyken M, Zeman W, Rusche T 1969 Hypokalemic periodic paralysis: Children with permanent myopathic weakness. Neurology (Minneapolis) 19: 691–699

Eberle E, Brinke J, Azen S, White D 1975 Early predictors of incomplete recovery in children with Guillain–Barré polyneuritis. Journal of Pediatrics 86: 356–359

Eeg-Olofsson O, Henriksson K-G, Thornell L-E, Wesstrom G 1983 Early infant death in nemaline (rod) myopathy. Brain and Development 5: 53–57

Egger J, Wilson J 1983 Mitochondrial inheritance in a mitochondrially mediated disease. New England Journal of Medicine 309: 142–146

Ek J I 1958 Cerebral lesions in arthrogryposis multiplex congenita. Acta Paediatrica Scandinavica 47: 302–316

Emery A E H 1971 The nosology of the spinal muscular atrophies. Journal of Medical Genetics 8: 481–495

Eng G D, Epstein B S, Engel W K, McKay D W, McKay R 1978 Malignant hyperthermia and central core disease in a child with dislocating hips: case presentation and review. Archives of Neurology 35: 189–197

Engel A G 1984 Myasthenia gravis and myasthenic syndromes. Annals of Neurology 16: 519–534

Engel A G, Gomez M R, Groover R V 1971 Multicore disease: a recently recognised congenital myopathy associated with multifocal degeneration of muscle fibres. Mayo Clinic Proceedings 10: 666–681

Engel A G, Angelini C, Gomez M R 1972 Fingerprint body myopathy. Mayo Clinic Proceedings 47:377

Engel A G, Lambert E H, Gomez M R 1977 A new myasthenic syndrome with end-plate acetylcholinesterase deficiency, small nerve terminals, and reduced acetylcholine release. Annals of Neurology 1: 315–330

Engel A G, Lambert E H, Mulder D M, Torres C F, Sahashi K, Bertorini T E, Whitaker J N 1982 A newly recognised congenital myasthenic syndrome attributed to a prolonged open time of the acetylcholine-induced ion channel. Annals of Neurology 11: 553–569

Engel W K, Gold G N, Karpati G 1968 Type I fiber hypotrophy and central nuclei. Archives of Neurology 18: 435–444

Fardeau M, Harpey J-P, Caille B, Lafourcade J 1975 Hyptonies neo-natales avec disproportion congénitale des differents types de fibre musculaire, et petitesse relative des fibres de type I: Demonstration du caractère familial de cette nouvelle entité. Archives Françaises de Pédiatrie 32: 901–914

Fardeau M, Tomé F M S, Derambure S 1976 Familial fingerprint body myopathy. Archives of Neurology 33: 724–725

Farkas-Bargeton E, Aicardi J, Arsenio-Nunes M L, Wehrle R 1978 Delay in the maturation of muscle fibers in infants with congenital hypotonia. Journal of the Neurological Sciences 39: 17–29

Favara B E, Vawter G F, Wagner R, Kevy S, Porter E G 1967 Familial paroxysmal rhabdomyolysis in children: A myoglobinuric syndrome. American Journal of Medicine 42: 196–207

Fear C N, Mutton D E, Berry A C, Heckmatt J Z, Dubowitz V 1985 Chromosome 15 in Prader–Willi syndrome. Developmental Medicine and Child Neurology 27: 305–311

Fenichel G M 1967 Abnormalities of skeletal muscle maturation in brain damaged children: A histochemical study. Developmental Medicine and Child Neurology 9:419

Fenichel G M 1978 Clinical syndromes of myasthenia in infancy and childhood: a review. Archives of Neurology 35: 97–103

Fenichel G M 1983 Myasthenia gravis. In: Emery A E H, Rimoin D L (eds) Principles and practice of medical genetics. Churchill Livingstone, Edinburgh, ch 34

Fenichel G M, Bazelon M 1966 Myopathies in search of a name: benign congenital forms. Developmental Medicine and Child Neurology 8: 532–538

Fidzianska A, Badurska B, Ryniewicz B, Dembek I 1981 'Cap disease': new congenital myopathy. Neurology (New York) 31: 1113–1120

Fishbein W N, Armbrustmacher V W, Griffin J L 1978 Monoadenylate deaminase deficiency: A new disease of muscle. Science 200: 545–548

Fisher R L, Johnstone W T, Fisher W H, Goldkamp O G 1970 Arthrogryposis multiplex congenita: A clinical investigation. Journal of Pediatrics 76: 255–261

Fleury P, Hageman G 1985 A dominantly inherited lower motor neuron disorder presenting at birth with associated arthrogryposis. Journal of Neurology, Neurosurgery and Psychiatry 48: 1037–1048

Ford F R 1966 Diseases of the nervous system in infancy, childhood and adolescence, 5th edn. Charles C Thomas, Springfield, Ill

Fowler M 1959 A case of arthrogryposis multiplex congenita with lesions in the nervous system. Archives of Disease in Childhood 34: 505–510

Frank J P, Harati Y, Butler I J, Nelson T E, Scott C I 1980 Central core disease and malignant hyperthermia syndrome. Annals of Neurology 7: 11–17

Frankenburg W K, Dodds J B 1967 The Denver developmental screening test. Journal of Pediatrics 71:181

French J H, Sherard E S, Lubell H, Brotz M, Moore C L

1972 Trichopoliodystrophy: 1. Report of a case and biochemical studies. Archives of Neurology 26: 229–244

Fried K, Beer S, Vure E, Algom M, Shapira Y 1979 Autosomal recessive sudden unexpected death in children probably caused by a cardiomyopathy associated with a myopathy. Journal of Medical Genetics 16: 341–346

Friedlander H L, Westin G W, Wood W L 1968 Arthrogryposis multiplex congenita. A review of 45 cases. Journal of Bone and Joint Surgery 50A: 89

Frischknecht W, Bianchi L, Pilleri G 1960 Familial arthrograyposis complex congenita. Neuro-arthromyodysplasia congenita. Helvetica Paediatrica Acta 15:259

Fukuyama Y, Sugiura S, Hirayama Y, Segawa M G 1973 The prognosis of myasthenia gravis in infancy and childhood. In: Kakulas B A (ed) Clinical studies in myology: Part II. Excerpta Medica, Amsterdam, p 552–559

Fukuyama Y, Ando T, Yokota J 1977 Acute fulminant myoglobinuric polymyositis with picornavirus-like crystals. Journal of Neurology, Neurosurgery and Psychiatry 40: 775–781

Fulthorpe J J, Gardner-Medwin D, Hudgson P, Walton J N 1969 Nemaline myopathy: a histological and ultrastructural study of skeletal muscle from a case presenting with infantile hypotonia. Neurology (Minneapolis) 19: 735–748

Gadoth N, Margalit D, Shapira Y 1978 Myopathy with multiple central cores: A case of hypersensitivity to pyrexia. Neuropädiatrie 9: 239–244

Gamstorp I, Hauge M, Helweg-Larsen H F, Mjönes H, Sagild U 1957 Adynamia episodica hereditaria: A disease clinically resembling familial periodic paralysis but characterised by increasing serum potassium during the paralytic attacks. American Journal of Medicine 23: 385–390

Gamstorp I, Sarnat H B (eds) 1984 Progressive spinal muscular atrophies. Raven, New York

Gardner-Medwin D, Walton J N 1969 Myokymia with impaired muscular relaxation. Lancet 1: 127–130

Gardner-Medwin D, Dale G, Parkin J M 1975 Lactic acidosis with mitochondrial myopathy and recurrent coma. In: Abstracts of the First International Congress of Child Neurology (Toronto) p 47

Geiger L R, Mancall E L, Penn A S, Tucker S H 1974 Familial neuralgic amyotrophy: Report of three families with review of the literature. Brain 97: 97–102

Gieron M A, Korthals J K 1985 Familial infantile myasthenia gravis: report of three cases with follow-up until adult life. Archives of Neurology 42: 143–144

Gil-Peralta A, Rafel E, Bautista J, Alberca R 1978 Myotonia in centronuclear myopathy. Journal of Neurology, Neurosurgery and Psychiatry 41: 1102–1108

Goebel H H, Zeman W, DeMyer W 1976 Peripheral motor and sensory neuropathy of early childhood, simulating Werdnig–Hoffmann disease. Neuropädiatrie 7: 182–195

Goebel H H, Lenard H G, Görke W, Kunze K 1977 Fibre type disproportion in the rigid spine syndrome. Neuropädiatrie 8: 467–477

Goebel H H, Muller J, Gillen H W, Merritt A D 1978 Autosomal dominant 'spheroid body myopathy'. Muscle and Nerve 1: 14–26

Goebel H H, Schloon H, Lenard H G 1981 Congenital myopathy with cytoplasmic bodies. Neuropediatrics 12: 166–180

Gomez M R, Clermont V, Bernstein J 1962 Progressive bulbar paralysis in childhood (Fazio–Londe's disease):

Report of a case with pathologic evidence of nuclear atrophy. Archives of Neurology 6: 317–323

Gonatas N K, Shy G M, Godfrey E H 1966 Nemaline myopathy: The origin of nemaline structures. New England Journal of Medicine 274: 535–539

Gordon A S, Rewcastle N B, Humphrey J G, Stewart B M 1974 Chronic benign congenital myopathy: finger print body type. Canadian Journal of Neurological Sciences 1: 106–113

Goto I, Nagasaka S, Nagara H, Kuroiwa Y 1979 Rigid spine syndrome. Journal of Neurology, Neurosurgery and Psychiatry 42: 276–279

Goutières F, Aicardi J, Farkas E 1977 Anterior horn cell disease associated with pontocerebellar hypoplasia in infants. Journal of Neurology, Neurosurgery and Psychiatry 40: 370–378

Guggenheim M A, Ringel S P, Silverman A, Grabert B E 1982 Progressive neuro-muscular disease in children with chronic cholestasis and vitamin E deficiency: diagnosis and treatment with alpha tocopherol. Journal of Pediatrics 100: 51–58

Hackett T N, Bray P F, Ziter F A, Nyhan W L, Creer K M 1973 A metabolic myopathy associated with chronic lactic acidemia, growth failure and nerve deafness. Journal of Pediatrics 83: 426–431

Hall J G 1983 Arthrogryposes (congenital contractures.) In: Emery A E H, Rimoin D L (eds) Principles and practice of medical genetics. Churchill Livingstone, Edinburgh, ch 55

Hall J G, Reed S D, Greene G 1982 The distal arthrogryposes: delineation of new entities — review and nosologic discussion. American Journal of Medical Genetics 11: 185–239

Hanson P A, Mastrianni A F, Post L 1977 Neonatal ophthalmoplegia with microfibers: A reversible myopathy? Neurology (Minneapolis) 27: 974–980

Harati Y, Butler I J 1985 Congenital hypomyelinating neuropathy. Journal of Neurology, Neurosurgery and Psychiatry 48: 1269–1276

Hardoff D, Sharf B, Berger A 1980 Myopathy as a presentation of coeliac disease. Developmental Medicine and Child Neurology 22: 781–783

Harriman D G F, Haleem M A 1972 Centronuclear myopathy in old age. Journal of Pathology 108: 237–248

Hart Z H, Chang C-H, Perrin E V D, Neerunjun J S, Ayyar R 1977 Familial poliodystrophy, mitochondrial myopathy and lactate acidemia. Archives of Neurology 34: 180–185

Hart Z, Sahashi K, Lambert E H, Engel A G, Lindstrom J M 1979 A congenital familial myasthenic syndrome caused by a presynaptic defect of transmitter resynthesis or mobilization. Neurology 29: 556–557

Hausmanowa-Petrusewicz I 1978 Spinal muscular atrophy: Infantile and juvenile type. National Science Foundation, Washington D C and National Centre for Scientific, Technical and Economic Information, Warsaw, Poland

Hawkes C H, Absolon M J 1975 Myotubular myopathy associated with cataract and electrical myotonia. Journal of Neurology, Neurosurgery and Psychiatry 38: 761–764

Haydar N A, Conn H L, Afifi A, Wakid N, Ballas S, Fawaz K, 1971 Severe hypermetabolism with primary abnormality of skeletal muscle mitochondria: Functional and therapeutic effects of chloramphenicol treatment. Annals of Internal Medicine 74: 548–558

Heckmatt J Z, Moosa A, Hutson C, Maunder-Sewry C A, Dubowitz V 1984 Diagnostic needle muscle biopsy: a practical and reliable alternative to open biopsy. Archives of Disease in Childhood 59: 528–532

Heckmatt J Z, Sewry C A, Hodes D, Dubowitz V 1985 Congenital centronuclear (myotubular) myopathy: a clinical, pathological and genetic study in eight children. Brain 108: 941–964

Heffernan L P, Rewcastle N B, Humphrey J G 1968 The spectrum of rod myopathies. Archives of Neurology 18: 529–542

Heffner R, Cohen M, Duffner P, Daigler G 1976 Multicore disease in twins. Journal of Neurology, Neurosurgery and Psychiatry 39: 602–606

Hoefnagel D, Jalberg E O, Publow D G, Richtsmeier A J 1978 Progressive fibrosis of the deltoid muscles. Journal of Pediatrics 92: 79–81

Hopkins I J 1974 A new syndrome: poliomyelitis-like illness associated with acute asthma in childhood. Australian Paediatric Journal 10: 273–276

Hopkins I J, Lindsey J R, Ford F R 1966 Nemaline myopathy. A long-term clinicopathologic study of affected mother and daughter. Brain 89:299

Hosking G P, Bhat U S, Dubowitz V, Edwards R H T 1976 Measurements of muscle strength and performance in children with normal and diseased muscle. Archives of Disease in Childhood 51: 957–963

Howes E L, Price H M, Pearson C M, Blumberg J M 1966 Hypokalemic periodic paralysis: Electronmicroscopic changes in the sarcoplasm. Neurology (Minneapolis) 16: 242–256

Hudgson P, Bradley W G, Jenkison M 1972 Familial 'mitochondrial' myopathy: A myopathy associated with disordered oxidative metabolism in muscle fibres. Journal of the Neurological Sciences 16: 343–370

Hurwitz L D, Carson N A J, Allen I V, Chopra J S 1969 Congenital ophthalmoplegia, floppy baby syndrome, myopathy and aminoaciduria. Journal of Neurology, Neurosurgery and Psychiatry 32:495

Huttenlocher P R, Gilles F H 1967 Infantile neuroaxonal dystrophy. Clinical, pathologic and histochemical findings in a family with 3 affected siblings. Neurology (Minneapolis) 17: 1174–1184

Ilett S J, Pugh R J, Smithells R W 1977 Poliomyelitis-like illness after acute asthma. Archives of Disease in Childhood 52: 738–740

Illingworth R S 1972 The development of the infant and young child, normal and abnormal, 5th edn. E & S Livingstone, Edinburgh

Ingram T T S 1955 The early manifestations and course of diplegia in childhood. Archives of Disease in Childhood 30:244

Inokuchi T, Umezaki H, Santa T 1975 A case of type I muscle fibre hypotrophy and internal nuclei. Journal of Neurology, Neurosurgery and Psychiatry 38: 475–482

Ionasescu V, Searby C, Rubenstein P, Sandra A, Cancilla P, Robillard J 1983 Giant axonal neuropathy: normal protein composition of neurofilaments. Journal of Neurology, Neurosurgery and Psychiatry 46: 551–554

Isaacs H 1961 A syndrome of continuous muscle fibre activity. Journal of Neurology, Neurosurgery and Psychiatry 24: 319–325

Isaacs H, Heffron J J A, Bandenhorst M 1975 Central core disease: A correlated genetic, histochemical, ultramicroscopic and biochemical study. Journal of Neurology, Neurosurgery and Psychiatry 38: 1177–1186

Jago R H 1970 Arthrogryposis following treatment of maternal tetanus with muscle relaxants. Archives of Disease in Childhood 45: 277–279

Jasper P L, Denny F W 1968 Sarcoidosis in children: with special emphasis on the natural history and treatment. Journal of Pediatrics 73: 499–512

Jenis E H, Lindquist R R, Lister R C 1969 New congenital myopathy with crystalline intranuclear inclusions. Archives of Neurology 20:281

Jerusalem F, Engel A G, Gomez M R 1973a Sarcotubular myopathy: A newly recognised, benign, congenital muscle disease. Neurology (Minneapolis) 23: 897–906

Jerusalem F, Angelini C, Engel A G, Groover R V 1973b Mitochondria-lipid-glyogen (MLG) disease of muscle: A morphologically recessive congenital myopathy. Archives of Neurology 29: 162–169

Johnson W G, Wigger H J, Karp H R, Glaubiger L M, Rowland L P 1982 Juvenile spinal muscular atrophy: a new hexosaminidase deficiency phenotype. Annals of Neurology 11: 11–16

Joosten E, Gabreëls F, Gabreëls-Festen A, Vrensen G, Korten J, Notermans S 1974 Electron-microscopic heterogeneity of onion-bulb neuropathies of the Déjerine-Sottas type: Two patients in one family with the variant described by Lyon (1969). Acta Neuropathologica (Berlin) 27: 105–118

Karch S B, Urich H 1975 Infantile polyneuropathy with defective myelination: An autopsy study. Developmental Medicine and Child Neurology 17: 504–511

Karpati G, Carpenter S, Wolfe L S, Sherwin A 1969 A peculiar polysaccharide accumulation in muscle in a case of cardioskeletal myopathy. Neurology (Minneapolis) 19: 553–564

Karpati G, Carpenter S, Nelson R F 1970 Type I muscle fibre atrophy and central nuclei: A rare familial neuromuscular disease. Journal of the Neurological Sciences 10: 489–500

Kasman M, Bernstein L 1974 Chronic progressive polyradiculoneuropathy of infancy. Neurology (Minneapolis) 24:367

Keeton B R, Moosa A 1976 Organic aciduria: Treatable cause of floppy infant syndrome. Archives of Disease in Childhood 51: 636–638

Kelemen J, Rice D R, Bradley W G, Munsat T L, DiMauro S, Hogan E L 1982 Familial myoadenylate deaminase deficiency and exertional myalgia. Neurology (New York) 32: 857–863

Kennedy W R, Sung J H, Berry J F 1977 A case of congenital hypomyelination neuropathy: Clinical, morphological and chemical studies. Archives of Neurology 34: 337–345

King J O, Denborough M A, Zapf P W 1972 Inheritance of malignant hyperthermia. Lancet 1: 365–370

Kinoshita M, Cadman T E 1968 Myotubular myopathy. Archives of Neurology 18: 265–271

Koch B M, Bertorini T E, Eng G D, Boehm R 1985 Severe multicore disease associated with reaction to anesthesia. Archives of Neurology 42: 1204–1206

Kohlschutter A, Sieg K, Schulte F J, Hayek H W, Goebel H H 1982 Infantile cardiomyopathy and neuromyopathy with β-galactosidase deficiency. European Journal of Pediatrics 139: 75–81

Kondo K, Yuasa T 1980 Genetics of congenital nemaline myopathy. Muscle and Nerve 3: 308–315

Krabbe K H 1958 Congenital generalised muscular atrophies. Acta Psychiatrica 33:94

Krugliak L, Gadoth N, Behar A J 1978 Neuropathic form of arthrogryposis multiplex congenita: report of 3 cases with complete necropsy, including the first reported case of agenesis of muscle spindles. Journal of the Neurological Sciences 37: 179–185

Kuitonnen P, Rapola J, Noponen A L, Donner M 1972 Nemaline myopathy. Report of 4 cases and review of the literature. Acta Paediatrica Scandinavica 61:353

Kuzuhara S, Chou S M 1981 Preservation of the phrenic motoneurons in Werdnig–Hoffmann disease. Annals of Neurology 9: 506–510

Lake B D, Wilson J 1975 Zebra body myopathy: Clinical, histochemical and ultrastructural studies. Journal of the Neurological Sciences 24: 437–446

Land J M, Morgan-Hughes J A, Clark J B 1981 Mitochondrial myopathy: biochemical studies revealing a deficiency of NADH-cytochrome b reductase activity. Journal of the Neurological Sciences 50: 1–13

Lapresle J M, Fardeau M, Godet-Guillain J 1972 Myopathie distale congénitale avec hypertrophie des mollets — Presence d'anomalies mitochondriales à la biopsie musculaire. Journal of the Neurological Sciences 17:87

Laurence B M 1967 Hypotonia, mental retardation, obesity and cryptorchidism associated with dwarfism and diabetes in children. Archives of Disease in Childhood 42:126

Lazaro R P, Fenichel G M, Kilroy A W, Saito A, Fleischer S 1980 Cramps, muscle pain and tubular aggregates. Archives of Neurology 37: 715–717

Lebenthal E, Shocket S B, Adam A et al 1970 Arthrogryposis multiplex congenita: Twenty-three cases in an Arab kindred. Pediatrics 46:891

Lecky B R F, Morgan-Hughes J A, Murray N M F, Landon D N, Wray D, Prior C 1986 Congenital myasthenia: further evidence of disease heterogeneity. Muscle and Nerve 9: 233–242

Lenard H G, Goebel H H 1975 Congenital fibre type disproportion. Neuropädiatrie 6: 220–231

Lenard H-G, Goebel H-H 1980 Congenital muscular dystrophies and unstructured congenital myopathies. Brain and Development 2: 119–125

Lesny I 1979 Follow up study of hypotonic forms of cerebral palsy. Brain and Development 1: 87–90

Lloyd-Roberts G C, Lettin A W F 1970 Arthrogryposis multiplex congenita. Journal of Bone and Joint Surgery 52B:494

Logothetis J, Constantoulakis M, Economidou J et al 1972 Thalassemia major (homozygous beta-thalassemia): a survey of 138 cases with emphasis on neurologic and muscular aspects. Neurology (Minneapolis) 22: 294–304

Löwenthal A 1954 Un groupe hérédodégénératif nouveau: les myoscléroses hérédofamiliales. Acta Neurologica et Psychiatrica Belgica 54: 155–165

Luft R, Ikkos D, Palmieri G, Ernster L, Afzelius B 1962 A case of severe hypermetabolism of nonthyroid origin with a defect in the maintenance of mitochondrial respiratory control: a correlated clinical, biochemical and morphological study. Journal of Clinical Investigation 41: 1776–1804

Lundberg A 1979 Dissociated motor development: Developmental patterns, clinical characteristics, causal factors and outcome, with special reference to late walking children. Neuropädiatrie 10: 161–182

Lyon G 1969 Ultrastructural study of a nerve biopsy from a case of early infantile chronic neuropathy. Acta Neuropathologica (Berlin) 13: 131–142

McGuire S A, Tomasovic J J, Ackerman N 1984 Hereditary continuous muscle fiber activity. Archives of Neurology 41: 395–396

Mac Keith R C, Polani P E, Clayton-Jones E 1960 English translation of: André-Thomas, Yves Chesni, St. Anne Dargassiess. The neurological examination of the infant. Spastics Society, Heinemann, London

McKinlay I A, Mitchell I 1976 Transient acute myositis in childhood. Archives of Disease in Childhood 51: 135–137

McLean W T, McKone R C 1973 Congenital myasthenia gravis in twins. Archives of Neurology 29: 223–226

McLeod J G, Baker W de C, Lethlean A K, Shorey C D 1972 Centronuclear myopathy with autosomal dominant inheritance. Journal of the Neurological Sciences 15: 375–387

McLeod J G, Baker W de C, Shorey C D, Kerr C B 1975 Mitochondrial myopathy with multisystem abnormalities and normal ocular movements. Journal of the Neurological Sciences 24: 39–52

McQuillen M P 1966 Familial limb-girdle myasthenia. Brain 89: 121–132

McWilliam R C, Gardner-Medwin D, Doyle D, Stephenson J B P 1985 Diaphragmatic paralysis due to spinal muscular atrophy: an unrecognised cause of respiratory failure in infancy? Archives of Disease in Childhood 60: 145–149

Martin J J, Clara R, Ceuterick C, Joris C 1976 Is congenital fibre type disproportion a true myopathy? Acta Neurologica Belgica 76: 335–344

Martyn C, Jellinek E H, Webb J N 1981 Lipid storage myopathy: successful treatment with propranolol. British Medical Journal 282: 1997–1999

Matsuoka Y, Gubbay S S, Kakulas B A 1974 A new myopathy with type II muscle fibre hypoplasia. Proceedings of the Australian Association of Neurologists 11: 155–159

Meier C, Voellmy W, Gertsch M, Zimmermann A, Geissbuhler J 1984 Nemaline myopathy appearing in adults as cardiomyopathy: a clinicopathologic study. Archives of Neurology 41: 443–445

Mellins R B, Hays A P, Gold A P, Berdon W E, Bowdler J D 1974 Respiratory distress as the initial manifestation of Werdnig–Hoffmann disease. Pediatrics 53: 33–40

Meyer-Betz F 1910 Beobachtungen an einem eigenartigen mit Muskellahmungen verbundenen Fall von Hamoglobinurie. Deutsches Archiv für klinische Medizin 101:85

Meyers K R, Golomb H M, Hansen J L, McKusick V A 1974 Familial neuromuscular disease with 'myotubes'. Clinical Genetics 5: 327–337

Midura T F, Arnon S S 1976 Infant botulism: Identification of Clostridium botulinum and its toxins in faeces. Lancet 2: 934–936

Millichap J G, Dodge P R 1960 Diagnosis and treatment of myasthenia gravis in infancy, childhood and adolescence. Neurology (Minneapolis) 10:1007

Mitsumoto H, Sliman R J, Schafer I A, Sternick C S, Kaufman B, Wilbourn A, Horwitz S J 1985 Motor neuron disease and adult hexosaminidase A deficiency in two families: evidence for multisystem degeneration. Annals of Neurology 17: 378–385

Miyabayashi S, Narisawa K, Iinuma K et al 1984 Cytochrome c oxidase deficiency in two siblings with Leigh encephalomyelopathy. Brain and Development 6: 362–372

Moosa A 1971 Peripheral neuropathy and ichthyosis in

Krabbe's leucodystrophy. Archives of Disease in Childhood 46:112

Moosa A, Dubowitz V 1970 Peripheral neuropathy in Cockayne's syndrome. Archives of Disease in Childhood 45: 674–677

Morgan-Hughes J A, Brett E M, Lake B D, Tomé F M S 1973 Central core disease or not? Observations on a family with non-progressive myopathy. Brain 96: 527–536

Morgan-Hughes J A, Darveniza P, Kahn S N, Landon D N, Sherratt R M, Land J M, Clark J B 1977 A mitochondrial myopathy characterised by a deficiency in reducible cytochrome b. Brain 100: 617–640

Morgan-Hughes J A, Lecky B R F, Landon D N, Murray N M F 1981 Alterations in the number and affinity of junctional acetylcholine receptors in a myopathy with tubular aggregates: a newly recognized receptor defect. Brain 104: 279–295

Murphy N P, Davidson D C, Bouton J 1985 Diaphragmatic paralysis due to spinal muscular atrophy. Archives of Disease in Childhood 60:495

Naveh Y, Ludatshcer C, Alon U, Sharf B 1985 Muscle involvement in progressive diaphyseal dysplasia. Pediatrics 76: 944–949

Neligan G, Prudham D 1969 Norms for four standard developmental milestones by sex, social class and place in family. Developmental Medicine and Child Neurology 11: 413–422

Nelson J S, Prensky A L 1972 Sporadic juvenile amyotrophic lateral sclerosis: a clinicopathological study of a case with neuronal cytoplasmic inclusions containing RNA. Archives of Neurology 27: 300–306

Newman D G, Pearn J, Barnes A, Young C M, Kehoe M, Newman J 1984 Norms for hand grip strength. Archives of Disease in Childhood 59: 453–459

Noble-Jamieson C M, Heckmatt J Z, Dubowitz V, Silverman M 1986 Effects of posture and spinal bracing on respiratory function in neuromuscular disease. Archives of Disease in Childhood 61: 178–181

Norman M G, Temple A R, Murphy J V 1970 Infantile quadriceps-femoris contracture resulting from intramuscular injections. New England Journal of Medicine 282: 964–966

Norman R M 1961 Cerebellar hypoplasia in Werdnig–Hoffmann disease. Archives of Disease in Childhood 3: 96–101

Oberklaid F, Hopkins I J 1976 'Juvenile' myasthenia gravis in early infancy. Archives of Disease in Childhood 51: 719–721

Oh S J, Meyers G J, Wilson E R, Alexander C B 1983 A benign form of reducing body myopathy. Muscle and Nerve 6: 278–282

Ohtani Y, Matsuda I, Iwamasa T, Tamari H, Origuchi Y, Miike T 1982 Infantile glycogen storage myopathy in a girl with phosphorylase kinase deficiency. Neurology (New York) 32: 833–838

Ortiz de Zarate J C, Maruffo A 1970 The descending ocular myopathy of early childhood. Myotubular or centronuclear myopathy. European Neurology 3:1

Osserman K E 1958 Myasthenia gravis. Grune & Stratton, New York

Paine R S 1963 The future of the 'floppy infant'. A follow up study of 133 patients. Developmental Medicine and Child Neurology 5:115

Parker D L, Mitchell P R, Holmes G L 1981 Poland-Möbius syndrome. Journal of Medical Genetics 18: 317–320

Parnes S, Karpati G, Carpenter S, Ng Ying Kin N M K, Wolfe L S, Suranyi L 1985 Hexosaminidase-A deficiency presenting as atypical juvenile-onset spinal muscular atrophy. Archives of Neurology 42: 1176–1180

Pasternak J F, Fulling K, Nelson J, Prensky A L 1982 An infant with chronic, relapsing polyneuropathy responsive to steroids. Developmental Medicine and Child Neurology 24: 504–524

Paulson G W 1970 The Landry–Guillain–Barré syndrome and childhood. Developmental Medicine and Child Neurology 12:604

Pavlakis S G, Phillips P C, DiMauro S, De Vivo D C, Rowland L P 1984 Mitochondrial myopathy, encephalopathy, lactic acidosis, and stroke-like episodes: a distinctive clinical syndrome. Annals of Neurology 16: 481–488

Pearn J H 1974 The use of motor milestones to determine retrospectively the clinical onset of disease. Australian Paediatric Journal 10: 147–153

Pearn J 1980 Classification of spinal muscular atrophies. Lancet 1: 919–922

Pearson C M 1964 The periodic paralyses. Differential features and pathology in permanent myopathic weakness. Brain 87:341

Pearson C M, Fowler W G 1963 Hereditary non-progressive muscular dystrophy inducing arthrogryposis syndrome. Brain 86:75

Peña C E, Miller F, Budzilovich G B, Feigen I 1968 Arthrogryposis multiplex congenita. Neurology (Minneapolis) 18:926

Peterman A F, Daly D D, Dion F R, Keith H M 1959 Infectious neuronitis (Guillain–Barré syndrome) in children. Neurology (Minneapolis) 9: 533–539

Peyronnard J-M, Charron L, Ninkovic S 1982 Type I fiber atrophy and internal nuclei: a form of centronuclear myopathy? Archives of Neurology 39: 520–524

Pickett J, Berg B, Chaplin E, Brunstetter-Shafer M-A 1976 Syndrome of botulism in infancy: Clinical and electrophysiologic study. New England Journal of Medicine 295: 770–772

Pierobon-Bormioli S, Armani M, Ringel S P, Angelini C, Vergani L, Betto R, Salviati G 1985 Familial neuromuscular disease with tubular aggregates. Muscle and Nerve 8: 291–298

Polani P E 1959 The natural clinical history of choreoathetoid cerebral palsy. Guy's Hospital Reports 108:32

Poskanzer D C, Kerr D N S 1961 A third type of periodic paralysis, with normokalemia and favourable response to sodium chloride. American Journal of Medicine 31: 328–342

Prader A, Labhart A, Willi H 1956 Ein Syndrome von Adipositas, Kleinwuchs, Kryptorchismus und Oligophrenie nach myatonieartigem Zustand im Neugeborenalter. Schweizerische medizinische Wochenschrift 86:1260

Pugh R C B, Dudgeon J A 1954 Fatal neonatal poliomyelitis. Archives of Disease in Childhood 29:381

Raifman M A, Berant M, Lenarsky C 1978 Cold weather and rhabdomyolysis. Journal of Pediatrics 93: 970–971

Rawles J M, Weller R O 1974 Familial association of metabolic myopathy, lactic acidosis and sideroblastic anemia. American Journal of Medicine 56: 891–897

Reik L, Steere A C, Bartenhagen N H, Shope R E, Malawista S E 1979 Neurologic abnormalities of Lyme disease. Medicine (Baltimore) 58: 281–294

Ricoy J R, Cabello A 1985 Hypotrophy of type 1 fibres with central nuclei: recovery 4 years after diagnosis. Journal of Neurology, Neurosurgery and Psychiatry 48: 167–171

Riddick M F, Winter R B, Lutter L D 1982 Spinal deformities in patients with spinal muscle atrophy: a review of 36 patients. Spine 7: 476–483

Riley D J, Santiago T V, Daniele R P, Schall B, Edelman N H 1977 Blunted respiratory drive in congenital myopathy. American Journal of Medicine 63: 459–465

Ringel S P, Neville H E, Duster M C, Carroll J E 1978 A new congenital neuromuscular disease with trilaminar muscle fibers. Neurology (Minneapolis) 28: 282–289

Robertson W C, Chun R W M, Kornguth S E 1980 Familial infantile myasthenia. Archives of Neurology 37: 117–119

Rohkamm R, Boxler K, Ricker K, Jerusalem F 1983 A dominantly inherited myopathy with excessive tubular aggregates. Neurology (Cleveland) 33: 331–336

Rondot P, Dalloz J-C, Tardieu G 1958 Mesure de la force des réactions musculaires a l'étirement passif aux cours des raideurs pathologiques par lésions cérébrales. Revue Française d'Études Cliniques et Biologiques 3:585

Rosing H S, Hopkins L C, Wallace D C, Epstein C M, Weidenheim K 1985 Maternally inherited mitochondrial myopathy and myoclonic epilepsy. Annals of Neurology 17: 228–237

Rosner F, Ong B H, Paine R S, Mahanand D 1965 Blood-serotonin activity in trisomic and translocation Down's syndrome. Lancet 1:1191

Rowland L P, Eskenazi A N 1956 Myasthenia gravis with features resembling muscular dystrophy. Neurology (Minneapolis) 6:667

Sahgal V, Sahgal S 1977 A new congenital myopathy: A morphological cytochemical and histochemical study. Acta Neuropathologica (Berlin) 37: 225–230

Salmon M A, Esiri M M, Ruderman N B 1971 Myopathic disorder associated with mitochondrial abnormalities, hyperglycaemia and hyperketonaemia. Lancet 2: 290–293

Sandbank U, Lerman P 1972 Progressive cerebral poliodystrophy — Alpers' disease: Disorganised giant neuronal mitochondria on electron microscopy. Journal of Neurology, Neurosurgery and Psychiatry 35: 749–755

Santavuori P, Leisti J, Kruus S 1977 Muscle, eye and brain disease: a new syndrome. Neuropädiatrie 8 (suppl):553

Savage D C L, Forbes M, Pearce G W 1971 Idiopathic rhabdomyolysis. Archives of Disease in Childhood 46: 594–604

Schapira D, Swash M 1985 Neonatal spinal muscular atrophy presenting as respiratory distress: a clinical variant. Muscle and Nerve 8: 661–663

Schneck L, Adachi M, Briet P, Wolintz A, Volk B W 1973 Ophthalmoplegia plus with morphological and chemical studies of cerebellar and muscle tissue. Journal of the Neurological Sciences 19:37

Schotland D L, DiMauro S, Bonilla E, Scarpa A, Lee C-P 1976 Neuromuscular disorder associated with a defect in mitochondrial energy supply. Archives of Neurology 33: 475–479

Seay A R, Ziter F A, Petajan J H 1977 Rigid spine syndrome: A type I fiber myopathy. Archives of Neurology 34: 119–122

Sengers R C A, Stadhouders A M, Jaspar H H J, Trijbels J M F, Daniels O 1976 Cardiomyopathy and short stature associated with mitochondrial and/or lipid storage myopathy of skeletal muscle. Neuropädiatrie 7: 196–208

Sengers R C A, ter Haar B G A, Trijbels J M F, Willems J L, Daniels O, Stadhouders A M 1975 Congenital cataract and mitochondrial myopathy of skeletal and heart muscle associated with lactic acidosis after exercise. Journal of Pediatrics 86: 873–880

Shafiq S A, Dubowitz V, Peterson H de C, Milhorat A T 1967 Nemaline myopathy: Report of a fatal case, with histochemical and electron miscroscopic studies. Brain 90:817–828

Shafiq S A, Sande M A, Carruthers R R, Killip T, Milhorat A T 1972 Skeletal muscle in idiopathic cardiomyopathy. Journal of the Neurological Sciences 15: 303–320

Shapira Y, Cividalli G, Szabo G, Rozin R, Russell A 1974 A myasthenic syndrome in childhood leukemia. Developmental Medicine and Child Neurology 16: 668–671

Shapira Y, Cederbaum S D, Cancilla P A, Nielsen D, Lippe B M 1975 Familial poliodystrophy, mitochondrial myopathy and lactate acidemia. Neurology (Minneapolis) 25: 614–621

Shapira Y, Amit R, Rachmilewitz E 1981 Vitamin E deficiency in Werdnig–Hoffmann disease. Annals of Neurology 10: 266–268

Sher J H, Rimalovski A B, Athanassiades T J, Aronson S M 1967 Familial myotubular myopathy: a clinical, pathological, histochemical and ultrastructural study. Journal of Neuropathology and Experimental Neurology 26:132

Shy G M, Engel W K, Somers J E, Wanko T 1963 Nemaline myopathy: a new congenital myopathy. Brain 86:793

Shy G M, Gonatas N K, Perez M 1966 Two childhood myopathies with abnormal mitochondria I. Megaconial myopathy. II. Pleoconial myopathy. Brain 89: 133–158

Shy G M, Magee K R 1956 A new congenital non-progressive myopathy. Brain 79:610

Sillence D O, Senn A S, Danks D M 1979 Genetic heterogeneity in osteogenesis imperfecta. Journal of Medical Genetics 16: 101–116

Smit L M E, Jennekens F G I, Veldman H, Barth P G 1984 Paucity of secondary synaptic clefts in a case of congenital myasthenia with multiple contractures: ultrastructural morphology of a developmental disorder. Journal of Neurology, Neurosurgery and Psychiatry 47: 1091–1097

Smit L M E, Veldman H, Jennekens F G I, Molenaar P C, Oen B S 1987 A congenital myasthenic disorder with paucity of secondary synaptic clefts: deficiency and altered distribution of acetylcholine receptors. Annals of the New York Academy of Sciences (in press)

Smith D W 1982 Recognisable patterns of human malformation, 3rd edn. Saunders, Philadelphia

Sobue I, Saito N, Iida M, Ando K 1978 Juvenile type of distal and segmental muscular atrophy of upper extremities. Annals of Neurology 3: 429–432

Sparkes R S, Graham C B 1972 Camurati–Engelmann disease: Genetics and clinical manifestations with a review of the literature. Journal of Medical Genetics 9: 73–85

Spiro A J, Shy G M, Gonatas N K 1966 Myotubular myopathy — persistence of fetal muscle in an adolescent boy. Archives of Neurology 14: 1–14

Spiro A J, Moore C L, Prineas J W, Strasberg P M, Rapin I 1970a A cytochrome-related inherited disorder of the nervous system and muscle. Archives of Neurology 23: 103–112

Spiro A J, Prineas J W, Moore C L 1970b A new

mitochondrial myopathy in a patient with salt craving. Archives of Neurology 22: 259–269

Stauber W T, Riggs J E, Schochet S S, Gutmann L, Crosby T W 1986 Nemaline myopathy; evidence of dipeptidyl peptidase 1 deficiency. Archives of Neurology 43: 39–41

Steiman G S, Rorke L B, Brown M J 1980 Infantile neuronal degeneration masquerading as Werdnig–Hoffmann disease. Annals of Neurology 8: 317–324

Stephenson J B P 1980 Prader–Willi syndrome: neonatal presentation and later development. Developmental Medicine and Child Neurology 22: 792–795

Stoessl A J, Hahn A F, Malott D, Jones D T, Silver M D 1985 Nemaline myopathy with associated cardiomyopathy: report of clinical and detailed autopsy findings. Archives of Neurology 42: 1084–1086

Sulaiman A R, Swick H M, Kinder D S 1983 Congenital fibre type disproportion with unusual clinico-pathological manifestations. Journal of Neurology, Neurosurgery and Psychiatry 46: 175–182

Swaiman K F, Wright F S 1979 Pediatric neuromuscular diseases. Mosby, St. Louis

Swash M, Schwartz M S 1981 Familial multicore disease with focal loss of cross-striations and ophthalmoplegia. Journal of the Neurological Sciences 52: 1–10

Takebe T, Koide N, Takahashi G 1981 Giant axonal neuropathy: report of two siblings with endocrinological and histological studies. Neuropediatrics 12: 392–404

Tan C T 1985 Juvenile muscular atrophy of distal upper extremities. Journal of Neurology, Neurosurgery and Psychiatry 48: 285–286

Taratuto A L, Sfaello Z M, Rezzonico C, Morales R C 1978 Multicore disease: Report of a case with lack of fibre type differentiation. Neuropädiatrie 9: 285–297

Tarlow M J, Lake B D, Lloyd J K 1973 Chronic lactic acidosis in association with myopathy. Archives of Disease in Childhood 48: 489–492

Telerman-Toppet N, Gerard J M, Coërs C 1973 Central core disease: A study of clinically unaffected muscle. Journal of the Neurological Sciences 19: 207–223

Thomas P K 1979 Chronic relapsing idiopathic inflammatory polyneuropathy. Neuropädiatrie 10 (suppl): 452–453

Thompson C E 1982 Infantile myositis. Developmental Medicine and Child Neurology 24: 307–313

Tizard J P M 1949 Osteogenesis imperfecta presenting with delay in walking. Proceedings of the Royal Society of Medicine 42:80

Tomé R M S, Fardeau M 1975 Congenital myopathy with 'reducing bodies' in muscle fibres. Acta Neuropathologica (Berlin) 31: 207–217

Touwen B 1976 Neurological development in infancy. Heinemann, London

Towbin A 1969 Latent spinal cord and brain stem injury in newborn infants. Developmental Medicine and Child Neurology 11:54

Tsairis P, Engel W K, Kark P 1973 Familial myoclonic epilepsy syndrome associated with skeletal muscle mitochondrial abnormalities. Neurology (Minneapolis) 23:408

Turnbull D M, Bartlett K, Johnson M A, Cullen M J, Gardner-Medwin D, Ashworth B 1986 Lipid storage myopathies associated with glutaric aciduria type II and ethylmalonic-adipic aciduria. Muscle and Nerve 9 (suppl): 193

Turner H D, Brett E M, Gilbert R J, Ghosh A C,

Liebeschuetz H J 1978 Infant botulism in England. Lancet 1: 1277–1278

Turner J W A, Lees F 1962 Congenital myopathy — a fifty-year follow up. Brain 85: 733–739

Vallat J M, Hugon J, Fressinaud C, Outrequin G, Dumas M, Vallat M 1985 Centronuclear myopathy, cataract and electrical myotonia: a new case. Muscle and Nerve 8: 807–809

Vanasse M, Dubowitz V 1979 Hereditary motor and sensory neuropathy type I in infancy and childhood: A clinical, electro-diagnostic, genetic and muscle biopsy study. Neuropädiatrie 10 (suppl): 454–455

Vanneste J A, Stam F C 1982 Autosomal dominant multicore disease. Journal of Neurology, Neurosurgery and Psychiatry 45: 360–365

van Wijngaarden G K, Bethlem J, Meijer A E F H, Hülsmann W C, Feltkamp C A 1967 Skeletal muscle disease with abnormal mitochondria. Brain 90:577

van Wijngaarden G K, Fleury P, Bethlem J, Meijer A E F H 1969 Familial 'myotubular' myopathy. Neurology (Minneapolis) 19:901

Verhiest W, Brucher J M, Goddeeris P, Lauweryns J, de Geest H 1976 Familial centronuclear myopathy associated with 'cardiomyopathy'. British Heart Journal 38: 504–509

Vincent A, Newsom-Davis J 1979 Absence of anti-acetylcholine receptor antibodies in congenital myasthenia gravis. Lancet 1: 441–442

Vincent A, Cull-Candy S G, Newsom-Davis J, Trautmann A, Moleaar P C, Polak R L 1981 Congenital myasthenia: end-plate acetylcholine receptors and electrophysiology in five cases. Muscle and Nerve 4: 306–318

Vital C, Vallat J-M, Martin F, LeBlanc M, Bergouignan M 1970 Étude clinique et ultrastructurale d'un cas de myopathie centronucléaire (myotubular myopathy) de l'adulte. Revue Neurologique 123: 117–130

Walker B A, Beighton P H, Murdoch J L 1969 The marfanoid hypermobility syndrome. Annals of Internal Medicine 71: 349–352

Walton J N 1956 Amyotonia congenita: a follow-up study. Lancet 1: 1023–1028

Walton J N 1957 The limp child. Journal of Neurology, Neurosurgery and Psychiatry 20: 144–154

Walton J N, Geschwind N, Simpson J A 1956 Benign congenital myopathy with myasthenic features. Journal of Neurology, Neurosurgery and Psychiatry 19:224

Wang P, Clausen T 1976 Treatment of attacks in hyperkalaemic familial periodic paralysis by inhalation of salbutamol. Lancet 1: 221–223

Watters G V, Barlow C F 1967 Acute and subacute neuropathies. Pediatric Clinics of North America 14:997

Weinberg A G, Kirkpatrick J B 1975 Cerebellar hypoplasia in Werdnig–Hoffmann disease. Developmental Medicine and Child Neurology 17: 511–516

Whiteley A M, Schwartz M S, Sachs J A, Swash M 1976 Congenital myasthenia gravis: clinical and HLA studies in two brothers. Journal of Neurology, Neurosurgery and Psychiatry 39: 1145–1150

Willems J A, Monnens L A H, Trijbels J M F, Veerkamp J H, Meyer A E F H, van Dam K, van Haelst U 1977 Leigh's encephalomyelopathy in a patient with cytochrome c oxidase deficiency in muscle tissue. Pediatrics 60: 850–857

Williams J, Hosking G 1985 Type V glycogen storage disease. Archives of Disease in Childhood 60: 1184–1186

Woolf A L 1960 Muscle biopsy in the diagnosis of the

'floppy baby' (infantile hypotonia). Cerebral Palsy Bulletin 2:19

Wynne-Davies R, Lloyd-Roberts G C 1976 Arthrogryposis multiplex congenita: Search for prenatal factors in 66 sporadic cases. Archives of Disease in Childhood 51: 618–623

Wynne-Davies R, Williams P F, O'Connor J C B 1981 The 1960s epidemic of arthrogryposis multiplex congenita: a survey from the United Kingdom, Australia and the United States of America. Journal of Bone and Joint Surgery 63B: 76–82

Yamaguchi M, Robson R M, Stromer M H, Dahl D S, Oda T 1982 Nemaline myopathy rod bodies: structure and composition. Journal of the Neurological Sciences 56: 35–56

Yudell A, Gomez M R, Lambert E H, Dockerty M B 1967 The neuropathy of sulfatide lipidosis (metachromatic leukodystrophy). Neurology (Minneapolis) 17:103

Yuill G M, Lynch P G 1974 Congenital non-progressive peripheral neuropathy with arthrogryposis multiplex. Journal of Neurology, Neurosurgery and Psychiatry 37: 316–323

Zellweger H, Schneider H J 1968 Syndrome of hypotonia–hypomentia–hypogonadism–obesity (O) or Prader–Willi syndrome. American Journal of Diseases of Children 115:588

Zlotogora J, Ben Ezra D, Livni N, Ashkenazi A, Cohen T 1983 A muscle disorder as presenting symptom in a child with mucolipidosis IV. Neuropediatrics 14: 104–105

The medical and psychological management of neuromuscular disease (including strategies for therapeutic trials)

INTRODUCTION

This chapter deals with the practical medical (including psychological) management of patients with neuromuscular diseases for which there is, as yet, no effective drug treatment. The muscular dystrophies, as a group of diseases to consider as an example, present a major challenge to research and a still greater burden for the sufferers and their families. Similar considerations apply to the spinal muscular atrophies and to many of the congenital myopathies. Although most are inherited, the muscular dystrophies raise questions about the extent in the pathogenesis to which events in postnatal life may have an important influence on the course of the disease. Examples of these changes following specific actions are the localised hypertrophy of muscle which may accompany increased use, or atrophy which may follow the immobilisation necessary for the healing of an injury to an adjacent bone or joint. What is *primary* is difficult to distinguish from what is *secondary*. Of particular scientific interest are the apparently exceptional circumstances of a benign course of Duchenne muscular dystrophy in a patient with growth hormone deficiency (Zatz & Frotta-Pessoa 1981, Zatz et al 1981). Clearly, in this instance, as in the interpretation of reports of apparently positive treatment trials, it is necessary to be convinced that the patients really had muscular dystrophy (as against a disease such as an inflammatory myopathy which could recover spontaneously) and, if so, which type (Duchenne or the more benign Becker type). In the clinical description of these diseases (Gardner-Medwin 1980) some of the appearances including the deformities may be more secondary to disuse (or neglect) rather than 'primary' or specific to the condition. These diseases are as yet *incurable* as far as the correction of the underlying genetic defect is concerned but they are eminently *treatable* (Siegel 1978) to a degree which can have profound effects on the quality of life for the sufferers and their families and indeed on life expectancy.

The approach followed in this chapter is to emphasise the benefits to patients and their families which can follow meticulous attention to detail in dealing promptly and efficiently with the treatable manifestations. Seeking underlying causes in such chronic incurable diseases is very difficult. For the physician-investigator responsible for such patients, it is essential to eliminate as many secondary complications of weakness, posture, or altered nutrition or energy exchanges so that the primary disorder can be kept in focus. For the patients and their families there is much support and benefit to be gained from involvement in a research programme.

The effect of the disease on family life

The presence in a family of a patient with Duchenne muscular dystrophy creates great stress and anxiety in addition to a host of practical problems (Firth 1983, Firth et al 1983). In more than a few families there are two brothers with the same diagnosis because the cause of delayed walking or muscle weakness in the elder boy had not been diagnosed by the time the second son was conceived. With the diagnosis confirmed in the index case it is usual for the second to be diagnosed at an earlier age, although this is scarcely a consolation or help. Mobilisation of family, neighbourhood and social resources usually follows, although some families remain isolated and disadvantaged. The Muscular Dystrophy Group of Great Britain and equivalent organisations in other countries provide an important practical source of education and support, as well as an opportunity to work towards the goal of rational treatment of the disease and, where possible, its prevention.

Through the ministrations and advice of the welfare services and other committees run by charity organisations, patients can share the experience of dealing with practical problems in everyday life. They also learn of the benefits of involvement in integrated treatment programmes which combine rational and critical trials of putative therapeutic agents while sustaining the highest standard of care. Muscular dystrophy clinics have a valuable role in giving a specialist diagnostic service and genetic counselling. Perhaps the greatest value of the muscular dystrophy charities is the way in which a greater awareness is created, as a result of fund-raising publicity as well as by specifically educational material, in what are admittedly rare diseases. Not surprisingly, the existing medical services are unfamiliar with the special problems of the disabled patient with muscular dystrophy. The patient's family doctor may be at a disadvantage because he or she has never had personal experience of managing the disease. Too often, in the past, families were frustrated by the time taken to secure a specialist opinion and thence a diagnosis. Then, when given the bad news, they gained the impression that nothing could be done and were left with the burden of caring while waiting for the premature death of their offspring. Here it is necessary to be sensitive in recommending literature for patients which describes the course and complications of the disease. Inevitably the literature needs to provide information which is relevant to the problems of patients at varying stages ('cross-sectional' information with regard to the population of patients). It is far more difficult (and potentially more hurtful for the family) to write about the progression, as the time course of the disease can vary from one patient to the next and, most importantly, depends on how vigorously the patient and his family determine to avoid complications. It can be helpful to remind the parents, on being informed of the diagnosis (first in a provisional form, to be confirmed after a period of observation) that their child has not changed at all *that day* as a consequence of the diagnosis.

Important psychological 'milestones' for the family

Suspicion. A family may suspect that a child is later in walking than other sibs or those of friends. On average 50 per cent of patients with Duchenne muscular dystrophy do not walk until after 18 months (Gardner-Medwin 1980). Later the child is seen to lag behind, tire easily or fall over while playing, so that comparison with other children creates anxiety that there may be a loco-motor disorder.

Diagnosis. The confirmation of the parents' suspicion by a specialist may leave them numbed and frightened with confused emotions of denial, rejection and perhaps several of those reactions through which the recently bereaved pass. For the parents of a child with muscular dystrophy, as for the bereaved, it is important to work through these emotions by articulating fears, resentments and worries to a sympathetic person who can explain in an honest but positive way what lies ahead, while suggesting means by which the family achieve a 'coping strategy'. What is *not* helpful, and indeed a dereliction of the medical advisor's duty, is to present the diagnosis and leave the family unsupported. It is illogical and unkind to change the attitudes of the parents to their child as a result of telling them of what may happen at some future date. For the time being the realisation that their child is not as others is the first step towards rational coping with their problem. The next is to ensure that they realise that what may happen in the future and, indeed, the time-scale over which deterioration can occur, is going to depend on how the problems of the present are dealt with from day to day. It is there-fore in a spirit of determination to face and over-come difficulties as they occur that the family can afford to be optimistic in their endeavours to support research for effective treatment. What is understandable, but less than satisfactory, is the wish for a 'cure' which will put all to rights without any effort on the part of the patient or his family to prevent or to correct complications.

Schooling. Considerable anxieties occur over the question of schooling. Ideally, the aim should be to provide schooling of the educational stan-dard which the patient's intellectual endowment allows him to attain, while sustaining the necessary care in the form of physiotherapy and orthotics. Important for the child's emotional development is the opportunity for him to take part in as many experiences as possible with normal children of similar age. Clearly impaired intellectual capacity (and there is a 20% downward shift in the distribution of intelligence quotients in Duchenne dystrophy) and increasing physical disability make it more difficult to attain these aims (Gardner-Medwin 1980). Nevertheless, some patients with severe disability show talent in drawing or other non-physically demanding activi-ties, such as computer studies, and this should be strongly encouraged.

Loss of walking capability. On average this occurs at 9.5 years of age (range 7–14, Gardner-Medwin 1980) but for some it occurs much earlier, particularly if there is an additional factor such as severe intercurrent illness, limb fracture or if the patient is overweight.

The handling of this anxiety and the realisation of deterioration demands sympathetic under-standing on the part of the medical advisors. The wheelchair, or perhaps the earlier attempts to maintain walking by long leg calipers, is seen as a threat and offends further the bruised image of the child's normality. For the child and the family a booklet such as Irwin Siegel's *Everybody's different, nobody's perfect* (Siegel 1982) is a helpful reminder that 'perfection', as a concept of body image of oneself or of one's offspring, is unreal-istic and potentially damaging. Rather than see one specific day when the patient takes to calipers or wheelchair, a more positive management strategy is to introduce a variety of aids to sustain a broad range of normal activities for as long as possible. Calipers are a means to the end of preventing contractures and sustaining upright standing posture, as well as for walking (Heckmatt et al 1985). When walking is not practical these provide the valuable alternative to a standing frame (or a 'hip guidance orthosis') which allows the patient to stand for several hours while participating in school work or recreational activi-ties such as drawing. The wheelchair is introduced as a means to improve mobility, to enable the patient to keep up with the family on outings and to reduce the effort of struggling to walk from place to place. It is this last point that has to be borne in mind when encouraging the patient to continue to persevere with such orthotic aids as are available. I well remember a boy who had been carefully managed with appropriate orthopaedic care (physiotherapy, tenotomy, calipers) and who had gone into a wheelchair some six months earlier. He was profoundly weak but had no contractures and I considered that with weight reduction (see below) he could well be able to stand again and possibly even walk with calipers. When this was put as a possible objective to him — he was then nine years of age — he made it very clear that he did not want to walk again because it was too much effort and he was afraid of falling. This last point cannot be ignored, because a fall in a patient who has been fitted with long leg calipers to overcome weakness in the lower limbs can result in a greater impact than when the legs simply give way, with the consequential risk of fracture of the long bones of the upper limbs and skull. The feeling of being insecure or of being at risk of falling is distressing for the patient. For strangers (even nurses or other paramedical professional staff) who want to help, sound advice is to ask the patient how he wishes to be moved or positioned and it is as well to observe how the family carries out transfers or other movements. This is important not only to avoid unnecessary discomfort but also to avoid embarrassment to the patient.

Possibility of corrective surgery for spinal deformity in Duchenne dystrophy

This important recent therapeutic intervention offers great advantages (Drennan 1984, Sussman 1984 and see Ch. 22) but also poses particular problems for the patient and the family. As a boy sees his contemporaries go forward for 'the operation' he is faced with the realisation that the way ahead for him is either going through with major surgery or letting the opportunity pass. (This is a relatively brief 'window' of perhaps 1–2 years between the time that there begins to be significant spinal curvature — usually after he has passed through the adolescent growth spurt at a mean age of about 12 years — and before deformity or deterioration in general physical condition, especially respiratory function (Rideau et al 1981, 1984, Kurtz et al 1983) precludes major surgery.) As never before, the patient is forced to consider his own disease and prognosis if he is to

participate (as he is entitled to) in the decision of whether or not to proceed to spinal surgery. Fortunately the Luque operation allows early mobilisation and patients do tolerate the surgery well. By now, the accumulated experience from personal diaries kept over the period and written after surgery, indicates that boys are pleased with the result because of improved head control, posture and appearance. These impressions are rapidly and clearly conveyed from the patient who has undergone the Luque procedure to those awaiting a decision and this gives encouragement.

The period in hospital, however, can be a very stressful one for the family, not least because not all the orthopaedic units at which the Luque procedure is carried out have the necessary nursing and ancillary experience as yet to cope with the special needs of patients with Duchenne dystrophy. (In contrast to those undergoing spinal surgery for idiopathic scoliosis.) In particular there are the difficulties with feeding, respiration and bowel and bladder care. Such procedures have been carried out in orthopaedic units with extensive experience of Harrington rod instrumentation for idiopathic scoliosis. The patients with the latter condition are usually otherwise fit and well with normal or near-normal muscle function and capabilities for feeding, coughing, and bowel and bladder action.

For the patient who is unwilling or unsuited for the operation, there is a continuing need to try to prevent spinal curvature by orthotic jackets (Falewski de Leon 1984, Young et al 1984) or moulded wheelchair inserts (Moseley 1984).

The later years. It is distressing for the patient to see his contemporaries deteriorating and eventually dying while he becomes aware of his own progressive weakness and further disability. So far, little has been done formally to explore the attitudes of the patient to his impending demise. My own discussions with individuals who have approached their end with more or less equanimity indicate a progressive weariness with the struggles of life. Occasionally there may be respiratory distress associated with respiratory muscle weakness or fatigue. Cardiac failure, which may dominate the final illness in a few patients, is liable to cause dyspnoea, orthopnoea and abdominal discomfort due to hepatic congestion. Spinal curvature and other deformities due to contracture formation can result in discomfort, e.g. between the lower ribs and the iliac crest on the concave side of the spinal curvature. Apart from these sources of discomfort or distress there is no pain and it is both kind and helpful to discuss this with the patient. To realise that the end may come as a sleep without waking is a comfort. To sleep and not to wake up is the end to be expected, as studies made recently indicate arterial desaturation associated especially with periods of REM sleep (Soudon et al 1985).

In *How briefly my son* Joan Neville described (Neville 1962) the last illness of her son with Duchenne muscular dystrophy, who died of pneumonia 12 days before he would have become 13 years of age. Today in the UK and other countries of Europe or North America there must be very very few patients with Duchenne muscular dystrophy who die as young as this. Thanks to antibiotics, physiotherapy, nursing care and spinal surgery, the life expectancy has increased by eight to 10 years, so much so that it would be unwise and unkind for the doctor to attempt to be too precise in predicting the eventual life expectancy. Rather, it is to be hoped that by dealing promptly and appropriately with each problem, the illness which could be the last may be averted to some future date. As with changes in the clinical features of the 'final illness', since the introduction of antibiotics, there may be a change in the near future owing to the introduction of the Luque operation to stabilise the spine: in consequence, cardiac failure may become a more important management problem in the older boys with Duchenne muscular dystrophy, as it is well recognised that the heart is affected to a greater or lesser degree (Danilowicz et al 1980, Hunter 1980, Nigro et al 1983) in this disease.

Pathogenesis of secondary changes in neuromuscular diseases

It is widely believed that there is a defect in the muscle cell membrane in most if not all forms of muscular dystrophy (Rowland 1984). This results in increased permeability with loss of cell components (notably creatine kinase) to the extracellular fluid and influx of calcium ions down the concentration gradient. The consequent rise in the intracellular calcium concentration (Jackson et al 1985a) can set in train a series of self-perpetuating processes which can result in cellular damage, activation of phospholipase A (Tagesson & Henriksson 1984), with resulting formation of prostaglandins which have not only further effects on cell membrane permeability but also, from animal studies, appear to influence protein synthesis and breakdown (Goldberg et al 1984). Free radicals may be formed as a consequence of the non-specific damage caused by calcium influx with the possibility of ensuing cell membrane damage (Jackson et al 1985b). These mechanisms appear to be capable of self-perpetuating damage to the muscle cell (Fig. 21.1) which responds well in the early stages by adaptive changes such as stimulating protein synthesis to meet the demands of increased protein breakdown — as indicated by the increased urinary excretion of 3-methyl-histidine (Mussini et al 1984). Failure of the muscle cell to continue to be successful with this adaptation leads to atrophy and at this stage there is a significant reduction in protein synthesis rate (Rennie et al 1982).

Compounding the damaging effect on muscle cell chemistry are the possible consequences of contractile activity. Further damage can affect sarcomere structure and cell membranes, particularly as a result of eccentric contraction — contraction made to resist a lengthening stress on the muscle as in stepping down or walking downhill (Newham et al 1983). The muscles most affected by this form of contraction (which is to be contrasted with less damaging 'concentric' contraction in which the muscle shortens, as in stepping up) are the proximal muscles controlling the posture of the axial skeleton and the shoulder and pelvic girdles against the forces of gravity and inertia (Edwards et al 1984c).

MANAGEMENT STRATEGIES

The aim is to prevent secondary complications in the hope that an effective drug therapy may become available in time to help the patient. Implicit in this approach is the recognition that,

PROPOSED MECHANISMS OF MUSCLE DAMAGE

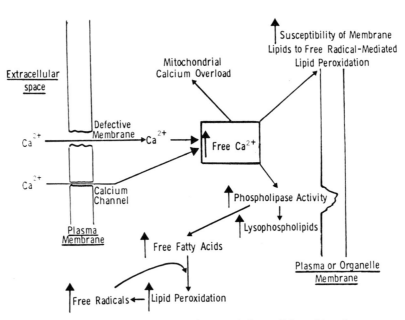

Fig. 21.1 Illustrative summary of current hypotheses on how increase in intracellular calcium ions may result in self-perpetuating damage to essential cellular processes (Jackson et al 1985b). Note that the original cause of the increase in calcium is not specified: the processes described might result if the increased membrane permeability were genetically determined or due to mechanical trauma (Edwards et al 1984c) or other environmental influence

should such a therapy be available tomorrow, it is the patients who are free from deforming contractures and spinal curvatures who would be most likely to benefit. Hence, there is still an important goal for the patients with advanced dystrophy and their families to aim for and that is to take advantage of any future agent which may reverse or ameliorate the dystrophic condition with a view to strengthening the respiratory muscles, e.g. with inspiratory muscle training, (DiMarco et al 1985, Ringel et al 1985) in the hope of sustaining life. The more advanced patients with dystrophy might thus be unable to look forward to walking again but they could expect to go on breathing.

As yet there is no agent which is known to reverse the pathological processes in muscular dystrophy; nevertheless, it is known that dystrophic muscle is not just dying tissue but, rather, shows evidence of regenerative activity of the kind which can be seen in successful recovery from severe muscle destruction, as in polymyositis (Edwards

et al 1979, 1981) or in animal muscle recovering from a nutritional myopathy (Jackson et al 1985b). Whether by seeking to correct the defective gene or its product, the search is on for a means of capitalising on this cellular potential for adaptation and repair (Edwards 1984b). Such research involves learning about the controlling mechanisms for regulating protein synthesis and degradation and for cellular growth and division. The choice of a putative therapeutic agent for trial is now usually a more or less rational attempt to influence a cellular process which is thought to be defective. So far the agents tried have been many and of widely different origin (Dubowitz & Heckmatt 1980). As these authors pointed out, the history of drug trials in muscular dystrophy is typically one of enthusiastic reporting of benefit of some agent used in a poorly controlled trial followed by refutation of the result after one or more better-controlled trials. Such was the recent history of allopurinol as a possible treatment of Duchenne muscular dystrophy (see Table 21.1).

Table 21.1 Classes of therapeutic agents tried in muscular dystrophy (Extended from the review of therapeutic trials presented by Dubowitz & Heckmatt 1980)

Agent or presumed indication	? effect in dystrophy
1 Aminoacids (glycine, leucine and various mixtures)	Protein metabolism in skeletal muscle
2 Anabolic steroids (testosterone or other synthetic derivative)	(as above)
3 Catecholamines (adrenaline)	Action of sympathetic on skeletal muscle
4 Calcium channel blockers (diltiazem, flunarizine, verapamil)	Intracellular calcium in skeletal muscle
5 Corticosteroids	Skeletal muscle damage (serum creatine kinase falls)
6 Dantrolene sodium	Calcium effects on muscle
7 Digitalis or related cardiac glycosides	Contractility of skeletal muscle
8 Energy-affecting agents (nucleotides, allopurinol, fructose D-ribose, L-carnitine, coenzyme Q)	Muscle ATP or substrates
9 Free radical protection agents (superoxide dismutase, vitamin E and selenium)	Damage by free radicals including oxidation
10 Lithium	Membrane stabilisation
11 Oestrogens	Reduce CK, ? anabolic
12 Penicillamine	Reduce collagen formation in dystrophic muscle
13 Thyroid (or synthetic analogue)	Reduce creatine kinase efflux
14 Vasodilators (serotonin antagonists, propranolol)	Reduce tissue ischaemia
15 Vitamins (B6, folic acid, vitamin E)	Nutrition
16 Zinc	Reduce protein breakdown, membrane stabilisation

Perhaps more important than the finding that the drug has no effect on the course of the disease has been the need to discover whether the initial premise (i.e. that there is a significant disorder of muscle energy metabolism) is correct and, if so, whether it is possible beneficially to alter the presumed disorder. In fact it was only the availability of magnetic resonance spectroscopy that made ethical, and therefore possible, a study (with strict double-blind control) which showed that energy metabolism is not greatly abnormal and that such changes that are seen cannot be corrected by allopurinol (Griffiths et al 1985). At this stage of our exploration of possible therapeutic avenues it is important not only to seek reliable criteria for recognising a significant positive result, but also to have clear, unequivocal evidence that a particular therapeutic avenue is, in fact, wrong in principle and not just in the dose of the drug used or in the particular derivative or representative of the class of drug chosen. To recognise the wrong therapeutic avenue is important as it can serve as a guide and a stimulus to seeking more promising alternatives. Unfortunately, very few of the many remedies listed in Table 21.1 are able to show reliable positive or negative results and this means that several of the hypotheses which motivated earlier trials are still 'open' and possibly worthy of further consideration with improved trial design and assessment techniques. In this connection it is worth remembering that Vitamin D is used therapeutically in two dosages which differ by more than two orders of magnitude (British National Formulary 1986). Thus a low dosage of 10 μg (400 units) daily can prevent nutritional osteomalacia in Asians living on unleavened bread or in the elderly living alone. Deficiency of Vitamin D due to intestinal malabsorption or chronic liver disease requires pharmacological doses of up to 1 mg (40 000 units) daily. Patients with renal osteodystrophy can require up to 5 mg (200 000 units) daily, as may patients with hypocalcaemia due to hypoparathyroidism. The possibility exists therefore, if this analogy is valid, that a negative or uncertain result for a substance already subjected to clinical trial may cause it to be eliminated from further consideration when it has not, in fact, been given a trial at an appropriate dosage or mode of administration. This consideration underlines the need for pursuing the pharmacology of any drug to be used in clinical trials (see below).

TRIAL STRATEGIES AND DESIGNS

The general process of drug development can be subdivided into four separate phases (based on Laurence & Black 1978 and Brown 1985): (1) pharmacological studies in human subjects to confirm the wanted effect and to determine the pharmacodynamics and pharmacokinetics; (2) studies in selected patients to confirm therapeutic effects and to study dose response and side-effects; (3) controlled double-blind trial on a larger scale to establish a significant benefit over a placebo or another preparation used previously to treat the condition; (4) a period of assessment after limited release for clinical trial to determine whether there are significant side effects and to give further guidance as to the correct dose utilisation for specific indications. Against this background it would seem that the present preoccupation with large-scale clinical trials is somewhat premature, particularly as there is no identifiable drug effect currently measurable. The methods of assessing disease progress are subject to criticism and debate (Brooke et al 1981, 1983, 1984, Angelini et al 1985). In the justifiable effort to improve the 'power' of clinical trials, clear criteria have been identified, such as the need to demonstrate a significant reduction of 75% in the rate of progress of the disease over a one-year period; to do this a double-blind trial would need to be carried out with with no fewer than 40 patients in each of the test and control groups. This poses real logistic and ethical problems which are well addressed (at no mean cost) in the USA. Behind such commendable scientific rigour is the human fact that the trials are restricted to the young and that half the patients in the trial are taking a placebo rather than a putatively active drug. This means that there are many patients who would like to participate in a treatment trial (and who might benefit physically and psychologically thereby) who are receiving placebo at any one time.

Another approach is to seek alternative yet statistically valid experimental designs (Armitage 1985, Bather 1985) and to follow the strategy that something can be learned from, and gained by, each and every patient by participation in research. Thus 'Care through Research' is a motto which is easy to understand but the exercise of a rigorous scientific approach to treatment trials is more difficult, although not impossible. In our studies (Edwards 1984b, Edwards et al 1984b), the aim is not so much to see short-term (one-year) effects on the course of the disease but to see if there are (objectively) measured changes in tissue or blood chemistry which can confirm a drug effect on a hypothesised cellular process of (presumed) relevance to the course of the disease. This means that studies of tissue chemistry may be made from various muscles (affected to different degrees) in the same subject with a view to seeing whether the effect, if any, of the drug action is dependent on a particular stage of the disease. Clearly this would be possible only by needle biopsy or magnetic resonance spectroscopy (Edwards 1984a). An example of the approach outlined above was a trial of anabolic steroids in adolescent and young adult patients with muscular dystrophy (Duchenne, Becker and 'limb-girdle'). The rationale for the trial was the observation (Rennie et al 1982) that there is a significantly reduced rate of muscle protein synthesis (measured by infusion of ^{13}C-leucine and determination of the incorporation of the label in needle biopsy samples of muscle) in these patients. The purpose of the trial was to see if an anabolic steroid (Stanozalol®) could increase synthesis rate and, if so, whether there were any observable clinical benefits. The study (Edwards et al 1984a) showed that there was indeed an improved synthesis rate but no increase was noticed in the strength of affected muscles, although some hypertrophy was noticed by one patient in a muscle which had not been thought to have been clinically affected. This raises the interesting question as to whether the possible beneficial effect of anabolic steroids on muscle protein metabolism is mediated through another regulatory mechanism for muscle protein homeostasis, namely the physiological response of hypertrophy to increased force demand as might be predicted from the combined effects of weight training and anabolic steroids in increasing muscle mass in the athletes who abuse these drugs.

It is therefore uncertain whether any of the agents tried (Table 21.1) are effective in achieving an increase in muscle strength and, if so, how this can best be recognised. The practical therapeutic benefits of weight reduction are not only obvious but potentially greater (i.e. improved power/weight ratio) and are seen sooner than the size of the change to be observed in a therapeutic trial. Now that there is evidence that restriction of dietary energy intake does not necessarily result in loss of muscle (Edwards et al 1984d) it can be argued that weight reduction should be included as an essential preliminary to drug evaluation. Certainly it is evident that early weight control, and therefore prevention of obesity, is easier than weight reduction. Our observations of chairbound teenage boys with Duchenne dystrophy suggest that they do not eat more than normal children but, because of their reduced capability for expending energy in physical movement, their requirements may be strikingly reduced. As a guide for estimating the target weight, the greatly reduced muscle mass can be quantitatively obtained from creatinine excretion and isotope dilution (Edmonds et al 1985) and applied to normal (weight) growth curves (Edwards et al 1984d). The result of achieving the appropriate weight is that the patient will appear 'thin' because of loss of subcutaneous and (according to CT observations) intramuscular fat.

PHYSIOTHERAPY IN NEUROMUSCULAR DISEASES

The commonsense principles of physiotherapy in these diseases are care of posture, prevention of contractures, maintenance of muscle strength and preservation of respiration, accompanied by more specific and skilled management with exercises and orthotic aids (Scott et al 1981). The role of exercise is a subject of discussion (de Lateur & Giaconi 1979, Dubowitz et al 1984, Vignos 1984) yet the evidence is to be seen in two ways: the assessment of active therapy, and consideration of possible adverse effects of inactivity or neglect of the basic principles of physiotherapy. In motor

neuron disease some more specific requirements result from the risk of aspiration (Burford & Pentland 1985, Norris et al 1985). Much of the writing on physiotherapy in muscular dystrophy refers to diseases of children but there are additional requirements in adults, not least because of the complicating factor of greater body weight.

PROSPECTS FOR TREATMENT IN MUSCLE DISEASES

This is a time when there are great and rapid advances in the search for the genetic defect in muscle diseases in general and Duchenne dystrophy in particular (Pembrey et al 1984, Bakker et al 1985, Monaco et al 1985). The prospects for reliable methods for carrier detection and antenatal diagnosis (Emery 1980) appear to be very promising: and once the appropriate gene probe is widely available, the problems are logistic and concern the effective provision of genetic advice to those who need it. A further advantage of this new development, more for research than for clinical service, is the opportunity of determining definitively whether patients with apparently similar clinical muscle diseases have, indeed, the same genetic disorder. Already there are indications that similar clinical appearances may be associated with widely different causes, e.g. neurogenic, myopathic and nutritional disorders, or 'mitochondrial myopathy', etc (Walton & Gardner-Medwin 1981, and see Ch. 15).

There are, perhaps, lessons to be learned from the veterinary literature. Recent efforts to improve the production of lean meat efficiently has stimulated research into the production of 'repartitioning agents' which can 'direct' food energy into the deposition of protein in skeletal muscle rather than as fat (Asato et al 1984). This raises the very interesting possibility that such a 'repartitioning' might be of therapeutic benefit in patients with muscular dystrophy; but more work is needed before such an agent can be tried in patients.

The prospect of effective treatment resulting from the new genetics research for existing sufferers seems to be remote. What is contemplated is the progress of this research as a form of 'reverse genetics', in contrast to conventional genetics where the defective gene associated with a well-characterised biochemical abnormality is identified. What is needed once the defective gene is identified and isolated in Duchenne dystrophy is to discover the 'gene product' and to elucidate its physiological function. In the meantime there is every reason to go on with guarded optimism that imaginatively but rigorously constructed therapeutic trials may yet prove effective in helping patients with Duchenne muscular dystrophy and

that the same philosophy applies for the time being in the case of other neuromuscular diseases (Wolf & Lewis 1985).

ACKNOWLEDGEMENT

The research underpinning the experience described in this chapter has been supported generously by the Muscular Dystrophy Group of Great Britain.

REFERENCES

Angelini C, Baron C, Bejato L et al 1985 Italian multicenter therapeutic trials in Duchenne muscular dystrophy III: Results of fructose diet and calcium antagonists. In: Carraro U, Angelini C (eds) Cell biology and clinical management in functional electrostimulation of neurones and muscles. Cleup Editore, Padova, p 235–239

Armitage P 1985 The search for optimality in clinical trials. International Statistical Review 53: 15–24

Asato G, Baker P K, Bass R T et al 1984 Repartitioning agents: 5-[1-Hydroxy-2-(isopropylamino) ethyl] — anthranilonitrile and related phenethanolamines; Agents for promoting growth, increasing muscle accretion and reducing fat deposition in meat producing animals. Agricultural Biological Chemistry 48: 2883–2888

Bakker E, Hofker M H, Goor N et al 1985 Prenatal diagnosis and carrier detection of Duchenne muscular dystrophy with closely linked RFLP's. Lancet i: 655–658

Bather J A 1985 On the allocation of treatments in sequential medical trials. International Statistical Review 53: 1–13

British National Formulary No 11 1986 British Medical Association and Pharmaceutical Society of Great Britain, p 308

Brooke M H, Griggs R C, Mendell J R, Fenichel G M, Shumate J B, Pellegrino R J 1981 Clinical trial in Duchenne muscular dystrophy. 1 The design of the protocol. Muscle and Nerve 4: 186–197

Brooke M H, Fenichel G M, Griggs R C et al 1983 Clinical investigation in Duchenne muscular dystrophy: 2 Determination of the 'power' of therapeutic trials based on the natural history. Muscle and Nerve 6: 91–103

Brooke M H, CIDD Group 1984 Therapeutic trials in Duchenne muscular dystrophy — the scientific difference between 'didn't' and 'doesn't'. Italian Journal of Neurological Sciences 1 (Suppl 3 Muscular dystrophy, facts and perspectives): 127–131

Brown M J 1985 Controlled clinical trials in the assessment of new therapies. Bone 2: 46–47

Burford K, Pentland B 1985 Management of motor neurone disease: the physiotherapist's role. Physiotherapy 71: 402–404

Danilowicz D, Rutkowski M, Myung D, Schively D 1980 Echocardiography in Duchenne muscular dystrophy. Muscle and Nerve 3: 298–303

de Lateur B J, Giaconi R M 1979 Effect on maximal strength of submaximal exercise in Duchenne muscular dystrophy. American Journal of Physical Medicine 56: 26–36

DiMarco A F, Kelling J S, DiMarco M S, Jacobs I. Shields R. Altose M D 1985 The effects of inspiratory resistive training on respiratory muscle function in patients with muscular dystrophy. Muscle and Nerve 8: 284–290

Drennan J C 1984 Surgical management of neuromuscular scoliosis. In: Serratrice S (ed) Neuromuscular diseases. Raven Press, New York, p 551–556

Dubowitz V, Heckmatt J 1980 Management of muscular dystrophy. Pharmacological and physical aspects. British Medical Bulletin 36: 139–144

Dubowitz V, Hyde S A, Scott O M, Goddard C 1984 Controlled trial of exercise in Duchenne muscular dystrophy. In: Serratrice G et al (eds) Neuromuscular diseases. Raven Press, New York, p 571–575

Edmonds C J, Smith T, Griffiths R D, Mackenzie, Edwards R H T 1985 Total body potassium and water, and exchangeable sodium, in muscular dystrophy. Clinical Science 68: 379–385

Edwards R H T 1984a Nuclear magnetic resonance and other new techniques for the study of metabolism in human muscular dystrophy. Italian Journal of Neurological Sciences 1 (Suppl 3 Muscular dystrophy, facts and perspectives): 75–90

Edwards R H T 1984b Exploratory approaches to metabolic treatment of human muscular dystrophy. Italian Journal of Neurological Sciences 1 (Suppl 3 Muscular dystrophy, facts and perspectives): 143–152

Edwards R H T, Wiles C M, Round J M, Jackson M J, Young A 1979 Muscle breakdown and repair in polymyositis: a case study. Muscle and Nerve 2: 223–228

Edwards R H T, Isenberg D A, Wiles C M, Young A, Snaith M L 1981 The investigation of inflammatory myopathy. Journal of the Royal College of Physicians of London 15: 19–24

Edwards R H T, Dworzack F, Gerber P P et al 1984a Anabolic steroids in patients with muscular dystrophy increase muscle protein synthesis measured in vivo with stable isotopes. Journal of Pharmacology and Therapeutics (Abstract)

Edwards R H T, Jones D A, Jackson M J 1984b An approach to treatment trials in muscular dystrophy with particular reference to agents influencing free radical damage. Medical Biology 62: 143–147

Edwards R H T, Newham D J, Jones D A, Chapman S J 1984c Role of mechanical damage in pathogenesis of proximal myopathy in man. Lancet i: 548–552

Edwards R H T, Round J M, Jackson M J, Griffiths R D,

Lilburn M F 1984d Weight reduction in boys with muscular dystrophy. Developmental Medicine and Child Neurology 26: 375–383

Emery A 1980 Duchenne muscular dystrophy — genetic aspects, carrier detection and antenatal diagnosis. British Medical Bulletin 36: 117–122

Falewski de Leon G H 1984 Orthotic jackets for scoliosis. In: Serratrice G et al (eds) Neuromuscular diseases. Raven Press, New York, p 539–543

Firth M A 1983 Diagnosis of Duchenne muscular dystrophy: experiences of parents of sufferers. British Medical Journal 286: 700–701

Firth M A, Gardner-Medwin D, Hosking G, Wilkinson E 1983 Interviews with parents of boys suffering from Duchenne muscular dystrophy. Developmental Medicine and Child Neurology 25: 466–471

Gardner-Medwin D 1980 Clinical features and classification of the muscular dystrophies. British Medical Bulletin 36: 109–115

Goldberg A L, Baracos V, Rodeman P, Waxman L, Dinarello C 1984 Control of protein degradation in muscle by prostaglandins, Ca^{2+}, and leukocytic pyrogen (interleukin 1) Federation Proceedings 43: 1301–1306

Griffiths R D, Cady E B, Edwards R H T, Wilkie D R 1985 Muscle energy metabolism in Duchenne dystrophy studied by 31P NMP: Controlled trials show no effect of allopurinol or ribose. Muscle and Nerve 8: 760–767

Heckmatt J Z, Dubowitz V, Hyde S A, Florence J, Gabain A C, Thompson N 1985 Prolongation of walking in Duchenne muscular dystrophy with lightweight orthoses: review of 57 cases. Developmental Medicine and Child Neurology 27: 149–154

Hunter S 1980 The heart in muscular dystrophy. British Medical Bulletin 36: 133–134

Jackson M J, Jones D A, Edwards R H T 1985a Measurements of calcium and other elements in muscle biopsy samples from patients with Duchenne muscular dystrophy. Clinica Chimica Acta 147: 215–221

Jackson M J, Jones D A, Edwards R H T 1985b Vitamin E and muscle diseases. Journal of Inherited and Metabolic Diseases 8 (Suppl 1): 84–87

Kurtz L T, Mubarak S J, Schultz P, Park S M, Leach J 1983 Correlation of scoliosis and pulmonary function in Duchenne muscular dystrophy. Journal of Pediatric Orthopedics 3: 347–353

Laurence D R, Black J W 1978 The medicine you take — benefits and risks of modern drugs. Collins, Glasgow, p 111–120

Monaco A P, Bertelson C J, Middlesworth W 1985 Detection of deletions spanning the Duchenne muscular dystrophy locus using a tightly linked DNA segment. Nature 316: 842–845

Moseley C F 1984 Natural history and management of scoliosis in Duchenne muscular dystrophy. In: Serratrice G et al (eds) Neuromuscular diseases. Raven Press, New York, p 545–549

Mussini E, Cornelio F, Colombo L et al 1984 Increased myofibrillar protein catabolism in DMD measured by 3-MH excretion in the urine. Muscle and Nerve 7: 388–391

Neville J 1962 So briefly my son. Hutchinson, London, p 1–80

Newham D J, Mc Phail G, Mills K R, Edwards R H T 1983 Ultrastructural changes after concentric and eccentric contractions of human muscle. Journal of the Neurological Sciences 61: 109–122

Nigro G, Comi L, Limongelli F M et al 1983 Prospective study of X-linked progressive muscular dystrophy in Campania. Muscle and Nerve 6: 253–262

Norris F H, Smith R A, Denys E H 1985 Motor neurone disease: towards better care. British Medical Journal 291: 259–262

Pembrey M E, Davies K E, Winter R M et al 1984 Clinical use of DNA markers linked to the gene for Duchenne muscular dystrophy. Archives of Disease in Childhood 59: 208–216

Rennie M J, Edwards R H T, Millward D J, Wolman S L, Halliday D, Matthews D E 1982 Effects of Duchenne muscular dystrophy on muscle protein synthesis. Nature 296: 165–167

Rideau Y, Jankowski L W, Grellet J 1981 Respiratory function in the muscular dystrophies. Muscle and Nerve 4: 155–164

Rideau Y, Glorion B, Delaubier A, Tarle O, Bach J 1984 The treatment of scoliosis in Duchenne muscular dystrophy. Muscle and Nerve 7: 281–286

Ringel S P, Martin R J, Libby L S 1985 Newer treatments of respiratory dysfunction in neuromuscular diseases. In: Carraro U, Angelini C (eds) Cell biology and clinical management in functional electrostimulation of neurones and muscles. Cleup Editore, Padova, p 217–221

Rowland L P 1984 The membrane theory of Duchenne dystrophy: Where is it? Italian Journal of Neurological Sciences 1 (Suppl 3 Muscular dystrophy, facts and perspectives): 13–28

Scott O M, Hyde S A, Goddard C, Dubowitz V 1981 Prevention of deformity in Duchenne muscular dystrophy — A prospective study of passive stretching and splintage. Physiotherapy 67: 177–180

Siegel I M 1978 The management of muscular dystrophy: a clinical review. Muscle and Nerve 1: 453–460

Siegel I M 1982 Everybody's different, nobody's perfect. Muscular Dystrophy Association America/Muscular Dystrophy Group of Great Britain, p 1–13

Sussman M D 1984 Advantage of early spinal stabilization and fusion in patients with Duchenne muscular dystrophy. Journal of Paediatric Orthopaedics 4: 532–537

Soudon P, Wouters A, Kulakowski S 1985 Transcutaneous monitoring during and ventilatory function in X-linked progressive muscular dystrophies. (Personal communication)

Tagesson C, Henriksson K G 1984 Elevated phospholipase A in Duchenne dystrophy. Muscle and Nerve 7: 260–261

Vignos P 1984 Exercise in neuromuscular disease: statement of the problem. In: Serratrice G et al (eds) Neuromuscular diseases. Raven Press, p 565–569

Walton J N, Gardner-Medwin D 1981 Progressive muscular dystrophy and the myotonic disorders. In: Disorders of voluntary muscle, 4th edn. Churchill Livingstone, Edinburgh, p 481–524

Wolf S, Lewis N J (eds) 1985 Clinical trials in chronic neuromuscular diseases. Muscle and Nerve 8: 453–492

Young A, Johnson D, O'Gorman E, Macmillan T, Chase A P 1984 A new spinal brace for use in Duchenne muscular dystrophy. Developmental Medicine and Child Neurology 26: 808–813

Zatz M, Betti R T B, Levy J A 1981 Benign Duchenne muscular dystrophy in a patient with growth hormone deficiency. American Journal of Medical Genetics 10: 301–304

Zatz M, Frota-Pessoa O 1981 Suggestion for a possible mitigating treatment of Duchenne muscular dystrophy. American Journal of Medical Genetics 10: 305–307

The orthopaedic management of neuromuscular disease

INTRODUCTION

The orthopaedic management of patients with neuromuscular disorders is aimed at obtaining the maximum quality of life by preventing deformity or treating it when it has occurred. It is also possible that in certain disorders the prevention and treatment of scoliosis may be associated with an improved prognosis, but orthopaedic treatment will not do anything for the underlying neuromuscular disorder.

The vast majority of patients treated are children, although adults (e.g., following a stroke) may also require orthopaedic management. That problem is beyond the scope of this chapter.

Multi-disciplinary approach

Ideally, the patient should be treated via a multi-disciplinary approach. The members of the team will depend on the disease, e.g., in spina bifida, a team could consist of a paediatric surgeon, neurologist, orthopaedic surgeon, physiotherapist, occupational therapist, orthotist and social worker; whereas in cerebral palsy essential members of the team include a paediatric neurologist or paediatrician, speech therapist, teacher, orthopaedic surgeon, orthotist, occupational therapist, physiotherapist, social worker and, depending on the associated abnormalities, the child may require help with hearing, vision or perceptual difficulties. For the dystrophies, other myopathies and spinal muscular atrophies, essential members of the team include a paediatric neurologist, orthopaedic surgeon, clinical geneticist, orthotist, occupational therapist and physiotherapist.

Diagnosis

Early diagnosis of the affected child is important: it relieves parental anxiety and allows early counselling, which is particularly important in hereditary conditions. The methods of diagnosis are beyond the scope of this chapter, but unfortunately, diagnosis is often delayed. Retrospective analysis of patients with Duchenne muscular dystrophy referred to our Muscle Clinic after a diagnosis had been made showed an average delay of two years (range 0–6 years). Many of these children had been 'treated' for clumsiness, abnormal gait and flat feet for months or years before the diagnosis was made (Read & Galasko 1986). The diagnosis of an underlying neuromuscular disorder should be considered in patients presenting with these non-specific complaints.

Assessment

Before embarking upon treatment, these children require a detailed assessment. This includes an assessment of their overall functional capability (Table 22.1), of their muscle power, the range of movement of each joint and measurement of any joint contractures. All deformities must be noted and the ability of the child to co-operate determined. This will depend on the intelligence of the child, his or her physical development, the psychological approach of the child and the

Table 22.1 Functional assessment in neuromuscular disease

Grade	Functional ability
1	Walks; climbs stairs without assistance
2	Walks; climbs stairs with aid of rail
3	Walks; unable to climb stairs; able to get out of chair
4	Walks unassisted; able to get out of chair
5	Walks with assistance of calipers
6	Stands in calipers; unable to walk with assistance or calipers
7	In wheelchair; can roll chair
8	In wheelchair; able to perform bed and chair activities
9	In wheelchair; sits erect with support. Minimal activities
10	In bed; unable to perform activities of daily living

family, and the age of the child. This assessment is usually carried out by the physiotherapist, and is repeated at regular intervals. As part of our initial assessment we obtain an erect antero-posterior X-ray of the spine, an X-ray of the pelvis and, in patients who can co-operate, lung function tests.

Deformity

The deformities vary in the different diseases (Galasko 1977) and will be discussed separately.

Several mechanisms may be involved in their development (Table 22.2).

Table 22.2 Mechanisms of development of deformity in neuromuscular disease

Muscle imbalance

Unequal growth of fibrotic muscle and adjacent bone

Gravity plus weak musculature

Pressure, e.g. bed clothes

Provided that the agonists and antagonists acting on a joint are balanced, deformity tends not to occur, irrespective of whether the muscles are hypertrophied, spastic, normal or weak. If there is imbalance between the power of the agonist and antagonist the joint will be pulled in the direction of the more powerful muscle. This occurs if one muscle is spastic and the other normal, one is normal and the antagonist is weak or both muscles are weak but to different degrees. The redundant capsule and ligaments fibrose on the contracted side of the joint, producing secondary joint contractures. At this stage, rebalancing the muscles will not correct the deformity: a soft-tissue release is also required. In the growing child, if the muscles are attached beyond a growth plate, the bone will tend to be deformed in the direction of the more powerful muscle. Treatment will depend on the stage of deformity but techniques include tendon division (tenotomy), elongation, transfer, soft tissue release, osteotomy and arthrodesis.

Fibrotic muscle grows more slowly than the adjacent bone. This may be responsible for the deformity, and probably is the main cause of recurrence. Before embarking upon surgical correction, the family, and the patient (if old enough), must appreciate that the deformity may recur and that the operation may have to be repeated before growth has ceased. Postoperatively, in most circumstances, the patient is provided with night splints in an attempt to prevent recurrence of the deformity, and ideally patients should wear the night splints until growth has ceased.

The aetiology of scoliosis, which is a common complication of many neuromuscular disorders, is not fully understood. One of the factors responsible for progressive scoliosis is the effect of gravity on a trunk with weak musculature. The process may be started by the patient leaning to one side to support his trunk. Gravity may also be partly responsible for the common development of equinovarus deformities in wheelchair-bound patients.

Local pressure on an area with gross muscle weakness may also produce deformity. The pressure of bedclothes may be sufficient to produce an equinus deformity in a flail foot.

The type of deformity varies in the different conditions and depends on which muscle groups are affected as well as the other factors discussed above. Table 22.3 contrasts the incidence of scoliosis treated by spinal fusion, dislocation of the hip and subluxation requiring surgery in patients with Duchenne dystrophy and cerebral palsy followed for one to five years.

Table 22.3 Comparison of spinal and hip surgery required in Duchenne muscle dystrophy and cerebral palsy

Disease	No. patients	No. undergone spinal fusion	No. patients with dislocated hips	No. patients requiring surgery for progressive subluxation of hip
Duchenne	138	19	0	0
Cerebral palsy	135	5	9	18 (bilateral in 9)

DUCHENNE MUSCULAR DYSTROPHY

This is the commonest of the neuromuscular disorders considered in this chapter. It is associ-

ated with progressive and rapid increase in weakness, most of the boys losing their ability to walk independently between the ages of eight and 11 years. Most die in their late teens from respiratory infection or cardiomyopathy.

Discussion with the parents of boys attending our Muscle Clinic indicated that there are four main areas of concern where orthopaedic management may help:

(1) Delay in diagnosis.
(2) Loss of independent ambulation.
(3) Scoliosis.
(4) Foot deformity.

Delay in diagnosis (see above)

Gardner-Medwin (1979) reported that in the UK the average age at diagnosis was 5.8 years, and in the US the average time which elapsed between initial parental concern and ultimate diagnosis was 3.0 years (range 1.5–5.5 years) (Crisp et al 1982). In our study (Read & Galasko 1986) the average age of diagnosis was 5.2 years (range 1.5 to 9 years). Although the condition is hereditary, many parents were not aware of their family background until the diagnosis was made in their son (Read & Galasko 1986).

The diagnosis is unlikely to be missed if the possibility of muscle dystrophy is considered when a boy is late in walking, is clumsy, has difficulty with climbing stairs or running, has a tendency to fall often or his walking deteriorates.

Mobility

Many parents stated that the morale of their son deteriorated significantly when he lost the ability to walk independently. Provision of calipers can maintain weight-bearing for several years (Spencer & Vignos 1962, Roy & Gibson 1970, Miller & Dunn 1982, Heckmatt et al 1985). However, the calipers must be fitted before the boy goes off his feet. It is extremely difficult to mobilise a child with Duchenne dystrophy once he is chairbound, in contrast to many other neuromuscular disorders. The orthoses are usually prescribed when the child is still able to walk on the flat, but cannot climb stairs or get out of a chair. The patient uses them for 20–30 minutes each day, and as he goes off his feet he gradually becomes more dependent upon them.

Several types of calipers are available, but they all rely on extending the hip, either with an elasticated strap or an ischial seat (Fig. 22.1). The patient leans back, tightening the Y ligament, stabilising the hips.

Frequently, these patients lose their independent ambulation after they have been confined to bed for an intercurrent illness, following an operation or as a result of injury. In general terms, they should not be confined to bed. Fractures should be treated by plaster of Paris or lightweight casts and immediate mobilisation. If a child is operated on in the morning, he should be stood with the help of the physiotherapist that afternoon. If surgery is carried out in the afternoon he should be stood the following morning.

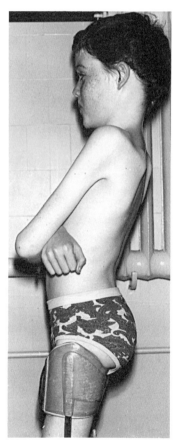

Fig. 22.1 The type of caliper most frequently used in Duchenne muscular dystrophy. The ischial-bearing moulded thigh piece allows the patient to lean back, extending and stabilising his hips. It also produces a lumbar lordosis

Not every child, nor every family, will accept calipers. They are cumbersome and slow the patient down. Some centres prefer to prescribe a wheelchair to allow the boy to keep up with his peers. Learning to use calipers requires a lot of effort and, unless the family co-operates, the child will not succeed.

Scoliosis

This is the most important and most serious deformity that can occur in these patients. It is not just a cosmetic deformity, but is associated with significant morbidity. In Duchenne dystrophy, like many other neuromuscular disorders, the scoliosis eventually involves the pelvis and results in an increasing pelvic obliquity. The patient can no longer sit squarely and weight is increasingly taken on one buttock and subsequently the lumbar spine. Sitting becomes uncomfortable and the patient is confined to bed, not because of the underlying neuromuscular disorder, but as a result of the progressive scoliosis. Hsu (1983) reported that progression of the curve beyond 40 degrees was associated with diminished sitting tolerance and use of the arms and hands to prop the body up when seated. Furthermore, the scoliosis continues to deteriorate after growth has ceased, probably due to the effect of gravity.

Progressive scoliosis is also associated with diminished lung function. Kurz and colleagues (1983) showed that the vital capacity peaked at approximately the age when standing ceased and then declined rapidly. Age and thoracic scoliosis together were better predictors of the forced vital capacity (FVC) than either one alone. The vital capacity deteriorated approximately 4% for each year of life after the patient became wheelchair bound. For every 10 degrees of thoracic scoliosis there was an additional 4% loss of vital capacity.

Obesity is another factor which may affect pulmonary function. It is important that the parents and the patient understand the complications of obesity. Because of the loss of muscle bulk, the ideal weight of these patients is less than the normal for their height and age (Edwards et al 1984).

Prevention. The scoliosis increases with increasing age (Gibson & Wilkins 1975). Under

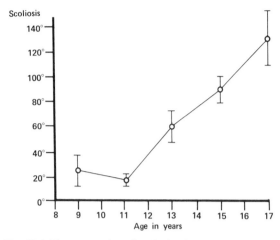

Fig. 22.2 The progression of scoliosis with increasing age in patients with Duchenne muscular dystrophy

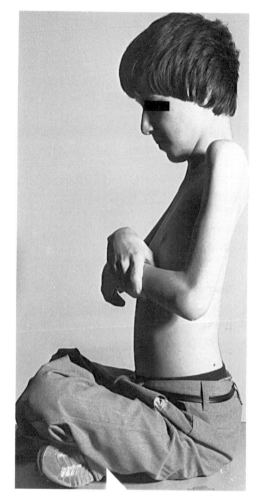

Fig. 22.3 Lordotic posture due to fibrotic extension contracture of the spine in a patient who was no longer ambulant

the age of eight years scoliosis is uncommon. This is thought to be due to the lordotic posture adopted by patients who are still mobile. Once the patient is confined to a wheelchair the curve deteriorates rapidly (Fig. 22.2). Very rarely, patients develop fibrotic extension contractures of the spine, with fixed lordosis and a mild scoliosis (Gibson & Wilkins 1975). Two of our 138 patients have developed such a contracture (Fig. 22.3). Provision of calipers not only maintains mobility, but also seems to maintain the lordotic posture (Fig. 22.1) and slows the development of scoliosis (Fig. 22.4). At the age of 13 years the mean curve in our chairbound patients was 62 ± 12 degrees, compared with 13 ± 3 degrees in patients who were still mobile in their orthoses.

Standing, even when the patient is no longer mobile, may protect the spine (Miller & Dunn 1982). We now encourage our patients to stand for two to three hours per day, even when they are no longer independently mobile in their calipers. When they are no longer stable in the calipers we provide them with a swivel walker or standing frame (Fig. 22.5).

Several centres have tried to modify the wheelchair to maintain a lordotic posture. If the back of the chair is made to recline at about 20–25 degrees, and is made from a soft material that surrounds the trunk when the child leans back, it may support the spine and hold it straight. Alternative designs include the use of a moulded lumbar lordosis in the reclined back (Gibson et al

1975). However, this design of chair has major disadvantages. Because the patient is reclining, he is further away from his work surfaces, both at school and at home. In practice it has proved extremely difficult to raise work surfaces to the patient's level, so that he has to lean forwards, adopting a kyphotic posture and putting his spine at risk. As a result, the use of these modified wheelchairs has been largely abandoned, as they have not controlled the progressive scoliosis (Fig. 22.6).

The arms of the wheelchair are sometimes removed to allow the child easier access to the wheels. This situation results in further lack of support to the trunk, the patient leaning to the

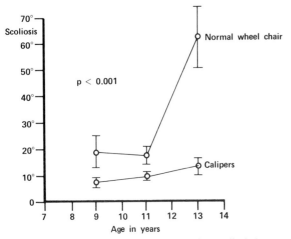

Fig. 22.4 The effect of calipers in preventing scoliosis in patients with Duchenne muscular dystrophy. Patients who wore calipers had a significantly smaller curve than those confined to a wheelchair

side, and may start the scoliotic process. It is essential that arm rests are fitted to the wheelchair to provide maximum support. These patients need powered chairs with a central control to obviate the necessity of leaning to one side (Fig. 22.7)

A variety of spinal orthoses have been tried. They may slow the scoliotic process, but there are inherent difficulties with these orthoses: because the patients are sedentary the orthoses are more difficult to fit and tend to ride up even if carefully moulded; they are often uncomfortable and, if they are too well fitting, may interfere with respiration; many patients will not use them regularly. Our results (Fig. 22.6) show that they slow the progression of the curve but do not prevent it; this may partly be due to lack of patient co-operation.

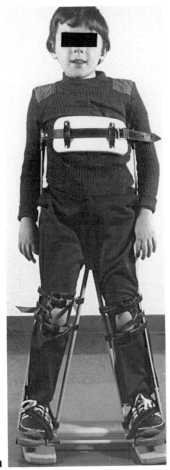
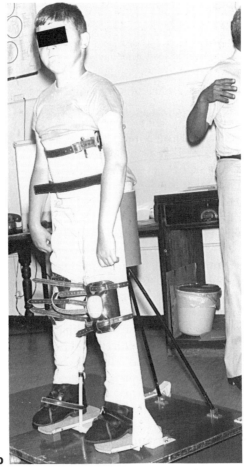

Fig. 22.5 a. Use of a swivel walker in a patient with Duchenne muscular dystrophy who is no longer able to stand with calipers. b. Modified swivel walker for use as a standing frame

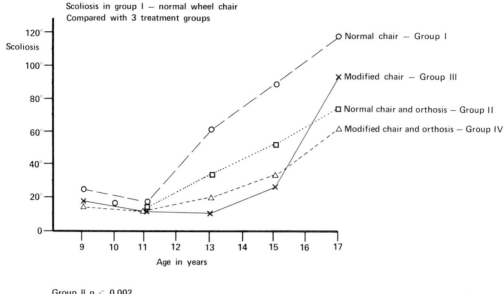

Scoliosis in group I — normal wheel chair
Compared with 3 treatment groups

○ Normal chair — Group I

✕ Modified chair — Group III

□ Normal chair and orthosis — Group II

△ Modified chair and orthosis — Group IV

Group I vs.
Group II p < 0.002
Group III p < 0.001
Group IV p < 0.001

Fig. 22.6 The effect of spinal orthoses and modified wheelchairs on the progression of scoliosis in Duchenne muscular dystrophy. Although there was some slowing of the rate of progression of the scoliosis, these forms of treatment did not prevent the development of a severe deformity

Treatment. Once a scoliosis has developed, the use of a modified chair or orthosis may slow the progression of the curve, but will not prevent it (Fig. 22.6). Seeger and colleagues (1984) reported that modular seats and custom-moulded seats had no effect on the rate of progression of the curve in patients of 14 years of age and older. Furthermore, once the curve has reached 45–50 degrees it deteriorates rapidly.

The optimum treatment for a progressive curve is surgical stabilisation of the spine. However, in Duchenne dystrophy the patient may no longer be fit for surgery because of rapid and progressive deterioration in lung function by the time he has developed a major curve. Fig. 22.8 shows the X-rays of a patient in whom spinal stabilisation was advised when the curve was 34 degrees and he was fit for surgery: the operation was refused as he had minimal side-effects from the curve. Nine months

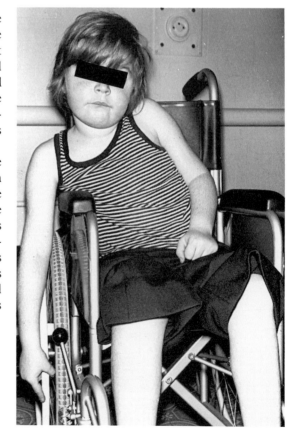

Fig. 22.7 With a manual chair the patient tends to lean to the side to propel the chair. This may start the scoliotic process, and is worsened if the arms of the chair are removed to provide easier access to the wheels. These patients should be provided with powered chairs, with a central control to obviate the necessity of leaning to one side

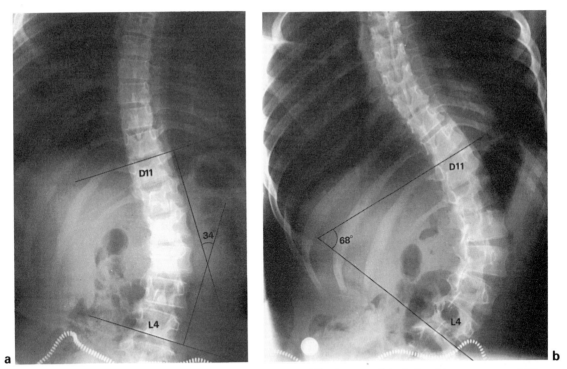

Fig. 22.8 Patient with Duchenne muscular dystrophy. a. Surgical stabilisation was advised when his curve measured 34 degrees, and he was fit for surgery. Operation was refused. b. Nine months later the curve had progressed to 68 degrees. Surgery was requested by the family, but the patient's pulmonary function had deteriorated to such an extent that he was no longer fit for the operation

later the curve had doubled, sitting was becoming awkward because of the associated pelvic obliquity, and surgery was requested; but he was no longer fit, his vital capacity having fallen to 19% of normal. The concept of 'prophylactic' surgery has therefore been developed, i.e. stabilisation of the spine when the patient is still fit for major surgery even though the curve is relatively small. The optimum time to stabilise the spine in a patient with Duchenne dystrophy is soon after he loses his ability to walk independently, when his lung function is adequate for major spinal surgery, before he has developed cor pulmonale or severe cardiomyopathy and when his curve is still mobile and preferably less than 30 degrees. Despite the risks of major surgery in these children it is the author's opinion that such prophylactic surgery is extremely worth while, in avoiding the problems associated with a late severe scoliosis.

The patients require a six-monthly erect X-ray of their spine and six-monthly lung function tests. Rapid deterioration in lung function or

progression of the curve suggests earlier stabilisation of the spine. We are also concerned about the cardiac status, and electrocardiograms and echocardiography are required before surgery. Provided that their cardiac status is reasonable, we have operated on patients whose vital capacity was only 23% of the expected normal for their age and arm span, although Swank and colleagues (1982), who reported on 14 boys with Duchenne dystrophy who had undergone spinal fusion with Harrington instrumentation, did not recommend surgery if the vital capacity was less than 40%, or the patient had a non-functional cough, symptoms due to cardiomyopathy, or rapidly progressive deterioration in muscle strength.

These patients must not be placed on a long waiting list, but must be given priority, to obviate the risk of them becoming unfit for the operation while waiting.

The operation is a major one. The spine is stabilised from the 3rd or 4th dorsal vertebra to the sacrum or pelvis. It is stabilised with two rods, each rod being fixed to each vertebra by sublaminal wires. The facet joints are excised and the spine grafted. The average operating time is (seven hours and the blood loss (average 3–4 l) is very much greater than in non-neuromuscular scoliosis, because of the length of the stabilisation and fusion, poor muscle contractility and the deliberate non-use of hypotensive anaesthesia in those patients with cardiac conduction defects (p. 742). Although the patients are weak they have normal sphincteric control and sensation. Spinal cord monitoring should be used to minimise the risk of damaging the spinal cord or cauda equina.

The postoperative regimen is critical. The patients require nursing in an intensive care unit for at least 24 hours, and they may require intubation for the first 12–24 hours. Analgesia is provided via an intravenous morphine drip, the drip rate being increased or decreased as required. Virtually all the patients develop a profound ileus and require nasogastric suction and intravenous feeding for three to four days.

We have stabilised the spine in 19 patients with Duchenne muscular dystrophy. The details of the first 11 are given in Tables 22.4 and 22.5 and the X-rays of two patients are shown in Figs. 22.9 and 22.10.

Treatment of the gross curve (Fig. 22.11) is unsatisfactory. At this stage the patients are unfit

Table 22.4 The effect of Luque segmental spinal stabilisation in 11 patients with Duchenne muscular dystrophy (Galasko 1987)

	Range	Average
Age	11 yrs. 8 months–15 yrs. 8 months	13 yrs 6 months
Preop. curve	10–82 °	43 °
Postop. curve	0–30 °	17 °
Correction	28.6%–100%	49.3%

Table 22.5 The effect of D4–sacrum stabilisation on pulmonary function in 11 patients with Duchenne muscular dystrophy. (Figures are mean and range) (Galasko 1987)

	Preop.	Postop. (2 months)
% FEV1	39.6 (26–36)	42.0 (36–54.6)
% FVC	37.1 (23–57)	37.4 (31.2–52.5)
% PEFR	39.2 (27.5–51)	32.9 (28.2–36.3)

for surgical correction. Attempts have been made to pad the chair or provide moulded inserts, but they usually fail and often the patient cannot be sat up without discomfort. Treatment must be aimed at preventing such gross curves and the consequential severe morbidity.

Foot deformity

Mobile patients. The development of an equinus deformity in an independently mobile patient makes walking even more difficult in a child with inherent muscle weakness (Fig. 22.12). Contractures should be avoided or minimised by physiotherapy in the form of gentle ankle stretching exercises and night ankle-foot orthoses (AFOs). The stretching exercises must be carefully carried out to avoid reflex contracture of the calf muscles. The parents should be taught the exercises so that they can be carried out daily. Once an equinus or equinovarus deformity has occurred, surgical correction should be considered (Williams et al 1984). The deformity can usually be corrected by simple elongation of the tendo Achilles, but it is essential not to overlengthen the tendon, as this may result in excessive dorsiflexion in the standing position with loss of balance. Some authors combine elongation of the tendo Achilles with a 'prophylactic' transfer of the tendon of tibialis posterior to the dorsum of the foot (Shapiro & Bresnan 1982).

Postoperatively the limbs are immobilised in below-knee plaster casts and the patients are mobilised, with the aid of the physiotherapist, within 12–16 hours of surgery. The plaster of Paris casts are changed at two to three weeks, when the sutures are removed and casts are taken for night splints, which are provided when the plaster casts are finally removed at approximately six weeks.

Patients in calipers. Equinus or equinovarus deformities must be corrected before a patient is fitted with calipers. Following surgery the limbs are immobilised in long leg casts and the patient is mobilised within 12–16 hours. The casts are usually changed at three weeks and the patients provided with calipers at six weeks, when the casts are removed.

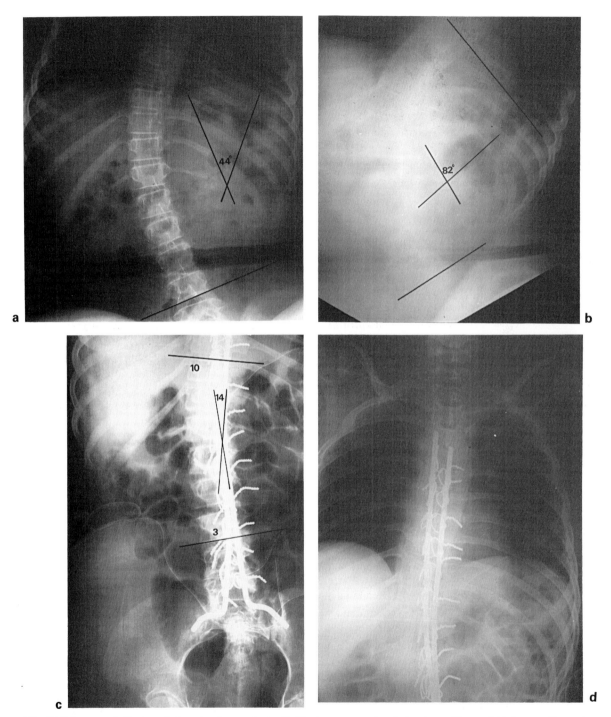

Fig. 22.9 Luque stabilisation of the spine in a patient with Duchenne muscular dystrophy. a. Curve of 44 degrees. Consent for surgical stabilisation was refused. b. One year later the curve had deteriorated to 82 degrees. Fortunately, the patient was still fit for surgery. c. Immediate postoperative X-ray showing the large bowel ileus, the fixation of the Luque rods into the pelvis and the drains. d. The Luque rods are fixed from L3 or 4 to the pelvis or sacrum

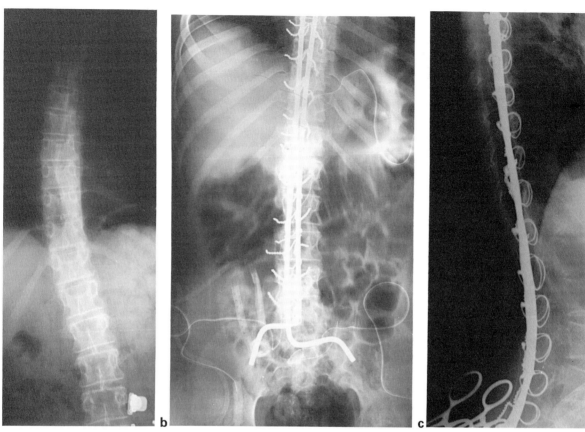

Fig. 22.10 Patient with Duchenne muscular dystrophy. a. Early progressive scoliosis. Ideally, spinal stabilisation should be carried out at this stage. b. Immediate postoperative X-ray showing the large bowel ileus and the drains. The fixation extended to D3. c. Lateral view indicating the lumbar lordosis moulded into the rods

Chairbound patients. Most of the equinus and equinovarus deformities occur after the patients have gone off their feet (Williams et al 1984, Fig. 22.13). Progressive equinovarus is often associated with pain which may be due to a stress fracture of an osteoporotic bone, pressure sores over bony prominences, or simply secondary to the contractures and inability to fit footwear. Attempts have been made to prevent the development of these deformities by providing adequate foot support by the wheelchair footplates, by modifying the footplate, the use of night AFOs and the provision of lightweight moulded day AFOs which fit into the shoes and hold the feet in a neutral or slightly dorsiflexed position (Galasko 1986, 1987).

If the deformity causes symptoms, surgical correction is indicated. Elongation of the tendo Achilles alone is usually insufficient and elongation or transfer of the tibialis posterior tendon with tenotomy of the tendons of flexor hallucis and flexor digitorum longus, and a posterior capsulotomy of the ankle joint, may be required (Williams et al 1984). The deformity tends to recur after surgical correction, but at a slower rate than in unoperated patients (Williams et al 1984). Transfer of the tibialis posterior tendon (Miller et al 1982) may prevent the recurrence. Siegel (1980) advised curettage of part of the cancellous bone from the head of the talus and distal calcaneus in equino-cavo-varus.

Postoperatively, the limb is immobilised in a below-knee plaster cast until the wounds have healed, after which day and night AFOs are worn.

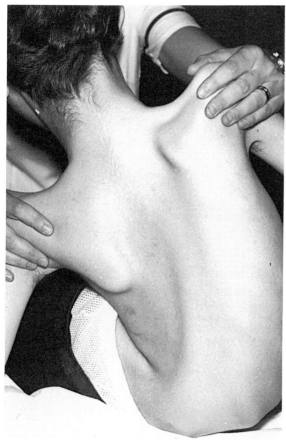

Fig. 22.11 A 16-year-old boy with Duchenne muscular dystrophy. He has progressive scoliosis with a rigid curve. He is unable to sit unsupported. When he sits, his weight is taken on the lumbar spine and his pelvis is almost vertical

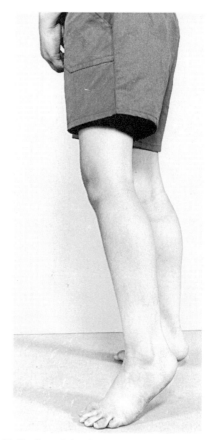

Fig. 22.12 Equinus deformity in an independently mobile patient with Duchenne muscular dystrophy

Contractures of the hip and knee

Contractures should be avoided or minimised in mobile patients by daily prone lying and stretching exercises. Contracture of the tensor fascia lata may affect the gait and require surgical release. Contractures must also be corrected before calipers are fitted; this is rarely required.

Flexion contractures of the hips and knees always develop in wheelchair-bound patients, but seem to be of little significance. Flexion of the hip is not associated with dislocation in Duchenne dystrophy, despite the pelvic obliquity (Fig. 22.14), and contractures of the hips or knees do not produce symptoms unless attempts are made forcibly to correct them. We have not found that surgical correction of these contractures was necessary in any of the 138 patients with Duchenne muscular dystrophy attending our Muscle Clinic.

Fractures

In our experience fractures are not a common complication of Duchenne muscular dystrophy although Matejczyk & Rang (1983) recorded an incidence of 18% during the course of the disease. Fractures of the long bones occur from falls out of a wheelchair as well as in ambulatory patients (Siegel 1977, Hsu 1979, Hsu & Garcia-Ariz 1981), the commonest site being the femoral supracondylar region (Matejczyk & Rang 1983). Patients in wheelchairs should have safety belts applied for transport over rough outdoor terrain. When a

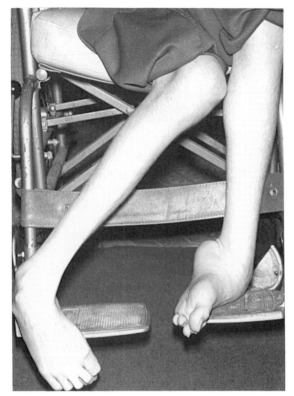

Fig. 22.13 Gross equinovarus deformities in a wheelchair-bound patient with Duchenne muscular dystrophy

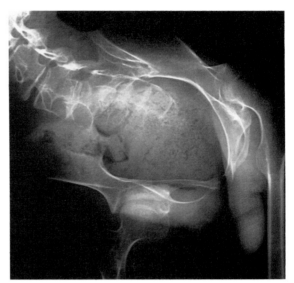

Fig. 22.14 Gross pelvic obliquity in a patient with Duchenne muscular dystrophy. Neither hip is dislocated; however, there is marked varus moulding of the more cranially situated femur. In many other forms of neuromuscular disorders, pelvic obliquity of this degree would have been associated with a dislocation of the more cranially sited hip joint

braced child falls, the calipers tend to protect his lower limbs from direct trauma (Siegel 1977).

The fractures heal rapidly and should be immobilised in the lightest possible cast. In the mobile child, fractures of the lower limbs should be treated in a weight-bearing cast and the patient may require admission to hospital so that intensive physiotherapy, including ambulation, can be supervised on a daily basis.

Anaesthesia

Complications of anaesthesia in children with Duchenne muscular dystrophy include sudden death (Boba 1970, Ellis 1980), anaesthesia-related cardiac arrest (Seay et al 1978), rhabdomyolysis (Miller et al 1978, Boltshauser et al 1980) and malignant hyperthermia (Oka et al 1982, Brownell et al 1983). Hyperpyrexia has also been described in other types of neuromuscular disease (Denborough et al 1973). Suxamethonium, a neural

blocking agent sometimes used in general anaesthesia, should be strictly avoided as it may be responsible for hyperkalaemic cardiac arrest and sudden death (Genever 1971).

In the later stage of the disease cardiomyopathy may occur, resulting in a lowering of cardiac reserve. This is not necessarily a contraindication to surgery, two of our patients undergoing foot surgery and three undergoing spinal stabilisation having shown these changes. Conduction defects occur most commonly. Most of our patients with Duchenne dystrophy had a bundle branch block or some other form of conductive cardiac abnormality at the time of spinal stabilisation. Congestive heart failure does not respond to conventional therapy and progresses rapidly (Mattioli & Melhorn 1982).

Table 22.6 shows our experience with cardiac and respiratory problems in patients with neuromuscular disease. Fifty patients have been operated upon for scoliosis. One patient with minicore disease (a congenital myopathy) had a cardiac arrest; he was successfully resuscitated but died four years later from cor pulmonale. One patient

Table 22.6 Cardiac and pulmonary complications in patients with neuromuscular disease undergoing spinal stabilisation

	No of patients
Duchenne dystrophy	19
Friedreich's ataxia	5
Spinal muscular atrophy	5
Cerebral palsy	5
Spina bifida	5
Congenital myopathy	3
Miscellaneous	8
Total	50

Cardiac and respiratory complications

Perioperative deaths	0	
Cardiac arrest (resuscitated)	1	(Minicore disease)
Postoperative death	1	(Friedreich's ataxia, cardiac failure 3 weeks postoperatively)
Died whilst awaiting surgery	1	(Nemaline myopathy)
Severe hypotension during inducation of anaesthesia. Operation cancelled	1	(Friedreich's ataxia)
Required serial postoperative bronchscopies	1	(Spinal muscle atrophy)
Required postoperative bronchoscopy for chest infection	1	(Duchenne muscle dystrophy)
Atrial flutter with 2:1 heart block	1	(Duchenne muscle dystrophy)

with Friedreich's ataxia died three weeks postoperatively from cardiac failure. One patient with nemaline myopathy died while awaiting surgery; she had nocturnal apnoea and was on nocturnal cuirasse ventilation. One patient with Friedreich's ataxia developed severe hypotension during induction of anaesthesia. She was resuscitated, but the operation was abandoned. One patient with spinal muscle atrophy required serial bronchoscopies and suction postoperatively as she was not able to co-operate with the physiotherapists and one patient with Duchenne muscular dystrophy required a bronchoscopy for a postoperative chest infection. One patient with Duchenne muscular dystrophy developed an atrial flutter with a 2:1 heart block.

OTHER DYSTROPHIES

This section covers a number of conditions which may require orthopaedic management, but perhaps less frequently than Duchenne dystrophy. The orthopaedic problems differ in the different disorders; e.g., congenital dystrophy is associated with a high incidence of scoliosis, hip dislocation which often is present at birth, severe talipes equinovarus and contractures (Jones et al 1979), whereas in the limb girdle dystrophies the main problem is abduction of the shoulders. The latter include a number of different syndromes, the primary condition often being spinal muscular atrophy. There is a slowly progressive weakness of the proximal upper and lower limb muscles, which is less rapid than in the muscle dystrophies and may become arrested (Walton 1983).

Patellar subluxation due to weakness of the quadriceps muscles is a recognised complication. It has been described in Becker dystrophy (Khan & MacNicol 1982), although this complication is not expected because isolated wasting of a single muscle group is rare in any form of muscle dystrophy.

Scoliosis

The optimum form of treatment is surgical stabilisation using segmental sublaminal wiring. As in Duchenne dystrophy, I prefer to stabilise the spine from D4 to the pelvis. Except for congenital dystrophy the other forms of muscular dystrophy seldom develop a significant scoliosis, presumably because their muscle weakness is mild during the growth period, e.g. in limb-girdle dystrophy.

Mobility

Where indicated, calipers should be used, but they are usually unnecessary.

Foot deformities

Equinus and equinovarus deformities occur commonly in many of these conditions. Contractures should be prevented by physiotherapy, if possible. If the tendo Achilles is tight, regular gentle stretching exercises and night AFOs are indicated. Established equinus deformity usually requires surgical correction, the extent of surgery depending on the severity of the deformity.

Hip and/or knee contractures

If the contractures interfere with gait, surgical release is required. This may include release of the hip flexors, ilio-tibial band and hamstrings.

Dislocation/subluxation of the hip

Dislocation of the hip should be avoided. Progressive subluxation of the hip should be treated by releasing soft tissue contractures, balancing the muscle pull across the hip joint and femoral and/or pelvic osteotomy. Usually the femoral neck is in valgus and a varus osteotomy is required. If the acetabulum is deficient a pelvic osteotomy will also be required. If the hip has already dislocated, and if the patient is grossly disabled (mentally and physically), or will not be expected to stand or walk (with or without the use of aids) and has no pain, treatment is usually not indicated. If the patient is likely to be able to stand or walk (with or without the provision of aids) the hip should be stabilised. The hip muscles must be balanced and the femoral head reduced into the acetabulum. As with subluxing hips, an upper femoral varus osteotomy is usually required and if acetabular development is poor, some form of pelvic osteotomy is needed. If the dislocated hip is painful, surgery is indicated: however, reduction of the hip may not reduce the pain, particularly if the femoral head is already deformed.

Loss of shoulder abduction

Many of these patients learn trick manoeuvres, but abduction of the shoulder can be helped by

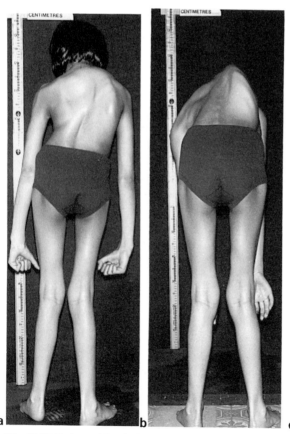
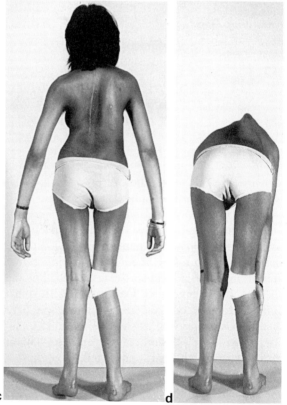

Fig. 22.15 Patient with spinal muscle atrophy. a, b. Rigid thoracic curve of 121 degrees. c, d. 12 months postoperatively. The curve has been corrected to 78 degrees. A long posterior fusion was carried out with Harrington instrumentation

stabilising the scapula to the chest wall. This minimises the winging of the scapula and allows the residual musculature optimum mechanical advantage. However, scapular stabilisation may be of little value if the deltoids are atrophied (Copeland & Howard 1978), and surgery should be postponed until growth is complete.

SPINAL MUSCULAR ATROPHY

Orthopaedic management is usually required in the intermediate variety, but only rarely is it indicated in the mild form (Kugelberg–Welander syndrome), where the children are ambulant and should be encouraged to remain so, or in the severe form (Werdnig–Hoffman disease), when the patient usually dies within the first year of life.

Mobility

Most of the children with intermediate spinal muscular atrophy are unable to walk when first seen. It is not usually possible to provide calipers until the child is three or four years old and during this period active physiotherapy is encouraged, provided that the child will co-operate. Most children will manage with cosmetic calipers, although occasionally a rollator is also needed with the younger child. Unlike Duchenne dystrophy patients with spinal muscular atrophy can sometimes be mobilised, even though they have been chairbound for some time. Recently we have used a reciprocating gait orthosis in some of these patients.

Scoliosis

As with Duchenne dystrophy, the most important deformity in these children is their scoliosis. A curve was already present in nearly half of our patients when first seen at our clinic. It is our policy to obtain an erect (sitting) antero-posterior X-ray of their spine at six-monthly intervals. Progressive curves, or curves of more than 20 degrees are braced until the patient is old enough for surgical stabilisation. Aprin and colleagues (1982) reported that bracing was ineffective in preventing the progression of scoliosis and recommended a long posterior fusion with

Harrington rod instrumentation (Fig. 22.15), but we now prefer segmental spinal stabilisation with sublaminal wiring, as this avoids the necessity for a postoperative plaster of Paris cast or spinal orthosis. However, these patients can tolerate a postoperative jacket and a posterior fusion with Harrington instrumentation or combined posterior and anterior correction and fusion (Riddick et al 1982) is feasible.

The type of bracing depends on the age of the child. In the first two to three years of life a plastazote jacket may suffice. In older children a moulded underarm orthosis is usually used, although curves greater than 70 degrees may require periods of immobilisation in a plaster cast. If bracing does not hold the curve, earlier surgery may be required.

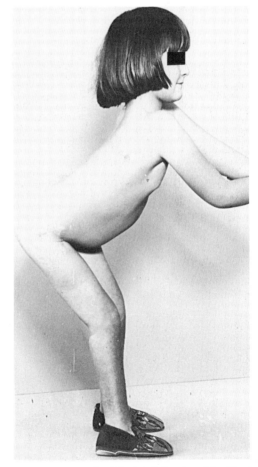

Fig. 22.16 90 degree fixed flexion deformity of the hips in a patient with spinal muscle atrophy. Following surgical release of the contractures, she regained her independent mobility

Hips

Unlike Duchenne dystrophy, dislocation of the hip does occur in patients with spinal muscular atrophy, although much less frequently than in spina bifida or cerebral palsy (Galasko 1986). Dislocation is secondary to muscle imbalance and is preceded by progressive subluxation. Serial X-rays will indicate which hips are at risk, and dislocation can usually be prevented by balancing the musculature (which usually requires release of the hip flexors and adductors) and a varus upper femoral osteotomy in hips which are progressively subluxing. Dislocated hips require open reduction and muscle-balancing procedures. If there is an associated scoliosis with pelvic obliquity, these should be corrected first before the hip is reduced.

Flexion contractures may be gross (Fig. 22.16), can interfere with mobility and may require surgical correction. Regular prone lying should be encouraged in an attempt to prevent these deformities.

Knees and feet

The principles of management are similar to those for Duchenne dystrophy. Regular stretching exercises are encouraged and, if the tendo Achilles are tight, night AFOs are provided. Surgical release is required for those deformities which interfere with ambulation, before the fitting of calipers and for symptomatic deformities.

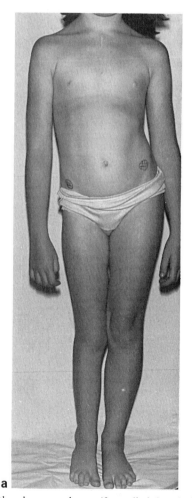
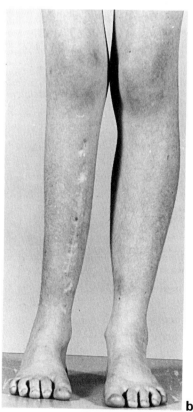

Fig. 22.17 Patient with polyneuropathy. a. 42 mm limb length discrepancy, the shortening being in the lower leg. The anterior superior iliac spines have been marked. b. Following tibial lengthening her discrepancy has been corrected

CONGENITAL MYOPATHY

This includes a variety of conditions: many are associated with a cardiomyopathy and preoperative cardiac investigations are essential. Anaesthesia carries the risk of malignant hyperpyrexia.

Most of the patients with a congenital myopathy are mobile, their commonest deformity being scoliosis. The principles of treatment are similar to those of spinal muscular atrophy, but the risk with anaesthesia is greater.

NEUROPATHIES AND ATAXIAS

Neuropathies

This group includes a variety of conditions. In hypertrophic neuropathy (peroneal muscular atrophy, Charcot–Marie–Tooth syndrome, HMSN type I), pes cavus is often noted in early childhood before the onset of symptoms. Later there is involvement of the hand with difficulty in fine manipulation. In the Dejerine–Sottas syndrome (hypertrophic neuropathy of infancy), the onset is usually in infancy with delay in early milestones and walking may be achieved only by the third or fourth year.

In the neuronal type of peroneal muscular atrophy (HMSN type 2), there is marked atrophy of muscle and there may be an associated pes cavus. The commonest early symptom is difficulty with walking, but the onset may not be until middle age and the patient may have excelled at sports in his youth.

The commonest orthopaedic problem is foot deformity. This usually is in the form of a pes cavus, but equinus and equinovarus deformities also occur. The latter are treated by soft tissue releases, whereas a significant cavus deformity requires wedge tarsectomy or triple arthrodesis.

Scoliosis may also occur in these conditions and the management is similar to that of spinal muscular atrophy. Asymmetrical lower limb involvement may result in limb length inequality (Fig. 22.17) and if this is greater than 3 cm, a limb-lengthening procedure may be required to improve the gait and to avoid the back pain which frequently is associated with significant limb length inequality.

Sensory neuropathies may present with trophic ulceration, osteomyelitis or septic arthritis (Fig. 22.18). These lesions also occur with congenital insensitivity to pain (Greider 1983).

It may not be possible to use spinal cord monitoring in patients with sensory neuropathy, because of the inability to stimulate a peripheral nerve (Arafa et al 1987).

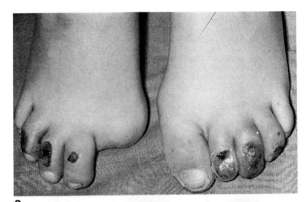
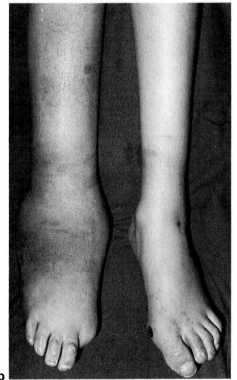

Fig. 22.18 Patient with a sensory neuropathy. a. Trophic ulceration affecting several of his toes. He already has had an amputation of his right great toe. b. Two years later he developed septic arthritis of his right ankle

Friedreich's ataxia

This is commonly associated with scoliosis and pes cavus. The scoliosis frequently requires surgical correction to allow for comfortable sitting (Figs. 22.19, 22.20). Cady & Bobechko (1984) suggested that bracing was of no value and recommended a long posterior spinal fusion as soon as the curve reached 40–50 degrees. In independently mobile patients, locomotion may be dependent on trunk movement and they may lose their mobility following upper thoracic to pelvic stabilisation. If the curve is still localised to the thoracic spine, a localised stabilisation should be carried out to preserve trunk mobility and allow for independent walking. If the curve

subsequently involves the lumbar spine, a secondary procedure may be required.

The cavus deformity may require treatment if the patient is ambulatory. A flexible deformity can be corrected by combining a Dwyer calcaneal osteotomy with a plantar release, but a triple arthrodesis is required if the cavus is rigid. Occasionally, talectomy may be necessary if the deformity is extremely severe and rigid.

Friedreich's ataxia may be associated with cardiac abnormalities (Table 22.6) and a careful cardiac assessment is required prior to major reconstructive surgery. Taddonio (1982) analysed segmental spinal stabilisation in 17 patients with a variety of neuromuscular disorders. The only death occurred 36 hours postoperatively in one of

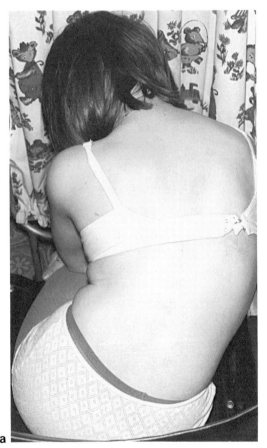
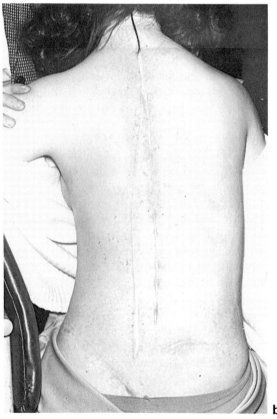

a   b

Fig. 22.19 17-year-old wheelchair-bound girl with Friedreich's ataxia. a. She was unable to sit for more than an hour at a time because of pain under her right buttock. b. Following spinal fusion using Harrington instrumentation. Routine evaluation at six months postoperatively revealed a pseudarthrosis and she required a supplementary bone graft. Following the fusion she was able to sit unsupported without pain

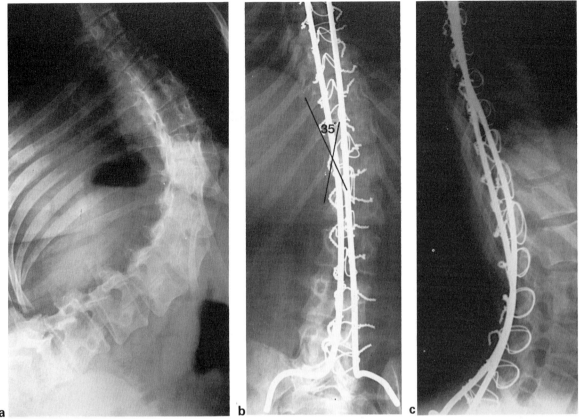

a   b   c

Fig. 22.20 32-year-old patient with Friedreich's ataxia. a. She had a 96 degree curve and associated pelvic obliquity. b. Following segmental stabilisation from D4 to the pelvis her curve has been corrected to 35 degrees and her pelvis is horizontal. c. Lateral view showing the lumbar lordosis, which is necessary for comfortable sitting

the two patients with Friedreich's ataxia, who also had cardiomyopathy. His series included two patients with Duchenne dystrophy, two with spinal muscular atrophy and one with congenital myopathy.

Hereditary telangiectatic ataxia is frequently associated with scoliosis, which may require surgical correction for comfortable sitting.

MISCELLANEOUS CONDITIONS

There are a variety of miscellaneous neurological and neuromuscular conditions which may require orthopaedic management, and which do not fit into any of the above categories. They include conditions such as hereditary spastic paraparesis,

where release of tight hip adductors for a scissoring gait, or elongation of the tendo Achilles for an equinus deformity may be beneficial; inflammatory myopathies, which may be associated with an equinus deformity or other contractures; myotonic syndromes where the patient may present with a scoliosis (Fig. 22.21) or foot deformity: and the rigid spine syndrome. In the latter condition, hyperextension of the cervical spine may be so severe as to create difficulties with deglutition. Release of the posterior spinal muscles is required but the deformity creates major anaesthetic difficulties. Cardiac muscle is frequently affected in dystrophia myotonica and in these patients thiopentone must be avoided. Congenital talipes equinovarus often occurs in this condition.

Arthrogryposis probably includes a number of

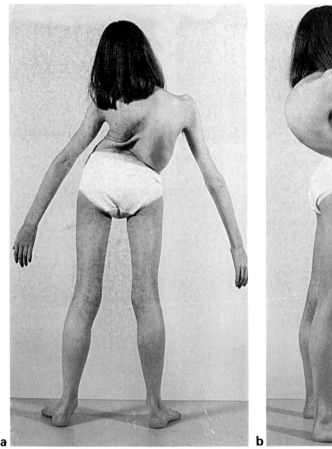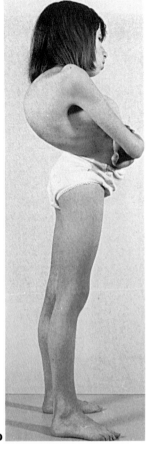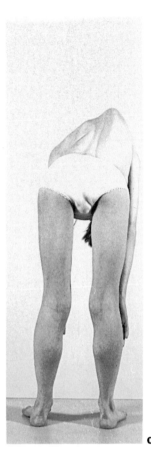

a   b   c

Fig. 22.21 Patient with myotonic dystrophy who has developed a gross scoliosis. Patients should be referred for orthopaedic management before they develop such severe deformities

conditions as yet not defined, where muscle is replaced by fibrous tissue. Multiple deformities may occur, especially talipes equinovarus, fixed flexion deformities of the knee (Fig. 22.22) and dislocation of the hip. Recurrence of the deformity following surgery is common, because the fibrotic muscle does not grow as rapidly as the adjacent bone.

SUMMARY

Deformities occur commonly in the dystrophies, myopathies, atrophies, neuropathies and ataxias. The incidence and type of deformity varies between the different conditions.

The most significant deformity is scoliosis.

Progressive neuromuscular scoliosis produces increasing respiratory insufficiency and increasing pelvic obliquity with loss of sitting balance. In Duchenne dystrophy it may be possible to control the scoliosis by prolonging standing. Irrespective of the underlying disorder, surgical stabilisation is indicated for a progressive curve, provided that the patient is fit enough for major surgery. At the moment, segmental stabilisation with sublaminal wiring appears to offer considerable advantages in that a postoperative plaster jacket or spinal orthosis is avoided. Ideally, the operation should not be carried out under the age of 11 or 12 years; however, if the curve is progressive and cannot be adequately controlled, earlier stabilisation may be necessary.

Contractures can occur in any joint. Contrac-

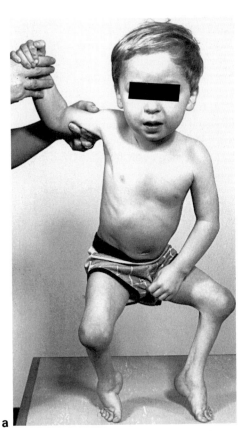 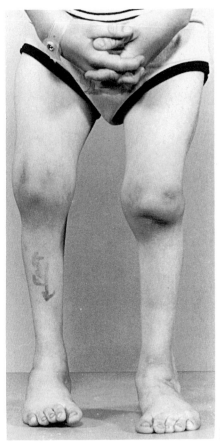

Fig. 22.22 Patient with arthrogryposis. a. Gross fixed flexion deformities of the knees. As a result the patient walked on his knees. Note the thickened skin over the front of the knees. b. Following bilateral femoral osteotomies to correct the deformities

tures of the upper limb rarely require surgical correction in this group of patients. Contractures occur most often in the feet and ankles, the commonest being equinus and equinovarus deformities, although any type of deformity can occur. Surgical correction is required if the contracture interferes with gait, interferes with the fitting of calipers or is symptomatic. Equinus or equinovarus deformities can be corrected by soft tissue release whereas a pes cavus deformity usually requires a wedge tarsectomy or a triple arthrodesis.

Contractures of the hips and knees occur less frequently. They always develop in children confined to a wheelchair, but under these circumstances rarely produce problems. Regular stretching exercises and prone lying may help prevent these

deformities. If contractures do occur, do not respond to physiotherapy and interfere with gait or the fitting of calipers, surgical correction is indicated.

Winging of the scapula and limb length discrepancy are other complications of specific neuromuscular conditions and may require surgery.

It must be emphasised that orthopaedic management is part of the continuing treatment of these patients. Orthopaedic management must be associated with a careful assessment, preoperative physiotherapy programme and detailed postoperative rehabilitation: it forms part of the overall management of the child.

Orthopaedic surgery can do nothing to cure the underlying neurological disorder: it is aimed at preventing and correcting deformity. Major reconstructive surgery in these patients is not undertaken purely for cosmetic reasons, but is used to aid mobility, to alleviate discomfort and to improve the quality of life of these patients.

ACKNOWLEDGEMENTS

I am grateful to my colleagues who have referred patients with neuromuscular diseases from a wide area. I am particularly grateful to my colleagues and the nursing staff at the Royal Manchester Children's Hospital, without whose skill and expertise the procedures described in this chapter could not have been carried out.

I wish to thank my Research Secretary, Mrs Margaret Powis, for typing the manuscript, the Department of Medical Illustration at Hope Hospital and the Royal Manchester Children's Hospital for the illustrations, and Blackwell Scientific Publications for permission to reproduce those already published.

REFERENCES

Aprin H, Bowen J R, MacEwen G D, Hall J E 1982 Spine fusion in patients with spinal muscular atrophy. Journal of Bone and Joint Surgery 64-A: 1179–1187

Arafa M, Morris P, Galasko C S B 1987 Spinal cord monitoring during surgery for scoliosis. In: Noble J, Galasko C S B (eds) Recent developments in orthopaedic surgery. Manchester University Press

Boba A 1970 Fatal postanaesthetic complications in two muscular dystrophic patients. Journal of Paediatric Surgery 5: 71–5

Boltshauser E, Steinmann B, Meyer A, Jerusalem F 1980 Anesthesia induced rhabdomyolysis in Duchenne muscular dystrophy. British Journal of Anaesthesia 52:559

Brownell A K W, Paasuke R T, Elash A, Fowlow S B, Seagram C G F, Diewold R J, Friesen C 1983 Malignant hyperthermia in Duchenne muscular dystrophy. Anesthesiology 58: 180–182

Cady R B, Bobechko W P 19841 Incidence, natural history and treatment of scoliosis in Friedreich's ataxia. Journal of Pediatric Orthopaedics 4: 673–676

Copeland S A, Howard R C 1978 Thoracoscapular fusion for facioscapulohumeral dystrophy. Journal of Bone and Joint Surgery 60-B: 547–551

Crisp D E, Ziter F A, Bray P F 1982 Diagnostic delay in Duchenne's muscular dystrophy. Journal of the American Medical Association 347: 478–480

Denborough M A, Dennett L, Anderson R M 1973 Central core and malignant hyperpyrexia. British Medical Journal 1: 272–273

Edwards R H, Round J M, Jackson M J, Griffiths R D, Lilburn M F 1984 Weight reduction in boys with muscular dystrophy. Developmental Medicine and Child Neurology 26: 384–390

Ellis F R 1980 Inherited muscle disease. British Journal of Anaesthesia 52: 153–164

Galasko C S B 1977 Incidence of orthopaedic problems in children with muscle disease. Israel Journal of Medicine Sciences 13: 165–176

Galasko C S B 1986 Orthopaedic management of children with neurological disorders. In: Gordon N, McKinlay I (eds) Neurologically handicapped child, treatment and management. Blackwell Scientific Publications, Oxford, p 109–147

Galasko C S B 1987 The orthopaedic management of the dystrophies, myopathies, atrophies, neuropathies and ataxias. In: Galasko C S B (ed) Neuromuscular problems in orthopaedics. Blackwell Scientific Publications, Oxford, p 83–105

Gardner-Medwin D 1979 Controversies about Duchenne muscular dystrophy: (1) Neonatal screening. Developmental Medicine and Child Neurology 21: 390–393

Genever E E 1971 Suxamethonium-induced cardiac arrest in unsuspected pseudohypertrophic muscular dystrophy: a case report. British Journal of Anaesthesia 43: 984–986

Gibson D A, Wilkins K E 1975 The management of spinal deformities in Duchenne muscular dystrophy. A new concept of spinal bracing. Clinical Orthopaedics and Related Research 108: 41–51

Gibson D A, Albisser A M, Koreska J 1975 Role of the wheelchair in the management of the muscular dystrophy patient. Canadian Medical Association Journal 113: 964–966

Greider T D 1983 Orthopaedic aspects of congenital insensitivity to pain. Clinical Orthopaedics and Related Research 172: 117–185

Heckmatt J Z, Dubowitz V, Hyde S A, Florence J, Gabain A C, Thompson N 1985 Prolongation of walking in Duchenne muscular dystrophy with lightweight orthoses: review of 57 cases. Developmental Medicine and Child Neurology 27: 149–154

Hsu J D 1979 Extremity fractures in children with neuromuscular diseases. The Johns Hopkins Medical Journal 145: 89–93

Hsu J D 1983 The natural history of spine curvature progression in the non-ambulatory Duchenne muscular dystrophy patient. Spine 8: 771–775

Hsu J D, Garcia-Ariz M 1981 Fracture of the femur in the Duchenne muscular dystrophy patient. Journal of Pediatric Orthopaedics 1: 203–207

Jones R, Khan R, Hughes S, Dubowitz V 1979 Congenital muscular dystrophy. The importance of early diagnosis and orthopaedic management in the long-term prognosis. Journal of Bone and Joint Surgery 61-B: 13–17

Khan R H, MacNicol M F 1982 Bilateral patellar subluxation secondary to Becker muscular dystrophy. Journal of Bone and Joint Surgery 64-A: 777–778

Kurz L T, Mubarak S J, Schultz P, Park S M, Leach J 1983 Correlation of scoliosis and pulmonary function in Duchenne muscular dystrophy. Journal of Pediatric Orthopaedics 3: 347–353

Matejczyk M B, Rang M 1983 Fractures in children with neuromuscular disorders. In: Houghton G R, Thompson

G D (eds) Problematic musculo-skeletal injuries in children. Butterworth, London, p. 178–192

Mattioli L, Melhorn M 1982 Duchenne's muscular dystrophy. The diagnosis and management of cardiac involvement. The Journal of the Kansas Medical Society 83: 115–121

Miller E D, Sanders D B, Rowlingson J C, Berry F A, Sussman M D, Epstein R M 1978 Anesthesia-induced rhabdomyolysis in a patient with Duchenne's muscular dystrophy. Anesthesiology 48: 146–148

Miller G, Dunn N 1982 An outline of the management and prognosis of Duchenne muscular dystrophy in Western Australia. Australian Paediatric Journal 18: 277–282

Miller G M, Hsu J D, Hoffer M M, Rentfro R 1982 Posterior tibial tendon transfer: a review of the literature and analysis of 74 procedures. Journal of Pediatric Orthopaedics 2: 363–370

Oka S, Igarashi Y, Takagi A, Nishida M, Sato K, Nakada K, Ikeda K 1982 Malignant hyperpyrexia and Duchenne muscular dystrophy. A case report. Canadian Anaesthetists' Society Journal 29: 627–629

Read L, Galasko C S B 1986 Delay in diagnosing Duchenne muscular dystrophy in orthopaedic clinics. Journal of Bone and Joint Surgery 68-B: 481–482

Riddick M F, Winter R B, Lutter L D 1982 Spinal deformities in patients with spinal muscle atrophy. A review of 36 patients. Spine 7: 476–483

Roy L, Gibson D A 1970 Pseudohypertrophic muscular dystrophy and its surgical management: review of 30 patients. Canadian Journal of Surgery 13: 13–21

Seay A R, Ziter F A, Thompson J A 1978 Cardiac arrest during induction of anaesthesia in Duchenne muscular dystrophy. Journal of Paediatrics 93: 88–90

Seeger B R, Sutherland A D'A, Clark M S 1984 Orthotic management of scoliosis in Duchenne muscular dystrophy. Archives of Physical Medicine and Rehabilitation 65: 83–86

Shapiro F, Bresnan M J 1982 Current concepts review: Orthopaedic management of childhood neuromuscular diseases. Part III: diseases of muscle. Journal of Bone and Joint Surgery 64-A: 1102–1107

Siegel I M 1977 Fractures of long bones in Duchenne muscular dystrophy. Journal of Trauma 17: 219–222

Siegel I M 1980 Maintenance of ambulation in Duchenne muscular dystrophy. The role of the orthopaedic surgeon. Clinical Paediatrics 19: 383–388

Spencer G E, Vignos P J Jr 1962 Bracing for ambulation in childhood progressive muscular dystrophy. Journal of Bone and Joint Surgery 44-A: 234–242

Swank S M, Brown J C, Perry R E 1982 Spinal fusion in Duchenne's muscular dystrophy. Spine 7: 484–491

Taddonio R F 1982 Segmental spinal instrumentation in the management of neuromuscular spinal deformity. Spine 7: 305–311

Walton J 1983 Changing concepts of neuromuscular diseases. Hospital Update 949–958

Williams E A, Read L, Ellis A, Galasko C S B, Morris P 1984 The management of equinus deformity in Duchenne muscular dystrophy. Journal of Bone and Joint Surgery 66-B: 546–550

Motor neurone diseases

INTRODUCTION

This chapter is concerned with human diseases of motor neurones of which the archetype is adult motor neurone disease (more often called amyotrophic lateral sclerosis, or ALS in the USA). Few, if any, of these clinical syndromes are exclusive to the motor system although in some diseases the non-motor involvement may be mild or subclinical. Furthermore, the motor system within the CNS may be selectively affected, with involvement of the upper or lower motor neurones at cerebral, brain-stem or spinal cord level, or even restricted with sparing of some neuronal group, e.g. the nucleus of Onufrowicz in the sacral cord supplying the external sphincteric muscles, or the oculomotor nuclei in the brain-stem which are motor to the external ocular musculature. Many of these conditions are inherited, a fact which indicates some, as yet unknown, genetically determined metabolic disorder of the motor neurones.

In recent years much research has been directed to studying neuronal function and metabolism, especially in relation to the role of various polypeptide neurotransmitters, to try to differentiate specific neuronal cell types. This would seem to be the key to characterising motor neurones and to determining the specific abnormalities related to individual motor neurone diseases. Only then are rational treatments likely to be feasible.

The neuronal cell body or soma undertakes a high level of protein synthesis, largely through ribosomes associated with the endoplasmic reticulum. These proteins, macromolecules, neurotransmitters and enzymes required by the axon and the target tissues are then conveyed by active transport into the nerve fibres to effect normal neuronal function. This involves primarily the conduction of the nerve impulse, neurotransmitter release and transport of neurotrophic factors, as well as maintaining the structure and functional integrity of the axonal membrane. Dyck and co-workers (Dyck et al 1971, Dyck & Lais 1973) showed that neuronal degeneration may give axonal atrophy, maximal distally, with myelin wrinkling, nodal lengthening and internodal demyelination causing slowing of impulse conduction. Attempts at remyelination by Schwann cell proliferation may lead to nerve hypertrophy. If the metabolic failure proceeds, then axonal degeneration spreads proximally (dying-back), leading to loss of the axon. Recovery of metabolic activity leads to restoration of axonal structure and function. Thus the rigid separation of motor neurone disease from peripheral neuropathy is not always possible (Dyck 1982). Wallerian degeneration is associated with a decline of the membrane potential and failure of excitability in the nerve distal to transection. The atrophy and other regressive changes in the target muscle cell after nerve section or block of axoplasmic transport indicate a failure to supply some (unknown) neurotrophic substances. Thus some motor neuronal diseases may be due to a deficiency of neurotropic substances or a defect of axoplasmic transport.

Fast axoplasmic transport is dependent on oxidative metabolism involving high-energy ATP provision, oxygen and calcium ions and takes place at a rate of approximately 400 mm/24 h (reviewed by Ochs 1984). Identified compounds carried down nerve fibres by fast transport include glycoproteins, glycolipids, lipids, cholesterol and acetylcholinesterase (AChE). Many studies have shown retrograde transport of labelled proteins, horseradish peroxidase (HRP), toxins, nerve growth factor (NGF) and viruses at roughly half the antegrade rate. This retrograde transport has been related to chromatolysis of the neurone cell body and an increased neuronal protein synthesis after nerve injury; the signal substance is unknown. It is not known whether there is a single or multiple transport mechanism.

It is postulated that some substances taken up from muscle and other cells by nerve terminals and carried back to the cell body may be required to maintain normal neuronal function. Interference with such processes or the uptake of abnormal substances such as chemicals or toxins, may be responsible for neuropathological changes in the motor unit (Ochs 1984). This might also be an explanation for the apparent loss of motor units in certain muscle diseases such as myotonic dystrophy (Ch. 16). How far axons of peripheral nerves rely on their satellite Schwann cells for metabolic support is not yet known.

The excitability and axoplasmic transport of mammalian nerves fail quickly under conditions of anoxia or ischaemia. Fast axoplasmic transport is related to the integrity of the microtubular system within the axon. Certain drugs, e.g. colchicine or vincristine, which cause a transport block, are associated with the disaggregation or reduction in the number of microtubules and in some cases an accumulation of neurofilamentous material in the axon. Abnormalities of axoplasmic transport have been described in motor neurone disease, both in man (Norris 1979, Bradley et al 1983) and in animal models (Griffin et al 1982).

Retrograde labelling of anterior horn cells (AHC) with HRP in experimental animals has permitted a direct correlation of neuronal size and nerve fibre diameter with nerve conduction velocity and the physiological characteristics of motor units (reviewed by Burke 1982). The largest motor neurones in the lateral part of the ventral grey matter (Rexed layer IX) innervate the Type II fast twitch motor units and the intermediate size cells innervate Type I slower twitch units. The smallest motor neurones of under 35 μm diameter are largely gamma cells innervating the muscle spindle. Campa & Engel (1970) showed that large AHC of >30 μm diameter had high phosphorylase and low succinic dehydrogenase histochemical activity, implying a mainly anaerobic metabolic pathway, compared with small < 30 μm motor neurones which had a reversed metabolic profile, that is, an aerobic pattern. Burke (1982) concluded that there is no clear histochemical difference between motor neurones that innervate the different types of extrafusal motor units, and there is no clear evidence of any affinity of specific disease processes for certain motor unit types in ALS.

The physiological effect of motor neurone disease may be motor overactivity or underactivity. Overactivity is commonly associated with muscle fasciculation and cramp, or less commonly focal myokymia or painful spasms, as in tetanus. Fasciculations may persist after nerve block or spinal anaesthesia (Forster & Alpers 1944, see Layzer 1982) suggesting that an independent peripheral process has been established; they are also triggered or exacerbated by anticholinesterase drugs. Underactivity of the motor unit commonly leads initially to abnormal fatiguability. Strength may be maintained for a time by the compensatory reinnervative activity of residual healthy motor neurones and axons. This leads to increased muscle fibre density within a motor unit but with variability of terminal nerve fibre branch conduction and depolarisation of individual muscle cells within the unit (Stålberg 1982). This conductive defect can be shown electrophysiologically by single-fibre electromyography (SFEMG) as 'jitter' and correlates with neuromuscular fatigue. Progressive neuronal loss leads to weakness and wasting of muscles. Such changes are seen to a degree as a natural consequence of ageing (Campbell et al 1973). Muscle wasting in the elderly, often selectively of type II units, correlates with measured loss of peripheral nerve fibres, ventral nerve roots and anterior horn cells (Tomlinson & Irving 1977, Kawamura et al 1981).

The differential diagnosis of motor neuronal diseases includes distinction from structural diseases of the spinal grey matter, as in intrinsic cord tumours or syringomyelia, compressive lesions of the spinal cord, particularly in the neck region, chronic polyradiculopathies or peripheral neuropathies and inflammatory muscle diseases (polymyositis). Cervical spondylosis may cause particular difficulty because of its frequent occurrence in the elderly, especially men, and because it often co-exists with motor neurone diseases.

The following account concerns those conditions where motor neuronal disease with neurogenic muscular atrophy and weakness are the predominant disorder leading to disability. Other conditions where amyotrophy, i.e. neurogenic muscular atrophy, is a significant secondary feature of more generalized disease are discussed briefly as study of such conditions has provided

Table 23.1 Motor neurone diseases

1. Adult motor neurone disease (ALS) includes:
   progressive muscular atrophy
   progressive bulbar palsy
   primary lateral sclerosis
   amyotrophic lateral sclerosis
   (a) Sporadic forms
   (b) Heredofamilial forms
   (c) Western Pacific types
2. Hereditary motor neuropathies
   (a) Spinal muscular atrophies (SMA)
   (b) Hereditary motor and sensory neuropathies (HMSN)
       including Charcot–Marie–Tooth disease
   (c) Spino-cerebellar ataxias
       including Familial spastic paraplegia with amyotrophy,
               Friedreich's ataxia
3. Infections
   including Poliomyelitis (and PPMA), tetanus, rabies,
           zoster, CJD
4. Metabolic disorders
   including Storage diseases, e.g. AMN, Pompe's disease,
           Hexosaminidase A deficiency
           Diabetes and hypoglycaemia
           Thyrotoxicosis
           Hyperparathyroidism
5. Toxicity — heavy metals, organophosphorus compounds
6. Ischaemic myelopathy including radiation injury
7. Trauma including electrical injury
8. Immune disorders
   including plasma cell dyscrasia with
           paraproteinaemias
           Cancers and lymphoma
9. Non-familial CNS degenerative disorders with amyotrophy
   including dementias, basal ganglia disease, Shy–Drager
           syndrome

clues to the metabolic disorders present in the primary diseases. A classification of motor neurone diseases is given in Table 23.1

ADULT MOTOR NEURONE DISEASE (ALS)

Adult motor neurone disease (MND) is a progressive degenerative disease of the motor system that encompasses several different clinical syndromes. It includes the features of progressive muscular atrophy (PMA), first described by Aran (1850), progressive bulbar palsy (PBP) (Duchenne 1860, Duchenne & Joffroy 1870) and primary lateral sclerosis (Charcot 1865), a purely upper motor neurone disorder. The descriptive term amyotrophic lateral sclerosis (ALS) coined by Charcot (1874) combines all these clinical features in single patients with the pathological findings in the disease. Hence motor neurone disease and amyotrophic lateral sclerosis have come to be used by some as synomyms identifying the same disease complex. It is generally agreed that there is a similar clinical picture in the sporadic and the rare hereditary forms and in the Western Pacific form of the disease. This is despite the various different genetic patterns that have been described for familial MND suggesting different abnormalities of neuronal metabolic pathways.

Clinical features

Progressive muscular atrophy

Progressive muscular atrophy of skeletal muscles reflects involvement of motor neurones in the anterior horn of the spinal grey matter. The disease most commonly presents in one or other upper limb (40%), usually with wasting and weakness of the muscles of one hand. The muscles of the thenar eminence are frequently involved and this prevents opposition and adduction of the thumb. Thus the patient complains of loss of fine finger control and difficulty in fastening buttons, turning keys, picking up small objects and writing. Alternatively, more proximal arm weakness may be associated with difficulty in lifting up heavier objects, especially shopping bags, cooking utensils or during occupations. Leg weakness may present with a limping gait, foot drop or difficulty in ascending steps or stairs. Frequently the weakness is preceded, often over several months, by symptoms of motor unit over-activity. Frequent muscle cramps are often accompanied by visible muscle fasciculation. Recurrent muscle cramps in the hand or forearm are almost diagnostic of MND. Progressive atrophy of the interossei and lumbrical muscles of the hand allows the unopposed action of the long extensor and flexor muscles causing clawing of the fingers. The atrophy and weakness commonly ascend progressively up the arm to the shoulder girdle muscles and then usually involve the contralateral hand and upper limb. The disease may then spread to the cranial musculature, as in bulbar palsy, or to the lower limbs and trunk musculature. The latter may lead to respiratory difficulty, which is discussed later.

The patchy asymmetrical wasting and weakness is associated with progressive weight loss. One hallmark of MND is the preservation or enhancement of tendon reflexes in the presence of signs of overt lower motor neurone disease. This is due to involvement of the upper motor neurones which later becomes more apparent in the fully manifest ALS picture. A pure progressive muscular atrophy picture with loss of tendon reflexes occurs in less than 10% of patients and should raise the question of an alternative diagnosis with a more favourable prognosis, e.g. hereditary spinal muscular atrophy or motor polyneuropathy.

Progressive bulbar palsy may be a presenting feature in 25% of patients, especially in elderly females, and often heralds a subacute disease. This causes difficulty with speech and swallowing. Indistinct or blurred speech is often the first symptom but inability to sing, whistle or speak rapidly or simply a change in tone or volume (dysphonia) may be the presenting complaint. Dysarthria arises from loss of speech muscle strength or co-ordination. This is a variable mixture of flaccid (LMN) and spastic (UMN) weakness depending on the chronology of the disease (see Aronson 1980). Dysphonia arises from altered muscle tone of the extra- and intralaryngeal muscles in addition to the weakness of the intercostal and diaphragmatic muscles: the former tends to affect the pitch and tone whereas the latter causes reduction of volume. Normal speech is said to require a tidal air volume of 500 ml (Aronson 1980). The dysphonia is accompanied by an increased frequency of respirations during speech and a decreased length of utterances. Spasticity may give glottal constriction and a strained harshness of the voice typical of the disorder. Pooling of secretions and food particles in the hypopharynx adds a telltale wet, gurgling component to speech, often with an occasional coughing or choking fit. Flaccidity of the hypopharyx and larynx gives adductor muscle weakness and dysphonia and often difficult, heavy breathing or inspiratory stridor. In addition, palatal weakness allows nasal escape of air with hypernasality and decreased intra-oral pressure, which reduces friction and plosion required for articulating some consonants, leading to blurring of speech. Articulation is dependent on the precise action of many muscles including those of the tongue, lips and cheeks. An early difficulty commonly arises from wasting and immobility of the tongue, especially of the tip (Colmant 1975). Dworkin et al (1980) showed considerable reduction of tongue protrusion force in ALS. Reduction of tongue strength and speed causes distortion of many consonants as the tongue is no longer able to make firm contact with the teeth and hard palate (Aronson 1980). Slowness of tongue movements and hence of speech is evident from the reduced number of syllables per second, from an average of six to a maximum of four (Dworkin et al 1980). With general weakness of the tongue the vowels 'u' and 'o' become progressively difficult to pronounce as these require subtle movements (Böhme 1974). Weakness of the circumoral musculature reduces lip mobility and seal pressure and lowers intra-oral pressure during speech: thus plosive sounds become difficult and then impossible (see Darley et al 1975). In the late stages all speech is lost (anarthria). In addition to the primary speech disorder there may be pathological laughter or crying from cortico-bulbar (pseudobulbar) involvement.

Difficulty with swallowing (dysphagia) may emanate from weakness of the tongue which normally controls the propulsion of the bolus in the oral phase and pushes it posteriorly into the oral pharynx. Masticatory muscle weakness causes difficulty in chewing and may even result in subluxation of the jaw, either spontaneously or during involuntary yawning. The soft palate should lift to prevent nasal regurgitation. Simultaneously the larynx should rise to assist with closure of the epiglottis and the pharyngeal constrictor muscles contract to move food down into the oesophagus. In the oesophagus reflex peristaltic waves move the food bolus down to the stomach. Bosma & Brodie (1969) have demonstrated several kinds of pharyngeal dysfunction in ALS, especially failure to prevent laryngeal penetration. Such penetration may not occur at the time of swallowing but during respiration afterwards. This is related to pooling of food particles in the hypopharynx, either as a result of flaccidity or due to hypertonicity of the cricopharyngeus muscle from UMN involvement.

Oesophageal motility has been studied by cinéradiological techniques and by measurement of intraluminar pressure using catheters connected to pressure transducers. Smith et al (1957) reported that, of 19 ALS patients studied, most had abnormalities of the middle and lower oesophagus with feeble contractions; some of their patients had weak upper and lower oesophageal sphincteric function. Smith et al (1980) reported that the low resting pressure seen in the upper sphincter could be augmented by administration of intravenous edrophonium chloride (Tensilon®) resulting in improved motility; however they found that lower oesophageal sphincter pressures were generally normal. Dysphagia is often aggravated by troublesome pooling of saliva, often resulting in drooling and a spluttering cough.

In some cases, visible wasting of the tongue with fasciculations may precede any bulbar symptoms. In others, physical signs in the bulbar musculature may not be apparent in the early stages and may lead erroneously to a diagnosis of hysteria. Later, wasting and fasciculation of the tongue, together with weak force and slowness of alternating movements, become obvious. Poor voluntary palatal or pharyngeal movement may be associated with a brisk gag reflex or jaw jerk from supranuclear (UMN) involvement.

Primary lateral sclerosis. This much-debated entity as described by Charcot (1865) is a rare presenting form of MND in less than 10% of cases. The insidious onset and slowly progressive symptoms of spasticity and weakness of the limbs, usually the lower extremities, together with pathologically brisk tendon reflexes, are the sole presenting clinical features (Stark & Moersch 1945). Its differentiation from other causes of spastic paraparesis or quadriparesis, e.g. multiple sclerosis or hereditary spastic paraplegia, is usually made by the appearance of visible fasciculations and wasting or by electrophysiological findings of LMN involvement. Some authors in the UK reserve the term amyotrophic lateral sclerosis for such cases in which the signs of upper motor neurone dysfunction predominate and evidence of involvement of involvement of lower motor neurones is slight. There have been few clinicopathological correlative studies describing complete preservation of anterior horn cells in such cases, but some have shown intracytoplasmine hyaline inclusions, as in familial ALS (Fisher 1977, Beal & Richardson 1981).

Amyotrophic lateral sclerosis (ALS). In a large series of MND patients Bonduelle (1975) found that 66% had ALS. This is the combined UMN and LMN disease state that is virtually always present terminally and is the commonest clinical syndrome. It is responsible for the common 'strained-strangled voice' disorder of bulbar involvement. Spasticity is rarely severe in the limbs, despite the very brisk reflexes and the extensor plantar (Babinski) responses. The clinical picture is one of steady progressive weakness of all limb and bulbar muscles, with increasing disability. Respiratory muscles are also involved, although dyspnoea is a late symptom. The diaphragm is the main muscle used in quiet breathing, and intercostal and accessory muscles can compensate for diaphragmatic weakness, but not during exertional breathing. Breathing difficulties may be apparent during speech. Very occasionally, alveolar hypoventilation can be a presenting symptom of MND (Parhad et al 1978, Sivak & Streib 1980). Spirometric studies have shown that the forced vital lung capacity (FVC) is the most useful measure of respiratory function in MND and correlates with the progression of the disease. It declines slowly until the terminal months when it falls below 50% of the predicted normal (Fallat et al 1979). The maximum expiratory pressure (MEP) or the peak flow rate (PFR) may be a more sensitive indication (Griggs et al 1980), but these are often difficult to record because of poor lip seal. The arterial blood gases are rarely abnormal even when the predicted FVC is less than 50% (Fallat & Norris 1980). Chronic respiratory failure often indicates co-existing lung disease. If it is present, it can only be treated with mechanical ventilatory support. Studies of autonomic nerve function, both of the vagal parasympathetic and sympathetic systems, have shown normal results (Sachs et al 1985). Some patients demonstrate breath-holding attacks in sleep (sleep apnoea) which may be responsible for respiratory arrest.

Respiratory complications are the most frequent terminal event. These include restricted ventilation causing chronic respiratory failure, pharyngeal or laryngeal weakness causing poor airway protection and bronchopulmonary aspiration, impaired cough response and inability to clear airway and sudden vagal arrest from choking or cough stimulation.

Familial forms of adult MND. The familial incidence of MND with pyramidal tract (UMN) signs, i.e. ALS, is 5–10% world-wide with a 1:1 sex distribution ratio and commonly with an autosomal dominant pattern of inheritance (Emery & Holloway 1982). The various forms of spinal muscular atrophy without UMN signs are dealt with below.

The clinical picture in general is similar to that in sporadic cases except for the earlier age of onset, mean 45.1 compared with 56.2 years for sporadic cases (Emery & Holloway 1982), the more frequent onset of weakness in the legs, especially in juvenile-onset cases, and the higher concurrence with other features of CNS disease, e.g. dementia, extrapyramidal disease (reviewed by Bonduelle 1975). Amyotrophy or motor neurone disturbance as part of multisystem degenerative disease is discussed later. Juvenile MND (ALS) is considered here, as a high proportion of cases are familial. Two separate forms appear to exist: an early childhood form, with bulbar features in 80% of cases, has an autosomal recessive pattern of inheritance; and a slowly progressive late juvenile form with autosomal dominant inheritance has early involvement of the legs and no bulbar signs (Emery & Holloway 1982). The latter might better be named familial spastic paraplegia with amyotrophy (Refsum & Skillicorn 1954).

The clinical course of familial MND varies widely, even among some family pedigrees. Overall there is a shorter duration to death (Engel et al 1959, Campbell 1979), but some familial cases, especially the juvenile forms, are extremely chronic (Horton et al 1976).

Western Pacific forms of adult MND. An abnormally high prevalence of MND is found in the indigenous Chamorro population of Guam and other Mariana islands (Reed & Brody 1975, Reed

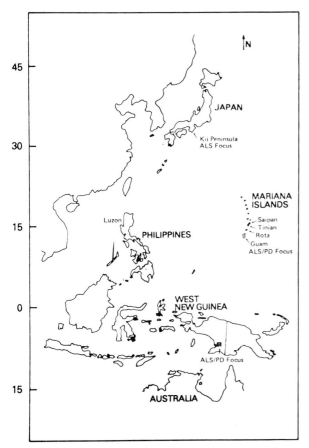

Fig. 23.1 Areas in the Western Pacific affected by a high incidence of adult MND

et al 1975), as well as in certain other foci: on the Kii peninsula of Honshu island, Japan (Kondo 1979), in West New Guinea (Gajdusek 1963, 1982) and in Groote Eylandt and the adjacent coastland of Northern Australia (Kiloh et al 1980) (Fig. 23.1). The clinical picture of MND in these high-incidence foci differs from the ubiquitous form in an earlier age of onset, the predominance of spasticity and leg involvement and the longer clinical course. There is also an inter-relationship with another high-incidence disease, the parkinsonism–dementia complex (P–D) which occurs in the Mariana islands. About 10% of MND patients on Guam show extrapyramidal or intellectual deficit (Kurland & Brody 1975); in the P–D complex about 30% of patients show evident muscle wasting. The epidemiological and pathological features of this form of disease are discussed later.

Unusual clinical features

Intellectual impairment or mental deficit have been described in a small proportion of typical MND patients, especially among familial cases (Wikstrom et al 1982); systematic investigation of cognitive function in a group of sporadic cases showed mild significant cognitive deficit but no memory impairment or behavioural disturbances (Gallassi et al 1985). The syndromes of ALS with dementia have been reviewed by Salazar et al (1983) in relation to transmissible Creutzfeldt-Jakob disease (CJD). Their review included 231 patients with dementia and early LMN signs: in these cases the clinical course was slower than that in CJD and there was little, if any, spongiform change in the brain at autopsy; only two out of 33 brains transmitted a spongiform change to inoculated primates. This is in contrast to the typical subacute transmissible CJD where LMN involvement occurs late in the course of the disease.

Ocular muscle involvement is seldom observed clinically in MND (Harvey et al 1979), although defective eye movements have been detected by electro-oculography (Leveille et al 1982) and nystagmus has also been observed in a few cases (Kushner et al 1984).

Sensory symptoms of numbness, deadness or tingling in the extremities are often mentioned by patients but routine sensory testing is normal even in those familial cases who are subsequently demonstrated to have spinal sensory tract degeneration. However, careful quantitative sensory testing has revealed a 40% incidence of impaired touch-pressure sensibility (Dyck et al 1975). Automated thermal sensory threshold studies have also shown mild abnormalities (Jamal et al 1985). This would correlate with the minor non-motor and sensory abnormalities which have been found in pathological studies (see Hirano et al 1969). Chronic pain has been described in MND but it is uncertain whether this is a primary disorder or secondary to the problems of immobility and pressure deformities (Drake 1983, Newrick & Hewer 1984). Pressure sores or other skin damage is unusual in MND and probably reflects normal autonomic function. Bladder, bowel and sexual dysfunction are unusual even in the terminal stages of the disease. The unaffected autonomic sphincter function correlates with the histological preservation of motor neurones in the nucleus of Onufrowicz area of the sacral spinal cord and of the external anal sphincteric muscle in ALS patients (Mannen et al 1982). Constipation may result from the enforced immobility and low-fibre dietary intake. This may account for the occasional urinary retention. Libido and sexual function can be retained up to the final weeks of the illness (Jokelainen & Palo 1976). Normal cardiovascular responses reflecting vagal nerve function have also been reported (Sachs et al 1985).

Clinical course and prognosis

The usual course of the disease is a relentless spread of wasting and weakness of all skeletal and cranial musculature towards total paralysis, with the exception of the extra-ocular muscles. Diaphragmatic paralysis is usually incomplete for the probable reason that respiratory failure, often complicated by lung infection, is the usual terminal event. A number of patients have an acute arrhythmia or myocardial ischaemia, some-times stimulated by troublesome coughing or choking. In some patients the course is unusually prolonged or even appears to arrest for several years (Mulder & Howard 1976, Norris et al 1980). Most studies have shown a better prognosis for those patients presenting with LMN disease as progressive muscular atrophy, but care must be taken in distinguishing late-onset forms of heredi-tary spinal muscular atrophy. A shorter mean survival occurs in cases of bulbar palsy and/or those patients with early-onset bulbar symptoms, with death within 12–18 months. Mulder & Howard (1976) reported a 50% survival of less than three years, but 20% survived five years and 10% survived 10 years from initial symptoms.

Epidemiology

Adult MND has been described world-wide and in Western countries is responsible for approxi-mately 1 in 1000 adult deaths, with a higher rate in men. The crude death rate is 0.5–1.1 per 100 000 population, centring near 0.8 (Kurtzke 1982). The age-adjusted mortality figure in the USA is 0.6–0.7, being 0.8 for men and 0.4 for women (Juergens & Kurland 1980). The age-specific mortality rates appear to increase steadily up to the 65+ age groups, especially in males, to 5–8 for men and 3–5 per 100 000 for women; recent studies suggest that there may not be a subsequent decline (Li et al 1985).

The annual incidence of MND (ALS) varies between 0.4 and 1.8 per 100 000 population, except in certain foci in the Western Pacific area where the incidence and prevalence are much higher. Recent studies for Rochester, Minnesota, USA, suggest that the age-specific incidence continues to rise with age up to 75+ like that of a degenerative or ageing disease (Juergens et al 1980), whereas earlier studies have shown a peak at 65–70 years with a subsequent decline. There is generally more variation in prevalence rates than reported for incidence, but an overall figure of 4–6 per 100 000 is an average figure (Kurtzke 1982): this would correspond to an average duration of MND of 3–4 years. Between 5% and 10% of cases in most countries are familial, with an equal sex distribution and an autosomal dominant pattern of inheritance (Kurland & Mulder 1955). Several foci of high incidence of MND (ALS) have been extensively reported in the Western Pacific area, starting with Guam. Initially, incidence and mortality rates there were 50–100 times greater than average world-wide figures; however, there has been a steady decline from these high rates to less than 5 per 100 000 population on Guam for 1980–82 (Garruto et al 1985). Similar declining rates have been reported for the Kii peninsula in Japan and a focus in West New Guinea. The significance of this rapid decline is discussed later, but it is inconsistent with a primary genetic origin.

Laboratory investigations

There are still no specific biochemical tests for MND but the most helpful findings are revealed by electro-diagnostic tests. Routine needle electro-myography (EMG) demonstrates scattered spon-taneous fibrillation and fasciculation potentials, and enlarged polyphasic volitional units in muscles from two or more extremities, indicative of dener-vative and reinnervative muscle disease. The spon-taneous motor unit discharges, or fasciculation potentials, are frequently polyphasic and discharge at a slower rate (average every 4–5) than in the benign fasciculation syndrome (Hjorth et al 1973, Trojaborg & Buchthal 1965 and see Ch. 14). The motor unit potentials (MUP) are often prolonged in duration and enlarged in amplitude, indicative of reinnervative activity with increased muscle-fibre density (FD). These changes are more easily seen with macro-EMG studies (Stålberg 1982). The enlarged MUP often has a variable shape or amplitude during consecutive discharges, indicating impaired transmission in new terminal nerve endings. This is best seen as abnormal jitter with single-fibre EMG (SFEMG) studies. An abnormal EMG picture including abnormal jitter in 30% of recordings can be found in clinically normal muscles in MND, or in patients with UMN signs only, but the abnormalities are maximal in the weakest muscles (Stålberg 1982). In slowly progressive disease a high FD (twice to four times the normal level) with high-amplitude macro MUPs (up to 15–20 times normal) and mild to moderate jitter is seen (Swash & Schwartz 1982). With moderately severe weakness the FD and MUP amplitudes are markedly elevated but the maximal reinnervative response is insufficient to compensate for motor unit loss. With increasing weakness the MUP amplitudes progressively decrease as the motor neurones are unable to maintain the maximal degree of reinnervation (Stålberg & Sanders 1983). A rapid clinical progression is associated with a moderately increased FD, normal or mildly increased macro EMG potentials but with very abnormal jitter and frequent impulse blocking on SFEMG (Swash & Schwartz 1982).

The fastest motor and sensory nerve conduction velocities (NCV) are frequently normal, except in severe denervation where the maximal evoked muscle response is less than 10% of normal (Lambert 1969). However, mild slowing and increased F-wave latencies were found in eight of 18 patients studied by Stålberg & Sanders (1983); sensory velocities were slightly abnormal in four patients. This probably reflects secondary demyelinative changes in degenerating axons. Abnormal neuromuscular transmission has been found in a high proportion of MND patients studied by repetitive nerve stimulation and is partly improved by anti-cholinesterase drug administration (Lambert & Mulder 1957, Mulder et al

1959, Denys & Norris 1979). This corresponds to the abnormal jitter found by SFEMG studies and is thought to relate to inefficient reinnervative sprouting rather than terminal fibre degeneration (Stålberg 1982). Slowing of electrical conduction in the central motor pathways of the brain and spinal cord has been demonstrated recently in MND (Ingram & Swash 1987). The changes were most marked in patients with UMN signs but a relative inexcitability of the motor cortex and spinal cord in other early cases was thought to reflect subclinical UMN cell loss, axonal degeneration and secondary demyelination in the central motor pathways. Similar findings of mild CNS slowing have been reported using the new technique of transcutaneous magnetic stimulation of the brain and spinal nerve roots (Barker et al 1985, Ingram et al 1987).

Routine blood investigations are generally normal apart from a mild to moderate increase in the serum creatine kinase (CK) activity in about 40% of MND patients (Williams & Bruford 1970, Harrington et al 1983). Increased serum CK cardiac isoenzyme (MB) has been described in more than one-half of all ALS patients and has been correlated with muscle-fibre regeneration, as seen histologically on muscle biopsy (Koller & Engel 1984). An abnormal blood glucose in response to a glucose loading test, together with a high circulating pyruvate level, has been repeatedly demonstrated in MND (Steinke & Tyler 1964). This was thought to be due to subnormal pancreatic insulin secretion (Gotoh et al 1972), or insulin resistance but this finding was not confirmed by others (Astin et al 1975). Similarly, earlier claims for an abnormal pancreatic exocrine function (Quick & Greer 1967) have not been substantiated.

Increased lead content in the blood and cerebrospinal fluid (CSF) has been reported in MND patients by Conradi and colleagues (see Conradi et al 1982) but has not been found by others (Manton & Cook 1979). A high incidence of radiographic abnormalities of the spine (Campbell et al 1970) has been found also by others and correlated with abnormalities of calcium metabolism in a proportion of MND patients. Abnormal blood calcium levels, usually high rather than low, and elevated concentrations of serum parathormone have been reported in 20% or more of ALS patients (Patten 1982). These changes are thought to represent a secondary hyperparathyroid reaction to hypocalcaemia but no improvement in the neurological state occurred with restoration of the calcium homeostasis. The reason for these changes remains unknown.

Blood group or histocompatibility (HLA) antigen studies have revealed no clear relationship with MND or ALS. Some reports have suggested an over-representation of A3 in ALS patients or an excess of B12 in slow progressive disease (Antel et al 1982, Kott et al 1979). Other studies have reported an excess of BW35 (Kott et al 1976, Bartfeld et al 1982b). Guamanian ALS patients with HLA-BW35 showed impaired cell-mediated immunity and T-cell mitogen reactivity, and a shorter disease duration, compared with Guamanian patients who lacked this antigen (Hoffman et al 1978). The total T-lymphocyte counts, and T-cell subset analyses and serum and CSF immunoglobulins have been unchanged from normal in most studies (Antel et al 1982, Bartfeld et al 1982a), but others have found decreased T-cell reactivity to non-specific mitogens (Hoffman et al 1977, Behan 1979, Aspin et al 1986). Kott et al (1979) reported increased cell- mediated immunity to pooled polio antigens and this has been confirmed by Bartfeld et al (1982a). Serological studies have not shown raised complement-fixing or neutralising antibodies to polio or other viruses in blood or CSF of MND patients (Kascsak et al 1982, Harter 1982). Virus-related antigens or nucleic acid sequences have not been identified in ALS tissue (see Fallis & Weiner 1982). Circulating immune complexes were reported by Oldstone and colleagues (1976) but were undetected in the CSF by Bartfeld et al (1982a); however, Digby et al (1985) reported that MND sera contain immunoglobulins that bind to spinal cord cells in culture. Studies of cell count and total protein levels in CSF are normal in MND.

Pathology

The gross pathological features described by Charcot (1874) have been little modified since (see recent review by Hughes 1982). The overall picture in the CNS is of selective neuronal loss with secondary motor tract degeneration in the brain stem and spinal cord maximal caudally. There may be substantial loss of the large pyramidal cells from layer V of the motor cortex plus corticospinal tract degeneration through the posterior limb of the internal capsule, the cerebral peduncles, brain stem and spinal cord. Such pyramidal tract degeneration is found even in cases without clinically detectable UMN involvement (Friedman & Freedman 1950). Neuronal loss and degeneration is seen in the motor nuclei of the brain stem, especially of the Vth, VIIth, Xth and XIIth cranial nerves. Mild changes may be seen in the oculomotor nuclei of the mid-brain. Degenerative changes include cell shrinkage and neuronophagia. In the spinal cord, neuronal changes are confined to the anterior horn neurones, especially at cervical and lumbar level but with selective sparing of motor neurones in the lateral parts of the sacral cord (nucleus of Onufrowicz) (Mannen et al 1982). The depletion of large neurones is associated with gliosis in the ventral grey matter. Chromatolysis and neurofilamentous accumulation may be found in the more acute cases. Spheroidal axonal swellings on the proximal nerve roots were first described by Wohlfart (1959) and were rediscovered by Carpenter (1968). Electron microscopy reveals that the swellings consist of bundles of 100 nm diameter filaments. Non-motor neurones and myelinated tracts may occasionally show minor degenerative changes in sporadic cases of MND or ALS, in contradistinction to familial MND cases (Hirano et al 1969). A familial form of the disease frequently includes degeneration of the posterior myelinated tracts and of the anterior and posterior spinocerebellar tracts, as well as of Clarke's column, despite the absence of clinical sensory involvement.

Histochemical studies of normal spinal cords show a heavy concentration of acetylcholinesterase (AChE), choline acetyltransferase (ChAT) and muscarinic cholinergic receptors in Rexed layer IX (Villiger & Faull 1985). In ALS, ChAT levels (Gillberg et al 1982) and muscarinic receptors (Whitehouse et al 1983) are markedly reduced. Various other polypeptide neurotransmitters have been studied: glycine levels are normal but glycine receptors are reduced (Hayashi et al 1981, Whitehouse et al 1983); aspartate and glutamate, excitatory transmitters, are normal (Patten et al 1982). Thyrotrophin releasing hormone (TRH) terminals, which are normally restricted to medial layer VII and layer IX (Hokfeld et al 1975, Schoenen et al 1985), are markedly reduced in ALS (Manaker et al 1985). Substance P (SP) studies have given variable results but SP fibres in layer IX of cervical and lumbar ALS cords have been reported as markedly reduced, even when degenerating motor neurones are inconspicuous (Schoenen et al 1985). ChAT activity in ALS peripheral nerves was reduced to 20% of control values and AChE to about 45%, with a greater loss distally (Bradley et al 1983).

Mann & Yates (1974) demonstrated decreased RNA content in the cytoplasm of anterior horn cells of two patients with ALS and postulated that the primary lesion was degeneration of neuronal nuclear DNA with secondary loss of RNA production. These findings have been confirmed by Hartmann & Davidson (1982) in both the cervical and lumbar motor neurones. Ribosomal RNA (rRNA) constitutes 80% of cellular RNA. The 40% reduction in RNA in motor but not in sensory neurones, presumably of rRNA, would deter neuronal protein synthesis.

The anterior nerve roots are thin and pale from depletion of axons and of large myelinated fibres, together with fibrosis. Smaller-diameter myelinated fibres, probably gamma efferents to the muscle spindles, are well preserved (Sobue et al 1981). These ventral root changes are maximal in the cervical and lumbar cord levels and correspond to the selective vulnerability of the large alpha motor neurones in MND (Kawamura et al 1981). Teased-fibre preparations of the ventral roots have demonstrated fibres undergoing axonal degeneration and, to a lesser extent, segmental demyelination (Hanyu et al 1981). The latter abnormality is probably a secondary Schwann-cell change and would correspond to the delayed F-wave nerve conduction seen in electrophysiological studies (Stålberg 1982). Similar degenerative changes have been demonstrated at proximal and distal levels of the phrenic nerve in keeping with a neuronopathy (Bradley et al 1983). Peripheral nerve trunks may appear normal because of the predominant large afferent sensory fibres, although

degeneration and demyelination of sensory fibres to a mild extent is well established in MND (Dayan et al 1969, Dyck et al 1975). These sensory nerve changes correlate with reports that neurones in the lumbar dorsal root ganglia are reduced to 46% of control numbers (Kawamura et al 1981). Degeneration and regenerative sprouting of motor nerve endings, together with denervated atrophic motor end-plates, are seen in muscle biopsy specimens (Bjornskov et al 1984, Tsujihata et al 1984). Skeletal muscles show the typical changes of chronic denervation with grouped fibre atrophy, often of the same histochemical type. Inflammatory changes are not present but occasional regenerating fibres may be seen, especially in rapidly progressive clinical cases.

Aetiology

Approximately 90–95% of cases of adult MND (ALS) seem to be sporadic. Familial cases of ALS show a greater degree of non-motor involvement pathologically but the motor neuronal changes are thought to be identical to those found in sporadic cases. The rapid decline in incidence of ALS on Guam and other foci in the Western Pacific area (Garruto et al 1985) is inconsistent with a primary genetic disease. The offspring of index cases have not shown an increased risk of developing ALS (Plato et al 1984). In addition, Chamorros on the neighbouring Mariana islands, Saipan and Tinian, do not have an increased incidence of ALS (Yanagihara et al 1983). Hence the earlier high incidence on Guam and the Kii peninsula of Japan has been suggested as resulting from environmental factors. The absence of any clear blood group or HLA association is also evidence against a genetically determined metabolic defect. Studies of motor neuropathies complicating known genetically determined metabolic disorders (e.g. hexosaminidase A deficiency or adrenomyeloneuropathy) have not been helpful so far.

Progressive neuronal loss occurs in the ventral horn of the spinal grey matter with normal ageing (Tomlinson & Irving 1977); this correlates with the finding of neurogenic muscular atrophy in skeletal muscles of the elderly (Tomlinson et al 1969) and electrophysiological evidence of progressive loss of motor units after the age of 60 years (Campbell et al 1973). Hence the suggestion has been made that MND is due to an accelerated ageing process (McComas et al 1973b). This suggestion would be more tenable if recent work suggesting an increasing incidence of MND with age were substantiated (Juergens et al 1980) rather than the more common finding of a peak incidence at about 65 years and a decline thereafter. The accelerated ageing could be due to exogenous factors, e.g. previous infection with polio or other viruses.

The observation of a low RNA content in motor neurones led Mann & Yates (1974) to postulate a primary defect of nuclear DNA with decreased RNA synthesis and subsequent protein synthesis. Such a theory is supported by the observation of a 30% reduction in RNA content and nuclear RNA synthesis in the spinal motor neurones of the wobbler mouse, an animal model of human MND (Murakami et al 1981). Actinomycin D, a specific RNA polymerase inhibitor that inhibits RNA and protein synthesis, and the 5-fluoropyrimidines that disturb biosynthesis of pyrimidine nucleotides, RNA and protein, when injected intrathecally into cats, both lead to neuronal degeneration (Koenig 1969). Thus there are several possible mechanisms for the reduced level of ribosomal RNA in ALS motor neurones, although Bradley & Krasin (1982) have postulated aberrant transcription caused by accumulation of unrepaired DNA damage arising from a deficiency of DNA repair enzymes.

The superficial similarity to PMA of various motor neuropathies attributable to intoxication with heavy metals, notably lead, has resulted in repeated searches for their involvement in MND; but it should be noted that an increased incidence of the disease has not been reported among lead or manganese workers. A higher incidence of exposure to the heavy metals, lead and mercury, participation in athletics and consumption of large quantities of milk, was reported for a group of 25 ALS patients (Felmus et al 1976). Several previous studies have reported failure of treatment with various chelating agents in MND or ALS patients who gave a history of exposure to lead, mercury or arsenic (Currier & Haerer 1968, Engel et al 1969, Campbell et al 1970). The reports by Conradi and colleagues (1982) of increased levels

of lead in blood and CSF of ALS patients have not been confirmed by others (Manton & Cook 1979), although a high level of lead in spinal cord tissue from ALS patients has been demonstrated (Kurlander & Patten 1979). The mode of entry of lead into the nervous system in ALS has not been established. The search for local environmental factors in the high-incidence Western Pacific areas have revealed a low calcium and magnesium concentration in garden soil and drinking water and a higher content of heavy or trace metals, e.g. manganese and aluminium (Yase 1972, 1984). Analyses of brain tissue from ALS cases on Guam and Japan have shown a high intra-neuronal content of calcium and aluminium (Garruto et al 1984) and also a high manganese level in spinal cord tissue (Miyata et al 1983). X-ray analysis has shown metal-related calcification in degenerating areas of the cervical cord in ALS (Yoshida 1977, 1979, quoted by Yanagihara 1982). Selective motor neurone involvement may occur because of the requirement for high levels of calcium ions. Yase (1984) has postulated that chronic nutritional deficiencies of calcium and magnesium may cause secondary hyperparathyroidism leading to increased bone resorption and release of calcium and other cations, as well as increased intestinal absorption of trace metals, thus leading to ectopic calcification and deposition of heavy metals. The deposition of heavy metals including manganese, aluminium and lead in the CNS may be a secondary phenomenon, as a consequence of an altered blood–brain barrier or as a result of neuronal degeneration and reactive gliosis (Mandýbur & Cooper 1979). However, Yase (1984) cites experiments with rats maintained on a low calcium and magnesium diet which results in ectopic calcification in kidney, muscle and the CNS, and is associated with increased gliosis and anterior horn cell degeneration in the spinal cord. Such changes are said to occur only in the presence of parathormone. Patients with primary or secondary hyperparathyroidism have been reported to have neuromuscular disorders and signs suggestive of MND (Patten 1982), but treatment of a number of typical MND patients with abnormal calcium metabolism showed no improvement in neurological function.

An alternative theory for a toxic cause of the

earlier high incidence and prevalence of ALS on Guam has been related to the dietary use of the Cycad nut. This was a major source of edible starch for the native Chamorros. It is known to contain certain neurotoxic compounds including cycasin, or methylazoxymethanol, a lathyrogenic factor (Kurland & Molgaard 1982). However, animal experiments have failed to produce a disease resembling ALS or human lathyrism. The decline in ALS on Guam has coincided with a striking reduction in the use of Cycad as the Chamorros have changed from a horticultural and fishing subsistence economy to a westernised culture (Garruto et al 1985).

A number of viruses selectively infect neurones and in some cases motor neurones, e.g. poliovirus. The production of new viral particles is the result of an ordered sequence of virus–cell interactions within the permissive cell. Susceptible cells may initiate translation of early viral proteins, but fail to form complete viruses, i.e., they are non-permissively infected. Non-permissive infections can lead to cell death, cell transformation or metabolic deficits, even though the infected cell does not contain infectious virus or morphologically discernible viral particles (Johnson RT 1982a). Polioviruses in man and the neurotrophic retrovirus in the mouse (Gardner et al 1973) both cause paralytic disease with acute pathological changes in the spinal motor neurones. Polio infection excites an intense inflammatory response with neuronal degeneration and an acute cytolytic reaction in some cells. In the retrovius infection in the mouse there is a long incubation period resulting in a chronic non-inflammatory infection with neuronal degeneration (Andrews & Gardner 1974. The selective involvement of motor neurones in poliomyelitis and MND has led to many attempts to isolate poliovirus, or to demonstrate virus structures, antigens or raised antibody responses in ALS patients, all with negative results. These studies were prompted by reports of a higher incidence of previous poliomyelitis infections in MND patients (Zilkha 1962, Poskanzer et al 1969). The situation has been complicated by the frequent description of chronic MND in patients occurring many years after acute paralytic poliomyelitis (Campbell et al 1969, Mulder et al 1972, Dalakas et al 1986). This disease, perhaps better

named post-poliomyelitis muscular atrophy (PPMA), becomes symptomatic some 15–54 years after acute poliomyelitis. The new weakness and muscular atrophy develops in muscles previously affected and fully or partly recovered, or in clinically unaffected muscles. Occasional fasciculations are seen but bulbar symptoms or UMN signs do not appear during the slow progressive course. Electrodiagnostic tests show the typical appearances of a very chronic denervation disorder with giant MUP, but abnormal jitter and frequent blocking are seen in most muscles (Dalakas et al 1986). This indicates poor function in the terminal nerve fibres and correlates with the old observations of myasthenic-like neuromuscular fatigue in surviving muscles (Hodes 1948). Histological studies of muscle biopsies from PPMA have shown scattered isolated angulated atrophic fibres and no grouped atrophy. This has been interpreted as indicative of degeneration of individual nerve terminals in the hypertrophied motor unit rather than as a result of complete motor unit loss from neuronal death (Dalakas et al 1986). It has been proposed that the motor neurone is unable to maintain the metabolic demands of the extended territory and target cells, i.e., it shows an accelerated ageing phenomenon. Cerebrospinal fluid studies have shown normal protein and IgG levels and no evidence of in situ antibody production to poliovirus. This does not entirely rule out the possibility of chronic or reactivated polio infection, as animal studies with Theiler's virus or murine poliomyelitis have shown a delayed immune response to the chronic mild inflammatory disease (Lipton & Dal Canto 1976). A case of chronic progressive poliomyelitis secondary to live virus vaccination has been reported in an immunodeficient child (Davis et al 1977). A search for other viruses in MND has produced no substantiated results. Repeated transmission studies of ALS material into primates have been negative (Gibbs & Gajdusek 1982). Similar negative results of attempts to isolate viruses in tissue culture from muscle were reported by Cremer et al (1973).

As mentioned in the section on investigations (p. 761–763), no strong link with an HLA antigen has been reported in MND: thus there is no evidence for a genetically determined immune responsiveness. Poliovirus antigens or other specific antigens have not been identified in the reported circulating immune complexes (Antel et al 1982). The report that MND sera contain immunoglobulins that bind to spinal cord cells in culture (Digby et al 1985) and the report of serum auto-antibodies directed against a muscle-derived growth factor for spinal neurones (Gurney et al 1984), add further evidence that ALS patients mount an immune response to the disease. The latter studies support earlier reports of a toxic effect of MND sera on spinal cord explants (Wolfgram & Myers 1973, Wolfgram 1976) and upon myelinated nerve cultures (Bornstein & Appel 1965, Field & Hughes 1969). The finding of an oncogenic retrovirus causing both lymphoma and chronic motor neuronal disease in mice (Gardner et al 1973) has raised the question of a relationship between cancer and MND. The rare reports of MND occurring in association with bronchial carcinoma probably represent a chance association (Barron & Rodichock 1982). There is a more direct link between plasma cell dyscrasias with paraproteinaemia and motor neuropathies. Plasma paraproteins of the IgG, IgM and IgA type have all been associated with LMN disease or a demyelinative neuropathy but only rarely with an ALS picture (Latov 1982). In any event, typical ALS patients do not normally show the presence of a paraprotein in the blood.

Treatment

Not surprisingly for a condition of unknown cause, many treatments have been tried, based on theories of the aetiology and generally with negative results. Initial anecdotal or uncontrolled studies have not been substantiated in clinical trials. The latter have been reviewed extensively elsewhere (Festoff & Crigger 1980) and this paper endeavours to summarize these and more recent reports. Some drugs do have an effect in modifying the symptoms or pathophysiological effects of the disease.

The early reports of ALS-like disorders associated with hypoglycaemia or insulinomas led to studies of glucose metabolism and then of pancreatic or gastrointestinal function. Pancreatic extract and tocopherol (vitamin E) have been tried

therapeutically but without benefit (Quick & Greer 1967, Brown & Kater 1969, Dorman et al 1969). Hydroxycobalamin (vitamin B_{12}) injections, either parenterally or intrathecally, were unhelpful (Peiper & Fields 1959). The reports of abnormal calcium metabolism in some ALS patients led to unsuccessful treatment with vitamin D preparations (Patten 1982). The association of ALS with parkinsonism on Guam led to unsuccessful therapeutic trials of levodopa in Guamanians and sporadic cases of ALS (Mendell et al 1971). Similarly, amantadine, an antiviral agent which also enhances dopamine release in the CNS, was unhelpful (Norris 1972a). Bovine brain gangliosides, which promote axonal sprouting, were not beneficial in two more recent trials (Bradley et al 1984, Harrington et al 1984).

The reports of abnormal exposure to lead or other heavy metals in MND patients led to several unsuccessful therapeutic trials with the chelating agents dimercaprol, EDTA and penicillamine (Kantarjian 1961, Campbell et al 1970, Conradi et al 1982). Reports of circulating neurotoxins (Wolfgram 1976) may have been the basis for treatment with modified snake neurotoxins (Sanders & Fellowes 1975) but initial enthusiasm was not borne out in controlled trials (Tyler 1979). Plasma exchange with or without immunosuppression has been ineffective in ALS patients (Silani et al 1980, Kelemen et al 1983).

The possible association of MND with polio or other virus infection has led to many negative studies with antiviral agents (Server & Wolinsky 1982). These have included idoxyuridine (Liversedge et al 1970), inosiplex (isoprinosine) (Percy et al 1971), amantadine (Norris 1972a), cytosine arabinoside (Ara-C) and guanidine (Norris et al 1974, Munsat et al 1981). Drugs which modify or improve the host defences against viral infection have also been tried unsuccessfully. These include levamisole (Olarte & Shafer 1985), interferons (Cook et al 1979, Rissanen et al 1980), tilorone (Olson et al 1978) polyinosinic-polycytidylic acid (Poly-ICIC) (Engel et al 1978), which are interferon-inducing drugs, and transfer factor (Olarte et al 1979). The corticosteroids and more powerful immunosuppressive drugs, including intrathecal hydrocortisone (Peiper & Fields 1959) and azathioprine, have also been tried with negative results in ALS. Plasmapheresis to remove any possible humoral factors has also given negative results (Olarte et al 1980).

The demonstration of low levels of TRH in spinal grey matter of ALS patients led to therapeutic trials. A transient improvement with intravenous therapy in large doses (Engel et al 1983) may be the result of modifying spasticity by an action on interneurones (Delwaide & Schoenen 1985). The results of further studies with intrathecal TRH infusions and with RX 77368, a long-acting TRH analogue, are being evaluated. Considerable benefit in relieving spasticity may be obtained from the synthetic GABA-like compound baclofen, but alternative treatment with the peripheral neuromuscular blocking agent dantrolene usually causes unacceptable enhancement of weakness and may precipitate respiratory failure. The earlier reports of benefit from an uncontrolled trial of guanidine therapy (Norris 1973) is probably related to its action in facilitating the release of acetylcholine at the neuromuscular junction (Otsuka & Endo 1960). Similar symptomatic benefits may be seen in some MND patients, especially with bulbar weakness, with the anticholinesterase drugs neostigmine and pyridostigmine. Unfortunately, the improvement is usually short-lived and may be masked by troublesome side effects of muscle cramps or increased salivation. The latter can be improved with anticholinergic compounds such as atropine or its synthetic analogues.

Management

The good management of a patient with MND or ALS requires considerable expertise in interpersonal relationships with the patient and his family, plus the support and help of other professional health care workers. A simple understanding of the nature of their progressive neuromuscular disorder leading to increasing disability must be imparted to the sufferers. This is helped by explaining the sparing of intellectual functioning and the absence of incontinence, together with a knowledge of the variable prognosis. In later stages of the disease, mood-elevating drugs may be necessary for the understandable depression. The need for attendance at special clinics is controversial but it is generally accepted that one medical adviser should undertake the supervision of care and co-ordination of various necessary aids. Contact with volunteer support organisations may be considered appropriate.

Many drug trials are taking place, as discussed previously, but essentially no effective treatment is available at present. Symptomatic treatment can be tried: for weakness, especially of bulbar musculature, pyridostigmine (Mestinon®) 60–90 mg 4-hourly; for spasticity, baclofen (Lioresal®) 10–30 mg 6-hourly; for hypersalivation, atropine sulphate 0.6–1.2 mg 6-hourly or benzhexol hydrochloride (Artane®) 2–5 mg 6-hourly, as well as appropriate psychotropic drugs.

The management of bulbar palsy involves treatment of dysphagia, of hypersalivation with drooling and of speech difficulty (Campbell & Enderby 1984). Dysphagia may be managed more successfully if positioning, texture of the diet, food supplements and a swallow routine are attended to by a therapist. In the case of more spastic difficulty, relaxation of muscles by sucking an ice cube prior to meals may facilitate swallowing. The drugs pyridostigmine or baclofen may be tried as detailed above. Progressive dysphagia may result in pooling of secretions and food in the hypopharynx, which predisposes to tracheo-bronchial aspiration. Benefits may be obtained from cricopharyngeal myotomy, which lowers the resting intrapharyngeal pressure (Mills 1973, Lebo et al 1976). Severe drooling, unresponsive to anticholinergic drugs, may be helped by salivary gland irradiation or denervation; division of the chorda tympani nerve by transtympanic surgery can be performed under local anaesthesia and can result in a 95% reduction of salivation (Zalin & Cooney 1974, Mullins et al 1979). Unfortunately, a drier mouth may have negative effects on speech, particularly if the tongue has LMN involvement causing generalised weakness. Occasionally tracheostomy and the use of a cuffed airway is necessary to prevent distressing choking or spluttering on natural secretions or food particles. Various means have been advocated for the treatment of severe dysphagia and maintenance of adequate nutrition, with additional food supplements being the primary course, but later surgical techniques including gastrostomy and cervical oesophagostomy may be considered. We favour the use of small-bore nasogastric tubes, which can be well tolerated for many months. Adequate nutrition will prevent some weight loss and will optimise strength.

Dyspnoea is a late symptom of ventilatory weakness in MND and usually arises only when the FVC is below 50% of the predicted normal, or where there is co-existing lung disease. Physiotherapy with inspiratory muscle training may improve ventilatory function in neuromuscular disease (Martin et al 1983). Some patients benefit from ventilatory support with a tracheostomy. This is best reserved for those patients who at least have good upper limb function which enables them to continue useful activities. Long-term management with portable mechanical ventilatory support at home is possible, provided that the necessary support of family or others is available. The physical and psychological problems associated with such long-term support have been discussed recently by Sivak and colleagues (1982), and by Tandan & Bradley (1985). In the terminal stages of MND with ventilatory weakness, the regular use of a small dose of opiate can be helpful; we advocate diamorphine 2.5 mg 4–6-hourly.

Physiotherapy for limb weakness is of limited value in MND but is helpful psychologically and allows evaluation of the needs for mechanical aids, such as foot drop splints, wrist supports, cervical collars for neck muscle weakness or suitable wheelchairs with adequate head rests or mobile arm supports. The help of an occupational therapist may prolong independence with dressing by the adaptation of clothing fasteners, or with eating by the provision of suitable large-handled cutlery and cups, or with writing by similar large-handled implements.

Speech therapy is useful on several counts. In the early stages of speech difficulty, deliberate slowing of the rate of speech may considerably aid intelligibility. More specific exercises, especially of the tongue, may help to overcome localised weakness for a short period. Modification of speech patterns may help to overcome hypernasality. In some cases a palatal lift incorporated into an upper denture will avoid nasal escape and increase intra-oral pressure. Relaxation exercises may help to overcome spasticity but the anti-spasmodic drug baclofen should also be tried, as mentioned above. Marked fatiguability of the voice with dysphonia may be eased by pyridostigmine therapy or by a simple amplifier. The availability of a portable suction apparatus may facilitate speech by removing excess secretions and distressing gurgling. Eventually, communication aids are required, ranging from a simple alphabet board to portable electronic communicators, or to more elaborately activated electronic display systems triggered by head or eye movements (Campbell & Enderby 1984). The latter may be incorporated into a comprehensive environmental control system (e.g. POSSUM) which opens doors, or operates controls of telephone, radio or television sets, etc.

The management of end-stage MND is concerned with maintaining a quality of life rather than prolonging misery and more suffering (Campbell 1980, Carey 1986). It is of prime importance that the patient and relatives do not feel abandoned at this stage. Rational symptomatic treatment, as described above, is insufficient and psychotropic drugs may be required to allay mental anguish. Narcotic medication, including opiates, is indicated rather than antibiotics or more supportive measures. We commonly use diamorphine 2.5 mg four to six-hourly, despite the increased risk of central respiratory depression, sleep apnoea and respiratory arrest.

HEREDITARY SPINAL MUSCULAR ATROPHIES

These are a heterogeneous group of heredofamilial disorders of the motor neurones, predominantly of the spinal cord but occasionally affecting the motor nuclei of the brain stem and without clinical evidence of involvement of sensory or UMN pathways (Harding 1984). The various types can generally be distinguished clinically by the distribution of weakness, the pattern of inheritance and by the age of onset. Family studies show virtually no overlap between the acute generalised, benign proximal, scapuloperoneal and distal forms of the disease, thus suggesting a different genetic cause (Emery 1971,

Pearn et al 1978a,c). Some overlap occurs in relation to age of onset and prognosis of the acute and chronic infantile forms (Pearn 1980, 1982).

Infantile spinal muscular atrophy (Werdnig–Hoffmann disease: SMA Type I)

It is agreed that there are two different forms of this severe generalised disease: an acute early form (SMA Type I) and a more chronic form (SMA Type II). Both are inherited as an autosomal recessive trait but there is some dispute as to whether one or several genes are involved. Pearn (1982) has claimed that, in his extensive studies, no family with the acute form of the disease had siblings with the milder chronic form.

The acute infantile form (SMA Type I) was first described by Sevestre (1899). It is characterised by its severe generalised muscle involvement and fatal outcome before three years of age (Brandt 1950, Byers & Banker 1961). In at least one-third of cases the disease is manifest, before or at birth, either by decreased fetal movements or by congenital skeletal deformities, usually of the chest, hips or feet. In a large study by Pearn & Wilson (1973a) the onset occurred before five months of age, and before three months in 95% of cases. Generalised weakness and hypotonia with areflexia was the commonest presenting feature in two-thirds, and feeding difficulties in 40% of cases. Breathing difficulties are usually responsible for the inevitably fatal outcome. Fasciculations may be evident in the wasted tongue but are generally invisible elsewhere. Buchthal & Olsen (1970) failed to find any true fasciculation potentials on EMG in the limbs but did document a unique finding of regularly discharging motor units every 5–15 seconds in relaxed muscles or during sleep. Other EMG features of severe denervation with a central motor neuropathy are commonly found. The mean age at death is six to nine months, depending on the pre- or postnatal onset, and 95% of infants died before 18 months of age.

Pathological studies of the brain and spinal cord show severe loss of motor neurones but some remaining cells are chromatolytic (Byers & Banker 1961, Chou & Fakadej 1971). The anterior motor roots are very atrophic and sensory roots and

spinal cord tracts appear normal, although careful studies have found mild abnormalities of the dorsal root ganglia and non-motor pathways (Carpenter et al 1978, Marshall & Duchen 1978). Histological studies of skeletal muscle show severe denervation changes with scattered small groups, or single hypertrophied fibres, usually of Type I and also apparent preservation of muscle spindles.

SMA Type II

The chronic infantile form (SMA Type II), first described by Werdnig (1891, 1894) and by Hoffmann (1893, 1897), is a more slowly progressive generalised disease with a variable prognosis. It appears to have a slightly later onset than SMA Type I and rarely presents before six months of age, but 75% are manifest in the first year (Pearn et al 1978b). Less than 25% of infants are ever able to sit unsupported and none learn to crawl or walk (Pearn & Wilson 1973b). Atrophy and fasciculation is seen in the tongue. Spontaneous tremor of the fingers may be evident and correlates with the EMG findings of spontaneous motor unit discharges (Buchthal & Olsen 1970). Tendon reflexes are depressed or absent, especially by two years of age. Clinical progression is slow or appears even to arrest, although sudden deterioration may be associated with intercurrent infection (Munsat et al 1969). All children, if untreated, develop scoliosis with further compromise of respiratory ventilation and increased risk of pneumonia. Life expectancy is very variable, ranging up to adult life in some cases.

The differentiation of this form from SMA Types I and III has been disputed. However, two studies have suggested that a single recessive gene accounts for over 90% of cases in Groups II and III (Bundey & Lovelace 1975, Pearn et al 1978c).

Chronic proximal spinal muscular atrophy (Kugelberg–Welander disease: SMA Type III)

Kugelberg & Welander (1954, 1956) and Wohlfart et al (1955) described a progressive proximal muscular weakness in young adults, clinically resembling a muscular dystrophy but showing fasciculations and investigational findings of a neuropathic disorder. Kugelberg (1975) later defined the clinical picture as proximal muscular atrophy and weakness especially in the legs, pseudohypertrophy of the calves, absent knee jerks with other tendon reflexes preserved, no pyramidal signs and normal intelligence. Patients are able to walk for more than 10 years after the onset and are capable of normal survival. Fasciculations in limb muscles are seen in at least 50% of cases, but are rarely evident in the tongue; bulbar involvement is rare. The usual presentation is difficulty in walking, especially up steps or stairs, together with a waddling gait. Later there is difficulty in lifting the arms and winging of the scapulae. The posture is hyperlordotic with a protuberant abdomen. Joint contractures and kyphoscoliosis are common later.

Kugelberg & Welander (1956) found EMG evidence of spontaneous fasciculations and chronic denervation changes with giant residual units. Muscle biopsy in five cases showed fibre-type grouping, both of the small atrophic and of the hypertrophied muscle fibres, thus indicating the neuropathic nature of the disease. Wohlfart (1942) had previously described two similar clinical cases, also with evident fasciculations, but on finding 'myopathic' changes in a muscle biopsy he ascribed the disease to a muscular dystrophy. He subsequently reassessed these two cases, together with seven others, and confirmed the findings of Kugelberg & Welander (Wohlfart et al 1955). The secondary myopathic abnormalities often found in muscle sections appear to correlate with the presence of 'myopathic' motor units on EMG studies (Gath et al 1969) and also with the frequent finding of an increased serum CK activity (Mastaglia & Walton 1971). The few autopsy reports have confirmed the spinal motor neuronal loss and have shown no evidence of corticospinal or sensory tract involvement (Gardner-Medwin et al 1967, Kohn 1968).

Juvenile proximal SMA was familial in about two-thirds of cases reviewed by Namba et al (1970). The majority of families have shown an autosomal recessive pattern of inheritance, but both dominant and X-linked recessive forms of the disease have been described (see Emery 1971). Adult onset of typical cases showing a benign cause was first described by Finkel (1962) and Wiesendanger (1962) and the clinical symptoms of

such patients resemble those in cases of Becker or limb-girdle muscular dystrophy (Pearn et al 1978c). However, the importance of their differentiation lies in distinguishing such cases from adult MND with its wretched prognosis.

Chronic distal spinal muscular atrophy

This group of disorders is very heterogeneous, both clinically and genetically. Sporadic and familial cases have been described with many different ages of onset. Autosomal dominant and recessive patterns of inheritance have been described. Atrophy and weakness usually start in the lower extremities and later spread to involve the hands and lower forearms (Dyck & Lambert 1968b, McLeod & Prineas 1971). However, Meadows & Marsden (1969) described three siblings with onset in the hands in childhood and with spread to the lower legs in later life. Pes cavus is more prominent in the early-onset cases. The condition is relatively benign and severe disability is uncommon. Some of the adult cases may be indistinguishable from early forms of the scapuloperoneal syndrome or the neuronal/axonal form of peroneal muscular atrophy (HMSN type II) (Harding & Thomas 1980). The latter condition is distinguished by the presence of minor sensory abnormalities found either clinically or on electrodiagnostic tests (Dyck & Lambert 1968b), whereas motor and sensory conduction velocities in distal SMA are normal.

Bulbo-spinal muscular atrophy

This disorder of late onset, which is clinically and genetically different from the proximal forms of spinal muscular atrophy (HMN), was first described by Kennedy et al al (1968). The age of onset varies but most cases occur at 20–40 years of age. Proximal weakness usually begins in the lower limbs, then spreads to the shoulder girdle, face and bulbar musculature. Fasciculation is prominent, especially in the face and tongue. Postural tremor of the outstretched hands occurs frequently (Harding 1984). Dysphagia and dysarthria develop some 10–20 years after the onset of weakness. Gynaecomastia is common and diabetes may also occur. Life expectancy may be normal.

Electrodiagnostic tests show evidence of severe denervation. Motor nerve conduction velocity is normal or slightly reduced; some cases have shown absent or reduced sensory potentials (Kennedy et al 1968, Stefanis et al 1975, Harding et al 1982).

In familial cases the condition is inherited as an X-linked recessive tract. Sporadic cases are also generally noted in males.

Scapuloperoneal form

The scapuloperoneal syndrome includes a variety of disorders giving rise to proximal weakness around the shoulders and distal weakness in the lower limbs. Some cases appear to be myopathic (see Kaeser 1975), generally with an onset around the shoulder girdle and with features resembling those of facioscapulohumeral muscular dystrophy except that the face is spared (see below). Kaeser (1964, 1965) reported the findings in 12 members of a family extending through five generations and with an autosomal dominant pattern of inheritance. The onset was in adult life with symmetrical weakness and wasting of the long extensor muscles of the toes and ankles. After many years the muscles around the shoulder girdle became involved, producing winging of the scapulae and difficulty in raising the arms. The weakness of the legs also spread to involve the calves and quadriceps muscles. In two cases, in the fourth and fifth generations, bulbar muscles became involved, resulting in dysphagia, dysphonia and facial weakness; extra-ocular weakness was present in one case. Tendon reflexes were diminished or absent; sensory examination revealed no abnormal findings. EMG studies in three affected members (Kaeser 1975) revealed abundant fibrillation and fasciculation potentials in some muscles. Severe denervation changes were evident in the legs but a mixed pattern was found in the facial muscles and in muscles around the shoulder girdle. Motor conduction velocities and sensory nerve studies were normal. Muscle biopsies from the lower extremities gave findings which were consistent with chronic denervation but specimens from the deltoid or triceps muscle were thought to be myopathic or pseudomyopathic. An autopsy study of one case showed clear evidence of degeneration of anterior horn cells and bulbar motor nuclei and a neurogenic type of muscle atrophy including muscles of the upper extremity.

Sporadic cases with a similar distribution of muscle involvement have been described in infancy (Feigenbaum & Munsat 1970). Zellweger & McCormick (1968) described a single congenital case with talipes equinovarus and progressive inspiratory stridor due to bilateral vocal cord paralysis. A family of three affected sibs with an onset in childhood and a mildly affected mother has been studied personally in conjunction with Dr B.Berg. The propositus presented with acute bulbar weakness and bilateral vocal cord paralysis requiring tracheostomy. She later developed a scapuloperoneal distribution of muscular atrophy which was evident in two of three brothers and in her mother. The EMG findings in this family, as in the other childhood cases, were those of chronic denervation with normal motor conduction velocities.

Facioscapulohumeral form

Conditions resembling facioscapulohumeral muscular dystrophy in the distribution of muscular atrophy and weakness have been described in a mother and daughter, with onset in adolescence but with pathological evidence of a neuropathy (Fenichel et al 1967). Facial weakness was the first symptom, followed by involvement of the proximal limb muscles. Two other sporadic cases with a similar picture were reported by Furukawa et al 1969). There are also some forms of the scapuloperoneal syndrome which could alternatively be included here (Kaeser 1975).

Progressive juvenile bulbar palsy (Fazio–Londe disease)

There appear to be two forms of this rare disease — the Vialetto–van Laere syndrome and Fazio–Londe disease. The Vialetto–van Laere syndrome is an autosomal recessive disorder usually presenting in the second decade with facial weakness, dysphagia and dysarthria, and associated with sensorineural deafness. The weakness later spreads to affect the limbs and sometimes the trunk, causing respiratory difficulty, sometimes with sleep apnoea (Vialetto 1936, van Laere 1966, Gallai et al 1981). Autopsy reports have described degeneration and atrophy of cranial nuclei VI to XII.

Cases of Fazio–Londe disease do not have deafness and generally begin in early childhood. Fazio (1892) described the disease in a mother and son, and Londe (1894) described a more rapid disease in two brothers. Excessive drooling from facial weakness, repeated respiratory infections and stridor are the usual presenting features. Dysphagia and ocular paresis as well as generalised limb weakness may follow. Death is usually from respiratory failure and/or infection. Autopsied cases have shown degeneration and atrophy of the brain-stem nuclei including the oculomotor nerves, and a variable loss of anterior horn cells in the cervical and dorsal spinal cord; the pyramidal tracts were normal (Gomez et al 1962, Alexander et al 1976).

Motor neuropathy with hexosaminidase A deficiency

Neurogenic muscular atrophy is a common feature of hexosaminidase deficiency diseases causing GM2-gangliosidosis but in two phenotypes motor neuropathy was the presenting manifestation (Johnson W G 1982). In one family a progressive adolescent-onset spinal muscular atrophy syndrome resembled Kugelberg–Welander disease (SMA type III) (Johnson et al 1982). There were no UMN findings or macular abnormality (cherry-red spot) and no dementia. Biochemically there was severe deficiency of hexosaminidase A (Hex. A). Rectal ganglion cells were filled with classic membranous cytoplasmic bodies. Presumably the spinal motor neurones were similarly affected. The second type concerns a single case of an ALS-like syndrome commencing in late adolescence with cramps, progressive proximal atrophy and weakness and dysarthria. Generally brisk tendon reflexes were accompanied by extensor plantar responses. The principal biochemical finding was of severe Hex. A deficiency. Rectal neurones were enlarged and contained membranous cytoplasmic bodies.

Juvenile muscular atrophy of one upper extremity

In 1959 Hirayama et al described a new clinical entity which they entitled 'juvenile muscular atrophy of unilateral upper extremity' and in 1987 Hirayama and his colleagues reported the first autopsy findings in a single case, noting that some 150 cases had been reported in the interim from Japan and many from other countries. The condition occurs predominantly in males aged 15–25 years, is usually sporadic and develops insidiously with muscular weakness and atrophy beginning in the hand and generally limited to the hand and forearm, ceasing to progress after one or two years. Pathologically they found atrophy of the anterior horns of the spinal cord at C5–T1 with degeneration of large and small nerve cells and some gliosis. The aetiology is unknown.

HEREDITARY MOTOR AND SENSORY NEUROPATHIES (HMSN)

A detailed description of all these conditions is outside the scope of this chapter and is dealt with more fully elsewhere (see Dyck 1984).

The separation of these conditions from hereditary spinal muscular atrophies especially in the distal forms is somewhat arbitrary. All have selective neuronal degeneration and atrophy but the conditions discussed here are not exclusive for motor neurones, that is both motor and sensory peripheral neurones are affected. The clinical features affect both sides of the body symmetrically and the course is chronic and fairly progressive. These are inherited disorders and hence are assumed to be related to inborn errors of metabolism; but in most cases the nature of this is unknown. The identification of biochemical abnormalities, and sometimes of the enzyme deficiency, has been made in a few cases, e.g. in Refsum's disease, metachromatic leucodystrophy and hexosaminidase A deficiency.

Many of these conditions are included in the peroneal muscular atrophy syndrome (Charcot–Marie–Tooth disease). This is a heterogeneous group, both clinically and genetically. All patients have predominant involvement of peripheral motor neurones, with lesser disease of peripheral sensory and autonomic neurones. The disorders are inherited, are slowly progressive and cause symmetrical distal muscular atrophy and weakness affecting the feet initially, together with some distal sensory loss (see Dyck 1984). Dejerine & Sottas (1893) described the pathological findings of hypertrophic interstitial neuritis in two siblings with typical features of HMSN. Subsequently it has been shown many times that nerve hypertrophy can be present in many different types of the disease, including the common form, HMSN type I. Dyck & Lambert (1968a) proposed a classification based on motor nerve conduction velocity measurements. In HMSN type I the conduction velocity is markedly slowed due to severe demyelinative and remyelinative changes along the degenerating axons. Type II HMSN was associated with normal or mildly slowed conduction related only to the minimal secondary demyelinative change in peripheral nerves. Subsequently, sub-groups based on the clinical picture and pattern of inheritance have been proposed (Dyck 1984).

HMSN type I includes the commonest clinical type inherited as an autosomal dominant trait as described by Charcot & Marie (1886) and concurrently by Tooth (1886). Separate rare autosomal recessive forms include those described by Dejerine & Sottas (1893) and Refsum (1946). The dominantly inherited form may be very variable in its severity and even asymptomatic. The onset is usually apparent in the second to fourth decades, with abnormalities of the feet, usually pes cavus, steppage gait and atrophy and weakness of the small muscles of the feet and peronei. Later cases show atrophy and clawing of the hands and sometimes wasting and weakness of the lower thigh muscles. Tendon reflexes are usually absent or severely diminished. Mild distal sensory loss is commonly found clinically. Severe disability and loss of walking ability are rare; life expectancy is normal. Kinships with identical features to those described above, but including tremor, were described by Roussy & Levy (1926). Pathological features of these diseases are confined to the spinal cord and peripheral nerves. Atrophy and loss of anterior horn cells are present, together with loss of myelinated fibres in the dorsal ascending tracts, especially in the cervical region.

HMSN type II has been called the neuronal form of peroneal muscular atrophy. It is inherited as an autosomal dominant trait but differs from HMSN type I in having a later onset of symptoms, more severe deformities of the feet and greater difficulties with balance and walking. There is less involvement of the hands. Fasciculations may be observed but peripheral nerve thickening is not a clinical feature. The motor and sensory nerve conduction velocities are normal or only mildly slowed. Digital sensory nerve action potentials are unobtainable or diminished, in contradistinction to the findings in the distal type of spinal muscular atrophy (HMN).

AMYOTROPHY IN THE HEREDITARY ATAXIAS

A detailed discussion of these diverse CNS disorders is outside the remit of this book. The classification of these conditions is difficult but has been considered in a recent monograph (Harding 1984). In general peripheral sensory neurones are affected more than lower motor neurones but neurogenic muscular atrophy (amyotrophy) is a feature in a number of these system degenerations (Rosenberg 1982). The purely peripheral diseases which present as hereditary motor neuropathies (SMA) or HMSN have already been discussed. The archetype of the spinal ataxic form is Friedreich's ataxia, although the spastic UMN forms comprise the various types of familial spastic paraplegia, some with prominent LMN involvement. Basal ganglia involvement occurs in the olivo-ponto-cerebellar ataxias and in certain dementias, e.g. Huntington's chorea.

The clinical and pathological features of Friedreich's ataxia as described in a series of papers between 1863 and 1877 by Friedreich, have been reviewed recently by Harding (1984). This is an autosomal recessive disorder, with onset usually by puberty, causing ataxia and dysarthria, associated with foot deformity, absent ankle jerks and extensor plantar responses. There is a progressive pyramidal-type weakness of the legs and sensory loss, usually of proprioception, together with generalised wasting of the lower limbs; distal amyotrophy is common in the hands.

Electrodiagnostic studies show normal or slightly reduced motor nerve conduction velocities (MNCV) and absent median and ulnar sensory action potentials (SAP) (Dyck & Lambert 1968b, McLeod 1971). Pathological studies show a small spinal cord with degeneration of the dorsal, pyramidal and spino-cerebellar tract, and also of the dorsal root ganglia. Some loss of AHC is seen, especially in the cervical cord. Mild degenerative changes are seen in the brain and cerebellum. Peripheral nerves show loss of large myelinated fibres to a greater extent distally than proximally, thus providing a pathological correlate for the 'dying-back' concept (Dyck & Lais 1973).

Two other forms of hereditary ataxia associated with peripheral neuropathy and muscle wasting are ataxia telangiectasia and xeroderma pigmentosa. Both are associated with abnormalities of DNA repair and increased risk of malignancies. Ataxia telangiectasia (Louis-Bar 1941) is associated with progressive cerebellar incoordination and choreo-athetosis but normal power until the later stages when general or distal weakness and atrophy occur. Tendon reflexes are depressed early and absent later (Sedgwick & Boder 1960, 1972). The spinal cord shows relatively few pathological changes (compared with Friedreich's ataxia), apart from some posterior column demyelination and mild loss of lumbar AHC and of neurones in the sensory and autonomic ganglia (Aguilar et al 1968).

Xeroderma pigmentosa is a skin condition with abnormal sensitivity to sunlight causing multiple skin cancers. Neurological disorder (de Sanctis–Cacchioni syndrome) occurs in 40% of cases. Mental subnormality, deafness, athetosis and ataxia are associated with areflexia and a variable sensorimotor polyneuropathy. Motor NCV is normal or slightly slowed, SAP are small or absent and muscle biopsy shows denervation atrophy (Thrush et al 1974).

Hereditary spastic paraplegia (HSP) in its pure form was first described by Strumpell (1880). This is inherited as an autosomal dominant trait with a variable age of onset and varying severity of weakness in the lower limbs. Distal amyotrophy, especially of the hands, is commoner in the older age group, who also show mild sensory loss. Normal MNCV and SAP studies have been reported, despite the wasting, distal sensory loss and ankle areflexia (McLeod et al 1977, Harding 1981). This has been explained on the basis of a central axonopathy and is supported by the report of absent or reduced somato-sensory evoked potentials (SSEP) in all of 18 patients, four of whom had sensory loss (Thomas et al 1981). Pathological studies have shown marked degeneration of the posterior sensory columns and pyramidal tracts, especially in the thoracic cord, despite the fact that the dorsal root ganglia and posterior roots appear normal. The AHC have appeared normal even in cases with distal amyotrophy (Van Bogaert 1952), giving further support for the concept of an axonopathy with 'dying-back'.

Some cases of HSP are associated with marked amyotrophy. Certain forms resemble peroneal muscular atrophy (HMSN type II) with pyramidal signs (Dyck & Lambert 1968b, Harding & Thomas 1984). Another autosomal recessive form, resembling ALS, was described by Refsum & Skillicorn (1954), with an early childhood onset of spastic paraparesis spreading to involve the arms and then, in adolescence, developing generalised wasting with fasciculations. The patients also developed bulbar symptoms.

Amyotrophy is often a late manifestation of olivo-ponto-cerebellar degeneration. Landis and colleagues (1974), in reviewing the family described by Schut (1950), found amyotrophy in 78% of cases and 50% with tongue wasting and fasciculations. Bulbar symptoms, especially dysphagia, may occur (see Harding 1984). Loss of AHC and sensory neurones have been described by several authors. Huntington's chorea may be associated with amyotrophy late in the disease. Pathological studies have shown involvement of the spinal cord, including pallor of the pyramidal tracts and some loss of AHC with occasional vacuolated cells (Bruyn et al 1979).

Typical motor neurone disease has been associated with familial parkinsonism (see Emery & Holloway 1982). The two disorders may show considerable variation in expressivity within families (Campbell 1979). Sporadic cases of Parkinson's disease with the late development of ALS have also been described (Bonduelle 1975). Several of these cases have followed encephalitis lethargica (Pallis 1976, Brait et al 1973). Some families, apart from those in the Western Pacific islands, have shown features of MND, parkinsonism and dementia with variable expression (see Tyler 1982).

Amyotrophy in non-familial CNS degenerative disorders

The association of MND with dementia has been reviewed recently by Salazar et al (1983) in relation to transmissible Creutzfeld–Jakob disease. In a review of more than 2000 cases they found 231 patients with dementia and early LMN signs causing amyotrophy. They showed that, in general, these cases had a much slower disease course and that pathological studies could not detect any spongiform change. In only two cases could the condition be transmitted to primates and these cases had the more typical subacute course, with myoclonus but presenting with amyotrophy (Allen et al 1971). Of the typical transmissible cases, approximately 15% showed fasciculations or amyotrophy late in the disease. Similarly, amyotrophy has been reported late in the course of Alzheimer's or Pick's disease. This may be simply an ageing phenomenon (Tomlinson et al 1969), as similar pathological changes have been found in elderly, non-demented patients (Jennekens et al 1971). The association of typical ALS with Alzheimer's or Pick's disease may be a chance association (reviewed by Brion et al 1980). Similarly, the association of parkinsonism–dementia and ALS in Guam is thought to be an overlap of two separate diseases which are common locally.

The presence of amyotrophy in sporadic cases of parkinsonism was mentioned previously. Other sporadic forms of basal ganglia disease may be associated with neurogenic muscular atrophy including pallido-nigral degeneration (Gray et al 1985), dystonia musculorum deformans (Tyler 1982), Hallervorden–Spatz disease (Seitelberger et al 1963), progressive supranuclear palsy (Steele et al 1964) and the Shy–Drager syndrome (Tyler 1982). Primary orthostatic hypotension (Shy–Drager syndrome) is said to be associated with mild amyotrophy, usually in the legs, in more than 50% of patients. Bulbar features have not been described. Mild changes of AHC degeneration including chromatolysis have been reported and

were indicated as the cause of the lax anal sphincter, as well as the distal limb wasting (Shy & Drager 1960).

MISCELLANEOUS DISEASES

Infections

Acute poliomyelitis is the archetype of a necrotising infection of the large motor neurones of the spinal cord, brain stem and cortex. Poliovirus is an enterovirus which may exist as a commensal in the bowel but causes a mild systemic upset only, without neurological features, in most cases. This may be associated with features of an aseptic meningitis. Paralytic disease occurs in less than 10% of infected individuals and may show a familial clustering, even at times of severe epidemics (Aycock 1942). This suggests a genetic predisposition to the development of poliomyelitis (Addair & Snyder 1942, Herndon & Jennings 1951). An association between HLA-A3 and poliomyelitis has been reported by Pietsch & Morris (1975) but denied by others (Lasch et al 1979).

After a prodromal illness for one to four days with fever, headache and neck stiffness, muscle stiffness with hyper-reflexia and fasciculations ensues, before the onset of asymmetrical muscle weakness and corresponding tendon reflex loss (Johnson RT 1982b). Maximum severity is reached within a few days and recovery may start within a week of the onset of paralysis. The brain-stem vital centres are involved in 10–15% of cases, especially the IXth and Xth cranial nuclei. Cardiorespiratory difficulties may develop, including hypertension and arrhythmias, but respiratory paralysis may also occur from peripheral involvement of the diaphragm and intercostal muscles. Fortunately, only a small proportion of affected muscles become permanently paralysed, but it is uncertain whether this implies that affected neurones are capable of recovery from viral infection and replication. The recovery of muscle power may be the result of sparing of individual motor neurones, but certainly electrophysiological studies demonstrate that reinnervative sprouting in surviving motor units occurs to produce greatly hypertrophied units (McComas et al 1971). It is probable that suboptimal conduction in these reinnervative terminal nerve fibres is responsible for the neuromuscular transmission defects which are demonstrable (Dalakas et al 1986). Pathological studies of acute fatal cases show inflammation and neuronal destruction, mainly in the spinal anterior horns, bulbar motor nuclei, reticular formation, thalamus and motor cortex (Bodian 1949). Treatment of acute paralytic poliomyelitis is supportive and may require tracheostomy and ventilatory assistance. The mortality appears to vary between 5% and 30%.

The clinical syndrome of paralytic poliomyelitis was caused initially almost exclusively by polioviruses. With the advent of widespread immunisation, other enteroviruses including Coxsackie and ECHO viruses, have rarely been associated with the syndrome, although 40% of the few cases in the USA are now associated with live vaccine virus infection (Johnson RT 1982b). Chronic progressive poliomyelitis has been reported secondary to vaccination in an immunodeficient child (Davis et al 1977). The encephalomyelitic picture which very occasionally complicates neoplastic disease, especially lymphomas, may also be attributable to viral infection, although full virological studies have not been undertaken (Walton et al 1968, Castleman 1970).

Herpes zoster or shingles is an acute viral infection of sensory ganglion cells, which produces a painful vesicular rash, but occasionally herpes simplex virus may be responsible. Very occasionally, the viral infection spreads to adjacent areas of the spinal cord to produce a segmental myelitis (Thomas & Howard 1972) and sometimes a generalised encephalomyelitis may occur (Gardner-Thorpe et al 1976). Segmental myelitis may be associated with local invasion and destruction of motor neurones, resulting in localised muscular atrophy and weakness. Such motor complications appear to occur more commonly with involvement of the lower spinal cord or cauda equina. Recovery from such weakness is possible but usually is incomplete. Cranial motor nerve involvement is also known, but may result from peripheral infection and swelling which is local rather than in the brain stem, e.g. oculomotor paralysis from orbital infection with ophthalmic zoster, or facial nerve paralysis from geniculate ganglion herpes (Ramsay Hunt syndrome).

Metabolic disorders with amyotrophy

Several workers have suggested an association between motor neurone disease and previous gastrectomy, but it seems probable that this is fortuitous (Norris 1975). A progressive muscle-wasting disorder has been described in patients having hypoglycaemic symptoms following partial gastrectomy (Williams 1955) but most cases of hypoglycaemic amyotrophy have been associated with insulin-secreting tumours (Silfverskiold 1946, Tom & Richardson 1951, Mulder et al 1956). Such patients commonly experience paraesthesiae although the sensory involvement has been minimal. Surgical removal of the tumour has led to disappearance of the paraesthesiae and at least to stabilisation of the muscle weakness, and in some cases electrophysiological evidence of improvement has been shown (Lambert et al 1960). The evidence that this disease is due to a neuronal disorder rather than to an axonopathy requires further study.

Diabetic amyotrophy is characterised by an asymmetrical proximal wasting and weakness of the legs, often accompanied by severe local pain in the anterior thighs and sometimes in the lumbar region or perineum. Garland & Taverner (1953) pointed out the frequent finding of extensor plantar responses and this, together with the appearance of fasciculations, can cause confusion with classic motor neurone disease. The patients are invariably middle-aged or elderly and the neuromuscular syndrome may be the presenting feature of maturity-onset diabetes. Good metabolic control may be associated with excellent recovery of function (Casey & Harrison 1972). Garland & Taverner (1953) initially attributed the disorder to a myelopathy but later were non-commital and coined the term diabetic amyotrophy (Garland 1955). The condition has been attributed to a local femoral neuropathy because of the prolonged latency of the knee jerk (Gilliatt & Willison 1962) and also a prolonged femoral conduction time (Chopra & Hurwitz 1968, Lamontagne & Buchthal 1970), but the frequent involvement of other muscle groups and the absence of sensory loss makes this an incomplete explanation. Pathological involvement of the femoral nerve has been shown in some cases (Raff et al 1968).

Chronic renal failure or uraemia is usually associated with a mixed motor and sensory poly-neuropathy. However, the motor involvement may predominate and may cause a distal weakness of the legs and, to a lesser extent, of the arms, with depressed tendon reflexes. Distal dysaes-thesiae are common, although rarely painful, and may be associated with muscle cramps and a 'rest-less legs' syndrome (Asbury 1984). There have been variable reports of benefits from long-term haemodialysis but rapid recovery has followed successful renal transplantation (Asbury 1984). Electrophysiological studies have shown mild slowing of motor and sensory conduction (Jebsen et al 1967). Recently, electrophysiological studies have shown that late responses using H-reflex and F-wave studies are abnormally slowed early in the disease course when MNCV is still normal (Knoll & Dierker 1980, Panayiotopoulos & Lagos 1980). Asbury and colleagues (1963), in an autopsy study of four cases of uraemic polyneuropathy, found a striking loss of nerve fibres in the distal parts of the nerves, with little or no involvement of the proximal portions or nerve roots. They also noted striking myelin breakdown. Central chromatolysis was noted in the spinal motor neurones. They concluded that the changes are those of an axonal degeneration. The demyelinative changes in fresh sural nerve biopsies have been stressed by some workers (Dinn & Crane 1970) but, in an elegant combined electrophysiological and histological study by Dyck and colleagues (1971), the demy-elination was shown to be non-random and present in nerve fibres undergoing axonal degeneration.

Chronic hepatic failure is commonly associated with mild muscle wasting and weakness. In many cases, mild abnormalities of peripheral nerve func-tion may be present but a frank neuropathy is unusual unless alcoholism or diabetes is also present (Kardel & Nielson 1974). Pathological studies on sural nerve biopsies have shown a mild, usually asymptomatic, demyelinating neuropathy in patients with liver disease, and this finding was not restricted to alcoholic cases (Dayan & Williams 1967). However, it is still not clear whether or not the demyelination is non-random and secondary to axonal degeneration. Electro-physiological studies have shown that there is a significant incidence of subclinical polyneur-opathy, affecting sensory fibres more than motor, including non-alcoholic cases (Seneviratne & Peiris 1970, Morgan et al 1979). The mild degree of slowing of nerve conduction suggests that this is primarily an axonal degenerative disorder similar to that observed in uraemia, but further studies are required to clarify this.

The muscle wasting in hyperthyroidism is generally thought to be a myopathic disorder, but histological studies have shown remarkably little abnormality in the majority of cases. Neither specific myopathic nor denervation changes have been described. McComas et al (1973a) have described electrophysiological findings of a revers-ible motor neuropathy in thyrotoxicosis, but this awaits independent confirmation. Hypothyroidism commonly results in local entrapment mono-neuropathy, especially in the carpal tunnel, but a polyneuropathy is rarely encountered. This is predominantly sensory with milder motor weak-ness (Dyck & Lambert 1970).

Muscle weakness may also be a feature of acro-megaly or gigantism caused by a pituitary tumour. In some cases this may be rapidly reversed with treatment of the tumour and lowering of the circulating growth hormone levels; no adequate explanation for this phenomenon has been given. The carpal tunnel syndrome is quite common in acromegaly and a diffuse hypertrophic neuropathy has been described very occasionally since the last century (Marie & Marinesco 1891). Histological studies have shown an increase of endoneural and perineural connective tissue with loss of myelinated nerve fibres (Stewart 1966) and recently Dinn (1970) described changes of a primary demyelinating disorder. However, nerve conduction is slowed only mildly in addition to the moderate reduction in nerve action potentials, which suggests a mainly axonal degeneration with non-random demyelination (Low et al 1974, Pickett et al 1975).

Hyperlipoproteinaemia has been associated with progressive muscular atrophy, but it is uncertain whether such cases represent an adult onset form of spinal muscular atrophy with an associated genetic abnormality of lipid metabolism (Quarfordt et al 1970).

Toxic motor neuropathies

Many exogenous toxins have been associated with peripheral neuropathies but few cause a predominantly motor syndrome. The possible association of chronic lead poisoning and motor neurone disease has been discussed earlier. Lead intoxication may affect the central nervous system or the peripheral nerves. Motor involvement predominates, although paraesthesiae and pain are common. The motor weakness is greatest in muscles receiving the most use: hence the wrist drop in painters intoxicated by lead paints. In children, the CNS involvement predominates, but foot drop may be evident in association with brisk reflexes and extensor plantar responses (Seto & Freeman 1964). Pathological studies have shown evidence of axonal degeneration and also demyelination, which is dose-dependent to a certain extent (Fullerton 1966).

Several other heavy metal intoxications have been associated with peripheral neuropathy. In arsenic poisoning, sensory involvement is prominent and causes painful dysaesthesiae in addition to distal weakness. In other metal intoxications the initial sensory disturbance may subside and produce a predominant distal motor weakness, e.g. in gold therapy of rheumatoid arthritis (Katrak et al 1980, Windebank et al 1984). It is not clear whether gold neuropathy is a direct neuronal toxicity or an immunologically mediated demyelinating polyradiculopathy.

The effects of mercury on the nervous system depend on the chemical state of the element. Inorganic mercuric chloride, when discharged into the sea of Minamata Bay, Japan, was converted to methylmercury by microorganisms, and then concentrated in the bodies of fish and shellfish. Mercury intoxication with organic compounds, e.g. methylmercury (Minamata disease) may affect the central nervous system and produce mental and extrapyramidal disorders (McAlpine & Araki 1958, Kurland et al 1960). Inorganic mercury intoxication, usually as a result of inhalation of vapour, generally causes a personality change and tremor, but a few cases of predominantly distal motor neuropathy have been described (Ross 1964, Swaiman & Flagler 1971, Windebank et al 1984). The significance of an ALS-like syndrome following chronic mercurialism reported by Kantarjian (1961) is uncertain.

Organophosphorus compounds have been widely used in industry, mainly as pesticides. They are powerful inhibitors of carboxylic esterase enzymes, including cholinesterase. In man, acute intoxication causes inhibition of acetylcholinesterase of the nervous system, resulting in accumulation of acetylcholine at the synapses and a paralytic cholinergic crisis. If respiratory paralysis is treated and the airway is protected from the excessive secretions, complete recovery occurs within 10 days (Namba et al 1971). Bidstrup et al (1953) described three cases of a delayed neuropathy after an acute cholinergic illness in workers manufacturing the compound 'Mipafox'. However, the delayed neuropathy in organophosphorus poisoning generally occurs without an antecedent cholinergic illness. Tri-orthocresyl phosphate (TOCP), a weak insecticide and a high-temperature industrial lubricant, has been responsible for the greatest number of cases of neuropathy in man. The largest outbreak of poisoning occurred in 1930–31 in the US when alcoholic extracts of ginger and rum were adulterated by TOCP and freely used as an alcoholic drink. An estimated 16 000 cases of polyneuropathy (ginger jake paralysis) occurred at that time (Namba et al 1971), and several other major outbreaks have resulted from contaminated cooking oil since then. The neuropathy develops after an interval of 7–21 days, beginning with paraesthesiae and swiftly followed by spreading distal weakness (Hopkins 1975). The paralysis progresses rapidly over a period of several days: the affected muscles waste; sensory loss is trivial or absent and the paraesthesiae disappear early in the course of the disease. The tendon reflexes may be lost, but sometimes are increased because of pyramidal tract involvement; spasticity may develop later. Recovery from the neuropathy attributable to organophosphorus poisoning is poor. Pathological studies in man and experimental animals have shown an axonal degeneration (present only in the distal ends of the motor nerves) and also changes in the spinal cord (Cavanagh 1964).

Ischaemic myelopathy

Acute occlusion of arteries supplying the spinal cord causes an initial paraplegia with sensory loss up to the level which is ischaemic, but in certain cases good sensory recovery has occurred, leaving a residual motor neuropathy (Dodson & Landau 1973). Less acute aortic disease has been associated with selective poliomyelomalacia, particularly of the ventral grey matter of the spinal cord (Herrick & Mills 1971) and a chronic motor neurone syndrome has been described in relation to arteriosclerosis or hypertension (Jellinger & Neumayer 1962, Hughes & Brownell 1966, Jellinger 1967). The latter is a progressive disease with a picture of weakness and wasting, mainly in the lower limbs, and mild but definite sensory impairment. The pathological changes are confined to the territory of the anterior spinal artery. Ischaemic lacunae are present in the spinal grey matter involving the motor nerve cells, and the lesions may extend laterally into the territory of the spinothalamic tracts or dorsally into the base of the posterior columns. Atherosclerosis does not appear to occur in the anterior spinal artery or its branches, but mesial thickening of the wall has been found, particularly in hypertensive patients. It seems unlikely that this disease state, which is largely restricted to the lower limbs, could be confused with MND. Its restriction to the territory of the anterior spinal artery is probably related to the architectural deficiency of the blood supply to the anterior two-thirds of the spinal cord, and its vulnerability to ischaemia (Jellinger & Neumayer 1969).

Radiation injury. The occasional chronic myelopathy with progressive muscle wasting and weakness which follows radiation therapy to the spinal region, including the spinal cord, is thought to be largely due to ischaemia. Prominent abnormalities of small and medium-sized arterioles are found in the damaged areas. Hyalinisation, fibrinoid necrosis and thrombosis of vessels are seen in relation to local necrosis and astrocytosis (Pennybacker & Russell 1948). Several authors have described a clinical syndrome of muscular atrophy and weakness in the lower extremities, with preserved sensation, which has occurred several months after irradiation (Greenfield & Stark 1948, Sadowsky et al 1976).

Trauma, including electrical injury

Cases of motor neurone disease with a previous history of significant trauma have been reported by many authors, but are thought to be chance associations (see Bonduelle 1975). However, a distinctive syndrome of benign posttraumatic amyotrophy developing several months after major local trauma has been described (Norris 1972b). The wasting was confined to the injured limb and after several months there was complete recovery; this is reminiscent of neuralgic amyotrophy or allergic brachial neuritis. A few cases of apparent posttraumatic MND were subsequently proved to be attributable to cervical arachnoiditis (Puech et al 1947, Kissel 1948).

The neurological effects of electrical trauma have been comprehensively reviewed by Panse (1970). Transient sensorimotor paralysis of limbs, persisting for up to two weeks, has been described in survivors of severe electrical trauma involving moderate or high energies (voltages of 1000 V or more and current in the range 25 mA–5 A) and also in those who have been struck by lightning. The site of damage has depended on the path taken by the electrical current through the body. Spinal amyotrophy following lightning accidents has been known for more than a century. It is also well known after passage of electricity from limb to limb, or trunk to limb. The muscular atrophy is commonly unilateral and is roughly confined to the neurological distribution of sensory dermatomes related to the point of contact. Hence, weakness and wasting around the shoulder and upper arm may develop after electrical burns to the thumb and index fingers. Not all victims show electrical burns or scars at the site of contact and roughly only one-half have suffered loss of consciousness at the time of injury. Apparently, the weakness may be immediate or delayed by as long as a few months and the atrophy can be progressive for a few months before becoming static or showing regression. Loss of the local tendon reflexes is the general rule, but sensory loss is usually slight. Spasticity or other pyramidal signs have been described and indicate more extensive damage to the spinal cord. There have been a few descriptions of typical clinical cases of MND following electrical trauma, but these are generally regarded as being coincidental. There have been no reports of electrophysiological or pathological studies of these cases of localised amyotrophy.

Plasma cell dyscrasias and motor neurone disease

The neuromuscular complications of plasma cell dyscrasias may be in the form of a spinal muscular atrophy, a motor polyneuropathy or as an ALS-like syndrome (Latov 1982). The plasma cell dyscrasia produces a paraproteinaemia in 80% of patients, usually IgG in about 50% and IgA in 20% of cases. The neurological disease may begin in association with an isolated plasmacytoma, but it is usually related to multiple myeloma by the time that the patient is seen. The disease may produce lambda light chains and cause amyloidosis but this is not thought to be the direct cause of the neuropathy in myeloma (McLeod et al 1984). Benign monoclonal gammopathy, where there is a monoclonal paraproteinaemia but no evidence of a malignant B-cell disorder, may be present in 6% of patients with peripheral neuropathy (Kelly et al 1981) and in an even higher proportion of elderly patients. IgG, IgM and IgA paraproteinaemia have been described.

Clinical sensorimotor neuropathy is present in about 15% of patients with multiple myeloma. Chazot et al (1976) demonstrated binding of paraproteins to the perineurium and endoneurium of peripheral nerves in IgA and IgG myeloma. Motor neurone syndromes (Patten 1984) and an ALS-like syndrome (Krieger & Melmed 1982) have been associated with paraproteinaemia. About 25% of patients with macroglobulinaemia have neurological complications, including neuropathies (Logothetis et al 1960). Sensory symptoms are usually prominent but the distal motor weakness and wasting may be very severe and often associated with fasciculations (Layani et al 1955, Saric et al 1967). Very occasionally the neuropathy may be acute, resembling a Guillain-Barré syndrome (Bing & Neel 1936, Logothetis et al 1960). A spinal muscular atrophy syndrome

(Peters & Clatanoff 1968) and a motor neurone syndrome have been described in association with IgM paraproteinaemia (Bauer et al 1977, Rowland et al 1982). Amyloidosis, either primary or secondary to myeloma, usually gives a polyneuropathy without CNS signs (Kyle & Greipp 1985) but UMN signs have been described in a recent case (Aberbanel et al 1986).

Non-metastatic carcinomatous neuromuscular disease

The various forms of neuromuscular disease occurring in association with lymphoma and cancer are discussed fully in Chapter 27. Reference here is limited to those cases where a direct involvement of motor neurones is apparent. Non-inflammatory degeneration of anterior horn cells and of dorsal ganglion cells has been described in sensorimotor polyneuropathies (Norris et al 1964, Victor 1965, Henson & Urich 1970). However, the direct association of cancer with a pure motor neurone disease state remains controversial and in most cases is coincidental (Norris & Engel 1965, Norris et al 1969, Brownell et al 1970).

Modern electrophysiological techniques have revealed evidence of subclinical neuropathy in up to 50% of cases of malignancy, usually lung cancer (McLeod 1984). These cases correspond to the carcinomatous 'neuromyopathy' of Brain & Henson (1958) and in some cases to the 'mild terminal neuropathy' which complicates known cancer (Croft et al 1967, Croft & Wilkinson 1969, Hawley et al 1980). This disorder presents with symmetrical, mainly proximal, limb weakness and wasting in association with minor sensory symptoms such as paraesthesiae or mild numbness. The examination findings are of depressed tendon reflexes and, frequently, occasional fasciculations or distal sensory loss, especially to vibration. Electromyography reveals a high incidence of chronic denervation changes together with spontaneous discharge of fibrillation and short-duration fasciculation potentials; active 'myopathic' units may also be found, particularly in proximal muscles (Trojaborg et al 1969, Campbell & Paty 1974). Motor conduction velocity is frequently normal but may be mildly slowed, especially in the terminal nerve segments. Sensory conduction is frequently impaired and sensory action potentials may be absent or markedly reduced. It has been suggested that the disorder is a progressive neuronal dysfunction with an involvement of motor to a greater extent than of sensory neurones (Campbell & Paty 1974).

The mechanism by which non-metastatic polyneuropathy and neuronal disease are produced is unknown. The possibility that they are caused by toxic factors released by the tumour has been suggested by many authors (Costa & Holland 1965). Certainly, the incidence of clinical neurological disease is apparently higher in association with undifferentiated cell tumours of the lung, which may produce a wide range of hormone-like compounds (Lebovitz 1965, Ross 1972). The possibility of neuronal damage from viral invasion was discussed earlier and this could be linked with an immune mechanism. Brain & Henson (1958) speculated on a crossed reaction to shared anti-genic sites between tumour and nervous tissue proteins. This was supported by the finding of anti-CNS antibodies in the serum of four patients with subacute sensory neuropathy but not in other forms of neuropathy (Wilkinson 1964). The demonstration of circulating lymphocytes sensitised to peripheral nervous tissue was thought, like the serum antibodies, to be a secondary phenomenon to sequestrated or damaged neural proteins (Paty et al 1974).

ACKNOWLEDGEMENTS

I would like to thank Dr Pam Enderby for her critical help on the sections about bulbar palsy and their management. My special thanks to Sue James and Margaret Watson for their secretarial assistance and to my wife, Patricia, for her forbearance.

REFERENCES

Abarbanel J M, Frisher S, Osimani A 1986 Primary amyloidosis with peripheral neuropathy and signs of motor neuron disease. Neurology 36: 1125–1127

Addair J, Snyder L H 1942 Evidence for an autosomal recessive gene for susceptibility to paralytic poliomyelitis. Journal of Heredity 33: 306–309

Aguilar M J, Kamoshita S, Landing B H, Boder E, Sedgewick R P 1968 Pathological observations in ataxia telangiectasia. Journal of Neuropathology and Experimental Neurology 27: 659–676

Alexander M P, Emery E S, Koerner F C 1976 Progressive bulbar paresis in childhood. Archives of Neurology 33:66

Allen I V, Dermott E, Connelly J H, Hurwitz L J 1971 A study of a patient with the amyotrophic form of Creutzfeld-Jakob disease. Brain 94:715

Andrews J M, Gardner M B 1974 Lower motor neuron degeneration associated with type C RNA virus infection in mice. Neuropathological features. Journal of Neuropathology and Experimental Neurology 33: 285–307

Antel J P, Noronha A B C, Oger J J F, Arnason B G W 1982 Immunology of amyotrophic lateral sclerosis, In: Rowland L P (ed) Human motor neuron diseases. Raven, New York, p 395–402

Aran F 1850 Recherches sur une maladie non encore décrite de système musculaire (atrophie musculaire progressive). Archives Générales de Médecin, Paris 24: 4–35

Aronson A E 1980 Definition and scope of the communication disorder. In: Mulder D W (ed) The diagnosis and treatment of amyotrophic lateral sclerosis. Houghton Mifflin, Boston, p 225–234

Asbury A K 1984 Uremic Neuropathy. In: Dyck P J, Thomas P K, Lambert E H, Bunge R (eds) Peripheral neuropathy. Saunders, New York, p 1811–1825

Asbury A K, Victor M, Adams R D 1963 Uremic polyneuropathy. Archives of Neurology 8:413

Aspin J, Harrison R, Jehanli A, Lunt G, Campbell M J 1986 Stimulation by mitogen and neuronal membranes of lymphocytes from patients with motor neurone disease. Journal of Neuroimmunology. 11: 31–40

Astin K J, Wilde C E, Davies-Jones G A B 1975 Glucose metabolism and insulin response in the plasma and cerebrospinal fluid in motor neurone disease. Journal of the Neurological Sciences 25: 205–210

Aycock W L 1942 Familial aggregation in poliomyelitis. American Journal of the Medical Sciences 203: 452–465

Barker A T, Jalinous R, Freeston I L 1985 Magnetic stimulation of the human brain. Lancet i: 1106–1107

Barron K D, Rodichock L D 1982 Cancer and disorders of motor neurons. In: Rowland L P (ed) Human motor neuron diseases. Raven, New York, p 267–272

Bartfeld H C, Dham H, Donnenfeld L et al 1982a Immunological profile of amyotrophic lateral sclerosis patients and their cell mediated immune responses to viral and CNS antigens. Clinical and Experimental Immunology 48: 137–147

Bartfeld H, Pollack M S, Cunningham-Rundles S, Donnenfeld H 1982b HLA frequencies in amyotrophic lateral sclerosis. Archives of Neurology 39: 270–271

Bauer M, Bergstrom R, Ritter B, Olsson Y 1977 Macroglobulinemia Waldenstrom and motor neuron syndrome. Acta Neurologica Scandinavica 55: 245–250

Beal M F, Richardson E P 1981 Primary lateral sclerosis. A case report. Archives of Neurology 39: 662–664

Behan P O 1979 Cell mediated immunity in motor neurone disease and poliomyelitis. In: Rose F Clifford (ed) Clinical neuroimmunology. Blackwell, London, p 259–272

Bidstrup P L, Bonnell J A, Beckett A G 1953 Paralysis following poisoning by a new organic phosphorus insecticide (mipafox). Report on two cases. British Medical Journal 1: 1068–1072

Bing J, Neel A V 1936 Two cases of hyperglobulinaemia with affection of the central nervous system on a toxic-infectious basis. Acta Medica Scandinavica 88:492

Bjornskov E R, Norris F H, Kirby-Mower J 1984 Quantitative axon terminal and end-plate morphology in amyotrophic lateral sclerosis. Archives of Neurology 41: 527–530

Bodian D. 1949 Poliomyelitis: Pathological anatomy. In: Poliomyelitis. Papers and discussion presented at the First International Poliomyelitis Conference. Lippincott, Philadelphia, p 62–84

Böhme G 1974 Stimm-, Sprech- und Hörstörungen. Aetiologie, Diagnostik, Therapie. Fischer Verlag, Stuttgart

Bonduelle M 1975 Amyotrophic lateral sclerosis. In: Vinken P J, Bruyn G W (eds) Handbook of clinical neurology, Vol. 22. North Holland, Amsterdam p 281–338

Bornstein M B, Appel S H 1965 Tissue culture studies of demyelination. New York Academy of Sciences 122: 280–286

Bosma J F, Brodie D R 1969 Disabilities of the pharynx in amyotrophic lateral sclerosis as demonstrated by cineradiography. Radiology 92: 97–103

Bradley W G, Krasin F 1982 A new hypothesis of the etiology of amyotrophic lateral sclerosis: the DNA hypothesis. Archives of Neurology 39–677–680

Bradley W G, Good P, Rassool C G, Adelman L S 1983 Morphometric and biochemical studies of peripheral nerves in amyotrophic lateral sclerosis. Annals of Neurology 14: 267–277

Bradley W G, Hedlund W, Cooper C et al 1984 A double-blind controlled trial of bovine brain gangliosides in amyotrophic lateral sclerosis. Neurology (Cleveland) 34: 1079–1082

Brain W R, Henson R A 1958 Neurological syndromes associated with carcinoma. Lancet 2:971

Brait K, Fahn S, Schwartz G A 1973 Sporadic and familial parkinsonism and motor neuron disease. Neurology 23: 990–1002

Brandt S 1950 Course and symptoms of progressive infantile muscular atrophy. A follow-up study of 112 cases in Denmark. Archives of Neurology and Psychiatry 63:218

Brion S, Psimzrus A, Chevalier J P et al 1980 Association of Pick's disease and amyotrophic lateral sclerosis. Encéphale 6: 259–286

Brown J C, Kater R M H 1969 Pancreatic function in patients with amyotrophic lateral sclerosis. Neurology (Minneapolis) 19: 1985–1989

Brownell D B, Oppenheimer D R, Hughes J T 1970 The central nervous system in motor neurone disease. Journal of Neurology, Neurosurgery and Psychiatry 33: 338–357

Bruyn G W, Bots G T A M, Dom R 1979 Huntington's chorea: Current neuropathological status. In: Chase T N, Wexler N S, Barbeau A (eds) Huntington's disease. Advances in Neurology 23: 83–93

Buchthal F, Olsen P Z 1970 Electromyography and muscle biopsy in infantile spinal muscle atrophy. Brain 93:15

Bundey, S, Lovelace R E 1975 A clinical and genetic study of chronic proximal spinal muscular atrophy. Brain 98: 455–472

Burke R E 1982 Motor units in cat muscles: Anatomical considerations in relation to motor unit types. In: Rowland L P (ed) Human motor neuron diseases. Raven, New York, p 31–46

Byers R K, Banker B Q 1961 Infantile muscular atrophy. Archives of Neurology 5: 140–164

Campa J F, Engel W K 1970 Histochemistry of motor neurons and interneurons in the cat lumbar spinal cord. Neurology 20: 559–568

Campbell A M G, Williams E R, Pearce J 1966 Late motor neuron degeneration following poliomyelitis. Neurology 19: 1101–1106

Campbell A M G, Williams E R, Barltrop D 1970 Motor neurone disease and exposure to lead. Journal of Neurology, Neurosurgery and Psychiatry 33: 872–885

Campbell M J 1979 Genetic aspects of motor neurone disease. In: Behan P O, Rose F C (eds) Progress in neurological research. Pitman, London, p 135–144

Campbell M J 1980 Management of patients with motor neurone disease. International Rehabilitation Medicine 2: 111–115

Campbell M J, McComas A J, Petito F 1973 Physiological changes in ageing muscle. Journal of Neurology, Neurosurgery and Psychiatry 36: 174–182

Campbell M J, Paty D W 1974 Carcinomatous neuromyopathy; an electrophysiological and immunological study of patients with carcinoma of the lung. I. Electrophysiological studies. Journal of Neurology, Neurosurgery and Psychiatry 37: 131–141

Campbell, M J, Enderby P M 1984 Management of motor neurone disease. Journal of the Neurological Sciences 64: 65–71

Carey J S 1986 Motor neuron disease — a challenge to medical ethics: discussion paper. Journal of the Royal Society of Medicine 79: 216–220

Carpenter S 1968 Proximal axonal enlargement in motor neuron disease. Neurology (Minneapolis) 18: 841–851

Carpenter S, Karpati G, Rothman S, Watters G, Andermann F 1978 Pathological involvement of primary sensory neurons in Werdnig-Hoffmann disease. Acta Neuropathologica 42: 91–97

Casey E B, Harrison M J G 1972 Diabetic amyotrophy: a follow-up study. British Medical Journal 1:656

Castleman B (ed) 1970 Case records of the Massachusetts General Hospital (case 42–1970). New England Journal of Medicine 283:806

Cavanagh J B 1964 Peripheral nerve changes in orthocresyl phosphate poisoning in the cat. Journal of Pathology and Bacteriology 87: 365–383

Charcot J M 1865 Sclérose de cords lateraux de la moelle spineuse chez une femme hysterique atteinte de contracture peiman de quatre menieres. Bulletin de la Societé Médicale des Hopitaux (Paris) 2 (suppl 2): 24–42

Charcot J M 1874 De la sclérose latérale amyotrophique. Progrès Médical (Paris) 2:325, 341, 453

Charcot J M, Marie P 1886 Sur une forme particulière d'atrophie musculaire progressive, souvent familiale, débutant par les pieds et les jambes et atteignant plus tard les mains. Revue de Médecine (Paris) 6: 97–138

Chazot G, Berger G, Carrier H et al Manifestations neurologiques des gammapathies monoclonales. Revue Neurologique 132:195

Chopra J S, Hurwitz L J 1968 Femoral nerve conduction in diabetes and chronic occlusive vascular disease. Journal of Neurology, Neurosurgery and Psychiatry 31: 28–33

Chou S M, Fakadej A V 1971 Ultrastructure of chromatolytic motoneurons and anterior spinal roots in a case of

Werdnig–Hoffmann disease. Journal of Neuropathology and Experimental Neurology 30:368

Colmant H J 1975 Progressive bulbar palsy in adults. In: Eds. Vinken P J, Bruyn G W (eds) Handbook of clinical neurology, Vol. 22. North Holland, Amsterdam, p 111–156

Conradi S, Ronnevi L–O, Norris F H 1982 Motor neuron disease and toxic metals. In: Rowland P (ed) Human motor neuron diseases. Raven, New York, p 201–231

Cook A W, Pertschuk L P, Gupta K et al 1979 The effect of antiviral agents on jejunal immunopathology in amyotrophic lateral sclerosis. In: Behan P O, Rose F C (eds) Progress in neurological research. Pitman, London, p 62–72

Costa G, Holland J F 1965 Systemic effect of tumors with special reference to the nervous system. In: Lord Brain, Norris F H (eds) The remote effects of cancer on the nervous system. Grune and Stratton, New York, p 125–133

Cremer N E, Oshiro L S, Norris F H, Lennette E H 1973 Cultures of tissues from patients with amyotrophic lateral sclerosis. Archives of Neurology 29: 331–333

Croft P B, Urich H, Wilkinson M 1967 Peripheral neuropathy of sensorimotor type associated with malignant disease. Brain 90: 31–66

Croft P B, Wilkinson M 1969 The course and prognosis in some types of carcinomatous neuropathy. Brain 92: 1–8

Currier R D, Haerer A F 1968 Amyotrophic lateral sclerosis and metallic toxins. Archives of Environmental Health 17: 712–719

Dalakas M C, Elder G, Hallett M et al 1986 A long-term follow-up study of patients with post-poliomyelitis neuromuscular symptoms. New England Journal of Medicine 314: 959–963

Darley F L, Aronson A E, Brown J R 1975 Motor speech disorders. Saunders, Philadelphia

Davis L E, Bodian D, Price D, Butler I J, Vickers J H 1977 Chronic progressive poliomyelitis secondary to vaccination of an immunodeficient child. New England Journal of Medicine 297: 241–245

Dayan A D, Williams R 1967 Demyelinating peripheral neuropathy and liver disease. Lancet 2: 133–134

Dayan A D, Graveson G S, Illis L S, Robinson P K 1969 Schwann cell damage in motor neuron disease. Neurology (Minneapolis) 19: 242–246

Dejerine J, Sottas J 1893 Sur la névrite interstitielle, hypertrophique et progressive de l'enfance. Comptes Rendus des Sceances de la Societé de Biologie et de ses filiales (Paris) 45:63

Delwaide P J, Schoenen J 1985 The effects of TRH on F waves recorded from antagonistic muscles in human subjects. Annals of Neurology 18: 366–367

Denys E H, Norris F H 1979 Amyotrophic lateral sclerosis. Impairment of neuromuscular transmission. Archives of Neurology 36: 202–205

Digby J, Harrison R, Jehanli A, Lunt G G, Rose F C 1985 Cultured rat spinal cord neurones: interaction with motor neurone disease immunoglobulins. Muscle and Nerve 8: 595–605

Dinn J J 1970 Schwann cell dysfunction in acromegaly. Journal of Clinical Endocrinology and Metabolism 31:140

Dinn J J, Crane D L 1970 Schwann cell dysfunction in uraemia. Journal of Neurology, Neurosurgery and Psychiatry 33:605

Dodson W E, Landau W M 1973 Motor neuron loss due to aortic clamping in repair of coarctation. Neurology (Minneapolis) 23: 539–542

Dorman J D, Engel W K, Fried D M 1969 Therapeutic trial in amyotrophic lateral sclerosis. Journal of the American Medical Association 209:257

Drake M E Jr 1983 Chronic pain syndrome in amyotrophic lateral sclerosis. Archives of Neurology 40: 453–454

Duchenne G 1860 Paralysie musculaire progressive de la langue, du voile du palais et des lèvres. Archives Générales de Médecine 16: 283–431

Duchenne G, Joffroy A 1870 De l'atrophie aigue et chronique des cellules nerveuses de la moelle et du bulbe rachidien, à propos d'une observation de paralysie glossolabio-laryngié. Archives de Physiologie 3:499

Dworkin J P, Aronson A E, Mulder D W 1980 Tongue force in normals and in dysarthric patients with amyotrophic lateral sclerosis. Journal of Speech and Hearing Research 23: 828–837

Dyck P J 1982 Are motor neuropathies and motor neuron diseases separable? In: Rowland L P (ed) Human motor neuron diseases. Raven, New York, p 105–114

Dyck P J 1984 Inherited neuronal degeneration and atrophy affecting peripheral motor, sensory and autonomic neurons. In: Dyck P J, Thomas P K, Lambert E H, Bunge R (eds) Peripheral neuropathy, 2nd edn. Saunders, Philadelphia, p 1600–1655

Dyck P J, Lais A C 1973 Evidence of segmental demyelination secondary to axonal degeneration in Friedreich's ataxia. In: Kakulas B A (ed) Clinical studies in myology. Excerpta Medica, Amsterdam, p 253–263

Dyck P J, Lambert E H 1968a Lower motor and primary sensory neuron diseases with peroneal muscular atrophy. I. Hereditary polyneuropathies. Archives of Neurology 18: 603–618

Dyck P J, Lambert E H 1968b Ibid. II Various neuronal degenerations. Archives of Neurology 18: 619–625

Dyck P J, Lambert E H 1970 Polyneuropathy associated with hypothyroidism. Journal of Neuropathology and Experimental Neurology 29:631

Dyck P J, Johnson W J, Lambert E H, O'Brien P C 1971 Segmental demyelination secondary to axonal degeneration in uremic neuropathy. Mayo Clinic Proceedings 46: 400–431

Dyck P J, Stevens J C, Mulder D W, Espinosa R E 1975 Frequency of nerve fiber degeneration of peripheral motor and sensory neurons in amyotrophic lateral sclerosis. Morphometry of deep and superficial peroneal nerves. Neurology (Minneapolis) 25: 781–785

Emery A E H 1971 The nosology of the spinal muscular atrophies. Journal of Medical Genetics 8: 481–495

Emery A E H, Holloway S 1982 Familial motor neuron diseases. In: Rowland L P (ed) Human motor neuron diseases. Raven, New York, p 139–147

Engel W K, Kurland L T, Klatzo I 1959 An inherited disease similar to amyotrophic lateral sclerosis with a pattern of posterior column involvement. An intermediate form? Brain 82: 203–220

Engel W K, Hogenhuis L A H, Collis W J, Schalch D S, Barlow M H, Gold E N, Dorman J D 1969 Metabolic studies and therapeutic trials in amyotrophic lateral sclerosis. In: Norris F H, Kurland L T (eds) Motor neuron diseases. Grune and Stratton, New York, p 199–208

Engel W K, Cuneo R A, Levy H B 1978 Polyinosinicytidylic acid treatment of neuropathy (letter). Lancet 1: 503–504

Engel W K, Siddique T, Nicoloff J T 1983 Effect on weakness and spasticity in amyotrophic lateral sclerosis of thyrotropin-releasing hormone. Lancet 2: 73–75

Fallat R J, Jewitt B, Bass M, Kamm B, Norris F H, Jr 1979 Spirometry in amyotrophic lateral sclerosis. Archives of Neurology 36: 74–80

Fallat R J, Norris F H Jr 1980 Respiratory problems. In: Mulder D W (ed) The diagnosis and treatment of amyotrophic lateral sclerosis. Houghton Mifflin, Boston, p 301–320

Fallis R J, Weiner L P 1982 Further studies in search of a virus in amyotrophic lateral sclerosis. In: Rowland L P (ed) Human motor neuron diseases. Raven, New York, p 363–393

Fazio M 1892 Ereditarieta della paralise bulbare progressiva. Riforma Medica 8:327

Feigenbaum J A, Munsat T L 1970 A neuromuscular syndrome of scapuloperoneal distribution. Bulletin of the Los Angeles Neurosurgical Society 35: 47–57

Felmus M T, Patten J P, Swanke D 1976 Antecedent events in amyotrophic lateral sclerosis. Neurology (Minneapolis) 26: 167–172

Fenichel G M, Emery E S, Hunt P 1967 Neurogenic atrophy simulating facio-scapulo-humeral dystrophy. A dominant form. Archives of Neurology 17: 257–260

Festoff B W, Crigger N J 1980 Therapeutic trials in amyotrophic lateral sclerosis; a review. In: Mulder D W (ed) The diagnosis and treatment of amyotrophic lateral sclerosis. Houghton Mifflin, Boston, p 337–349

Field E J, Hughes D 1969 Toxicity of serum from motor neuron disease for myelin and glial cells in tissue culture. In: Norris F H, Kurland L T (eds) Motor neuron diseases. Grune and Stratton, New York, p 179–182

Finkel N 1962 A forma pseudomiopatica tardia da atrophia muscular progressiva heredo-familial. Archives de Neuropsiquiatria 4:307

Fisher C M 1977 Pure spastic paralysis of corticospinal origin. Canadian Journal of Neurological Sciences 4:252

Forster F M, Alpers B J 1944 Site of origin of fasciculations in voluntary muscle. Archives of Neurology and Psychiatry 51: 264–267

Friedman A P, Freedman D 1950 Amyotrophic lateral sclerosis. Journal of Nervous and Mental Disease 111: 1–18

Fullerton P M 1966 Chronic peripheral neuropathy produced by lead poisoning in guinea-pigs. Journal of Neuropathology and Experimental Neurology 25:214

Furukawa T, Tsukagoshi H, Sugita H, Toyokura Y 1969 Neurogenic muscular atrophy simulating facioscapulohumeral muscular dystrophy. Journal of the Neurological Sciences 9:389

Gajdusek D C 1963 Motor neuron disease in natives of New Guinea. New England Journal of Medicine 268: 474–476

Gajdusek D C 1982 Foci of motor neurone disease in high incidence in isolated populations of East Asia and the Western Pacific. In: Rowland L P (ed) Human motor neuron diseases. Raven, New York, p 363–395

Gallai V, Hockaday J M, Hughes J T, Lane D J, Oppenheimer D R, Rushworth G 1981 Ponto-bulbar palsy with deafness (Brown–Vialetto–van Laere syndrome). A report on 3 cases. Journal of the Neurological Sciences 50:250

Gallassi R, Montagua P, Ciardulla C, Lorusso S, Mussuto V,

Stracciari A 1985 Cognitive impairment in MND. Acta Neurologica Scandinavica 71: 480–484

Gardner M B, Henderson B E, Officer J E et al 1973 A spontaneous lower motor neuron disease apparently caused by indigenous Type-C RNA virus in wild mice. Journal of the National Cancer Institute 51: 1243–1254

Gardner-Medwin D, Hudgson P, Walton J N 1967 Benign spinal muscular atrophy arising in childhood and adolescence. Journal of the Neurological Sciences 5: 121–158

Gardner-Thorpe C, Foster J B, Barwick D D 1976 Unusual manifestations of herpes zoster: A clinical and electrophysiological study. Journal of the Neurological Sciences 28: 427–447

Garland H 1955 Diabetic amyotrophy. British Medical Journal 2:1287

Garland H, Taverner D 1953 Diabetic myelopathy. British Medical Journal 1:1405

Garruto R M, Yanagihara R, Gajdusek D C, Arion D M 1984 Concentrations of heavy metals and essential minerals in garden soil and drinking water in the Western Pacific. In: Chen K M, Yase Y (eds) Amyotrophic lateral sclerosis in Asia and Oceania. National Taiwan University, Taipei, p 265–330

Garruto R M, Yanagihara R, Gajdusek D C 1985 Disappearance of high-incidence amyotrophic lateral sclerosis and parkinsonism-dementia on Guam. Neurology 35: 193–198

Gath I, Sjaastad O, Loken A C 1969 Myopathic electromyographic changes correlated with histopathology in Wohlfart–Kugelberg–Welander disease. Neurology (Minneapolis) 19:344

Gibbs C J, Gajdusek D C 1982 An update on long-term in vivo and in vitro studies designed to identify a virus as the cause of amyotrophic lateral sclerosis, parkinsonism-dementia and Parkinson's disease. In: Rowland L P (ed) Human motor neuron diseases. Raven, New York, p 343–353

Gillberg P G, Aquilonius S M, Eckernas S A 1982 Choline acetyltransferase and substance P-like immunoreactivity in the human spinal cord: changes in amyotrophic lateral sclerosis. Brain Research 250: 394–397

Gilliatt R W, Willison R G 1962 Peripheral nerve conduction in diabetic neuropathy. Journal of Neurology, Neurosurgery and Psychiatry 25:11

Gomez M R, Clermont V, Bernstein J 1962 Progressive bulbar palsy in children (Fazio–Londe's disease). Archives of Neurology and Psychiatry 6:317

Gotoh F, Kitamura A, Koto A, Kataoka K, Atsuji H 1972 Abnormal insulin secretion in amyotrophic lateral sclerosis. Journal of the Neurological Sciences 16:201

Gray F, Eizenbaum J F, Ghervardi R, Degos J D, Poirier J 1985 Luyso-pallido nigral atrophy and amyotrophic lateral sclerosis. Acta Neuropathologica 66: 78–82

Greenfield J G, Stark F M 1948 Post-irradiation neuropathy. American Journal of Roentgenology, Radium Therapy and Nuclear Medicine 60: 617–622

Greenfield J G, Matthews W B 1954 Post-encephalitic parkinsonism and amyotrophy. Journal of Neurology, Neurosurgery and Psychiatry 17:50

Griffin J W, Cork L C, Adams R J, Price D L 1982 Axonal transport in hereditary canine spinal muscular atrophy (HCSMA). Journal of Neuropathology and Experimental Neurology 41:370

Griggs R C, Donohue K M, Utell M J, Goldblatt D, 1980

Pulmonary function testing. In: Mulder D W (ed) The diagnosis and treatment of amyotrophic lateral sclerosis. Houghton Mifflin, Boston, p 291–299

Gurney M E, Belton A C, Cashman N, Antel J P 1984 Inhibition of terminal axon sprouting by serum from patients with amyotrophic lateral sclerosis. New England Journal of Medicine 311: 933–939

Hanyu N, Oguchi K, Yangisawa N, Tsukagoshi H 1981 Degeneration and regeneration of ventral root motor fibers in amyotrophic lateral sclerosis. Journal of the Neurological Sciences 55: 99–115

Harding A E 1981 Hereditary 'pure' spastic paraplegia: a clinical and genetic study of 22 families. Journal of Neurology, Neurosurgery and Psychiatry 44: 871–883

Harding A E 1984 The hereditary ataxias and related disorders. Churchill Livingstone, Edinburgh

Harding A E, Thomas P K 1980 Hereditary distal spinal muscular atrophy. A report on 34 cases and a review of the literature. Journal of the Neurological Sciences 45: 337–348

Harding A E, Thomas P K, Baraitser M, Bradbury P G, Morgan-Hughes J A, Ponsford J R 1982 X-linked recessive bulbospinal neuronopathy: a report of ten cases. Journal of Neurology, Neurosurgery and Psychiatry 45: 1012–1019

Harding A E, Bradbury P G, Murray N M F 1983 Chronic asymmetrical spinal muscular atrophy. Journal of the Neurological Sciences 59: 69–83

Harding A E, Thomas P K 1984 Peroneal muscular atrophy with pyramidal features. Journal of Neurology, Neurosurgery and Psychiatry 47: 168–172

Harrington H, Hallet M, Tyler H R 1984 Ganglioside therapy for amyotrophic lateral sclerosis: a double-blind controlled trial. Neurology (Cleveland) 34: 1083–1085

Harrington T M, Cohen M D, Batheson J D, Ginsburg W W 1983 Elevation of creatine kinase in amyotrophic lateral sclerosis. Potential confusion with polymyositis. Arthritis and Rheummatism 26: 201–205

Harter D H 1982 Viruses other than poliovirus in human amyotrophic lateral sclerosis. In: Rowland L P (ed) Human motor neuron diseases. Raven, New York, p 339–342

Hartmann H A, Davidson T J 1982 Neuronal RNA in motor neuron disease. In: Rowland L P (ed) Human motor neuron diseases. Raven, New York, p 89–103

Harvey D, Torack R, Rosenbaum H 1979 Amyotrophic lateral sclerosis with ophthalmoplegia: a clinicopathologic study. Archives of Neurology 36: 615–617

Hawley R J, Cohen M H, Saini N, Armbrustmacher V M 1980 The carcinomatous neuromyopathy of oat-cell lung cancer. Annals of Neurology 7:65

Hayashi H, Suga M, Satake M, Tsubaki T 1981 Reduced glycine receptor in the spinal cord in amyotrophic lateral sclerosis. Annals of Neurology 9: 292–294

Henson R·A, Urich H 1970 Peripheral neuropathy associated with malignant disease. In: Vinken P J, Bruyn G W (eds) Handbook of clinical neurology, Vol. 8. North Holland, Amsterdam, p 131–148

Herndon C N, Jennings R G 1951 A twin-family study of susceptibility to poliomyelitis. American Journal of Human Genetics 3: 17–46

Herrick M K, Mills P E 1971 Infarction of the spinal cord. Archives of Neurology 24:228

Hirano A, Malamud N, Kurland L T, Zimmerman H W 1969 A review of the pathological findings in amyotrophic lateral sclerosis. In: Norris F H, Kurland L T, (eds)

Motor neuron diseases. Grune and Stratton, New York, p 51–60

Hirayama K, Toyokura Y, Tsubaki T 1959 Juvenile muscular atrophy of unilateral upper extremity: a new clinical entity. Psychiatry Neurology Japan 61:2190

Hirayama K, Tomonaga M, Kitano K, Yamada T, Kojima S, Arai K 1987 Focal cervical poliopathy causing juvenile muscular atrophy of distal upper extremity: a pathological study. Journal of Neurology, Neurosurgery and Psychiatry 50:285

Hjorth R J, Walsh J C, Willison R G 1973 The distribution and frequency of spontaneous fasciculations in motor neurone disease. Journal of the Neurological Sciences 18: 469–474

Hodes R 1948 Electromyographic study of defects of neuromuscular transmission in human poliomyelitis. Archives of Neurology and Psychiatry 60:457

Hoffmann J 1893 Uber chronische spinale Muskelatrophie im Kindesalter, auf familiarer Basis. Deutsche Zeitschrift für Nervenheilkunde 3:427

Hoffmann J 1897 Weiter Beitrag zur Lehre von der hereditaren progressiven spinalen. Muskelatrophie im Kindesalter. Deutsche Zeitschrift für Nervenheilkunde 10:292

Hoffman P M, Robbins D S, Gibbs C J, Gajdusek D C, Garruto R M, Terasaki P I 1977 Histocompatability antigens in amyotrophic lateral sclerosis and parkinsonism-dementia on Guam. Lancet 2:717

Hoffman P M, Robbins D S, Nolte M T, Gibbs C J, Gajdusek D C 1978 Cellular immunity in Guamanians with amyotrophic lateral sclerosis and parkinsonism-dementia. New England Journal of Medicine 299: 680–685

Hokfeld T, Fuxe K, Johansson O et al 1975 Distribution of thyrotrophin releasing hormone (TRH) in the central nervous system as revealed with immunohistochemistry. European Journal of Pharmacology 34: 389–392

Hopkins A 1975 Toxic neuropathy due to industrial agents. In: Dyck P J, Thomas P K, Lambert E H (eds) Peripheral neuropathy. Saunders, New York, p 1207–1226

Horton W A, Eldridge R, Brody J A 1976 Familial motor neuron disease: evidence for at least three different types. Neurology (Minneapolis) 26: 460–465

Hughes J T 1982 Pathology of amyotrophic lateral sclerosis. In: Rowland L P (ed) Human motor neuron diseases. Raven, New York, p 61–74

Hughes J T, Brownell D B 1966 Spinal cord ischaemia due to arteriosclerosis. Archives of Neurology 15: 189–202

Ingram D A, Swash M 1987 Central motor conduction is abnormal in motor neurone disease. Journal of Neurology, Neurosurgery and Psychiatry 50: 159–166

Ingram D A, Thompson A J, Swash M 1987 Abnormalities of central motor conduction in multiple sclerosis revealed by transcutaneous magnetic stimulation of the brain. Journal of Neurology, Neurosurgery and Psychiatry 50 (in press)

Jamal G A, Hansen S, Weir A I, Ballantyne J P 1985 An improved automated method for the measurement of thermal thresholds in patients with peripheral neuropathy. Journal of Neurology, Neurosurgery and Psychiatry 48: 361–366

Jebsen R H, Tenckhoff H, Honet J C 1967 Natural history of uremic polyneuropathy and effects of dialysis. New England Journal of Medicine 277:327

Jellinger K 1967 Arteriosclerosis of the spinal cord and progressive vascular myelopathy. Journal of Neurology, Neurosurgery and Psychiatry 30: 195–206

Jellinger K, Neumayer E 1962 Myelopathie progressive d'origine vasculaire. Revue Neurologique 106:666

Jellinger K, Neumayer E 1969 Intermittent claudication of the cord and cauda equina. In: Vinken P J, Bruyn G W (eds) Handbook of clinical neurology, Vol. 13. North Holland, Amsterdam, p 507

Jennekens F G I, Tomlinson B E, Walton J N 1971 Data on the distribution of fibre types in five human limb muscles. An autopsy study. Journal of the Neurological Sciences 14: 245–257

Johnson R T 1982a Selective vulnerability of neural cells to viral infection. In: Rowland L P (ed) Human motor neuron diseases. Raven, New York, p 331–338

Johnson R T 1982b Viral infections of the nervous system. Raven, New York

Johnson W G 1982 Hexosaminidase deficiency: A cause of recessively inherited motor neuron diseases. In: Rowland L P (ed): Human motor neuron diseases. Raven, New York, p 159–164

Johnson W G, Wigger H J, Karp H R et al 1982 Juvenile spinal muscular atrophy; a new hexosaminidase deficiency phenotype. Annals of Neurology 11: 11–16

Jokelainen M, Palo J 1976 Amyotrophic lateral sclerosis and autonomic nervous system (letter). Lancet 1:1246

Juergens S M, Kurland L T 1980 Epidemiology. In: Mulder D W (ed) The diagnosis and treatment of amyotrophic lateral sclerosis. Houghton Mifflin, Boston, p 35–51

Juergens S M, Kurland L T, Okazaki H, Mulder D W 1980 ALS in Rochester, Minnesota, 1925–1977. Neurology (New York) 30: 463–470

Kaeser H E 1964 Die familiare scapulo-peroneale Muskelatrophie. Deutsche Zeitschrift für Nervenheilkunde 186:379

Kaeser H E 1965 Scapuloperoneal muscular atrophy. Brain 88:407

Kaeser H E 1975 Scapulo-peroneal syndrome. In: Vinken P J, Bruyn G W (eds) Handbook of clinical neurology, Vol. 22. North Holland, Amsterdam, p 57–65

Kantarjian A D 1961 A syndrome clinically resembling amyotrophic lateral sclerosis following chronic mercurialism. Neurology (Minneapolis) 11:639

Kardel T, Nielson V K 1974 Hepatic neuropathy, a clinical and electrophysiological study. Acta Neurologica Scandinavica 50:513

Kascsak R J, Carp R I, Vilcek J T et al 1982 Virological studies in amyotrophic lateral sclerosis. Muscle and Nerve 5: 93–101

Katrak S M, Pollock M, O'Brien C P et al 1980 Clinical and morphological features of gold neuropathy. Brain 103:671

Kawamura Y, Dyck P J, Shimono M et al 1981 Morphometric comparison of the vulnerability of peripheral motor and sensory neurons in amyotrophic lateral sclerosis. Journal of Neuropathology and Experimental Neurology 40: 667–675

Kelemen J, Hedlund W, Orlin J B, Berkman E M, Munsat, T L 1983 Plasmapheresis with immunosuppression in amyotrophic lateral sclerosis. Neurology 40: 752–753

Kelly J J, Kyle R A, Miles J M, O'Brien P C, Dyck P J 1981 The spectrum of peripheral neuropathy in myeloma. Neurology (New York) 31:24

Kennedy W R, Alter M, Sung J H 1968 Progressive proximal spinal and bulbar muscular atrophy of late onset; a sex-linked recessive trait. Neurology (Minneapolis) 18:671

Kiloh K G, Lethlean A K, Morgan G, Cawte J E, Harris M 1980 An endemic neurological disorder in tribal Australian aborigines. Journal of Neurology, Neurosurgery and Psychiatry 43: 661–668

Kissel P 1948 Syndrome de sclérose latérale amyotrophique avec paralysie labio-glosso-laryngée par arachnoidite cervicale post-traumatique. Verification operatoire. Revue Neurologique 80: 771–3

Knoll O, Dierker E 1980 Detection of uremic neuropathy by reflex response latency. Journal of the Neurological Sciences 47:305

Koenig H 1969 Neurobiologic effects of agents which alter nucleic acid metabolism. In: Norris F H, Kurland L T (eds) Motor neuron diseases: Research on amyotrophic lateral sclerosis and related disorders. Grune & Stratton, New York, p 347–368

Kohn R 1968 Postmortem findings in a case of Wohlfart–Kugelberg–Welander disease. Confinia Neurologica 30:253

Koller M, Engel W K 1984 Increased serum creatine kinase (CK) MB isozyme and alkaline phosphate positive (AP + ve) regenerative muscle fibers in amyotrophic lateral sclerosis (abst). Neurology (Cleveland) 34:84

Kondo K 1979 Population dynamics of motor neuron disease. In: Tsubaki T, Toyokura Y (eds) Amyotrophic lateral sclerosis. University Park Press, Baltimore, p 61–103

Kott E, Livni E, Zamir R, Kuritzky A 1976 Amyotrophic lateral sclerosis: Cell-mediated immunity to polio virus and basic myelin protein in patients with high frequency of HLA-BW35. Neurology (Minneapolis) 26: 376–377

Kott E, Livni E, Zamir R, Kuritzky A 1979 Cell-mediated immunity to polio and HLA antigens in amyotrophic lateral sclerosis. Neurology (Minneapolis) 29: 1040–1044

Krieger C, Melmed K A 1982 A case of amyotrophic lateral sclerosis and paraproteinemia. Neurology (New York) 32: 896–898

Kugelberg E 1975 Chronic proximal (pseudomyopathic) spinal muscular atrophy. Kugelberg–Welander syndrome. In: Vinken P J, Bruyn G W (eds) Handbook of clinical neurology, Vol. 22(11). Elsevier, New York, p 67–80

Kugelberg E, Welander L 1954 Familial neurogenic (spinal?) muscular atrophy simulating ordinary proximal dystrophy. Acta Psychiatrica Scandinavica 29: 42–43

Kugelberg E, Welander M 1956 Heredofamilial juvenile muscular atrophy simulating muscular dystrophy. Archives of Neurology and Psychiatry 75:500

Kurland L T, Mulder D W 1955 Epidemiologic investigations of amyotrophic lateral sclerosis: 2 Familial aggregations indicative of dominant inheritance. Neurology 5: 192–196, 249–268

Kurland L T, Faro S N, Siedler H 1960 Minamata disease: the outbreast of a neurological disorder in Minamata, Japan, and its relationship to the ingestion of seafood contaminated by mercuric compounds. Neurology (Minneapolis) 1:370

Kurland L T, Brody J A 1975 Amyotrophic lateral sclerosis Guam type. In: Vinken P J, Bruyn G W (eds) Handbook of clinical neurology, Vol. 22. Elsevier, New York, p 339–347

Kurland L T, Molgaard C A 1982 Guamanian ALS: Hereditary or acquired? In: Rowland L P (ed) Human motor neuron diseases. Raven, New York, p 165–172

Kurlander H M, Patten B M 1979 Metals in spinal cord tissue of patients dying of motor neuron disease. Annals of Neurology 6: 21–24

Kurtzke J F 1982 Epidemiology of amyotrophic lateral sclerosis. In: Rowland L P (ed) Human motor neuron diseases. Raven, New York, p 281–302

Kushner M J, Parrish M, Burke A et al 1984 Nystagmus in motor neuron disease: clinicopathological study of two cases. Annals of Neurology 16: 71–77

Kyle R A, Greipp P R 1985 Amyloidosis. Clinical and laboratory features in 229 cases. Mayo Clinic Proceedings 58: 665–683

Lambert E H 1969 Electromyography in amyotrophic lateral sclerosis. In: Norris F H, Kurland L T (eds) Motor neuron diseases. Grune and Stratton, New York, p 135–153

Lambert E H, Mulder D W 1957 Electromyographic studies in amyotrophic lateral sclerosis. Proceedings of the Staff Meetings of the Mayo Clinic 32: 441–447

Lambert E H, Mulder D W, Bastron J A 1960 Regeneration of peripheral nerves and hyperinsulin neuronopathy. Neurology (Minneapolis) 10: 851–854

Lamontagne A, Buchthal F 1970 Electrophysiological studies in diabetic neuropathy. Journal of Neurology, Neurosurgery and Psychiatry 33:442

Landis D M, Rosenberg R N, Landis S C, Schut L, Nyhan W L 1974 Olivopontocerebellar degeneration. Archives of Neurology 31: 295–307

Lasch E E, Joshua K, Gazit E, El Nasri M, Marcus O, Zamir R 1979 Study of the HLA antigens in Arab children with paralytic poliomyelitis. Israel Journal of Medical Sciences 15: 12–13

Latov N 1982 Plasma cell dyscrasia and motor neuron disease. In: Rowland L P (ed) Human motor neuron diseases. Raven, New York, p 273–279

Layani F, Asehkenasy A, Bengui A 1955 Macroglobulinémie avec lesions du squelette. Presse Médicale 63:44

Layzer R B 1982 Diagnostic implications of clinical fasciculation and cramps. In: Rowland L P (ed) Human motor neuron diseases. Raven, New York, p 23–30

Lebo C P, U K S, Norris F H Jr 1976 Cricopharyngeal myotomy in amyotrophic lateral sclerosis. Laryngoscope 86: 862–868

Lebovitz H E 1965 Endocrine-metabolic syndromes associated with neoplasms. In: Brain Lord, Norris F H Jr (eds) Remote effects of cancer on the nervous system. Grune and Stratton, New York, p 104–111

Leveille A, Kiernan J, Goodwin J A, Antel J 1982 Eye movements in amyotrophic lateral sclerosis. Archives of Neurology 39: 684–686

Li T M, Swash M, Alberman E 1985 Morbidity and mortality in motor neurone disease; comparison with multiple sclerosis and Parkinson's disease; age and sex specific rates and cohort analyses. Journal of Neurology, Neurosurgery and Psychiatry 48: 320–327

Lipton H L, Dal Canto M C 1976 Theiler's virus-induced CNS disease in mice. In: Andrews J M, Johnson R T, Brazier M (eds) Amyotrophic lateral sclerosis. Recent research trends. Academic Press, New York, p 263–277

Liversedge L A, Swinburn W R, Yuill G M 1970 Idoxuridine and motor neurone disease. British Medical Journal 1:755

Logothetis J, Silverstein P, Coe J 1960 Neurologic aspects of Waldenstrom's macroglobulinemia. Archives of Neurology 3:564

Londe P 1894 Paralysie bulbaire progressive infantile et familiale. Revue Médicale 14:212

Louis-Bar D 1941 Sur un syndrome progressif comprenant des telangiectasies capillaires, cutanées et conjonctivales symmetriques, a disposition naevoide et des troubles cerebelleux. Confinia Neurologica (Basel) 4: 32–42

Low P A, McLeod J G, Turtle J R, Donnelly P, Wright R G 1974 Peripheral neuropathy in acromegaly. Brain 97: 139–152

McAlpine D, Araki S 1958 Minamata disease: an unusual neurological disorder caused by contaminated fish. Lancet 2:629

McComas A J, Sica R E P, Campbell M J, Upton A R M 1971 Functional compensation in partially denervated muscles. Journal of Neurology, Neurosurgery and Psychiatry 34: 453–460

McComas A J, Sica R E P, McNabb A R, Goldberg W, Upton A R M (1973a) Neuropathy in thyrotoxicosis. New England Journal of Medicine 289: 219–220

McComas A J, Upton A R M, Sica R E P 1973b Motor neurone disease and aging. Lancet 2: 1474–1480

McLeod J G 1971 An electrophysiological and pathological study of peripheral nerves in Friedreich's ataxia. Journal of the Neurological Sciences 12: 333–349

McLeod J G 1984 Carcinomatous neuropathy. In: Dyck P J, Thomas P K, Lambert E H, Bunge R (eds) Peripheral neuropathy. 2nd edn. Saunders, New York, p 2180–2191

McLeod J G, Prineas J W 1971 Distal type of chronic spinal muscular atrophy: clinical, electrophysiological and pathological studies. Brain 94: 703–714

McLeod J G, Morgan J A, Reye C 1977 Electrophysiological studies in familial spastic paraplegia. Journal of Neurology, Neurosurgery and Psychiatry 40: 611–615

McLeod J G, Walsh J C, Pollard J D 1984 Neuropathies associated with paraproteinemias and dysproteinemias. In: Dyck P J, Thomas P K, Lambert E H, Bunge R (eds) Peripheral neuropathy. Saunders, New York, p 1847–1865

Manakar S, Shulman L H, Winokur A, Rainbow T C 1985 Autoradiographic localisation of thyrotrophin releasing hormone receptors in amyotrophic lateral sclerosis spinal cord. Neurology 35: 1650–1653

Mandybur T I, Cooper G P 1979 Increased spinal cord lead content in amyotrophic lateral sclerosis — possibly a secondary phenomenon. Medical Hypotheses 5: 1313–1315

Mann D M A, Yates P O 1974 Motor neurone disease: the nature of the pathogenic mechanism. Journal of Neurology, Neurosurgery and Psychiatry 37: 1036–1046

Mannen T, Iwata M, Toyokura Y, Nagashima K 1982 The Onuf's nucleus and the external anal sphincter muscle in amyotrophic lateral sclerosis and Shy-Drager syndrome. Acta Neuropathologica (Berlin) 58: 255–260

Manton W J, Cook J D 1979 Lead content of cerebrospinal fluid and other tissue in amyotrophic lateral sclerosis (ALS). Neurology (New York) 29: 611–612

Marie P, Marinesco G 1891 Sur l'anatomie pathologique de l'acromegalie. Archives de médecine experimental et d'anatomie Pathologique (Paris) 3:539

Martin R J, Sufit R L, Ringel S P et al 1983 Respiratory improvement by muscle training in adult-onset acid maltase deficiency. Muscle and Nerve 6: 201–203

Marshall A, Duchen L W 1978 Sensory system involvement in infantile spinal muscular atrophy. Journal of the Neurological Sciences 26: 349–359

Mastaglia F L, Walton J N 1971 Histological and histochemical changes in skeletal muscle from cases of chronic juvenile and early adult spinal muscular atrophy (the Kugelberg–Welander syndrome). Journal of the Neurological Sciences 12:15

Meadows J C, Marsden C D 1969 A distal form of chronic spinal muscular atrophy. Neurology (Minneapolis) 19:53

Mendell J R, Chase T N, Engel W K 1971 Amyotrophic lateral sclerosis. A study of central monamine metabolism and a therapeutic trial of levodopa. Archives of Neurology 25:320

Mills C P 1973 Dysphagia in pharyngeal paralysis treated by cricopharyngeal sphincterotomy. Lancet 1: 455–457

Miyata S, Nakamura S, Nagata H, Kameyama M 1983 Increased manganese level in spinal cords of amyotrophic lateral sclerosis determined by radiochemical neutron activation analysis. Journal of the Neurological Sciences 61: 283–293

Morgan M H, Read A E, Campbell M J 1979 Clinical and electrophysiological studies of peripheral nerve function in patients with chronic liver disease. Clinical Science 57: 31–37

Mulder D W, Howard F M 1976 Patient resistance and prognosis in amyotrophic lateral sclerosis. Mayo Clinic Proceedings 51: 537–541

Mulder D W, Bastron J A, Lambert E H 1956 Hyperinsulin neuropathy. Neurology (Minneapolis) 6: 627–635

Mulder D W, Lambert E H, Eaton L M 1959 Myasthenic syndrome in patients with amyotrophic lateral sclerosis. Neurology (Minneapolis) 9:627

Mulder D W, Rosenbaum R A, Layton D D 1972 Late progression of poliomyelitis or forme fruste amyotrophic lateral sclerosis? Mayo Clinic Proceedings 47:756

Mullins W M, Gross C W, Moore J M 1979 Long-term follow-up of tympanic neurectomy for sialorrhoea. Laryngoscope 89: 1219–1223

Munsat T L, Woods R, Fowler W, Pearson C M 1969 Neurogenic muscular atrophy of infancy with prolonged survival. Brain 92: 9–24

Munsat T L, Easterday C S, Levy S, Wolff S M, Hiett R 1981 Amantadine and guanidine are ineffective in ALS. Neurology 31: 1054–1055

Murakami T, Mastaglia F L, Mann D M A, Bradley W G 1981 Abnormal RNA metabolism in spinal motor neurons in the wobbler mouse. Muscle and Nerve 4: 407–412

Namba T, Aberfeld D C, Grob D 1970 Chronic proximal spinal muscular atrophy. Journal of the Neurological Sciences 11:401

Namba T, Nolte C T, Jackrel J, Grob D 1971 Poisoning due to organophosphate insecticides. Acute and chronic manifestations. American Journal of Medicine 50: 475–492

Newrick P G, Hewer R L 1984 Motor neuron disease: can we do better? A study of 42 patients. British Medical Journal 289: 539–542

Norris F H 1972a Amantadine in Jakob–Creutzfeld disease. British Medical Journal 2:349

Norris F H 1972b Benign post-traumatic amyotrophy. Archives of Neurology 27: 269–270

Norris F H 1973 Guanidine in amyotrophic lateral sclerosis. New England Journal of Medicine 288:690

Norris F H 1975 Adult spinal motor neuron disease. In: Vinken P J, Bruyn G M (eds) Handbook of clinical neurology, Vol. 22. North Holland, Amsterdam, p 156

Norris F H 1979 Moving axon particles of intercostal nerve terminals in benign and malignant ALS. In: Tsubaki T, Toyokura Y (eds) Amyotrophic lateral sclerosis. University Park Press, Baltimore, p 375–385

Norris F H, Rudolf J H, Barney M 1964 Carcinomatous neuropathy. Neurology (Minneapolis) 14:202

Norris F H, Engel W K 1965 Carcinomatous amyotrophic lateral sclerosis. In: Brain W R, Norris F H (eds) The remote effects of cancer on the nervous system. Grune and Stratton, New York, p 24–34

Norris F H, McMenemey W H, Barnard R O 1969 Anterior horn cell pathology in carcinomatous neuromyopathy compared with other forms of motor neurone disease. In: Norris F H, Kurland L T Motor neurone diseases. Grune and Stratton, New York, p 100

Norris F H, Calanchini P R, Fallat R J, Panchari R P T, Jewett B 1974 The administration of guanidine in amyotrophic lateral sclerosis. Neurology (Minneapolis) 24: 721–728

Norris F H, Denys E H, U K S 1980 Differential diagnosis of adult motor neuron disease. In: Mulder D W (ed) The diagnosis and treatment of amyotrophic lateral sclerosis. Houghton Mifflin, Boston, p 53–78

Ochs S 1984 Basic properties of axoplasm transport. In: Dyck P J, Thomas P K, Lambert E H, Bunge R (eds) Peripheral neuropathy, 2nd edn. Saunders, New York p 453–476

Olarte M R, Gersten J C, Zabriskie J, Rowland L P 1979 Transfer factor is ineffective in amyotrophic lateral sclerosis. Annals of Neurology 5: 385–388

Olarte M R, Schoenfeldt R S, McKiernan G, Rowland L P 1980 Plasmapheresis in amyotrophic lateral sclerosis. Annals of Neurology 8: 644–645

Olarte M R, Shafer S R 1985 Levamisole is ineffective in the treatment of amyotrophic lateral sclerosis. Neurology 35: 1063–1066

Oldstone M B A, Perrin L H, Wilson C B, Norris F H 1976 Evidence for immune-complex formation in patients with 'ALS'. Lancet 2:169

Olson W H, Simons J A, Halaas G W 1978 Therapeutic trial of tilorone in ALS. Lack of benefit in a double-blind placebo-controlled study. Neurology (Minneapolis) 28: 1293–1295

Otsuka M, Endo M 1960 The effect of guanidine on neuromuscular transmission. Journal of Pharmacology and Experimental Therapeutics 128:273

Pallis C 1976 In: Rose F C (ed) Motor neurone disease. Pitman, London

Panayiotopoulos C P, Lagos G 1980 Tibial nerve H-reflex and F-wave studies in patients with uremic neuropathy. Muscle and Nerve 3:423

Panse F 1970 Electrical lesions of the nervous system. In: Vinken P J, Bruyn G W (eds) Handbook of clinical neurology, Vol. 7. North Holland, Amsterdam p 344–387

Parhad I M, Clark A W, Barron K D, Staunton S B 1978 Diaphragmatic paralysis in motor neuron disease: report of two cases and a review of the literature. Neurology (New York) 28: 18–22

Patten B M 1982 Phosphate and parathyroid disorders associated with the syndrome of amyotrophic lateral sclerosis. In: Rowland L P (ed) Human motor neuron diseases. Raven, New York, p 181–200

Patten B M 1984 Neuropathy and motor neuron syndromes associated with plasma cell disease. Acta Neurologica Scandinavica 69: 47–61

Patten B M, Kurlander H M, Evans B 1982 Free amino acid concentrations in spinal tissue from patients dying of motor neuron disease. Acta Neurologica Scandinavica 66: 594–599

Paty D W, Campbell M J, Hughes D 1974 Carcinomatous neuromyopathy; an electrophysiological and immunological study of patients with carcinoma of the lung. II Immunological studies. Journal of Neurology, Neurosurgery and Psychiatry 37: 142–151

Pearn J 1980 Classification of spinal muscular atrophies. Lancet I: 919–922

Pearn J 1982 Infantile motor neuron diseases. In: Rowland L P (ed) Human motor neuron diseases. Raven, New York, p 121–130

Pearn J H, Wilson J 1973a Acute Werdnig–Hoffmann disease. Archives of Disease in Childhood 48: 425–430

Pearn J H, Wilson J 1973b Chronic generalised spinal muscular atrophy of infancy and childhood. Archives of Disease in Childhood 48: 768–774

Pearn J H, Bundey S, Carter C O, Wilson J, Gardner-Medwin D Walton J N 1978a A genetic study of subacute and chronic spinal muscular atrophy in childhood — A nosological analysis of 124 index patients. Journal of the Neurological Sciences 37: 227–248

Pearn J, Gardner-Medwin D, Wilson J 1978b A clinical study of chronic childhood spinal muscular atrophy. A review of 141 cases. Journal of the Neurological Sciences 38: 23–37

Pearn J, Hudgson P, Walton J N 1978c A clinical and genetic study of adult-onset spinal muscular atrophy. The autosomal recessive form as a discrete disease entity. Brain 101: 591–606

Peiper S J, Fields W S 1959 Failure of amyotrophic lateral sclerosis to respond to intrathecal steroid and vitamin B 12 therapy. Archives of Neurology 9:522

Pennybacker J, Russell D S 1948 Necrosis of the brain due to radiation therapy. Journal of Neurology, Neurosurgery and Psychiatry 11: 183–198

Percy A K, Davis L E, Johnston D M, Drachman D B 1971 Failure of isoprinosine in amyotrophic lateral sclerosis. New England Journal of Medicine 285:689

Peters H A, Clatanoff D V 1968 Spinal muscular atrophy secondary to macroglobulinemia. Neurology (Minneapolis) 18: 101–108

Pickett J B E, Layzer R B, Levin S R, Schneider V, Campbell M J, Sumner A J 1975 Neuromuscular complications of acromegaly. Neurology (Minneapolis) 25: 638–645

Pietsch M C, Morris P J 1975 An association of HLA 3 and HLA 7 with paralytic poliomyelitis. Tissue Antigens 4:50

Plato C C, Garruto R M, Fox K M 1984 Familial and epidemiological studies of amyotrophic lateral sclerosis and parkinsonism-dementia of Guam. A twenty-five year prospective patient control study. American Journal of Epidemiology 120:478

Poskanzer D C, Cantor H M, Kaplan G S 1969 The frequency of preceding poliomyelitis in amyotrophic lateral sclerosis. In: Norris F H, Kurland L T (eds) Motor neuron diseases. Grune & Stratton, New York, p 286

Puech P, Grossiard A, Brun M, Denis J P 1947 Tableau clinique de sclérose latérale amyotrophique. Arachnoidite cervicale en virole à l'intervention. Revue Neurologique 79: 358–359

Quarfordt S H, Devino D C, Engel W K, Levy R I, Fredrickson D S 1970 Familial adult-onset proximal spinal muscular atrophy. Archives of Neurology 22: 541–549

Quick D T, Greer M 1967 Pancreatic dysfunction in amyotrophic lateral sclerosis. Neurology (Minneapolis) 17:112

Raff M C, Sangalang V, Asbury A K 1968 Ischemic mononeuropathy multiplex associated with diabetes mellitus. Archives of Neurology 18:487

Reed D A, Brody J A 1975 Amyotrophic lateral sclerosis and parkinsonism-dementia on Guam, 1945–1972. I. Descriptive epidemiology. American Journal of Epidemiology 101(4): 287–301

Reed D A, Torres J M, Brody J A 1975 Amyotrophic lateral sclerosis and parkinsonism-dementia on Guam, 1945–1972. II Familial and genetic studies. American Journal of Epidemiology 101(4): 302–310

Refsum S 1946 Heredopathia atactica polyneuritisformis: a familial syndrome not hitherto described. Acta Psychiatrica Scandinavica (Suppl) 38:1

Refsum S, Skillicorn S A 1954 Amyotrophic familial spastic paraplegia. Neurology (Minneapolis) 4:40

Rissanen A, Palo J, Myllyla G, Cantell K 1980 Interferon therapy for ALS. Annals of Neurology 7:392

Rosenberg R N 1982 Amyotrophy in multisystem genetic diseases. In: Rowland L P (ed) Human motor neuron diseases. Raven, New York, p 149–158

Ross A T 1964 Mercuric polyneuropathy with albumino-cytologic dissociation and eosinophilia. Journal of the American Medical Association 188:830

Ross E J 1972 Endocrine and metabolic manifestations of cancer. British Medical Journal 1: 735–738

Roussy G, Levy G 1926 Sept cas d'une maladie familiale particulière. Revue Neurologique 1:427

Rowland L P, Defendini R, Sherman W et al 1982 Macroglobulinemia with peripheral neuropathy simulating motor neuron disease. Annals of Neurology 11: 532–536

Sachs C, Conradi S, Kaijsu 1985 Autonomic function in ALS: a study of cardiovascular responses. Acta Neurologica Scandinavica 71: 373–378

Sadowsky C H, Sachs E, Ochoa J 1976 Post-radiation motor neuron syndrome. Archives of Neurology 33: 786–788

Salazar A M, Masters C L, Gajdusek D C, Gibbs C J, Jr 1983 Syndromes of amyotrophic lateral sclerosis and dementia: relation to transmissible Creutzfeldt–Jakob disease. Annals of Neurology 14: 17–26

Sanders M, Fellowes J 1975 Use of detoxified snake neurotoxin as a partial treatment for amyotrophic lateral sclerosis. Journal of Cancer and Cytology 15: 26–30

Saric R, Moreau F, Tignol J 1967 Neuropathie précédant de loin une maladie de Waldenstrom: effet du traitement prolongé par le melphalan. Journal Médicale Bordeaux 114:1301

Schoenen J, Resnik M, Delwaide P J, Vanderhaeghen J J 1985 Etude immunocytoclinique de la distribution spinale de sub. P., des encéphalines, de cholecystokinene et de serotonine dans la sclérose latérale amyotrophique. Comptes Rendus des Sceances de la Societé de Biologie et de ses Filiales (Paris) 179: 528–534

Schut J W 1950 Hereditary ataxia: clinical study through six generations. Archives of Neurology and Psychiatry (Chicago) 63: 535–568

Sedgwick R P, Boder E, 1960 Progressive ataxia in childhood with particular reference to ataxia-telangiectasia. Neurology 10: 705–715

Sedgwick R P, Boder E 1972 Ataxia-telangiectasia. In: Vinken P J, Bruyn G W (eds) Handbook of clinical neurology, vol. 14. North Holland, Amsterdam, p 267–339

Seitelberger F, Gootz E, Gross H, 1963 Beitrag zur spatinfantilen Hallevorden-Spatzchen Krankheit. Acta Neuropathologica (Berlin) 3: 16–28

Seneviratne K N, Peiris O A 1970 Peripheral nerve function in chronic liver disease. Journal of Neurology, Neurosurgery and Psychiatry 33:609

Seto D S Y, Freeman J M 1964 Lead neuropathy in

childhood. American Journal of Diseases of Children 107:337

Server A C, Wolinsky J S 1982 Approaches to antiviral therapy. In: Rowland L P (ed) Human motor neuron diseases. Raven, New York, p 519–546

Sevestre M 1899 Paralysie flasque des quatre membres et des muscles du tronc (sauf le diaphragme) chez un nouveau-né. Bulletin des Sociétés Pédiatriques Paris 1–2: 7–13

Shy G M, Drager G A 1960 A neurological syndrome associated with orthostatic hypotension. Archives of Neurology 2: 511–527

Silani V, Scarlato G, Valli G, Marconi M 1980 Plasma exchange ineffective in amyotrophic lateral sclerosis. Archives of Neurology 37: 511–513

Silfverskiold B P 1946 Polyneuritic hypoglycaemia. Late peripheral paresis after hypoglycemic attacks in two insulinoma patients. Acta Medica Scandinavica 125: 502–504

Sivak E D, Streib E W 1980 Management of hypoventilation in motor neuron disease presenting with respiratory insufficiency. Annals of Neurology 7: 188–191

Sivak E D, Gipson W T, Hanson M R 1982 Long-term management of respiratory failure in amyotrophic lateral sclerosis. Annals of Neurology 12: 18–23

Smith A W M, Mulder D W, Code C F 1957 Esophageal motility in amyotrophic lateral sclerosis. Proceedings of the Staff Meetings of the Mayo Clinic 32: 438–440

Smith R A, Dawson A, Foroozan P 1980 Pharmacology and surgical modalities. In: Mulder D W (ed) The diagnosis and treatment of amyotrophic lateral sclerosis. Houghton Mifflin, Boston, p 241–257

Sobue G, Matsuoka Y, Mukai E et al 1981 Pathology of myelinated fibers in cervical and lumbar ventral spinal roots in amyotrophic lateral sclerosis. Journal of the Neurological Sciences 50: 413–421

Stålberg E 1982 Electrophysiological studies of reinnervation in ALS. In: Rowland L P (ed) Human motor neuron diseases. Raven, New York, p 47–59

Stålberg E, Sanders D B 1984 The motor unit in ALS studied with different electrophysiological techniques. In: Rose F C (ed) Progress in motor neurone disease. Pitman, London

Stark F M, Moersch F P 1945 Primary lateral sclerosis. Journal of Nervous and Mental Disorders 102: 332–337

Steele J C, Richardson J C, Olszewski J 1964 Progressive supranuclear palsy. Archives of Neurology 10: 333–359

Stefanis C, Papapetropoulos T, Scarpalezos S, Lygidarkis G Panayiotopoulos C P 1975 X-linked spinal and bulbar muscular atrophy of late onset. Journal of the Neurological Sciences 24:493

Steinke J, Tyler R H 1964 The association of amyotrophic lateral sclerosis (motor neuron disease) and carbohydrate intolerance, a clinical study. Metbolism 13:1376

Stewart B M 1966 The hypertrophic neuropathy of acromegaly: a rare neuropathy associated with acromegaly. Archives of Neurology 14:107

Strumpell A 1880 Beitrage zur Pathologie des Ruckenmarks. Archiv für Psychiatrie und Nervenkrankheiten 10: 676–717

Swaiman K F, Flagler D G 1971 Penicillamine therapy of the Guillain–Barré syndrome caused by mercury poisoning. Neurology 21:456

Swash M, Schwartz M S 1982 A longitudinal study of changes in motor units in motor neurone disease. Journal of the Neurological Sciences 56: 185–197

Tandan R, Bradley W G 1985 Amyotrophic lateral sclerosis: Part 1. Clinical features, pathology and ethical issues in management. Part 2. Etiopathogenesis. Annals of Neurology 18: 271–280, 419–431

Thomas J E, Howard F M 1972 Segmental zoster paresis: A disease profile. Neurology (Minneapolis) 22: 459–466

Thomas P K, Jefferys J G R, Smith I S, Loulakakis D 1981 Spinal somatosensory evoked potentials in hereditary spastic paraplegia. Journal of Neurology, Neurosurgery and Psychiatry 44: 243–246

Thrush D C, Holti G, Bradley W G, Campbell M J, Walton J N 1974 Neurological manifestations of xeroderma pigmentosum in two siblings. Journal of the Neurological Sciences 22: 91–104

Tom M I, Richardson J C 1951 Hypoglycaemia from islet cell tumour of pancreas with amyotrophy and cerebrospinal nerve cell changes. Journal of Neurology, Neurosurgery and Psychiatry 10: 51–66

Tomlinson B E, Walton J N, Rebeiz J J 1969 The effects of ageing and of cachexia upon skeletal muscle. A histopathological study. Journal of the Neurological Sciences 9:321

Tomlinson B E, Irving D 1977 The numbers of limb motor neurons in the human lumbosacral cord throughout life. Journal of the Neurological Sciences 34:213

Tooth H H 1886 The peroneal type of progressive muscular atrophy. H K Lewis, London

Trojaborg W, Buchthal F 1965 Malignant and benign fasciculations. Acta Psychiatrica et Neurologica Scandinavica (Suppl 13) 41: 251–254

Trojaborg W, Frantzen E, Andersen I 1969 Peripheral neuropathy and myopathy associated with carcinoma of the lung. Brain 92: 71–82

Tsujihata M, Hazama R, Yoshimura T, Sotch A, Moir M, Nagataki S 1984 The motor end-plate fine structure and intrastructural localisation of acetylcholine receptors in amyotrophic lateral sclerosis. Muscle and Nerve 7: 243–249

Tyler H R 1979 Double-blind study of modified neurotoxin in motor neurone disease. Archives of Neurology 29: 77–81

Tyler H R 1982 Nonfamilial amyotrophy with dementia or multisystem degeneration and other neurological disorders. In: Rowland L P (ed) Human neuron diseases. Raven, New York, p 173–180

Van Bogaert L 1952 Etudes sur la paraplégie spasmodique familiale V. Acta Neurologica et Psychiatrica Belgica 52: 795–807

Van Laere J 1966 Paralysie bulbo-pontine chronique progressive familiale avec surdité. Revue Neurologique 115:289

Vialetto E 1936 Contributo alla forma ereditaria della paralisi bulbare progressiva. Rivista Spir di Fren. 40:1

Victor M 1965 The effects of nutritional deficiency on the nervous system. A comparison with the effects of carcinoma. In: Brain Lord, Norris F H (eds) The remote effects of cancer on the nervous system. Grune and Stratton, New York, p 134–161

Villiger J W, Faull R L 1985 Muscarinic cholinergic receptors in the human spinal cord: differential localization of (3H). Brain Research 14: 196–199

Walton J N, Tomlinson B E, Pearce G W 1968 Subacute 'poliomyelitis' and Hodgkin's disease. Journal of the Neurological Sciences 6: 435–445

Werdnig G 1891 Zwei fruhinfantile hereditare Fälle von progressiver Muskelatrophie unter dem bilde der Dystrophie, aber auf neurotischer Grundlag. Archiv Psychiatrie und Nervenkrankheiten 22: 437–480

Werdnig G 1894 Die fruh-infantile progressive spinale Amyotrophie. Archives of Psychiatry 26:706

Whitehouse P J, Wamsley J K, Zarbin M A et al 1983 Amyotrophic lateral sclerosis: alterations in neurotransmitter receptors. Annals of Neurology 14: 8–16

Wiesendanger M 1962 Uber die hereditare, neurogene proximale Amyotrophie (Kugelberg–Welander). Archiv der Julius Klaus-Stiftung für Vererungsforschung 37:147

Wikstrom J, Paetau A, Palo J et al 1982 Classic amyotrophic lateral sclerosis with dementia. Archives of Neurology 39: 681–683

Wilkinson P C 1964 Serological findings in carcinomatous neuropathy. Lancet 1: 1301–1303

Williams C J 1955 Amyotrophy due to hypoglycaemia. British Medical Journal 1: 707–708

Williams E R, Bruford A 1970 Creatine phosphokinase in motor neurone disease. Clinical Chimica Acta 27:53

Windebank A J, McCall J T, Dyck P J 1984 Metal neuropathy. In: Dyck P J, Thomas P K, Lambert E H, Bunge R (eds) Peripheral neuropathy. Saunders, New York, p 2133–2161

Wohlfart G 1942 Zwei Fälle von Dystrophia musculorum progressiva mit fibrillaren Zuckungen und atypischen Muskelbefund. Deutsche Zeitschrift für Nervenheilkuncle 153:189

Wohlfart G 1959 Degenerative and regenerative axonal changes in the ventral horns, brain stem and cerebral cortex in amyotrophic lateral sclerosis. Acta Universitatis Lundensis (New Series 2): 56, 1–13

Wohlfart G, Fex J, Eliasson S 1955 Hereditary proximal spinal muscle atrophy simulating progressive muscular dystrophy. Acta Psychiatrica et Neurologica 30:395

Wolfgram F 1976 Blind studies on the effect of amyotrophic lateral sclerosis sera on motor neurons in vitro. In: Andrews J M, Johnson R T, Brazier M (eds) Amyotrophic lateral sclerosis. Recent research trends. Academic Press, New York, p 145–149

Wolfram F, Myers L 1973 Amyotrophic lateral sclerosis: Effect of serum on anterior horn cells in tissue culture. Science 179: 579–580

Yanagihara R 1982 Heavy metals and essential minerals in motor neuron disease. In: Rowland L P (ed) Human motor neuron diseases. Raven, New York, p 233–247

Yanagihara R T, Garruto R M, Gajdusek D C 1983 Epidemiological surveillance of amyotrophic lateral sclerosis and parkinsonism-dementia in the Commonwealth of the Northern Mariana Islands. Annals of Neurology 13: 79–86

Yase Y 1972 The pathogenesis of amyotrophic lateral sclerosis. Lancet 2: 292–296

Yase Y 1984 Environmental contribution to the amyotrophic lateral sclerosis process. In: Serratrice G, Desnuelle C, Pellissier J–F et al (eds) Neuromuscular disease. Raven, New York, p 335–339

Yoshida S 1977 X-ray microanalytic studies on amyotrophic lateral sclerosis. I Metal distribution compared with neuropathological findings in cervical spinal cord. Rinsho Shinkeigaku 17: 299–309

Yoshida S 1979 X-ray microanalytic studies on amyotrophic lateral sclerosis. III Relationship of calcification and degeneration found in cervical spinal cord of ALS. Rinsho Shinkeigaku 19: 641–652

Zalin H, Cooney T C 1974 Chorda tympani neurectomy — a new approach to sub-mandibular salivary obstruction. British Journal of Surgery 61: 391–394

Zellweger H, McCormick W F 1968 Scapuloperoneal dystrophy and scapuloperoneal atrophy. Helvetica Paediatrica Acta 6:643

Zilkha K J 1962 Contribution to discussion on motor neurone disease. Proceedings of the Royal Society of Medicine 55:1028

Peripheral nerve diseases

INTRODUCTION

This book deals with disorders of voluntary muscle, and the primary symptom of such disorders is weakness. Weakness may also be caused by disorders of the neuromuscular junction, peripheral nerve, anterior horn cell and central nervous system. Voluntary effort is required for muscle contraction and therefore simulated weakness can be due to malingering or a complaint of weakness can be related to psychiatric disorders. This chapter provides an outline of disorders of the peripheral nerves as they enter into the differential diagnosis of disorders of skeletal muscle.

CLINICAL PATTERNS OF PERIPHERAL NERVE DISEASE

Anatomy

The nervous system is divided into two parts, comprising the brain and spinal cord, in which oligodendroglial cells are responsible for myelination, and the peripheral nervous system, consisting of the cranial nerves (with the exception of the second), the spinal nerve roots and sensory ganglia, the peripheral nerves and the autonomic nerves and their ganglia. The limits of the peripheral nervous system are defined by the association of axons with Schwann cells. This distinction has a rational basis in terms of many of the diseases which separately affect the two parts of the nervous system. Two neuronal systems, however, lie in both the central and the peripheral nervous systems. In the efferent systems, the perikarya and proximal axons of the anterior horn cells (alpha and gamma motor neurones), cranial nerve motor nuclei and preganglionic parasympathetic and sympathetic neurones lie within the central nervous system, whereas their distal axons run in the peripheral nerves. Similarly, the centrally directed axons of the primary sensory neurones run in the central nervous system, while their cell bodies and peripheral axons lie within the peripheral nervous system.

The peripheral nervous system is divided into the somatic motor, the sensory and the autonomic systems. The motor system innervates the skeletal (alpha motor neurones) and fusimotor (gamma motor neurones) muscle fibres. The sensory nerves run from free nerve endings or specialised receptors in the skin, subcutaneous tissue, muscles, joints, ligaments and bones to the spinal cord, predominantly via the posterior roots. The autonomic nervous system provides motor innervation to glands, the smooth muscle of the eyes and viscera, blood vessels, and the sweat glands and erector pili muscles of the skin. The autonomic nervous system is divided into two separate subdivisions. The preganglionic fibres of the sympathetic nervous system leave the spinal cord from the T1–L2 segments and pass to the sympathetic chain. Postganglionic fibres then join visceral plexuses and peripheral nerves to innervate the distal structures. The preganglionic fibres of the parasympathetic nervous system run in the third, seventh and tenth cranial nerves and in the sacral nerves, to reach the eyes, glands and the viscera, where they synapse on short postganglionic neurones.

The perikarya and axons of neurones of the different components of the peripheral nervous system are of different sizes. The alpha motor neurones tend to be large, and their axons are all myelinated. The sensory axons have a very wide range of diameters from the largest myelinated A-alpha fibres, through the smaller myelinated A-delta fibres, to the unmyelinated C fibres, the latter two categories conveying pain and temperature sensation. The autonomic preganglionic fibres are myelinated, and the postganglionic axons are of small diameter and unmyelinated. The structure of the mammalian body results in some nerve fibres, such as those going to the hands and feet, being extremely long, while others, such as those in most of the cranial nerves, are extremely short (e.g. those to the external ocular muscles).

The anatomical arrangement of the peripheral nervous system is based upon the segmental development of the embryo, with a series of dermatomes and myotomes, and a bilaterally symmetrical pattern. The distal arrangements of the nerve fibres, however, show a dazzling array of plexiform interchanges both in the upper and lower limb plexuses and in the individual nerve fasciculi themselves.

The structural characteristics of the peripheral nervous system explain many of the features of peripheral nerve disorders. Both the neurone and the Schwann cell are cells under considerable metabolic stress. The axons of many of the neurones of the peripheral nervous system are extremely long for their diameter. Moreover all of the protein of the neurone has to be synthesised by the Nissl substance within the perikaryon. An indication of the geometric asymmetry of the neurone can be gauged from the following analogy. The perikaryon of a human S1 anterior horn cell is approximately 100 μm in diameter. An axon running from the sacral spinal cord to the extensor digitorum brevis muscle of the foot is about 1 m long, and about 10 μm in diameter. If the neurone were magnified so that the perikaryon became the size of a man's head, it would be 1.3 km high, and 1.2 cm in diameter. The volume of axoplasm in the axon is at least 150 times that of the perikaryon. It is for this reason that the neurones have such abundant Nissl substance, and such a high rate of protein synthesis. The axoplasmic transport of material down the axon is an energy-dependent and very important process. Impairment of either perikaryal synthesis of macromolecules or of their axoplasmic transport may underlie the distal degeneration of axons in many neuropathies. The Schwann cell is under a different form of metabolic stress from the neurone. It is a very thin cell with little cytoplasm and a very large surface area. This would be clear if a Schwann cell from a large myelinated fibre could be unwrapped and laid flat. The Schwann cell covers approximately 1 mm of the axon, and is about 3 mm long when unwrapped. Only a thin sliver of about 2 μm diameter of Schwann cell cytoplasm is present around the complete periphery of the cell, with lesser amounts of Schwann cell cytoplasm connecting the outer and inner portions of cytoplasm and corresponding to the Schmidt–Lanterman clefts. All the remainder of the Schwann cell consists of two apposed layers of Schwann cell plasmalemma, which comprises the myelin sheath. In the case of the Schwann cell, the surface-to-volume ratio is approximately 75 while that of a lymphocyte is less than one. Thus the Schwann cell has a great deal of immunogenic cell membrane, which it has to keep continually maintained metabolically. This explains the vulnerability of the myelin sheath, and the frequency of demyelinating neuropathies.

The peripheral neuropathies can be motor, sensory or autonomic or any combination of these. Single or multiple nerves or nerve roots can be involved. Disorders may affect only large or small fibres, or long or short fibres. Disease processes may lead to the loss of nerve cell bodies as well as their axons (neuronopathies), the distal axons only (axonopathies), or the Schwann cells and the myelin derived from them (demyelinating neuropathies).

Clinical patterns of disorders

There is an extremely wide range of patterns of disorders of the peripheral nerves. The distribution may be distal, proximal, restricted to the cranial nerves or diffuse. The pattern may be symmetrical or asymmetrical. It may involve single nerves (mononeuropathy), multiple single nerves (multiple mononeuropathy), nerve roots (radiculopathy), nerve plexuses (plexopathy) or affect the peripheral nervous system diffusely (polyneuropathy). A polyneuropathy may be distal, proximal or generalised. The involvement may be motor, sensory, autonomic or a combination of any of these. The development of the disorder may be acute (over a few days), subacute (over several weeks) or chronic. Motor or predominantly motor neuropathies, especially those with a symmetrical proximal distribution or, less importantly, a symmetrical distal distribution,

must be considered in the differential diagnosis of myopathic disorders.

PATTERNS OF PERIPHERAL NERVE DISEASE WHICH ENTER INTO THE DIFFERENTIAL DIAGNOSIS OF DISORDERS OF SKELETAL MUSCLE
(See Table 24.1)

Distal symmetrical motor polyneuropathy

The longest and often the largest diameter motor nerves are affected in a number of different disorders of peripheral nerves, with consequent distal amyotrophy, muscle weakness and loss of tendon reflexes. The clinical picture can be very similar to that of a distal spinal muscular atrophy, progressive muscular atrophy or a distal myopathy. Peripheral nerve diseases which can produce this pattern of clinical involvement include peroneal muscular atrophy (Charcot–Marie–Tooth disease, hereditary motor and sensory neuropathy), chronic inflammatory polyneuropathy, toxic neuropathy, many of the peripheral nerve disorders associated with metabolic diseases, vitamin deficiencies and neoplasms such as carcinoma, lymphoma and paraproteinaemia. In many such cases no cause can be identified and the disease has to be classified as a cryptogenic or idiopathic polyneuropathy. Disorders of the peripheral nerves usually involve some abnormality of sensation which is a helpful diagnostic point. Anterior horn cell disorders and less commonly axonopathies are often associated with muscle fasciculations. Full laboratory investigation is frequently required to separate the possible diseases responsible for the clinical picture of a distal symmetrical motor polyneuropathy.

Proximal symmetrical motor polyneuropathy

In a small number of disorders of the peripheral nerves, there is a predominantly proximal motor neuropathy, producing proximal muscle weakness and sometimes wasting. Such a pattern is much more commonly produced by muscular dystrophy,

Table 24.1 The main patterns of muscle weakness and their differential diagnosis

Distribution of muscle weakness	Differential diagnosis	
	Peripheral nerve disorders	Muscle, motor neurone, and neuromuscular junction disorders
Distal symmetrical weakness and wasting	Peroneal muscular atrophy (Charcot–Marie–Tooth disease) Chronic inflammatory polyneuropathy Chronic polyneuropathy of many aetiologies or idiopathic	Distal myopathy Distal spinal muscular atrophy Progressive muscular atrophy Dystrophia myotonica
Chronic proximal symmetrical weakness (± wasting)	Chronic inflammatory polyneuropathy	Muscular dystrophies Polymyositis Motor neurone disorders (ALS, Spinal muscular atrophy) Neuromuscular junction disorders (Myasthenia gravis, myasthenic syndrome)
Acute severe diffuse muscle weakness	Acute inflammatory polyneuropathy (Guillain–Barré) Porphyric neuropathy Toxic neuropathy Diphtheritic neuropathy	Acute polymyositis Rhabdomyolysis Toxic myopathy Periodic paralysis Myasthenia gravis
Cranial muscle weakness	Acute inflammatory polyneuropathy Diphtheritic neuropathy Bell's palsy Sarcoidosis and other structural lesions around base of skull	Ocular myopathy Oculopharyngeal muscular dystrophy Dystrophia myotonica Facioscapulohumeral muscular dystrophy Myasthenia gravis Congenital myopathies Motor neurone diseases
Asymmetrical muscle weakness (± wasting)	Vasculitic neuropathy Proximal diabetic plexopathy Other plexopathies Focal inflammatory polyneuropathy	Motor neurone diseases (spinal muscular atrophy, progressive muscular atrophy) Muscular dystrophies

polymyositis, spinal muscular atrophy or even a disorder of neuromuscular transmission such as myasthenia gravis. The disorders of the peripheral nerves causing such a pattern of involvement include the neuropathy of acute intermittent porphyria, acute inflammatory polyneuropathy (Guillain–Barré syndrome) and chronic inflammatory polyneuropathy. Many cases have some degree of sensory involvement, most often distal or diffuse, and rarely proximal, which can be helpful in separating the neuropathies from the other conditions. The distribution of muscle involvement in the muscular dystrophies is usually specific in that it severely involves some muscles and, to a large extent, spares others. Polymyositis may be associated with muscle tenderness in about one-quarter of the cases and with a skin rash in 40% of cases (dermatomyositis). Anterior horn cell disorders are often associated with visible fasciculations which can be increased by neostig-

mine. In myasthenia gravis, the muscle fatiguability may be evident from the history or on examination and wasting is not usually pronounced.

Acute severe diffuse motor polyneuropathies

Acute severe muscle weakness can be produced by a number of disorders of the peripheral nerves including acute inflammatory polyneuropathy (Guillain–Barré syndrome), the neuropathy of acute intermittent and variegate porphyria, diphtheritic neuropathy and sometimes neuropathies related to pharmaceutical and environmental neurotoxins such as thallium and various industrial solvents. The condition can simulate acute polymyositis, rhabdomyolysis, toxic myopathy, periodic paralysis and myasthenia gravis. The severity of the patient's condition can sometimes make it difficult to recognise minor sensory involvement in such acute neuropathies.

The release of creatine kinase into the blood and myoglobin into the urine can help to point to conditions damaging muscles rather than nerves. Relapses and remissions and variability can point towards a diagnosis of periodic paralysis or myasthenia gravis.

Cranial neuropathies

The cranial motor nerves are affected in a number of local and general conditions. Symmetrical cranial muscle weakness can occur in the descending form of acute inflammatory polyneuropathy (the Miller Fisher syndrome), diphtheritic neuropathy and sarcoidosis. The distribution of muscle weakness may suggest a motor neuropathy, but ocular myopathy, facioscapulohumeral muscular dystrophy and myasthenia gravis will often enter into the differential diagnosis. Many of the cranial neuropathies involve both sensory and motor nerves, which can help to clarify the differential diagnosis.

Asymmetrical motor neuropathies and plexopathies

The peripheral nerves can be damaged by various focal phenomena, including nerve compression in anatomical tunnels such as the carpal tunnel, or can be damaged by adjacent tumours or fractures. Focal nerve ischaemia can occur with disorders that affect the vasa nervorum, such as polyarteritis nodosa and other vasculitides, or diabetic vasculopathy. A focal form of chronic inflammatory polyneuropathy can produce multiple asymmetrical mononeuropathies and plexopathies. Generally, the anatomical distribution, the presence of sensory abnormalities and pain can help to separate these conditions from the disorders of anterior horn cells and muscles which can initially present with asymmetrical focal weakness and wasting.

INVESTIGATIONS TO SEPARATE PERIPHERAL NERVE DISORDERS FROM OTHER CAUSES OF MUSCLE WEAKNESS

Clinical examination and laboratory investigations can help to distinguish disorders of the peripheral nerves from other causes of muscle weakness. The presence of significant sensory abnormality, in the absence of any other cause, suggests that the weakness is due to peripheral nerve dysfunction. Needle electromyography (see Ch. 30) is a powerful tool for separating conditions causing denervation of muscle from primary disorders of muscle, although the changes are similar in peripheral neuropathy and in anterior horn cell disorder. Single-fibre EMG and repetitive nerve stimulation studies are particularly helpful for the diagnosis of disorders of the neuromuscular junction.

Studies of sensory and motor nerve conduction, including the latency of late waves, can usually be demonstrated to be abnormal in peripheral neuropathies. If there is severe demyelination, conduction velocity will be markedly reduced and the phenomenon of multifocal block may be observed. The latter is demonstrated by the evoked muscle action potential on proximal nerve stimulation being less than 50% of the amplitude of that on distal stimulation. Sensory nerve action potentials may be desynchronised and of reduced amplitude because of temporal dispersion of conduction. Motor neuronopathies and axonopathies cause loss of nerve fibres, with consequent reduction in amplitude of evoked compound muscle action potentials. In mixed neuropathies sensory nerve action potentials will also be reduced in amplitude, or lost. There is, however, a wide range of normal amplitudes for sensory and motor evoked action potentials, and small degrees of loss of axons may not be appreciated by this technique. The routinely applied clinical electrophysiological studies examine only the largest (fastest-conducting) axons, and disease of small myelinated and unmyelinated axons can go undetected by these techniques.

Repetitive nerve-stimulation studies are of help in demonstrating neuromuscular junction failure, such as occurs in myasthenia gravis, and the changes associated with the Lambert–Eaton myasthenic syndrome.

Cerebrospinal fluid examination may show raised CSF protein concentrations in patients with demyelinating neuropathies, particularly where the nerve roots are involved. Biopsy of a skeletal muscle, studied with histochemistry, can be of diagnostic help in separating myopathy and myositis from chronic denervating conditions including peripheral neuropathy. At times a biopsy of a nerve may be required, but nerve biopsy is usually undertaken to establish the nature of, rather than the presence of, neuropathy. Biopsies are usually taken from the sural or terminal radial nerves, which are both sensory, but fascicular biopsies may be taken from mixed motor nerves. This is rarely indicated for clinical diagnosis, and has a significant potential morbidity.

DISEASES OF PERIPHERAL NERVES

A list of many of the causes of peripheral neuropathy is given in Chapter 14. This section provides an outline of the clinical and electrophysiological features of the main disorders of peripheral nerves which have to be considered in the differential diagnosis of skeletal muscle weakness. These conditions may all cause a virtually pure motor neuropathy, although in many patients there will also be some degree of sensory nerve involvement.

Acute inflammatory polyneuropathy (Guillain–Barré–Strohl syndrome)

Landry (1859) described a group of patients with acute ascending paralysis, now recognised to embrace patients with both inflammatory polyneuropathy and transverse myelitis. Guillain et al (1916) collected a series of patients with acute polyradiculoneuritis, stressing the albuminocytological dissociation in the cerebrospinal fluid. Many such patients have been described since and much is known about the aetiology of the condition, although the criteria for diagnosis still remain difficult to define. A spectrum of disease is seen, ranging from the acute with a relatively good prognosis, to subacute· and chronic cases where continuing activity of the disease causes a worsening of the prognosis. In order to achieve a group with a relatively homogeneous clinical course and prognosis, it is important to establish criteria for the diagnosis (Ad Hoc NINCDS Committee 1978). Emphasis is particularly given to the duration between the onset and peak of the

weakness, and generally four weeks is the maximum accepted for the diagnosis.

The following gives an outline of the *clinical pattern* of the condition drawn from several reviews of large numbers of patients (Ravn 1967, Cambier & Brunet 1970, Prineas 1970). Over 50% of patients give a history of some preceding viral infection two to four weeks before the onset of the neuropathy. Over one-quarter begin with paraesthesiae in the feet, spreading proximally and then involving the hands. Over one-third have moderately severe pains, particularly in the back and limbs, which may cause diagnostic difficulties. Sensory loss is usually slight and may be absent in one-third of patients, while motor involvement is the most striking feature. In one-half of the patients, weakness is diffuse from the onset, whereas in the remainder it spreads from the lower limbs to involve the upper limbs, the respiratory and then bulbar muscles in the most severe cases. On average the condition progresses for two to four weeks and, at its maximum, respiratory support is required in about 10–20% of cases. In terms of a peripheral neuropathy, such a progress is *acute*.

For the average patient, the paresis is at its maximum for one to four weeks, and thereafter there is gradual recovery, although it may take three to six months. The range of duration of severe disability is wide. About 3–6% of patients have relapses.

The cerebrospinal fluid protein concentration is raised in almost all patients at some time during the illness. The maximum rise is seen from the tenth to twentieth day and the level may rise to 20 g/l. The proportion of gamma globulin is raised in most cases. Although Guillain et al (1916) emphasised the albuminocytological dissociation, about one-quarter of patients have a raised cell count in the CSF, although rarely to more than 40 cells/mm³. Inflammatory infiltration with lymphocytes and segmental demyelination involve both the roots and the peripheral nerves. Involved nerves may show either complete or partial conduction block, or may show a decrease of maximum conduction velocity of up to 50% of normal; but studies undertaken early in the condition may give entirely normal results. Investigation of the late (F and H) waves of the evoked motor action potential may help to demonstrate proximal nerve and root involvement.

The overall prognosis for recovery is good, considering the poor state of some patients. Most series have a mortality rate of more than 10%, mainly in respirator-dependent patients. About 18% of patients followed for more than three years have some permanent residual signs and symptoms. In children, this figure surprisingly rises to 26% (Ravn 1967). Those more severely paralysed have a worse prognosis. Of those on a respirator, 17% remain severely disabled and an additional 10% have residual signs but lead a normal life (Hewer et al 1968).

An uncommon variant of this condition affects predominantly the cranial nerves, including the extraocular muscles. Ataxia and areflexia are usually the sole indication of peripheral nerve involvement (Fisher 1956, Elizan et al 1971). Autonomic involvement can also occur in the Guillain–Barré–Strohl syndrome (Appenzeller & Marshall 1963, Birchfield & Shaw 1964). Orthostatic hypotension on tipping patients on a respirator is common, but spontaneous episodes of hypotension, hypertension and cardiac dysrrhythmia may also occur (Hewer et al 1968, Davies & Dingle 1972). These may result from partial blockage of the afferent and efferent portions of the cardiovascular reflexes.

Aetiology. Uncertainty still exists concerning the exact aetiology of this condition. Although it is clear that a preceding viral or other infection is often important, a wide variety of organisms have been implicated and the condition may occur following other precipitants such as surgical operations (Arnason & Asbury 1968) and immunising procedures (Schonberger et al 1981). The histological features suggest a cell-mediated disorder and there is evidence of accompanying disturbances of cellular immunity (Knowles et al 1969, Cook et al 1970, Currie & Knowles 1971). It has been suggested that patients with a higher proportion of reactive lymphocytes in the peripheral blood at the onset of the disease have a worse prognosis (Cook et al 1970). Nevertheless, there is also evidence that humoral factors may be implicated (Melnick & Flewett 1964, Cook et al 1971). The immunological mechanisms involved

in acute inflammatory polyneuropathy are still obscure but have been reviewed by Hughes (1979) and Arnason (1984).

An experimental model of this condition is available, namely experimental allergic neuritis (EAN) produced by the injection of peripheral nerve antigens together with Freund's adjuvant (Waksman & Adams 1955). This is a T-cell-mediated delayed hypersensitivity reaction (Linington et al 1984). The principal antigen involved is myelin P_2 protein (Kadlubowski et al 1980).

Many of the details of the immunological mechanisms still require elucidation, in particular, the factors involved in the natural termination of the disease. An antibody-mediated experimental neuropathy has also been produced in rabbits by hyperimmunisation with galactocerebroside (Saida et al 1979).

Treatment. If acute inflammatory polyneuropathy were an autoimmune disease, treatment with immunosuppressive agents might be appropriate. There is, however, argument as to the effectiveness of these agents. Some patients appear to respond to corticosteroid therapy, but others show no response. Uncontrolled and retrospective controlled series have failed to establish the efficacy of corticosteroids. Controlled trials of ACTH and prednisolone have produced conflicting results (McQuillen 1971, Hughes et al 1978) but the current evidence gives little encouragement for the use of corticosteroid treatment in acute cases. Some authors have reported a beneficial effect of cytotoxic immunosuppressive therapy (Yuill et al 1970, Heathfield & Dallos 1970). A multicentre controlled trial of plasma exchange in over 200 patients with severe acute inflammatory polyneuropathy has demonstrated the efficacy of this treatment if given within the first 14 days of the illness (McKhann et al 1985).

Chronic inflammatory polyneuropathies

These have much more diverse clinical presentations than the acute syndrome. Some have a picture resembling acute inflammatory polyneuropathy but the disorder continues to progress for more than four weeks. Some have a relapsing

– remitting course; others, usually with a later age of onset, have a chronic progressive picture, which is generally distal or diffuse, but may rarely be proximal. A hypertrophic neuropathy with thickened nerves may develop; nerve biopsies show onion bulbs from chronic repetitive segmental demyelination and remyelination. In all these conditions there may be inflammatory cell infiltration maximal in the proximal parts of the nerves, together with segmental demyelination and remyelination (Thomas et al 1969, Dyck et al 1975). Particularly in the chronic cases, distal axonal degeneration is frequent, explaining the relatively poor response to immunosuppressive therapy in such cases. These syndromes are predominantly motor, although in most there is some degree of sensory involvement. Peripheral nerve conduction velocity is reduced and multifocal block may be demonstrable in nerve conduction studies. In the later stages, axonal loss may become extensive. Like acute inflammatory polyneuropathy, the chronic syndrome appears to be an autoimmune disorder, although the immunopathogenetic mechanisms are not established for either.

Treatment with immunosuppressive agents appears more effective in this condition than in acute inflammatory polyneuropathy, especially in patients with a relapsing–remitting course and major degrees of demyelination. High-dose corticosteroids have been effective in many cases (Austin 1958), although relapses may occur if the dose is reduced too rapidly after the condition has been brought under control. Cytotoxic drugs such as azathioprine and plasma exchange have been beneficial in a number of patients, usually combined with corticosteroid therapy.

Acute intermittent porphyria

Acute intermittent porphyria may produce severe episodes of abdominal pain, psychiatric disorders and peripheral neuropathies. It is an acute, severe and chiefly motor neuropathy leading to flaccid paralysis and loss of reflexes (Ridley 1969). There often is a *proximal* predominance, the upper limbs being involved more than the lower. The cranial nerves, trunk and respiratory muscles and sphincters are also often involved. In about 50% of patients there is some sensory impairment, which may be either proximal or distal and which affects all modalities. The most classic picture is of a proximal muscle weakness with sensory loss in a bathing trunk distribution, and paradoxical preservation of the ankle jerks. Muscle wasting is rapid.

Pathological changes are predominantly of axonal degeneration, which in the motor nerves affects particularly the distal parts of the larger fibres in the intramuscular nerves and in the sensory fibres affects predominantly the centrally directed axons of the dorsal roots (Cavanagh & Ridley 1967). In both instances there is, therefore, a 'dying-back' distribution in individual axons, although the longest fibres are not involved as is usual in the 'dying-back' type of condition. It has been suggested that the effects fall particularly on those fibres with the largest motor units, although this appears unlikely in view of the similar distribution of damage in the sensory fibres. In some cases there may be segmental demyelination.

In severe attacks, respiratory and bulbar paralysis may cause death, and artificial ventilation is often required. A few patients make a rapid recovery (Hierons 1957), although in most the recovery is relatively slow, as might be expected after axonal degeneration. Sorensen & With (1971) reviewed 95 patients with acute intermittent porphyria, 41 of whom had suffered from paralytic episodes. Of these 41, 17 had died, and 12 of the 24 survivors had residual paralyses after three years which, in most cases, remained permanent thereafter. Recovery was less rapid and complete in males.

Attacks of acute intermittent porphyria occur either spontaneously or are precipitated by drugs, such as alcohol in excess, barbiturates and sulphonamides. The disease has a dominant mode of inheritance with incomplete penetrance (Pratt 1967). It has been shown that the attacks are associated with the induction of high levels of delta-aminolaevulinic acid synthetase in the liver causing increased excretion of delta-aminolaevulinic acid and porphobilinogen in the urine (Cavanagh & Ridley 1967, Sweeney et al 1970). The enzyme requires pyridoxal-5-phosphate as its co-enzyme, and it has been suggested that the induction of this enzyme causes a deficiency of pyridoxine, which produces the neuropathy. However the picture of porphyric neuropathy differs from that of deficiency of pyridoxine, and there is no correlation between the pyridoxal-5-phosphate level and the neuropathy (Hamfelt & Wetterberg 1968). The mechanism of production of the neuropathy remains obscure. Early diagnosis is vital in order to prevent the administration of drugs that aggravate the condition. Often, the diagnosis of conversion hysteria may be made because of associated psychiatric features, or the predominant motor symptomatology and the proximal distribution of the weakness may lead to an erroneous diagnosis of an acute polymyositis. Confirmation of acute intermittent porphyria is obtained by estimating red cell uroporphyrinogen-I-synthetase (porphobilinogen deaminase).

Treatment with glucose and haematin appears to be helpful in aborting an attack of porphyric neuropathy; the haematin probably produces feedback inhibition of the abnormally increased enzymes of the early parts of the pathway for haem synthesis (Bosch et al 1977).

Diphtheritic neuropathy

Diphtheria was once a scourge in many parts of the world, but immunisation in early childhood and the frequent use of antibiotics have now made it a rare disease in developed countries. It was first described by Trousseau & Lassegue (1851). Kinnier Wilson's textbook (Wilson 1954) gives a full review. The responsible organism is *Corynebacterium diphtherii*, which usually causes an acute pharyngitis characterised by a grey membrane, but which can infect a skin wound. The dangerous complications are delayed and are due to a cardiotoxin and a neurotoxin. In experimental animals, the severity of the disease is proportional to the dose of neurotoxin used. However, the amount of neurotoxin produced by the *Corybacterium* varies from strain to strain. In human infections it is therefore impossible to predict the severity of the delayed complications.

The major nerve damage due to the neurotoxin is usually delayed for 15–40 days after the onset of pharyngitis. Occasionally a precocious paralysis may develop three to 10 days after infection, being limited to the local area, particularly the palate, and being relatively benign. The major paralysis often begins in the palate but rapidly spreads into a generalised neuropathy, motor involvement predominating. The patient may require assisted ventilation, because of paralysis of bulbar and respiratory muscles.

The toxin is rapidly fixed in the body; one hour after injection into experimental animals its effect can no longer be neutralised by an injection of massive doses of antitoxin. The toxin is a potent inhibitor of elongation factor 2 and therefore of protein synthesis. It causes segmental demyelination by damaging the Schwann cells of the peripheral nerves in a patchy fashion. There is breakdown of the myelin sheaths, but the axons remain intact unless the neuropathy is very severe. This produces slowing of nerve conduction or a complete conduction block and paralysis. However, remyelination occurs quickly and the paralysis disappears in 15–30 days if death from complications does not supervene. In the experimental animal, clinical recovery occurs at a stage when nerve conduction remains slowed.

Exogenous toxins

A wide range of chemical agents may damage the peripheral nervous system (see Table 24.2). Most cause a sensorimotor distal polyneuropathy affecting the longest and largest axons. However, others such as lead may produce a pure muscle weakness. A diligent search for intoxication in a patient may allow withdrawal of the source of the neuropathy and hence recovery.

Care is required before accepting all reports of neuropathies due to toxic substances, particularly those recording uncommon reactions to drugs. The neuropathy may in fact be due to the underlying disease for which the drug was first given, or the association may be fortuitous. Moreover, allergic immunological reactions to almost any agent can occur. The agent acts as a hapten and binds to protein, which then becomes an antigen against which the body reacts. Such reactions are usually no more common with one agent than another, the 'allergic predisposition' being more a characteristic of the individual.

Other idiosyncratic reactions may indicate an underlying metabolic abnormality. Isoniazid

Table 24.2 Some causes of toxic neuropathy

Metals:	Lead, arsenic, mercury, thallium, gold
Industrial organic compounds:	*Solvents*: n-hexane, methyl-n-butyl-ketone, trichlorethylene, carbon disulphide *Insecticides and herbicides*: dichlorophen-oxyacetic acid *Others*: TOCP, acrylamide, dimethylamino-dipropionitrile, ethylene oxide
Drugs:	*Anticonvulsants*: phenytoin *Chemotherapeutic*: isoniazid, furans (nitrofurantoin, furaltadone), dapsone, metronidazole, ethambutol, clioquinol *Antimitotic*: Vinca alkaloids (vincristine, vinblastine), *cis*-platinum *Sedatives*: thalidomide, glutethimide *Others*: disulfiram, hydrallazine, stilbamidine, nitrofurazone, misonidazole, pyridoxine
Foods:	Cyanogens (cassava, cycasin), alcohol, lathyrogens
Bacterial and viral:	Diphtheria

intoxication occurs particularly in slow inactivators of the drug. In these individuals hepatic acetylation is slow and, consequently, blood levels are abnormally high, the major mechanism for drug elimination being urinary excretion (Evans et al 1960, Evans 1963). This tendency is inherited as an autosomal recessive trait, heterozygotes showing intermediate rates of inactivation.

Poisons may affect multiple sites and are rarely entirely specific, although many have a predilection for certain parts of the peripheral nervous system. Botulinum toxin blocks the release of transmitter vesicles at the neuromuscular junctions (Duchen 1970). Saxitoxin and tetrodotoxin block the depolarisation of axonal and neuronal membranes (Evans 1969). Diphtheria toxin has a particular effect on the Schwann cells (see above) causing demyelination with relative sparing of the axons. However, in most cases of toxic neuropathies the agent acts mainly on the perikaryon and axon, producing axonal degeneration. In triorthocresyl phosphate (TOCP) (Cavanagh 1964) and acrylamide neuropathies (Fullerton 1969) this has been particularly well studied. Frequently, the pattern of degeneration is the 'dying-back' type, affecting the distal parts of the largest fibres.

Vitamin deficiencies

Peripheral nerve damage occurs in a number of vitamin deficiencies, those with the greatest degree of motor involvement being in beriberi and alcoholism. Leaving aside the deficiency of vitamin B_{12}, deficiencies of other vitamins usually occur in the setting of malnutrition, where multiple deficiencies coexist. In experimental work it has been difficult to prove the requirement of an individual vitamin for peripheral nerve function, with the exception of thiamine (Victor 1965). For an extensive review of this problem the reader is referred to Victor (1984).

Thiamine — vitamin B_1. The active form of this vitamin is thiamine pyrophosphate which is the co-enzyme for at least three important enzymes of carbohydrate metabolism — pyruvate decarboxylase, alpha-ketoglutarate decarboxylase and transketolase. Deficiency causes an accumulation of pyruvate and lactate, with an impairment of energy metabolism in both the neurone and in Schwann cells. Although starvation alone in the presence of vitamin therapy may cause a peripheral neuropathy, a typical setting for thiamine deficiency was that occurring in the Japanese prisoner-of-war camps in the Second World War. The diet consisted predominantly of polished rice, which contains carbohydrate but not vitamins because of the removal of the rice husks. The result was damage to the peripheral nerves (dry beriberi) and to the heart with congestive cardiac failure (wet beriberi). The incidence of symptomatic neuropathy depended upon the severity of deprivation. Most of the patients showed signs of a distal, symmetrical polyneuropathy, which in 50% was mixed sensorimotor, in 30% mainly sensory, and in 20% mainly motor (Cruickshank 1952). Treatment with thiamine at a dose of more than 100 mg/day led to a slow recovery which often took more than six months. Those who had suffered prolonged and severe starvation made a lesser degree of recovery, residual dysaesthesiae being particularly common.

Vitamin B$_{12}$ is involved in the metabolism of methyl units, in nucleic acid metabolism, and probably in cell-membrane synthesis. Deficiency is most commonly due to loss of intrinsic factor produced by the gastric mucosa and required for the intestinal absorption of vitamin B$_{12}$; this is usually due to autoimmune damage to the gastric parietal cells by circulating autoantibodies. There is a familial tendency and the disease usually presents in middle age. More rarely there is congenital absence of transcobalamin II, a serum protein that carries vitamin B$_{12}$, and the disease presents in the infant. Other causes of malabsorption of vitamin B$_{12}$ include the bowel blind loop syndrome, ileal resection, the fish tapeworm and the dietary habits of vegans. The mechanism of damage of the peripheral nerves in vitamin B$_{12}$ deficiency is not certain. Clinically, the central nervous system changes predominate, particularly those in the spinal cord, with progressive signs of damage to the pyramidal tracts and dorsal columns. In addition, many patients have paraesthesiae in the hands and feet and a mild glove and stocking impairment of the modalities of sensation conveyed by the larger fibres, together with loss of ankle jerks.

There is slowing of the maximum motor and sensory conduction velocities by 10–20% of normal in the distal parts of the peripheral nerves, with no change in the proximal parts (Mayer 1965). The response to treatment with intramuscular vitamin B$_{12}$ at a dose of 1000 μg/day is relatively quick, the paraesthesiae sometimes disappearing within a few days and the distal reflexes returning within one or two months. Similarly, the distal nerve conduction velocity returns to normal within one month (Mayer 1965). However, the spinal cord disease is much less responsive to therapy, and the prognosis is entirely dependent upon this. Physiological studies suggest that the neuropathy is a 'dying-back' type of axonal degeneration, and this suggestion is supported by pathological studies in man, there being loss of the larger myelinated fibres in distal sensory nerves with the changes of axonal degeneration in teased single fibres (McLeod et al 1969). However, in experimental vitamin B$_{12}$ deficiency in monkeys, segmental demyelination apparently predominates (Torres et al 1971).

Malabsorption and other causes of vitamin deficiencies. Several different types of nervous and muscular syndromes have been reported in association with diseases causing malabsorption, a progressive symmetrical distal mixed polyneuropathy being the commonest, with sensory ataxia, paraesthesiae and spontaneous pains (Cooke & Smith 1966, Cooke et al 1966, Erbsloh & Abel 1970). Malabsorptions of all types may cause deficiencies, particularly of the fat-soluble vitamins and folic acid. Supplementation with all the known vitamins, together with replacement of pancreatic enzymes or the institution of a gluten-free diet as required, will still not correct some of the neuropathies. Pathological changes are axonal and distal; however, more studies are required of this interesting group of conditions (Cooke et al 1966). Some are related to chronic vitamin E deficiency (Harding et al 1982) and, in these, there may be accompanying evidence of myopathy.

Alcoholics. These subjects frequently have a peripheral neuropathy similar in presentation to that of thiamine deficiency, and have been shown to have deficiencies of thiamine, folic acid, pyridoxine, pantothenic acid and riboflavine (Fennely et al 1964), with evidence of malabsorption of thiamine (Tomasulo et al 1968). The high calorie intake in the form of alcohol, with deficiency of thiamine, may be responsible for the nerve damage in many. Some, however, fail to improve with replacement of vitamins of the B group, and the direct toxic effect of alcohol and the possible effect of liver damage must also be considered.

Pyridoxine (vitamin B$_6$). Deficiency of pyridoxine, of which the active derivative pyridoxal-5-phosphate is a co-enzyme for many decarboxylases and transaminases, experimentally produces a peripheral neuropathy (Follis & Wintrobe 1945, Vilter et al 1953). This is predominantly a distal, symmetrical sensory polyneuropathy, although central nervous system changes also occur. In the pig it is probably mainly an axonal degeneration, although single-fibre studies have not been undertaken (Follis & Wintrobe 1945). Isoniazid produces an essentially identical neuropathy by interfering with pyridoxine metabolism, probably with the formation of the isonicotinyl hydrazone of pyridoxine (Aspinall 1964). The pathological changes of axonal degeneration in isoniazid neuropathy are well described (Cavanagh 1967, Ochoa 1970). Excessive (greater than 1 g/day) doses of pyridoxine produce a distal sensory polyneuropathy (Schaumburg et al 1983).

In pellagra, which is due to *nicotinic acid* deficiency, a painful burning distal symmetrical sensory polyneuropathy may occur, although the central nervous system changes predominate (Erbsloh & Abel 1970). The burning-feet syndrome may at times be due to *riboflavine* deficiency (Lai & Ransome 1970).

Ischaemic neuropathies and connective tissue disorders. Although the peripheral nerves have an extensive plexus of blood vessels, occlusion of several major feeding vessels or of many smaller vasa nervorum can cause a neuropathy. This is usually asymmetrical, acute and predominantly motor. Large artery disease causes symptoms which are due to ischaemia of muscles (intermittent claudication) or gangrene of the whole limb, but 63% of patients with symptomatic arterial disease showed paraesthesiae, 87.5% had sensory abnormalities, 41% had depressed ankle jerks, 51% had weakness of one or both legs, and 31% had muscle wasting which was frequently asymmetrical (Eames & Lange 1967). Pathological examination often showed severe loss of myelinated fibres with both Wallerian degeneration and segmental demyelination (Eames & Lange 1967, Chopra & Hurwitz 1968). An acute asymmetrical mononeuropathy may occur in subacute bacterial endocarditis because of embolisation of the major feeding vessels (Jones & Seikert 1968). The proximal ischaemic mononeuropathy of diabetes is described below.

Most of the collagen-vascular diseases can damage the nerves by ischaemia. A review of this group of conditions was published by Glaser (1970). The incidence of peripheral nerve involvement is highest in polyarteritis nodosa in which up to 20–30% of patients have a neuropathy (Lovshin & Kernohan 1948, Bleehen et al 1963). The picture is usually that of multiple mononeuropathies with acute lesions of several individual nerves, although later it may blend into a progressive distal symmetrical sensorimotor polyneuropathy. Individual vascular lesions of the nerve are often painful. The treatment of polyarteritis nodosa with corticosteroids alone is not completely effective, and combination with cytotoxic immunosuppressive agents is often required.

The incidence of involvement of the peripheral nervous system in systemic lupus erythematosus varies from 3 to 13% (Dubois 1966, Johnson & Richardson 1968), central nervous system involvement being considerably more frequent. Again the pattern is usually that of multiple mononeuropathies, although in some patients there is a distal symmetrical sensorimotor polyneuropathy. Occasionally a picture resembling an acute inflammatory polyneuropathy may develop. A peripheral neuropathy can occur in giant cell arteritis (Warrell et al 1968), scleroderma (Richter 1954, Kibler & Rose 1960), dermatomyositis (McEntee & Mancall 1965) and Wegener's granulomatosis (Stern 1970).

Several types of clinically symptomatic peripheral neuropathy have been described in rheumatoid arthritis. They are best classified into four types (modified from Pallis & Scott 1965):

Lesions of the major nerves of the upper and lower limbs (37%);
Distal symmetrical sensory polyneuropathy of the lower limbs (35%);
Digital neuropathy (22%);
Distal mixed sensorimotor polyneuropathy of upper and lower extremities.

This last category is the smallest group (6%) but is the most severe and has the poorest prognosis. It often presents initially with multiple mononeuropathies before progressing to a distal symmetrical sensorimotor polyneuropathy. The course is relatively rapid over a few months, and most patients die within two years from a widespread vasculitis.

Pathological studies have generally shown a diffuse vasculitis with occlusion of the vasa nervorum, more marked in the fourth type of neuropathy than in the second. Nerve fibre loss occurs, particularly at upper arm and mid-thigh levels, involving the centre of the fasciculi, and these areas may constitute 'watershed territories' in the peripheral nerves (Dyck et al 1972a). The nerves may show segmental demyelination, although Wallerian degeneration predominates, particularly in the more severe cases (Haslock et al 1970, Weller et al 1970, Dyck et al 1972b). Treatment is extremely difficult. In the fourth type of neuropathy, cytotoxic immunosuppressive agents are worthy of trial because of the poor prognosis. D-penicillamine may also be of value (Golding 1971).

Motor syndromes in diabetic neuropathy

The commonest type of peripheral neuropathy related to diabetes mellitus is a distal symmetrical sensory and autonomic polyneuropathy. There may be coexistent electromyographic evidence of denervation in peripheral muscles (Fagerberg et al 1963) or sometimes mild distal muscle wasting and weakness. Less commonly, syndromes occur in which motor deficits predominate.

Focal cranial and limb neuropathies.
These are most frequently encountered in the older age groups. Among cranial mononeuropathies, the third and seventh are most common and usually have an abrupt onset. They are likely to have a vascular basis (Asbury et al 1970).

Focal neuropathies affecting the limbs and the thoracoabdominal wall are commoner in patients with diabetes than is generally recognised. Those of acute onset again probably have a vascular cause. Others occur at sites of entrapment or external compression, and it is likely that there is an increased susceptibility to pressure palsies in diabetes.

Diabetic amyotrophy.
A proximal lower limb motor neuropathy may develop, usually in the older diabetic, and can be the presenting feature in maturity-onset cases of noninsulin-dependent diabetes. Very occasionally the proximal muscles in the upper limbs are involved. Lower limb proximal motor neuropathy was originally recognised by Bruns (1890) but interest in the condition

was reawakened by Garland (Garland & Taverner 1953, Garland 1955) who introduced the term 'diabetic amyotrophy' after initially referring to this condition as 'diabetic myelopathy' in view of the presence of extensor plantar responses in three out of the five original cases. Electromyography demonstrates denervation, and conduction time in the femoral nerve is prolonged (Chopra & Hurwitz 1968), clearly indicating a motor neuropathy. The site of damage is probably not only in nerve trunks, including the femoral (Skanse & Gydell 1956), but also in the lumbrosacral plexus (Linden 1962).

Some cases are unilateral and of acute onset. They may recover, only to be followed by the same sequence on the opposite side. The onset is frequently associated with pain which may persist for several weeks and which is particularly troublesome at night. The territory of the femoral nerve is most often affected but muscles innervated by other lower limb nerves may also be involved simultaneously. The distribution often indicates lumbosacral plexus rather than nerve trunk involvement. The knee jerk is frequently lost but sensory impairment tends to be slight unless there is an accompanying distal sensory polyneuropathy. In other patients there is bilateral symmetrical or asymmetrical lower limb weakness of insidious onset, especially quadriceps muscle weakness. The prognosis for recovery is less satisfactory in this situation. As for other types of proximal motor neuropathy, confusion with myopathic disorders not infrequently occurs.

The basis for instances where there is an acute onset is probably vascular and there is evidence of the occurrence of ischaemic lesions in the nerves to affected muscles (Raff et al 1968). It has been suggested that cases with an insidious onset and symmetrical distribution have a metabolic basis (Asbury 1977), but this clinical picture could be related to the cumulative effects of multiple small ischaemic lesions.

Peroneal muscular atrophy, Charcot–Marie–Tooth disease and hypertrophic neuropathy

The history of peroneal muscular atrophy goes back to the descriptions by Charcot & Marie

(1886) and Tooth (1886) with progressive distal wasting and weakness producing a 'stork-leg' appearance, with motor involvement later spreading to the hands and relatively little involvement of the sensory nerves. That of hypertrophic neuropathy goes back to the original descriptions of Dejerine & Sottas (1893) and Dejerine & André-Thomas (1906) of a brother and sister presenting in childhood and adolescence with a relatively rapidly progressive distal sensorimotor neuropathy, and in whom the peripheral nerves were hypertrophied with 'onion-bulb' formation. It is only in recent times that the relationship between these diseases and a number of other conditions with a similar clinical and pathological picture has been elucidated. This was initiated by the seminal work of Dyck & Lambert (1968a, b) and has been elaborated in numerous later studies.

It is clear that the clinical syndrome of peroneal muscular atrophy is genetically complex. In some cases there is a pure motor syndrome, constituting a hereditary distal spinal muscular atrophy (Harding & Thomas 1980a). In the remainder there is associated sensory involvement, although motor phenomena predominate. They have been categorised as hereditary motor and sensory neuropathy (HMSN) and are again subdivisible on clinical and genetic grounds (Harding & Thomas 1980b).

(1) Hereditary motor and sensory neuropathy, type I (hypertrophic form of Charcot–Marie–Tooth disease). This group includes kinships similar to those described by Charcot & Marie (1886), and Roussy & Levy (1926). Symptoms most often begin during the first decade. The earliest sign is usually pes cavus, and some gait disturbance often appears by the second decade due to progressive atrophy of the anterior tibial group of muscles. A progressive foot-drop develops, and later there is difficulty in manipulating the fingers. Significant sensory impairment appears late, affects especially the large fibre modalities, and is less severe than the motor involvement. Some relatives with no symptoms show marked slowing of nerve conduction (Bradley & Aguayo 1969). The condition is very slowly progressive and many patients can still walk with aids 30 years after the onset. The maximum motor and sensory nerve

conduction velocities are 5–20 m/s, and the nerve shows extensive segmental demyelination and hypertrophy with 'onion-bulb' formation. Signs of spinal cord dysfunction are sometimes present, resulting from compression by hypertrophic nerve roots (Symonds & Blackwood 1962).

The inheritance is usually autosomal dominant, but pedigrees with autosomal recessive and possibly X-linked inheritance also occur. Recently, linkage in some of the dominantly inherited families with the Duffy blood group, the locus for which is on chromosome I, has been demonstrated (Bird et al 1982, Guiloff et al 1982).

(2) Hereditary motor and sensory neuropathy, type II (neuronal form of Charcot–Marie–Tooth disease). The clinical pattern in this condition is similar to that in type I, but the onset is commonest in the second decade and is sometimes delayed to middle or late life; in addition, there is less hand and more leg involvement, and no enlargement of the peripheral nerves. Sensory loss is mild compared with motor impairment. Nerve conduction velocity is normal or modestly reduced. Sensory nerve biopsies show loss of the larger myelinated nerve fibres, little segmental demyelination and virtually no onion bulbs. The disorder probably represents a primary degeneration of anterior horn and primary sensory neurones. Inheritance is usually autosomal dominant.

(3) Hereditary motor and sensory neuropathy, type III (hypertrophic neuropathy of Dejerine–Sottas type). The onset is usually in the first few years of life with delayed walking. The condition progresses slowly so that the patient becomes wheelchair-bound by 20–30 years of age. There is a progressive symmetrical glove-and-stocking loss of sensation. The peripheral nerves are thickened and nerve conduction velocity is severely reduced, usually to less than 10 m/s. Nerve biopsies show hypertrophic changes and hypomyelination (Dyck et al 1971). Inheritance is autosomal recessive.

The limits of HMSN are not yet fully defined and current classifications will have to be modified as individual genes are identified. Some families do not fit easily into the present scheme, such as those described by Madrid et al (1977), Bradley et al (1977) and Davis et al (1979) with nerve conduction velocity values that lie mainly in the upper part of the HMSN I range but which overlap with HMSN II, and which show 'intermediate' pathological features. Others, described by Ouvrier et al (1981) resemble HMSN II, but have an early onset and an aggressive clinical course. Yet others show clinical features such as pyramidal signs (Harding & Thomas 1984), in addition to peroneal muscular atrophy.

Hypertrophic neuropathy also occurs in *Refsum's disease* (Cammermeyer 1956) in which inheritance is autosomal recessive. The disease was originally described by Refsum (1946), under the title of *heredopathia atactica polyneuritiformis*. Symptoms usually appear in the first and second decades of life, with the development of a chronic progressive symmetrical distal sensorimotor polyneuropathy which may show relapses and remissions. There is cerebellar dysfunction with ataxia and nystagmus, and a pigmentary retinopathy which lacks the classic 'bone corpuscle' pigment cells of typical retinitis pigmentosa. The cerebrospinal fluid protein concentration is raised, and there are often anosmia, nerve deafness, ichthyosis, and cardiac and pupillary abnormalities. The condition is rare, but is important because of a knowledge in part of the underlying biochemistry of the condition and its treatment. There is an increased amount of the long-chain fatty acid, phytanic acid (3, 7, 11, 15-tetramethyl-hexadecanoic acid) in the blood and many tissues of the body (Klenk & Kahlke 1963); this accumulation is due to impaired metabolism of dietary phytol. The exclusion of phytol from the diet (Steinberg et al 1970), and plasma exchange to remove phytanic acid may produce considerable improvement.

Chronic cryptogenic polyneuropathy

In a significant proportion of the patients with a chronic progressive peripheral neuropathy referred to a neurologist, no aetiology is found. In such cases the condition is usually termed chronic cryptogenic (idiopathic) polyneuropathy, and about half of these are predominantly motor in type. Dyck and coworkers (1981) found that very detailed investigation of the patients themselves and of their family members demonstrated that about one-half of these patients have a familial neuropathy. A further quarter probably have chronic inflammatory polyneuropathy, although the response to corticosteroids in this group is poorer than in cases with a more acute or relapsing–remitting picture. Some are related to a paraproteinaemia.

CONCLUSIONS

Disorders of the peripheral nerves frequently enter into the differential diagnosis of conditions affecting skeletal muscle, the neuromuscular junction and the anterior horn cells. Careful clinical examination, full laboratory investigation and knowledge of the anatomy of the musculoskeletal system and the diseases which affect it allow the separation and identification of these conditions in most patients.

REFERENCES

Ad Hoc NINCDS Committee 1978 Criteria for diagnosis of Guillain–Barré syndrome. Annals of Neurology 3(6): 565–566

Appenzeller O, Marshall J 1963 Vasomotor disturbance in Landry–Guillain–Barré syndrome. Archives of Neurology 9:368

Arnason B G 1984 Acute inflammatory demyelinating polyradiculoneuropathies. In: Dyck P J, Thomas P K, Lambert E H, Bunge R (eds) Peripheral neuropathy, 2nd edn. W B Saunders, Philadelphia, p 2050–2100

Arnason B G, Asbury A K 1968 Idiopathic polyneuritis after surgery. Archives of Neurology 18:500

Asbury A K 1977 Proximal diabetic neuropathy. Annals of Neurology 2: 179–180

Asbury A K, Aldredge H, Herschberg R, Fisher C M 1970 Oculomotor palsy in diabetes mellitus: a clinico-pathological study. Brain 93: 555–566

Aspinall D L 1964 Multiple deficiency state associated with isoniazid therapy. British Medical Journal 2:1177

Austin J H 1958 Recurrent polyneuropathies and their corticosteroid treatment. Brain 81:157

Birchfield R J, Shaw C M 1964 Postural hypotension in the Guillain–Barré syndrome. Archives of Neurology 10:149

Bird T D, Ott J, Giblett E R 1982 Evidence for linkage of Charcot-Marie-Tooth neuropathy to the Duffy locus on chromosome I. American Journal of Human Genetics 34: 288–394

Bleehen S S, Lovelace R E, Cotton R E 1963 Mononeuritis

multiplex in polyarteritis nodosa. Quarterly Journal of Medicine 32:193

Bosch E P, Pierach C A, Bossenmaier I, Cardinal R, Thorson M 1977 Effect of hematin in porphyric neuropathy. Neurology (Minneapolis) 27:1053

Bradley W G, Aguayo A 1969 Hereditary chronic neuropathy. Electrophysiological and pathological studies in an affected family. Journal of the Neurological Sciences 9:131

Bradley W G, Madrid R, Davis C J F 1977 The peroneal muscular atrophy syndrome. Part 3: Clinical, electrophysiological and pathological correlations. Journal of the Neurological Sciences 32:123

Bruns L 1890 Über neuritische Lahmungen beim Diabetes mellitus. Berlinen klinische Wochenschrift 27:509

Cambier J, Brunet P 1970 Le syndrome de Guillain et Barré. Ballière, Paris

Cammermeyer J 1956 Neuropathological changes in hereditary neuropathies: manifestations of the syndrome of heredopathia atactica polyneuritiformis in the presence of interstitial hypertrophic polyneuropathy. Journal of Neuropathology and Experimental Neurology 15:340

Cavanagh J B 1964 Peripheral nerve changes in orthocresyl phosphate poisoning in the cat. Journal of Pathology and Bacteriology 87:365

Cavanagh J B 1967 Pattern of change in peripheral nerves produced by isoniazid intoxication in rats. Journal of Neurology, Neurosurgery and Psychiatry 30:26

Cavanagh J B, Ridley A R 1967 The nature of the neuropathy complicating acute intermittent porphyria. Lancet 2:1023

Charcot J M, Marie P 1886 Sur une forme particulière d'atrophie musculaire progressive souvent familial débutant par les pieds et les jambes et atteignant plus tard les mains. Revue de médecine (Paris) 6:97

Chopra J S, Hurwitz L J 1968 Femoral nerve conduction in diabetes and chronic occlusive vascular disease. Journal of Neurology, Neurosurgery and Psychiatry 31:28

Cook S D, Dowling P C, Whitaker J N 1970 The Guillain–Barré syndrome. Relationship of circulating immunocytes to disease activity. Archives of Neurology 22:470

Cook S D, Dowling P C, Murray M R, Whitaker J N 1971 Circulating demyelinating factors in acute idiopathic polyneuritis. Archives of Neurology 24:136

Cooke W T, Smith W T 1966 Neurological disorders associated with adult coeliac disease. Brain 89:683

Cooke W T, Joynson A G, Woolf A L 1966 Vital staining and electron microscopy of the intramuscular nerve endings in the neuropathy of adult coeliac disease. Brain 89:663

Cruikshank E K 1952 Dietary neuropathies. Vitamins and Hormones 10:1

Currie S, Knowles M 1971 Lymphocyte transformation in the Guillain–Barré syndrome. Brain 94:109

Davies A G, Dingle H R 1972 Observations on cardiovascular and neuroendocrine disturbances in the Guillain–Barré syndrome. Journal of Neurology, Neurosurgery and Psychiatry 35:176

Davis C J F, Bradley W G, Madrid R 1979 The peroneal muscular atrophy syndrome. 1: Clinical, genetic, and electrophysiological findings and classification. Journal de Génétique Humaine 26:311

Dejerine J, André-Thomas 1906 Sur la névrite interstitielle et hypertrophique de l'enfance (Observation suivie d'autopsie). Nouvelle Iconographie de la Salpêtrière 19:477

Dejerine J, Sottas J 1893 Sur la névrite interstitielle, hypertrophique et progressive de l'enfance. Comptes Rendus des Seances de la Societé de Biologie et de ses Filiales 45:63

Dubois E L (ed) 1966 Lupus erythematosus. McGraw Hill, New York

Duchen L W 1970 Changes in motor innervation and cholinesterase localization induced by botulinum toxin and skeletal muscle of the mouse: difference between fast and slow muscles. Journal of Neurology, Neurosurgery and Psychiatry 33:40

Dyck P J, Lambert E H 1968a Lower motor and primary sensory neuron diseases with peroneal muscular atrophy. I: Neurologic, genetic and electrophysiologic findings in hereditary polyneuropathies. Archives of Neurology 18:603

Dyck P J, Lambert E H 1968b II: Neurologic, genetic and electrophysiologic findings in various neuronal degenerations. Archives of Neurology 18:619

Dyck P J, Lambert E H, Sanders K, O'Brien P C 1971 Severe hypomyelination and marked abnormality of conduction in Dejerine-Sottas hypertrophic neuropathy: myelin thickness and compound action potential of sural nerve in vitro. Mayo Clinic Proceedings 46:433

Dyck P J, Conn D L, Okazaki H 1972a Necrotizing angiopathic neuropathy. Mayo Clinic Proceedings 47:461

Dyck P J, Schultz P W, O'Brien P C 1972b Quantitation of touch-pressure sensation. Archives of Neurology 26:465

Dyck P J, Lais A C, Ohta M, Bastron J A, Okazaki H, Groover R V 1975 Chronic inflammatory polyneuropathy. Mayo Clinic Proceedings 50: 621–637

Dyck P J, Oviatt K F, Lambert E H 1981 Intensive evaluation of referred unclassified neuropathies yields improved diagnosis. Annals of Neurology 10:222

Eames R A, Lange L S 1967 Clinical and pathological study of ischaemic neuropathy. Journal of Neurology, Neurosurgery and Psychiatry 30:215

Elizan T S, Spire J P, Andiman R M, Baughman F A, Lloyd-Smith D L 1971 Syndrome of acute idiopathic ophthalmoplegia with ataxia and areflexia. Neurology (Minneapolis) 21:281

Erbsloh F, Abel M 1970 Deficiency neuropathies. In: Vinken P J, Bruyn G W (eds) Handbook of clinical neurology, vol 7. North Holland, Amsterdam, p. 558–663

Evans D A P 1963 Pharmacogenetics. American Journal of Medicine 34:639

Evans D A P, Manley K A, McKusick V A 1960 Genetic control of isoniazid metabolism in man. British Medical Journal 2:485

Evans M H 1969 Mechanism of saxitoxin and tetrodotoxin poisoning. British Medical Bulletin 25:263

Fagerberg S E, Petersen I, Steg G, Wilhelmsen L 1963 Motor disturbances in diabetes mellitus. A clinical study using electromyography and nerve conduction determination. Acta Medica Scandinavica 174: 711–719

Fennely J, Frank O, Baker H, Leevy C M 1964 Peripheral neuropathy of the alcoholic. Aetiologic role of aneurin and other B-complex vitamins. British Medical Journal 2:1290

Fisher C M 1956 An unusual variant of acute idiopathic polyneuritis (syndrome of ophthalmoplegia, ataxia and areflexia). Journal of Medicine 255:57

Follis R H Jr, Wintrobe M M 1945 A comparison of the effects of pyridoxine and pantothenic acid deficiency on nervous tissue of swine. Journal of Experimental Medicine 81:539

Fullerton P M 1969 Electrophysiological and histological

observations on peripheral nerves in acrylamide poisoning in man. Journal of Neurology, Neurosurgery and Psychiatry 32:186

Garland H 1955 Diabetic amyotrophy. British Medical Journal 2:1287

Garland H, Taverner D 1953 Diabetic myelopathy. British Medical Journal 1:1405

Glaser G H 1970 Neuropathies in collagen diseases. In: Vinken P J, Bruyn G W (eds) Handbook of clinical neurology, vol 8. North Holland, Amsterdam, p 118–130

Golding D N 1971 Rheumatoid neuropathy. British Medical Journal 2:169

Guillain G, Barré J, Strohl H 1916 Sur un syndrome de radiculonévrite avec hyperalbuminose du liquide cephalo-rachidien sans réaction cellulaire. Bulletin et memoires de la Societe médicale des hôpitaux de Paris 1462

Guiloff R J, Thomas P K, Contreras M, Schwarz G, Sedgwick E M 1982 Linkage of autosomal dominant type I hereditary motor and sensory neuropathy to the Duffy locus on chromosome I. Journal of Neurology, Neurosurgery and Psychiatry 45: 669–674

Hamfelt A, Wetterberg L 1968 Neuropathy in porphyria. Lancet 1:50

Harding A E, Thomas P K 1980a Hereditary distal spinal muscular atrophy. A report on 34 cases and a review of the literature. Journal of the Neurological Sciences 45: 337–338

Harding A E, Thomas P K 1980b The clinical features of hereditary motor and sensory neuropathy, types I and II. Brain 103: 259–280

Harding A E, Muller D P R, Thomas P K, Willison H J 1982 Spinocerebellar degeneration secondary to chronic intestinal malabsorption: a vitamin E deficiency syndrome. Annals of Neurology 12: 419–424

Harding A E, Thomas P K 1984 Peroneal muscular atrophy with pyramidal features. Journal of Neurology, Neurosurgery and Psychiatry 47: 169–172

Haslock D I, Wright V, Harriman D G F 1970 Neuromuscular disorders in rheumatoid arthritis. A motor-point biopsy study. Quarterly Journal of Medicine 39:335

Heathfield K, Dallos V 1970 Treatment of polyneuropathy with azathioprine. Lancet 2:1030

Hewer R L, Hilton P J, Crampton-Smith A, Spalding J M K 1968 Acute polyneuritis requiring artificial respiration. Quarterly Journal of Medicine 37:479

Hierons R 1957 Changes in the nervous system in acute porphyria. Brain 80:176

Hughes R A C 1979 Acute inflammatory polyneuropathy. In: Rose F C (ed) Clinical neuroimmunology. Blackwell, Oxford, p 170–184

Hughes R A C, Newsom-Davis J M, Perkin J D, Pearce J M 1978 Controlled trial of prednisolone in acute polyneuropathy. Lancet 2:750

Johnson R T, Richardson E P 1968 The neurological manifestations of systemic lupus erythematosus. Medicine (Baltimore) 47:333

Jones H R, Siekert R G 1968 Embolic mononeuropathy and bacterial endocarditis. Archives of Neurology 19:535

Kadlubowski M, Hughes R C, Gregson N A 1980 Experimental allergic neuritis in the Lewis rat: characterization of the activity of peripheral myelin and its major basic protein, P_2. Brain Research 184: 439–454

Kibler R F, Rose F C 1960 Peripheral neuropathy in the 'collagen diseases'. A case of scleroderma neuropathy. British Medical Journal 1:1781

Klenk E, Kahlke W 1963 Über das Vorkommen, der 3, 7, 11, 15-tetramethyl-Hexadecansaure in den Cholisterniestern und anderen Lipoid fraktionen der Organe bein einem Krankheitsfall unbebannter Genese (Verdacht auf Heredopathia atactica polyneuritiformis [Refsum-Syndrom]). Hoppe-Seyler's Zeitschrift für physiologische Chemie 333:133

Knowles M, Saunders M, Currie S, Walton J N, Field E J 1969 Lymphocyte transformation in the Guillain–Barré syndrome. Lancet 2:1168

Lai C S, Ransome G A 1970 Burning feet syndrome: a case due to malabsorption and responding to riboflavin. British Medical Journal 2:151

Landry O 1859 Note sur la paralysie ascendante aigue. Gazette hebdomadaire de Médecine et de Chirurgie 6: 472–486

Linden L 1962 Amyotrophia diabetica. Svenska Läkertidningen 59:3368

Linington C, Izumo S, Suzuki M, Uyemura K, Meyermann R, Wekerle H 1984 A permanent rat T-cell line that mediates experimental allergic neuritis in the Lewis rat in vivo. Journal of Immunology 133: 1946–50

Lovshin L L, Kernohan J W 1948 Peripheral neuritis in periarteritis nodosa. Archives of Internal Medicine 82:321

McEntee W J, Mancall E L 1965 Neuromyositis: a reappraisal. Neurology (Minneapolis) 15:69

McKhann G (The Guillain–Barré Study Group) 1985 Plasmapheresis and acute Guillain-Barré syndrome. Neurology (Cleveland) 35:1096

McLeod J G, Walsh J C, Little J M 1969 Sural nerve biopsy. Medical Journal of Australia ii:1092

McQuillen M P 1971 Idiopathic polyneuritis: several studies of nerve and immune functions. Journal of Neurology, Neurosurgery and Psychiatry 34:607

Madrid R, Bradley W G, Davis C J F 1977 The peroneal muscular atrophy syndrome. Part 2: Observations on the pathological changes in sural nerve biopsies. Journal of the Neurological Sciences 32:91

Mayer R F 1965 Peripheral nerve function in vitamin B_{12} deficiency. Archives of Neurology 13:355

Melnick S C, Flewett T H 1964 Role of infection in the Guillain-Barré syndrome. Journal of Neurology, Neurosurgery and Psychiatry 27:395

Ochoa J 1970 Isoniazid neuropathy in man. Quantitative electron microscopic study. Brain 93:831

Ouvrier R A, McLeod J G, Morgan G J, Wise G A, Conchin T E 1981 Hereditary motor and sensory neuropathy of neuronal type with onset in early childhood. Journal of the Neurological Sciences 51: 181–197

Pallis C A, Scott J T 1965 Peripheral neuropathy in rheumatoid arthritis. British Medical Journal 1:1141

Pratt R T C 1967 The genetics of neurological disorders. Oxford University Press, London

Prineas J 1970 Polyneuropathies of undetermined cause. Acta Neurologica Scandinavica (Suppl) 44:1

Raff M C, Sangalang V, Asbury A K 1968 Ischaemic mononeuropathy multiplex associated with diabetes mellitus. Archives of Neurology 18:487

Ravn H 1967 The Landry–Guillain–Barré syndrome. Acta Neurologica Scandinavica (Suppl) 30:1

Refsum S 1946 Heredopathia atactica polyneuritiformis: familial syndrome not hitherto described. Acta Psychiatrica et Neurologica Scandinavica 38

Richter R B 1954 Peripheral neuropathy and connective

tissue disease. Journal of Neuropathology and Experimental Neurology 13:168

Ridley A 1969 The neuropathy of acute intermittent porphyria. Quarterly Journal of Medicine 38:307

Roussy G, Lévy G 1926 Sept cas d'une maladie familiale particulière: Trouble de la marche, pied bots et aréfléxie tendineuse généralisée, avec accessoirement, légère maladresse des mains. Revue Neurologique 1:427

Saida T, Saida K, Dorfman S H et al 1979 Experimental allergic neuritis induced by sensitisation with galactocerebroside. Science 204: 1103–1106

Schaumburg H, Kaplan J, Windebank A, Vick N, Rasmus S, Pleasure D, Brown M J 1983 Sensory neuropathy from pyridoxine abuse. New England Journal of Medicine 309(8): 445–448

Schonberger L B, Hurwitz E S, Katona P, Holman R C, Bergman D J 1981 Guillain–Barré syndrome: its epidemiology and associations with influenza vaccination. Annals of Neurology 9 (Suppl): 31–38

Skanse B, Gydell K 1956 A rare type of femoral sciatic neuropathy in diabetes mellitus. Acta Medica Scandinavica 155:463

Sørensen A W S, With T K 1971 Persistent paresis after porphyric attacks. Acta Medica Scandinavica 190:219

Steinberg D, Mize C E, Herndon J H Jr., Fales H M, Engel W K, Vroom F Q 1970 Phytanic acid in patients with Refsum's syndrome and response to dietary treatment. Archives of Internal Medicine 125:75

Stern G 1970 The peripheral nerves in Wegener's granulomatosis. In: Vinken P J, Bruyn G W (eds) Handbook of clinical neurology. North Holland, Amsterdam, p 112–117

Sweeney V P, Pathak M A, Asbury A K 1970 Acute intermittent porphyria: increased ALA-synthetase activity during an acute attack. Brain 93:369

Symonds C P, Blackwood W 1962 Spinal cord compression in hypertrophic neuritis. Brain 85:251

Thomas P K, Lascelles R G, Hallpike J F, Hewer R L 1969 Recurrent and chronic relapsing Guillain-Barré polyneuritis. Brain 92: 589–606

Tomasulo P A, Kater R M H, Iber F L 1968 Impairment of thiamine resorption in alcoholism. American Journal of Clinical Nutrition 21:1340

Tooth H H 1886 The peroneal type of progressive muscular atrophy (Thesis, University of London) H K Lewis, London

Torres I, Smith W T, Oxnard C E 1971 Peripheral neuropathy associated with vitamin B_{12} deficiency in captive monkeys. Journal of Pathology 105:125

Trousseau A, Lassegue G 1851 Du nassonnement de la paralysie du voile de palais. L'Union Médicale 5:471

Victor M 1965 The effects of nutritional deficiency on the nervous system. A comparison of the effects of carcinoma. In: Lord Brain, Norris F H Jr (eds) The remote effects of cancer on the nervous system. Grune and Stratton, New York, p 134–161

Victor M 1984 Polyneuropathy due to nutritional deficiency and alcoholism. In: Dyck P J, Thomas P K, Lambert E H, Bunge R (eds) Peripheral neuropathy, 2nd edn. W B Saunders, Philadelphia, p 1899–1940

Vilter R W, Muller J F, Glazer H S, Jarrold T, Abraham J, Thompson C, Hawkins V R 1953 The effect of vitamin B_6 deficiency produced by desoxypytridoxine in human beings. Journal of Laboratory and Clinical Medicine 42:335

Waksman B H, Adams R D 1955 Allergic neuritis: an experimental disease of rabbits induced by injection of peripheral nervous tissue and adjuvants. Journal of Experimental Medicine 102:213

Warrell D A, Godrey S, Olsen E G J 1968 Giant-cell arteritis with peripheral neuropathy. Lancet 1:1010

Weller R O, Bruckner F E, Chamberlain M A 1970 Rheumatoid neuropathy: a histological and electrophysiological study. Journal of Neurology, Neurosurgery and Psychiatry 33:592

Wilson S K A 1954 In: Bruce A N (ed) Neurology, 2nd edn. Butterworth, London, p 738

Yuill G M, Swinburn W R, Liversedge L A 1970 Treatment of polyneuropathy with azathioprine. Lancet 2:854

Metabolic and endocrine myopathies

THE PERIODIC PARALYSES

It is convenient to classify the periodic paralyses as primary or secondary and, according to associated changes in the serum K level, as hypo-kalaemic, normokalaemic or hyperkalaemic. The different types of periodic paralysis share several common features. Paralytic attacks may last from less than one hour to several days. Weakness can be localised or generalised. The deep tendon reflexes are diminished or lost in the course of the attacks. The muscle fibres become unresponsive to either direct or indirect electrical stimulation during attacks. The generalised attacks usually begin in proximal muscles and then spread to distal ones. Respiratory and cranial muscles tend to be spared but eventually may also be paralysed. Rest after exercise tends to provoke weakness of the muscles that had been exercised, but continued mild exercise may abort attacks. Exposure to cold may provoke weakness in the primary forms of the disease. Complete recovery usually occurs after initial attacks. Permanent weakness and irreversible pathological changes in muscle can develop after repeated attacks.

Primary hypokalaemic periodic paralysis

The disease is transmitted by an autosomal dominant gene with reduced penetrance in women. Sporadic cases, especially in men, have also been reported (Talbott 1941, Sagild 1959). The attacks typically begin in the first or second decade and about 60% of the patients are affected before the age of 16 years. Initially the attacks tend to be infrequent, but eventually may recur daily. Diurnal fluctuations in strength may then appear, so that the patient shows the greatest weakness during the night or in the early morning hours and gradually gains strength as the day passes (Allott & McArdle 1938, Engel et al 1965). In major attacks the serum potassium level decreases, but not always to below normal, and there is urinary retention of sodium, potassium, chloride and water (Biemond & Daniels 1934, Aitken et al 1937, Allott & McArdle 1938, Ferrebee et al 1938). Oliguria or anuria develop during such attacks and the patients tend to be constipated. Sinus bradycardia and electrocardiographic (ECG) signs of hypokalaemia (U waves in leads II, V-2, V-3, and V-4, progressive flattening of T waves and depression of ST segment) appear when the serum potassium falls below normal (Van Buchem 1957, Weisler 1961). In the fourth and fifth decades the attacks become less frequent and may cease altogether. However, repeated attacks may leave the patient with permanent residual weakness (Bekeny 1961, Pearson 1964, Engel et al 1965, Howes et al 1966, Odor et al 1967). The metabolic defect of this type of disease can be exacerbated or provoked by a high dietary intake of sodium or carbohydrate and by emotional excitement (Aitken et al 1937, Ferrebee et al 1938, Talbott 1941, McArdle 1956, Rowley Kliman, 1960, Shy et al 1961, Engel et al 1965).

The diagnosis is supported by a positive family history and a low serum potassium during major attacks. Depressed serum potassium levels between attacks suggest secondary rather than primary hypokalaemic paralysis. Provocative tests can be done to confirm the diagnosis. The oral administration of glucose, 2 g/kg body weight, combined with 10–20 units of crystalline insulin given subcutaneously may provoke an attack within 2–3 h. If this test fails to induce an attack in adults, it may be repeated after exercise and salt loading (2 g sodium chloride in aqueous solution given orally every hour for a total of four doses). Depression of the serum potassium level during the induced attack and a favourable response to 2.5–7.5 g of potassium chloride given orally must be demonstrated. Negative results do not exclude the diagnosis because patients may, at times, be refractory to such tests (Chen 1959). Glucose and insulin must never be given to patients already hypokalaemic and potassium must not be given unless patients have an adequate renal and adrenal reserve. The intra-arterial epinephrine test is particularly useful (Engel et al 1965). Two μg/min of epinephrine is infused into the brachial artery for 5 min and the amplitude of the evoked compound muscle action potential is recorded from perfused small hand muscles at intervals before, during and for 30 min after the infusion. The test, which is positive when the amplitude of the evoked action potential decreases by more than 30% within 10 min after the infusion, is essentially specific for primary hypokalaemic period paralysis.

Thyrotoxic periodic paralysis

This type resembles the primary hypokalaemic form with regard to changes in serum and urinary electrolytes during attacks and in its response to glucose, insulin and potassium. However, it is six times more common in males than in females, approximately 75% of the cases occur in Orientals, 85% of the patients first exhibit the attacks between the ages of 20 and 39 years, 95% of cases are sporadic and, in all, the attacks cease when the euthyroid state is restored (Engel 1961). A predisposing genetic factor in Chinese patients is suggested by an increased association with certain HLA haplotypes (Yeo et al 1978). Natural or induced recurrence of the hypermetabolic state causes recurrence of the paralytic attacks (Dunlap & Kepler 1931, Robertson 1954, Okihiro & Nordyke 1966).

Hypokalaemic periodic paralysis secondary to urinary or gastrointestinal potassium wastage

Potassium depletion may be associated with generalised weakness or, less frequently, with periodic paralysis. The latter usually does not occur unless the serum potassium falls to below 3 mmol/l. During the attack the potassium decreases further (Owen & Verner 1960, River et al 1960, Staffurth 1964). The relationship of attacks to excessive ingestion of carbohydrate or sodium has not been clearly established. The diagnosis of excessive urinary potassium loss may be made if, with an average daily intake of sodium or potassium, the daily urinary potassium excretion exceeds 20 mmol on several consecutive days while the serum potassium remains less than 3 mmol/l at different times of the day (Mahler & Stanbury 1956, Brooks et al 1957). The normal daily faecal potassium excretion is usually small (10 mmol) (Danowsky & Greenman 1953). Because the serum potassium is already decreased, provocative tests that may lower it further are contraindicated.

Various conditions to be considered in differential diagnosis are listed in Table 25.1. In addition to periodic or non-periodic weakness, the non-specific effects of chronic potassium depletion may also be present. These include hyposthenuria, polydypsia, and vasopressin-resistant polyuria (Conn 1955, Dustan et al 1956, Milne et al 1957, Manitius et al 1960). Chronic pyelonephritis and secondary hypertension leading to secondary aldosteronism and further potassium depletion

Table 25.1 Differential diagnosis of secondary hypokalaemic periodic paralysis

---

Thyrotoxic periodic paralysis

Paralysis secondary to urinary potassium wastage
  Hypertension, alkaline urine, metabolic alkalosis
    Primary hyperaldosteronism (Conn 1955)
    Liquorice intoxication (Salassa et al 1962)
    Excessive thiazide therapy for hypertension (Cohen 1959)
    Excessive mineralocorticoid therapy of Addison's disease
  Normotension, alkaline urine, metabolic alkalosis
    Hyperplasia of juxtaglomerular apparatus with hyperaldosteronism (Bryan et al 1966)
  Alkaline urine, metabolic acidosis
    Primary renal tubular acidosis (Owen & Verner 1960)
    Fanconi's syndrome (Milne et al 1952)
  Acid urine, metabolic acidosis
    Chronic ammonium chloride ingestion (Goulon et al 1962)
    Recovery phase of diabetic coma (Nabarro et al 1952)
    Bilateral ureterocolostomy (Sataline & Simonelli 1961)
    Recovery phase of acute renal tubular necrosis (Bull et al 1950)

Paralysis secondary to gastrointestinal potassium wastage

  Nontropical sprue.
  Laxative abuse (Schwartz & Relman 1953)
  Pancreatic gastrin-secreting adenoma with severe diarrhoea (Verner & Morrison 1958)
  Villous adenoma of the rectum (Keyloun & Grace 1967)
  Severe or chronic diarrhoea (Keye 1952)
  Draining gastrointestinal fistula
  Prolonged gastrointestinal intubation or vomiting

Barium-induced periodic paralysis

---

may develop (Owen & Verner 1960, Caroll & Davies 1964). Latent or manifest tetany can occur in several types of potassium depletion (Engel et al 1949, Fourman 1954, Conn 1955, Owen & Verner 1960, Caroll & Davies 1964). Growth retardation and proportional dwarfism occur in patients whose potassium has been depleted since infancy (Van Buchem et al 1956, Caroll & Davies 1964, Bryan et al 1966).

Barium-induced periodic paralysis

The accidental ingestion of absorbable barium salts, such as barium carbonate, induces a haemorrhagic gastroenteritis, hypertension, cardiac arrhythmias, muscle twitching, convulsions, hypokalaemia and muscle paralysis. Barium blocks muscle potassium channels and thereby reduces potassium efflux from muscle; potassium uptake by muscle, mediated by the Na–K pump, continues and hypokalaemia results (Lewi & Bar-Khayim 1964, Gallant 1983).

Primary hyperkalaemic periodic paralysis

The disease is transmitted by an autosomal dominant gene with high penetrance in both sexes (Helweg-Larsen et al 1955, Gamstorp 1956, McArdle 1962, Layzer et al 1967a). Rare sporadic cases have been reported (Dyken & Timmons 1963). Attacks usually begin in childhood and may be brief or last several days (Layzer et al 1967a). Myalgias (McArdle 1962), release of enzymes from muscle into serum and creatinuria (Mertens et al 1964, Hudson et al 1967) can occur during or after paralysis and a permanent myopathy may develop after repeated attacks (French & Kilpatrick 1957, Hudson 1963, MacDonald et al 1968). During attacks the serum potassium increases (French & Kilpatrick 1957, Egan & Klein 1959, Van Der Meulen et al 1961, McArdle 1962, Gamstorp 1956, Samaha 1965, Hudson et al 1967, Layzer 1967a) but may not exceed the normal range, and precordial T waves in the ECG increase in amplitude (French & Kilpatrick 1957, Egan & Klein 1959). Potassium, water and possibly sodium diuresis occurs during major attacks and the patient may complain of urinary urgency (Gamstorp 1956, Egan & Klein 1959, Klein et al 1960,

Carson & Pearson 1964, Mertens et al 1964). Hypocalcaemia was found during the paralysed state in three patients but their urinary calcium excretion was not studied (Dyken & Timmons 1963, Layzer et al 1967a). The metabolic defect is worsened by exposure to cold, fasting, pregnancy or by potassium administration (Gamstorp 1956, Drager et al 1958, McArdle 1962, Van't Hoff 1962, Herman & McDowell 1963, Hudson 1963, Layzer et al 1967a).

Myotonic phenomena have been demonstrated in some patients and are especially prone to be present in levator palpebrae and other external ocular muscles and in facial, lingual, thenar and finger extensor muscles (French & Kilpatrick 1957, Drager et al 1958, McArdle 1962, Van't Hoff 1962, Hudson 1963, Carson & Pearson 1964, Layzer et al 1967a). However, no myotonia was found in some patients who had all the other typical features of primary hyperkalaemic periodic paralysis (Gamstorp 1956, 1963), although there was abnormal electrical irritability of the muscle fibres (Buchthal et al 1958). A positive Chvostek sign is frequently observed in attacks (Gamstorp 1956).

The diagnosis of primary hyperkalaemic periodic paralysis is based on the family history, myotonic phenomena (if present) and the provocative effects of orally administered potassium chloride (2–10 g, given in an unsweetened solution just after exercise, in the fasting state). The test is contraindicated in subjects already hyperkalaemic and unless there is adequate renal and adrenal reserve. An abnormally high serum potassium between attacks suggests secondary rather than primary hyperkalaemic periodic paralysis.

Paramyotonia congenita

Myotonic hyperkalaemic periodic paralysis and paramyotonia congenita share several common features. The hallmarks of paramyotonia congenita, as described by Eulenburg (1886) and by Rich (1894) were: (1) dominant inheritance with high penetrance; (2) myotonia provoked especially by exposure to cold; (3) predilection of the myotonia for facial, lingual, neck and hand muscles; and (4) attacks of weakness upon exposure to cold and also after exercise. Subsequently, some patients

with features of paramyotonia congenita were also found to fulfil the diagnostic criteria of primary hyperkalaemic periodic paralysis, suggesting that the two disorders were, in fact, a single nosological entity (French & Kilpatrick 1957, Drager et al 1958, Van der Meulen et al 1961).

However, as mentioned above, even a careful electromyographic search disclosed no myotonia in some cases of hyperkalaemic periodic paralysis. Further, in some patients diagnosed as having paramyotonia congenita, potassium loading did not provoke paralytic attacks (Marshall 1952, Gamstorp 1963, Garcin et al 1966). Accentuation rather than improvement of the myotonia on repeated muscle contraction ('myotonia paradoxa') has also been cited as a distinguishing feature of paramyotonia (Magee 1963, Garcin et al 1966). Cold-induced muscle stiffness associated with electrical silence can occur in paramyotonia congenita, but is not a feature of myotonic and non-myotonic hyperkalaemic periodic paralysis (Magee 1966, Nielsen et al 1982). Finally, recent studies, discussed below, suggest that different membrane ion channel abnormalities operate in paramyotonia congenita and myotonic hyperkalaemic periodic paralysis.

Secondary hyperkalaemic periodic paralysis

This is associated with renal or adrenal insufficiency and may occur when the serum potassium exceeds 7 mmol/l. Males tend to be affected more often than females. Rest after exercise provokes weakness as it does in other types of periodic paralysis (Bull et al 1953, Marks & Feit 1953, Richardson & Sibley 1953, Pollen & Williams 1960, Faw & Ewer 1962, Bell et al 1965, Daughaday & Rendleman 1967). Paraesthesiae in the distal extremities tend to occur when the serum potassium level exceeds 7.5 mmol/l. ECG abnormalities (T wave elevation, disappearance of P waves and, eventually, a sinusoidal tracing) evolve as the serum potassium rises from 7 mmol/l to 9.5 mmol/l (Keith et al 1942, Finch et al 1946, Pollen & Williams 1960). The diagnosis is suggested by the very high serum potassium during the attack, persistent hyperkalaemia between attacks and by the associated primary disorder.

Normokalaemic, sodium-responsive familial periodic paralysis

A third type of primary periodic paralysis was described by Poskanzer & Kerr (1961). The disease is transmitted by dominant inheritance with high penetrance in both sexes. Paralytic attacks began during the first decade of life and were exacerbated or provoked by rest after exercise, exposure to cold, alcohol in excess and by potassium loading. Large doses of sodium improved the weakness. Glucose administration had no effect on the disease. No consistent changes of serum electrolytes occurred in attacks but there was increased sodium excretion and potassium retention. A family described by Meyers et al (1972) suffered from a similar illness but attacks were not provoked by large doses of potassium.

Periodic paralysis with cardiac arrhythmia

Periodic paralysis associated with extrasystoles and tachycardia that is often bidirectional has been described in several patients. The disorder is transmitted by dominant inheritance. The cardiac symptoms are provoked or worsened by hypokalaemia or digitalis, are refractory to disopyramide phosphate, propranolol or phenytoin, but may respond to imipramine. Syncopal attacks and sudden death can occur in the course of the disease. Dysmorphic features, such as short stature, clinodactyly and microcephaly, occur in some cases (Klein et al 1963, Andersen et al 1971, Stubbs 1976, Levitt et al 1972, Gould et al 1985). The disorder was hyperkalaemic and associated with myotonia in some families (Gould et al 1985), hypokalaemic in one patient (Levitt et al 1972), and normokalaemic in others (Klein et al 1963).

Histopathological alterations in periodic paralysis

The histopathological hallmark of the syndrome is a vacuolar myopathy (Goldflam 1895). This can be seen in either primary or secondary periodic paralysis, but more often in the former than in the latter. The vacuolation is more consistently associated with the permanent myopathy which develops after repeated attacks, than with the acute paralysis (Klein et al 1960, McArdle 1963, Samaha 1965, Resnick & Engel 1967, Engel 1977). The vacuoles are typically centrally situated in the muscle fibres and usually one vacuole, but at times several, appear in a fibre in a single plane of sectioning. Some vacuoles are limited by a delicate membrane, some are loculated, and some contain finely granular material staining positively for glycogen.

Numerous ultrastructural studies in the primary and thyrotoxic periodic paralyses can be summarised as follows. Dilatation and proliferation of sarcoplasmic reticulum (SR) components and abundant networks of transverse tubular (T) system origin have been observed in the muscle fibres (Shy et al 1961, Howes et al 1966, Engel 1966a, Gruner 1966, Odor et al 1967, MacDonald et al 1968, Schutta & Armitage 1969, Bergman et al 1970). The larger and light-microscopically visible vacuoles were thought to arise by coalescence of dilated SR components (Shy et al 1961, Odor et al 1967), from fusion of T system networks (Biczyskowa et al 1969), or to be the end-result of focal fibre destruction (MacDonald et al 1968, Schutta & Armitage 1969). In view of these divergent results, Engel (1970a) re-examined the morphological sequence of fibre vacuolation in the primary hypokalaemic disorder. The steps identified were: (1) evolving vacuole; (2) intermediate-stage vacuole; (3) mature vacuole; and (4) remodelling. Abnormal fibre regions arise containing myriad dilated and at times mineralised SR vesicles, masses of bizarre tubules or osmiophilic lamellae of T system origin, or varied cytoplasmic degradation products (evolving vacuole). The T system proliferates and acts as a membrane source for trapping components of the evolving vacuole. These components are degraded by an autophagic mechanism and a membrane-bound space is formed containing remnants of the trapped organelles which are now embedded in an amorphous matrix (intermediate-stage vacuole). When all trapped components have undergone lysis, the entire vacuole is filled with matrix (mature vacuole). The intermediate-stage and mature vacuoles communicate with the extracellular space via T tubules and T networks and there is prompt ingress of peroxidase-labelled extracellular fluid into the matrix compartment. Because these vacuoles are the prevalent ones, most of the vacuolar volume is filled with extracellular fluid. Intermediate-stage and mature vacuoles are remodelled by invaginations of the vacuolar membrane by glycogen-containing sarcoplasm. When the invaginated membrane ruptures, extracellular fluid enters the myofilament space causing fibre injury. Non-vacuolated fibre regions contain numerous focal dilatations of T tubules, T networks and dilated SR vesicles. Subsequent studies also showed that the ultrastructural changes in the different types of periodic paralysis are virtually identical, that electrical inexcitability of a muscle fibre can occur without associated ultrastructural change, and that the morphological changes are reactive, representing delayed consequences of the physiological abnormality (Engel 1977).

Pathophysiological mechanisms in the periodic paralyses

In primary hypokalaemic periodic paralysis there is a shift of potassium, sodium, chloride and phosphate ions and of water into muscle during generalised attacks. The ionic shifts are reflected by decreased urinary excretion of these ions and by decreased serum potassium levels (Aitken et al 1937, Ferrebee et al 1938, Zierler & Andres 1957, Shy et al 1961, Engel et al 1965). The fluid and electrolyte movements must be caused by a muscle membrane abnormality or an increased intracellular demand, or both, and probably occur to maintain osmotic, electrical and Donnan equilibria (Boyle & Conway 1941).

In thyrotoxic periodic paralysis the fluid and electrolyte shifts are similar to those noted in the primary hypokalaemic form. In periodic paralysis caused by renal or gastrointestinal potassium wastage the hypokalaemia and body potassium depletion are more marked and episodic paralysis appears when the exchangeable body potassium has fallen to approximately one-half normal levels (Staffurth 1964). The paroxysmal nature of the attacks is unexplained and it is not known whether the ionic shifts during the attacks are the same as in the primary hypokalaemic form.

In primary hyperkalaemic periodic paralysis the movements of potassium are the opposite of those which occur in the primary hypokalaemic type: the hyperkalaemia is associated with enhanced urinary excretion of potassium (Gamstorp 1956, Klein et al 1960, Creutzfeldt 1961, Carson & Pearson 1964). Careful studies have demonstrated a decreased serum sodium level and urinary sodium excretion, and a decreased or unaltered serum chloride level (Streeten et al 1971, Clausen et al 1980). These findings are consistent with the egress of potassium and the entry of sodium and possibly of chloride into muscle cells during attacks. Fluid and electrolyte shifts have not been investigated during paroxysmal attacks of secondary hyperkalaemic periodic paralysis.

Abnormalities of carbohydrate metabolism, such as a block in hexose phosphate utilisation (McArdle 1956) or in glycogen synthesis (Shy et al 1961) were postulated to account for the adverse effects of carbohydrate loading in primary hypokalaemic periodic paralysis. Biochemical studies by Engel et al (1967) did not confirm these hypotheses. From a different viewpoint, the opposite effects of carbohydrate loading in the primary hypokalaemic and hyperkalaemic syndromes could be related to ionic movements associated with cellular glucose uptake and utilisation because potassium movements follow the carbohydrate cycle from muscle to liver and back. Such movements could provoke or correct a defect which is not one of carbohydrate metabolism but which resides in the electrical and biophysical properties of the muscle fibre surface membrane.

Several lines of evidence implicate the muscle fibre surface membrane in the pathogenesis of the attacks. The resting membrane potential is abnormally low during and even between attacks in both the primary hypokalaemic and primary hyperkalaemic syndromes (Creutzfeldt et al 1963, Riecker & Bolte 1966, McComas et al 1968, Bradley 1969, Brooks 1969, Hofmann & Smith 1970). On the basis of the Goldman constant field equation for the membrane potential (Goldman 1943), the hypopolarisation in the different types of periodic paralysis can be attributed to increased sodium permeability, decreased chloride permeability, or both. A decrease in the resting membrane potential itself can block the action potential mechanism because sodium activation fails below a resting potential of 60 mV, while potassium activation and membrane repolarisation cannot occur below a resting potential of 40 mV (Jenerick 1959). Resting membrane potentials lower than 60 mV have, in fact, been recorded during paralytic attacks (Creutzfeldt et al 1963). A lower than normal membrane input resistance, consistent with increased sodium permeability, has also been observed in the primary hypokalaemic disease by Elmqvist, Engel and Lambert (cited by Engel 1977) and in the primary hyperkalaemic disease by McComas et al (1968). There are no reports of membrane potential measurements in the secondary types of periodic paralysis.

Recent studies of the properties of muscle membrane ion channels by the voltage clamp technique have provided new insights into the membrane abnormalities in the different types of primary paralyses. In each instance the abnormalities involve the sodium channel. In primary hypokalaemic periodic paralysis Rüdel et al (1984) found that even a small decrease in extracellular potassium causes marked membrane depolarisation (in healthy fibres this induces hyperpolarisation). The paradoxical depolarisation in the low-potassium medium stems from an abnormally high steady state sodium conductance. Further, even a small depolarisation (i.e. to −70 mV) causes failure of action potential propagation, suggesting abnormal sodium channel inactivation. In myotonic hyperkalaemic periodic paralysis Lehmann-Horn and co-workers (1983) found that a high-potassium medium (7 Meq/L) caused an abnormal increase in sodium conductance and abnormally large depolarisation. The depolarisation was reversed by tetrodotoxin and was not associated with increased chloride conductance. Muscle fibres from a patient with non-myotonic hyperkalaemic periodic paralysis were also depolarised in a high-potassium medium but became inexcitable at a resting membrane potential at which normal muscle fibres remained excitable, indicating an abnormal sensitivity of the sodium channel to inactivation by small depolarisations. In paramyotonia congenita Lehmann-Horn et al (1981) showed that cooling of the muscle fibres to 27 °C

caused an abnormal increase in both sodium and chloride conductance and the fibres became depolarised. The depolarisation could be prevented but not reversed by tetrodotoxin.

These studies implicate the surface membrane of the muscle fibre in the pathogenesis of the attacks, but do not exclude an abnormality of the contractile mechanism. However, Engel & Lambert (1969) found that direct application of calcium to the myofilament space of electrically inexcitable fibres readily activated the contractile mechanism. This established that the block in excitation-contraction coupling resided in the membranous components of the fibre (the surface membrane, T system, the SR, or all three. Both the surface membrane and the T tubules may fail to conduct the action potential during attacks, but failure of transverse impulse conduction would be relatively unimportant if the surface membrane were unresponsive.

Treatment of periodic paralyses

Primary hypokalaemic periodic paralysis. Acute attacks are treated with 2.0–10.0 g of potassium chloride, given by mouth as an unsweetened 10–25% solution. This dose may be repeated, if necessary, after 3–4 h (Talbott 1941, McArdle 1963). Intravenous administration of potassium salts is seldom, if ever, required. Utmost care must be exercised in giving potassium intravenously in order to avoid life-threatening hyperkalaemia, and intravenous fluids must contain no glucose or sodium. The patient's strength and serum potassium must be frequently monitored during treatment of major attacks.

Preventive therapy of the primary hypokalaemic form of the disease consists of a relatively low sodium (2.3 g per day) and low carbohydrate (60–80 g per day) diet, avoidance of exposure to cold and over-exertion, and supplemental doses of potassium chloride, 2.5–7.5 g, as a 10% aqueous solution taken two to four times daily. The dosage must be adjusted according to attack frequency and severity. Because severely affected patients awaken paralysed, a dose may have to be taken at 0200 h (2 a.m.). The serum potassium should not exceed 6 mmol/l during therapy. Acetazolamide

(Diamox®) is also highly effective in preventing paralytic attacks. Up to 2 g per day of the drug can be used instead of the other preventive measures. The drug probably acts by inducing a mild metabolic acidosis, which prevents an intracellular shift of potassium (Griggs et al 1970, Riggs & Griggs 1979).

Thyrotoxic periodic paralysis. Treatment consists of antithyroid therapy. Until the patient becomes euthyroid, preventive measures and the treatment of the acute attacks are the same as in the primary hypokalaemic form. Acetazolamide is ineffective, but propranolol (40 mg q.i.d.) may prevent attacks (Yeung & Tse 1974).

Other forms of secondary hypokalaemic periodic paralysis. Therapy is directed at the primary disorder and potassium is replaced to compensate for both the static deficits and the dynamic losses. Additional treatment is directed against the metabolic acidosis or alkalosis and other associated electrolyte abnormalities that may be present.

Primary sodium-responsive normokalaemic periodic paralysis. In the family studied by Poskanzer & Kerr (1961), therapy with large doses of sodium chloride, or with 0.1 mg 9-α-fluorohydrocortisone and 250 mg acetazolamide per day was effective in preventing attacks.

Primary hyperkalaemic periodic paralysis. Acute attacks in established cases can be treated with 2 g/kg glucose by mouth and 15–20 units of crystalline insulin subcutaneously, but severe attacks may fail to respond to these measures (Gamstorp 1956, Sagild 1959). Calcium gluconate, 0.5–2 g administered intravenously, has been reported to terminate attacks in some cases (Gamstorp 1956, Van der Meulen et al 1961, Van't Hoff 1962), but not in others (McArdle 1962). The inhalation of beta-adrenergic agents, such as 1.3 mg metaproterenol every 15 min for three doses, has also aborted acute attacks (Benheim et al 1985). Preventive therapy consists of frequent meals of high carbohydrate content, avoidance of fasting or of exposure to cold and over-exertion, and use of diuretics promoting kaliuresis, such as

acetazolamide or chlorothiazide. The lowest dose of diuretic required to prevent attacks should be used and the amount given should not lower the serum potassium level below 3.7 mmol/l or the serum sodium below 135 mmol/l (McArdle 1962, Carson & Pearson 1964, Samaha 1965). Daily treatment with small doses of albuterol has also prevented attacks (Clausen et al 1980, Benheim et al 1985).

Tocainide, a frequency-dependent antiarrhythmic drug, can prevent weakness and myotonia induced by cold in paramyotonia congenita and in myotonic hyperkalaemic periodic paralysis. The drug does not prevent hyperkalaemic weakness in myotonic hyperkalaemic periodic paralysis (Ricker et al 1983).

Secondary hyperkalaemic periodic paralysis. Therapy is again aimed at the primary disorder and should include restriction of dietary potassium intake until the primary cause can be corrected. Intravenous insulin and glucose therapy can temporarily decrease the serum potassium level. In patients with renal failure, severe hyperkalaemia is an indication for haemodialysis.

THE GLYCOGEN STORAGE DISEASES

Cori (1957) assigned numbers to the glycogen storage diseases in the sequence in which they were discovered. However, those glycogenoses discovered after 1957 were not numbered consistently and recently discovered diseases have been named after the enzyme that is deficient. Skeletal muscle is directly involved in glycogenoses caused by deficiency of acid maltase (type II) (glucan 1,4-d-glucosidase; EC 3.2.1.3), debranching enzyme (type III) (α-dextrin endo-1,6-d-glucosidase; EC 3.2.1.41), branching enzyme (type IV) (1,4-α-glucan branching enzyme, EC 2.4.1.18), myophosphorylase (type V; EC 2.4.1.1), 6-phosphofructokinase (type VII) (EC 2.7.1.11), phosphoglycerate kinase (EC 2.7.2.3), phosphoglycerate mutase (EC 5.4.2.1), and lactate dehydrogenase (EC 1.1.1.28); and is indirectly involved in glucose-6-phosphatase (EC 3.1.3.9) deficiency (type I). All glycogenoses are autosomal recessive disorders except phosphoglycerate kinase deficiency, which is an X-linked recessive. By now, considerable genetic heterogeneity has been observed in each recognised glycogenosis. There are also other glycogen or polysaccharide storage syndromes of muscle for which no enzymatic basis has been uncovered to date.

Glucose-6-phosphatase deficiency

The enzyme normally occurs in liver, kidney and small intestine but not in muscle. Deficiency of the enzyme causes no glycogen excess in muscle but profound hypotonia can occur in affected infants. The metabolic fault prevents the release from liver of glucose derived from glycogenolysis or gluconeogenesis. The consequences are severe fasting hypoglycaemia, lactic acidosis and excessive mobilisation of fat from adipose tissue. Chronic lactic acidosis causes osteoporosis and interferes with the renal excretion of uric acid, resulting in hyperuricaemia and secondary gout. Fat mobilisation leads to marked hyperlipidaemia, fatty infiltration of liver and xanthoma formation. A haemorrhagic tendency occurs in many patients. All manifestations of the disease tend to improve with age (Moses & Gutman 1972, Huijing 1975, Howell 1978).

Acid maltase deficiency

Acid maltase, a lysosomal enzyme, hydrolyses both 1,4-and 1,6-α-glycosidic linkages. It is optimally active between pH 4 and 5 and is capable of degrading glycogen completely. The biosynthesis of acid maltase resembles that of other lysosomal enzymes: a high-molecular-weight precursor synthesised by ribosomes enters the endoplasmic reticulum where it acquires a high-mannose carbohydrate; it then moves to the Golgi apparatus where it becomes phosphorylated, glycosylated and fitted with a special mannose-6-phosphate recognition marker that allows the enzyme to bind to membrane receptors. From the Golgi apparatus the enzyme is exported to lysosomes where it is further modified by proteolysis and stabilised to prevent autolysis (Callahan & Lowden 1981, Barranger & Brady 1984). The synthesis of acid maltase follows the above scheme. An enzyme of molecular weight 110 000

daltons, that already carries the mannose-6-phosphate marker, can be detected in human urine (Oude Elferink et al 1984). In cultured fibroblasts the precursor enzyme is processed through a number of intermediates to become a glycoprotein of molecular weight 76 000 daltons (Hasilik & Neufeld 1980). Although acid maltase deficiency (AMD) was the first lysosomal disorder to be identified (Hers 1963), the precise metabolic role of the enzyme is still enigmatic. That massive amounts of glycogen, and at times acid mucopolysaccharides, accumulate in cells lacking the enzyme attest to its biological significance, yet severe deficiency of the enzyme can exist in some cells and tissues without glycogen excess or functional impairment. The disease originally described by Pompe (1932) was a generalised glycogenosis invariably fatal in infancy (Sant'Agnese 1959). Subsequently, milder forms of AMD, presenting as myopathy, have been observed in children (Hers & van Hoof 1968) and adults (Engel & Dale 1968, Hudgson et al 1968, Engel 1970b). All three forms of the disease are transmitted by autosomal recessive inheritance (Williams 1966, Nitowsky & Grunfeld 1967, Engel & Gomez 1970) and, with few exceptions (Busch et al 1979), the disease breeds true in each family.

Infantile AMD presents within the first few months of life with generalised and rapidly progressive weakness and hypotonia, and enlargement of the heart, tongue and liver. Respiratory and feeding difficulties are common and death is usually due to cardiorespiratory failure before the age of two years. The ECG typically shows a short P-R interval, high QRS voltage and left ventricular hypertrophy (Sant' Agnese 1959, Caddell & Whitemore 1962, Engel et al 1973). Massive amounts of glycogen accumulate in skeletal muscle, heart and liver. Microscopic examination also shows widespread glycogen deposition in smooth muscle, endothelial and renal tubular cells and in both neural and glial elements of the central nervous system. Most cells of the brain and spinal cord are affected but cerebellar cortical nerve cells are spared. Motor neurones in the brain stem and spinal cord are most severely involved (Mancall et al 1965, Hogan et al 1969). Glycogen also accumulates in Schwann cells in peripheral nerves (Gambetti et al 1971). In addition to glycogen, acid mucopolysaccharides also accumulate in skeletal muscle (Martin et al 1973, Engel et al 1973) and have been noted in muscle, liver, heart, leucocytes and cultured fibroblasts (Nitowsky & Grunfeld 1967, Danzis et al 1969, Brown et al 1970) but not in kidney (Steinitz & Rutenberg 1967). However, the renal enzyme probably differs from lysosomal acid maltase (Steinitz & Rutenberg 1967, Salafsky & Nadler 1971, Koster et al 1976, De Burlet & Sudaka 1977). A sensitive fluorometric assay, using an artificial substrate, reveals that there is no residual enzyme activity in affected tissues in infantile AMD (Mehler & DiMauro 1977). Catalytically inactive enzyme protein could not be detected by immunological techniques in some patients (De Barsy et al 1972, Reuser et al 1978), but such a protein was abundantly present in at least one infant (Beratis et al 1978). This indicates that even infantile AMD, which seems to be clinically homogeneous, is genetically heterogeneous.

The childhood type of AMD presents clinically in infancy or early childhood as a myopathy. Motor milestones are delayed and weakness is usually greater in proximal than distal limb muscles. Respiratory muscles tend to be selectively severely affected. Calf enlargement can also occur resulting in a clinical picture which simulates muscular dystrophy (Hers & van Hoof 1968, Swaiman et al 1968, Engel et al 1973). The disease progresses relatively slowly and death usually occurs from respiratory failure after repeated bouts of pneumonia. Few patients survive beyond the second decade. Liver, heart or tongue enlargement occur relatively infrequently. Glycogen excess in muscle is less marked and more variable than in infantile AMD. Autopsy studies reveal little if any increase of glycogen in heart, liver, skin and nervous system (Smith et al 1966, 1967, Engel et al 1973, Martin et al 1976b). The enzyme is deficient in muscle, heart and liver (Hers & Van Hoof 1968, Angelini & Engel 1972, Mehler & DiMauro 1977), cultured fibroblasts (Koster et al 1972) and inconsistently in leucocytes (Brown & Zellweger 1966). Residual acid maltase activity is detected in muscle, liver and heart (Angelini & Engel 1972, Mehler & DiMauro 1977).

The adult form of AMD presents after the age of 20 years. The symptoms can be those of a slowly progressive myopathy which clinically mimics polymyositis or limb-girdle dystrophy (Engel & Dale 1968, Hudgson et al 1968, Engel 1970b, Carrier et al 1975, Gullotta et al 1976, Martin et al 1976a, Karpati et al 1977, DiMauro et al 1978b, Bertagnolio et al 1978). However, one-third of the cases present with respiratory failure which may overshadow other manifestations (Rosenow & Engel 1978). Respiratory muscle involvement eventually occurs in all and respiratory failure is the usual cause of death. Heart and liver enlargement does not occur and cardiac manifestations, if present, are those of cor pulmonale secondary to the respiratory failure. Glycogen accumulates in clinically affected muscles but seldom exceeds 5%. In some muscles with histological abnormalities the muscle glycogen content is surprisingly normal. No glycogen excess is found in tissues other than muscle. Acid mucopolysaccharides, which accumulate in muscle in infants and children with AMD, are sparse or absent from muscle in affected adults. Deficiency of the enzyme has been found in muscle (Engel & Dale 1968, Hudgson et al 1968), liver (Engel 1970b, Engel et al 1973), heart and central nervous system (DiMauro et al 1978b) as well as in cultured fibroblasts (Angelini et al 1972) and cultured muscle cells (Askanas et al 1976). A lower than normal leucocyte acid maltase level and a depressed acid/neutral maltase ratio were found by Angelini & Engel (1972) and by Koster et al (1974), but not by Bertagnolio et al (1978). Residual acid maltase activity is detectable in muscle and other tissues (Engel et al 1973, Mehler & DiMauro 1977).

Serum enzymes of muscle origin (creatine kinase (EC 2.7.3.2), aspartate aminotransferase (EC 2.6.1.1) are increased in all three types of AMD, but the increases are usually less than 10-fold over the normal upper limit. Electromyographic findings indicate a myopathy in all three types. The abnormalities are more widespread in infants than in older patients. In children and adults, some muscles show no electrical abnormalities whereas others have motor unit potentials of abnormally short duration as well as some of normal duration. Abnormal insertional activity and myotonic discharges (without clinically detectable myotonia) occur in all patients. Other forms of abnormal activity (fibrillation potentials, positive waves and bizarre repetitive discharges) also occur at rest. In adults, the myotonic discharges are less widely distributed and less intense and appear especially in the paraspinal muscles (Engel et al 1973).

The common light-microscopic feature in all cases of AMD is a vacuolar myopathy. In infants, virtually all muscle fibres contain large vacuoles. In children, vacuolation tends to be less marked and some fibres or muscles are spared. In adults, almost all fibres in severely affected muscles show vacuoles. In less severely affected muscles the vacuolation involves 25–75% of the fibres whereas clinically unaffected muscles show few, if any, such fibres. The vacuoles have a high glycogen content and are strongly reactive for acid phosphatase. Abnormal increases of acid phosphatase activity also occur in fibres with no vacuoles detectable light-microscopically.

Ultrastructural studies show that glycogen accumulates in muscle fibres in four types of space: (1) dispersed in the sarcoplasm, displacing, replacing or compressing normal organelles; (2) in sac-like structures, limited by continuous or discontinuous single or double membranes; (3) in ordinary autophagic vacuoles, containing glycogen and miscellaneous cytoplasmic degradation products; (4) in spaces representing transitions between the above. The limiting membranes are generated by proliferating T-system networks and by the Golgi system. Acid hydrolases are delivered to the vacuoles by vesicles arising from T-system networks (Engel 1970b, Engel et al 1973). Because many vacuoles are membrane-bound and contain acid hydrolases and cytoplasmic degradation products, they represent secondary lysosomes.

Diagnostic clues in AMD consist of organomegaly in infants and children; the firm consistency of the weak muscles; the selectively severe involvement of respiratory muscles, and also of the hip adductor muscles, in some of the adults; the abnormal electrical irritability, including myotonic discharges without clinical myotonia, in the EMG; and a vacuolar myopathy with high glycogen content and acid phosphatase activity of the vacuoles. However, none of the clinical and morphological findings are specific, and

confirmatory enzyme studies are essential for diagnosis. Acid maltase can be readily assayed in muscle, cultured fibroblasts and urine (Salafsky & Nadler 1973, Mehler & DiMauro 1976). Prenatal diagnosis is possible by enzyme assays on cultivated amniotic fluid cells obtained during the 14th and 18th weeks of pregnancy (Galjaard et al 1973).

The marked clinical variability of AMD between infants, children and adults is unexplained. Biochemical differences exist between and within the different clinical types of AMD. Total absence of enzyme activity, with or without the presence of an inactive enzyme protein occurs in infantile AMD. However, similar biochemical phenotypes also occur in some childhood and adult cases. In some adults, enzyme activity and enzyme protein are proportionately reduced (De Barsy et al 1972, Beratis et al 1983, Ninomiya et al 1984, Miranda et al 1985). Thus, the different clinical types cannot be readily explained by the remaining residual enzyme activity. Studies of cultured fibroblasts from patients with different types of AMD have revealed five different biochemical defects: (1) no synthesis of the enzyme precursor; (2) reduced synthesis of an enzyme precursor which then matures normally; (3) normal synthesis of an enzyme precursor, most of which is degraded before it is processed by the Golgi apparatus; (4) a defect in the phosphorylation of the enzyme precursor; (5) a defect in the proteolytic processing of the glycosylated and phosphorylated enzyme (Reuser & Kroos 1982, Steckel et al 1982, Reuser et al 1985). However, no consistent correlation has been demonstrated between the biochemical and clinical phenotypes. Finally, there is no explanation for the fact that, in childhood or adult AMD, glycogen content in muscle can vary from normal to moderately high from patient to patient, in different muscles of the same patient, and even in different regions of the same muscle.

Apart from symptomatic management of cardiac and respiratory insufficiency, there is no satisfactory treatment for AMD. Respiratory support with an oscillating bed during the night, and eventually during the day, may prolong life for some years in affected adults. Replacement therapy with fungal or human placental acid maltase has been attempted but delivery of adequate amounts of the enzyme to the tissues without sensitisation of the host, is still impractical (Badhuin et al 1964, Hug & Schubert 1967, De Barsy et al 1973). A low-carbohydrate diet combined with adrenaline administration has been tried in some adults with AMD (Engel 1970b, Rosenow & Engel 1978). Despite transient improvement in the strength of selected limb muscles, the course of the disease was not significantly altered.

Debranching enzyme deficiency

Debranching enzyme is bifunctional: it hydrolyses glycogen branch points (amylo-1, 6-glucosidase activity) and transfers those three glucose residues adjacent to the branch points which resist cleavage by phosphorylase (oligo-1,4→1,4-glucan transferase; EC 2.4.1.18) activity (Brown & Illingworth 1962). The two activities are located at separate catalytic sites on the same molecule (Gillard & Nelson 1977). Deficiency of the enzyme leads to the accumulation of glycogen with abnormally short outer chains which resembles limit dextrin (Illingworth & Cori 1952, Illingworth et al 1956). The enzyme is normally present in all tissues and can be assayed in leucocytes, erythrocytes, cultured fibroblasts, muscle, liver and heart (Huijing 1964, Van Hoof 1967, Justice et al 1970). The disease is transmitted by autosomal recessive inheritance but is genetically heterogeneous. This is evidenced by the existence of subgroups of the disease according to whether the enzyme deficiency involves some or all tissues, the reactivity of the enzyme toward different substrates and the clinical patterns of the disease.

Van Hoof & Hers (1967) determined debranching enzyme activity with four different substrates in tissues of 45 patients. In 34 cases, debranching enzyme activity was very low in muscle, liver and erythrocytes with each method of assay, the glycogen content of the same tissues was high and the outer chains of glycogen were abnormally short. In the remaining 11 cases, enzyme activity was normal or only moderately reduced in one or more tissues with at least one method of assay, and in most cases the muscle glycogen content was normal. In another series investigated by Brown & Brown (1968), seven of 34 patients had normal glycogen content and enzyme activity in muscle.

In other cases enzyme activity was absent from liver and muscle but was preserved in leucocytes or erythrocytes (Brandt & De Luca 1966, Williams & Field 1968, Deckelbaum et al 1972).

Two major clinical patterns of the disease have been recognised. In the more common form, the metabolic disturbance secondary to the hepatic enzyme deficiency dominates the clinical picture. Hepatomegaly, growth retardation and fasting hypoglycaemia, present since infancy, are the usual findings. In some cases there is also cardiomegaly (Huijing 1975, Howel 1978, Moses & Gutman 1972). The hypoglycaemia causes increased mobilisation and utilisation of fat, hyperlipidaemia and a tendency to develop ketosis (Fernandes & Pikaar 1969, 1972). Because the outer chains of glycogen can still contribute to blood glucose homeostasis and glucose derived from gluconeogenesis or glycogenolysis can freely leave the liver, the metabolic disturbance is less profound than in type I glycogenosis. The hepatomegaly and fasting hypoglycaemia diminish or disappear after puberty (Brown & Brown 1968, Cohn et al 1975, Howell 1978). Despite glycogen storage in muscle, the myopathic features are seldom disabling (Levin et al 1967).

In a smaller group of patients there is a clinically significant myopathy (Oliner et al 1961, Sidbury 1965, Brunberg et al 1971, Murase et al 1973, DiMauro et al 1978c). In these there may be a history of protuberant abdomen in childhood, decreasing in adolescence, and muscle fatigue or aching on heavy exertion since an early age. Progressive muscle weakness begins in childhood or, more commonly, in adult life and may involve both proximal and distal muscles. Selectively severe involvement of distal forearm muscles occurs in some patients. Persistent hepatomegaly is found in most cases. The ECG revealed biventricular hypertrophy in all of five cases studied by DiMauro et al (1978c) and in two of these there was also congestive heart failure. Serum enzymes of muscle origin are increased from twice to more than 10 times the upper limit of normal. The EMG shows changes consistent with myopathy. Increased insertional activity, myotonic discharges and fibrillation potentials can also occur (Brunberg et al 1971, DiMauro et al 1978c). The muscle glycogen concentration varies between 3 and 6%

and the iodine absorption spectrum of glycogen resembles that of limit dextrin. Histopathological studies show a vacuolar myopathy. The abnormal spaces are filled with glycogen which displaces and replaces normal organelles but is not membrane-bound (Neustein 1969, Brunberg et al 1971, Murase et al 1973, DiMauro et al 1978c). Glycogen excess was also found in erythrocytes in the five cases studied by DiMauro et al (1978c).

The diagnostic clues in this myopathy consist of a history of hepatic enlargement, and possibly of hypoglycaemic episodes, during childhood; persistent mild hepatomegaly; cardiomyopathy in some patients; easy fatiguability on heavy exertion; a diminished or absent glycaemic response to adrenaline or glucagon; an impaired or absent rise of lactic acid in venous blood flowing from muscles after ischaemic exercise (Brunberg et al 1971, DiMauro et al 1978c); abnormal electrical irritability of the muscle fibres in the EMG; and a vacuolar myopathy. Confirmatory biochemical studies include glycogen assay and structural analysis and biochemical determination of debranching enzyme activity by more than one method of assay (van Hoof & Hers 1967, Di-Mauro et al 1978c).

There is no effective treatment of the myopathy. Therapy in younger patients consists of prevention of hypoglycaemia by frequent meals of high protein content. After the age of one year, a diet with 45% of the calories from carbohydrate, 20% from fat and the rest from protein is beneficial (Fernandes & Pikaar 1969). Vigorous exercise, which can provoke arrhythmias in patients with cardiomyopathy, should be avoided.

Branching enzyme deficiency

The enzyme introduces branch points into glycogen through its α-1,4-glucan: α-1,4-glucan 6-glycosyl transferase activity. Deficiency of the enzyme was predicted by Illingworth & Cori (1952) on the basis of structural analysis of glycogen isolated from the liver of an affected boy. This glycogen had abnormally long inner and outer chains and fewer than normal branch points, resembling amylopectin. Andersen (1956) described the clinical aspects of this case and the predicted enzyme deficiency was confirmed by Brown &

Brown (1966). As the defect is in the synthetic pathway, glycogen storage would not be expected, but in some cases the liver glycogen content is abnormally high. This is probably due to the poor solubility of the abnormal polysaccharide in the cytosol, which may also explain the hepatocellular injury characteristic of the disease. The abnormal glycogen still contains branch points and is heterogeneous in composition (Reed et al 1968, Mercier & Whelan 1973). Thus, there must be an alternative mechanism for introducing branch points into glycogen: an additional enzyme not detected by the usual assay for branching enzyme (Brown & Brown 1966), or debranching enzyme acting in reverse (Huijing et al 1970).

The disease is transmitted by autosomal recessive inheritance (Legum & Nitowsky 1969, Howell et al 1971). Abnormal glycogen deposits occur in liver, spleen and lymph nodes and, occasionally, in muscle, kidney, adrenals and the central nervous system (Howell et al 1971, Schochet et al 1970). Deficiency of the enzyme has been observed in liver, leucocytes and cultured fibroblasts (Brown & Brown 1966, Fernandes & Huijing 1968, Howell et al 1971) but, thus far, not in muscle. However, the enzyme was not determined in muscle in those cases in which the presence of abnormal glycogen in muscle was documented.

The disorder presents during the first year of life with progressive enlargement of liver and spleen and failure to thrive. The abnormal polysaccharide in liver induces nodular cirrhosis, hepatoparenchymal insufficiency and portal hypertension. Carbohydrate tolerances remain normal. Muscle weakness and atrophy appear in some patients (Sidbury et al 1962, Levin et al 1968, Hollerman 1966, Reed et al 1968, Zellweger et al 1972), but not in others (Brown & Brown 1966). Death occurs in infancy or early childhood due to hepatic or cardiac failure.

The abnormal polysaccharide stains positively with periodic acid-Schiff (PAS), alcian blue and colloidal iron, gives a brown-blue colour with iodine and resists diastase digestion. It consists of finely filamentous and granular material which intermingles with normal glycogen particles in affected tissues. The presence of normal glycogen particles again suggests that an alternative mechanism for glycogen synthesis is still operative. Deposits in the central nervous system, conspicuous in astroglial cells, resemble Lafora bodies. Different muscles are affected to different extents, but the tongue appears to be particularly severely affected (Schochet et al 1970).

The diagnosis of this enzyme deficiency is suggested by progressive hepatosplenomegaly and failure to thrive in infancy, muscle weakness (if present), and PAS-postive, diastase-fast deposits in affected tissues. Enzyme assays and structural analysis of glycogen are confirmatory. Antenatal diagnosis is possible by enzyme assays on fibroblasts cultured from amniotic fluid cells (Howell et al 1971).

Therapy with fungal α-glucosidase was attempted in two cases (Fernandes & Huijing 1968, Huijing et al 1973). Although liver glycogen content was reduced, the course of the disease was not altered.

Myophosphorylase deficiency

McArdle in 1951 described the clinical features of the disease and attributed them to a deficiency of muscle phosphorylase. This prediction was confirmed by Schmid & Mahler (1959) and by Mommaerts et al (1959).

Phosphorylase catalyses the cleavage of 1,4-α-glucosidic linkages, releasing glucose-1-phosphate from non-reducing ends of exposed glycogen chains. Its action comes to a halt when chain length is reduced to four glucose residues which are then removed by the debranching enzyme complex. In resting muscle, phosphorylase is mostly in an inactive *b* form which phosphorylase *b* kinase converts to an active *a* form. Activation of the kinase, and hence of phosphorylase, is mediated by cyclic AMP via activation of adenyl cyclase by adrenaline (in muscle and liver) or glucagon (in liver). Electrical stimulation or exercise activate phosphorylase, probably through calcium release from the sarcoplasmic reticulum (Ozawa et al 1967). Phosphorylase *a* is reconverted to phosphorylase *b* by a specific phosphatase which, in turn, is inhibited by cyclic AMP (for reviews see Huijing 1975, Howell 1978).

Different tissues contain different phosphorylase isoenzymes, and different structural genes code for the isoenzymes present in skeletal muscle, liver and smooth muscle. Cardiac muscle contains isoenzymes found in smooth and skeletal muscle as well as hybrid isoenzymes (Yunis et al 1962, Davis et al 1967). Deficiency of muscle phosphorylase occurs independently of other isoenzymes and only skeletal muscle is affected clinically. The syndrome, however, is genetically heterogeneous. This is evinced by subgroups of the disease defined according to mode of inheritance, clinical patterns, and the presence or absence of catalytically inactive enzyme protein in muscle.

In most instances the disease is transmitted by autosomal recessive inheritance, but there is an unexplained preponderance of males (Huijing 1975). Possibly, some females remain undiagnosed, being less likely to engage in the type of exercise which provokes symptoms. Autosomal dominant transmission of phosphorylase deficiency was reported in one family (Chui & Munsat 1976).

Symptoms may date from early childhood, but more typically the capacity for exercise is unimpaired until the second half of the second decade. In contrast to this common pattern, a fatal infantile case, with death due to respiratory insufficiency at the age of 13 weeks, has been reported (DiMauro & Hartlage 1978); and 'late-onset' cases have been described in a brother and sister who did not develop symptoms until their fiftieth year (Engel et al 1963) and in a patient who presented with muscle weakness at the age of 74 years (Hewlett & Gardner-Thorpe 1978).

Catalytically inactive enzyme protein is present in some cases but not in others. The inactive protein has been detected by immunological tests (Dreyfus & Alexandre 1971) or by SDS polyacrylamide electrophoresis (Feit & Brooke 1976, Koster et al 1979). In one case, the electrophoretic method detected inactive enzyme protein when the immunological method did not (Koster et al 1979).

The typical symptoms consist of muscular pain, weakness and stiffness during slight to moderate exertion. Pain on exercise, which is the most prominent feature, can occur in any muscle, even those of the jaw. Rest rapidly relieves the symptoms after moderate exercise, but the more severe or protracted the exercise, the longer symptoms persist (McArdle 1951). The pain may disappear with continued exercise if stiffness has not developed. This 'second wind' is related to increased muscle blood flow, and the augmented utilisation by muscle of plasma free fatty acids (Pernow et al 1967) and amino acids (Wahren et al 1973) as energy sources. A frequent and characteristic symptom is inability to extend the fingers fully after sustained gripping movements against resistance; full recovery may take many minutes. After severe exercise, muscle pain, weakness and swelling may persist for several days. Myoglobinuria after exercise occurs at least once in the course of the disease in one-half to two-thirds of cases (Dawson et al 1968, Fattah et al 1970). Muscle weakness and atrophy are detected in about one-third and are usually mild. Muscles of the pectoral girdle are more likely to be affected than those of the pelvic girdle, and calf muscle bulk may be larger than normal. Moderate exercise provokes the typical muscle symptoms as well as tachycardia, dyspnoea, exhaustion and rarely nausea and vomiting. Ischaemic exercise of forearm muscles results in rapid fatigue and shortening of forearm flexors which may persist for some minutes after return of the circulation. It is not a true cramp but a physiological contracture during which affected muscles remain electrically silent (McArdle 1951, Rowland et al 1966). To perform the test, a blood-pressure cuff is placed on the upper arm and is maximally inflated to occlude arterial blood flow. Exercise is by squeezing a rubber bulb against a fixed resistance at a rate of one per second. Normal subjects can readily do this for a minute. In occasional patients, weakness develops during the test, preventing them from exercising to the point of developing a contracture. Because the muscles cannot degrade glycogen to lactic acid during the exercise, there is no rise in lactate in venous blood taken from forearm muscles after release of the circulation (McArdle 1951). Normal subjects exhibit a three-fold to five-fold increase of lactate within 5 min of the end of exercise and the lactate level returns to baseline in about 30 min.

The mechanism of the electrically silent muscle contractures is not understood. One possible explanation would be a deficiency of ATP required for the operation of the sarcoplasmic reticulum (SR) calcium pump. However, Rowland et al (1965) could not demonstrate a decrease of ATP in muscle during a contracture induced by ischaemic exercise. On the other hand, Gruener et al (1968) found that micro-applications of a calcium-containing solution to skinned muscle fibres elicited prolonged contractures, and Brody et al (1970) noted that isolated SR vesicles accumulated calcium normally in the presence of ATP. The latter two studies are consistent with the view that the SR calcium pump fails when ATP becomes unavailable. However, ^{31}P-nuclear magnetic resonance studies show normal levels of ATP but a reduced concentration of phosphocreatine in fatigued myophosphorylase deficient muscle (Ross et al 1981).

The serum levels of muscle enzymes are usually raised at rest. Following exercise, these levels increased markedly within a few hours (Hammett et al 1966). EMG studies may show alterations in motor unit potentials indicative of a myopathy and there is electrical silence of muscle fibres during contracture. Repetitive stimulation of motor nerves at 18 Hz was reported to produce an abnormal decrement of the amplitude of the evoked compound muscle action potential (Dyken et al 1967) but this finding has not been confirmed.

Muscle glycogen is usually raised, often to between 2 and 5%, but very occasionally it is normal. Glycogen accumulates subsarcolemmally in blebs and between myofibrils, especially adjacent to I bands (Schotland et al 1965). Small pockets of glycogen may also become invaginated into mitochondria (Gruener et al 1968). Lack of phosphorylase can be demonstrated histochemically in cryostat sections of fresh-frozen muscle. Characteristically, enzyme activity is absent from muscle fibres but is preserved in the smooth muscle cells of blood vessels. The histochemical demonstration of phosphorylase in muscle depends on the presence of glycogen primer, and the enzyme cannot be demonstrated even in normal muscle depleted of glycogen as, e.g., after prolonged storage of a muscle specimen at room temperature, or after death. Biochemical assay of the enzyme is independent of the muscle glycogen content. Although mature skeletal muscle fibres of affected patients lack phosphorylase, regenerating fibres and muscle cells cultured in vitro do show enzyme activity (Roelofs et al 1971). This has been attributed to the synthesis of a fetal isozyme by immature muscle cells (Sato et al 1977, DiMauro et al 1978a). Synthesis of the fetal isozyme is repressed by the time of birth.

The diagnosis of myophosphorylase deficiency is suggested by weakness, pain and contractures of muscle on exertion, a history of myoglobinuria, failure to form lactic acid on ischaemic exercise and by histochemical studies of the muscle biopsy specimen. Biochemical assay of the enzyme is required to confirm the diagnosis.

The ingestion of glucose or fructose increases exercise tolerance, but their long-term use has proved disappointing. They are awkward to take, predispose to obesity, and fructose may cause colicky pain. All patients should be advised to keep within the limits of exertion causing significant pain and, as far as possible, to precede vigorous exertion by a period of more gentle activity.

Muscle phosphofructokinase deficiency

Phosphofructokinase (PFK) is a tetrameric enzyme under the control of three structural genes located on chromosomes 1, 10 and 21 which encode muscle-type (M), liver-type (L), and fibroblast- or platelet-type (P) subunits respectively. The three genes are differentially expressed in various tissues, resulting in tissue-specific isozyme patterns. The various homotetrameric and heterotetrameric enzymes can be distinguished by subunit-specific monoclonal antibodies and ion-exchange chromatography (reviewed by Vora 1983). Muscle and liver contain homotetramers M_4 and L_4 respectively, whereas erythrocytes contain five isozymes made up of M and L subunits in various combinations (Vora et al 1983). Cultured muscle fibres express all three subunits and contain multiple homotetrameric and heterotetrameric isozymes (Davidson et al 1983).

Muscle PFK deficiency was first described by Tarui et al (1965); a second case was investigated by Layzer et al (1967b). More than 20 cases of the disease have been described to date (reviewed by Rowland et al 1986).

The enzyme catalyses the conversion of fructose-6-phosphate to fructose-1,6-diphosphate. The reaction requires ATP and is irreversible. Absence of the enzyme completely inhibits the Embden–Meyerhof pathway and blocks glucose utilisation. Glucose-1-phosphate and glucose-6-phosphate levels are increased, and fructose-1,6-diphosphate is markedly reduced in muscle (Tarui et al 1965). There is an associated partial enzyme deficiency in erythrocytes which lack the M isoenzyme (Tarui et al 1965, Layzer et al 1967b, Tarui et al 1969).

The clinical picture can be similar to that seen with myophosphorylase deficiency and the ischaemic exercise test is positive. In addition, there is a mild haemolytic disease, secondary to the partial erythrocyte enzyme defect (Tarui et al 1969). Hyperuricaemia and gout occur in a proportion of the patients. This may be related to the accelerated erythropoiesis, or to the stimulation of nucleotide metabolism by another mechanism. Exercise results in an abnormal rise of inosine, hypoxanthine, uric acid and ammonia in venous blood flowing from exercised muscle (Kono et al 1986). Autosomal recessive inheritance operates in some families (Tarui et al 1965, Layzer et al 1967b, Dupond et al 1977) but, in the family reported in Serratrice et al (1969), the trait was probably autosomal dominant. In the latter family, the propositus was also atypical in that he had hepatomegaly and suffered from progressive muscle weakness.

Other 'atypical' cases of PFK deficiency have also been observed, attesting to the heterogeneity of the syndrome. In two sibs (Guibaud et al 1978) and in an isolated case (Danon et al 1981a) of PFK deficiency, muscle weakness and joint contractures were present from birth. Two of the three patients died in infancy or early childhood.

Some patients have partial erythrocyte PFK deficiency and a haemolytic syndrome but no muscle symptoms and produce lactate normally on ischaemic exercise. This syndrome has been attributed to an unstable or deficient L subunit or to kinetically abnormal M or L subunits (Vora 1983, Vora et al 1983, Rowland et al 1986).

The subsarcolemmal glycogen deposits in muscle resemble those seen in myophosphorylase deficiency. Structurally abnormal glycogen, resembling amylopectin that accumulates in branching enzyme deficiency, has also been observed in some muscle fibres in a few patients (Agamanolis et al 1980, Hays et al 1981). Absence of phosphofructokinase can be demonstrated histochemically (Bonilla & Schotland 1970) but the diagnosis is best established by biochemical assay of the enzyme in muscle. Cultured muscle cells express the M, L and P subunits of PFK in multiple tetrameric combinations. However, the M subunit is catalytically inactive in muscle cells cultured from patients with PFK deficiency (Davidson et al 1983). This suggests a structural mutation involving the catalytic site of the M subunit.

Defects in the distal glycolytic pathway

Deficiencies of phosphoglycerate kinase (PGK), phosphoglycerate mutase (PGAM), and lactate dehydrogenase (LDH) have been recognised to date. The three disorders share certain common features (reviewed by DiMauro & Bresolin 1986): (1) As in myophosphorylase and PFK deficiencies, severe exercise is poorly tolerated and provokes attacks of myoglobinuria; (2) there is mild or no glycogen accumulation in the muscle fibres; (3) the ischaemic exercise test is either positive, or there may be a modest (less than two-fold) rise of lactate in venous blood flowing from the ischaemically exercised muscles; (4) residual enzyme activity can be detected in the muscle fibres.

Phosphoglycerate kinase deficiency

This is the only glycogenosis transmitted by X-linked recessive inheritance. PGK is a monomer; tissue-specific PGK isozymes are lacking, and the enzyme defect is expressed in cultured cells. Mutations involving PGK are asymptomatic, or result in severe haemolytic anaemia associated with neurological deficits (reviewed by DiMauro & Bresolin 1986), or produce a myopathy with the features described above (Rosa et al 1982, DiMauro et al 1983a). Mutant PGKs differ in their kinetic and physical properties. The mutant enzyme studied by DiMauro et al (1983a) had reduced substrate affinity, altered electrophoretic mobility, and an abnormal pH profile. Muscle contained reduced amounts of the immunologically recognisable but abnormal enzyme protein (Bresolin et al 1984). The mutant enzyme observed by Rosa et al (1982) had increased affinity for ATP, increased heat lability and abnormal electrophoretic mobility. As PGK has no tissue-specific isozymes, the fact that a given mutation affects either erythrocytes, or muscle fibres, or neither, remains unexplained.

Phosphoglycerate mutase deficiency

This is an autosomal recessive disorder. PGAM is a dimeric enzyme composed of muscle (M) and brain (B) subunits giving rise to MM, MB and BB isozymes (reviewed by DiMauro & Bresolin 1986). The expression of the various isozymes in different tissues is developmentally regulated. In mature muscle, the MM isozyme predominates. Only a few patients with a deficiency of the M subunit of PGAM, and with the clinical features described above, have been reported to date (DiMauro et al 1982, Bresolin et al 1983, Kissel et al 1985). The residual enzyme activity detected in muscle corresponded to the amount of the BB isozyme found in normal muscle. Cultured muscle fibres had enzyme activity associated with the BB isozyme. Although heart contains substantial amounts of the MB and MM isozymes, the patients had no clear evidence of a cardiomyopathy.

Lactate dehydrogenase deficiency

This is also an autosomal recessive disorder. LDH is a tetrameric enzyme composed of various combinations of muscle (M) and heart (H) subunits. As in the case of PGAM, the expression of the various isozymes in different tissues is developmentally regulated. The M_4 form predominates in mature muscle. A deficiency of the M subunit was reported in a Japanese man who had exercise intolerance associated with pigmenturia. Ischaemic exercise resulted in a reduced rise of lactate and a greater than normal rise of pyruvate in venous blood flowing from exercised muscles (Kanno et al 1980, Nishimura et al 1983).

Other glycogenoses

Other glycogenoses have been reported, some affecting muscle, in which only a single patient or a single family have been described, or in which the enzymic disorder has been insufficiently defined. An example was the disorder described by Satoyoshi & Kowa (1967) in two brothers. Both, when 35 years old, developed muscle pain, stiffness and weakness occurring a few hours after moderately heavy exercise. Blood lactate failed to rise after ischaemic exercise except following fructose ingestion. Biopsy studies showed an apparent block at the level of phosphohexoseisomerase (glucose-6-phosphate isomerase; EC 5.3.1.9), thought to be due to inhibition of the enzyme, associated with a decreased activity of phosphofructokinase. Exercise tolerance improved considerably following fructose, but not glucose, ingestion.

Another example was the eight-year-old boy with pains on exercise, described by Strugalska-Cynowska (1967); he had a very delayed rise in blood lactate following ischaemic exercise. This was attributed, on histochemical grounds, to a disturbance in the activity of phosphorylase-*b*-kinase (EC 2.7.1.38) which converts phosphorylase from the inactive to the active form.

Another glycogenosis was noted in the four-year-old boy described by Thomson et al (1963) with a mild myopathy and marked contracture of his calves, having only a slight rise in blood lactate after ischaemic exercise. His muscles were loaded with glycogen of normal structure. It was thought that there was a partial deficiency of phosphoglucomutase and possibly other glycolytic enzymes.

Holmes et al (1960) studied a female patient who presented at the age of 21 with symptoms of a myopathy and died at the age of 31 years. Cardiac and skeletal muscle contained basophilic, PAS-positive, diastase-fast polysaccharide deposits. Similar material was found in hepatocytes and in the lumen of the convoluted tubules. Enzyme assays and structural analysis of the polysaccharide were not performed. A similar disorder was reported by Karpati et al (1969) in a male patient who died of cardiac failure at the age of 19 years. Post-mortem examination was restricted to muscle and liver. The abnormal polysaccharide had filamentous fine structure and was especially abundant in type II muscle fibres.

A cardioskeletal lysosomal glycogenosis without acid maltase deficiency has been observed in chil-dren and young adults (Danon et al 1981b, Riggs et al 1983). Mental retardation and abnormal liver functions are variable associated features. The cardiomyopathy distinguishes the disorder clinically from adult AMD. An infantile variant of this syndrome may also exist (Atkin et al 1984). All patients described to date were male. The mode of inheritance is still uncertain.

DISORDERS OF LIPID METABOLISM

Long-chain fatty acids taken up by skeletal muscle are utilised for energy metabolism or esterified to triglycerides and incorporated into lipid droplets. It is now known that these fatty acids are the major substrate for oxidation by skeletal muscle at rest and during sustained exercise (Andres et al 1956, Hagenfeldt & Wahren 1968, Tancredi et al 1976, Zierler 1976). The main steps in the oxidation of long-chain fatty acids, reviewed by Ontko (1986), are as follows: (1) fatty acids are esterified with coenzyme (CoA), catalysed by long-chain fatty acyl-CoA synthase (EC 2.3.1.86); (2) acyl CoA is converted to acylcarnitine by carnitine palmityl transferase I (EC 2.3.1.21), located on the outer surface of the inner mitochondrial membrane barrier, permitting passage of acyl carnitine esters through the inner mitochondrial membrane barrier; (3) acyl carnitine esters are transported by exchange diffusion through the inner mitochondrial membrane by carnitine-acylcarnitine translocase; (4) acyl carnitine esters are reconverted to acyl-CoA by carnitine palmityl transferase II, located on the inner surface of the inner mitochondrial membrane; (5) intra-mitochondrial β-oxidation of acyl-CoA units; (6) utilisation of acetyl-CoA via the citric acid cycle; (7) the inner mitochondrial membrane is impermeable to acyl-CoAs, but the intramitochondrial CoAs are in equilibrium with the cytosolic carnitine pool via carnitine acyltranferases and carnitine-acylcarnitine translocase. The long, medium- and short-chain carnitine acyltransferases in the mitochondrial inner compartment can convert acyl-CoAs of various chain lengths, and branched-chain acyl-CoA derivatives of leucine, isoleucine and valine, to their corresponding carnitine esters and the translocase shuttles carnitine and acylcarnitines between the mitochondria and the cytosol along the respective concentration gradients. Consequently, carnitine, carnitine acyltransferases and carnitine-acylcarnitine translocase jointly regulate the intramitochondrial CoA concentration and the CoA/acyl-CoA ratio. Impairment of any step in this scheme may result in triglyceride accumulation within muscle fibres, or could cause symptoms due to lack of fatty acid substrate for energy metabolism. In addition, depending on the defect, an abnormally low intramitochondrial CoA/acyl-CoA ratio can result and this, in turn, can secondarily inhibit energy utilisation from glucose, the citric acid cycle and branched chain amino acids.

Not all defects in fatty acid oxidation are associated with a lipid storage myopathy. A lipid storage myopathy is defined as one in which lipid accumulation in muscle fibres is the predominant, or a predominant, pathological feature. Most lipid storage myopathies are associated with carnitine deficiency, and most carnitine deficiency syndromes are secondary to another metabolic disorder.

From a historical standpoint it is of interest to note that a lipid storage myopathy was first described in a young adult by Bradley et al (1969). The biochemical basis of the disorder was not defined. In 1970 W. K. Engel, and co-workers described two patients (identical twins) who had lipid excess in muscle without weakness, cramping pain after exercise, fasting or ingestion of a high-fat, low-carbohydrate diet, and who had previous attacks of myoglobinuria. The twins could form no ketone bodies after fasting or after ingesting long-chain fatty acids, but could produce ketone bodies from short-chain or medium-chain fatty acids. The basic biochemical defect in these patients was not discovered. In 1972, A. G. Engel & Siekert observed a young woman with progressive muscle weakness and lipid excess in muscle, whose symptoms responded favourably to prednisone. In 1973, A. G. Engel & Angelini found that this patient suffered from muscle carnitine deficiency. Also in 1973, DiMauro & DiMauro described a patient with intermittent myoglobinuria but without lipid excess in muscle, who suffered from muscle carnitine palmityltransferase (CPT) deficiency. In 1975, Chanarin et al

reported a further disorder associated with congenital ichthyosis and neutral lipid excess in muscle, liver, gastrointestinal mucosa, leucocytes and cultured fibroblasts. Another patient suffering from a similar illness, but also having steatorrhoea and muscle weakness, was reported by Miranda et al in 1979. The biochemical basis of this disorder remains unsolved.

Carnitine deficiency syndromes

Carnitine (γ-trimethylamino-β-hydroxybutyrate) is present in many foods but the daily human requirements are met only by additional biosynthesis. The two main precursors are lysine and methionine. The synthesis involves the formation of ε-N-trimethyllysine, oxidative cleavage of this to glycine and υ-trimethylaminobutyrate followed by β-hydroxylation of the latter compound to carnitine (Haigler & Broquist 1974, Tanphaichitr & Broquist 1974, Hulse et al 1978). In man, all the enzymes required for carnitine biosynthesis are found in liver, kidney and brain. Cardiac and skeletal muscle can also participate in biosynthesis but lack the final enzyme, γ-trimethylaminobutyrate hydroxylase (Rebouche & Engel 1980). Carnitine formed by liver and kidney is delivered to the other tissues by the circulation. Cardiac and skeletal muscle carnitine levels greatly exceed the serum level, and uptake into these tissues is by an active transport mechanism (Rebouche, 1977, Willner et al 1978). In a 70 kg adult the total body carnitine store is close to 100 mmol. Of this, 98% is in muscle, 0.6% in extracellular fluid and 1.6% in liver and kidney (Rebouche & Engel 1984). In normal subjects the renal plasma excretory threshold for free carnitine is close to the plasma level (about 50 μM) (Engel et al 1981). Acylcarnitines have much lower excretory thresholds than free carnitine (Carroll et al 1981a, Ohtani et al 1984). The turnover times for carnitine in extracellular fluid, muscle and the whole are 1.1 h, 8 days and 66 days, respectively (Rebouche & Engel 1984).

After the discovery of muscle carnitine deficiency (Engel & Angelini 1973, Engel et al 1974), a syndrome of systemic carnitine deficiency was described by Karpati et al (1975). Their patient, an 11-year-old male, had suffered recurrent attacks of Reye's syndrome since the age of three years and progressive muscle weakness since the age of 10 years. Carnitine was reduced in the patient's muscle, liver and serum. Between 1973 and 1981 some 40 cases of carnitine deficiency were reported (reviewed by Engel 1986): 16 of these were classified as myopathic and 24 as systemic deficiencies.

The 16 myopathic cases all had muscle weakness, muscle carnitine deficiency and lipid excess in muscle. The weakness appeared between 18 months and 38 years of age. Serum enzymes of muscle origin were increased in 12. Five also had cardiomyopathy and three had recurrent episodes of myoglobinuria. In systemic carnitine deficiency the initial symptoms presented between eight months and 38 years of age. Among the 24 patients with systemic disease 13 had one or more crises resembling Reye's syndrome, and eight of the 13 died during a crisis; 14 had muscle weakness; three had cardiomyopathy. All had lipid excess in muscle and other tissues in one stage of illness or at death. During the crises all patients had hepatic dysfunction and enlargement. Tissue carnitine levels were low when measured, but serum carnitine levels were normal in two patients who were terminally ill.

In four other cases (Smyth et al 1975, Whitaker et al 1977, Di Donato et al 1978a, b, Dusheiko et al 1979) with systemic or muscle carnitine deficiency, the clinical or laboratory features strongly suggested another associated metabolic disorder. In addition, by 1981, reduced carnitine levels were found in muscle in patients undergoing chronic haemodialysis (Bohmer et al 1978), in serum, liver and muscle in patients with cirrhosis and cachexia (Rudman et al 1977), and in muscle in severe and chronic myopathies (Borum et al 1977).

The marked clinical heterogeneity in both myopathic and systemic carnitine deficiency, the mixed features in some patients and the associated but divergent metabolic abnormalities in others presaged the recognition of a variety of metabolic errors causing carnitine deficiency. Between 1981 and 1986 numerous inborn errors of metabolism causing carnitine deficiency syndromes were identified, and some cases previously diagnosed as primary carnitine deficiency were then shown to

be secondary to another metabolic lesion, such as medium chain acyl-CoA dehydrogenase deficiency (Coates et al 1984, Hale et al 1985a), multiple acyl-CoA dehydrogenase deficiency (Di Donato et al 1984a), and mitochondrial ATPase deficiency (Clark et al 1984). It now appears that some myopathic and most systemic carnitine deficiencies are secondary to other metabolic errors.

Secondary carnitine deficiency syndromes

Table 25.2 lists the currently recognised secondary carnitine deficiency syndromes. Except for short-chain acyl-CoA dehydrogenase deficiency (Turnbull et al 1984), organic acidurias causing carnitine deficiency are associated with recurrent crises resembling the Reye syndrome and probably account for most cases of systemic carnitine deficiency. Defects in the mitochondrial respiratory chain or energy utilisation can be associated with exercise intolerance, resting or exertional lactacidaemia and variable decreases in serum and muscle carnitine. Some of the so-called mixed carnitine deficiencies may fall into this group. In most inherited syndromes the transmission is autosomal recessive, but some mitochondrial respiratory chain defects can also be transmitted by maternal mitochondrial inheritance.

Acyl-CoA dehydrogenase deficiencies. Acyl-CoA dehydrogenases consist of four subunits of identical size and range from 160 000 to 180 000 in molecular weight. Short-chain acyl-CoA dehydrogenase acts nearly exclusively on butyryl-CoA; the medium-chain and the long-chain enzyme dehydrogenate C_6–C_{10} and C_{14}–C_{22} acyl-CoAs, respectively. A branched-chain acyl-CoA dehydrogenase acts on isovaleryl-CoA and another on isobutyryl CoA. Finally, glutaryl-CoA dehydrogenates and decarboxylates its substrate. Reducing equivalents from all these enzymes are accepted by an electron-transferring flavoprotein (ETF; EC 1.3.99.2–3), which, in turn, is oxidised by ETF:ubiquinone oxidoreductase (ETF:QO). Flavin adenine dinucleotide (FAD) is a cofactor for the three straight-chain acyl-CoA dehydrogenases, ETF and ETF:QO (Gregersen 1985, Ikeda et al 1983, 1985).

Table 25.2 Secondary carnitine deficiency syndromes

Organic acidurias with acyl-CoA dehydrogenase deficiencies
　Long-chain acyl-CoA dehydrogenase deficiency[a]
　Medium-chain acyl-CoA dehydrogenase deficiency[b]
　Short-chain acyl-CoA dehydrogenase deficiency[c]
　Multiple acyl-CoA dehydrogenase deficiency[d]

Organic acidurias with defects in branched-chain amino acid metabolism
　Isovaleryl-CoA dehydrogenase deficiency[e]
　Propionyl-CoA carboxylase deficiency[f]
　Methylmalonyl-CoA mutase deficiency[g]
　β-hydroxy-β-methylglutaric-CoA lyase deficiency[h]

Defects in mitochondrial respiratory chain or energy utilisation
　Block at NADH-Coenzyme Q reductase[i]
　Block at succinate-cytochrome c reductase[j]
　Cytochrome c oxidase deficiency[k]
　Mitochondrial ATPase deficiency[l]

Other metabolic disorders
　Methylenetetrahydrofolate reductase deficiency[m]
　Kearns–Sayre syndrome[n]

Miscellaneous disorders
　Idiopathic Reye syndrome[o]
　Valproate therapy[p]
　Renal Fanconi syndrome[q]
　Chronic renal failure treated by haemodialysis[r]
　Kwashiorkor[s]
　Cirrhosis with cachexia[t]
　Chronic severe myopathies[u]

[a]　Hale et al 1985b
[b]　Stanley et al 1983a, Coates et al 1985, Roe et al 1984b
[c]　Turnbull et al 1984
[d]　Dusheiko et al 1979, Gregersen et al 1982, Mooy et al 1984
[e]　Stanley et al 1983b, Roe et al 1984b. Note that this enzyme is also an acyl-CoA dehydrogenase
[f]　Roe & Bohan 1982, Di Donato et al 1984b, Roe et al 1984a
[g]　Seccombe et al 1982, Roe et al 1982, Chalmers et al 1984, Millington et al 1984, Di Donato et al 1984b
[h]　Chalmers et al 1984
[i]　Busch et al 1981, Clark et al 1984
[j]　Sengers et al 1983
[k]　Müller-Höcker et al 1983b, Barth et al 1983
[l]　Clark et al 1984
[m]　Allen et al 1980
[n]　Allen et al 1983
[o]　Millington et al 1984
[p]　Ohtani et al 1982, Böhles et al 1982, Murphy et al 1985, Keene et al 1982
[q]　Netzloff et al 1981, Bernardini et al 1985
[r]　Bohmer et al 1978
[s]　Khan & Bamji 1977
[t]　Rudman et al 1977
[u]　Borum et al 1977

Long-chain Acyl-CoA dehydrogenase deficiency (LC-ACD) (Hale et al 1985b). This syndrome is characterised by a neonatal onset, frequent gastrointestinal upsets, aketotic, hypoglycaemic, encephalopathic crises, hepatomegaly, hypertrophic cardiomyopathy, weakness and hypotonia. Dicarboxylic aciduria occurs on fasting or in crises. Carnitine deficiency has been demonstrated in serum and liver. LC-ACD has been demonstrated in leucocytes, fibroblasts and liver. A high-carbohydrate, low-fat diet and carnitine supplements (100 mg/kg/day) may mitigate the clinical course.

Medium-chain acyl-CoA dehydrogenase deficiency (MC-ACD) (Stanley et al 1983a, Roe et al 1985, Coates et al 1985). This syndrome presents between the ages of five and 25 months, usually with aketotic metabolic crises resembling Reye attacks. Muscle weakness appears or becomes worse during attacks. Between attacks the patients are well or have mild weakness, easy fatiguability and mild hepatomegaly. Slight to moderate lipid excess is found in muscle between attacks. The serum carnitine fluctuates from low to normal; muscle and liver carnitine levels are low between attacks. There is an abnormal renal loss of both free and acyl carnitines and the renal plasma excretory threshold for these substances is lower than normal (Engel et al 1981, Engel 1986). MC-ACD can be demonstrated in liver, muscle, fibroblasts and leucocytes. Octanoylcarnitine is always present in urine and is diagnostic of MC-ACD even between crises. Other dicarboxylic acids such as adipic, suberic and sebacic acids, appear in the urine. The organic aciduria increases markedly during crises. A high-carbohydrate low-fat diet and carnitine supplements may help. Crises can be prevented by avoiding fasting and maintaining alimentation at all times, and especially in the course of febrile illnesses.

Short-chain acyl-CoA dehydrogenase deficiency (SC-ACD). (Turnbull et al 1984). A single patient with this disorder has been described. The illness was characterised by weakness and exercise intolerance beginning in adult life. The patient had muscle carnitine deficiency, a lipid storage myopathy, lactacidaemia on even mild exertion, and increased ketogenesis without hypoglycaemia on fasting. Serum acylcarnitines and the urinary excretion of acylcarnitines and of ethylmalonate and methylsuccinate were increased. Carnitine therapy was clinically ineffective. Because the patient formed ample ketone bodies on fasting, one can infer that hepatic short-chain acyl-CoA dehydrogenase activity was preserved.

Multiple acyl-CoA dehydrogenase deficiency (MU-ACD) (Di Donato et al 1984b, Dusheiko et al 1979, Gregersen et al 1982, Mooy et al 1984). In this disease (previously referred to as glutaric aciduria type II) there is a block in electron transport at the ETF or ETF:QO level so that the activity of all acyl-CoA dehydrogenases is impaired. A severe neonatal form, with or without congenital malformations and cardiomyopathy, and milder, late-onset cases have been described. Carnitine deficiency has been documented in the late-onset cases, but probably also exists in the severe neonatal cases. The late-onset cases present with ketoacidotic, hypoglycaemic Reye's syndrome-like crises and can be associated with marked lipid excess in liver and muscle (Dusheiko et al 1979, Di Donato et al 1984b). Treatment consists of riboflavine and carnitine supplements and a low-fat, low-protein and high-carbohydrate diet.

Defects in branched-chain amino acid metabolism. Carnitine depletion has now been documented in deficiencies of isovaleryl-CoA dehydrogenase, propionyl-CoA carboxylase, methylmalonyl-CoA mutase and β-hydroxy-β-methylglutaric-CoA lyase (references listed in Table 25.2). All these enzymes are in the degradative pathways of branched-chain amino acids. Each disease is associated with hypoglycaemic, ketoacidotic, hyperammonaemic encephalopathic crises resembling Reye's syndrome and with abnormal urinary excretion of short-chain acylcarnitines. The urinary acylcarnitine profile reflects the site of the metabolic block and the operation of alternative degradative pathways (Chalmers et al 1983, 1984, Millington et al 1984). Muscle biopsy studies have not been reported in these diseases. Muscle weakness has been observed in methylmalonic aciduria and may have been overlooked in other syndromes. Treatment consists of dietary management and carnitine supplements.

Defects in mitochondrial respiratory chain or oxidative phosphorylation. Abnormal fatiguability and lactacidaemia on exertion are non-specific features. Marked lipid excess in muscle, muscle carnitine depletion, and muscle weakness occur in a minority of patients with a defect in the NADH–ubiquinone reductase (NADH dehydrogenase (ubiquinone); EC 1.6.5.3) portion of the respiratory chain (Morgan-Hughes 1986). Slight muscle carnitine deficiency was found in a two-year-old boy with neurodegenerative disease and progressive weakness whose muscle mitochondria failed to oxidise pyruvate normally and showed reduced succinate-cytochrome c reductase activity (Sengers et al 1983). Marked mitochondrial, lipid and glycogen excess can occur in muscle with defects in the cytochrome oxidase system even without carnitine deficiency (Morgan-Hughes 1986). Slight to moderate decreases in total carnitine and increased acylcarnitine have been noted in muscle in a few patients with defects of this portion of the respiratory chain (References cited in Table 25.2).

A patient with mitochondrial ATPase deficiency had basal ganglia calcification, seizures, high-tone hearing loss, increased spinal fluid protein, muscle weakness, exertional lactacidaemia and frequent vomiting but no acute episodes of encephalopathy. Carnitine treatment improved the patient's strength, but he developed dementia, peripheral neuropathy, ataxia and retinopathy (Smyth et al 1975, Clark et al 1984). Markesbery (1979) observed a clinically similar disorder in a 27-year-old man but did not assay mitochondrial enzymes or carnitine.

Methylenetetrahydrofolate reductase deficiency (Allen et al 1980). This was noted in a one-month-old infant who had leucoencephalopathy associated with homocystinuria, hypomethionaemia, reduced free carnitine in serum and muscle, and a lipid storage myopathy. Treatment with folate, methionine and carnitine resulted in dramatic clinical and metabolic improvement. The carnitine deficiency was attributed to diminished availability of *S*-adenosylmethionine for carnitine biosynthesis.

Idiopathic Reye's syndrome. The acute episodes in secondary carnitine deficiency syndromes associated with genetic defects in organic acid metabolism resemble idiopathic Reye's syndrome attacks. In idiopathic Reye's syndrome the urinary acetylcarnitine excretion is markedly increased suggesting massive release of this compound from muscle and liver (Millington et al 1984). These findings imply a block in the mitochondrial utilisation of acetyl-CoA and suggest that acetylcarnitine exits from the mitochondria and the cells to buffer the intramitochondrial CoA/acetyl-CoA ratio. Eventually, with conversion of most carnitine to acetylcarnitine and depletion of free carnitine, even this mechanism would fail (Stumpf et al 1985).

Valproate therapy. This drug decreases the serum free carnitine and increases the serum ammonia level (Ohtani et al 1982). A few children on this medication had fatal Reye's attacks, and at least one had a markedly decreased free serum carnitine level (Böhles et al 1982). The carnitine deficiency may be secondary to detoxification of valproyl-CoA and its derivatives as carnitine esters.

Renal Fanconi syndrome. One child with idiopathic renal Fanconi's syndrome had severe systemic carnitine deficiency, an attack of Reye's syndrome, muscle weakness and lipid storage myopathy (Netzloff et al 1981). In other patients with renal Fanconi's syndrome the muscle carnitine levels are only slightly reduced although the fractional excretions of free carnitine and acylcarnitines are increased (Bernardini et al 1985).

Current status of the carnitine deficiency syndromes. Because so many metabolic errors can cause secondary carnitine deficiency, primary carnitine deficiency should not be diagnosed unless all currently recognised causes of secondary carnitine deficiency have been adequately excluded. Further, even those carnitine deficiency cases that are still considered to be primary (Di Donato et al 1984a, Duran et al 1984) show marked heterogeneity, suggesting that additional biochemical causes of carnitine deficiency will be discovered.

Primary muscle carnitine deficiency is still considered to be the diagnosis in the first recognised case of human carnitine deficiency (Engel & Angelini 1973, Engel et al 1974). This patient had no Reye's syndrome attacks, nor organic aciduria, showed appropriate ketogenesis on fasting, and had normal liver carnitine levels. Her muscle short-chain, medium-chain and long-chain acyl-CoA dehydrogenase activities were normal (Zierz et al 1986). She had no renal carnitine leak (Engel et al 1981). Kinetic compartment analysis in vivo demonstrated impaired carnitine transport into her muscle (Rebouche & Engel 1984).

Carnitine deficiencies associated with familial cardiomyopathy. A syndrome of familial cardiomyopathy, tissue carnitine depletion, and a favourable response to carnitine replacement therapy may represent a distinct clinical entity (Chapoy et al 1980, Tripp et al 1981, Waber et al 1982). A renal carnitine leak was demonstrated in the patients studied by Waber et al (1982). However, even this syndrome may be secondary, for LC-ACD and MUL-ACD can be associated with cardiomyopathy and a renal carnitine leak exists in MC-ACD (Engel 1986, Hale et al 1985a). Another syndrome has been observed in fraternal twins (Glasgow et al 1983). In these patients ketone body production was impaired and the carnitine deficiency was associated with an absolute increase of long-chain acylcarnitines. The cardiomyopathy and myopathy did not respond to carnitine therapy but was improved by a medium-chain triglyceride diet. The findings suggest a defect in the utilisation of long-chain fatty acids.

Mechanisms of carnitine depletion. Several mechanisms have been identified. (1) An excessive release of acylcarnitines from tissues and their subsequent excretion by the kidney is an important mechanism in the organic acidurias. The abnormal release is triggered by the intramitochondrial accumulation of acyl-CoAs. This stimulates the intramitochondrial formation of acylcarnitines, which then exit from the mitochondrion and from the cell and are preferentially excreted by the kidney. (2) An abnormal renal excretion of carnitine also has a role in MC-ACD, in the renal Fanconi's syndrome, and in some familial cardiomyopathies with carnitine deficiency. (3) A defect in the active transport of carnitine into muscle cells has been demonstrated in the first reported case of muscle carnitine deficiency (Rebouche & Engel 1984).

A dietary carnitine deficiency reduces tissue carnitine stores in premature infants (Penn et al 1980). It appears, however, that dietary carnitine deficiency in itself does not cause clinical symptoms unless carnitine metabolism is also compromised by another mechanism, such as severe cirrhosis combined with protein malnutrition (Rudman et al 1977), or by an associated inborn error of metabolism (Slonim et al 1983). A defect in intestinal carnitine transport or in carnitine biosynthesis might also contribute to carnitine depletion, but convincing evidence for such defects has not been published to date.

The metabolic crises in carnitine deficiency syndromes. The acute crises of systemic carnitine deficiency begin with vomiting followed by deepening stupor and coma, increase in serum liver enzymes, hepatomegaly, hypoglycaemia, hypoprothrombinaemia, hyperammonaemia and lipid accumulation in hepatocytes. Thus, they resemble attacks of Reye's syndrome (DeVivo & Keating 1976). Crises occur in all systemic carnitine deficiencies associated with organic acidurias except in SC-ACD. They are aketotic in LC-ACD and MC-ACD but are ketotic in MUL-ACD and in those with defects of branched-chain amino-acid metabolism. Crises can also occur in systemic carnitine deficiency not associated with other recognisable metabolic disease (Di Donato et al 1984a) and in carnitine deficiency caused by a renal carnitine leak (Netzloff et al 1981). The encephalopathy is mediated by hypoglycaemia and/or toxic organic acids (Kim et al 1984). Hyperammonaemia and ketoacidosis, when present, may also contribute. A vicious circle comprising four steps operates in the crises and can begin at any one of the steps: (1) fatty acid oxidation is reduced by decreased entry of acylcarnitines into the mitochondria; (2) increased utilisation of carbohydrate for energy depletes glycogen stores, and gluconeogenesis is inhibited by lack of acetyl-CoA and ATP (Hers & Hue 1983); (3) abnormal intramitochondrial accumulation of acyl-CoAs decreases the intramitochondrial CoA level and the CoA/acyl-CoA ratio and carnitine is lost from the cells in the form of acylcarnitines; (4) the CoA lack and the low CoA/acyl-CoA ratio further inhibit fatty acid oxidation, amino-acid oxidation and the citric acid cycle.

Diagnosis of carnitine deficiency. All carnitine deficiency syndromes, with or without crises or other systemic manifestations, should be considered secondary until all currently known causes of secondary carnitine deficiency are excluded. Carnitine deficiency should be suspected in any patient with one or more of the following: (1) lipid storage myopathy, with or without hepatomegaly; (2) Reye's syndrome attacks, especially if recurrent or familial; (3) recurrent episodes of hypoglycaemia provoked by exertion, infection, fasting or pregnancy; (4) myalgias, abnormal fatiguability and lactacidaemia on exertion; (5) hypertrophic cardiomyopathy; (6) organic aciduria.

Accurate measurements of total and acylcarnitines in tissues and tissue fluids are essential for the diagnosis (Rebouche & Engel 1983). For the diagnosis of secondary carnitine deficiency syndromes the reader is referred to the references listed in Table 25.2. The following general principles apply: (1) analysis of plasma and urinary metabolites by the technique of gas chromatography-mass spectrometry is an important aid in the diagnosis of an enzyme defect in organic acidurias; (2) the abnormal metabolites in the tissue fluids increase during crises; (3) the identification of acylcarnitines in tissue fluids by fast atom bombardment-mass spectrometry is a powerful method for identifying the metabolite accumulating at the site of the metabolic block; further, oral carnitine loading increases the amount of the abnormal acylcarnitine in urine (Roe et al 1985, Millington et al 1984); (4) whenever possible, the diagnosis is to be confirmed by specific enzyme assays, such as determination of acyl-CoA dehydrogenases or measurement of the activities of respiratory chain enzymes, utilising fibroblasts, leucocytes, liver or muscle.

Treatment of carnitine deficiency syndromes. Replacement therapy consists of 50–100 mg/kg/day of L-carnitine taken orally in divided doses. Higher dosages and parenteral administration of L-carnitine may be required in crises. Avoidance of fasting, frequent meals of high carbohydrate content, a low-fat diet and, depending on the site of the metabolic block, a medium-chain triglyceride diet may be of benefit. Some patients not responding to carnitine replacement therapy have responded to prednisone (Engel & Siekert 1972, VanDyke et al 1975), high doses of riboflavine (Carroll et al 1981b), or propranolol (Isaacs et al 1976). It is interesting to note that in some patients responding to carnitine therapy the low tissue carnitine levels have remained unchanged (Angelini et al 1976, Matsuishi et al 1985). In only a few patients has carnitine treatment replenished the muscle stores nearly completely (Di Donato et al 1984a). The varying clinical and tissue responses to carnitine and the efficacy of various forms of therapy can be explained by the clinical and biochemical heterogeneity of the carnitine deficiency syndromes.

Clinically distinct genetic defects of fatty acid oxidation

The acyl-CoA dehydrogenase deficiencies were considered in the preceding sections. Three other inherited syndromes associated with putative defects in long-chain fatty acid oxidation but without carnitine deficiency have been described. The first of these, observed in identical twins by W. K. Engel et al (1970) has been considered above.

An autosomal recessive syndrome associated with life-long slowly progressive weakness, myalgias, electrical myotonia, lipid accumulation in leucocytes and muscle, and a slight delay in ketogenesis on fasting was described by Snyder et al (1982). Therapy with prednisone relieved the myalgia without improvement in strength. Treatment with carnitine and a medium-chain triglyceride diet improved the myopathy and in one patient also abolished the electrical myotonia.

A lipid storage neuromyopathy was described in a mother and her two sons. The patients had a life-long history of muscle weakness and intolerance to fatty foods. All three had electrical myotonia. Abnormal mitochondria and lipid excess were found in muscle. Lipid droplets, zebra bodies and abnormal mitochondria were noted in most Schwann cells. Treatment with a medium-chain triglyceride diet resulted in remarkable clinical and morphological improvement (Askanas et al 1985).

Carnitine palmityl transferase (CPT) deficiency

Since the original report of this disorder by Di-Mauro & DiMauro in 1973, about 45 cases have been reported in the literature (Bank et al 1975, Cumming et al 1976, Herman & Nadler 1977, Layzer et al 1977, Carroll et al 1978, Di Donato et al 1978b, Hostetler et al 1978, Reza et al 1978, Brownell et al 1979, Patten et al 1979, Scholte et al 1979; Zierz & Engel 1985, DiMauro & Papadimitriou 1986). The male:female ratio is close to 8:2. Transmission is probably by autosomal recessive inheritance with markedly reduced penetrance in women. Intermittent symptoms begin during the first or second decade of life. Muscle aching and fatiguability occur on sustained exertion. There are recurrent attacks of myoglobinuria, usually, but not invariably, after sustained exertion and especially if exercise is during caloric deprivation or exposure to cold. Severe muscle aching and stiffness precede the myoglobinuria by a few hours and marked muscle weakness can develop in the course of the attack. Renal failure may complicate the myoglobinuria (Bank et al 1975, Di Donato et al 1978b, Brownell et al 1979). Serum enzymes of muscle origin increase greatly during attacks, but may also rise after exercise which does not precipitate overt myoglobinuria. Between attacks, patients are of normal strength and show no EMG abnormality. Muscle biopsy at such times shows either no lipid excess or only slight lipid excess (Engel et al 1979, DiMauro & Papadimitriou 1986). Fasting for 38–72 h is associated with a delayed rise of serum ketone bodies in some patients (Bank et al 1975, Cumming et al 1976, Hostetler et al 1978, Patten et al 1979), but not in others (Patten et al 1979, Scholte et al 1979). The serum creatine kinase (CK) level increases abnormally during fasting in some patients, but not in others (Scholte et al

1979). Increased basal serum triglyceride and cholesterol levels which rose further on fasting were noted in two brothers studied by Bank et al (1975) but not in other patients.

Depending on the assay system used, CPT activities in the patients ranged from not detectable to 45–60% of normal (reviewed by Zierz & Engel 1985). Several attempts to attribute the syndrome to selective deficiency of CPT I (Di-Mauro & DiMauro, 1973, Hoppel et al 1980) or CPT II (Patten et al 1979, Scholte et al 1979, Trevisan et al 1984) gave further conflicting results. These discrepancies might stem from biochemical heterogeneity or methodological problems with the CPT assay. In all reported cases, CPT deficiency in muscle was established by the isotope exchange assay or by the backward assay (in which palmityl-CoA is formed from palmityl-carnitine). Decreased enzyme activity in the forward assay (in which palmitylcarnitine is formed from palmityl-CoA) was found only in the presence of high substrate concentration or detergent (reviewed by Zierz & Engel 1985). In studies of sonicated homogenates of previously frozen muscle (in which both CPT 1 and CPT 2 are assayed) obtained from 12 non-weak controls and seven cases of CPT deficiency, Zierz & Engel (1985) found the following: (1) although all patients had severe CPT deficiency in the isotope exchange assay, the enzyme deficiency disappeared when concentration of the substrate (L-palmitylcarnitine) was reduced from 0.5 to 0.05 mM; (2) normal enzyme activity was obtained in all patients in the forward assay in the presence of 0.1% albumin and 0.08 mM palmityl-CoA; (3) omission of albumin, increasing the substrate concentration, the addition of small amounts (0.025 to 0.2 mM) of palmitylcarnitine, or 0.4% Triton® X-100 abnormally inhibited enzyme activity in the forward assay in all seven patients. Thus, the mutant CPT was abnormally inhibited by its own substrate or product in both the forward and isotope exchange assays. Subsequent studies also demonstrated abnormal inhibition of the enzyme in the backward assay by palmitylcarnitine and palmityl-CoA (S. Zierz and A. G. Engel, unpublished observations). These data imply that CPT deficiency is caused by the altered regulatory properties of a mutant enzyme, or altered interaction between the enzyme and its membranous environment, rather than by lack of catalytically active CPT I, II or both. Further, the mutant enzyme would be most vulnerable to substrate/product inhibition when lipid metabolism is stressed. These data readily explain why the symptoms of CPT deficiency are intermittent, why they differ from those of carnitine deficiency, and why so much less lipid accumulates in muscle in CPT than in carnitine deficiency (Zierz & Engel 1985).

The diagnosis of the disease is based on the history of exercise intolerance, recurrent myoglobinuria, the normal rise of lactate in venous blood flowing from ischaemically exercised muscles and demonstration of CPT deficiency in muscle by the isotope exchange assay in the presence of 0.5 mM palmitylcarnitine. Treatment consists of a high-carbohydrate, low-fat diet, frequent feeding and extra carbohydrate intake before and during sustained exertion (Cumming et al 1976, Reza et al 1978, Patten et al 1979).

MITOCHONDRIAL MYOPATHIES

The term 'mitochondrial myopathies' has been applied to muscle diseases in which mitochondria have abnormal structure, function or both. The typical morphological alteration consists of unusually large or excessively abundant mitochondria, often with bizarre cristae and with inclusions of various types. Such organelles usually occur in type I and sometimes in type IIA muscle fibres in which they form subsarcolemmal and inter-myofibrillar aggregates. The affected fibres often also contain an excess of small lipid droplets and the mitochondrial aggregates are usually surrounded by glycogen granules. On the basis of their light-microscopic appearance in trichromatically stained sections, the term 'ragged red' has been applied to such fibres (Olson et al 1972). A purely morphological definition of mitochondrial myopathies is unsatisfactory, however. In certain disorders with a definite abnormality of mitochondrial metabolism, as in CPT deficiency (DiMauro & DiMauro 1973) or in certain types of exertional lactic acidosis (Sussman et al 1970) there are no structural abnormalities of muscle mitochondria. Conversely, abnormal mitochondria have been found in diseases in which a primary mitochondrial abnormality seems unlikely, as in adult acid maltase deficiency (Engel & Dale 1968), a few cases of polymyositis (Chou 1967, Shafiq et al 1967) and in certain cases of denervation atrophy (Gruner 1963, Shafiq et al 1967). Finally, similar mitochondrial structural alterations can be associated with divergent abnormalities of mitochondrial function. For these reasons, a biochemical classification of mitochondrial myopathies, even if tentative, is preferable. The classification proposed by Morgan-Hughes et al (1979) will be adopted in this chapter: (1) transport or enzymatic defects of mitochondria causing impaired substrate utilisation; (2) defective mitochondrial energy conservation; (3) specific deficiency of one or more mitochondrial respiratory chain components. The biochemical abnormalities are not necessarily confined to the muscle mitochondria and, in a number of disorders, the myopathy represents but one facet of a multisystem disease. Other features shared by many, but not all, mitochondrial myopathies are: slowly progressive weakness involving proximal and distal muscle and/or external ocular muscles; transiently increased weakness after sustained exertion; and lactic acidaemia after exercise or even at rest. Several recent reviews deal with mitochondrial myopathies (Sengers et al 1984a, DiMauro et al 1985, Morgan-Hughes 1986, Petty et al 1986).

Mitochondrial disorders associated with transport and enzymatic defects causing impaired substrate utilisation

These syndromes include the carnitine deficiencies, the acyl-CoA dehydrogenase deficiencies, CPT deficiency and defects of the pyruvate dehydrogenase complex. As the carnitine, acyl-CoA dehydrogenase and CPT deficiencies were discussed under Disorders of Lipid Metabolism (p. 828), this section will deal only with defects of the pyruvate dehydrogenase complex. The complex has three components; pyruvate decarboxylase (E_1), dihydrolipoyl transacetylase (E_2) and dihydrolipoyl dehydrogenase (E_3). E_1 exists in an active and inactive form. Formation of the inactive form is catalysed by an ATP-dependent pyruvate dehydrogenase kinase. Inactive E_1 is converted to active E_1 by a calcium- and magnesium-stimulated pyruvate dehydrogenase phosphatase (Robinson

& Sherwood 1975). In most patients with a deficiency of the pyruvate dehydrogenase complex the clinical picture is dominated by central nervous system involvement (reviewed by Blass 1979, Sengers et al 1984a, Morgan-Hughes 1986).

Pyruvate decarboxylase deficiency. A patient with this disorder was reported by Blass et al (1970). A nine-year-old boy had suffered from attacks of choreoathetosis and ataxia provoked by fever or excitement, from 16 months of age. Blood, urine and cerebrospinal fluid pyruvate levels were abnormally high but lactate levels were rarely abnormal. The enzyme deficiency was demonstrated in cultured fibroblasts and leucocytes. The oxidation of pyruvate was impaired but that of glutamate, acetate and palmitate was normal. Muscle specimens revealed an excess of small lipid droplets, especially in type I fibres, but the patient was not weak (Blass et al 1971).

Another patient with a deficiency of the pyruvate dehydrogenase complex (in cultured fibroblasts) was a three-year-old girl with microcephaly, hypotonia, spasticity and with persistent pyruvic and lactic acidaemia (Blass et al 1972). As the cultured cells showed subnormal oxidation not only of pyruvate but also of citrate and palmitate, the metabolic defect was probably not confined to the pyruvate dehydrogenase complex. No muscle biopsy was taken.

Pyruvate decarboxylase deficiency associated with Leigh's subacute necrostising encephalomyelopathy and signs of myopathy was described by Evans (1981) and by Toshima et al (1982).

Pyruvate dehydrogenase phosphatase deficiency. This disorder, described by Robinson & Sherwood (1975), caused congenital and chronic lactic acidosis and death in the first year of life. During life, serum lactate, pyruvate, free fatty acid and ketone body levels were increased and there was an associated metabolic acidosis. The enzyme deficiency was demonstrated post mortem in muscle, liver and brain. Muscle histopathology was not described.

Dihydrolipoyl dehydrogenase (E_3) deficiency. This was observed by Robinson et al (1978) in a floppy male infant with congenital and chronic lactic, pyruvic, 2-oxoglutaric and branched-chain aminoacidaemia. Hypoglycaemia was intermittently present. The enzyme deficiency was demonstrated post mortem in all tissues. Muscle histopathology was not described.

Mitochondrial disorders associated with defective energy conservation

Hypermetabolic myopathy. The first case of this disorder was described in detail by Luft et al in 1962. A 35-year-old woman had exhibited profuse perspiration, heat intolerance, polydipsia without polyuria, hyperphagia and progressive asthenia since early childhood. Her BMR varied between +140 and +210%. Thyroid function studies excluded hyperthyroidism. Morphological studies of muscle revealed a mitochondrial myopathy (the first ultrastructural description) with abundant and large mitochondria harbouring crystalloid and other inclusions. Biochemical studies showed loosely coupled oxidative phosphorylation. Basal ATPase activity was abnormally high and not further stimulated by uncoupling agents. A second case was reported by Afifi et al (1972). Biochemical studies in this case by Di-Mauro et al (1976) confirmed the observations made by Luft et al (1962) and also revealed subnormal accumulation of calcium by the isolated muscle mitochondria. This was attributed to an abnormal release of calcium and it was suggested that the continued recycling of calcium between mitochondria and the cytosol was responsible for the sustained stimulation of respiration and loose coupling.

Mitochondrial myopathies with defective respiratory control without hypermetabolism. The disorders in this group are clinically heterogeneous and it is likely that the loose coupling is secondary to another, but still undefined, abnormality of mitochondrial respiration. Muscle specimens in each instance showed a typical mitochondrial myopathy and lactacidaemia was present at rest or on exertion. The patients studied by Hülsmann et al (1967), Van Wijngaarden et al (1967), Schellens & Ossentjuk (1969) and by Worsfold et al (1973) fall in this group.

Another clinical pattern was reported by Spiro et al (1970a). This was the case of a boy who had craved salt since infancy, had non-progressive weakness since the age of eight years and experienced three episodes of transient, severe generalised weakness lasting several hours, at the age of 13 years. The clinical features resembled those of a child with 'pleoconial myopathy' described by Shy et al (1966). However, no biochemical studies were reported by Shy et al (1966).

Another disorder with a defective mitochondrial energy supply was described by Schotland et al (1976). A 37-year-old patient had suffered from non-progressive muscle weakness of limb and torso muscles since early childhood. The electrocardiogram showed biventricular hypertrophy. Mitochondrial respiratory rate and control were markedly reduced with pyruvate-malate, succinate plus rotenone and palmitylcarnitine, but phosphorylative efficiency was normal. The basal, as well as the magnesium stimulated and 2,4-dinitrophenol-stimulated mitochondrial ATPase activities were also greatly decreased. Thus, the defect involved energy transfer at a level common to all three coupling sites of the respiratory chain, yet, surprisingly, the clinical symptoms were relatively mild. Another case of mitochondrial ATPase deficiency associated with neurodegenerative disease, described by Clark et al (1984), was discussed in the section on secondary carnitine deficiency syndromes (p. 830).

Defective respiratory control with α-glycerophosphate, but not with other substrates, has been observed in mitochondria isolated from muscles of a patient with oculocraniosomatic muscle weakness (DiMauro et al 1973). Muscle glycogen content was also increased but the glycolytic pathway was intact. A similar biochemical abnormality was reported in a 30-year-old man, with slowly progressive muscle weakness since the age of 12 years, who had no ocular or cranial muscle weakness (Black et al 1975).

Disorders associated with specific deficiencies of one or more mitochondrial respiratory chain components

The components of the respiratory chain include NADH:ubiquinone oxidoreductase (complex I), succinate:ubiquinone oxidoreductase (complex II; EC 1.3.5.1), ubiquinol:cytochrome c reductase (complex III; EC 1.10.2.2) and ferrocytochrome c:oxygen oxidoreductase (or cytochrome c oxidase; EC 1.9.3.1) (complex IV). ATP synthase (complex V; EC 3.6.1.3) is concerned with energy conservation. Ubiquinone (coenzyme Q) carries electrons from complex I and II to complex III, and cytochrome c carries electrons from complex III to complex IV.

Complex I contains flavin adenine mononucleotide (FAM), Fe-S clusters and 25 polypeptide subunits. Complex II contains FAD, Fe-S clusters, a species of cytochrome b and four or five polypeptide subunits. Complex III consists of an Fe-S cluster, two species of cytochrome b, cytochrome c_1 and 9–10 polypeptide subunits. Complex IV is composed of cytochromes a and a_3 associated with Cu_a and Cu_{a3}, respectively, and at least eight polypeptide subunits. Complex V includes adenine nucleotides, Mg^{2+}, and 12–14 polypeptide subunits (reviewed by Hatefi 1985). Six subunits of complex I, one subunit of complex III, the three catalytic subunits of complex IV, and two subunits of complex V are now known to be encoded by mitochondrial DNA (Chonym et al 1985, Kuhn-Nentwig & Kadenbach 1985, Hatefi 1985). Mutations involving these subunits are transmitted by vertical maternal inheritance to more than 50% of offspring of either sex. The remaining subunits of the complexes are encoded by nuclear DNA and mutations of these subunits are transmitted by Mendelian inheritance. It now also appears likely that tissue-specific isozymes of the complexes exist because of differences in the expression of nuclear DNA-encoded subunits in different tissues. Immunological differences between the nucleus-encoded subunits of complex IV derived from liver, kidney, brain, heart and skeletal muscle support this notion. Further, nucleus-encoded subunits of complex III in some fetal tissues differ from the corresponding subunits in the corresponding adult tissues. This implies the existence of fetal isozymes and the developmental regulation of the complex (Kuhn-Nentwig & Kadenbach 1985). The presence of multiple subunits in a complex, each encoded by a different gene, and the existence of tissue-specific subunits can explain the clinical heterogeneity seen with defects in a given complex and the tissue-specific expressions of a given defect in any one complex.

Defects in complex I. Eighteen patients with complex I deficiency have been investigated by Morgan-Hughes and co-workers (Morgan-Hughes et al 1979, Land et al 1981, Morgan-Hughes et al 1982, Morgan-Hughes 1986, Petty et al 1986). Eleven patients had skeletal muscle involvement with weakness, exercise intolerance, exertional lactacidaemia and ragged red muscle fibres. Among these 11 patients three also had external ophthalmoplegia and three had muscle carnitine deficiency and lipid storage myopathy. Eight patients had predominantly central nervous system manifestations, such as headaches, visual failure, hemiparesis, dysphasia, dementia, dystonia and cerebral atrophy. Biochemical studies revealed low or absent mitochondrial respiration with NAD-linked, but not other, substrates. The cytochrome spectra, mitochondrial NAD content, and substrate dehydrogenase and citrate synthase activities were normal. The oxidation of NAD-linked substrates by muscle homogenates was also impaired in a four-year-old boy with lactacidaemia after glucose loading, progressive dementia, ataxia, myoclonus, spastic quadriparesis and eventually fatal liver failure (Prick et al 1981).

Defects in complex II. A defect in complex II was postulated in one of two siblings with myoclononus, seizures, short stature, low intelligence and a mitochondrial myopathy (Riggs et al 1984).

Defects in complex III. Eight patients with abnormalities in complex III have been studied in detail (Spiro et al 1970b, Morgan-Hughes et al 1977, 1982, Hayes et al 1984, Kennaway et al 1984, Morgan-Hughes 1986). Muscle weakness, exercise intolerance, exertional lactacidaemia and structurally abnormal mitochondria in muscle were consistent findings. Five of the eight patients also had external ophthalmoplegia (Spiro et al 1970b, Hayes et al 1984, Morgan-Hughes 1986). Neurodegenerative features, such as dementia, myoclonus, ataxia, corticospinal tract signs and loss of proprioception were present in three patients (Spiro et al 1970b, Morgan-Hughes et al 1982). In one patient the defect was localised to the coenzyme Q-cytochrome bc_1 segment of the respiratory chain (Morgan-Hughes 1986). In another patient the defect may have involved the Fe-S cluster in complex III (Morgan-Hughes 1986). Deficiency of reducible cytochrome b was shown by spectral analysis in four patients (Spiro et al 1970b, Morgan-Hughes et al 1977, 1982). Low levels of reduced cytochrome b and c_1 were detected in one patient (Hayes et al 1984). In another patient, a 17-year-old woman, spectral analysis of muscle mitochondria indicated a low level of reduced cytochrome b and further analysis with subunit specific antibodies revealed greatly diminished levels of core proteins, Fe-S protein and of subunit VI, suggesting that complex III was not assembled in muscle mitochondria (Darley-Usmar et al 1983, Kennaway et al 1984). ^{31}p NMR studies of this patient's muscle showed an abnormally low phosphocreatine to inorganic phosphate ration that became even lower on exercise (Eleff et al 1984). Treatment with menadione (10 mg every 6 h) and ascorbate (1 g every 6 h), which could function as electron transfer mediators instead of complex III, improved the patient's exercise tolerance and the phosphocreatine to inorganic phosphate ration in muscle (Eleff et al 1984).

Defects in complex IV. Several distinct syndromes have been recognised in this group (reviewed by DiMauro et al 1985). A fatal infantile mitochondrial myopathy presents at birth or within the first few months of life and death ensues a few weeks or months after the onset. Severe muscle weakness and hypotonia are associated with lactacidaemia. Seven patients in this group also had features of the DeToni–Fanconi syndrome (hypophosphataemia, hyperphosphaturia, generalised aminoaciduria, glycosuria and polyuria) (Van Biervliet et al 1977, DiMauro et al 1980, Heimann-Patterson et al 1982, Minchom et al 1983, Müller-Höcker et al 1983b, Zeviani et al 1985). Two patients had no renal involvement but had cardiomyopathy (Sengers et al 1984b, Rimoldi et al 1982). Three patients had neither renal nor cardiac involvement (Trijbels et al 1983, Boustany et al 1983, Bresolin et al 1985), but one of these had hepatopathy (Bresolin et al 1985). The histological changes in muscle consisted of accumulation of structurally abnormal mitochondria and, in some patients, also of lipid and

glycogen, except in the patient studied by Rimoldi et al (1982) who did not have a mitochondrial myopathy by morphological criteria. Cytochrome oxidase deficiency was demonstrated by one or more of the following tests: oxygen electrode studies of mitochondrial respiration with appropriate substrates; spectrophotometric assay of cytochrome c oxidase; analysis of the cytochrome spectra, and enzyme cytochemical and immunochemical studies. Spectral analysis in some patients demonstrated a deficiency not only of cytochrome aa_3, which is associated with complex IV, but also of cytochrome b (Van Biervliet et al 1977, DiMauro et al 1980, Bresolin et al 1985). The variability in tissue involvement in the fatal syndrome could be accounted for by the existence of tissue-specific subunits of complex IV (Kuhn-Nentwig & Kadenbach 1985).

A benign infantile mitochondrial myopathy associated with a reversible deficiency of cytochrome c oxidase has now been recognised. The disorder presents in the neonatal period with profound weakness of all but the extraocular muscles, hyporeflexia, hepatoglossomegaly and severe lactacidaemia. Muscle specimens contain mild glycogen but marked lipid and mitochondrial excess. Spontaneous improvement begins after six months of age and only mild weakness is present after the age of two years. The clinical recovery is associated with a return of biochemically and enzyme cytochemically detectable cytochrome c oxidase activity. However, immunoreactivity for complex IV (with polyclonal antibody) is present at all ages (DiMauro et al 1983b, 1985). This disorder resembles, clinically and morphologically, the mitochondria–lipid–glycogen myopathy described by Jerusalem and co-workers in 1973. A plausible explanation of the regressive character of this syndrome would be that an abnormal fetal subunit of complex IV is replaced by a normal adult-type subunit during infancy (Kuhn-Nentwig & Kadenbach 1985).

Cytochrome c oxidase deficiency associated with a partial deficiency of the pyruvate dehydrogenase complex was reported by Monnens et al (1975) in an eight-year-old patient with diffuse muscle weakness, nerve deafness, reduced visual acuity and chronic lactic acidaemia. Serum alanine levels were raised. This disorder appears to be clinically and genetically different from that described by Van Biervliet et al (1977).

Cytochrome c oxidase deficiency was also reported in Leigh's disease (subacute necrotising encephalomyelopathy) (Willems et al 1977). The patient had recurrent vomiting, hypotonia, motor and mental retardation and ataxia since infancy and died at the age of six years of respiratory failure. Serum pyruvate and lactate levels were slightly increased. The enzyme defect was observed in muscle but not in liver. Partial enzyme deficiency was noted in heart. Skeletal muscle mitochondria were structurally abnormal. Cytochrome c oxidase deficiency in muscle, liver, brain and fibroblasts was described in two sibs whose clinical course and neuropathological findings were consistent with Leigh's disease (Miyabayashi et al 1983). Defects involving thiamine metabolism, pyruvate carboxylase and pyruvate dehydrogenase had been previously reported in different cases of Leigh's disease (reviewed by Willems et al 1977).

A deficiency of terminal mitochondrial respiration due to decreased levels of cytochrome a + a_3 in muscle, liver and heart has been reported in trichopoliodystrophy (Menkes' disease) (French et al 1972). However, in two other cases of Menkes' disease, DiMauro et al (1985) have found normal or only slightly decreased cytochrome c oxidase activity in muscle although there was a marked decrease in enzyme activity in brain. This disorder may be related to maldistribution of body copper (Danks et al 1972). The clinical features include sparse, coarse, stiff hair with twisted, beaded and fragile shafts, microcephaly, micrognathia, developmental regression and muscle hypotonia.

Defects in cytochromes c_1, c, b and aa_3 associated with mild muscle carnitine deficiency, mitochondrial myopathy and cardiomyopathy were described in an infant by Barth et al 1983. Similar abnormalities in the cytochrome system were noted by Neustein et al (1979) in a patient with mitochondrial myopathy and cardiomyopathy. The inheritance in these patients was X-linked recessive.

Histochemical lack of cytochrome oxidase reactivity in isolated muscle fibres has been described in some patients with progressive external ophthalmoplegia (Johnson et al 1983, Müller-

Höcker et al 1983a). This interesting observation will need to be correlated with appropriate biochemical and immunocytochemical studies of complex IV and other respiratory chain enzymes.

Miscellaneous syndromes of unknown aetiology associated with mitochondrial myopathy and lactic acidaemia

Rawles & Weller (1974) observed excessive fatiguability, slight generalised weakness, sideroblastic anaemia, congestive heart failure and lactic acidaemia in a 19-year-old man with symptoms persisting since he was 12 years old. The patient's father had asymptomatic lactic acidaemia. Sengers et al (1975) described congenital cataracts, mitochondrial myopathy, obstructive cardiomyopathy and exercise-induced lactic acidaemia in a 14-year-old boy with symptoms from the age of eight years.

Kearns–Sayre syndrome. The syndrome described by Kearns & Sayre (1958) was that of retinitis pigmentosa, heart block and external ophthalmoplegia. In 1977 Bolthauser et al found a wider spectrum of abnormalities in the 60 cases published since 1958: increased spinal fluid protein in 66%; ataxia, hearing loss and short stature in 66, 57 and 53%; muscle weakness and mental changes in 40%; corticospinal tract signs in 17%; and hypogonadism and diabetes in 21 and 14%, respectively. The findings of Berenberg et al (1977) were similar. The onset is before the age of 15 years. Morphological abnormalities in mitochondria in many organs and increased serum and spinal fluid lactate and pyruvate levels suggest mitochondrial dysfunction (Lou & Reske-Nielsen 1976, Shy et al 1967, Karpati et al 1973, Schneck et al 1973, Kuriyama et al 1984a, Ogasahara et al 1986). It is noteworthy that in this syndrome there are no acute episodes involving the central nervous system and the family history is typically negative (DiMauro et al 1985). Ogasahara et al (1986) reported an increase in mitochondrial protein but a decrease in the specific activity of respiratory chain enzymes in muscle, and a decrease in coenzyme Q levels in muscle and serum. Prolonged treatment with 120–150 mg coenzyme Q_{10} per day improved mitochondrial respiration in muscle, cardiac conduction and the neurological symptoms, and decreased the spinal fluid protein content.

Myoclonus, generalised seizures, cerebellar syndrome, mitochondrial myopathy and lactacidaemia. This syndrome has been repeatedly described. It is frequently associated with short stature, dementia, hearing loss, and optic atrophy; less commonly it occurs with spasticity, central hypoventilation, endocrine abnormalities and peripheral neuropathy (Tsairis et al 1973, Fukuhara et al 1980, Fitzsimmons et al 1981, Roger et al 1982, Feit et al 1982, Holliday et al 1983, Sasaki et al 1983, Nakano et al 1982, Riggs et al 1984, Kuriyama et al 1984b, Rosing et al 1985). Early development is normal. The symptoms present in childhood or adult life. The family history is often positive and, in at least one large kinship, there was evidence for maternal mitochondrial inheritance (Rosing et al 1985). The clinical boundaries of the syndrome are not entirely distinct. Myoclonus, cerebellar ataxia and seizures are elements of the Ramsay–Hunt syndrome. A fluctuating clinical course, cortical lesions resembling infarctions but not corresponding to the territories of main blood vessels and basal ganglia calcifications, all features of MELAS (see below), were also present in the patient reported by Kuriyama et al (1984b). The biochemical basis of the syndrome is also unclear. In most cases reported under the rubric of myoclonus epilepsy with ragged red fibres, mitochondrial metabolism has not been thoroughly investigated. In some cases the findings are similar to those noted with complex I deficiency (Holliday et al 1983, Petty et al 1986) or complex III deficiency (Morgan-Hughes et al 1982), and in one of two affected sibs the findings suggested complex II deficiency (Riggs et al 1984).

Mitochondrial myopathy, encephalopathy, lactic acidosis and stroke-like episodes (MELAS). The main distinction between this syndrome and the preceding one is the occurrence of stroke-like episodes associated with intermittent vomiting (Pavlakis et al 1984). Areas of encephalomalacia not in the territories of the main blood vessels and of low density on the computerised tomogram appear during the acute episodes. Other associated features include limb weakness, small stature, seizures, hearing loss, progressive dementia, macular degeneration and ferrocalcific deposits in the basal ganglia. Early development is normal and the family history is often positive (Shapira et al 1975, Hart et al 1977, Askanas et al 1978, Skoglund 1979, Yamamoto et al 1984, Pavlakis et al 1984). The clinical boundaries of this syndrome are also uncertain, e.g. the patient studied by Kuriyama et al (1984b) could fit in this group or the preceding one. Mitochondrial metabolism has not been thoroughly investigated in most cases of MELAS. Of the four patients in whom respiratory chain enzymes were studied, two had partial deficiencies of cytochrome c oxidase (49 and 67% of the control mean); one had a lower than normal (36% of the control mean) activity of succinate-cytochrome c reductase; and one of these patients also had muscle carnitine deficiency (Pavlakis et al 1984). Two patients were treated with prednisone. This improved the central nervous system symptoms and fatiguability and reduced the lactacidaemia and serum CK activity (Shapira et al 1975, Skoglund et al 1979).

MALIGNANT HYPERTHERMIA

Since its recognition (Denborough & Lovell 1960), this syndrome has aroused great interest among anaesthetists. The current status of the disorder is summarised in reviews by Stephen (1977), Britt (1979), Harriman (1979) and Gronert (1980, 1986). In most cases, susceptibility to the disorder is thought to be transmitted by autosomal dominant inheritance with variable penetrance. The reaction is triggered by potent inhalation anaesthetics (halothane, ether, cyclopropane, methoxyflurane, enflurane) or succinylcholine. Premonitory signs include tachycardia, tachypnoea, dysrhythmias, skin mottling, cyanosis, rising body temperature, muscle rigidity, sweating and unstable blood pressure. Failure to obtain muscle relaxation with adequate doses of succinylcholine can also be an early warning sign. The fully developed syndrome is associated with a rapid rise of body temperature (up to 1 °C every 5 min); rapidly evolving metabolic acidosis with lactic acidaemia; often, also, respiratory acidosis due to carbon dioxide overproduction; muscle rigidity in 75% of the cases; hyperkalaemia; variable alterations of the serum calcium; very high serum CK activity; myoglobinaemia and myoglobinuria. Despite wide awareness of the syndrome and symptomatic therapy, and the mortality rate remains high.

The postulated pathophysiological factor is a failure of calcium homeostasis in the muscle fibre. Cytoplasmic calcium concentration may increase because of abnormal calcium release from the sarcoplasmic reticulum or possibly because the muscle fibre plasma membrane is rendered abnormally permeable to calcium by provocative agents. A high intracellular calcium level activates phosphorylase b kinase and myosin ATPase, inhibits troponin and overloads mitochondria with calcium. These events, in turn, cause accelerated glycogenolysis and glycolysis, ATP splitting, uncontrolled muscle contraction, uncoupling of oxidative phosphorylation and excessive production of heat, lactic acid and carbon dioxide. An animal model of the disease has been described and investigated in Landrace or Poland China pigs (Hall et al 1966, Gronert 1980). The idea that intracellular calcium homeostasis is lost during the attacks is now supported by studies of mitochondrial calcium uptake in susceptible pigs (Stadhouders et al 1984) and by an increase of ionised calcium in muscles of susceptible humans between attacks (Lopez et al 1985).

Treatment of the acute syndrome consists of termination of anaesthesia, body cooling, intravenous hydration, sodium bicarbonate administration to combat metabolic acidosis, mechanical hyperventilation to decrease the respiratory acidosis, and mannitol or frusemide, as needed, to maintain urine flow. More specific treatment consists of dantrolene, given intravenously, 1–2 mg/kg, which may be repeated each 5–10 min, up to 10 mg/kg (Faust et al 1979, Gronert 1980).

Screening of relatives of affected patients for susceptibility to malignant hyperthermia is important. 70% of the cases at risk have increased serum CK activities (Britt et al 1976). Without this finding, in vitro testing of muscle strips for an abnormal contracture response to halothane, caffeine or a combination of both agents can be done. The technique and interpretation of the test are not fully standardised, but the test has been valuable in detecting patients at risk (reviewed by Gronert 1980, 1986).

An association of malignant hyperthermia with myotonic dystrophy or myotonia congenita (King et al 1972), branchial hypertrophic myopathy (Lambert & Young 1976) and central core disease (Denborough et al 1973, Eng et al 1978), has been reported. It is not yet known what proportion of patients with these disorders is, in fact, at risk. The disease can also occur in a congenital myopathy associated with short stature, cryptochordism and skeletal abnormalities which is transmitted by autosomal recessive inheritance (King et al 1972). Muscle biopsy studies by Harriman (1979) in 105 patients revealed a number of mild and non-specific myopathic changes in two-thirds; increased central nuclei, small angulated fibres, focal decreases in oxidative enzyme activity, focal myofibrillar alterations and, rarely, regenerating fibres. Typical central cores, spanning the entire fibre length, were not observed. No myopathic changes were seen in children under the age of five years. However, there is now good evidence that central core disease and Duchenne dystrophy sometimes involve susceptibity to malignant hyperthermia (Frank et al 1980, Gronert 1986).

MUSCLE AMP DEAMINASE DEFICIENCY

AMP deaminase (EC 3.5.4.6) converts AMP to IMP with liberation of ammonia. The biological role of the enzyme is not understood; possibly it participates in regulation of ATP levels in muscle. In 1978, Fishbein et al found deficiency of the muscle enzyme in five young men with complaints, often since childhood, of muscle weakness or cramping after exercise. Three patients had mild increases in serum CK and two had abnormal EMGs. Muscle histology was normal except for mild type I fibre atrophy in one case. Erythrocyte enzyme activity was normal. Ammonia levels failed to rise but lactate values rose normally in venous blood flowing from ischaemically exercised muscles. Muscle AMP deaminase deficiency had also been reported in a single case of primary hypokalaemic periodic paralysis (Engel et al 1964). Fishbein (1985, 1986) now distinguishes between inherited and acquired forms of AMP deaminase deficiency. The primary deficiency is transmitted by autosomal recessive inheritance and may or may not manifest clinically in adult life with muscle cramping and exercise intolerance. The prognosis is benign. The secondary type, in which residual enzyme activity is higher (1–10%) than in the primary type, can occur in a variety of neurogenic and myopathic disorders. In view of the marked clinical heterogeneity, the significance of muscle AMP deaminase deficiency remains uncertain.

NUTRITIONAL AND TOXIC MYOPATHIES

Nutritional deficiencies

Although malnutrition is common in many parts of the world, its effects on skeletal muscle have not been thoroughly investigated. The negative nitrogen balance and lack of essential nutrients can be expected to cause muscle weakness and wasting, but their relative significance is not clearly understood.

Vitamin E deficiency has now been shown to cause a disorder associated with progressive gait and limb ataxia, sensorimotor neuropathy, extra-ocular muscle paresis, and a myopathy in which giant abnormal lysosomes accumulate in muscle. The cause is a malabsorption syndrome, as in chronic cholestasis or with cystic fibrosis of the pancreas (Blanc et al 1958, Tomasi 1979, Burck et al 1981, Neville et al 1983, Werlin et al 1983). The patient with giant lysosomes in muscle, peripheral neuropathy and hyperparathyroidism studied by Gomez et al (1972) was also subsequently shown to have vitamin E deficiency (M. R. Gomez & A. G. Engel, unpublished observations). Malabsorption of vitamin E also occurs in abetalipoproteinaemia and treatment with high doses of vitamin E arrests the neuropathy and myopathy in this disease (Hegele & Angel 1985).

The muscle weakness in nutritional osteo-

malacia has been attributed partly to disuse and partly to malnutrition (Dastur et al 1975). The myopathy of osteomalacia is discussed together with the myopathy of hyperparathyroidism (p. 849).

Myopathy in chronic alcoholism

Alcohol may have a direct toxic effect on muscle, or its effects can be mediated by malnutrition and fluid and electrolyte disturbances. Song & Rubin (1972) found that ingestion of ethanol (42% of calories) without malnutrition induced increased serum CK activity and non-specific ultrastructural changes in muscle in human volunteers. In ethanol-fed rats, mitochondria show reduced ability to oxidise various substrates, energy production with NAD-dependent substrates, calcium uptake, activity of several enzymes and cytochrome content. These effects may be mediated by acetaldehyde rather than ethanol (Cederbaum & Rubin 1975).

Two types of clinically distinct myopathy, acute and subacute, have been described in chronic alcoholics. The acute type (Hed et al 1962) occurs after a bout of acute drinking. In these patients, muscle swelling and tenderness are associated with weakness and myoglobinuria. Hyperkalaemia and renal insufficiency develop in the more severely affected. A painless variety of acute alcoholic myopathy associated with severe hypokalaemia, marked serum CK elevation, vacuolar myopathy and focal fibre necrosis has been also described (Rubenstein & Wainapel 1977). The hypokalaemia may be secondary to the combined effects of sweating, vomiting, diarrhoea or renal potassium wastage. The hypokalaemia may be followed by hyperkalaemia as rhabdomyolysis, myoglobinuria and secondary renal failure develop. Histochemical studies in acute alcoholic myopathy reveal focal decreases in oxidative enzyme activity in type I muscle fibres and in necrotic fibres. Ultrastructural changes occur in mitochondria, but some of these changes are secondary to fibre necrosis (Martinez et al 1973). Other causes of severe hypokalaemia can also produce a necrotising myopathy (reviewed by Victor 1986). The subacute alcoholic myopathy described by Ekbom et al (1964) is associated with symmetrical proximal weakness with little loss of muscle bulk, EMG changes and increased serum levels of muscle enzymes. In some alcoholics, serum enzyme and EMG abnormalities occur without muscle weakness. However, Faris & Reyes (1971) suggest that the sub-clinical group is neuropathic rather than myopathic. Alternatively, a chronic, mild neuropathy can exist in alcoholics who also develop a myopathy. The subacute syndrome is reversible within a few months of alcohol withdrawal.

Perkoff et al (1966) drew attention to impaired production of lactate by ischaemically exercised muscle in chronic alcoholics within 48 hours after intoxication. Muscle phosphorylase activity was reduced or low normal in six of seven biopsies. Muscle symptoms, when present, resembled those of phosphorylase deficiency. For an extensive review of acute and chronic alcoholic myopathy the reader is referred to Victor (1986).

Chloroquine myopathy

This quinoline derivative, introduced as an anti-malarial drug but useful in the treatment of amoe-biasis and certain collagen-vascular diseases, causes undesirable side effects involving the macula, cornea, skeletal muscle and peripheral nerves. The first cases of myopathy were described by Whisnant et al (1963). Most of those patients who became weak during chloroquine treatment received 500 mg of the drug per day for a year or longer. Pathologically, it is a vacuolar myopathy mainly affecting type I fibres (Garcin et al 1964, MacDonald & Engel 1970, Hughes et al 1971). The vacuoles contain cytoplasmic degra-dation products and are autophagic in character. In an experimental study, MacDonald & Engel (1970) found that the initial ultrastructural change was a proliferation of the internal membrane system (both T system and SR) and the encircle-ment of small cytoplasmic areas. Larger vacuoles arose by fusion of smaller ones. The entrapped membranous organelles were degraded by myeloid structures. The limiting membranes of the vacuoles were derived from tubules and labyrin-thine networks of T-system origin, and the degraded vacuolar contents reacted strongly for acid phosphatase. Exocytosis of vacuolar contents and frequent fibre splitting occurred after other pathological changes were well established. Chlor-oquine myopathy is a prototype for those muscle disorders in which an autophagic mechanism becomes excited.

Emetine myopathy

Emetine, an ipecac alkaloid used in the treatment of amoebiasis, inhibits protein synthesis in many cell types (Grollman 1968). Side effects include cardiotoxicity and muscle weakness (Klatskin & Friedman 1948). In experimental animals the drug induces focal decreases in muscle mitochondria, associated with focal myofibrillar degeneration in type I fibres (Duane & Engel 1970). The lesions in type I fibres resemble those observed in multi-core disease (Engel et al 1971). More advanced pathological changes induced by emetine include muscle fibre necrosis (Bradley et al 1976). A reversible myopathy has been observed in patients with major eating disorders who abuse ipecac to induce vomiting (Mateer et al 1985, Palmer & Guay 1985) and in chronic alcoholics receiving emetine (about 500 mg over 11–14 days) for aver-sion therapy (Sugie et al 1984). The pathological findings resembled those described in exper-imental animals.

DISEASES ASSOCIATED WITH MYOGLOBINURIA

Myoglobin is a 17 000 dalton protein with a pros-thetic haem group and the muscle concentration is about 1 mg/g (Kagen & Christian 1966). The appearance of myoglobin in the urine is both an indication of severe and acute muscle injury, and a warning that renal damage may result. Any injury to muscle fibres which abnormally increases the permeability or disrupts the integrity of the surface membrane entails leakage of myoglobin into the plasma. The renal threshhold for myoglobin is relatively low (Koskelo et al 1967) but massive and relatively synchronous injury to muscle (rhabdomyolysis) is required before brown discoloration of urine, caused by myoglobin plus metmyoglobin, is observed. The urinary pigment reacts positively with benzidine. If there is no haemoglobinaemia and no haematuria, the test strongly suggests myoglobinuria. However, microhaematuria can also develop with myoglobinuria. Positive identification of myoglobin requires specific chemical, spectrophotometric or immunological tests. The last are the most sensitive and the immunoprecipitation assay is both quantitative and simple (Markowitz & Wobig 1977).

Acute attacks of myoglobinuria are characterised by the onset, over a few hours, of muscle weakness, swelling and pain. In addition to myoglobin, phosphate, potassium, creatine, creatinine and muscle enzymes are released into the circulation. The haem pigment in the glomerular filtrate and myoglobin casts in renal tubules may cause proteinuria, haematuria and renal tubular necrosis. Renal failure is more likely if the attack is complicated by hypovolaemia, hypotension or metabolic acidosis. With increasing renal insufficiency, hyperphosphataemia with secondary hypocalcaemia and tetany, and life-threatening hyperkalaemia may develop (Hed 1955, Bowden et al 1956, Pearson et al 1957, Savage et al 1971, Rowland & Penn 1972, Penn 1986). Death can result from renal or respiratory failure. If the patient survives, the myoglobinuria and proteinuria tend to disappear by the third to fifth day after the onset of the attack; marked hyperenzymaemia, present initially, subsides more gradually; muscle strength returns relatively slowly after major attacks. EMG abnormalities (fibrillation potentials, increased insertional activity and motor unit potential alterations) may persist for several months after severe attacks (Haase & Engel 1960).

The syndrome has many known causes but in many cases the aetiology remains elusive. The immediate biochemical mechanism which disrupts the plasma membrane remains to be determined. For descriptive purposes, it is convenient to classify the syndrome as metabolic, post-infectious, toxic, ischaemic and/or traumatic, secondary to inflammatory or other myopathies, and idiopathic.

Metabolic. The common denominator is impaired substrate utilisation for energy metabolism, or a critical substrate deficiency in the face of excessive demands for energy. Most diseases in this group were considered earlier in this chapter.

Phosphorylase, phosphofructokinase, phosphoglycerate kinase, phosphoglycerate mutase, and lactate dehydrogenase deficiencies block anaerobic glycolysis, and carnitine palmityltransferase deficiency impairs oxidation of long-chain fatty acids. Rare instances of muscle carnitine deficiency may also be associated with myoglobinuria (W. K. Engel et al 1980). Impaired utilisation of fatty acids probably played a part in the recurrent myoglobinuria of the twin sisters who had a lipid storage myopathy due to an unknown biochemical defect (Engel et al 1970).

Critical substrate deficiency in the face of excessive demands for energy probably accounts for the myoglobinuria which occurs in malignant hyperthermia. Substrate deficiency may also cause the myoglobinuria which occurs after unusually severe exercise in untrained but otherwise healthy individuals, as in military recruits (Demos et al 1974) or conga drummers (Furie & Penn 1974).

Myoglobinuria also occurs with marked muscle rigidity and hyperthermia in the malignant neuroleptic syndrome (Guzé & Baxter 1985) and in some patients with parkinsonism when drug therapy is abruptly withdrawn (Friedman et al 1985).

Post-infectious. Myoglobinuria has been reported after infections with influenza A, herpes simplex, Epstein-Barr and Coxsackie viruses (Simon et al 1970, DiBona & Morens 1977, Schlesinger et al 1978). Virus-like structures have been demonstrated by electron microscopy in affected muscle by Fukuyama et al (1977) and by Gamboa et al (1979). The latter workers were also able to isolate influenza B virus from muscle of a patient who had a fatal attack. The muscle biopsy in this individual showed inflammatory changes as well as perifascicular atrophy. The precise mechanism by which viral infections cause rhabdomyolysis is not understood. Myoglobinuria can also occur with bacterial infections accompanied by high fever and sepsis and with muscle gangrene caused by clostridial infection (Penn 1986).

Toxic. Myoglobinuria complicating chronic alcoholism was considered above. Almost any other extreme metabolic insult may produce it. These include carbon monoxide poisoning, extreme hypoglycaemia, severe hypokalaemia, hypernatraemia or water intoxication, diabetic acidosis, barbiturate, narcotic and amphetamine intoxication and uraemic hyperparathyroidism (reviewed by Penn 1986). In Haff's disease the eating of fish contaminated by an unidentified toxin induced an epidemic of myoglobinuria along the Baltic coast (Berlin 1948). In Malayan waters, fisherman bitten by the sea snake *Enhydrina schistosa* develop myalgias, flaccid paralysis, trismus and myoglobinuria (Reid 1961).

Ischaemic and traumatic. Prolonged massive ischaemia of muscle from whatever cause results in necrosis of muscle fibres and can induce myoglobinuria and renal failure (Bywaters et al 1941, Bywaters & Stead 1945). Localised ischaemic necrosis of muscle and occasionally myoglobinuria may occur in severe forms of the anterior tibial syndrome.

Secondary to other myopathies. Myoglobinuria has been described in dermatomyositis (Kessler et al 1972), and in fulminant polymyositis (Fukuyama et al 1977, Sloan et al 1978, Gamboa et al 1979). In some such patients, the myoglobinuria could have been related to a concurrent or underlying viral infection (Fukuyama et al 1977, Gamboa et al 1979). Recurrent myoglobinuria was observed by the author in one patient with classic systemic lupus erythematosus. Finally, anaesthesia-induced myoglobinuria without rigidity or hyperthermia was reported in a patient with Duchenne dystrophy (Miller et al 1978).

Idiopathic. It is likely that at least some cases initially classified as idiopathic will eventually be shown to have a metabolic or post-infectious aetiology.

ENDOCRINE DISORDERS OF MUSCLE

Muscle disorders associated with hyperthyroidism

Some of these disorders are a direct consequence of the endocrinopathy: others occur more often with thyroid dysfunction than predicted by chance and may or may not be affected by the altered endocrine state. Thyrotoxic myopathy, thyrotoxic hypokalaemic periodic paralysis, myasthenia gravis and exophthalmic ophthalmoplegia are the currently recognised neuromuscular diseases associated with hyperthyroidism. Thyrotoxic hypokalaemic periodic paralysis was considered above.

Thyrotoxic myopathy. Both acute and chronic forms have been described but it is doubtful that the rare acute type exists as a distinct entity. More likely, it represents cases of acute myasthenia gravis associated with severe thyrotoxicosis (Millikan & Haines 1953).

Muscle weakness occurs in about 80% of untreated cases of hyperthyroidism (Ramsay 1965). Men are affected more often than women and the average duration of muscle symptoms before diagnosis is about six months. Proximal muscle weakness is present in about two-thirds, and both proximal and distal muscle weakness in another one-fifth of the cases. The thyrotoxicosis is relatively mild and of long duration, or present for only a few weeks before the onset of weakness. The weakness is often out of proportion to visible muscle atrophy, although severe atrophy can occur. The deep tendon reflexes are usually normal or hyperactive, only seldom decreased or absent. The serum CK is not increased as a rule (in contrast to myxoedema in which it is usually increased, but weakness is uncommon) (Ramsay 1965, 1968, Fleisher et al 1965). EMG abnormalities are found in about 90% of patients with hyperthyroidism (Havard et al 1963, Ramsay 1965). These abnormalities consist of a decrease in the mean duration of motor unit potentials and an increase in the incidence of polyphasic potentials. Spontaneous electrical activity (fibrillation potentials, fasciculation, or repetitive discharges) is absent as a rule. After correction of the hyperthyroidism, the EMG reverts to normal.

Light-microscopic studies of muscle may show no abnormality or varying degrees of fatty infiltration and fibre atrophy. Ultrastructural studies have revealed mitochondrial hypertrophy; focal loss of mitochondria from muscle fibres; focal myofibrillar degeneration beginning at the Z disc; focal dilatations of the transverse tubular system; sub-sarcolemmal glycogen deposits; and papillary projections of the surface of the muscle fibres, probably resulting from fibre atrophy (Engel 1966b, 1972). None of the ultrastructural changes are specific for thyrotoxic myopathy.

The mechanism of the muscle weakness remains obscure. Physiological investigations have demonstrated shortening of the duration of the active state (Takamori et al 1971) and reduced surface membrane excitability (Gruener et al 1975). The latter is associated with lower than normal resting membrane potential, and impaired action potential generation on repetitive stimulation secondary to membrane depolarisation and marked after-hyperpolarisation. Biochemical studies have demonstrated a significant decrease in high-energy phosphate compounds in muscle (Satoyoshi et al 1963). The original notion that oxidative phosphorylation was uncoupled by the hyperthyroid state was not substantiated by Ernster et al (1959). Further, Stocker et al (1968) found that mitochondria from human thyrotoxic muscle were tightly coupled and had normal respiratory control rates. Other possible causes of the weakness might be related to accelerated protein degradation (Yates et al 1981), an abnormally active plasma membrane sodium pump, attributed to an increased number of pump units in the membrane (Philipson & Edelman 1977), or to an increased number of catecholamine receptor sites in the muscle cell membrane (Williams et al 1977, Tsai & Chen 1977). It seems probable that muscle weakness in thyrotoxic myopathy results from several different effects rather than from a single action of thyroxine.

Thyroid dysfunction and myasthenia gravis. Incidence of thyroid disorders is much greater in patients with myasthenia gravis than could occur by chance: 5.7% of myasthenic patients are hyperthyroid, 5.3% hypothyroid and 2.1% have non-toxic goitre. Further, about 17% of euthyroid and 40% of thyrotoxic myasthenic patients have circulating antibodies directed against thyroid cell antigens (Osserman et al 1967). The association of the two diseases is not surprising for both are now recognised to be of autoimmune origin. Careful case studies (Millikan & Haines 1953) and the experimental induction of hyperthyroidism in myasthenic patients (Engel 1961) show that the

hyperthyroidism has an adverse effect on the myasthenia. A plausible explanation for this was adduced by Hofmann & Denys (1972) who found a decrease in the size of miniature end-plate potentials in hyperthyroid animals.

Myasthenia gravis seldom occurs with spontaneous myxoedema but 19% of myasthenic patients, compared with less than 1% of the general population, have evidence of thyroiditis at autopsy (Becker et al 1964).

Exophthalmic ophthalmoplegia (Graves' ophthalmopathy). This aspect of Graves' disease may pursue a course independent of the metabolic state. Hyperthyroidism was present in 23 of 50 cases studied by Brain (1959) and in nine there was no history or evidence of thyrotoxicosis. The immediate cause of the exophthalmos is an increase in orbital contents with infiltration of external ocular muscles, lacrimal glands and loose connective tissue. The orbital exudate is composed of lymphocytes, plasma cells, polymorphonuclear leucocytes and a fluid rich in mucoproteins and mucopolysaccharides. The infiltration and subsequent atrophy of ocular muscles results in weakness of ocular movements. The two main symptoms are exophthalmos, usually painful, of one or both eyes and diplopia. Levators and abductors of the globe are most often affected, and ptosis sometimes occurs. The ophthalmoplegia tends to be proportionate to the exophthalmos. This varies in degree and when severe can be associated with chemosis and marked eyelid oedema. Corneal ulceration, papilloedema, optic atrophy and blindness may ensue.

The pathogenesis is complex (Havard 1972). Recent evidence supports the assumption that it involves a delayed hypersensitivity response directed against orbital contents. Thyroglobulin can be detected on normal human orbital muscle. Antibodies directed against this protein may instigate a cell-mediated immune reaction, since patients with Graves' ophthalmopathy consistently demonstrate delayed hypersensitivity to thyroglobulin (Mullin et al 1977).

The disease is initially subacute but tends to be self-limiting. Therapy is mandatory when there is a threat to vision. Prednisone treatment, with or without azathioprine, irradiation of orbital contents behind the lens and surgical decompression of the orbit represent current modes of therapy. Full recovery is rare and some degree of exophthalmos usually remains. Residual diplopia may require operative treatment (Dresner & Kennerdell 1985).

Muscular disorders in hypothyroidism

The main manifestations of the various types of muscle disorder described in hypothyroidism are weakness, cramps, aching or painful muscles, sluggish movements and reflexes, myoidema (i.e. ridging of muscle on percussion) and in some an increase in muscle bulk. The reflex changes are seen in most cases, myoidema and myalgia are less common and weakness occurs in but a few. The serum CK activity is typically elevated even if there are no other clinical symptoms of muscle involvement (Fleisher et al 1965). Electrical recording of the slow contraction and relaxation of the tendon reflex (Lambert et al 1951) and of the myoidema (Salick & Pearson 1967) would suggest that it is the contractile mechanism of the muscle that is predominantly involved. It seems possible that many enzyme systems are affected, the pattern of involvement determining the clinical type. There is some evidence to suggest impaired glycogenolysis (reduced acid maltase levels in muscle and impaired lactic acid formation on ischaemic exercise) (McDaniel et al 1977).

Muscle hypertrophy, with weakness and slowness of movement, constitute the syndrome of Debré–Semelaigne (Debré & Semelaigne 1935) which occurs predominantly in cretinous children; when accompanied by painful spasms it is given the name of Hoffmann's syndrome and is then seen in myxoedematous adults. However, the two conditions tend to merge into each other and may even occur, although at different times, in the same patient (Wilson & Walton 1959, Norris & Panner 1966). Slow relaxation and myoidema are prominent features of Hoffmann's syndrome; superficially, therefore, it resembles myotonia congenita or the very rare cases of true myotonia associated with myxoedema, either iatrogenic or resulting from disease. In the two patients reported by Jarcho & Tyler (1958) the myxoedema probably exacerbated a pre-existing mild myotonia,

because symptomless myotonia was demonstrated in some relatives. The occasional association of a girdle myopathy causing mild proximal weakness and atrophy has been described by Åström et al (1961). Morphological studies reveal non-specific alterations in hypothyroid myopathy. These include fibre enlargement, increased central nuclei, glycogen and mitochondrial aggregates, dilated SR and proliferating T-system profiles, and focal myofibrillar degeneration (Norris & Panner, 1966, Afifi et al 1974, Emser & Schimrigk 1977). The muscle disorders respond favourably to therapy of the hypothyroid state.

Muscle disorders associated with hyperparathyroidism and with osteomalacia

Parathormone and biologically active forms of vitamin D are important regulators of calcium metabolism and of the serum calcium level. Parathormone mobilises calcium from bone, increases the reabsorption of calcium and excretion of phosphate by the kidney, and stimulates the renal conversion of 25-hydroxycholecalciferol to 1,25-dihydroxycholecalciferol, a highly potent form of vitamin D. Biologically active vitamin D promotes intestinal calcium absorption and facilitates mineralisation of osteoid and of newly formed enchondral bone (Haussler & McCain 1977, Habener & Potts 1978). Studies in vitamin D-deficient animals also suggest that vitamin D has a direct effect on muscle in augmenting SR and mitochondrial calcium uptake, protein synthesis, ATP stores and force generation (Curry et al 1974, Birge & Haddad 1975, Pleasure et al 1979).

Muscle weakness can occur in primary and secondary hyperparathyroidism and in osteomalacia. Further, conditions that lead to osteomalacia, such as vitamin D deficiency, renal tubular acidosis or chronic renal failure, are also typically associated with secondary hyperparathyroidism. Vicale in 1949 observed a distinctive syndrome in two cases of primary hyperparathyroidism and in one case of renal tubular acidosis. It was characterised by symmetrical weakness and fatiguability involving especially the proximal muscles, pain on muscular effort, slow, waddling gait, muscle atrophy, creatinuria, weight loss, hyperactive deep tendon reflexes, guarding against passive movement of limbs and tenderness of bone. The EMG showed no fibrillations or fasciculations. Subsequent reports confirmed the existence of the syndrome in both primary hyperparathyroidism and in osteomalacia (Murphy et al 1960, Bischoff & Esslen 1965, Prineas et al 1965, Smith & Stern 1967, Frame et al 1968, Cholod et al 1970, Schott & Wills 1975). The serum alkaline phosphatase level is usually raised; the serum calcium is typically increased in primary hyperparathyroidism but is low or normal in osteomalacia; the serum phosphate tends to be low, except in the presence of chronic renal failure.

Muscle biopsy studies have revealed simple atrophy (Bischoff & Esslen 1965), minimal vacuolar change (Cholod et al 1970), type II fibre atrophy and changes which might suggest mild denervation atrophy (Patten et al 1974, Mallette et al 1975). The latter works speculate that the muscle involvement in both primary and secondary hyperparathyroidism is neuropathic.

A clearly myopathic and highly malignant syndrome may occur in uraemic hyperparathyroidism. Here, metastatic calcification of vessel walls is associated with intimal proliferation, causing ischaemia of tissues. This results in gangrenous skin lesions arising on ulcerating areas of livedo reticularis, a necrotising myopathy with hyperenzymaemia, myoglobinuria, and visceral infarcts (Richardson et al 1969, Goodhue et al 1972).

Therapy of the various syndromes is directed at removal of the primary cause. When this is not possible, as in chronic renal failure with secondary hyperparathyroidism, long-term treatment with small doses of 1,25-dihydroxycholecalciferol, or its analogue, 1-α- hydroxycholecalciferol, can improve the bone disease and increase muscle strength (Henderson et al 1974, Davie et al 1976).

Myopathy associated with hypoparathyroidism

This endocrine disorder is not definitely known to be associated with a myopathy. Increased serum CK activity, but normal muscle histology, has been observed in a few cases by Hower & Struck (1972) and by Shane et al (1980). Cape (1969) found histochemical deficiency of phosphorylase *a*, but not of phosphorylase *b*, in a case of pseudohypoparathyroidism.

Diseases of the pituitary and suprarenal

Acromegaly and hypopituitarism. Acromegaly in its earlier stages can cause increased muscle bulk and strength, especially if its onset precedes cessation of growth. Later it results in generalised muscle weakness and wasting. Mastaglia et al (1970) noted mild weakness in six of 11 acromegalics with raised serum CK activity in five. The EMG showed a decrease in the mean duration of motor unit potentials. Muscle biopsy studies revealed segmental fibre degeneration, foci of small round cell infiltration, thickening of capillary basement membranes, variable hypertrophy and atrophy involving either type I or type II fibres, lipofuscin accumulation, large nuclei with prominent nucleoli and prominent Golgi systems (Mastaglia et al 1970, Mastaglia 1973). Pickett et al (1975) found clinical and EMG evidence of myopathy in nine of 17 acromegalics. Carpal tunnel syndrome was a frequent associated finding. They found no abnormalities in muscle biopsies of three patients and no patient had increased serum CK activity. The weakness improved slowly after surgical therapy of the acromegaly.

Idiopathic hypopituitarism in children gives rise to dwarfism and poor muscle development. The reduced mass (when related to age) has been attributed to diminished replication of nuclear DNA (Cheek et al 1966), a process that can be reversed by giving human growth hormone.

Cushing's syndrome and steroid myopathy. Muscle weakness develops in 50–80% of patients suffering from Cushing's syndrome (Plotz et al 1952, Müller & Kugelberg 1959, Golding et al 1961) and can also occur as a complication of glucocorticoid hormone treatment (Golding et al 1961, Perkoff et al 1959, Williams 1959, Byers et al 1962, Coomes 1965, Askari et al 1976). Fluorinated steroids (dexamethasone, triamcinolone) appear to be more pathogenetic for muscle than non-fluorinated ones (prednisone, cortisone) but the latter also cause myopathy in sufficiently high dosages. The lowest dosage which can induce myopathy is not known for any steroid, and considerable individual variation must exist. However, for a given dose of prednisone, women are more susceptible than men (Bunch et al 1980).

The onset of steroid myopathy is usually insidious, but occasionally it can be sudden and accompanied by diffuse myalgia (Askari et al 1976). Muscles of the pelvic girdle are affected earlier and more severely than those of the pectoral girdle. Proximal muscles are typically weaker than distal, but relatively severe weakness of anterior tibial muscles can occur. Normal muscle bulk was found in Cushing's syndrome by Müller & Kugelberg (1959) but muscle atrophy can occur in steroid myopathy (Engel 1966b). EMG studies have not shown a consistent pattern (reviewed by Askari et al 1976) but typically there is no spontaneous electrical activity. The serum CK activity is not increased but creatinuria is constant (Askari et al 1976). The muscle biopsy in Cushing's syndrome shows type II fibre atrophy (Pleasure et al 1970). Many light-microscopic abnormalities have been described in human steroid myopathy (reviewed by Askari et al 1976) but earlier reports, based on paraffin sections, included descriptions of artefacts. Type II fibre atrophy, focal increases and decreases in oxidative enzyme activity and focal myofibrillar degeneration were observed by the author (A.G.E.) in human steroid myopathy. Of these, type II fibre atrophy represents the most consistent finding. Ultrastructural studies demonstrate mitochondrial alterations (proliferation, aggregation, degeneration and disappearance), increased numbers of lipid droplets and sub-sarcolemmal glycogen deposits (Engel 1966b, Afifi et al 1968).

The diagnosis of steroid myopathy poses no problem when the drug is given for diseases which cause no muscle weakness, such as asthma or psoriasis. However, in polymyositis and in other collagen-vascular diseases treated by steroids, weakness may result from the primary diseases as well as the treatment. In such cases, the following favour the diagnosis of steroid myopathy: a temporal relationship between the exacerbation of the weakness and the appearance of other manifestations of hypercortisonism; increased weakness within a few weeks of the time when steroid dosage was raised; absence of spontaneous electrical activity in the EMG; normal serum CK activity but significant creatinuria; and type II fibre atrophy but no inflammation in the muscle biopsy. In practice, the differential diagnosis is difficult because none of the criteria are entirely reliable: high doses of steroids are often started when the primary disease itself becomes more severe, and weakness due to the primary disease and due to steroids can coexist.

The pathogenesis of steroid myopathy is not fully understood. Morphological studies in experimental animals have shown type II fibre atrophy (Vignos & Greene 1973), mitochondrial proliferation followed by mitochondrial disappearance and focal myofibrillar degeneration (Tice & Engel 1967). Electrophysiological studies of rat extensor digitorum longus have revealed decreased resting membrane potentials and reduced membrane excitability which could be prevented by phenytoin treatment (Gruener & Stern 1972). Biochemical studies in rabbits have demonstrated impaired oxidation of different substrates which correlated with the proportion of type II fibres in the muscle studied (Vignos & Greene 1973) but mitochondria isolated from rat hind limbs had normal oxidative respiration (Peter et al 1970). Glucocorticoids also inhibit protein synthesis (Rannels et al 1978, Kelly et al 1986), may accelerate protein degradation (Clark & Vignos 1979), and enhance lysosomal protease activity (Clark & Vignos 1981) in muscle. These effects are greater on type II than type I fibres. Impaired calcium uptake and binding by the SR has been noted in steroid myopathy in humans and rabbits (Shoji et al 1976) but not in rats (Peter et al 1970).

Therapy of steroid myopathy requires withdrawal, if possible, of the offending hormone, or use of the minimum effective dose of a non-fluorinated preparation for control of the primary disease. Muscle strength returns to normal within one to four months of cessation of steroid therapy (Askari et al 1976).

Primary hyperaldosteronism. The periodic

paralysis occurring in this condition was discussed earlier in the chapter.

Myopathy and pigmentation after adrenalectomy for Cushing's syndrome. Prineas et al (1968) reported a series of patients who developed diffuse pigmentation and severe myopathy accompanied by lipid excess in muscle fibres after adrenalectomy for Cushing's syndrome. The pathogenesis remains obscure.

Addison's disease. Generalised weakness is a characteristic feature of Addison's disease. It is closely related to plasma and muscle water and electrolyte changes and possibly to the associated hypotension. When these are adequately treated, the weakness rapidly disappears. Joint contractures, especially of the knees, have been observed in Addison's disease. They may be caused by a disorder of tendon and fascia rather than by a primary disease of muscle (Thorn 1949).

REFERENCES

Afifi A K, Bergman R A, Harvey J C 1968 Steroid myopathy. Clinical, histologic and cytologic observations. Johns Hopkins Medical Journal 123:158

Afifi A K, Ibrahim M Z M, Bergman R A et al 1972 Morphologic features of hypermetabolic mitochondrial disease. A light microscopic, histochemical and electron microscopic study. Journal of the Neurological Sciences 15:271

Afifi A K, Najjar S S, Mire-Salman J, Bergman R A 1974 The myopathy of the Kocher-Debré-Semelaigne syndrome. Electromyography, light and electron-microscopic study. Journal of the Neurological Sciences 22:445

Agamanolis D P, Askari A D, DiMauro S, Hays A, Kumar K, Lipton M, Raynor A 1980 Muscle phosphofructokinase deficiency: Two cases with unusual polysaccharide accumulation and immunologically active enzyme protein. Muscle and Nerve 3:456

Aitken R S, Allott E N, Castleden L I M, Walker M 1937 Observations on a case of familial periodic paralysis. Clinical Science and Molecular Medicine 3:47

Allen R J, Wong P, Rothenberg S P, DiMauro S, Headington J T 1980 Progressive neonatal leukoencephalopathy due to absent methylenetetrahydrofolate reductase, responsive to treatment. Annals of Neurology 8:211 (abst)

Allen R J, DiMauro S, Coulter D L 1983 Kearns-Sayre syndrome (KSS): A possible disorder of folate and carnitine metabolism. Pediatric Research 17:286A (abst)

Allott E N, McArdle 8 1938 Further observations on familial periodic paralysis. Clinical Science and Molecular Medicine 3:229

Andersen D H 1956 Familial cirrhosis of the liver with storage of abnormal glycogen. Laboratory Investigation 5:11

Andersen E D, Krasilnikoff P A, Overvad H 1971 Intermittent muscular weakness, extrasystoles, and multiple developmental anomalies. Acta Paediatrica Scandinavica 60:559

Andres R, Cader G, Zierler K L 1956 The quantitatively minor role of carbohydrate in oxidative metabolism by skeletal muscle in intact man in the basal state. Journal of Clinical Investigation 35:671

Angelini C, Engel A G 1972 Comparative study of acid maltase deficiency. Archives of Neurology 26:344

Angelini C, Engel A G, Titus J L 1972 Adult acid maltase deficiency. Abnormalities in fibroblasts cultured from patients. New England Journal of Medicine 287:948

Angelini C, Lücke S, Cantarutti F 1976 Carnitine deficiency of skeletal muscle: Report of a treated case. Neurology 26:633

Askanas V, Engel W K, DiMauro S, Brooks D R, Mehler M 1976 Adult onset acid maltase deficiency. Morphological and biochemical abnormalities reproduced in cultured muscle. New England Journal of Medicine 294:573

Askanas V, Engel W K, Britton D E, Adornato B T, Eiben R M 1978 Reincarnation in cultured muscle of mitochondrial abnormalities. Two patients with epilepsy and lactic acidosis. Archives of Neurology 35:801

Askanas V, Engel W K, Kwan H H et al 1985 Autosomal dominant syndrome of lipid neuromyopathy with normal carnitine: Successful treatment with long-chain fatty-acid-free diet. Neurology 35:66

Åström K E, Kugelberg E, Muller R 1961 Hypothyroid myopathy. Archives of Neurology 5:472

Atkin J, Snow J W, Zellweger H, Rhead W J 1984 Fatal infantile cardiac glycogenosis without acid maltase deficiency presenting as congenital hydrops. European Journal of Pediatrics 142:150

Badhuin P, Hers H G, Loeb H 1964 An electron microscope and biochemical study of type II glycogenosis. Laboratory Investigation 13:1139

Bank W J, DiMauro S, Bonilla E, Capuzzi D M, Rowland L P 1975 A disorder of muscle lipid metabolism and myoglobinuria. Absence of carnitine palmityl transferase. New England Journal of Medicine 292:443

Barranger J A, Brader R O (eds) 1984 Molecular basis of lysosomal storage disorders. Academic Press, New York

Barth P G, Scholte H R, Berden J A et al 1983 An X-linked mitochondrial disease affecting cardiac muscle, skeletal muscle and neutrophil leucocytes. Journal of the Neurological Sciences 62:327

Becker K L, Titus J H, McConahey W M, Wollner L B 1964 Morphologic evidence of thyroiditis in myasthenia gravis. Journal of the American Medical Association 187:994

Bekeny G 1961 Über irreversible Muskelveränderungen, bei der paroxysmalen Lähmung auf grund bioptischer Muskeluntersuchungen. Deutsche Zeitschrift für Nervenheilkunde 182:119

Bell H, Hayes W L, Vosburgh J 1965 Hyperkalemic paralysis due to adrenal insufficiency. Archives of Internal Medicine 115:418

Benheim P E, Reale E O, Berg B O 1985 β-adrenergic treatment of hyperkalemic periodic paralysis. Neurology 35:746

Beratis N G, Labadie G U, Hirschhorn K 1978
Characterization of the molecular defect in infantile and
adult acid a-glucosidase deficiency in fibroblasts. Journal of
Clinical Investigation 62:1264

Beratis N G, LaBadie G U, Hirschhorn K 1983 Genetic
heterogeneity in acid alpha-glucosidase deficiency.
American Journal of Human Genetics 35:21

Berenberg R A, Pellock J M, DiMauro S et al 1977
Lumping or splitting? 'Ophthalmoplegia plus' or Kearns-
Sayre syndrome? Annals of Neurology 1:37

Bergman R A, Afifi A K, Dunkle L M, Johns R J 1970
Muscle pathology in hypokalemic periodic paralysis with
hyperthyroidism. Bulletin of the Johns Hopkins Hospital
126:100

Berlin R 1948 Haff disease in Sweden. Acta Medica
Scandinavica 129:560

Bernardini I, Rizzo W B, Dalakas M, Bernar J, Gahl W A
1985 Plasma and muscle free carnitine deficiency due to
renal Fanconi syndrome. Journal of Clinical Investigation
75:1124

Bertagnolio S, Di Donato S, Peluchetti D, Rimoldi M,
Storchi G, Cornelio F 1978 Acid maltase deficiency in
adults. Clinical, morphological and biochemical study of
three patients. European Neurology 17:193

Biczyskowa W, Fidzianska A, Jedrzejowska H 1969 Light
and electron microscopic study of the muscles in
hypokalemic periodic paralysis. Acta Neuropathologica
12:329

Biemond A, Daniels A P 1934 Familial periodic paralysis
and its transition into spinal muscular atrophy. Brain
57:91

Birge S J, Haddad J G 1975 25-Hydroxycholecalciferol
stimulation of muscle metabolism. Journal of Clinical
Investigation 56:1100

Bischoff A, Esslen E 1965 Myopathy with primary
hyperparathyroidism. Neurology (Minneapolis) 15:64

Black J T, Judge D, Demers L, Gordon S 1975. Ragged-red
fibres. A biochemical and morphological study. Journal of
the Neurological Sciences 26:479

Blanc W A, Reid J D, Andersen D H 1958 Avitaminosis E
in cystic fibrosis of the pancreas. A morphologic study of
gastrointestinal and striated muscle. Pediatrics 22:494

Blass J P 1979 Disorders of pyruvate metabolism. Neurology
29:280

Blass J P, Avigan J, Uhlendorf B W 1970 A defect in
pyruvate decarboxylase in a child with an intermittent
movement disorder. Journal of Clinical Investigation 49:423

Blass J P, Kark A P, Engel W K 1971 Clinical studies of a
patient with pyruvate decarboxylase deficiency. Archives of
Neurology 25:449

Blass J P, Schulman D, Young D S, Horn E 1972 An
inherited defect affecting the tricarboxylic acid cycle in a
patient with congenital lactic acidosis. Journal of Clinical
Investigation 51:1845

Böhles H, Richter K, Wagner-Thiessen E, Schafer H 1982
Decreased serum carnitine in valproate induced Reye
syndrome. European Journal of Pediatrics 139:185

Bohmer T, Bergrem H, Eiklid K 1978 Carnitine deficiency
induced during intermittent haemodialysis for renal failure.
Lancet 1:126

Bolthauser E, Jerusalem F, Niemeyer G, Huber C 1977
Kearns-Syndrom. Progressive externe Ophthalmoplegie,
Pigmentdegeneration der Retina und kardiale
Reizleitungsstörungen. Schweizerische Medizinische
Wochenschrift 107:1880

Bonilla E, Schotland D L 1970 Histochemical diagnosis of
muscle phosphofructokinase deficiency. Archives of
Neurology 22:8

Borum P R, Broquist H P, Roelofs R I 1977 Muscle
carnitine levels in neuromuscular disease. Journal of the
Neurological Sciences 34:279

Boustany R N, Aprille J R, Halperin J, Levy H, DeLong
G R 1983 Mitochondrial cytochrome deficiency presenting
as a myopathy with hypotonia, external ophthalmoplegia,
and lactic acidosis in an infant and as fatal hepatopathy in
a second cousin. Annals of Neurology 14:462

Bowden D H, Fraser D, Jackson S H, Walker N F 1956
Acute recurrent rhabdomyolysis (paroxysmal
myohaemoglobunaria). Medicine (Baltimore) 35:335

Boyle P J, Conway E J 1941 Potassium accumulation in
muscle and associated changes. Journal of Physiology
100:1

Bradley W G 1969 Adynamia episodica hereditaria. Brain
92:345

Bradley W G, Fewings J D, Harris J B, Johnson M A 1976
Emetine myopathy in the rat. British Journal of
Pharmacology 57:29

Bradley W G, Hudgson P, Gardner-Medwin D, Walton J N
1969 Myopathy associated with abnormal lipid metabolism
in skeletal muscle. Lancet 1:495

Brain W R 1959 Pathogenesis and treatment of endocrine
exophthalmos. Lancet 1:109

Brandt I K, De Luca V A 1966 Type III glycogenosis: A
family with unusual tissue distribution of the enzyme
lesion. American Journal of Medicine 40:779

Bresolin N, Ro Y-I, Reyes M, Miranda A F, DiMauro S
1983 Muscle phosphoglycerate mutase (PGAM) deficiency:
A second case. Neurology 33:1049

Bresolin N, Miranda A F, Chang H W, Shanske S, Di-
Mauro S 1984 Phosphoglycerate kinase deficiency
myopathy: Biochemical and immunological studies of the
mutant enzyme. Muscle and Nerve 7:542

Bresolin N, Zeviani M, Bonilla et al 1985 Fatal infantile
cytochrome c oxidase deficiency: Decrease of
immunologically detectable enzyme in muscle. Neurology
35:802

Britt B A 1979 Etiology and pathophysiology of malignant
hyperthermia. Federation Proceedings 38:44

Britt B A, Endrenyi L, Peters P L 1976 Screening of
malignant hyperthermia susceptible families by creatine
phosphokinase measurement and other clinical
investigations. Canadian Anaesthetists' Society Journal
23:263

Brody I A, Gerber C J, Sidbury J B 1970 Relaxing factor in
McArdle's disease. Calcium uptake by sarcoplasmic
reticulum. Neurology (Minneapolis) 20:555

Brooks J E 1969 Hyperkalemic periodic paralysis. Archives
of Neurology 20:13

Brooks R V, McSwiney R R, Prunty T F G, Wood F J Y
1957 Potassium deficiency of renal and adrenal origin.
American Journal of Medicine 23:391

Brown B I, Brown D H 1966 Lack of an α-1,4-glucan:α-1,4-
glucan:α-1, 4-glucan 6-glycosyl transferase in a case of
type IV glycogenosis. Proceedings of the National
Academy of Sciences USA 56:725

Brown B I, Brown D H 1968 Glycogen storage diseases:
Types I, III, IV, V, VII and unclassified glycogenosis. In:
Dickens F, Randle P J, Whelan W J (eds) Carbohydrate
metabolism and its disorders, Vol 2. Academic Press, New
York, p 123

Brown B I, Zellweger H 1966 α-1,4-glucosidase activity in leukocytes from the family of two brothers who lack this enzyme in muscle. Biochemical Journal 101:16c

Brown B I, Brown D H, Jeffrey P L 1970 Simultaneous absence of α-1,4-glucosidase and α-1,6-glucosidase activities (pH 4) in tissues of children with type II glycogen storage disease. Biochemistry 9:1423

Brown D H, Illingworth B 1962 The properties of an oligo-1,4→1,4 glucantransferase from animal tissues. Proceedings of the National Academy of Sciences USA 48:1783

Brownell A K W, Severson D L, Thomson C D, Fletcher T 1979 Cold induced rhabdomyolis in carnitine palmityltransferase deficiency. Canadian Journal of Neurological Sciences 6:367

Brunberg J A, McCormick W F, Schochet S S 1971 Type III glycogenosis. An adult with diffuse weakness and muscle wasting. Archives of Neurology 25:171

Bryan G T, MacCardle R C, Bartter F C 1966 Hyperaldosteronism, hyperplasia of the juxtaglomerular complex, normal blood pressure, and dwarfism. Pediatrics 37:43

Buchthal F, Engbaek L, Gamstorp I 1958 Paresis and hyperexcitability in adynamia episodica hereditaria. Neurology (Minneapolis) 8:347

Bull G M, Carter A B, Lowe K G 1953 Hyperpotassaemic paralysis. Lancet 2:60

Bull G M, Joekes A M, Lowe K G 1950 Renal function studies in acute tubular necrosis. Clinical Science 9:379

Bunch T W, Worthington J W, Combs J J, Ilstrup D M, Engel A G 1980 Azathioprine with prednisone for polymyositis. A controlled clinical trial. Annals of Internal Medicine (in press)

Burck U, Goebel H H, Kuhlendahl H D, Meier C, Goebel K M 1981 Neuromyopathy and vitamin E deficiency in man. Neuropediatrics 12:267

Busch H F M, Koster J F, Van Weerden T W 1979 Infantile and adult-onset acid maltase deficiency occurring in the same family. Neurology (Minneapolis) 29:415

Busch H F M, Scholte H R, Arts W F, Luyt-Houwen I E M 1981 A mitochondrial myopathy with a respiratory chain defect and carnitine deficiency. In: Busch H F M, Jennekens F G I, Scholte H R (eds) Mitochondria and muscle diseases. Mefar, Netherlands, p 207

Byers R K, Bergman A B, Joseph M C 1962 Steroid myopathy: Report of five cases occurring during treatment of rheumatic fever. Pediatrics 29:26

Bywaters E G L, Stead J K 1945 Thrombosis of the femoral artery with myoglobinuria and low serum potassium concentration. Clinical Science 5:195

Bywaters E G L, Delory G E, Rimington C, Smiles J 1941 Myohaemoglobin in the urine of the air raid casualties with crushing injury. Biochemical Journal 35:1164

Caddell J, Whitemore R 1962 Observations on generalised glycogenosis with emphasis on electrocardiographic changes. Pediatrics 29:743

Callahan J W, Lowden J A (eds) 1981 Lysosomes and lysosomal storage diseases. Raven Press, New York

Cape C A 1969 Phosphorylase a deficiency in pseudohypoparathyroidism. Neurology (Minneapolis) 19:167

Caroll D, Davies P 1964 Renal tubular acidosis presenting with muscle weakness. Journal of Neurology, Neurosurgery and Psychiatry 27:5

Carrier H, Lebel M, Mathieu M, Pialat J, Oevic M 1975

Late familial pseudo-myopathic muscular glycogenosis with α-1,4-glucosidase deficiency. Pathologica Europea (Bruxelles) 10:51

Carroll J E, Brooke M B, De Vivo D, Kaiser K R, Hagberg J M 1978 Biochemical and physiological consequences of carnitine palmityltransferase deficiency. Musle and Nerve 1:103

Carroll J E, Brooke M H, Shumate J B, Janes N J 1981a Carnitine intake and excretion in neuromuscular diseases. American Journal of Clinical Nutrition 34:2693

Carroll J E, Shumate J B, Brooke M H, Hagberg J M 1981b Riboflavin-responsive lipid myopathy and carnitine deficiency. Neurology 31:1557

Carson M J, Pearson C M 1964 Familial hyperkalemic periodic paralysis with myotonic features. Journal of Pediatrics 64:853

Cederbaum A I, Rubin E 1975 Molecular injury to mitochondria produced by ethanol and acetaldehyde. Federation Proceedings 34:2045

Chalmers R A, Roe C R, Tracey B M, Stacey T E, Hoppel C L, Millington D S 1983 Secondary carnitine insufficiency disorders of organic acid metabolism: Modulation of acyl-CoA/CoA ratios by L-carnitine in vivo. Biochemical Society Transactions 11:724

Chalmers R A, Stacey T E, Tracey B M et al 1984 L-carnitine insufficiency in disorders of organic acid metabolism: Response to L-carnitine by patients with methylmalonic aciduria and 3-hydroxy-3-methylglutaric aciduria. Journal of Inherited Metabolic Disease 7 (Suppl 2):109

Chanarin I, Patel A, Slavin G, Wills E J, Andrews T M, Stewart G 1975 Neutral lipid storage disease: A new disorder of lipid metabolism. British Medical Journal 1:553

Chapoy P R, Angelini C, Brown W J, Stiff J E, Shug A L, Cederbaum S D 1980 Systemic carnitine deficiency. A treatable inherited lipid-storage disease presenting as Reye's syndrome. New England Journal of Medicine 303:1389

Cheek D B, Brasel J A, Elliott D, Scott R 1966 Muscle cell size and number in normal children and in dwarfs (pituitary, cretins and primordial) before and after treatment. Bulletin of the Johns Hopkins Hospital 119:46

Chen R.F 1959 Familial periodic paralysis. Archives of Neurology 1:475

Cholod E J, Haust M D, Hudson A J, Lewis F N 1970 Myopathy in primary familial hyperparathyroidism. Clinical and morphologic studies. American Journal of Medicine 48:700

Chomyn A, Mariottini P, Cleeter M W et al 1985 Six unidentified reading frames of human mitochondrial DNA encode components of the respiratory-chain NADH dehydrogenase

Chou S 1967 Myxovirus-like structures in a case of chronic human polymyositis. Science 158:1453

Chui L A, Munsat T L 1976 Dominant inheritance of McArdle syndrome. Archives of Neurology 33:636

Clark A F, Vignos P J 1979 Experimental corticosteroid myopathy: Effect on myofibrillar ATPase activity and protein degradation. Muscle and Nerve 2:265

Clark A F, Vignos P J 1981 The role of proteases in experimental glucocorticoid therapy. Muscle and Nerve 4:219

Clark J B, Hayes D J, Morgan-Hughes J A, Byrne E 1984 Mitochondrial myopathies: Disorders of the respiratory chain and oxidative phosphorylation. Journal of Inherited Metabolic Disease 7 (Suppl 1):62

Clausen T, Wang P, Orskov H, Kristensen O 1980 Hyperkalemic periodic paralysis: Relationship between changes in plasma water, electrolytes, insulin and catecholamines during the attacks. Scandinavian Journal of Clinical and Laboratory Investigation 40:211

Coates P M, Hale D E, Stanley C A, Glasgow A M 1984 Systemic carnitine deficiency simulating Reye syndrome. Journal of Pediatrics 105:679

Coates P M, Hale D E, Stanley C A, Corkey B E, Cortner J A 1985 Genetic deficiency of medium-chain acyl coenzyme A dehydrogenase: Studies in cultured skin fibroblasts and peripheral mononuclear leukocytes. Pediatric Research 19:671

Cohen T 1959 Hypokalemic muscle paralysis associated with administration of chlorothiazide. Journal of the American Medical Association 170:2083

Cohn J, Wang P, Hauge M, Henningsen K, Jensen B, Sveigaard A 1975 Amylo-1,6-glucosidase deficiency (glycogenosis type III) in the Faroe Islands. Human Heredity 25:115

Conn J W 1955 Presidential address. I. Painting background. II. Primary aldosteronism. Journal of Laboratory and Clinical Medicine 45:3

Coomes E N 1965 Corticosteroid myopathy. Annals of Rheumatic Diseases 24:465

Cori G T 1957 Biochemical aspects of glycogen deposition diseases. Modern Problems in Paediatrics 3:344

Creutzfeldt O D 1961 Die episodiche Adynamie (Adynamia episodica hereditaria Gamstorp) eine familiäre hyperkalämische Lähmung. Fortschritte der Neurologie, Psychiatrie und Irhe Grenzgebiete 29:529

Creutzfeldt O D, Abbott B C, Fowler W M, Pearson C M 1963 Muscle membrane potentials in episodic adynamia. Electroencephalography and Clinical Neurophysiology 5:1508

Cumming W J K, Hardy M, Hudgson P, Walls J 1976 Carnitine palmityl-transferase deficiency. Journal of the Neurological Sciences 30:247

Curry O B, Basten J F, Francis M J O, Smith R 1974 Calcium uptake by sarcoplasmic reticulum of muscle from vitamin D-deficient rabbits. Nature 249:83

Danks D M, Stevens B J, Campbell P E et al 1972 Menkes' kinky hair syndrome. Lancet 1:1100

Danon M J, Carpenter S, Manaligod J R, Schliselfeld L H 1981a Fatal infantile glycogen storage disease: Deficiency of phosphofructokinase and phosphorylase b kinase. Neurology 31:1303

Danon M J, Oh S J, Di Mauro S et al 1981b Lysosomal glycogen storage with normal acid maltase. Neurology 31:51

Danowski T S, Greenman L 1953 Changes in fecal and serun constituents during ingestion of cation and anion exchange. Annals of the New York Academy of Sciences 57:273

Danzis J, Hutzler J, Lynfield J, Cox R P 1969 Absence of acid maltase in glycogenosis type II (Pompe's disease) in tissue culture. American Journal of Diseases of Children 117:108

Darley-Usmar V M, Kennaway N G, Buist N R M, Capaldi R A 1983 Deficiency of ubiquinone cytochrome c reductase in a patient with mitochondrial myopathy and lactic acidosis. Proceedings of the National Academy of Sciences USA 80:5103

Dastur D K, Gagrat B M, Wadia N H, Desai M M, Bharucha E P 1975 Nature of muscular change in osteomalacia: Light and electronmicroscope observations. Journal of Pathology 117:221

Daughaday W H, Rendleman D 1967 Severe symptomatic hyperkalemia in an adrenalectomized woman due to enhanced mineralocorticoid requirement. Annals of Internal Medicine 66:1197

Davidson M, Miranda A F, Bender A N, DiMauro S, Vora S 1983 Muscle phosphofructokinase deficiency. Biochemical and immunological studies of phosphofructokinase isozymes in muscle culture. Journal of Clinical Investigation 72:545

Davie M W J, Chalmers T M, Hunter J O, Pelc B, Kodicek E 1976 1-Alpha-hydroxycholecalciferol in chronic renal failure: Studies of the effect of oral doses. Annals of Internal Medicine 84:281

Davis C H, Schliselfeld L H, Wolf D P, Leavitt C A, Krebs E G 1967 Interrelationships among glycogen phosphorylase isoenzymes. Journal of Biological Chemistry, 242:4824

Dawson D M, Spong F Z, Harrington J F 1968 McArdle's disease: Lack of muscle phosphorylase. Annals of Internal Medicine 69:229

De Barsy T, Jacquemin P, Devos P, Hers H G 1972 Rodent and human acid α-glucosidase: Purification, assay and inhibition by antibodies. Investigations in type II glycogenosis. European Journal of Biochemistry 31:156

De Barsy T, Jacquemin P, Van Hoof F, Hers H G 1973 Enzyme replacement in Pompe's disease: An attempt with purified human α-glucosidase. Birth Defects 9:184

Debré R, Semelaigne G 1935 Syndrome of diffuse muscular hypertrophy in infants causing athletic appearance. Its connection with congenital myxedema. American Journal of Diseases of Children 50:1351

De Burlet G, Sudaka P 1977 Properties catalitiques de l'α-glucosidase neutre du rein humain. Biochimie 59:7

Deckelbaum R J, Russell A, Shapira E, Cohen T, Agam G, Gutman G 1972 Type III glycogenosis: Atypical enzyme activities in blood cells in two siblings. Journal of Pediatrics 81:955

Demos M A, Gitin E L, Kagen L J 1974 Exercise myoglobinemia and acute exertional rhabdomyolysis. Archives of Internal Medicine 134:669

Denborough M A, Lovell R R H 1960 Anaesthetic deaths in a family. Lancet 2:45

Denborough M A, Dennett X, Anderson R McD 1973 Central core disease and malignant hyperpyrexia. British Medical Journal 1:272

DeVivo D C, Keating J P 1976 Reye's syndrome. Advances in Pediatrics 22:175

DiBona F J, Morens D M 1977 Rhabdomyolysis associated with influenza A. Report of a case with unusual fluid and electrolyte abnormalities. Journal of Pediatrics 91:943

Di Donato S, Cornelio F, Balestrini M R, Bertagnolio B, Peuchetti D 1978a Mitochondria-lipid-glycogen myopathy, hyperlactacolisdemia, and carnitine deficiency. Neurology (Minneapolis) 28:1110

Di Donato S, Cornelio F, Pacini L, Peluchetti D, Rimoldi M, Spraefico S 1978b Muscle carnitine palmityltransferase deficiency. A case with enzyme deficiency in cultured fibroblasts. Annals of Neurology 4:465

Di Donato S, Peluchetti D, Rimoldi M, Mora M, Garavaglia B, Finocchiaro G 1984a Systemic carnitine deficiency: Clinical, biochemical, and morphological cure with L-carnitine. Neurology 34:157

Di Donato S, Rimoldi M, Garavaglia B, Uziel G 1984b
Propionylcarnitine excretion in propionic and
methylmalonic acidurias: A cause of carnitine deficiency.
Clinica Chimica Acta 139:13

DiMauro S, DiMauro P P M 1973 Muscle carnitine
palmityltransferase deficiency and myoglobinuria. Science
182:929

DiMauro S, Schotland D L, Bonilla E, Lee C P, Gambetti
P, Rowland L P 1973 Progressive ophthalmoplegia,
glycogen storage and abnormal mitochondria. Archives of
Neurology 29:170

DiMauro S, Bonilla E, Lee C P et al 1976 Luft's disease.
Further biochemical and ultrastructural studies of skeletal
muscle in the second case. Journal of the Neurological
Sciences 27:217

DiMauro S, Hartlage P L 1978 Fatal infantile form of
muscle phosphorylase deficiency. Annals of Neurology
28:1124

DiMauro S, Arnold S, Miranda A, Rowland L P 1978a
McArdle disease: The mystery of reappearing
phosphorylase activity in muscle culture — a fetal
isozyme. Annals of Neurology 3:60

DiMauro S, Stern L Z, Mehler M, Nagle R B, Payne C
1978b Adult-onset acid maltase deficiency: A postmortem
study. Muscle and Nerve 1:27

DiMauro S, Hartwig G B, Hays A et al 1978c Debrancher
enzyme deficiency: Neuromuscular disorder in 5 adults.
Annals of Neurology 5:422

DiMauro S, Mendell J R, Sahenk Z et al 1980 Fatal
infantile mitochondrial myopathy and renal dysfunction
due to cytochrome-C oxidase deficiency. Neurology
(Minneapolis) 30:795

DiMauro S, Miranda A F, Olarte M, Friedman R, Hays
A P 1982 Muscle phosphoglycerate mutase deficiency.
Neurology 32:584

DiMauro S, Dalakas M, Miranda A F 1983a
Phosphoglycerate kinase (PGK) deficiency: A new cause of
recurrent myoglobinuria. Annals of Neurology 13:11

DiMauro S, Nicholson J F, Hays A P et al 1983b Benign
infantile mitochondrial myopathy due to reversible
cytochrome c oxidase deficiency. Annals of Neurology
14:226

DiMauro S, Bonilla E, Zeviani M, Nakagawa M, De Vivo
D C 1985 Mitochondrial myopathies. Annals of Neurology
17:521

DiMauro S, Bresolin N 1986 Newly recognized defects in
distal glycolysis. In: Engel A G, Banker B O (eds)
Myology. McGraw-Hill, New York, p 1619

DiMauro S, Papadimitriou A 1986 Carnitine
palmityltransferase deficiency. In: Engel A G, Banker B O
(eds) Myology. McGraw-Hill, New York, p 1697

Drager G A, Hammill J F, Shy G M 1958 Paramyotonia
congenita. Archives of Neurology 80:1

Dresner S C, Kennerdell J S 1985 Dysthyroid orbitopathy.
Neurology 35:1628

Dreyfus J C, Alexandre Y 1971 Immunological studies on
glycogen storage disease type III and V. Demonstration of
the presence of an immunoreactive protein in one case of
muscle phosphorylase deficiency. Biochemical and
Biophysical Research Communications 44:1364

Duane D D, Engel A G 1970 Emetine myopathy. Neurology
(Minneapolis) 20:733

Dunlap H F, Kepler E J 1931 Occurrence of periodic
paralysis in the course of exophthalmic goiter. Proceedings
of the Staff Meetings of the Mayo Clinic 6:272

Dupond J L, Robert M, Carbillet J P, Leconte Des Floris R
1977 Glycogénose musculaire et anémie hémolytique par
déficit enzymatique chez aux germains. La Nouvelle Presse
Médicale 6:2665

Duran M, deKlerk J B C, Wadman S K, Scholte H R,
Beekman R P, Jennekens F G I 1984 Systemic carnitine
deficiency: Benefit of oral carnitine supplements vs.
persisting biochemical abnormalities. European Journal of
Pediatrics 142:224

Dusheiko G, Kew M C, Joffe B I, Lewin J R, Mantagos S,
Tanaka K 1979 Recurrent hypoglycemia associated with
glutaric aciduria type II in an adult. New England Journal
of Medicine 301:1405

Dustan H P, Corcoran A C, Page I H 1956 Renal function
in primary aldosteronism. Journal of Clinical Investigation
35:1357

Dyken M L, Timmons G D 1963 Hyperkalemic periodic
paralysis with hypocalcemic episode. Archives of
Neurology 9:508

Dyken M L, Smith D M, Peake R L 1967 An
electromyographic diagnostic screening test in McArdle's
disease and a case report. Neurology (Minneapolis) 17:45

Egan T J, Klein R 1959 Hyperkalemic familial periodic
paralysis. Pediatrics 24:761

Ekbom K, Hed R, Kirstein L, Åström K E 1964 Muscular
affections in chronic alcoholism. Archives of Neurology
10:449

Eleff S, Kennaway N G, Buist N R M et al 1984 ^{31}P NMR
study of improvement in oxidative phosphorylation by
vitamins K$_3$ and C in a patient with a defect in electron
transport at complex III in skeletal muscle. Proceedings of
the National Academy of Sciences USA 81:3529

Emser W, Schimrigk K 1977 Myxedema myopathy: A case
report. European Neurology 16:286

Eng G D, Epstein B S, Engel W K, McKay D W, McKay
R 1978 Malignant hyperthermia and central core disease
with congenital dislocating hips. Archives of Neurology
35:189

Engel A G 1961 Thyroid function and periodic paralysis.
American Journal of Medicine 30:327

Engel A G 1966a Electron microscopic observations in
primary hypokalemic and thyrotoxic periodic paralysis.
Mayo Clinic Proceedings 41:797

Engel A G 1966b Electron microscopic observations in
thyrotoxic and corticosteroid-induced myopathies. Mayo
Clinic Proceedings 41:785

Engel A G 1970a Evolution and comment on vacuoles in
primary hypokalemic periodic paralysis. Mayo Clinic
Proceedings 45:774

Engel A G 1970b Acid maltase deficiency in adults: Studies
in four cases of a syndrome which may mimic muscular
dystrophy or other myopathies. Brain 93:599

Engel A G 1972 Neuromuscular manifestations of Graves'
disease. Mayo Clinic Proceedings 47:919

Engel A G 1977 Hypokalemic and hyperkalemic periodic
paralysis. In: Goldensohn E S, Appel S H (eds) Scientific
approach to clinical neurology. Lea and Febiger,
Philadelphia, p 1742

Engel A G 1986 Carnitine deficiency syndromes and lipid
storage myopathies. In: Engel A G, Banker B Q (eds)
Myology. McGraw-Hill, New York, p 1663

Engel A G, Potter C S, Rosevear J W 1964 Nucleotides and
adenosine monophosphate deaminase activity of muscle in
primary hypokalemic periodic paralysis. Nature 292:670

Engel A G, Lambert E H, Rosevear J W, Tauxe W N 1965

Clinical and electromyographic studies in a patient with primary hypokalemic periodic paralysis. American Journal of Medicine 38:626

Engel A G, Potter C S, Rosevear J W 1967 Studies on carbohydrate metabolism and mitochondrial respiratory activities in primary hypokalemic periodic paralysis. Neurology (Minneapolis) 17:329

Engel A G, Dale A J D 1968 Autophagic glycogenesis of late onset with mitochondrial abnormalities: Light and electron microscopic observations. Mayo Clinic Proceedings 43:233

Engel A G, Lambert E H 1969 Calcium activation of electrically inexcitable muscle fibers in primary hypokalemic periodic paralysis. Neurology (Minneapolis) 19:851

Engel A G, Gomez M R 1970 Acid maltase levels in human heterozygous acid maltase deficiency and in non-weak and neuromuscular disease controls. Journal of Neurology, Neurosurgery and Psychiatry 33:801

Engel A G, Gomez M R, Groover R V 1971 Multicore disease. A recently recognized congenital myopathy with multifocal degeneration of muscle fibers. Mayo Clinic Proceedings 46:666

Engel A G, Siekert R G 1972 Lipid storage myopathy responsive to prednisone. Archives of Neurology 27:174

Engel A G, Angelini C 1973 Carnitine deficiency of skeletal muscle with associated lipid storage myopathy: A new syndrome. Science 173:899

Engel A G, Gomez M R, Seybold M E, Lambert E H 1973 The spectrum and diagnosis of acid maltase deficiency. Neurology (Minneapolis) 23:95

Engel A G, Angelini C, Nelson R A 1974 Identification of carnitine deficiency as a cause of human lipid storage myopathy. In: Milhorat A T(ed) Exploratory concepts in muscular dystrophy II. Excerpta Medica, Amsterdam, p 601

Engel A G, Santa T, Stonnington H H et al 1979 Morphometric study of skeletal muscle ultrastructure. Muscle and Nerve 2:229

Engel A G, Rebouche C J, Wilson D M, Glasgow A M, Romshe C A, Cruse R P 1981 Primary systemic carnitine deficiency: II. Renal handling of carnitine. Neurology 31:819

Engel F L, Martin S P, Taylor H 1949 On the relation of potassium to the neurological manifestations of hypocalcemic tetany. Bulletin of the Johns Hopkins Hospital 84:285

Engel W K, Eyerman E L, Williams H E 1963 Late-onset type of skeletal muscle phosphorylase deficiency. New England Journal of Medicine 268:135

Engel W K, Vick N A, Glueck C J, Levy R I 1970 A skeletal muscle disorder associated with intermittent symptoms and a possible defect of lipid metabolism. New England Journal of Medicine 282:697

Engel W K, Prokopis L D, Askanas V et al 1980 Nearly fatal lipid laden myopathy with myoglobinuria and myo-deficiency of carnitine. Neurology (Minneapolis) 30:368

Ernster L, Ikkos D, Luft R 1959 Enzymatic activities of human skeletal muscle mitochondria: A tool in clinical metabolic research. Nature 184:1851

Eulenberg A 1886 Uber eine familiäre durch 6 Generationen verfolgbere form congenitaler Paromyotonie. Neurologisches Zentralblatt 5:265

Evans O B 1981 Pyruvate decarboxylase deficiency in subacute necrotizing encephalomyelopathy. Archives of Neurology 38:515

Faris A A, Reyes M G 1971 Reappraisal of alcoholic myopathy. Clinical and biopsy study on chronic alcoholics without muscle weakness or wasting. Journal of Neurology, Neurosurgery and Psychiatry 34:86

Fattah S M, Rubulis A, Faloon W W 1970 McArdle's disease: Metabolic studies in a patient and review of the syndrome. American Journal of Medicine 48:693

Faust D K, Gergis S D, Sokoll M D 1979 Management of suspected hyperpyrexia in an infant. Anesthesia and Analgesia 58:33

Faw M L, Ewer R W 1962 Intermittent paralysis and chronic adrenal insufficiency. Annals of Internal Medicine 57:461

Feit H, Brooke M H 1976 Myophosphorylase deficiency: Two different molecular forms of etiology. Neurology (Minneapolis) 26:963

Feit H, Kirkpatrick J, Van Woert M H, Pandian G 1983 Myoclonus, ataxia and hypoventilation: Response to L-5-hydroxytryptophan. Neurology 33:109

Fernandes J, Huijing F 1968 Branching enzyme deficiency glycogenosis: Studies in therapy. Archives of Diseases in Childhood 43:347

Fernandes J, Pikaar N A 1969 Hyperlipidemia in children with liver glycogen disease. American Journal of Clinical Nutrition 22:617

Fernandes J, Pikaar N A 1972 Ketosis in hepatic glycogenosis. Archives of Diseases of Childhood 47:41

Ferrebee J W, Atchley D W, Loeb R F 1938 A study of the electrolyte physiology in a case of familial periodic paralysis. Journal of Clinical Investigation 17:504

Finch C A, Sawyer C G, Flynn J M 1946 Clinical syndrome of potassium intoxication. American Journal of Medicine 1:337

Fishbein W N 1985 Myoadenylate deaminase deficiency: Inherited and acquired forms. Biochemical Medicine 33:158

Fishbein W N 1986 Myoadenylate deaminase deficiency. In: Engel A G, Banker B Q (eds) Myology. McGraw-Hill, New York, p 1745

Fishbein W N, Armbrustmacher V W, Griffin J L 1978 Myoadenylate deaminase deficiency: A new disease of muscle. Science 200:545

Fitzsimmons R B, Clifton-Bligh B, Wolfenden W H 1981 Mitochondrial myopathy and lactic acidaemia with myoclonic epilepsy, ataxia and hypothalamic infertility: A variant of Ramsay-Hunt syndrome? Journal of Neurology, Neurosurgery and Psychiatry 44:79

Fleisher G A, McConahey W M, Pankow M 1965 Serum creatine kinase, lactic dehydrogenase and glutamic-oxaloacetic transaminase in thyroid diseases and pregnancy. Mayo Clinic Proceedings 40:300

Fourman P 1954 Experimental observations on the tetany of potassium deficiency. Lancet 2:525

Frame B, Heine E G, Block M A 1968 Myopathy in primary hyperparathyroidism. Observations in 3 patients. Annals of Internal Medicine 68:1022

Frank J P, Harati Y, Butler I J, Nelson T E, Scott C I 1980 Central core disease and malignant hyperthermia syndrome. Annals of Neurology 7:11

French E G, Kilpatrick R 1957 A variety of paramyotonia congenita. Journal of Neurology, Neurosurgery and Psychiatry 20:40

French J H, Sherard E S, Lubell H, Brotz M, Moore C L 1972 Trichopoliodystrophy. I. Report of a case and biochemical studies. Archives of Neurology 26:229

Friedman J H, Feinberg S F, Feldman R G 1985 A neuroleptic malignant syndrome due to levodopa therapy withdrawal. Journal of the American Medical Association 254:2792

Fukuhara N, Tokiguchi S, Shirakawa K, Tsubaki T 1980 Myoclonus epilepsy associated with ragged-red fibres (mitochondrial abnormalities). Disease entity or a syndrome? Journal of the Neurological Sciences 46:117

Furie B, Penn A S 1974 Pigmenturia from conga drumming. Annals of Internal Medicine 80:727

Galjaard H, Menkes M, De Josselin de Jong J E, Niermeijer M F 1973 A method for rapid prenatal diagnosis of glycogenosis II (Pompe's disease). Clinica Chimica Acta 49:361

Gallant E M 1983 Barium-treated mammalian skeletal muscle: Similarities to hypokalaemic periodic paralysis. Journal of Physiology (London) 335:577

Gambetti P L, Di Mauro S, Baker L 1971 Nervous system in Pompe's disease. Journal of Neuropathology and Experimental Neurology 30:412

Gamboa E T, Eastwood A B, Hays A P, Maxwell J, Penn A S 1979 Isolation of influenza virus from muscle in myoglobinuric polymyositis. Neurology (Minneapolis) 29:1323

Gamstorp I 1956 Adynamia episodica hereditaria. Acta Paediatrica Scandinavica 45:1

Gamstorp I 1963 Adynamia episodica hereditaria and myotonia. Acta Neurologica Scandinavica 39:41

Garcin R, Rondot P, Fardeau M 1964 Sur les accidents neuromusculaires et en particulier sur une 'myopathie vacuolaire' observés au cours d'un traitement prolongé par la chloroquine. Amélioration rapid apres arrêt du médicament. Revue Neurologique (Paris) 111:117

Garcin R, Legrain M, Rondot P, Fardeau M 1966 Étude clinique et métabolique d'une observation de paramyotonie congénitale d'Eulenberg. Documents ultrastructuraux concernant la biopsie musculaire. Revue Neurologique 115:295

Gillard B K, Nelson T E 1977 Amylo-1,6-glucosidase/4-α-glucano-transferase: Use of reversible substrate model inhibitors to the binding and active sites of rabbit muscle debranching enzyme. Biochemistry 16:3978

Glasgow A M, Engel A G, Bier D M et al 1983 Hypoglycemia, hepatic dysfunction, muscle weakness, cardiomyopathy, free carnitine deficiency and long-chain acylcarnitine excess responsive to medium chain triglyceride diet. Pediatric Research 17:319

Goldflam S 1895 Weitere Mittheilung über die paroxysmale, familiäre Lähmung. Deutsche Zeitschrift für Nervenheilkunole 7:1

Golding D N, Murray S M, Pearce G W, Thompson M 1961 Corticosteroid myopathy. Annals of Physical Medicine 6:171

Goldman D E 1943 Potential, impedance and rectification in membranes. Journal of General Physiology 27:37

Gomez M R, Engel A G, Dyck P J 1972 Progressive ataxia, retinal degeneration, neuromyopathy, and mental subnormality in a patient with true hypoparathyroidism, dwarfism, malabsorption and cholelithiasis. Neurology (Minneapolis) 22:849

Goodhue W W, Davis J N, Porro R S 1972 Ischemic myopathy in uremic hyperparathyroidism. Journal of the American Medical Association 221:911

Gould R J, Steeg C N, Eastwood A B, Penn A S, Rowland L P, De Vivo D 1985 Potentially fatal cardiac dysrythmia and hyperkalemic periodic paralysis. Neurology 35:1208

Goulon M, Rapin M, Lissac J, Pocidolo J J, Mantel O 1962 Quadriplegia with hypokalemia and hypokalemic acidosis secondary to the absorption of ammonium chloride over a three-year period. Bulletin de la Societé des Hôpitaux Médicales de Paris 113

Gregerson N 1985 The acyl-CoA dehydrogenation deficiencies. Scandinavian Journal of Clinical and Laboratory Investigation 45 (Suppl 174): 1

Gregerson N, Wintzensen H, Christensen S K E, Christensen M F, Brandt N J, Rasmussen K 1982 C16-C110-Dicarboxlyic aciduria: Investigations of a patient with riboflavin responsive multiple acyl-CoA dehydrogenation defects. Pediatric Research 16:861

Griggs R C, Engel W K, Resnick J S 1970 Acetazolamide treatment of hypokalemic periodic paralysis. Annals of Internal Medicine 73:39

Grollman A P 1968 Inhibitors of protein biosynthesis. V. Effects of emetine on protein and nucleic acid biosynthesis in HeLa cells. Journal of Biological Chemistry 243:4089

Gronert G A 1980 Malignant hyperthermia. Anesthesiology 53:395

Gronert G A 1986 Malignant hyperthermia. In: Engel A G, Banker B Q (eds) Myology. McGraw Hill, New York, p 1763

Gruener R, McArdle B, Ryman B E, Weller R O 1968 Contracture of phosphorylase deficient muscle. Journal of Neurology, Neurosurgery and Psychiatry 31:268

Gruener R G, Stern L Z 1972 Diphenylhydantoin reserves membrane in steroid myopathy, Nature New Biology 235:41

Gruener R G, Stern L Z, Payne C, Hannapel L 1975 Hyperthyroid myopathy. Intracellular electrophysiological measurements in biopsied human intercostal muscle. Journal of the Neurological Sciences 24:339

Gruner J E 1963 Sur quelques anomalies mitochondriales observées au cours d'affections musculaires variées. Comptes Rendus des Seances de la Société de Biologie et de ses Filiales 157:181

Gruner J E 1966 Anomalies du réticulum sarcoplasmique et prolifération de tubules dans le muscle d'une paralysie périodique familiale. Comptes Rendus des Seances de la Société de Biologie et de ses Filiales 160:193

Guibaud P, Carrier H, Mathieu M et al 1978 Observation familiale de dystrophie musculaire congenitale par deficit en phosphofructokinase. Archives Françaises de Pédiatrie (Paris) 35:1105

Gullotta F, Stefan H, Mattern H 1976 Pseudodystropohische Muskelglykogenose im Erwachsenenalter (Saure-Maltase-Mangle-Syndrome). Journal of Neurology 213:199

Guzé B H, Baxter L R 1985 Neuroleptic malignant syndrome. New England Journal of Medicine 313:163

Haase G R, Engel A G 1960 Paroxysmal recurrent rhabdomyolysis. Archives of Neurology 2:410

Habener J F, Potts J T 1978 Parathyroid physiology and primary hyperparathyroidism. In: Avioli L V, Krane S M (eds) Metabolic bone disease, Vol 2. Academic Press, New York, p 1

Hagenfeldt L, Wahren J 1968 Human forearm muscle metabolism during exercise. II. Uptake, release and oxidation of individual FFA and glycerol. Scandinavian Journal of Clinical and Laboratory Investigation 21:263

Haigler H T, Broquist H P 1974 Carnitine synthesis in rat tissue slices. Biochemical and Biophysical Research Communications 56:676

Hale D E, Cruse R P, Engel A G 1985a Familial systemic carnitine deficiency. Archives of Neurology 42:1133

Hale D E, Batshaw M L, Coates P M et al 1985b Long chain acyl coenzyme A dehydrogenase deficiency: An inherited cause of nonketotic hypoglycemia. Pediatric Research 19:666

Hall L W, Woolf N, Bradley J W, Jolly D W 1966 Unusual reactions to suxamethonium chloride. British Medical Journal 2:1305

Hammett J F, Bale P, Basser L S, Neale F C 1966 McArdle's disease: Three cases in an Australian family. Proceedings of the Australian Association of Neurologists 4:21

Harriman D G F 1979 Preanesthetic investigation of malignant hyperthermia: Microscopy. International Anesthesiology Clinics 17:97

Hart Z W, Chang C, Perrin E V D, Neerunjun J S, Ayyar R 1977 Familial poliodystrophy, mitochondrial myopathy and lactate acidemia. Archives of Neurology 34:180

Hasilik A, Neufeld E F 1980 Biosynthesis of lysosomal enzymes in fibroblasts: Phosphorylation of mannose residues. Journal of Biological Chemistry 255:4946

Hatefi Y 1985 The mitochondrial electron transport and oxidative phosphorylation system. Annual Reviews of Biochemistry 54:1015

Haussler M R, McCain T A 1977 Basic and clinical concepts related to vitamin D metabolism and action. New England Journal of Medicine 297:974

Havard C W H 1972 Clinical endocrinology: Endocrine exophthalmos. British Medical Journal 1:360

Havard C W H, Campbell E D R, Ross H B, Spence A W 1963 Electromyographic and histological findings in the muscles of patients with thyrotoxicosis. Quarterly Journal of Medicine 32:145

Hayes D J, Lecky B R F, Landon D N, Morgan-Hughes J A, Clark J B 1984 A new mitochondrial myopathy. Biochemical studies revealing a deficiency in the cytochrome b-c$_1$ complex (complex III) of the respiratory chain. Brain 107:1165

Hays A, Hallett M, Delf J et al 1981 Muscle phosphofructokinase deficiency: Abnormal polysaccharide in a case of late-onset myopathy. Neurology 31:1077

Hed R 1955 Myoglobinuria in man, with special reference to familial form. Acta Medica Scandinavica (Suppl 303) 151:1

Hed R, Lundmark C, Fahlgren H, Orell S 1962 Acute muscular syndrome in chronic alcoholism. Acta Medica Scandinavica 171:585

Hegele A R, Angel A 1985 Arrest of neuropathy and myopathy in a-betalipoproteinemia with high-dose vitamin E therapy. Canadian Medical Association Journal 132:41

Heiman-Patterson T D, Bonilla E, Di Mauro S, Foreman J, Schotland D L 1982 Cytochrome c oxidase deficiency in a floppy infant. Neurology 32:898

Helweg-Larsen H F, Hauge M, Sagild U 1955 Hereditary transient muscular paralysis in Denmark. Acta Geneticae Medicae et Gemmellologiae (Rome) 5:263

Henderson R G, Ledingham J G G, Oliver D O et al 1974 Effects of 1,25-dihydroxycholecalciferol on calcium absorption, muscle weakness, and bone disease in chronic renal failure. Lancet 1:379

Herman J, Nadler H L 1977 Recurrent myoglobinuria and muscle palmityl-transferase deficiency. Journal of Pediatrics 91:247

Herman R G, McDowell M K 1963 Hyperkalaemic paralysis (adynamia episodica hereditaria). American Journal of Medicine 35:749

Hers H G 1963 α-Glucosidase deficiency in generalized glycogen storage disease (Pompe's disease). Biochemical Journal 86:11

Hers H G, Van Hoof F 1968 Glycogen storage diseases: Type II and type VI glycogenosis. In: Dickens F, Randle P J, Whelan W J (eds) Carbohydrate metabolism and its disorders Vol 2. Academic Press, New York, p 151

Hers H G, Hue L 1983 Gluconeogenesis and related aspects of glycolysis. Annual Review of Biochemistry 52:617

Hewlett R H, Gardner-Thorpe C 1978 McArdle's disease — What limit to the age of onset? South African Medical Journal 53:60

Hofman D D, Denys E H 1972 Effects of thyroid hormone at the neuromuscular junction. American Journal of Physiology 223:283

Hofman W W, Smith R A 1970 Hypokalemic periodic paralysis studied in vitro. Brian 93:445

Hogan G R, Gutmann L, Schmidt R, Gilbert E 1969 Pompe's disease. Neurology (Minneapolis) 19:894

Holleman L W J, Van Der Haar J A, De Vaan G A M 1966 Type IV glycogenosis. Laboratory Investigation 15:357

Holliday P L, Climie A R W, Gilroy J, Mahmud M Z 1983 Mitochondrial myopathy and encephalopathy: Three cases — A deficiency of NADH-CoQ dehydrogenase? Neurology 33:1619

Holmes J M, Houghton C R, Woolf A L 1960 A myopathy presenting in adult life with features suggestive of glycogen storage disease. Journal of Neurology, Neurosurgery and Psychiatry 23:302

Hoppel C, Genuth S, Brass E, Fuller R, Hostetler K 1980 Carnitine and carnitine palmitoyltransferase in metabolic studies. In: Frenkel R A, McGarry J D (eds) Carnitine biosynthesis, metabolism and function. Academic Press, New York, p 287

Hostetler K Y, Hoppel C L, Romine J S, Sipe J C, Gros S R, Higginbottom P A 1978 Partial deficiency of muscle carnitine palmityl-transferase with normal ketone production. New England Journal of Medicine 298:553

Howell R R 1978 The glycogen storage diseases In: Stanbury J B, Wyngaarden J B, Frederickson D S (eds) The metabolic basis of inherited disease, 4th edn. McGraw-Hill, New York, p 137

Howell R R, Kaback M M, Brown B I 1971 Type IV glycogen storage disease: Branching enzyme deficiency in skin fibroblasts and possible heterozygote detection. Journal of Pediatrics 78:638

Hower J, Struck H 1972 CPK activity in hypo-parathyroidism (Letter to the editor). New England Journal of Medicine 287:1096

Howes E L, Price H M, Blumberg J M 1966 Hypokalemic periodic paralysis. Neurology (Minneapolis) 16:242

Hudgson P, Gardner-Medwin D, Worsfold M, Pennington R J T, Walton J N 1968 Adult myopathy from glycogen storage disease due to acid maltase deficiency. Brain 91:435

Hudson A J 1963 Progressive neurological disorder and myotonia congenita associated with paramyotonia. Brain 86:811

Hudson A J, Strickland K P, Wilensky A J 1967 Serum enzyme studies in familial hyperkalemic periodic paralysis. Clinica Chimica Acta 17:331

Hug G, Schubert W K 1967 Lysosomes in type II glycogenosis: Changes during administration of extract from Aspergillus niger. Journal of Cell Biology 35:C1

Hughes J T, Esiri M, Oxbury J M, Whitty C W M 1971

Chloroquine myopathy. Quarterly Journal of Medicine 40:85

Huijing F 1964 Amylo-1,6-glucosidase activity in normal leukocytes and in leukocytes of patients with glycogen storage disease. Clinica Chimica Acta 9:269

Huijing F 1975 Glycogen metabolism and glycogen storage diseases. Physiological Reviews 55:609

Huijing F, Lee E Y C, Carter J H, Whelan W J 1970 Branching action of amylo-1,6-glucosidase/oligo 1,4→1,4-glucantransferase. FEBS Letters 7:251

Huijing F, Waltuck B L, Whelan W J 1973 α-Glucosidase administration: Experiences in two patients with glycogen-storage disease compared with animal experiments. Birth Defects (Original Article Series 9) No. 2:191

Huise J D, Ellis S R, Henderson L M 1978 Carnitine biosynthesis. β-Hydroxylation of trimethyllysine by an α-ketoglutarate dependent mitochondrial dioxygenase. Journal of Biological Chemistry 253:1654

Hulsmann W C, Bethlem J, Meijer A E F H, Fleury P, Schellens J P A 1967 Myopathy with abnormal structure and function of mitochondria. Journal of Neurology, Neurosurgery and Psychiatry 30:519

Ikeda Y, Dabrowski C, Tanaka K 1983 Separation and properties of five distinct acyl-CoA dehydrogenases from rat liver mitochondria. Journal of Biological Chemistry 258:1066

Ikeda Y, Okamura-Ikeda K, Tanaka K 1985 Purification and characterization of short-chain, medium-chain and long-chain acyl-CoA dehydrogenases from rat liver mitochondria. Journal of Biological Chemistry 260:1311

Illingworth B, Cori G T 1952 Structure of glycogen and amylopectins: III. Normal and abnormal human glycogen. Journal of Biological Chemistry 199:653

Illingworth B, Cori G T, Cori C F 1956 Amylo-1,6 glucosidase in muscle tissue in generalized glycogen storage disease. Journal of Biological Chemistry 213:123

Isaacs H, Heffron J J A, Badenhorst M, Pickering A 1976 Weakness associated with pathological presence of lipid in skeletal muscle: A detailed study of a patient with carnitine deficiency. Journal of Neurology, Neurosurgery and Psychiatry 39:1114

Jarcho L W, Tyler F H 1958 Myxedema, pseudomyotonia and myotonia congenita. Archives of Internal Medicine 102:357

Jenerick H 1959 The control of membrane ionic currents by the membrane potential of muscle. Journal of General Physiology 42:923

Jerusalem F, Angelini C, Engel A G, Groover R V 1973 Mitochondria-lipid-glycogen (MLG) disease of muscle. A morphologically repressive congenital myopathy. Archives of Neurology 29:162

Johnson M A, Turnbull D M, Dick D J, Sherratt H S A 1983 A partial deficiency of cytochrome c oxidase in chronic progressive external ophthalmoplegia. Journal of the Neurological Sciences 60:31

Justice P, Ryan C, Hsia D Y, Kromptik E 1970 Amylo-1,6-glucosidase in human fibroblasts: Studies in type III glycogen-storage disease. Biochemical and Biophysical Research Communications 39:301

Kagen L J, Christian C L 1966 Immunologic measurements of myoglobin in human and fetal skeletal muscle. American Journal of Physiology 211:656

Kanno T, Sudo K, Takeuchi I et al 1980 Hereditary deficiency of lactate dehydrogenase M subunit. Clinica Chimica Acta 108:267

Karpati G, Carpenter S, Labrisseau A, La Fontaine R 1973 The Kearns-Shy syndrome. Journal of the Neurological Sciences 19:133

Karpati G, Carpenter S, Wolfe L S, Sherwin A 1969 A peculiar polysaccharide accumulation in muscle in a case of cardioskeletal myopathy. Neurology (Minneapolis) 19:553

Karpati G, Carpenter S, Engel A G et al 1975 the syndrome of systemic carnitine deficiency: Clinical, morphologic, biochemical and pathophysiologic features. Neurology (Minneapolis) 25:16

Karpati G, Carpenter S, Eisen A, Aube M, DiMauro S 1977 The adult form of acid maltase (α-1,4-glucosidase) deficiency. Annals of Neurology 1:276

Kearns T P, Sayre G P 1958 Retinitis pigmentosa, external ophthalmoplegia and complete heart-block. Archives of Ophthalmology 60:280

Keene D L, Humphreys P, Carpenter B, Fletcher J P 1982 Valproic acid producing a Reye-like syndrome. Canadian Journal of Neurological Sciences 9:435

Keith N M, Osterberg A E, Burchell H B 1942 Some effects of potassium salts in man. Annals of Internal Medicine 16:879

Kelly F J, McGrath J A, Goldspink D F, Cullen M J 1986 A morphological/biochemical study of the actions of corticosteroids on rat skeletal muscle. Muscle and Nerve 9:1

Kennaway N G, Buist N R, Darley-Usmar V M et al 1984 Lactic acidosis and mitochondrial myopathy associated with deficiency of several components of complex III of the respiratory chain. Pediatric Research 18:991

Kessler E, Weinberger I, Rosenfeld J B 1972 Myoglobinuric acute renal failure in a case of dermatomyositis. Israel Journal of Medical Sciences 8:978

Keye J D 1952 Death in potassium deficiency. Circulation 5:766

Keyloun V E, Grace W J 1967 Villous adenoma of the rectum associated with severe electrolyte imbalance. American Journal of Digestive Diseases 12:104

Khan L, Bamji M S 1977 Plasma carnitine levels in children with protein-calorie malnutrition before and after rehabilitation. Clinica Chimica Acta 75:163

Kim C S, Dorgan D R, Roe C R 1984 L-Carnitine: Therapeutic strategy for metabolic encephalopathy. Brain Research 310:149

King J O, Denborough M A, Zapf P W 1972 Inheritance of malignant hyperpyrexia. Lancet 1:365

Kissel J T, Beam W, Bresolin N, Gibbons G, Di Mauro S, Mendell J R 1985 The physiologic assessment of a newly described metabolic myopathy, phosphoglycerate mutase deficiency, through incremental exercise testing. Neurology 35:828

Klatskin G, Friedman H 1948 Emetine toxicity in man: Studies on the nature of early toxic manifestations, their relationship to the dose level, and their significance in determining safe dosage. Annals of Internal Medicine 28:892

Klein R, Egan T, Usher P 1960 Changes in sodium, potassium and water in hyperkalemic familial periodic paralysis. Metabolism 9:1005

Klein R, Ganelin R, Marks J F, Usher P, Richards C 1963 Periodic paralysis with cardiac arrythmia. Journal of Pediatrics 62:371

Kono N, Mineo I, Shimizu T et al 1986 Increased plasma uric acid after exercise in muscle phosphofructokinase deficiency. Neurology 36:106

Koskelo P, Kekki M, Wager O 1967 Kinetic behaviour of ^{131}I-labelled myoglobin in human beings. Clinica Chimica Acta 17:339

Koster J F, Slee R G, Hulsmann W C, Neimeijer M F 1972 The electrophoretic pattern and activities of acid and neutral maltase of cultivated fibroblast and amniotic fluid cells from controls and patients with the variant of glycogen storage disease type II (Pompe's disease). Clinica Chimica Acta 40:294

Koster J F, Slee R G, Hulsmann W C 1974 The use of the leukocytes as an aid in the diagnosis of glycogen storage disease type II (Pompe's disease). Clinica Chimica Acta 51:319

Koster J F, Slee R G, Van Der Klei-Van Moorsel J M, Rietra P J G M, Lucas C J 1976 Physicochemical and immunologic properties of acid α-glucosidase from various human tissues in relation to glycogenosis type 1I (Pompe's disease). Clinica Chimica Acta 68:49

Koster J F, Slee R G, Jennekens F G I, Wintzen A R, Van Berkel T J C 1979 McArdle's disease: A study of the molecular basis of two different etiologies of myophosphorylase deficiency. Clinica Chimica Acta 94:229

Kuhn-Nentwig L, Kadenbach B 1985 Isolation and properties of cytochrome c oxidase from rat liver and identification of immunological differences between isozymes from various rat tissues with subunit-specific antisera. European Journal of Biochemistry 149:147

Kuriyama M, Suehara M, Marume N, Osame M, Igata A 1984a High CSF lactate and pyruvate content in Kearns-Sayre syndrome. Neurology 34:253

Kuriyama M, Umezaki H, Fukuda et al 1984b Mitochondrial encephalomyopathy with lactate-pyruvate elevation and brain infarctions. Neurology 34:72

Lambert C D, Young J R B 1976 Hypertrophy of branchial muscles. Journal of Neurology, Neurosurgery and Psychiatry 39:810

Lambert E H, Underdahl L O, Beckett S, Mederos L O 1951 A study of the ankle jerk in myxedema. Journal of Clinical Endocrinology and Metabolism 11:1186

Land J N, Morgan-Hughes J A, Clark J B 1981 Mitochondrial myopathy. Biochemical studies revealing a deficiency of NADH-cytochrome b reductase activity. Journal of Neurological Sciences 50:1

Layzer R G, Lovelace R E, Rowland L P 1967a Hyperkalemic periodic paralysis. Archives of Neurology 16:455

Layzer R G, Rowland L P, Ranney H M 1967b Muscle phosphofructokinase deficiency. Archives of Neurology 17:512

Layzer R B, Havel R J, Becker N, McIlroy M B 1977 Muscle carnitine palmityltransferase deficiency: A case with diabetes and ketonuria. Neurology (Minneapolis) 27:379 (abst)

Legum C P, Nitowsky H M 1969 Studies on leukocyte brancher enzyme activity in a family with type IV glycogenosis. Journal of Pediatrics 74:84

Lehmann-Horn F, Rüdel R, Dengler R, Lorkovic H, Hass A, Ricker K 1981 Membrane defects in paramyotonia congenita with and without myotonia in a warm environment. Muscle and Nerve 4:396

Lehmann-Horn F, Rüdel R, Ricker K, Lorkoniv H, Dengler R, Hopf H C 1983 Two cases of adynamia episodica hereditaria: In vitro investigation of muscle cell membrane and contraction parameters. Muscle and Nerve 6:113

Levin B, Burgess E A, Mortimer P E 1968 Glycogen-storage disease type IV, amylopectinosis. Archives of Diseases in Childhood 43:548

Levin S, Moses S W, Chayoth R, Jagoda N, Steinitz K 1967 Glycogen storage disease in Israel. Israel Journal of Medical Sciences 3:397

Levitt L P, Rose L I, Dawson D M 1972 Hypokalemic periodic paralysis with arrhythmia. New England Journal of Medicine 286:253

Lewi Z, Bar-Khayim Y 1964 Food poisoning from barium carbonate. Lancet 2:342

Lopez J R, Alamo L, Caputo C, Wikinski J, Ledezma D 1985 Intracellular ionized calcium concentrations in muscles from humans with malignant hyperthermia. Muscle and Nerve 8:355

Lou H C, Reske-Neilsen E 1976 Progressive external ophthalmoplegia: evidence for a disorder in pyruvate-lactate metabolism. Archives of Neurology 33:455

Luft R, Ikkos D, Palmieri G, Ernster L, Afzelius B 1962 A case of severe hypermetabolism of nonthyroid origin with a defect in the maintenance of mitochondrial respiratory control: a correlated clinical, biochemical and morphological study. Journal of Clinical Investigation 41:1776

MacDonald R D, Engel A G 1970 Experimental chloroquine myopathy. Journal of Neuropathology and Experimental Neurology 29:479

MacDonald R D, Rewcastle N B, Humphrey J G 1968 The myopathy of hyperkalemic periodic paralysis. Archives of Neurology 19:274

McArdle B 1951 Myopathy due to a defect in muscle glycogen breakdown. Clinical Science 10:13

McArdle B 1956 Familial periodic paralysis. British Medical Bulletin 12:226

McArdle B 1962 Adynamia episodica hereditaria and its treatment. Brain 85:121

McArdle B 1963 Metabolic myopathies. American Journal of Medicine 35:661

McComas A J, Mrozek K, Bradley W G 1968 The nature of the electrophysiological disorder in adynamia episodica. Journal of Neurology, Neurosurgery and Psychiatry 31:448

McDaniel H, Pittman C S, Oh S J, Di Mauro S 1977 Carbohydrate metabolism in hypothyroid myopathy. Metabolism 26:867

Magee K R 1963 A study of paramyotonia congenita. Archives of Neurology 8:461

Magee K R 1966 Paramyotonia congenita: Association with cutaneous cold sensitivity and description of peculiar sustained posture after muscle contraction. Archives of Neurology 14:590

Mahler R F, Stanbury S W 1956 Potassium-losing renal disease. Quarterly Journal of Medicine 25:21

Mallette L E, Patten B M, Engel W K 1975 Neuromuscular disease in secondary hyperparathyroidism. Annals of Internal Medicine 82:474

Mancall E L, Aponte G E, Berry R G 1965 Pompe's disease (diffuse glycogenosis) with neuronal storage. Journal of Neuropathology and Experimental Neurology 24:85

Manitius A, Levitin H, Beck D, Epstein F H 1960 On the mechanism of impairment of renal concentrating ability in potassium deficiency. Journal of Clinical Investigation 39:684

Markesbery W R 1979 Lactic acidemia, mitochondrial myopathy, and basal ganglia calcification. Neurology (Minneapolis) 29:1057

Markowitz H, Wobig G H 1977 Quantitative method for estimating myoglobin in urine. Clinical Chemistry 23:1689

Marks L J, Feit E 1953 Flaccid quadriplegia, hyperkalemia and Addison's disease. Archives of Internal Medicine 91:56

Marshall J 1952 Observations on a case of myotonia paradoxa. Journal of Neurology, Neurosurgery and Psychiatry 15:206

Martin J J, De Barsy T, Van Hoof F, Palladini G 1973 Pompe's disease: An inborn lysosomal disorder with storage of glycogen. A study of brain and striated muscle. Acta Neuropathologica (Berlin) 23:229

Martin J J, De Barsy T, Den Tandt W R 1976a Acid maltase deficiency in non-identical adult twins. A morphological and biochemical study. Journal of Neurology 213:105

Martin J J, De Barsy T, De Schrijver R, LeRoy J G, Palladini G 1976b Acid maltase deficiency (type II glycogenosis). Morphological and biochemical studies of a childhood type. Journal of the Neurological Sciences 30:155

Martinez A J, Hooshmand H, Faris A A 1973 Acute alcoholic myopathy. Enzyme histochemistry and electron microscopic findings. Journal of the Neurological Sciences 20:245

Mastaglia F L 1973 Pathological changes in skeletal muscle in acromegaly. Acta Neuropathologica (Berlin) 24:273

Mastaglia F L, Barwick D D, Hall R 1970 Myopathy in acromegaly. Lancet 2:907

Mateer J E, Farrell B J, Chou S S, Gutmann L 1985 Reversible ipecac myopathy. Archives of Neurology 42:188

Matsuishi T, Hirata K, Terasawa K et al 1985 Successful carnitine treatment in two siblings having lipid storage myopathy with hypertrophic cardiomyopathy. Neuropediatrics 16:6

Mehler M, Di Mauro S 1976 Late-onset acid maltase deficiency. Detection of patients and heterozygotes by urinary enzyme assay. Archives of Neurology 33:692

Mehler M, Di Mauro S 1977 Residual acid maltase activity in late-onset acid maltase deficiency. Neurology (Minneapolis) 27:178

Mercier C, Whelan W J 1973 Further characterization of glycogen from type IV glycogen-storage disease. European Journal of Biochemistry 40:22

Mertens H G, Schimrigk K, Volkwein U, Voigt K D 1964 Elekrolyt- und Adlosteronestoffwechsel bei der Adynamia episodica hereditaria, der hyperkaliämschen Form der periodischen Lähmung. Klinische Wochenschrift 42:65

Meyers K R, Gilden D H, Rinaldi C F, Hansen J L 1972 Periodic muscle weakness, normokalemia and tubular aggregates. Neurology (Minneapolis) 22:269

Miller E D, Sanders D B, Rowlinson J C, Berry F A, Sussman M D, Epstein R M 1978 Anesthesia-induced rhabdomyolysis in a patient with Duchenne's muscular dystrophy. Anesthesiology 48:146

Millikan C H, Haines S F 1953 The thyroid gland in relation to neuromuscular disease. Archives of Internal Medicine 92:5

Millington D S, Roe C R, Maltby D A 1984 Application of high resolution fast atom bombardment and constant B/E ratio linked scanning to the identification and analysis of acylcarnitines in metabolic disease. Biomedical Mass Spectrometry 11:236

Milne M D, Muehrcke R C, Heard B E 1957 Potassium deficiency and the kidney. British Medical Bulletin 13:15

Milne M D, Stanbury S W, Thomson A E 1952 Observations on Fanconi syndrome and renal hyperchloremic acidosis in adults. Quarterly Journal of Medicine 21:61

Minchom P E, Dormer R L, Hughes I A et al 1983 Fatal infantile mitochondrial myopathy due to cytochrome c oxidase deficiency. Journal of the Neurological Sciences 60:453

Miranda A, Di Mauro S, Eastwood A et al 1979 Lipid storage myopathy, ichthyosis and steatorrhea. Muscle and Nerve 2:1

Miranda A F, Shanske S, Hays A P, Di Mauro S 1985 Immunocytochemical analysis of normal and acid maltase-deficiency muscle cultures. Archives of Neurology 42:371

Miyabayashi S, Narisawa K, Tada K, Sakai K, Kobayashi K, Kobayashi Y 1983 Two siblings with cytochrome c oxidase deficiency. Journal of Inherited Metabolic Disease 6:121

Mommaerts W F H M, Illingworth B, Pearson C M, Guillory R J, Seraydarian K 1959 A functional disorder of muscle associated with the absence of phosphorylase. Proceedings of the National Academy of Sciences USA 46:791

Monnens L, Gabreels F, Willems J L 1975 A metabolic myopathy associated with chronic lactic acidosis, growth failure and nerve deafness. Journal of Pediatrics 86:983

Mooy P D, Przyrembel H, Giesberts M A H, Scholte H R, Blom W, van Gelderen H H 1984 Glutaric aciduria type II: Treatment with riboflavine, carnitine and insulin. European Journal of Pediatrics 143:92

Morgan-Hughes J A 1986 The mitochondrial myopathies. In: Engel A G, Banker B Q (eds) Myology. McGraw-Hill, New York, p 1709

Morgan-Hughes J A, Darveniza P, Kahn S N et al 1977 A mitochondrial myopathy characterized by a deficiency of reducible cytochrome b. Brain 100:617

Morgan-Hughes J A, Darveniza P, Landon D N, Land J M, Clark J B 1979 A mitochondrial myopathy with deficiency of respiratory chain NADH-CoQ reductase activity. Journal of the Neurological Sciences 43:27

Morgan-Hughes J A, Hayes D J, Clark J B et al 1982 Mitochondrial encephalomyopathies. Biochemical studies in two cases revealing defects in the respiratory chain. Brain 105:553

Moses S W, Gutman A 1972 Inborn error of glycogen metabolism. Advances in Pediatrics 19:95

Müller R, Kugelberg E 1959 Myopathy in Cushing's syndrome. Journal of Neurology, Neurosurgery and Psychiatry 22:314

Müller-Hocker J, Pongratz D, Hubner G 1983a Focal deficiency of cytochrome c oxidase in skeletal muscle of patients with progressive external ophthalmoplegia. Virchows Archiv. B. Cell Pathology (Berlin) 42:61

Müller-Hocker J, Pongratz D, Deufel T, Trijbels J M F, Endres W, Hubner G 1983b Fatal lipid storage myopathy with deficiency of cytochrome c oxidase and carnitine. Virchows Archiv. A. Pathological Anatomy and Histopathology (Berlin) 399:11

Mullin B R, Levinson R E, Friedman A, Henson D R, Winand R J, Kohn L D 1977 Delayed hypersensitivity in Graves' disease and exophthalmos. Identification of thyroglobulins in normal human orbital muscle. Endocrinology 100:351

Murase T, Ikeda H, Muro T, Nakao K, Sugita H 1973 Myopathy associated with type III glycogenosis. Journal of the Neurological Sciences 20:287

Murphy T R, ReMine W H, Burbank M H 1960 Hyperparathyroidism: Report of a case in which a parathyroid adenoma presented primarily with profound muscular weakness. Proceedings of the Staff Meetings of the Mayo Clinic 35:629

Murphy J V, Marquardt K M, Shug A L 1985 Valproic acid associated abnormalities of carnitine metabolism. Lancet 1:820

Nabarro J D N, Spencer A G, Stowers J M 1952 Treatment of diabetic ketoacidosis. Lancet 1:983

Nakano T, Sakai H, Amano N, Yagishita S, Ito Y 1982 An autopsy case of degenerative type myoclonus epilepsy associated with Friedreich's ataxia and mitochondrial myopathy. Brain and Nerve (Tokyo) 34:321

Netzloff M L, Kohrman A F, Jones M A, Emaus R K, Bieber L L, DiMauro S 1981 Carnitine deficiency associated with renal Fanconi syndrome. Journal of Neuropathology and Experimental Neurology 40:351 (abst)

Neustein H B 1969 Fine structure of skeletal muscle in type III glycogenosis. Archives of Pathology (Chicago) 88:130

Neustein H B, Lurie P R, Dahms B, Takahasi M 1979 An X-linked recessive cardiomyopathy with abnormal mitochondria. Pediatrics 64:24

Neville H E, Ringel S R, Guggenheim M A, Wehling C A, Starcevich J M 1983 Ultrastructural and histochemical abnormalities of skeletal muscle in patients with chronic vitamin E deficiency. Neurology 33:483

Nielsen V K, Friis M L, Johnsen T 1982 Electromyographic distinction between paramyotonia congenita and myotonia congenita: effect of cold. Neurology (Minneapolis) 32:827

Ninomiya N, Matsuda I, Matsuoka T, Iwamasa T, Nonaka I 1984 Demonstration of acid alpha-glucosidase in different types of Pompe disease by use of an immunochemical method. Journal of the Neurological Sciences 66:129

Nishimura Y, Honda N, Oyama K, Ichiyama A, Yanagisawa M, Sudo K, Kanno T 1983 Lactate dehydrogenase: a subunit deficiency. In: Rattazzi M C, Scandalios J G, Whitt G S (eds) Isoenzymes: Current topics in biological and medical research, Vol. II. Alan Liss, New York, p 51

Nitowski H M, Grunfeld A 1967 Lysosomal α-glucosidase activity in type II glycogenosis: Activity in leukocytes and cell cultures in relation to genotype. Journal of Laboratory and Clinical Medicine 69:742

Norris F H, Panner B J 1966 Hypothyroid myopathy. Archives of Neurology 14:574

Odor D L, Patel A N, Pearce L A 1967 Familial hypokalemic periodic paralysis with permanent myopathy. Journal of Neuropathology and Experimental Neurology 26:98

Ogasahara S, Nishikawa Y, Yorifuki S et al 1986 Treatment of Kearns-Sayre syndrome with coenzyme Q_{10}. Neurology 36:45

Ohtani Y, Endo F, Matsuda I 1982 Carnitine deficiency and hyperammonemia associated with valproic acid therapy. Journal of Pediatrics 101:782

Ohtani Y, Nishiyama S, Matsuda I 1984 Renal handling of free and acylcarnitine in secondary carnitine deficiency. Neurology 34:977

Okihiro M M, Nordyke R A 1966 Hypokalemic periodic paralysis. Journal of the American Medical Association 198:949

Oliner L, Schulman M, Larner J 1961 Myopathy associated with glycogen deposition from generalized lack of amylo-1,6-glucosidase. Clinical Research 9:243

Olson W, Engel W K, Walsh G O, Einaugler R 1972 Oculocraniosomatic neuromuscular disease with 'ragged-red' fibres. Archives of Neurology 26:193

Ontko J A 1986 Lipid metabolism in muscle. In: Engel A G, Banker B Q (eds) Myology. McGraw-Hill, New York, p 697

Osserman K E, Tsairis P, Weiner L B 1967 Myasthenia gravis and thyroid disease: Clinical and immunological correlation. Mount Sinai Journal of Medicine (New York) 34:469

Oude Elferink R P J, Brouwer-Kelder E M Surya I 1984 Isolation and characterization of a precursor form of lysosomal alpha-glucosidase from human urine. European Journal of Biochemistry 139:489

Palmer E P, Guay A T 1985 Reversible myopathy secondary to abuse of ipecac in patients with major eating disorders. New England Journal of Medicine 313:1457

Patten B M, Bilezikian J P, Mallette L E, Prince A, Engel W K, Aurbach G D 1974 Neuromuscular disease in primary hyperparathyroidism. Annals of Internal Medicine 80:182

Patten B M, Wood J M, Harati Y, Hefferan P, Howell R R 1979 Familial recurrent rhabdomyolysis due to carnitine palmityltransferase deficiency. American Journal of Medicine 67:167

Pavlakis S G, Phillips P C, Di Mauro S, DeVivo D C, Rowland L P 1984 Mitochondrial myopathy, encephalopathy, lactic acidosis, and strokelike episodes: A distinctive clinical syndrome. Annals of Neurology 16:481

Pearson C M 1964 The periodic paralyses. Brain 87:341

Pearson C M, Beck W S, Blahd W H 1957 Idiopathic paroxysmal myoglobinuria. Archives of Internal Medicine (Chicago) 99:376

Penn A S 1986 Myoglobinuria. In: Engel A G, Banker B Q (eds) Myology. McGraw-Hill, New York, p 1785

Penn D, Schmidt-Sommerfeld E, Wolf H 1980 Carnitine deficiency in pre-mature adults receiving total parental nutrition. Early Human Development 4:23

Perkoff G T, Hardy P, Velez-Garcia E 1966 Reversible acute muscular syndrome in chronic alcoholism. New England Journal of Medicine 274:1277

Perkoff G T, Silber R, Tyler F H, Cartwright G E, Wintrobe M M 1959 Studies on disorders of muscle XII. Myopathy due to the administration of therapeutic amounts of 17-hydroxycorticosteroids. American Journal of Medicine 26:891

Pernow B B, Havel R J, Jennings D B 1967 The second-wind phenomenon in McArdle's syndrome. Acta Medica Scandinavica (Suppl) 472:294

Peter J B, Verhaag D A, Worsfold M 1970 Studies of steroid myopathy. Examination of the possible effect of triamcinolone on mitochondria and sarcotubular vesicles of rat skeletal muscle. Biochemical Pharmacology 19:1627

Petty R K H, Harding A E, Morgan-Hughes J A 1986 The clinical features of mitochondrial myopathy. Brain 109:915

Philipson K D, Edelman I S 1977 Thyroid hormone control of Na-K-adenosine triphosphatase and K-dependent phosphatase in rat heart. American Journal of Physiology 232:C 196

Pickett J B E, Layzer R B, Levin S R, Schneider V, Campbell M J, Sumner A J 1975 Neuromuscular complications of acromegaly. Neurology (Minneapolis) 25:638

Pleasure D E, Walsh G O, Engel W K 1970 Atrophy of skeletal muscle in patients with Cushing's syndrome. Archives of Neurology 22:118

Pleasure D, Wyszynski B, Sumner D et al 1979 Skeletal muscle calcium metabolism and contractile force in vitamin D-deficient chicks. Journal of Clinical Investigation 64:1157

Plotz C M, Knowlton A I, Ragan C 1952 The natural history of Cushing's syndrome. American Journal of Medicine 13:597

Pollen R H, Williams R H 1960 Hyperkalemic neuromyopathy in Addison's disease. New England Journal of Medicine 262:273

Pompe J C 1932 Over idiopatsche hypertrophie van het hart. Nederlands Tijdschrift voor Geneeskunde 76:304

Poskanzer D C, Kerr D N S 1961 A third type of periodic paralysis with normokalemia and favourable response to sodium chloride. American Journal of Medicine 31:328

Prick M I J, Gabreels F J M, Renier W O, Trijbels J M F, Sengers R C A, Sloof J L 1981 Progressive infantile poliodystrophy. Association with disturbed pyruvate oxidation in muscle and liver. Archives of Neurology 38:767

Prineas J W, Hall R, Barwick D D, Watson A J 1968 Myopathy associated with pigmentation following adrenalectomy for Cushing's syndrome. Quarterly Journal of Medicine 37:63

Prineas J W, Mason A S, Henson R A 1965 Myopathy in metabolic bone disease. British Medical Journal 1:1034

Ramsay I D 1965 Electromyography in thyrotoxicosis. Quarterly Journal of Medicine 34:255

Ramsay I D 1968 Thyrotoxic muscle disease. Postgraduate Medical Journal 44:385

Rannels S R, Rannels D E, Pett A E, Jefferson L S 1978 Glucocorticoid effects on peptide chain initiation in skeletal muscle and heart. American Journal of Physiology 253:E134

Rawles J M, Weller R O 1974 Familial association of metabolic myopathy, lactic acidosis and sideroblastic anemia. American Journal of Medicine 56:891

Rebouche C J 1977 Carnitine movement across muscle cell membranes. Studies in isolated rat muscle. Biochimica et Biophysica Acta 471:145

Rebouche C J, Engel A G 1980 Tissue distribution of carnitine biosynthetic enzymes in man. Biochemica et Biophysica Acta 630:22

Rebouche C J, Engel A G 1983 Carnitine metabolism and deficiency syndromes. Mayo Clinic Proceedings 58:533

Rebouche C J, Engel A G 1984 Kinetic compartmental analysis of carnitine metabolism in the human carnitine deficiency syndromes: Evidence for alterations in tissue carnitine transport. Journal of Clinical Investigation 73:857

Reed G B, Dixon J F P, Neustein H B, Donnell G N, Landing B H 1968 Type IV glycogenosis: Patient with absence of a branching enzyme α-1,4-glucan 6-glucosyl transferase. Laboratory Investigation 19:546

Reid H A 1961 Myoglobinuria in sea-snake-bite poisoning. British Medical Journal 1:1284

Resnick J S, Engel W K 1967 Myotonic lid lag in hyperkalaemic periodic paralysis. Journal of Neurology, Neurosurgery and Psychiatry 30:478

Reuser A J J, Koster J F, Hoogeveen A, Galjaard H 1978 Biochemical, immunochemical and cell genetic studies in glycogenosis type II. American Journal of Human Genetics 30:132

Reuser A J J, Kroos M 1982 Adult forms of glycogenosis type II: A defect in an early stage of alpha-glucosidase realization. FEBS Letters 146:361

Reuser A J J, Kroos M, Oude Elferink R P J, Tager J M 1985 Defects in synthesis, phosphorylation, and maturation of acid alpha-glucosidase in glycogenosis type II. Journal of Biological Chemistry 260:8336

Reza J M, Kar N C, Pearson C M, Kark R A P 1978 Recurrent myoglobinuria due to muscle carnitine palmityltransferase deficiency. Annals of Internal Medicine 88:610

Rich E C 1894 A unique form of motor paralysis due to cold. Medical News 65:210

Richardson G O, Sibley J C 1953 Flaccid quadriplegia associated with hyperpotassemia. Canadian Medical Association Journal 69:504

Richardson J A, Herron G, Reitz R, Layzer R 1969 Ischemic ulcerations of the skin and necrosis of muscle in azotemic hyperparathyroidism. Annals of Internal Medicine 71:129

Ricker K, Böhlen R, Rohkamm R 1983 Different effectiveness of tocainide and hydrochlorothiazide in paramyotonia congenita with hyperkalemic episodic paralysis. Neurology 33:1615

Riecker G, Bolte H D 1966 Membranpotentiale einzelner Skeletmuskelzellen bei periodischer Muskelparalyse. Klinische Wochenschrift 44:894

Riggs J E, Griggs R C 1979 Diagnosis and treatment of the periodic paralyses. In: Klawans H L (ed) Clinical neuropharmacology, Vol 4. Raven Press, New York, p 123

Riggs J E, Schochet S S, Gutmann L, Shanske S, Neal W A, Di Mauro S 1983 Lysosomal glycogen storage disease without acid maltase deficiency. Neurology 33:873

Riggs J E, Schochet S S, Fakadej A V et al 1984 Mitochondrial encephalomyopathy with decreased succinate-cytochrome c reductase activity. Neurology 34:48

Rimoldi M, Bottacchi E, Rossi L, Cornelio F, Uziel G, Di Donato S 1982 Cytochrome c oxidase deficiency in muscles of a floppy infant without mitochondrial myopathy. Journal of Neurology 227:201

River G L, Kushner D S, Armstrong S H, Dubin A, Sodki S J, Cutting H O 1960 Renal tubular acidosis with hypokalemia and muscular paralysis. Metabolism 9:118

Robertson E G 1954 Thyrotoxic periodic paralysis. Australian and New Zealand Journal of Medicine 3:182

Robinson B H, Sherwood W G 1975 Pyruvate dehydrogenase phosphatase deficiency. A cause of congenital lactic acidosis in infancy. Pediatric Research 9:935

Robinson B H, Taylor J, Sherwood W G 1978 Deficiency of dihydrolipoyl dehydrogenase (a component of pyruvate and α-ketoglutarate dehydrogenase complexes). A cause of congenital lactic acidosis. Pediatric Research 11:1198

Roe C R, Bohan T P 1982 L-Carnitine therapy in propionicacidemia. Lancet 1:1411

Roe C R, Hoppel C L, Stacey T E, Chalmers R A, Tracey B M, Millington D S 1983 Metabolic response to carnitine in methylmalonic aciduria. Archives of Disease in Childhood 58:916

Roe C R, Millington D S, Maltby D, Bohan T P, Hoppel C L 1984a L-carnitine enhances excretion of propionyl coenzyme A as propionylcarnitine in propionic acidemia. Journal of Clinical Investigation 73:1785

Roe C R, Millington D S, Maltby D A, Kahler S G, Bohan T P 1984b L-Carnitine therapy in isovaleric acidemia. Journal of Clinical Investigation 74:2290

Roe C R, Millington D S, Maltby D A, Bohan T P, Kahler S G, Chalmers R A 1985 Diagnostic and therapeutic implications of medium-chain acylcarnitines in the medium-chain acyl-CoA dehydrogenase deficiency. Pediatric Research 19:459

Roelofs R I, Engel W K, Chauvin P 1971 Demonstration of myophosphorylase activity in muscle grown in tissue culture from patients with muscle phosphorylase deficiency (McArdle's disease). Journal of Histochemistry and Cytochemistry 19:715

Roger J, Pellissier J F, Dravet C, Bureau-Paillas M, Arnoux M, Larrieu J L 1982 Dégénerescence spino-cérébelleuse — atrophie optique — épilepsie — myoclonies — myopathie mitochondriale. Revue Neurologique (Paris) 138:187

Rosa R, George C, Fardeau M, Calvin M C, Rapin M, Rosa J 1982 A new case of phosphoglycerate kinase deficiency: PGK Creteil associated with rhabdomyolysis and lacking hemolytic anemia. Blood 60:84

Rosenow E C, Engel A G 1978 Acid maltase deficiency in adults presenting as respiratory failure. American Journal of Medicine 64:485

Rosing H S, Hopkins L C, Wallace D C, Epstein C M, Weidenheim K 1985 Maternally inherited mitochondrial myopathy and myoclonic epilepsy. Annals of Neurology 17:228

Ross B D, Radda G K, Gadian D G, Rocker G, Esiri M, Falconer-Smith J 1981 Examination of a case of suspected McArdle's syndrome by ^{31}P nuclear magnetic resonance. New England Journal of Medicine 304:1338

Rowland L P, Penn A S 1972 Myoglobinuria. Medical Clinics of North America 56:1233

Rowland L P, Araki S, Carmel P 1965 Contracture in McArdle's disease. Archives of Neurology 13:541

Rowland L P, Lovelace R E, Schotland D L, Araki S, Carmel P 1966 The clinical diagnosis of McArdle's disease. Identification of another family with deficiency of muscle phosphorylase. Neurology (Minneapolis) 16:93

Rowland L P, Di Mauro S, Layzer R B 1986 Phosphofructokinase deficiency. In: Engel A G, Banker B Q (eds) Myology. McGraw-Hill, New York, p 1603

Rowley P T, Kliman B 1960 The effect of sodium loading and depletion on muscular strength and aldosterone excretion in familial periodic paralysis. American Journal of Medicine 28:376

Rubenstein A E, Wainapel S F 1977 Acute hypokalemic myopathy in alcoholism. A clinical entity. Archives of Neurology 34:553

Rüdel R, Lehmann-Horn F, Riker K, Küther G 1984 Hypokalemic periodic paralysis: In vitro investigation of muscle fiber membrane parameters. Muscle and Nerve 7:110

Rudman D, Sewell C W, Ansley J D 1977 Deficiency of carnitine in cachectic cirrhotic patients. Journal of Clinical Investigation 60:716

Sagild U 1959 Hereditary transient paralysis. Ejnar Munksgaard, Copenhagen

Salafsky I S, Nadler H L 1971 Alpha-1,4-glucosidase activity in Pompe's disease. Journal of Pediatrics 79:794

Salafsky I S, Nadler H L 1973 Deficiency of acid alpha-glucosidase in the urine of patients with Pompe's disease. Journal of Pediatrics 82:294

Salassa R M, Mattox V R, Rosevear J W 1962 Inhibition of the 'mineralo-corticoid' activity of licorice by spironolactone. Journal of Clinical Endocrinology and Metabolism 22:1156

Salick A I, Pearson C M 1967 Electrical silence of myoedema. Neurology (Minneapolis) 17:899

Samaha F J 1965 Hyperkalemic periodic paralysis. Archives of Neurology 12:145

Sant'Agnese P A 1959 Diseases of glycogen storage with special reference to the cardiac type of generalized glycogenosis. Annals of the New York Academy of Sciences 72:439

Sasaki H, Kuzuhara S, Kanazawa I, Nakanishi T, Ogata T 1983 Myoclonus, cerebellar disorder, neuropathy, mitochondrial myopathy, and ACTH deficiency. Neurology 33:1288

Sataline L R, Simonelli J M 1961 Potassium paresis following ureterosigmoidostomy. Journal of Urology 85:559

Sato K, Imai F, Hatayama I, Roelofs R I 1977 Characterization of glycogen phosphorylase isenzymes present in cultured skeletal muscle from patients with McArdle's disease. Biochemical and Biophysical Research Communications 78:663

Satoyoshi E, Murakami K, Kowa H 1963 Myopathy in thyrotoxicosis: With special emphasis on an effect of potassium ingestion on serum and urinary creatine. Neurology (Minneapolis) 13:645

Satoyoshi E, Kowa H 1967 A myopathy due to glycolytic abnormality. Archives of Neurology 71:248

Savage D C L, Forbes M, Pearce G W 1971 Idiopathic rhabdomyolysis. Archives of Disease in Childhood 46:594

Schellens J P M, Ossentjuk E 1969 Mitochondrial ultrastructure with crystalloid inclusions in an unusual type of human myopathy. Virchow Archiv B. Cell Pathology 4:21

Schlesinger J J, Gandara D, Bensch K G 1978 Myoglobinuria associated with herpes-group viral infection. Archives of Internal Medicine 138:422

Schmid R, Mahler R 1959 Chronic progressive myopathy with myoglobinuria: Demonstration of a glycogenolytic defect in the muscle. Journal of Clinical Investigation 38:1044

Schneck L, Adachi M, Brieti P, Wolintz A, Volk B W 1973 Ophthalmoplegia plus with morphological and clinical studies of cerebellar and muscle tissue. Journal of the Neurological Sciences 19:37

Schochet S S Jr, McCormick W F, Zellweger H 1970 Type IV glycogenosis (amylopectinosis). Archives of Pathology 90:354

Scholte H R, Jennekens F G I, Bouvy J J B J 1979 Carnitine palmityl-transferase II deficiency with normal carnitine palmityltransferase I in skeletal muscle and leukocytes. Journal of the Neurological Sciences 40:39

Schotland D L, Spiro D, Rowland L P, Carmel P 1965 Ultrastructural studies of muscle in McArdle's disease. Journal of Neuropathology and Experimental Neurology 24:629

Schotland D L, Di Mauro S, Bonilla F, Scarpa A, Lee C P 1976 Neuromuscular disorder associated with a defect in mitochondrial energy supply. Archives of Neurology 33:475

Schott G D, Wills M R 1975 Myopathy and hypophosphoataemic osteomalacia presenting in adult life. Journal of Neurology, Neurosurgery and Psychiatry 38:297

Schutta H S, Armitage J L 1969 Thyrotoxic hypokalemic periodic paralysis. Journal of Neuropathology and Experimental Neurology 28:321

Schwartz W R, Relman A S 1953 Metabolic and renal studies in chronic potassium depletion resulting from overuse of laxatives. Journal of Clinical Investigation 32:258

Seccombe D W, Snyder F, Parsons H G 1982 L-Carnitine for methylmalonic acidemia. Lancet 2:1401

Sengers R C A, Ter-Haar B G A, Trijbels J M F, Willems J L, Daniels O, Stadhouders A M 1975 Congenital cataract and mitochondrial myopathy of skeletal and heart muscle associated with lactic acidosis after exercise. Journal of Pediatrics 86:873

Sengers R C A, Fischer J C, Trijbels J M F et al 1983 A mitochondrial myopathy with a defective respiratory chain and carnitine deficiency. European Journal of Pediatrics 140:332

Sengers R C A, Stadhouders A M, Trijbels J M F 1984a Mitochondrial myopathies. Clinical, morphological and biochemical aspects. European Journal of Pediatrics 141:192

Sengers R C A, Trijbels J M, Bakkeren J A et al 1984b Deficiency of cytochromes b and aa$_3$ in muscle from a floppy infant with cytochrome oxidase deficiency. European Journal of Pediatrics 141:178

Serratrice G, Monges A, Roux H, Aquaron R, Gambarelli D 1969 Myopathic form of phosphofructokinase deficit. Revue Neurologique 120:271

Shafiq S A, Milhorat A T, Gorycki M A 1967 Giant mitochondria in human muscle with inclusions. Archives of Neurology 17:666

Shane E, McClane K A, Olarte M R, Bilezikian J P 1980 Hypoparathyroidism and elevated muscle enzymes. Neurology 30:192

Shapira Y, Cederbaum S D, Cancilla P A, Neilsen D, Lippe B M 1975 Familial poliodystrophy, mitochondrial myopathy and lactate acidemia. Neurology (Minneapolis) 25:614

Shoji S, Takagi A, Sugita H, Toyokura Y 1976 Dysfunction of sarcoplasmic reticulum in rabbit and human steroid myopathy. Experimental Neurology 51:304

Shy G M, Wanko T, Rowley P T, Engel A G 1961 Studies in familial periodic paralysis. Experimental Neurology 3:53

Shy G M, Gonatas N K, Perez M 1966 Two childhood myopathies with abnormal mitochondria. I. Megaconial myopathy. II. Pleoconial myopathy. Brain 89:133

Shy G M, Silberberg D H, Appel S H, Mishkin M M, Godfrey E H 1967 A generalised disorder of nervous system, skeletal muscle and heart resembling Refsum's disease and Hurler's syndrome. I. Clinical, pathologic and biochemical characteristics. American Journal of Medicine 42:163

Sidbury J B 1965 The genetics of the glycogen storage diseases. Progress in Medical Genetics 4:32

Sidbury J B Jr, Mason J, Burns W B Jr, Ruebner B H 1962 Type IV glycogenosis: Report of a case proven by characterization of glycogen and studies at necropsy. Bulletin of the Johns Hopkins Hospital 57:157

Simon N M, Rovner R N, Berlin B S 1970 Acute myoglobinuria with type A2 (Hong Kong) influenza. Journal of the American Medical Association 212:1704

Skoglund R R 1979 Reversible alexia, mitochondrial myopathy, and lactic acidemia. Neurology 29:717

Sloan M F, Franks A J, Exley K A, Davison A M 1978 Acute renal failure due to polymyositis. British Medical Journal 1:1457

Slonim A E, Borum P R, Mrak R E, Najjar J, Richardson D, Diamond M P 1983 Nonketotic hypoglycemia: An early indicator of systemic carnitine deficiency. Neurology 33:29

Smith H L, Amick L D, Sidbury J B Jr 1966 Type II glycogenosis: Report of a case with four-year survival and absence of acid maltase associated with an abnormal glycogen. American Journal of Diseases of Children 111:475

Smith J, Zellweger H, Afifi A K 1967 Muscular form of glycogenosis, type II (Pompe): Report of a case with unusual features. Neurology (Minneapolis) 17:537

Smith R, Stern G 1967 Myopathy, osteomalacia and hyperparathyroidism. Brain 90:593

Smyth D P L, Lake B D, MacDermot J, Wilson J 1975 Inborn error of carnitine metabolism ('carnitine deficiency') in man. Lancet 1:1198

Snyder T M, Little B W, Roman-Campos G, McQuillen J B 1982 Successful treatment of familial idiopathic lipid storage myopathy with L-carnitine and modified lipid diet. Neurology 32:1106

Song S K, Rubin E 1972 Ethanol produces muscle damage in human volunteers. Science 175:327

Spiro A J, Prineas J W, Moore C L 1970a A new mitochondrial myopathy in a patient with salt craving. Archives of Neurology 22:259

Spiro A J, Moore C L, Prineas J W, Strasberg P M, Rapin I 1970b A cytochrome related inherited disorder of the nervous system and muscle. Archives of Neurology 23:103

Stadhouders A M, Viering W A L, Verburg M P, Ruitenbeek W, Sengers R C A 1984 In vivo induced malignant hyperthermia in pigs. III. Localization of calcium in skeletal muscle mitochondria by means of electron microscopy and electron probe analysis. Acta Anaesthesiologica Scandinavica 28:1426

Stanley C A, Hale D E, Coates P M 1983a Medium-chain acyl-CoA dehydrogenase deficiency in children with non-ketotic hypoglycemia and low carnitine levels. Pediatric Research 17:877

Stanley C A, Hale D E, Whiteman D E H et al 1983b Systemic carnitine deficiency in isovaleric acidemia. Pediatric Research 17:296A (abs)

Staffurth J S 1964 The total exchangeable potassium in patients with hypokalemia. Postgraduate Medical Journal 40:4

Steckel F, Gieselmann V, Waheed A 1982 Biosynthesis of acid alpha-glucosidase in late-onset forms of glycogenosis type II (Pompe's disease). FEBS Letters 150:69

Steinitz K, Rutenberg A 1967 Tissue α-glucosidase activity and glycogen content in patients with generalized glycogenosis. Israel Journal of Medical Sciences 3:411

Stephen C R 1977 Malignant hyperpyrexia. Annual Review of Medicine 28:153

Stocker W W, Samaha F J, De Groot L J 1968 Coupled oxidative phosphorylation in muscle of thyrotoxic patients. American Journal of Medicine 44:900

Streeten D H P, Dalakos T G, Fellerman H 1971 Studies on hyperkalemic periodic paralysis: Evidence of changes in plasma Na and Cl and induction of paralysis by adrenal glucocorticosteroids. Journal of Clinical Investigation 50:142

Stubbs W A 1976 Bidirectional ventricular tachycardia in familial hypokalaemic periodic paralysis. Proceedings of the Royal Society of Medicine 69:223

Stumpf D A, Parker W D, Angelini C 1985 Carnitine deficiency, organic acidemias, and Reye's syndrome. Neurology 35:1041

Strugalska-Cynowska M 1967 Disturbances in the activity of phosphorylase-b-kinase in a case of McArdle myopathy. Folia Histochemica et Cytochemica 5:151

Sugie H, Russin R, Verity M A 1984 Emetine myopathy:

Two case reports with pathobiochemical analysis. Muscle and Nerve 7:54

Sussman K E, Alfrey A, Kirsch W M, Zweig P, Felig P, Messner F 1970 Chronic lactic acidosis in an adult. A new syndrome associated with an altered redox state of certain NAD/NADH coupled reactions. American Journal of Medicine 48:104

Swaiman K F, Kennedy W R, Sauls H S 1968 Late infantile acid maltase deficiency. Archives of Neurology 18:642

Takamori M, Gutmann L, Shane S R 1971 Contractile properties of human skeletal muscle: Normal and thyroid disease. Archives of Neurology 25:535

Talbott J H 1941 Periodic paralysis. Medicine (Baltimore) 20:85

Tancredi R G, Dagenais G R, Zierler K L 1976 Free fatty acid metabolism in the forearm at rest: Muscle uptake and adipose tissue release of free fatty acids. Johns Hopkins Medical Journal 138:167

Tanphaichitr V, Broquist H P 1974 Site of carnitine biosynthesis in the rat. Journal of Nutrition 104:1669

Tarui S, Kono N, Nasu T, Nishikawa M 1969 Enzymatic basis for coexistence of myopathy and hemolytic disease in inherited muscle phosphofructokinase deficiency. Biochemical and Biophysical Research Communications 34:77

Tarui S, Okuno G, Ikura Y, Tanaka T, Suda M, Nishikawa M 1965 Phosphofructokinase deficiency in skeletal muscle. A new type of glycogenosis. Biochemical and Biophysical Research Communications 19:517

Thomson W H S, MacLaurin J C, Prineas J W 1963 Skeletal muscle glycogenosis: An investigation of two dissimilar cases. Journal of Neurology, Neurosurgery and Psychiatry 26:60

Thorn G W 1949 The diagnosis and treatment of adrenal insufficiency. Thomas, Springfield, Illinois, p 44

Tice L W, Engel A G 1967 The effects of glucocorticoids on red and white muscles in the rat. American Journal of Pathology 50:311

Tomasi L G 1979 Reversibility of human myopathy caused by vitamin E deficiency. Neurology (Minneapolis) 29:1183

Toshima K, Kuroda Y, Hashimoto T et al 1982 Enzymologic studies and therapy of Leigh's disease associated with pyruvate decarboxylase deficiency. Pediatric Research 16:430

Trevisan C P, Angelini C, Freddo L, Isaya G, Martinuzzi A 1984 Myoglobinuria and carnitine palmityltransferase (CPT) deficiency: Studies with malonyl-CoA suggest absence of only CPT-II. Neurology 34:353

Trijbels F, Sengers R, Monnens L et al 1983 A patient with lactic acidaemia and cytochrome oxidase deficiency. Journal of Inherited Metabolic Disease 6 (Suppl 2):127

Tripp J E, Katcher M L, Peters H A et al 1981 Systemic carnitine deficiency presenting as familial endocardial fibroelastosis. A treatable cardiomyopathy. New England Journal of Medicine 305:385

Tsai J S, Chen A 1977 L-triiodothyronine increases the level of β-adrenergic receptor in cultured myocardial cells. Clinical Research 25:303A

Tsairis P, Engel W K, Kark P 1973 Familial myoclonic epilepsy syndrome associated with skeletal muscle mitochondrial abnormalities. Neurology 23:408 (abst)

Turnbull D M, Bartlett K, Stevens D L et al 1984 Short-chain acyl-CoA dehydrogenase deficiency associated with a lipid-storage myopathy and secondary carnitine deficiency. New England Journal of Medicine 311:1232

Van Biervliet J P G M, Bruinvis L, Ketting D et al 1977 Hereditary mitochondrial myopathy with lactic acidemia, a De Toni-Fanconi-Debré syndrome, and a defective respiratory chain in voluntary striated muscles. Pediatric Research 11:1088

Van Buchem F S P 1957 The electrocardiogram and potassium metabolism. American Journal of Medicine 23:376

Van Buchem F S P, Doorenbos H, Elings H S 1956 Conn's syndrome, caused by adrenocortical hyperplasia. Acta Endocrinologica 23:313

Van Der Meulen J P, Gilbert G J, Kane C A 1961 Familial hyperkalemic paralysis with myotonia. New England Journal of Medicine 264:1

VanDyke D H, Griggs R C, Markesbery W, DiMauro S 1975 Hereditary carnitine deficiency of muscle. Neurology 25:154

Van Hoof F 1967 Amylo-1,6-glucosidase activity and glycogen content of the erythrocytes of normal subjects, patients with glycogen-storage disease and heterozygotes. European Journal of Biochemistry 2:271

Van Hoof F, Hers H G 1967 The subgroups of type III glycogenosis. European Journal of Biochemistry 2:271

Van't Hoff W 1962 Familial myotonic periodic paralysis. Quarterly Journal of Medicine 31:385

Van Wijngaarden G K, Bethlem J, Meijer A E F H, Hülsmann W C, Feltkamp C A 1967 Skeletal muscle disease with abnormal mitochondria. Brain 90:577

Verner J V, Morrison A B 1958 Islet cell tumor and a syndrome of refractory watery diarrhea and hypokalemia. American Journal of Medicine 25:374

Vicale C T 1949 The diagnostic features of a muscular syndrome resulting from hyperparathyroidism, osteomalacia owing to renal tubular acidosis and perhaps to related disorders of calcium metabolism. Transactions of the American Neurological Association 74:143

Victor M 1986 Toxic and nutritional myopathies. In: Engel A G, Banker B Q (eds) Myology. McGraw-Hill, New York, p 1807

Vignos P J, Greene R 1973 Oxidative respiration of skeletal muscle in experimental corticosteroid myopathy. Journal of Laboratory and Clinical Medicine 81:365

Vora S 1983 Isozymes of human phosphofructokinase. Biochemical and genetic aspects. In: Ratazzi J G, Scandalios J G, Whitt G S (eds) Isozymes: Current topics in biological and medical research, Vol II. Alan Liss, New York, p 3

Vora S, Davidson M, Seaman C et al 1983 Heterogeneity of the molecular lesions in inherited phosphofructokinase deficiency. Journal of Clinical Investigation 72:1995

Waber L J, Valle D, Neill C, DiMauro S, Shug A 1982 Carnitine deficiency presenting as familial cardiomyopathy: A treatable defect in carnitine transport. Journal of Pediatrics 101:700

Wahren J, Felig P, Havel R J, Jorfeldt L, Pernow B, Saltin B 1973 Amino acid metabolism in McArdle's syndrome. New England Journal of Medicine 288:774

Weisler M J 1961 The electrocardiogram in periodic paralysis. Chest 4:217

Werlin S L, Harb J M, Swick H, Bank E 1983 Neuromuscular dysfunction and ultrastructural pathology in children with chronic cholestasis and vitamin E deficiency. Annals of Neurology 13:291

Whisnant J P, Espinosa R E, Kierland R R, Lambert E H 1963 Chloroquine neuromyopathy. Proceedings of the Staff Meetings of the Mayo Clinic 38:501

Whitaker J N, DiMauro S, Solomon S S, Sabesin S, Duckworth W C, Mendell J R 1977 Corticosteroid-responsive skeletal muscle disease associated with partial carnitine deficiency. Studies of liver and metabolic alterations. American Journal of Medicine 63:805

Willems J L, Monnens A H, Trijbels J M F et al 1977 Leigh's encephalomyopathy in a patient with cytochrome c oxidase deficiency of muscle tissue. Pediatrics 60:850

Williams C, Field J B 1968 Studies in glycogen-storage disease: Limit dextrinosis, a genetic study. Journal of Pediatrics 72:214

Williams H E 1966 α-Glucosidase activity in human leukocytes. Biochimica et Biophysica Acta 124:34

Williams L T, Lefkowitz R J, Watanabe A M 1977 Thyroid hormone regulation of β-adrenergic receptor number. Journal of Biological Chemistry 252:2787

Williams R S 1959 Triamcinolone myopathy. Lancet 1:698

Willner J H, Ginsburg S, Di Mauro S 1978 Active transport of carnitine into skeletal muscle. Neurology (Minneapolis) 28:721

Wilson J, Walton J N 1959 Some muscular manifestations of hypothyroidism. Journal of Neurology, Neurosurgery and Psychiatry 22:320

Worsfold M, Park D C, Pennington R J 1973 Familial 'mitochondrial' myopathy. A myopathy associated with disordered oxidative metabolism in muscle fibres. Part 2, Biochemical findings. Journal of the Neurological Sciences 19:261

Yamamoto T, Beppu H, Tsubaki T 1984 Mitochondrial encephalomyopathy. Fluctuating symptoms and CT. Neurology 34:1456

Yates R O, Connor H, Woods H F 1981 Muscle breakdown in thyrotoxicosis assessed by urinary 3-methylhistidine excretion. Annals of Nutrition and Metabolism 25:262

Yeo P P B, Chan S H, Lui K F, Wee G B, Lim P, Cheah J S 1978 HLA and thyrotoxic periodic paralysis. British Medical Journal 2:930

Yeung R T T, Tse T F 1974 Thyrotoxic periodic paralysis. Effect of propranolol. American Journal of Medicine 59:584

Yunis A A, Fischer E H, Krebs E G 1962 Comparative studies on glycogen phosphorylase. Purification and properties of rabbit heart phosphorylase. Journal of Biological Chemistry 237:2809

Zellweger H, Mueller S, Ionasescu V, Schochet S S, McCormick W F 1972 Glycogenosis IV: A new cause of infantile hypotonia. Journal of Pediatrics 80:842

Zeviani M, Nonaka I, Bonilla E et al 1985 Fatal infantile mitochondrial myopathy and renal dysfunction due to cytochrome c oxidase deficiency: Immunological studies in a new patient. Annals of Neurology 17:414

Zierler K L 1976 Fatty acids as substrates for heart and skeletal muscle. Circulation Research 38:459

Zierler K L, Andres R 1957 Movement of potassium into skeletal muscle during spotaneous attacks in family periodic paralysis. Journal of Clinical Investigation 28:376

Zierz S, Engel A G 1985 Regulatory properties of a mutant carnitine palmityltransferase in human skeletal muscle. European Journal of Biochemistry 149:207

Zierz S, Engel A G, Romshe C A 1986 Assay of acyl-CoA dehydrogenases in muscle and liver and identification of four new cases of medium-chain acyl-CoA dehydrogenase deficiency associated with systemic carnitine deficiency. Abstracts of the VIIth International Congress of Muscle Disease, Los Angeles

Genetic aspects of neuromuscular disease

INTRODUCTION

All the disorders discussed in this chapter are
genetic. This means that in each case the basic
defect resides within the genes which are
composed of deoxyribonucleic acid (DNA). The
latter consists of two chains of nucleotides
arranged in a double helix. Each nucleotide is
composed of a nitrogenous base, a sugar molecule
(deoxyribose) and a phosphate molecule. The
backbone of each nucleotide chain is formed by
sugar-phosphate molecules, and the two chains are
held together by hydrogen bonds between the
nitrogenous bases which point inward towards the
centre of the helix. There are four bases: adenine,
thymine, guanine and cytosine. The arrangement
of bases in each strand of the DNA molecule is
not random but is in the form of triplet codes,
each triplet specifying a particular amino acid.
The latter join together to form polypeptides and
proteins such as enzymes or structural proteins
(e.g. membranes).

Genetic information in DNA is transmitted to
a particular form of ribonucleic acid (RNA)
referred to as messenger-RNA (mRNA). This
process is called *transcription*. The mRNA then
migrates from the nucleus into the cytoplasm
and the process whereby genetic information from
mRNA is transformed into protein synthesis
within the ribosomes is called *translation*. Developments in recombinant DNA technology (genetic
engineering) have revealed a great deal about the
fine structure of genes, the molecular pathology
of a variety of disorders and many of the details
of transcription and translation. It now seems
clear that over 90% of the DNA does *not* code for
protein. Some of this latter DNA is concerned

with gene regulation, so-called 'promoter' sequences (e.g. the thymine, adenine, thymine, adenine (TATA) sequences situated 'upstream' from functional genes), and some is concerned with the synthesis of RNA molecules, but the function of most is unknown. In addition, sequences of noncoding DNA also exist *within* genes. These are called intervening sequences or *introns* to distinguish them from the transcribed portions of the gene which are called *exons*. RNA transcription from DNA proceeds in the direction from the 5' (upstream) to the 3' (downstream) end of the RNA molecule. During transcription a 'cap' of methyl residues is added to the 5' end, then the entire gene (both introns and exons) is transcribed into precursor or heterogeneous nuclear RNA, and ultimately a 'tail' of adenine residues is added at the 3' end. The 'cap' and 'tail' are believed to stabilise the RNA molecule. The region of the precursor RNA transcribed from the introns is then excised and does not form functional mRNA. On the other hand, the precursor RNA from exons is not excised and is spliced together to form a definitive mRNA which specifies the gene product. It should be noted that the first two bases at the 5' end of each intron are invariably guanine (G) and thymine (T) and the last two bases are adenine (A) and guanine (G) and this arrangement is essential for accurate excision and splicing (Fig. 26.1).

In such a complicated process it is understandable that errors (mutations) could occur in a number of different ways. Detailed studies of the

molecular pathology of the haemoglobinopathies and a few other disorders have now revealed that disease-producing mutations can occur in promoter sequences and in exons (point mutations) and also in introns affecting splicing. With regard to the inherited neuromuscular disorders, a molecular defect has so far only been identified in some cases of Duchenne muscular dystrophy in which there is a small gene deletion (Monaco et al 1985).

MODES OF INHERITANCE

At the clinical level it is convenient to consider genetic disorders as being autosomal dominant, autosomal recessive or X-linked. For each particular genetic trait an individual possesses two genes which may be alike, in which case the individual is said to be homozygous, or they may be different in which case he is said to be heterozygous. A trait manifest in the heterozygote is dominant, whereas one which is manifest only in the homozygote is recessive. A classic dominant disorder affects both males and females and is transmitted from one generation to another. There is a 1 in 2 chance that any child of an affected parent will inherit the mutant gene and will therefore be affected.

Dominant disorders often show considerable variation in severity, sometimes referred to as expressivity. Occasionally a trait may not be manifest in all heterozygotes. In those who appear to be unaffected the gene is said to be non-penetrant. For any dominant disorder the proportion of heterozygotes who are affected (even if only minimally) is referred to as the 'penetrance' of the gene. Thus in epiloia penetrance is reduced to about 80% because in 20% of heterozygotes the trait is apparently not manifest.

Recessive disorders also affect both males and females but in this case only sibs are affected and these disorders are not transmitted from one generation to another. The risk of recurrence after one affected child is 1 in 4. Affected individuals themselves can usually be reassured regarding the risks to their children because their children will be affected only if the affected parent marries a heterozygote which, in the case of an unrelated person, is very unlikely with a rare disorder.

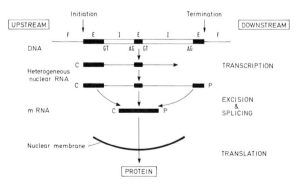

Fig. 26.1 Diagrammatic representation of transcription of a gene consisting of introns (I) and exons (E). Both ends are untranslated flanking regions (F). 'C' is the methyl cap and 'P' the poly-A tail (From Emery 1984)

X-linked disorders are caused by mutant genes on the X chromosome. Almost all such disorders are recessive and therefore female heterozygotes (or carriers) are usually normal and only males (who are hemizygous) are affected. In the case of a carrier female there is a 1 in 2 chance that any of her sons will be affected and a 1 in 2 chance that any of her daughters will be carriers. In the case of an affected male, none of his sons will be affected because they inherit their father's Y chromosome, but all his daughters will be carriers because they inherit their father's X chromosome which has the mutant gene.

As there is no effective treatment for the vast majority of the inherited neuromuscular disorders the only approach to the problem is prevention. This is possible through genetic counselling and prenatal diagnosis. Genetic counselling involves explaining the nature of the disorder, its prognosis and the chances of recurrence. Important advances in this field in the last few years have been the development of tests for detecting preclinical cases of certain genetic disorders such as myotonic dystrophy, and methods for identifying healthy female carriers of various X-linked disorders such as Duchenne muscular dystrophy. In those disorders where the basic biochemical defect is known (e.g. Pompe's disease) prenatal diagnosis is possible from the biochemical study of cultured amniotic fluid cells obtained by transabdominal amniocentesis carried out at about the 16th–18th week of gestation. If the fetus proves to be affected the parents can be offered therapeutic abortion. In the case of X-linked recessive disorders where the basic biochemical defect is not yet known (e.g. Duchenne muscular dystrophy) it is possible to sex the fetus in utero and, through selective abortion of any male fetuses, guarantee that a mother who is a carrier will have a daughter who will not be affected. However, the advent of recombinant DNA technology has opened up several new approaches to prenatal diagnosis which will be discussed later.

PROGRESSIVE MUSCULAR DYSTROPHY

Until Walton & Nattrass (1954) attempted a classification based on genetic considerations, studies were handicapped by the use of categories which embraced a conglomeration of genetic entities. Some of the modifications in classification which clarify further the separation of genetic entities include suggestions made by Becker (1953, 1964), Lamy & de Grouchy (1954), Becker & Kiener (1955), Kloepfer & Talley (1958), Chung & Morton (1959), Morton & Chung (1959), Rotthauwe & Kowalewski (1965) and Emery & Walton (1967).

Duchenne and Becker muscular dystrophy

Stevenson (1953, 1958), in his series of 27 families of Duchenne-type muscular dystrophy, excluded affected individuals and families in which the gene was not X-linked, the onset was not early, and progression was not rapid. Other investigators have included families with muscular dystrophy in which the gene was X-linked, but in which onset age was later and progression was slower. Becker & Kiener (1955) defined the severe form as having an age of onset before 10 years, inability to walk usually by age 11 years, and death by age 20, while the mild form usually has onset age after 10 years, ability to walk in maturity, and death after age 25. The severe and mild forms of X-linked muscular dystrophy never occur in the same family (Blyth & Pugh 1959). From the X-linked pedigrees of Walton (1955, 1956) it would seem that about 9 out of 10 pedigrees represent the rapidly progressive Duchenne type.

Clinically severe X-linked recessive Duchenne type of muscular dystrophy. This form of muscular dystrophy (reviewed in detail by Emery 1987) is characterised by: (1) transmission as an X-linked recessive trait; (2) expression limited to males except occasionally in carrier females (Emery 1963) and in females with Turner's syndrome (Walton 1957a, Ferrier et al 1965) or an X-autosome translocation (Emanuel et al 1983); (3) onset usually in the first five years of life; (4) symmetrical involvement first of pelvic girdle muscles, later of the shoulder girdle; (5) pseudohypertrophy, particularly of the calf, in about 80% of cases; (6) steady and rapid progression leading usually to inability to walk by 11 years of age and subsequently causing progressive deformity with muscular contractures; (7) occasional facial weakness in terminal stages; (8) serum creatine kinase levels elevated except in terminal stages with high levels even at birth (Heyck et al 1966); (9) death from inanition or respiratory infection, usually in the second decade.

It has been generally assumed that the gene for Duchenne muscular dystrophy is 100% penetrant in hemizygous (XY) males. However, there have been reports which suggest that occasionally males may be hemizygous for the mutant gene and yet do not have clinical symptoms of the disease (Thompson et al 1962, Richterich et al 1963). In a proportion of apparently unaffected male sibs and in some fathers of affected boys, slight abnormalities in serum creatine kinase levels, electromyography and even muscle histology have been reported (Beckmann & Jerusalem 1966, Smith et al 1966). However, Emery & Spikesman (1970), using carefully matched controls, concluded that slightly elevated serum creatine kinase levels in male relatives were not associated with a subclinical form of X-linked Duchenne muscular dystrophy or with the heterozygous state of autosomal recessive Duchenne muscular dystrophy.

We have reviewed the findings in a number of studies of the incidence of Duchenne muscular dystrophy which have been carried out over the last 30 years (Stephens & Tyler 1951, Walton 1955, Stevenson 1958, Blyth & Pugh 1959, Moser et al 1964, Kuroiwa & Miyazaki 1967, Gardner-Medwin 1970, Prot 1971, Lawrence et al 1973, Brooks & Emery 1977). Out of 1532 218 male births, 324 were affected, which gives an overall mean incidence ($\pm$ S.E.) of $21.1 \pm 1.2 \times 10^{-5}$ or approximately 1 in 4800 male births (Emery 1977). Incidences in fact ranged from 1 in 7689 to 1 in 3067, probably because of different degrees of ascertainment in different populations. In our own studies in S.E. Scotland over the period 1953–68 the incidence was 26.5×10^{-5} or approximately one in 3774 male births (Brooks & Emery 1977).

In an X-linked recessive condition in which affected males do not survive to have children, the mutation rate is one-third the birth incidence. Using the overall mean incidence of 21.1×10^{-5} the mutation rate is therefore 70×10^{-6}. This figure is higher than values obtained for other X-linked disorders, possible explanations being that the gene is very large (different mutations within it producing the same disease) or that a cluster of several genes is present.

Clinically milder X-linked recessive types of muscular dystrophy. A milder X-linked form of muscular dystrophy was recognised first by Becker (1955, 1957, 1962). This is clinically similar to the Duchenne-type muscular dystrophy but differs in that the disease usually manifests itself in the teens or early twenties and affected individuals usually survive at least to the third decade. Other investigators have also reported families with X-linked muscular dystrophy in which the onset was later and the progression slower than in the classic Duchenne type of muscular dystrophy (Levison 1951, Lamy & de Grouchy 1954, Walton 1955, 1956, Blyth & Pugh 1959, Rotthauwe & Kowalewski 1966a, Zellweger & Hanson 1967, Markand et al 1969, Radu & Stenzel 1969a, Conomy 1970). From a detailed study of 10 extensive families with benign (Becker type) X-linked muscular dystrophy, Emery & Skinner (1976) have defined the clinical features of this disease and the differences from Duchenne muscular dystrophy. Both disorders are characterised by predominantly proximal muscle weakness with pseudohypertrophy of the calf muscles. However, unlike Duchenne muscular dystrophy, in Becker muscular dystrophy there is no evidence of right ventricular preponderance on electrocardiography and cardiac involvement, when present, is a late manifestation. The best criterion for distinguishing between the two disorders is the age of becoming chair-bound: nearly 97% of boys with Duchenne muscular dystrophy become chair-bound *before* the age of 11 whereas 97% cent of patients with Becker muscular dystrophy become chair-bound *after* the age of 11 (Emery & Skinner 1976). In both diseases the serum level of creatine kinase is raised, particularly in the early stages, and in this way preclinical cases may be indentified.

Mabry et al (1965) have described a large family with a benign X-linked form of muscular dystrophy which appears to differ from the Becker type in age of onset and the greater degree of disability which it produces. Emery & Dreifuss

Table 26.1 X-linked muscular dystrophies

Type	Onset	Course	Weakness	Pseudohypertrophy	Myocardial involvement	Contractures (early)
Duchenne	<5	severe	proximal	+++	+	−
Becker	3–25	benign	proximal	+++	−	−
Mabry	11–13	benign	proximal	+++	+	−
Emery-Dreifuss	<10	benign	scapulo-humeral-peroneal	−	+	+

(1966) have described another benign form of muscular dystrophy in which there was no pseudohypertrophy and muscular contractures were an *early* and prominent feature. Similar families have also been described (Cammann et al 1974, Rowland et al 1979). Interestingly the gene causing this form of muscular dystrophy has now been located on the distal part of the long arm of the X-chromosome (Xq 28) and is not therefore allelic with the Duchenne and Becker types (Hodgson et al 1986). The main distinguishing features between the various forms of X-linked muscular dystrophy are summarised in Table 26.1.

The locus for Duchenne muscular dystrophy has been shown not to be within measurable distance of the loci for colour blindness (Emery 1966, Greig 1977), glucose-6-phosphate dehydrogenase (G6PD) deficiency (Zatz et al 1974) or the Xg blood group (Blyth et al 1965). Studies on rare females with X-autosome translocations indicate that the locus is located on the short arm of the X (at Xp 21) and linkage with DNA markers indicates that the genes for Duchenne and Becker muscular dystrophy are allelic, that is at the same locus (Kingston et al 1983).

Autosomal recessive Duchenne type of muscular dystrophy. Stevenson (1953) suggested that the name Duchenne be limited to that type of muscular dystrophy which affects boys and has early onset and rapid progression. However, many investigators have found the Duchenne clinical description useful whether or not affection is limited to males (Becker 1953). Lamy & de Grouchy (1954) found the Duchenne clinical description applicable to cases inherited as an autosomal recessive trait in about one out of 10 pedigrees in their series of 102 families totalling 160 cases. Walton (1955) included two girls among his 56 cases of Duchenne type with the comment

that they 'have shown no significant difference in clinical manifestations and course from several of the boys'. Kloepfer & Talley (1958) studied the occurrence of Duchenne-type muscular dystrophy (three males and four females) in four related sibships in which all eight parents had a common ancestor. There was no doubt that an autosomal recessive pattern of inheritance was involved. Age of onset ranged from five to 13 years. Blyth & Pugh (1959) accepted this category and Dubowitz (1960) presented a pedigree. Jackson & Carey (1961) reported 14 affected individuals (including five girls) distributed in seven related sibships with clinical stigmata typically similar to the Duchenne type which they found to be transmitted as an autosomal recessive trait. Age of onset was from five to 13 years. Milhorat (1961) reported the occurrence of 25 females clinically similar to 185 X-linked recessive males of the Duchenne type. Others have also studied and commented upon the occurrence of muscular dystrophy in young girls (Johnston 1964, Radu & Stenzel 1969b, Penn et al 1970). A relatively high incidence in Tunisia has been reported, possibly related to the high degree of consanguinity in that country (Ben Hamida et al 1983). However, at least in Britain, this is an uncommon condition and many of the cases reported in the past probably had spinal muscular atrophy and not muscular dystrophy.

Facioscapulohumeral muscular dystrophy

Facioscapulohumeral muscular dystrophy is characterised as follows: (1) transmission as an autosomal dominant trait; (2) expression in either sex; (3) onset usually in adolescence, but possibly at any age from childhood until 'late adult life; (4) occurrence of abortive or mildly affected cases is common; (5) initial involvement, sometimes asymmetrical, of facial and scapulohumeral muscles, usually with spread within 20 or 30 years to the pelvic muscles; (6) rare pseudohypertrophy; (7) slow insidious progression with periods of long arrest of the disease; (8) rarely severe disability and usually slight skeletal changes; (9) a relatively good prognosis; (10) usually normal or slightly raised serum creatine kinase levels.

All extensive studies of this entity including those of Bell (1943), Boyes et al (1949), Tyler & Stephens (1950), Becker (1953), Walton & Nattrass (1954) and Morton et al (1963), are in agreement that transmission is as a dominant trait which is completely penetrant (Morton & Chung 1959) in both sexes. However, expression of the gene may be so mild that the condition goes unrecognised. For example Walton (1955) emphasised the unreliability of family histories when he said 'The affected girls in generation III were examined on two occasions and each time II.4 was interviewed. It was only at a late stage of the second interview that the author's suspicions of facial involvement in II.4 were aroused and examination subsequently revealed that she was undoubtedly an abortive case. She had insisted previously that all her sibs were well; however, when they, too, agreed to be examined it was discovered that II.9 was another abortive case, and that II.7 was quite severely affected.' In some cases facial weakness may be the most prominent or even the only feature (Hanson & Rowland 1971).

Morton & Chung (1959) found the incidence rate of facioscapulohumeral muscular dystrophy to be 38×10^{-7} when determined from their own Wisconsin data and 92×10^{-7} when based on pooled data. From these same data prevalence rates were 23×10^{-7}, and 56×10^{-7}, respectively. In the studies of Tyler & Stephens (1950), Walton (1955), Race (1955), and Stevenson et al (1955) data were insufficient to establish linkage between the gene for facioscapulohumeral muscular dystrophy and genes for the ability to taste phenylthiocarbamide (PTC), for blood groups, and the secretor factor.

Limb-girdle muscular dystrophy

This form of muscular dystrophy, according to Walton & Nattrass (1954) and Morton et al (1963), is characterised by: (1) transmission as an autosomal recessive trait in 59% cent of the cases, and sporadic occurrence in the remaining 41%; (2) expression in either sex; (3) onset usually late in the first or in the second or third decades, but occasionally in middle age; (4) primary involvement of the shoulder girdle muscles (usually) or of the pelvic girdle (rarely) with spread to other areas after a variable period; (5) only rare occurrence of muscular pseudohypertrophy; (6) rare occurrence of abortive cases; (7) variable severity and rate of progression, intermediate between the Duchenne and facioscapulohumeral forms; (8) in most cases severe disability in middle life and death at a younger than normal age; (9) occasional slight facial weakness in late stages; (10) usually normal or slightly raised serum creatine kinase levels.

Many investigators, including Bell (1943), Becker (1953), Stevenson (1953), Walton (1955, 1956), Morton & Chung (1959), and Morton et al (1963), have found limb-girdle muscular dystrophy to be inherited as an autosomal recessive trait which is probably 100% penetrant in both sexes in the homozygous genotype. Autosomal recessive limb-girdle dystrophy with onset in adult life and affecting *predominantly the upper limbs* is now believed to be a rare condition (Yates & Emery 1985). Cases with predominantly lower limb involvement prove to have a variety of other disorders including Kugelberg–Welander spinal muscular atrophy, benign X-linked muscular dystrophy and a variety of myopathies. Early estimates of the incidence of this disorder therefore have to be accepted with caution.

Limb-girdle muscular dystrophy clearly inherited as an autosomal dominant trait has been described but appears to be very rare (Schneiderman et al 1969, Bacon & Smith 1971). In one such family, linkage with the Pelger–Huet anomaly has been reported (Schneiderman et al 1969). In some families there has been a preponderance of females (Henson et al 1967), in others, males (De Coster et al 1974).

Manifesting carriers of X-linked muscular dystrophy. It has been estimated that about 8% of all female carriers of X-linked Duchenne muscular dystrophy may have varying degrees of muscle weakness (Moser & Emery 1974). In its more extreme form this weakness may resemble limb-girdle muscular dystrophy. The distinction between these two conditions is important because in limb-girdle muscular dystrophy an affected woman (or her unaffected sister) is most unlikely to have affected children, but in the case of a manifesting carrier of X-linked Duchenne muscular dystrophy there is a 1 in 2 chance that any son she has will be affected and her sister may also be at risk of having affected sons. Some distinguishing features between these two conditions are summarised in Table 26.2.

Table 26.2 Some distinguishing features between manifesting female carriers of X-linked Duchenne muscular dystrophy and limb-girdle muscular dystrophy

Features	Manifesting carriers	Limb-girdle dystrophy
Pseudohypertrophy	80%	rare
Asymmetrical weakness	60%	rare
ECG abnormalities	5–10%	—
Serum creatine kinase increased	>95% often very high	60% rarely high

Distal muscular dystrophy

This characteristically benign disease begins in the small muscles of the hands, feet and legs. From 78 propositi Welander (1951) examined 249 individuals with distal muscular dystrophy who were distributed in 72 pedigrees. The age of onset ranged from 20 to 77 with a mean of 47 years. Transmission was as an autosomal dominant trait which was about 80% penetrant in males and 69% penetrant in females. As prevalence in the population studied was as high as one in 55 for individuals who were 65 years or older, it was possible to observe a mating between two affected parents who had 15 offspring, of whom two were severely affected and therefore considered to be homozygous for the dominant gene (Welander 1957). Walton (1963) studied six cases of distal muscular dystrophy, and although there was no evidence of the disease in any of their relatives they were all severely affected in a way comparable to Welander's patients whom she considered to be homozygotes. Distal muscular dystrophy has been described in a large English family (Sumner et al 1971) and in a North American family (Markesbery et al 1974). However, the disorder in Europe

and North America appears to be rare, most cases are sporadic and, although the distribution of muscle weakness is similar to that in the Swedish cases, the disease may be less benign. There is also an autosomal dominant form of the disease with onset in childhood (Bautista et al 1978).

Ocular muscular dystrophy

When extrinsic ocular muscles are affected by ocular muscular dystrophy, the clinical symptoms begin with ptosis or diplopia and progress to complete bilateral ophthalmoplegia. Upper facial muscles are usually weak and atrophy of neck, trunk and limb muscles may also occur. The disease usually begins in early adult life but may be manifest even in infancy.

Although the disease frequently follows an autosomal dominant mode of inheritance, the large number of isolated cases described in various reports and reviewed by Kiloh & Nevin (1951) and by Lees & Liversedge (1962) suggest either that penetrance is often reduced, or the mutation rate is high, or that the condition may be due to more than one gene and that whereas one such gene is clearly an autosomal dominant others may be recessive.

The so-called 'oculopharyngeal' type of muscular dystrophy, in which the onset is in middle age (Bray et al 1965) and progressive dysphagia is a prominent feature, is a distinct entity. A large proportion of cases with this type of muscular dystrophy have been of French-Canadian extraction (Taylor 1915, Victor et al 1962, Hayes et al 1963, Peterman et al 1964, Murphy & Drachman 1968). A similar condition, but with somewhat earlier onset, has been reported in Israel in an Ashkenazi Jewish family, but here it was inherited as an autosomal recessive trait (Fried et al 1975).

Congenital myopathies

The syndrome of generalised muscular hypotonia, feebleness of voluntary movements and depressed or absent tendon reflexes present at birth or manifest during early infancy, has been variously referred to as amyotonia congenita, myatonia congenita or Oppenheim's disease. Batten (1910) was the first to recognise that the syndrome could be myopathic in origin or result from a lesion in the anterior horn cells of the spinal cord (infantile spinal muscular atrophy or Werdnig–Hoffmann disease). In fact, more recent studies have shown that the syndrome may result from many causes (Brandt 1950, Walton 1957b) although Werdnig–Hoffmann disease and congenital myopathies, of one form or another, account for most cases. The congenital myopathies themselves are a heterogeneous group of disorders although they all have in common muscular weakness dating from birth or early infancy. A classification of the congenital myopathies is given in Table 26.3, details of which have been discussed elsewhere (Emery & Walton 1967). Zellweger (1966), Dubowitz (1978) Baraitser (1982), Heckmatt & Dubowitz (1983) and Bundey (1985) have reviewed their differential diagnosis in detail and provide extensive bibliographies.

The proposed classification is based largely on histological appearances and leaves much to be desired, and in many instances the mode of inheritance is far from clear. An understanding of the pathogenesis and biochemical basis of these disorders is therefore urgently needed, both for genetic counselling and for determining the prognosis in the individual case.

Carrier detection in muscular dystrophy

From the point of view of genetic counselling carrier detection is more important in X-linked than in autosomal recessive disorders. With regard to carriers of X-linked Duchenne muscular dystrophy, a small proportion of such women have enlarged calves and some may even have quite marked muscle weakness (Emery 1963). It has been estimated that about 8% of carriers exhibit some degree of weakness (Moser & Emery 1974) which may mimic limb-girdle muscular dystrophy (see p. 874). However, the majority of carriers are symptom-free and their detection is important for genetic counselling. The simplest and most reliable test has proved to be estimation of the serum level of creatine kinase first employed by Okinaka et al in 1959. Results from many centres have shown that about two-thirds of carriers have significantly elevated levels of serum creatine kinase (Emery 1980). Attempts have been made to improve the detection rate by studying the

Table 26.3 Proposed classification of the congenital myopathies

1. *Congenital muscular dystrophies proper*
   Muscle histology characteristic of dystrophy
   Serum enzymes usually normal
   Autosomal recessive inheritance probable
   A. Rapidly progressive
      Death in infancy or early childhood.
   B. Slowly progressive

2. *Exceptional early onset in forms of muscular dystrophy which usually begin in childhood.*
   e.g. Duchenne muscular dystrophy
   Myotonic dystrophy

3. *Congenital 'myopathies'*
   Abnormal muscle histology with special staining techniques or on electron microscopy
   Serum enzymes usually normal
   A. Central core disease
      Autosomal dominant
   B. Nemaline myopathy
      Autosomal recessive (usual)
      Autosomal dominant
   C. Myotubular (centronuclear) myopathy
      Autosomal recessive
      Autosomal dominant
      X-linked recessive
   D. Minicore (multicore) disease
      ? Autosomal recessive
   E. Congenital fibre type disproportion
      ? Autosomal dominant
   F. Mitochondrial myopathies
      Luft disease
      Kearns–Sayre syndrome
      Other forms
         (Autosomal recessive or dominant)
   G. Miscellaneous
      Sarcotubular myopathy
      Fingerprint body myopathy
      Inclusion body myopathy, etc.

4. *Arthrogryposis multiplex congenita*
   (myopathic form)
   ? Autosomal recessive

5. *Muscle carnitine deficiency*
   Autosomal recessive

effects of controlled exercise on serum enzyme levels (Emery 1967) or by other methods, but none of these has so far proved superior to the serum level of creatine kinase (Emery 1987).

Other abnormalities reported in a proportion of carriers include electrocardiographic changes (Emery 1969, Hausmanowa-Petrusewicz et al 1971) and certain electromyographic changes (Caruso & Buchthal 1965, Gardner-Medwin et al 1971, Moosa et al 1972). Abnormalities have also been observed in muscle histology by light microscopy (Dubowitz 1963, Emery 1963, 1965, Pearson et al 1963, Macciotta et al 1964, Stephens & Lewin 1965, Kowalewski et al 1966, Pearce et al 1966, Smith et al 1966), by electron microscopy (Roy & Dubowitz 1970) and by histochemical studies (Morris & Raybould 1971). Various biochemical abnormalities in muscle tissue from carriers have been reported, including a significant reduction in LDH-5 (Emery 1964, Mannucci et al 1965, Johnston et al 1966, Pearson & Kar 1966), and increased protein synthesis (Ionasescu 1975). A reduction in lymphocyte capping has also been reported in a proportion of carriers (Pickard et al 1978). None of these various techniques has, however, replaced the serum level of creatine kinase as being the most practical and sensitive test for the carrier state in Duchenne muscular dystrophy. Carriers of Becker muscular dystrophy also have elevated levels of serum creatine kinase (Rotthauwe & Kowalewski 1966b, Emery et al 1967) and about 60% have levels which exceed the normal 95th percentile (Skinner et al 1975). In both Duchenne and Becker types of muscular dystrophy there is therefore, the problem of counselling a suspected carrier whose serum creatine kinase level falls within the normal range. Simple statistical techniques have been devised which can be applied in such situations and which take into account enzyme levels, not only in the potential carrier, but also in her sisters and mother, and also include information on normal brothers and sons (Emery 1986, Emery & Holloway 1977). In these various calculations we assume that the mutation rates in male and female germ lines are equal, from which it follows, according to classic genetic theory, that one-third of all cases of Duchenne muscular dystrophy are the result of new mutations and their mothers are not, therefore, carriers. This is borne out by various epidemiological and statistical techniques (Davie & Emery 1978, Emery 1987).

In calculating the probability of a woman being a carrier it is necessary to know the distribution of serum creatine kinase activities in known carriers as well as in normal women, and this is best determined for each laboratory. Our results in 200 controls and 80 definite carriers are given in Table 26.4.

Table 26.4 Relative probabilities of normal homozygosity to heterozygosity (h) for various serum levels of creatine kinase expressed in International Units (From Emery 1986)

Serum creatine kinase (IU/l)	Controls No.	% (Y_1)	Carriers No.	% (Y_2)	h (Y_1/Y_2)
11–30	26	13.0	2	2.5	5.20
31–50	112	56.0	10	12.5	4.48
51–70	47	23.5	8	10.0	2.35
71–90	6	3.0	10	12.5	0.24
91–100	3	1.5	6	7.5	0.20
111–170	6	3.0	16	20.0	0.15
>170	0	0.0	28	35.0	—
Total	200	100.0	80	100.0	—

The relative probabilities of normal homozygosity to heterozygosity (Y_1/Y_2 or h) for various enzyme activities are determined, which in turn are used in estimating a woman's likelihood of being a carrier (Emery 1986).

A major development in recent years has been the introduction of DNA markers for carrier detection and prenatal diagnosis in various genetic disorders (see reviews by Emery 1984, 1987), and the way in which such information can be used deserves special consideration.

Linkage with DNA markers. There are normal variations in base sequences of the DNA molecule which have no apparent effects on the individual, are inherited in a Mendelian fashion and occur once in about every 100 base pairs. They are detected by enzymes called restriction endonucleases: these enzymes cut DNA at sequence-specific sites but, because of variations in base sequences, the restriction site for a particular enzyme may be altered and the fragments so produced by the enzyme will be of different lengths in different individuals. They are therefore referred to as restriction fragment length polymorphisms (RFLPs). DNA samples are extracted from peripheral blood leucocytes obtained at venepuncture. The extracted DNA is then exposed to a restriction enzyme and the resultant fragments detected on an electrophoretic gel by hybridisation with an appropriate DNA probe (so-called Southern blot). A DNA probe is a radioactively labelled DNA fragment which will hybridise with, and thereby detect and locate, complementary sequences among DNA fragments on a gel. These points are illustrated in Fig. 26.2.

Here it is assumed that there is a polymorphism at restriction site B; the absence of the site is called allele-1 and the presence of the site is allele-2. When the restriction enzyme cuts the DNA in one chromosome at sites A and C it generates a single fragment of size 10 kilobases (1 kb = 1000 base pairs) which corresponds to allele-1. If the enzyme cuts the DNA not only at sites A and C but also at B, two fragments will now be generated of sizes 7 kb and 3 kb, which corresponds to allele-2. Polymorphic genotypes can therefore be deduced from the pattern of bands on an electrophoretic gel. In this example the mother is not only heterozygous for the X-linked disorder but

also for the polymorphism (1–2). Both her affected sons (II_1 and II_3) have inherited her allele-2, whereas her daughter (II_2) has inherited her allele-1.

The importance of RFLPs is that, if close linkage can be found with a disease locus, then this can be useful for preclinical and prenatal diagnosis and, in X-linked disorders, the detection of female carriers. This information is most valuable when the polymorphism actually occurs within the disease locus itself. However, if the polymorphism is some distance from the disease locus then the possibility of crossing-over (recombination) has to be taken into account. In the above hypothetical example, the risks to any subsequent child would depend on the polymorphic allele he or she inherited from the mother and the possibility of recombination occurring. Thus if the next child inherits allele-2 from mother then it will be affected, if a son, or be a carrier, if a daughter, unless crossing-over occurs. Distances between genes are measured in centiMorgans, where 1 cM represents 1% recombination between two loci; therefore, if in this example the disease locus and RFLP were 10 cM apart, the risks of a son being affected or a daughter being a carrier should they inherit allele-2 would be 90%; or if they inherited allele-1 the risks would be 10%. Using RFLPs which lie on either side (flank) a disease locus reduces the risks of misdiagnosis in such a situation (Bakker et al 1985, Monaco et al 1985). In carrier detection, information from linked RFLPs may also be combined with serum creatine kinase data; details are given by Harper et al (1983) and Pembrey et al (1984). However, when information from *flanking* markers is used the calculations can become complicated (Emery 1986) and an appropriate computer program may be necessary (Winter 1985).

So far, linked DNA markers have been found only for the X-linked Duchenne, Becker and Emery–Dreifuss forms of muscular dystrophy and myotonic dystrophy, but it is only a matter of time before useful linkages are also found for other muscular dystrophies.

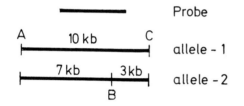

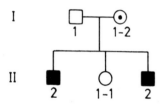

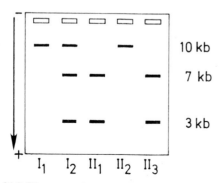

Fig. 26.2 Diagrammatic representation of an X-linked RFLP (above), its inheritance within a family in which two males (II_1, and II_3) are affected (middle), and the appearance of the resultant restriction fragments on a Southern blot (below)

Prenatal diagnosis. Over the last few years a number of abnormalities have been reported in muscle specimens from male fetuses at risk for Duchenne muscular dystrophy. Morphometry of cryostat sections has revealed increased mean fibre diameter, increased variation in fibre size, and an increase in the proportion of eosinophilic fibres and calcium-positive fibres as early as the second trimester of pregnancy (Brambati et al 1980, Emery & Burt 1980). These observations indicate that an early and significant biochemical abnormality in Duchenne muscular dystrophy is an increase in intracellular calcium. However, although these findings may help our understanding of pathogenesis, they cannot be used for prenatal diagnosis. Until recently the only possibility in X-linked Duchenne muscular dystrophy was fetal screening from cytogenetic studies on cultured amniotic fluid cells obtained at amniocentesis carried out at around 16–18 weeks' gestation. If the fetus proved to be a male then the mother could be offered pregnancy termination. Nevertheless, this is an unsatisfactory solution to the problem because a proportion of aborted male fetuses will be normal. Fetal blood samples can be obtained using fetoscopy, but unfortunately fetal serum creatine kinase activity has not proved sufficiently reliable as a method of prenatal diagnosis. However, DNA can be extracted either from amniotic fluid cells or even from chorionic tissue obtained transcervically as early as 10 weeks gestation. From linkage with DNA markers it is then possible to assess the likelihood of the male fetus being affected (Bakker et al 1985).

When an RFLP is found to be closely linked to a disease locus, then this opens up the possibility of eventually isolating the defective gene itself. By DNA sequencing and in vitro translation studies it may then become possible to identify the molecular defect. Part of the Duchenne gene has already been isolated (Monaco et al 1985) and is now being characterised. Already it is clear that between 5 and 10% of cases have a small gene deletion (Monaco et al 1985) which can be familial.

MYOTONIA

Myotonia is a failure of voluntary muscle to relax immediately following contraction. Morton et al (1963) agree with the conclusions of Bell (1947), Thomasen (1948), Stephens (1953) and de Jong (1955) that myotonia congenita, dystrophia myotonica, and paramyotonia are clinically and genetically distinct.

Myotonia congenita

This condition is usually present at birth and is characterised by stiffness which is accentuated by cold and relieved by exercise. Generalised muscular hypertrophy is common. A dominant gene with high penetrance in both sexes is the typical pattern of inheritance for myotonia congenita (Birt 1908, Bell 1947, Thomasen 1948). Becker (1977), however, has shown that the disease may also be inherited as an autosomal recessive trait. In the dominant form, myotonia is less severe and muscle weakness less common than in the recessive form.

Dystrophia myotonica

Dystrophia myotonica (Steinert 1909, Batten & Gibb 1909) typically begins in adult life with myotonia localised to the small hand muscles, forearms and tongue. Other manifestations include cataract, frontal baldness in males, gonadal atrophy, mental retardation, facial myopathy, sternomastoid weakness and progressive myopathy of peripheral distribution in the limbs. All studies, including those of Maas & Paterson (1943), Bell (1947), Thomasen (1948), de Jong (1955) and Lynas (1957), have reported transmission by an autosomal dominant gene which is over 90% penetrant and which reduces fertility to around 75% (Harper 1979). The prevalence of the disorder is approximately 5×10^{-5}. Klein (1958) observed cataract in 97.9% of his cases, testicular atrophy in 70% of the males, and sexual disorders in 47% of the females. A congenital form of myotonic dystrophy, characterised by hypotonia, mental retardation and various congenital abnormalities, has been described in the offspring of mothers with myotonic dystrophy, probably attributable to the combination of a genetic predisposition and as yet unidentified 'humoral' factors (Harper 1975).

The original claim of an additional small acrocentric chromosome in a proportion of cells in some patients with dystrophia myotonica (Fitzgerald & Caughey 1962), has been disproved (Jackson 1965). However, Mutton & Gross (1965) have reported a significantly higher frequency of chromatid and isochromatid breaks in some patients with this disease.

It has been shown that the loci (on chromosome 19) for dystrophia myotonica and ABH secretion are linked, being about 10 cM apart (Harper 1979). The detection of preclinical cases of this disease is important in genetic counselling. In this regard, the linkage with secretor status may be helpful in some families, and preclinical detection might also be accomplished by a combination of electromyography and careful slit-lamp examination for cataracts (Bundey et al 1970, Pescia & Emery 1976). However, these methods are now being supplanted by linkage with RFLPs. For example, an apolipoprotein CII probe detects an RFLP which is only 2–4 cM from the myotonic dystrophy gene (Shaw et al 1985, Pericak-Vance et al 1986). Even closer linkages will no doubt be found in future for use in both preclinical and prenatal diagnosis.

Paramyotonia

Paramyotonia (Eulenburg 1886) resembles myotonia congenita except that myotonia appears only after exposure to cold and is followed by severe generalised weakness like that of periodic paralysis. The pattern of inheritance is that of an autosomal dominant trait (Stephens 1953, de Jong 1955, Hudson 1963) which is almost 100% penetrant in heterozygotes of both sexes.

PERIODIC PARALYSIS

This condition may be subdivided into three genetic categories primarily because affected individuals within kindreds are typically hypokalaemic, hyperkalaemic or normokalaemic (Pearson 1964). However, normokalaemic cases are comparatively rare and as this sub-variety seems closely related to the hyperkalaemic type it will not be considered separately here.

Hypokalaemic periodic paralysis

Mitchell et al (1902) and Holtzapple (1905) recommended administration of potassium in periodic paralysis on purely empirical grounds, and Biemond & Daniels (1934) demonstrated that serum potassium was decreased during attacks, which could be provoked by the administration of glucose (Aitken et al 1937, Jantz 1947, McQuarrie & Ziegler 1952). The age of onset of attacks ranged from age four to 40 years with a median of about 15 years, and the frequency of attacks ranged from one to 200 per year (Oliver et al 1944). Duration of attacks varied from one to 96 h with an average of 12 h (Meyers 1949) and they usually occurred at night (Cerny & Katzonstein-Sutro 1952). Most family studies (Gaupp 1940, Meyers 1949, Sagild & Helweg-Larsen 1955) show transmission as an autosomal dominant trait which, according to the pedigrees of Helweg-Larsen et al (1955), is almost 100% penetrant in males and about 8% penetrant in females.

Hyperkalaemic periodic paralysis

From a review of the literature and personal examination of 68 cases (17 in hospital) Gamstorp (1956) found that serum potassium was typically increased during attacks of this type of periodic paralysis which could be provoked by the administration of potassium. She called this condition 'adynamia episodica hereditaria'. The age of onset ranged from one to 31 years with an average of six years and the frequency of attacks was usually once a week with a duration typically about one hour. Attacks occurred usually during the day. The condition may be associated with myotonia and even muscle wasting (Saunders et al 1968). Transmission is as an autosomal dominant trait which is completely penetrant in both sexes. Data were insufficient for Tyler et al (1951) to find linkage relations between the gene for this condition and genes for the blood groups or for PTC detection.

OTHER DISEASES OF MUSCLE
Myasthenia gravis

An abnormal degree of fatiguability of skeletal muscle, which may be reversed by anticholinesterase drugs, characterises myasthenia gravis. There appear to be at least three forms of this disease. A neonatal form, which occurs in about one in 10 newborn babies of myasthenic mothers, is transient and lasts only a few weeks. This is not genetic but is the result of antibodies to acetylcholine receptors traversing the placental barrier. Secondly, there is an inherited recessive form, beginning usually in childhood (Bundey 1972) which has a relatively better prognosis than the commoner adult form. Although adult familial cases are rare (Jacob et al 1968), when they are reported the high frequency of occurrence over two generations rather than one generation and the absence of consanguinity in the parents (Wilson & Stoner 1944, Stone & Rider 1949, Foldes & McNell 1960) is compatible with transmission by an autosomal dominant gene with low penetrance or more likely multifactorial inheritance. In a review of 1873 cases, Namba et al (1971) found a family history of secondary cases in 64 (3.4%).

Myosclerosis

Familial information about myosclerosis, characterised by progressive sclerosis of intramuscular connective tissue, is limited to a study by Löwenthal (1954) in which one male and three female sibs were affected in one family and in another family four individuals were affected in three generations. A dominant gene with reduced penetrance probably accounts for the occurrence of myosclerosis in these families if only one genotype is involved.

Myoglobinuria

In individuals who have not had a crush injury (Bywaters et al 1941) or polymyositis (Walton & Adams 1958), familial myoglobinuria (Meyer-Betz 1911) is characterised by paroxysmal attacks of generalised muscular pains, often after exercise, accompanied by myoglobinuria which is sometimes associated with permanent muscular wasting. Evidence for the role of genetic factors in this condition is limited to the observation of two affected sibs by Acheson & McAlpine (1953) and of three brothers by Hed (1955). Most reported

cases have been sporadic (Reiner et al 1956). This information suggests an autosomal recessive pattern of inheritance but the available data is insufficient to rule out other possibilities. There is increasing evidence to suggest that at least some cases may be due to carnitine palmityl transferase deficiency (see Ch. 25).

Myositis ossificans

Progressive sclerosis of intramuscular connective tissue which is followed by deposition of bone, characterises myositis ossificans (Mair 1932). Bone is laid down directly without an intermediate stage of calcification. Most cases show congenital anomalies of the great toes and thumbs (van Creveld & Soeters 1941). Evidence that this condition may be transmitted as a dominant trait with reduced penetrance is suggested by its occurrence in a father and son (Burton-Fanning & Vaughan 1901) and in a two-generation family (Gaster 1905). The condition has also been observed in two pairs of monozygotic twins (Vastine et al 1948, Eaton et al 1957). Finally, there is a paternal age effect in sporadic cases which also suggests dominant inheritance (Tünte et al 1967). The clinical and genetic features of this disorder, also known as fibrodysplasia ossificans progressiva, have recently been reviewed in detail by Connor & Evans (1982a, b) who studied 44 patients.

NEUROMUSCULAR DISEASES

Motor neurone disease

Motor neurone disease (MND) may present in one of three forms: progressive bulbar palsy, progressive muscular atrophy and amyotrophic lateral sclerosis. MND may run a rapidly progressive course leading to death within a year or so from the onset. Most cases are non-familial and the cause is obscure. In 10 studies of the familial occurrence of motor neurone disease, 32 secondary cases have been found among 1008 relatives, compared with a prevalence of about 50×10^{-6} in the general population (Pratt 1967). Families in which the disease is clearly inherited as an autosomal dominant trait, however, have been described, but are uncommon (Kurland & Mulder 1955, Engel et al

Table 26.5 A proposed classification of the primary motor neurone diseases
(AD = autosomal dominant; AR = autosomal recessive)

I *Classic MND*
  A. Sporadic
    1. Adult-onset
    2. Juvenile-onset
  B. Familial
    1. Adult-onset (AD)
    2. Juvenile-onset (AD, AR)
II *MND with parkinsonism*
  A. Sporadic
  B. Familial (AD)
III *MND with dementia*
  A. Sporadic
  B. Familial
    1. Adult-onset (AD)
    2. Juvenile-onset (AR)
IV *Guam MND*

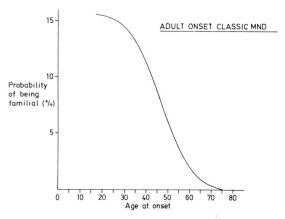

Fig. 26.3 Probability that a case of classic adult onset MND is familial depending on age at onset

1959, Roe 1964). On the basis of a series of personal cases, as well as a detailed review of 48 reported studies in the literature involving over a thousand affected individuals, a clinico-genetic classification has been proposed (Emery & Holloway 1982, Table 26.5).

By far the commonest form of MND is the classic, adult-onset form. About 5% of these cases are familial. Differentiation of sporadic from familial cases can be achieved to some extent on the basis of age at onset — the earlier the age at onset, the more likely it is to be inherited (as an autosomal dominant trait). Thus, if the age at onset is 30 years, the chances of this being familial are about 15% and therefore the risk to any offspring is about 8%. However, if onset is at 60 years, the chance of this being familial is at most 2%, and the risk to any offspring therefore less than 1% (Fig. 26.3).

Because sporadic cases of MND with onset before adulthood are very rare, if onset is before the age of 20 years this is likely to be familial, especially if the disease began in the lower limbs and spasticity is a predominant feature. Such cases are more likely to be inherited as a recessive than as a dominant trait if onset is in *early* childhood and if there is bulbar involvement (Emery & Holloway 1982). MND associated with parkinsonism or dementia and the Guam form are discussed in detail elsewhere (see Ch. 23).

Spinal muscular atrophy

The spinal muscular atrophies (SMA) may be defined as a group of inherited disorders in which the primary defect is degeneration of the anterior horn cells of the spinal cord and often of bulbar motor nuclei, but with no evidence of peripheral nerve or long tract involvement. When so defined, motor neurone disease and its variants and the various forms of 'amyotrophy' are excluded, as are congenital abnormalities of the spinal cord and traumatic, toxic, infective and neoplastic causes of anterior horn cell degeneration (see Ch. 23).

In an international collaborative study of SMA involving over 500 established cases (Emery et al 1976a) there was considerable variation in age of onset, although in over three-quarters onset was before four years of age and in these cases the prognosis was much worse than where onset was after this age. A febrile episode, often of viral origin, was occasionally noted at the time of onset and might possibly be of aetiological signifi-cance, perhaps by precipitating the disease in a genetically predisposed individual. Proximal limb muscles were predominantly affected and cranial nerves were rarely affected. Almost 10% of cases were reported as being mentally retarded. Muscle fasciculations were present in about half the cases. Electromyography and muscle histology were the most reliable diagnostic tests, the serum level of creatine kinase rarely being high and in more than half the cases it was normal (Emery et al

Table 26.6 A clinicogenetic classification of the spinal muscular atrophies

I *Proximal SMA*
  A. Infantile
     Autosomal recessive
     1. Without arthrogryposis multiplex congenita
     2. With arthrogryposis multiplex congenita
  B. Intermediate
     Autosomal recessive
  C. Juvenile
     1. Autosomal recessive
        a. Usual form (Kugelberg–Welander)
        b. 'Ryukyuan' SMA
        c. With microcephaly and mental subnormality
     2. Autosomal dominant
  D. Adult
     1. Autosomal recessive
     2. Autosomal dominant
     3. X-linked recessive
II *Distal SMA*
     1. Autosomal recessive
     2. Autosomal dominant
III *Juvenile progressive bulbar palsy*
     Autosomal recessive
     1. Usual form (Fazio–Londe)
     2. With nerve deafness (Van Laere)
IV *Scapuloperoneal SMA*
     1. Autosomal dominant
     2. Autosomal recessive
V *Facioscapulohumeral SMA*
     Autosomal dominant

1976a). Most of the cases dealt with in this particular study were of the childhood types of proximal SMA (see below).

Analysis of the genetic data suggested that the majority of these cases were attributable to at least one (but probably several) autosomal recessive genes, very few being inherited as a dominant trait, and in only one out of the 403 families was there any suggestion of X-linked inheritance (Emery et al 1976b).

A classification of the spinal muscular atrophies based on clinical and genetic differences has been proposed previously (Emery 1971, 1973) and will be adopted in the following discussion (Table 26.6). The subject has recently been reviewed in detail by Pearn (1983).

Proximal SMA. The spinal muscular atrophies with predominantly proximal muscle involvement are much commoner than other forms, and can be further subdivided according to age of onset, clinical severity and certain other features (Table 26.7).

Not all investigators agree that proximal SMA can be so subdivided and some suggest that there is a 'spectrum of clinical variation' ranging from the severe infantile to the more benign forms. If distinct forms exist, there should be little variation within a family. We have analysed the clinical and genetic data in 24 published reports involving 201 families of patients with proximal SMA with onset before adulthood (Emery 1973). The results indicated that there was a high degree of correlation in age of onset and various clinical features within families. Reported families showing considerable clinical variation in different affected members are therefore the exception and are probably highly selective.

Infantile Werdnig–Hoffmann disease. Although mild contractures are frequently found in infants with the infantile (Werdnig 1891, Hoffmann 1893) form of proximal SMA, the reported association with arthrogryposis multiplex congenita may well represent a distinct clinical entity. *Both* disorders have been described in several sibs in the same

Table 26.7 Distinguishing features of the various forms of proximal spinal muscular atrophy

Type	Age (usual)		Ability to sit without support*	Fasciculations of skeletal muscles	Serum creatine kinase
	onset	survival			
Infantile	<9 months	<4 years	never	+/−	normal
Intermediate	3–18 months	>4 years	usually	+/−	usually normal
Juvenile	>2 years	adulthood	always	++	often raised
Adult	>30 years	50 years +	always	++	often raised

* At some time during the course of the illness

family (Frischknecht et al 1960, Bargeton et al 1961).

Intermediate. It has been suggested that an autosomal recessive form of SMA intermediate in severity between the infantile (Werdnig–Hoffmann) and juvenile (Wohlfart–Kugelberg–Welander) forms may exist (Fried & Emery 1971, Emery 1971, 1973). Although there is some overlap in age of onset with the infantile form, patients with the intermediate type survive longer, even into the late teens.

Juvenile. Clinical features of the usual autosomal recessive form of juvenile, Wohlfart–Kugelberg–Welander SMA (Wohlfart et al 1955, Kugelberg & Welander 1956) have been well documented. Possible variants include the autosomal recessive form described in an inbred community in the Ryukyuan islands off Japan, the clinical features of which include pes cavus and scoliosis (Kondo et al 1970). An autosomal recessive form of juvenile proximal SMA associated with microcephaly and mental subnormality has been described by Spiro et al (1967) in three brothers. An autosomal dominant form of juvenile proximal SMA has also been described (Kugelberg & Welander 1956).

Adult. The adult form of proximal SMA may be inherited in different families as an autosomal recessive, autosomal dominant or X-linked recessive trait. The gene responsible for the X-linked recessive variety has now been located on the proximal part of the long arm of the X chromosome and an RFLP (DXY S1) is sufficiently closely linked (about 4 cM) to be useful for carrier detection and prenatal diagnosis (Fischbeck et al 1986).

Distal SMA is a relatively benign condition transmitted either as an autosomal recessive or autosomal dominant trait. Onset is usually in early childhood (Meadows & Marsden 1969). Clinically, the condition resembles peroneal muscular atrophy. However, in the latter condition the legs are typically more severely affected than the arms, peripheral sensory abnormalities can usually be detected if carefully sought, motor nerve conduc-

tion velocities are usually reduced and the pathology of peripheral nerves is abnormal, features not found in distal SMA.

Juvenile progressive bulbar palsy (Fazio–Londe's disease) is inherited as an autosomal recessive trait and is characterised by progressive cranial nerve paralyses usually dating from early childhood (Gomez et al 1962). The association with bilateral perceptive deafness (Van Laere's syndrome) appears to be a different disorder (Boudin et at 1971) but is also inherited as an autosomal recessive trait.

Scapuloperoneal muscular atrophy. Most cases of scapuloperoneal SMA are inherited as an autosomal dominant trait but instances of autosomal recessive inheritance have also been described (Feigenbaum & Munsat 1970, Emery 1971). The weakness is mainly localised to the pectoral girdle musculature and the peroneal muscles. It may be myopathic or neuropathic (SMA) in origin and the latter group itself is probably heterogeneous as the onset in some cases is in the second or third decade of life, but in others it begins in childhood.

Facioscapulohumeral muscular atrophy. This clinically resembles facioscapulohumeral muscular dystrophy, from which it can be differentiated only on the basis of muscle histology and electromyography. This rare form of SMA can apparently be inherited as an autosomal dominant trait (Fenichel et al 1967).

GENERAL CONCLUSIONS

All neuromuscular disorders have a genetic component to their aetiology although this is relatively less important in some disorders, such as mature-onset myasthenia gravis, than in others such as Duchenne muscular dystrophy. The recognition of genetic heterogeneity within what clinically may appear to be a single disorder is important for a number of reasons. Disorders inherited differently presumably have a different biochemical basis, they may have different prognoses and might conceivably respond differently to a particular treatment should such become available. However, the most important reason for understanding the genetic basis of a particular neuromuscular disorder is for reliable genetic counselling. Hereditary disorders, including neuromuscular disorders, are invariably serious, rarely treatable and never curable. The only approach is therefore prevention through genetic counselling and prenatal diagnosis. This is likely to become increasingly effective in the future when the basic biochemical defects in these disorders are better understood and with the increasing utilisation of DNA markers and gene-specific probes.

REFERENCES

Acheson D, McAlpine D, 1953 Muscular dystrophy associated with paroxysmal myoglobinuria and excessive excretion of ketosteroids. Lancet 2:327

Aitken R S, Allott E N, Castleden L I M, Walker M 1937 Observations on a case of familial periodic paralysis. Clinical Science 3:479

Bacon P A, Smith B 1971 Familial muscular dystrophy of late onset. Journal of Neurology, Neurosurgery and Psychiatry 34:93

Bakker E, Hofker M H, Goor N et al 1985 Prenatal diagnosis and carrier detection of Duchenne muscular dystrophy with closely linked RFLPs. Lancet 1:655

Baraitser M 1982 The genetics of neurological disorders. Oxford University Press, p 273

Bargeton E, Nezelof C, Guran P, Job J C 1961 Étude anatomique d'un cas d'arthrogrypose multiple congénitale et familiale. Revue Neurologique (Paris) 104:47

Batten F E 1910 Critical review: The myopathies or muscular dystrophies. Quarterly Journal of Medicine 3:313

Batten F E, Gibb H P 1909 Myotonia atrophica. Brain 32:187

Bautista J, Rafel E, Castilla J M, Alberca R 1978 Hereditary distal myopathy with onset in early infancy. Journal of the Neurological Sciences 37:149

Becker P E 1953 Dystrophia musculorum progressiva. Eine genetische und klinische Untersuchung der Muskeldystrophien. Georg Thieme, Stuttgart

Becker P E 1955 Zur Genetik der Myopathien. Deutsche Zeitschrift für Nervenheilkunde 173:482

Becker P E 1957 Neue Ergebnisse der Genetik der Muskeldystrophien. Acta genetica et statistica medica (Basel) 7:303

Becker P E 1962 Two new families of benign sex-linked recessive muscular dystrophy. Revue canadienne de biologie 21:551

Becker P E 1964 Myopathien. In: Becker P E (ed) Humangenetik, Ein Kurzes Handbuch, Vol 3. Georg Thieme, Stuttgart

Becker P E 1977 Myotonia congenita and syndromes associated with myotonia. Georg Thieme, Stuttgart

Becker P E, Kiener F 1955 Eine neue X chromosomale Muskeldystrophie. Zeitschrift für Neurologie 193:427

Beckmann R, Jerusalem F 1966 Male carriers of Duchenne-type muscular dystrophy? Lancet 2:1138

Bell J 1943 Nervous diseases and muscular dystrophies. On pseudohypertrophic and allied types of progressive muscular dystrophy. Treasury of Human Inheritance 4 (Part IV): 283

Bell J 1947 On dystrophia myotonica, myotonia congenita and paramyotonia. Treasury of Human Inheritance 4 (Part V): 343

Ben Hamida M, Fardeau M, Attia N 1983 Severe childhood muscular dystrophy affecting both sexes and frequent in Tunisia. Muscle and Nerve 6:469

Biemond A, Daniels A P 1934 Familial periodic paralysis and its transmission into spinal muscular atrophy. Brain 57:91

Birt A 1908 A study of Thomsen's disease (congenital myotonia) by a sufferer from it. Montreal Medical Journal 37:771

Blyth H, Pugh R J 1959 Muscular dystrophy in childhood. The genetic aspect. Annals of Human Genetics 23:127

Blyth H, Carter C O, Dubowitz V et al 1965 Duchenne's muscular dystrophy and the Xg blood groups: A search for linkage. Journal of Medical Genetics 2:157

Boudin G, Pepin B, Vernant J C, Gautier J C, Gouerou H 1971 Cas familial de paralysie bulbopontine chronique progressive avec surdité. Revue Neurologique (Paris) 124:90

Boyes J W, Fraser F C, Lawler S D, Mackenzie H J 1949 A pedigree of progressive muscular dystrophy. Annals of Eugenics 15:46

Brambati B, Cornelio F, Dworzak F, Dones I 1980 Calcium positive muscle fibres in fetuses at risk for Duchenne muscular dystrophy. Lancet 2:969

Brandt S 1950 Werdnig-Hoffman's infantile progressive muscular atrophy. Opera ex domo biologiae hereditariae humanae Universitatis hafniensis, vol 22

Bray G M, Kaarsoo M, Ross R T 1965 Ocular myopathy with dysphagia. Neurology (Minneapolis) 15:678

Brooks A P, Emery A E H 1977 The incidence of Duchenne muscular dystrophy in the south-east of Scotland. Clinical Genetics 11:290

Bundey S 1972 A genetic study of infantile and juvenile myasthenia gravis. Journal of Neurology, Neurosurgery and Psychiatry 35:41

Bundey S 1985 Genetics and neurology. Churchill Livingstone, Edinburgh, p 133

Bundey S, Carter C O, Soothill J F 1970 Early recognition of heterozygotes for the gene for dystrophia myotonica. Journal of Neurology, Neurosurgery and Psychiatry 33:279

Burton-Fanning F W, Vaughan A L 1901 A case of myositis ossificans. Lancet 2:849

Bywaters E G L, Delory G E, Rimington C, Smiles J 1941 Myohaemoglobin in the urine of air raid casualties with crushing injury. Biochemical Journal 35:1164

Cammann R, Vehreschild T, Ernst K 1974 Eine neue Sippe von X-chromosomaler benigner Muskeldystrophie mit Frühkontrakturen (Emery-Dreifuss). Psychiatrie Neurologie und medizinische Psychologie (Leipzig) 26:431

Caruso G, Buchthal F 1965 Refractory period of muscle and electromyographic findings in relatives of patients with muscular dystrophy. Brain 88:29

Cerny A, Katzenstein-Sutro, E 1952 Die paroxysmale

Lahmung. Schweizer Archiv für Neurologie und Psychiatrie 70:259

Chung C S, Morton N E 1959 Discrimination of genetic entities in muscular dystrophy. American Journal of Human Genetics 11:339

Connor J M, Evans D A P 1982a Fibrodysplasia ossificans progressiva: The clinical features and natural history of 34 patients. Journal of Bone and Joint Surgery 64:76

Connor J M, Evans D A P 1982b Genetic aspects of fibrodysplasia ossificans progressiva. Journal of Medical Genetics 19:35

Conomy J P 1970 Late-onset slowly progressive sex-linked recessive muscular dystrophy. Military Medicine 135:471

Davie A, Emery A E H 1978 Estimation of the proportion of new mutants among cases of Duchenne muscular dystrophy. Genetics 15:339

De Coster W, De Reuck J, Thiery E 1974 A late autosomal dominant form of limb-girdle muscular dystrophy: A clinical, genetic and morphological study. European Neurology 12:159

Dubowitz V 1960 Progressive muscular dystrophy of the Duchenne type and its mode of inheritance. Brain 83:432

Dubowitz V 1963 Myopathic changes in muscular dystrophy carriers. Proceedings of the Royal Society of Medicine 56:810

Dubowitz V 1978 Muscle disorders in childhood. Saunders, London

Eaton W L, Conkling W S, Daeschner C W 1957 Early myositis ossificans progressiva occurring in homozygotic twins; a clinical and pathological study. Journal of Pediatrics 50:591

Emanuel B S, Zackai E H, Tucker S H 1983 Further evidence for Xp21 location of the Duchenne muscular dystrophy (DMD) locus: X;9 translocation in a female with DMD. Journal of Medical Genetics 20:461

Emery A E H 1963 Clinical manifestations in two carriers of Duchenne muscular dystrophy. Lancet 1:1126

Emery A E H 1964 The electrophoretic pattern of lactic dehydrogenase in carriers and patients with Duchenne muscular dystrophy. Nature 201:1044

Emery A E H 1965 Muscle histology in carriers of Duchenne muscular dystrophy. Journal of Medical Genetics 2:1

Emery A E H 1966 Genetic linkage between the loci for colour blindness and Duchenne type muscular dystrophy. Journal of Medical Genetics 3:92

Emery A E H 1967 The use of serum creatine kinase for detecting carriers of Duchenne muscular dystrophy. In: Milhorat A T (ed) Exploratory concepts in muscular dystrophy and related disorders. Excerpta Medica, International Congress ser 147, Amsterdam, p 90

Emery A E H 1969 Abnormalities of the electrocardiogram in female carriers of Duchenne muscular dystrophy. British Medical Journal 2:418

Emery A E H 1971 The nosology of the spinal muscular atrophies. Journal of Medical Genetics 8:481

Emery A E H 1973 The nosology of the spinal muscular atrophies. In: Kakulas B A (ed) Clinical studies in myology. Excerpta Medica, Amsterdam, p 439

Emery A E H 1977 Genetic considerations in the X-linked muscular dystrophies. In: Rowland L P (ed) Pathogenesis of human muscular dystrophies. Excerpta Medica, Amsterdam, p 42

Emery A E H 1980 Duchenne muscular dystrophy: genetic aspects, carrier detection and antenatal diagnosis. British Medical Bulletin 36: 117

Emery A E H 1984 An Introduction to recombinant DNA. John Wiley, Chichester

Emery A E H 1986 Methodology in medical genetics — An introduction to statistical methods, 2nd edn. Churchill Livingstone, Edinburgh

Emery A E H 1987 Duchenne muscular dystrophy. Oxford University Press, Oxford

Emery A E H, Dreifuss F E 1966 Unusual type of benign X-linked muscular dystrophy. Journal of Neurology, Neurosurgery and Psychiatry 29:338

Emery A E H, Walton J N 1967 The genetics of muscular dystrophy. In: Steinberg A G, Bearn A G (eds) Progress in medical genetics vol 5. Grune and Stratton, New York, p 116

Emery A E H, Clack E R, Simon S, Taylor J L 1967 Detection of carriers of benign X-linked muscular dystrophy. British Medical Journal 4: 522

Emery A E H, Spikesman A 1970 Evidence against the existence of a subclinical form of X-linked Duchenne muscular dystrophy. Journal of the Neurological Sciences 10:523

Emery A E H, Skinner R 1976 Clinical studies in benign (Becker type) X-linked muscular dystrophy. Clinical Genetics 10:189

Emery A E H, Davie A M, Holloway S, Skinner R 1976a International collaborative study of the spinal muscular atrophies Part 2. Analysis of genetic data. Journal of the Neurological Sciences 30:375

Emery A E H, Hausmanowa-Petrusewicz I, Davie A M, Holloway S, Skinner R 1976b International collaborative study of the spinal muscular astrophies. Part 1. Analysis of clinical and laboratory data. Journal of the Neurological Sciences 29:83

Emery A E H, Holloway S 1977 Use of normal daughters' and sisters' creatine kinase levels in estimating heterozygosity in Duchenne muscular dystrophy. Human Heredity 27:118

Emery A E H, Burt D 1980 Intracellular calcium and pathogenesis and antenatal diagnosis of Duchenne muscular dystrophy. British Medical Journal 280:355

Emery A E H, Holloway S 1982 Familial motor neuron diseases. In: Rowland L P (ed) Human motor neuron diseases. Raven Press, New York, p 139

Engel W K, Kurland L T, Klatzo I 1959 An inherited disease similar to amyotrophic lateral sclerosis with a pattern of posterior column involvement. An intermediate form? Brain 82:203

Eulenburg A 1886 Ueber eine familiare, durch 6 Generationen verfolgbare form congenitaler Paramiotonie. Neurologisches Zentralblatt 5:265

Feigenbaum J A, Munsat T L 1970 A neuromuscular syndrome of scapuloperoneal distribution. Bulletin of the Los Angeles Neurological Society 35:47

Fenichel G M, Emery E S, Hunt P 1967 Neurogenic atrophy similating facioscapulohumeral dystrophy. Archives of Neurology 17:257

Ferrier P, Bamatter F, Klein D 1965 Muscular dystrophy (Duchenne) in a girl with Turner's syndrome. Journal of Medical Genetics 2:38

Fischbeck K H, Ionasescu V, Ritter A W et al 1986 Localization of the gene for X-linked spinal muscular atrophy. Neurology 36:1595

Fitzgerald P H, Caughey J E 1962 Chromosome and sex

chromatin studies in cases of dystrophia myotonica. New Zealand Medical Journal 61:410

Foldes F C, McNell P G 1960 Unusual occurrence of myasthenia gravis. Journal of the American Medical Association. 174:418

Fried K, Arlozorov A, Spira R 1975 Autosomal recessive oculopharyngeal muscular dystrophy. Journal of Medical Genetics 12:416

Fried K, Emery A E H 1971 Spinal muscular atrophy type II. Clinical Genetics 2:203

Frischknecht W, Bianchi L, Pilleri G 1960 Familiare Arthrogryposis multiplex congenita Neuro-arthro-myodysplasia congenita. Helvetica Paediatrica Acta 15:259

Gamstorp I 1956 Adynamia episodica hereditaria. Acta Paediatrica (Stockholm) suppl 108

Gardner-Medwin D 1970 Mutation rate in Duchenne type of muscular dystrophy. Journal of Medical Genetics 7:334

Gardner-Medwin D, Pennington R J, Walton J N 1971 The detection of carriers of X-linked muscular dystrophy genes. A review of some methods studied in Newcastle upon Tyne. Journal of the Neurological Sciences 13:459

Gaster D 1905 A case of myositis ossificans. West London Medical Journal 10:37

Gaupp R 1940 Erblichkeitsuntersuchungen beiparoxysmaler Lahmung. Zeitschrift für die gesamte Neurologie und Psychiatrie 170:108

Gomez M R, Clermont V, Bernstein J 1962 Progressive bulbar paralysis in childhood (Fazio-Londe's disease). Archives of Neurology 6:317

Greig D N H 1977 Family in which Duchenne's muscular dystrophy and protan colour blindness are segregating. Journal of Medical Genetics 14:130

Hanson P A, Rowland L P 1971 Möbius syndrome and facioscapulohumeral muscular dystrophy. Archives of Neurology 24:31

Harper P S 1975 Congenital myotonic dystrophy in Britain. II. Genetic basis. Archives of Disease in Childhood 50:514

Harper P S 1979 Myotonic dystrophy. Saunders, Philadelphia

Harper P S, O'Brien T, Murrray J M, Davies K E, Pearson P, Williamson R 1983 The use of linked DNA polymorphisms for genotype prediction in families with Duchenne muscular dystrophy. Journal of Medical Genetics 20:252

Hausmanowa-Petrusewicz I, Prot J, Dobosz I et al 1971 Further studies concerning the detection of carriership in the Duchenne type of dystrophy. European Neurology 5:186

Hayes R, London W, Siedman J, Embree L 1963 Oculopharyngeal muscular dystrophy. New England Journal of Medicine 268:163

Heckmatt J Z, Dubowitz V 1983 Congenital myopathies. In: Emery A E H, Rimoin D (eds) Principles and practice of medical genetics. Churchill Livingstone, Edinburgh, p 367

Hed R 1955 Myoglobinuria in man. Norstedt, Stockholm

Helweg-Larson H F, Hauge M, Sagild E 1955 Periodic paralysis. Acta Genetica et Statistica Medica (Basel) 5:263

Henson T E, Muller J, De Myer W E 1967 Hereditary myopathy limited to females. Archives of Neurology 17:238

Heyck H, Laudahn G, Carsten P M 1966 Enzymaktivitätsbestimmungen bei Dystrophia musculorum progressiva. IV. Die Serumenzymkinetik im präklinischen Stadium des Typus Duchenne während der ersten 2 Lebensjahre. Klinische Wochenschrift 44:695

Hodgson S, Boswinkel E, Cole C et al 1986 A linkage study of Emery-Dreifuss muscular dystrophy. Human Genetics 74:409

Hoffman J 1893 Ueber chronische spinale Muskelatrophie im Kindesalter auf familiarer basis. Deutsche Zeitschrift für Nervenheilkunde 3:427

Holtzapple G E 1905 Periodic paralysis. Journal of the American Medical Association 45:1224

Hudson A J 1963 Progressive neurological disorder and myotonia congenita associated with paramyotonia. Brain 86:811

Ionasescu V 1975 Distinction between Duchenne and other muscular dystrophies by ribosomal protein synthesis. Journal of Medical Genetics 12:49

Jackson C E, Carey J N 1961 Progressive muscular dystrophy; autosomal recessive type. Pediatrics 28:77

Jackson J F 1965 Chromosomes in dystrophia myotonica. Lancet 1:1225

Jacob A, Clack E R, Emery A E H 1968 Genetic study of sample of 70 patients with myasthenia gravis. Journal of Medical Genetics 5:257

Jantz H 1947 Stoffwechsel untersuchungen bei paroxysmaler Lähmung. Nervenarzt 18:360.

Johnston H A 1964 Severe muscular dystrophy in girls. Journal of Medical Genetics 1:79

Johnston H A, Wilkinson J H, Withycombe W A, Raymond S 1966 Alpha-hydroxybutyrate dehydrogenase activity in sex-linked muscular dystrophy. Journal of Clinical Pathology 19:250

de Jong J G Y 1955 Myotonia. Van Gorcum, Assen

Kiloh L G, Nevin S 1951 Progressive dystrophy of the external ocular muscles. Brain 74:115

Kingston H M, Thomas N S T, Pearson P L, Sarfarazi M, Harper P S 1983 Genetic linkage between Becker muscular dystrophy and a polymorphic DNA sequence on the short arm of the X chromosome. Journal of Medical Genetics 20:255

Klein D 1958 La dystrophie myotonique (Steinert) et la myotonie congénitale (Thomsen) en Suisse. Journal de Génétique Humaine (suppl) 7:1

Kloepfer H W, Talley C 1958 Autosomal recessive inheritance of Duchenne-type muscular dystrophy. Annals of Human Genetics 22:138

Kondo K, Tsubaki T, Sakamoto F 1970 The Ryukyuan muscular atrophy. An obscure heritable neuromuscular disease found in the islands of Southern Japan. Journal of the Neurological Sciences 11:359

Kowalewski S, Rotthauwe H W, Mölbert E, Mumenthaler M 1966 Female carriers of muscular dystrophy. Lancet 1:1216

Kugelberg E, Welander L 1956 Heredofamilial juvenile muscular atrophy simulating muscular dystrophy. Archives of Neurology and Psychiatry 75:500

Kurland L T, Mulder D W 1955 Epidemiologic investigations of amyotrophic lateral sclerosis — familial aggregations indicative of dominant inheritance. Neurology (Minneapolis) 5:182

Kuroiwa Y, Miyazaki T 1967 Epidemiological study of myopathy in Japan. In: Milhorat A T (ed) Exploratory concepts in muscular dystrophy. Excerpta Medica, Amsterdam, p 98

Lamy M, de Grouchy J 1954 L'hérédité de la myopathie (formes basses). Journal de Génétique Humaine 3:219

Lawrence E F, Brown B, Hopkins J I 1973 Pseudohypertrophic muscular dystrophy of childhood: An epidemiological survey in Victoria. Australian and New Zealand Journal of Medicine 3:142

Lees F, Liversedge L A 1962 Descending ocular myopathy. Brain 85:701

Levison H 1951 Dystrophia musculorum progressiva; clinical and diagnostic criteria; inheritance. Acta Psychiatrica et Neurologica (suppl) 76:1

Löwenthal A 1954 Myosclérose familiale. Études presentées à la Ire reunion neurologique Belgo-Suisse, Vevey, p 62

Lynas M 1957 Dystrophia myotonica with special reference to Northern Ireland. Annals of Human Genetics 21:318

Maas O, Paterson A S 1943 Genetic and familial aspects of dystrophia myotonica. Brain 66:55

Mabry C C, Roeckel I E, Munich R L, Robertson D 1965 X-linked pseudohypertrophic muscular dystrophy with a late onset and slow progression. New England Journal of Medicine 273:1062

Macciotta A, Costa V, Cao A, Sforza F, Scano V 1964 Studio istologica sul tessuto muscolare die genitori di un bambino con Miodistrofia pelvi-femorali tipo Duchenne. Annali Italian di Pediatria 17:1

Mair W E 1932 Myositis ossificans progressiva. Edinburgh Medical Journal 29:13, 69

Mannucci P M, Idéo G, Cao A, Macciotta A 1965 Gli isoenzimi della latticodeidrogenasi (LDH) e della transaminasi glutammico-ossalacetica (TGO) nel muscolo fetale, adulto, e di Sogetti affetti da distrofia muscolare, progressiva tipo Duchenne. Rassegna medica Sarda 68:287

Markand O N, North R R, D'Agostino A M, Daly D D 1969 Benign sex-linked muscular dystrophy. Neurology (Minneapolis) 19:617

McQuarrie I, Ziegler M R 1952 Hereditary periodic paralysis; effects of fasting and of various types of diet on occurrence of paralytic attacks. Metabolism 1:129

Markesbery W R, Griggs R C, Leach R P, Lapham L W 1974 Late onset hereditary distal myopathy. Neurology (Minneapolis) 24:127

Meadows J C, Marsden C D 1969 A distal form of chronic spinal muscular atrophy. Neurology (Minneapolis) 19:53

Meyer-Betz F 1911 Zur vergleichenden Pathologie der paroxysmalen Hemoglobinurie. Deutsches Archiv für Klinische Medizin 103:150

Meyers W A 1949 Familial periodic paralysis as traced in one family for five generations. Pennsylvania Medical Journal 52:1060

Milhorat A T 1961 Clinico-genetic aspects of muscular dystrophy. 2nd International Conference of Human Genetics, Rome, p 83

Mitchell J K, Flexner S, Edsall D L 1902 A brief report of the clinical, physiological and chemical study of three cases of family periodic paralysis. Brain 25:109

Monaco A P, Bertelson C J, Middlesworth W et al 1985 Detection of deletions spanning the Duchenne muscular dystrophy locus using a tightly linked DNA segment. Nature 316:842

Monaco A P, Neve R L, Colletti-Feener C, Bertelson C J, Kurnit D M, Kunkel L M 1986 Isolation of candidate cDNAs for portions of the Duchenne muscular dystrophy gene. Nature 323:646

Moosa A, Brown B H, Dubowitz V 1972 Quantitative electromyography: Carrier detection in Duchenne type muscular dystrophy using a new automatic technique. Journal of Neurology, Neurosurgery and Psychiatry 35:841

Morris C J, Raybould J A 1971 Histochemically demonstrable fibre abnormalities in normal skeletal muscle and in muscle from carriers of Duchenne muscular dystrophy. Journal of Neurology, Neurosurgery and Psychiatry 34:348

Morton N E, Chung C S 1959 Formal genetics of muscular dystrophy. American Journal of Human Genetics 11:360

Morton N E, Chung C S, Peters H A 1963 Genetics of muscular dystrophy. In: Bourne G H, Golarz N (eds) Muscular dystrophy in man and animals. Karger, Basel

Moser H, Wiesmann U, Richterich R, Rossi E 1964 Progressive muskeldystrophie VI. Häufigkeit, Klinik und Genetik der Duchenne-Form. Schweizerische medizinische Wochenschrift 94:1610

Moser H, Emery A E H 1974 The manifesting carrier in Duchenne muscular dystrophy. Clinical Genetics 5:271

Murphy S F, Drachman D B 1968 The oculopharyngeal syndrome. Journal of the American Medical Association 203:1003

Mutton D E, Gross N 1965 Chromosomes in dystrophia myotonica. Lancet 2:289

Namba T, Brunner N G, Brown S B, Muguruma M, Grob D 1971 Familial myasthenia gravis. Archives of Neurology 25: 49

Okinaka S, Sugita H, Momoi H et al 1959 Serum creatine phosphokinase and aldolase activity in neuromuscular disorders. 84th annual meeting of the American Neurological Association, Atlantic City

Oliver C P, McQuarrie I, Ziegler M 1944 Hereditary periodic paralysis in a family showing varied manifestations. American Journal of Diseases of Children 69:308

Pearce G W, Pearce J M S, Walton J N 1966 The Duchenne type muscular dystrophy: histopathological studies of the carrier state. Brain 89:109

Pearn J 1983 Spinal muscular atrophies. In: Emery A E H, Rimoin D (eds) Principles and practice of medical genetics. Churchill Livingstone, Edinburgh, p 414

Pearson C M 1964 The periodic paralyses: Differential features and pathological observations in permanent myopathic weakness. Brain 87:341

Pearson C M, Kar N C 1966 Isoenzymes: General considerations and alterations in human and animal myopathies. Annals of the New York Academy of Sciences 138:293

Pearson C M, Fowler W M, Wright S W 1963 X-chromosome mosaicism in females with muscular dystrophy. Proceedings of the National Academy of Sciences USA 50:24

Pembrey M E, Davies K E, Winter R M et al 1984 Clinical use of DNA markers linked to the gene for Duchenne muscular dystrophy. Archives of Disease in Childhood 59:208

Penn A S, Lisak R P, Rowland L P 1970 Muscular dystrophy in young girls. Neurology (Minneapolis) 20:147

Pericak-Vance M A, Yamaoka L H, Assunder L I F et al 1986 Tight linkage of apolipoprotein C2 to myotonic dystrophy on chromosome 19. Neurology 36:1418

Pescia G, Emery A E H 1976 Valeur et limites de l'examen biomicroscopique du cristallin dans la detection des heterozygotes pour la dystrophie myotonique. Journal de Génétique Humaine 24:227

Peterman A F, Lillington G A, Jamplis R W 1964 Progressive muscular dystrophy with ptosis and dysphagia. Archives of Neurology 10:38

Pickard N A, Gruemer H D, Verrill H L et al 1978

Systemic membrane defect in the proximal muscular dystrophies. New England Journal of Medicine 299:841

Pratt R T C 1967 The genetics of neurological disorders. Oxford University Press, London

Prot J 1971 Genetic-epidemiological studies in progressive muscular dystrophy. Journal of Medical Genetics 8:90

Race R R 1955 On the inheritance of muscular dystrophy. A note on the blood groups. Annals of Human Genetics 20:13

Radu H, Stenzel K 1969a Beiträge zum Studium der pseudohypertrophischen Muskeldystrophien I. Gutartige pseudohypertrophische Muskeldystrophie. Deutsche Zeitschrift für Nervenheilkunde 196:92

Radu H, Stenzel K 1969b Beiträge zum Studium der pseudohypertrophischen Muskeldystrophien II. Pseudohypertrophische Muskeldystrophie bei Mädchen. Deutsche Zeitschrift für Nervenheilkunde 196:116

Reiner L R, Konikoff N, Altschule M D, Dammin G J, Merrill J P 1956 Idiopathic paroxysmal myoglobinuria: Report of 2 cases and evaluation of syndrome. Archives of Internal Medicine 97:537

Richterich R, Rosin S, Aebi U, Rossi E 1963 Progressive muscular dystrophy V. The identification of the carrier state in the Duchenne type by serum creatine kinase determination. American Journal of Human Genetics 15:133

Roe P F 1964 Familial motor neurone disease. Journal of Neurology, Neurosurgery and Psychiatry 27:140

Rotthauwe H W, Kowalewski S 1965 Klinische und biochemische Untersuchungen bei Myopathien I. Serumenzyme bei progressiver Muskeldystrophie (Typ I, II, IIIa). Klinische Wochenschrift 43:144

Rotthauwe H W, Kowalewski S 1966a Gutartige recessiv X-chromosomal vererbte Muskeldystrophie I. Untersuchungen bei Merkmalsträgern. Humangenetik 3:17

Rotthauwe H W, Kowalewski S 1966b Gutartrige recessiv X-chromosomal vererbte Muskeldystrophie II. Untersuchungen bei Konduktorinnen. Humangenetik 3:30

Rowland L P, Fetell M, Olarte M, Hays A, Singh N, Wanat F E 1979 Emery-Dreifuss muscular dystrophy. Annals of Neurology 5:111

Roy S, Dubowitz V 1970 Carrier detection in Duchenne muscular dystrophy. A comparative study of electron microscopy, light microscopy and serum enzymes. Journal of the Neurological Sciences 11:65

Sagild U, Helweg-Larsen H F 1955 Clinical picture of hereditary transitory muscular paralysis: Periodic adynamia and periodic paralysis. Nordisk Medicin 53:981

Saunders M, Ashworth B, Emery A E H, Benedikz J E G 1968 Familial myotonic periodic paralysis with muscle wasting. Brain 91:295

Schneiderman L J, Sampson W I, Schoene W C, Haydon G B 1969 Genetic studies of a family with two unusual autosomal dominant conditions: Muscular dystrophy and Pelger-Huet anomaly. American Journal of Medicine 46:380

Shaw D L, Meredith A L, Sarfarazi M et al 1985 The apolipoprotein C II gene: Subchromosomal localisation and linkage to the myotonic dystrophy locus. Human Genetics 70:271

Skinner R, Emery A E H, Anderson A J B, Foxall C 1975 The detection of carriers of benign (Becker-type) X-linked muscular dystrophy. Journal of Medical Genetics 12:131

Smith H L, Amick L D, Johnson W W 1966 Detection of subclinical and carrier states in Duchenne muscular dystrophy. Journal of Pediatrics 69:67

Spiro A J, Fogelson M H, Goldberg A C 1967 Microcephaly and mental subnormality in chronic progressive spinal muscular atrophy of childhood. Developmental Medicine and Child Neurology 9:594

Steinert H 1909 Myopathologische Seitrage. Deutsche Zeitschrift für Nervenheilkunde 37:58

Stephens F E 1953 Inheritance of diseases primary in the muscle. American Journal of Medicine 15:558

Stephens F E, Tyler F H 1951 Studies in disorders of muscle. V. The inheritance of childhood progressive muscular dystrophy in 33 kindreds. American Journal of Human Genetics 3:111

Stephens J, Lewin E 1965 Serum enzyme variations and histological abnormalities in the carrier state in Duchenne dystrophy. Journal of Neurology, Neurosurgery and Psychiatry 28:104

Stevenson A C 1953 Muscular dystrophy in Northern Ireland. I. An account of 51 families. Annals of Eugenics (London) 18:50

Stevenson A C 1958 Muscular dystrophy in Northern Ireland. IV. Some additional data. Annals of Human Genetics 22:231

Stevenson A C, Cheeseman E A, Huth M C 1955 Muscular dystrophy in Northern Ireland. III. Linkage data with particular reference to autosomal limb-girdle muscular dystrophy. Annals of Human Genetics 19:165

Stone C T, Rider J A 1949 Treatment of myasthenia gravis. Journal of the American Medical Association 141:107

Sumner D, Crawfurd M D A, Harriman D G F 1971 Distal muscular dystrophy in an English family. Brain 94:51

Taylor E W 1915 Progressive vagus-glossopharyngeal paralysis with ptosis. A contribution to the group of family diseases. Journal of Nervous and Mental Disease 42:129

Thomasen E 1948 'Myotonia' vol 17. Hereditarae Humanae Universitates Hafniensis, Aarhus

Thompson M W, Ludvigsen B, Monckton G 1962 Some problems in the genetics of muscular dystrophy. Revue canadienne de biologie 21:543

Tünte W, Becker P E, Knorre G 1967 Zur Genetik der Myositis ossificans progressiva. Humangenetik 4:320

Tyler F H, Stephens F E 1950 Studies in disorders of muscle. II. Clinical manifestations and inheritance of facioscapulohumeral dystrophy in a large family. Annals of Internal Medicine 32:640

Tyler F H, Stephens F E, Gunn F D, Perkoff G T 1951 Studies in disorders of muscle. VII. Clinical manifestations and inheritance of periodic paralysis without hypopotassemia. Journal of Clinical Investigation 30:492

van Creveld S, Soeters J M 1941 Progressive myositis ossificans. American Journal of Diseases of Children 62:1000

Vastine J H, Vastine M F, Arango O 1948 Myositis ossificans progressiva in homozygotic twins. American Journal of Roentgenology 59:204

Victor M, Hayes R, Adams R D 1962 Oculopharyngeal muscular dystrophy. A familial disease of late life characterized by dysphagia and progressive ptosis of the eyelids. New England Journal of Medicine 267:1267

Walton J N 1955 On the inheritance of muscular dystrophy. Annals of Human Genetics 20:1

Walton J N 1956 The inheritance of muscular dystrophy: Further observations. Annals of Human Genetics 21:40

Walton J N 1957a The inheritance of muscular dystrophy. Acta Genetica et Statistica Medica (Basel) 7:318

Walton J N 1957b The limp child. Journal of Neurology, Neurosurgery and Psychiatry 20:144

Walton J N 1963 Clinical aspects of human muscular dystrophy. In: Bourne G H, Golarz Ma Nelly (eds) Muscular dystrophy in man and animals. Hafner, New York, p 263

Walton J N, Nattrass F J 1954 On the classification, natural history and treatment of the myopathies. Brain 77:169

Walton J N, Adams R D 1958 Polymyositis. Livingstone, Edinburgh

Welander L 1951 Myopathia distalis tarda hereditaria; 249 examined cases in 72 pedigrees. Acta Medica Scandinavica 141 (suppl 265):41

Welander L 1957 Homozygous appearance of distal myopathy. Acta Genetica et Statistica Medica (Basel) 7:321

Werdnig G 1891 I Zwei fruhinfantile hereditare Falle von progressiver Muskelatrophie unter dem bilde der Dystrophie aber auf neurotischer Grundlage. Archiv für Psychiatrie und Nervenkrankheiten 22:437

Wilson A, Stoner H B 1944 Myasthenia gravis: a consideration of its causation in a study of 14 cases. Quarterly Journal of Medicine 13:1

Winter R M 1985 The estimation of recurrence risks in monogenic disorders using flanking marker loci. Journal of Medical Genetics 22:12

Wohlfart G, Fex J, Eliasson S 1955 Hereditary proximal spinal muscular atrophy — a clinical entity simulating progressive muscular dystrophy. Acta Psychiatrica et Neurologica 30:395

Yates J R W, Emery A E H 1985 A population study of adult onset limb-girdle muscular dystrophy. Journal of Medical Genetics 22:250

Zatz M, Itskan S B, Sanger R, Forta-Pessoa O, Saldanha P H 1974 New linkage data for the X-linked types of muscular dystrophy and G6PD variants, colour blindness and Xg blood groups. Journal of Medical Genetics 11:321

Zellweger H 1966 Congenital myopathies and their differential diagnosis. Pädologie Fortibildungskurse 18:105

Zellweger H, Hanson J W 1967 Slowly progressive X-linked recessive muscular dystrophy (Type IIIb). Archives of Internal Medicine 120:525

The clinical features of some miscellaneous neuromuscular disorders

INTRODUCTION

Several disorders of the spinal cord or nerve roots and trunks present no problem of pathogenesis, and yet are important because of their frequency in clinical practice. Although affecting voluntary muscles secondarily, they should be considered in any comprehensive treatise on disorders of muscle. Denervation atrophy is the resulting change in muscle affected by lesions of its motor nerve supply and the histological changes of neurogenic atrophy are non-specific, regardless of the cause. These changes have been considered in detail elsewhere (Ch. 5). Any disorder of the motor neurone may result in this type of change, whether that disorder is of the axons themselves or of their cells of origin, produced either by direct implication in a pathological process or because of ischaemia or compression arising from some extraneuronal lesion.

Tetanus

Traumatic inoculation with the bacillus *Clostridium tetani* is followed after a variable incubation period of one, two or more weeks by restlessness leading to stiffness of muscles and the noise-induced spasms of classic clinical tetanus. The exotoxin of the bacillus is fatal to man in a dose of 0.22 mg and, although spasm is often maximal in muscles closely related to the point of entry, there is general agreement that the toxin reaches the central nervous system by the blood stream, where it possibly acts by blocking the Renshaw cell inhibitory system (Eccles 1957). There is no consistent or specific neuropathological change in muscle or neural tissue in the fatal cases, even when prolonged spasm has resulted in tonic contracture of skeletal muscle (Adams et al 1962). However, many patients recovering from the illness suffer irritability, fits and myoclonus, sleep disturbances, decreased libido and postural hypotension. These features may be reflected in abnormalities in the electroencephalogram (Illis & Taylor 1971). Recent clinical interest in the management of cases of tetanus has been concerned with the establishment of centres for its treatment and, more specifically, the control of spasms by early tracheostomy, the use of muscle-relaxant drugs, often with a total paralysis regimen, and positive pressure respiration.

NERVE ROOT LESIONS

Neuralgic amyotrophy and serum neuropathy

After the injection of antitetanus serum, or other sera containing foreign protein, a syndrome of arthralgia, rash and fever may appear and may be associated with extensive weakness and, later, wasting of the muscles of one (or rarely both) shoulder girdle and upper limb. The prognosis of the muscle weakness and of the serum sickness itself is good, but occasional focal pareses persist, e.g. paresis of serratus anterior. Closely allied to serum neuropathy is the syndrome of neuralgic amyotrophy, a shoulder-girdle neuritis in which some 10–14 days after a specific or non-specific illness, or sometimes without obvious precipitant, severe pain in the shoulder on one side or both is followed after a few days' interval by weakness and, later, wasting of muscle. The muscles innervated by the fifth and sixth cervical roots are usually affected and there is often some sensory impairment within the distribution of the axillary nerve, i.e. over the lower belly and insertion of the deltoid. Paralysis of serratus anterior is common and often associated with weakness of the deltoid and spinati. Less commonly, groups innervated by the sixth and seventh roots, i.e. in the forearm, may be involved. This disorder affects young adults and was first clearly delineated as an entity during wartime (Parsonage & Turner 1948). It is curiously common in the UK and European countries. The prognosis is excellent but recovery of

the paralysed muscle may be extremely slow, taking up to 18 months. There appears to be no equivalent disorder involving the lumbosacral roots and plexus and, when such a syndrome of pain and weakness of the lower limbs presents, then some pathological process other than one of the putative allergic monoradiculopathy must be considered.

PERIPHERAL NERVE

Restless legs syndrome

Formication, prickling and crawling sensations in the legs, felt particularly between the knee and ankle, often relieved by movement, form the clinical syndrome of restless legs. First described by Thomas Willis in 1685, the clinical features have been reviewed by Beard (1880), Oppenheimer (1923), Norlander (1954), Wittmach (1961) and Gorman et al (1965), with a definitive review by Ekbom (1960), whose name is now frequently associated with the syndrome.

The symptoms may spread into the thighs and feet and, rarely, the hands and arms may be involved. The symptoms occur most frequently in bed at night and prevent sleep. It was Ekbom's initial belief that the symptoms had a vascular pathogenesis but this has not been substantiated. Although in most cases there is no evident pathology, these symptoms which constitute Ekbom's syndrome have been described in association with drug therapy, notably prochlorperazine, with barbiturate withdrawal, prolonged exposure to cold, carcinoma, iron deficiency anaemia and avitaminosis, diabetic neuropathy, prostatitis and uraemic neuropathy (Callaghan 1966). The syndrome has also been reported in association with chronic pulmonary disease (Spillane 1970). The paraesthesiae are more frequent in women, especially in pregnancy, and are not accompanied by evidence of polyneuropathy; it has been suggested that the basic pathology lies in the spinal cord (Ask-Upmark 1954). There is a strikingly high incidence of psychoneurotic symptoms, especially anxiety, tension and depression, in patients suffering from this syndrome. Myokymia is present in some affected individuals, but distressing sensory symptoms differentiate 'restless legs' from other disorders where myokymia is a feature; e.g. the syndrome of continuous muscle fibre activity (Isaacs 1961), or quantal squander myokymia (McComas 1977) (see below).

When the sensation in the legs is pain, there may be an associated spontaneous movement of the toes (Spillane et al 1971). Recent work suggests that in this distinctive disorder the lesion responsible is in the afferent fibres of the posterior nerve roots (Nathan 1978).

Although there is no recognisable pathogenesis in the spontaneously occurring cases, treatment with phenothiazines or diazepam may be successful. Chlorpromazine 50 mg given last thing at night may alleviate the troublesome nocturnal symptoms. In otherwise refractory cases relief has been obtained by using procaine hydrochloride i.v., in a dose of 500 mg in 0.5 litre of normal saline infused over a period of 30–40 min on three consecutive days.

NEUROMUSCULAR JUNCTION

Botulism

Rapid death from bulbar paralysis results from the injection of the exotoxin of *Clostridium botulinum*. The bacillus is strictly anaerobic and is found in all soils and animal faeces; outbreaks of botulism have usually been associated with improperly prepared canned and bottled foods. The toxin is the most powerful poison recognised, 0.05 mg being fatal to man. It has a specific action in blocking terminal motor nerve filaments (Brooks 1956). Experimental botulinus paralysis in the rabbit is due to a block of cholinergic fibres (Ambache 1949) with a specific action of blocking the terminal nerve filaments at the presynaptic level and of interfering with acetylcholine release. The neuromuscular block differs from that due to curare in that, although paralysed muscle will no longer respond to nerve stimulation, it contracts after the intra-arterial injection of acetylcholine. Symptoms appear two to 36 hours after ingestion. The paralysis is first confined to the bulbar muscles with diplopia, ptosis, irritability and

giddiness, then spreads to give respiratory failure of both central and peripheral type. Sensation is not affected (Lamanna 1959).

Repetitive nerve stimulation shows a defect of neuromuscular transmission similar to that seen in myasthenia gravis and in the Eaton–Lambert syndrome. Motor nerve conduction velocity and sensory latencies are not affected. As guanidine has been used with benefit in the Eaton–Lambert syndrome (Lambert & Rooke 1965), Cherington & Ryan (1969) used the compound successfully in botulism in doses of 35–50 mg/kg body weight. Guanidine acts by enhancing the release of acetylcholine (Otsuka & Endo 1960) and its salts can inactivate botulinum toxin directly (Stefanye et al 1964). Polyvalent antitoxin and neostigmine are ineffective, but further experience with guanidine in botulism has shown that it is of value.

Infant botulism. Botulism can be a cause of an acute illness leading to death in infancy and Arnon (1980) has estimated that some 500 cases occur annually in the USA. The first case recorded in the UK was in a 24–week–old girl reported by Turner et al (1978). Other cases have been reported from Australia by Shield and colleagues (1978) but the condition seems to be especially common in Western America.

The clinical presentation is one of poor sucking and difficulty with feeding, poor ability to cry with loss of head control and bilateral ptosis with generalised flaccid paralysis. Arnon (1980) reports that 30% of infants with botulism suffer a final respiratory arrest. Sonnabend et al (1981) describe a four-month-old infant dying unexpectedly at home in the company of four adults. A type-G toxin was present in the serum in three cases. They describe botulism as a cause of sudden unexplained death recognised at autopsy among 40 infants and 55 adults. This suggests that as many as 10% of pathologically unexplained sudden deaths in infants may be due to botulism (Layzer 1985).

As far as treatment is concerned, immediate access to an intensive care unit is essential as respiratory arrest and aspiration is a usual cause of death and supportive care is the key to the treatment of any infant suspected of suffering from botulism. The administration of botulinum antitoxin does not appear to affect the course of the disease (Turner et al 1978).

Myokymia, continuous muscle fibre activity

Three forms of myokymia have been described in clinical practice. One of these takes the form (Harman & Richardson 1954) of continuous undulating movement in the muscles of the face (facial myokymia) or sometimes in those of the limbs and trunk. Electromyographically, in these cases there are stereotyped groups of from two to over 200 motor unit potentials (multiplets) occurring at intervals of about 20 ms. Facial myokymia is occasionally a manifestation of multiple sclerosis (Matthews 1966) or even of pontine tumour, but the variety which affects the limbs and trunk and which may be particularly prominent in calf muscles is usually benign.

Another form of myokymia, known as 'live flesh', takes the form of a brief series of twitches of the lower eyelid or of a calf muscle, often related to fatigue and again of no pathological significance.

The third variety, first described by Gamstorp & Wohlfart (1959) and later by Isaacs (1961), under the title of 'continuous muscle fibre activity and spasm', is characterised by diffuse coarse fasciculation and muscle stiffness and cramps with impaired relaxation after contraction which are transiently improved by repeated contraction. Sometimes there is marked stiffness of gait and movement and some patients develop laryngeal and other localised spasms or occasionally progressive deformity of the feet. Hyperhidrosis is common and some patients go on to develop atrophy of distal limb muscles (Gardner-Medwin & Walton 1969).

The electromyogram shows continuous spontaneous repetitive discharges of potentials resembling motor unit potentials, but myotonic discharges are usually absent from the EMG and as a rule no fibrillation potentials are seen. Peripheral nerve block has no influence upon the activity but neuromuscular block abolishes it. Ultrastructural studies of motor end-plates have given normal findings (Sigwald et al 1966), although Mertens & Zschocke (1965), who entitled the

same disorder 'neuromyotonia', thought that there were minor end-plate abnormalities in methylene blue preparations. Isaacs (1961) suggested that the condition was a functional anomaly of the distal part of the motor nerve fibres and postulated excessive release of acetylcholine at motor end-plates ('quantal squander'). However, other evidence suggests a postsynaptic defect with increasing sensitivity of the muscle fibre membrane to acetylcholine. The condition is almost specifically relieved by phenytoin and by other membrane-stabilising drugs (Isaacs & Heffron 1974), although in the more severe cases the muscular atrophy may prove to be progressive even if the myokymia is relieved.

The continuous muscle fibre activity (which is sometimes referred to as the Isaacs-Mertens syndrome) has usually presented sporadically. However, Auger et al (1984) reported six patients in two unrelated families who suffered generalised myokymia and muscle cramps with no clinical or electromyographic evidence of peripheral neuropathy. In 1984 Stephen and colleagues described a family with this problem appearing in an autosomal dominant pattern with mother and son developing muscle stiffness and rigidity in early childhood. They were distinguished from hereditary cases of 'stiff-man syndrome' where no myokymia is seen and the rigidity is obscured by sleep.

Ashizawa et al (1983) have described an autosomal dominant form of continuous muscle fibre activity in a seven-year-old girl and four other members of the family. In these patients the symptoms appeared in childhood, tended to improve later and were almost confined to the lower limbs.

MUSCLE

Acute muscle compartment compression syndromes

Severe boring pain in the tibialis anterior muscle may occur in male adults, and especially those who undertake unaccustomed exercise (tibialis anticus syndrome). The pain is also recognised in athletes with gross hypertrophy of the anterior crural group of muscles and is thought to be ischaemic. Exercise of the anterior crural group encased in their osseofibrous sheath results in swelling and increased vascularity. Oedema followed by ischaemic necrosis within the anterior crural compartment may also be due to arterial embolism or thrombosis, direct trauma or even fracture of the tibia and fibula. The resultant damage to the muscle and the anterior tibial nerve results in foot-drop and impaired walking. Most patients with the anterior tibial syndrome are able to obtain complete relief by resting, but occasionally the pain persists and decompression of the anterior crural compartment has been recommended in order to prevent permanent muscle damage (Sirbou et al 1944). The long flexors of the toes lying in the deep posterior compartment of the lower leg are also susceptible to compression necrosis, usually following fracture of the tibia. Such a fracture may damage the posterior tibial or peroneal arteries with subsequent necrosis and fibrosis of the long flexor muscles.

Volkmann's ischaemic contracture

Post–ischaemic fibrosis of the long flexors of the fingers, first described in 1881 by Volkmann, is specifically associated with supracondylar fractures of the humerus in childhood. The onset is often rapid, accompanied by burning pain in the hand and forearm. Diminution of the radial pulse may be observed, and paralysis of the long flexor muscles develops without sensory loss. After the oedema has settled, the atrophic muscles become fibrosed and essentially useless. Similar post-ischaemic contraction may follow arterial embolism. Thus the syndrome is very similar to that occurring in the anterior and posterior crural compartments, ischaemia being followed by infarction and consequent fibrosis.

Myositis ossificans

In the literature there are reports of some 350 patients, mostly children, often suffering from a congenital anomaly of their great toes or other digits, in whom sclerosis of muscle connective tissue is followed by the deposition of bone — fibrodysplasia ossificans progressiva (McKusick

1956) or progressive myositis ossificans. There is some evidence that this disorder may be transmitted by a dominant gene (Gaster 1905, Eaton et al 1957) or may be due to autosomal dominant mutations exposed to strong selection pressure, i.e. almost all cases are new mutants (Tunte et al 1967), but its pathogenesis is unknown. Chromosome studies show a normal karyotype (Viparelli 1963). Children or young adults are affected, with the involvement of aponeuroses, tendons and fascia in addition to the connective tissue of the muscle itself. Commonly, the child presents with a swelling or swellings in the neck, mimicking congenital torticollis. These may be fluctuant or hard and tend to vary in size and consistency but ultimately become hardened as the bone is deposited. Although they are frequently painless, in some cases the swellings are very tender and this picture, together with swelling of joints and fever, may superficially resemble acute rheumatism. Ulceration of the tense, overlying skin may expose the ossified muscle and result in secondary infection. Although almost any voluntary muscle may be involved, in most cases the most severely affected muscles are those of the back, shoulder and pelvic girdles. Ultimately, large groups of muscles become ossified and the bone tends to conform to the shape of the muscle involved. Although the diaphragm itself is very rarely affected, the general fixation of the ribs results in a terminal aspiration pneumonia and death from infection and/or asphyxia. Corticotrophin and steroids have been used in treatment and a diphosphonate, disodium etidronate, has been recommended following its use in preventing ectopic calcification in the experimental animal (Russel et al 1972).

Direct and indirect trauma to muscle with resulting rupture, contusion or frank haemorrhage is common in industrial accidents and in various sports. In most cases, treatment results in complete clinical recovery. In a few, however, the traumatic incident is followed by increasing stiffness in the muscle over the next one to four weeks and the development of a firm, painful calcified mass, palpable at the site of the injury. Similar calcification or ossification, particularly in thigh muscles and in the region of the hip joints, may be seen in cases of paraplegia or paraparesis, as after partial recovery from transverse myelitis. Radiography will indicate calcification of a feathery pattern in the swelling (Howard 1946) where a haematoma has dissected along the fasciculae, or a more common irregular circumscribed area of variable density where a solitary haematoma is calcified. Post-traumatic inflammatory change in connective tissue is replaced by islands of cartilage and eventually by bone in the thickened septa. The clinical disability which results is largely dependent upon the precise situation of the new bone: that close to joints may cause, by direct mechanical interference, the most severe disability, whereas an area of bone formation in the belly of a muscle at a distance from its origin or insertion may scarcely be discernible to the patient except perhaps for pain and stiffness in the muscle itself.

Less common than the myositis ossificans circumscripta is the ossification of specific muscles as a result of their repeated involvement in the trauma of certain exercises or occupations. Riders and infantrymen have suffered from local ossification in the adductors of the thighs (rider's bone) and the deltoid and pectorals (drill bone) respectively. Fencers, and athletes throwing a weapon or weight, may develop ossification in biceps, brachialis and brachioradialis of the arm involved. Traumatic ossifying myositis may not be evident to the victim and may be discovered on routine radiology, but in the majority of cases the new bone is tender and restricts normal movement. Spontaneous reabsorption is reported on cessation of the provocative activity, but most cases come to surgery. The histological appearance of the muscles is similar in both the acute and subacute varieties.

Tumours of muscle

Primary muscle tumours are rare, although direct invasion of muscle tissue by adjacent carcinoma or other malignant neoplasm is relatively uncommon, a notable exception being the infiltration of the pectoral muscles by adjacent malignant breast carcinoma. Direct invasion causes muscle atrophy from compression and the histological changes are those of the invasive tumour itself. Despite the fact that muscle is a highly vascular tissue and makes up 40% of body weight, metastatic cancer to muscle is surprisingly rare, even at autopsy, perhaps because of some local change in pH or metabolism which does not allow implantation and development of tumour emboli. However, Pearson (1959) examined the muscles histologically post-mortem in 38 cases and found tumour emboli and growths in six (16%); three of the patients suffered lymphosarcoma or leukaemia. Fourteen muscles were involved out of a total of eight to nine muscles examined in each of the 38 cases. This work suggests that tumour embolisation to muscle is not as rare as we formerly believed. However, in the terminal stages of malignancy it is very unlikely that such small metastatic deposits would be clinically recognisable or would exert an influence to be distinguished from the generalised cachexia of the primary disease. A recent case of lymphatoid granulomatosis involving several muscles has been described by Schmalzi et al (1982). In addition, a generalised subacute myopathy was reported to be due to more diffuse infiltration by metastatic carcinoma by Fowler & Doshi (1983). One patient improved with tamoxifen where the primary site had been breast. Patients with visceral carcinoma, especially carcinoma of the gastrointestinal tract, may suffer a migrating monomyositis multiplex (Heffner 1971) caused by systemic emboli from non-bacterial thrombotic endocarditis The condition mimics polymyositis but is more focal, with severe pains of sudden onset lasting for a few days. The muscles of the lower leg are preferentially affected, and the underlying pathology is embolic infarction of muscle tissue.

A tumour or swelling in the substance of voluntary muscle does not necessarily imply new growth, and abscess formation due either to aerobic or anaerobic organisms is seen in various conditions, notably diabetes mellitus or tropical myositis. Frequently, the cardinal signs of acute inflammation are absent and the abscess has to be distinguished from old haematoma or localised nodular myositis (see Ch. 17). Of the tumours of supporting tissues, angioma is uncommon, whether of cavernous, capillary or arteriovenous type, but dermoid tumours and benign fibrous growths are more common and particularly involve the anterior abdominal wall. They may be associated with dull, aching pain and are evident on palpation. In the limbs, neurofibromata may cause severe pain aggravated by contraction of the surrounding muscle and often provoked by palpation of the tumour itself. There is frequently a curious wasting of the surrounding muscle, perhaps because of disuse, a wasting which frequently recovers after surgical removal of the lesion. Rupture of a tendon (e.g. of biceps brachii) or a muscle hernia (through the deep fascia) may give an appearance of local swelling which can be misconstrued by the unwary.

Primary tumours of muscle are fortunately uncommon and fall into three distinct histological groups:

Rhabdomyoma. These rare tumours of skeletal muscle may be circumscribed, diffuse, solitary or multiple. A distinctive form is seen as a congenital tumour of cardiac muscle often associated with tuberous sclerosis.

The rhabdomyosarcoma is an extremely malignant tumour estimated by Stout (1946) to be associated with a less than 4% survival at five years. It tends to occur in the muscles of the extremities, especially the legs and involves patients between the ages of 40 and 60 in particular. The tumour presents as a deep-seated muscle swelling which is relatively immobile and spreads by local invasion. Unfortunately, the tumour is not particularly radiosensitive and only radical surgery can offer a better prognosis, 35% survival at five years (Pack & Ariel 1958).

Mid-line teratomas whatever their situation, may contain elements of striated muscle and the clinical features here are largely determined by the situation of the lesion. Particularly common are those involving the genital organs, where primitive muscle tissue may form a sarcomatous mass (sarcoma botryoides in the female or a malignant rhabdomyoma of the prostate in the male).

The granular cell myoblastoma is an uncommon tumour; 30% appear in the tongue, others in the skin, subcutaneous tissues or breast. Surgical treatment with total extirpation is often feasible.

Stiff-man syndrome

From the Mayo Clinic in 1956 Moersch & Woltman reported 14 patients who had suffered a progressive, fluctuating muscle rigidity and spasm resembling a chronic form of tetanus: they used the term stiff-man syndrome to describe these patients. Since then some 40 further reports have appeared in the neurological literature describing patients, almost all males, suffering from similar stiffness and rigidity and, in a critical survey of the literature, Gordon et al (1967) laid down certain criteria for the diagnosis. The sporadic disorder is more common in men and tends to affect adults in middle life, persisting for many years. The first symptoms are brief episodes of aching and tightness of the axial muscles; after some weeks, these episodes become more persistent and eventually involve the limb girdles and limb muscles, producing a symmetrical continuous stiffness of the systemic musculature. The muscles become board-like and rigid and any attempt at passive movement or sudden noise may precipitate excruciatingly painful muscle spasms causing the patient to cry out; they are associated with adrenergic concomitants such as tachycardia and sweating. The spasms may be initiated by talking, chewing, swallowing or attempted voluntary movement. The muscle involvement is unselective in that agonists and antagonists are equally involved, so that the patient becomes rigid in extension. In some patients dysphagia has been described, and in others the facial muscles have been involved by similar rigidity. Patients are described in whom the respiratory muscles have also shown this stiffness, with resulting difficulty in breathing. During sleep the muscles relax and, indeed, general anaesthesia will produce complete relaxation (Price & Allott 1958). In those cases accepted by Gordon and his colleagues as fulfilling these clinical criteria there were no neurological abnormalities, apart from the extreme rigidity. Corticospinal signs were absent and there was no sensory impairment. Intellectually, these patients are intact and electromyographic examination of the involved muscles shows these to be in persistent tonic contraction, even at rest. The action potentials are normal (Moersch & Woltman 1956, Trethowan et al 1960, Howard 1963). The spasm can be abolished by spinal anaesthetic (Werk et al 1961) and by procaine infiltration around an appropriate nerve trunk (Gordon et al 1967). Myoneural blocking agents, e.g. curare (Brage 1959), tubocurarine (Stuart et al 1960) and succinylcholine (Werk et al 1961) have all been shown to relieve the spasms. In 1963 Howard described the use of diazepam (Valium®) following the demonstration that the drug blocked strychnine-induced convulsions in mice and spinal reflexes in cats. He was able with this drug to induce electromyographic silence when the involved muscles were at rest. More recently, the effectiveness of baclofen, clonazepam and diazepam has been assessed, and the ineffectiveness of dipropylacetate has been confirmed (Martinelli et al 1978).

There has been much conjecture about the pathogenesis of this strange and rare disorder. Gordon and his colleagues (1967) suggested that the persisting α-neurone bombardment of the muscle is probably maintained by abnormal γ-motor system activity, perhaps initiated from higher centres. The pain of the spasms is thought to be due to further intensification of the contraction resulting from exteroceptive and enteroceptive stimuli and emotional factors. In their case, the presence of a reducing substance other than glucose in the urine suggested a possible metabolic factor. An association between this disease, nocturnal myoclonus and epilepsy has recently been suggested (Martinelli et al 1978). However, in our current stage of knowledge the pathogenesis still remains unresolved. One report (Kasperek & Zebrowski 1971) described a patient whose clinical signs were characteristic and in whom, at autopsy some 11 months after the onset of the stiffness, changes of a subacute encephalomyelitis, presumed to be viral, were found. Most of the pathological abnormalities were in the brain stem and spinal cord. On the basis of pharmacological evidence it has been suggested that the syndrome depends upon an imbalance between the cholinergic and GABA systems (Martinelli et al 1978), giving excessive activity in interneurones in the spinal cord.

Diagnosis from other organic disorders of the nervous system is not usually difficult. Cervical spondylosis with myelopathy may produce severe cortico-spinal rigidity. Extra-pyramidal disease such as torsion dystonia, Wilson's disease and parkinsonism may all produce a somewhat similar clinical picture, but usually give rise to little diagnostic difficulty. Chronic tetanus, McArdle's myopathy, myotonia and dermatomyositis have all mimicked the stiff-man syndrome, and severe generalised arthritis with resulting muscle spasm has also been confused with it. However, in the stiff-man syndrome the pain and stiffness are confined to the muscles and are not periarticular, as they would be in a diffuse arthropathy.

Occasionally the spasms are severe enough to cause spontaneous fractures and gross deformity of the limbs (Asher 1958) and it is not, therefore, surprising that several biopsy reports have described changes in the muscles. However, occasional degenerative foci, nerve-sprouting and slight fibrosis could all result from the intense spasms themselves, producing, as they must, relative ischaemia of muscle. In most biopsies, however, the muscle fibres, the myomesium and the intramuscular nerve endings show no consistent abnormality.

The absence of objective organic change in these patients has led to the suggestion that many of the spasms may be 'hysterical'. However, the personality of the patient suffering from this syndrome does not conform to that of the true hysteric and the extreme distress, immobility and eventual bed-dependence do not support this suggestion.

In a recent report Alberca et al (1982) described a female patient with permanent axial muscle rigidity similar to that of the stiff-man syndrome, together with axial myoclonus very similar to that seen in the patient of Leigh et al (1980) where the association of a 'stiff-man syndrome' with myoclonus suggested that a 'jerking stiff-man syndrome' may exist. The most recent review by Meinck et al (1984) showed that exteroceptive reflexes, especially those elicited from the skin, were excessively enhanced. It was found that clomipramine given by injection severely aggravated the clinical symptoms but that diazepam, clonidine and tizanidine decreased both the muscular stiffness and the abnormal exteroceptive reflexes. They suggested that the stiff-man syndrome is a disorder of descending brain-stem systems which exert a net inhibitory control on axial and limb girdle muscle tone as well as exteroceptive reflex transmission.

Epidemic myalgia, pleurodynia (Bornholm disease)

The first clinical descriptions of this disease are found in the Norwegian literature (Daae 1872, Homann 1872) and in 1934 Sylvest published his classic monograph on the subject from Copenhagen.

It is now recognised that viruses of the Coxsackie Group B are responsible for the clinical picture of headache, fever, and pain in the lower chest and abdomen, of sudden onset. The pain is made worse by respiratory movements and frequently pleural friction can be heard, with tenderness and skin hyperaesthesia over the lower chest wall (Curnen et al 1949, Kilbourne 1950, Weller et al 1950). B-1 types of virus and also strains of B-3 have been recovered from patients with pleurodynia and the condition has been associated with B-4 infection in South Africa (Patz et al 1953, Wilkins et al 1955), so that many B strains of virus have been implicated but Group A viruses are not responsible.

Focal inflammatory and necrotic foci similar to those seen in the muscle of infected mice have been seen in the few recorded biopsies from human cases. The disease is short-lived; its main clinical interest lies in its epidemic qualities and, when endemic, in its differentiation from more significant pleural and peritoneal inflammatory disorders.

Epidemic myalgic encephalomyelitis

At the Royal Free Hospital in London in 1955 an outbreak of this disease affected more than 300 people. The disorder tends to occur in the summer months and affects young people who suffer headache, muscle pains, occasional lymphadenopathy and fever. Neurological signs have been detected, e.g. nystagmus, myoclonus, and weakness of the bulbar muscles together with generalised muscle weakness and hyporeflexia. The majority of the patients complain of peripheral paraesthesiae and peripheral sensory loss is often described. The disease is associated with a feeling of generalised fatigue, and the frequent psychiatric disturbance has suggested to some that the disease is not organically determined. The exact nosology of this disorder is still in doubt, and terms such as neuromyasthenia have been suggested. An organic basis is supported by the abnormal lymphocytes found in the peripheral blood of some patients (Wallis 1957). During an outbreak in London a high incidence of serum anticomplementary activity together with ill-defined aggregates on electron microscopy of acute phase sera was described (Dillon et al 1974). However, many observers of this disorder would regard most of the clinical manifestations as hysterical and psychogenic, perhaps encouraged by medical personnel (May et al 1980). This is to some extent borne out by the almost invariable association of irritability, weeping spells and mood swings together with nightmares in addition to the more organic symptoms of vertigo, tinnitus, diplopia and muscle pain, headache and fatigue. The condition is sometimes referred to now as the post-viral fatigue syndrome.

NEUROMUSCULAR DISORDERS ASSOCIATED WITH NEOPLASTIC DISEASES

The muscular wasting encountered in patients with malignant disease is due to a variety or combination of factors, including cachexia, malnutrition, disuse, infection, toxaemia, arthropathy and old age. It is well known that nonspecific pathological abnormalities are found in post-mortem specimens of muscle from patients with or without malignant disease, and Pearson, (1959) discovered such changes in 54 out of 110 routine autopsies; the lesions are presumably attributable to different or multiple factors, including those mentioned above, but the loss of muscle protein during starvation is not fully understood. Muscular atrophy and weakness deriving from involvement of the lower motor neurones is relatively uncommon and so are the myopathies, such as the myasthenic syndrome and dermatomyositis, described below.

Direct involvement of neural tissues

Local infiltration of neural tissue may occur in the leptomeningeal compartment. There may be dural and extradural involvement affecting not only spinal nerve roots but also cranial nerves, individually or collectively, the spinal nerves themselves and also the brachial or lumbar plexus or the peripheral nerves. The commonest type of peripheral nerve lesion encountered in malignant disease is compression or infiltration of individual nerve roots or nerve plexuses by neoplastic tissue deriving from neighbouring growths, either primary or secondary. However, considering the high incidence of carcinoma, sarcoma and the reticuloses, clinical manifestations of nervous lesions of this type are relatively uncommon. Willis (1952) commented on the way in which nerves escape invasion when enveloped by growth; when invasion does occur, nerve degeneration may not follow. Once infiltration of a nerve takes place there is longitudinal permeation via the perineurium, endoneurium and perineural lymphatics; if nerve damage results, there will be muscular wasting and weakness in the distribution of the affected nerve. Familiar examples of this process include lesions of the brachial plexus in Pancoast's tumour, of the lumbar plexus in retroperitoneal lymphosarcoma and of the sacral plexus in pelvic carcinoma.

Diffuse infiltration of peripheral nerves. Diffuse malignant infiltration of peripheral nerves must be extremely rare in any type of carcinoma; indeed, Russell & Rubinstein (1959) knew of no authentic cases in which peripheral nerves or ganglia, other than the trigeminal, were the seat of metastases in carcinoma. However, diffuse infiltration of nerves has been recorded in cases of myeloma, leukaemia, myeloid metaplasia and lymphoma (Barron et al 1960, Cairncross & Posner 1980, Spaar 1980, Yuill 1980). The first symptoms may be those of a peripheral neuropathy due to the malignant invasion, possibly via the vasa nervorum or from the leptomeningeal seedlings in which case the 'peripheral neuropathy' could be associated with an abnormal cerebrospinal fluid. Such cases, however, are seen much less frequently than those associated with paraneoplastic mechanisms. Leptomeningeal infiltration producing carcinomatous meningitis allows a very characteristic syndrome of headache with signs of meningeal irritation and multiple focal

neurological signs, both due to cranial nerve involvement and involvement of the spinal nerves. Root pain, focal muscle weakness and atrophy and sensory impairment in root distribution together with focal depression of reflexes constitute the clinical pattern. Almost invariably the CSF will show raised pressure, increased protein content with a low glucose and a pleocytosis, often with malignant cells being readily identified by the cytologist. It has been suggested that levels of β-glucuronidase are increased in cases of leptomeningeal carcinoma but not in those where the meninges are infiltrated with lymphoma (Schold et al 1979). Tumour invasion of the brachial and lumbosacral plexuses produces severe pain, dysaesthesiae and sensory impairment with weakness and wasting of the muscles innervated by the nerve trunks involved. Breast carcinoma commonly spreads into the brachial plexus and the lumbosacral plexus is frequently involved by direct invasion of carcinoma from cervix, prostate, bladder or rectum.

Non-metastatic neurological manifestations of malignant disease

In 1948 Denny-Brown described a form of sensory neuropathy in two patients with carcinoma of the lung and, although earlier in the century dermatomyositis had been recognised in association with various malignancies, it fell to Brain to introduce the terms 'carcinomatous neuropathy' and 'neuromyopathy' to describe involvement of the central or peripheral nervous system and muscle by non-metastatic processes in patients with cancer. The extensive studies undertaken by Brain's colleagues at the London Hospital have led to a greater understanding of the clinical features, prevalence and prognosis of the various forms of non-metastatic neurological neuromyopathies. Henson (1970) preferred to use the general diagnosis of 'non-metastatic neurological manifestations of malignant disease', specifying the type of nervous or muscular disorder present. His reasons included the fact that important non-invasive neurological syndromes occur in the reticuloses as well as in carcinoma.

The important neurological disorders associated with malignant disease include encephalomyelitis with carcinoma (Henson et al 1965), cerebellar degeneration, progressive multifocal leucoencephalopathy, peripheral neuropathy and a variety of myopathies. It has been estimated that the combined incidence of symptomatic peripheral neuropathy and encephalomyelitis with carcinoma of the lung was of the order of 1–2% in an unselected group. The cases of peripheral neuropathy rated second in incidence to cases of Guillain–Barré syndrome in his department of the London Hospital. However, others (McLeod 1975) would regard diabetic, alcoholic and nutritional neuropathies as having a higher incidence. The 'pick-up' rate in the neoplastic group has increased with the increasing use of electrophysiological studies (Moody, 1965). In a prospective study, Wilkinson et al (1967) found that 6.6% of 1465 cases of carcinoma showed clinical evidence of non-metastatic nervous or neuromuscular disorder. The highest incidence in their series was in patients with carcinoma of the lung, ovary and stomach: 15% of the males with lung cancer were so affected; this figure falls to approximately 6% if the less well-defined neuromuscular and muscular syndromes are excluded. Signs of peripheral neuropathy were discovered in 5.3% of 316 patients with lung carcinoma; 2.8% of patients with carcinoma of stomach and 1.2% of those with growths of the breast and large bowel were affected.

Recent electrodiagnostic studies have shown a high yield of abnormalities in patients with lung cancer who made no neurological complaints. These subclinical neuromyopathies were found by Campbell & Paty (1974) in 21 out of 26 patients. The term neuromyopathy is used advisedly here as the abnormalities found reflected disorder in both muscle and nerve in the majority. Muscle weakness was a prominent symptom in 3.6% of patients in a series studied by Paul et al (1978) — a group of 195 Indian patients with untreated cancers of various types — but generalised weakness and wasting of non-metastatic origin was present in 22%. Lenman et al (1981) compared 50 lung cancer patients with 50 controls and in them found no evidence of non-metastatic neuromuscular disease, although in two patients there were EMG abnormalities of myopathic type. In only five patients was the serum creatine kinase

(CK) activity elevated and motor and nerve conduction tests were only rarely abnormal. Despite discrepancies in the various series reported, nevertheless a distinct syndrome of proximal muscle weakness and wasting with depressed reflexes and EMG abnormalities, without definite abnormality of motor nerve conduction or neuromuscular transmission, has been defined and conveniently labelled 'carcinomatous neuromyopathy' (Campbell & Paty 1974).

Peripheral neuropathy. A predominantly sensory form of neuropathy was the first to be described as a complication of carcinoma but a sensorimotor type of neuropathy is more common.

Sensory neuropathy. The dominant symptoms of this sensory form of paraneoplastic neuropathy comprise distal numbness with dysaesthesiae and paraesthesiae with a distal–proximal spread. The neuropathy may be ataxic and may be accompanied by pain in the limbs. Although usually symmetrical, the neuropathy may be asymmetrical and may become very severe. Physical examination reveals little muscle wasting and weakness except in the late stages of the disease, but the tendon reflexes are greatly diminished or absent and the peripheral sensory loss affects all modalities, with severe involvement of proprioceptive sensibility. Thus the ataxic neuropathy is often accompanied by pseudoathetosis. Occasionally there are cranial nerve abnormalities. It has long been recognised that the neuropathic symptoms may precede the clinical presentation of the underlying neoplasm, usually by some six to 15 months, although cases are reported of a much longer delay. The disorder progresses rapidly in the majority of cases. The mean survival rate is about 14 months (Croft & Wilkinson 1965).

Sensorimotor neuropathy. Croft & Wilkinson (1965) felt that this form of neuropathy was one of the more common neurological manifestations of carcinoma and occurred more frequently than the pure sensory type. Similar observations were made by Morton et al (1967), with primary carcinoma of lung being the most common underlying tumour. However, cases have been described where stomach, breast, colon, rectum, pancreas, uterus, cervix, kidney and thyroid, together with prostate and testis, have harboured the underlying neoplasm. McLeod (1975) would divide the sensorimotor neuropathies secondary to carcinoma into three distinct clinical groups: a subacute or chronic neuropathy with predominantly distal features, with distal weakness, sensory impairment and diminished reflexes; an acute peripheral neuropathy resembling the Guillain–Barré syndrome, and a remitting or relapsing neuropathy which may long precede or antedate the clinical presentation of the neoplasm. The electrophysiological studies of such patients usually show denervation with spontaneous fibrillation, reduction in the number of motor units and an increased number of polyphasic units. In the sensory neuropathies, sensory action potentials are absent although motor conduction velocities are normal. In the subacute and chronic types of sensorimotor neuropathy, an increased terminal motor latency has been described in the acute or subacute neuropathy and in some cases of the relapsing form the motor conduction velocities may be significantly slowed.

Examination of pathological material in carcinomatous neuropathy has frequently shown severe degenerative change in the posterior columns of the cord secondary to dorsal nerve root degeneration. There may be degenerative changes in the anterior horn cells and in the dorsal root ganglia, profound loss of neurones with loss of fibres in the peripheral nerves, a reduction in the number of myelinated fibres of all diameters and occasional segmental demyelination but, most often, axonal degeneration.

Motor neurone disease. Brain et al (1965) described a group of patients in whom there was an association between neoplasm and a neurological disorder similar to motor neurone disease. The clinical course was relatively benign compared with that of classic motor neurone disease. There was no evidence of a significant incidence of classic motor neurone disease in patients with carcinoma. Brain suggested the term 'diffuse polioencephalopathy' to emphasise the involvement of central and peripheral nervous structures and this has come to include the cerebellar syndromes, dementia, sensory neuropathy, upper

and lower motor neurone abnormalities and brainstem disturbances. In some cases this lower motor neurone deterioration has been the most significant feature in the clinical picture and a case of amyotrophic lateral sclerosis showing a coincidental carcinoma suggested a possible link. Norris & Engel (1965) described 13 patients who suffered a carcinoma in a consecutive series of 130 cases of motor neurone disease (ALS). However, many continue to regard the association as chance. Mitchell & Olczak (1979) described a patient suffering from a large-cell carcinoma of the lung who presented with upper and lower motor neurone signs which resolved after resection of the carcinoma. In this case there may have been a causal relationship between the motor neurone disease and the carcinoma. However, a subacute motor neuropathy has been described in patients suffering from lymphomas and reticuloses with patchy muscle weakness and atrophy together with evidence of denervation. Some such patients have been found to be suffering from Hodgkin's disease (Schold et al 1979) and similar changes are seen in Waldenstrom's macroglobulinaemia.

Encephalomyelitis with carcinoma. This condition is usually linked with an oat cell bronchial carcinoma, and is characterised pathologically by inflammatory changes with nerve cell destruction in the limbic lobes, brain stem, spinal cord and posterior root ganglia (Henson et al 1965). The clinical manifestations depend upon the distribution and intensity of lesions and vary from those of limbic encephalitis (Corsellis et al 1968) to an extreme form of sensory neuronopathy (Denny Brown 1948). Brain-stem involvement is reflected in ataxia, vertigo, nystagmus, external ophthalmoplegia and bulbar palsy. Disturbances of tone, involuntary movements, increased tendon reflexes and extensor plantar responses may be noted. Spinal cord symptoms are usually limited to muscular wasting and weakness stemming from damage to anterior horn cells; fasciculation may be seen in the affected musculature.

When neuromuscular symptoms are predominant the clinical picture can resemble that of motor neurone disease, but thorough examination of the material available to Henson & Urich (1979) always revealed evidence of brain-stem involvement, such as nystagmus, vertigo and ataxia, or posterior root ganglion lesions. Cord involvement may be patchy or localised; e.g. in one patient seen by Henson the weakness was limited to muscles of the neck and shoulder girdles.

The cerebrospinal fluid protein is often raised in the active stage and there may be a mild lymphocytic pleocytosis. The most important laboratory finding was Wilkinson's discovery of brain-specific complement-fixing antibodies in blood and cerebrospinal fluid in four successive patients (Croft et al 1965); however, the immunological significance of this finding has been questioned. Henson & Urich (1979) have reviewed the problem of aetiology.

Muscular disorders. The paraneoplastic syndromes affecting muscle can be classified under four headings: (1) direct involvement of muscle tissue itself; (2) disorders of neuromuscular transmission; (3) inflammatory muscle disease, dermatomyositis and polymyositis; (4) the endocrine and metabolic myopathies.

Carcinomatous myopathy. Consideration has already been given to the wasting and cachexia of cancer which is associated with marked muscle weakness of the proximal muscles and, occasionally, acute muscle necrosis. It is generally agreed that there is a separate and distinct syndrome of proximal muscle weakness with elevated serum CK levels occurring without any significant neural component. The true nature of this syndrome is uncertain and although the term 'carcinomatous myopathy' was first introduced by Henson et al (1954) to describe these cases, the site and nature of the lesion has not been fully established. Shy & Silverstein (1965), Campbell & Paty (1974) and Warmolts et al (1975) have confirmed the original clinical observations and suggest that this is the commonest remote effect of cancer. The complaint is of weakness affecting the proximal muscles without a myasthenic element and may occur in patients who are otherwise well. It has been suggested by Warmolts et al (1975) that the muscle atrophy is predominantly of type II fibres and the suggestion has been made after EM examination that degenerative changes occur in the

intramuscular nerve twigs (Barron & Heffner 1978).

Acute necrotising myopathy. In 1969 Smith described material showing acute necrosis of skeletal muscle in biopsies from patients suffering carcinoma of the colon, breast and stomach. In further cases widespread muscle necrosis has been seen with minimal inflammatory reaction and it was thought that the entity was different from polymyositis and that the link was directly with that of underlying carcinoma.

It is still not altogether clear whether there are separate clearly definable disorders of voluntary muscle and peripheral nerve in association with underlying carcinoma: whereas the cases reported and reviewed to date suggest this distinction, often in clinical practice there appears to be a spectrum of disorders from peripheral neuropathy through to myopathy with, in some cases, the main functional abnormality appearing to be in the peripheral nerve and in others in the muscle tissue itself.

Dermatomyositis and polymyositis. For many years clinicians have recognised the association between inflammatory muscle disease and underlying malignant disease, especially in the older patient groups. One study in the literature found more than 50% of dermatomyositis patients to be suffering from occult cancer (Arundell et al 1960). However, Bohan & Peter in 1975 concluded that the association had not been clearly defined. When carcinoma is found it is usually in the lung, breast, ovary or gastrointestinal tract but inflammatory muscle disease may also occur in association with thymomas. De Vere & Bradley (1975) reviewed the Newcastle cases collected over a 20-year period, including 21 cases of dermatomyositis and 97 cases of polymyositis. In the older age groups 40% of those suffering from dermatomyositis harboured an occult cancer whereas only 3.4% of the older patients with polymyositis had cancer. Layzer (1985) reviewed the records of 20 patients over the age of 40 suffering from dermatomyositis seen in the University of California Medical Center, San Francisco: 11 proved to have cancer, i.e. an incidence of some 55%, and the tumours in these patients were in the lung (4), the pelvis (5), colon (1) and breast (1). Thus although there has been some suggestion that the association is fortuitous, most clinicians now accept the association and in any adult patient suffering dermatomyositis or polymyositis a careful search for an underlying carcinoma is undertaken. The clinical and pathological features are similar to those found in dermatomyositis uncomplicated by the presence of malignant disease (see Ch. 17). The course of the muscular disorder is not modified by the presence of the cancer although remissions do occur. The treatment of dermatomyositis and polymyositis is considered in Chapter 17.

Metabolic and endocrine myopathies. Abnormal electrolyte levels and abnormal endocrine function can both severely influence muscle metabolism and muscle function. Elsewhere in this book (Ch. 25) there are descriptions of the myopathies associated with disease of the thyroid gland. These include hypothyroid myopathy, the thyrotoxic myopathy which occurs in thyrotoxicosis, myokymia, acute bulbar myopathy, hypocalcaemic paralysis, perhaps a motor polyneuropathy and ocular myopathy. In that thyrotoxicosis has been recorded as a paraneoplastic complication of oat cell lung cancer, it is possible but not (to my knowledge) yet reported, that such a patient could also develop one of the myopathic complications of hyperthyroidism.

Patients suffering from hyponatraemia (as e.g., those suffering from Addison's disease) show generalised muscle weakness which quickly responds to treatment with 9-alpha-fluorohydrocortisone or saline infusions. Patients with carcinoma of the bronchus may similarly show hyponatraemia mimicking the metabolic myopathy of primary adrenal failure.

Hypercalcaemic states due to benign or malignant tumours of the parathyroid gland are associated with profound muscular weakness, pain and wasting. Prineas et al (1965) and Smith & Stern (1967) have shown that the myopathy associated with primary hyperparathyroidism can occur independently of plasma calcium concentration. In such cases osteomalacia is often present and it has been suggested that the muscle disorder might well be linked to a deranged vitamin D metabolism. The myopathic syndrome shown by these patients is similar, whether the cause is hypercalcaemia or metabolic bone disease. Quite

characteristically the reflexes are brisk, and bone pain and tenderness may be prominent.

The myopathy associated with acromegaly was first described by Pierre Marie (1886). In Cushing's disease, especially where the patients have been treated with a bilateral total or subtotal adrenalectomy, the hyperpigmented patients may complain of severe muscular weakness or excessive tiredness on effort. Muscle biopsy has shown an accumulation of fat droplets under the sarcolemma of both type I and type II fibres but without any other distinctive ultrastructural or histological abnormalities. Thus in this so-called 'Nelson's syndrome', the hyperpigmentation and secondary pituitary tumour may be associated with a distinctive myopathy.

Berry et al (1974) and Swash et al (1975) have reported single examples of myopathy in patients suffering from argentaffin carcinoma with metastases. Swash's patient developed severe muscle tenderness, 10 years after resection of the associated primary tumour in the ileum; secondary deposits had been seen in the liver at operation. In both cases muscle biopsy showed advanced atrophy of type II muscle fibres, scattered necrotic fibres and central nuclei. In Swash's patient, type I fibres were smaller than normal and the diameters of both type I and II fibres were abnormally variable. Electromyography showed a reduced interference pattern with numerous short-duration low-amplitude polyphasic potentials.

The serotonin and histamine antagonist, cyproheptadine, improved muscle strength in both cited cases when given in addition to methysergide. The dose of cyproheptadine was 24 mg daily. Although muscle weakness in patients with the carcinoid syndrome could develop from intestinal malabsorption, or hypercalcaemia due to bony metastases or, possibly, due to the release of other active substances by the tumour, the clinical evidence suggests that the cause is circulating serotonin. This view is supported by experimental evidence derived from serotonin-induced myopathy (Parker & Mendell 1974, Patten et al 1974).

Disorders of neuromuscular transmission. Much more clearly defined than the neuromyopathies are the disorders of neuromuscular transmission associated with underlying cancer. Eaton & Lambert in 1957 described a disorder of neuromuscular transmission associated with cancer in some 70% of cases. Curiously, the neoplasm is almost invariably a carcinoma of the bronchus of small-cell type but occasional cases have been reported where no carcinoma has been discovered; in some of these there has been an association with hypothyroidism, pernicious anaemia, vitiligo and coeliac disease (Gutmann et al 1972, Lang et al 1981). As with the other non-neoplastic complications, the symptoms often precede the symptoms of the underlying cancer, sometimes by many months. The majority of the patients are men who complain of weakness and fatiguability resembling true myasthenia gravis. This causes difficulty in walking, as the muscles affected are usually systemic; however, occasionally ocular and bulbar forms are described. Sometimes there are peripheral paraesthesiae. The characteristic feature of these cases is that muscle strength improves with sustained effort and the tendon reflexes are initially depressed or absent but will return on strong voluntary contraction. The patients are extremely susceptible to muscle relaxants so that, frequently, the disease is first noted after a surgical procedure. The muscles are extremely sensitive to the paralysing action of decamethonium.

The most important abnormalities are discovered in the electrophysiological examination. The EMG frequently shows no abnormality and no increase in spontaneous muscle activity. Nerve conduction is normal both in motor and sensory nerves but repetitive motor nerve stimulation shows the characteristic incremental response at rates of stimulation of from 10 to 150 Hz which may reach 20 times the initial amplitude.

It has been found that the defect of neuromuscular transmission lies in the release of acetylcholine from the nerve terminals (Elmqvist & Lambert 1968). It is suggested that the defect may involve the calcium-mediated release of acetylcholine in the nerve terminals.

The Eaton–Lambert syndrome must be distinguished from the simple myopathy of cachexia, from true myasthenia gravis, from polymyositis and from other myopathies of late onset. True myasthenia occurs predominantly in females with a lower age incidence than that of the Eaton–Lambert syndrome and the distribution of the weakness is dissimilar. There is, as a rule, no loss of tendon reflexes in early cases of myasthenia and the electrophysiological changes are diagnostic and distinctive. The clinical features of the Eaton–Lambert syndrome often resemble those of polymyositis but, again, electrophysiological testing separates the two syndromes; muscle biopsy will show the distinctive features of the inflammatory muscle disease.

Treatment. Unlike the majority of the paraneoplastic complications of carcinoma, the Eaton–Lambert syndrome does respond to treatment. Guanidine hydrochloride has been moderately effective in many patients treated with 15–30 mg per kg body weight in divided dosage. Often this drug produces nausea and vomiting together with distal paraesthesiae and some authors have suggested a combination of pyridostigmine and guanidine. Subsequently, it was suggested that 3, 4-diaminopyridine would prove safer and more effective (Lundh et al 1977).

Removal of the underlying carcinoma has often resulted in considerable improvement in the neuromuscular disorder and more recently it has been suggested that plasma exchange or treatment with immunosuppressive drugs such as azathioprine and prednisolone may prove helpful (Newsom-Davis et al 1982).

Myasthenia gravis. There is, as yet, no acceptable evidence that true myasthenia gravis is associated with carcinoma, except where the neoplasm lies in the thymus gland. Approximately 30% of patients with a thymoma will suffer from clinical myasthenia gravis. Some 15% with clinical myasthenia gravis will be found to have an underlying thymoma, two-thirds of these tumours will be found to be encapsulated and one-third will be invasive. Those myasthenic patients who submit to thymectomy have a worse prognosis if there is a thymoma. Slater et al (1978) reported a 50% five-year survival of patients with an invasive thymoma as against 70% five-year survival in those whose tumours were non-invasive.

Neuromuscular disorders in the reticuloses

The lymphomas comprising Hodgkin's disease, lymphosarcoma, reticulum cell sarcoma and follicular lymphoma will be associated with nervous system involvement in some 10–25% of cases. Local deposits of tissue may occur in the brain, spinal cord, or the cranial and peripheral nerves and there are, as with carcinoma, obscure forms of encephalomyelitis, progressive multifocal leucoencephalopathy, cerebellar degeneration and peripheral neuropathy and polymyositis. Usually the neural structures are affected by direct compression or lymphomatous meningitis. The peripheral effects are usually attributable to peripheral nerve invasion or plexus involvement but several types of peripheral neuropathy have been recognised, e.g. sensory neuropathy and an acute sensorimotor neuropathy both of demyelinative and axonal type. In all such cases the muscle weakness and wasting is secondary to the involvement of the peripheral nerves. An acute polyneuropathy similar to the Guillain–Barré syndrome has been reported complicating lymphoma and, as in carcinoma, there will also be subacute and chronic neuropathies and relapsing and remitting neuropathies. Occasionally a myasthenic syndrome has been reported in reticulum cell carcinoma (Rooke et al 1960) and dermatomyositis may complicate myeloma, lymphoproliferative disease and leukaemia.

REFERENCES

Adams R D, Denny-Brown D, Pearson C M 1962 Diseases of muscle; a study in pathology, 2nd edn. Hoeber, New York

Alberca R, Romero M, Chaparro J 1982 Jerking stiff-man syndrome. Journal of Neurology, Neurosurgery and Psychiatry 45: 1159–60

Ambache N 1949 The peripheral action of Cl botulinum toxin. Journal of Physiology 108:127

Arundell F D, Wilkinson R D, Haserick J K 1960 Dermatomyositis and malignant neoplasms in adults. Archives of Dermatology 82: 772–775

Asher R A 1958 A woman with stiff-man syndrome. British Medical Journal 1:265

Ashizawa T, Bulter I J, Harati Y 1983 A dominantly inherited syndrome with continuous motor neuron discharges. Annals of Neurology 13: 285–290

Ask-Upmark E 1954 Contribution to the pathogenesis of the syndrome of restless legs. Acta Medica Scandinavica 164:231

Auger R G, Daube J R, Gomez M R, Lambert E H 1984 Hereditary form of sustained muscle activity of peripheral nerve origin causing generalized myokymia and muscle stiffness. Annals of Neurology 15: 13–21

Barron K D, Rowland L P, Zimmerman H M 1960 Neuropathy with malignant tumor metastases. Journal of Nervous and Mental Disease 131: 10–31

Barron S A, Heffner R R 1978 Weakness in malignancy: Evidence for a remote effect of tumor on distal axons. Annals of Neurology 4: 268–274

Beard G M 1880 A practical treatise in nervous exhaustion. W Wood, New York, p 41

Berry E M, Maunder C, Wilson M 1974 Carcinoid myopathy and treatment with cyproheptadine (Periactin®). Gut 15:34

Bohan A, Peter J B 1975 Polymyositis and dermatomyositis. New England Journal of Medicine 292:344 (1st of two parts)

Brain Lord, Croft P B, Wilkinson M 1965 Motor neurone disease as a manifestation of neoplasm. Brain 88: 479–500

Brage D 1959 Stiff-man syndrome. Revista Clinica Espanola 72:30

Brooks V B 1956 The action of botulinum toxin on motor-nerve filaments. Journal of Physiology 134:264

Cairncross J G, Posner J B 1980 Neurological complications of malignant lymphoma. In: Vinken P J, Bruyn G W (eds) Handbook of clinical neurology, vol 39. North-Holland, Amsterdam, p 27–62

Callaghan N 1966 Restless legs syndrome in uraemic neuropathy. Neurology (Minneapolis) 16: 359–361

Campbell M J, Paty D W 1974 Carcinomatous neuromyopathy. Journal of Neurology, Neurosurgery and Psychiatry 37: 131–141

Cherington M, Ryan D W 1969 Botulism and guanidine. New England Journal of Medicine 278:931

Corsellis J A N, Goldberg G J, Norton A R 1968 'Limbic encephalitis' and its association with carcinoma. Brain 91: 481–496

Croft P B, Wilkinson M 1965 The incidence of carcinomatous neuromyopathy with special reference to carcinoma of the lung and the breast. In: Brain W R, Norris F H (eds) The remote effects of cancer on the nervous system. Grune and Stratton, New York, p 44–54

Croft P B, Henson R A, Urich H, Wilkinson M 1965 Sensory neuropathy with bronchogenic carcinoma: a study of four cases showing serological abnormalities. Brain 88: 501–514

Curnen E C, Shaw E W, Melnick J L 1949 Diseases resembling nonparalytic poliomyelitis associated with a virus pathogenic for infant mice. Journal of the American Medical Association 141:894

Daae A 1872 Epidemi i drangedal af miskel — reumatisme udbredt ved smitte. Norsk magazin fau Laegevidenskaben 2:409

Denny-Brown D 1948 Primary sensory neuropathy with muscular changes associated with carcinoma. Journal of Neurology, Neurosurgery and Psychiatry 1:73

De Vere R, Bradley W G 1975 Polymyositis: Its presentation, morbidity and mortality. Brain 98: 637–666

Doshi R, Fowler T 1983 Proximal myopathy due to discrete carcinomatous metastases to muscle. Journal of Neurology, Neurosurgery and Psychiatry 46: 358–360

Dillon M J, Marshall W C, Dudgeon J A et al 1974 Epidemic neuromyasthenia: Outbreak in nurses at a children's hospital. British Medical Journal 1: 301–305

Eaton L M, Lambert E H 1957 Electromyography and electric stimulation of nerves in diseases of the motor units. Journal of the American Medical Association 163: 1117–1124

Eaton W L, Conkling W S, Daeschner C W 1957 Early myositis ossificans progressiva occurring in homozygotic twins; a clinical and pathological study. Journal of Pediatrics 50:591

Eccles J C 1957 In: The physiology of nerve cells. Oxford University Press, London

Ekbom K A 1960 Restless legs syndrome. Neurology (Minneapolis) 10:868

Elmqvist D, Lambert E H 1968 Detailed analysis of neuromuscular transmission in a patient with the myasthenic syndrome sometimes associated with bronchogenic carcinoma. Mayo Clinic Proceedings 43: 689–713

Gamstorp I, Wohlfart G 1959 A syndrome characterised by myokymia, myotonia, muscular wasting and increased perspiration. Acta Psychiatrica et Neurologica 34:181

Gardner-Medwin D, Walton J N 1969 Myokymia with impaired muscular relaxation. Lancet 1:127

Gaster D 1905 A case of myositis ossificans. West London Medical Journal 10:37

Gordon E E, Janusko D M, Kaufman L 1967 A critical survey of the stiff-man syndrome. American Journal of Medicine 42:582

Gorman C A, Dyck P J, Pearson J S 1965 Symptoms of restless legs. Archives of Internal Medicine 155:155

Guttman L, Crosby T W, Takamore M et al 1972 The Eaton-Lambert syndrome and autoimmune disorders. American Journal of Medicine 53: 354–536

Harman J B, Richardson A T 1954 Generalised myokymia in thyrotoxicosis: Report of a case. Lancet 2:473

Heffner R R 1971 Myopathy of embolic origin in patients with carcinoma. Neurology (Minneapolis) 21: 840–846

Henson R A 1970 Non-metastatic neurological manifestations of malignant disease. In: Williams D (ed) Modern trends in neurology, 5. Butterworth, London, p 209

Henson R A, Russell D S, Wilkinson M 1954 Carcinomatous neuropathy and myopathy. Brain 77: 82–121

Henson R A, Hoffman H L, Urich H 1965 Encephalomyelitis with carcinoma. Brain 88: 449–464

Henson R A, Urich H 1979 Remote effects of malignant disease: certain intracranial disorders. In: Vinken P J, Bruyn G W (eds) Handbook of clinical neurology, vol 38. North-Holland, Amsterdam, Ch 26, p 625–668

Homann C 1872 Om en i Kragero Laegedistrikt Lerskende Smitsom Febersygdom. Norsk magazin fau Laegevidenskaben 2:542

Howard C 1946 Traumatic ossifying myositis. United States Naval Medical Bulletin 46:724

Howard F M 1963 A new and effective drug in the treatment of stiff-man syndrome. Mayo Clinic Proceedings 38:203

Illis L S, Taylor F M 1971 Neurological and electroencephalographic sequelae of tetanus. Lancet 1:826

Isaacs H 1961 A syndrome of continuous muscle-fibre activity. Journal of Neurology, Neurosurgery and Psychiatry 24: 319–325

Isaacs H, Heffron J J A 1974 The syndrome of 'continuous muscle-fibre activity' cured: further studies. Journal of Neurology, Neurosurgery and Psychiatry 37: 1231–1235

Kasperek S, Zebrowski S 1971 Stiff-man syndrome and encephalomyelitis. Archives of Neurology 24:22

Kilbourne E D 1950 Diverse manifestations of infection with a strain of Coxsackie virus. Federation Proceedings 9:581

Lamanna C 1959 Most poisonous poison. Science 130:763

Lambert E H, Rooke E D 1965 Myasthenic state and lung cancer. In: Brain Lord, Norris F H (eds) The remote effects of cancer on the nervous system. Proceedings of a symposium. Grune and Stratton, New York

Lang B, Wray D, Newsom-Davis J et al 1981 Autoimmune aetiology for myasthenic (Eaton-Lambert) syndrome. Lancet ii: 224–226

Layzer R B 1979 Motor unit hyperactivity states. In: Vinken P J, Bruyn G W (eds) Handbook of clinical neurology, vol 41. North Holland, Amsterdam, p 295–316

Layzer R B 1985 Neuromuscular manifestations of systemic disease. F A Davis, Philadelphia, p 266

Leigh P N, Rothwell J C, Traub M, Marsden C D 1980 A patient with reflex myoclonus and muscle rigidity: 'jerking stiff-man syndrome'. Journal of Neurology, Neurosurgery and Psychiatry 43: 1125–1131

Lundh H, Nilsson O, Rosen I 1977 4-Aminopyridine — A new drug tested in the treatment of Eaton-Lambert syndrome. Journal of Neurology, Neurosurgery and Psychiatry 40: 1109–1112

Lenman J A R, Fleming A M, Robertson M A H et al 1981 Peripheral nerve function in patients with bronchial carcinoma. Comparison with matched controls and effects of treatment. Journal of Neurology, Neurosurgery and Psychiatry 44: 54–61

McComas A 1977 Neuromuscular functions and disorders. Butterworth, London, p 213–214

McGuire S A, Tomasovic J J, Ackerman N jr 1984 Hereditary continuous muscle fiber activity. Archives of Neurology 41: 395–396

McKusick, V 1956 Heritable disorders of connective tissue. Mosby, St. Louis, p 184

McLeod J G 1975 Carcinomatous neuropathy. In: Dyck P J, Thomas P K, Lambert E H (eds) Peripheral neuropathy. W B Saunders, Philadelphia, p 1301–1313

Martinelli P, Pazzaglia P, Montagna P, Coccagna G, Rizzuto N, Simonati S, Lugaresi E 1978 Stiff-man syndrome associated with nocturnal myoclonus and epilepsy. Journal of Neurology, Neurosurgery and Psychiatry 41: 458–462

Marie P 1886 Sur deux cas d'acromegalie hypertrophie singulière non congénitale, des extremités supérieures, inférieures et céphalique. Revue de Médecine (Paris) 6: 297–333

May P G R, Ashton J R, Donnan S P B et al 1980 Personality and medical perception in benign myalgic encephalomyelitis. Lancet ii: 1122–1124

Matthews W B 1966 Facial myokymia. Journal of Neurology, Neurosurgery and Psychiatry 29: 35–39

Meinck H M, Ricker K, Conrad B 1984 The stiff-man syndrome. Journal of Neurology, Neurosurgery and Psychiatry 47: 280–287

Mertens H G, Zschocke S 1965 Neuromyotonia. Klinische Wochenschrift 43:917

Mitchell D M, Olczak S A 1979 Remission of a syndrome indistinguishable from motor neurone disease after resection of bronchial carcinoma. British Medical Journal 2: 176–177

Moersch F P, Woltman H W 1956 Progressive fluctuating muscular ridigity and spasm (stiff-man syndrome). Proceedings of the Staff of the Mayo Clinic 31:421

Moody J F 1965 Electrophysiological investigations into the neurological complications of carcinoma. Brain 88:1023

Morton D L, Itabashi H H, Grimes D F 1967 Nonmetastatic neurological complications of bronchogenic carcinoma. The carcinomatous neuromyopathies. Journal of Thoracic and Cardiovascular Surgery 51:14

Nathan P W 1978 Painful legs and moving toes: evidence on the site of the lesion. Journal of Neurology, Neurosurgery and Psychiatry 41: 934–939

Newsom-Davis J, Murray N, Wray D et al 1982 Lambert-Eaton myasthenic syndrome: Electrophysiological evidence for a humoral factor. Muscle and Nerve 5: S17–S20

Norlander N B 1954 Restless legs. British Journal of Physical Medicine 17:160

Norris F H jr, Engle W K 1965 Carcinomatous amyotrophic lateral sclerosis. In: Brain W R, Norris F H jr (eds) The remote effects of cancer on the nervous system. Grune and Stratton, New York, p 81–82

Oppenheimer H 1923 Lehrbuch der Nervenkrankheiten. S Karger, Berlin, p 1774

Otsuka M, Endo M 1960 Effect of guanidine on neuromuscular transmission. Journal of Pharmacology and Experimental Therapeutics 128:273

Pack G T, Ariel I M 1958 Tumours of the soft somatic tissues; a clinical treatise. Hoeber, New York

Parker J M, Mendell J R 1974 Proximal myopathy induced by 5 HT-imipramine simulates Duchenne dystrophy. Nature 247:103

Parsonage M J, Turner J W A 1948 Neuralgic amyotrophy, the shoulder girdle syndrome. Lancet 1:973

Patten B M, Oliver K L, Engel W K 1974 Serotonin-induced muscle weakness. Archives of Neurology 31: 347–349

Patz I M, Measroch V, Gear J 1953 Bornholm disease, pleurodynia or epidemic myalgia: outbreak in Transvaal associated with Coxsackie virus infection. South African Medical Journal 27:397

Paul T, Katiyar B C, Misra S et al 1978 Carcinomatous neuromuscular syndromes. A clinical and quantitative electrophysiological study. Brain 101: 53–63

Pearson C M 1959 The incidence and type of pathologic alterations observed in muscles in a routine autopsy survey. Neurology (Minneapolis) 9:757

Price T M L, Allott E H 1958 The stiff-man syndrome. British Medical Journal 1:682

Prineas J W, Mason A S, Henson R A 1965 Myopathy in metabolic bone disease. British Medical Journal 1:1034

Rooke E D, Eaton L M, Lambert E H, Hodgson C H 1960 Myasthenia and malignant intrathoracic tumor. Medical Clinics of North America 44:977

Russell D S, Rubinstein L J 1959 Pathology of tumours of the nervous system. Arnold, London

Russel R G G, Smith R, Bishop M C, Price D A, Squire C M 1972 Treatment of myositis ossificans progressiva with a diphosphonate. Lancet 1: 10–12

Schmalzi F, Gasser R W, Weiser G et al 1982 Lymphomatoid granulomatosis with primary manifestation in the skeletal muscular system. Klinische Wochenschrift 60: 311–316

Schold S C, Cho E S, Somasundaram M et al 1979 Subacute motor neuronopathy: A remote effect of lymphoma. Annals of Neurology 5: 271–287

Shy G M, Silverstein I 1965 A study of the effects upon the motor unit by remote malignancy. Brain 88: 515–528

Sigwald J, Raverdy P, Fardeau M, Gremy F, Mace de Lepinay A, Bouttier D, Danic M 1966 Pseudo-myotonie.

Forme particulière d'hypertonie musculaire à prédominance distale. Revue Neurologique 115:1003

Sirbou A B, Murphy M J, White A S 1944 Soft tissue complications of fractures of the leg. California and Western Medicine 60:63

Slater G, Papatestas A E, Genkins G 1978 Thymomas in patients with myasthenia gravis. Annals of Surgery 188: 171–174

Smith B 1969 Skeletal muscle necrosis associated with carcinoma. Journal of Pathology 97:207

Smith R, Stern G 1967 Myopathy, osteomalacia and hyperparathyroidism. Brain 90: 593–602

Spaar R W 1980 Paraproteinaemias and multiple myeloma. In: Vinken P J, Bruyn G W (eds) Handbook of clinical neurology, vol 39. North Holland, Amsterdam, p 131–179

Spillane J D 1970 Restless legs in chronic pulmonary disease. British Medical Journal 4:796

Spillane J D, Nathan P W, Kelley R E, Marsden C D 1971 Painful legs and moving toes. Brain 94: 541–574

Stefanye K, Iwamasa R T, Schantz E J, Spero L (1964) Effect of guanidium salts on toxicity of botulinum toxin. Biochemica et Biophysica Acta 86:412

Stephen A, McGuire M C, Tomasovic M C, Ackerman N Jr 1984 Hereditary continuous muscle fibre activity. Archives of Neurology 41: 395–396

Stout A P 1946 Rhabdomyosarcoma of the skeletal muscles. Annals of Surgery 123:447

Stuart F S, Henry M, Holley H L 1960 The stiff-man syndrome. Arthritis and Rheumatism 3:229

Swash M, Fox K P, Davidson A R 1975 Carcinoid myopathy. Serotonin-induced muscle weakness in man? Archives of Neurology 32:572

Sylvest E 1934 Epidemic myalgia: Bornholm disease. Levin and Munksgaard, Copenhagen

Trethowan W H, Allsop J L, Turner B 1960 The stiff-man syndrome. Archives of Neurology 3:448

Tunte W, Becker P E, Knorre G V 1967 Zur Genetik der Myositis ossificans progressiva. Humangenetik 4:320

Turner H D, Brett E M, Gilbert R J, Ghosh A C, Liebeschuetz H J 1978 Infant botulism in England. Lancet i: 1277–1278

Viparelli V 1963 La miosite ossificante progressiva. Annali de Neuropsichiatria e Psicoanalisi 9:297

Volkmann R 1881 Die ischaemischen Muskellahmungen und Kontrakturen. Zentralblatt fur Chirurgie 8:801

Wallis A L 1957 M D thesis (Edinburgh University) cited by British Medical Journal, leading article 1978 1:1436

Warmolts J R, Re P K, Lewis R J, Engel W K 1975 Type II muscle fibre atrophy (II atrophy). An early systemic effect of cancer. Neurology (Minneapolis) 25:374

Weller T H, Enders J F, Buckingham M, Finn J J jr 1950 The aetiology of epidemic pleurodynia; a study of two viruses isolated from a typical outbreak. Journal of Immunology 65:337

Werk E E, Sholiton L J, Monell R J 1961 The stiff-man syndrome and hyperthyroidism. American Journal of Medicine 31:647

Wilkins A J W, Kotze D M, Melvin J, Gear J, Prinsloo F R, Kirsch Z 1955 Meningo-encephalitis due to Coxsackie B virus in Southern Rhodesia. South African Medical Journal 29:25

Wilkinson M, Croft P B, Urich H 1967 The remote effects

of cancer on the nervous system. Proceedings of the Royal Society of Medicine 60:683

Willis T 1685 The London practice of physic. Barsett and Cooke, London, p 404

Willis R A 1952 The spread of tumours in human body. Butterworth, London

Wittmach T 1961 Pathologie und Therapie der sensibilitat-Neurosen. E Shafer, Leipzig p 459

Yuill G M 1980 Leukaemia: Neurological involvement. In: Vinken P J, Bruyn G W (eds) Handbook of clinical neurology, vol 39. North-Holland, Amsterdam, p 1–26

Neuromuscular disease in animals

INTRODUCTION

The equivalent chapter of the last edition of this book concentrated on the presentation of accounts of a wide range of myopathies of non-primate mammals. In this chapter we have modified our approach by reducing the descriptions of animal myopathies without human counterpart and by condensing the information into tables. We recommend consultation of the previous edition for expanded descriptions of the tabulated conditions.

We have revised and expanded those sections describing myopathies of relevance to the human subject including those used as experimental models of human diseases. A new section on avian myopathies including chicken dystrophy, is contributed by one of us (EAB) together with brief commentaries upon several other myopathies affecting the quail, duck and turkey. Previously we excluded from our discussions neurogenic muscle diseases of which there are a large number. However, because in man the spinal muscular atrophies and motor neurone diseases commonly enter into the differential diagnosis of primary myopathies, some related conditions in animals are described. We must point out that the additional text is not intended to give a comprehensive account of either the full range of avian myopathies or of neurogenic muscle diseases. An account of peripheral neuropathies of domestic animals with emphasis on dog, cat and horse is given by Duncan & Griffiths (1984). As previously, we have excluded reference to primate and piscine myopathies, to neoplasia and to inflammatory myopathies, some of which are of considerable economic importance. Adequate descriptions can be found in the texts of Hadlow (1962), Nieberle & Cohrs (1967), Jones & Hunt (1983) and Jubb et al (1985).

An attempt has been made to simplify the classification of the myopathies; this, however, is not precise. Probably in some instances the primary defect leading to a myopathy develops during gestation, and yet clinical manifestations may not appear until some days or weeks after birth. Thus because of gaps in knowledge about the genesis of some diseases in this category some classified as neonatal may be congenital. Classification by aetiology is potentially a sound method with clinical value. Unfortunately the causes of many animal myopathies are unknown or complex. Despite this we can make some generalisations: all disease has a genetic component and conversely all disease has an environmental component; thus many or probably most myopathies have a mixed aetiology with relatively few having a predominantly hereditary or predominantly environmental cause.

In some instances the question of heritability has been a problem. We have classified a myopathy as heritable where it has been established that this aspect of phenotypic variation is due to additive gene effects. Otherwise, where a myopathy has been detected in a small number of animals which had a common parent or where it affects a single breed, we have classified it as familial, provided that the condition does not occur in other animals of the same species, reared in the same environment at the same time. Such considerations quickly lead to the concept of 'liability' and the acceptance that all diseases have a genetic element.

As with studies of human myopathies the counterparts in animals have been investigated by veterinary pathologists using histological, histochemical, ultrastructural and biochemical techniques. At the clinical level patient co-operation and economic factors dictate the extent to which myopathies in animals may be investigated. Consequently the number of centres at which expertise and equipment are available for diagnostic purposes is limited, with most investigations carried out on horses or dogs.

Acute myopathies are usually diagnosed clinically with biochemical support. As in human myopathies (see Ch. 15, 17, 18, 20 and 25), as a result of the impairment of membrane function and integrity, enzymes normally present in muscle such as creatine kinase (CK, EC 2.7.3.2.) escape and can be detected in increased amounts in the blood. This enzyme is one of the most useful indicators of acute muscle damage. The plasma activity of CK varies in normal animals within small limits with age, sex and physical fitness and larger limits as a result of exercise, prolonged recumbency, physical restraint and minor manipulative procedures or treatment. Activities have relatively short half-lives in the blood (four hours for CK in cattle, Anderson et al 1976).

Recent investigations have established that, under physiological conditions, 3-methyl histidine is in some species a valid index of muscle protein degradation (Harris et al 1977). During myofibrillar protein catabolism it may be rapidly excreted in the urine. Urinary excretion of 3-methyl histidine is not a reliable measure of muscle protein degradation in sheep (Harris & Milne 1977) or pigs (Milne & Harris 1978), but it may be a valid index of muscle protein degradation in cattle (Harris & Milne 1978). The usefulness of this metabolite as an indicator of myopathy remains to be explored (Ward & Buttery 1978). In horses and dogs, and for experimental study in a wide range of species, muscle biopsies are used for diagnostic or research purposes although to a much lesser extent than in human medicine. There are a number of major differences in approach to the study of myopathies in man and in animals and it is important for the medical practitioner to bear these in mind when reading the accounts that follow.

The veterinary myopathologist is commonly involved with many species which differ from man in the length of gestation. Their rates of fetal growth are greater, when expressed as a function of maternal body weight (Blaxter 1964). There is a wide range in litter size and neonates may be relatively immature and helpless, or well developed and active. Regardless of the number of offspring or their state of development at birth, lower animals grow more rapidly than man, and reach maturity at an earlier age. These characteristics have been exaggerated by genetic selection in farm animals bred for production. This intensification has led to the unmasking of hitherto unsuspected nutritional deficiencies or limiting factors, as greater growth rates are achieved; this is particularly apparent when the animals are housed, and fed on locally grown crops. Examples of nutritional myopathies so induced are discussed below.

When the product is meat, intended to suit modern tastes, selection and husbandry have tended to favour the well-muscled animal, free from excess fat. As a consequence, there seems to have been an inadvertent selection of somewhat doubtful virtues of 'doubling muscling' in cattle (deliberately pursued in parts of continental Europe), and the associated occurrence of unwanted characteristics such as susceptibility to the porcine stress syndrome in 'improved' pigs. Livestock may also be subjected to long distance driving or transportation and may thereby suffer metabolic stresses resulting in 'transport myopathy', while the horse bred for work is susceptible to the notorious condition of paralytic myoglobinuria. These myopathies may be compared with their human counterparts, so-called 'Boot Camp Disease' or 'March Myoglobinuria'.

The physiological specialisation of muscle cell types is similar in farm animals to that of the extensively studied laboratory animals, and fibre-typing is usually based on standard histochemical methods. The alkali-stable myosin ATPase reaction (Guth & Samaha 1970) is particularly useful, and is the basis for the type I, intermediate and type II system of classification we have adopted in this chapter (except in the section on avian myopathy where subtyping of type II fibres is often used (Barnard et al 1982).

The subtyping of type II fibres, as in human muscle (IIA, IIB, IIC) using histochemical methods, has been used in dogs (Tunell & Hart 1977, Braund et al 1978, Braund & Lincoln 1981) and in horses (Essen et al 1980). However Snow et al (1982a), using histochemical, immunocytochemical and myosin heavy chain peptide-mapping methods in canine muscle, were unable to demonstrate 'classic' type II B fibres. The histochemical subtyping techniques are not consistently reliable in other species and are not frequently reported. In farm animal muscle, although type I cells can

be consistently identified, type II cells reacted for alkali-stable ATPase may show a range of density of reaction product. The acid lability or stability of myosin ATPase in these cells can be determined but again there is often a spectrum of reaction which enables only partial sub-classification. The intermediate type encompasses a range of type II cells, some possibly in a transitional state. Cells classed as type II without suffix are for the most part equivalent to human type IIB. The intermediate type II fibre is not confined to animal muscle. In the human *M. masseter* Ringqvist (1973) also used an intermediate cell classification. Similar problems arise when using oxidative enzyme reactions (Spurway 1981). These complications of fibre type identification arising presumably as a result of real differences in myocyte metabolism may be compounded when the technical procedures used in the ATPase methods are imprecisely controlled, especially with respect to temperature and pH. As immunocytochemical and peptide-mapping methods for myosin heavy chains are further developed and exploited for identification of the different forms of myosin some of these difficulties may be resolved. Table 28.1 shows three systems of fibre-type nomenclature and the corresponding physiological, biochemical and main histochemical features. We accept, however, that the functional state of a muscle cell is dynamic: it can change with age and training, and is dependent on normal innervation.

There are species differences, such as the graduation according to body size, from mouse to horse, that occurs in the proportion of fast-twitch aerobic cells in the diaphragm (Davies & Gunn 1972). Furthermore, some muscles of pigs have, as a normal feature, intrafascicular groups of type I cells, giving an appearance which deceptively resembles the pathological change known as fibre-type grouping. Individual muscles vary in fibre–type proportion (van den Hoven et al 1985) at different depths, perhaps because of the differing functions in relation to posture, locomotion and mechanical advantage.

Muscles differ in function and therefore structure and this is clearly reflected in their histochemistry. One expects to find a different structure in the *M. masseter* of a cud-chewing

Table 28.1 The relationship between physiological, biochemical and histochemical parameters and three systems of cell-type nomenclature

Contraction speed	ATPase pH 10.4 reaction	Energy method	NADH-TR reaction or haemoglobin content		Type		
Slow	[Low]	Oxidative (aerobic)	[High]	SO	I	β red
Fast	[Intermediate]	Oxidative/glycolytic (combined)	[Intermediate]	FOG	INT	α red
Fast	[High]	Glycolytic (anaerobic)	[Low]	FG	II	α white

ruminant than in a carnivore, and this is indeed the case with the *M. masseter* which in the ox and sheep appears to have the histochemical characteristics appropriate to a functional demand for slow sustained work (Suzuki 1977). We might also expect a change in structure to occur as a result of change in function. Thus the *M. masseter* of a new-born or veal calf may well differ from that of a cud-chewing adult or contemporary.

Such observations serve to confirm the importance of the dynamic state of skeletal muscle and permit its exploitation for athletic and meat-producing performance. Within species there may be wide ranges in phenotype and use. This is most obvious in dogs but is of great economic importance in cattle bred for beef production, on the one hand, or milk on the other. Comprehensive differences between breeds within a species have also been described (Gunn 1975) and significant differences may also exist between individuals when athletic ability is considered, e.g. the thoroughbred racehorse and racing greyhound are clearly equipped for athletic prowess. The fundamental basis for this is related partly to body size, bone length (and thereby mechanical advantage of muscles working over specific joints) but also to muscle fibre number and histochemical type proportion. As with human athletes, the hereditary factors which control these features determine the nature of the event which most suits the individual: some may be best equipped for sprinting, others for endurance. As the skills of trainers become more scientifically based, training régimes are produced for individuals with a view to fulfilling the potential for the optimal aerobic or anaerobic metabolism a specific event demands.

Biopsies are therefore potentially useful for assessing the suitability of individual animals for particular events and in genetic selection for breeding.

With regard to pathology, the reactions of muscle cells are limited. In particular, myocyte necrosis (myodegeneration) is the end result of a process common to many animal and human myopathies. In all species, dystrophic or injured muscle cells are either abnormally permeable, or suffer total structural breakdown. Loss of normal membrane function tends to result in leakage of potassium from, and entry of sodium and calcium ions into, the muscle cells, irrespective of the cause of the injury. Wrogemann & Pena (1976) have suggested that the increased net influx of Ca^{2+} resulting in mitochondrial calcium overload is the basis of a final common pathogenic mechanism for muscle necrosis in a wide variety of muscle disorders, independent of their aetiology. The histological appearance is exhibited as a hyaline, floccular and granular change. The other main features of myocyte alteration in disease relate to changes in size and shape (atrophy and hypertrophy) and to altered internal structure as determined by histochemical and ultrastructural study. These features include virtually the full range of those seen in human muscle disease. As in muscle disease in man, the geometrical distribution of degenerative change within a particular transverse section such as fibre-type grouping, small or large group atrophy may be important in disease definition. Finally, it has long been recognised in animals that disease of skeletal muscle is commonly and importantly associated with disease of cardiac muscle which should not be neglected in investigations of myopathies. This is particularly true in some toxic and nutritionally induced myopathies and is vital because, whereas damaged skeletal muscle can recover, cardiac muscle cannot.

FAMILIAL OR HEREDITARY MYOPATHIES INCLUDING MYOTONIA

These are listed by species in Table 28.2. Glycogen storage myopathies, type II cell deficiency of the Labrador retriever, muscular dystrophies of mink, mouse and hamster and myotonia have importance as models for the equivalent diseases of man and these will be amplified below. Some further information is given also about four farm animal myopathies — two in cattle, one each in sheep and pigs — because of their unique nature and potential value for study to elucidate specific myopathic problems.

Farm animal myopathies

Double muscling is a condition of cattle, sheep and pigs (although the term is commonly applied only to cattle) in which there is bilateral muscle enlargement especially of the proximal limbs, back and neck (Johnson 1981) due to myofibre hyper-

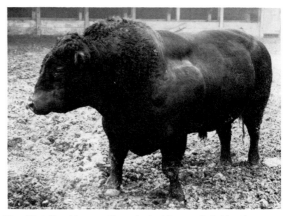

Fig. 28.1 Double muscling. A double-muscled Aberdeen Angus bull

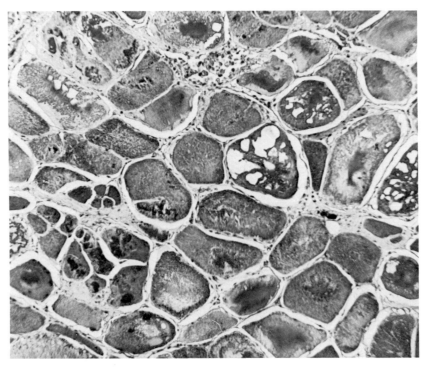

Fig. 28.2 Diaphragm myopathy. Diaphragm muscle of a Meuse-Rhine-Yssel cow affected with diaphragm myopathy. Many muscle cells show vacuolar change, target or targetoid formation and splitting. There is also an increase in endomysial connective tissue. Masson's trichrome, ×85 (section supplied by courtesy of Dr S. A. Goedegebuure)

Table 28.2 Familial or hereditary myopathy

Species	Condition	Breed	Mode of inher.	Onset	Signs	Pathology	Notes	Key ref.
O	DOUBLE MUSCLING	Many	AR (VE)	Congenital Neonatal	Generalised muscle hypertrophy (Fig. 28.1)	Myocyte hyperplasia	Cause of dystocia. Stress susceptibility. Good muscle:bone ratio and low fat carcase	King & Menissier 1982
O	LIMBER LEGS	Jersey	Semi-lethal AR	Congenital	Splayed limbs. Abnormal joint posture	No lesions in bone or muscle		Lamb et al 1976
O	DIAPHRAGM MYOPATHY	Meuse-Rhine-Yssel	F	2–10 y (Mean 5 y)	Progressive. Bloat, dyspnoea, asphyxia	Diaphragm myocyte CCV, vacuolation, degeneration, splitting and cores (Fig. 28.2)	No lesions in PNS/CNS. Mm. intercostales also affected	Goedegebuure et al 1983
O	MYOPATHY + HYDROCEPHALUS	Hereford	AR	Congenital	Generalised progressive	Myocyte CCV, degeneration, fibrosis. No regeneration (Fig. 28.3)	Primary myopathy. Ventral horn cells normal	Hadlow 1973
O	GLYCOGENOSIS TYPE II	(a) Shorthorn (b) Brahman	(a) AR (b) F	(a) 3–5 m or 9–12 m (b) 2–3 m	Muscular weakness + inco-ordination	Glycogen deposits in neurones, cardiac and skeletal myocytes (Fig. 28.4)	(a) Infantile and late onset forms equivalent to Pompe's disease	(a) Howell et al 1981 (b) O'Sullivan et al 1981
S	DOUBLE MUSCLING	Merino/others	F	Congenital but rare	Muscle hypertrophy	Myocyte hyperplasia	Causes dystocia	Naerland 1940 Swatland 1974
S	DAFT LAMB DISEASE	Border Leicester	AR	Congenital	Abnormal gait and neck posture	Type I hypertrophy. Type II hypotrophy (Fig. 28.5)	Clinically improves with age. Myopathy not apparent until 3 months	Bradley & Terlecki 1977
S	PRIMARY MYOPATHY	Merino	AR	1 m	Rocking horse gait when driven	Rounded fibres. Int nuc. Connective tissue ↑ Sarcoplasmic masses. Vacuoles (Fig. 28.6)		McGavin & Baynes 1969

Table 28.2 (*Cont'd*)

Species	Condition	Breed	Mode of inher.	Onset	Signs	Pathology	Notes	Key ref.
S	GLYCOGEN STORAGE DISEASE	Corriedale	F	6–10 m	Lethargy. Inco-ordination. May be fatal	Glycogen stored in brain stem neurones and all types of myocytes	Resembles Pompe's disease in man	Manktelow & Hartley 1975
P	DOUBLE MUSCLING	Pietrain and others	AR (Halothane sensitivity)	Congenital	Generalised muscle hypertrophy	Myocyte hyperplasia	Associated with halothane sensitivity and susceptibility to stress (qv)	Bradley & Done 1986
P	PIETRAIN CREEPER	Pietrain	F	3 w	Initial tremor and reluctance to stand. Creeping gait. Recumbent by 12 w	CCV. Int nuc. Focal myodegeneration/regeneration (Fig. 28.7)		Bradley & Wells 1980
DGH	MYOTONIA	(See Table 28.3)						
D	CONGENITAL MYASTHENIA GRAVIS	(a) Jack Russell terrier; (b) Springer spaniel; (c) Fox terrier	AR; F; F	6–8 w	Weakness. Dysphagia	(a & b) Due to low insertion rate of acetylcholine receptors in postsynaptic membrane	May provide animal models of some forms of congenital myasthenia gravis in man	Oda et al 1984
D	TYPE II FIBRE DEFICIENCY	Labrador retriever	AR	3–6 m	Mm atrophy. Exercise intolerance	Variable: includes small group atrophy, Type II fibre deficiency, Int nuc. Fibre splitting, necrosis & regeneration	Resembles limb girdle dystrophy of man	Kramer et al 1976 McKerrell et al 1984
D	X-LINKED MYOPATHY	(a) Irish terrier; (b) Golden retriever	XR	6–8 w	Dysphagia. Stiff gait. Slowly progressive	Muscle necrosis & degeneration	HFD on EMG resembling myotonia. (See Table 28.3) Mitochondrial abnormalities	(a) Wentink et al 1972, 1974b; (b) Kornegay 1984
D	MITOCHONDRIAL MYOPATHY	(a) Clumber spaniel; (b) Sussex spaniel	F; F	When first lead-exercised (3–4 m)	Severe exercise intolerance. Acidosis. Collapse. Possible death	Not reported	Shown to be defect in PDH complex	(a) Herrtage & Houlton 1979; (b) Houlton & Herrtage 1980

	Disease	Breed/strain	Inheritance	Age	Clinical signs	Pathology	Comments	References
D	GLYCOGENOSIS TYPE III	Alsatian	F	2 m	Progressive loss of weight. Muscular weakness and hepatomegaly	Glycogen storage in hepatocytes, neurones, all types of myocyte	Equivalent to Cori's disease in man. (See also Mostafa 1970 re Pompe's disease in the dog)	Ceh et al 1976, Rafiquzzaman et al 1976
C	GLYCOGENOSIS TYPE II	Domestic short haired	F	12 m	Progressive weakness and Mm atrophy. Retarded growth	PAS positive material in and necrosis of Mm fibres	Resembles Pompe's disease of man	Sandström et al 1969
MIN	MUSCULAR DYSTROPHY	Commercial brown	AR	2 m	Muscle weakness and atrophy. Dysphagia	Degeneration. Fibrosis. CCV. Int nuc	Resembles limb girdle, facioscapulohumeral and childhood autosomal recessive dystrophies of man	Hegreberg 1979
HAM	DYSTROPHY-LIKE MYOPATHY	Syrian B10 1.50 (Whitney)	AR	60–200 d	Progressive muscle weakness. Death due to cardiomyopathy	CCV. Fibre atrophy & fragmentation. Necrosis Int nuc (Fig. 28.8)	Of particular use as a model of cardiomyopathy	Caulfield 1972, Homburger 1979
M	MUSCULAR DYSTROPHY	Bar Harbor 129/Re	AR (a) dy (b) dy^{2J}	2 w	Progressive muscular weakness	CCV. Necrosis. Abortive regeneration. Int nuc	Used as model of Duchenne dystrophy	(a) Michelson et al 1955 (b) Meier & Southard 1970
		C57BL/10	XR (c)mdx	12 m	Slight locomotor abnormalities	CCV. Necrosis. Degeneration. Int nuc. Cardiac involvement	—	(c) Bulfield et al 1984
M	MUSCULAR DYSGENESIS	Inbred tailless	AR (mdg)	Congenital	Def. of skeletal muscle. Fatal	—	—	Pai 1965a, b

C = cat   D = dog   G = goat   GP = guinea pig   HAM = hamster   H = horse   MIN = mink   M = mouse   O = ox   S = sheep   P = pig   RAB = rabbit   d = days   w = weeks   m = months   y = years   AD = Autosomal dominant   AR = Autosomal recessive   F = Familial   VE = Variable expressivity   XR = Sex linked recessive   BHFD = Bizarre high frequency discharge   CCV = cell calibre variation   LMN = Lower motor neurone   MND = Motor neurone disease   HFD = high-frequency discharge   Int nuc = Internal nuclei   M(m) = muscle(s)
↑ = increase   ↓ = decrease   → = resulting in

plasia (Fig. 28.1). In cattle it is a condition of considerable commercial importance. In the UK the artificial insemination authorities select against it because of the associated problems of dystocia resulting from relative fetal oversize. On the other hand in Belgium, France, Italy and Spain the condition is exploited for beef production in local areas or breeds. Carcasses can contain as much as 18% more muscle (meat), virtually no fat and have a more advantageous muscle-to-bone ratio than normal animals of the same breed. Double-muscled animals tend to be stress susceptible; this is, however, of greater importance in the pig (see Porcine Stress syndrome). There are no myopathic changes in affected muscles.

Diaphragm myopathy of Meuse–Rhine–Yssel (MRY) cattle. This unique disease was first described by Hoebe (1975) and subsequently by Goedegebuure & Hoebe (1976) and Goedegebuure et al (1983).

It occurs in MRY cattle in Eastern Holland where the breed forms half the population. About 60 female cattle between two and ten years old (mean five years) have been affected. Anorexia, reduced rumination and eructation and recurrent rumenal tympany are the main clinical symptoms. Electromyography of the diaphragm reveals a decreased duration of action potentials and in four out of seven cows the number of polyphasic potentials was increased. Animals die within two to ten weeks from asphyxia. Gross lesions affect only the *M. diaphragma*. The muscular part is pale, swollen and hard. Histological lesions are diffuse and include rounded myocytes, hypertrophic and atrophic type II myocytes, cell splitting and an increase in range of cell calibre. There is no change in cell type distribution but intramyocyte nuclei increase. Myodegeneration with vacuolation is common. Partial degeneration of myocytes and core and target fibre formation are particular features seen with special stains (Fig. 28.2). A histiocyte response and some fibrosis occurs. Brain, spinal cord, nerves and end-plates are normal. *Mm. interterostales externi et interni* also show partial degeneration of myocytes and cell calibre variation. Milder changes have been seen in other muscles including the tongue and heart. After a thorough study, Goedegebuure et al (1983)

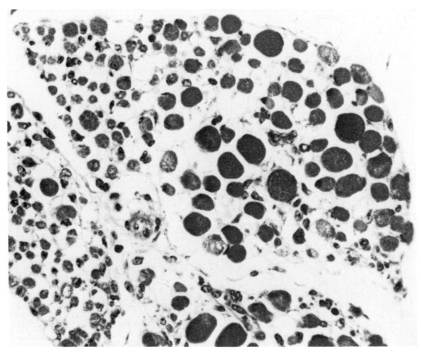

Fig. 28.3 Myopathy associated with hydrocephalus in Hereford cattle. There is a wide variation in cell size and many cells are hypotrophic. H & E, ×275 (section supplied by courtesy of Dr W. J. Hadlow)

conclude that the disease is an inherited progressive muscular dystrophy.

Primary myopathy of Merino sheep. A progressive myopathy of Merino lambs, inherited as an autosomal recessive trait, was described by McGavin & Baynes (1969) and McGavin (1974) (see also White et al 1978). Clinically, signs of stiffness are usually detected when the lambs are about one month old. When driven, affected lambs develop a 'rocking-horse' type of gait because they are unable to extend the stifle and flex the hock joints. The condition is progressive and, under range conditions, results in death from starvation.

Lesions sometimes occur in the *M. triceps brachii*, always in the *M. quadriceps femoris* and consistently in the *M. vastus intermedius*. Lesions are bilaterally symmetrical and visible to the naked eye as white areas, or indeed whole white muscles, because of replacement of muscle fibres with fat cells.

The histological lesions are distinctive. In lambs aged six weeks, the muscle cells are rounded in cross section and vary from 15 to 100 μm in diameter. Some have central and peripheral sarcoplasmic masses, while others are vacuolated (Fig. 28.6). There is an increase in muscle cell nuclei which may be vesicular, and may occur internally in long chains. There is a slight increase in, or condensation of, endomysial connective tissue. Type I cells are particularly affected; the *M. vastus intermedius* of Merino sheep is composed entirely of this type of cell.

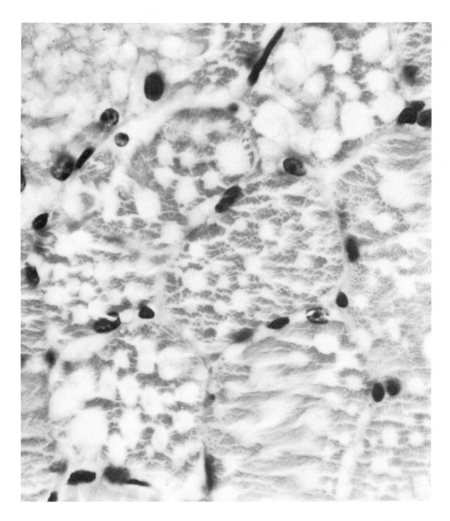

Fig. 28.4 Glycogenosis type II. Skeletal muscle from a yearling Beef Shorthorn showing multiple vacuoles in muscle cells. H & E, ×900 (section supplied by courtesy of Dr R. B. Richards)

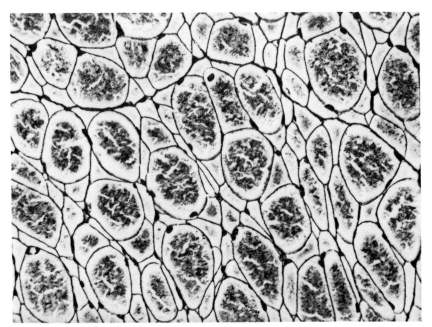

Fig. 28.5 'Daft lamb' disease. *M. splenius* of a 3-month-old 'daft lamb' showing a wide variation in cell size, with large intrafascicular cells. Gomori's reticulin stain, ×275

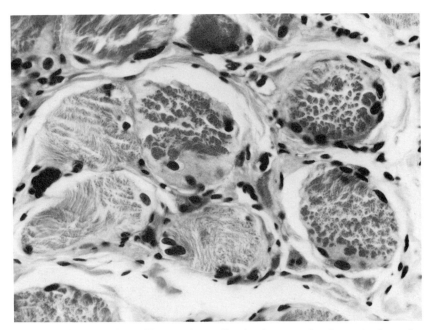

Fig. 28.6 Primary myopathy of Merino sheep. *M. vastus intermedius* showing sarcoplasmic masses, internal nuclei and a slight increase or condensation of endomysial connective tissue. H & E, ×275 (section supplied by courtesy of Dr R. B. Richards)

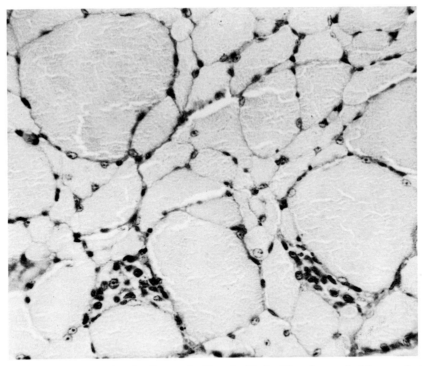

Fig. 28.7 Pietrain creeper syndrome. *M. semitendinosus* of a 12-week-old pig. There is a marked increase in the range of cell size with some focal myodegeneration. A few cells contain internal nuclei. Collagen/elastin, ×275

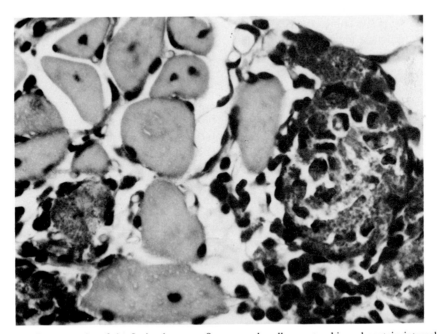

Fig. 28.8 Dystrophy-like myopathy of the Syrian hamster. Some muscle cells are atrophic and contain internal nuclei. Myodegeneration and phagocytosis are prominent. H & E, ×400

As the lambs age there is a reduction in the number of muscle cells. These are progressively replaced with fat cells until, at five years, more than 90% of an affected muscle may be replaced with fat. Significant lesions have not been found in the central or peripheral nervous system.

Pietrain creeper syndrome (PCS) is a familial, presumed inherited, progressive primary myopathy of the Pietrain pig — a breed particularly well muscled (double-muscled) and prone to the porcine stress syndrome (PSS), q.v. However, the clinical signs of PCS usually develop before animals develop age susceptibility either to PSS or to halothane. A comprehensive account of the disease and its pathology is given by Bradley & Wells (1980). PCS has been recognised in the UK in one pure-bred herd in which selection for susceptibility to the porcine stress syndrome has been practised for experimental purposes and in one commercial herd; it has also occurred in Pietrain pigs in continental Europe. Usually only two or three pigs in each affected litter show the characteristic clinical features.

The pigs appear to be normal until they are about three weeks old, when initially they develop static tremor in fore and hind quarters when standing, and are reluctant to stand for more than a few seconds. The condition is progressive. Although the pigs grow well at first, after four or five weeks recumbency becomes almost continuous, brief periods of standing being accompanied by carpal flexion. By 10–12 weeks, carpal extension is restricted and infrequent movement is limited to a creeping type of gait. Macroscopically, affected muscles appear atrophic.

Histological examination shows that all major muscles are affected but the severity of pathological change varies between muscles. The proximal limb muscles are most affected. The main pathological features are a wide variation in muscle-cell diameter (Fig. 28.7), an increase in the number of internal nuclei and focal myodegeneration and regeneration in excess of the focal myopathic changes observed in normal Pietrain pig muscle (Muir 1970) (see Focal myopathy). Both type I and type II muscle fibres are involved, and there are marked changes in the normal distribution pattern of muscle fibre types. Target

cells do not occur, but there is an abnormal distribution of histochemical enzyme reaction products within the cells. Significant abnormalities have not been detected in the central or peripheral nervous systems, the motor end-plates or the neuromuscular spindles.

Since the account of this disease was given in the last edition a breeding experiment has been conducted, but without resolution of the mode of inheritance. Furthermore, some clinically affected pigs have recovered and some apparently normal littermate pigs have revealed lesions similar to, but milder than, those of clinically affected animals. These additional complexities have not been satisfactorily explained.

Myopathy due to storage disease

Glycogen storage disease. A generalised glycogen storage disease occurring in Corriedale sheep has been recognised in New Zealand (Manktelow & Hartley 1975). Between six and 10 months of age, the animals became lethargic and inco-ordinated, and lost condition. Some collapsed and died on exertion. There was an accumulation of glycogen in skeletal, cardiac and smooth muscle cells, and in nerve cells of the brain stem; Manktelow and Hartley suggested that the disease was comparable with Pompe's disease of man (type II glycogenosis or acid maltase (α-1,4-glucosidase, EC 3.2.1.3) deficiency.

Richards et al (1977) described the clinical, biochemical and pathological features of hereditary glycogenosis type II in cattle. The affected animals were part of a group of yearling Shorthorn beef cattle in Western Australia. The clinical signs were muscle weakness, inability to rise normally and inco-ordination of gait. Stored intracytoplasmic glycogen was demonstrated in the central nervous system, heart and skeletal muscle (Fig. 28.4).

Additional information on field cases has been given by Edwards & Richards (1979). O'Sullivan et al (1981) have described a very similar glycogenosis in Brahman cattle in Australia.

Howell et al (1981) described the clinico-pathological findings of infantile- (3–7 months) and later-(>9 months) onset forms of glycogenosis type II in a single experimental herd of cattle.

Diagnosis of affected, carrier or normal animals can be made on the day of birth by measurement of lymphocyte acid maltase activity and muscle biopsy. ECG tracings were abnormal with tall broad QRS complexes. In the infantile form cardiomegaly is a feature. Glycogen deposition is widespread and particularly severe in cardiac and skeletal muscle and nervous tissue. Despite the presence of nervous lesions neurological signs are curiously absent. Glycogen is aggregated in cells in membrane-bound structures derived from lysosomes. The disease is inherited as an autosomal recessive trait.

Type II glycogenosis has also been recorded in dogs and cats. Rafiquzzaman et al (1976) discussed glycogen storage diseases in domestic animals and described, in detail, glycogenosis in four female Alsatian (German Shepherd) dogs. They consider the disease to be similar to Cori's disease in man (type III glycogenosis). A comparative account of this glycogenosis with the human disease and its usefulness as a model is given by Svenkerud & Hauge (1978). Biochemical investigation of one of these animals by Ceh et al (1976) provided further evidence that the disease was similar to Cori's disease and was associated with deficiency of the debranching enzyme amylo-1,6-glucosidase (EC 3.2.1.33).

Hegreberg & Norby (1973) reported an inherited storage disease of cats, which was accompanied by growth retardation, progressive muscular weakness and atrophy. The changes particularly involved the hind limb musculature. Periodic acid-Schiff positive material occurred in reticulo-endothelial cells, liver and muscle cells. There was focal necrosis of muscle and increased serum creatine kinase (CK) activity.

Dystrophic conditions of small animals with relevance to human muscular dystrophy

Murine muscular dystrophy first appeared as a spontaneous mutation in the Bar Harbor strain 129/Re mouse in 1951. This mutation was named *Dystrophia muscularis* and later shown to be inherited via an autosomal recessive gene (gene symbol *dy*) (Michelson et al 1955). Subsequently a milder progressive myopathy was discovered by Meier & Southard (1970) and shown to be an

allele of the *dy* gene (gene symbol *dy²ᴶ*) and recently a third allele (symbol *dyᵏ*) has been described in an unrelated colony of SM mice (Hayakawa & Tsuji 1985). Although differing in some respects from human forms of dystrophy (Mendell et al 1979) the *dy* and *dy²ᴶ* mutants have been studied and used extensively as experimental models of muscular dystrophy.

In the *dy* mouse symptoms are first recognised at approximately two weeks of age. Affected animals are low in body weight and less active than normal. Generalised atrophy of skeletal muscle is accompanied by rapidly progressive muscular weakness. Functional control of the hind limbs is lost first and in some individuals muscular tremors, head nodding and gasping respiration are seen. Kyphosis and contractures develop later and most affected animals die at about four months of age.

In man Duchenne dystrophy is characterised by elevated serum creatine kinase (CK) activity, but in dystrophic mice there have been conflicting reports regarding serum CK levels. Nicholson & Matheson (1981) showed that dystrophic mouse muscle does leak the MM isoenzyme of CK but that the defect is mild compared with that seen in Duchenne dystrophy. Shivers & Atkinson (1984) suggested that these elevated levels might result either from the escape of enzymes from necrotic cells or from extravasation along avenues provided by the hyperplastic membrane caveolae; in contrast to other studies, they found no evidence for focal lesions in the sarcolemma of viable dystrophic cells.

Because of the early onset and severity of signs, normal breeding from affected *dy* mice is not possible. However, techniques such as transplantation of *dy/dy* ovaries and artificial insemination of young dystrophic females with sperm from dystrophic males have allowed all-dystrophic litters to be produced.

The less severely affected *dy²ᴶ* mutants have a longer life-span and may breed successfully. Meier & Southard (1970) showed that the differences between *dy* and *dy²ᴶ* mutants were those only of degree, and later MacPike & Meier (1976) demonstrated that on the same genetic background the two alleles are essentially the same, indicating that the remainder of the genome exerts a major influence on the expression of murine muscular dystrophy.

The histological features of both mutants include marked variations in fibre size, segmental necrosis with phagocytosis of debris and the presence of numerous enlarged internal nuclei, often in prominent rows (Pearce & Walton 1963, Banker 1967). Longitudinal splitting is often found, involving many fibres (Isaacs et al 1973). Proliferation of connective tissue is relatively mild and there is relatively little fat replacement. Evidence of early regeneration is present but tends to be abortive, particularly when there is proliferation of connective tissue.

In a study of postnatal growth and differentiation of dystrophic muscle fibres, Wirtz et al (1983) demonstrated that development is normal in the immediate postnatal period. This is followed first by severe necrosis involving all fibre types in the second week of life and then by a wave of regeneration which is insufficient to restore fibre numbers. By four or five months of age, dystrophic mice have a reduction of 40–70% in the number of muscle fibres in many muscles when compared with normal animals of equivalent age.

Ultrastructural studies have revealed various abnormalities (Banker 1967) including significant changes in both the pre- and postsynaptic regions of the end-plate (Banker et al 1979), similar to those seen in Duchenne dystrophy.

In both the *dy* and *dy*[2J] mutants the predominant lesion in the nervous system is the presence in both dorsal and ventral nerve roots of large groups of amyelinated fibres. The number of myelinated fibres in these areas may be reduced to 5% of normal (Bradley & Jaros 1979) and similar lesions are seen in the proximal parts of cranial nerves (Biscoe et al 1975).

Bradley & Jaros (1979) suggested that a loss of Schwann cells occurs in these areas as, despite showing a normal ability to proliferate, Schwann cell numbers gradually fall to approximately 50% of those seen in normal adults. However, the reduction in the number of myelinated fibres in dystrophic roots is much greater than can be explained by the deficency in Schwann cells alone and it has been suggested that they may be unable to establish a normal relationship with the axon or that the axons themselves may be incapable of providing the necessary stimulus for myelination (Bradley & Jaros 1979).

John & Purdom (1984) showed that there is a reduction in collagen in dystrophic nerves and roots and suggested that, since it is probable that there must be a minimum amount of type I collagen in the extracellular matrix for ensheathment to occur, the greatly decreased levels of type I collagen might explain the amyelination of axons in these areas.

Morphologically, the axons themselves appear normal although functional abnormalities have been demonstrated. The amount of protein conveyed by fast transport systems (Bradley & Jaros 1979) is increased and that conveyed at slower rates decreased.

Because Dystrophia-muscularis is a progressive necrotising myopathy it was initially thought that it would provide a good model for human forms of muscular dystrophy. The presence of morphological, functional and electrophysiological abnormalities in the nervous system of both the *dy* and *dy*[2J] dystrophic mouse, however, has caused the value of these lines as models for human dystrophy to be questioned, as there is no indication of central or peripheral nerve involvement in human cases.

In view of this controversy, the appearance of an X-linked degenerative myopathy in the mouse is of considerable interest (Bulfield et al 1984). This mutant (mdx) produces viable homozygous animals with high serum activities of muscular enzymes and exhibits histological lesions similar to those seen in muscular dystrophy in man.

Clinically, the mice are very mildly affected. Young animals show virtually no sign of the disease and are able to breed normally. In yearling mice slight locomotor abnormalities may be encountered including muscular tremors. Histological features include fibre-size variation, internal nuclei, degeneration, necrosis and phagocytosis. There are areas of regeneration but little replacement of muscle with fat cells, and only mild fibrosis (Bulfield et al 1984). Recently it has been shown that cardiac muscle is affected (L R Bridges, personal communication) but to date no abnormalities have been demonstrated in either the peripheral or central nervous system.

Ultrastructural changes include dilatation of sarcoplasmic reticulum, mitochondrial degeneration and disruption of normal myofibrillar architecture.

As in other forms of murine dystrophy there are some morphological differences between the muscle lesions seen in the mdx mutant and those characteristic of human dystrophy. A further point of difference from Becker and Duchenne dystrophies is the late onset of clinical signs in the mdx mutant. Whether these variations are due to species differences or indicate a different aetiology or pathogenesis, is not yet clear.

In common with the human condition, the mdx mice share various histological features, involvement of cardiac muscle, elevated levels of CK and, of particular interest, linkage to the X-chromosome, all of which may make this particular mouse mutant a valuable animal model for future studies. However, Dangain & Vrbová (1984) found that three-to four-week-old mice had suffered acute episodes of muscle degeneration and subsequently recovered. They therefore suggested that, although this mutant may be useful in the study of muscle destruction and repair, it is unlikely to be related to Duchenne dystrophy and should be used with caution.

Dystrophy-like myopathy of the Syrian hamster was first recognised and described in an inbred line B10.1.50 (Whitney) strain by Homburger and his colleagues. It was demonstrated that the condition was inherited via an autosomal recessive gene and, although the original strain has now been lost, several other lines with variable clinical severity and life expectancy have been maintained (Homburger 1979).

Onset of signs is gradual, with muscular weakness becoming apparent between 60 and 200 days of age. Cardiomyopathy occurs in all affected animals and causes congestive heart failure resulting in death about halfway through the normal life span. Death from cardiac involvement thus occurs too soon to allow the pathological changes in the skeletal muscles to reach the advanced stage seen in dystrophic mice. Diagnosis is suspected when plasma CK activity is abnormally high (often markedly increased by 30 days of age). Confirmation is by histological examination of cheek pouch retractor muscle biopsy. At

necropsy, tongue muscles show pathognomonic myolysis and calcification from 55 days onwards. The presence of disease in young animals showing no other clinical signs can also be demonstrated by subjecting them to forced swimming which reveals weakness of the adductor hindlimb muscles (Homburger 1972).

Homburger et al (1965) reported that the earliest morphological change seen in muscle from affected animals is the appearance of a perinuclear halo around some subsarcolemmal nuclei. Later in the disease process the histology resembles that seen in murine dystrophy with marked fibre-calibre variation, loss of muscle fibres from fragmentation and atrophy, degeneration, coagulation necrosis and phagocytosis of debris (Fig. 28.8). There is an increase in the number of myocyte nuclei, some of which are internal and occur in long chains, and nucleoli are prominent. Some evidence of regeneration occurs and there is some increase in connective tissue and fat, although these are not conspicuous features. Both fibre types are involved.

Homburger (1972) emphasised the similarity between these lesions and the changes seen in Duchenne dystrophy. Karpati et al (1982) have shown that denervation of dystrophic hamster muscle prevents muscle fibre necrosis, and also demonstrated that hypophysectomy mitigates skeletal muscle fibre damage (Karpati et al 1985). Ultrastructural lesions are non-specific and include degeneration and disintegration of Z and I bands, condensation of cells, mineralisation of mitochondria and dilatation of the sarcotubular system (Caulfield 1966, 1972). An advantage of the hamster as an animal model of muscular dystrophy is the relatively late onset of disabling signs, preceded by increased serum enzyme levels, calcification of the tongue and changes in the muscle detectable on biopsy. The hamster has been a particularly useful model of cardiomyopathy, as heart muscle involvement occurs early.

Muscular dystrophy of mink is a progressive degenerative condition of skeletal muscle which has a familial pattern suggesting an autosomal recessive mode of inheritance (Hegreberg et al 1975). Onset of clinical signs occurs at two months of age and the disease follows a progressive course, resulting in muscle weakness, hypotonia, atrophy and dysphagia. The condition is generalised with particular involvement of proximal limb musculature and the temporal and masseter muscles of the head. Serum enzymes of muscle origin are markedly raised in affected animals (Hamilton et al 1974).

Histological examination of affected muscles reveals a wide range of changes including marked fibre-size variation, internal nuclei (up to 15%), fibre splitting, degeneration, including hyaline change and necrosis, increase in endomysial and perimysial connective tissue and attempts at regeneration (Hegreberg et al 1974). Both fibre types I and II are involved (Hamilton et al 1974).

Although several of these changes are features of dystrophy in man and other animals, the histology of mink muscular dystrophy does differ from that in other species in several respects. In contrast to the myopathy of the Syrian hamster, perinuclear halos and severe myonecrosis have not been reported; there is no evidence of the long chains of central nuclei which are a feature of murine muscular dystrophy and no reports of the vacuolation, fat deposition or ringed fibres characteristic of chicken dystrophy.

No major changes have been noted in either the central or peripheral nervous system (Hegreberg et al 1974). A further point of difference from Duchenne dystrophy of man is the slower onset and more gradual progression. However, it has been suggested that the course of the condition does resemble the limb-girdle, facioscapulo-humeral and childhood autosomal recessive dystrophies (Hegreberg 1979) and may therefore provide an animal model of this group of dystrophies.

Muscular dystrophy in the dog is rare. Isolated cases of progressive muscular dystrophy in adult dogs have been recorded (Innes 1951, Meier 1958, Whitney 1958, Funkquist et al 1980). Chrisman (1982) reported signs consistent with muscular dystrophy in a litter of Old English sheepdog puppies. It has been suggested that the sex-linked inherited degenerative myopathy of Golden retrievers (de Lahunta 1983) and Irish terriers (Wentink et al 1972) may represent a canine condition analogous to Duchenne dystrophy in man (Kornegay 1984).

In both breeds only males are affected, with signs developing at about six to eight weeks of age. Affected puppies show a stiff gait, difficulty in swallowing, enlargement of the tongue and atrophy of skeletal musculature. Hypertrophy of some muscle groups has been observed. Tone is increased in affected muscles and on electromyography bizarre high-frequency discharges are recorded. Serum enzymes of muscle origin are markedly elevated.

Histological features of affected muscles include fibre-calibre variation, areas of extensive necrosis with phagocytosis and calcification together with evidence of regenerative change. Ultrastructural examination of material from the Irish terriers showed abnormalities in mitochondria which were later confirmed by biochemical studies (Wentink et al 1974b, see p. 932).

Cardiac involvement has not been reported as a feature of the degenerative myopathy in either the Golden retriever or Irish terrier. However, persistent atrial standstill associated with a muscular dystrophy-like condition has been observed in the English springer spaniel. In some cases, atrial myocarditis was reported, in other affected animals there was evidence of an associated facioscapulohumeral type of muscular dystrophy (Bonagura & O'Grady 1983, Tilley 1985). Atrial standstill has been described in man in association with various forms of muscular dystrophy, particularly facioscapulohumeral. This newly described condition of the dog may therefore prove to be of comparative interest.

Myotonia in animals

Myotonia is characterised by the continued active contraction of skeletal muscle which persists after voluntary effort, or stimulation, has ceased (Ch. 14 and 16). Myotonia has been reported in several animal species (see Table 28.3) and may, as in man, be seen alone or as part of a more complex disorder. In the account which follows, most emphasis is placed on those conditions which provide useful models of myotonia in man.

Myotonia in the goat. The myotonic goat represents the earliest known animal model of an inherited skeletal muscle disorder of man. All myotonic goats are descended from a strain which first appeared in central Tennessee around 1880 and evidence from breeding studies suggests that the condition is inherited as an autosomal dominant trait with the variability of phenotype which suggests incomplete penetrance (Atkinson et al 1981, Atkinson & Le Quire 1985). Affected animals show no stiffness and no abnormal response to percussion during the first 14 days of life, although it is possible to demonstrate electromyographic abnormalities in utero and in newborn kids (Bryant 1979). Onset of signs therefore occurs after two weeks of age and varies in severity between individuals from day to day (Bryant et al 1968).

Attacks may be provoked by startling affected animals, whereupon the anxiety and sudden initial movement to escape result in stiffness. In the most severely affected animals the stiffness may be so profound that the goat falls to the ground, with limbs abducted and extended and the neck and back held in a position of opisthotonos. The diaphragm may become fixed causing cessation of respiration, but consciousness is not lost and in less than a minute the animal is able to regain its feet. There are no reports of death due to respiratory dysfunction and the life span of affected animals is not shortened.

In mildly affected individuals the only detectable sign may be stiffness of gait involving the hindlimbs. Muscular stiffness is alleviated by exercise and by water deprivation, and disappears in affected pregnant females around the time of parturition. Repeated attempts to precipitate an attack also result in progressively milder symptoms (the 'warm-up' phenomenon). Conversely, exposure to cold markedly worsens the severity of the signs (Atkinson & Le Quire 1985).

Mechanical percussion of affected muscles produces a local area of contraction, the so-called 'percussion dimple'. Electromyographically, the features of myotonia in the goat are identical to those seen in patients with myotonia congenita and consist of high-frequency repetitive discharges which persist following administration of curare.

Histological examination of skeletal muscle reveals only mild changes, which may include hypertrophy of muscle fibres and an increase in central nuclei. Ultrastructural changes include proliferation of sarcotubular elements, increased density of T tubules and degenerative changes in the mitochondria (Atkinson & Le Quire 1985).

There are striking similarities in clinical signs, electromyographic features and muscle pathology between myotonia in the goat and the dominantly inherited (Thomsen's) type of myotonia congenita in man (Atkinson & Le Quire 1985). This has led to the use of the myotonic goat as an animal model where its principal value has been in investigation of the underlying electrophysiological defects in myotonic muscle and in examination of other aspects of excitation–contraction coupling. It has been shown that the major membrane defect in muscle fibres from affected goats is a reduction in chloride conductance (Bryant 1979), due to a decrease in the number of chloride channels present. It now seems likely that the same pathophysiological mechanism exists in the Thomsen type of congenital myotonia but that different defects may exist in the Becker (recessive) type and in other myotonic syndromes in man and animals (Rüdel & Lehmann-Horn 1985).

Myotonia in the dog.

Chow Chow. Griffiths & Duncan (1973) reported myotonia in four dogs, one of which was a five-month-old Chow Chow. Since that report, a congenital form of canine myotonia has been shown to exist in this breed and cases have been reported in Britain, Holland, New Zealand and Australia (Griffiths & Duncan 1973, Wentink et al 1974a, Jones et al 1977, Farrow & Malik 1981 respectively).

Affected dogs show signs of stiffness and abnormal gait from two to three months of age. Affected muscles are hypertrophied and may dimple on percussion. Electromyography reveals characteristic myotonic discharges.

Strong circumstantial evidence points to a familial or inherited aetiology but this has not yet been proved conclusively. It is of interest to speculate that Chow Chows, which were originally bred for meat, may have been selected over the

Table 28.3 Myotonic syndromes in animals

Species	Breed	Inheritance	Clinical Features	EMG	Pathology (muscle)	Mechanism	Notes	References
(A) CONGENITAL MYOTONIA								
G	All from a strain originating in central Tennessee	A D (incomplete penetrance)	Muscular stiffness. Worsened by cold. Improved with exercise. Percussion dimple. Variable severity. Lifespan normal	Myotonic discharges	Minimal changes on light microscopy. EM: proliferation & dilatation of sarcotubular elements. Mitochondrial degeneration	↓ chloride conductance. Inability of SR to regulate calcium	Clinically identical to M. congenita in man. Widely used animal model in physiol/biochem. studies of myotonia	Bryant 1979 Atkinson & Le Quire 1985
H	Reported in several breeds	Unknown	Stiff gait. Worsened by cold. Percussion dimple. Outcome variable	Myotonic discharges	CCV. Central nuclei. Some degeneration and necrosis. May be ↑ Type I and ↓ Type II fibres	No evidence of abnormal chloride conductance	—	Steinberg & Botelho 1962 Farnbach 1982 Ronéus et al 1983
D	Chow Chow	F	Stiff gait. Improved with exercise. Percussion dimple. Worsened by cold	Myotonic discharges	Variable. Mild to moderate CCV. Myocyte hypertrophy. Focal necrotic fibres. Int nuc & chains of nuclei	not reported	Seen in UK Holland N. Zealand Australia	Griffiths & Duncan 1973 Wentink et al 1974a Jones et al 1977 Farrow & Malik 1981
D	Stafford-shire terrier	F	Stiff gait. Improved with exercise. Secondary skeletal abnormalities. Percussion dimple	Myotonic discharges	Overall increase in type IIA fibres	not reported	Seen in USA	Shires et al 1983
(B) MYOTONIA–LIKE SYNDROMES								
D	Rhodesian Ridgeback	One case	Normal gait. Dysphagia. Percussion dimple. Progressive wasting.	Myotonic BHFDs which ↓ slowly in amplitude	↓ CCV. Int nuc. Connective tissue. Focal necrosis, phagocytosis. Fibre splitting	—	Resembles dystrophia myotonica	Simpson & Braund 1985

	Breed	Inheritance	Clinical signs	EMG	Histopathology	Aetiology	References
D	Irish terrier	XR	Stiffness. ↑ Muscle tone. Muscle atrophy. No dimpling ↑ CK Large tongue	Myotonia-like discharges	CCV. Degeneration. Phagocytosis. Calcification of fibres. Cellular infiltration Abnormal mitochondria	—	Wentink et al 1974b
D	Golden retriever	XR	Stilted gait. Muscle atrophy & hypertrophy. Large tongue. CK	BHFD pseudomyotonic (no waxing/waning)	Necrosis, mineralisation. Regenerating clusters. Some int nuclei	—	Kornegay 1984
D	Labrador retriever	AR	Stilted gait. ↓ muscle tone. Worse on exercise. Worse in cold weather. No percussion dimple	BHFD pseudomyotonic	Variable, includes: Small group atrophy, Type II fibre deficiency, Int nuc, fibre splitting, necrosis, regeneration	—	Kramer et al 1976 McKerrell et al 1984
O	Friesland	One calf	—	Abnormal action potentials		—	Van Niekerk & Jaros 1970
S	Shropshire	F(?)	Fall over when startled. Stiff, waddling gait. Double muscled	Myotonia-like	Hypertrophy & degeneration	—	Rings et al 1976

These 2 conditions thought to be identical. Some similarity to Duchenne dystrophy

(See inherited myopathies Table 28.2)

(See type II fibre def. Table 28.2)

Resembles Thomsen's myotonia

(C) ACQUIRED MYOTONIA

	Breed	Inheritance	Clinical signs	EMG	Histopathology	Aetiology	References
D	Many breeds	None. Associated with Cushing's disease	Stiffness. Muscle hypertrophy + signs of Cushing's disease	Pseudomyotonic and myotonic	Varied, includes group atrophy, Int nuc, target fibres, necrosis	Unknown ? neurogenic	Duncan et al 1977 Greene et al 1979

For key to abbreviations see foot of Table 28.2

years for an increased volume of skeletal muscle. A well-muscled appearance and stilted gait are regarded as desirable characteristics in this breed.

Myotonia in the Chow resembles myotonia congenita (Thomsen's disease) of man in both clinical and electrophysiologic features. However, whereas in man serum CK activities usually fall within the normal range, the serum CK of affected dogs is frequently elevated (Jones et al 1977). Differences also exist in the pathology of the skeletal muscle. In man the changes are generally mild with some fibre hypertrophy and occasional internal nuclei (Swash & Schwartz 1984). In contrast, affected dogs show a wide variation in pathological features ranging from very mild to severe myopathic changes. Changes tend to be more severe in older dogs, with biopsies showing greatly increased numbers of central nuclei (Duncan & Griffiths 1983).

Affected dogs show no evidence of abnormalities in other systems and, even when severe, the muscle histology does not closely resemble that of human myotonic dystrophy. It is probably not justifiable to regard this condition as a model of any human disorder although it seems to resemble Thomsen's disease most closely.

Staffordshire terrier. Congenital canine myotonia has also been recognised in the Staffordshire terrier in the USA (Shires et al 1983).

Affected dogs first show signs of stiffness at between eight and 16 weeks of age. Orthopaedic injuries and skeletal deformities may arise due to abnormal stresses placed on the developing skeleton. As the animals mature they develop marked hypertrophy of skeletal muscle, stiffness which decreases with exercise and respiratory stridor. Percussion of skeletal muscle, or the tongue, gives rise to a myotonic dimple and electromyography reveals myotonic high-frequency discharges.

Histologically, no myopathic or neurogenic features have been reported in muscle from affected dogs, but an overall increase in the percentage of type IIA fibres was noted (Shires et al 1983). Breeding studies have indicated that although the condition is genetically determined it is not inherited as a simple dominant or recessive trait (Nafe & Shires 1984). Again, it is of interest that the Staffordshire terrier has been

bred for a heavily muscled appearance, and hence this may have led to the inadvertent selection of myotonia in this breed.

Others. Individual cases of myotonia have been described in various other breeds including the West Highland White terrier (Giffiths & Duncan 1973), Samoyed, Dachshund (Cardinet & Holliday 1979). Labrador retriever (Duncan & Griffiths 1983) and the Rhodesian Ridgeback (Simpson & Braund 1985). Jones & Johnstone (1982) described an unusual condition in a nine-month-old Cavalier King Charles spaniel which could not withdraw the tongue and had difficulty in eating and drinking. Myotonic discharges and percussion dimpling were demonstrated in the tongue, but convincing morphological lesions were not found in the skeletal musculature.

In addition myotonic and myotonia-like discharges have been recorded during electromyographic (EMG) examination of muscles of dogs with inherited myopathies such as the X-linked degenerative myopathy of Irish terriers and Golden retrievers (see Wentink et al 1972, Kornegay 1984) and Labrador retrievers with type II fibre deficiency (Kramer et al 1976). These findings may equate with the pseudomyotonic discharges well known to occur in human dystrophies, spinal muscular atrophy and metabolic myopathies.

An acquired form of myotonia may also be seen in dogs with hyperadrenocorticism (Duncan et al 1977, Greene et al 1979). Affected dogs show muscle stiffness, hypertrophy and myotonic discharges in the EMG. In some cases a percussion dimple may be elicited. In addition, signs characteristic of canine Cushing's disease are present.

Myotonia in the horse. Steinberg & Botelho (1962) described a case of myotonia in a thoroughbred filly. Since then there have been sporadic reports of myotonia in the horse (Farnbach 1982, Ronéus et al 1983).

The signs of myotonia and its progression in the horse are variable. Age of onset ranges from three weeks to several months and the first signs are usually lameness associated with stiffness and hypertrophy of affected muscles. In most cases the abnormalities appear most prominent in the hind-quarters with the head, neck and forelimbs apparently unaffected. Percussion of skeletal muscle results in dimpling and on electromyographic examination characteristic myotonic discharges are recorded.

Histological examination of affected muscle has shown fibre-size variation, increased numbers of central nuclei and evidence of degeneration and necrosis. Ronéus et al (1983) reported an increase in the proportion of type I fibres and a decrease in type II fibres.

In those animals in which membrane chloride conductance has been examined, no abnormality was detected and there is so far insufficient evidence available regarding inheritance to suggest that this condition is analogous to any of the congenital forms of myotonia seen in man or other species.

Myotonia in sheep. A myotonia-like condition in Shropshire lambs was described by Rings et al (1976). The lambs were normal at birth but developed signs of myopathy at three months of age when they appeared double muscled and had a waddling gait. When startled they fell into lateral recumbency with the limbs rigidly extended.

Both plasma CK and lactate dehydrogenase activities (LDH) were raised and EMG of skeletal muscles revealed possible myotonic discharges. At necropsy, enlargement of the diaphragm, heart and skeletal muscles was found and there was histological evidence of both hypertrophy and hyperplasia of muscle fibres and possibly some degenerative change. No breeding records were available.

Mitochondrial myopathies

Various myopathic conditions have been described in man, in which mitochondrial abnormalities occur. These may include alterations in mitochondrial structure and/or function, and may be primary or secondary features of the disease (see Ch. 5, 8, 20 and 25).

In the veterinary literature there have been reports of similar conditions in animals. Maltin et al (1983a) described histochemical and ultrastructural abnormalities in mitochondria of cardiac and skeletal muscle in vitamin B_{12}-deficient sheep and there have been sporadic reports of inherited myopathies associated with abnormal mitochondria in the dog.

Mitochondrial myopathies in dogs. In 1979, a mitochondrial myopathy associated with a potentially fatal acidosis was described in the Clumber spaniel (Herrtage & Houlton 1979). Affected puppies were eager to exercise but tired rapidly, sinking into sternal recumbency within 100 m. After 10–15 min they were able to rise but remained depressed for up to an hour after collapsing. During the period of collapse, excessive panting and pronounced tachycardia were observed. Arterial blood samples revealed a severe post-exercise acidosis with levels of lactate and pyruvate dramatically increased. Subsequent sampling showed that resting levels were higher in affected than in normal dogs. No abnormal muscle pathology was reported but the mitochondria were unable to oxidise pyruvate, due to an abnormality in function of the pyruvate dehydrogenase complex.

Although there is strong circumstantial evidence to indicate that this condition may be inherited, it has not been demonstrated conclusively. However, the condition has more recently been recognised in the Sussex spaniel (Houlton & Herrtage 1980), a breed known to have been interbred with the Clumber in the past. Other canine myopathies have been reported in which morphological changes were evident in the mitochondria.

Through the courtesy of Dr N. Edington of the Royal Veterinary College, London, one of us (RB) examined a hitherto undescribed myopathy in a West Highland terrier. Clinical signs were muscle atrophy, progressive weakness, muscle tremors and ataxia. In this case the histological lesions were striking and included marked variation in fibre diameter, replacement of muscle by fat, proliferation of capillaries and nerve fibres and the presence of densely stained central areas in many muscle cells (Fig. 28.9). These had the appearance of unstructured central cores and were particularly well demonstrated by trichrome and Heidenhain's haematoxylin stains. Ultrastructurally these areas consisted of disarrayed actin and myosin filaments

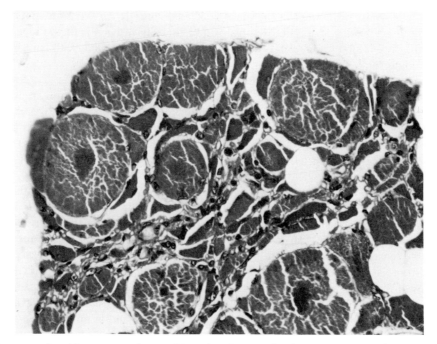

Fig. 28.9 Canine myopathy with unstructured cores. *M. semimembranosus* showing severe atrophy of muscle cells, increase in intrafascicular fat cells and central cores in some of the larger muscle cells. Picro-Mallory, ×275 (section supplied by courtesy of Dr N. Edington)

and Z-disc material. The mitochondria in this case contained bar-like inclusions.

Mitochondrial abnormalities were also demonstrated in the muscle of Irish terriers with degenerative X-linked myopathy (Wentink et al 1972) (see p. 926). Ultrastructural abnormalities were described in the mitochondria and it was shown that although they appeared to have normal oxidative phosphorylation they lacked respiratory control (loosely coupled mitochondria) (Wentink et al 1974b).

Hereditary type II fibre deficiency in the Labrador retriever

This condition was first reported by Kramer et al (1976). Since then there have been further reports of a clinically identical disease in America (Simpson et al 1982, Hoskins & Root 1983) and Great Britain (McKerrell et al 1984), and it has been shown to be inherited as an autosomal recessive trait (Kramer et al 1981).

Onset of signs generally occurs between three and six months of age. Affected puppies show a stiff, stilted gait, decreased exercise tolerance and marked atrophy of skeletal muscle which is most pronounced in the proximal limb musculature and in the muscles of the head. Affected muscles are hypotonic. Patellar and triceps jerks are generally reduced or absent.

Progression of the condition is slow and in many cases the clinical signs appear to stabilise at about one year of age although subsequent exacerbations may occur, usually as a result of exposure to cold or concurrent illness.

Electromyographic examinations have revealed the presence of spontaneous activity including fibrillation potentials, positive sharp waves and bizarre high-frequency discharges. These high-frequency discharges do not wax or wane and may be also referred to as pseudomyotonic. There is no evidence of a myotonic dimple on percussion of affected muscles.

Despite the similarity of the clinical signs in the various reports, muscle pathology has been varied. In their initial description Kramer et al (1976) described a deficiency of type II fibres in affected muscles together with variation in fibre diameter and increased amounts of fibrous connective tissue. It is possible therefore that this condition may be similar to fibre-type disproportion in humans. However, type II fibre deficiency has not been a feature in all subsequent reports of the condition (Simpson et al 1982, McKerrell et al 1984).

Additional changes which may be seen include scattered angular atrophic fibres of both fibre types, small and large group atrophy, increased numbers of internal nuclei, fibre splitting, evidence of necrosis and regeneration and occasional fibre-type grouping.

The features therefore are not entirely typical of a myopathy. Some are more suggestive of neurogenic atrophy. Nevertheless, no abnormalities have been demonstrated in either the central or peripheral nervous systems.

Labrador retriever 'myopathy' shares many clinical and histological features with some forms of limb girdle dystrophy in man and with muscular dystrophy of mink. It is also clinically similar to benign spinal muscular atrophy. As the underlying pathophysiology of this condition is not yet clear, it illustrates the difficulty, which may exist in animals as in man, in distinguishing between the milder dystrophies and more benign neurogenic disorders.

MYOPATHY DUE TO TRANSITORY DEFECTS OF CELL METABOLISM

The definition of this section is imprecise. Because of the dynamic nature of the skeletal myocyte, stresses placed upon it may have different effects in different circumstances. Training to develop either aerobic or anaerobic capacity in the muscle cells for sporting purposes enables it to resist some stresses and to become more vulnerable to others. The protection provided by training is reversible, as is susceptibility. The muscular stiffness which may follow over-exertion in the human after the first tennis match of the season is equivalent to that in animals which follows turn out to pasture in the spring after a long period of winter housing (Anderson et al 1977). The clinical, biochemical and pathological changes which do occur are usually mild and transitory.

The popularity of Greyhound and Thoroughbred racing, and other equine riding pursuits have stimulated some to analyse the changes that occur in muscle and other tissue at the cellular level following exertional events. As a result of such studies, which include analysis of muscle fibre-type proportion and capacity for aerobic/anaerobic metabolism, animals can be more suitably matched to events and trained in appropriate ways to perform at an optimal level.

Not only does such knowledge benefit man but it also improves the welfare of the participating animals. Comparable investigations including physiological studies in man have revolutionised athletic training schedules. Selection of individuals for specific events rather than acting on the whim of the individual has secured better and better performances at the highest levels of competition. This knowledge, apart from benefiting leisure pursuits, has a spin-off in improving the quality of life of those individuals unfortunate enough to be suffering from some of the crippling neuro-muscular diseases. It is beyond the scope of this section to say more, but the physiology and pathophysiology of muscle is an important field of study which may lead to improved control of some of these depressing illnesses.

It is important for medical practitioners and veterinarians to appreciate the dynamic nature of muscle and also to improve the knowledge possessed by the population at large to ensure that sudden changes in work pattern and load on muscles are avoided. These include changes in physical work, postural strain (e.g. unaccustomed standing for long periods) or exposure to cold. Training for these activities may reduce some of the exertional myopathies which are currently commonplace. For further information with regard to man see Edwards (1979), Prince et al (1981), Staron et al (1981, 1984), Warhol et al (1985) and in animals Gunn (1975), Guy & Snow (1977, 1981), Snow & Guy (1980), Taylor & Brassard (1981), Snow et al (1981, 1982b).

Some exertional myopathies, because their aetiology is obscure, are covered in a later section of this chapter (see Table 28.8). Transport stress is another common insult to the well-being of animals, which has effects on skeletal and cardiac muscle. For a review see Hails (1978).

Table 28.4 Myopathy due to transitory defects of cell metabolism (Bradley & Fell 1981, Hulland 1985)

Species	Condition	Breed/Type	Clinical features	Pathology
H O	(a) PARALYTIC MYOGLOBINURIA (Azoturia)	(a) Draft type mainly	(a) Severe. Typically occurs very soon after exercise or work following a period of 2–5 days rest. Symptoms: collapse, sweating, pain, muscular weakness myoglobinuria and death	(a,b) Skeletal myodegeneration (especially type II cells), principally of gluteal and lumbar muscles (a) Haemoglobinuric nephrosis ± myocardial necrosis. Myonecrosis is probably due to rapid lactic acid production and failure to metabolise or remove (Fig. 28.10)
H D	(b) TYING-UP (Set fast)	(b) Thoroughbred and riding horses. Racing greyhound	(b) Mild but recurrent with recovery. Symptoms: muscular stiffness, pain. Gluteal and lumbar muscles hard. Reversible. Relates to march haemoglobinuria in man	
O	EXERCISE MYOPATHY	Yearling cattle	Occurs irrespective of vitamin E/selenium status on the day following turn out to pasture. Transient plasma CK rise. Very mild or non-detectable postural or locomotor deficits	Reversible myodegeneration of distal flexor muscles of fore limbs
P	PORCINE STRESS SYNDROME (PSS)	Especially Pietrain, Landrace and Poland China at slaughter weight	A naturally-occurring condition resulting in sudden death precipitated by stress. Sudden collapse resultant on metabolic acidosis with pyrexia, dyspnoea and muscular rigidity	In PSS muscles especially. Mm longissimus and semitendinosus are pale soft and exudative (PSE). Separation of fibres by oedema, fluid contraction bands and floccular change (Fig. 28.11)
P	BACK MUSCLE NECROSIS	Stress susceptible pigs at slaughter weight	A specific, usually non-lethal form of PSS in which either one or both longissimus muscles and Mm multifidi are affected. Symptoms: pain, back swelling and kinking with convexity towards affected side — 'banana krankheit'	Acute lesions are identical with those in PSS but muscle haemorrhage is also a feature. Chronic cases show muscle atrophy, fibrosis and a degree of repair (Fig. 28.12)

For key to abbreviations see foot of Table 28.2

Important and fairly clearly defined animal myopathies attributable to transitory defects of cell metabolism are listed in Table 28.4. Those affecting the draught horse (Fig. 28.10) or ox are now of less importance than formerly, because of the decline in the use of these animals in developed countries. The increase in popularity of riding in all its forms has, however, resulted in the mild form of paralytic myoglobinuria ('tying up') becoming more frequent. This condition is clinically similar to 'March myoglobinuria' (Boot Camp disease) of untrained army recruits when stressed by a long march, while carrying unaccustomed loads in inclement weather. To a considerable extent these diseases are avoidable.

Porcine stress syndrome

Of greater significance economically has been the evolution of the porcine stress syndrome (PSS) as rapid genetic improvement in muscularity (at the expense of fat) has been achieved. Such pigs may be regarded as 'double muscled' and the phenotypic expression of the gene(s) involved is to reduce fat and increase muscle bulk (especially of ham, back and shoulder) by myocyte hyperplasia;

additionally, the cell-type proportion of type II cells in hypertrophied muscles is increased. In contrast to the myopathies previously discussed in this section, susceptibility to the PSS is inherited. The susceptibility is, however, converted to overt disease by environmental stresses such as transportation, excitement or exposure to high environmental temperature and usually results in sudden death.

There are three principal manifestations of PSS, two of commercial importance and one important as a model for study of human malignant hyperpyrexia. The first is sudden death during transport or in lairage before slaughter. The second is the occurrence of poor-quality pale, soft and exudative (PSE) meat in stress-susceptible (SS) animals that survive to the point of slaughter. The main reason for this second phenomenon is a very rapid postmortem glycolysis in the muscle which reduces the pH to below pH 6.0 within 45 min of death while the carcase temperature is still high. This results in denaturation of sarcoplasmic and myofibrillar proteins, their precipitation on the structural components of the muscle cell and a loss of water-binding capacity. This leads to drip, loss of carcase weight and, in some

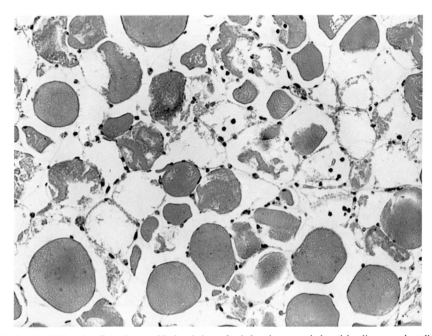

Fig. 28.10 Paralytic myoglobinuria of the horse. *M. longissimus dorsi* showing rounded and hyaline muscle cells, floccular change, empty endomysial tubes and a minimal infiltration of inflammatory cells. H & E, ×125

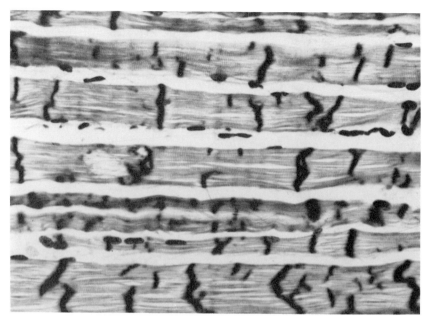

Fig. 28.11 Porcine stress syndrome. *M. longissimus dorsi* of a pig dying as a result of stress and showing extensive contraction band necrosis. Heidenhain's iron haematoxylin, ×275

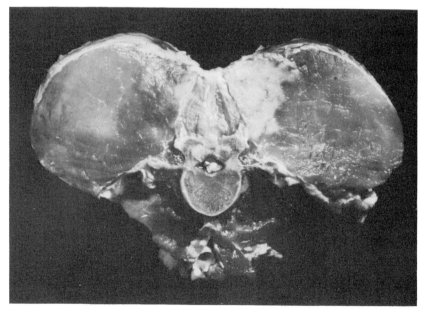

Fig. 28.12 Acute back-muscle necrosis. Section through the back of a pig at the level of the last rib showing pale areas of necrosis in *Mm. longissimus dorsi* and *multifidi*

instances, economic loss. The muscles particularly exhibiting the PSE appearance are those with high proportions of type II cells such as the Mm *longissimus* and *semitendinosus*.

The third manifestation is malignant hyperpyrexia which occurs when SS pigs are exposed to depolarising agents such as succinylcholine or the anaesthetic halothane. This condition is equivalent to the human condition of the same name. Halothane sensitivity in pigs is, however, largely inherited as an autosomal recessive trait controlled by a single gene ('n') (Carden et al 1983). The equivalent normal gene is 'N'. Thus heterozygotes are carriers (Nn) and should not react to halothane. Unfortunately varying proportions of Nn pigs (depending on breed) do react positively, making their detection by this means unreliable and thus gene elimination becomes impossible (Webb et al 1985)

General anaesthesia of pigs is less frequently performed than in humans since the economic costs of surgery exceed the value of the patient in all but valuable breeding stock. However, halothane is used in pigs around eight weeks of age to test for halothane sensitivity, exposure being for three minutes (Webb & Jordan 1978). Pigs developing rigidity of the hind limb muscles within three minutes of the exposure period are scored as halothane positive or stress susceptible (SS). Once muscular rigidity is detected, the halothane is stopped to avoid progression to fatal malignant hyperthermia (hyperpyrexia) (Gronert 1980). The purpose of this testing is to detect SS pigs at an early age so that decisions can be made in breeding programmes. It is also used experimentally in research strategies for the control of the gene in national pig herds. Seeler et al (1983) consider that a more sensitive test for use in pigs negative after their standard five minutes (3 min induction + 2 min maintenance) test is to continue halothane for a further three minutes and also to administer succinylcholine i.v.

Sensitivity to halothane is age related, an increasing proportion of known nn pigs becoming positive to the test from three to nine weeks of age. It is also breed related: most strains of Duroc and Large White are virtually 100% resistant and Belgian Pietrain and Landrace over 80% sensitive, with other Landrace strains being variably intermediate. Recent detection of halothane-positive Large White pigs led Webb et al (1985) to hypothesise that in this breed a natural suppressor mechanism might operate in the presence of the gene, the latter being progressively uncovered by continued selection for lean meat.

Currently, because of the incomplete detection of all heterozygotes by halothane testing, the only certain method of eliminating the gene is by test mating to positive nn homozygotes. This is very expensive, six litters being required. Other potentially useful methods (Webb et al 1985) include blood typing, CK activity measurement after a standard stress (higher in nn pigs), biochemical analysis of muscle biopsy (serious disadvantages), mitochondrial calcium efflux measurement (Cheah et al 1984), erythrocyte fragility testing and assessment of sensitivity to succinylcholine.

Future developments include detection of changes in the DNA in the region of the gene on the chromosome (Webb et al 1985) using restriction endonucleases and similar techniques. The restriction fragment length polymorphisms (RFLPs) (Botstein et al 1980) hold promise in this field. Another development will be in the separation of the beneficial and harmful effects of the gene and, determining whether such effects are due to one or several adjacent genes. It may be that the effects of harmful genes could be modified.

Pre-existing myopathy in unstressed SS pigs akin to that described for humans has not been described. Muir (1970), Venable (1973) and Bradley & Wells (1978) have recorded a non-specific focal myopathy (see Fig. 28.13) but this is of little diagnostic value. Swatland & Cassens (1972) demonstrated differences in the terminal innervation of skeletal muscle from SS and stress-resistant (SR) pigs.

Palmer et al (1977) studied Mm biceps femoris and longissimus from halothane-negative and -positive pigs and found a higher proportion of supercontracted myocytes in the latter. The M. longissimus also contained a larger number of internal nuclei. In humans the presence of fibre-calibre variation and much higher proportions of internal nuclei appear to be more consistently found (Harriman et al 1978).

In SS pigs dying from stress the lesions are consistent but dependent upon the time elapsing from death to necropsy and fixation. If necropsy is delayed the muscle is pale, soft and exudative, particularly in the normally 'white' muscles. For results of histological examination of acutely affected muscle see Table 28.4 and Fig. 28.11.

If death is delayed, myodegenerative changes including phagocytosis occur (Fig. 28.14). In the occasional animal that recovers (e.g. after cooling

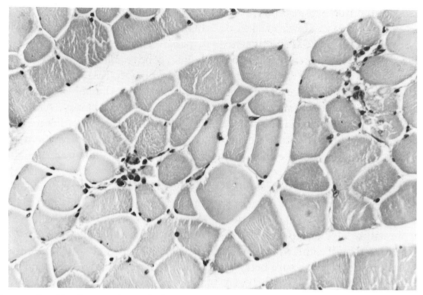

Fig. 28.13 Focal myopathy. Myodegeneration and phagocytosis occur focally within 2 fascicles. H & E, ×125

by immersion in cold water), regeneration occurs with possible fibrosis depending on the severity of the muscle damage. These changes are similar to those occuring in MH in man (Weitz & Hübner 1980). Bergmann (1974, 1975a,b), Wesemeier (1974) and Wesemeier & Bergmann (1972) have described the muscle ultrastructure in PSE meat. Johannsen et al (1982) have made similar studies in unstressed SS and SR pigs and in such pigs after movement over 40 m and electric anaesthesia. Mitochondrial alterations were described in each case after stress.

For accounts of the biochemical events occurring at the cellular level in MH/PSS see Cheah & Cheah (1981a,b) and Meijer (1983). For discussion of myocardial involvement in this syndrome see Bradley & Fell (1981), Johansson & Jönsson (1977) and Jönnson et al (1984).

Back muscle necrosis of pigs may be regarded as a specific clinical manifestation of the PSS which is not usually fatal in the short term. It is well recognised on the European mainland and more recently in Britain. The clinical and pathological features are described by Bradley et al (1979).

Clinical signs occur suddenly: pigs are reluctant to rise and have bi- or unilateral swellings in the back; skin sensation is lost over the affected areas. In severe non-fatal cases, repair of the muscles leads to atrophy giving a dished appearance to the affected area; in unilateral cases the lateral kink of the back that develops has given rise to the name 'Banana krankheit'.

Gross lesions consistently occur in the Mm *longissimus dorsi* and *multifidi* (Fig. 28.12) and in acute cases consist of haemorrhages between muscle fascicles and variable muscle pallor. The histological features are as for PSS (qv) but haemorrhage is a frequent complication in the acute phase.

Post–anaesthetic myonecrosis in horses

Equine post–anaesthetic forelimb lameness is a well recognised sequel in horses maintained in lateral recumbency for extended periods (>2 hours). The muscles in contact with the supporting surface are most vulnerable and include Mm *masseter, triceps, deltoid, pectoral*, lateral thigh and flank. If restrained in dorsal recumbency, the *gluteal* and back muscles are affected. Muscles become hard, hot, painful and swollen. Plasma CK activity is increased and myoglobinuria, associated with acute skeletal myodegeneration, may occur. Mild cases recover spontaneously in a few days. The more affected animal may suffer severe pain, develop further self-inflicted injury or suffer irreversible muscle damage leading to atrophy and fibrosis, so that the horse has to be put down humanely. Sometimes renal failure occurs and is associated with tubular nephrosis and glomerular capillary thrombosis.

For lengthy surgery in the horse, a variety of pre-medicants are used followed by inhalation anaesthesia, usually with halothane. The myonecrosis produced is characterised by oedema, haemorrhage, hyaline and floccular change, mineralisation and also thrombosis and fibrinoid necrosis of blood vessels (Friend 1981). Factors which may be involved in inducing the condition include the weight and fitness of the animal, the patient position, the nature of the padding of the supporting surface, the duration of the procedure and the nature of the drugs and anaesthetic used (Lindsay et al 1980).

Experimental results suggest an ischaemic basis for the lesions. Lindsay et al (1980) recorded intracompartmental muscle pressures in upper and lower forelimb muscles during prolonged anaesthesia of horses held in lateral recumbency. They found increased haematocrit, plasma potassium blood lactate and serum inorganic phosphate and reduced plasma chloride values; intra-compartmental pressures were highest in the lower limb muscles. They concluded that local hypoxia caused by restricted local capillary blood flow was implicated in the aetiology: thus, this may be primarily a 'Compartmental syndrome' condition the basis of which is ischaemic (see Hulland 1985 for further information).

A generalised bilaterally symmetrical post-anaesthetic myopathy has also been reported in horses (Anderson 1983). This is essentially similar but differs in two respects. First, the contralateral (in lateral recumbency) or opposing (in dorsal recumbency) muscles not in contact with the supporting surface are equally affected. Secondly, muscles from such patients demonstrate increased sensitivity to caffeine and in vitro halothane. This is perhaps more specifically a halothane sensitivity and occurs when the depth of anaesthesia is unstable; it is accompanied also by cardiovascular depression, hyperpyrexia, muscle rigidity, tremors and pain.

MYODEGENERATION DUE TO NUTRITIONAL DEFICIENCIES

This is probably the most economically important group of myopathies affecting farm animals world wide. Within the group the most important are those resulting from nutritional deficiencies of selenium and vitamin E and/or excesses of dietary polyunsaturated fatty acids (PUFA). Apart from the default in nutrition, other environmental factors are often involved in precipitating clinical disease: these include turning ruminants out to pasture or suddenly increasing the exercise of untrained animals.

Death frequently results either from myocardial necrosis or from widespread skeletal myodegeneration. In animals myopathies due to nutritional deficiency are both preventable and treatable but, despite the availability of this knowledge, the diseases continue to recur in different guises as new management and nutritional systems are developed. Table 28.5 lists myodegenerations of animals due to nutritional deficiencies. Expanded accounts were given in the last edition of this book and the essential histological features of nutritional myodegeneration are shown in Fig. 28.14. There are no direct human counterparts to this group of myopathies. However, Keshan disease is described briefly below because of its relationship to selenium-responsive disease of animals.

Keshan disease (Chen et al 1980)

This is an endemic cardiomyopathy first recognised in Keshan County of north-east China in 1935 (Zhu 1982). Since then, foci of disease have occurred in mountainous areas in a belt-like zone of the country from north-east to south-west. Children under 15 and women of childbearing age are affected. The main, but probably not the only, factor involved in the aetiology is dietary selenium deficiency related to soil and crop selenium deficiency. Skeletal myopathy is not reported.

If Keshan disease is specifically related to selenium deficiencies (as distinct from being selenium-responsive) and if no skeletal lesions exist, then elucidation of the mechanisms of skeletal myocyte protection would be both interesting and valuable.

Table 28.5 Nutritional myopathies of animals

Species	Age	Main muscle groups affected	Associated factors	Associated pathology
(A) DUE TO DEFICIENCIES OF VITAMIN E/SELENIUM (Bradley & Fell 1981, Hulland 1985)				
H	0–12 w	(a) Shoulder, neck, thigh (b) Masticatory and tongue	Poor nutrition	Steatitis sometimes Cardiac myodegeneration
O	0–6 m	Shoulder, proximal hind limbs. Sometimes only Mm. diaphragma/intercostales	Increasing physical activity (turning to pasture). Bad weather	Cardiac myodegeneration Hepatic/pulmonary congestion
		Proximal hind limbs especially M. gluteus medius	As above and feeding of unsupplemented propionic acid-treated grain	—
	Parturient cows	Proximal hind limbs	Parturition (muscle anoxia due to circulation failure often complicates)	Cardiac myodegeneration
S G	0–3 m (3 m — adult)	Shoulder, proximal hind limb, back, neck and respiratory muscles	Bad weather. Increased physical activity. Inadequate ewe feeding	Cardiac myodegeneration. Hepatic/pulmonary congestion
P	0–10 d	Widespread	Vitamin E deficient sow. Piglets prophylactically injected with iron-dextrose to prevent anaemia (= Iron-catalysed lipid peroxidation)	Cardiac myodegeneration
P	6–20 w	Widespread but often not grossly obvious	Feeding oxidised lipids, peas, newly harvested grain. Contaminating minerals e.g. Ag, Cu, Cd, Co, V, T, Zn. in diet	Massive hepatic necrosis (Hepatosis dietetica) May occur alone. Cardiac myodegeneration (Mulberry Heart disease) May occur alone
GP RAB	Any	Widespread	None	Cardiac myodegeneration
MIN	Any	Widespread	Oxidised dietary lipids especially fish oils	steatitis
D	—	Localised	Selenium responsive	—
WILD especially zebra, antelope, rottnest quokka, wallabies	—	Widespread	Stress of capture or confinement/release	Cardiac myodegeneration

(B) DUE TO DEFICIENCIES OF COBALT/VITAMIN B12 (Fell 1981, Maltin et al 1983a)

Species	Age	Lesions	Associated lesions	Key references
S	Adults	Ultrastructural and histochemical evidence of mitochondrial myopathy especially of M. extensor digiti longus	Enlarged and distorted hepatocyte mitochondria	

(C) DUE TO DEFICIENCIES OF ZINC

Species/Breed	Lesions	Key references
SQUIRREL MONKEY	Atrophy of tongue muscles	Barney et al 1967
S — DORSET HORN	(Experimental lambs) Parakeratosis of tongue with myodegeneration, atrophy, fibrosis. Thinning of myelin, abnormal nerve endings and degeneration of arterio-venous shunts	Mann et al 1974
R	Change in Type I and II fibre proportion in M. soleus. ↑ in intermediate ↓ in type II fibres & ↑ in lipid in M. diaphragma	Maltin et al 1983b

(D) DUE TO DEFICIENCIES OF SULPHUR CONTAINING AMINO ACIDS

Species	Clinical signs	Lesions	Key references
P	Congenital splayleg	Unknown	Cunha 1968, Ward 1978

For key to abbreviations see foot of Table 28.2

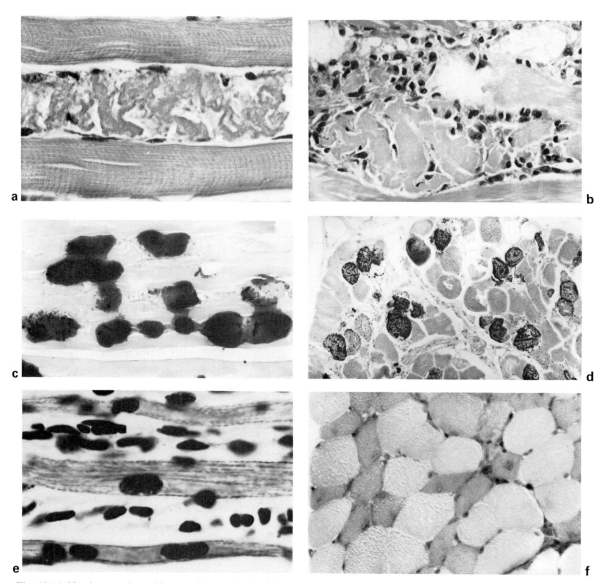

Fig. 28.14 Myodegeneration with an aetiology principally involving nutritional deficiency of vitamin E and/or selenium, but involving metabolic and non-nutritional environmental factors. a. Floccular change. H & E, ×280. b. Phagocytosis of necrotic cell contents. H & E, ×180. c. Cellular calcification. Nuclear fast red, ×70. d. Mitochondrial calcification. Notice that the distribution of necrotic cells is similar to the distribution of type I cells in normal muscle. H & E, ×70. e. Regeneration showing myotubes with central nuclei and peripheral myofibrils. Loyez's haematoxylin, ×480. f. Regeneration showing darkly staining small cells, many of which have internal nuclei. These are regenerating cells rich in RNA. Quinolic phthalocyanin, ×220

The effect of selenium intake on myocardial necrosis induced by Coxsackie B4 virus in mice (Bai et al 1982) has been studied experimentally. The heart lesions resembled those in Keshan disease and were reduced in severity by administration of selenium. This experimentally produced condition may provide a useful animal model of the human disease.

Although conditions of this kind are uncommon in man, the medical practitioner should be aware of the potential for humans to develop nutritionally-induced skeletal or cardiac myopathy. These may be expected in the nutritionally deprived or in those relying on dietary ingredients from restricted sources or from nutritional fads of the moment. Thus people relying on the locally grown food where soil selenium deficiencies exist (as in Keshan disease), those in famine areas, old people restricting their diet for economic reasons, suckling infants or those following (excessively) advice to reduce the intake of saturated fats may be inadvertently increasing the intake of PUFA to dangerous levels. Much of this is, perhaps, speculation but selenium deficiency has been implicated in the sudden infant death syndrome (cot death) (Kendeel & Ferris 1977) and the potential for development of mild reversible or even fatal myodegeneration does exist in the population at large.

TOXIC MYOPATHIES

These are of importance in local geographical areas where plants containing toxic principles are available to, and eaten by, livestock. Of particular interest are *Cassia* spp. which may occur in abundance in the pasture in some southern states of the USA: they may be consumed by yearling cattle and result in inco-ordination, prostration, myoglobinuria and death. The lesions, believed to be caused by a myotoxin, are restricted to skeletal muscle; they are myodegenerative and resemble those of myopathies responsive to selenium/vitamin E. A potential use of this plant is in the preparation of standard toxic extracts which could be of value in the study of myodegenerative processes under variable conditions of nutrition and muscle training in farm animals or, in appropriate cases, in laboratory animals.

In grazing animals, exposure to toxic plants does not always mean that these will be consumed: consumption is more likely if there is a drought and thus a deficiency of grass or other edible pasture plants. Toxicity is often related to the age of the plant, the stage of growth and the parts eaten. In some circumstances, human error may permit access of animals to toxic plant waste such as tobacco-plant stalks (Crowe & Pike 1973). The poisoning of livestock due to consumption of seleniferous plants containing either organic

selenium compounds or insoluble protein-bound selenium is well recognised in specific geographical locations, but is not a significant problem. These compounds cause so-called 'blind staggers' or 'alkali disease' respectively and result in, among other things, myocardial necrosis.

Once a deficiency state is recognised and its cause identified, it is usually not long before incidents of toxicity due to accidental prophylactic or treatment overdosage are reported: such is the case with selenium. Shortridge et al (1971) report myocardial lesions in cattle from a field incident whereas MacDonald et al (1981) experimentally found only skeletal myositis at the injection site. In pigs, skeletal myodegeneration occurs (Van Vleet et al 1974). Of some veterinary importance is the association of the antibiotic monensin with toxicity in a wide range of farm animals. Toxicity can result from frank overdosage or by a reduction in the normally rapid excretion. The latter can result from diminished hepatic detoxifying capacity due to liver disease and/or the simultaneous administration of therapeutic doses of sulphonamides in cattle (Simpson 1984), chloramphenicol in turkeys (Weisman et al 1984) or tiamulin in pigs (Stansfield & Lamont 1981). The toxic moiety variously affects skeletal and/or cardiac muscle. In the former, type I cells predominantly are affected. The pathogenesis is presumed to be related to the Na^+-selective properties of the ionophore monensin. It produces an intramyocyte influx of Na^+ and Ca^{2+} ions and this results in mitochondrial calcium overload and resultant myonecrosis. A fuller explanation is given by Van Vleet & Ferrans (1984) who also produce a useful table of toxic chemical, plant and drug-induced myonecrosis in various species, including man.

It is important that cognisance is given to the study of muscle in drug safety testing, because it has been widely neglected. It is a sensitive indicator of toxic actions on aerobic or anaerobic pathways generally and on contraction processes in particular. It would seem essential that such studies should include muscle enzyme histochemical, ultrastructural and conventional light microscopical investigation, as appropriate.

Table 28.6 lists plants and ions responsible for myotoxicity, together with the essential clinical

Table 28.6 Toxic myopathies (Bradley & Fell 1981)

Species	Name/Cause	Clinical and pathological features	Key reference
(A) DUE TO CONSUMPTION OF TOXIC PLANTS OR THEIR PRODUCTS			
O	CASSIA MYOPATHY (a) *Cassia occidentalis* (b) *Cassia obtubifolia* (Senna/coffee senna)	Cattle readily eat plant after first frosts of winter. Occurs in southern USA. Symptoms: diarrhoea, muscular weakness, ataxia, recumbency and death. Lesions; cardiac and skeletal myodegeneration	Mercer et al 1967
P	GOSSYPOL MYOTOXICITY Yellow polyphenol from cottonseed	Chronic toxicity occurs in pigs at levels >10% of diet after 1 month. Eliminated now by effective control of feed preparation	
S	HUMPY BACK *Solanum esuriale*	Disorder of Merino sheep in W. Queensland. Occurs when adult sheep are mustered for shearing. Symptoms: lethargy, dragging hind feet, knuckling, lowered head and arched back. Lesions are severe myodegeneration of hind limbs and accompanying spinal Wallerian degeneration	O'Sullivan 1976
H O S P	MONENSIN TOXICITY (*Streptomyces cinnamonensis*)	Monensin is an antibiotic ionophore used as a coccidiostat. It also has growth promoting activities in ruminants. Monogastrics have a low toxicity tolerance. Symptoms: lethargy, stiffness, muscle weakness and recumbency after a single toxic dose. Lesions; cardiac and skeletal myodegeneration with minimal mineralisation	Hulland 1985

(B) DUE TO METALLIC AND OTHER IONS

Species	Ion	Clinical and pathological features	Key references
S	COBALT	Implicated in cardiac failure of beer drinkers in man. Chronic cumulative toxicity can occur rarely in sheep. In man lesions are of diffuse hydropic myocardial degeneration	Anon 1968
S	COPPER	In sheep copper toxicity is not uncommon and a rise in plasma CK activity has been reported at the stage of haemolytic crisis. The morphological changes have not been described	Thompson & Todd 1974 Howell 1978
R	IODINE	In rats induces muscular rigidity, motor disturbances and thyrotoxic-type myopathy in Mm intercostales, triceps brachii, quadriceps and the intrinsic laryngeal muscles	Cantin 1967
P	IRON	In neonatal piglets given prophylactic iron (as iron dextrose) lethal skeletal and myocardial degeneration occur. Improved formulations have virtually eliminated this once common toxicity	(see Nutritional myopathies)
RAB	MOLYBDENUM	In rabbits severe hind limb muscle and cardiac muscle degeneration occurred experimentally, possibly as a result of antagonism between molybdenum and copper	Valli et al 1969

Table 28.6 (*Cont'd*)

Species	Name/Cause	Clinical and pathological features	Key reference
MANY	SELENIUM	Occurs in well-defined geographical areas due to ingestion of highly seleniferous plants which convert insoluble selenium to soluble selenates. Therapeutic overdosage can also occur in treating deficiency states. Lesions include cardiac and skeletal and vascular smooth muscle degeneration especially in myocardial and pulmonary arteries	Van Vleet et al 1974 Bradley 1975 Anderson et al 1985
MANY	CADMIUM, MERCURY, SILVER, SULPHUR, TELLURIUM, THALLIUM, ZINC	These have all been implicated experimentally in producing skeletal and/or cardiac myodegeneration. They probably all act finally via the system of mitochondrial calcium overload as described in the introduction (qv)	Van Vleet et al 1981

For key to abbreviations see foot of Table 28.2

and pathological features and key references; few are of direct relevance to disease in man.

LOWER MOTOR NEURONE (LMN) DISEASES IN ANIMALS

Introduction

In this section, muscle dysfunction resulting from lesions in the LMN in animals is discussed. The LMN includes the cell body (perikaryon), axon (ventral root, spinal nerve and peripheral nerve) and the axonal part of the motor end-plate. The presence of a lesion at one or more of these sites may result in LMN dysfunction and give rise to all the signs of neurogenic muscle disease: these include muscle weakness, decreased tone, absent or reduced spinal reflexes and neurogenic atrophy.

In animals, as in man, many potential aetiological agents and pathogenic mechanisms may produce lesions of the LMN. The large number of conditions which, therefore, exist in the various domestic animal species precludes a detailed description of each, but some relevant examples will be mentioned. The reader is referred to Palmer (1976), de Lahunta (1983) and Duncan & Griffiths (1984), for more detailed accounts. We have added short descriptions of a few well-characterised conditions affecting different parts of the LMN, concentrating on those which are of particular comparative interest.

Diseases with the main lesions in the LMN cell body

The ventral horn cells of the spinal cord may be damaged or destroyed in any condition in which focal myelopathy is produced as part of the pathological process. Neurogenic muscle atrophy may therefore be seen in a wide variety of conditions, ranging from protozoal encephalomyelitis in the horse to fibrocartilagenous embolism in the dog.

LMN disease due to viruses. Viral disease may result in damage to ventral horn cells. In man, one such condition of particular importance is poliomyelitis. In pigs, the term Teschen–Talfan disease (or polioencephalomyelitis) is used to embrace a group of well-documented encephalomyelitides caused by a group of closely related enteroviruses (Mills & Nielsen 1968). Clinically, Teschen–Talfan disease bears some resemblance to human poliomyelitis: young pigs show signs of a febrile illness which is followed by the development of flaccid paralysis, particularly of the hind legs. Pathological features include widespread necrosis of the nerve cells in the diencephalon, brain stem, spinal cord and dorsal root ganglia, together with focal proliferation of microglia and perivascular cuffing.

It has been suggested that viruses may also be involved in the aetiology of chronic progressive motor neurone diseases such as amyotrophic lateral sclerosis (ALS) although at present there is little direct evidence to support this hypothesis (see Ch. 23).

Recently, the endogenous murine leukaemia virus (MuLV) has been shown to cause both tumours and LMN disease in a population of wild mice. The virus is acquired by 'maternal congenital infection' and, in a proportion of animals, paralysis due to lower motor neurone damage develops after a long incubation period of between eight months and two years (Gardner 1978). Experimental studies have shown that virus expression and disease development are suppressed in some strains of laboratory mouse. However, inoculation of virus into mice known to have an inherited degenerative condition of lower motor neurones (wobbler mice), has shown that these animals are abnormally susceptible to the virus, succumbing to illness after a very short incubation period (Ch. 23). These observations may be of interest when considering the possible role of viruses in the development of chronic motor neurone diseases, as they indicate the involvement of genetic factors which control the expression of the disease in different individuals.

Any consideration of virus diseases which give rise to lower motor neurone signs should include a mention of rabies and canine distemper. Although both diseases are more usually thought of as resulting in encephalitis, myelitis and resulting LMN signs are common features in both conditions.

LMN disease due to nutritional factors. A well-recognised example of LMN disease associated with nutritional deficiency is enzootic ataxia (delayed swayback), seen in young sheep and goats and red deer. Chromatolysis and degeneration of the large neurones of the brain stem and spinal cord result in LMN signs. Although the condition is known to be associated with low copper status, the underlying pathophysiological mechanisms are not yet fully understood (Sullivan 1985).

Inherited and familial LMN disease. Of particular comparative interest are those conditions in which ventral horn cell degeneration is familial or inherited. Several such entities have

been described in animals and these are listed in Table 28.7. Wobbler mice are mutants in which lower motor neurone degeneration with muscle weakness is inherited via an autosomal recessive gene. The weakness is more pronounced proximally than distally and is particularly evident in forelimb and shoulder muscles. Rounding and enlargement of the motor neurone may be seen late in the course of the disease and there may be vacuolation of the cytoplasm.

In dogs, several inherited LMN degenerative conditions have been described. Recently, dominantly inherited bilateral laryngeal paralysis of Bouvier de Flandres dogs has been shown to be a degenerative neurogenic disease. Histological examination of the recurrent laryngeal nerves of affected Bouviers revealed Wallerian degeneration throughout the length of both right and left nerves. This strongly indicated that the primary lesion is in the cell bodies of the vagus nerves in the nucleus ambiguus of the medulla (Venker-van Haagen 1980). Subsequent examination of this nucleus showed degeneration and loss of motor neurones. Occasional cases of laryngeal paralysis resulting from degenerative neurogenic disease have been reported in man (Holinger et al 1979) but laryngeal hemiplegia involving the left recurrent laryngeal nerve ('roaring') is particularly important in the horse where it has been recognised for several centuries. Although there is a higher incidence of the condition in certain types of horse, especially large heavy hunters, there has been no conclusive demonstration of genetic involvement. Examination of the nucleus ambiguus in a number of horses revealed no changes and, although many theories have been proposed as to its aetiology, the cause of the condition remains unknown.

Hereditary canine spinal muscular atrophy in Brittany spaniels

Hereditary canine spinal muscular atrophy (HCSMA) is a progressive motor neurone disease of the Brittany spaniel which is characterised by progressive muscle weakness and atrophy, particularly of proximal limb and paraspinal muscles (Lorenz et al 1979).

Three distinct phenotypes are recognised: these

Table 28.7 Inherited or Familial (F) Lower Motor Neurone Conditions

Species	Condition	Breed	Mode of inher.	Onset	Signs	Pathology	Comparative notes	Key ref.
D	NEURONAL ABIOTROPHY	Swedish Lapland	AR	5–7 w	Progressive muscle weakness and atrophy resulting in tetraplegia. Survive up to 18 m	Neuronal degeneration in CNS. Degeneration of axons and myelin in dorsal & ventral roots. Wallerian degeneration in peripheral nerve	Mainly historic interest	Sandeveldt et al 1976
	CANINE SPINAL MUSCULAR ATROPHY	Brittany spaniel	AD	(a) 6 w–3 m	3 phenotypes: (a) Tetraplegia by 3–4 m (accelerated) (Fig. 28.15)	(a) Many neurofilamentous swellings in proximal axons. Degeneration of neurones (Fig. 28.16)	Good animal model of MND (a) ?≡Werdnig-Hoffman disease	Cork et al 1980
				(b) 6 m–3 y	(b) Tetraplegia by 2–3 y (intermediate)	(b) Reduced numbers of motor neurones, fewer axonal swellings	(b) ?≡Kugelberg-Welander disease	
				(c) >1 y	(c) Survive well into adult life (chronic)	(c) No pathology yet available	(c) Similar course to Amyotrophic lateral sclerosis	
	STOCKARD'S PARALYSIS	Great Dane ×Bloodhound and Great Dane × St. Bernard	F	3 m	Paralysis of distal pelvic limb muscles. Progression rapid over 3–5 m	Central chromatolysis, microgliosis & neuronophagia of motor nerves of the lumbar spinal cord	Mainly of historic interest	Stockard 1936

Table 28.7 (*Cont'd*)

Species	Condition	Breed	Mode of inher.	Onset	Signs	Pathology	Comparative notes	Key ref.
	HEREDITARY PROGRESSIVE NEUROGENIC MUSCULAR ATROPHY	Pointer	F	4–5 m	Muscle weakness & atrophy. Progresses to complete tetraplegia by 9 m	Muscle pathology & EMG suggestive of denervation. Degeneration of axons in PNS and ventral roots. Zebra bodies in LMN hypoglossal and spinal accessory nuclei	Clinical similarities to progressive SMA in man	Inada et al 1978 Izumo et al 1983
C	LMN DISEASE	Domestic Short Haired	1 Case	3–4 w	Progressive weakness resulting in tetraplegia by 6 w	Neuronal degeneration in spinal cord. Abnormal proliferation of 10 nm neurofilaments. Wallerian degeneration in ventral roots & peripheral nerve		Vandevelde et al 1976
RAB	LMN DISEASE	New Zealand White × Californians	F	6–8 w	Inco-ordination & weakness. Progressing to tetraplegia in 3–4 w	Neuronal degeneration and loss in ventral horn cells, and brain stem. Excess 10 nm neurofilaments in perikarya. Type II fibre atrophy of muscle		Shields & Vandevelde 1978

	Name	Breed	Inheritance	Onset	Clinical signs	Pathology	Comparison to human disease	Reference
M	WOBBLER MOUSE		AR (wr gene)	10–30 d	Muscular weakness. May die in 2–3 m or lifespan may be normal	Degeneration of lower motor neurones in brain stem & spinal cord	Distribution of lesions similar to that in Kugelberg-Welander disease & Werdnig-Hoffman disease	Duchen & Strich 1968
O	SHAKER CALVES	Horned Herefords	F	Birth	Difficulty standing. Generalised tremor. Wobbly gait. Aphonia	Neuronal degeneration. Excess neurofilaments (12 nm diameter) in neurones of CNS, PNS, ANS & retina. Wallerian degeneration in nerve roots	Some similarities to forms of MND & spinocerebellar degenerations of man	Rousseaux et al 1985
P	LMN DISEASE	Yorkshire	F	5 w	Bilateral posterior ataxia progressing to tetraplegia by 10 w	Neuronal chromatolysis, degeneration & loss in ventral horns of spinal cord, medulla & mid brain. Wallerian degeneration in cord & ventral roots. Neurogenic muscle atrophy. Accumulations of 10 nm neurofilaments in motor neurones		Higgins et al 1983

For key to abbreviations see foot of Table 28.2

are distinguishable by their age of onset and rate of progression and are termed accelerated, intermediate and chronic. Recent breeding studies have indicated that the condition is inherited via an autosomal dominant gene (Sack et al 1984). Animals homozygous for the gene develop the accelerated form in which signs are first seen between six weeks and three months of age and there is rapid progression to tetraparesis (Fig. 28.15). Heterozygous animals may develop the intermediate condition. In these cases, weakness usually becomes apparent during the first six months of life and progresses to tetraparesis by two or three years of age. However, a few heterozygotes have developed a chronic form characterised by late onset, slow progression and survival well into adult life. The factors which determine whether the intermediate or chronic form occurs in heterozygous dogs are not yet clear.

In all three phenotypes the first clinical sign is muscular weakness. This is most severe in the muscles of the limb girdles and trunk, resulting in an abnormal gait and reduced exercise tolerance. Affected dogs are alert and remain so throughout the course of the disease. There are no upper motor neurone signs, no evidence of sensory deficits and no indication of autonomic involvement. Tendon reflexes are reduced in significantly atrophied muscles but intact in those which are relatively unaffected.

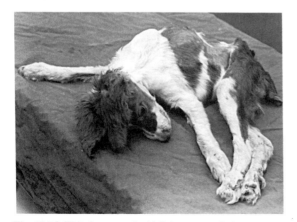

Fig. 28.15 This four-month-old Brittany pup is homozygous for the autosomal dominant trait for Hereditary Canine Spinal Muscular Atrophy. Muscle weakness was first noted in proximal muscles between six and eight weeks of age and progressed to tetraparesis as shown here (Figure supplied by courtesy of Dr L. C. Cork)

Electromyographically there are fibrillation potentials and fasciculations, particularly in axial muscles. There is no decremental response to repetitive nerve stimulation and nerve conduction velocities are normal (Lorenz et al 1979).

Sequentially collected muscle biopsies from affected dogs have shown that muscle pathology appears first and is most severe in the proximal musculature. The earliest evidence of denervation atrophy is the presence of small fibres. The proportion of these increases as the disease progresses and is accompanied by some hypertrophy of both type I and II fibres. Late in the course of the condition group atrophy is a feature but fibre-type grouping does not appear to occur at any stage (Cork et al 1979).

The pathology of the nervous system varies in the different forms of the disease. In accelerated HCSMA the most striking feature is swelling in the proximal portion of almost all the motor axons, which are filled with maloriented arrays of neurofilaments (Fig. 28.16). Other changes include neuronophagia, chromatolysis and the presence of glial bundles in axons of the proximal ventral roots.

In the intermediate phenotype a few axonal swellings are present and there are reduced numbers of motor neurones in the spinal cord. The proximal axonal swellings which are characteristic of this disease closely resemble those seen in ALS of man. Similar swellings are also known to be produced by experimental administration of β,β'-iminodipropionitrile (IDPN), a toxin which impairs slow axonal transport. As neurofilaments are carried by this slow axonal transport system it was suggested that a transport abnormality may exist in HCSMA and in other motor neurone diseases (Cork et al 1980). Subsequent examination of affected dogs has shown that slow transport of all cytoskeletal proteins is, indeed, impaired (Griffin et al 1982).

The clinical and pathological similarities of HCSMA to various forms of human motor neurone disease make it a valuable animal model. Further studies on the pathophysiology of this disease may therefore be important in elucidating some of the mechanisms involved in the development of degenerative changes in the motor neurone in both man and animals.

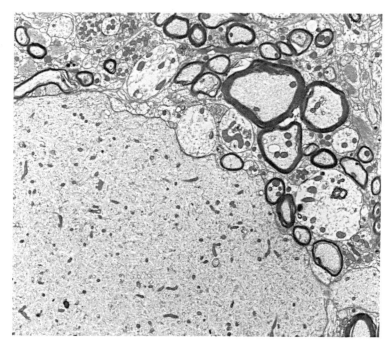

Fig. 28.16 This thinly myelinated axon internode from the spinal cord of a dog with Hereditary Canine Spinal Muscular Atrophy is distended with maloriented neurofilaments. Transport of neurofilament triplet proteins is impaired in dogs with HCSMA. ×6,850 (Figure supplied by courtesy of Dr L. C. Cork)

Diseases with the main lesion in the axon of the LMN

Nerve roots and peripheral nerves may be damaged by compression or traumatic injury or may be involved in inflammatory processes, as seen in acute polyradiculoneuritis in the dog.

This condition is also known as coonhound paralysis, as the onset of the signs usually occurs 10–14 days after a racoon bite. Affected dogs rapidly develop a bilaterally symmetrical flaccid tetraplegia which may result in death attributable to paralysis of respiratory muscles. In other instances, recovery may occur although return to normal function may take up to six months. Cases have been recorded in which no exposure to racoons has occurred and the actual mechanism of pathogenesis remains unknown. The lesion of coonhound paralysis is similar to that seen in experimentally produced allergic neuritis in dogs and there are clinical and pathological similarities to the acute polyneuritis which is seen in man in the Landry–Guillain–Barré syndrome (Duncan & Griffiths 1984).

In the horse, chronic inflammation of the extradural roots of the cauda equina causes signs which include urinary incontinence, faecal retention, tail paralysis and hindlimb weakness; this syndrome is known as neuritis of the cauda equina. However, detailed examination of the nervous system has shown that the inflammatory changes are more widespread, affecting also the cranial and peripheral roots and nerves. The cause is unknown but again it has been suggested that this disease represents an example of allergic neuritis. In contrast to the Guillain–Barré syndrome, the course of the disease is more chronic and unremitting and there are differences in the distribution of the lesions (Cummings et al 1979).

Griffiths & Duncan (1979) described a condition of dogs in which generalised degeneration of the most distal portion of the motor axons resulted in flaccid paralysis. The condition is termed distal denervating disease and results in quadriparesis. Typical neurogenic muscle atrophy and/or quadriplegia develops, but affected dogs usually make a complete recovery after a few weeks. It has been suggested that some kind of toxin might be responsible for the condition but, so far, none has been demonstrated.

Various toxins are known to cause degeneration of peripheral nerve. The fruits of the Coyotillo plant (*Karwinskia humboldtiana*), when eaten by cattle, goats or sheep, give rise to both segmental demyelination and Wallerian degeneration, especially of the long motor fibres: this results in weakness, particularly of the hind limbs (Charlton et al 1970). Posterior paralysis in cattle is also associated with ingestion of *Melochia pyramidata*, which results in fibre degeneration in the inferior cerebellar peduncle and spinocerebellar tracts, the cervical and thoracic cord and in the sciatic nerve (Palmer & Woodham 1975). The nerve degeneration results in neurogenic atrophy of the muscles.

Organophosphate compounds such as those commonly used as anthelmintics in farm animals may also give rise to delayed neurotoxicity and consequent LMN signs. Paraplegia or ataxia of the hindlimbs has occurred in pigs nine to 26 days after dosing with particular formulations of haloxon (now withdrawn from the market). Lesions of both the CNS and PNS occur: in particular, there is degeneration of the more distal parts of the long myelinated fibre tracts and resultant extensive muscle fibre atrophy (Wells & Bradley 1977) (Fig. 28.17).

Diseases with the main lesions at the neuromuscular junction

Some neurotoxins act by specifically altering the function of the neuromuscular junction. Botulinum toxin produced by *Clostridium botulinum* causes a flaccid paralysis which may cause death because of respiratory paralysis. The toxin is generally ingested in contaminated food although it may gain entry via open wounds. Many species, including man, may be affected by botulism although species susceptibility varies. There may be different degrees of severity associated with toxins from different strains of bacteria. Botulinum toxin acts at the neuromuscular junction by interfering with release of acetylcholine.

In the murine mutant with motor end-plate disease (med) a state of functional denervation appears to exist, because of an inherited failure of neuromuscular transmission. Signs of progressive muscle weakness are first apparent at 10 days of age and as the disease progresses the muscle fibres become severely atrophied. Affected mice die at

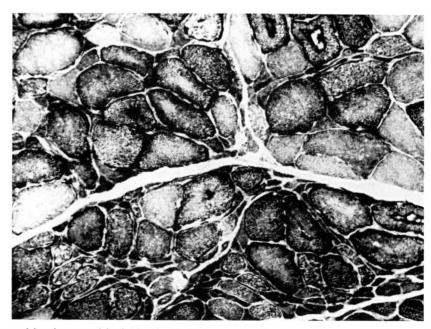

Fig. 28.17 Haloxon delayed neurotoxicity in the pig *M. diaphragma*. Small group atrophy, target and targetoid fibres. Atrophic myocytes show high reaction for aerobic enzymes. NADH-Tetrazolium reductase. ×160

three to four weeks of age (Duchen et al 1967).

The weakness and fatigue following exercise characteristic of myasthenia gravis is also due to functional disturbance at the neuromuscular junction. Both congenital and acquired forms of myasthenia are seen in animals and, because these conditions are of considerable comparative interest, they are discussed in more detail below.

Myasthenia gravis

Myasthenia gravis has been reported both in dogs and in cats. In dogs, acquired and congenital forms of myasthenia gravis occur spontaneously.

Acquired canine myasthenia was first reported in 1961 (Ormrod 1961). Subsequently there have been further reports (Palmer & Barker 1974, Lennon et al 1981) with most cases occurring in adults of large breeds. Onset may occur after a bout of febrile illness. Clinical signs are primarily those of severe muscle weakness which characteristically improves with rest, and is often most noticeable in the forelimbs. As the animal exercises, the stride shortens and the head is lowered until eventually the dog collapses or refuses to continue. In many instances there is difficulty in raising the head and in prehending and swallowing food. The swallowing defects are frequently associated with the presence of mega-oesophagus; this is a common feature of acquired myasthenia gravis in the dog, probably because of the high proportion of striated muscle present throughout the length of the oesophagus in this species. When present, mega-oesophagus may result in the development of secondary complications such as inhalation pneumonia.

Autoantibodies to acetylcholine receptors have been found in 50% of dogs with a clinical diagnosis of idiopathic mega-oesophagus suggesting that this entity in many instances is a manifestation of a restricted form of autoimmune myasthenia gravis (V. Lennon, personal communication). Diagnosis of acquired myasthenia is based on clinical signs, together with the response to short-acting anticholinesterase drugs administered intravenously. The response is generally dramatic, with immediate restoration of normal exercise tolerance lasting several minutes. Electro-

diagnostic techniques such as those used in man may also be used. Repetitive stimulation of peripheral nerve results in a decremental response which is abolished by short-acting anticholinesterases.

As in man, circulating antibodies to acetylcholine receptor are detectable. The condition is therefore considered to be of autoimmune aetiology, and may be found in association with thymoma. Histological examination shows that there is little muscle pathology (Palmer & Barker 1974), although in one case non-specific degenerative changes were found in the muscles of the head and larynx, associated with isolated foci of lymphocytic infiltration (Darke et al 1975). Ultrastructural examination of the neuromuscular junction of one affected dog showed marked widening of the primary and secondary synaptic clefts (Zacks et al 1966).

Treatment of acquired myasthenia gravis involves the oral administration of long-acting anticholinesterase drugs. In many cases spontaneous remission and complete recovery may result, although complications such as inhalation pneumonia or inadvertent overdose of anticholinesterases may be fatal.

Congenital canine myasthenia gravis was first described in the Jack Russell terrier in 1974 (Palmer & Barker 1974), and has since been reported in the Springer spaniel and the Smooth Haired Fox terrier (Johnson et al 1975, Jenkins et al 1976). The condition is believed to be inherited as an autosomal recessive trait (Wallace & Palmer 1984).

Signs of weakness are first noticed at six to eight weeks of age. Severely affected puppies are unable to stand or raise their heads, have difficulty in eating, and may have mega-oesophagus. Diagnosis, as in cases of acquired myasthenia gravis, is based on the clinical picture and the response to short-acting anticholinesterases. Prognosis is generally poor although, with treatment using small doses of oral preparations of long-acting anticholinesterase drugs, it has proved possible to keep affected animals alive for up to two years.

There are no circulating antibodies to acetylcholine receptors present in congenital canine myasthenia gravis. However, in all three affected breeds it has been shown that there is a reduction in density of acetylcholine receptors in the post-synaptic membrane, which remains at a constant low level throughout life. Recent studies indicate that the defect may be due to a low insertion rate of acetylcholine receptors in the postsynaptic membrane (Oda et al 1984).

Trojaborg & Flagstad (1982) described an inherited disease of neuromuscular transmission in the Gammel Dansk Honsehund breed. It is as yet unknown whether the cause of failure of neuro-muscular transmission in these dogs is pre- or postsynaptic. Four incidents of myasthenia gravis have been reported in cats but the pathology has not been described (Dawson 1970, Mason 1976, Indrieri et al 1983).

MYOPATHIES OF COMPLEX OR UNRESOLVED AETIOLOGY

Some of the conditions dealt with in this section have some or even great relevance to analogous conditions in man and are dealt with in the text: these include congenital articular rigidity and porcine splayleg. The remainder have little relevance to myopathies of man or are insufficiently well documented pathologically to permit such comparison. They are listed in Table 28.8. together with the main distinguishing features and sources of further information. (Also please consult the last edition of this book.) The weaver

syndrome of Brown Swiss cattle (Leipold et al 1973), previously considered to be a myopathy has now been defined as a myelo-encephalopathy (Stuart & Leipold 1985) and is not considered further.

Congenital articular rigidity (CAR)

CAR is a term used to indicate a congenital dysfunction of one or more joints. When this causes joints to be fixed in flexion the condition is synonymous with arthrogryposis. The condition was reviewed in farm animals generally by Swatland (1974), in cattle by Done (1976) and in pigs by Bradley & Wells (1978) and Wells & Bradley (1987).

CAR is one of the more common developmental defects of cattle. It is sometimes accompanied by other defects such as hydrocephalus, spinal dysraphism and cleft palate. An inherited form of arthrogryposis/palatoschisis occurs in the Charolais breed (Russell et al 1985). However most incidents in all species are attributable to environmental teratogens: viruses, phytotoxins (e.g. *Lupinus* and *Cassia* sp. and locoweed) or chemical toxins are the most frequently implicated. Of particular interest to the medical practitioner is the CAR that occurs in pigs due to exposure of the pregnant sow to the tobacco plant (*Nicotiana tabacum*) (Crowe & Pike 1973): the teratogenic chemical is believed to be anabasine and not nicotine (Keeler et al 1981).

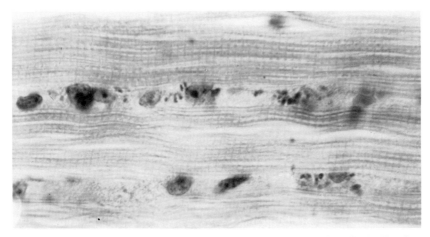

Fig. 28.18 Xanthosis. *M. masseter* of an aged Ayrshire cow. There is an accumulation of lipofuscin-like pigment close to the nuclear poles. H & E, ×675

Table 28.8 Myopathies of complex or unresolved aetiology

Species	Condition	Breed	Clinical signs	Pathology	Key references
O	SPASTIC PARESIS	Friesian mainly	Progressive from calfhood. Non-fatal. Locomotor impairment. Straightening of pelvic limb(s) moved in pendulum fashion	Unknown	Baird et al 1974 Bradley & Wijeratne 1980 Keith 1981
O	XANTHOSIS	Ayrshire mainly	Discoloration of white areas of body coat in adults. Most severe cases are old	Paranuclear lipofuscinosis of skeletal and cardiac myocytes sometimes with a vacuolar myopathy (Fig. 28.18)	Bradley & Duffell 1982
O	PRIMARY MYOPATHY WITH ABSENCE OF Z DISCS AND MYOFIBRILLAR HYPOPLASIA	Friesian solitary case	Neonatal onset. Progressive muscle weakness	Myofibrillar hypoplasia, abnormal nuclear morphology, absence of Z discs, sarcoplasmic inclusions	Bradley 1979
O S P	MUSCULAR STEATOSIS (Lipomatous atrophy)	Any	Nil	Muscle replaced with fat. Myocytes replaced with lipocytes (Fig. 28.19)	Hulland 1985
O (S)	TRANSPORT MYOPATHY	Any	Following droving, chasing or long journeys. Transitory gait abnormalities or sudden death	Acute myodegeneration	Bradley & Fell 1981
WILD	CAPTURE MYOPATHY (Exertional rhabdomyolysis)	Mostly ruminants	Following the chase — muscle stiffness, respiratory distress, collapse and death	Severe metabolic acidosis, myoglobinuria nephrosis. Acute cardiac and skeletal oedema and degeneration (Fig. 28.20)	Bartsch et al 1977 Hulland 1985
S	MYOPATHY OF THE ABDOMINAL MUSCLE OF PREGNANT EWES	Finnish Landrace × Dorset Horn	Not reported	Type I cell hypertrophy and increase in proportion. Later degeneration and chronic change (Fig. 28.21)	Wilson et al 1978

Table 28.8 (*Cont'd*)

Species	Condition	Breed	Clinical signs	Pathology	Key references
S	POLYMYOPATHY ASSOCIATED WITH SCRAPIE	Any adult	Progressive fatal neuromuscular symptoms. Muscle atrophy. Ataxia, faulty eye movements and difficulty in raising the head	Myopathy similar to human dermatomyositis and muscular dystrophy in pelvic limbs, extrinsic eye and neck muscles	Bosanquet et al 1956 Parry 1983
P	ASYMMETRIC HINDQUARTER SYNDROME	Often Large White type	Progressive asymmetrical development of hind quarters from three months. Otherwise asymptomatic (Fig. 28.22)	Asymmetry due to unequal distribution of subcut. fat and myocytes in the posterior thigh muscles of the two sides (Fig. 28.23)	Done et al 1975 Bradley & Wells 1978
P	CHRONIC MYOPATHY WITH CYTOPLASMIC BODIES	Landrace × large white	Mild hind limb weakness	M. longissimus type II cells contain cytoplasmic bodies, PAS positive material and glycogen- metabolising enzymes	Scarlato & Meola 1978
P	FOCAL MYOPATHY	Pietrain (and other, stress susceptible pigs)	None	Focal myodegeneration particularly in muscles prone to produce pale soft and exudative meat (Fig. 28.13)	Muir 1970 Bradley & Wells 1978
P	SPLAYLEG (see text)	Pietrain and Landrace mainly	Transient congenital limb adductor muscle weakness	Not yet defined. Myofibrillar hypoplasia often reported as the lesion is a normal feature of neonatal piglet muscle (Fig. 28.24)	Ward 1978 Ward & Bradley 1979, 1980 Bradley 1980 Bradley et al 1980
D	ABNORMAL DEVELOPMENT OF THE PECTINEUS MUSCLE	Alsatian and mongrel	Those associated with hip dysplasia	Retarded type II cell growth and compensatory type I cell hypertrophy of M. pectineus only	Cardinet et al 1969
D	MYOSITIS OF MASTICATORY MUSCLES (a) Eosinophilic myositis (b) Atrophic myositis	(a) Alsatians mainly (b) Any dolocephalic breed	Repetitive episodes of pain, swelling and mandibular immobility terminating in jaw fixation and muscle atrophy	Bilaterally symmetrical acute, eosinophilic in (a) or chronic myositis, predominantly masticatory muscles. Possibly immune mediated (Fig. 28.25)	Oghiso et al 1976 Hulland 1985

GP	NECROTISING MYOPATHY	—	Not recorded	Limb and trunk muscle atrophy with myonecrosis and mononuclear invasion with regeneration	Webb 1970
R	SENILE MYOPATHY		Onset at >2y. Waddling gait progressing to posterior postural collapse over 2 months. Loss of weight and death	Myodegeneration and regeneration with myocyte ceroid pigmentation	Berg 1956
RAB	RESTRAINT MYOPATHY	New Zealand	Reversible decreased hind limb mobility with or without lumbar kyphosis following restraint in stocks for 6h/d for 3 m	Diffuse or focal Wallerian degeneration and myelin disintegration of sciatic nerves. Unconnected focal myonecrosis of trunk, fore and hind limb muscles	Mendlowski 1975
H O S P G	CONGENITAL ARTICULAR RIGIDITY (Arthrogryposis)	—	Permanent congenital fixation of limb and/or other joints. Often results in dystocia and and/or death of the newborn	Variable but often reduced muscle bulk. Myocytes substituted with lipocytes (brown fat). Fibrosis. Myocyte hypoplasia (Fig. 28.26)	Swatland 1974 Done 1976 Bradley & Wells 1978, 1987
O P G D C	HAFFKRANKHEIT	—	Imprecise neuromuscular symptoms probably of toxic (alkyl-mercury compounds) or deficiency (Thiamine/vitamin E/selenium) causation	Skeletal myodegeneration including calcification. Cardiac Purkinje fibre degeneration in cattle	Innes & Saunders 1962 Gardner 1967

For key to abbreviations see foot of Table 28.2

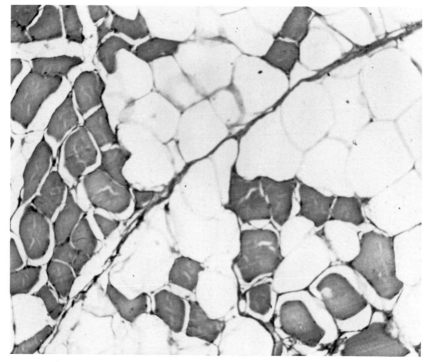

Fig. 28.19 Muscular steatosis. Hind-quarter muscle of a beef carcass showing high proportion of fat cells within muscle fascicles of normal architecture. Lillie's allochrome, ×85

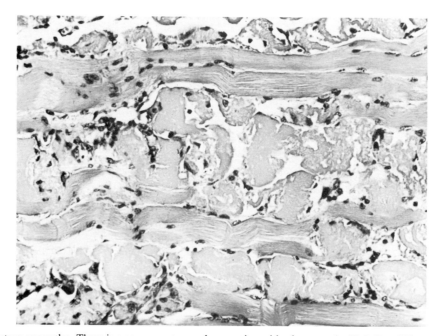

Fig. 28.20 Capture myopathy. There is a severe acute myodegeneration with phagocytosis. H & E, ×125

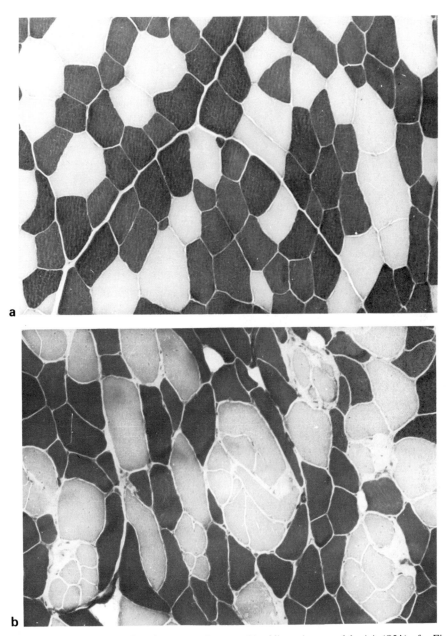

Fig. 28.21 Myopathy of abdominal muscles of pregnant sheep. a. *M. obliquus internus abdominis* (OIA) of a Finnish Landrace × Dorset Horn ewe after two pregnancies at pasture. b. *M*. OIA of Finn × Dorset ewe after 7 pregnancies of intensive breeding. Type I cells show variable cross sectional areas, cell splitting and focal necrosis. Alkali-stable myosin ATPase, ×120

In Akabane virus infection of the pregnant ruminant, CAR can reach epidemic proportions as in Israel, Japan and Australia. This is related to viral transmission by a biting fly which is seasonally on the wing during the period of gestation. The effect on the fetus depends on the stage of

pregnancy, the immune state of the dam and probably the infecting dose. Other viral causes include bluetongue, border disease, Rift Valley fever and Wesselbron disease viruses.

The mechanism of CAR has not been clearly established for each cause. In many instances

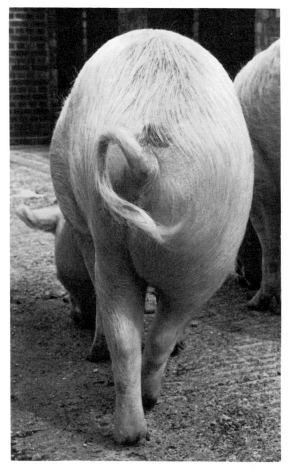

Fig. 28.22 Asymmetric hindquarter syndrome. An affected pig

neuronal failure is certain (Mayhew 1984) or probable, but skeletal, connective or muscular tissue targets for gene expression or teratogenic effects are also possible. In several instances in which the muscle has been examined, the findings are of a normal fascicular architecture with myocytes being completely or partly replaced by adipose cells (see Fig. 28.26). Neuromuscular spindles, blood vessels and, curiously, intramuscular nerves appear morphologically normal.

On gross inspection such muscles are atrophic, yellowish brown and float in formalin. CAR is an important and common condition of farm animals, resulting in economic loss by fetal or neonatal death and effects of dystocia. A mild reversible CAR of pastern joints of lambs, calves and foals (Gunn 1976, McLaughlin & Doige 1981, Mason 1981) of unknown cause also occurs.

Splayleg

Splayleg is a transient clinical syndrome of the improved pig in which the newborn animal is unable to support its body weight as a result of a failure of adduction, particularly of the hind limbs. This is a condition of considerable economic importance because there is an associated 50% mortality rate, principally as a result of overlaying by the sow. The aetiology and pathogenesis are not known. Recovery in uncomplicated cases occurs within the first week of life.

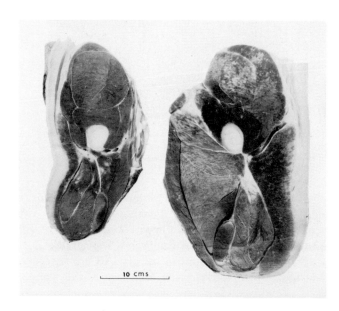

10 cms

Fig 28.23 Asymmetric hindquarter syndrome. Transverse section mid-femur level of the hind limbs of the pig illustrated in Fig. 28.22. The quadriceps muscles (top) are similar in size but the muscle mass of the posterior thigh on the left side is conspicuously reduced

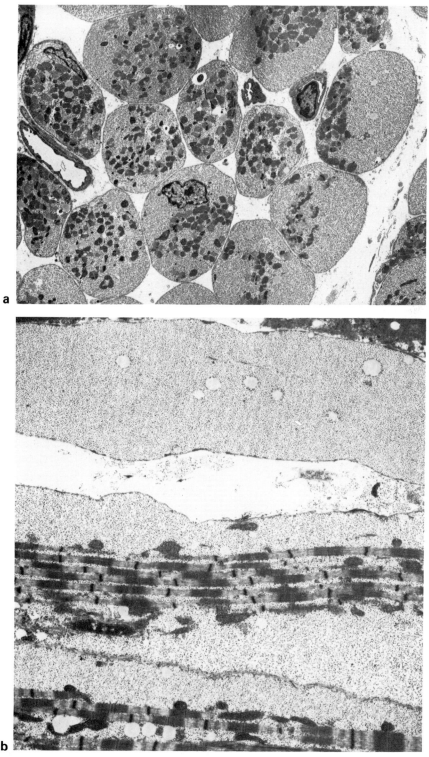

Fig. 28.24 Myofibrillar hypoplasia. a. *M. sartorius* of a newborn piglet, showing muscle cells exhibiting myofibrillar hypoplasia. The areas not occupied by myofibrils contain granular material, ×2000. b. Longitudinal section of a similar area. Myofibrils have a normal sarcomere structure, but do not fill the sarcoplasmic space, ×2500

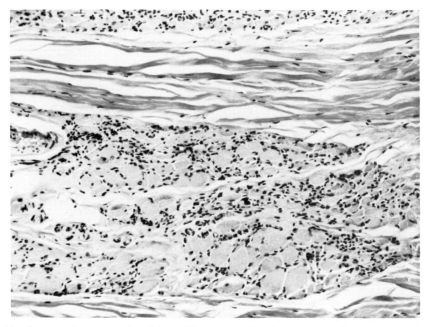

Fig. 28.25 Myositis of the masticatory muscles of dogs. *M. temporalis* showing severe atrophy of muscle cells and fibrosis in the perimysium. H & E, ×85

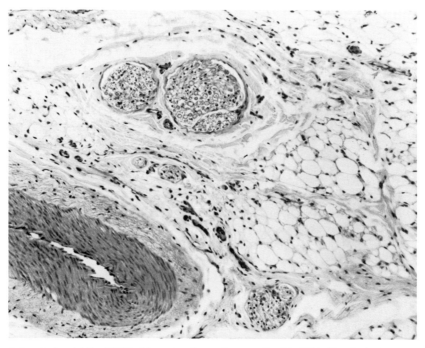

Fig. 28.26 Congenital articular rigidity (CAR). *M. semitendinosus* from a calf with CAR. The fascicular architecture is normal but the cells that compose the fascicles are adipose cells. Some contain single large lipid droplets; others contain variable numbers of smaller lipid droplets. The intramuscular nerves and vasculature appear normal. H & E, ×85

Of particular interest is the presence in the newborn pig, both normal and splay-legged, of the phenomenon of myofibrillar hypoplasia (mfh) (see Fig. 28.24). The extra-myofibrillar space is filled with material which has the morphology and staining reactions of glycogen. By the end of the first week of life the muscle cells have a more conventional appearance, mfh is no longer apparent, glycogen is reduced and intramyocyte fat is plentiful. The use of the splayleg pig as a model for the floppy infant syndrome is described by Ward & Bradley (1979).

AVIAN MYOPATHIES

Introduction

Because of the extensive breeding of enormous numbers of domesticated birds in order to improve the meat qualities of their muscles, this group of animals has furnished favourable material for the detection of inherited myopathies and their propagation for research purposes. Most work of this type has been performed on the chicken, *Gallus domesticus*, but domesticated turkeys, ducks and quails have also yielded examples of interest. Muscular dystrophy of the chicken is of particular interest in that it appears similar in some of its features to human muscular dystrophy; there is, therefore, extensive documentation of this model, which is reviewed only in outline here.

Inherited chicken muscular dystrophy

This condition was identified in 1956 and was isolated by selective breeding within a commercial flock of New Hampshire chickens (Asmundson & Julian 1956). Genetic analysis through many generations confirmed that a single genetic locus is mutant in this condition, this gene being co-dominant (Chung et al 1960). This gene has since been propagated in a variety of chicken genetic backgrounds; homozygotes are obtained by artificial insemination, and so far four breeding flocks maintained thus have been established, namely at the University of Davis, California, USA (B. W. Wilson), at the University of Connecticut, Storrs, USA (L. Pierro), jointly at Imperial College, London and a Medical Research

Council (MRC) Unit Cambridge, UK (P. J. Barnard and E. A. Barnard) and at the Nippon Institute for Biological Science, Yamanashi, Japan (M. Mizutani and K. Kondo). The commonest strains currently in use are the dystrophic 'early-onset' Davis line 413 and its genetically related normal control line 412 (Wilson et al 1979).

Features. The principal features of this disease in all of the dystrophic chicken strains can be summarised as follows:

1. Muscle weakness with histopathological change which spares the grossly red muscles and largely affects the white muscles, the fast-twitch (type II) fibres being affected first. Of the muscles containing (in the normal bird) essentially only type II fibres, the most commonly studied in the dystrophic chicken are the pectoral and the posterior latissimus dorsi (PLD) muscles (Barnard et al 1982).

2. Progressive changes in structure in the affected muscles, including formation of a wide range of fibre sizes and shapes, with later fibre splitting, vacuolation, atrophy, infiltration by adipose tissue and pronounced fibrosis.

3. Modifications of the muscle fibre-type pattern, as shown by histochemical enzyme staining and measurement of overall muscle enzyme contents, e.g. an increase in high-oxidative fibres and lower glycolytic activities (Barnard et al 1982), although no strictly uniform pattern of fibre type involvement emerges. Glycogen phosphorylase and glycogen in the sarcoplasmic reticulum are greatly increased in the dystrophic muscles (Sokolove 1985).

4. An increase in blood plasma creatine kinase (CK) activity, progressing with the disease and reaching extremely high levels (10–15 000 mU/ml at the peak, compared with about 300 mU/ml in the normal chicken); and similarly, substantial increases in plasma pyruvate kinase (PK) activity and in certain other enzymes.

5. A concomitant decrease in the content of some, but not all, of those plasma- elevated enzymes in the muscles.

6. Abnormal isoform distributions of certain muscle proteins, with some co-existence of embryonic and mature forms in the adult.

7. Abnormal electromyograms, showing increased excitability and prolonged repetitive firing (Entrikin et al 1982). In the intact muscles the twitch tension is significantly reduced in the dystrophic chicken (Hoekman 1976).

8. Decreasing action potential generation in the muscle cell membrane in response to repetitive low-frequency neural stimulation (Warnick et al 1979).

9. Abnormal endocytosis of the dystrophic muscles in vivo (Libelius et al 1979).

On the other hand, some important systems relating to skeletal muscle have been shown to be unaffected in chicken dystrophy, at least until after gross pathological change in the muscle is well established. The sensitivity to focally applied acetylcholine (ACh) and the frequency of the miniature end-plate potentials are not significantly different between normal and dystrophic chick muscles; there is no substantial abnormality of membrane depolarisation or the input resistance in the latter, and the end-plate potential waveform is unchanged in the dystrophic muscle (Warnick & Albuquerque 1979, Yeagle & Albuquerque 1984). In the earlier stages of the disease the end-plate ultrastructure is generally normal and the mean number of acetylcholine receptors on the postsynaptic membrane is unchanged (Porter & Barnard 1976). Another system that appears normal is that of axonal transport in the nerves to these muscles, at least as far as recognisable markers of the rates of such transport are concerned (Di Giamberardino et al 1979).

However, a few of the motor end-plates in certain muscles have been seen to be abnormal in the early stages of dystrophic chicken growth and this increases with age: at eight weeks of age about 25% of the motor nerve terminals are anomalously small and more highly branched than normal (Gunther & Letinsky 1985). The dystrophic fibres show evidence of enhanced innervation, including a significant incidence of nerve terminal sprouting and multiple innervation (Gunther & Letinsky 1985), the repetitive firing of directly elicited muscle action potentials and an enhanced reinnervation after nerve crush in vivo (Yeagle & Albuquerque 1984).

Measurement of muscular incapacity. A feature unique to birds is the ease of applying a 'performance test', i.e. a test of muscular disability in the living animal as shown in an unequivocal performance which can be scored quantitatively. This is the Flip Test in which the dystrophic bird, when placed on its back, is seen to be unable to right itself. A bird must use its wings for assistance in rising from this position, and incapacity from any cause affecting the muscles involved in these movements is readily perceived in the righting performance. For obvious anatomical reasons, an equivalent Flip Test is not applicable in a dystrophic mammal.

In the test, the bird is placed on its back five times and allowed to rise. A normal bird invariably scores a Flip Number (FN) of 5 out of five successful attempts, rising in a rapid co-ordinated movement. As muscular dystrophy develops, the chicks have increasing difficulty, struggling up fewer and fewer times, and eventually will score 0/5. The progression of the FN with age, in the line 413 chickens homozygous for dystrophy, is shown in Fig. 28.27. From about 20 days of age the FN declines in the line 413 birds and by 60 days is close to its final value. Normal chickens,

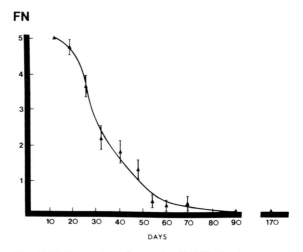

FN

DAYS

Fig. 28.27 Progression of muscular disability in the dystrophic chick as measured by the Flip Number (FN). The righting ability is scored out of five consecutive attempts. The means and SD bars for groups of 30 line 413 male chicks are shown. Normal chicks always score 5 from day 10 onwards

in contrast, always show 100% performance (scoring 5) from about day 10 onwards.

Despite the simplicity of this measurement, the FN is a surprisingly reliable guide to the progress of the disease. Different observers, testing blind and with a suitable recovery interval, the same birds with developing dystrophy, find identical values and each bird shows a steady progression in FN along the general form of the curve shown, although there is, of course, individual variation in the rate of decline within this period.

Histological markers in dystrophic chicken muscles. Progressive changes occur in the proximal fast-twitch muscles, in which the regular polygonal fibre shape becomes rounded or extended and some fibres become clearly enlarged in cross section. This hypertrophy is accompanied by the presence of many unusually small fibres, arising mainly from longitudinal fibre splitting but also from attempted regeneration — the latter phenomenon occurring visibly, however, only in 1% of the fibre population in 50-day-old line 413 chickens (Pizzey & Barnard 1983a). The result is, therefore, that a histogram of fibre areas shows a much greater spread and a more skewed character than the relatively narrow distribution in the normal muscle (Fig. 28.28). The mean fibre area

increases in the normal chicken muscles, of course, with age and likewise in dystrophic muscles; the mean area for the dystrophic muscle fibres is often only slightly greater than that for a normal muscle of the same age but the standard deviation of the mean fibre area (SD) is always very significantly increased. Hence the SD or the coefficient of variation of the mean fibre area is a much better index than the mean itself (Pizzey & Barnard 1983a).

Related changes, which become appreciable only after about four weeks of age, are the occurrence of foci of necrosis and of phagocytosis. Vacuolation of fibres can occur, being more obvious in sections studied with the electron microscope. Connective tissue infiltration is progressive and is pronounced after two months of age; it is accompanied by fat deposits and adipose tissue infiltration (Pizzey & Barnard 1983b).

At the electron-microscopic level a disruption of the myofibrillar pattern is seen focally, with an increase in vesicles near the transverse tubules (Libelius et al 1979). A prominent feature is disorganisation and great proliferation of the transverse tubules and (to a lesser degree) of the sarcoplasmic reticulum membranes (Beringer 1978, Crowe & Baskin 1979). The transverse tubules open extracellularly in normal avian muscles via sarcolemmal caveolae and in the dystrophic muscles these structures lose their characteristic marked banding arrangement, increase in number and become irregular in profile, as seen in quantitative freeze-fracture studies (McLean et al 1986). Similar changes distinguish the sarcolemmae of muscles from normal human subjects and those with Duchenne dystrophy (Bonillo et al 1981, Appleyard et al 1982). The loss of caveolar patterning is uniformly developed by seven weeks of age in the dystrophic chicken, when there is still relatively little muscle necrosis but marked clinical weakness. This has been taken to support the hypothesis that in both man and the chicken a muscle membrane defect initiates the abnormalities (through e.g. Ca^{2+} entry) in the internal membrane system (McLean et al 1986).

The position of the muscle cell nuclei is one of the diagnostic features of human dystrophic

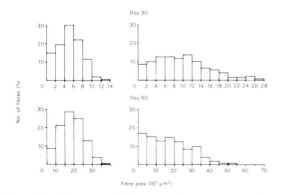

Fig. 28.28 Histograms of fibre area of pectoral muscle from normal (left-hand plots) and dystrophic (right-hand plots) chicks. The fibre area unit used is one hundred square microns. The distribution of fibre areas in the dystrophic muscle is characteristically skewed and hypertrophy is evident. (Note the change of scale for the older birds.) The increase in the smallest fibre-size group in the 60-day dystrophic birds is due to fibre splitting and to small regenerating fibres (From Pizzey & Barnard 1983b)

muscle, changing from predominantly peripheral to central. In affected chicken muscles there is always a considerable increase in the number of nuclei. A change in their position is found in some muscle types but in the reverse direction to the human case. In the normal chicken posterior latissimus dorsi (PLD) muscle the distribution of the nuclei is about 70% peripheral and remains so when their number increases due to the dystrophy. In the pectoral and some other 'white' muscles the normal position of the nuclei is predominantly internal and the proportion of peripheral nuclei in these muscles increases sharply in dystrophy (Pizzey & Barnard 1983b).

All of these changes can be expressed as quantitative parameters (Pizzey & Barnard 1983a). Also easily measured are the fractions of the muscle area occupied by (a) muscle fibres, (b) connective tissue and (c) fatty material, the ratios b/a and c/a being useful indices. These and the fibre area measurements are conveniently made with a digitiser–computer system.

The progression of pathological change. The rate of development of overt pathological signs can be much affected by the genetic background of the dystrophic chicken strain. The Davis line 413 has been bred for rapid myopathic development, whereas other lines develop similar abnormalities much more slowly (Wilson et al 1979). Hence a marked effect of genetic environment on the dystrophy gene is evident in avian dystrophy. In the line 413 birds, fibre hypertrophy (in the pectoral muscles) and the changes in nuclei become discernable four days after hatching, and from that stage they progress to the extremely skewed area distributions seen (Fig. 28.28) by 30 days (Pizzey & Barnard 1983b). By about one year of age, 80% of the dystrophic pectoral muscle is fat and connective tissue, as is 36% of the dystrophic PLD muscle (Pizzey & Barnard 1983b). Even by seven weeks of age, the dystrophic pectoral muscle has five times the normal collagen content (Fujii et al 1983), and an increased stiffness seen in the relaxed myofibres may be attributable to this (Feit et al 1985).

Some changes are detectable even in the embryonic stages. Thus, the numbers of fibroblasts and of muscle satellite cells are increased in the dystrophic 20-day embryonic pectoral muscle (Pizzey & Barnard 1983b). Indications of muscle deterioration, notably vesiculation, were detected as early as 17 days in vivo in the line 413 pectoral muscle (Allen & Murphy 1979). Ultrastructural abnormalities in the fibroblasts occurred here as early as embryonic day 13 and were marked at day 19 (Sweeny 1983). Fibroblast lysosomes also developed and the collagen fibril diameters were reduced. These features were remarkably similar to those seen in the connective tissue elements of muscles from young patients with congenital muscular dystrophy (Fidzianska et al 1982). Defective connective tissue differentiation, which affects myotube differentiation, is, therefore, another possible aetiological factor. Feit et al (1985) have reported evidence that an abnormal form of collagen, which is excessively cross-linked, is produced in the avian dystrophic muscle; a fuller investigation of this hypothesis is now desirable.

The muscle satellite cell increase detected in dystrophic chick embryos is maintained in post-hatch development (Yorita et al 1980, Pizzey & Barnard 1983a). In the dystrophic pectoral muscle their number is moderately raised above normal even after several months.

Involvement of fast and slow muscles in the disease. This issue has been the subject of much enquiry in the human muscular dystrophies, as discussed elsewhere in this volume; it is readily addressed in the dystrophic chicken developing under controlled conditions, because in birds there is much more segregation of the fibre types in different muscles than there is in mammals.

Normal chicken muscle fibres can be classified, by histochemical and morphological criteria, into fast-twitch (type IIA, oxidative–glycolytic and type IIB, glycolytic), slow-twitch (type I, which are oxidative and multiply innervated) and tonic (type III, oxidative and highly multiply innervated, giving sustained tonic contractions). These are fully described, across a range of muscles, by Barnard et al (1982). Tonic muscle fibres are very rare in man and are very resistant to muscular dystrophy (Gardner-Medwin 1980). They are common in birds, always occurring in a pure tonic muscle.

These tonic muscles are completely spared in the dystrophic chicken, as has been observed in the anterior latissimus dorsi (ALD) muscle (Cosmos & Butler 1967, Wilson et al 1979) and the plantaris and adductor profundus muscles (Barnard et al 1982) and likewise the metapagialis latissimus dorsi, a small tonic cutaneous muscle (Pizzey et al 1983). The type IIB fibres in twitch muscles show pathological changes in these birds (Cosmos & Butler 1967, Ashmore & Doerr 1971). This is invariably the case in muscles where these fibres predominate; they are then affected in the earliest stages of the disease (Pizzey & Barnard 1983b). However, when type IIB fibres occur as a minority in the fibre population of a normal mixed-type fast-twitch muscle (e.g. the red sartorius), they are essentially unaffected by the disease (Barnard et al 1982). The type IIA fast-twitch fibres show a much slower development of the pathological changes (Beringer 1978) and when they constitute the great majority of the fibres in a muscle (as in the adductor superficialis muscle) they become extremely resistant (Barnard et al 1982).

Involvement of the slow-twitch type I fibres has been much studied in the human muscular dystrophies. In the avian model there are several interesting findings (Pizzey et al 1983). In the PLD muscle, only a few of these type I fibres are present and these are resistant to the disease, despite the great changes occurring in their type IIB neighbours. However, in the serratus metapagialis (SMP) muscle, which has a similar overall fibre composition to the PLD, *both* the type IIB and the type I fibres show severe progressive histopathological transformations from the earliest stages of development (Pizzey et al 1983). These findings have been confirmed in freeze-fracture studies (McLean et al 1986), where the sarcolemmal caveolae (see above) do not show the dystrophic change in the type I fibres of the PLD but do show it in the type I fibres of the SMP.

These results of differential expression are of interest for two reasons. First, they demonstrate that slow-twitch chicken muscles do not possess an inherent genetic resistance to the dystrophic process. Secondly, they suggest that the probability of overt pathological change in a dystrophic chicken muscle fibre is determined by its neighbours *or* by its degree of use. A hypothesis which can encompass all of the variations noted is that chronic disuse or infrequent exercise renders the muscle fibres more susceptible to the action of the dystrophic gene. The postural function of the tonic muscles means that these are consistently in a stimulated state, and those fibres are resistant. The muscles which are used in some aspect of flight or wing movement in other birds are mostly disused in this flightless species: this feature would explain the rapid deterioration of the pectoral, biceps, PLD, SMP and similar muscles in the dystrophic chicken. A minority of slow-twitch fibres in one of these fast-twitch muscles may or may not receive much natural stimulation, depending upon the size and position of the muscle itself. The type II fibres in the leg muscles of the chicken, and the muscles rich in type I fibres, get much more use and are more retarded in their pathological change.

Moderate, repetitive exercise has, in fact, been shown to delay pathological changes in the dystrophic chicken (Entrikin et al 1978). There have been claims for such an effect in human muscular dystrophy, too, as noted by Dubowitz & Heckmatt (1980). A related effect may underlie the beneficial results of chronic low-frequency electrical stimulation upon the dystrophic chicken muscle (Barnard et al 1986). After about three weeks of stimulation (by a totally implanted device) of the PLD muscle in vivo at 10 Hz, extensive correction is observed in the histopathology, fibre-type changes, nucleus distribution and enzymic content of the dystrophic muscle.

Enzymic changes. Almost all of the enzymes and other proteins which are in any way characteristic of skeletal muscle have been examined at some time for possible changes in this genetic myopathy. Four types of change have been detected:

1. Some enzymes appear in abnormally high amounts in the blood plasma. These include creatine kinase, pyruvate kinase (EC 2.7.1.40) (Liu et al 1980), phosphoglycerate mutase (EC 5.4.2.1) (Chown et al 1984), aldolase (fructose-biphosphate aldolase, EC 4.1.2.13), and alkaline phosphatase (EC 3.1.3.1). Often the enzymes concerned

are undetectable in the plasma in the normal state. Glutamate oxaloacetic transaminase (aspartate aminotransferase, EC 2.6.1.1), however, is present in normal chicken plasma, and shows only a modest though significant increase (less than doubled) in the dystrophic plasma (Bhargava et al 1977). The typical time course for the accumulation of this group of enzymes in the plasma is exemplified by the rise of plasma pyruvate kinase which increases between three and 10 weeks of age to reach a plateau (3000–4000 U per ml plasma) and later declines slowly (Liu et al 1980).

2. A number of enzymes are significantly reduced below their usual amounts in the dystrophic muscles, generally to the order of one-third to one-half of the normal muscle content by four to six weeks of age (before the changes in the composition of the tissue complicate concentration measurements). This loss applies only to those muscles that will show gross pathological changes, and is found with most of the enzymes which appear anomalously in the blood, suggesting the obvious possibility that this loss is due to a simple escape from defective muscle cells. Enzymes declining significantly and persistently in the dystrophic muscle include creatine kinase, pyruvate kinase, aldolase, lactate dehydrogenase (EC 1.1.1.28) (Chown et al 1983) and phosphoglycerate mutase (EC 5.4.2.1) (Chown et al 1984).

3. A few enzymes, in contrast, increase in amount in the dystrophic muscle. Increases in the muscle, starting after hatching and soon reaching a stable level of several hundred per cent of the normal value, have been found for the isozyme III of carbonic anhydrase (carbonate dehydratase, EC 4.2.1.1) and for glucose-6-phosphate dehydrogenase (EC 1.1.1.49) (Chown et al 1983). A smaller increase, in older dystrophic birds, has been reported for muscle hexokinase (EC 2.7.1.1) (Woodward et al 1979).

4. Some of the enzymes which undergo one of the aforementioned changes exist in the dystrophic muscle in part in abnormal isoforms, generally showing a persistence of the embryonic type into the adult stage. These include CK, carbonic anhydrase (Chown et al 1983), phosphoglycerate mutase and acetylcholinesterase (AChE EC 3.1.1.7) (Lyles et al 1979, 1982).

A special feature of chicken muscular dystrophy, discovered by B. W. Wilson and colleagues is the large increase in acetylcholinesterase which occurs in the affected muscles and its concurrent appearance in large quantities in the plasma, see Wilson et al 1979. The time course of these changes, in the muscle and blood, of the production of anomalous forms of the enzyme has been charted in detail (Lyles et al 1979, 1980). These changes begin in the late embryonic stage. The more severe the pathological change in a muscle type in the dystrophic chicken, the greater these effects upon the muscle acetylcholinesterase (Lyles et al 1982). No changes occur in this enzyme in cardiac muscle or in nerves.

Not all of the enzymes which decline in the dystrophic muscle accumulate in the plasma. Lactate dehydrogenase is such an exception (Bhargava et al 1977); phosphorylase (EC 2.4.1.1) is another. Very different rates of accumulation of the various enzymes in the blood are seen. This must be due at least in part to different susceptibilities to destruction in the blood and to clearance therefrom. In some cases the muscle origin of the elevated plasma enzyme has been established by demonstrating that it is a tissue-specific isozyme.

Inherited myopathies in other birds

Ducks. A mutant strain of the White Pekin duck (*Anas platyrhynchis*) was shown by Rigdon (1966) to inherit a progressive myopathy. The clinical features include loss of ambulation by the age of three weeks, low body weight and a shortened life span. Contractures of the leg muscles commonly develop. Histopathological change develops rapidly in this mutant, the muscles showing extensive necrosis and fibrosis by one month (Gopalakrishnakone & Voon 1985). Fatty degeneration appears, but is less than that in human Duchenne dystrophy (Rigdon 1966). As in chicken muscular dystrophy, electron-microscopic examination shows that, even in the early stages, there is disorientation and proliferation of the transverse tubules and dilatation of the sarcoplasmic reticulum. A large number of vacuoles appear beneath the sarcolemma and around the transverse tubules, and Z-line thickening followed by the disruption of the myofilaments develops. A feature more specific for the duck myopathy is a large accumulation of glycogen in the presynaptic terminals of the end-plates: this has been attributed to a secondary degenerative change in this species (Gopalakrishnakone & Voon 1985).

Turkeys. A relatively common myopathy in commercial flocks of breeder turkeys, deep pectoral myopathy or Oregon disease (Harper et al 1975), is genetically determined but environmental factors control its expression. In gross appearance, this lesion starts with reddish discoloration of the breast musculature, followed by oedema and swelling, and later a necrotic, hard-textured centre develops with a characteristic green colour (Siller et al 1979). By about 40 weeks the condition is apparent externally. It is unusual in being confined almost exclusively to a single muscle, the supracoracoid, which is adjacent to the larger pectoralis muscle.

The green colour and the oedema are attributable to haemorrhagic infarction of this muscle. The histological picture (Henrichs et al 1979, Swash et al 1980) is consistent with this. The intramuscular capillaries have disappeared in the lesioned zone and other blood vessels are generally empty. Endomysial tissue is fragmented or lost, the nuclei disappear and necrosis spreads from the centre.

It appears that genetic selection in the commercial stocks of turkeys, in which heavily hypertrophied muscles are sought in the breeding, has led to an overdevelopment of the supracoracoid muscle without a matched increase in its vascular supply (Henrichs et al 1979). In some pedigrees this can be extreme enough to produce this ischaemia when some sudden exercise is given, e.g. the wing-flapping which occurs when the birds are weighed (Siller et al 1979). In confirmation, electrical stimulation of the motor nerves to the breast muscles produces the supracoracoid lesions in these genetically susceptible birds (Wight et al 1979). The restriction to the supracoracoid, among the over-developed muscles, has been explained as due to its oxidative fibre type and to the more distal branching of arterial supply to, and the inelastic fascial sheath around, this particular muscle, giving a local pressure rise after exercise (Henrichs et al 1979, Swash et al 1980).

Quail. A myopathy which has been characterised and maintained in this species by a group of workers in Japan (Murakami et al 1982) is of interest because it is one of the rare cases in which a genetic storage myopathy has been maintained in a breeding colony of mutant animals, and is the only avian storage disorder yet known.

The disorder is a deficiency of acid maltase (Type II glycogenosis) and occurred spontaneously in a Japanese quail, which developed difficulty in wing-lifting at six weeks of age. A breeding colony of these quails was established, in which the inheritance of the trait is autosomal recessive. In the extent and tissue distribution of the glycogen increase, the clinical course and the histopathology, this avian defect provides a close model for the late-onset form of Pompe's disease in man. In the homozygotes the skeletal muscle weakness first develops at about six weeks of age (Fujita et al 1986) and is progressive, leading to wing dysfunction at about three months, severe wing contractures and emaciation. The lifespan is about half that of the normal quail under comparable conditions. By three months the affected muscle fibres develop numerous glycogen-rich vacuoles, as well as glycogen deposits elsewhere in the muscle fibre. Many fibres are increased in size, and adipose replacement subsequently predominates (Murakami et al 1982).

The glycogen content of the first-affected muscles is increased three- to four-fold compared with the normal (Murakami et al 1982). However, the accumulations in the heart and liver of the mutant quail were greater still (in contrast to the human disorder). The pathology is largely confined to the skeletal muscles.

The content of the skeletal muscle acid α-glucosidase is always abnormally low in the mutants. This enzyme has a residual activity of 10–15% of the normal, and this is true from day 14 of embryonic life (Usuki et al 1986). The glycogen content of the mutant embryonic muscle is, however, normal and this has been attributed to the activity of the embryonic form of neutral α-glucosidase, also present and normal.

COMPARISONS OF AVIAN AND OTHER MYOPATHIES

The chicken myopathy described above will be seen to have a number of features which resemble those of human X-linked muscular dystrophies. The mutation is autosomal in the chicken, but this does not per se exclude similarity in the molecular origin: in birds the chromosomal pattern of sex determination is reversed relative to that of mammals, and the total number of chromosomes is approximately doubled in the birds. These factors make it impossible at present to predict where a gene present on the X-chromosome in man is likely to be located in a bird. Further, because of the very different developmental patterns, the effects of a given mutation at an equivalent locus in the two cases would not be expected to agree in all respects.

Similar comments apply to the duck myopathy described above. This has a great deal in common with the chicken muscular dystrophy, but diverges in some important points of detail: thus, the contractures, hind-limb deformation and subsequent paralysis are much more prominent in the duck. Some significant differences remain between avian myopathy and human Duchenne muscular dystrophy (DMD) (e.g. some points of histopathology differ; the time course of plasma CK appearance shows a delayed peak in the avian forms but a progressive decline from the earliest stages in DMD; AChE is little changed in DMD but greatly increased in chicken dystrophy). The general question remains, therefore, as to whether inherited myopathies with many features in common, but with some differences, can be determined to be due to differential expression of a mutation or deletion at a truly equivalent locus, or whether convergence in myopathic development can occur from origins in entirely different mutant genetic loci. Molecular genetic approaches have not yet been extended to the avian myopathies.

In this context, illustrations of how quite similar skeletal muscle pathologies can arise from diverse aetiologies are brought to our attention by some of the nutritionally-induced myopathies. Deprivation in chickens or ducks of vitamin E or of selenium produces a myopathy which is similar in many features to the genetic forms described above (Sweeny et al 1972, Sweeny & Brown 1981) but differs from them in that these changes are reversed specifically by the missing nutrient, whereas the vitamin E or selenium administration has no significant beneficial effect on the inherited forms.

The disease in the turkey appears to be of a quite different character from that in the chicken and duck, and to be due to an inherited susceptibility to muscle ischaemia. The peculiarities of the genetic overdevelopment of the breast muscles and the anatomical enclosure of the supracoracoid muscle produce a special effect in this case. It has been noted by Henrichs et al (1979) that there is a marked similarity of turkey Oregon disease to a human myopathy, namely the anterior tibial compartment syndrome. In both disorders, the anatomical compartmentalisation of the single target muscle, provocation by unusual exercise stress and ischaemic pathology are important factors.

The glycogen storage myopathy of the Japanese quail shows striking resemblances to the human Type II glycogenosis or Pompe's disease. Here the basic defect appears to be essentially the same, i.e. a mutation producing very low activity of acid α-(1,4) glucosidase. Most of the features of the disease are the same in the two species but again some details differ, as can be expected.

It is of interest to compare the pattern in which different muscles are affected by disease, in the metabolic and the dystrophic defects in the two related species, the chicken and the quail. In the glycogen storage myopathy, the pectoral is affected the most severely and the femoral considerably. The PLD and ALD muscles are also affected, about equally, more slowly than the pectoral but still strongly (Murakami et al 1982). In chicken muscular dystrophy, the pectoral and (rather more slowly) the PLD muscles are very strongly affected, the femoral much more slowly and the ALD and other tonic muscles not at all (Barnard et al 1982). Hence the avian slow-twitch and tonic muscle fibres are not immune to the progressive changes of myopathic degeneration, if the causative factor (glycogen storage) is sufficiently general.

It can be concluded that the well characterised avian genetic myopathies are of interest in understanding the mechanisms of muscle disease pathogenesis and, due to the favourable embryonic accessibility in birds, they have a potential for experimentation which can be relevant to some related human myopathies.

CONCLUDING REMARKS

Although this review has covered a wider range of species and conditions than in the previous edition, it is not intended to be a complete coverage of the subject of animal neuromuscular disease: we have concentrated on conditions of relevance to human disease. Our attempts to classify the animal myopathies have highlighted the frequent overlap in their aetiologies, particularly with regard to the impact of nutritional and stress factors of various types. The reactions of muscle to injury are rather restricted and therefore it is not surprising that the lesions seen in the acute myopathies, in which myodegeneration is a main feature, are similar whereas the initiating factors vary widely, as in selenium/vitamin E-responsive myopathies of the ruminant, PSS, capture myopathies and equine 'tying up'.

We have at various points drawn attention to the fact that, in animals, skeletal myopathies are accompanied by equivalent or even more serious lesions in the myocardium. Nowhere is this more important than in the selenium/vitamin E-responsive myopathies of ruminants. Thus it may be that such geographically isolated diseases as Keshan disease, which is primarily a cardiomyopathy, could have a skeletal component which so far has not been reported. It is not yet known why sometimes cardiac and sometimes skeletal muscle is apparently resistant to disease whereas on other occasions both are susceptible.

The potential for regeneration in damaged muscle is well exemplified in the nutritional and exertional myopathies of animals. However, there are relatively few pathological studies demonstrating the results of repair in relation to fibre-type distribution. What happens to the terminal axon, motor end-plate and cell type of a myocyte that is destroyed but replaced? How similar is this to the effects of denervation followed by reinnervation?

Another area of possible value for future exploitation is the potential of satellite cells to regenerate myocytes, utilising the remaining endomyseal tube as a preformed template to assure correct orientation and growth. Transplantation of such cells from one muscle to another within an individual should avoid rejection problems. Could they not also be used in damaged cardiac muscle which has little or no powers of regeneration following injury due to the absence of satellite cells?

It is very clear that the study of animal myopathies has great relevance to human muscle disease. This is particularly true for malignant hyperpyrexia in man and pigs. The pig is a very useful and under-utilised model for human disease. It has similar omnivorous eating habits and a simple and similar alimentary tract. It has a relatively short gestation (114 days), large litter size (c15), it grows rapidly and healthy animals can be used for human consumption. It is surprising, therefore, that it is not utilised more as an experimental model. At the same time, however, we must always be cautious in relating findings from one species to another. In the pig there is a wide variation of cell-type proportion in different muscles or even in different parts of the same muscle. Myocytes in 'improved' adults are larger than those of most if not all other species. Type I cells in some normal muscles occur in island groups suggestive to the uninitiated of type-grouping resultant upon denervation atrophy. To the muscle researcher these differences can be exploited as they have been in the past by the cross-innervation studies between white and red muscles.

Various forms of myotonia and storage myopathies have counterparts in animals and there is a growing number of spinal muscular atrophy-like conditions in animals of potential value as models. A number of these affect companion animals and there is growing resentment in some parts of the population when such animals are needlessly used for experimentation. We have a responsibility as serious scientific researchers to avoid the use of animals where this is unnecessary; but to resolve some of the areas of deficient knowledge there appears as yet to be no satisfactory alternative. In the future, muscle culture techniques and biotechnology in all its forms may well lead to progress without resorting to animal experimentation. In the meantime the medical researcher should be aware of the magnitude of the range of animal myopathies, selecting for study those of promise as animal models of human diseases. As reported by Done (1976), it is unrealistic to seek an exact replica of a disease in man which would clarify all the problems of the analogous human condition. Rather, we should recognise that the genetic diversity of the animal population contributes greatly to the scope of the model system and we should use these models to study the mechanisms involved in this most crippling group of diseases of man.

ACKNOWLEDGEMENTS

We are indebted to numerous colleagues in our respective Institutes and around the world including Dr B F Fell, the co-author of this chapter in the previous edition, and Dr A C Palmer of the Cambridge Veterinary School. We are particularly grateful for the generous gifts of tissues, sections, photographs and unpublished literature that has enabled us to study unfamiliar diseases at first hand. Special acknowledgement has been given under the respective figures. At the Central Veterinary Laboratory we thank particularly Dr P H Anderson and Mr G A H Wells for provision of material and access to data, Mrs R Baldwin, Mrs J Pink and Mrs P Francis for secretarial work and Mrs N Pascoe and Mrs J Cox for typing services. We also thank Dr L R Bridges of Charing Cross and Westminster Medical School and Professor Vanda A Lennon of Mayo Medical School for their personal communications and Dr Linda C Cork of the Johns Hopkins University School of Medicine for provision of the new figures of canine spinal muscular atrophy.

All the illustrations in this chapter are Crown Copyright and we are grateful to the Ministry of Agriculture, Fisheries and Food for permission to reproduce them here.

REFERENCES

Allen E R, Murphy B J 1979 Early detection of inherited muscular dystrophy in chickens. Cell and Tissue Research 197:165

Anderson I 1983 The pathophysiology of post-anaesthetic myopathy and related disease. In: Alley M R (ed) Diseases of muscle and peripheral nerve. Proceedings of the 13th annual meeting of the New Zealand society for veterinary and comparative pathology. Massey University, Palmerston North, p 37

Anderson P H, Berrett S, Patterson D S P 1976 The significance of elevated plasma creatine phosphokinase activity in muscle disease of cattle. Journal of Comparative Pathology 86:531

Anderson P H, Bradley R, Berrett S, Patterson D S P 1977 The sequence of myodegeneration in nutritional myopathy of the older calf. British Veterinary Journal 133:160

Anderson P H, Berrett S, Parker B N J 1985 Suspected selenium poisoning in lambs. Veterinary Record 116:647

Anon 1968 Epidemic cardiac failure in beer drinkers. Nutrition Reviews 26:173

Appleyard S T, Witkowski J A, Shotton D M, Dubowitz V 1982 Distribution of caveolae in Duchenne muscle membranes: a freeze-fracture study. Biology of the Cell 45:273

Ashmore C R, Doerr L 1971 Postnatal development of fiber types in normal and dystrophic skeletal muscle of the chick. Experimental Neurology 30:431

Asmundson V S, Julian L M 1956 Inherited muscle abnormality in the domestic fowl. Journal of Heredity 47:248

Atkinson J B, LeQuire V S 1985 Animal models of human disease. Myotonia congenita. Comparative Pathology Bulletin 17 (No 2):3

Atkinson J B, Swift, L L, Le Quire V S 1981 Myotonia congenita. A histochemical and ultrastructural study in the goat: comparison with abnormalities found in human myotonia dystrophica. American Journal of Pathology 102:324

Bai J, Ge K, Deng X, Wu S, Wang S, Xue A, Su C 1982 The effect of selenium intake on myocardial necrosis induced by Coxsackie viral infection in mice. Yingyang Xuebao 4:235

Baird J D, Johnston K G, Hartley W J 1974 Spastic paresis in Friesian calves. Australian Veterinary Journal 50:239

Banker B Q 1967 A phase and electron microscopic study of dystrophic muscle. 1. The pathological changes in the two-week-old Bar Harbor 129 dystrophic mouse. Journal of Neuropathology and Experimental Neurology 26:259

Banker B Q, Hirst N S, Chester C S, Fok R Y 1979 Histometric and electron cytochemical study of muscle in the dystrophic mouse. Annals of the New York Academy of Sciences 317:115

Barnard E A, Lyles J M, Pizzey J A 1982 Fibre types in chicken skeletal muscles and their changes in muscular dystrophy. Journal of Physiology 331:333

Barnard E A, Barnard P J, Jarvis J C, Lai J 1986 Low frequency chronic electrical stimulation of normal and dystrophic chicken muscle. Journal of Physiology 376:377

Barney G H, Macapinlac M P, Pearson W N, Darby W J 1967 Parakeratosis of the tongue — a unique histopathologic lesion in the zinc-deficient squirrel monkey. Journal of Nutrition 93:511

Bartsch R C, McConnell E E, Imes G D, Schmidt J M 1977 A review of exertional rhabdomyolysis in wild and domestic animals and man. Veterinary Pathology 14:314

Berg B N 1956 Muscular dystrophy in aging rats. Journal of Gerontology 11:134

Bergmann V 1974 Zur Ultrastruktur der Mitochondrien in der Skelettmuskulatur des Schweines: ein Beitrag zur Pathogenese des PSE-Fleisches. Archiv für Experimentelle Veterinärmedizin 28:225

Bergmann V 1975a Vergleich postmortaler Veränderungen der Ultrastruktur im M. masseter und M. longissimus dorsi bei Schweine mit PSE-Fleisch. Archiv für Experimentelle Veterinärmedizin 29:717

Bergmann V 1975b Die Ultrastruktur von PSE-Muskulatur vor und nach der Schlachtung. Monatshefte für Veterinärmedizin 30:285

Beringer T 1978 Stereologic analysis of normal and dystrophic avian αW myofibers. Experimental Neurology 61:380

Bhargava A K, Barnard E A, Hudecki M S 1977 Effects of serotonin antagonists on the development of inherited muscular dystrophy in the chicken. Experimental Neurology 55:583

Biscoe T J, Caddy K W T, Pallot D J, Pehrgon U M M 1975 Investigation of cranial and other nerves in the mouse with muscular dystrophy. Journal of Neurology, Neurosurgery and Psychiatry 38:391

Blaxter K L 1964 Protein metabolism and requirements in pregnancy and lactation. In: Munro H N, Allison, J B (eds) Mammalian protein metabolism, vol 2. Academic Press, New York, p 173

Bonagura J D, O'Grady M 1983 ECG of the month: Muscular dystrophy with involvement of sinoatrial and atrioventricular nodal tissues. Journal of the American Veterinary Medical Association 183:658

Bonillo E, Fischbeck K, Schotland D L 1981 Freeze-fracture studies of muscle caveolae in human muscular dystrophy. American Journal of Pathology 104:167

Bosanquet F D, Daniel P M, Parry H B 1956 Myopathy in sheep. Its relationship to scrapie and to dermatomyositis and muscular dystrophy. Lancet 2:737

Botstein D, White R L, Skolnick M, Davis R W 1980 Construction of a genetic linkage map in man using restriction fragment length polymorphisms. American Journal of Human Genetics 32:314

Bradley R 1975 Selenium deficiency and bovine myopathy. In: Grunsell C S G, Hill F W G (eds) The Veterinary Annual, 15th issue. (Wright-Scientechnica, Bristol), p 27

Bradley R 1979 A primary bovine skeletal myopathy with absence of Z discs, sarcoplasmic inclusions, myofibrillar hypoplasia and nuclear abnormality. Journal of Comparative Pathology 89:381

Bradley R 1980 What do we know about splayleg? Pig Farming 28:51

Bradley R, Terlecki S 1977 Muscle lesions in hereditary 'Daft lamb' disease of Border Leicester sheep. Journal of Pathology 123:225

Bradley R, Wells G A H 1978 Developmental muscle disorders of the pig. The Veterinary Annual, 18th issue (Wright-Scientechnica, Bristol) p 144

Bradley R, Wells G A H, Gray L J 1979 Back muscle necrosis of pigs. Veterinary Record 104:183

Bradley R, Wells G A H 1980 The pietrain 'creeper' pig: a primary myopathy. In: Clifford Rose F, Behan P O (eds) Animal models of neurological disease. Pitman Medical, Tunbridge Wells, p 34

Bradley R, Wijeratne W V S 1980 A locomotor disorder clinically similar to spastic paresis in an adult Friesian bull. Veterinary Pathology 17:305

Bradley R, Ward P S, Bailey J 1980 The ultrastructural morphology of the skeletal muscles of normal pigs and pigs with splayleg from birth to one week of age. Journal of Comparative Pathology 90:433

Bradley R, Fell B F 1981 Myopathies in animals. In: Walton J (ed) Disorders of voluntary muscle, 4th edn. Churchill Livingstone, Edinburgh, p 824

Bradley R, Duffell S J 1982 The pathology of the skeletal and cardiac muscles of cattle with xanthosis. Journal of Comparative Pathology 92:85

Bradley R, Done J T 1986 Nervous and muscular systems. In: Leman A D, Straw B, Glock R D, Mengeling W L, Penny R H C, Scholl E (eds) Diseases of swine, 6th edn. Iowa State University Press, Ames Ch 4

Bradley R, Wells G A H 1987 Developmental skeletal disorders of the pig. The Veterinary Annual, 27th issue (Wright-Scientechnica, Bristol) p 120

Bradley W G, Jaros E 1979 Involvement of peripheral and central nerves in murine dystrophy. Annals of the New York Academy of Sciences 317:132

Braund K G, Hoff E J, Richardson K E Y 1978 Histochemical identification of fiber types in canine skeletal muscle. American Journal of Veterinary Research 39:561

Braund K G, Lincoln C E 1981 Histochemical differentiation of fiber types in neonatal canine skeletal muscle. American Journal of Veterinary Research 42:407

Bryant S H 1979 Myotonia in the goat. Annals of the New York Academy of Sciences 317:314

Bryant S H, Lipicky R J, Herzog W H 1968 Variability of myotonic signs in myotonic goats. American Journal of Veterinary Research 29:2371

Bulfield G, Siller W G, Wight P A L, Moore K J 1984 X-chromosome-linked muscular dystrophy (mdx) in the mouse. Proceedings of the National Academy of Sciences USA 81:1189

Cantin M 1967 Skeletal muscle lesions in iodine-treated rats. Archives of Pathology 83:500

Carden A E, Hill W G, Webb A J 1983 The inheritance of halothane susceptibility Genetique Selection Evolution 15:65

Cardinet G H, Wallace L J, Feede M R, Guffy M M, Bardens J W 1969 Developmental myopathy in the canine with type II muscle fibre hypotrophy. Archives of Neurology 21:620

Cardinet G H, Holliday T A 1979 Neuromuscular diseases of domestic animals: A summary of muscle biopsies from 159 cases. Annals of the New York Academy of Sciences 317:290

Caulfield J B 1966 Electron microscopic observations on the dystrophic hamster muscle. Annals of the New York Academy of Sciences 138:151

Caulfield J B 1972 Striated muscle lesions in dystrophic hamsters. Progress in Experimental Tumor Research 16:274

Ceh L, Hauge J G, Svenkerud R, Strande A 1976 Glycogenosis type III in the dog. Acta Veterinaria Scandinavica 17:210

Charlton K M, Claborn L D, Pierce K R 1970 A neuropathy in goats caused by experimental coyotillo (Karwinskia humboldtiana) poisoning: clinical and neurophysiologic studies. American Journal of Veterinary Research 32:1381

Cheah K S, Cheah A M 1981a Mitochondrial calcium transport and calcium-activated phospholipase in porcine malignant hyperthermia. Biochimica et Biophysica Acta 634:70

Cheah K S, Cheah A M 1981b Skeletal muscle mitochondrial phospholipase A_2 and the interaction of mitochondria and sarcoplasmic reticulum in porcine malignant hyperthermia. Biochimica et Biophysica Acta 638:40

Cheah K S, Cheah A M, Crosland A R, Casey J C, Webb A J 1984 Relationship between Ca^{2+} release, sarcoplasmic Ca^{2+}, glycolysis and meat quality in halothane-sensitive and insensitive pigs. Meat Science 10:117

Chen X, Yang G, Chen J, Chen X, Wen Z, Ge K 1980 Studies on the relations of selenium and Keshan disease. Biological Trace Element Research 2:91

Chown P, Moyle S, Jeffrey S, Carter N D, Barnard E A, Barnard P J 1983 Elevations of muscle carbonic anhydrase III and glucose-6-phosphate dehydrogenase during dystrophic chicken development. Neurochemical Pathology 1:279

Chown P, Barnard E A, Barnard P J, Liu P K S, Carter N D 1984 Plasma phosphoglycerate mutase as a marker of muscular dystrophy. Journal of the Neurological Sciences 65:201

Chrisman C L 1982 Problems in small animal neurology. Lea and Febiger, Philadelphia, p 345

Chung L S, Morton N E, Peters J A 1960 Serum enzymes and genetic carriers in muscular dystrophy. American Journal of Human Genetics 12:52

Cork L C, Griffin J W, Munnell J F, Lorenz M D, Adams R J, Price D L 1979 Hereditary canine spinal muscular atrophy. Journal of Neuropathology and Experimental Neurology 38:209

Cork L C, Griffin J W, Adams R J, Price D L 1980 Hereditary canine spinal muscular atrophy. American Journal of Pathology 100:599

Cosmos E, Butler J 1967 Differentiation of fiber types in muscle of normal and dystrophic chickens. In: Milhorat A T (ed) Exploratory concepts in muscular dystrophy and related disorders. Excerpta Medica, Amsterdam, p 197

Crowe L M, Baskin R J 1979 Stereologic analysis of dystrophic chicken muscle. American Journal of Pathology 95:295

Crowe M W, Pike H T 1973 Congenital arthrogryposis associated with ingestion of tobacco stalks by pregnant sows. Journal of the American Veterinary Medical Association 162:453

Cummings J F, de Lahunta A, Timoney J F 1979 Neuritis of the cauda equina, a chronic idiopathic polyradiculoneuritis in the horse. Acta Neuropathologica (Berlin) 46:17

Cunha T J 1968 Spraddled hind legs may be a result of choline deficiency. Feedstuffs (Minneapolis) 40: No. 10, 25

Dangain J, Vrbová G 1984 Muscle development in mdx mutant mice. Muscle and Nerve 7:700

Darke P G G, McCullagh K G, Geldart P H 1975 Myasthenia gravis, thymoma and myositis in a dog. Veterinary Record 97:392

Davies A S, Gunn H M 1972 Histochemical fibre types in the mammalian diaphragm. Journal of Anatomy 112:41

Dawson J R B 1970 Myasthenia gravis in a cat. Veterinary Record 86: 562–563

de Lahunta A 1983 Veterinary neuro-anatomy and clinical neurology, 2nd edn. W B Saunders, Philadelphia, p 87

Di Giamberardino L, Couraud J Y, Barndard E A 1979 Normal axonal transport of acetylcholinesterase forms in peripheral nerves of dystrophic chickens. Brain Research 160:196

Done J T 1976 Developmental disorders of the nervous system in animals. Advances in Veterinary Science and Comparative Medicine 20:69

Done J T, Allen W M, Bailey J, De Gruchy P H, Curran, M K 1975 Asymmetric hindquarter syndrome (AHQS) in the pig. Veterinary Record 96:482

Dubowitz V, Heckmatt J 1980 Management of muscular dystrophy. British Medical Bulletin 36:139

Duchen L W, Strich S J 1968 An hereditary motor neurone disease with progressive denervation of muscle in the mouse: the mutant 'Wobbler'. Journal of Neurology, Neurosurgery and Psychiatry 31:535

Duchen L W, Searle A G, Strich S J 1967 An hereditary motor end-plate disease in the mouse. Journal of Physiology (London) 189:4

Duncan I D, Griffiths I R 1983 Myotonia in the dog. In: Kirk R W (ed) Current veterinary therapy VIII. Small animal practice. Saunders, London, p 686

Duncan I D, Griffiths I R 1984 Peripheral neuropathies of domestic animals. In: Dyck P J, Thomas P K, Lambert E H, Bunge R (eds) Peripheral neuropathies, vol 1. Saunders, London, p 707

Duncan I D, Griffiths I R, Nash A S 1977 Myotonia in canine Cushing's disease. Veterinary Record 100:30

Edwards J R, Richards R B 1979 Bovine generalised glycogenosis type II: a clinico-pathological study. British Veterinary Journal 135:338

Edwards R H T 1979 Physiological and metabolic studies of the contractile machinery of human muscle in health and disease. Physics in Medicine and Biology 24:237

Entrikin R K, Patterson G T, Weidoff P M, Wilson B W 1978 Righting ability and skeletal muscle properties of phenytoin-treated dystrophic chickens. Experimental Neurology 61:650

Entrikin R K, Randall W R, Wilson B W 1982 Myotonic electromyographic activity in complexus muscles of normal and dystrophic chicks. Muscle and Nerve 5:396

Essen B, Lindholm A, Thornton J 1980 Histochemical properties of muscle fibre types and enzyme activities in skeletal muscles of standardbred trotters of different ages. Equine Veterinary Journal 12:175

Farnbach G C 1982 Myotonia. In: Marsmann, McAllister, Pratt (eds) Equine medicine and surgery, 3rd edn. American Veterinary Publications, California, vol II, p 935

Farrow B R H, Malik R 1981 Hereditary myotonia in the Chow Chow. Journal of Small Animal Practice 22:451

Feit H, Kawai M, Schulman M I 1985 Stiffness and contractile properties of normal and dystrophic avian muscle bundles as measured by sinusoidal length perturbations. Muscle and Nerve 8:503

Fell B F 1981 Pathological consequences of copper deficiency and cobalt deficiency. Philosophical Transactions of the Royal Society (London) Series B 294:153

Fidzianska A, Goebel H H, Lenard H G, Heckmann C 1982 Congenital muscular dystrophy (CMD-A collagen formative disease). Journal of the Neurological Sciences 55:79

Friend S C E 1981 Postanesthetic myonecrosis in horses. Canadian Veterinary Journal 22:367

Fujii H, Murota K, Tanzer M I 1983 Abnormal collagen synthesis in skeletal muscle of dystrophic chicken. Biochemical and Biophysical Research Communications III:933

Fujita T, Nonaka I, Takagi A, Sugita H 1986 Muscle histochemistry in Japanese quail with Type 2 glycogenesis (Pompe's disease). Muscle and Nerve 9 (Suppl):186

Funkquist B, Haraldsson I, Stahre L 1980 Primary

progressive muscular dystrophy in the dog. Veterinary Record 106:341

Gardner D E 1967 Skeletal myonecrosis in a cat. New Zealand Veterinary Journal 15:211

Gardner M B 1978 Lower motor neuron disease in wild mice caused by endogenous murine leukaemia virus (MuLV). Comparative Pathology Bulletin 10 (No 2):3

Gardner-Medwin D 1980 Clinical features and classification of muscular dystrophies. British Medical Bulletin 36:109

Goedegebuure S A, Hoebe H P 1976 Zwerchfells-myopathie bei MRY-Rindern. Vortag für die 25. Tagung der Europäischen Gesellschaft für Veterinärpathologie: Freiburg, 8 June 1976

Goedegebuure S A, Hartman W, Hoebe H P 1983 Dystrophy of the diaphragmatic muscles in adult Meuse-Rhine-Yssel cattle: electromyographical and histological findings. Veterinary Pathology 20:32

Gopalakrishnakone P, Voon F C T 1985 Muscular dystrophy in the duck. Laboratory Animals 19:368

Greene C E, Lorenz M D, Munnell J F, Prasse K W, White N A, Bowen J M 1979 Myopathy associated with hyperadrenocorticism in the dog. Journal of the American Veterinary Medical Association 174:1310

Griffin J W, Cork L C, Adams R J, Price D L 1982 Axonal transport in hereditary canine spinal atrophy (HCSMA). Journal of Neuropathology and Experimental Neurology 41:370

Griffiths I R, Duncan I D 1973 Myotonia in the dog: A report of four cases. Veterinary Record 93:184

Griffiths I R, Duncan I D 1979 Distal denervating disease: a degenerative neuropathy of the distal motor axon in dogs. Journal of Small Animal Practice 20:579

Gronert G A 1980 Malignant hyperthermia. Anaesthesiology 53:35

Gunn H M 1975 Adaptations of skeletal muscle that favour athletic ability. New Zealand Veterinary Journal 23:249

Gunn H M 1976 Morphological aspects of the deep digital flexor muscle in horses having rigid flexion of their distal forelimb joints at birth. Irish Veterinary Journal 30:145

Gunther J S, Letinsky M S 1985 Structure of motor nerve terminals in chickens with hereditary muscular dystrophy. Muscle and Nerve 8:568

Guth L, Samaha F J 1970 Procedure for the histochemical demonstration of actomyosin ATPase. Experimental Neurology 28:365

Guy P S, Snow D H 1977 The effect of training and detraining on muscle composition in the horse. Journal of Physiology (London) 269:33

Guy P S, Snow D H 1981 Skeletal muscle fibre composition in the dog and its relationship to athletic ability. Research in Veterinary Science 31:244

Hadlow W J 1962 Diseases of skeletal muscle. In: Innes J R M, Saunders L Z (eds) Comparative neuropathology. Academic Press, New York, p 147

Hadlow W J 1973 Myopathies of animals. In: Pearson C M, Mostofi F K (eds) The striated muscle. International Academy of Pathology. Monograph No. 12. Williams & Wilkins, Baltimore, p 364

Hails M R 1978 Transport stress in animals: a review. Animal Regulation Studies 1:289

Hamilton M J, Hegreberg G A, Gorham J R 1974 Histochemical muscle fibre typing in inherited muscular dystrophy of mink. American Journal of Veterinary Research 35:1321

Harper J A, Bernier P E, Helfer D H, Schmitz J A 1975 Degenerative myopathy of the deep pectoral muscle in the turkey. Journal of Heredity 66:362

Harriman D G F, Summer D W, Ellis F R 1978 Malignant hyperpyrexia myopathy. Quarterly Journal of Medicine 42:639

Harris C I, Milne G 1977 The unreliability of urinary 3-methyl-histidine excretion as a measure of muscle protein degradation in sheep. Proceedings of the Nutrition Society 36:138A.

Harris C I, Milne G, Lobley G E, Nicholas G A 1977 3-methyl histidine as a measure of skeletal-muscle protein catabolism in the adult New Zealand white rabbit. Biochemical Society Transactions 5:706

Harris C I, Milne G 1978 Urinary excretion of 3-methyl histidine in cattle as a measure of muscle protein degradation. Proceedings of the Nutrition Society 38:11A.

Hayakawa J, Tsuji S 1985 A new mutant at the dystrophia muscularis (dy) locus in the SM strain of mice. Laboratory Animals 19:1

Hegreberg G A, & Norby D E 1973 An inherited storage disease of cats. Federation Proceedings. Federation of American Societies for Experimental Biology 32:821

Hegreberg G A 1979 Mink muscular dystrophy. In: Andrews, Ward, Altman (eds) Spontaneous animal models of human disease. Academic Press, New York, vol 2 p 96

Hegreberg G A, Comacho Z, Gorham J R 1974 Histopathologic description of muscular dystrophy of mink. Archives of Pathology 97:225

Hegreberg G A, Padgett G A, Prieur D J, Johnson M I 1975 Genetic studies of a muscular dystrophy of mink. Journal of Heredity 66:63

Henrichs K J, Jones J M, Berry C L, Swash M 1979 Pathogenesis of ischaemic pectoral myopathy in the turkey. British Veterinary Journal 135:286

Herrtage M E, Houlton J E F 1979 Collapsing Clumber spaniels. Veterinary Record 105:334

Higgins R J, Rings D M, Fenner W R, Stevenson S 1983 Spontaneous lower motor neuron disease with neurofibrillary accumulation in young pigs. Acta Neuropathologica (Berlin) 59:288

Hoebe H P 1975 Diaphragm myopathy in Meuse-Rhine-Ijssel cattle. Tijdschrift voor diergeneeskunde 100:1201

Hoekman T B 1976 Isometric contractile properties of the posterior latissimus dorsi muscle in normal and genetically dystrophic chickens. Experimental Neurology 53:729

Holinger P C, Vuckovich D M, Holinger L D, Holinger P H 1979 Bilateral abductor vocal cord paralysis in Charcot–Marie–Tooth disease. Annals of Otology, Rhinology and Laryngology 88:205

Homburger F 1972 Disease models in Syrian hamsters. Progress in Experimental Tumor Research 16:69

Homburger F 1979 Myopathy in the Syrian hamster. In: Andrews, Ward, Altman (eds) Spontaneous animal models of human disease. Academic Press, New York, vol 2 p 94

Homburger F, Baker J R, Nixon C W, Wilgram G, Harrop J 1965. The early histopathological lesion of muscular dystrophy in the Syrian golden hamster. Journal of Pathology and Bacteriology 89:133

Hoskins J D, Root C R 1983 Myopathy in a Labrador retriever. Veterinary Medicine and Small Animal Clinician 78:1387

Houlton J E F, Herrtage M E 1980 Mitochondrial myopathy in the Sussex spaniel. Veterinary Record 106:206

Howell J McC 1978 The pathology of chronic copper

poisoning in sheep. In: Kirchgessner M (ed) Trace element metabolism in man and animals 3. Arbeitskreis für Tierernährungsforschung Weihenstephan, p 536

Howell J McC, Dorling P R, Cook R D, Robinson W F, Bradley S, Gawthorne J M 1981 Infantile and late onset form of generalised glycogenosis type II in cattle. Journal of Pathology 134:267

Hulland T J 1985 Muscles and tendons. In: Jubb K V F, Kennedy P C, Palmer N (eds) Pathology of domestic animals, 3rd edn. Academic Press, Orlando, vol 1 p 139

Inada S, Sakamoto H, Haruta K, Miyazono Y, Sasaki M 1978 A clinical study on hereditary progressive neurogenic muscular atrophy in Pointer dogs. Japanese Journal of Veterinary Science 40:539

Indrieri R J, Creighton S R, Lambert E H, Lennon V A 1983. Myasthenia gravis in two cats. Journal of the American Veterinary Medical Association 182:57

Innes J R M 1951 Myopathies in animals. British Veterinary Journal 107:131

Innes J R M, Saunders L Z 1962 Comparative neuropathology. Academic Press, New York

Isaacs E R, Bradley W G, Henderson G 1973 Longitudinal fibre splitting in muscular dystrophy: a serial cinematographic study. Journal of Neurology, Neurosurgery and Psychiatry 36:813

Izumo S, Ikuta F, Igata A, Osame M, Yamauchi C, Inada S 1983 Morphological study on the hereditary neurogenic amyotrophic dogs: accumulation of lipid compound-like structures in the lower motor neuron. Acta Neuropathologica (Berlin) 61:270

Jenkins W L, van Dyk E, McDonald C B 1976 Myasthenia gravis in a Fox Terrier litter. Journal of the South African Veterinary Association 47:59

Johannsen U, Menger S, von Lengerken G 1982 Comparative studies into ultrastructure of skeletal muscles (M. longissimus dorsi) in pig breeds with differentiated resistance to stress — comparison between Duroc and Pietrain. Archiv für experimentelle Veterinärmedizin 36:372

Johansson G, Jönsson L 1977 Myocardial cell damage in the porcine stress syndrome. Journal of Comparative Pathology 87:67

John H A, Purdom I F 1984 Myelin proteins and collagen in the spinal roots and sciatic nerves of muscular dystrophic mice. Journal of the Neurological Sciences 65:69

Johnson E R 1981 Carcass composition of double-muscled cattle. Animal Production 33:31

Johnson R P, Watson A D J, Smith J, Cooper B J 1975. Myasthenia in Springer Spaniel littermates. Journal of Small Animal Practice 16:641

Jones B R, Anderson L J, Barnes G R G, Johnstone A C, Juby W D 1977 Myotonia in related Chow Chow dogs. New Zealand Veterinary Journal 25:217

Jones B R, Johnstone A C 1982 An unusual myopathy in a dog. New Zealand Veterinary Journal 30:119

Jones T C, Hunt R D 1983 Veterinary pathology, 5th edn. Lea and Febiger, Philadelphia, p 1792

Jönsson L, Karlsson S, Thoren-Tolling K, Johansson G, Häggendal J 1984 Cardiac and skeletal muscle changes at transport stress and experimental restraint stress in pigs. In: Mansson I (ed) Proceedings of the 5th International Conference on Production Disease in Farm Animals, August 10–12 1983. Uppsala, Sweden, p 374

Jubb K V F, Kennedy P C, Palmer N 1985 Pathology of domestic animals, 3rd edn. Academic Press, Orlando, vol 1 p 139

Karpati G, Carpenter S, Prescott S 1982 Prevention of skeletal muscle fiber necrosis in hamster dystrophy. Muscle and Nerve 5:369

Karpati G, Jacob P, Carpenter S, Prescott S 1985 Hypophysectomy mitigates skeletal muscle fibre damage in hamster dystrophy. Annals of Neurology 17:60

Keeler R F, Balls L D, Panter K 1981 Teratogenic effects of Nicotiana glauca and concentrations of anabasine, the suspect teratogen in plant parts. Cornell Veterinarian 71:47

Keith J R 1981 Spastic paresis in beef and dairy cattle. Veterinary Medicine and Small Animal Clinician 76:1043

Kendeel S R M, Ferris J A J 1977 Sudden infant death syndrome: a review of literature. Journal of the Forensic Science Society (Harrogate) 17:223

King J W B, Menissier F (eds) 1982 Muscle hypertrophy of genetic origin and its use to improve beef production. Nijhoff, The Hague p 658

Kornegay J N 1984 Golden retriever myopathy. Proceedings of the XII Annual Scientific program of the American College of Veterinary Internal Medicine May 17–20 1984, Washington DC

Kramer J W, Hegreberg G A, Bryan G M, Meyers K, Ott R L 1976 A muscle disorder of Labrador retrievers characterised by deficiency of type II muscle fibres. Journal of the American Veterinary Medical Association 169:817

Kramer J W, Hegreberg G A, Hamilton M J 1981 Inheritance of a neuromuscular disorder of Labrador retriever dogs. Journal of the American Veterinary Medical Association 179:380

Lamb R C, Arave C W, Shupe J L 1976 Inheritance of limber legs in Jersey cattle. Journal of Heredity 67:241

Leipold H W, Blaugh B, Huston K, Edgerly C G M, Hibbs C M 1973 Weaver syndrome in Brown Swiss Cattle: clinical signs and pathology. Veterinary Medicine and Small Animal Clinician 68:645

Lennon V A, Lambert E H, Palmer A C, Cunningham J G, Christie T R 1981 Acquired and congenital myasthenia gravis in dogs — a study of 20 cases. In: Satoyoshi E (ed) Myasthenia gravis: pathogenesis and treatment. University of Tokyo Press, Tokyo, p 41

Libelius R, Jirmanova I, Lundquist I, Thesleff S, Barnard E A 1979 T-tubule endocytosis in dystrophic chicken muscle and its relation to muscle fiber degeneration. Acta Neuropathologica 48:31

Lindsay W A, McDonell W, Bignell W 1980 Equine postanesthetic forelimb lameness: Intracompartmental muscle pressure changes and biochemical patterns. American Journal of Veterinary Research 41:1919

Liu P K S, Barnard E A, Barnard P J 1980 Blood plasma pyruvate kinase as a marker of muscular dystrophy — Properties in dystrophic chickens and hamsters. Experimental Neuropathy 67:581

Lorenz M D, Cork L C, Griffin J W, Adams R J, Price D L 1979 Hereditary spinal muscular atrophy in Brittany Spaniels: clinical manifestations. Journal of the American Veterinary Medical Association 175:833

Lyles J M, Silman I, Barnard E A 1979 Developmental changes in levels and forms of cholinesterases in muscles of normal and dystrophic chickens. Journal of Neurochemistry 33:727

Lyles J M, Barnard E A, Silman I 1980 Changes in the levels and forms of cholinesterases in the blood plasma of normal and dystrophic chickens. Journal of Neurochemistry 34:978

Lyles J M, Silman I, Di Giamberardino L, Couraud J–Y, Barnard E A 1982 Comparison of the molecular forms of the cholinesterases in tissues of normal and dystrophic chickens. Journal of Neurochemistry 38:1007

MacDonald D W, Christian R G, Strausz K I, Roff J 1981 Acute selenium toxicity in neonatal calves. Canadian Veterinary Journal 22: 279–281

McGavin M D 1974 Progressive ovine muscular dystrophy. Comparative Pathology Bulletin VI:3

McGavin M D, Baynes I D 1969 A congenital progressive ovine muscular dystrophy. Pathologia Veterinaria, 6:513

McKerrell R E, Anderson J R, Herrtage M E, Littlewood J D, Palmer A C 1984 Generalised muscle weakness in the Labrador Retriever. Veterinary Record 115:276

McLaughlin B G, Doige C E 1981 Congenital musculoskeletal lesions and hyperplastic goitre in foals. Canadian Veterinary Journal 22:130

McLean B, Mazen-Lynch L, Shotton D M 1986 Quantitative freeze-fracture studies of membrane changes in chicken muscular dystrophy. Muscle and Nerve 9:501

MacPike A D, Meier H 1976 Comparison of dy and dy²ᴶ, two alleles expressing forms of muscular dystrophy in the mouse. Proceedings of the Society for Experimental Biology and Medicine 151:670

Maltin C A, Duncan L, Wilson A B 1983a Mitochondrial abnormalities in muscle from vitamin B_{12}-deficient sheep. Journal of Comparative Pathology 93:429

Maltin C A, Duncan L, Wilson A B, Hesketh J E 1983b Effect of zinc deficiency on muscle fibre type frequencies in the post-weanling rat. British Journal of Nutrition 50:597

Manktelow B W, Hartley W J 1975 Generalized glycogen storage disease in sheep. Journal of Comparative Pathology 85:139

Mann S O, Fell B F, Dalgarno A C 1974 Observations on the bacterial flora and pathology of the tongue of sheep deficient in zinc. Research in Veterinary Science 17:91

Mason K V 1976 A case of myasthenia gravis in a cat. Journal of Small Animal Practice 17:467

Mason T A 1981 A high incidence of congenital angular limb deformities in a group of foals. Veterinary Record 109:93

Mayhew I G 1984 Neuromuscular arthrogryposis multiplex congenita in a thoroughbred foal. Veterinary Pathology 21:187

Meier H 1958 Myopathies in the dog. Cornell Veterinarian 48:313

Meier H, Southard J L 1970 Muscular dystrophy in the mouse caused by an allele at the dy-locus. Life Sciences 9:137

Meijer A E F H 1983 The histochemical demonstration of loosely coupled mitochondria in human skeletal muscle. Histochemical Journal 15:331

Mendell J R, Higgins R, Sahenk Z, Cosmos E 1979 Relevance of genetic animal models of muscular dystrophy to human muscular dystrophies. Annals of the New York Academy of Sciences 317:409

Mendlowski B 1975 Neuromuscular lesions in restrained rabbits. Veterinary Pathology 12: 378:386

Mercer H D, Neal F C, Himes J A, Edds G T 1967 Cassia occidentalis toxicosis in cattle. Journal of the American Veterinary Medical Association 151:735

Michelson A M, Russell E S, Harman P J 1955 Dystrophia Muscularis: A hereditary primary myopathy in the house mouse. Proceedings of the National Academy of Sciences 41:1079

Mills J H L, Nielsen S W 1968 Porcine polioencephalomyelitides. Advances in Veterinary Science 12:33

Milne G, Harris C I 1978 The inadequacy of urinary 3-methylhistidine excretion as an index of muscle protein degradation in the pig. Proceedings of the Nutrition Society 37:18A

Mostafa I E 1970 A case of glycogenic cardiomegaly in a dog. Acta Veterinaria Scandinavica 11:197

Muir A R 1970 Normal and regenerating skeletal muscle fibres in Pietrain pigs. Journal of Comparative Pathology 80:137

Murakami H, Takagi A, Nonaka I, Ishiura S, Sugita H Mizutani M 1982 Type 2 glycogen storage disease in Japanese quails. In: Ebashi S (ed) Muscular dystrophy. University of Tokyo Press, Tokyo, p 37

Naerland G 1940 Forekommer dobbelenderkarakteren hos andre husdyrarter enn storfe? Universell hyperplasi av stammens og lemmens muskulatur hos sau. Skandinavisk Veterinärtidskrift 30:813

Nafe L A, Shires P K 1984 Myotonia in the dog. Proceedings of the XII Annual Scientific Program of the American College of Veterinary Internal Medicine May 17–20 1984, Washington DC

Nicholson G A, Matheson E 1981 Plasma creatine kinase isoenzymes in the Bar Harbor dystrophic mouse. Journal of the Neurological Sciences 51:3

Nieberle K, Cohrs P 1967 Textbook of the special pathological anatomy of domestic animals, 1st English edn. Pergamon Press, Oxford, p 881

Oda K, Lennon V A, Lambert E H, Palmer A C 1984 Congenital myasthenia gravis II: Acetylcholine receptor metabolism. Muscle and Nerve 7:717

Oghiso Y, Kubokawa K, Lee Y–S, Fujiwara K 1976 Clinical and pathological studies on a spontaneous case of canine systemic atrophic myositis. Japanese Journal of Veterinary Science, 38:553

Ormrod A N 1961 Myasthenia gravis in a Cocker Spaniel. Veterinary Record 73:489

O'Sullivan B M 1976 Humpy back of sheep, clinical and pathological observations. Australian Veterinary Journal 52:414

O'Sullivan B M, Healy P J, Fraser I R, Nieper R E, Whittle R J, Sewell C A 1981 Generalised glycogenosis in Brahman cattle. Australian Veterinary Journal 57:227

Pai A C 1965(a) Developmental genetics of a lethal mutation, muscular dysgenesis (mdg) in the mouse. I Genetic analysis and gross morphology. Developmental Biology 11:82

Pai A C 1965(b) Developmental genetics of a lethal mutation, muscular dysgenesis (mdg) in the mouse. II Developmental analysis. Developmental Biology 11:93

Palmer A C 1976 Introduction to Animal Neurology. 2nd edn. Blackwell Scientific Publications Oxford

Palmer A C, Barker J 1974 Myasthenia in the dog. Veterinary Record 95:452

Palmer A C, Woodham C B 1975 Derrengue, a paralysis of cattle in El Salvador ascribed to ingestion of Melochia pyramidata. Veterinary Record 96:547

Palmer E G, Topel D G, Christian L L 1977 Microscopic observations of muscle from swine susceptible to malignant hyperthermia. Journal of Animal Science 45:1032

Parry H B 1983 Scrapie disease in sheep. Academic Press, London, p 127

Pearce G W, Walton J N 1963 A histological study of muscle

from the Bar Harbor strain of dystrophic mice. Journal of Pathology and Bacteriology 86:25

Pizzey J A, Barnard E A 1983a Structural change in muscles of the dystrophic chicken. I. Quantitative indices. Neuropathology and Applied Neurobiology 9:21

Pizzey J A, Barnard E A 1983b Structural change in muscles of the dystrophic chicken. II. Progression of the histopathology in the pectoralis muscle. Neuropathology and Applied Neurobiology 9:149

Pizzey J A, Barnard E A, Barnard P J 1983 Involvement of fast and slow twitch muscle fibres in avian muscular dystrophy. Journal of the Neurological Sciences 61:217

Porter C W, Barnard E A 1976 Ultrastructural studies on the acetylcholine receptor at motor endplates of normal and pathological muscles. Annals of the New York Academy of Sciences 274:85

Prince F P, Hikida R S, Hagerman F C, Staron R S, Allen W H 1981 A morphometric analysis of human muscle fibers with relation to fiber types and adaptations to exercise. Journal of the Neurological Sciences 49:165

Rafiquzzaman M, Svenkerud R, Strande A Hauge J G 1976 Glycogenosis in the dog. Acta Veterinaria Scandinavica 17:196

Richards R B, Edwards J R, Cook R D, White R R 1977 Bovine generalised glycogenosis. Neuropathology and Applied Neurobiology 3:45

Rigdon R H 1966 Hereditary myopathy in the White Pekin duck. Annals of the New York Academy of Sciences 138:28

Ringqvist M 1973 Histochemical enzyme profiles of fibres in human masseter muscles with special regard to fibres with intermediate myofibrillar ATPase reaction. Journal of the Neurological Sciences 18:133

Rings D M, Hoffsis G F, Donham J C 1976 A myotonia-like syndrome in sheep. Speculum 28:13

Ronéus B, Lindholm A, Jönsson L 1983 Myotoni hos häst. Svensk Veterinartidning 35:217

Rousseaux C G, Klavano G G, Johnson E S, Shnitka T K, Harries W N, Snyder F F 1985 'Shaker' calf syndrome: a newly recognized inherited neurodegenerative disorder of horned Hereford calves. Veterinary Pathology 22:104

Rüdel R, Lehmann-Horn F 1985 Membrane changes in cells from myotonia patients. Physiological Reviews 65:310

Russell R G, Doige C E, Oteruelo F T, Hare D, Singh E 1985 Variability in limb malformations and possible significance in the pathogenesis of an inherited congenital neuromuscular disease of Charolais cattle (syndrome or arthrogryposis and palatoschisis). Veterinary Pathology 22:2

Sack G H, Cork L C, Morris J M, Griffin J W, Price D L 1984 Autosomal dominant inheritance of hereditary canine spinal muscular atrophy. Annals of Neurology 15:369

Sandefeldt E, Cummings J F, de Lahunta A, Bjorck G, Krook L P 1976 Hereditary neuronal abiotrophy in Swedish Lapland dogs. American Journal of Pathology 82:649

Sandström B, Westman J, Ockerman P A 1969 Glycogenosis of the central nervous system in the cat. Acta Neuropathologica (Berlin) 14:194

Scarlato G, Meola G 1978 Chronic myopathy with cytoplasmic bodies in the pig. Journal of Comparative Pathology 88:31

Seeler D C, McDonell W N, Basrur P K 1983 Halothane and halothane/succinylcholine induced malignant

hyperthermia (Porcine stress syndrome) in a population of Ontario boars. Canadian Journal of Comparative Medicine 47:284

Shields R P, Vandevelde M, 1978 Spontaneous lower motor neuron disease in rabbits (Oryctolagus cuniculus). Acta Neuropathologica 44:55

Shires P K, Nafe L A, Hulse D A 1983 Myotonia in a Staffordshire terrier. Journal of the American Veterinary Medical Association 183:229

Shivers R R, Atkinson B G 1984 The dystrophic murine skeletal muscle cell plasma membrane is structurally intact but 'leaky' to creatine phosphokinase. A freeze-fracture analysis. American Journal of Pathology 116:482

Shortridge E H, O'Hara P J, Marshall P M 1971 Acute selenium poisoning in cattle. New Zealand Veterinary Journal 19:47

Siller W G, Wight P A L, Martindale L 1979 Exercise-induced deep pectoral myopathy in broiler fowls and turkeys. Veterinary Science Communications 2:331

Simpson S T, Braund K G 1985 Myotonic dystrophy-like disease in a dog. Journal of the American Veterinary Medical Association 186:495

Simpson S T, Braund K G, Sorjonen D C 1982 Muscular dystrophy of Labrador Retrievers. Proceedings of the Annual Scientific meeting of the American College of Veterinary Internal Medicine, p 78

Simpson V R 1984 Toxicity of ionophores. Veterinary Record 114:434

Snow D H, Guy P S 1980 Muscle fibre type composition of a number of limb muscles in different types of horse. Research in Veterinary Science 28:137

Snow D H, Baxter P, Rose R J 1981 Muscle fibre composition and glycogen depletion in horses competing in an endurance ride. Veterinary Record 108:374

Snow D H, Billeter R, Mascarello F, Carpene E, Rowlerson A, Jenny E 1982a No classical type IIB fibres in dog skeletal muscle. Histochemistry 75:53

Snow D H, Kerr M G, Nimmo M A, Abbot E M 1982b Alterations in blood, sweat, urine and muscle composition during prolonged exercise in the horse. Veterinary Record 110:377

Sokolove P M 1985 Altered membrane association of glycogen phosphorylase in the dystrophic chicken. Biochimica et Biophysica Acta 841:232

Spurway N 1981 Interrelationship between myosin-based and metabolism-based classifications of skeletal muscle fibers. Journal of Histochemistry and Cytochemistry 29:87

Stansfield D G, Lamont M H 1981 Monensin–tiamulin interactions in pigs. Veterinary Record 109:545

Staron R S, Hagerman F C, Hikida R S 1981 The effects of detraining on an elite power lifter — a case study. Journal of the Neurological Sciences 51:247

Staron R S, Hikida R S, Hagerman F C, Dudley G A, Murray T F 1984 Human skeletal muscle fiber type adaptability to various workloads. Journal of Histochemistry and Cytochemistry 32:146

Steinberg S, Botelho S 1962 Myotonia in a horse. Science 137:979

Stockard C R 1936 An hereditary lethal for localised motor and preganglionic neurones with resulting paralysis in the dog. American Journal of Anatomy 59:1

Stuart L D, Leipold H W 1985 Lesions in bovine progressive degenerative myeloencephalopathy ('Weaver') of Brown Swiss cattle. Veterinary Pathology 22:13

Sullivan N D 1985 The nervous system. In: Jubb K V F, Kennedy P C, Palmer N (eds) Pathology of domestic animals, 3rd edn. Academic Press, Orlando, vol 1 p 201

Suzuki A 1977 A comparative histochemical study of the masseter muscle of the cattle, sheep, swine, dog, guinea pig and rat. Histochemistry 51:121

Svenkerud R, Hauge J G 1978 Animal models of human disease — glycogenosis type III. Comparative Pathology Bulletin 10 (No 2):2

Swash M, Henrichs K J, Berry C L, Jones J M 1980 Deep pectoral myopathy (Oregon Disease) in the turkey. In: Rose F C, Behan P O (eds) Animal models of neurological disease. Pitman Medical, Tunbridge Wells, p 3

Swash M, Schwartz M S 1984 Biopsy pathology of muscle. Chapman and Hall, London, p 111

Swatland H J 1974 Developmental disorders of skeletal muscle in cattle, pigs and sheep. Veterinary Bulletin 44:179

Swatland H J, Cassens R G 1972 Peripheral innervation of muscle from stress-susceptible pigs. Journal of Comparative Pathology 82:229

Sweeny P R, Buchanan-Smith J R, deMille F, Pettit J R Moran E T 1972 Ultrastructure of muscular dystrophy. II. A comparative study in lambs and chickens. American Journal of Pathology 68:493

Sweeny P R, Brown R G 1981 Ultrastructural studies on the gastrocnemius tendon of selenium deficient ducklings. American Journal of Pathology 103:210

Sweeny P R 1983 Ultrastructure of the developing myotendinous junction of genetic dystrophic chickens. Muscle and Nerve 6: 207–217

Taylor A W, Brassard L 1981 Skeletal muscle fiber distribution and area in trained and stalled standardbred horses. Canadian Journal of Animal Science 61:601

Thompson R H, Todd J R 1974 Muscle damage in chronic copper poisoning of sheep. Research in Veterinary Science 16:97

Tilley L P 1985 Essentials of canine and feline electrocardiography, 2nd edn. Lea and Febiger, Philadelphia, p 164

Trojaborg W, Flagstad A 1982 A hereditary neuromuscular disorder in dogs. Muscle and Nerve 5:830

Tunell G L, Hart M N 1977 Simultaneous determination of skeletal muscle fiber, Types I, IIA, and IIB by histochemistry. Archives of Neurology (Chicago) 34:171

Usuki F, Ishiura S, Sugita H 1986 Developmental study of α-glucosidases in Japanese quails with acid maltase deficiency. Muscle and Nerve 9:537

Valli V E O, McCarter A, McSherry B J, Robinson G A 1969 Hematopoiesis and epiphyseal growth zones in rabbits with molybdenosis. American Journal of Veterinary Research 30:435

van den Hoven R, Wensing T, Breukink H J, Meijer A E, Kruip T A 1985 Variation of fiber types in the triceps brachii, longissimus dorsi, gluteus medius and biceps femoris of horses. American Journal of Veterinary Research 46:939

Vandevelde M, Greene C E, Hoff E J 1976 Lower motor neuron disease with accumulation of neurofilaments in a cat. Veterinary Pathology 13:428

Van Niekerk I J M, Jaros G G 1970 Myotonia in the calf: a case report. South African Medical Journal 44:898

Van Vleet J F, Meyer K B, Olander H J 1974 Acute selenium toxicosis induced in baby pigs by parenteral administration of selenium–vitamin E preparations. Journal of the American Veterinary Medical Association 165:543

Van Vleet J F, Ferrans V J 1984 Ultrastructural alterations in skeletal muscle of pigs with acute monensin myotoxicosis. American Journal of Pathology 114:461

Van Vleet J F, Boon G D, Ferrans V J 1981 Induction of lesions of selenium–vitamin E deficiency in weanling swine fed silver, cobalt, tellurium, zinc, cadmium and vanadium. American Journal of Veterinary Research 42:789

Venable J H 1973 Skeletal muscle structure in Poland China pigs suffering from malignant hyperthermia. In: Gordon R A, Britt B A, Kalors W (eds) International symposium on hyperthermia. Thomas, Springfield, p 208

Venker-van Haagen A J 1980 Investigations on the pathogenesis of hereditary laryngeal paralysis in the Bouvier. Doctoral Thesis, University of Utrecht, p 86

Wallace M E, Palmer A C 1984 Recessive mode of inheritance in myasthenia gravis in the Jack Russell terrier. Veterinary Record 114:350

Ward L C, Buttery P J 1978 N^t-Methylhistidine — an index of the true rate of myofibrillar degradation? An appraisal. Life Sciences 23:1103

Ward P S 1978 The splayleg syndrome in new-born pigs: a review. Part I and Part II. Veterinary Bulletin 48: 279, 381

Ward P S, Bradley 1979 Floppy infants, porcine splayleg, and myofibrillar hypoplasia. In: Andrews E J, Ward B C, Altman N H (eds) Spontaneous animal models of human disease, vol II. Academic Press, New York, p 97

Ward P S, Bradley R 1980 The light microscopical morphology of the skeletal muscles of normal pigs and pigs with splayleg from birth to one week of age. Journal of Comparative Pathology 90:421

Warhol M J, Siegel A J, Evans W J, Silverman L M 1985 Skeletal muscle injury and repair in marathon runners after competition. American Journal of Pathology 118:331

Warnick J E, Albuquerque E X 1979 Changes in genotypic expression development, and the effects of chronic penicillamine treatment on the electrical properties of the posterior latissimus dorsi muscle in two lines of normal and dystrophic chickens. Experimental Neurology 63:135

Warnick J E, Lebeda F J, Albuquerque E X 1979 Junctional and extrajunctional aspects of inherited muscular dystrophy in chickens: development and pharmacology. Annals of the New York Academy of Sciences 317:263

Webb A J, Jordan C H C 1978 Halothane sensitivity as a field test for stress-susceptibility in the pig. Animal Production, 26:157

Webb A J, Simpson S P, Southwood O I 1985 Porcine stress syndrome — recent advances. In: Animal health and productivity (Proceedings of an International Symposium). Royal Agricultural Society of England, London, p 143

Webb J N 1970 Naturally occurring myopathy in guinea pigs. Journal of Pathology 100:155

Weisman Y, Shkap I, Egyed M N, Shlosberg A 1984 Chloramphenicol induced monensin toxicity in turkeys. Refuah Veterinarith 41:3

Weitz H, Hübner G 1980 Rhabdomyolysis in a severe case of malignant hyperthermia — a light and electron microscopical study. Pathology Research and Practice 169:276

Wells G A H, Bradley R 1977 Haloxon neurotoxicity in the pig. Neuropathology and Applied Neurobiology 3:218

Wells G A H, Bradley R, 1987 Developmental skeletal

disorders of the pig. Veterinary Annual, 26th issue. (Wright-Scientechnica, Bristol) p 120

Wentink G H, van der Linde-Sipman J S, Meijer A E F H, Kamphuisen H A C, van Vorstenbosch C J A H V, Hartman W, Hendricks H J 1972 Myopathy with a possible recessive X-linked inheritance in a litter of Irish terriers. Veterinary Pathology 9:328

Wentink G H, Hartman W, Koeman J P 1974a Three cases of myotonia in a family of Chows. Tijdschrift voor Diergeneeskunde 99:729

Wentink G H, Meijer A E F H, van der Linde-Sipman J S, Hendricks H J 1974b Myopathy in an Irish terrier with a metabolic defect of the isolated mitochondria. Zentralblatt für Veterinärmedizin 21A:62

Wesemeier H 1974 Elektronenmikroskopische Untersuchungen an der Skelett-muskulatur von unbelasteten sowie experimentell belasteten Fleischschweinen: ein Beitrag zur Ätiologie und Pathogenese des blassen, wässrigen Schweinefleisches (PSE-Fleisch) Archiv für Experimentelle Veterinarmedizin 28:329

Wesemeier H, Bergmann V 1972 Elektronenmikroskopische Untersuchungen am M. longissimus dorsi bei Fleischschweinen nach experimenteller Belastung. Archiv für Experimentelle Veterinärmedizin 26:477

White N A, McGavin M D, Smith J E 1978 Age-related changes in percentage of fiber types and mean fiber diameters of the ovine quadriceps muscle. American Journal of Veterinary Research 39:1297

Whitney J C 1958 Progressive muscular dystrophy in the dog. Veterinary Record 70:611

Wight P A L, Siller N G, Mastindale L, Filshie J H 1979 Induction by muscle stimulation of a deep pectoral myopathy in the fowl. Avian Pathology 8:115

Wilson A B, Duncan L, Wrottesley M G, Fell B F 1978 Hypertrophy of the internal oblique abdominal muscle of ewes bred intensively. Journal of Comparative Pathology 88:345

Wilson B W, Randall W R, Patterson G T, Entrikin R K 1979 Major physiologic and histochemical characteristics of inherited dystrophy of the chicken. Annals of the New York Academy of Sciences 317:224

Wirtz P, Loermans H M Th, Peer P G M, Reintjes A G M 1983 Postnatal growth and differentiation of muscle fibres in the mouse II. A histochemical and morphometrical investigation of dystrophic muscle. Journal of Anatomy 137:127

Woodward J, Park J H, Colowick S P 1979 The increase in hexokinase activity in hereditary avian muscular dystrophy. Biochimica et Biophysica Acta 586:641

Wrogemann K, Pena S D J 1976 Mitochondrial calcium overload: a general mechanism for cell-necrosis in muscle diseases. Lancet 1:672

Yeagle S P, Albuquerque E X 1984 Reinnervation of normal and dystrophic skeletal muscle. Experimental Neurology 86:1

Yorita T, Nakamura H, Nonaka I 1980 Satellite cells and muscle regeneration in the developing dystrophic chicken. Experimental Neurology 70:567

Zacks S I, Shields D R, Steinberg S A 1966 A myasthenic syndrome in the dog: a case report with electron microscopic observations on motor end plates and comparisons with the fine structure of end plates in myasthenia gravis. Annals of the New York Academy of Sciences 135:79

Zhu L 1982 Keshan Disease. In: Gawthorne J M, Howell J McC, White C L (eds) Trace element metabolism in man and animals. Proceedings of the 4th International Symposium on Trace Element Metabolism in Man and Animals (TEMA-4) held in Perth, Australia, 1981. Springer, Berlin p 514

Drug-induced neuromuscular disorders in man

INTRODUCTION

An increasing number of drugs has been recognised to have effects on the neuromuscular system when used therapeutically in man. Some have a selective effect on the structure and function of muscle (Lane & Mastaglia 1978), while others interfere with neuromuscular transmission or are neurotoxic. Certain drugs such as vincristine and chloroquine are both myotoxic and neurotoxic.

The frequency of drug-induced neuromuscular disorders in clinical practice is difficult to establish because the association with drug therapy is not always recognised and subclinical forms are probably commoner than is generally appreciated. The recognition of such iatrogenic forms of neuromuscular disease is important, because early withdrawal of the offending agent often results in complete reversal of symptoms, while failure to do so may lead to serious disability. Awareness of the possibility of drug effects on the neuromuscular system is also of importance as the range of therapeutic agents introduced into clinical practice continues to expand. The increasing recognition of neuromuscular effects of drugs in widespread clinical use also has important implications with regard to the adequacy of laboratory testing of new therapeutic agents before they are released for general use.

MYOPATHIES

Muscle damage may result from the local effects of drugs administered by intramuscular injection, or from a more widespread effect on the skeletal muscles. The resulting clinical syndromes vary in

Table 29.1 Features of drug-induced myopathies

	Drug implicated	Clinical features	Serum[†] enzymes	Myoglobinuria	Electromyography findings	Pathology
Focal myopathy	IM injections of various drugs	—	may be ↑	—	—	Focal necrosis
Muscle fibrosis and contractures	antibiotics pethidine pentazocine heroin	Induration and contracture of injected muscles	Normal may be ↑	—	BSAPPs; variable spontaneous activity	Marked fibrosis and myopathic changes in injected areas
Acute/subacute painful proximal myopathy Toxic effect	clofibrate EACA emetine heroin	Muscle pain, tenderness, proximal or generalised weakness; reflexes usually preserved	↑ ↑	+/−	BSAPPs; spontaneous potentials may be prominent	Necrosis/ regeneration
	vincristine	Proximal pain, atrophy, weakness, absent reflexes	?	—	?	?
	clofibride isoetherine danazol cimetidine metolazone bumetadine lithium salbutamol mercaptopropionyl glycine suxamethonium labetalol nifedipine D-penicillamine gold	Myalgia/cramps/ myokymia/ weakness	?	?	?	?
Hypokalaemia	diuretics purgatives liquorice carbenoxolone amphotericin B	Weakness may be periodic; reflexes may be depressed or absent	↑ ↑	+/−	BSAPPs	Vacuolar myopathy ± necrosis/ regeneration
Inflammatory myopathy	D-penicillamine procainamide levodopa phenytoin penicillin cimetidine	Proximal muscle pain, weakness ± skin changes	↑ ↑	—	Myopathic features	Necrosis/ regeneration/ inflammation
Acute rhabdomyolysis	heroin methadone amphetamine barbiturates diazepam meprobamate isoniazid amphotericin B phenformin fenfluramine carbenoxolone vasopressin phenylpropano-lamine loxapin	Severe muscle pain, swelling flaccid quadriparesis, areflexia, renal failure	↑ ↑ ↑	+ + +	BSAPPs; prominent spontaneous discharges	Severe necrosis; regeneration

Table 29.1 (*Cont'd*)

	Drug implicated	Clinical features	Serum[†] enzymes	Myoglobinuria	Electromyography findings	Pathology
Subacute or chronic painless proximal myopathy	corticosteroids	Predominantly proximal, atrophy and weakness	Normal	—	BSAPPs	Type II fibre atrophy
	chloroquine	Reflexes may be lost due to associated neuropathy	Normal	—	Myopathic/ neuropathic; spontaneous discharges may be prominent	Vacuolar myopathy
	heroin perhexiline amiodarone					Nonspecific myopathic changes
	squill oxymel (cardiac glycoside)	Proximal weakness + myasthenic features	↑ ↑ ↑	— (see above)	Myopathic/ neuropathic	Necrosis
	*Drugs causing ↑ K+					
Myotonic syndrome	20, 25-diazacholesterol and analogues	Muscle cramps, weakness, myotonia			Myotonic and other spontaneous discharges	
	suxamethonium propranolol pindolol fenterol ritodrine	May aggravate myotonia	Normal	—		
Malignant hyperpyrexia	suxamethonium halothane diethyl ether cyclopropane chloroform methoxyflurane ketamine enflurane	Rigidity, hyperpyrexia, acidosis, hyperkalaemia, disseminated intra-vascular coagulation, renal failure	↑ ↑ ↑ (↑ in some cases at risk)	+ + +	Variable myopathic changes in survivors and family members at risk	Necrosis (variable abnormalities in cases at risk)

† Creatine kinase, aldolase, aspartate transminase
BSAPPs: brief duration, small amplitude, polyphasic ('myopathic') motor unit action potentials

severity, mode of onset and rate of progression. Some are acute or subacute and are associated with muscle pain, while others are more protracted and painless (Table 29.1). Muscle involvement is usually widespread and symmetrical, the proximal muscles often being most severely affected, while those innervated by the cranial nerves are usually spared. The mechanisms involved may be either direct myotoxicity or indirect muscle damage through drug-induced electrolyte disturbances, immunological abnormalities, ischaemia, neural activation or muscle compression in drug-induced coma (Mastaglia 1982).

Focal myopathy

Intramuscular injections produce localised areas of muscle damage as a result of needle insertion ('needle myopathy') and local effects of the agent injected. Creatine kinase (CK) activity in the serum may be increased after injection of a variety of drugs including diazepam, lidocaine and digoxin; histological examination of the injection site in animals has shown extensive necrosis after injection of such drugs, but not after injection of saline (Steiness et al 1978). Other drugs which have a local toxic effect include chloroquine (Aguayo & Hudgson 1970), and the opiates and chlorpromazine which are thought to cause damage by inducing histamine release (Cohen 1972, Brumback et al 1982). Some drugs such as paraldehyde and cephalothin sodium, which are particularly irritant, may cause more severe tissue damage leading to abscess formation (Lane & Mastaglia 1978, Greenblatt & Allen 1978). These focal forms of muscle damage are usually of little clinical consequence apart from the fact that the finding of elevated serum enzyme activities may be misleading in patients with suspected myocardial infarction, unless isoenzyme studies are performed (Marmor et al 1978).

Marked muscle fibrosis leading to progressive induration and contractures may occur as a result of repeated intramuscular injections. This complication has occurred particularly in children who have had intramuscular injections of antibiotics (Saunders et al 1965, Battacharrya 1966, Hagen 1968), and in adults addicted to pethidine (Mastaglia et al 1971) or pentazocine (Steiner et al 1973, Levin & Engel 1975, Adams et al 1983, Roberson & Dimon 1983). The quadriceps femoris and deltoid muscles have been most commonly affected but more widespread involvement has been reported in some drug addicts (Aberfeld et al 1968, Mastaglia et al 1971, Steiner et al 1973, Choucair & Ziter 1984). Repeated needle trauma, toxic effects of the drug, haemorrhage and low-grade infection may all be contributory factors.

Acute or subacute painful proximal myopathy

A number of drugs may cause a rapidly evolving syndrome characterised by muscle pain, tenderness and weakness involving the proximal limb and axial muscles most severely. This may be due to a direct toxic effect of the drug on muscle or to the development of hypokalaemia or of an inflammatory myopathy. The tendon reflexes are usually preserved unless the myopathy is profound or is associated with a peripheral neuropathy. Serum activities of CK and other enzymes are usually considerably raised and myoglobinuria may occur. Electromyography (EMG) shows the typical changes of primary muscle disease (see Ch. 30) and spontaneous potentials may be prominent (Lane et al 1979).

Toxic myopathy. The drugs which most frequently produce this syndrome as a result of a direct toxic effect are clofibrate, epsilon-aminocaproic acid (EACA) and emetine, all of which cause a necrotising myopathy (Fig. 29.1a). An identical syndrome has also been reported in heroin addicts (Richter et al 1971) and alcoholics (Perkoff et al 1966).

Clofibrate. At least 45 patients with clofibrate myopathy have been reported and were recently reviewed by Rimon et al (1984). The myopathy appears to be dose-dependent; it is uncommon when the drug is administered in conventional therapeutic doses but is more likely to develop in patients with renal failure (Pierides et al 1975), the nephrotic syndrome (Bridgeman et al 1972) or hypothyroidism, probably because plasma levels of the unbound drug are high in these conditions (Rumpf et al 1976). However 20 patients with normal renal function also developed this complication. Five patients with clofibrate-induced myopathy continued to take the drug at lower doses and all of them recovered. Symptoms develop quite abruptly, usually within three weeks of the start of therapy, possibly when the concentration of the drug in the blood reaches a critical level (Teravainen et al 1977). In almost all patients muscle enzyme activity in the serum was increased. The mechanism whereby clofibrate causes muscle necrosis is uncertain, but the observation that the drug causes a significant increase in muscle lipoprotein-lipase activity may be relevant (Lithell et al 1978). Disturbances in muscle energy metabolism were found in rats treated with clofibrate (Paul & Abidi 1979).

Epsilon-aminocaproic acid. The development of a myopathy is a well-recognised but uncommon complication of treatment with this antifibrinolytic agent. Brown et al (1982) reviewed 19 reported cases. This myopathy usually develops abruptly after three to six weeks of treatment with daily doses of 10–30 g, suggesting that it is due to a cumulative dose-related effect of the drug (Lane et al 1979). It has been reported most frequently in patients with hereditary angioneurotic oedema (Korsan-Bengsten et al 1969) or subarachnoid haemorrhage (Lane et al 1979). The myopathy

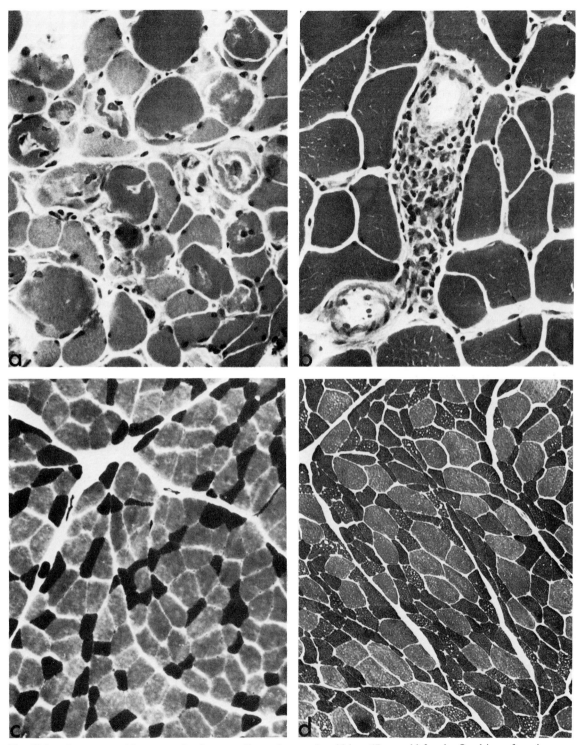

Fig. 29.1 a. Severe necrotising myopathy due to epsilon-aminocaproic acid in a 67-year-old female. Quadriceps femoris biopsy; H & E, ×320. b. Interstitial perivascular mononuclear cell infiltrate in a 54-year-old man with a procainamide-induced lupus-like syndrome. Quadriceps femoris biopsy; H & E, ×320. c. Type II fibre atrophy in a 26-year-old female treated with corticosteroids for systemic lupus erythematosus (SLE). Quadriceps femoris biopsy; myofibrillar ATPase (pH 9.4), ×125. d. Vacuolar myopathy with predominant involvement of intermediate and type II fibres in a 55-year-old female with suspected SLE who was treated with chloroquine. Quadriceps femoris biopsy; myofibrillar ATPase (pH 7.2), ×160

may be severe and acute rhabdomyolysis with renal failure has been recorded (Brodkin 1980). It has been suggested that complement abnormalities and lysine deficiency may possibly be predisposing factors. Active muscle regeneration occurs and complete recovery over a period of weeks is the rule (Lane et al 1979, Brown et al 1982). The mechanism of the myopathy is unclear. Histological evidence of capillary occlusion was reported in some (Cullen & Mastaglia 1980, Kennard et al 1980) but not all cases (Britt et al 1980). Attempts to reproduce this myopathy in animals have been unsuccessful.

Emetine. Patients treated with the anti-amoebic agent emetine hydrochloride frequently develop generalised muscle weakness during (Klatskin & Friedman 1948) or after a course of treatment (Young & Tudhope 1926). This is usually reversible, but the outcome may be fatal, particularly when there is an associated cardiomyopathy (Fewings et al 1973). Although emetine myopathy is usually painful and is associated with elevated serum CK activity, a painless case with no change in serum CK was described (Bennett al 1982). Overdose of emetine may be responsible for a myopathy developing in some patients treated with ipecac syrup to induce emesis (Bennett al 1982). Early clinical reports suggested that there were both 'neuritic' and 'myositic' forms of emetine toxicity. However, experimental studies have shown a pure myotoxic effect with mitochondrial and myofibrillar changes followed by necrosis and regeneration (Duane & Engel 1970, Bradley et al 1976) and no evidence of damage to intramuscular nerves or motor end-plates.

Vincristine. A painful proximal necrotising myopathy may occur in some patients treated with vincristine in association with the severe polyneuropathy caused by the drug (Bradley et al 1970). Electron-microscopic studies in man (Bradley et al 1970) and in the experimental animal (Anderson et al 1967, Bradley 1970) have shown that the drug has a profound effect on membrane systems and causes severe autophagic degeneration of muscle fibres.

Other drugs. A number of other drugs including lithium carbonate (Ghose 1977), cimetidine (Wade 1977), labetalol (Teicher et al 1981), nifedipine (Keidar et al 1982), gold (Mitsumoto et al 1982), D-penicillamine (Pinals 1983), mercaptopropionyl glycine (Hales et al 1982), clofibride, danazol, isoetherine, metolazone, bumetanide, cytotoxic agents (Dukes 1977) and salbutamol (Palmer 1978) have been reported to cause myalgia, muscle cramps, myokymia or weakness in some patients. The mechanisms involved have not been investigated. Muscle pain following suxamethonium, usually after minor surgical procedures, is a relatively common complaint (Dottori et al 1965, Brodsky & Ehrenwerth 1980).

Myositis. A painful drug-induced inflammatory myopathy may develop in some patients (Mastaglia & Argov 1982). In the case of procainamide, an interstitial form of myositis occurs (Fig. 29.1b), usually as part of a lupus- like syndrome and may be a manifestation of an arteritic process (Dubois 1969, Blomgren et al 1972, Fontiveros et al 1980). A similar type of myopathy has been described in a patient on levodopa therapy for parkinsonism (Wolf et al 1976). In one case myositis was suspected to result from phenytoin therapy (Harney & Glasberg 1983) but penicillin was also administered in this case. There is one report of a possible association between penicillin and myositis (Hayman et al 1956). A case of myositis in a patient taking cimeditine has been reported (Watson et al 1983) but the role of the drug in this case has been questioned (Hawkins et al 1983). The possibility that cimetidine may induce muscle damage has also been reported by others (Feest & Read 1980).

A number of patients with rheumatoid arthritis or Wilson's disease treated with D-penicillamine in daily doses up to 700 mg have developed acute or subacute polymyositis (Schraeder et al 1972, Bettendorf & Neuhaus 1974, Cucher & Goldman 1976, Halla et al 1984) or dermatomyositis (Fernandes et al 1977, Wojnarowska 1980, Lund & Nielsen 1983). Three of the reported cases, two fatal, had associated myocardial involvement (Bettendorf & Neuhaus 1974, Cucher & Goldman 1976, Doyle et al 1983). Spontaneous recovery can occur after withdrawal of the drug but in several cases steroid therapy was required to induce remission (Halla et al 1984). This complication has been reported less frequently than the immuno-logically mediated myasthenic syndrome which develops in other patients treated with penicillamine.

Hypokalaemic myopathy. Widespread muscle weakness, which may be painful, and which may be associated with depressed or absent tendon reflexes and a marked increase in serum CK activity and myoglobinuria, may result from hypokalaemia in patients taking diuretics (Jensen et al 1977), purgatives (Basser 1979), liquorice (Gross et al 1966), carbenoxolone (Mohamed et al 1966), or amphotericin B which causes renal tubular damage (Drutz et al 1970). Histological studies in such cases usually show a vacuolar myopathy but, in severe cases, necrosis and regeneration may be present.

Acute rhabdomyolysis

Although a number of drugs already discussed may cause a severe necrotising myopathy and myoglobinuria, the features of the potentially fatal condition referred to as acute rhabdomyolysis are sufficiently distinctive to merit special consideration. It is characterised by the abrupt onset of severe generalised muscle pain, tenderness and flaccid areflexic paralysis, often with severe muscle swelling which may require fasciotomy. Gross myoglobinuria usually leads to acute oliguric renal failure which may be responsible for death. Serum levels of CK and of other enzymes are markedly raised and the EMG reveals myopathic changes, often with prominent spontaneous discharges. Muscle biopsy shows widespread necrosis with mild reactive inflammatory changes, and regenerative activity may be profuse. Recovery usually occurs over a period of weeks, but full muscle power may not be restored for several months.

Acute rhabdomyolysis has occurred in association with amphotericin B (Drutz et al 1970), carbenoxolone therapy (Mohamed et al 1966), intravenous vasopressin (Affarah et al 1984) and high doses of the appetite suppressant phenylpropanolamine (Swenson et al 1982). Intoxication with barbiturates, meprobamate and diazepam (Nicolas et al 1970, Penn et al 1972, Wattel et al 1978), phencyclidine (Cogen et al 1978), loxapin

(Tam et al 1980) and its analogue amoxapin (Abreo et al 1982), amphetamine poisoning (Grossman et al 1974), combined overdosage with phenformin and fenfluramine (Palmucci et al 1978), alcoholism (Perkoff et al 1966) and heroin and methadone addiction (Richter et al 1971) can all lead to rhabdomyolysis. The mechanisms of myotoxicity in these situations have not been investigated and it remains to be determined whether a direct toxic drug effect is involved, or whether individual idiosyncracy or other predisposing factors play a part.

Less severe forms of rhabdomyolysis have been recognised in apparently normal individuals (Gibbs 1978, Hool et al 1984) and in patients with Duchenne muscular dystrophy (Watters et al 1977) following administration of suxamethonium during anaesthesia.

Subacute or chronic painless proximal myopathy

This is probably the commonest form of drug-induced myopathy encountered in clinical practice and occurs most frequently in patients on long-term corticosteroid therapy.

Corticosteroids. Myopathy occurs particularly in patients treated with the fluorinated steroids triamcinolone (Williams 1959), betamethasone and dexamethasone (Golding & Begg 1960), and has also been associated with cortisone, prednisone, prednisolone and methylprednisolone therapy (Askari et al 1976). Myopathy is more likely to develop in patients maintained on high doses of these drugs for prolonged periods (Askari et al 1976) and is unlikely to occur if the daily dose of steroid is kept down to 10 mg or less of prednisone or its equivalent (Yates 1970). Severe myopathy may occasionally follow parenteral treatment with high doses of hydrocortisone (MacFarlane & Rosenthal 1977), and may even complicate topical steroid therapy (M. D. Rawlins, personal communication). Severe myopathy is uncommon but the true frequency of the condition is difficult to determine because mild forms may be overlooked, particularly in patients with an underlying disorder such as rheumatoid arthritis, which may also cause muscle weakness and wasting. Quantitative studies of muscle function in such patients have shown significant reductions in muscle performance (Rothstein et al 1983, Khaleeli et al 1983). Electromyographic findings indicate that subclinical myopathy is common (Coomes 1965a, Yates 1970).

In the typical case there is symmetrical involvement of proximal limb muscles, particularly those of the pelvic girdle, and atrophy and weakness of the quadriceps femoris are prominent. Muscle pain is not a feature and the tendon reflexes are usually preserved. Serum enzyme levels are normal and, if found to be elevated, should suggest the possibility of active inflammatory muscle disease. Creatinuria occurs and urinary creatine levels have been held to be useful in diagnosis and in monitoring progress (Askari et al 1976). The EMG shows the typical changes of primary muscle disease, particularly in proximal groups, spontaneous discharges usually being absent. In contrast to experimental corticosteroid myopathy (see Ch. 12), the histological changes in steroid myopathy in man are relatively inconspicuous. Muscle biopsy shows an atrophic process with particular involvement of the type II fibres (Fig. 29.1c), and necrosis, regeneration and vacuolar change are not usually found. The myopathy is usually reversible on stopping the drug or, to some extent, on substituting prednisone for the offending steroid (Williams 1959, Walton 1977). Anabolic agents do not prevent the development of the myopathy (Coomes 1965b).

Although usually subacute or chronic, steroid myopathy can also be acute. There have been reports of patients with status asthmaticus who were treated with high doses of intravenous hydrocortisone, who developed a severe generalised myopathy with involvement of the respiratory muscles and elevation of serum CK activity (MacFarlane & Rosenthal 1977, Van Marle & Woods 1980, Mastaglia 1982). Biopsy showed vacuolar changes in both fibre types with evidence of regeneration. These features resembled experimental steroid myopathy in rabbits (Afifi & Bergman 1969). Recovery was slow in these cases.

The mechanism of steroid-induced myopathy has been clarified by experimental studies which have shown that specific steroid receptor proteins are present in muscle (Shoji & Pennington 1977a), and that steroids interfere with oxidative metabolism (Koski et al 1974), enhance glycogen synthesis (Shoji et al 1974) and inhibit protein synthesis (Shoji & Pennington 1977b).

Chloroquine. A severe myopathy may result from the prolonged administration of chloroquine (Whisnant et al 1963). It may be indistinguishable clinically from steroid myopathy and there may be difficulty in deciding which drug is responsible, in patients receiving both chloroquine and corticosteroids (Mastaglia et al 1977). As the drug may also cause a mild peripheral neuropathy, sensory changes, reflex depression and abnormal nerve conduction may be found (Whisnant et al 1963). In contrast to steroid myopathy, spontaneous potentials, including myotonic discharges, are commonly found in the EMG, in addition to the typical changes of primary muscle disease (Mastaglia et al 1977). Biopsy shows a vacuolar myopathy, type I fibres usually being more severely affected, although in some cases there is predominant involvement of intermediate or type II fibres (Fig. 29.1d) (Mastaglia et al 1977). Electron-microscopic studies of human and experimental animal material have shown that the drug has a profound effect on intracellular membrane systems, leading to the formation of a variety of membranous bodies, and to autophagic degeneration of muscle fibres (MacDonald & Engel 1970, Mastaglia et al 1977). The myopathy is reversible after withdrawal of the drug, but recovery is protracted (Mastaglia et al 1977).

A similar myopathy may be induced experimentally in animals by a number of drugs which are all amphiphilic cationic compounds (Drenckhahn & Lullman-Rauch 1979). These drugs have high affinity for polar lipids and form non-digestible drug-lipid complexes within lysosomal structures. The abnormal lysosomes form the lamellated membrane bodies which may also be present in other tissues, resulting in a drug-induced lipidosis (Lullman et al 1978). Perhexiline (Fardeau et al 1979) and amiodarone (Meier et al 1979), which are usually implicated as causing drug-induced neuropathy, can also lead to a myopathy of a similar nature in man.

Other drugs. Some of the drugs already mentioned, such as heroin and those causing hypokalaemia, may also produce a painless proximal or generalised myopathy. Such a syndrome has also been ascribed to other drugs, including perhexiline (Tomlinson & Rosenthal 1977), colchicine (Kontos 1962) and rifampicin (Jenkins & Emerson 1981) but such cases have not usually been investigated fully.

Patients treated with beta-adrenergic blockers frequently complain of muscle weakness associated with fatigue (Stone 1979). It is not clear whether such drugs induce a myopathy (Forfar et al 1979) or interfere with energy metabolism of muscle by partial inhibition of glycogenolysis.

A severe, reversible proximal myopathy with high serum CK activities has been reported in individuals consuming large quantities of linctus codeine and has been attributed to the squill constituent which is a cardiac glycoside (Kennedy 1981, Kilpatrick et al 1982).

Myotonia

Drug-induced myotonia is now no longer encountered in clinical practice. The classic example of a drug-induced myotonic syndrome was that produced by the hypocholesterolaemic agent 20,25-diazacholesterol (Somers & Winer 1966). Patients taking the drug in daily doses of 25–50 mg developed muscle spasms and weakness with clinical and EMG evidence of myotonia. Complete recovery occurred over a period of two to three months after withdrawal of the drug. A comparable syndrome occurs in rats and goats after administration of the drug or of its analogues. Accumulation of desmosterol has been demonstrated in the serum and sarcolemma (Winer et al 1966) and the altered sterol composition and enzyme activity of the sarcolemma are thought to be the basis for the myotonia (Peter & Fiehn 1973). Myotonia which resembles human myotonia congenita can also be induced in animals by other compounds, such as noncarboxylic aromatic acids, triparanol and clofibrate (Kwiecinski 1981). Clofibrate myotoxicity in humans is not associated with clinical or electrical myotonia.

A number of drugs may precipitate or exacerbate myotonia in patients with dystrophia myotonica or other myotonic disorders. These include the beta-blockers propranolol (Blessing

& Walsh 1977) and pindolol (Ricker et al 1978), the beta-adrenergic agonists fenoterol (Ricker et al 1978) and ritodrine (Sholl et al 1985), and the depolarising muscle relaxant suxamethonium (Mitchell 1978). In contrast, non-depolarising muscle relaxants do not have this effect in patients with dystrophia myotonica (Mitchell et al 1978). A number of diuretics including furosemide and acetazolamide may be considered harmful in myotonic disorders because they have been shown to induce myotonic potentials in vitro (Bretag et al 1980).

Myotonic discharges may be found, together with other high-frequency ('pseudomyotonic') discharges, in some of the drug-induced syndromes already discussed, such as chloroquine neuromyopathy (Mastaglia et al 1977) and EACA myopathy (Lane et al 1979), and may occasionally be associated with clinical myotonia (Blomberg 1965).

Malignant hyperpyrexia

In this serious condition, various anaesthetic agents and other drugs may precipitate a potentially fatal state characterised by generalised muscular rigidity, severe hyperpyrexia, metabolic acidosis and myoglobinuria (King & Denborough 1973a, Britt 1979, Gronert 1983). The condition is usually familial, being inherited by an autosomal dominant mechanism, and susceptible individuals have either a clinically apparent or, more frequently, a subclinical myopathy (King et al 1972, Harriman et al 1973). Those who are clinically normal may be identified by the finding of elevated serum CK activities (King et al 1972, Ellis et al 1975), focal myopathic changes in the EMG (F. L. Mastaglia, unpublished observations), or, most reliably, by the demonstration of abnormal sensitivity of muscle tissue to anaesthetic agents in vitro (Ellis et al 1972). A second group of individuals with this susceptibility are young males of short stature with a progressive congenital myopathy, skeletal abnormalities and other dysmorphic features similar to those seen in the Noonan syndrome, and in whom an autosomal recessive mechanism of inheritance is probably involved (King & Denborough 1973b, Kaplan et al 1977). Malignant hyperpyrexia may rarely also occur in cases of myotonia congenita, myotonic dystrophy, Duchenne muscular dystrophy, central core disease and in osteogenesis imperfecta (Rowland 1980, Mastaglia 1982).

The drugs which may precipitate malignant hyperpyrexia in susceptible individuals include halothane, suxamethonium, diethyl ether, cyclopropane, chloroform, methoxyflurane (Newson 1972), ketamine (Page et al 1972) and enflurane (Knape 1977). Tricyclic antidepressants and monoamine oxidase inhibitors have also been reported to precipitate a similar syndrome (Newson 1972). A safe anaesthetic regime for muscle biopsy in susceptible individuals comprises oral premedication with diazepam followed by thiopentone, fentanyl citrate and nitrous oxide (Ellis et al 1975). D-Tubocurarine and local, regional or spinal anaesthesia and neuroleptalgesia may also be used with safety (Denborough 1977).

The mechanism of the reaction to anaesthetic agents has been clarified by studies in man and in certain inbred strains of swine which suffer from an apparently identical syndrome (Hall et al 1966). On the basis of such studies it has been concluded that, in susceptible individuals, there is an intrinsic abnormality of the excitation–contraction coupling mechanism in muscle, exposure to these agents causing excessive release of Ca^{2+} ions into the myoplasm and sustained myofibrillar contraction (Denborough 1977, Britt 1979).

Various drugs have been used in the treatment of the acute fulminant hyperpyrexia syndrome with the aim of reducing myoplasmic Ca^{2+} levels. These include procaine, procainamide, hydrocortisone, dexamethasone and dantrolene sodium which blocks excitation–contraction coupling and enhances Ca^{2+} uptake by the sarcoplasmic reticulum and is now the drug of choice (Nelson & Flewellen 1983, Gronert 1983).

Neuroleptic malignant syndrome. This is a severe form of drug-induced extrapyramidal disorder occurring in patients treated with drugs belonging to the phenothiazine, butyrophenone or thioxanthene groups (Knezevic et al 1984a, Gibb & Lees 1985). It is characterised by pyrexia, severe rigidity and akinesia and bulbar muscle dysfunction. The serum CK activity is often increased and overt myoglobinuria and renal

failure have been reported in some cases (Hashimoto et al 1984).

DISORDERS OF NEUROMUSCULAR TRANSMISSION

A variety of drugs, in addition to the neuromuscular blocking agents used in anaesthesia, may interfere with neuromuscular transmission in man (Argov & Mastaglia 1979a, Kaeser 1984). Drug-induced neuromuscular block may manifest clinically in the following ways.

Clinical presentations

Drug-induced myasthenic syndrome. As shown in Table 29.2, a number of drugs have been implicated in causing a myasthenic syndrome in patients with no evidence of pre-existing myasthenia gravis (MG). The disorder has usually developed within a short period of starting treatment and has been reversible after withdrawal of the drug. In spite of this, the possibility remains that, in at least some of these cases, a subclinical disorder of neuromuscular transmission was unmasked by the effects of the drug. This is a relatively uncommon complication of treatment with these drugs, probably because of the high safety factor for neuromuscular transmission which exists under normal circumstances (Desmedt 1973, Stalberg et al 1975). Clinically manifest neuromuscular block probably occurs only when this safety margin is reduced, as in hypocalcaemia or other electrolyte disturbances (Katz 1966), or when high blood levels of the drug develop, as in patients with renal failure (Lindesmith et al 1968).

With drugs such as the antibiotics, which have a direct effect at the neuromuscular junction, the onset is relatively acute and respiratory paralysis with variable involvement of other muscle groups is the rule. On the other hand, in the case of D-penicillamine, which induces neuromuscular block through an immunological mechanism, symptoms usually develop only after a period of months or years, are generally less acute in onset and the resulting clinical syndrome resembles more closely classical MG.

Table 29.2 Clinical symptoms of drug-induced neuromuscular blockade and drugs implicated

Clinical pesentation	Antibiotics	Antirheumatic drugs	Cardiovascular drugs	Anticonvulsants	Psychotropic drugs	Anaesthetics	Other drugs
Drug-induced myasthenic syndrome	neomycin streptomycin kanamycin gentamycin polymyxin B colistins	D-penicillamine	oxprenolol practolol trimetaphan	trimethadione phenytoin			bulsulfan (?) oral contraceptive (?) DL-carnitine
Aggravation or unmasking of myasthenia gravis	streptomycin kanamycin colistin rolitetracycline oxytetracycline gentamycin ampicillin	chloroquine	quinidine procainamide propranolol	phenytoin	lithium chlorpromazine		Methoxyflurane ACTH corticosteroids thyroid hormones ACh-esterase inhibitors timolol magnesium? iodinated contrast media
Postoperative respiratory depression							
Antibiotic-induced respiratory arrest syndrome	neomycin streptomycin kanamycin colistin lincomycin clindamycin						
Potentiation of muscle relaxants		chloroquine	quinidine trimetaphan		lithium promazine phenelzine	diazepam ketamine propanidid ether	oxytocin Trasylol® cholinesterase inhibitors procaine lidocaine timolol magnesium

Aggravation or unmasking of myasthenia gravis. It is well known that certain drugs may lead to clinical deterioration when administered to previously stable myasthenic patients (Table 29.2). This is probably caused by a further reduction in the already lowered safety margin for transmission in such patients (Desmedt 1973), because of the effects of the drug at the neuromuscular junction. In patients in whom an irreversible myasthenic syndrome develops, it is likely that the drug has unmasked previously undeclared MG.

Postoperative respiratory depression. This is perhaps the commonest manifestation of drug-induced neuromuscular blockade. As shown in Table 29.2, a number of drugs may cause respiratory depression, during or after anaesthesia, through an effect on neuromuscular transmission. This may be due to a direct effect of the drug itself, to enhancement of the blockade induced by muscle relaxants, or to a combination of these effects. The commonest example is the respiratory depression which may occur in patients given certain antibiotics in the preoperative period or during operation. In addition, some patients are unduly susceptible to the neuromuscular blocking action of certain drugs administered in the immediate postoperative period. For example, respiratory depression may occur following the administration of quinidine in patients who have recovered from the effects of muscle relaxants and have already been extubated, a phenomenon which has been referred to as 'recurarisation' (Way et al 1967). Electrophysiological study has shown that partial curarisation in the postoperative period is common (Lennmarken & Lofstrom 1984) explaining why drug-induced neuromuscular block has been described frequently as a postanaesthetic complication.

Mechanisms of drug-induced neuromuscular block

Drugs may interfere with neuromuscular transmission through a presynaptic local anaesthetic-like action at the nerve terminal, a postsynaptic curariform action, a combined pre- and postsynaptic action, or by a separate effect on the muscle fibre membrane (Fig. 29.2). The mechanism of

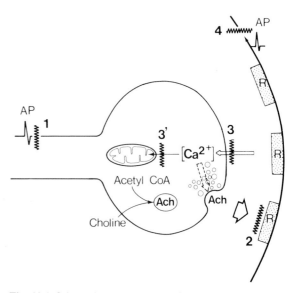

Fig. 29.2 Schematic representation of neuromuscular junction showing the possible sites of action of the drugs discussed. 1 — Presynaptic local anaesthetic-like effect on propagation of nerve action potential (AP); 2 — Postsynaptic receptor (R) blockade; 3,3' — interference with acetylcholine (ACh) release through inhibition of entry of Ca^{2+} ions into the nerve terminal (3) and into mitochondria (3'); 4 — Impairment of muscle action potential propagation

action of some of the drugs to be discussed has been determined by experimental studies, while that of others is still conjectural.

Presynaptic local anaesthetic-like action. A number of drugs with local anaesthetic properties are suspected to reduce transmitter release by interfering with the generation of the nerve terminal action potential (Table 29.3). Confirmation of such an action would require simultaneous extracellular recording of the nerve terminal potential and the end-plate current produced by nerve stimulation (Katz & Miledi 1965).

Postsynaptic curariform block. A number of drugs exert their effect by competing for acetylcholine (ACh) receptor binding sites on the postsynaptic membrane (Table 29.3). Some of these drugs possess an ionised ammonium group which is thought to be the active binding site to the receptor (Koelle 1975). Such an effect has been demonstrated in vitro by the finding of a reduced end-plate electrical response to iontophoretically applied ACh (Werman & Wislicki 1971), or of a

Table 29.3 Mechanisms of action of drugs which cause neuromuscular blockade

Mechanism	Antibiotics	Antirheumatic drugs	Cardiovascular drugs	Anticonvulsants	Psychotropic drugs	Anaesthetics	Other drugs
Presynaptic local anaesthetic-like action (1)*	clindamycin lincomycin	chloroquine	propranolol		lithium imipramine		
Postsynaptic curare-like action (2)*	Polymyxin B roliteracycline lincomycin clindamycin	chloroquine	propranolol		amphetamines	ketamine ether halothane	emetine D,L-carnitine
Pre- and postsynaptic membrane stabilising action (2, 3)*	neomycin streptomycin gentamicin polymyxins			phenytoin	chlorpromazine amitriptyline droperidolol haloperidol barbiturates	methoxyflurane	ACTH (?) diphenydramine
Inhibition of muscle membrane conductance (4)*	polymyxin B (?) lincomycin (?)				imipramine		amantadine
Other mechanisms	colistin		ajmaline				
Immunological		D-penicillamine		trimethadione			busulfan (?)

* Refer to Figure 29.2

rapid reduction in miniature end-plate potential (mepp) amplitude after addition of the drug (Gissen et al 1966). The in vivo demonstration of potentiation of neuromuscular block by D-tubo-curarine and reversal by neostigmine, although less conclusive, have been the basis for establishing a curare-like action of certain drugs such as the amphetamines (Skau & Gerald 1978), and procainamide (Galzigna et al 1972).

The neuromuscular block which occurs in patients who develop myasthenia during treatment with D-penicillamine is also postsynaptic in nature. ACh receptor antibodies have been demonstrated in the serum of such patients (Masters et al 1977, Vincent et al 1978, Russell & Lindstrom 1978) and mepp amplitude is reduced (Vincent et al 1978), presumably because of binding of antibody to the receptor as occurs in classic MG (Shibuya et al 1978).

Combined pre- and postsynaptic block. A number of drugs have been shown to have both a presynaptic inhibitory effect on transmitter release and a postsynaptic curariform action. In the case of drugs with so-called 'membrane-stabilising' properties, the presynaptic effect has been shown to be due to interference with the movement of Ca^{2+} ions into and within the nerve terminal (Fig. 29.2). Such drugs include phenytoin (Yaari et al 1977), chlorpromazine (Argov & Yaari 1979), and the aminoglycoside antibiotics (Elmqvist & Josefsson 1962, Dretchen et al 1973, Fiekers 1983a,b).

Interference with muscle membrane conductance. Certain drugs, such as amantadine, imipramine, and possibly polymyxin B and lincomycin, produce a postsynaptic block by interfering directly with ionic conductance across the muscle end-plate membrane rather than by binding to receptor sites. This has been demonstrated conclusively in the case of amantadine using the voltage clamp technique (Albuquerque et al 1978).

Specific drugs

Antibiotics

Aminoglycosides. Various antibiotics may interfere with neuromuscular transmission (Pittinger et al 1970). The most severe forms of neuromuscular block have occurred in patients treated with the aminoglycosides neomycin (Pridgeon 1956), kanamycin (Mullet & Keats 1961), streptomycin (Bodley & Brett 1962) and gentamycin (Warner & Sanders 1971). This complication has developed either following introduction of one of these drugs into the peritoneal or pleural cavities during surgery, or after oral or parenteral administration of the drug, leading to postoperative respiratory depression. This has usually been seen as a delay in recovery of spontaneous respiration, both in patients in whom muscle relaxants had been administered and in some in whom inhalational anaesthetics alone were used (Pridgeon 1956, Bennetts 1964). In some cases, respiratory depression has occurred some time after apparently complete recovery from the effects of muscle relaxants (Pinkerton & Munro 1964). Involvement of the respiratory muscles has been the only, or predominant, manifestation of the neuromuscular block in some cases, while in others there was more generalised weakness. Some patients have had associated pupillary dilatation, blurring of vision, depression of corneal reflexes and paraesthesiae (McQuillen et al 1968).

Neomycin (Percy & Saef 1967), streptomycin (Loder & Walker 1959) and kanamycin (Ream 1963) may also produce a myasthenic syndrome unrelated to surgery, or may lead to transient deterioration in patients with MG (Hokkanen 1964). Gentamycin can severely aggravate MG (Argov & Abramsky 1982) and of the currently used antibiotics is probably the most hazardous in this disorder. Streptomycin and neomycin have been shown to interfere with neuromuscular transmission by a combined pre- and postsynaptic effect (Elmqvist & Josefsson 1962, Tamaki 1978, Fiekers 1983a,b) and it is likely that the other closely related drugs act in a similar way.

Polypeptide antibiotics. Polymyxin B (Lindesmith et al 1968), colistin (Hokkanen 1964) and colistin methosulphonate (Perkins 1964, Zaunder et al 1966) may have similar effects to the aminoglycosides, but their mechanism of action has not been as well clarified. Colistin has been shown to reduce mepp amplitude and it has been suggested that this is due to a reduction in quantum size

(McQuillen & Engbaek 1975). However, as these drugs have an ionised ammonium group at physiological pH, a postsynaptic effect seems more likely (Wright & Collier 1976a). Indeed a recent study has shown that these drugs have a predominantly postsynaptic action with an additional presynaptic effect (Viswanath & Jenkins 1978).

Other antibiotics. Oxytetracycline and rolitetracycline have been reported to aggravate MG in some patients (Gibbels 1967, Wullen et al 1967). The mechanism of action has been studied in the case of rolitetracycline, which has been shown to have a postsynaptic curare-like effect (Wright & Collier 1976a). Lincomycin (Duignan et al 1973, Samuelson et al 1975) and its derivative clindamycin (Fogdall & Miller 1974) have been shown to prolong the action of muscle relaxants in some patients. These drugs have been shown to have a postsynaptic effect and also a presynaptic local anaesthetic-like action in higher concentrations (Wright & Collier 1976b, Rubbo et al 1977). It has been suggested that ampicillin and erythromycin may produce a Lambert–Eaton type of disorder of neuromuscular transmission on the basis of an electromyographic and repetitive nerve stimulation study (Herishanu & Taustein 1971). Argov et al (1985) have reported two myasthenic patients who deteriorated after ampicillin administration. They also showed that high doses of this drug can aggravate experimental myasthenia.

Antirheumatic drugs

D-penicillamine. A syndrome resembling classic MG may develop in patients with rheumatoid arthritis on long-term D-penicillamine therapy; this is now a well-recognised complication of treatment with the drug (Seitz et al 1976, Bucknall 1977). Although commonly reported in rheumatoid arthritis, D-penicillamine-induced myasthenia has also been reported in Wilson's disease (Czlonkowaska 1975), primary biliary cirrhosis (Marcus et al 1984) and progressive systemic sclerosis (Torres et al 1980); most reported cases were women. Involvement of the ocular muscles has usually been an early manifestation of such cases, and some have subsequently developed more widespread involvement. The duration of treatment before the appearance of myasthenic symp-

toms in the cases reported was between four months and five years. In about two-thirds of affected patients spontaneous recovery occurred after withdrawal of the drug, while the remainder required continuing anticholinesterase therapy or thymectomy; one death has been recorded (Delrieu et al 1976, Delamere et al 1983).

It has been suggested that this complication may be more likely to develop in patients with rheumatoid arthritis, because most of the cases reported have been in patients with this condition (Bucknall 1977, Mastaglia & Argov 1982). That an immunological mechanism is involved has been shown by the finding of raised ACh receptor antibody levels in the serum in most cases (Masters et al 1977, Russell & Lindstrom 1978, Vincent et al 1978). In addition, antibody levels have been shown to fall with clinical improvement after withdrawal of the drug, suggesting that the antibody is directly involved in the pathogenesis of the disorder (Vincent et al 1978, Fawcett et al 1982). The association of HLA A1, B8 and DR3 found in classic MG has been found in only some patients with the drug-induced disorder (Bucknall 1977, Russell & Lindstrom 1978). In a recent study of 18 cases, HLA Dr1 was increased in frequency and HLA Dr3 was absent (Delamere et al 1983). An association with thymoma has not been reported. It has been suggested that the development of myasthenia may be due to an independent effect of the drug on the immune system rather than to unmasking of subclinical MG.

The mechanism is not clear; D-penicillamine may stimulate B cells to secrete anti-acetylcholine receptor antibodies (Fawcett et al 1982), change the equilibrium between helper and suppressor T cells (Mastaglia & Argov 1982) or alter antigenic properties of the acetylcholine receptor (Bever et al 1982). A direct effect of D-penicillamine on neuromuscular transmission has also been found in animal studies (Burres et al 1979, Aldrich et al 1979).

Chloroquine has also been reported to aggravate or unmask MG (Robinson 1959). In addition, respiratory depression has occurred in the immediate postoperative period in 14% of a series of 67 patients in whom the drug was introduced into the peritoneal cavity during abdominal surgery to prevent the formation of adhesions (Jui-Yen 1971). Experimental studies have shown that the drug may have both a presynaptic local anaesthetic-like effect (Vartanian & Chinyanga 1972) and a postsynaptic curariform action (Jui-Yen 1971).

Cardiovascular drugs. Quinidine, procainamide and a number of the beta-adrenergic blockers possess neuromuscular blocking properties. Quinidine has been reported to aggravate or to unmask MG in some patients (Weisman 1949, Kornfeld et al 1976). In addition this drug may interact with muscle relaxants and has been reported to cause delayed respiratory depression in the postoperative period (Grongono 1963, Schmidt et al 1963, Way et al 1967). The mechanism of action of the drug has not been fully investigated. Procainamide, which has been shown to have a postsynaptic blocking effect on neuromuscular transmission (Galzigna et al 1972), has also been reported to aggravate MG (Drachman & Skom 1965, Kornfeld et al 1976, Niakan et al 1981).

Propranolol, oxprenolol and practolol have been reported to induce a myasthenic syndrome or to unmask MG (Herishanu & Rosenberg 1975, Hughes & Zacharias 1976). Interestingly, eye drops containing the potent beta-adrenergic blocker timolol have also been reported to unmask (Coppeto 1984) or aggravate MG (Shaivits 1979). Experimental studies with propranolol (Werman & Wislicki 1971) have shown that, in concentrations comparable to those achieved during therapy, the drug has a postsynaptic curariform action, while at higher concentrations it has an additional presynaptic anaesthetic-like effect. Pindolol has both a pre- and a postsynaptic action (Larsen 1978).

Trimetaphan, which has postsynaptic curariform blocking properties (Gergis et al 1977), has been reported to induce a myasthenic syndrome (Dale & Schroeder 1976) or to increase the neuromuscular block produced by curare derivatives in man (Wilson et al 1976, Nakamura et al 1980).

Anticonvulsants. Phenytoin and trimethadione have been reported to induce myasthenia, prob-

ably through different mechanisms. In the case of trimethadione, this was associated with an SLE-like syndrome and high titres of antimuscle antibodies and antinuclear factor, suggesting that the myasthenia was part of a drug-induced autoimmune disorder (Peterson 1966, Booker et al 1970). A myasthenic syndrome has been reported in patients with evidence of phenytoin intoxication and it is not clear whether or not this complication may also occur with well-controlled therapy (Norris et al 1964, Regli & Guggenheim 1965, Brumlik & Jacobs 1974). The effects of phenytoin on neuromuscular transmission have been studied in detail and the drug has been shown to have both a postsynaptic curariform and a presynaptic action, the latter being thought to predominate (Yaari et al 1977, 1979).

Psychotropic drugs. Lithium carbonate may unmask MG (Neil et al 1976, Granacher 1977) and has also been shown to prolong the neuromuscular blockade induced by pancuronium (Borden et al 1974) and suxamethonium (Hill et al 1976). The action of the drug is probably mainly a presynaptic one, resulting from substitution of Li^+ for Na^+ ions at the nerve terminal (Crawford 1975), but a postsynaptic effect has also been demonstrated (Onodera & Yamakawa 1966). Chlorpromazine, which has been shown in experimental studies to interfere with transmitter release and to have a lesser postsynaptic curare-like effect (Argov & Yaari 1979), may also aggravate MG (McQuillen et al 1963). Promazine (Regan & Aldrete 1967) and phenelzine (Bodley et al 1969) may potentiate the effect of suxamethonium. In the case of phenelzine this has been shown to be associated with reduced blood pseudocholinesterase levels.

Anaesthetic agents. Methoxyflurane has been reported to unmask subclinical MG (Elder et al 1971) and has been shown experimentally to have a combined pre- and postsynaptic action, the latter predominating (Kennedy & Galindo 1975). Ketamine and propanidid have been shown to potentiate the neuromuscular blocking effect of suxamethonium (Clarke et al 1967, Bovill et al 1971) and diazepam that of gallamine (Feldman & Crawley 1970).

Carnitine. Four anuric patients on chronic haemodialysis who received D,L-carnitine developed a myasthenic syndrome with involvement of skeletal and bulbar but not of ocular muscles (De Grantis et al 1980). The condition resolved when D,L-carnitine was withdrawn and did not recur when L-carnitine alone was administered (Bazzato et al 1981). The mechanism of carnitine-induced myasthenia is not clear. Carnitine has been found to interfere competitively with neuromuscular transmission (Blum et al 1971) and to cause a presynaptic block (Bazzato et al 1981) in different preparations. The tendency for D-carnitine to accumulate selectively in renal insufficiency may explain the differential response to D,L and L-carnitine administration in the same patient.

Magnesium salts. Magnesium is known to block neuromuscular transmission through a presynaptic interference with calcium-mediated acetylcholine release. Thus, the use of magnesium-containing drugs in any situation where the synaptic safety factor is reduced, should be closely monitored. Reports that magnesium may potentiate neuromuscular blocking drugs (Ghoneim & Long 1970), interact with aminoglycosides to produce neuromuscular block (L'Hommedieu et al 1983), or aggravate the Lambert–Eaton syndrome (Gutmann & Takamori 1973, Streib 1977) have been published but there are no reports of adverse effects in MG. However, it is apparent that magnesium salts are potentially hazardous in this disorder.

Other drugs. A number of other drugs have been shown to have an effect on neuromuscular transmission when used therapeutically. These include oxytocin (Hodges et al 1959), Trasylol® (aprotinin) (kallikrein-trypsin inactivator) (Chasapakis & Dimas 1966), procaine and lidocaine (Usubiaga et al 1967) and eye drops containing potent anticholinesterases (Gesztes 1966), all of which have been reported to cause postoperative respiratory depression through potentiation of muscle relaxants. Intravenous iodinated contrast agents may precipitate a myasthenic crisis (Canal & Franceschi 1983, Chagnac et al 1985). There have been single reports of the development of myasthenic syndromes in patients

taking the oral contraceptive pill (Bickerstaff 1975) or busulphan (Djaldetti et al 1968) but these are difficult to evaluate. Thyroid hormones in doses affecting the basal metabolic rate may also aggravate MG (Engel 1961, Drachman 1962). Acetazolamide has been shown to prevent the increment induced by edrophonium in myasthenic patients and to have a similar action in vitro (Carmignani et al 1984). It is well known that corticosteroids, ACTH and the anticholinesterases which are used in the treatment of MG may interfere with neuromuscular transmission in their own right and lead to exacerbation of the myasthenic state. This is discussed further in Chapter 19.

A number of other drugs which have not been implicated clinically, have been shown to interfere with neuromuscular transmission in experimental studies. The inhalational anaesthetics halothane and ether have been shown to have a postsynaptic curariform action (Watland et al 1957, Gissen et al 1966). The barbiturates (Proctor & Weakly 1976), amitriptyline (Lermer et al 1970), haloperidol and droperidol (Sokoll et al 1974, Boucher & Katz 1977) and certain of the antihistamines (Abdel-Aziz & Bakry 1973) have been shown to have combined pre- and postsynaptic blocking properties while the amphetamines (Skau & Gerald 1978) and emetine (Salako 1970) have a postsynaptic curariform action. Imipramine is thought to have a presynaptic anaesthetic-like effect (Chang & Chuang 1972). Amantadine has been shown to interfere with muscle membrane conductance (Albuquerque et al 1978) and ajmaline is thought to interfere with neuromuscular transmission by combining with ACh (Manani et al 1970).

Management. Recognition and withdrawal of the offending drug are the most important measures in the management of drug-induced neuromuscular block. Treatment of acute severe blockade, as in patients with antibiotic-induced postoperative respiratory depression, involves assisted respiration and other supportive measures, as well as pharmacological attempts to reverse the block (Argov & Mastaglia 1979a, Sokoll & Gergis 1981). Calcium infusions may be effective in reversing presynaptic block and 4-aminopyridine may also be helpful in this situation. In the case of drugs with a primarily post-synaptic action, neostigmine should be administered parenterally. In many instances the block is of the combined form and both calcium and neostigmine are required. If the respiratory muscles are not affected, discontinuation of the drug responsible and close monitoring of the patient will usually suffice. The form of myasthenia induced by D-penicillamine is usually slowly reversible after withdrawal of the drug but treatment with oral anticholinesterases or corticosteroids may be required until remission occurs.

PERIPHERAL NEUROPATHIES

Over 50 drugs used in clinical practice have been reported over the past 30 years to cause peripheral nerve damage in man (Le Quesne 1970, 1984, Argov & Mastaglia 1979b). Prompt recognition of this complication of drug therapy is clearly of importance if severe neurological deficits are to be avoided. Mild forms of neuropathy are easily over-looked and subclinical involvement is not uncommon.

Clinical presentations

The common clinical forms of drug-induced neuropathy are shown in Table 29.4. While in most instances specific drugs produce fairly consistent and characteristic syndromes, this is not always the case and some drugs may cause either a sensorimotor neuropathy or a pure motor or sensory neuropathy.

Paraesthesiae and sensory neuropathy. A variety of drugs cause acroparaesthesiae, suggesting a disturbance of sensory nerve function, but clinical examination and electrophysiological studies fail to show objective evidence of peripheral nerve damage (Table 29.4). Some, such as acetazolamide and cytosine arabinoside, cause unpleasant and even painful paraesthesiae. Others, such as streptomycin and stilbamidine, cause facial paraesthesiae or other unpleasant sensations in the upper part of the body (Collard & Hargreaves 1947, Janssen 1960). A number of other drugs produce a sensory neuropathy with clinical and electrophysiological evidence of damage to sensory nerve fibres (Table 29.4). The resulting clinical syndrome is that of a symmetrical distal sensory disturbance, initially with paraesthesiae, and subsequently impairment, particularly of superficial sensory modalities, with relative sparing of vibration and proprioceptive sensation. The tendon reflexes are usually preserved but may be depressed or absent in some cases, presumably due to involvement of afferent fibres from the muscle spindles.

Sensorimotor neuropathy. Most cases of drug-induced neuropathy fall into this category (Table 29.4). Sensory manifestations usually appear first and are followed by motor involvement at a later stage only if the drug is not stopped. The onset and clinical progression of the disorder are usually gradual, but may be relatively acute in some cases, and may even resemble the Guillain–Barré form of post-infective polyneuropathy. Sensory and motor involvement is usually distal and symmetrical and, with occasional exceptions in which there is predominant involvement of the upper limbs (Bruun & Hermann 1942), the lower limbs are usually involved first and most severely. Muscle pain and cramps may be prominent in some cases (Le Quesne 1984). The tendon reflexes are usually depressed or absent even when motor involvement is absent or inconspicuous (Casey et al 1973). Exaggerated tendon reflexes in some cases suggest concomitant involvement of central motor pathways (Le Quesne 1984). Some drugs such as dapsone cause a motor neuropathy with absent or inconspicuous sensory abnormalities (Saquenton et al 1969, Epstein & Bohm 1976), while others such as nitrofurantoin, which usually produces a sensorimotor neuropathy, may rarely cause a pure motor neuropathy (Toole & Parrish 1973).

Localised neuropathies. Involvement of peripheral nerve trunks may occur as a complication of intramuscular injections of drugs, attributable either to direct needle trauma or to a local toxic effect of the drug itself. The best-known example is the sciatic nerve damage which may occur with injections into the buttock. Peripheral nerve involvement may also occur as a

Table 29.4 Drug-induced peripheral neuropathies (clinical syndromes and drugs implicated)

Clinical presentation	Antimicrobial drugs	Antineoplastic drugs	Antirheumatic drugs	Hypnotics and psychotropics	Cardiovascular drugs	Other drugs
Sensory neuropathy	ethionamide chloramphenicol thiamphenicol diamines	procarbazine nitrofurazone misonidazole cisplatinum	sulindac	thalidomide		calcium carbimidine sulfoxone, ergotamine propylthiouracil, pyridoxine almitraine
Paraesthesiae only	colistin streptomycin nalidixic acid	cytosine-arabinoside		phenelzine	propranolol	sulthiame, chlorpropamide methysergide, acetazolamide
Sensorimotor neuropathy	isoniazid ethambutol streptomycin nitrofurantoin clioquinol metronidazole	vincristine podophyllin chlorambucil laetrile cisplatinum hexamethyl-melamine	gold indomethacin colchicine chloroquine phenylbutazone	thalidomide methaqualone glutethimide amitriptyline lithium	perhexiline hydrallazine amiodarone disopyramide clofibrate	phenytoin, disulfiram carbutamide, tolbutamide chlorpropamide methimazole methylthiouracil, cimetidine D-penicillamine, tetanus toxoid, streptokinase
Predominantly motor	sulphonamides amphotericin B streptomycin dapsone	azathioprine	sulindac	imipramine		

result of haemorrhage into confined spaces in patients on poorly controlled oral anticoagulant therapy. The femoral nerve trunk and the lumbosacral roots are most frequently affected in this way when the haemorrhage is retroperitoneal, but other peripheral nerves such as the median may also be involved (Dhaliwal et al 1976). Localised forms of neuropathy may also occur after intra-arterial perfusion of cytotoxic agents such as nitrogen mustard or ethoglucid in the treatment of malignancy (Scholes 1960, Westbury 1962, Bond et al 1964). In addition, local damage to nerves in the cubital fossa may occur as a result of intravenous infusions of certain drugs (Utz et al 1957). Of particular interest is the occasional occurrence of brachial plexus neuropathy following penicillin injections into the buttock (Kolb & Gray 1946), presumably on an 'allergic' basis.

Cranial neuropathies. Certain cranial nerves may be involved, either selectively or as part of a more generalised drug-induced neuropathy. The optic, trigeminal and eighth cranial nerve are the most commonly affected.

Pathogenesis

The mechanisms involved in the production of drug-induced neuropathies are, in general, not well understood. Experimental animal studies have clarified the mechanism of action of certain drugs such as vincristine (Bradley 1970) and nitrofurantoin (Klinghardt 1967) while that of others remains to be determined. Few histological studies of peripheral nerve have been performed in patients with drug-induced neuropathy, but axonal degeneration appears to be the principal process in most cases. A predominantly demyelinating process has been described in some patients with neuropathy due to perhexiline (Said 1978) or amiodarone (Aronson 1978).

In general, the drugs which cause peripheral neuropathy do so either by interfering with axonal or Schwann cell metabolism or through a vascular effect. The neuropathy in which the nature of the metabolic disturbance is best understood is probably that caused by isoniazid in which peripheral nerve damage is secondary to an effect of the drug on pyridoxine metabolism (Beihl & Nimitz 1954, Biehl & Vilter 1954, McCormick & Snell 1959). Vitamin deficiency may also play a part in other drug-induced neuropathies, e.g. it has been shown that prolonged administration of chloramphenicol in the rat may lead to vitamin B_{12} deficiency, which in turn may play a part in causing the neuropathy which occasionally develops in patients treated with the drug (Satoyoshi & Wakata 1978). Thalidomide is thought to inhibit riboflavine (Leck & Millar 1962) and to interfere with pyruvate metabolism (Buckle 1963), while the nitrofurans interfere with pyruvate oxidation by competing with thiamine pyrophosphate (Paul et al 1954). Preliminary work has suggested that a disturbance of lipid metabolism may underlie the neuropathy caused by perhexiline (Pollet et al 1977). Vincristine and colchicine are neurotubular toxins (Schochet et al 1968, Rasmussen 1970). The neuropathy caused by laetrile is probably due to cyanide intoxication (Kalyanaraman et al 1983).

Some drugs cause peripheral nerve damage by an effect on neural blood vessels. This may result either from severe vasospasm, as in chronic ergotism (Merhoff & Porter 1974), or from a vasculitic process (Stafford et al 1975). The possibility that certain drugs may produce a true allergic polyneuropathy has been considered (Cohen 1970), especially when a Guillain–Barré-like syndrome develops, but evidence for this is tenuous. Drugs reported to induce neuropathy via such mechanisms are cimetidine (Walls et al 1980), D-penicillamine (Knezevic et al 1984b), streptomycin (Janssen 1960), streptokinase (Leaf et al 1984), sulindac (Lending et al 1984), tetanus toxoid (Halliday & Bauer 1983) and the antidepressant drug zimeldine (Fagius et al 1985).

Predisposing factors

Some drugs such as amitriptyline, clofibrate and disopyramide cause peripheral neuropathy only rarely and the possibility therefore arises that certain individuals are unduly susceptible to the effects of such drugs. By contrast, other drugs such as vincristine are highly neurotoxic and will consistently cause peripheral nerve damage if administered for long enough in high enough doses (Bradley et al 1970).

The best-known example of a genetic predisposition is the striking susceptibility of the Japanese to clioquinol neurotoxicity. The syndrome of subacute myelo-opticoneuropathy (SMON) developed in 17% of Japanese patients who took the drug (Sobue et al 1971, Tsubaki et al 1971) whereas very few cases were reported from other parts of the world where the drug was also freely used (Selby 1972, Le Quesne 1984). Variations in the pharmacokinetics of certain drugs may also modify the susceptibility to neurotoxic effects. Impaired renal function may lead to toxic blood levels of drugs such as nitrofurantoin which are excreted through the kidneys, and thereby increase the likelihood of neuropathy developing (Ellis 1962). Similarly, it is well known that slow acetylators of isoniazid are more likely to develop peripheral neuropathy if pyridoxine supplements are not given (Hughes et al 1954). Strenuous exercise was thought to predispose to the development of neuropathy in patients treated with the older sulphonamides (Bruun & Hermann 1942).

The underlying disease process may itself modify the susceptibility to drug-induced neuropathy, e.g. patients with lymphoma develop neuropathy more frequently when treated with vincristine than those with other forms of malignancy (Watkins & Griffin 1978). Hypomagnesaemia induced by cisplatinum is thought to increase the chances of developing cisplatinum neuropathy (Ashraf et al 1983). Whether or not drug-induced neuropathy is more likely to occur in patients with cancer, diabetes, vitamin deficiency or alcoholism, situations in which the peripheral nervous system may already be affected, is uncertain.

Specific drugs

It is beyond the scope of this chapter to discuss in detail each drug involved. Brief mention of the more important ones with relevant references will be given here.

Antimicrobial agents. Over a dozen drugs used in the treatment of bacterial and protozoal infections over the past 35 years have been recognised to cause peripheral neuropathy (Snavely & Hodges 1984).

Isoniazid. The occurrence of peripheral neuropathy in patients treated with this antituberculous agent was first recognised soon after its introduction (Gammon et al 1953). The incidence of neuropathy was found to be dose-dependent, being as high at 17% in patients taking 400 mg of the drug per day, and 35% during a second course of treatment (Mandel 1959). As indicated previously, the neuropathy has been shown to be due to the development of pyridoxine deficiency (Biehl & Vilter 1954), being more likely to occur in individuals who inactivate the drug at slow rates in the liver, and being preventable when adequate supplements of vitamin B_6 are administered with the drug (10 mg per 100 mg of isoniazid) (Cohen 1970, Le Quesne 1984).

Other anti-tuberculous agents. Ethambutol may also cause a sensorimotor neuropathy (Cohen 1970, Tugwell & James 1972) which responds favourably to withdrawal of the drug. Ethionamide, which is structurally similar to isoniazid, is also known to cause a mild sensory neuropathy (Poole & Schneeweiss 1961) and to have other neurotoxic effects (Brouet et al 1959). Streptomycin has been reported to cause a peripheral neuropathy (Janssen 1960), but this is much less common than its ototoxic effects.

Nitrofurantoin. Peripheral neuropathy was a relatively frequent complication of treatment with this drug. A review of the literature by Toole & Parrish in 1973 disclosed 137 reported cases. With the exception of two patients who had a pure motor neuropathy (Morris 1966), the majority of cases presented with distal sensory symptoms followed after a few days by pain and muscle weakness, the latter being profound in some cases and contributing to a fatal outcome (Rubenstein 1964, Yiannikas et al 1981).

Sulphonamides. Peripheral neuropathy was a well-recognised complication of treatment with sulphonamides in the 1940s. The clinical features were well documented in two Scandinavian reviews of over 100 patients, most of whom were treated with sulphanyldimethylsulfanilamide (Uliron®) (Bruun & Hermann 1942, Muller 1945). Although transient paraesthesiae occurred in some cases, the neuropathy was predominantly motor and usually developed one to three weeks after completion of treatment. The mechanism of the neuropathy remains uncertain, but it has been suggested that in some cases it is due to a toxic effect of the drug, while in others it may be allergic in nature (Le Quesne 1970). None of the sulphonamides in current clinical use are known to have toxic effects on the peripheral nervous system (Weinstein et al 1974).

Clioquinol. The SMON syndrome, which was characterised by abdominal pain and the subsequent development of a neurological disorder involving the optic nerves, spinal cord and peripheral nerves, was prevalent in Japan during the 1950s and 1960s. Kono reviewed a total of 7856 probable cases of this syndrome in 1971. The association with clioquinol was recognised in 1971 (Tsubaki et al 1971), when it was found that 96% of a series of 969 affected patients had taken the drug before the onset of neurological symptoms.

Metronidazole. There have been a number of reports of a sensory neuropathy developing in patients with various conditions who were treated with this drug for prolonged periods (Ramsay 1968, Ingham et al 1975, Ursing & Kamme 1975, Coxon & Pallis 1976, Bradley et al 1977). Motor involvement has not been apparent clinically, but mild prolongation of distal motor latencies was found in one case (Bradley et al 1977). Misonidazole and related compounds, which are chemically similar to metronidazole, and are used as radio-sensitising agents in cancer therapy, can also induce a sensory neuropathy (Paulson et al 1984, Dische et al 1981).

Anti-neoplastic agents
Vinca alkaloids. These drugs, which have been used in the treatment of various malignancies, are extremely neurotoxic. Vincristine is particularly toxic and most patients who are on the drug for long enough will develop signs of peripheral nerve damage. The clinical features of vincristine neuropathy are well documented (Warot et al 1965, Bradley et al 1970, Casey et al 1973). Distal paraesthesiae, which are usually the earliest symptom, may involve the hands before the feet

and may antedate sensory or motor deficits for long periods. Muscle cramps may be a prominent symptom which accompanies the onset of motor involvement. The latter shows a predilection for the forearm extensor muscles in some cases (Casey et al 1973). The tendon reflexes are lost at an early stage, particularly in the lower limbs. Autonomic involvement may also occur and postural hypotension and constipation may be early symptoms (Warot et al 1965). Recovery may occur if the drug is stopped or even if the dose is reduced, but mild sensory impairment and reflex depression often persist.

Other cytotoxic drugs. A number of other drugs used in the treatment of malignancy may cause neuropathy. An extensive review of the neurotoxic effects of cancer therapy should be consulted for details (Kaplan & Wiernik 1982). Procarbazine, which is structurally similar to isoniazid, has occasionally been associated with a sensory neuropathy (Weiss et al 1974) as have nitrofurazone, a congener of nitrofurantoin which was used in the treatment of testicular carcinoma (Le Quesne 1975) and cytosine arabinoside (Russell & Powles 1974). Podophyllin derivatives, which have been used in the treatment of disseminated malignancies, and which are also constituents of certain laxative preparations and topical agents, may cause a mild or severe peripheral neuropathy (Falkson et al 1975, Langman 1975, Filley et al 1982, Dobb & Edis 1984). Chlorambucil has also been reported to cause a sensorimotor neuropathy occasionally (Sandler & Gonsalkorale 1977). A primarily sensory neuropathy, with subtle motor involvement, may occur in patients treated with cisplatinum. Nerve biopsy has shown combined axonal and myelin damage in such cases (Thompson et al 1984, Roelofs et al 1984).

Antirheumatic drugs
Gold. Peripheral neuropathy is a well-recognised complication of gold therapy in rheumatoid arthritis (Endtz 1958), occurring in 0.5–1% of patients treated in this way (Hartfall et al 1937, Doyle & Cannon 1950). Motor involvement is usually prominent and may be asymmetrical, and sensory signs may be inconspicuous. The onset may be abrupt and progression rapid, mimicking

the Guillain–Barré form of postinfective poly-neuropathy, particularly in some patients who also develop facial diplegia and have elevated cerebro-spinal fluid protein levels (Le Quesne 1970, Katrak et al 1980). Fever and a skin rash may be associated with the neuropathy, indicating a more generalised reaction in some cases (Doyle & Cannon 1950).

Chloroquine. Evidence of peripheral nerve involvement has been found in some patients who developed a vacuolar myopathy while being treated with chloroquine (Loftus 1963, Whisnant et al 1963, Hicklin 1968).

Other anti-inflammatory drugs. Indomethacin has also been implicated in causing a neuropathy (Eade et al 1975). There are occasional reports of peripheral neuropathy developing in patients treated with colchicine (Prescott 1975) or D-peni-cillamine (Meyboom 1977), the latter drug being known to have an antipyridoxine effect (Jaffe et al 1964).

Hypnotics and psychotropic drugs
Thalidomide. This drug was first reported to cause neuropathy in 1960, five years after it was introduced into clinical use (Florence 1960). Although the drug was withdrawn from the market two years later, victims of its teratogenic and neurotoxic effects are still seen. The charac-teristics of thalidomide neuropathy were reviewed by Fullerton & Kremer (1961) and Fullerton & O'Sullivan (1968). The drug is now in exper-imental use in dermatology and there have been reports of patients developing a neuropathy (Clemmensen et al 1984).

Methaqualone. A number of reports have raised suspicion that methaqualone may be neurotoxic. At least 11 cases of a sensorimotor neuropathy have now been reported in patients taking 200–600 mg of methaqualone nightly for periods of a few days to two years, either alone or with diphenhydramine, diazepam, meprobamate or promazine (McQuaker & Bruggen 1963, Finke & Spiegelberg 1973, Hoaken 1975, Markes & Sloggen 1976).

Glutethimide. Reports of two patients with sensory symptoms and areflexia after prolonged high-dose treatment with this drug (Bartholomew 1961), and of a suspected case of neuropathy in a glutethimide addict (Lingle 1966) raised suspicion that the drug, which has structural simi-larities to thalidomide, may be neurotoxic.

Other drugs. There have been occasional reports of a predominantly motor neuropathy developing in patients treated with imipramine (Collier & Martin 1960, Miller 1963, Cohen 1970) and lithium carbonate (Uchigata et al 1981).

Cardiovascular drugs
Perhexiline. The occurrence of neuropathy in patients treated with this coronary vasodilator is now well recognised (Bousser et al 1976, Lher-mitte et al 1976, Fraser et al 1977, Gerand et al 1978, Sebille 1978). It has been claimed that clini-cally manifest neuropathy occurs in about 0.1% of patients treated with the drug and that subclinical involvement is even commoner (Sebille 1978). Sensory symptoms, which are usually prominent, may appear as early as three weeks after commencement of treatment (Robinson 1978) and are followed by distal motor involvement in the limbs.

Amiodarone. There have been a number of reports of a demyelinating sensorimotor poly-neuropathy developing in patients treated with this anti-arrhythmic agent (Robinson 1975, Aronson 1978, Meier et al 1979, Martinez-Arizala et al 1983, Lim et al 1984, Pellissier et al 1984, Anderson et al 1985, Fraser et al 1985, Jacobs & Costa-Jussa 1985).

Hydrallazine. A number of cases of a mixed but predominantly sensory peripheral neuropathy have been reported in patients treated with this drug (Kirkendall & Page 1958, Le Quesne 1970, Perry 1973). The neuropathy appears to be unre-lated to the lupus-like syndrome induced by the drug.

Clofibrate. Clinical and electrophysiological evidence of peripheral nerve involvement was found in two patients with clofibrate myopathy

(Gabriel & Pearce 1976, Pokroy et al 1977). However, there is some doubt as to the cause of the neuropathy in these cases and further evidence is required before accepting that the drug is neurotoxic.

Other drugs

Phenytoin. The occurrence of a mild peripheral neuropathy in patients on long-term phenytoin treatment is well recognised (Finkleman & Arieff 1942, Lovelace & Horwitz 1968). Sensory symptoms are present in some patients but most are asymptomatic, being found to have reflex depression or sensory impairment on clinical examination (Lovelace & Horwitz 1968). The frequency of polyneuropathy appears to increase with the duration of therapy (Lovelace & Horwitz 1968, Eisen et al 1974).

Disulfiram. The occurrence of a sensorimotor polyneuropathy in alcoholics treated with this drug is well established (Hayman & Wilkins 1956, Bradley & Hewer 1966, Gardner-Thorpe & Benjamin 1971, Nukada & Pollock 1981, Ansbacher et al 1982) although in some cases it has been difficult to be certain of the extent to which alcohol or nutritional deficiencies may have contributed to the neuropathy.

Dapsone. This drug, which has been used in the treatment of leprosy and of a number of dermatological conditions, is known to cause an almost exclusively motor form of peripheral neuropathy (Saquenton et al 1969, Epstein & Bohm 1976, Gehlmann et al 1977). This has usually developed after prolonged high-dose therapy but has also occurred with lower doses of the drug (Rapoport & Guss 1972). Electrophysiological studies have shown mild impairment of motor conduction (Saquenton et al 1969, Fredericks et al 1976) with normal sensory conduction (Wyatt & Stevens 1972, Fredericks et al 1976).

Antithyroid agents. Several drugs which were used in the treatment of thyrotoxicosis have been associated with neurotoxic side effects. Methimazole was reported to cause acute motor neuropathy (Accetta et al 1954) or sensory neuropathy (Roldan & Nigrin 1972) in single case records. Propyl-thiouracil caused sensory neuropathy (Crile 1947, Frawley & Koeppe 1950), while methylthiouracil was claimed to be responsible for widespread sensorimotor neuropathy in a case report (Barfred 1947).

Pyridoxine. Megadoses of pyridoxine, which in low doses is used to protect against isoniazid neuropathy, can cause a sensory neuropathy (Schaumburg et al 1983).

Almitrine. Almitrine bismesylate, a drug which has been used in patients with cerebrovascular disease and chronic obstructive pulmonary disease, has recently been reported to cause a sensory polyneuropathy (Chedru et al 1985).

CONCLUSIONS

It will be seen from the present review that drugs used in various clinical situations may interfere with neuromuscular function. The possibility of such a complication should be considered in any patient who complains of muscle pain, weakness, fatiguability or sensory disturbances while on drug therapy: patients complaining of such symptoms should be subjected to a careful neurological examination and EMG study. In view of their potentially reversible nature, drug-induced disorders should enter into the differential diagnosis in any patient presenting with a myopathy, neuropathy or myasthenic syndrome and full details of drug therapy should be obtained in all such patients. The possibility of drug effects should be considered, particularly in patients with a pre-existing neuromuscular disorder, who may be more susceptible to, and less able to compensate for, such effects.

In addition to their diagnostic role, electrophysiological and pathological studies of patients with drug-induced neuromuscular disorders will help to provide a clearer indication of the true incidence of such complications. Such studies will also contribute to the understanding of the pathogenesis and pathophysiology of toxic forms of neuropathy and myopathy and of the basic pathological reactions of peripheral nerve and muscle.

Experimental studies in vivo and in vitro have

elucidated the mechanisms whereby a number of drugs interfere with neuromuscular function. However, because of various differences between the experimental and human situations, the results of such studies have not always been directly applicable to man. Thus in the case of certain drugs such as amantadine, an effect on neuromuscular transmission has been identified in in vitro studies but has not been manifest clinically. Nevertheless, such studies are clearly of importance for the screening of newly introduced

therapeutic agents and will serve to alert the clinician to possible effects on neuromuscular function.

ACKNOWLEDGEMENTS

The authors are grateful to Miss M. Jenkison who prepared the photomicrographs and provided technical assistance, and to Mrs. P. McBryde for secretarial assistance.

REFERENCES

Abdel-Aziz A, Bakry N 1973 The action and interaction of diphenhydramine (Benadryl) hydrochloride at the neuromuscular junction. European Journal of Pharmacology 22:169

Aberfeld D C, Bienenstock H, Shapiro M S, Namba T, Grob D 1968 Diffuse myopathy related to meperidine addiction in a mother and daughter. Archives of Neurology 19:384

Abreo K, Shelp W D, Kosseff A, Thomas S 1982 Amoxapin-associated rhabdomyolysis and acute renal failure: Case report. Journal of Clinical Psychiatry 43:426

Accetta G S, Fitzmorris A O, Wettingfeld R F 1954 Toxicity of methimazole. Journal of the American Medical Association 155:253

Adams E M, Horowitz H W, Sundstrom W R 1983 Fibrous myopathy in association with pentazocine. Archives of Internal Medicine 143:2203

Affarah H B, Mars R L, Someren A, Smith H W B, Heymsfield S B 1984 Myoglobinuria and acute renal failure associated with intravenous vasopressin infusion. Southern Medical Journal 77:918

Afifi A K, Bergman R A 1969 Steroid myopathy — a study of the evolution of the muscle lesion in rabbits. Johns Hopkins Medical Journal 124:66

Aguayo A J, Hudgson P 1970 The short-term effects of chloroquine on skeletal muscle: An experimental study in the rabbit. Journal of the Neurological Sciences 11:301

Albuquerque E X, Eldefrawi A T, Eldefrawi M E, Mansour N, Tsai M C 1978 Amantadine: neuromuscular blockade by suppression of ionic conductance of the acetylcholine receptor. Science 199:788

Aldrich M S, Kim Y I, Sanders D B 1979 Effects of D-penicillamine on neuromuscular transmission in rats. Muscle and Nerve 2:180

Anderson N E, Lynch N M, O'Brien K P 1985 Disabling neurological complications of amiodarone. Australian and New Zealand Journal of Medicine 15:300

Anderson P J, Song S K, Slotwiner P 1967 The fine structure of spheromembranous degeneration of skeletal muscle induced by vincristine. Journal of Neuropathology and Experimental Neurology 26:15

Ansbacher L E, Bosch E P, Cancilla P A 1982 Disulfiram neuropathy: a neurofilamentous distal axonopathy. Neurology (NY) 32:424

Argov Z, Mastaglia F L 1979a Disorders of neuromuscular

transmission caused by drugs. New England Journal of Medicine 301:409

Argov Z, Mastaglia F L 1979b Drug-induced peripheral neuropathies. British Medical Journal 1:663

Argov Z, Yaari Y 1979 The action of chlorpromazine at an isolated cholinergic synapse. Brain Research 164:227

Argov Z, Abramsky D 1982 Antibiotic treatment in myasthenia gravis. Harefuah 10:225

Argov Z, Brenner T, Abramsky D 1986 Ampicillin may aggravate clinical and experimental myasthenia. Archives of Neurology 43:255

Aronson J K 1978 Cardiac glycosides and drugs used in dysrhythmias. In: Dukes M N G (ed) Side effects of drugs. Excerpta Medica, Amsterdam, II, p 163

Ashraf M, Scotchel P L, Krall J M, Flink E B 1983 Cis-platinum-induced hypomagnesemia and peripheral neuropathy. Gynecologic Oncology 16:309

Askari A, Vignos P J, Moskowitz R W 1976 Steroid myopathy in connective tissue disease. American Journal of Medicine 61:485

Barfred A 1947 Methylthiouracil in the treatment of thyrotoxicosis. American Journal of Medical Sciences 214:349

Bartholomew A A 1961 (in correspondence) British Medical Journal 2:1570

Basser L S 1979 Purgatives and periodic paralysis. Medical Journal of Australia 1:47

Battacharrya S 1966 Abduction contracture of the shoulder from contracture of the intermediate part of the deltoid. Report of three cases. Journal of Bone and Joint Surgery 46B:127

Bazzato G, Coli U, Landini S, Mezzina C, Ciman M 1981 Myasthenia-like syndrome after D,L- but not L-carnitine. Lancet i:1209

Bennett H S, Spiro A J, Pollack M A, Zucker P 1982 Ipecac-induced myopathy simulating dermatomyositis. Neurology 32:91

Bennetts F E 1964 Muscular paralysis due to streptomycin following inhalation anaesthesia. Anaesthesia 19:93

Bettendorf U, Neuhaus R 1974 Penicillamin-induzierte polymyositis. Deutsche Medizinische Wochenschrift 99:2522

Bever C T, Chang H W, Penn A S, Jaffe I A, Bock E 1982 Penicillamine-induced myasthenia gravis: effects of penicillamine on acetylcholine receptor. Neurology 32:1077

Bickerstaff E R 1975 Neurological complications of oral contraceptives. Clarendon Press, London, p 93

Biehl J P, Nimitz H J 1954 Studies on the use of a high dose of isoniazid. American Review of Tuberculosis 70:430

Biehl J P, Vilter R W 1954 Effects of isoniazid on pyridoxine metabolism. Journal of the American Medical Association 156:1549

Blessing W, Walsh J C 1977 Myotonia precipitated by propranolol therapy. Lancet i:73

Blomberg L H 1965 Dystrophia myotonica probably caused by chloroquine. Acta Neurologica Scandinavica (Suppl) 13:647

Blomgren S E, Condemi J J, Vaughan J H 1972 Procainamide-induced lupus erythematosus. American Journal of Medicine 52:338

Blum K, Seifter E, Seifter J 1971 The pharmacology of D- and L-carnitine. Comparison with choline and acetylcholine. Journal of Pharmacology and Experimental Therapeutics 178:331

Bodley P O, Brett J E 1962 Post-operative respiratory inadequacy and the part played by antibiotics. Anaesthesia 17:438

Bodley P O, Halwax K, Potts L 1969 Low pseudocholinesterase levels complicating treatment with phenelzine. British Medical Journal 3:510

Bond M R, Clark S D, Neal F E 1964 Use of ethoglucid in treatment of advanced malignant disease. British Medical Journal 1:951

Booker H E, Chun R W M, Sanguino M 1970 Myasthenia gravis syndrome associated with trimethadione. Journal of the American Medical Association 212:2262

Borden H, Clarke M T, Katz H 1974 The use of pancuronium bromide in patients receiving lithium carbonate. Canadian Anaesthetic Society Journal 21:79

Boucher S D, Katz N L 1977 Effects of several 'membrane stabilizing' agents on frog neuromuscular junction. European Journal of Pharmacology 42:139

Bousser M G, Bouche P, Brochard C, Herreman G 1976 Sept neuropathies périphériques après traitement par maleate de perhexiline. La Nouvelle Presse Médicale 5:652

Bovill J G, Dundee J W, Coppel D L, Moore J 1971 Current status of ketamine anaesthesia. Lancet 1:1285

Bradley W G 1970 The neuropathy of vincristine in the guinea pig. An electrophysiological and pathological study. Journal of the Neurological Sciences 10:133

Bradley W G, Hewer R L 1966 Peripheral neuropathy due to disulfiram. British Medical Journal 1:449

Bradley W G, Lassman L P, Pearce G W, Walton J N 1970 The neuromyopathy of vincristine in man. Clinical, electrophysiological and pathological findings. Journal of the Neurological Sciences 10:107

Bradley W G, Fewings J D, Harris J B, Johnson M A 1976 Emetine myopathy in the rat. British Journal of Pharmacology 57:29

Bradley W G, Karlsson I J, Rasool C G 1977 Metronidazole neuropathy. British Medical Journal 2:610

Bretag A H, Dawe S R, Kerr D I B, Moskwa A G 1980 Myotonia as a side effect of diuretic action. British Journal of Pharmacology 71:467

Bridgeman J F, Rosen A M, Thorp J M 1972 Complications during clofibrate treatment of nephrotic syndrome hyperlipoproteinaemia. Lancet 2:502

Britt B A 1979 Etiology and pathophysiology of malignant hyperthermia. Federation Proceedings 38:44

Britt C W, Light R R, Peters B H, Schochet S S 1980

Rhabdomyolysis during treatment with epsilon-aminocaproic acid. Archives of Neurology 37:187

Brodkin H M 1980 Myoglobinuria following epsilon-aminocaproic acid (EACA) therapy. Journal of Neurosurgery 53:690

Brodsky J B, Ehrenwerth J 1980 Postoperative muscle pains and suxamethonium. British Journal of Anaesthesia 52:215

Brouet G, Marche J, Rist N, Chevallier J, Le Meur G 1959 Observation on the antituberculous effectiveness of alpha-ethyl-thioisonicotinamide in tuberculosis in humans. American Review of Tuberculosis 79:6

Brown J A, Wollmann R L, Mullan S 1982 Myopathy induced by epsilon-aminocaproic acid. Journal of Neurosurgery 57:130

Brumback R A, Empting L, Susag M E, Staton R D 1982 Muscle fibrosis associated with intramuscular chlorpromazine administration: A preliminary report. Journal of Pharmacy and Pharmacology 34:526

Brumlik J, Jacobs R S 1974 Myasthenia gravis associated with diphenyl hydantoin therapy for epilepsy. Canadian Journal of Neurological Sciences 1:127

Bruun E, Hermann K 1942 Polyneuritis after treatment with sulfonamide preparations. Acta Medica Scandinavica 111:261

Buckle R M 1963 Blood pyruvic acid in thalidomide neuropathy. British Medical Journal 2:973

Bucknall R C 1977 Myasthenia associated with D-penicillamine therapy in rheumatoid arthritis. Proceedings of the Royal Society of Medicine 70 (Suppl 3):114

Burres S A, Richman D P, Crayton J W, Arnason B G W 1979 Penicillamine-induced myasthenia responses in the guinea pig. Muscle and Nerve 2:186

Canal N, Franceschi M 1983 Myasthenic crisis precipitated by iothalmic acid. Lancet i:1288

Carmignani M, Scoppetta C, Ranelletti F O Tonali P 1984 Adverse interaction between acetazolamide and anticholinesterase drugs at the normal and myasthenic neuromuscular junction level. International Journal of Clinical Pharmacology, Therapeutics and Toxicology 22:140

Casey E B, Jellife A M, Le Quesne P M, Millett Y L 1973 Vincristine neuropathy, clinical and electrophysiological observations. Brain 96:69

Chagnac Y, Hadani M, Goldhammer Y 1985 Myasthenic crisis after intravenous administration of iodinated contrast agent. Neurology 35: 1219

Chang C C, Chuang S T 1972 Effects of desipramine and imipramine on the nerve, muscle and synaptic transmission of rat diaphragms. Neuropharmacology 11:777

Chasapakis G, Dimas C 1966 Possible interaction between muscle relaxants and the kallikrein-trypsin inactivator Trasylol. British Journal of Anaesthesia 38:838

Chedru F, Nodzenski R, Dunand J F et al 1985 Peripheral neuropathy during treatment with almitrine. British Medical Journal 290:896

Choucair A K, Ziter F 1984 Pentazocine abuse masquerading as familial myopathy. Neurology 34:524

Clarke R S J, Dundee J W, Hamilton R C 1967 Interaction between induction agents and muscle relaxants. Anaesthesia 22:235

Clemmensen O J, Olsen P Z, Andersen K E 1984 Thalidomide neuro-toxicity. Archives of Dermatology 120:338

Cogen F C, Rigg G, Simmons J L, Domino E F 1978

Phencyclidine-associated acute rhabdomyolysis. Annals of Internal Medicine 88:210

Cohen L 1972 CPK test — effect of intramuscular injection in myocardial infarction. Journal of the American Medical Association 219:625

Cohen M M 1970 Toxic neuropathies. In: Vinken P J, Bruyn G W (eds) Handbook of clinical neurology vol 7. North Holland, Amsterdam, p 527

Collard P J, Hargreaves W H 1947 Neuropathy after stilbamidine treatment of kala-azar. Lancet 2:686

Collier G, Martin A 1960 Les effects sécondaires du tofranil. Revue générale à propos de trois cas de polynévrite des membres inferieurs. Annales Medicopsychologiques 118:719

Coomes E N 1965a Corticosteroid myopathy. Annals of Rheumatic Diseases 24:465

Coomes E N 1965b The rate of recovery of reversible myopathies and the effects of anabolic agents. Neurology (Minneapolis) 15:523

Coppeto J 1984 Timolol-associated myasthenia gravis. American Journal of Ophthalmology 98:244

Coxon A, Pallis C A 1976 Metronidazole neuropathy. Journal of Neurology, Neurosurgery and Psychiatry 39:403

Crawford A C 1975 Lithium ions and the release of transmitter at the frog neuromuscular junction. Journal of Physiology 246:109

Crile G 1947 Treatment of hyperthyroidism. Canadian Medical Association Journal 57:359

Cucher B G, Goldman A L 1976 D-Penicillamine-induced polymyositis in rheumatoid arthritis. Annals of Internal Medicine 85:615

Cullen M J, Mastaglia F L 1980 Myopathy due to epsilon aminocaproic acid. Neuropathology and Applied Neurobiology 6:78

Czlonkowaska A 1975 Myasthenia syndrome during peincillamine treatment. British Medical Journal 2:726

Dale R C, Schroeder E T 1976 Respiratory paralysis during treatment of hypertension with trimetaphan camsylate. Archives of Internal Medicine 136:816

De Grantis D, Mezzina C, Fiaschi A, Pinelli P, Bazzato G, Morachiello M 1980 Myasthenia due to carnitine treatment. Journal of the Neurological Sciences 46:365

Delamere J P, Jobson S, Mackintosh L P, Wells, Walton K W 1983 Penicillamine-induced myasthenia in rheumatoid arthritis: its clinical and genetic features. Annals of the Rheumatic Diseases 42:500

Delrieu F, Menkes C J, Sainte-Croix A, Baninet P, Chesneau A M, Delbarre F 1976 Myasthénie et thyroidite auto-immune au course du traitement de la polyarthrite rhumatoide par la D-penicillamine. Annales de Médecine Interne 127:739

Denborough M A 1977 Malignant hyperpyrexia. Medical Journal of Australia 2:757

Desmedt J E 1973 The neuromuscular disorder in myasthenia gravis. In: Desmedt J E (ed) New developments in electromyography and clinical neurophysiology vol 1. Karger, Basel, p 305

Dhaliwal G S, Schlagenhauff R E, Megahed S M 1976 Acute femoral neuropathy induced by oral anticoagulation. Diseases of the Nervous System 37:539

Dische S, Saunders M I, Stratfort M R 1981 Neurotoxicity with desmethylmisonidazole. British Journal of Radiology 54:156

Djaldetti M, Pinkhas J, De Vries A, Kott E, Joshua H, Dollberg L 1968 Myasthenia gravis in a patient with chronic myeloid leukemia treated by busulfan. Blood 32:336

Dobb G J, Edis R H 1984 Coma and neuropathy after ingestion of herbal laxative containing podophyllin. Medical Journal of Australia 140:495

Dottori O, Lof B A, Yagge H 1965 Muscle pains after suxamethonium chloride. Acta Anaesthesiologia Scandinavica 9:247

Doyle D R, McCurly T L, Sergent J S 1983 Fatal polymyositis in D-penicillamine-treated rheumatoid arthritis. Annals of Internal Medicine 98:327

Doyle J B, Cannon E F 1950 Severe polyneuritis following gold therapy for rheumatoid arthritis. Annals of Internal Medicine 33:1468

Drachman D A, Skom J H 1965 Procainamide — a hazard in myasthenia gravis. Archives of Neurology 13:316

Drachman D B 1962 Myasthenia gravis and the thyroid gland. New England Journal of Medicine 266:330

Drenckhahn D, Lullmann-Rauch R 1979 Experimental myopathy induced by amphiphilic cationic compounds including several psychotropic drugs. Neuroscience 4:549

Dretchen K L, Sokoll M D, Gergis S D, Long J P 1973 Relative effects of streptomycin on motor nerve terminal and endplate. European Journal of Pharmacology 22:10

Drutz D J, Fan J H, Tai T Y, Cheng J T, Hsieh W C 1970 Hypokalaemic rhabdomyolysis and myoglobinuria following amphotericin B therapy. Journal of the American Medical Association 211:824

Duane D D, Engel A G 1970 Emetine myopathy. Neurology (Minneapolis) 20:733

Dubois E L 1969 Procainamide induction of a systemic lupus erythematosus-like syndrome. Medicine (Baltimore) 48:217

Duignan N, Andrews J, Williams J D 1973 Pharmacological studies with lincomycin in late pregnancy. British Medical Journal 3:75

Dukes M N G 1977 Side effects of drugs; Annual 1. Excerpta Medica, Amsterdam, p 118, 181, 292, 331, 339

Eade O E, Acheson E D, Cuthbert M F, Hawkes C H 1975 Peripheral neuropathy and indomethacin. British Medical Journal 2:66

Eisen A A, Woods J F, Sherwin A L 1974 Peripheral nerve function in long-term therapy with diphenylhydantoin. Neurology (Minneapolis) 24:411

Elder B F, Beal H, De Wald W, Cobb S 1971 Exacerbation of subclinical myasthenia by occupational exposure to anaesthetic. Anesthesia and Analgesia Current Researches 50:383

Ellis F G 1962 Acute polyneuritis after nitrofurantoin therapy. Lancet 2:1136

Ellis F R, Keaney N P, Harriman D G F et al 1972 Screening for malignant hyperpyrexia. British Medical Journal 3:559

Ellis F R, Clarke, I M C, Modgill M, Currie S, Harriman D G F 1975 Evaluation of creatine phosphokinase in screening patients for malignant hyperpyrexia. British Medical Journal 3:511

Elmqvist D, Josefsson J O 1962 The nature of the neuromuscular block produced by neomycin. Acta Physiologica Scandinavica 54:105

Endtz L J 1958 Complications nerveuses du traitement aurique. Revue Neurologique 99:395

Engel A G 1961 Thyroid function and myasthenia gravis. Archives of Neurology 4:663

Epstein F W, Bohm M 1976 Dapsone-induced peripheral neuropathy. Archives of Dermatology 112:1761

Fagius J, Osterman P O, Sidén A, Wiholm B-E 1985 Guillain-Barré syndrome following zimeldine. Journal of Neurology, Neurosurgery and Psychiatry 48:65

Falkson G, van Dyk J J, van Eden E B, van der Merwe A M, van der Bergh J A, Falkson H C 1975 A clinical trial of the oral form of 4'-demethyl-epipodophyllotoxin-B-D ethylidene glucose (NSC 141540) VP 16–213. Cancer 35:1141

Fardeau M, Tomé F M S, Simon P 1979 Muscle and nerve changes induced by perhexiline maleate in man and mice. Muscle and Nerve 2:24

Fawcett P R W, McLachlan S M, Nicholson L V B, Argov Z, Mastaglia F L 1982 D-Penicillamine-associated myasthenia gravis: immunological and electrophysiological studies. Muscle and Nerve 5:328

Feest T G, Read D J 1980 Myopathy associated with cimetidine? British Medical Journal 281:1284

Feldman S A, Crawley B E 1970 Interaction of diazepam with the muscle-relaxant drugs. British Medical Journal 2:336

Fernandes L, Swinson D R, Hamilton E B D 1977 Dermatomyositis complicating penicillamine treatment. Annals of Rheumatic Diseases 36:94

Fewings J D, Burns, R J, Kakulas B A 1973 A case of acute emetine myopathy. In: Kakulas B A (ed) Clinical studies in myology. Excerpta Medica, Amsterdam, p 594

Fiekers J F 1983a Effects of the aminoglycoside antibiotics, streptomycin and neomycin, on neuromuscular transmission. 1. Presynaptic considerations. Journal of Pharmacology and Experimental Therapeutics 225:487

Fiekers J F 1983b Effects of the aminoglycoside antibiotics, streptomycin and neomycin, on neuromuscular transmission. II. Postsynaptic considerations. Journal of Pharmacology and Experimental Therapeutics 225:496

Filley C M, Graff-Radford N R, Lacy J R, Heitner M A, Earnest M P 1982 Neurologic manifestations of podophyllin toxicity. Neurology (New York) 32:308

Finke J, Spiegelberg U 1973 Polyneuropathy nach methaqualone. Nervenarzt 44:104

Finkelman I, Arieff A J 1942 Untoward effects of phenytoin sodium in epilepsy. Journal of the American Medical Association 118:1209

Florence A L 1960 Is thalidomide to blame? British Medical Journal 2:1954

Fogdall R P, Miller R D 1974 Prolongation of pancuronium induced neuromuscular block by clindamycin. Anesthesiology 41:407

Fontiveros E S, Cumming W J K, Hudgson P 1980 Procainamide-induced myositis. Journal of the Neurological Sciences 45:143

Forfar J C, Brown G J, Cull R E 1979 Proximal myopathy during beta-blockade. British Medical Journal ii:1331

Fraser A G, McQueen I N F, Watt A H, Stephens M R 1985 Peripheral neuropathy during longterm high-dose amiodarone therapy. Journal of Neurology, Neurosurgery and Psychiatry 48:576

Fraser D M, Campbell I W, Miller H C 1977 Peripheral and autonomic neuropathy after treatment with perhexiline maleate. British Medical Journal 2:75

Frawley T F, Koeppe G F 1950 Neurotoxicity due to thiouracil and thiourea derivatives. Journal of Clinical Endocrinology 10:623

Fredericks E J, Kugelman T P, Kirsch N 1976 Dapsone-induced motor polyneuropathy. Archives of Dermatology 112:1158

Fullerton P M, Kremer M 1961 Neuropathy after intake of thalidomide (Distaval). British Medical Journal 2:855

Fullerton P M, O'Sullivan D J 1968 Thalidomide neuropathy: a clinical, electrophysiological, and histological follow-up study. Journal of Neurology, Neurosurgery and Psychiatry 31:543

Gabriel R, Pearce J M S 1976 Clofibrate–induced myopathy and neuropathy. Lancet 2:906

Galzigna L, Manani G, Mammano S, Gasparetto A, Deana R 1972 Experimental study on the neuromuscular blocking action of procain amide. Agressologie 13:107

Gammon G D, Burge F W, King G 1953 Neural toxicity in tuberculous patients treated with isoniazid (isonicotinic acid hydrazine). Archives of Neurology and Psychiatry 70:64

Gardner-Thorpe C, Benjamin S 1971 Peripheral neuropathy after disulfiram administration. Journal of Neurology, Neurosurgery and Psychiatry 34:253

Gehlmann L K, Koller W C, Malkinson F D 1977 Dapsone-induced neuropathy. Archives of Dermatology 113:845

Geraud G, Caussanel J P, Jauzac P H, Arbus L, Bes A 1978 Peripheral neuropathy after perhexiline maleate therapy. 4th International Congress on Neuromuscular Diseases, Montreal, Canada, Abstract 81

Gergis S D, Sokoll M D, Rubbo J T 1977 Effect of sodium nitro-prusside and trimetaphan on neuromuscular transmission in the frog. Canadian Anaesthetists Society Journal 24:220

Gesztes T 1966 Prolonged apnoea after suxamethonium injection associated with eye drops containing an anticholinesterase agent. British Journal of Anaesthesia 38:408

Ghoneim M M, Long J P 1970 The interaction between magnesium and other neuromuscular blocking agents. Anesthesiology 32:23

Ghose K 1977 Lithium salts: therapeutic and unwanted effects. British Journal of Hospital Medicine 18:578

Gibb W R G, Lees A J 1985 The neuroleptic malignant syndrome — a review. Quarterly Journal of Medicine 220:421

Gibbels E 1967 Weitere beobachtungen zur Nebenwirkung intravenoser reverin-gaben bei Myasthenia gravis pseudoparalytica. Deutsche Medizinische Wochenschrift 92:1153

Gibbs J M 1978 A case of rhabdomyolysis associated with suxamethonium. Anaesthesia and Intensive Care 6:141

Gissen A J, Karis J H, Nastuk W L 1966 Effect of halothane on neuromuscular transmission. Journal of the American Medical Association 197:116

Golding D N, Begg T B 1960 Dexamethasone myopathy. British Medical Journal 2:1129

Granacher R P 1977 Neuromuscular problems associated with lithium. American Journal of Psychiatry 134:702

Greenblatt D J, Allen D 1978 Intramuscular injection-site complications. Journal of the American Medical Association 240:542

Gronert G A 1983 Malignant hyperthermia. Anesthesiology 53:395

Grongono A W 1963 Anaesthesia for atrial defibrillation. Effects of quinidine on muscular relaxation. Lancet 2:1039

Gross E G, Dexter J D, Roth R G 1966 Hypokalemic myopathy with myoglobinuria associated with licorice ingestion. New England Journal of Medicine 74:602

Grossman R A, Hamilton R W, Morse B M, Penn A S,

Goldberg M 1974 Nontraumatic rhabdomyolysis and acute renal failure. New England Journal of Medicine 291:807

Gutmann L, Takamori M 1973 Effects of Mg^{++} on neuromuscular transmission in the Eaton–Lambert syndrome. Neurology 23:977

Hagen R 1968 Contracture of the quadriceps muscle. A report of 12 cases. Acta Orthopaedica Scandinavica 39:565

Hales D S M, Scott R, Lewi H J E 1982 Myopathy due to mercaptopropionyl glycine. British Medical Journal 285:939

Hall L W, Woolf N, Bradley J W P, Jolly D W 1966 Unusual reaction to suxamethonium chloride. British Medical Journal 2:1305

Halla J T, Fallahi S, Koopman W J 1984 Penicillamine-induced myositis. American Journal of Medicine 77:719

Halliday P L, Bauer R B 1983 Polyradiculoneuritis secondary to immunization with tetanus and diphtheria toxoids. Archives of Neurology 40:56

Harney J, Glasberg M R 1983 Myopathy and hypersensitivity to phenytoin. Neurology 33:790

Harriman D G F, Sumner D W, Ellis F R 1973 Malignant hyperpyrexia myopathy. Quarterly Journal of Medicine 42:639

Hartfall S J, Garland H G, Goldie W 1937 Gold treatment of arthritis. A review of 900 cases. Lancet 2:838

Hashimoto F, Sherman C B, Jeffery W H 1984 Neuroleptic malignant syndrome and dopaminergic blockade. Archives of Internal Medicine 144:629

Hawkins R A, Eckhoff P J, MacCarter D K, Harmon C E 1983 Cimetidine and polymyositis. New England Journal of Medicine 309:187

Hayman I, Abresman C E, Terplan K L 1956 Dermatomyositis following penicillin injections. Neurology 6:63

Hayman M, Wilkins P A 1956 Polyneuropathy as a complication of disulfiram therapy of alcoholism. Quarterly Journal of Studies in Alcohol 17:601

Herishanu Y, Taustein I 1971 The electromyographic changes induced by antibiotics. A preliminary study. Confinia Neurologica 33:41

Herishanu Y, Rosenberg P 1975 β-Blockers and myasthenia gravis. Annals of Internal Medicine 83:834

Hicklin J A 1968 Chloroquine neuromyopathy. Annals of Physical Medicine 9:189

Hill G, Wong K C, Hodges M R 1976 Potentiation of succinylcholine neuromuscular blockage by lithium carbonate. Anesthesiology 44:439

Hoaken P C S 1975 Adverse effect of methaqualone. Canadian Medical Association Journal 112:685

Hodges R J H, Bennett J R, Tunstall M E 1959 Effects of oxytocin on the response to suxamethonium. British Medical Journal 1:413

Hokkanen E 1964 The aggravating effect of some antibiotics on the neuromuscular blockade in myasthenia gravis. Acta Neurologica Scandinavica 40:346

Hool G J, Lawrence P J, Sivaneswaran N 1984 Acute rhabdomyolytic renal failure due to suxamethonium. Anaesthesia and Intensive Care 12:360

Hughes H B, Biehl J P, Jones, A P, Schmidt L H 1954 Metabolism of isoniazid in man as related to the occurrence of peripheral neuritis. American Review of Tuberculosis 70:266

Hughes R O, Zacharias F J 1976 Myasthenic syndrome during treatment with practolol. British Medical Journal 1:460

Ingham H R, Selkon J B, Hale J H 1975 The antibacterial activity of metronidazole. Journal of Antimicrobial Chemotherapy 1:355

Jacobs J M, Costa-Jussa F R 1985 The pathology of amiodarone neurotoxicity. II. Peripheral neuropathy in man. Brain 108:753

Jaffe I A, Altman K, Merryman P 1964 Antipyridoxine effect of penicillamine in man. Journal of Clinical Investigation 43:1869

Janssen P J 1960 Peripheral neuritis due to streptomycin. American Review of Respiratory Diseases 81:726

Jenkins P, Emerson P A 1981 Myopathy induced by rifampicin. British Medical Journal 283:105

Jensen O B, Mosdal C, Reske-Nielsen E 1977 Hypokalaemic myopathy during treatment with diuretics. Acta Neurologica Scandinavica 55:465

Jui-Yen T 1971 Clinical and experimental studies on mechanism of neuromuscular blockade by chloroquine cliorotate. Japanese Journal of Anesthesia 20:491

Kaeser H E 1984 Drug-induced myasthenic syndromes. Acta Neurologica Scandinavica 70:39

Kalayanaraman U P, Kalayanaraman K, Cullinan S A, McLean J M 1983 Neuromyopathy of cyanide intoxication due to 'laetrile' (amygdalin). Cancer 51:2126

Kaplan A M, Bergeson P S, Gregg S A, Curless R G 1977 Malignant hyperthermia associated with myopathy and normal muscle enzymes. Journal of Pediatrics 91:431

Kaplan R S, Wiernik P H 1982 Neurotoxicity of antineoplastic drugs. Seminars in Oncology 9:103

Katrak S M, Pollock M, O'Brien C P et al 1980 Clinical and morphological features of gold neuropathy. Brain 103:671

Katz B 1966 Nerve, muscle and synapse. McGraw-Hill, New York

Katz B, Miledi R 1965 Propagation of electric activity in motor nerve terminals. Proceedings of the Royal Society of London B161:453

Keidar S, Binenboim C, Palant A 1982 Muscle cramps during treatment with nifedipine. British Medical Journal 285:1241

Kennard C, Swash M, Henson R A 1980 Myopathy due to epsilon amino-caproic acid. Muscle and Nerve 3:202

Kennedy M 1981 Cardiac glycoside toxicity. An unusual manifestation of drug addiction. Medical Journal of Australia 2:686

Kennedy R D, Galindo A D 1975 Comparative site of action of various anaesthetic agents at the mammalian myoneural junction. British Journal of Anesthesia 47:533

Khaleeli A A, Edwards R H T, Gohil K et al 1983 Corticosteroid myopathy: A clinical and pathological study. Clinical Endocrinology 18:155

Kilpatrick C, Braund W, Burns R 1982 Myopathy with myasthenic features possibly induced by codeine linctus. Medical Journal of Australia 2:410

King J O, Denborough M A, Zapf P W 1972 Inheritance of malignant hyperpyrexia. Lancet 1:365

King J O, Denborough M A 1973a Malignant hyperpyrexia in Australia and New Zealand. Medical Journal of Australia 1:525

King J O, Denborough M A 1973b Anesthetic-induced malignant hyperpyrexia in children. Journal of Pediatrics 83:37

Kirkendall W M, Page E B 1958 Polyneuritis occurring during hydralazine therapy. Journal of the American Medical Association 167:427

Klatskin G, Friedman H 1948 Emetine toxicity in man:

studies on the nature of early toxic manifestations, their relation to the dose level, and their significance in determining safe dosage. Annals of Internal Medicine 28:892

Klinghardt G W 1967 Schadigungen des nervensystems durch nitrofurane bei der ratte. Acta Neuropathologica (Berlin) 9:18

Knape H 1977 In: Dukes M N G (ed) Side effects of drugs, vol 1. Excerpta Medica, Amsterdam, p 103

Knezevic W, Mastaglia F L, Lefroy R B, Fisher A 1984a Neuroleptic malignant syndrome. Medical Journal of Australia 140:28

Knezevic W, Quintner J, Mastaglia F L, Zilko P J 1984b Guillain–Barré syndrome and pemphigus foliaceus associated with D-penicillamine therapy. Australian and New Zealand Journal of Medicine 14:50

Koelle G B 1975 Neuromuscular blocking agents. In: Goodman L S, Gilman A (eds) The pharmacological basis of therapeutics, 5th edn. Macmillan, New York, p 577

Kolb L C, Gray S J 1946 Peripheral neuritis as a complication of penicillin therapy. Journal of the American Medical Association 132:323

Kono R 1971 Subacute myelo-optico-neuropathy, a new neurological disease prevailing in Japan. Japanese Journal of Medical Science and Biology 24:195

Kontos H A 1962 Myopathy associated with chronic colchicine toxicity. New England Journal of Medicine 266:38

Kornfeld P, Horowitz S H, Genkins G, Papatestas A E 1976 Myasthenia gravis unmasked by antiarrhythmic agents. Mount Sinai Journal of Medicine 43:10

Korsan-Bengsten K, Ysander L, Blohme G, Tibblin E 1969 Extensive muscle necrosis after long-term treatment with aminocaproic acid (EACA) in a case of hereditary periodic oedema. Acta Medica Scandinavica 185:341

Koski C L, Rifenberick D H, Max S R 1974 Oxidative metabolism of skeletal muscle in steroid atrophy. Archives of Neurology 31:407

Kwiecinski H 1981 Myotonia induced by chemical agents. CRC Critical Reviews in Toxicology 8:279

Lane R J M, Mastaglia F L 1978 Drug-induced myopathies in man. Lancet 2:562

Lane R J M, McLelland N J, Martin A M, Mastaglia F L 1979 Epsilon aminocaproic acid (EACA) myopathy. Postgraduate Medical Journal 55:282

Langman M J S 1975 Gastrointestinal drugs. In: Dukes M N G (ed) Meyler's side-effects of drugs, vol 8. Excerpta Medica, Amsterdam, p 795

Larsen A 1978 On the neuromuscular effects of pindolol and sotalol in the rat. Acta Physiologica Scandinavica 102:35

Leaf D A, MacDonald I, Kliks B, Wilson R, Jones S R 1984 Streptokinase and the Guillain–Barré syndrome. Annals of Internal Medicine 100:617

Leck I M, Millar E L M 1962 Incidence of malformation since the introduction of thalidomide. British Medical Journal 1:16

Le Quesne P M 1970 Iatrogenic neuropathies. In: Vinken P J, Bruyn G W (eds) Handbook of clinical neurology, North Holland, Amsterdam, p 527

Le Quesne P M 1975 Neuropathy due to drugs. In Dyck P J, Thomas P K, Lambert E H (eds) Peripheral neuropathy. Saunders, Philadelphia, p 1263

Le Quesne P M 1984 Neuropathy due to drugs. In: Dyck P J, Thomas P K, Lambert E H, Bunge R (eds) Peripheral neuropathy, 2nd edn. Saunders, Philadelphia, p 2162

Lending R E, Gall E P. Buchsbaum H W, Foote R A 1984 Hypersensitivity reaction to sulindac (Clinoril). Archives of Internal Medicine 144:2259

Lennmarken C, Lofstrom J B 1984 Partial curarization in the postoperative period. Acta Anaesthesiologica Scandinavica 28:260

Lermer H, Avni J, Bruderman I 1970 Neuromuscular blocking action of amitriptyline. European Journal of Pharmacology 13:266

Levin B E, Engel W K 1975 Iatrogenic muscle fibrosis. Arm levitation as an initial sign. Journal of the American Medical Association 234:621

Lhermitte F, Fardeau M, Chedru F, Mallecourt J 1976 Polyneuropathy after perhexiline maleate therapy. British Medical Journal 1:1256

L'Hommedieu C S, Huber P A, Rasche D K 1983 Potentiation of magnesium-induced neuromuscular weakness by gentamycin. Critical Care Medicine 11:55

Lim P K, Trewby P N, Storey G C A, Holt D W 1984 Neuropathy and fatal hepatitis in a patient receiving amiodarone. British Medical Journal 288:1638

Lindesmith L A, Baines R D, Bigelow D B, Petty T L 1968 Reversible respiratory paralysis associated with polymyxin therapy. Annals of Internal Medicine 68:318

Lingle F A 1966 Irreversible effects of glutethimide addiction. Journal of Psychiatry 123:349

Lithell H, Boberg J, Hellsing K, Lundqvist G, Vessby B 1978 Increase in the lipoprotein-lipase activity in human skeletal muscle during clofibrate administration. European Journal of Clinical Investigation 8:67

Loder R E, Walker G F 1959 Neuromuscular-blocking action of streptomycin. Lancet 1:812

Loftus L R 1963 Peripheral neuropathy following chloroquine therapy. Canadian Medical Association Journal 89:917

Lovelace R E, Horwitz S J 1968 Peripheral neuropathy in long-term diphenylhydantoin therapy. Archives of Neurology 18:69

Lullman H, Lullman-Rauch R, Wassermann O 1978 Lipidosis induced by amphiphilic cationic drugs. Biochemical Pharmacology 27:1103

Lund H I, Nielsen M 1983 Penicillamine-induced dermatomyositis. Scandinavian Journal of Rheumatology 12:350

McCormick D B, Snell E E 1959 Pyridoxal kinase of human brain and its inhibition by hydrazine derivatives. Proceedings of the National Academy of Sciences USA 45:1371

MacDonald R D, Engel A G 1970 Experimental chloroquine myopathy. Journal of Neuropathology and Experimental Neurology 29:479

MacFarlane I A, Rosenthal F D 1977 Severe myopathy after status asthmaticus. Lancet 2:615

McQuaker W, Bruggen P 1963 Side-effects of methaqualone. British Medical Journal 1:749

McQuillen M P, Gross M, Johns R J 1963 Chlorpromazine-induced weakness in myasthenia gravis. Archives of Neurology 8:286

McQuillen M P, Cantor H E, O'Rourke J R 1968 Myasthenic syndrome associated with antibiotics. Archives of Neurology 18:402

McQuillen M P, Engbaek L 1975 Mechanism of colistin-induced neuromuscular depression. Archives of Neurology 32:235

Manani G, Gasparetto A, Bettini V, Caldesi Valeri V,

Galzigna G L 1970 Mechanism of action of ajmaline on neuromuscular junction. Agressologie 11:275

Mandel W 1959 Pyridoxine and the isoniazid induced neuropathy. Diseases of the Chest 36:293

Marcus S N, Chadwick D, Walker R 1984 D-Penicillamine-induced myasthenia gravis in primary biliary cirrhosis. Gastroenterology 86:166

Markes P, Sloggen J 1976 Peripheral neuropathy caused by methaqualone. American Journal of the Medical Sciences 272:323

Marmor A, Alpan G, Keider S, Grenadier E, Palant A 1978 The MB isoenzyme of creatine kinase as an indicator of severity of myocardial infarction. Lancet 2:812

Martinez-Arizala A, Sobol S M, McCarty G E, Nichols B R, Rakita L 1983 Amiodarone neuropathy. Neurology 33:643–645

Mastaglia F L 1982 Adverse effects of drugs on muscle. Drugs 24: 304–321

Mastaglia F L, Argov Z 1982 Immunologically-mediated drug-induced neuromuscular disorders. In: Dukor P, Kallos P, Schlumberger H D, West G B (eds) Pseudo-allergic reactions — involvement of drugs and chemicals, vol 3, Cell mediated reactions. Karger, Basel, p 1–24

Mastaglia F L, Gardner-Medwin D, Hudgson P 1971 Muscle fibrosis and contractures in a pethidine addict. British Medical Journal 4:532–533

Mastaglia F L, Papadimitriou J M, Dawkins R L, Beveridge B 1977 Vacuolar myopathy associated with chloroquine, lupus erythematosus and thymoma. Journal of the Neurological Sciences 34:315

Masters C L, Dawkins R L, Zilko P J, Simpson J A, Leedman R J, Lindstrom J 1977 Penicillamine-associated myasthenia gravis, antiacetylcholine receptor and antistriatal antibodies. American Journal of Medicine 63:689

Meier C, Kauer B, Muller U, Ludin H P 1979 Neuro-myopathy during chronic amiodarone treatment. A case report. Journal of Neurology 220:231

Merhoff G C, Porter J M 1974 Ergot intoxication: Historical review and description of unusual clinical manifestation. Annals of Surgery 180:773

Meyboom R H B 1977 Heavy metal antagonists. In: Dukes M N G (ed) Side effects of drugs, vol 1. Excerpta Medica, Amsterdam, p 192

Miller M 1963 Neuropathy, agranulocytosis and hepatotoxicity following imipramine therapy. American Journal of Psychiatry 120:185

Mitchell M M, Ali H H, Savarese J J 1978 Myotonia and neuromuscular blocking agents. Anesthesiology 49:44

Mitsumoto H, Wilbourne A J, Subramony S H 1982 Generalized myokymia and gold therapy. Archives of Neurology 39:449

Mohamed S D, Chapman R S, Crooks J 1966 Hypokalaemia, flaccid quadriparesis, and myoglobinuria with carbenoxolone (Biogastrone). British Medical Journal 1:1581

Morris J S 1966 Nitrofurantoin and peripheral neuropathy with megaloblastic anemia. Journal of Neurology, Neurosurgery and Psychiatry 29:224

Muller R 1945 Polyneuritis following sulfanilamide therapy. Acta Medica Scandinavica 121:95

Mullet R D, Keats A S 1961 Apnea and respiratory insufficiency after intraperitoneal administration of kanamycin. Surgery 49:530

Nakamura K, Koide M, Imanaga T, Ogasawara H,

Takahashi M, Yoshikawa M 1980 Prolonged neuromuscular blockade following trimetaphan infusion. Anaesthesia 35:1202

Neil J F, Himmelhoch J M, Licata S 1976 Emergence of myasthenia gravis during treatment with lithium carbonate. Archives of General Psychiatry 33:1090

Nelson T E, Flewellen E H 1983 The malignant hyperthermia syndrome. New England Journal of Medicine 309:416

Newson A J 1972 Malignant hyperthermia: Three case reports. New England Journal of Medicine 75:138

Niakan E, Bertorini T E, Acchiatdo S R, Werner M F 1981 Procainamide-induced myasthenia-like weakness in a patient with peripheral neuropathy. Archives of Neurology 38:378

Nicolas F, Baron D, Dixneuf B, Visset J, Dubigeon P 1970 Les nécroses musculaires au cours des intoxications aigues. Presse Médicale 78:751

Norris F H, Colella J, McFarlin D 1964 Effect of diphenylhydantoin on neuromuscular synapse. Neurology (Minneapolis) 14:869

Nukada H, Pollock M 1981 Disulfiram neuropathy. A morphometric study of sural nerve. Journal of the Neurological Sciences 51:51–67

Onodera K, Yamakawa K 1966 The effects of lithium on the neuromuscular junction of the frog. Japanese Journal of Physiology 16:541

Page P, Morgan M, Loh L 1972 Ketamine anaesthesia in paediatric procedures. Acta Anaesthesiologica Scandinavica 16:155

Palmer K N V 1978 Muscle cramp and oral salbutamol. British Medical Journal 3:833

Palmucci L, Bertolotto A, Schiffer D 1978 Acute muscle necrosis after chronic overdosage of phenformin and fenfluramine. Muscle and Nerve 1:245

Paul H S, Abidi S A 1979 Paradoxical effects of clofibrate on liver and muscle metabolism in rats. Journal of Clinical Investigation 64:405

Paul M F, Paul H E, Kopko F, Bryuson M J, Harrington C 1954 Inhibition by furacin of citrate formation in testis preparations. Journal of Biological Chemistry 206:491

Paulson O B, Melgaard B, Hansen H S et al 1984 Misonidazole neuropathy. Acta Neurologica Scandinavica (Suppl) 100:133

Pellissier J F, Pouget J, Cros D, De Victor B, Serratrice G, Toga M 1984 Peripheral neuropathy induced by amiodarone chlorhydrate. Journal of the Neurological Sciences 63:251

Penn A S, Rowland L P, Fraser D W 1972 Drugs, coma and myoglobinuria. Archives of Neurology 26:336

Percy A K, Saef E C 1967 An unusual complication of retrograde pyelography: neuromuscular blockade. Pediatrics 39:603

Perkins R L 1964 Apnea with intramuscular colistin therapy. Journal of the American Medical Association 190:421

Perkoff G T, Hardy P, Velez-Garcia E 1966 Reversible acute muscular syndrome in chronic alcoholism. New England Journal of Medicine 274:1277

Perry H M 1973 Late toxicity to hydralazine resembling systemic lupus erythematosus or rheumatoid arthritis. American Journal of Medicine 54:58

Peter J B, Fiehn W 1973 Diazacholesterol myotonia: Accumulation of desmosterol and increased adenosine triphosphatase activity of sarcolemma. Science 179:910

Peterson H C 1966 Association of trimethadione therapy and

myasthenia gravis. New England Journal of Medicine 274:506

Pierides A M, Alvarez-Ude F, Kerr D N S, Skillen A W 1975 Clofibrate-induced muscle damage in patients with renal failure. Lancet 2:1279

Pinals R S 1983 Diffuse fasciculations induced by D-penicillamine. Journal of Rheumatology 10: 809–810

Pinkerton H A, Munro J R 1964 Respiratory insufficiency associated with the use of streptomycin. Scottish Medical Journal 9:256

Pittinger C B, Eryasa Y, Adamson R 1970 Antibiotic-induced paralysis. Anesthesia and Analgesia Current Researches 49:487

Pokroy N, Ress S, Gregory M C 1977 Clofibrate-induced complications in renal disease. South African Medical Journal 52:806

Pollet S, Hauw J J, Escourolle R, Baumann N 1977 Peripheral nerve lipid abnormalities in patients on perhexiline maleate. Lancet 1: 1258

Poole G W, Schneeweiss J 1961 Peripheral neuropathy due to ethionamide. American Review of Respiratory Diseases 84:890

Prescott L F 1975 Anti-inflammatory analgesics and drugs used in rheumatoid arthritis and gout. In: Dukes M N G (ed) Meyler's side effects of drugs, vol 8. Excerpta Medica, Amsterdam, p 228

Pridgeon J E 1956 Respiratory arrest thought to be due to intra-peritoneal neomycin. Surgery 40:571

Proctor W R, Weakly J N 1976 A comparison of the presynaptic and post-synaptic actions of pentobarbitone and phenobarbitone in the neuromuscular junction of the frog. Journal of Physiology 258:257

Ramsay I D 1968 Endocrine ophthalmopathy. British Medical Journal 4:706

Rapoport A M, Guss S B 1972 Dapsone-induced peripheral neuropathy. Archives of Neurology 27:184

Rasmussen H 1970 Cell communication, calcium ion and cyclic adenosine monophosphate. Science 170:404

Ream C R 1963 Respiratory and cardiac arrest after intravenous administration of kanamycin with reversal of toxic effects by neostigmine. Annals of Internal Medicine 59:384

Regan A G, Aldrete J A 1967 Prolonged apnea after administration of promazine hydrochloride following succinylcholine infusion. Anesthesia and Analgesia Current Researches 46:315

Regli F, Guggenheim P 1965 Myasthenisches syndrom als seltene komplikation unter hydantoinbehandlung. Nervenartz 36:315

Richter R W, Challenor Y B, Pearson J, Kagen L J, Hamilton L L, Ramsey W H 1971 Acute myoglobinuria associated with heroin addiction. Journal of the American Medical Association 216:1172

Ricker K, Haass A, Glotzner F 1978 Fenoterol precipitating myotonia in a minimally affected case of recessive myotonia congenita. Journal of Neurology 219:279

Rimon D, Ludatscher R, Cohen L 1984 Clofibrate-induced muscular syndrome. Israel Journal of Medical Sciences 20:1082

Roberson J R, Dimon J H 1983 Myofibrosis and joint contractures caused by injections of pentazocine. Journal of Bone and Joint Surgery 65:1007

Robinson B F 1975 Drugs acting on the cardiovascular system. In: Dukes M N G (ed) Meyler's side effects of drugs, vol 8. Excerpta Medica, Amsterdam, p 447

Robinson B F 1978 Anti-anginal and beta adreno-receptor blocking drugs. In: Dukes M N G (ed) Meyler's side effects of drugs, vol 2. Excerpta Medica, Amsterdam, p 173

Robinson R G 1959 Leucotrichia totalis from chloroquine. Medical Journal of Australia 2:460

Roelofs R I, Hrushesky W, Rogin J, Rosenberg L 1984 Peripheral sensory neuropathy and cisplatin chemotherapy. Neurology 34:934

Roldan E C, Nigrin G 1972 Peripheral neuritis after methimazole therapy. New York State Journal of Medicine 72:2898

Rothstein J M, Delitto A, Sinacore D R, Rose S J 1983 Muscle function in rheumatic disease patients treated with corticosteroids. Muscle and Nerve 6:128

Rowland L P 1980 Malignant hyperpyrexia — A reply. Muscle and Nerve 3:443

Rubbo J T, Gergis S D, Sokoll M D 1977 Comparative neuromuscular effects of lincomycin and clindamycin. Current Researches in Anesthesia and Analgesia 56:329

Rubenstein C J 1964 Peripheral neuropathy caused by nitrofurantoin. Journal of the American Medical Association 187:647

Rumpf K W, Alberts R, Scheler F 1976 Clofibrate-induced myopathy syndrome. Lancet 1:249

Russell A S, Lindstrom J M 1978 Penicillamine-induced myasthenia gravis associated with antibodies to acetylcholine receptor. Neurology (Minneapolis) 28:847

Russell J A, Powles R L 1974 Neuropathy due to cytosine arabinosine. British Medical Journal 4:652

Said G 1978 Perhexiline neuropathy: A clinicopathological study. Annals of Neurology 3:259

Salako L A 1970 Inhibition of neuromuscular transmission in the intact rat by emetine. Journal of Pharmaceutics and Pharmacology 22:69

Samuelson R J, Giesecke A H, Kallus F T, Stanley V F 1975 Lincomycin–curare interaction. Current Researches in Anesthesia and Analgesia 54:103

Sandler R M, Gonsalkorale M 1977 Chronic lymphatic leukemia, chlorambucil and sensorimotor peripheral neuropathy. British Medical Journal 2:1265

Saquenton A C, Lorinz A L, Vick N A, Hamer R D 1969 Dapsone and peripheral motor neuropathy. Archives of Dermatology 100:214

Satoyoshi E, Wakata N 1978 Chloramphenicol neuropathy and vitamin B_{12} deficiency. 4th International Congress on Neuromuscular Diseases, Montreal, Canada, Abstract 89

Saunders F P, Hoefnagel D, Staples O S 1965 Progressive fibrosis of the quadriceps muscle. Journal of Bone and Joint Surgery 47A:380

Schaumburg H, Kaplan J, Windebank A et al 1983 Sensory neuropathy from pyridoxine abuse. New England Journal of Medicine 309:445

Schmidt J L, Vick N A, Sadove M S 1963 The effect of quinidine on the action of muscle relaxants. Journal of the American Medical Association 183:669

Schochet S S, Usar M C, Lampert P W 1968 Neuronal changes induced by intrathecal vincristine sulfate. Journal of Neuropathology and Experimental Neurology 27:645

Scholes D M 1960 Pelvic perfusion with nitrogen mustard for cancer: a neurological complication. American Journal of Obstetrics and Gynecology 80:481

Schraeder P L, Peters H A, Dahl D S 1972 Polymyositis and penicillamine. Archives of Neurology 27:456

Sebille A 1978 Prevalence of latent perhexiline neuropathy. British Medical Journal 1:1321

Seitz D, Hopf H C, Janzen R C W, Meyer W 1976 Penicillamin induzierte Myasthenie bei chronischer Polyarthritis. Deutsche Medizinische Wochenschrift 101:1153

Selby G 1972 Subacute myelo-optic neuropathy in Australia. Lancet 1:123

Shaivits S A 1979 Timolol and myasthenia gravis. Journal of the American Medical Association 242:1611

Shibuya N, Mori K, Nakazawa Y 1978 Serum factor blocks neuromuscular transmission in myasthenia gravis: electrophysiologic study with intracellular microelectrodes. Neurology (Minneapolis) 28:804

Shoji S, Takagi A, Sugita H, Toyokura Y 1974 Muscle glycogen metabolism in steroid-induced myopathy of rabbits. Experimental Neurology 45:1

Shoji S, Pennington R J T 1977a Binding of dexamethasone and cortisol to cytosol receptors in rat extensor digitorum longus and soleus muscles. Experimental Neurology 57:342

Shoji S, Pennington R J T 1977b The effect of cortisone on protein breakdown and synthesis in rat skeletal muscle. Molecular and Cellular Endocrinology 6:159

Sholl J S, Hughey M J, Hirschmann R A 1985 Myotonic muscular dystrophy associated with ritodrine tocolysis. American Journal of Obstetrics and Gynecology 151:83

Skau K A, Gerald M C 1978 Curare-like effects of the amphetamine isomers on neuromuscular transmission. Neuropharmacology 17:271

Snavely S R, Hodges G R 1984 The neurotoxocity of antibacterial agents. Annals of Internal Medicine 101:92

Sobue I, Ando K, Iida M, Takayanagi T, Yamamura Y, Matsuoka Y 1971 Myeloneuropathy with abdominal disorders in Japan. Neurology (Minneapolis) 21:168

Sokoll M D, Gergis S D, Post E L, Cronnelly R, Long J P 1974 Effects of droperidol on neuromuscular transmission and muscle membrane. European Journal of Pharmacology 28:209

Sokoll M D, Gergis S D 1981 Antibiotics and neuromuscular function. Anesthesiology 55:148

Somers J E, Winer N 1966 Reversible myopathy and myotonia following administration of a hypocholesterolaemic agent. Neurology (Minneapolis) 16:761

Stafford C R, Bogdanoff B M, Green L, Spector H B 1975 Mononeuropathy multiplex as a complication of amphetamine angiitis. Neurology (Minneapolis) 25:570

Stalberg E, Schiller H H, Schwartz M S 1975 Safety factor in single human motor end-plates studied in vivo with single fibre electromyography. Journal of Neurology, Neurosurgery and Psychiatry 38:799

Steiner J C, Winkelman A C, De Jesus P V 1973 Pentazocine-induced myopathy. Archives of Neurology 28:408

Steiness E, Rasmussen F, Svendsen O, Nielsen P 1978 A comparative study of serum creatine phosphokinase (CPK) activity in rabbits, pigs and humans after intramuscular injection of local damaging drugs. Acta Pharmacologica et Toxicologica 42:357

Stone R 1979 Proximal myopathy during beta-blockade. British Medical Journal 2:1583

Streib E W 1977 Adverse effects of magnesium salt cathartics in a patient with the myasthenic syndrome (Lambert–Eaton syndrome). Annals of Neurology 2:175

Swenson R D, Golper T A, Bennett W M 1982 Acute renal failure and rhabdomyolysis after ingestion of phenylpropanolamine-containing diet pills. Journal of American Medical Association 248:1216

Tam C W, Olin B R, Ruiz A E 1980 Loxapin-associated rhabdomyolysis and acute renal failure. Archives of Internal Medicine 140:975

Tamaki M 1978 The effect of streptomycin on the neuromuscular junction of the frog. 4th International Congress on Neuromuscular Diseases, Montreal, Canada, Abstract 48

Teicher A, Rosenthal T, Kinnin E, Sarova I 1981 Labetalol-induced toxic myopathy. British Medical Journal 282:1824

Teravainen H, Larsen A, Hillbom M 1977 Clofibrate-induced myopathy in the rat. Acta Neuropathologica (Berlin) 39:135

Thompson S W, Davis L E, Korenfeld M, Hilgers R D, Standefer J C 1984 Cisplatin neuropathy. Cancer 54:1269

Tomlinson I W, Rosenthal F D 1977 Proximal myopathy after perhexiline maleate treatment. British Medical Journal 2:1319

Toole J F, Parrish M L 1973 Nitrofurantoin polyneuropathy. Neurology (Minneapolis) 23:554

Torres C F, Griggs R C, Baum J, Penn A S 1980 Penicillamine-induced myasthenia gravis in progressive systemic sclerosis. Arthritis and Rheumatism 23:505

Tsubaki T, Honma Y, Hoshi M 1971 Neurological syndrome associated with clioquinol. Lancet 1:696

Tugwell P, James S L 1972 Peripheral neuropathy with ethambutol. Postgraduate Medical Journal 48:667

Uchigata M, Tanabe H, Hasue I, Kurihara M 1981 Peripheral neuropathy due to lithium intoxication. Annals of Neurology 9:414

Ursing B, Kamme C 1975 Metronidazole for Crohn's disease. Lancet 1:775

Usubiaga J E, Wikinski J A, Morales R L, Usubiaga L E J 1967 Interaction of intravenously administered procaine, lidocaine and succinylcholine in anesthetized subjects. Current Researches in Anesthesia and Analgesia 46:39

Utz J P, Louria D B, Feder N, Emmons C W, McCullough N B 1957 A report of clinical studies on the use of amphotericin in patients with systemic fungal diseases. Antibiotics Annals 65

Van Marle W, Woods K L 1980 Acute hydrocortisone myopathy. British Medical Journal 281:271

Vartanian G A, Chinyanga H M 1972 The mechanism of acute neuromuscular weakness induced by chloroquine. Canadian Journal of Physiology and Pharmacology 50:1099

Vincent A, Newsom Davis J, Martin V 1978 Antiacetylcholine receptor antibodies in D-penicillamine-associated myasthenia gravis. Lancet 1:1254

Viswanath D V, Jenkins H J 1978 Neuromuscular block of the polymixin group of antibiotics. Journal of Pharmaceutical Sciences 67:1275

Wade A 1977 Martindale — the extra pharmacopoeia, 27th edn. Pharmaceutical Press, London, p 1295

Walls T J, Pearce S J, Venables G S 1980 Motor neuropathy associated with cimetidine. British Medical Journal 281:974

Walton J N 1977 Brain's diseases of the nervous system, 8th edn. Oxford University Press, Oxford, p 1032

Warner W A, Sanders E 1971 Neuromuscular blockage associated with gentamycin therapy. Journal of the American Medical Association 215:1153

Warot P, Goudemand M, Habay D 1965 Troubles neurologiques provoqués par les alcaloïdes de Vinca rosea (la polynévrite de la pervenche). Revue Neurologique 113:464

Watkins S M, Griffin J P 1978 High incidence of vincristine-induced neuropathy in lymphomas. British Medical Journal 1:610

Watland D C, Long J P, Pittinger C B, Cullen S C 1957 Neuromuscular effects of ether, cyclopropane, chloroform and fluothane. Anesthesiology 18:883

Watson A J S, Dalbow M H, Stachura I et al 1983 Immunologic studies in cimetidine-induced nephropathy and polymyositis. New England Journal of Medicine 308:142

Wattel F, Chopin C, Durocher A, Berzin B 1978 Rhabdomyolyses au cours des intoxications aigues. La Nouvelle Presse Médicale 7:2253

Watters G, Karpati G, Kaplan B 1977 Post-anesthetic augmentation of muscle damage as a presenting sign in three patients with Duchenne muscular dystrophy. Canadian Journal of Neurological Sciences 4:228 .

Way W L, Katzung B G, Larson C P 1967 Recurarization with quinidine. Journal of the American Medical Association 200:163

Weinstein L, Madoff M A, Samet C M 1974 The sulfonamides. New England Journal of Medicine 291:793

Weisman S L 1949 Masked myasthenia gravis. Journal of the American Medical Association 141:917

Weiss H D, Walker M D, Wiernik P H 1974 Neurotoxicity of commonly used antineoplastic agents. New England Journal of Medicine 291:127

Werman R, Wislicki L 1971 Propranolol, a curariform and cholinomimetic agent at the frog neuromuscular junction. Comparative General Pharmacology 2:69

Westbury G 1962 Treatment of advanced cancer by extracorporeal perfusion and continuous intra-arterial infusion. Proceedings of the Royal Society of Medicine 55:643

Whisnant J P, Espinosa R E, Kierland R R, Lambert E H 1963 Chloroquine neuromyopathy. Proceedings of the Mayo Clinic 38:501

Williams R S 1959 Triamcinolone myopathy. Lancet 1:698

Wilson S L, Miller R N, Wright C, Haas D 1976 Prolonged neuromuscular blockade associated with trimetaphan: A case report. Current Researches in Anesthesia and Analgesia 55:353

Winer N, Klachko D M, Baer R D, Langley P L, Burns T W 1966 Myotonic response induced by inhibitors of cholesterol biosynthesis. Science 153:312

Wojnarowska F 1980 Dermatomyositis induced by penicillamine. Journal of the Royal Society of Medicine 73:884

Wolf S, Goldberg L S, Verity A 1976 Neuromyopathy and periarteriolitis in a patient receiving levodopa. Archives of Internal Medicine 136:1055

Wright J M, Collier B 1976a The site of the neuromuscular block produced by polymyxin B and rolitetracycline. Canadian Journal of Physiology and Pharmacology 54:926

Wright J M, Collier B 1976b Characterization of the neuromuscular block produced by clindamycin and lincomycin. Canadian Journal of Physiology and Pharmacology 54:937

Wullen F, Kast G, Bruck A 1967 Uber nebenwirkungen bei tetracyclin-verabreichung an Myastheniker. Deutsche Medizinische Wochenschrift 92:667

Wyatt E H, Stevens C 1972 Dapsone induced peripheral neuropathy. British Journal of Dermatology 86:521

Yaari Y, Pincus J H, Argov Z 1977 Depression of synaptic transmission by diphenylhydantoin. Annals of Neurology 1:334

Yaari Y, Pincus J H, Argov Z 1979 Phenytoin and transmitter release at the neuromuscular junction of the frog. Brain Research 160:479

Yates D A H 1970 Steroid myopathy. In: Walton J N, Canal N, Scarlato G (eds) Muscle diseases. Excerpta Medica, Amsterdam, p 482

Yiannikas C, Pollard J D, McLeod J G 1981 Nitrofurantoin neuropathy. Australian and New Zealand Journal of Medicine 11:400

Young W A, Tudhope G R 1926 The pathology of prolonged emetine administration. Transactions of the Royal Society of Tropical Medicine and Hygiene 30:93

Zaunder H L, Barton N, Benetts E J, Lore J 1966 Colistimethate as a cause of post-operative apnoea. Canadian Anesthetic Society Journal 13: 607

The clinical physiology of neuromuscular disease

INTRODUCTION

An important property of muscle fibres is their ability to generate small voltages or action potentials forming an essential link in the chain of events leading to contraction of the muscle fibre. Clinical electromyography (EMG), which is concerned with the recording and analysis of these electrical events in human muscle, effectively dates from the introduction by Adrian & Bronk (1929) of the coaxial or concentric needle electrode (CNEMG). Subsequent development of EMG as a clinical tool was carried out principally by workers in Scandinavia who defined the characteristics of the electrical signals derived from normal and diseased muscle. Studies in the laboratories of Kugelberg and of Buchthal did much to establish the foundation of CNEMG which remains the most widely used technique. Recently there have been considerable developments in clinical neurophysiology, partly due to technological advances in electronics and particularly the availability of low-cost microcomputers. These have facilitated data acquisition, analysis and presentation, leading to improved quantitation, particularly in CNEMG. The introduction of several new recording techniques (single-fibre EMG, scanning EMG and Macro EMG) has revealed new information about the organisation and function of the lower motor neurone in health and disease.

The anatomy and physiology of the motor unit are described in Chapter 1; only a brief recapitulation is given here. The motor unit (Sherrington 1926) consists of a lower motor neurone and all the individual muscle fibres innervated by its branches. It forms the smallest element of a muscle capable of separate volitional activation when all of the constituent muscle fibres are excited almost synchronously. The number of muscle fibres innervated by a single neurone (the innervation ratio) has been estimated to vary from about six in the extraocular muscles to 400–17 000 in normal limb muscles (Feinstein et al 1955, Christensen 1959).

Motor unit territory is the cross-sectional area over which the muscle fibres of a single motor unit are dispersed. In a normal muscle the diameter of the motor unit territory is less than 10 mm (Buchthal et al 1954a, Stålberg et al 1976, Stålberg & Antoni 1980). Individual muscle fibres of the unit are widely distributed throughout the territory and only rarely are two or three fibres found in propinquity (Edström & Kugelberg 1968). The sub-unit theory (Buchthal 1961), which suggested an arrangement within the territory of closely packed groups of 10–30 muscle fibres as subunits, has been abandoned (Buchthal & Rosenfalk 1973). Each motor unit territory is extensively overlapped by those of other motor units. The diameter of individual muscle fibres shows some variation within a muscle; mean diameters are largest in the lower limbs (50–60 μm) and only 20–30 μm in the facial muscles (Polgar et al 1973). Normally each muscle fibre has a single neuromuscular junction, located in the central portion of the fibre. In many muscles the end-plates are distributed in a distinct area known as the endplate zone. The muscle fibres of an individual motor unit are responsible for the motor unit action potential (MUP), the dimensions of which depend on a number of variables. The first of these is the form of the action potentials arising in individual muscle fibres. Parallel studies of intracellullar and extracellular recordings of the single-fibre action potential have been carried out in animals (Håkansson 1957, Katz & Miledi 1965). The extracellular recording resembles the second derivative of the intracellular action potential (Clark & Plonsey 1966, 1968). The extracellular action potential amplitude increases in proportion to 1.7 times the fibre diameter (Håkansson 1957). Muscle is a physical space permeable to electric currents; the spread of current in such a medium is termed volume conduction. In a homogeneous volume conductor (e.g. Ringer's solution) the amplitude of the extra-

cellularly recorded action potential falls off linearly with the logarithm of the distance of the electrode from the fibre. When electrode-to-fibre distances exceed 0.15 mm the amplitude decreases with increasing distance by the power of −1.3. Whereas the intracellular action potential is monophasic, the extracellular single fibre action potential is biphasic (Håkansson 1957). Volume conduction in muscle is more complex as muscle is neither isotropic nor homogeneous. Various elements in the muscle tissue have different electrical resistivity. Anisotropy is also present, with the radial resistivity being some two to ten times that parallel to the longitudinal axis of the muscle fibres in mammalian muscle (Geddes & Baker 1967).

Volume conduction of the action potentials of single fibres in human muscle has been studied by Gath & Stålberg (1977, 1978). The amplitude attenuation with distance was greater than predicted by mathematical models and, although the discrepancy between forecast and actual results was greater for slow components, the fast components showed the greatest decline. In the biceps brachii the mean distance over which the action potential declined to 90% of its original amplitude was 191 μm (s.e. (mean) 20 μm) when recorded with a 25 μm diameter electrode (Gath & Stålberg 1978).

Single-fibre action potentials summate to form the MUP and this summation depends upon the degree of synchronisation of muscle fibre action potentials as recorded at the electrode employed. According to Buchthal et al (1957), the anatomical dispersion of the end-plate zone in the muscle has the major role in determining the total duration of the MUP. Muscle fibre propagation velocity, terminal axonal velocity and neuromuscular transmission times are relatively unimportant in normal muscle.

The form of the electrical activity recorded when a motor unit is excited, depends to a considerable extent on the type of electrode which is used to study the potential changes. These various electrodes are mentioned below.

Technical considerations

The technical specifications of amplifiers suitable for CNEMG recording have been detailed in a report by the Special Committee on EMG Instrumentation (Guld et al 1970). A recent review of the topic and an outline of the safety precautions required in EMG systems can be found in Kimura's textbook (Seaba & Walker 1983).

COMPARISON OF DIFFERENT RECORDING TECHNIQUES

Concentric needle electromyography (CNEMG)

The concentric needle is the most widely used electrode, consisting of a stainless steel cannula resembling a hypodermic needle, through the centre of the shaft of which an insulated platinum (or nichrome silver) core is inserted (Fig. 30.1a). The usual central core diameter is 0.1 mm, while the outer diameter of the shaft is about 0.5 mm. Recordings are made between the core tip and the cannula. A separate earth (ground) electrode is required during the recording process. The oblique, oval recording surface has an exposed tip area of the order of 150 μm × 580 μm (0.007 mm²). The electrode is relatively selective and has an effective pick-up area about 1 mm in diameter, within which only a portion of the activity of the whole motor unit is registered. The leading-off surface is large in relation to the muscle fibres, resulting in pronounced shunting of the electrical field, producing an average value of the isopotential lines crossing the electrode surface (Ståalberg & Trontelj 1979). The recording electrode itself has marked directional properties, registering activity mainly from fibres situated in front of the bevelled surface (Nakao et al 1965).

Dorfman et al (1985) have examined the electrical characteristics of a variety of commercial CNEMG electrodes, and demonstrated the value of electrolytic treatment. Untreated electrodes show considerable variation both in impedance and broadband-noise characteristics, even between electrodes from the same manufacturer. Electrolytic treatment reduces impedance by a factor of up to four and reduces the variability. Broadband-noise is also reduced, often down to the level of the instrumentation. Distortion is usually negligible but line interference from nearby power cables is suppressed only when the recording cables are fully shielded and the electromyo-

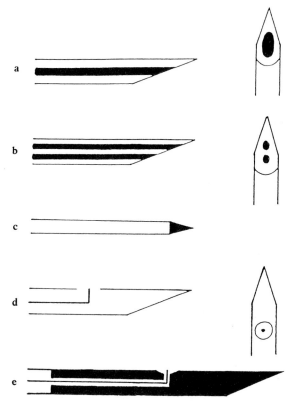

Fig. 30.1 Different types of intramuscular needle electrodes. a. Concentric needle electrode (CNE); active recording surface 150 × 580 μm in bevel — cannula reference. b. Bipolar needle electrode; recordings derived between the two surfaces in the bevel. c. Monopolar electrode; recordings derived between the electrode tip and a remote reference electrode. d. Single fibre electrode; active recording surface 25 μm in diameter placed in side-port behind tip of electrode — cannula reference. e. Macro electrode; recordings derived between exposed terminal 15 mm portion of cannula and remote subcutaneous electrode. Separate SFEMG electrode 7.5 mm behind tip (Modified from Stålberg & Trontelj 1979)

grapher earthed. The effect of electrolytic treatment is short-lived but repeatable.

The CNEMG electrode is inserted into a relaxed muscle and the presence or absence of insertional and spontaneous activity is determined. During gentle voluntary contraction, the MUPs of early recruiting motor units from a number of separate sites in the muscle can be examined and their firing rates and wave-form recorded. A delay-line which allows display of the triggering MUP in the centre of the screen facilitates examination of MUP parameters. Various oscilloscope sweep-speeds are employed so that late components occurring many ms after the main MUP are detected. Fast sweep-speeds and a 500 Hz high-pass filter enable MUP stability to be assessed. Increasing force of contraction results in the appearance of MUPs from more motor units firing asynchronously and rapidly building up to a pattern in which superimposed activity completely obscures the oscilloscope base-line, producing an 'interference pattern', the amplitude and density of which is noted.

Bipolar needle electrodes consist of two insulated wires with exposed tips inserted into a steel cannula which can act as the earth electrode (Fig. 30.1b). Potential changes are registered between the two wire tips and provide a relatively selective electrode. Activity from more distant sources arriving at the two recording surfaces simultaneously is not registered because of the common-mode rejection of the differential amplifier. As a consequence the initial and terminal elements of the MUP are cancelled and MUP duration is only 75% of the values obtained in CNEMG (Guld 1951, Buchthal et al 1954b). These electrodes are used for special purposes, where some selectivity of recording or stimulation is required.

The monopolar needle electrode is a solid steel needle insulated with varnish and bared at the tip (Fig. 30.1c). Recordings are made from the tip referred to a distant surface electrode or a subcutaneous needle electrode. They are less selective than the CNEMG electrodes, and MUP duration and amplitude as measured with the monopolar electrodes tend to be somewhat greater than those determined in CNEMG (Guld 1951). These electrodes are used in EMG in similar situations to the CNEMG electrode and are less expensive but also less easy to standardise.

Scanning electromyography

This recently introduced technique combines the technologies of CNEMG and SFEMG. Briefly, the SFEMG is used to lock-on to a single muscle fibre action potential in a gently contracting muscle. At the same time a CNEMG electrode (the scanning electrode) is positioned between 10 and 20 mm from the SFEMG electrode. The position of the former is then adjusted so that it records a MUP

synchronous with the single fibre action potential (i.e. from the unit to which the single fibre belongs). By appropriate delay-line settings the MUP is displayed in the centre of a 15 ms sweep of the oscilloscope. The scanning electrode is then advanced a further 10 mm into the muscle and scanning can begin. Gentle muscular contraction is required to give a constant, low firing rate. At the same time the electrode is pulled through the motor unit using a specially designed step-motor (linear actuator) to produce small, reproducible increments of movement of 50 μm. Between 150 and 400 sweeps are obtained by the procedure and

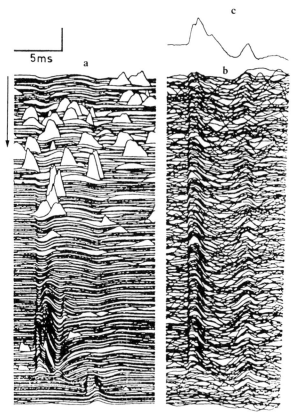

Fig. 30.2 a. Scanning EMG recording from normal tibialis anterior muscle (deepest position at top of the plot). b. Simultaneous recording between cannula and remote reference electrode. c. Averaged recording from (b) with the needle at its deepest position; this corresponds to the Macro EMG. The plot shows that the cannula is also recording activity from the motor unit. This is seen as a 'trough' in the scan (a) which 'announces' the fibres before the action potentials are recorded at the tip of the electrode. Amplitude calibration: a = 200 μV; b = 100 μV; c = 50 μV (from Stålberg & Antoni 1980)

a computer or microprocessor is used to create a graphical display of the data on an XY plotter (utilising a special-purpose programme) as a contour map of the motor unit (Fig. 30.2a).

Single-fibre electromyography (SFEMG)

The electrode is a steel hypodermic needle with a 0.5 mm cannula diameter in which 25 μm diameter leading-off surfaces of between one and 15 platinum-wire recording electrodes are mounted in a side port opposite the bevel of the cannula (Fig. 30.1d). The small recording surface makes this a highly selective electrode. The SFEMG needle is inserted into the muscle at right angles to the long axis of the muscle fibres and its position adjusted so as to record a single muscle fibre action potential (Fig. 30.3). Recordings use a fast oscilloscope sweep, trigger and delay-line so that the delayed potentials can be centrally displayed on the oscilloscope. Recording selectivity may be further increased by using a 500 Hz high-pass filter which restricts activity from more distant fibres, attenuating their low-frequency components. An upper limit of 16 KHz is normally used. These settings are unsuitable for studies of the form of individual single-fibre

potentials: they distort the shape of the action potential even from the close fibres; settings for study of the shape of the potential should be from 2 Hz to 16 KHz.

Macro electromyography

The recording electrode is relatively non-selective and consists of a modified SFEMG electrode in which the single-fibre recording surface is exposed in a side port some 7.5 mm from the tip (Stålberg 1980a, Stålberg & Fawcett 1982). The steel cannula of 0.55 mm diameter is insulated to within 15 mm of the tip: the single-fibre aperture is thus at the mid-point of the cannula recording surface (Fig. 30.1e). The electrode is placed in a muscle so that a single fibre from a motor unit can be recorded. If the fibre lies near the centre of the unit, the Macro electrodes should span the whole motor unit territory in healthy as well as in diseased muscle. Macro MUPs are obtained by

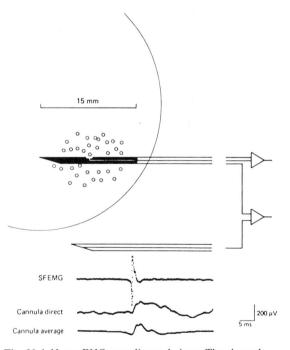

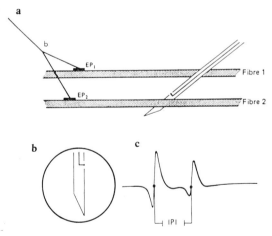

Fig. 30.3 Single-fibre EMG recording technique. a. shows the SFEMG needle (insert b) recording from two muscle fibres. c. shows the two fibre action potentials. The interpotential interval (IPI) is the time taken for the two nerve impulses from the branching point in the axon (b), transmission across the two motor end-plates (EP 1 & 2) and conduction of the two muscle-fibre action potentials up to the electrode

Fig. 30.4 Macro EMG recording technique. The electrode position is adjusted in order to record the action potential of a single muscle fibre with the small SFEMG recording surface. This triggers the oscilloscope and averager and the cannula signal is delayed and then averaged to extract the Macro motor unit potential (Macro MUP) (After Stålberg 1980a)

electronically averaging those potentials recorded by the Macro electrode time-locked to the single fibre trigger. It is possible to record a variety of different motor units selecting different single fibres to act as triggers (Fig. 30.4). The Macro MUP represents the total activity of the individual motor unit. Considerable attenuation occurs of high-frequency components arising from muscle fibres close to the cannula, compared with more distant fibres, so that recorded amplitudes are smaller than those seen in CNEMG and very much smaller than in SFEMG. The wave-form corresponds to the findings in scanning EMG (Fig. 30.2b) and the major peaks and troughs seen in the latter technique can usually be identified in an attenuated form in the Macro EMG (Fig. 30.2) (Stålberg 1983, Stålberg & Fawcett 1982).

Ocular electromyography

A monopolar needle electrode was introduced by Björk (1952) and by Björk & Kugelberg (1953), the shaft of which is insulated and the tip left bare. An indifferent electrode is required which can be either a surface electrode placed on the tip of the nose or forehead or a blepharostat (lid retractor) fixed to the eyelid. Concentric needles of small diameter have also been used (Breinin 1957). The needle has a diameter of 0.25 mm and leading-off surface of 0.08 mm. The electrode is 2.5–3 cm in length, although a much longer electrode is needed to reach the superior oblique muscle. The needle electrode is inserted subconjunctivally after·topical anaesthesia of the eye in a supine patient. The procedure is usually well tolerated but requires full patient co-operation. As adequate knowledge of the anatomy of the extraocular muscles is essential and as the possible complication of penetration of the globe of the eye is so serious, studies should be carried out with an ophthalmologist who positions the electrode. Less serious complications of the procedure are corneal exposure and subconjunctival haemorrhage.

The innervation ratio of the ocular muscles is very low, ranging from six to about 20 muscle fibres per motor unit (Breinin 1962). Unlike other voluntary muscles, extraocular muscles are not electrically silent in the waking state. With the eye in the primary position, continuous tonic discharge in the muscles is required to maintain eye position. Increasing discharge rates are seen in the agonist muscles on eye movement, whereas the antagonists show relative or complete electrical silence, due to reciprocal inhibition. Because of the muscle fibre size, ranging in diameter from 10 to 50 μm, and the low innervation ratio of the extraocular muscles, MUPs are brief and of low voltage and polyphasic potentials are rare. The average amplitude is 200 μv and the average duration is 1.5 ms (Breinin 1962). Björk & Kugelberg (1953) found a maximum discharge rate of up to 200 Hz.

Ocular EMG is useful in detecting denervation, myopathy or defects in neuromuscular transmission; it is also of value in assessing abnormalities of gaze.

Surface electromyography

In the past, surface EMG has appeared to have little value for diagnostic electromyography and found its major application in long-term monitoring of muscle activity in kinesiology. High-frequency components tend to be lost and individual motor unit potentials are difficult to detect.

Surface electrodes are used in the technique of motor unit counting (McComas et al 1971b), described fully in Chapter 31. Special multiple surface electrodes were used by Hjorth et al (1973) to document the distribution and rate of occurrence of fasciculation potentials in motor neurone disease. Surface electrodes have been used in conjunction with SFEMG and averaging techniques to record single motor units (Milner-Brown & Stein 1975).

A series of special surface electrodes has been used to study the location of the neuromuscular junction and MUP propagation (Nishizono et al 1979, Masuda et al 1983, 1985). Nishizono et al used a fine wire electrode inserted in the middle of the belly of the biceps in healthy volunteers and a series of small, 8 mm diameter surface electrodes linearly disposed at 20 mm intervals on the longitudinal axis of the muscle. Computer averaging techniques were applied to the extraction of the contribution made by a single motor unit (recorded by a wire electrode) to the surface recording during gentle maintained voluntary contraction. A conduction velocity of 4.6 m/s (s.e. (mean) 0.5 m/s) was found. Masuda et al (1983) used an elaborate array of surface electrodes consisting of 15 stainless steel wires parallel to each other with a 5 mm interelectrode gap and, in conjunction with computer analysis, studied the sites of neuromuscular junctional activity in the biceps in relation to muscular exertion. A still more elaborate surface electrode system was used by Hilfiker & Meyer (1984) to study normal and myopathic MUP propagation. During isometric contraction of the biceps brachii, using an array of 30 surface electrodes parallel to the long axis and centred on the end-plate zone, a computer programme was used to display the action potentials and to analyse their propagation pattern.

Wire electrodes

Using a hypodermic needle, one can insert wire electrodes into a muscle where they may remain for long periods and are used in kinesiology (Basmajian & Stecko 1962). Wire electrodes have also been used for SFEMG studies. Very small recording surfaces can be obtained by using a spark to break through the insulation of a fine wire. Although selectivity is high, there are problems in the standardisation of recording surface size and impedance; in addition, the form of the single-fibre action potential is liable to distortion and fine adjustments to the electrode position are difficult (Stålberg & Trontelj 1979).

CLINICAL ELECTROMYOGRAPHY

CNEMG

Insertional activity. Injury to muscle fibres caused by movement of the exploring electrode evokes potentials referred to as insertion activity (Weddell et al 1944, Kugelberg & Petersén 1949). Brief bursts of short-duration high-frequency spikes occur with each movement of the electrode, hardly outlasting the movement (Fig. 30.5a). The spike cluster is mainly positive and is due to the mechanical stimulation or injury of muscle fibres by the needle (Wiechers 1977). Where fibrous replacement of muscle has occurred in chronic

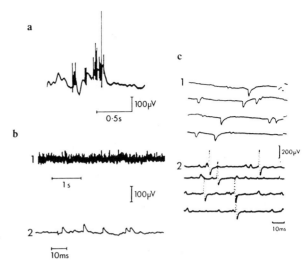

Fig. 30.5 CNEMG recordings. a. Insertion activity recorded following needle movement. b. Recordings from the region of the motor end-plate zone: (1) end-plate 'noise' recorded at a slow sweep speed; (2) miniature end-plate potentials recorded at faster sweep speed. showing characteristic initial sharp negative deflection and slow decay. c. Positive sharp waves (1) and fibrillation potentials (2) recorded outside the end-plate zone

atrophic disorders, insertional activity is reduced or absent. Increased insertional activity occurs when muscle fibres are abnormally excitable, as in denervation, myotonia, myositis, etc.

End-plate potentials. Spontaneous activity is recorded when the electrode is placed close to the end-plate zone (Fig. 30.5b). Often this appears as low-voltage irregularities of the baseline of 10–40 μv and is called end-plate noise. With fine adjustment of the electrode position it is possible to record monophasic negative potentials of 50–100 μv in amplitude and 0.5–5 ms duration occurring at high frequency and somewhat irregularly (Rosenfalck & Buchthal 1962). These spontaneous negative discharges are recorded when the CNEMG electrode tip is very close to the end-plate (Weiderholt 1970), and they correspond to miniature end-plate potentials as recorded intracellularly with a micro-electrode (Buchthal & Rosenfalck 1966).

Also in the end-plate zone, biphasic spontaneous spike potentials (end-plate spikes) of 100–200 μv amplitude and 3–5 ms duration, firing irregularly at 5–50 Hz may be seen (Jones et al 1955). This activity initially was thought to originate from small intramuscular nerve bundles, but it now appears that it is attributable to the firing of one or several muscle fibres activated by mechanical irritation of their intramuscular nerve terminals by the recording electrodes. These spikes have an initial negative deflection, unlike fibrillation potentials (Buchthal & Rosenfalck 1966). However, small positive potentials may be recorded in the end-plate zone and represent cannula pick-up of end-plate spikes with consequent reversed polarity and amplitude attenuation (Pickett & Schmidley 1980).

Spontaneous activity

Positive sharp waves. This activity is evoked by needle movement and consists of positive potentials, varying in voltage (50–400 μV) and duration 10–100 ms). They discharge at 2–50 Hz and have an abrupt positive initial deflection followed by a slow, almost exponential negative decay (Kugelberg & Petersén 1949, Jasper & Ballem 1949). A series of positive waves has a typical 'saw-tooth' appearance (Fig. 30.5c). The potential arises from the spontaneous or (more often) mechanical excitation of a non-propagated action potential at a damaged region of a single muscle fibre, and is led-off from currents spreading from the inside of the fibre to the surrounding conducting tissue. Positive sharp waves are not seen when recording from normal muscle (Buchthal & Rosenfalck 1966), although they appear in the intrinsic foot muscles in apparently healthy subjects (Falk & Alaranta 1983) where they are probably related to the presence of a traumatic neuropathy. Positive waves are closely associated with fibrillation potentials and appear as frequently as fibrillations in the presence of complete denervation. With a partial lesion they occur only one-third as often as fibrillation (Buchthal & Rosenfalck 1966). They precede by a day or two the appearance of fibrillation following nerve section (Wiechers 1977).

Fibrillation potentials. Spontaneous fibrillation potentials are bi- or tri-phasic waves of amplitude 20–300 μV, often less than 2 ms and not more than 5 ms in duration (Fig. 30.5c). They discharge either regularly or irregularly at rates varying from 2 to 20 Hz and are derived from the

excitation of single muscle fibres (Denny-Brown & Pennybacker 1938, Jasper & Ballem 1949). While electrode insertion may produce profuse fibrillation, mechanical stimulation is not required for their production as they are recorded with subcutaneous electrodes (Rosenfalck & Buchthal 1962). Fibrillation potentials recorded in the endplate region have an initial negative phase (Buchthal & Rosenfalck 1966). They may be detected in this region in normal individuals and the finding of an isolated fibrillation potential outside the end-plate zone is not considered to be abnormal (Buchthal & Rosenfalck 1966). Falk & Alaranta (1983) have shown that fibrillation in the intrinsic foot muscles is seen in many apparently healthy individuals. In older subjects this may be due to an age-related neuropathy and in younger people the fibrillation is confined to the extensor digitorum brevis and may be due to local nerve trauma from footwear.

In denervation, the development of fibrillation potentials is closely associated with the timecourse of Wallerian degeneration and the fibrillations appear on average 10–21 days after nerve section. Denervated muscle shows an abnormal sensitivity to acetylcholine (ACh) (Denny-Brown 1949) and Denny-Brown & Pennybacker (1938) suggested that circulating ACh might excite the abnormally sensitive fibre. Axelson & Thesleff (1959) have demonstrated the appearance of extrajunctional cholinergic receptors following denervation. Fibrillation potentials continue to occur in the presence of curare and other neuromuscular blocking agents (Belmar & Eyzaguirre 1966). Recent evidence suggests that ACh is not directly involved in the generation of fibrillations, which can be recorded from muscle in tissue culture where no ACh is present (Purves Sakmann 1974, Thesleff 1982). In the denervated muscle fibre a number of potentially reversible physical, biochemical and physiological changes occur, resulting from the synthesis of new protein and its insertion into the fibre membrane (Fambrough 1979). These changes appear as the nerve terminals degenerate and they can be prevented in vitro by protein-synthesis inhibitors.

There are physiological differences in the genesis of regular, rhythmically discharging fibrillations and those which occur irregularly (Thesleff

1963, Thesleff & Ward 1975, Smith & Thesleff 1976). Rhythmical fibrillation tends to be maximal early in denervation, the irregular type appearing later. Fibrillation appears in a cyclical fashion in any one fibre and at any one time only a minority of denervated fibres are fibrillating (Smith & Thesleff 1976). Regular fibrillation is due to spontaneous biphasic oscillations of the membrane potential which increase in amplitude and, on reaching a critical value, trigger an action potential in the muscle fibre which in turn initiates repetitive firing at a regular frequency of about 10 Hz (Li et al 1957). Although the precise cause of the oscillations is uncertain, it appears to be related to changes in sodium channels and resultant effects on sodium activation and inactivation. The reduction in resting membrane potential affects the threshold at which the oscillations generate an action potential (Thesleff 1982). Depolarisations responsible for the action potentials of irregularly discharging fibrillations occur randomly, arising in the region of the former end-plate. Their origin relates to alterations in sodium and potassium conductance in the transverse tubular system, generating local discrete triggering depolarisations. These irregularly summate to reach threshold for the propagation of a fibrillation potential. This process appears less related to the level of the resting membrane potential than that generating rhythmical fibrillation (Thesleff 1982). Fibrillation will continue only as long as these mechanisms remain functional and, in prolonged denervation, fibre atrophy results in the cessation of recurrent spontaneous action potentials.

Fibrillation and positive sharp-wave activity are widespread and easy to detect in recently denervated muscle but also occur in other situations, such as botulism (Josefsson 1960), and in a variety of hereditary and acquired myopathies. Fibrillation seen in these conditions may be generated by mechanisms other than those responsible for the spontaneous activity in denervation (Desmedt 1978). For example, the transient profuse fibrillation occurring in paramyotonia congenita on exposure to cold, the activity accompanying the onset of a paralytic attack in adynamia episodica hereditaria and the fibrillation sometimes seen in neuromyotonia, show a clearly different electrogenesis (see below).

Fasciculation potentials. Fasciculation is the often visible muscle twitching accompanying the spontaneous contraction of some or all of the constituent fibres of motor units (Fig. 30.6). It occurs in healthy subjects, especially in the orbicularis oculi, and may be seen in conditions such as thyrotoxicosis, tetany and debilitating disorders. These fasciculation potentials are 'benign', i.e. they are not associated with a progressive lower motor neurone disorder. Fasciculation potentials are often a striking feature of anterior horn cell diseases, e.g. motor neurone disease, where they have a 'malignant' connotation. SFEMG evidence suggests that benign fasciculations are of primary myogenic origin whereas malignant fasciculations arise at various points in the nerve supply to the muscle (Stålberg & Trontelj 1982).

Fasciculation in motor neurone disease was first studied by Denny-Brown & Pennybacker (1938) who described it recurring at intervals of 2–10 s, apparently involving motor units still under

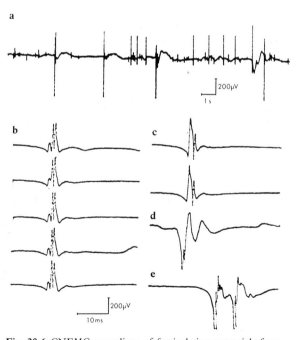

Fig. 30.6 CNEMG recordings of fasciculation potentials from a patient with motor neurone disease. a. Displayed at slow sweep speed to show irregularity of discharge. b, c, d. show examples of different fasciculation potentials which have a polyphasic shape. The potentials in b and c are relatively stable in successive discharges. e. Fasciculation potential discharging as a doublet

voluntary control. Fasciculation is reduced but not abolished by peripheral nerve procaine block (Forster & Alpers 1944, Denny-Brown 1949) and persists for three to five days following motor nerve division (Forster et al 1946). Fasciculations are reduced to about one-half by spinal anaesthesia (Swank & Price 1943). These observations suggest both a central and a peripheral neuronal origin for the fasciculation of motor neurone disease.

Conradi et al (1982) examined the fasciculations of motor neurone disease and showed that antidromic impulses occurred in the axons of fasciculating units as demonstrated by a collision technique. Lignocaine motor nerve blockade did not abolish fasciculation, which was enhanced by neostigmine administration and abolished by a non-paralytic dose of a synthetic curare derivative. The fasciculation of motor neurone disease resembles that induced by cholinergic and anticholinesterase drugs (Meadows 1971). The mechanism of these drugs is to act on ACh receptors in the motor axon terminals, generating action potentials at these sites. Conradi et al (1982) postulate a similar site of origin in motor neurone disease.

The view that most neurogenic fasciculations have an extremely peripheral origin in the axon terminal or preterminal has received much support (Stålberg & Trontelj 1970, Roth 1982, Conradi et al 1982). Distal ectopic excitation sites generate impulses which antidromically invade, and thus excite, the rest of the peripheral branches of the motor unit. The pattern of recruitment of the individual muscle fibres within the unit may differ, often considerably, from that seen when the motor unit is activated centrally. If a fasciculation potential is generated at a single ectopic site, its waveform should be constant: many fasciculations have unstable waveforms, due to the presence of multiple excitation sites or to variable axonal blocking in the preterminal neuronal network (Stålberg Trontelj 1982). This may explain the different conclusions regarding the question of fasciculating motor units being, or not being, capable of voluntary recruitment; with the use of CNEMG, the shape of the action potential is a cardinal factor in its identification.

Fasciculations in the lower limb muscles have been reported in patients with cervical spondylotic myelopathy (King & Stoops 1973). These resolved following decompression in some patients and were attributed to impaired inhibitory influences.

The benign fasciculations of myogenic origin have been shown by SFEMG studies to be due to a hyperexcitable muscle fibre which fires spontaneously and which ephaptically activates neighbouring muscle fibres which may belong to other motor units in the same fascicle. Although there is a low jitter value between the fibres activated in the fasciculation when examined with SFEMG, suggesting ephaptic excitation, different muscle fibres may take part in the process on successive occasions, so that these fasciculations may also appear unstable when recorded with CNEMG (Stålberg & Trontelj 1982). Fasciculation in normal muscle differs from that of motor neurone disease in having a shorter mean interval between successive potentials (Trojaborg & Buchthal 1965). The average interval between successive fasciculation potentials in motor neurone disease was 3.5 s (s.e. (mean) 2.5 s) whereas in benign fasciculation the interval was 0.8 s (s.e. (mean) 0.8 s). Distinction between benign fasciculation and that associated with progressive neurogenic lesions by study of the form and discharge rate of the potentials using CNEMG remains difficult in an individual case. Using special surface electrodes, Hjorth et al (1973) studied the spatial and temporal distribution of fasciculations in motor neurone disease. They found that fasciculations occurred very irregularly at rates as slow as one per min. The significance of fasciculation is best determined by the co-existence of fibrillation potentials or other signs of denervation.

Another form of spontaneous motor unit activity of uncertain nosology has been described by Buchthal & Olsen (1970) as the most consistent abnormality in the EMG in infantile spinal muscular atrophy. The units discharged regularly at rates from 5–15 Hz even during sleep, but the same units could be activated during voluntary contraction. The finding has been confirmed by Hausmanowa-Petrusewicz & Karwanska (1986).

High-frequency repetitive discharges (bizarre high-frequency discharges). Rapid discharges of constant frequency, amplitude and usually polyphasic wave form (Fig. 30.7b) may occur in muscle disease, particularly polymyositis (Walton & Adams 1958,

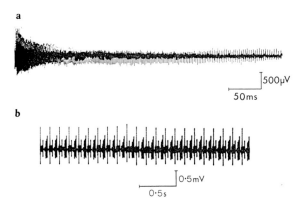

Fig. 30.7 a. CNEMG recording of a myotonic discharge in a patient with dystrophia myotonica. b. CNEMG recording of a repetitive high-frequency discharge in a patient with a chronic neurogenic disorder

Barwick & Walton 1963) and also in neurogenic atrophy, especially anterior horn cell disease (Eisen & Karpati 1971). The discharge frequency, although constant for an individual train, may vary from 5 to 100 Hz. Repetitive discharges are evoked by needle movement and generally start and stop abruptly. They were previously called 'pseudomyotonic discharges,' a term no longer approved. SFEMG studies have shed light on the genesis of this form of abnormal activity (see below).

Myotonic discharges. Myotonia is a sustained contraction of muscle fibres caused by repetitive depolarisation of their membranes (McComas & Johns 1981), recognised clinically by delayed muscular relaxation following a maintained contraction or twitch. The phenomenon may be elicited by movement of the exploring EMG electrode and by external percussion of the muscle. Myotonia is usually worsened by cooling and diminished by exercise. The hereditary myotonias include dystrophia myotonica, myotonia congenita and paramyotonia congenita. The condition may be acquired as the result of the administration of diazocholesterol and monocarboxylic acid groups of drugs and may be a manifestation of hypothyroidism (Somers & Winer 1966, Venables et al 1978, Okuno et al 1981). Myotonia also occurs in hyperkalaemic periodic paralysis, malignant hyperpyrexia, acid maltase deficiency (Engel et al 1973) and chloroquine myopathy (Mastaglia et al

1977). The CNEMG shows prolonged trains of potentials occurring in profusion in response to electrode movement (Fig. 30.7a). Their frequency may reach 150 Hz, dropping subsequently to 20 or 30 Hz. They may resemble fibrillation potentials, positive sharp potentials or may be larger and more complex. An initial increase in frequency and amplitude is rapidly followed by a diminution in both, giving rise to a characteristic sound when the signal is relayed over a loudspeaker. The sound, increasing and decreasing in pitch, resembles the noise of a dive-bomber.

Myotonic activity is reduced by drugs such as phenytoin, quinine and procaine amide, which interfere with voltage-dependent sodium channels. Extracellular electrolyte changes such as a rise in sodium or potassium concentration or a fall in calcium or magnesium, may increase the severity of the myotonia. Myotonic discharges arise from the repetitive activity of the single fibres or a number of muscle fibres, independent of neuronal activation as shown by the persistence of myotonia after curarisation (Landau 1952).

The underlying abnormalities in the myotonic muscle fibre membrane are discussed in detail elsewhere in this volume (Ch. 10). Reduced chloride conductance, either from a reduction in the number of chloride channels or a disorder of the channels themselves, appears to have a central role in myotonia congenita and monocaroboxylic-acid-induced myotonia. Theoretical considerations suggest that a fall in chloride conductance of only 10% would induce repetitive firing in the muscle fibre membrane (Barchi 1975, 1982, Bryant 1982). In dystrophia myotonica an abnormality of sodium ion channel function appears to be the major cause of the myotonia (Hoffmann & DeNardo 1968, Rüdel & Lehmann-Horn 1985). The sodium ion channel kinetics show an abnormal temperature dependence in paramyotonia which is responsible for the depolarisation and paralysis of that disorder (Lehmann-Horn et al 1981). A disturbance of sodium ion channels is also found in hyperkalaemic periodic paralysis (Lehmann-Horn et al 1983). The response to supramaximal stimulation of the motor nerve in the myotonias is discussed below.

Neuromyotonia. Delayed muscular relaxation

following a voluntary contraction, deriving from abnormal impulse generation in nerve rather than muscle, is called neuromyotonia to differentiate it from true myotonia related to muscle fibre membrane abnormalities. The clinical disorders reported under this rubric are a heterogeneous group of conditions, having in common a tendency to muscle stiffness and failure of muscle relaxation. Frequently, muscle cramps and excessive sweating are seen and postural abnormalities may develop in severe generalised neuromyotonia. Other names applied to these disorders include neurotonia, pseudomyotonia and the syndrome of continuous muscle fibre activity (Bergmans 1982). The cases reported have often been isolated and the extent to which the underlying pathophysiology has been elucidated varies considerably. Some instances of neuromyotonia occur in sporadic or hereditary peripheral neuropathy; in other patients, evidence of neuropathic involvement is more subtle. Although some reports indicate the presence of clinical myotonia as well as typical CNEMG myotonic trains, these are abolished by curare, indicating their origin proximal to the muscle fibre membrane. Other associated electrical change consists of continuous high-frequency asynchronous motor unit discharges, often at 100–300 Hz. There is a marked decrement in the amplitude of these high-frequency trains, indicating a failure to keep abreast of the rapidly firing nerve impulses. Myokymia (see below) is also often present, as is fasciculation. Although fibrillation may be seen, unlike the fibrillation of denervation, it is abolished by curare and appears to be due to ectopic impulses arising in the terminal axon exciting single muscle fibre; and positive waves are not usually seen.

Extra discharges occasionally occur in normal motor units and are most common following initial recruitment of the unit or after an isolated electrical stimulus to the nerve. In neuromyotonia, extra discharges are a striking feature and doublets, triplets and multiplets are seen (Fig. 30.8). Doublets or triplets may be recognised by the fact that the second or subsequent discharges have a form similar to that of the first, and that the amplitude depends on the time interval between the initial and extra discharge, decreasing as this falls below 10 ms due to refractoriness in the

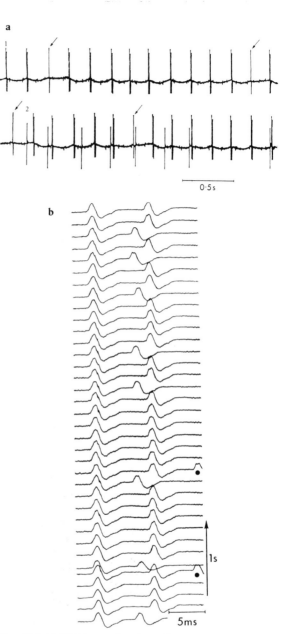

Fig. 30.8 CNEMG recording from tibialis anterior muscle in patient with peripheral neuropathy and neuromyotonia. a. Spontaneously discharging units (1 & 2). Except for four occasions, indicated by arrows, unit 1 fires as a doublet or triplet (b, closed circle). b. shows that the extra discharge in the doublet has two preferred intervals after the original discharge, suggesting that the extra discharges may originate at separate sites along the axon

muscle fibres. The interval between the first and second potentials is from 4 to 10 ms and that between the second and third from 15 to 30 ms

(Stålberg & Trontelj 1982). They may be evoked by electrical stimulation of the nerve (Warmolts & Mendell 1980), particularly by polarising currents, and may also be provoked by the mechanical stimulation of tapping over the motor point; they are often seen in short spontaneous bursts. In addition to their occurrence in the neuromyotonias, multiple discharges are seen in tetany, motor neurone disease and some forms of polyneuropathy. They form grouped or repetitive motor unit discharges, formerly called 'iterative' discharges.

Neuromyotonic activity is at first accentuated, and later abolished, by ischaemia (Mertens & Zschocke 1965, Bergmans 1982). The effect is as pronounced when the cuff is applied distally as proximally, suggesting that the activity is generated at a distal site in the axon. This contrasts with the effects of ischaemia in normal individuals where the generators which will produce transient repetitive activity are predominantly proximal in situation (Kugelberg 1948). The neuromyotonic activity is abolished by curare (Harman & Richardson 1954); it persists during general anaesthesia and is uninfluenced by spinal anaesthesia or brachial anaesthetic nerve block, but is progressively reduced as peripheral nerve block is induced more distally. These features exclude origin of the activity in the muscle fibre, the spinal cord or supraspinally and indicate that the proximal axon is not involved. Membrane stabilisers such as phenytoin and carbamazepine reduce or abolish the activity in some but not all cases. The site of origin of the high-frequency spontaneous activity probably lies in the distal portion of the motor axon. Isaacs (1961, 1967) believed that there was an excessive release of acetylcholine at the motor end-plate and coined the term 'quantal squander' but micro-electrode studies of EPPs from a biopsy of intercostal muscles showed no such excess (Lambert 1978). Apart from the presence of neuromyotonia in overt peripheral neuropathy (Gamstorp & Wohlfart 1959, Welch et al 1972, Lance et al 1979), patients with minor electrophysiological and histological abnormalities of distal motor nerve have been reported (Isaacs 1967, Hudson et al 1978, Lublin et al 1979, Bergmans 1982). Spontaneous activity in neuromyotonia may be generated in the distal motor

axon which is in a hyperpolarised state, repetitive discharges being generated by a breakdown in nerve accomodation (Bergmans 1982). In a significant minority of patients, sensory symptoms, typically peripheral paraesthesiae, have been present (Welch et al 1972). Microneurography (Lance et al 1979) in a single case demonstrated sensory as well as motor axonal hyperexcitability and sural nerve biopsy has indicated axonal degeneration in both myelinated and non-myelinated fibres (Wallis et al 1970, Welch et al 1972, Lance et al 1979).

Myokymia. The 'benign' fasciculations of myokymia are observable clinically as undulating contractions of narrow strips of a muscle along its long axis, likened to a subcutaneous 'bag of worms'. Myokymia has been reported in thyrotoxicosis, peripheral neuropathy, multiple sclerosis, post-irradiation damage to the spinal cord or nerve plexus, facial palsy, ischaemic neuropathy, diffuse vasculitis and the carpal tunnel syndrome (Daube et al 1979, Albers et al 1981, Auger et al 1984). The term has also been applied to the more transient fasciculations appearing around the eye or in the calf muscles in normal individuals (the benign myogenic fasciculations to which reference has already been made). Unfortunately, 'myokymia' is also used by some workers to categorise patients who, on electrophysiological grounds, appear to have neuromyotonia or other disorders of muscular relaxation. The most widely studied form of myokymia affects the facial muscles, often in multiple sclerosis. The EMG shows groups of potentials with intervening periods of silence, the activity recurring in a quasi-rhythmical fashion producing a distinctive form of activity (Gamstorp & Wohlfart 1959). Considerable variation occurs in the number of individual discharges per burst, in the discharge frequency (usually 50 Hz or less) and in the duration and frequency of occurrence of each group. The activity in neuromyotonia shows a considerably higher discharge rate (200 Hz or more) and does not occur in the rhythmical or semi-rhythmical pattern of myokymia. The activity may resemble grouped motor unit discharge but is not susceptible to voluntary alteration and persists in sleep. Unlike myotonia, the discharges are not influenced by needle movement or percussion and may be reduced or abolished by peripheral nerve block. Daube et al (1979) propose the term 'myokymic discharge' for activity of this type and suggest that classification should be on neurophysiological grounds. The myokymic discharge may be recorded in the absence of visible muscular abnormality, especially in radiation plexopathies, but not in malignant infiltration of the plexus (Auger et al 1984). Although the exact origin of myokymia is not known, it often appears to be more proximal than the origin of the neuromyotonias. In the carpal tunnel syndrome the origin appears to be at the wrist (Auger et al 1984) and ectopic impulse generation in a damaged nerve, plexus or root seems likely (Auger et al 1984). The status of the various myokymia and neuromyotonia syndromes is still subject to debate and there is no universal agreement on the neurophysiological or clinical nosology of these disorders (DeJong et al 1951, Harman & Richardson 1954, Greenhouse et al 1967, Gardner-Medwin & Walton 1969, Hughes & Matthews 1969, Daube et al 1979, Lublin et al 1979, Albers et al 1981, Bergmans 1982, Auger et al 1984).

Stiff-man syndrome. Spontaneous activity occurring in the stiff-man syndrome (Moersch & Woltman 1956) resembles physiological cramps but is widespread and continuous. CNEMG reveals a sustained interference pattern in affected muscles with normal individual MUPs. Sleep, and general, spinal and local anaesthetic nerve block, abolish the muscle fibre activity, suggesting a central origin (Price & Allott 1958, Werk et al 1961, Gordon et al 1967). Agents which suppress activity in spinal and supra-spinal intraneurones, such as diazepam, baclofen and clonazepam, are effective therapies (Howard 1963, Martinelli et al 1978). Some similarities to tetanus have been remarked upon (Moersch & Woltman 1956, Gordon et al 1967). Excessive excitability of the motor neurone pool may develop because of a failure of recurrent inhibition, perhaps due to disturbed Renshaw interneurone function. The silent period is normal in the stiff-man syndrome, unlike the situation in tetanus, where it is lost (Stohr & Heckl 1977). Clomipramine, which

inhibits the re-uptake of serotonin and noradrenaline, producing increased central serotoninergic and noradrenergic activity, severely aggravates the activity (Meink et al 1984). The presence of grossly exaggerated responses to exteroceptive stimuli and abnormally short transmission times with excessive reflex excitatory phases in face and limb muscles has been demonstrated (Meink et al 1984). The suggestion has been made that the disorder is the result of transmission of descending noradrenergic impulses from disordered medial brain-stem pathways impinging on the alpha motor neurone.

In tetanus, the toxin may impair Renshaw cell activity, resulting in alpha motor neurone hyperexcitability (Brooks et al 1957). Renshaw cell failure would also explain the absence of the silent period. The spontaneous activity in the EMG is abolished by sleep, general and spinal anaesthesia and peripheral nerve block. The peripheral nerves have been shown to be affected by the disease (Shahani et al 1979) and the motor end-plate is also abnormal (Duchen 1973). It is not yet clear how these peripheral defects contribute to the clinical picture.

When the serum ionised calcium is low, spontaneous muscular activity occurs (Kugelberg 1948). Ischaemia, hyperventilation or nerve percussion evoke or accentuate the muscular activity (Layzer & Rowland 1971). Increased sodium conductance is produced by low extracellular calcium leading to repetitive nerve excitation and there is loss of nerve accommodation (Kugelberg 1948). The CNEMG shows groups of MUPs often firing asynchronously at rates of 5–30 Hz, either in brief bursts or longer trains, with periods of relative silence between them. Many repetitive firing units show doublets, triplets and multiplets. The ectopic impulses appear to arise at a variety of levels in the motor axon and some may occur in muscle fibres (Stålberg & Trontelj 1982). Cramps and painful involuntary sustained contractions of muscles are associated with high-frequency motor unit discharges at 200–300 Hz. Synchronous involvement of large areas of muscle is usual (Layzer Rowland 1971). Recurrent muscle cramps are often present in motor neurone disease and there are syndromes in which cramps are a major feature, including the familial and sporadic muscle pain and fasciculation syndromes (Jusic et al 1972, Lazaro et al 1981). Mild abnormalities of nerve conduction are sometimes found but CNEMG is normal apart from the cramps. A syndrome has been described, mainly affecting women, where cramps are associated with diarrhoea and alopecia; later, painful muscle spasms resembling tetany develop but the serum calcium is normal (Satoyoshi 1978).

Motor unit action potential (MUP)

Description, definition and methods of analysis. The MUP is the summation of the individual action potentials of its constituent muscle fibres. MUPs recorded with CNEMG electrodes (Fig. 30.9) appear as spikes, with one or more phases. Phases are defined as one more than the number of base-line crossings. Smaller changes in polarity failing to cross the base-line are called turns. The spikes are derived from the action potentials of two to 12 muscle fibres of the motor unit lying within a 1 mm radius of the electrode's leading-off surface (Thiele & Böhle 1978). Because of their distance from the recording electrode, action potentials from more remote muscle fibres in the unit may appear only in the smaller lower-frequency initial or terminal portions of the MUP. Because the individual muscle fibres of the

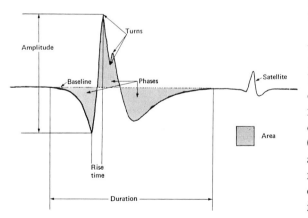

Fig. 30.9 Diagram of a motor unit potential (MUP) recorded with a CNEMG electrode. The duration, amplitude and number of phases are the most widely measured parameters. The satellite potential is excluded for measurement of the duration. Determination of the area requires the use of a computer

motor unit are dispersed and the concentric electrode has directional properties (Nakao et al 1965), MUP configuration varies with needle position. The degree of asynchrony between the arrival of individual muscle fibre action potentials at the electrode determines the number of phases or turns in the MUP recorded at a particular site. MUP duration varies less with changes in electrode position than the amplitude, the number of phases and the phase-relationships of the potential.

In up to 10% of MUPs in normal muscle, spikes separated from the main action potential are seen and are termed variously linked, late, parasite or satellite components (Lang & Partanen 1976) (Fig. 30.9). They generally follow, but may occasionally precede, the main portion of the MUP; they are usually generated by single muscle fibres. Linked components are usually excluded from MUP duration measurements but their presence should be noted because they have important pathological implications, frequently being seen in neurogenic and certain myopathic conditions.

Most MUPs have amplitudes of from 250 μV to 2–4 mV and have diphasic or triphasic forms, with durations of 4–12 ms. In the majority of normal limb muscles up to 10% of units may be polyphasic (Caruso & Buchthal 1965), although in deltoid 25% may have a polyphasic shape. The time interval between the initial positive peak and the subsequent negative peak is the MUP risetime and relates to the proximity of the electrode to the active muscle fibres.

The mean MUP duration of voluntary muscles varies with the muscle examined. Petersén & Kugelberg (1949) found a mean MUP duration in biceps brachii of 7.56 ms (s.e. (mean) 0.14 ms) compared with 2.28 ms (s.e. (mean) 0.03 ms) in facial muscles. In the external ocular muscles the duration is even shorter, 1.60 ms (s.e. (mean) 0.06 ms) (Björk & Kugelberg 1953). Scattering of arrival times of individual action potentials making up the MUP depends on the distribution of motor end-plates. Normally these are arranged in one (or sometimes two) zones (Coërs & Woolf 1959), extending for about 1% of the total muscle length: e.g. in the biceps brachii there is a 20–30 mm longitudinal spread of the site of the end-plates and therefore of the origin of the muscle fibre action potentials. MUPs recorded deep within the muscle have durations comparable with those obtained with monopolar needle electrodes and are longer than those recorded close to the surface (Buchthal et al 1954b). The CNEMG cannula is not inert: it is a conductor which takes on a potential equal to the mean value of the tissue potential along its length. Thus the deeper the electrode is inserted, the lower is the cannula potential (Pollak 1971). When the electrode is superficial, the cannula potential is high and MUP durations no longer approximate to those found with a monopolar system.

In infants, mean MUP duration is shorter than in adults and in the elderly it is prolonged. The increase in duration occurring with maturation from infancy to adulthood is attributed to widening of the end-plate zones with growth, while that associated with advancing years appears to relate to an increased muscle fibre density within the motor units due to age-related denervation and reinnervation (Sacco et al 1962). MUP duration is also increased by cooling by about 5% for each degree Celsius fall; the amplitude of the potential drops between 2 and 5% and the number of polyphasic potentials rises by 1% (Buchthal et al 1954c). Differential cooling causes desynchronisation which more than offsets the facilitatory effect of cooling on the muscle fibre membrane. MUP amplitude has been shown to be greater in men than in women in the biceps brachii and tibialis anterior (Pertanan & Lang 1982) but duration values appear to be the same in both sexes (Kaiser & Petersén 1965).

Quantification of MUP dimensions has a long history. Initial studies involved recording early-recruiting units on long lengths of film, and MUPs identified as repeating free of artefact or interference from other units on at least three occasions were measured; this method ensures that polyphasic potentials are single MUPs and not superimpositions of more than one potential, as can occur, for instance, in tremor. This laborious procedure was made easier by the introduction of the delay-line. It is necessary to measure at least 20 separate randomly recorded MUPs in order to derive the mean MUP duration (Buchthal & Rosenfalk 1955). When the same biceps brachii was examined on 20 separate occasions to validate the reproducibility of mean duration measure-

ments based on a sample of about 20 different MUPs, a significant shortening occurred only on the final examination, attributed to the repeated needling (Buchthal et al 1954b). Because of variations in MUP amplitude with needle position, a much larger sample is needed if reproducible mean MUP amplitude measurements are to be made. The other feature studied is the percentage of polyphasic potentials (i.e. those with five or more phases) present. Manual determinations of MUP parameters may differ between individual electromyographers measuring the same material, and biased selection of MUPs can occur during the recording process if random electrode repositioning is not strictly observed (Barwick & Gardner-Medwin 1967, Falk 1983).

Automatic and semiautomatic measurements of MUP characteristics have been introduced; in addition, methods of interference pattern analysis have been developed (Ch. 32). In many automated methods of MUP measurement the electromyographer still controls the selection of the units measured, first by siting the recording electrode and, in some methods, by choosing to accept or reject the particular action potential. Most systems require display of a delayed action potential after it has triggered the oscilloscope sweep. A window discriminator allows selection of a potential of a certain amplitude or slope in the presence of other activity, so that several different MUPs may be recorded at a single site. The electrode should be repositioned at a transverse distance of at least 10 mm in order to ensure that the same motor unit is not recorded twice from different parts of its territory. In smaller distal muscles this may not be possible and MUPs from different fractions of the same unit are registered. Electronic averaging makes it simpler to measure the dimensions of the motor unit potential free from noise or interference from other active units. Amplitude, phases, turns and rise-time are straightforward but problems in defining duration remain. MUP onset may be abrupt or more gradual when determination of its beginning may be difficult. The terminal portion of the MUP, due to volume conduction of action potentials travelling away from the recording site and towards the tendon, gradually disappears into the baseline. Its termination is particularly difficult to define and is a function of the gain in the recording system (Falk 1983). The automated methods so far reported (Bergmans 1971, Lee & White 1973, Kopeć et al 1973, Kopeć & Hausmanowa-Petrusewicz 1976) use arbitrary threshold levels of what constitutes a significant departure from the baseline. The lower this threshold is set, the longer will the MUP duration appear.

Four main methods for the identification of MUPs which are to be subject to automatic analysis have been described. First, the electromyographer selects the action potential and only then is the computer used to make the measurements. Second, there is the template technique in which the computer identifies one or more template MUPs and stores them. Each subsequent MUP is compared with the template until a predetermined number of identical MUPs have been collected; these are averaged and parameters defined by the particular programme used are analysed and displayed (Bergmans 1971, 1973, Tanzi et al 1979, Hynninen et al 1979). Third, an individual MUP may be isolated using a suitable trigger, such as a peak-window or an adjustable-level trigger (Lang et al 1971). The operator then decides, after the potentials have been averaged and displayed, whether to accept them for further analysis by the programme. Fourth, a SFEMG port on the side of a CNEMG electrode is used to select a single-fibre potential from the unit and locks on to this while the MUP is registered on the second channel (Lang & Falk 1980).

The Polish minicomputer ANOPS 100 forms the basis of a MUP analysis system, the subject of several reports (Kopeć & Hausmanowa-Petrusewicz 1969, 1976, 1983, Kopeć et al 1973, Singh & Lovelace 1979, Wagner et al 1979). All potentials exceeding 100 μV are accepted for measurement and an amplitude criterion is used to measure duration. (The onset and termination are 20 μV above the baseline.) Peak-to-peak amplitude is also determined but the analysis of phases is unconventional. Phases are defined as polarity changes of over 50 μV rather than the number of baseline crossings plus one, so that some 'turns' are counted as phases. Recordings are made at 16 different sites and 64 signals from each site are subjected to analysis. Although this method is criticised because it may well analyse the same

MUP several times and because it treats superimposed units as separate single MUPs (Ludin 1980), the values obtained for MUP amplitude and duration in normal subjects, using this technique, correspond with those obtained manually (Wagner et al 1979). Moreover, there is a satisfactory differentiation between normal control values and those obtained in various neuromuscular diseases (Singh & Lovelace 1979).

The values obtained with automatic systems generally compare well with those obtained by manual measurements of the same material (Hirose et al 1974, Fugelsang-Frederiksen et al 1976, 1977). It has been pointed out (Sica et al 1978) that the durations established by Buchthal et al (1957) may differ from those produced by the automated methods. The analysis programmes vary (Rathjen et al 1968, Bergmans 1971, 1973, Kunze 1971, 1973, Lee & White 1973, Kopeć & Hausmanowa-Petrusewicz 1976, Tanzi et al 1979, Hynninen et al 1979, Stålberg & Antoni 1981, Falk 1983). There are now a number of commercial systems providing microprocessor-based automatic analysis of the standard motor unit potential parameters. Various workers have produced programmes which will carry out the analysis on standard microcomputers to which many modern electromyographs can be linked (Rathjen et al 1968, Stålberg & Antoni 1981). Using such devices it is possible to analyse many parameters that are not readily assessable manually, such as MUP area, duration and area of the spike component(s), spike slope, etc. The clinical utility of such extra measurements has yet to be demonstrated.

INTERPRETATION OF THE EMG

CNEMG

In healthy muscle at rest, with the exploring electrode outside the end-plate zone, no electrical activity can be detected. In the end-plate zone occur the electrical changes already described, including MEPPs and fibrillations. Electrical activity accompanying movement of the needle is brief. The initiation of volitional activity is associated with the recruitment of one or a small number of MUPs firing at low frequency with

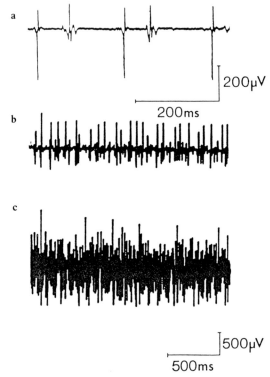

200μV

200ms

500μV

500ms

Fig. 30.10 CNEMG recordings of motor unit recruitment at different levels of activity in normal muscle. a. Gentle contraction showing individual motor unit potentials. b. Moderate contraction showing some overlap of potentials. c. Maximal contraction showing an interference pattern

asynchrony between the units when more than one is present (Fig. 30.10a). The early-recruiting units are generally smaller than those which appear at higher tensions and they recruit in an orderly fashion. The smallest anterior horn cells are responsible for the early units — the 'size principle' (Henneman 1957). Increasing force of contraction is associated with a rising firing rate of the early-recruited units and the appearance of additional MUPs (Fig. 30.10b). Initial firing rates are usually from 5–10 Hz and these rise considerably before it becomes impossible to follow individual MUPs and an interference pattern develops (Fig. 30.10c).

Upper motor neurone lesions. In upper motor neurone paralysis, physiological hypertrophy of muscle and in the wasting of disuse atrophy, the EMG recorded with a CNEMG electrode was thought to remain normal, apart from some

increase in polyphasic potentials reported in the latter condition (Pinelli & Buchthal 1953).

Considerable controversy has developed over the changes occurring in pyramidal tract lesions. Goldkamp (1967) reported fibrillations in approximately two-thirds of the paretic mucles examined in a series of 116 hemiplegics. Spontaneous activity was more pronounced in distal muscles. This finding has been confirmed in a number of other studies (Johnson et al 1975, Segura & Sahgal 1981). Similar spontaneous activity has been reported in the lower limbs of paraplegics after spinal cord injuries (Van Alphen et al 1962, Spielholz et al 1972, Taylor et al 1974). There is argument as to the cause of these findings: it has been suggested that they are secondary to various compression or traction injuries to peripheral nerves or plexuses consequent upon the paresis and immobility. Although it is likely that such peripheral factors do play a part, the very widespread fibrillation recorded in some studies and its early onset between the second and fifth week after the development of the hemiplegia, suggest that unrecognised lower motor neurone pathology is not the only cause. Considerable changes in the physiological properties of the motor unit occur in upper motor neurone lesions (Edström 1970, McComas et al 1973, Young & Rowley 1982). McComas et al reported a loss of 50% of motor units in hemiplegic muscle, and histological evidence of denervation in hemiplegic muscle has been reported (Segura Sahgal 1981). A greater decrement in the compound muscle action potential in response to repetitive stimulation in muscles on the hemiplegic side has been found (Brown & Wynn-Parry 1981). Trans-synaptic degeneration was proposed by McComas et al (1973) as the cause of these features. For a fuller discussion of this controversial but important area see Brown (1984).

Lower motor neurone lesions. After complete nerve section, total electrical silence of the denervated muscle ensues outside the end-plate zone. Fibrillations appear, following the time-course of Wallerian degeneration, and so take longer to appear in distal muscles when the nerve section is proximal (Luco & Eyzaguirre 1955). Positive sharp waves followed by fibrillation are seen, at first in relation to the mechanical stimulation of electrode movement and later spontaneously. By three weeks, fibrillation potentials and positive sharp waves are easily detected. Volitional potentials are absent from the time of onset of the nerve section. End-plate potentials eventually disappear from completely denervated muscle (Miledi & Slater 1963, Weiderholt 1970, Buchthal 1982).

The retention of some volitional MUPs in a lower motor neurone lesion indicates that the lesion is incomplete, an important finding in peripheral nerve injuries. Absence of MUPs indicates total dysfunction of the nerve, some of which may be axonal in type but conduction-block due to demyelination may also contribute. The complete absence of excitability of the nerve distal to the site of injury may not indicate total section: the nerve sheath may remain intact, despite complete degeneration of its axonal content. Evidence of continuity may have to await the orderly return of motor unit activity consequent upon axonal regeneration at approximately 1–2 mm per day.

Fibrillations are profuse in acute and severe neurogenic lesions but may be less easy to identify in more chronic processes. Their absence can only be presumed after an exacting search. Buchthal (1982) reports being unable to detect fibrillation in one-quarter to one-third of partially denervated muscles. In longstanding partial denervation, absence of fibrillation may be due to reinnervation of many denervated fibres by collateral sprouting and severe atrophy of the remainder.

Incomplete lower motor neurone lesions cause a reduction of volitional MUPs which may preclude the development of an interference pattern on full volition. The interference pattern is deemed to be reduced when the base-line of the oscilloscope sweep is not continuously obscured by MUP activity but individual MUPs cannot be identified. More severe lesions result in the presence of so few units in the pick-up area of the CNEMG electrode that the beam returns to the isoelectric line between individual MUPs which can be identified; this is called discrete activity (Fig. 30.11a). The loss of motor units results in abnormally high firing-rates of the recruited surviving units. In severe partial denervation, the fall-out of motor units may be so extreme that a

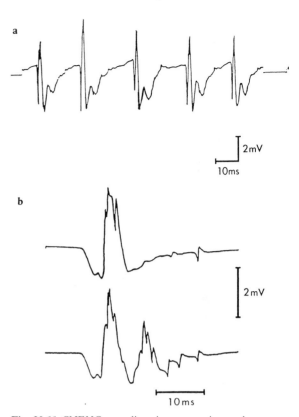

Fig. 30.11 CNEMG recordings in neurogenic atrophy. a. Discrete motor unit activity at maximal effort in patient with old poliomyelitis. The motor unit is firing at a frequency of about 60 Hz. b. Motor unit potential of prolonged duration and with late components. In the lower trace there is an extra discharge of the motor unit

single MUP recurring at rates of 50–60 Hz may represent maximal effort.

Changes occur in MUP morphology when partial denervation has been present for some time. Collateral sprouts from intramuscular nerve twigs of surviving motor units reinnervate adjacent muscle fibres. This first results in small late or satellite potentials of the MUP showing an unstable connection to the parent unit, evident with a delay-line and superimposition techniques (Borenstein & Desmedt 1973). The lateness of the component relates to slow conduction through an immature axon sprout; its frequent absence is due to transmission failure ('impulse blocking') at an immature end-plate. These small spikes may follow the main MUP by 40–80 ms; later, the connections become more mature and the components appear with less delay and more stability.

Collateral reinnervation results in increased fibre density (FD) as large numbers of muscle fibres are incorporated into the motor unit (Kugelberg 1973). When FD is increased in that part of the motor unit close to the leading-off surface of the recording electrode and there is close synchronisation between muscle fibre excitation, a large amplitude MUP results (Fig. 30.11b). These MUPs have been called 'giant' motor units as they commonly reach amplitudes of 10 or even 20 mV. This terminology is no longer approved; measurement of peak-to-peak amplitude and comparison with normal ranges for the particular muscle explored is preferred.

Prolonged MUP duration in reinnervation is mainly due to the increase in the number of fibres within the pick-up area of the electrode. Collateral sprouting widens the innervation zone, leading to increased temporal dispersion of the muscle fibre action potentials, adding to MUP duration as well as increasing the number of polyphasic potentials (Buchthal & Clemmesen 1941). The collateral reinnervation capacity appears to be an important property of healthy anterior-horn cells (McComas et al 1971a).

Nerve conduction studies and EMG complement each other in the assessment of peripheral neuropathies. In acute axonal neuropathies, fibrillation and positive sharp waves in distal muscles appear before reduction in CMAP amplitude or other conduction abnormalities can be identified confidently (Thage et al 1963, Trojaborg et al 1969). In severe post-infectious demyelinating neuropathy there is profound slowing of conduction, but ultimately the prognosis depends upon the amount of axonal damage associated with the demyelination (Eisen & Humphreys 1974). During recovery from axonal damage, the EMG may show the presence of long-duration (15–30 ms) polyphasic MUPs consisting of many short spikes, due to axonal regeneration and reinnervation (Buchthal 1970).

The process of compensatory reinnervation may be complete in a year and remains stable thereafter if caused by a non-progressive lesion (Hakelius & Stålberg 1974). With ongoing disease, collateral reinnervation occurs but the disorder's progression ultimately causes its failure. A useful function of the EMG is to indicate the tempo and extent of the denervating process. Although SFEMG plays a major part in this, CNEMG may be useful. If profuse fibrillations and positive sharp waves accompany evidence of widespread remodelling of motor units with many unstable MUPs, a fairly rapidly evolving disease process is likely. If denervation is slowly progressive, florid spontaneous activity is less likely to be found, and the proportion of unstable MUPs may suggest the rate of progression. Complex high-amplitude or long-lasting but stable MUPs suggest that denervation and reinnervation has occurred but that the disorder is currently inactive. Using a CNEMG electrode and a 500 Hz high-pass filter, the stability of individual motor units can be assessed. With a delay-line and a fast sweep speed, the time-relationships of individual spikes in the MUP can be observed. Although it is not possible to measure jitter accurately, instability of the MUP and blocking of individual components can be identified. The technique provides an intermediate stage between CNEMG and SFEMG (Payan 1978).

Synchronisation of motor unit activity. The smoothness of muscular contraction is mainly due to asynchronous recruitment of motor units; however, there is some apparent grouping of the MUPs which characteristically occurs at a frequency of about 9 Hz and is most striking during fatigue. The suggested cause for this is oscillation in the stretch reflex servo-loop, which may account in part for physiological tremor (Lippold et al 1957). Apparent grouping of motor unit activity can occur in deafferented muscle so that not all grouping has a reflex basis. There is evidence (Taylor 1962) that under normal conditions a significant amount of grouping is a random occurrence.

In patients who have muscle weakness as a result of anterior horn cell disease such as poliomyelitis, action potentials can be recorded simultaneously from widely separated electrodes in the same muscle (Buchthal & Clemmesen 1941). The finding was regarded as evidence of a central (spinal cord) disorder. Denny-Brown (1949) suggested that there was a loss of the smaller earlier-recruiting motor units in anterior horn cell diseases and that the apparent synchronisation was due to the uncovering of larger units which in normal individuals were lost in the interference pattern.

Synchronous potentials are more frequent in muscle affected by anterior horn cell disease than in peripheral nerve lesions (Buchthal & Madsen 1950). This may indicate an interaction between motor neurones leading to periods of synchronous firing (Simpson 1962, 1966, Norris 1965). Synchronisation may be due to the fact that each Renshaw interneurone receives fewer recurrent collateral fibres when there is a reduced anterior horn cell population promoting synchronous firing (Simpson 1966). There are alternative explanations: e.g. ephaptic excitation could occur proximally in the cord or motor root to explain the finding of synchronous motor unit activity in different muscles innervated by the same spinal segment, in advanced motor neurone disease, as reported by Norris (1965).

Aberrant reinnervation and synkinesis. Regeneration and reinnervation after nerve damage is often misdirected, especially when the internal architecture of the nerve has been disrupted by the causative lesion. The axonal regrowth may result in the reinnervation of muscle fibres in quite separate muscles (such as the circumoral and circumocular muscles) following Bell's palsy, resulting in a permanent synchronisation (synkinesis) between different parts of what are pathologically dispersed single motor units. Aberrant reinnervation may also result in the presence of abnormal axon reflexes.

While studying axon reflex latencies in normal individuals to determine the sites of axonal branching, Stålberg & Trontelj (1979) found evidence suggesting that the branching began more proximally than was previously suspected, some 10–15 cm proximal to the innervation zone. In chronic compressive nerve lesions, reinnervating axonal branches may occur distal to the site of the lesion, allowing the possibility of widespread synkinesis (Fullerton & Gilliatt 1965). Esslen (1960) demonstrated synchronous 'volitional' motor unit activity in different muscles after aberrant reinnervation in facial and peripheral nerve lesions. Periodic recruitment of MUPs in the deltoid or biceps brachii, in phase with respiration, may develop after injuries to the brachial plexus and is due to aberrant reinnervation by axons of the phrenic nerve (Swift et al 1980). Obstetric brachial plexus injury may cause extensive synkinesis and axon reflexes, sometimes involving antagonistic muscles (De Grandis et al 1979).

Primary myopathies. High-frequency discharges, positive sharp waves and fibrillations occur in some myopathies. McComas & Mrozek (1968) suggested that fibrillation in muscular dystrophy was due to functional denervation occurring when segmental necrosis separates a viable portion of a muscle fibre from its end-plate. Regenerating muscle fibres without an innervation may also discharge spontaneously. Because such fibres have a very small diameter their spontaneous discharges will be of low amplitude compared with fibrillations seen in recent denervation. The genesis of fibrillation potentials in myopathy is obscure but may be different from those mechanisms responsible for fibrillation in denervated muscle. Florid fibrillations may be recorded in polymyositis (particularly in the acute and subacute forms), which suggests that secondary involvement of the terminal branches by the inflammatory process might be responsible (Richardson 1956). Functional denervation may also play a part as may increased membrane irritability (Bohan et al 1977). In Duchenne dystrophy, fibrillation can be more easily recorded if the patient exercises before the examination (Buchthal & Rosenfalck 1966).

The alterations in CNEMG-recorded MUP parameters in myopathy are, first, a reduction in mean MUP duration (Kugelberg 1947). This is the most characteristic change and to be considered significant, the reduction should be greater than 20% of that recorded from the same muscle of a normal subject of similar age. Secondly, there may be an increase in the number of polyphasic potentials present (Fig. 30.12a) and when this increase is combined with the finding of shortening of the mean MUP duration, the probability of myopathy is high. MUP amplitude may be reduced, but this is a less pronounced and more variable feature. The reduced MUP duration and amplitude seen in myopathy may have several causes. In myopathy the resting membrane poten-

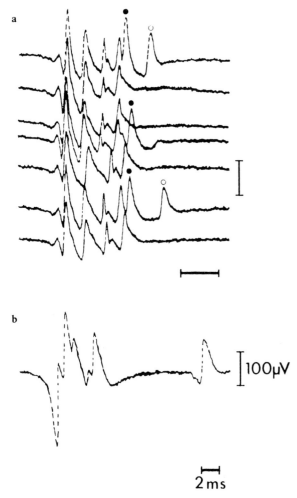

Fig. 30.12 CNEMG recordings in myopathy. a. Polyphasic motor unit potential recorded from biceps in a patient with mitochondrial myopathy. Two potentials (closed and open circles) show increased jitter and blocking. b. Recording from biceps in another patient with mitochondrial myopathy showing a polyphasic potential containing a late component 15 ms after the onset of the potential (From Fawcett et al 1982a)

processes including muscle fibre regeneration and reinnervation, fibre splitting, and perhaps closer packing of atrophied fibres. There is marked variation of fibre diameters resulting in increased scatter of action potential propagation velocities, causing desynchronisation of component spikes and temporal dispersion, leading to the presence of late components (Fig. 30.12b). Local increase in FD and the presence of hypertrophied fibres may account for the occasional high-amplitude potentials. Restriction of volume conduction due to fibrosis and fatty infiltration may result in an increase in the recorded amplitude of individual muscle fibre action potentials and hence an increased MUP amplitude (Stålberg & Trontelj 1979). Polyphasic potentials probably derive from the wider range of conduction velocities in immature nerve sprouts and smaller muscle fibres. In some recordings the effective MUP duration when all the satellite or late potentials are included may be prolonged to values of 40 to 80 ms (Lang & Partanen 1976).

The fall in mean interference pattern amplitude may be explained by loss of individual muscle fibres within the units, combined with fibrosis and fatty replacement which may alter the volume conduction characteristics of the muscle. The loss of muscle fibres, which would have contributed to the contractile process, accounts for the recruitment of more units to develop a given tension, resulting in an increased interference pattern density. As indicated above, in more severely affected dystrophic muscles individual MUPs may have an excessively complex form and prolonged duration, so that rapid discharge of a few such potentials will result in overlapping of the complexes. Thus, a full interference pattern may be recorded at only moderate contractions and it is of reduced amplitude. The finding of small, brief, often polyphasic MUPs, recruiting early in large numbers in myopathy, contrasts with MUPs of large amplitude and long duration showing reduced recruitment seen in chronic neurogenic disease.

Differentiation of myopathy from neurogenic lesions may be less straightforward than suggested above (Gath et al 1969). Several neurogenic processes may result in an excess of low amplitude

tial may be reduced in amplitude (Lenman 1965) and consequently the action potential amplitude is also reduced. Extracellularly recorded action potentials from narrow-diameter fibres are of low amplitude (Håkansson 1957). The initial and terminal portions of the MUP are of low amplitude and disappear into the baseline earlier.

Primary muscle disease may cause local increases in FD as a result of a number of polyphasic short-duration MUPs. In the early phase of reinnervation, neural connection may be established with a few muscle fibres within the motor unit. The resulting MUPs will resemble those found in myopathy, although conduction in the immature terminal innervation will be slow (Engel 1975). In distal neuropathy the sick axon may be unable to sustain innervation of all its muscle fibres and an apparently random drop-out could produce a picture suggestive of myopathy.

Both histological and electrophysiological changes suggestive of a myopathy may be seen in long-standing partial denervation (Drachman et al 1967). In addition, in what appears to be a myopathic process, changes suggestive of denervation may occur and may be regarded as secondary neuropathic changes (Guy et al 1950). In muscles severely and chronically affected by myopathy or denervation, it may be impossible to decide, in the presence of findings suggestive of both a myopathic and neurogenic process, which of these is primary. The selection of mildly or moderately involved muscles for study is likely to be more profitable than examining those which are severely affected.

Scanning EMG

Normal muscle. The basis of this technique has already been mentioned. The biceps brachii and tibialis anterior have been studied most often. For any one position of the needle electrode, the MUP form remains relatively constant, the major spikes occurring at the same point along the sweep in successive recordings. Movement of the electrode through the motor unit territory gives information concerning the spatial and temporal distribution of the muscle fibres and their action potentials. MUPs which contain spike components are distributed over a distance of 5–10 mm for the biceps brachii and tibialis anterior muscles (Fig. 30.13a). In normal muscle there are usually no gaps or silent areas in the cross-section. A collection of adjacent spikes is called a 'peak'. In

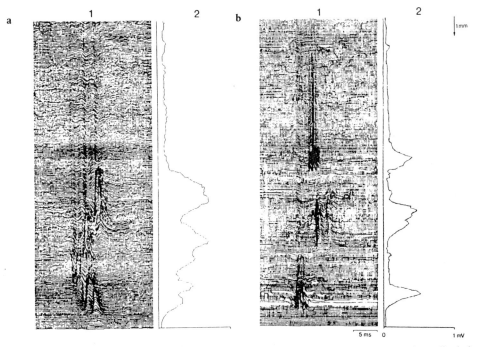

Fig. 30.13 Scanning EMG in tibialis anterior. a. Normal muscle; b. FSH dystrophy. The peak-to-peak amplitude in each sweep is measured and indicated to the right of the scans (a2, b2). Note in this example that the total length of the territory is slightly longer in the dystrophic muscle, but that the unit activity is interrupted by silent areas (Reproduced with permission from Hilton-Brown & Stålberg 1983b)

biceps brachii and tibialis anterior a single major negative peak is found in about 50% of recordings. Less often two, three or more rarely four peaks may be found, separated in the temporal domain by up to 9 ms. This appears to depend upon differing arrival-times of the muscle fibre action potentials at the electrode. Typically, the inter-peak interval is about 3 ms. These individual peaks derive from groups of muscle fibres called 'motor unit fractions'. They either have separate end-plate zones or may be innervated from different major axonal branches occurring relatively proximally. Each branch may have a different conduction time. The motor unit fraction concept should not be confused with the sub-unit theory (Buchthal 1961). There is no suggestion of anatomical sub-units, the muscle fibres in each fraction being randomly scattered and intermingled with fibres of other motor units. The relationship of muscle fibres within the fraction is temporal rather than spatial.

Lower motor neurone lesions. Recordings with scanning EMG (Stålberg 1982) show those features characteristic of the findings in CNEMG in neurogenic disease. These are increased mean duration, amplitude and number of phases of the MUP. As in normal muscle, the electrical front of MUPs within the whole motor unit is dispersed. There is no definite alteration from the normal temporal dispersion of the fractions. Some increase in the transverse distance over which spike components can be recorded is sometimes found. Because of volume conduction of action potentials of higher amplitude than normal, slow components of the motor unit can be recorded over a larger distance than is found in normal muscle. Synchronous activity, when found, only occurs within that area of muscle corresponding to the motor unit territory and there is no abnormally dispersed synchrony.

Primary myopathies. In primary myopathies, a normal or slightly reduced spatial dispersion is found in scanning EMG. In addition, there may be silent areas in the territory (Fig. 30.13b). Individual action potentials recorded show either a reduced duration (due to fibre loss) or increased duration (due to the presence of late components).

An increase in duration is particularly striking in Duchenne dystrophy (Stålberg 1977, Hilton-Brown & Stålberg 1983a,b).

Single-fibre EMG

The appearance of a single-fibre action potential recorded by SFEMG electrodes has distinctive characteristics (Ekstedt 1964, Ekstedt & Stålberg 1973, Stålberg & Trontelj 1979). Single-fibre potentials consist of smooth biphasic spikes, usually with an initial positive phase. The mean amplitude of single-fibre potentials ranges from just under 1 mV to over 25 mV. A steep fall-off in the amplitude of the potentials occurs as distance between the electrode and muscle fibre increases. The rise time of single muscle-fibre action potential is brief, ranging from 75 μs to 200 μs and the total duration is about 1 ms.

Jitter. At about one in three sites where a single-fibre potential is recorded, a second potential clearly separate from the triggering spike is seen. The second wave form is not identical to the first, indicating that it is a separate muscle-fibre action potential, not a repetitive discharge. The second spike fires with a fairly constant time relationship to the first, indicating that they both derive from a single motor unit. However, small variations in the time relationships occur between the two potentials, which are termed 'jitter' (see Fig. 30.23 & 24a). The jitter value or interpotential interval variation relates to the safety-factor of neuromuscular transmission at the two neuromuscular junctions (see Part 2, p. 1060).

Jitter may be expressed as the mean of consecutive differences (MCD) of successive interpotential intervals (see Part 2). In normal muscle it varies between 5 and 50 μs MCD. Jitter of less than 5 μs between two action potentials, and not increased by neuromuscular blocking agents, strongly suggests that the recordings come from a split portion of a single muscle fibre (Ekstedt & Stålberg 1969b). Similar low jitter values occur when one muscle fibre ephaptically excites another. Ephapsis is an insecure process and continued recording may demonstrate a sudden transmission failure, distinguishing the phenomenon from that due to fibre splitting. Jitter in excess of 100 μs MCD is usually associated with transmission failure at one of the end-plates, manifesting as intermittent blocking of one of the spike components (see Fig. 30.24c, p. 1062).

Fibre density (FD). Single-fibre electrodes are used to measure FD, the mean number of single muscle–fibre spikes per recording site, at a minimum of 20 separate sites. Because two single-fibre action potentials are recorded relatively infrequently at any one site, FD measured by this method is usually about 1.4–1.5 (Gath & Stålberg 1982). There is some increase in FD with age, and a marked increase in the neurogenic disorders. In many myopathies muscle fibre degeneration, regeneration and reinnervation increase FD (Stålberg & Trontelj 1979, Hilton-Brown & Stålberg 1983). The SFEMG electrode can also be used to deduce the presence of conduction block in motor axons. Thus SFEMG provides important insights into what has been termed the 'microphysiology' of the motor unit.

Muscle fibre propagation velocity. With a multilead SFEMG electrode the propagation velocity in single muscle fibres can be measured, as the action potential of one muscle fibre can be recorded at two sites along the electrode about 200 μm apart (Stålberg 1966). The conduction time between the two recording sites can be accurately assessed and the propagation velocity calculated. The major factor governing fibre velocity appears to be fibre size, the velocity being greater in larger fibres. Values range from 1.5 to 6.5 m/s, averaging about 3.5 m/s. In most muscle fibres the velocity is also related to activity. The velocity falls during continuous activation and recovers after a brief rest. The relationship of velocity to prior activation is called the velocity recovery function (VRF). Two stimuli can be delivered to the fibre at different intervals and changes in response to the second or test stimulus can be observed. The muscle fibre is refractory for intervals of less than 3 ms. With interstimulus intervals of 3–10 ms the velocity in response to the test impulse is 80–100% of that of the conditioning stimulus. When interstimulus intervals from 10 to 500 ms are used, the test response velocity rises above that of the conditioning response, reaching a maximum of 120% with intervals of from 50 to 100 ms. The VRF reflects the process of repolarisation and provides information about the muscle-fibre membrane characteristics, whereas the velocity value gives an indirect measure of fibre diameter.

Lower motor neurone lesions. In denervated muscle, SFEMG shows that spontaneous fibrillations are the action potentials of single muscle fibres. At times, one denervated muscle fibre may trigger another by ephaptic excitation (Stålberg & Trontelj 1979, 1982). Using an intramuscular needle electrode to stimulate a denervated fibre electrically, ephaptic excitation of one or more muscle fibres adjacent to the stimulated fibre can be demonstrated. This explains the occasional more complex fibrillations sometimes recorded in CNEMG. SFEMG recordings have revealed the mechanisms underlying the generation of high-

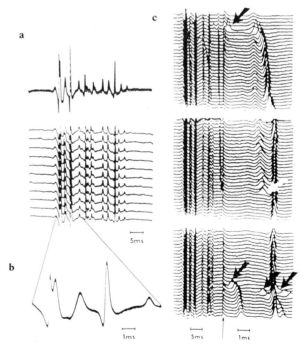

Fig. 30.14 Bizarre high-frequency repetitive discharges recorded by SFEMG. a. Superimposed and rastered display of a complex containing 16 separate spikes. b. Part of the recording presented at fast sweep speed to show abnormally low jitter (< 5 μs MCD) between components. c. Complex showing recruitment of new components (black arrows) and blocking of one component (white arrow). Gaps in sequence correspond to interruptions in the recording

frequency repetitive discharges. The discharges originate in an abnormally excitable 'pacemaker' muscle fibre which drives ephaptically one or several adjacent fibres and is itself re-excited to continue the discharge until the onset of subnormal excitability in the pacemaker causes the cycle to halt abruptly (Stålberg & Trontelj 1982). The presence of ephaptic transmission is recognised by the finding of jitter of less than 5 μs MCD between individual spike components (Fig. 30.14a). This process may also cause the recruitment of a new muscle fibre or fibres during the discharge (Fig. 30.14b). Other fibres or groups of fibres may suddenly drop out, the high discharge rate having resulted in the development of subnormal excitability.

Reinnervation. Increased fibre density (FD) occurs in partial denervation (Stålberg et al 1975, Schwartz et al 1976). The FD reflects the balance

between regenerative and degenerative processes and increases in FD of two to five times normal are seen in chronic neurogenic disorders; smaller increases occur in more rapidly evolving states. Increased jitter and impulse blocking are characteristic of active neurogenic disorders, reflecting abnormal neuromuscular transmission at newly formed functionally immature motor end-plates (Fig. 30.15a). Abnormal jitter and blocking are less striking in patients with slowly progressive diseases.

In chronic spinal muscular atrophy there is usually a marked increase in FD. Many complex potentials are present, often of prolonged duration (Fig. 30.15e–g). The final component of the complex may be 15–50 ms after the first. Extremely late potentials may result from slow conduction in new axonal sprouts, excessively long collaterals, end-plate formation at a distance from the main end-plate zone or to low propagation

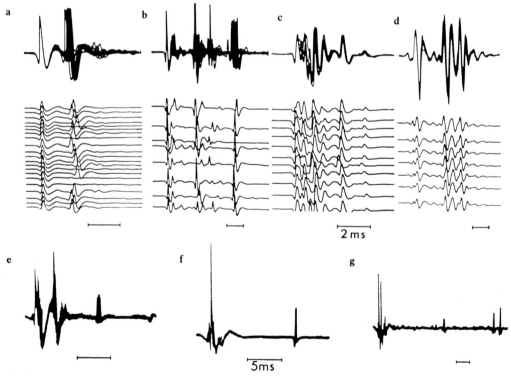

Fig. 30.15 SFEMG recordings in spinal muscular atrophy (SMA). a–d. 14-year-old girl with advanced disease: a and b respectively show relatively simple and more complex potentials with increased jitter and blocking in all but the triggering spikes, indicating recent reinnervation of these muscle fibres. c. Increased jitter in early components but no blocking, suggesting a more mature phase of reinnervation. d. All the components are stable, indicating completed reinnervation. e–g. 24-year-old man with chronic SMA. Complex potentials showing prolonged durations of between 14 and 44 ms

velocity in a reinnervated, atrophic muscle fibre. Marked increase in jitter and blocking are commonly seen in these complexes. The degree of jitter may vary in different complexes within the same muscle, being high with frequent blocking in some (Fig. 30.15a,b), consistent with recent reinnervation, and more moderate with less blocking in others (Fig. 30.15c) suggesting more advanced reinnervation. In yet other complexes (Fig. 30.15d) jitter is normal, indicating that reinnervation has been completed (Stålberg & Fawcett 1984).

In the relatively rapidly progressive condition of motor neurone disease, FD is generally higher in muscles which are weak or showing wasting, but it is also increased in clinically normal muscles (Stålberg 1982). When symptoms present initially in the upper limb, they are associated with higher FD values, but individual values for different upper limb muscles do not differ significantly from one another (Swash 1980). An increase in FD is associated with reduced available muscle force suggesting that the reinnervation process is being outstripped by the rate of denervation.

In more slowly progressive neurogenic disorders, e.g. syringomyelia (Schwartz et al 1980), the action potential complexes show greater stability than those found in motor neurone disease. Depending on the muscle sampled, differing jitter values may be obtained. Higher values, often with blocking, occur in distal muscles of the arm where clinical weakness and wasting is more likely. High jitter and frequent blocking is present in late components, being more marked the greater the delay in the late component.

Various peripheral neuropathies have been studied by SFEMG (Thiele & Stålberg 1975); e.g. in the Guillain–Barré syndrome increased jitter may be found in a minority of patients as early as 14 days into the illness, before regeneration is established. The jitter is attributed to demyelination causing uncertain impulse transmission in the axon. If there is no associated axonal degeneration, there is no increase in FD, as collateral reinnervation will not take place without antecedent denervation. Axonal involvement is quite frequent and is signalled by the appearance of fibrillation. During recovery, FD increases with marked jitter at recently connected end-plates.

In chronic progressive peripheral neuropathies such as hereditary sensorimotor neuropathy type I, both increased FD and jitter have been demonstrated (Thiele & Stålberg 1975). Surprisingly, in view of the clinically mainly distal nature of the condition, increased FD occurs in the biceps brachii associated with increased jitter and impulse blocking. However, greater abnormality is present in the more distal tibialis anterior; here, excess jitter can be seen in 25–50% of recordings and blocking in 5–20%. In other neuropathies such as those related to alcohol and diabetes, similar changes in FD and jitter are found.

During reinnervation when the SFEMG electrode is leading-off three or more spike components from one motor unit, two or more of them may disappear simultaneously (Fig. 30.16). This

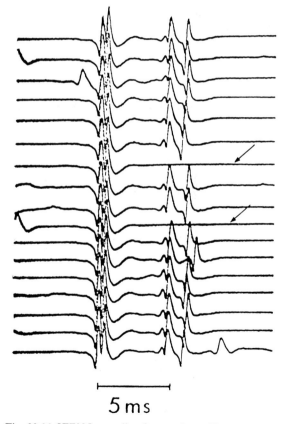

5 ms

Fig. 30.16 SFEMG recording from patient with motor neurone disease showing concomitant (paired) blocking of two components (arrows). Jitter between a pair of blocking spikes is also increased, indicating that the concomitant blocking is occurring in the axon prior to the branching point to these fibres

phenomenon is called concomitant blocking and appears to be due to transmission failure in a terminal nerve branch. Components showing concomitant blocking also share a common jitter value in relation to the other components recorded, called concomitant jitter. At low innervation rates, concomitant jitter is more likely; as the innervation rate increases, concomitant blocking is manifest. The block may be improved by the injection of edrophonium chloride. Concomitant blocking can cause a fall in amplitude of the CMAP in response to repetitive nerve stimulation, simulating a defect in neuromuscular transmission when the actual defect is in the axon. At times, one or more late spike components occur with two latencies related to the remainder of the action-potential complex. This phenomenon, which is called bimodal jitter, appears to relate to two differing transmission times along a single nerve branch, perhaps due to alternations between saltatory and continuous conduction along the fibre, occurring at a particular stage of axonal remyelination (Thiele & Stålberg 1974). The presence of an extra discharge of the motor unit within a brief interval has been noted in various lower motor neurone disorders (Fig. 30.17). These are usually followed by a compensatory pause at the next discharge. The site of the generation of the extra discharge is thought to be at a point of hyperexcitability in the axon, possibly in an immature axonal sprout (Stålberg 1982).

Primary myopathies. SFEMG has contributed substantially to the understanding of disturbances in the function of the motor unit brought about by primary muscle disease. The technique provides information concerning alterations in the anatomical arrangement of muscle fibres within the motor unit territory. Pathophysiological disturbances of neuromuscular transmission and muscle fibre function can be assessed.

The muscular dystrophies. SFEMG abnormalities have been described in all the commoner dystrophies including the Duchenne, Becker, facioscapulohumeral (FSH) and limb-girdle forms (Stålberg 1977, Hilton-Brown & Stålberg 1983a, Fawcett et al 1985a). FD is increased in Duchenne dystrophy from two to two and a half times

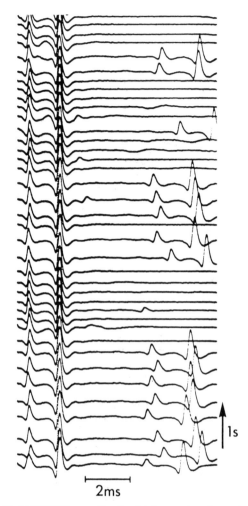

2ms

Fig. 30.17 SFEMG recording in tibialis anterior of a patient with HMSN type I showing extra discharges of a potential pair. The inter-discharge interval is prolonged following an extra discharge, helping to distinguish it from concomitant blocking. The interpotential interval is greater in the extra discharge than in the original discharge, due to the effects of refractoriness

normal (Stålberg 1977). Multiple compound spikes are encountered in many recordings and may contain three to six or more rarely 10–15 separate action potentials derived from fibres in the same motor unit. In more advanced disease FD may decrease but remains above the normal range. The complex duration is prolonged and averages about 10 ms with a range of up to 40–50 ms between the first and last components. Unlike chronic neurogenic disorders, individual spikes tend to be well dispersed throughout the

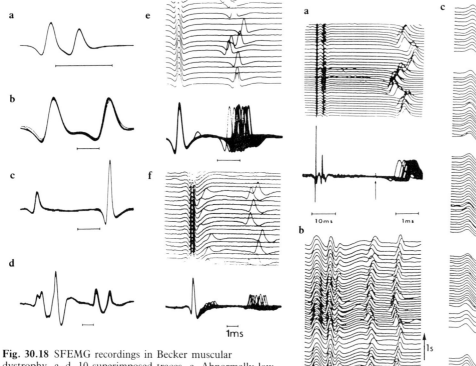

Fig. 30.18 SFEMG recordings in Becker muscular dystrophy. a–d. 10 superimposed traces. a. Abnormally low jitter, probably from a split muscle fibre. b and c. Normal jitter. d. Complex potential with five components and slightly increased duration (6.5 ms). e. Increased jitter (235 μs MCD) and blocking (80%). f. Concomitant jitter and blocking; relative jitter between pair is slightly increased (80 μs MCD), suggesting that the blocking is occurring in the nerve-

Fig. 30.19 SFEMG recordings in Becker muscular dystrophy. a. Potential with a total duration of 22 ms. Influence of irregular discharge rate on IPI causing increased jitter in late component. b. Multispike potential showing parallel changes in latencies to later components related to the discharge rate. c. Recruitment of a third component, initially with high jitter and blocking and eventually normal jitter. Gaps in the sequence correspond to interruptions in the recording

complex, resulting in an increase in the mean interspike interval (MISI) of 1–3 ms (normal 0.6 ms). In Becker, FSH and limb-girdle dystrophies, FD is either normal or shows a mild to moderate increase and the mean duration of complex potentials and MISI are less prolonged (Fig. 30.18, 30.19).

Increased jitter and blocking are commonly seen in Duchenne and Becker dystrophy with 20–40% of potentials showing increased jitter and 5–10% exhibiting blocking (Fig. 30.18e). In some recordings the magnitude of jitter may depend on the interdischarge interval (Fig. 30.19a). This effect tends to be particularly marked in later components and results in slow trends, simultaneously affecting several elements of the multispike potential (Fig. 30.19b). This phenomenon probably relates to the propagation VRF and may be quite pronounced for the later spikes which tend to be

generated by smaller muscle fibres. Rarely, blocking may occur in the presence of normal jitter; more usually, blocking of individual spikes is associated with very high jitter values. Concomitant jitter is seen occasionally and at times concomitant blocking of two or more spikes occurs. This may result from failure of axonal conduction (Fig. 30.18f) or from transmission failure at an end-plate supplying a split muscle fibre. A rare occurrence is the recruitment of an additional fibre into the complex (Fig. 30.19c): this tends to be seen at high discharge rates with disappearance of the spike as the rate decreases. Abnormally low jitter of less than 5 μs MCD, suggestive of split muscle fibres, may be seen in

2–16% of recordings from dystrophic muscle and are particularly common in Duchenne and Becker dystrophy (Hilton-Brown & Stålberg 1983a, Fawcett et al 1985a) (Fig. 30.18a).

Various factors may underlie the increase in FD in the muscular dystrophies (Hilton-Brown et al 1985). Closer packing of atrophic fibres may lead to an increase of their number within the pick-up zone, although this effect will be countered by the fact that small fibres generate smaller action potentials which may not meet the required dimensions for inclusion in FD measurements. Most of the increase is probably accounted for by reinnervation of sequestered segments of fibres undergoing segmental necrosis and innervation of regenerated fibres originating from satellite cells (Hilton-Brown & Stålberg 1983). Reinnervation and the resultant immature end-plates may also explain the presence of increased jitter in a proportion of the recordings. Split muscle fibres and fibres recruited by the process of ephaptic transmission also contribute to the increase in local FD within the motor unit.

Polymyositis. SFEMG findings vary between patients and even within the same patient in this condition, depending upon the stage and severity of the disease at the time of the investigation. In the early phases FD is usually only slightly increased and jitter is abnormal in many of the recordings, probably reflecting attempts at repair by the process of fibre regeneration and reinnervation. Neurogenic concomitant blocking and extra discharges occur, suggesting neural involvement, most probably in newly formed and immature axonal sprouts. In the later stages, more complex potentials may be recorded which tend to have increased durations. With successful treatment and recovery the FD increases and jitter improves, while the spike components of complex potentials become more synchronised and duration and MISI gradually shorten (Henriksson & Stålberg 1978).

Macro EMG

Normal muscle. An example of a Macro EMG recording from vastus lateralis in a normal subject is shown in Fig. 30.20. Normal values for Macro MUP amplitudes and areas have been obtained for the biceps brachii, vastus lateralis and tibialis anterior muscles in healthy subjects of various ages (Stålberg & Fawcett 1982). A strong positive correlation is found between amplitude and area

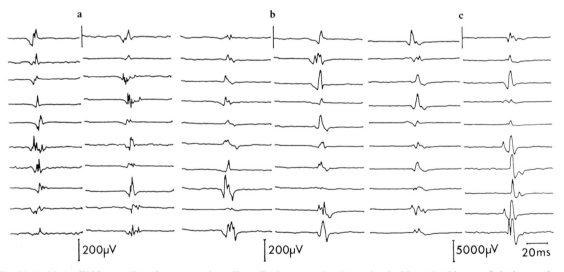

Fig. 30.20 Macro EMG recordings from vastus lateralis. a. Becker muscular dystrophy. b. Normal subject. c. Spinal muscular atrophy (SMA). Note different amplitude calibration for SMA recording. Macro MUPs in dystrophic muscle are slightly smaller and tend to contain more peaks than normal. In SMA, Macro MUPs are frequently very large with amplitudes in this case of between four and 50 times the normal median value for the decade. Median Macro MUP amplitude values: Becker 105 μV, normal 117 μV, SMA 2345 μV

measurements: for this reason, amplitude values are used because they can be determined manually if computer facilities are not available. In each individual a fairly wide scatter of values may be obtained, frequently with a positively skewed distribution: consequently, the median value is calculated in preference to the mean. The most important factor accounting for the wide range of amplitude values is that motor unit size is related to its recruitment threshold (size principle). This relationship is found in Macro EMG recordings (P. R. W. Fawcett, E. Stålberg & P. Hilton-Brown, unpublished results). Values in women appear to be slightly smaller than those for men. Macro MUP configuration is different in the three muscles, those in the biceps having a relatively simple shape with single or double peaks; in tibialis anterior two or more peaks are quite frequent. Most variation occurs in vastus lateralis where complex potentials are common. Despite this, no significant difference is seen in the interval between the furthest peaks within each action potential. Mean interpeak interval is the same, being of the order of 3 ms. The median amplitude of the Macro MUPs varies from muscle to muscle and tends to increase with age over 60 years, particularly in vastus lateralis and tibialis anterior, probably reflecting age-related denervation and compensatory reinnervation.

Lower motor neurone lesions. In slowly progressive or longstanding partial denervation such as chronic spinal muscular atrophy, the Macro MUP is typically increased in amplitude (Stålberg & Fawcett 1984, Fawcett et al 1986) (Fig. 30.20). In more rapidly progressive denervating processes, the Macro potential may remain of normal size despite SFEMG evidence of increased FD, indicating local collateral reinnervation. In adult motor neurone disease, increased amplitudes are found and there is an inverse correlation of amplitude with the degree of muscle weakness. Amplitudes of 10 times normal have been recorded from some motor units (Stålberg 1982).

Primary myopathies. In muscular dystrophy the Macro MUP is usually either normal or slightly reduced in amplitude (Hilton-Brown &

Stålberg 1983b) (Fig. 30.20). Only occasionally is an increase in amplitude detected. The largest Macro MUPs are recorded in young patients with facioscapulohumeral dystrophy and may reflect compensatory hypertrophy. The relative preservation of the Macro MUP in dystrophy relates to the interaction of a variety of different pathophysiological processes as well as to inherent properties of the electrode. Loss of some muscle fibres and atrophy of others due to the dystrophy would be expected to reduce Macro MUP amplitude. The presence of fibres of widely differing diameters and different propagation velocities leading to desynchronisation of the motor unit would have a similar effect. Shrinkage of the muscle with closer packing of muscle fibres may increase the amplitude of the Macro MUP. The formation of new muscle fibres, fibre splitting and ephaptic transmission between muscle fibres will also increase Macro amplitude. Because there is a major contribution of relatively low-frequency components to the Macro MUP, the electrode is relatively insensitive to alterations in volume conduction related to increased fibrosis or fatty infiltration.

Correlation between EMG and histology

Muscle and nerve biopsy may be employed in the investigation of neuromuscular disease and a number of reports have appeared in which the findings of muscle biopsy and EMG have been compared (Buchthal & Olsen 1970, Hausmanowa-Petrusewicz & Jedrzejowska 1971, Black et al 1974, Schwartz et al 1977, Schimrigk 1978, Buchthal & Kamieniecka 1982, Shields 1984). Hausmanowa-Petrusewicz & Jedrzejowska (1971) discuss the different roles of the EMG and biopsy; with the former it is possible to sample many muscles whereas biopsy is usually from a single site. A retrospective comparison of muscle biopsy, CNEMG and clinical data in 105 patients (Black et al 1974) showed, in the 63 in whom both EMG and biopsy were needed to attempt a diagnosis, that the overall agreement was greater than 90% with spinal muscular atrophy causing most difficulty. In a study of quantitative EMG and biopsy — with histology, histochemistry or both — EMG agreed with clinical diagnosis in 87% of patients with myopathy and 91% with neurogenic pathology (Buchthal & Kamieniecka 1982). Muscle biopsy gave similar results but was more specific in identifying particular pathologies. When SFEMG is carried out with open muscle biopsy, correlations between FDs and histochemical evidence of fibre grouping is possible (Schwartz et al 1977). CNEMG has been used in a rather similar fashion (Petajan & Thurman 1981) with the use of an emulsion to localise the site of recording. Abnormal MUP duration, amplitude and recruitment intervals were seen to correlate with neurogenic atrophy in the biopsy.

Comparisons between SFEMG fibre density and quantitative estimates of histological fibre-type grouping (Enclosed Fibre Count, EFC) in patients with various neuromuscular disorders showed a close correlation between FD and EFC in those with reinnervation (Fawcett et al 1985b). FD was found to be more sensitive to minor disturbances of motor unit architecture in myopathies and mild neurogenic states.

EMG findings in various myopathies

It is not suggested that these abnormalities necessarily allow differentiation between different disease entities.

Findings in Duchenne dystrophy depend on the stage of the disease at which the examination is made. Insertion activity may be increased early in the disease, together with fibrillation and positive sharp waves (Buchthal & Rosenfalck 1966). In clinically weak muscle, short-duration, low-voltage, excessively polyphasic MUPs are seen (Kugelberg 1949, Pinelli & Buchthal 1953, Buchthal & Rosenfalck 1963). Complex long-duration polyphasic potentials with variable or stable late components can be seen.

The use of a trigger and delay-line in CNEMG and information gained from SFEMG and other techniques allows a better understanding of the changes occurring in dystrophic muscle. Originally it was felt that the short-duration potentials indicated a marked loss of fibres from the motor unit. The increased FD and relatively normal Macro MUP amplitudes are at odds with this view, but scanning EMG has shown the probable explanation to be a redistribution of muscle fibres

within the unit territory giving rise to local concentrations of fibres separated by silent areas (Hilton-Brown & Stålberg 1983). The occasional high-amplitude MUP may be due to a hypertrophied fibre close to the electrode, to restriction of volume conduction due to local fibrosis or, most often, to a locally increased FD. Increased recruitment at low tension is often a striking feature (Buchthal & Rosenfalck 1963). Macro MUP amplitudes are normal or reduced in contrast to the increased sizes seen in chronic neurogenic diseases. As the disease progresses, fatty replacement and fibrosis result in a reduction in insertional activity and spontaneous potentials become harder to find. Eventually, in severely affected muscle, the fall-out of fibres is such that there are many silent areas in the territory seen in the scanning EMG and the spatial dispersion of the unit is reduced. At this stage an isolated small-amplitude potential may be the only activity seen at any one CNEMG recording site.

The suggestion in 1963 by Barwick and by Van den Bosch that some female carriers of the gene responsible for Duchenne muscular dystrophy showed minor CNEMG abnormalities, aroused considerable interest in detecting evidence of a mild myopathy in these subjects. The need to quantify small deviations from normal provided an impetus to refining existing methods and to the development of new methods of EMG analysis (Willison 1968). There is a shortening of muscle refractory period in a proportion of carriers (Caruso & Buchthal 1965) and there are changes in the individual MUP parameters which allow identification of 50–70% of definite carriers (Davey & Woolf 1965, Emery et al 1966, Smith et al 1966, Willison 1967, Gardner-Medwin 1968, Hausmanowa-Petrusewicz et al 1968, Moosa et al 1972). However, CNEMG has always played a subservient role to biochemical studies in carrier detection and recent developments in recombinant DNA technology should soon consign these observations to history.

In the Becker-type muscular dystrophy (Bradley et al 1978) spontaneous fibrillation and positive waves are commonly recorded. Volitional activity consists of both low-amplitude, short-duration and high-amplitude, longer-duration units. Interference pattern density and amplitude are often reduced and occasional high-frequency and myotonic discharges occur. Symmetrical involvement of proximal muscles is the rule and the paraspinal muscles often show complex repetitive discharges (Kimura 1983). SFEMG and Macro EMG studies (Fawcett et al 1985a) show a mild to moderate FD increase and abnormal jitter affecting around 10% of potential pairs. Blocking is seen in up to 5% and low jitter suggesting fibre splitting in about 6–13% of pairs. Concomitant jitter and blocking are infrequent. Both abnormally large and small Macro MUPs occur but most of the amplitudes are normal. There is little evidence of a neurogenic component other than that related to muscle-fibre regeneration and reinnervation. Carrier detection in Becker dystrophy is less satisfactory than in Duchenne and only a minority of carriers have CNEMG abnormalities (Gardner-Medwin 1968).

The term 'limb-girdle syndrome' has been used to describe a heterogeneous group of disorders having in common proximal muscle weakness and a sporadic or autosomal recessive pattern of occurrence. As well as a hereditary primary myopathy (dystrophy), diseases such as polymyositis, metabolic myopathies, some congenital myopathies and spinal muscular atrophy may present in this way. CNEMG may help to distinguish neurogenic causes for the syndrome. Inflammatory myopathy tends to produce more florid EMG abnormalities than those seen in limb-girdle dystrophy, which resemble those found in Duchenne dystrophy but are generally milder. SFEMG shows increased FD and jitter (Hilton-Brown & Stålberg 1983). Scanning EMG shows silent areas in the motor unit territories but the corridors examined are of normal extent.

Facioscapulohumeral dystrophy may similarly be mimicked clinically by spinal muscular atrophy, inflammatory and metabolic myopathies. CNEMG may aid in identifying neurogenic disorders but at present has a lesser role in distinguishing between the various myopathies. Facioscapulohumeral dystrophy shows CNEMG, SFEMG and scanning EMG abnormalities very similar to those of limb-girdle dystrophy (Hilton-Brown & Stålberg 1983).

Oculopharyngeal dystrophy may resemble myasthenia clinically, with ptosis and dysphagia

developing in late life, but the CMAP, although sometimes of low amplitude, shows no significant alteration on repetitive stimulation. CNEMG shows brief, often polyphasic, low-amplitude MUPs and no spontaneous activity in proximal upper-limb muscles (Murphy & Drachman 1968, Bosch et al 1979).

Hereditary distal myopathy (Welander 1951) is a dominantly inherited or occasionally sporadic disorder, affecting mainly or exclusively distal limb muscles. CNEMG shows almost total loss of MUPs in the most severely affected muscles with abundant positive waves, fibrillation and scanty fasciculation. These findings suggest a neuropathy, but distal motor and sensory nerve conduction is normal. Profuse recruitment of small complex brief potentials in less affected muscles points to a myopathy, confirmed pathologically (Miller et al 1979). In the more severe sporadic form, similar, less florid CNEMG abnormalities also occur in proximal muscles (Markesbury et al 1974a).

Myotonic dystrophy is a dominantly inherited disorder which may be detected shortly after birth as congenital myotonic dystrophy or may present in later life. Infants present with neonatal hypotonia without clinical myotonia which is absent until later childhood (Zellweger & Ionasescu 1973, Harper 1975, Swift et al 1975, Lazaro et al 1979). EMG myotonia is less distinct and easy to detect in the presence of prominent end-plate activity due to the multiple end-plates on single muscle fibres and the larger percentage of total muscle occupied by the end-plate zone in neonates. Infantile myotonic discharge is of lower voltage, briefer duration and shows less frequency variation than that seen in adults. Nerve conduction is in the normal range for the age of the infant. Only occasionally are low-voltage polyphasic MUPs found in infants and children; usually, MUP parameters are normal (Zellweger & Ionasescu 1973). In childhood the electrophysiological expression of the disease is variable so that the absence of myotonic discharge in a child at risk does not exclude the diagnosis (Dodge et al 1965).

Myotonic discharges occur in all affected adults and also appear in roughly one-half of the relatives at risk, who have sub-clinical or mild disease (Bundey et al 1970, Polgar et al 1972), although an incomplete syndrome in which some individuals do not show myotonia has been reported in Labrador (Pryse-Phillips et al 1982). In adults, MUP abnormalities are found in distal muscles, polyphasic potentials being produced by regeneration and reinnervation. MUP amplitude may show progressive reduction when an isolated unit is followed with the delay-line as sarcolemmal membrane changes cause progressive inactivation of individual muscle fibres of the unit. Recovery of MUP amplitude takes place with rest, although very gradual recovery may accompany continuing exertion. The effect of repetitive stimulation is discussed in Part 2. Abnormal nerve conduction has been reported in older patients, the changes being variable in severity (Messina et al 1976, Panayiotopoulos & Scarpalezos 1976, McComas et al 1978, Roohi et al 1981). Suggested causes for the neuropathy have included premature age-dependent neuropathy, the presence of associated disturbances such as alveolar hypoventilation and diabetes, as well as the idea that the neuropathy is an integral part of the disease.

In myotonia congenita and paramyotonia, no abnormalities in individual MUPs are seen and nerve conduction is normal. Myotonia is widespread, both clinically and electrophysiologically. Other spontaneous activity, such as fibrillation and positive discharges, is also evident. In paramyotonia, exposure to cold has dramatic effects: it may produce increasing muscular stiffness and, in some families, this is paradoxical, being aggravated by muscular activity. The slow relaxation is not myotonic, there being no EMG after-discharge. Cooling to 30–25°C results in the disappearance of clinical and electrical myotonia and the falling temperature is associated with transient intense fibrillation. Flaccid muscle paralysis follows this phase, outlasting rewarming by several hours (Haas et al 1981). In vitro studies have shown a progressive depolarisation of paramyotonic muscle fibres from -80 to -40 mV: this is the probable explanation of the transient fibrillation, muscle weakness and paralysis, as depolarisation first passes the electrical threshold and procedes into inexcitability (Lehmann-Horn et al 1981). Cooling increases sodium conductance, possibly by a failure of proper closure of Na^+ channels after they open in the cold. Muscular activity accelerates the process by allowing Na^+ channel opening (Lehmann-Horn et al 1981). The lignocaine derivative, tocainide, a Na^+ channel blocker, may prevent paramyotonic symptoms (Ricker et al 1980). The reason for the development of the muscle stiffness remains obscure. In myotonia congenita, exposure to cold has no such effect: the severity of the myotonia is increased (Ricker et al 1977, Nielson et al 1982), but no paralysis or non-myotonic muscle stiffness occurs. Thomsen's disease is an autosomal dominant disorder but Becker (1977) has described a recessive form which he called recessive generalised myotonia. In this condition EMG may be helpful in genetic counselling, as myotonic discharges may be present without clinical myotonia in heterozygotes (Harel et al 1979, Zellweger et al 1980). Decremental CMAP changes with repetitive stimulation and progressive reduction of individual MUP amplitudes with exercise are a feature of the recessive (Becker) variety of myotonia congenita (Aminoff et al 1977) (see Fig. 30.22). SFEMG shows that the MUP is reflecting similar changes in single-fibre action potentials as the defective repolarisation capacity of the sarcolemmal membrane causes an extra negativity during the decaying phase of the potential (Stålberg 1977) (Fig. 30.21b). During high-frequency discharges there are continuous changes in the shape of the action potentials, often with an initial increase in amplitude followed by a fall and prolongation of their rise-time and duration (Stålberg & Trontelj 1979) (Fig. 30.21a,b).

Although myotonic discharges are said to occur in the Schwartz–Jampel syndrome (Aberfeld et al 1956), recent reports suggest that the activity is not truly myotonic (Taylor et al 1972, Fowler et al 1974, Cao et al 1978). Continuous widespread low-voltage activity is present; no tendency to wax and wane is seen. The activity accounts for the persistent muscle contraction observed clinically and both continue during sleep and general and local anaesthesia. D-tubocurarine abolishes the discharge in most instances but persistence after inadvertent denervation in a single case suggests that an abnormality of the muscular component of the neuromuscular junction is responsible. Phenytoin reduces the discharges but procaine amide, quinidine and diazepam are ineffective. There is evidence of hyperirritability of the muscle-fibre membrane but the bursts produced

a

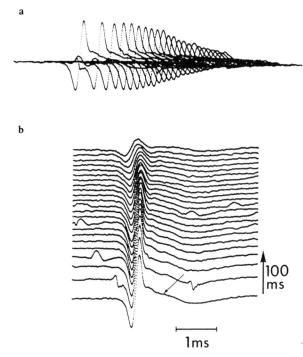

b

100 ms

1ms

Fig. 30.21 a. Myotonic discharge recorded by SFEMG showing progressive decline of the single muscle-fibre action potential. b. Faster display of same discharge. Note the extra negativity during the decaying phase (arrow) which probably corresponds to defective repolarisation of the muscle fibre membrane. The fall in amplitude is accompanied by prolongation of the rise time and total duration of the action potential

by needle movement are of constant frequency and cease abruptly, unlike those of myotonia (Taylor et al 1972). Nerve conduction velocities are normal and volitional MUPs have been described as small and brief or normal.

Congenital fibre-type disproportion is a genetically determined cause of infantile hypotonia, often with associated contractures and skeletal deformities. CNEMG findings are variable, being normal in many patients; others show short-duration, low-amplitude and polyphasic MUPs with no spontaneous activity and in some the striking feature is fibrillation, positive waves and complex high-frequency discharges (Kimura 1983).

Myotubular or centronuclear myopathy is a rare disorder which may present as infantile hypotonia. Striking spontaneous activity occurs: fibrillations, positive waves, high-frequency repetitive activity and even myotonic discharges are present. MUPs

are of low voltage, polyphasic and of brief duration (Munsat et al 1969, Hawkes & Absolon 1975, Radu et al 1977, Gil-Peralta et al 1978, Bill et al 1979). Clinical myotonia is a rare accompaniment (Gil-Peralta et al 1978). These abnormalities are much more florid than those seen in other congenital myopathies.

Central core disease may also cause infantile hypotonia or may be recognised in later life. There may be mild neurogenic features such as reduced CMAP amplitude, slight slowing of nerve conduction and the terminal innervation ratio is increased. No spontaneous activity is present and MUPs are often small, with excessive early recruitment but large polyphasic units also occur. An increased number of MUP late components is seen and SFEMG reveals increased FD (Mrozek et al 1970, Isaacs et al 1975, Coërs et al 1976, Cruz Martinez et al 1979, Lopez-Terradas & Conde Lopez 1979).

Nemaline myopathy is another cause of a relatively non-progressive hypotonia evident early in life, often first suspected because of associated dysmorphism. CNEMG reveals no spontaneous or abnormal insertion activity with short-duration MUPs and increased polyphasia (Shy et al 1963, Kuitonen et al 1972, Radu & Ionasescu 1972).

Acid maltase deficiency may present as a fatal infantile hypotonia and in childhood or in later life as a limb-girdle myopathy. Pathologically there is anterior-horn cell involvement and a vacuolar myopathy. CNEMG shows the most florid changes in paraspinal and gluteal muscles, with increased insertion activity, fibrillation, complex repetitive discharges and true myotonic discharges but no clinical myotonia. MUPs are of low voltage, recruit early and are generally brief, with increased polyphasia. No disturbance of neuromuscular transmission has been found and nerve conduction is normal (Hogan et al 1969, Engel 1970, Engel et al 1973).

Debrancher enzyme deficiency causes hypotonia, failure to thrive, hepatomegaly and hypoglycaemia with a proximal myopathy. CNEMG reveals spontaneous activity which is often profuse, and small brief MUPs (Brunberg et al 1971, DiMauro et al 1979).

Mitochondrial myopathies are an extremely heterogeneous group of disorders and may be familial, varying in mode of inheritance and clinical expression. A progressive external ophthalmoplegia with additional features may be seen and a facioscapulohumeral syndrome has been reported. CNEMG shows shortened MUP duration without spontaneous activity and SFEMG reveals increased FD and increased jitter in complex potentials and normal nerve conduction (Hudgson et al 1972, Olson et al 1972, Mechler et al 1981, Fawcett et al 1982a). The presence of increased jitter in patients with fatiguability and ptosis should not, therefore, be automatically taken to indicate a diagnosis of myasthenia gravis and in equivocal cases a muscle biopsy may be indicated to exclude the possibility of a mitochondrial myopathy.

Lipid storage myopathies include those attributable to carnitine palmityl transferase deficiency and other defects of fatty-acid oxidation. Recurrent myoglobinuria and painful muscle cramps are the clinical features of carnitine palmityl transferase deficiency. Nerve conduction and CNEMG are normal between attacks (Engel et al 1970). Other lipid storage disorders result in progressive weakness of limb-girdle muscles, with or without episodes of muscle pain and myoglobinuria. CNEMG shows spontaneous fibrillation in more than half of those affected. MUPs are brief, small with excessive early recruitment and nerve conductions are usually normal. The occasional presence of a neuropathy has been described (Markesbury et al 1974b).

Polymyositis and dermatomyositis are the commonest forms of inflammatory myopathy. In untreated patients with the acute condition, fibrillation and positive sharp waves are abundant and are most obvious in superficial layers of the paraspinal muscles. Fragility of the muscle fibre membrane as a result of inflammation is suggested as a reason for the very large numbers of positive sharp waves sometimes present (Streib et al 1979). Other spontaneous activity, high-frequency repetitive discharge in particular, together with myotonic discharge may be found. CNEMG examination reveals markedly polyphasic MUPs, initially of short duration. Regeneration and reinnervation result in long polyphasic units with variable late components. The excessive spontaneous activity tends to disappear with treatment but may recur with flare-ups in the disorder (Mechler 1974, Bohan et al 1977). In patients receiving cortico-steroid drugs, increasing clinical weakness without EMG evidence of muscle fibre irritability should raise suspicion of a steroid myopathy (Sandstedt et al 1982). Response to corticosteroid treatment can be monitored by serial quantitative EMG study as increase in amplitude and duration of MUPs accompanies clinical improvement but polyphasia improves much more slowly (Mechler 1974, Sandstedt et al 1982). In acute myositis the EMG changes may be more localised within a single muscle than is the case in dystrophy; focal forms of myositis have also been recorded. SFEMG shows increased jitter and blocking where immature connections have been made with early regenerating muscle fibres and FD is increased. It is still not clear whether the denervation and reinnervation in this disease are simply due to muscle regeneration or whether damage to the terminal innervation by inflammation is a significant factor (Henriksson & Stålberg 1978).

CMAPs may show decrement or, more rarely, an incremental response on repetitive stimulation. Chronic polymyositis results in long-duration often relatively stable MUPs (Mechler 1974). Fibrosis causes the development of silent areas with increased resistance to electrode movement and an apparent reduction in CNEMG recruitment may occur in advanced disease. CNEMG abnormalities are more widespread and uniform in advanced disease. Occasional large-amplitude potentials may be generated by local FD increase. Polymyositis may complicate connective tissue disorders and may be relatively mild with CNEMG changes limited to the paraspinal muscles. In these collagen diseases, peripheral neuropathy or mononeuritis may occur with reduced CMAP amplitude, altered nerve conduction and reduced or absent recruitment together with fibrillation.

Inclusion body myositis is relatively benign and often mainly distal in distribution so that EMG changes similar to those of polymyositis are seen. Parasitic and sarcoid myopathies show more scattered and more localised involvement than is usual in polymyositis. At the sites of involvement CNEMG abnormalities, including evidence of local hyperirritability of muscle, can be seen.

Various disorders of muscular function occur in endocrine disease. In hypothyroidism, muscular manifestations are common (Rao et al 1980).

Myoidema is a localised knot of contracting muscle occurring in response to percussion of the muscle or other direct mechanical stimulation. Brief contractions can be seen in normal subjects but gross and prolonged contractions occur in hypothyroidism (Salick & Pearson 1967). An initial short burst of action potentials accompanies the percussion, and the whole fascicle tightens and remains in a state of electrically silent contraction for 30–60s and then slowly disappears (Denny-Brown & Pennybacker 1938). This form of electrically silent contraction, called a contracture, may be due to a prolongation of the active state due to excessive release or to slow reaccumulation of calcium by the sarcoplasmic reticulum (Mizusawa et al 1983). Enlargement of muscle may gradually develop in patients with myxoedema, and pain and muscular stiffness are commonly present (Wilson & Walton 1959, Norris & Panner 1966). Evidence of muscular irritability with increased insertional activity, fibrillation, positive sharp activity and high-frequency discharges may be recorded (Åström et al 1961) and true clinical and electromyographic myotonia has been observed (Venables et al 1978). Quantitive CNEMG of an unselected group of hypothyroid patients revealed shortened MUP duration in proximal muscles in 70% and excessive polyphasic potentials in 90%, although only 20% of the patients had significant muscular weakness (Rao et al 1980).

Thyrotoxic myopathy (Sanderson & Adey 1952) is a relatively infrequent presentation of thyrotoxicosis; nevertheless, in hyperthyroidism quantitative CNEMG is almost always abnormal and the changes are most marked in patients with clinical weakness (Ramsay 1965, Buchthal 1970, Puvanendran et al 1979). Shortening of the mean MUP duration and an increased proportion of polyphasic MUPs are found. Spontaneous activity is infrequent.

Proximal myopathy is often a prominent feature of Cushing's syndrome and the CNEMG shows shortening of MUP duration without spontaneous activity (Muller & Kugelberg 1959). The iatrogenic disorder associated with the use of synthetic corticosteroids, especially triamcinolone, shows similar CNEMG changes (Williams 1959, Yates 1963, Coomes 1965).

Addison's disease is characterised by generalised muscular weakness which may be associated with shortened mean MUP duration (Buchthal 1970). Nelson's syndrome (increasing cutaneous pigmentation following adrenalectomy for Cushing's syndrome) may be associated with proximal muscle weakness. A pituitary tumour secreting high levels of ACTH is present and, in the patients with weakness, Prineas et al (1968) demonstrated the presence of a lipid storage myopathy with quantitative CNEMG studies showing reduced mean MUP duration, increased percentage of polyphasic MUPs and hyperirritability of the muscle with high-frequency discharges, fibrillations and positive sharp waves.

Patients with acromegaly often complain of muscular weakness and of easy fatiguability: these complaints are due to a myopathy (Mastaglia et al 1970, Lundberg et al 1970). Mastaglia et al (1970) demonstrated a striking reduction in mean MUP duration in proximal muscles in more than one-half of a group of acromegalics including some without overt weakness. Spontaneous activity was not a feature of the CNEMG.

Vicale (1949) drew attention to the mild proximal weakness present in some patients with hyperparathyroidism. Other workers (Bischoff & Esslen 1965, Frame et al 1968) confirmed these observations and showed that there were changes in the CNEMG suggestive of a myopathy without spontaneous activity. Hudson et al (1970) described the familial variety of this disorder. Many diseases in which osteomalacia develops are associated with proximal muscle weakness and myopathic EMG abnormalities (Skaria et al 1975).

Although neuropathy is well recognised in chronic renal failure and in patients receiving regular haemodialysis, there are some in whom gross proximal weakness is due to a myopathy (Lindholm 1968, Floyd et al 1974, Hudgson & Barwick 1974) with shortening of the mean MUP duration and increased numbers of polyphasic potentials without spontaneous activity. Improvement in muscle function followed renal allografts and improvement was also produced by vitamin D therapy in undialysed patients.

Axonal neuropathy is the commonest toxic complication of alcoholism affecting the neuromuscular system but several types of myopathy may be seen. Acute muscular necrosis occurs in some chronic alcoholics during a drinking bout

(Hed et al 1962). CNEMG shows copious spontaneous activity, reduced MUP duration and polyphasia. A syndrome of chronic proximal weakness and atrophy can also be seen in chronic alcoholism when signs of a neuropathy are absent or mild (Ekbom et al 1964, Perkoff et al 1967, Rossouw et al 1976). The CNEMG showed shortened MUP duration without spontaneous activity. Similar changes are seen in chronic alcoholics without overt clinical muscle involvement (Ekbom et al 1964, Faris & Reyes 1971). Another problem is the occasional development of acute hypokalaemic paralysis during an alcoholic debauch (Rubenstein & Wainapel 1977). This paralysis develops progressively over several days and spares the respiratory and bulbar muscles. The EMG abnormalities are florid with numerous spontaneous fibrillations resolving rapidly with potassium replacement.

The clinical features and the nature of the underlying defect in periodic paralysis are discussed elsewhere in this volume (see Ch. 25). The EMG changes seen in hyperkalaemic periodic paralysis are as follows. Between attacks there may be increased insertional activity with myotonic discharges and high-frequency complex repetitive activity. In attacks there is an increase in the myotonic activity and transient copious fibrillations occur in some patients (Morrison 1960) but neither mechanical nor electrical stimuli will excite the muscle. Jitter is usually normal between attacks but shows a significant increase as an attack begins and blocking rapidly develops. The abnormalities are increased by cooling and, when the myotonia is pronounced, repetitive nerve stimulation may result in a decremental response (Lundberg et al 1974). A permanent myopathy sometimes develops. Recent in vitro studies (Lehmann-Horn et al 1983) suggest that the depolarisation of the fibre membrane associated with the paralytic attacks is connected with an increased sodium ion conductance.

In hypokalaemic periodic paralysis there is a reduction in the number of motor units available for voluntary recruitment and a reduced or absent muscle response to motor nerve stimulation (Gordon et al 1970). An incremental response to nerve stimulation at 10–25 Hz may be seen in muscles only mildly affected but does not occur in the weaker muscles (Grob et al 1957, Campa

& Sanders 1974). Permanent progressive myopathy with associated EMG abnormalities occurs in some patients (Pearson 1964). Rüdel et al (1984) suggest, on the basis of in vitro studies, that the basic defect lies in a reduced membrane excitability and an increased sodium conductance and that both these defects are aggravated when the extracellular potassium concentration falls.

Chronic painless proximal myopathy is the commonest form of drug-induced myopathy and a particularly severe form occurs in some patients receiving chloroquine medication. In contrast to most other drug-induced myopathies, spontaneous activity abounds: fibrillations, positive waves, high-frequency repetitive activity and even true myotonic discharges are seen. In addition, the typical volitional changes of a myopathy are seen and the presence of a neuropathy which may also complicate this therapy is revealed by abnormal nerve conduction (Mastaglia et al 1977).

Neuromuscular transmission defects. Normal fatigue during voluntary contraction is accompanied by drop-out of motor unit potentials rather than change in their form. Lindsley (1935) found that the fatigue of myasthenia was accompanied by a marked fluctuation in amplitude of individual MUPs. Mean MUP duration is significantly shortened in myasthenia gravis (Oosterhuis et al 1972) especially in clinically weak muscles. Examination of MUPs isolated by use of a delay-line displays alterations in motor unit dimensions during sustained recruitment, as more and more individual end-plates show conduction block. A high-pass filter (Payan 1978) assists in the demonstration of unstable motor units in the presence of abnormal neuromuscular transmission but CNEMG results are difficult to quantify and SFEMG and/or the response to repetitive nerve stimulation may be preferred. Studies of nerve conduction have shown an increase in terminal latency and prolongation of the CMAP at the end of a train of tetanic stimuli, greater than that which occurs in normal subjects. In some severely affected cases there is significant slowing of the motor conduction velocity during a tetanus (Preswick 1965). The distal latency of the CMAP may sometimes be prolonged in the resting state (Slomic et al 1968).

PART II

TESTING OF NEUROMUSCULAR TRANSMISSION

INTRODUCTION

Primary disorders of neuromuscular transmission, such as myasthenia gravis and the myasthenic (Eaton–Lambert) syndrome, are uncommon. However, recent advances in understanding of their pathophysiology have led to improvements in management and prognosis. Early and accurate diagnosis is important if the patient is to benefit. Many treatments, e.g. long-term immunosuppression using steroids or other drugs, thymectomy and plasmapheresis; carry risks, so that diagnostic techniques must not only be sensitive but also objective and reliable.

The anatomy and physiology of the normal neuromuscular junction have been fully detailed elsewhere (Ch. 1 & 6). Normal and abnormal pharmacology of neuromuscular transmission has also been considered (Ch. 3). Methods available for the study of neuromuscular transmission in man are described here and the results obtained both in the normal and in various disease states are discussed. Neuromuscular transmission defects may be divided into two broad groups according to whether the defect is presynaptic or postsynaptic. In the former, the problem may lie in the synthesis, storage, availability and release from the nerve terminal of acetylcholine (ACh); postsynaptic disorders include abnormalities of ACh receptors, the phase of end-plate potential depolarisation, initiation of the muscle fibre action potential and ACh removal.

METHODS FOR STUDYING NEUROMUSCULAR TRANSMISSION IN MAN

In vitro microelectrode studies on muscle biopsy specimens

Much of our knowledge of the pathophysiology of various defects of neuromuscular transmission derives from intracellular recordings in the region of the motor end-plate. Microelectrodes inserted into resting muscle in this situation reveal intermittent small depolarisations across the post synaptic membrane, so-called minature end-plate potentials (MEPPs). These correspond to the random release of quanta of ACh, each of which is derived from one of the many vesicles situated in the presynaptic portion of the nerve terminal. In normal human muscle, MEPP frequency is of the order of 0.2 Hz (Elmqvist 1973), while MEPP amplitude is about 1 mV, much lower than the threshold for initiation of an action potential. Invasion of the terminal by a nerve impulse results in a marked increase in the number of quanta of ACh released, producing a much larger depolarisation called the end-plate potential (EPP) which reaches threshold and gives rise to an action potential in the adjacent muscle fibre membrane.

The amplitude of the EPP is variable and is influenced by preceding activity. During a high-frequency train of stimuli the first few EPPs show increasing amplitude (facilitation), soon followed by a progressive decline, or depressive phase (Katz 1966). At slower impulse rates, e.g. 1–3 Hz, there is no early increase; instead, a steady reduction of EPP amplitude occurs and eventually reaches a plateau. A few seconds after a tetanic train or period of intense activity, a longer lasting increase in EPP amplitude develops, corresponding to the phase of post-tetanic potentiation which may persist for 1–2 min. Subsequently, during a period of depression (post-tetanic exhaustion), the EPP amplitude gradually falls. The mechanisms underlying these events are not fully understood, but both facilitation and potentiation may relate to accumulation of calcium ions in the presynaptic region, leading to elevated ACh mobilisation by increasing vesicle fusion with the nerve terminal (Katz & Miledi 1968). Desensitisation of the ACh receptors has been suggested as the cause of the phase of exhaustion (Gage 1976), but the presence of normal-size MEPPs would seem to be against this theory.

In normal muscle these fluctuations in EPP size are of no consequence because they remain well above the threshold for the generation of action potentials, reflecting the high safety factor for neuromuscular transmission. However, in pathological states in which the safety factor is lowered, either by reduced availability of ACh (presynaptic) or reduced effect of transmitter (postsynaptic), these normal phenomena become significant, resulting in defective neuromuscular transmission (Elmqvist et al 1964).

Repetitive stimulation techniques

The observation by Harvey & Masland (1941) that repetitive nerve stimulation resulted in a decline in the amplitude of the compound muscle action potential (CMAP) in patients with myasthenia gravis, led to its development as a clinical neurophysiological test of disorders of neuromuscular transmission. Since its introduction, various modifications of the technique have been described, designed to increase its sensitivity when used in patients with localised or subclinical disease.

Supramaximal motor nerve stimulation is carried out as in the determination of motor conduction velocity (see Ch. 29). Conventional surface stimulating electrodes are satisfactory but must be very securely applied, as close as possible to the underlying nerve to ensure stimulation of the whole nerve trunk without using unduly high and unpleasant stimulus intensities. As it is essential that the stimulus remains supramaximal throughout the stimulus train, an intensity of 1.5 times maximal is used. This allows for the occurrence of any slight electrode movement in relation to the nerve, during the course of the muscle contraction. Preparation of the overlying skin with spirit and mild abrasion will improve conductance and will slightly lower the required stimulus intensity. Some authors (Slomic et al 1968) prefer subcutaneous needle electrodes inserted close to the nerve, reducing the stimulus strength needed and the degree of discomfort to the patient. A surface silver disc electrode may be placed over the motor point of the target muscle, where the muscle action potential has a sharp negative onset, together with a reference electrode over the tendon (often referred to as belly-tendon recording). The CMAP so recorded is an indication of the number of muscle fibres contributing to the response by summation relatively synchronously when stimulated. When the stimuli are repeated, changes in the CMAP may indicate a rise or fall in the number of muscle fibres responding.

Before coming to conclusions as to normal or abnormal behaviour of the muscle, it is vital to exclude artefacts. Electrode movement is a common problem with a surface electrode over an activated muscle; movement can also occur during the delivery of a long train of stimuli. Slomic et al (1968) prefer subcutaneous needle electrodes which are less prone to produce artefacts but most workers appear to prefer immobilisation of the stimulated muscle. At faster rates of stimulation of the nerve, an initial progressive increase in the size of the responses is due to shortening of the muscle fibres and improved synchronisation of the individual muscle fibre action potentials. The increase in amplitude is accompanied by a reduction in response duration, but little or no change in the CMAP area, indicating that this is a technical artefact or pseudofacilitation. Meticulous attention to technique is essential and results should be validated by the demonstration of their reproducibility in repeated trials.

Another factor requiring attention is temperature, as a lowering of the temperature at the endplate improves the efficiency of impulse transmission (Borenstein & Desmedt 1974). Attempts should be made to maintain the temperature above 35°C, particularly when studying distal muscles. At higher temperatures the amplitude of the EPPs is reduced despite an increase in MEPP frequency (Hubbard et al 1969). The timing and dosage of medications affecting neuromuscular transmission should be recorded and, if possible, these should be withheld before the testing session.

A variety of muscles are available for study: in myasthenia gravis, muscles showing clinical fatiguability are most likely to give positive results on repetitive stimulation; these are often proximal or facial muscles. In botulism there may be a similar restriction of neurophysiological and clinical abnormalities to certain muscle groups in contrast to the myasthenic syndrome where the changes are usually widespread. Kimura (1983) indicates those muscles commonly studied and suggests appropriate electrode placements.

After suitable amplification, the CMAP is displayed either on a storage oscilloscope, from which permanent photographic records may be obtained, or recorded directly on to light-sensitive paper. The amplitude of the negative phase of each response can then be measured. In some laboratories, the signals are fed directly into a computer which stores and displays the data in digital form and calculates the amplitude and area of the negative portion of the response.

A number of different stimulation paradigms may be used to test neuromuscular transmission; these are briefly considered in turn, below.

Paired stimuli may be delivered with short interstimulus intervals of 2.5 ms, 15 ms and 25 ms. When using the shortest of these intervals in a normal subject, the second response is reduced as it arrives during the relative refractory period for nerve and muscle. Similar responses are likely to be found in patients suffering from myasthenia gravis. In the .myasthenic syndrome, however, the first response will be of subnormal amplitude while the second response may be up to double the first. The defective ACh release in this condition results in small sub-threshold EPPs which fail to produce an action potential in most muscle fibres with the first shock. The arrival of the second stimulus allows the EPPs to summate, exciting muscle fibres not responsive to the initial shock. A similar response often occurs in botulism and may very occasionally be seen in myasthenia gravis (Cherington 1973).

Paired stimuli with longer interstimulus intervals such as 15–100 ms will result in no change in the second potential in normal individuals, in myasthenia and botulism. In the myasthenic syndrome true facilitation is to be expected when stimulating in this range. The decremental response to paired stimuli in myasthenia is best seen when interstimulus intervals of 100–700 ms are applied.

Repetitive stimulation at slow rates. Stimuli delivered at slow rates are generally well tolerated by patients and technically satisfactory records are more easily obtained than with faster or tetanic rates. Stimulation at rates of 2–3 Hz should produce an identical series of responses in normal subjects. It is usual to compare the amplitude of the smallest of the first five responses with the first of a train. The largest percentage decrement usually occurs in the second response but, as the process continues, the largest absolute change in amplitude is evident when the fourth or fifth response is compared with the first. When a reproducible percentage decrement between the first and fifth response of 10% or more can be obtained, the result is considered to be abnormal (Slomic et al 1968) (see Fig. 30.22). If the abnormality can be reversed or reduced by drugs such as edrophonium or neostigmine, which block the action of acetylcholinesterase, then the diagnosis of myasthenia is probable. A number of other diseases may produce abnormalities of neuromuscular transmission which give rise to decremental responses at slow stimulus rates. Motor neurone disease, botulism, multiple sclerosis, the myasthenic syndrome and reinnervating nerve have all been reported as showing decremental responses (Mulder et al 1959, Gilliatt 1966, Eisen et al 1978). Both botulism and the myasthenic syndrome are usually associated with small-amplitude responses to initial stimuli and a further fall in amplitude is usual.

Repetitive stimulation at faster rates. Here the effects of stimulation at rates of 20–30 Hz are considered. At these rates of stimulation the safety factor for neuromuscular transmission in the normal individual is sufficiently large for the amplitude of the response to be maintained throughout the train. In the myasthenic syndrome the initial response is of low amplitude but there is a striking increase in the size of the response to the succeeding train: the amount of the increment at the end of the train is several times that of the first response, reflecting excitation of all or nearly all the muscle fibres in the muscle (Lambert et al 1961). In myasthenia gravis, particularly during steroid therapy or during spontaneous deterioration, a less striking incremental response may be detected and a similar slight increment may occur in botulism, both being more likely when the amplitude of the first response is normal (Mayer & Williams 1974, Pickett et al 1976). Prolonged stimulation is uncomfortable for the patient and is associated with increasing problems of artefact due to muscle contraction and electrode movement, particularly when proximal muscles are studied.

When the force of muscle contraction (twitch tension) is also measured in normal muscle subjected to a prolonged train of low frequency (1–2 Hz stimuli) there is a slow progressive increase in the force of muscle twitch over the first minutes (positive staircase phenomenon); a less marked fall in twitch tension (negative staircase

phenomenon) precedes the development of the positive staircase in about 50% of cases (Slomic et al 1968). This mechanical response is not accompanied by alteration in the size of the evoked action potential and its cause is uncertain but it appears to be independent of the number of active muscle fibres.

When patients with myasthenia are subjected to an isolated supramaximal stimulus to the motor nerve the twitch tension is often normal, although in those with moderate to severe disease there may be some reduction (Lambert et al 1961, Slomic et al 1968). When subjected to a slow train of stimuli, however, the positive staircase response is said to be absent or reduced in myasthenics (Slomic et al 1968). However, Grob & Namba (1976) found that the staircase phenomenon was present and usually normal in the myasthenic patients whom they studied. The position of the staircase phenomenon in myasthenia awaits further appraisal.

Tetanic stimulation. Shocks delivered at 50 Hz for 30 s will produce brief tetanic contractions of the muscle. Such stimulation is generally perceived as being most uncomfortable and few patients tolerate it for more than short periods. Because of this, many laboratories no longer employ this rate and utilise the effect of exercise. However, the main features of interest are not the responses during the train but the changes in function over a period of up to 15 min after the tetany.

Post-tetanic potentiation is seen during the first 2 min. The response to an initial isolated supramaximal shock is compared with a similar response obtained shortly after a tetanic train has been delivered; post-tetanic potentiation occurs when the second response is clearly greater than the first. As all of the fibres in a normal muscle are excited by supramaximal stimulation there is no change in the response size (i.e. there is no post-tetanic potentiation). Where there is a defect in ACh availability, the initial response would be smaller than normal and the tetany will increase the mobilisation of ACh; thus the amplitude of the post-tetanic response will exceed that of the first response. This is the case in the myasthenic

ADM

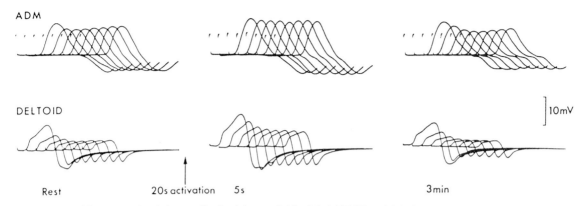

DELTOID

]10mV

Rest   20s activation   5s   3min

Fig. 30.22 Repetitive nerve stimulation studies in abductor digiti minimi (ADM) and deltoid in a patient with generalised myasthenia gravis. 3 Hz trains of stimuli at rest, 5 s and 3 min after 20 s maximal contraction. In both muscles a significant decrement (5th compared with 1st) occurred at rest (24% ADM, 53% deltoid). The decrement was abolished immediately after activation in ADM and was reduced in deltoid (33%) (post-activation potentiation); it was the same in ADM but more marked in deltoid 3 min later (59%) (post-activation exhaustion)

syndrome where the second response may show an increment of up to 200%.

In myasthenia gravis a smaller degree of potentiation may occur or the level of decrement may be less during the first 2 min, due to the opposite effects of ACh depletion and post-tetanic potentiation. Instead of receiving an uncomfortable tetanic train, the patient can be asked to make a strong voluntary contraction over a time period of 20–30 s and this is the preferred routine in the authors' laboratory (Fig. 30.22). Activation of motor units at rates of up to 50 Hz can be achieved by most patients. Post-tetanic exhaustion appears after potentiation, usually 2–4 min after the tetany or exercise.

After the stimulation it is usual to deliver single test shocks at 10 s and at 1 min or 2 min intervals over the succeeding 15 min. There is a large safety margin in normal muscle so that although there has been a marked reduction in the available store of ACh, the response to supramaximal shocks is maintained. The immature end-plates of the premature or newborn infant do not possess the same safety margin and post-tetanic exhaustion can be detected. Typically, patients with myasthenia gravis show progressively more impairment of neuromuscular transmission during the period: this is thought to be due to failure of mobilisation of ACh to cope with the demand during the tetanus/exercise leading to post-tetanic exhaustion.

In the myasthenic syndrome post-tetanic exhaustion produces responses of even lower amplitude than the first abnormally reduced action potential.

Additional stimulation techniques

Double step ischaemia. As patients with mild generalised myasthenia or ocular myasthenia may not show any definite abnormality when tested by the methods noted above, modifications of the test conditions have been introduced to increase diagnostic sensitivity. It has long been known that under ischaemic conditions there is a rapid increase in the amount of decrement to repetitive stimulation in patients with myasthenia gravis and that prolonged ischaemia causes failure of neuromuscular transmission in normal subjects (Harvey & Masland 1941).

A double-step ischaemic test has been described by Desmedt & Borenstein (1977a). The initial phase consists of recording the CMAP from the hypothenar muscles during a 4 min period of continuous supramaximal stimulation of the ulnar nerve at a rate of 3 Hz. Thereafter, further brief trains of 3 Hz stimuli are delivered at 30 s intervals and the presence or absence of decremental responses within each train is determined. If this first phase does not produce definite evidence of a defect, then the second, ischaemic step is introduced. An occlusive cuff inflated to above arterial pressure is secured about the arm proximal to the site of nerve stimulation in order to induce ischaemia. The stimulation paradigm is then repeated.

In some normal subjects a progressive reduction of the CMAP amplitude may occur after 2–3 min of stimulation. Whereas in others the action potential amplitude remains unchanged (Desmedt & Borenstein 1977a). However, the subsequent short test periods of stimulation at 3 Hz produce no progressive decrement even in those individuals who had shown a diminution of the amplitude during the continuous conditioning period of ischaemic stimulation. Desmedt & Borenstein (1977a) suggest that the reduction in amplitude which occurs in some normal subjects is due to the production of a temporary conduction block in some of the nerve fibres by the ischaemia. If ischaemia is much more prolonged, to 7–15 min, a decremental response to the 3 Hz test stimuli is seen in normal individuals.

In patients with myasthenia gravis, evidence of a failure of neuromuscular transmission may be seen in the first step — that of 'exercise' induced by continuous 3 Hz stimulation. Where mild or mainly ocular disease is present, this first phase may not reveal any abnormality. When stressed by both prolonged stimulation and ischaemia, many patients will show decremental responses during the initial ischaemic exercise period and more will show defects in transmission during the subsequent test periods.

Regional curare sensitivity. The use of neuro-muscular blocking agents together with repetitive stimulation provides a further means of revealing mild disturbances of transmission by reducing the safety-factor. The neuromuscular blocking drug D-tubocurarine is used for the procedure. In patients with ocular myasthenia the systemic injection of one-tenth of the normal curarising dose will often result in the development of weakness in previously clinically unaffected limb muscles (Rowland et al 1961). Such systemic injections are hazardous as they may induce respiratory failure and protracted generalised paralysis in myasthenic individuals. In order to overcome this danger, the small dose of curare may be injected into a forearm vein subsequent to the total occlusion of

the circulation by inflating an occlusive cuff proximal to the injection site (Horowitz et al 1975, Horowitz & Sivak 1978). Alterations in CMAP amplitude produced by a stimulation programme are then assessed (Brown & Charlton 1975, Brown et al 1975). The concentration of curare at the neuromuscular junction varies from patient to patient because of differing diffusion through the volume of tissue in the occluded region: in consequence, there may be difficulties in separating normal from pathological responses (Hertel et al 1977). Extra sensitivity to curare is not solely a feature of myasthenia: it is also seen in muscular weakness caused by certain antibiotics (Pittinger & Adamson 1972) and in motor neurone disease (Mulder et al 1959). There is also some risk of curare reaching the systemic circulation and affecting the respiratory muscles, after release of the tourniquet (Hertel et al 1977). For these reasons many investigators see no place for this test in most myasthenic patients as the diagnosis can be reached using the safer methods available (Özdemir & Young 1976).

Ocular electromyography

The technique of ocular electromyography has already been mentioned. Because of the very frequent involvement of the extraocular muscles in myasthenia gravis, ocular EMG can be useful; presumably the subjective unpleasantness of the technique, the logistics of close collaboration between ophthalmologist and neurophysiologist and the difficulty in acquiring control data from normal subjects have prevented its wider application. The presence of motor unit fatigue and recovery occurring with rest can be readily demonstrated with the recording electrode in the frequently affected levator palpebrae. An edro-phonium hydrochloride (Tensilon®) test is simple to assess in a muscle showing underactivity. During a sustained attempt to raise the eyelid with the needle in situ, an intravenous injection of 2 mg of edrophonium is administered: a marked increase in motor unit recruitment and elevation of the eyelid may develop within seconds. Equi-vocal or apparently negative clinical responses to the standard Tensilon® test in ocular myasthenia are not uncommon but the presence of a definite increase in the amount of recruiting motor units is almost always demonstrable with ocular EMG (Breinin 1962), although it may be necessary to administer up to 20 mg of the drug. A positive response to edrophonium is not seen in normal extraocular muscle or in other causes of ocular palsies.

Permanent myopathic change may develop in myasthenia gravis and, when it develops in the extraocular muscles, it may be demonstrated by ocular EMG (Breinin 1957, 1962).

Single-fibre electromyography (SFEMG)

Methods

The identification of disordered neuromuscular transmission depends upon demonstrating a failure of transmission during muscular activity. That failure appears in SFEMG as impulse blocking but abnormally high jitter values can indicate the presence of a disturbance before blocking develops. Thus, positive findings may be present in muscles which appear to be clinically unaffected (Ekstedt & Stålberg 1965, Stålberg & Ekstedt 1973, Stålberg et al 1974, Stålberg 1980b). Two different techniques are available — electrical stimulation and voluntary activation.

Electrical stimulation. A single-fibre action potential evoked by repetitive supramaximal stimulation of its motor nerve shows, in successive appearances, small latency variations of the order of tens of microseconds. This phenomenon is due to variations in transmission times between the stimulus and recording sites. Normally, neither the nerve action potential nor muscle fibre contribute to the variation by more than 3 μs, the major source being the neuromuscular junction (Stålberg & Trontelj 1979). The term 'jitter' has been coined for this phenomenon and is derived from technical electronic terminology, used to indicate the presence of instability in an oscilloscope display, as a result of varying trigger level or instability in the time-base generator. Two principal causes for jitter at the end-plate have been suggested: first, the steepness of the rising slope of the EPP may change, because of small alterations in amplitude with successive EPPs, causing variations in the time that a muscle fibre

action potential can be triggered; second, there may be temporal variations in the muscle-fibre firing threshold, leading to differing neuromuscular transmission times in the presence of constant-amplitude EPPs.

Stimulation of the nerve trunk can be performed and is useful in unconscious or very young patients. A number of methodological factors are important when testing neuromuscular function in this way. Supramaximal stimulus strength for the axon to the single fibre should be employed. This is ensured by the absence of further reduction in jitter with increments of stimulus intensity. The stimuli must not result in activation, in adjacent motor units, of single-fibre potentials with similar latency to the target single-fibre potential, as false values for jitter would result from the 'rogue' fibre. At high rates of stimulation, nerve threshold may increase and a constant stimulus strength employed becomes subliminal, resulting in progressive increase in jitter and blocking. This phenomenon may be recognised and corrected by increasing the stimulus intensity which returns jitter to its former value and abolishes blocking (Stålberg & Trontelj 1979).

Intramuscular nerve stimulation may be employed and gives similar results. Care is necessary to avoid direct muscle fibre stimulation, which may be suspected in the presence of abnormally low jitter values of under 5 μs.

Voluntary activation. During gentle voluntary activation of a muscle (often the extensor digitorum communis (EDC)) the SFEMG electrode is sited so that it records the action potentials of a pair of fibres belonging to the same motor unit. One of the action potentials triggers the oscilloscope sweep and is used as a reference; the other potential appears with a variable interval in relation to the triggering potential. In this situation the jitter represents the variability of neuromuscular transmission at both motor end-plates and may be expressed mathematically as

$$jitter = \sqrt{jitter\ 1^2 + jitter\ 2^2}.$$

For the assessment of jitter in an individual muscle at least 20 pairs are recorded and the jitter value in each pair is measured. In normal subjects, one of the potential pairs may show increased jitter or impulse blocking, but the remainder should have jitter values within the normal range of 5–55 μs; individual muscles have smaller ranges (Stålberg & Trontelj 1979). Considerable variation exists in the jitter found at normal end-plates, both within single motor units and in muscles as a whole. The recording site does not influence the magnitude of jitter, which is the same when recording near the insertion or end-plate region. Jitter in normal muscle is increased by a fall in intramuscular temperature below 35°C but increase in temperature up to 38°C has no effect. Individuals over 70 years of age show age-related increases in jitter in EDC but there is evidence of earlier increases in other muscles, usually accompanied by an increase in FD and thought to have a neurogenic origin (Stålberg & Trontelj 1979). Continuous recording over several hours from a normal potential pair, utilising firing rates of 10–15 Hz, shows stable jitter. Fatigue prevents protracted recording at higher rates, such as over 30 Hz, but no change occurs with up to 10 min activation at these rates.

Jitter in a number of potential pairs within a single motor unit has been studied using a two-needle technique. The first needle is positioned in proximity to a single-fibre potential which acts as the trigger throughout the study. The second electrode is moved to a series of positions where potentials time-locked to the trigger are detected. These potentials belong to the same motor unit and in this way the function of up to seven neuromuscular junctions in a single motor unit has been studied (Stålberg et al 1976). The range of values for jitter determined for the muscle as a whole are the same as those within the single motor unit.

Quantifying neuromuscular jitter. Variation of the interpotential interval can be expressed in terms of the standard deviation (SD) of the mean interpotential interval (MIPI). However, during the recording of potential pairs, slow trends in the IPI quite frequently occur because of minor alterations in electrode position affecting action potential shape and short-term variability in neuromuscular transmission timing (Stålberg &

Trontelj 1979), which renders the SD invalid as an accurate measure of jitter. Thus another method which measures the mean value of consecutive differences (MCD) of the IPIs is recommended (Stålberg et al 1971) (Fig. 30.23a). In certain situations, especially those where the velocity recovery function of the muscle fibre comes into play, the IPI is affected by the preceding interdischarge interval (IDI): in such circumstances the MCD includes a spurious variability not due to end-plate jitter. To overcome this problem, the measured interpotential intervals are sorted in increasing order, according to the magnitude of the preceding interdischarge intervals, following which the mean value of consecutive differences of this new sequence is estimated. This new value is called the mean sorted-data difference (MSD). In practice, in order to determine in which way the data should be reported, an index is used: this is the ratio MCD/MSD. A ratio of more than 1.25 is an indication that interdischarge intervals have so affected the variability that jitter should be expressed by the MSD. With ratios below 1.25 the results should be reported as the MCD.

Manual methods of jitter analysis. Manual methods of analysis consist of measurement of latency differences of baseline intersection points of the earliest- and latest-occurring second potential when the first has been used to trigger the oscilloscope. A total of at least 50 successive discharges of the pair are recorded and super-imposed on to photographic paper, either in 10 groups of five or five groups of 10. An oscilloscope sweep speed of at least 200 μs/cm should be used. The range of variations of the IPI in each group of recordings is measured between identical points on the rising positive–negative slope of the action potentials (Fig. 30.23b). The mean range from all of the groups of superimpositions is determined and converted into the MCD value using an appropriate conversion factor (0.49 for five and 0.37 for 10 superimpositions). The manual method is unable to assess the effects of irregular discharge rates on jitter and, in order to reduce this problem, the patient should attempt to main-tain a constant firing rate throughout the recording.

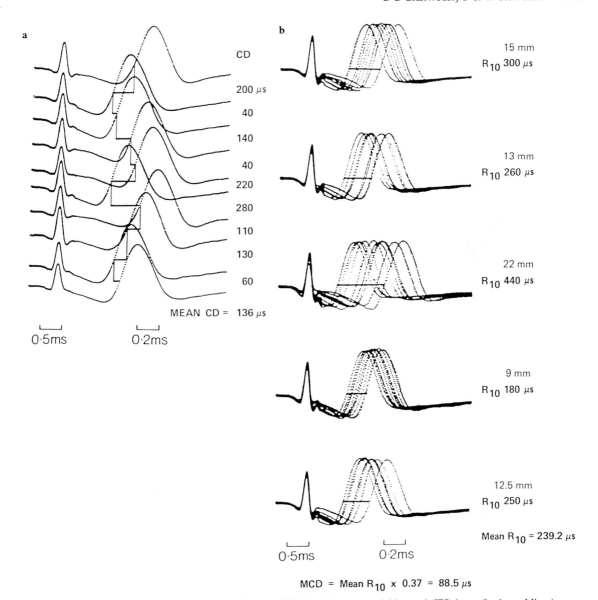

Fig. 30.23 Jitter measurement. a. Consecutive differences (CD) in the interpotential interval (IPI) in μs (horizontal lines). b. Manual method for jitter measurement using five groups of 10 superimposed sweeps

Automated methods of jitter analysis. As well as manual methods of SFEMG analysis, a number of automated methods have been described utilising mini- or microcomputers, and are incorporated into some of the recently developed commercial EMG systems. All systems use a triggering device to isolate the two potentials, and either a hardware interval counter or real-time clock within the computer to measure the IPIs accurately. The firing rate or IDI can also be measured and the effect of IDI on jitter may be automatically assessed by determining the MSD value, after which the MCD/MSD index is obtained. The use of minicomputers and the storage capacity of hard-disc drives allows virtually continuous analysis and updating of both normal and pathological parameters for the SFEMG laboratory. Where such comprehensive facilities are lacking, the recording on to reel-to-reel or cassette tape of the studies carried out provides a means of subsequent off-line analysis and comparison of individual results.

SFEMG findings in myasthenia gravis. In the presence of myasthenia gravis a 20-potential study may show some pairs with jitter values within the normal range, others with abnormal jitter and some where impulse blocking is present (Stålberg et al 1974, 1976) (Fig. 30.24). Blocking occurs in pairs showing higher jitter values and usually manifests itself when jitter has reached 100 μs. When a series of 50 consecutive discharges from a potential pair showing intermittent blocking is analysed, the range between minimal and maximal interpotential interval could be up to 4000 μs. Even when myasthenia is mild and restricted clinically, usually more than 30% of pairs show either increased jitter or blocking. Continuous activation, especially when accompanied by rising firing rates, will increase jitter and blocking at an affected neuromuscular junction. With a fall in firing rate, the proportion of blockings and magnitude of jitter decline. Occasionally the

reverse will be true, with a fall in jitter and impulse blocking as the firing rate increases. If an end-plate appears to have been spared, as indicated by an initial normal jitter, attempts to evoke an abnormality by continuous activity and increasing firing rate are usually fruitless. Although in myasthenia there is usually a variety of degrees of involvement of different end-plates in a muscle, from normal jitter at one to impulse blocking at another, this is not apparently due to selective involvement or sparing of individual motor units.

When a muscle shows clinical weakness at the time of the SFEMG study and jitter is normal, the diagnosis of myasthenia gravis is excluded (Stålberg & Trontelj 1979). In a minority of myasthenic patients (up to 30%) a recording from the EDC may be normal or show equivocal changes; these are usually patients with ocular myasthenia (Stålberg et al 1976, Sanders et al 1979). In this situation, SFEMG of the facial muscles will give an abnormal result in about 85% of patients (Stålberg 1980b). Conditions other than myasthenia may be associated with disturbed neuromuscular transmission and give rise to abnormal jitter values.

Jitter in normal muscle is unaffected by the

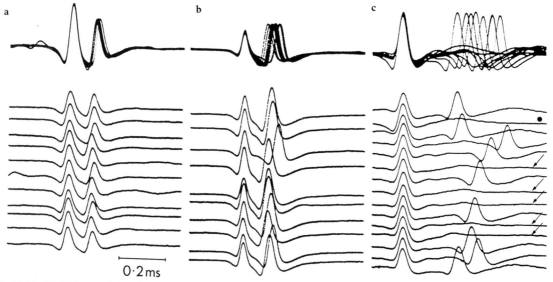

Fig. 30.24 SFEMG recordings from extensor digitorum communis muscle in a patient with myasthenia gravis. Upper trace — 10 superimposed sweeps, lower traces — faster display of successive sweeps. a. Normal jitter (33 μs MCD); b. increased jitter (80 μs MCD); c. increased jitter associated with intermittent blocking of second potential (arrows) and first potential (closed circle)

injection of edrophonium hydrochloride whereas, in myasthenia, blocking may be abolished and jitter reduced. In patients receiving anticholinesterase therapy, some potential pairs may show the reverse effect with edrophonium, with increases in jitter and impulse blocking. These 'cholinergic crises' at isolated end-plates are an indication of the variations in severity of the disorder when looked at microphysiologically in an individual muscle (Stålberg & Trontelj 1979). Despite this, there is good overall correlation between severity of SFEMG changes and the clinical severity of the myasthenia (Sanders et al 1979). The number of potential pairs showing blocking matches the clinical fatiguability both in untreated patients and in those receiving anticholinesterase or steroids. Serial studies in individual patients should show parallel changes in SFEMG abnormality and variations in clinical severity.

A minority of patients in remission occurring spontaneously after thymectomy or during corticosteroid therapy, show no SFEMG abnormality (Sanders et al 1979). In remission, impulse blocking is exceptional but abnormal numbers of pairs show elevated jitter levels. Where maintenance therapy with anticholinesterase preparations appears to have achieved complete control of the disorder clinically, the SFEMG remains unequivocally abnormal (Stålberg & Trontelj 1979). There is no need to discontinue therapy prior to SFEMG in a suspected case already on treatment.

Normal individuals receiving anticholinesterase drugs, in the therapeutic range employed in the treatment of myasthenia, do not develop abnormal jitter. Chronic medication of this type fails to produce SFEMG abnormalities in normal subjects and people erroneously diagnosed and treated as myasthenics have been identified (Stålberg & Trontelj 1979).

The SFEMG in apparently normal first-degree relatives of patients with myasthenia is of interest. Stålberg et al (1976) have examined a number of the relatives of patients with juvenile myasthenia and found abnormalities in one-third of them. Increased jitter was found in 25% of the pairs examined and blocking in about 15%; overall, 25% of all the recordings were abnormal whereas

in the clinically affected juveniles the abnormality rate was 75%.

SFEMG may be used to determine FD in patients with myasthenia and other disorders of neuromuscular transmission. Hilton-Brown et al (1982) reported the results of a study of 71 myasthenic patients and found a significant increase in FD compared with controls. Neither severity nor duration of the disease were correlated with the change in FD. Those individuals receiving anticholinesterase drugs had significantly higher FD values than untreated patients and controls. As many subjects in the study had a repeated examination, care was taken to avoid the possibility that needle injury to the muscle was a factor in the production of the FD increase. The problem of myasthenic drop-out of single fibres affecting FD was also addressed. The possibility of muscle fibre shrinkage leading to closer packing of the fibres appeared to be excluded by muscle biopsy. A direct effect of medication on the terminal innervation, producing functional denervation and subsequent reinnervation, appears to be possible. Morphological and physiological changes induced by anticholinesterase drugs administered experimentally to animel species, discussed elsewhere (Ch. 3), support this hypothesis.

Stapedius reflex

In 1965 Blomberg & Persson described a new test for myasthenia gravis which depended on fatiguing the stapedius muscle. The stapedius muscle contracts reflexly in response to sound and prevents hyperacusis. Its contraction alters the acoustic impedance of the middle ear so that it is easy to monitor its contraction by impedance audiometry. In normal individuals, sustained contractions in response to sound stimuli 70–100 dB above threshold at frequencies from 250 to 100 Hz can be maintained for up to 1 min; in contrast, the myasthenic stapedius shows a rapid decrement and is unable to sustain reflex contraction, resulting in the rapid onset of hyperacusis. The response may be reversed, or at least improved, by intravenous edrophonium (Blom & Zakrisson 1974). The test appears to be well tolerated and in some myasthenics may be the only electrophysiological abnormality (Warren et al 1977). It may therefore be of value not only as a diagnostic procedure but also as an easy means of monitoring the response to treatment (Kramer et al 1981, Stålberg & Sanders 1981).

Saccadic eye movements

A number of methods of measuring the development of fatigue in the extraocular muscles, by recording the fall-off in the velocity of angular movement during oculokinetic nystagmus or other eye movements (Baloh & Keesey 1976, Yee et al 1976), have been reported. In patients with myasthenia gravis there may be a fall-off in eye-movement velocities, which can be improved by the administration of edrophonium. These tests require the co-operation of the patient and may be difficult to quantify.

NEUROPHYSIOLOGICAL FINDINGS IN THE VARIOUS DISORDERS OF NEUROMUSCULAR TRANSMISSION

Myasthenia gravis

Patients with myasthenia gravis may vary from those with mild restricted disease to those with severe widespread involvement, which, by virtue of affecting bulbar and respiratory muscles, may threaten life. The ease with which the diagnosis is made relates to the severity of the condition at presentation. Methods of repetitive stimulation are most widely available but will prove positive in only one-quarter of patients with mild or restricted disease if distal muscles are tested. When the disease has resulted in moderate or severe weakness, the diagnostic yield reaches 90%. Utilising proximal muscles for repetitive stimulation studies produces positive results in 65–70% of all myasthenics. The double-step ischaemic test increases the detection rate dramatically, even in mildly affected patients. Regional curare sensitivity now has no part to play in the routine diagnosis of myasthenia. Where SFEMG is available, examination of jitter and blocking in the EDC muscle will give abnormal results in 95% of myasthenics. If the patient has ocular myasthenia and shows no abnormality in EDC, then SFEMG

studies in the frontalis will demonstrate abnormal neuromuscular transmission in over 80% of these patients (Stålberg & Sanders 1981). Less widely available are the stapedius-reflex fatigue test which appears very sensitive, and tests of intraocular tension, ocular muscle fatigue and ocular EMG (Kelly et al 1982). Levels of antibody to ACh receptor are elevated in about 75–80% of myasthenics. The antibody level does not correlate with clinical severity, which is better shown by the jitter in SFEMG studies (Konishi et al 1981).

Neonatal myasthenia. In about 15% of infants born to myasthenic mothers, a transient disorder of neuromuscular transmission is seen (Greer & Schotland 1969). The condition appears to be due to the presence of ACh receptor antibodies which have been independently synthesised by the affected infants rather than, as previously thought, to the transplacental passive transfer of maternal antibodies (Lefvert & Osterman 1983). The main signs of the disorder are feeding difficulties, respiratory problems and hypotonia appearing within three days of birth, responding to anticholinesterase treatment. The neurophysiological findings (Desmedt & Borenstein 1977b) are identical with those of true myasthenia gravis and may still be present after apparent clinical recovery.

Congenital myasthenic syndromes

At least four of these rare disorders of neuromuscular transmission have been characterised and it is likely that other defects are still to be delineated (see Ch. 19, 20). The first to be described was the myasthenic syndrome associated with end-plate ACh esterase deficiency, small nerve terminals and reduced ACh release (Engel et al 1977). After isolated nerve stimulation, the CMAP appears repetitively and there is a decremental response at all frequencies when trains of stimuli are delivered. Only a single case has been described and in vitro studies of a biopsy showed reduced MEPP frequencies but preservation of MEPP amplitude. The time course of the MEPP was prolonged. There was a reduced quantal content of the EPP and a reduction in the stores of ACh immediately available for release. A total absence of ACh esterase at the end-plate was demonstrated and normal numbers of acetylcholine receptors were present. The prolonged MEPP duration and repetitive firing appear to be due to the absence of ACh esterase.

A familial congenital myasthenic syndrome, possibly attributable to a presynaptic defect in transmitter resynthesis or mobilisation, was first described by Hart et al in 1979. Further cases have been reported and the disorder is most often seen in the newborn but can affect older patients (Engel 1980, Lambert 1982). When stimuli are applied to the nerve at 2 Hz there is a decrement in the CMAP only in muscles which are weak. Exercise or a tetanic train induces a significant decrement in the CMAP in other muscles. The only in vitro abnormality is the presence of a marked fall in MEPP and EPP amplitudes when stimulated at 10 Hz, which is similar to the effect when normal muscle is treated with hemicholinium and suggests the presence of a defect in ACh synthesis. The congenital myasthenic syndrome, attributable to a prolonged open time of the ACh-sensitive ion channels, or 'slow channel syndrome', was described by Engel et al in 1982. The disease may begin in infancy or appear later and is associated with the presence of repetitive discharges of the CMAP in response to single stimuli. In vitro studies have revealed the presence of very prolonged decay of the MEPPs and EPPs and prolonged MEP currents together with a reduction in MEPP amplitude. Other structural abnormalities which are thought to be secondary to the primary ion channel defect, include a reduction in the numbers of ACh receptors, decrease in the size of the nerve terminals and focal degeneration of the postjunctional folds. Small groups of atrophic muscle fibres and degenerative changes in the muscle fibres were also noted (Engel 1980, Engel et al 1982). The MEP currents are produced by opening of ACh-induced ion channels in response to a single quantum of transmitter; their prolonged decay in the presence of normal acetylcholinesterase activity suggests that the channels remain open too long. The effect of this could be to allow an excessive calcium influx into the muscle cell which, in turn, could lead to the degenerative changes observed.

A familial myasthenic syndrome with possible abnormalities in the synthesis of ACh receptor or its insertion into the postsynaptic membrane was described by Vincent et al (1981) and by Lambert (1982). The results of neuromuscular testing in these patients were similar to those in myasthenia gravis, although no antibodies to ACh receptors are present.

Eaton–Lambert syndrome

In vitro studies (Elmqvist & Lambert 1968, Elmqvist 1973, Sanders et al 1980) demonstrate a defect in ACh release from nerve terminals. Spontaneously occurring MEPPs are normal in frequency and amplitude, demonstrating a normal postsynaptic response to a single ACh 'packet' and a normal ACh content of the packet. In the myasthenic syndrome EPP amplitude is reduced as, instead of the usual 50 quanta of ACh being released in response to the nerve impulse, the EPPs are generated by only 2–10 quanta. The majority of the EPPs do not reach the level needed to initiate muscle-fibre action potentials and some nerve impulses fail to produce an EPP. When stimulated repetitively, an increase in EPP amplitude restores neuromuscular transmission. The resting MEPP frequency, for reasons that are not clear at present, is about twice that seen in normal subjects. The findings on neuromuscular testing in the Eaton–Lambert syndrome may be summarised as follows. In distal limb muscles the response to an isolated supramaximal stimulus is a very low-voltage CMAP. Repetitive stimulation at low rates (2 or 3 Hz) is accompanied by a further decline in the amplitude of the response (Fig. 30.25a). A train of shocks at 10 Hz may result in an initial decline followed by recovery to the original amplitude (Fig. 30.25b). At 20 Hz and, more strikingly, at 50 Hz there is a rapid increase in CMAP amplitude to normal or nearly normal (Fig. 30.25 c,d). Single shocks delivered immediately after such a train result in a much enhanced CMAP but the effect is short lived. Similar results are produced by voluntary exercise for 30 s. CNEMG often reveals MUP instability similar to that seen in myasthenia gravis. There is no evidence of fibrillation, positive sharp waves or nerve conduction defects to suggest denervation. SFEMG shows that, in contrast to myas-

ADM

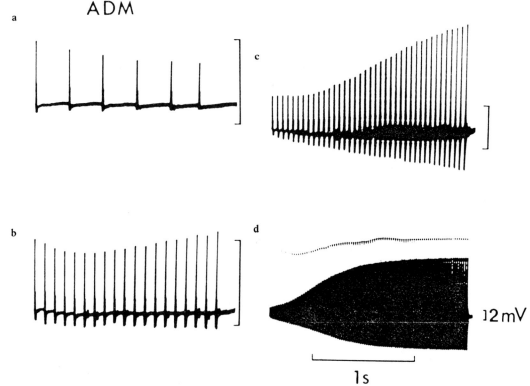

Fig. 30.25 Eaton-Lambert syndrome. Repetitive nerve stimulation studies at different frequencies in the abductor digiti minimi (ADM) muscle. Note low amplitude of the initial CMAP in train. a. 3 Hz, showing a decrement of 25% at the 5th response; b. 10 Hz, showing an initial decrement followed by slight increment; c. 20 Hz; d. 50 Hz, progressive increment of responses reaching 371% and 943% respectively

thenia gravis, jitter and impulse blocking are less at higher discharge rates and increase as the firing rate falls (Fig. 30.26). The maximum jitter (MCD) can be as high as 500 μs and the range of interpotential intervals for 50 discharges may reach 2000 μs (Stålberg & Trontelj 1979). The first impulse blocking tends to appear at somewhat higher jitter values than is the case with myasthenia gravis. Blocking is more probable if the preceding interpotential interval is long. Edrophonium chloride produces improvement, as do guanidine hydrochloride and the less toxic 3,4-diaminopyridine, but anticholinesterase drugs are not very effective.

Botulism

The clinical features of the rapidly developing paralysis attributable to the blocking action on ACh release from motor nerve terminals caused by the exotoxin of *Clostridium botulinum* are described

elsewhere (Ch. 27). In affected individuals CNEMG examination of weak muscles shows short-duration low-amplitude MUPs with reduced recruitment on effort (Cornblath et al 1983). When patients are examined approximately 14 days after the onset of paralysis, fibrillations are seen; these are believed to be due to the severity of the damage to the presynaptic region and they disappear as the patient recovers (De Jesus et al 1973). Conduction velocity in motor nerves is normal and CMAP amplitude is normal or reduced in those muscles mildly involved. With rapid repetitive stimuli some facilitation may occur. In weak muscles, CMAP amplitude to single shocks is low and falls further with 3 Hz stimulation; no facilitation is seen with rapid trains (Cherington 1973, 1974, 1982, Oh 1977). The duration of post-tetanic facilitation is prolonged, lasting for 10–15 min after a conditioning stimulus train, much longer than in myasthenia or the Eaton–Lambert syndrome (Cull-Candy et al 1976, Gutmann &

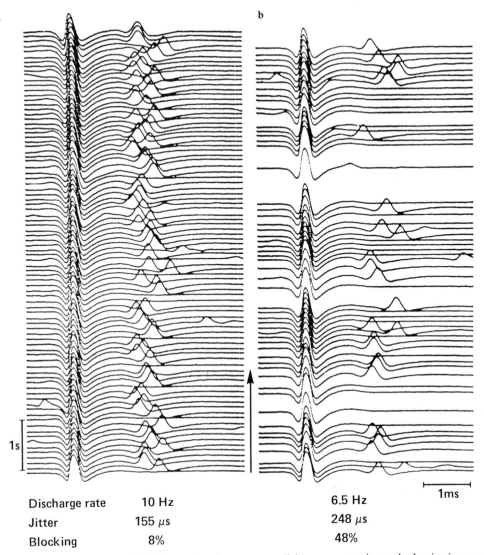

	a	b
Discharge rate	10 Hz	6.5 Hz
Jitter	155 μs	248 μs
Blocking	8%	48%

Fig. 30.26 Eaton-Lambert syndrome. SFEMG recordings from extensor digitorum communis muscle showing increased jitter and blocking. Jitter and blocking are less marked at higher discharge (a) than lower discharge rates (b)

Pratt 1976). Administration of guanidine or calcium gluconate may increase CMAP amplitudes (Oh 1977, Messina et al 1979). SFEMG studies in two patients revealed increased jitter and impulse blocking which were less pronounced at higher discharge frequencies (Schiller & Stålberg 1978).

Drug-induced myasthenic syndromes

D-Penicillamine-induced myasthenia is a reversible disorder of neuromuscular transmission seen in patients receiving penicillamine treatment for rheumatoid arthritis, Wilson's disease or sclero derma. Anti-ACh receptor antibodies can often be detected in these patients and the disorder is neurophysiologically identical to myasthenia gravis (Stålberg & Trontelj 1979, Fawcett et al 1982b).

Antibiotics affect neuromuscular transmission and, especially in patients with renal failure, myasthenia gravis or other disorders of neuromuscular transmission, they may cause weakness lasting for hours or days. The mechanism whereby the weakness is produced varies with the antibiotic used and is detailed elsewhere (Ch. 29). Other drugs such as anticonvulsants, procainamide, quinidine, adrenergic blockers and lithium may also impair neuromuscular transmission.

Curare combines with the ACh receptors and reduces the number available for interaction with ACh. Clinically, curare in non-paralytic doses but in amounts sufficient to produce diplopia and ptosis is associated with increased jitter and impulse blocking, developing with jitter of the order of 70 μs. Muscle-fibre conduction velocity is unaffected (Ekstedt & Stålberg 1969a).

Transmission disorders in other neuromuscular diseases

Motor neurone disease is often associated with disordered neuromuscular transmission (Lambert & Mulder 1957, Mulder et al 1959, Simpson 1966, Lambert 1969, Brown & Jaatoul 1974, Bernstein & Antel 1981). A decrementing CMAP is found at low stimulus rates, such as 1 Hz or less, improving only slightly with anticholinesterase administration. Slight decremental responses may occur at higher stimulus rates. SFEMG shows increased jitter and blocking, especially in rapidly progressive disease (Stålberg et al 1975). Although transmission may be abnormal at the end-plates of anterior horn cells which are starting to degenerate, it is the presence of many immature junctions due to the abundant collateral reinnervation process that provides a situation where the uncertainty of neuromuscular transmission is increased. Neurogenic block due to intermittent axonal conduction is seen in 5–10% of potentials in motor neurone disease (Stålberg & Thiele 1972). In situations where nerve regeneration can be studied it can be shown that decremental responses to nerve stimulation occur frequently, especially in the early period of reinnervation.

Peripheral neuropathies such as the Guillain–Barré syndrome, diabetic neuropathy, chronic idiopathic neuropathy and ' post-herpetic motor neuropathy' have been shown to give a decremental response to stimulation (Simpson & Lenman 1959, Simpson 1966). No abnormalities in neuromuscular transmission were detected by SFEMG in uraemic or diabetic neuropathy but increased jitter and blocking were found in alcoholic neuropathy. With stimulus frequencies of up to 500 Hz, a decline in CMAP amplitude occurs earlier, and is more marked in patients with diabetes mellitus than in normal subjects. This is the case even where there is no clinical evidence of a neuropathy (Miglietta 1971). In view of the high stimulus frequencies used, the presence of segmental demyelination of peripheral nerve in diabetes, and the absence of SFEMG abnormality, the finding may be attributable to defective axonal conduction. At present it is uncertain where the blocking occurs in these disorders and to what extent neurogenic rather than neuromuscular blocking is responsible (Thiele & Stålberg 1975).

Clinical fatigue, partly relieved by administration of anticholinesterase drugs and associated with 'a decremental response to repetitive stimulation, has been reported in some patients with multiple sclerosis (Patten et al 1972, Eisen et al 1978). There may be evidence of denervation and reinnervation, and jitter may be increased. Involvement of motor axons within the spinal cord in the ventral horns may account for the denervation seen.

In Duchenne-type muscular dystrophy, SFEMG examination has shown increased jitter in about 30% of recordings and sometimes blocking in about 10% of those recordings where the largest jitter had been seen (Stålberg & Trontelj 1979). This is probably due to the presence on regenerated muscle fibres of immature neuromuscular junctions where the safety factor for neuromuscular transmission remains reduced for several months (Stålberg & Trontelj 1979). A high incidence of late unstable linked potentials lends support to this hypothesis (Desmedt & Borenstein 1976, Stålberg 1977). Stålberg & Trontelj (1979) found a high incidence of concomitant blocking and a common value for jitter in two muscle fibres in relation to the rest of the complex: this suggests that the problem of transmission is situated in the terminal nerve twig. Another frequent finding was the presence of interdischarge interval-dependent jitter particularly affecting the later components giving rise to the accordion phenomenon (see Fig. 30.19). The presence of abnormally small jitter values has been taken to indicate recording from a split muscle fibre.

In limb-girdle dystrophy (Stålberg & Trontelj

1979) jitter is increased in over 50% of sites in clinically affected muscle but blocking averaged only 4%. Similar findings were described in patients with facioscapulohumeral dystrophy.

In the myotonic disorders, particularly myotonia congenita, there is a decremental response to repetitive stimulation caused by increasing muscle fibre membrane refractoriness (Brown 1974, Özdemir & Young 1976, Aminoff et al 1977). This response differs from that of myasthenia in several respects (Fig. 30.27): first, it is steadily progressive with no evidence of a tendency to plateau or recover at the fifth or sixth stimulus; second, the decremental response develops later in the train than in myasthenia and is greater with higher stimulus frequencies; third, the response can be obtained when the muscle is stimulated directly, indicating that neuromuscular transmission is not involved. There is no decremental response when the stimulus frequency is 5 Hz. The response to single stimuli following exercise or a rapid train is reduced because most of the muscle fibres are refractory and it takes about 15–30 s for resting amplitudes to reappear.

In polymyositis, Henriksson & Stålberg (1978) showed that increased jitter and impulse blocking are frequent. When increased jitter was found on gentle contraction, a further rise in jitter and the development of blocking was produced by continuous activity and correlated with the presence of clinical fatiguability. Low jitter values suggesting fibre splitting may be seen and concomitant blocking indicating impaired nerve conduction of the impulse is also present.

In McArdle's disease (myophosphorylase deficiency) a significant decremental response occurs at a stimulus frequency of 19 Hz accompanying the cramp after exercise (Dyken et al 1967). Even in the absence of cramp, a decrement develops provided that the stimulus train is continued for over 4 s (Delwaide et al 1968).

Systemic disorders

In thyroid disease, weakness due to defective neuromuscular transmission is an occasional occurrence. A decremental response similar to that of myasthenia gravis is most common, the association between these disorders being well recognised. However, marked facilitation at rapid stimulus rates in a patient with thyrotoxicosis has been reported (Norris 1966). Changes characteristic of the Eaton–Lambert syndrome in a patient with myxoedema have been documented (Takamori et al 1972). A decremental response has been noted in patients with both thyrotoxicosis and myxoedema who were not clinically weak (Drechsler & Lastoukay 1969). The neurophysiological features of both the myasthenic syndrome and of myasthenia gravis have been detected in different muscles in a patient with hyperthyroidism (Mori & Takamori 1976). A significant decremental response to repetitive stimulation, particularly at rates of 20–30 Hz, has been found in a proportion of patients with intrinsic asthma (Basomba et al 1976). SFEMG studies have shown an increase in the jitter phenomenon in patients in both the acute and convalescent phases of viral illnesses (Schiller et al 1977). The considerable functional reserve of the neuromuscular junction ensures that transmission is unaffected in most systemic illnesses. Disuse of muscle is associated with an abnormal decline in CMAP at rapid stimulus frequencies; it is therefore unsafe to infer that such changes are due to the effects of systemic illness on the neuromuscular junction.

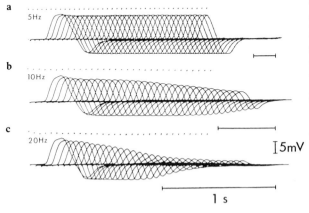

Fig. 30.27 Myotonia congenita (recessive Becker type). Repetitive nerve stimulation studies in abductor digiti minimi. a. No change in amplitude at 5 Hz. b. Progressive decline in amplitude at 10 Hz. c. More rapid and marked decrement at 20 Hz to almost absence of response

REFERENCES

Aberfeld D C, Hinterbuchner L P, Schneider M 1956 Myotonia, dwarfism, diffuse bone disease and unusual ocular and facial abnormalities (a new syndrome). Brain 88:313

Adrian E D, Bronk D V 1929 Discharges of impulses in motor nerve fibres. Journal of Physiology 67:119

Albers J W, Allen A A, Bastron J A, Daube J R 1981 Limb myokymia. Muscle and Nerve 4:494

Aminoff M J, Layzer R B, Satya-Murti S, Faden A I 1977 The declining response of muscle to repetitive nerve stimulation in myotonia. Neurology 27:812

Åstrom K E, Kugelberg E, Muller R 1961 Hypothyroid myopathy. Archives of Neurology 5:472

Auger R G, Daube J R, Gomez M R, Lambert E H 1984 Hereditary form of sustained muscle activity of peripheral nerve origin causing generalised myokymia and muscle stiffness. Annals of Neurology 15:13

Axelson J, Thesleff S 1959 A study of supersensitivity in denervated mammalian muscle. Journal of Physiology 147:178

Baloh R W, Keesey J C 1976 Saccadic fatigue and response to edrophonium for the diagnosis of myasthenia gravis. Annals of the New York Academy of Science 274:631

Barchi R L 1975 An evaluation of the chloride hypothesis. Archives of Neurology 32:175

Barchi R L 1982 A mechanistic approach to the myotonic syndrome. Muscle and Nerve (Suppl) 5:60

Barwick D D 1963 Investigations of the carrier state in the Duchenne type dystrophy. In: Proceedings of the 2nd Symposium on Research in Muscular Dystrophy. Pitman, London

Barwick D D, Walton J N 1963 Polymyositis. American Journal of Medicine 35:645

Barwick D D, Gardner-Medwin D 1967 Observer bias in the measurement of motor unit action potentials. Electroencephalography and Clinical Neurophysiology 23:490

Basmajian J V, Stecko G 1962 A new bipolar electrode for electromyography. Journal of Applied Physiology 17:849

Basomba A, Permuy J, Pelaez A, Campos A. Villamanzo I G 1976 Myasthenia-like electrophysiological response in intrinsic bronchial asthma. Lancet 2:968

Becker P E 1977 Myotonia congenita and syndromes associated with myotonia. Thieme, Stuttgart

Belmar J, Eyzaguirre C 1966 Pacemaker site of fibrillation potentials in denervated mammalian muscle. Journal of Neurophysiology 29:425

Bergmans J 1971 Computer assisted on-line measurement of motor unit parameters in human electromyography. Electromyography and Clinical Neurophysiology 11:161

Bergmans J 1973 Computer assisted measurement of the parameters of single motor unit potentials in human electromyography. In: Desmedt J (ed) New developments in electromyography and clinical neurophysiology, vol 2. Karger, Basel

Bergmans J 1982 Repetitive activity induced in human motor axons: a model for pathological repetitive activity. In: Culp W J, Ochoa J (eds) Abnormal nerves and muscles as impulse generators. Oxford University Press, Oxford

Bernstein L P, Antel J P 1981 Motor neurone disease: decremental responses to repetitive nerve stimulation. Neurology 31:202

Bill P L A, Cole G, Proctor N S F 1979 Centrinuclear

myopathy. Journal of Neurology Neurosurgery and Psychiatry 42:548

Bischoff A, Esslen E 1965 Myopathy with primary hyperparathyroidism. Neurology (Minneapolis) 15:64

Björk A, 1952 Electrical activity of human extrinsic eye muscles. Experientia 8:226

Björk A, Kugelberg E 1953 Motor unit activity in the human extra-ocular muscles. Electroencephalography and Clinical Neurophysiology 5:271

Black J T, Bhatt G P, DeJesus P V, Schotland D L, Rowland L P 1974 Diagnostic accuracy of clinical data, quantitive electromyography and histochemistry in neuromuscular disease. Journal of the Neurological Sciences 21:59

Blom S, Zakrisson J E 1974 The stapedius reflex in the diagnosis of myasthenia gravis. Journal of the Neurological Sciences 21:71

Blomberg L H, Persson T 1965 A new test for myasthenia gravis. Acta Neurologica Scandinavica 41 (suppl) 13:363

Bohan A, Peter J B, Bowman R L, Pearson C M 1977 Computer-assisted analysis of 153 patients with polymyositis and dermatomyositis. Medicine 56:255

Borenstein S, Desmedt J E 1973 Electromyographical signs of collateral reinnervation. In: Desmedt J E (ed) New developments in electromyography and clinical neurophysiology. Karger, Basel

Borenstein S, Desmedt J E 1974 Local cooling in myasthenia. Improvement of neuromuscular failure. Archives of Neurology 32:152

Bosch E P, Gowans J D C, Munsat T 1979 Inflammatory myopathy in oculopharyngeal dystrophy. Muscle and Nerve 2:73

Bradley W G, Jones M Z, Mussini J-M. Fawcett P R W 1978 Becker-type muscular dystrophy. Muscle and Nerve 1:111

Breinin G M 1957 Electromyography — a tool in ocular neurogenic diagnosis. II. Muscle palsies. Archives of Ophthalmology 57:165

Breinin G M 1962 The electrophysiology of extraocular muscle. University Press, Toronto

Brooks V B, Curtis D R, Eccles J C 1957 The action of tetanus toxin on the inhibition of motoneurones. Journal of Physiology 135:655

Brown J C 1974 Muscle weakness after rest in myotonic disorders: an electrophysiological study. Journal of Neurology, Neurosurgery and Psychiatry 37:1336

Brown J C, Charlton J E 1975 Study of sensitivity to curare in certain neurological disorders using a regional technique. Journal of Neurology, Neurosurgery and Psychiatry 38:34

Brown J C, Charlton J E, White D J K 1975 A regional technique for the study of sensitivity to curare in human muscle. Journal of Neurology, Neurosurgery and Psychiatry 38:18

Brown J C, Wynn-Parry C B 1981 Neuromuscular stimulation and transmission. In: Walton J N (ed) Disorders of voluntary muscle. 4th edn. Churchill Livingstone, Edinburgh

Brown W F 1984 The physiological and technical basis of electromyography. Butterworth, London

Brown W F, Jaatoul N 1974 Amyotrophic lateral sclerosis. Electrophysiological study (number of motor units and rate of decay of motor units). Archives of Neurology 30:242

Brunberg J A, McCormick W F, Schochet S S 1971 Type III glycogenosis. An adult with diffuse weakness and muscle wasting. Archives of Neurology 25:71

Bryant R H 1982 Abnormal impulse production in myotonic muscle. In : Culp W J, Ochoa J (eds) Abnormal nerves and muscles as impulse generators. Oxford University Press, Oxford

Buchthal F 1961 The general concept of the motor unit. Research Publications of the Association of Nervous and Mental Diseases 38:3

Buchthal F 1970 Electrophysiological abnormalities in metabolic myopathies and neuropathies. Acta Neurologica Scandinavica (suppl) 43:129

Buchthal F 1982 Fibrillations: clinical electrophysiology. In: Culp W J, Ochoa J (eds) Abnormal nerves and muscles as impulse generators. Oxford University Press, New York

Buchthal F, Clemmesen B 1941 On the differentiation of muscle atrophy by electromyography. Acta Psychiatrica et Neurologica Scandinavica 16:143

Buchthal F, Kamieniecka Z 1982 The diagnostic yield of quantified electromyography and quantified muscle biopsy in neuromuscular disorders. Muscle and Nerve 5:265

Buchthal F, Madsen A 1950 Synchronous activity in normal and atrophic muscle. Electroencephalography and Clinical Neurophysiology 2:425

Buchthal F, Olsen P Z 1970 Electromyography and muscle biopsy in infantile spinal muscular atrophy. Brain 93:15

Buchthal F, Rosenfalck P 1955 Action potential parameters in different human muscles. Acta Psychiatrica Scandinavica 30:216

Buchthal F, Rosenfalck P 1963 Electrophysiological aspects of myopathy with particular reference to progressive muscular dystrophy. In: Bourne G H, Golarz M (eds) Muscular dystrophy in man and animals. Karger, New York

Buchthal F, Rosenfalck P 1966 Spontaneous electrical activity of human muscles. Electroencephalography and Clinical Neurophysiology 20:321

Buchthal F, Rosenfalck P 1973 On the structure of motor units. In: Desmedt J E (ed) New developments in electromyography and clinical neurophysiology. Karger Basel

Buchthal F, Erminio F, Rosenfalck P 1954a Motor unit territory in different human muscles. Acta Physiologica Scandinavica 54:72

Buchthal F, Guld C, Rosenfalck P 1954b Action potential parameters in normal human muscle and their dependence on physical variables. Acta Physiologica Scandinavica 32:200

Buchthal F, Pinelli P, Rosenfalck P 1954c Action potential parameters in normal human muscle and their physiological determinants. Acta Physiologica Scandinavica 32:219

Buchthal F, Guld C, Rosenfalck P 1957 Multielectrode study of the territory of a motor unit. Acta Physiologica Scandinavica 39:83

Bundey S, Carter C O, Solthill J F 1970 Early recognition of heterozygotes for the gene for dystrophia myotonica. Journal of Neurology, Neurosurgery and Psychiatry 33:279

Campa J F, Sanders D B 1974 Familial hypokalemic periodic paralysis. Local recovery after nerve stimulation. Archives of Neurology 31:110

Cao A, Cianchetti C, Calisti L, de Virgiliis S, Ferreli A, Tangheroni W 1978 Schwartz–Jampel syndrome: clinical, electrophysiological and histopathological study of a severe variant. Journal of the Neurological Sciences 35:175

Caruso G, Buchthal F 1965 Refractory period of muscle and electromyographic findings in relatives of patients with muscular dystrophy. Brain 88:29

Cherington M 1973 Botulism: electrophysiological and therapeutic observations. In: Desmedt J (ed) New developments in electromyography and clinical neurophysiology. Karger, Basel

Cherington M 1974 Botulism. Ten year experience. Archives of Neurology 30:432

Cherington M 1982 Electrophysiological methods as an aid in diagnosis of botulism: a review. Muscle & Nerve 5:s28

Christensen E 1959 Topography of terminal motor innervation in striated muscles from stillborn infants. American Journal of Physical Medicine 38:17

Clark J, Plonsey R 1966 A mathematical evaluation of the core conductor model. Biophysical Journal 6:95

Clark J, Plonsey R 1968 The extracellular potential field of the single active nerve fibre in a volume conductor. Biophysical Journal 8:842

Coërs C, Woolf A L 1959 The innervation of muscle. Blackwell, Oxford

Coërs C, Telerman-Toppet N, Gerard J M. Szliwowski H, Bethlem J, Wijngaarden G K V 1976 Changes in motor innervation and histochemical patterns in some congenital myopathies. Neurology (Minneapolis) 26:1046

Conradi S, Grimby L, Lundemo G 1982 Pathophysiology of fasciculation in ALS as studied by electromyography of single motor units. Muscle and Nerve 5:202

Coomes E N 1965 Corticosteroid myopathy. Annals of the Rheumatic Diseases 24:465

Cruz Martinez A, Ferrer M T, Lopez-Terradas J M, Pascual-Castroviejo I, Mingo P 1979 Single fibre electromyography in central core disease. Journal of Neurology, Neurosurgery and Psychiatry 42:662

Cornblath D R, Sladky J T, Sumner A J 1983 Clinical electromyography of infantile botulism. Muscle and Nerve 6:448

Cull-Candy S G, Lundh H, Thesleff S 1976 Effects of botulism toxin on neuromuscular transmission in the rat. Journal of Physiology 260:177

Daube J R, Kelly J J, Martin R A 1979 Facial myokymia with polyradiculoneuropathy. Neurology 29:662

Davey M R, Woolf A L 1965 An electromyographic study of carriers of muscular dystrophy. In: Proceedings of the 6th International Congress of Electroencephalography and Clinical Neurophysiology. Weiner Medizinische Akademie. Vienna

De Grandis D, Fiaschi A. Michieli G, Mezzina C 1979 Anomalous reinnervation as a sequel to obstetric brachial plexus palsy. Journal of the Neurological Sciences 43:127

DeJesus P V, Slater R, Spitz L K, Penn A S 1973 Neuromuscular physiology of wound botulism. Archives of Neurology 29:425

DeJong H H, Matzner I A, Unger A A 1951 Clinical and physiological studies in a case of myokymia. Archives of Neurology and Psychiatry 65:181

Delwaide P J, Lemaire R, Reznik M 1968 EMG findings in a case of McArdle's myopathy. Electroencephalography and Clinical Neurophysiology 25:414

Denny-Brown D 1949 Interpretation of the electromyogram. Archives of Neurology and Psychiatry 61:99

Denny-Brown D, Pennybacker J B 1938 Fibrillation and fasciculation in voluntary muscle. Brain 61:311

Desmedt J E 1978 Muscular dystrophy contrasted with denervation: different mechanisms underlying spontaneous fibrillation. Electroencephalography and Clinical Neurophysiology (suppl) 34:531

Desmedt J E, Borenstein S 1976 Regeneration in Duchenne muscular dystrophy. Archives of Neurology 33:642

Desmedt J E Borenstein S 1977a Double–step nerve stimulation test for myasthenic block: sensitisation of post-activation exhaustion by ischaemia. Annals of Neurology 1:55

Desmedt J E, Borenstein S 1977b Time course of neonatal myasthenia gravis and unexpectedly long duration of neuromuscular block in distal muscles. New England Journal of Medicine 296:633

DiMauro S, Hartwig G B, Hays A et al 1979 Debrancher deficiency: Neuromuscular disorder in five adults. Annals of Neurology 5:422

Dodge P R, Gamstorp I, Byers R K, Russell P 1965 Myotonic dystrophy in infancy and childhood. Pediatrics 35:3

Dorfman L J, McGill K C, Cummins K L 1985 Electrical properties of commercial concentric EMG electrodes. Muscle and Nerve 8:1

Drachman D B, Murphy S R, Nigam M, Hill J R 1967 'Myopathic' changes in chronically denervated muscles. Archives of Neurology 16:14

Drechsler B, Lastoukay M 1969 An electrophysiological study of patients with thyriopathy. Electroencephalography and Clinical Neurophysiology 26:234

Duchen L W 1973 The effects of tetanus toxin on the motor end-plates of the mouse. Journal of the Neurological Sciences 19:160

Dyken M L, Smith D M, Peak R L 1967 An electromyographic screening test in McArdle's disease and a case report. Neurology (Minneapolis) 17:45

Edström J, Kugelberg E 1968 Histochemical composition, distribution of fibres and fatiguability of single motor units. Journal of Neurology, Neurosurgery and Psychiatry 31:424

Edström L 1970 Selective changes in the size of red and white muscle fibres in upper motor lesions and parkinsonism. Journal of the Neurological Sciences 11:537

Eisen A, Karpati G 1971 Spontaneous electrical activity in muscle. Description of two patients with motor neurone disease. Journal of the Neurological Sciences 12:137

Eisen A, Humphreys P 1974 The Guillain-Barré syndrome: a clinical and electrodiagnostic study of 25 cases. Archives of Neurology 30:438

Eisen A, Yufe R, Trop D, Campbell I 1978 Reduced neuromuscular transmission safety factor in multiple sclerosis. Neurology 28:598

Ekbom K, Hed R, Kirstein L, Åstrom K E 1964 Muscular affections in chronic alcoholism. Archives of Neurology 10:449

Ekstedt J 1964 Human single muscle fibre action potentials. Acta Physiologica Scandinavica 61 (Suppl) 226:1

Ekstedt J, Stålberg E 1965 The diagnostic use of single muscle fibre recordings and the neuromuscular jitter in myasthenia gravis. In: The 6th International Congress of Electroencephalography and Clinical Neurophysiology Communications. Weiner Medizinische Akademie, Vienna

Ekstedt J, Stålberg E 1969a The effect of non-paralytic doses of D-tubocurarine on individual motor end-plates in man, studied with a new electrophysiological method.

Electroencephalography and Clinical Neurophysiology 27:557

Ekstedt J, Stålberg E 1969b Abnormal connections between skeletal muscle fibres. Electroencephalography and Clinical Neurophysiology 27:607

Ekstedt J, Stålberg E 1973 Single fibre electromyography for the study of the microphysiology of the human muscle. In: Desmedt J E (ed) New developments in electromyography and clinical neurophysiology. Karger, Basel

Elmqvist D 1973 Neuromuscular transmission defects. In: Desmedt J E (ed) New developments in electromyography and clinical neurophysiology. Karger, Basel

Elmqvist D, Lambert E H 1968 Detailed analysis of neuromuscular transmission in a patient with the myasthenic syndrome sometimes associated with bronchogenic carcinoma. Mayo Clinic Proceedings 43:689

Elmqvist D, Hofmann W W, Kugelberg E, Quastel D M J 1964 An electrophysiological investigation of neuromuscular transmission in myasthenia gravis. Journal of Physiology 174:417

Emery A E H, Teasdall R D, Coombes E N 1966 Electromyographic studies in carriers of Duchenne muscular dystrophy. Bulletin of the Johns Hopkins Hospital 118:439

Engel A G 1970 Acid maltase deficiency in adults: Studies in four cases of syndrome which may mimic muscular dystrophy or other myopathies. Brain 93:599

Engel A G 1980 Morphologic and immunopathalogic findings in myasthenia gravis and in congenital myasthenic syndromes. Journal of Neurology, Neurosurgery and Psychiatry 43:577

Engel A G, Gomez M R, Seybold M E, Lambert E H 1973 The spectrum and diagnosis of acid maltase deficiency. Neurology (Minneapolis) 27:95

Engel A G, Lambert E H, Gomez M R 1977 A new myasthenic syndrome with end-plate acetylcholinesterase deficiency, small nerve terminals and reduced acetylcholine release: Annals of Neurology 1:315

Engel A G, Lambert E H, Mulder D M, Torres C F, Sahashi K, Bertorini T E, Whitaker J N 1982 A newly recognised congenital myasthenic syndrome attributed to a prolonged open time of the acetylcholine induced ion channel. Annals of Neurology 11:553

Engel W K 1975 Brief small, abundant motor unit action potentials. A further critique of electromyographic interpretation. Neurology 25:173

Engel W K, Vick N A, Glueck C J, Levy R I 1970 A skeletal muscle disorder associated with intermittent symptoms and a possible defect of lipid metabolism. New England Journal of Medicine 282:697

Esslen E 1960 Electromyographic findings in two types of misdirection of regenerating axons. Electroencephalography and Clinical Neurophysiology 12:738

Falk B 1983 Automatic analysis of individual motor unit potentials recorded with a special two channel electrode. Academic Dissertation, University of Turku, Kirjapaino Pika Oy-Turku

Falk B, Alaranta H 1983 Fibrillation potentials, positive sharp waves and fasciculation in the intrinsic muscles of the feet of healthy subjects. Journal of Neurology, Neurosurgery and Psychiatry 46:681

Fambrough D M 1979 Control of acetyl choline receptors in skeletal muscle. Physiological Reviews 59:165

Faris A A, Reyes M G 1971 Reappraisal of alcoholic

myopathy. Clinical and biopsy study on chronic alcoholics without muscle weakness or wasting. Journal of Neurology, Neurosurgery and Psychiatry 34:86

Fawcett P R W, Mastaglia F L, Mechler F 1982a Electrophysiological findings including single fibre EMG in a family with mitochondrial myopathy. Journal of the Neurological Sciences 53:397

Fawcett P R W, McLachlan S M, Nicholsen L B V, Argov Z, Mastaglia F L 1982b D-Penicillamine-associated myasthenia gravis: immunological and electrophysiological studies. Muscle and Nerve 5:328

Fawcett P R W, Dick D J, Schofield I S 1985a SFEMG and Macro EMG in Becker muscular dystrophy. Electroencephalography and Clinical Neurophysiology 61:3 (S76)

Fawcett P R W, Dick D J, Schofield I S 1986 Single fibre EMG and Macro EMG in spinal muscular atrophy. Electroencephalography and Clinical Neurophysiology 63:33P

Fawcett P R W, Johnson M A, Schofield I S 1985b Comparison of electrophysiological and histochemical methods for assessing the spatial distribution of muscle fibres of a motor unit within muscle. Journal of the Neurological Sciences 69:67

Feinstein B, Lindegard B, Nyman E, Wohlfart G 1955 Morphologic studies of motor units in normal human muscles. Acta Anatomica 23:127

Floyd M, Ayyar D R, Barwick D D, Hudgson P, Weightman D 1974 Myopathy in chronic renal failure. Quarterly Journal of Medicine 53:509

Forster F M. Alpers B J 1944 The site of origin of fasciculation in voluntary muscle. Archives of Neurology and Psychiatry 51:254

Forster F M, Borkowski W J, Alpers B J 1946 Effects of denervation on fasciculation in human muscle. Archives of Neurology 56:276

Fowler W M, Layzer R B, Taylor R G et al 1974 The Schwartz–Jampel syndrome: Its clinical, physiological and histological expression. Journal of the Neurological Sciences 22:127

Frame B, Heinze E G Jr, Block M A, Manson G A 1968 Myopathy in primary hyperparathyroidism. Observations in three patients. Annals of Internal Medicine 68:1022

Fugelsang-Frederiksen A, Scheel U, Buchthal F 1976 Diagnostic yield of analysis of the pattern of electrical activity and of individual motor unit potentials in myopathy. Journal of Neurology, Neurosurgery and Psychiatry 39:742

Fugelsang-Frederiksen A, Scheel U, Buchthal F 1977 Diagnostic yield of the analysis of the pattern of electrical activity of muscle and of individual motor unit potentials in neurogenic involvement. Journal of Neurology, Neurosurgery and Psychiatry 40:544

Fullerton P M, Gilliatt R W 1965 Axonal reflexes in human motor nerve fibres. Journal of Neurology, Neurosurgery and Psychiatry 28:1

Gage P W 1976 Generation of end-plate potentials. Physiology Reviews 56:177

Gamstorp I, Wohlfart G 1959 Syndrome characterised by myokymia, myotonia, muscular wasting and increased perspiration. Acta Psychiatrica Scandinavica 34:181

Gardner-Medwin D 1968 Studies on the carrier state of the Duchenne type of muscular dystrophy. 2. Quantitive electromyography as a method of carrier detection. Journal of Neurology, Neurosurgery and Psychiatry 31:124

Gardner-Medwin D, Walton J N 1969 Myokymia with impaired muscle relaxation. Lancet 1:127

Gath I, Sjaastad O, Løken A C 1969 Myopathic electromyographic changes correlated with histopathology in Wohlfart-Kugelberg-Welander disease. Neurology (Minneapolis) 19:344

Gath I, Stålberg E 1977 On the volume conduction in human muscle: in situ measurements. Electroencephalography and Clinical Neurophysiology 43:106

Gath I, Stålberg E 1978 The calculated radial decline of extracellular action potential compared with in situ measurements in the human brachial biceps. Electroencephalography and Clinical Neurophysiology 4:547

Gath I, Stålberg E 1982 On the measurement of fibre density in human muscles. Electroencephalography and Clinical Neurophysiology 54:699

Geddes L A, Baker L E 1967 The specific resistance of biologic material — A compendium for the biomedical engineer and physiologist. Medical Biological Engineering 5:271

Gilliatt R W 1966 Applied electrophysiology in nerve and muscle disease. Proceedings of the Royal Society of Medicine 59:989

Gil-Peralta A, Rafel E, Bautista J, Alberrca R 1978 Myotonia in centrinuclear myopathy. Journal of Neurology, Neurosurgery and Psychiatry 41:1102

Goldkamp O 1967 Electromyography and nerve conduction studies in 116 patients with hemiplegia. Archives of Physical Medicine 48:59

Gordon A M, Green J R, Lagunoff D 1970 Studies on a patient with hypokalemic familial periodic paralysis. American Journal of Medicine 48:185

Gordon E E, Jauszko D M, Kaufman L 1967 A critical survey of the stiff-man syndrome. American Journal of Medicine 42:582

Greenhouse A H, Bicknell J M, Pesch R N, Seelinger D F 1967 Myotonia, myokymia, hyperhidrosis and wasting of muscle. Neurology (Minneapolis) 17:263

Greer M, Schotland M 1969 Myasthenia in the newborn. Paediatrics 26:101

Grob D, Johns R J, Liljestrand A 1957 Potassium movement in patients with familial periodic paralysis. American Journal of Medicine 23:356

Grob D, Namba T 1976 Characteristics and mechanism of neuromuscular block in myasthenia gravis. Annals of the New York Academy of Science 274:143

Guld C 1951 On the influence of the measuring electrodes on the duration and amplitude of muscle action potentials. Acta Physiologica Scandinavica (suppl) 89:30

Guld C, Rosenfalck A, Willison R G 1970 Technical factors in recording electrical activity of muscle & nerve in man. Electroencephalography and Clinical Neurophysiology 28:399

Gutmann L, Pratt L 1976 Pathophysiologic aspects of human botulism. Archives of Neurology 33:175

Guy E, Lefebvre J, Lerique J, Scherrer J 1950 Les signes electromyographiques des dermatomyosites. Etude de 9 cas. Revue Neurologique 83:278

Haas A, Ricker K, Rüdel R, Lehmann-Horn F, Böhlen R, Dengler R, Mertens H G 1981 Clinical study of paramyotonia congenita with and without myotonia in a warm environment. Muscle and Nerve 4:388

Hakelius L, Stålberg E 1974 Electromyographical studies of

free autogenous muscle transplants in man. Scandinavian Journal of Plastic and Reconstructive Surgery 8:211

Håkansson C H 1957 Action potentials recorded intra and extracellularly from the isolated frog muscle fibre in Ringer's solution and in air. Acta Physiologica Scandinavica 39:291

Harel S, Chui L A, Shapira Y 1979 Myotonia congenita (Thomsen's disease): Early diagnosis in infancy. Acta Pediatrica Scandinavica 68:225

Harman J B, Richardson A T 1954 Generalised myokymia in thyrotoxicosis. Report of a case. Lancet 2:473

Harper P S 1975 Congenital myotonic dystrophy in Britain. 1. Clinical aspects. Archives of Disease in Childhood 50:505

Hart Z H, Sahashi K, Lambert E H, Engel A G, Lindstrom J M 1979 A congenital, familial myasthenic syndrome caused by a presynaptic defect of transmitter resynthesis or mobilisation. Neurology 29:556

Harvey A M, Masland R L 1941 A method for the study of neuromuscular transmission in human subjects. Bulletin of the Johns Hopkins Hospital 69:1

Hausmanowa-Petrusewicz I, Prot J, Niebrój-Dobsoz I, et al 1968 Studies of healthy relatives of patients with Duchenne muscular dystrophy. Journal of the Neurological Sciences 7:465

Hausmanowa-Petrusewicz I, Jedrzejowska H 1971 Correlation between electromyographic findings and muscle biopsy in cases of neuromuscular disease. Journal of the Neurological Sciences 13:85

Hausmanowa-Petrusewicz I, Karwanska A 1986 Electromyographic findings in different forms of infantile and juvenile proximal spinal muscular atrophy. Muscle and Nerve 9:37

Hawkes C H, Absolon M J, 1975 Myotubular myopathy associated with cataract and electrical myotonia. Journal of Neurology, Neurosurgery and Psychiatry 38:761

Hed R, Lundmark C, Fahlgren H, Orell S 1962 Acute muscular syndrome in chronic alcoholism. Acta Medica Scandinavica 171:585

Henneman E 1957 Relation between size of neurons and their susceptibility to discharge. Science 126:1345

Henriksson K G, Stålberg E 1978 The terminal innervation pattern in polymyositis: a histological and SFEMG study. Muscle and Nerve 1:3

Hertel G, Ricker K, Hirsch A 1977 The regional curare test in myasthenis gravis. Journal of Neurology 24:257

Hilfiker P, Meyer M 1984 Normal and myopathic propagation of surface motor unit action potentials. Electroencephalography and Clinical Neurophysiology 57:21

Hilton-Brown P, Stålberg E, Osterman P O 1982 Signs of reinnervation in myasthenia gravis. Muscle and Nerve 5:215

Hilton-Brown P, Stålberg E, 1983a The motor unit in muscular dystrophy, a single fibre EMG and scanning EMG study. Journal of Neurology, Neurosurgery and Psychiatry 46:981

Hilton-Brown P, Stålberg E 1983b Motor unit size in muscular dystrophy, a Macro EMG and Scanning EMG study. Journal of Neurology, Neurosurgery and Psychiatry 46:996

Hilton-Brown P, Stålberg E, Trontelj J, Mihelin M 1985 Causes of the increased fibre density in muscular dystrophies studied with single fibre EMG during electrical stimulation. Muscle and Nerve 8:383

Hirose K, Uono M, Sobue I 1974 Quantitative electromyography; comparison between manual values and computer ones on normal subjects. Electromyography and Clinical Neurophysiology 14:315

Hjorth R J, Walsh J C, Willison R G 1973 The distribution and frequency of spontaneous fasciculations in motor neurone disease. Journal of the Neurological Sciences 18:469

Hofmann W W, DeNardo G L 1968 Sodium flux in myotonic muscular dystrophy. American Journal of Physiology 214:330

Hogan G R, Gutmann L, Schmidt R, Gilbert E 1969 Pompe's disease. Neurology (Minneapolis) 19:894

Horowitz S H, Genkins G, Kornfeld P, Papatestas A E 1975 Regional curare test in evaluation of ocular myasthenia. Archives of Neurology 32:84

Horowitz S H, Sivak M 1978 The regional curare test and electrophysiologic diagnosis of myasthenia gravis: further studies. Muscle and Nerve 1:432

Howard F M 1963 A new and effective drug in the treatment of the stiff-man syndrome. Proceedings of the staff of the Mayo Clinic 38:203

Hubbard J I, Llinas R, Quastel D M J 1969 Electrophysiological analysis of synaptic transmission. Edward Arnold, London

Hudgson P, Bradley W G, Jenkison M 1972 Familial 'mitochondrial' myopathy — A myopathy associated with disordered oxidative metabolism in muscle fibres. Journal of the Neurological Sciences 16:343

Hudgson P, Barwick D D 1974 Myopathy in chronic renal failure. 3rd International Congress on Muscle Diseases, Excerpta Medica, Amsterdam 334:172

Hudson A J, Cholod E J, Haust M D 1970 Familial hyperparathyroid myopathy. In: Walton J N, Canal C, Scarlato G (eds) Muscle disease. Excerpta Medica, Amsterdam

Hudson A J, Brown W F, Gilbert J J 1978 The muscular pain–fasciculation syndrome. Neurology 28:1105

Hughes R C, Matthews W B 1969 Pseudomyotonia and myokymia. Journal of Neurology, Neurosurgery and Psychiatry 32:11

Hynninen P, Philipson L, Manderson B, Elmqvist D 1979 Computer based method for automatic motor unit potential analysis. Acta Neurologica Scandinavica 60 (suppl) 73:300

Isaacs H 1961 A syndrome of continuous muscle-fibre activity. Journal of Neurology, Neurosurgery and Psychiatry 24:319

Isaacs H 1967 Continuous muscle fibre activity in an Indian male with additional evidence of terminal motor fibre abnormality. Journal of Neurology, Neurosurgery and Psychiatry 30:126

Isaacs H, Heffron J J A, Badenhorst M 1975 Central core disease. Journal of Neurology, Neurosurgery and Psychiatry 38:1177

Jasper H, Ballem G 1949 Unipolar electromyograms of normal and denervated human muscle. Journal of Neurophysiology 12:231

Johnson E W, Denny S T, Kelley J P 1975 Sequence of electromyographic abnormalities in stroke syndrome. Archives of Physical Medicine and Rehabilitation 56:468

Jones R V, Lambert E H, Sayre G P 1955 Source of a type of 'insertion activity' in electromyography with evaluation of a histologic method of localisation. Archives of Physical Medicine 36:301

Josefsson I O 1960 An electromyographic study of botulism

intoxicated skeletal muscle. Acta Physiologica Scandinavica 49: (suppl) 172

Jusic A, Dogan S, Stojanovic V 1972 Hereditary persistent distal cramps. Journal of Neurology, Neurosurgery and Psychiatry 35:379

Kaiser E, Petersen I 1965 Muscle action potentials studied by frequency analysis and duration measurement. Acta Neurologica Scandinavica 41 (suppl) 13:213

Katz B 1966 Nerve, muscle and synapse. McGraw-Hill, New York

Katz B, Miledi R 1965 Propagation of electrical activity in motor nerve terminals. Proceedings of the Royal Society B 161:453

Katz B, Miledi R 1968 The role of calcium in neuromuscular facilitation. Journal of Physiology 195:481

Kelly J J, Daube J R, Lennon V A, Howard F M, Younge B R 1982 The laboratory diagnosis of mild myasthenia. Annals of Neurology 12:238

Kimura J 1983 Electrodiagnosis in diseases of nerve and muscle: principles and practice. Davis, Philadelphia

King R B, Stoops W L 1973 Cervical myelopathy with fasciculations in the lower extremity. Journal of Neurosurgery 20:945

Konishi T, Nishitani H, Matsubara F, Ohta M 1981 Myasthenia gravis: relation between jitter in single fibre EMG and antibody to acetylcholine receptor. Neurology (New York) 31:386

Kopeć J, Hausmanowa-Petrusewicz I 1969 Histogram of muscle potentials recorded automatically with the aid of the averaging computer 'Anops'. Electromyography and Clinical Neurophysiology 9:36

Kopeć J, Hausmanowa-Petrusewicz I 1976 On-line computer application in clinical quantitative electromyography. Electromyography and Clinical Neurophysiology 16:49

Kopeć J, Hausmanowa-Petrusewicz I 1983 Computeranalyse des EMG und klinishe Ergebensse. EEG-EMG 14:28

Kopeć J, Hausmanowa-Petrusewicz I, Rawaki M, Wolynski M 1973 Automatic analysis in electromyography. In: Desmedt J (ed) New developments in electromyography and clinical neurophysiology, volume 2. Karger, Basel

Kramer L D, Ruth R A, Johns M E, Sanders D B 1981 A comparison of stapedial reflex fatigue with repetitive stimulation and single fibre EMG in myasthenia gravis. Annals of Neurology 9:531

Kugelberg E 1947 Electromyogram in muscular disorders. Journal of Neurology, Neurosurgery and Psychiatry 10:122

Kugelberg E 1948 Activation of human nerves by ischaemia. Archives of Neurology and Psychiatry 60:140

Kugelberg E 1949 Electromyography in muscular dystrophy. Journal of Neurology, Neurosurgery and Psychiatry 10:122

Kugelberg E 1973 Properties of the rat hind-limb motor units. In: Desmedt J E (ed) New developments in electromyography and clinical neurophysiology Vol 1. Karger, Basel

Kugelberg E, Petersén I 1949 'Insertion activity' in electromyography. Journal of Neurology, Neurosurgery and Psychiatry 12:268

Kuitonnen P, Rapola J, Noponen A L, Donner M 1972 Nemaline Myopathy. Report of 4 cases and review of the literature. Acta Paediatrica Scandinavica 61:353

Kunze K 1971 Die automatische Analyse in der klinischen Electromyographie. Nervenarzt 42:275

Kunze K 1973 Quantitative EMG analysis in myogenic and neurogenic muscle disease. In: Desmedt J (ed) New

developments in electromyography and clinical neurophysiology, vol 2. Karger, Basel

Lambert E H 1969 Electromyography in amyotrophic lateral sclerosis. In: Norris F H, Kurland L T (eds) Motor neurone disease. Grune and Stratton, New York

Lambert E H 1978 Muscle spasms, cramps and stiffness. American Academy of Neurology (Special Course) 17

Lambert E H 1982 Electrophysiological studies of the myasthenic syndrome and congenital neuromuscular syndromes. In: Didactic programme, 29th annual meeting. American Association of Electromyography and Electrodiagnosis, Minneapolis

Lambert E H, Mulder D W 1957 Electromyography studies in amyotrophic lateral sclerosis. Proceedings of the Staff Meetings of the Mayo Clinic 32:441

Lambert E H, Rooke E D, Eaton L M, Hodgson C H 1961 Myasthenic syndrome occasionally associated with bronchial neoplasm–neurophysiologic studies. In: Viet H R (ed) Myasthenia gravis. Thomas, Springfield, Illinois, p 362

Lance J W, Burke D, Pollard J 1979 Hyperexcitability of motor neurones in neuromyotonia. Annals of Neurology 5:523

Landau W M 1952 The essential mechanism in myotonia. Neurology (Minneapolis) 2:369

Lang A H, Nurkkanen P, Vaahtoranta K M 1971 Automatic sampling and averaging of electromyographic unit potentials. Electroencephalography and Clinical Neurophysiology 31:404

Lang A H, Partanen V S J 1976 'Satellite' potentials and the duration of motor unit potentials in normal, neuropathic and myopathic muscles. Journal of the Neurological Sciences 27:513

Lang A H, Falk B 1980 A two-channel method for sampling, averaging and quantifying motor unit potentials. Journal of Neurology 223:199

Layzer R B, Rowland L P 1971 Cramps. New England Journal of Medicine 285:31

Lazaro R P, Fenichel G M, Kilroy A W 1979 Congenital muscular dystrophy: case reports and reappraisal. Muscle and Nerve 2:349

Lazaro R P, Rollinson R D, Fenichel G M 1981 Familial cramps and muscle pain. Archives of Neurology 38:22

Lee R G, White D G 1973 Computer analysis of motor unit action potentials in routine clinical electromyography. In: Desmedt J (ed) New developments in electromyography and clinical neurophysiology. Karger, Basel

Lefvert A K, Osterman P O 1983 New-born infants to myasthenic mothers: a clinical study and an investigation of acetylcholine receptor antibodies in 17 children. Neurology 33:133

Lehmann-Horn F, Rüdel R, Dengler R, Lorković H, Haass A, Ricker K 1981 Membrane defects in paramyotonia with and without myotonia in a warm environment. Muscle and Nerve 2:109

Lehmann-Horn F, Rüdel R, Ricker K, Lorković H, Dengler R, Hopf H C 1983 Two cases of adynamia episodica hereditaria: in vitro investigation of muscle cell membrane and contraction parameters. Muscle and Nerve 6:113

Lenman J A R 1965 Effect of denervation on the resting membrane potential of healthy and dystrophic muscle. Journal of Neurology, Neurosurgery and Psychiatry 28:525

Li C Y, Shy G M, Wells J 1957 Some properties of mammalian skeletal muscle fibres with particular reference to fibrillation potentials. Journal of Physiology 135:522

Lindholm T 1968 The influence of uraemia and electrolyte disturbances on muscle action potentials and motor nerve conduction in man. Acta Medica Scandinavica (suppl) 491:81

Lindsley D B 1935 Electrical activity of human motor units during voluntary contraction. American Journal of Physiology 114:90

Lippold O C J, Redfern J W T, Vuco J 1957 The rhythmical activity of groups of motor units in the voluntary contraction of muscle. Journal of Physiology 137:473

Lopez-Terradas J M, Conde Lopez M 1979 Late components of motor units in central core disease. Journal of Neurology, Neurosurgery and Psychiatry 42:461

Lublin F D, Tsairis P, Streletz L J, Chambers R A, Riker F, VanPosnak A, Duckett S W 1979 Myokymia and impaired muscular relaxation with continuous motor unit activity. Journal of Neurology, Neurosurgery and Psychiatry 42:557

Luco J V, Eyzaguirre C 1955 Fibrillation and hypersensitivity to ACh in denervated muscle: effect of length of degenerating nerve fibre.

Ludin H P 1980 Electromyography in practice. Thieme Verlag, Stuttgart

Lundberg P O, Osterman P O, Stålberg E 1970 Neuromuscular signs and symptoms in acromegaly. In: Walton J N, Canal N, Scarlato G (eds) Muscle diseases. Excerpta Medica, Amsterdam

Lundberg P O, Stålberg E, Thiele B 1974 Paralysis periodica myotonica. A clinical and neurophysiological study. Journal of the Neurological Sciences 21:309

McComas A J, Mrozek K 1968 The electrical properties of muscle fibre membranes in dystrophia myotonica and myotonia congenita. Journal of Neurology, Neurosurgery and Psychiatry 31:441

McComas A J, Sica R E P, Campbell M J 1971a 'Sick motor neurones', a unifying concept of muscle disease. Lancet 1:321

McComas A J, Fawcett P R W, Campbell M J, Sica R E P 1971b Electrophysiological estimates of the number of motor units within a human muscle. Journal of Neurology, Neurosurgery and Psychiatry 34:121

McComas A J, Sica R E P, Upton A R M, Aguilera N 1973 Functional changes in motoneurones of hemiparetic patients. Journal of Neurology, Neurosurgery and Psychiatry 36:183

McComas A J, Sica R E P, Toyonaga K 1978 Incidence, severity and time-course of moto-neurone dysfunction in myotonic dystrophy. Journal of Neurology, Neurosurgery and Psychiatry 41:882

McComas A J, Johns R F 1981 Potential changes in the normal and diseased muscle cell. In: Walton J N (ed) Disorders of voluntary muscle, 4th edn. Churchill Livingstone, Edinburgh

Markesbery W R, Griggs R C, Leach R P, Lapham L W 1974a Late onset hereditary distal myopathy. Neurology (Minneapolis) 24:127

Markesbery W R, McQuillen M P, Procopis P G, Harrison A R, Engel A G 1974b Muscle carnitine deficiency. Association with lipid myopathy, vacuolar neuropathy and vacuolated leucocytes. Archives of Neurology 31:320

Martinelli P, Pazzaglia P, Montagna P, Coccagna G, Rizzuto N, Simonati S, Lugaresi E 1978 Stiff-man syndrome associated with nocturnal myoclonus and epilepsy. Journal of Neurology, Neurosurgery and Psychiatry 41:58

Mastaglia F L, Barwick D D, Hall R 1970 Myopathy in acromegalics. Lancet 2:907

Mastaglia F L, Papadimitriou J M, Dawkins R L, Beveridge B 1977 Vacuolar myopathy associated with chloroquine, lupus erythematosus and thymoma. Journal of the Neurological Sciences 34:315

Masuda T, Miyano H, Sadoyama T 1983 The propagation of motor unit action potentials and the location of the neuromuscular junction by surface electrode array. Electroencephalography and Clinical Neurophysiology 55:594

Masuda T, Miyano H, Sadoyama T 1985 A surface electrode array for detecting action potential trains of single motor units. Electroencephalography and Clinical Neurophysiology 60:435

Mayer R F, Williams I R 1974 Incrementing responses in myasthenia gravis. Archives of Neurology 31:24

Meadows J C 1971 Fasciculation caused by suxamethonium and other cholinergic agents. Acta Neurologica Scandinavica 47:381

Mechler F 1974 Changing electromyographic findings during the chronic course of polymyositis. Journal of the Neurological Sciences 23:237

Mechler F, Fawcett P R W, Mastaglia F L, Hudgson P 1981 Mitochondrial myopathy. A study of clinically affected and asymptomatic members of a six-generation family. Journal of Neurology, Neurosurgery and Psychiatry 50:191

Meink H M, Ricker K, Conrad B 1984 The stiff-man syndrome: new pathophysiological aspects from abnormal exteroceptive reflexes and the response to clomipramine, clonidine and tizanide. Journal of Neurology, Neurosurgery and Psychiatry 47:280

Mertens H G, Zschocke S 1965 Neuromyotonia. Klinische Wochenschrift 43:917

Messina C, Tonali P, Scopetta C 1976 The lack of deep reflexes in myotonic dystrophy: a neurophysiological study. Journal of the Neurological Sciences 30:303

Messina C, Dattola R, Ginlanda P 1979 Effect of guanidine on the neuromuscular block of botulism. An electrophysiological study. Acta Neurologica Napoli 34:459

Miglietta O E 1971 Myasthenic-like response in patients with neuropathy. American Journal of Physical Medicine 50:1

Miledi R, Slater C R 1963 A study in rat nerve-muscle junctions after degeneration of the nerve. Journal of Physiology 151:1

Miller R G, Blank N K, Layzer R B 1979 Sporadic distal myopathy with early adult onset. Annals of Neurology 5:220

Milner-Brown H S, Stein R B 1975 The relation between the surface electromyogram and muscular force. Journal of Physiology 246:549

Mizusawa H, Takagi A, Sugita H, Toyokura Y 1983 Mounding phenomenon: an experimental study in vitro. Neurology 33:90

Moersch F P, Woltman H W 1956 Progressive fluctuating muscular rigidity and spasm ('stiff man' syndrome): report of a case and some observations on 13 other cases. Proceedings of the Staff Meetings of the Mayo Clinic 31:421

Moosa A, Brown B H, Dubowitz V 1972 Quantitative electromyography: carrier detection in Duchenne type muscular dystrophy using a new automatic technique. Journal of Neurology, Neurosurgery and Psychiatry 35:841

Mori M, Takamori M 1976 Hyperthyroidism and myasthenic

gravis with features of Eaton–Lambert syndrome. Neurology (Minneapolis) 26:882

Morrison J B 1960 The electromyographic changes in hyperkalaemic familial periodic paralysis. Annals of Physical Medicine 5:153

Mrozek K, Strugalska M, Fidzianska A A 1970 A sporadic case of central core disease. Journal of the Neurological Sciences 10:339

Mulder D W, Lambert E H, Eaton L M 1959 Myasthenic syndrome in patients with amyotrophic lateral sclerosis. Neurology (Minneapolis) 9:627

Muller R, Kugelberg E 1959 Myopathy in Cushing's syndrome. Journal of Neurology, Neurosurgery and Psychiatry 22:314

Munsat T L, Thompson L R, Coleman R F 1969 Centrinuclear ('myotubular') myopathy. Archives of Neurology 20:120

Murphy S F, Drachman D B 1968 The oculopharyngeal syndrome. Journal of the American Medical Association 203:1003

Nakao K, Nakanishi T, Tsubaki T 1965 Action potentials recorded by co-axial needle electrodes in Ringer's solution. Electroencephalography and Clinical Neurophysiology 18:412

Nielson V K, Friis M L, Johnsen T 1982 Electromyographic distinction between paramyotonia congenita and myotonia congenita: effect of cold. Neurology 32:827

Nishizono H, Saito Y, Miyshita M 1979 The estimation of conduction velocity in human skeletal muscle in situ with surface electrodes. Electroencephalography and Clinical Neurophysiology 46:659

Norris F H 1965 Central mechanisms of fasciculations. Proceedings of the 6th International Congress of Electroencephalography and Clinical Neurophysiology. Wiener Zinosche Akademie, Wien

Norris F H, Panner B J 1966 Hypothyroid myopathy, clinical, electromyographic and ultrastructural observations. Archives of Neurology 14:574

Oh S J 1977 Botulism: electrophysiological studies. Annals of Neurology 1:481

Okuno T, Mori K, Furomi K, Takeoka T Kondo K 1981 Myotonic dystrophy and hypothyroidism. Neurology 31:91

Olson W W K, Engel W K, Walsh G O, Einaugler R 1972 Oculocraniosomatic neuromuscular disease with 'ragged-red' fibres. Archives of Neurology 26:193

Oosterhuis H J G H, Hoostmans W J M, Veenhuyzen H B, Van Zadelhoff 1972 The mean duration of motor unit potentials in patients with myasthenia gravis. Electroencephalography and Clinical Neurophysiology 12:697

Özdemir C, Young R R 1976 Electrical testing in myasthenia gravis. Annals of the New York Academy of Sciences 274:203

Panayiotopoulos C P, Scarpalezos S 1976 Dystrophia myotonica: peripheral nerve involvement and pathogenetic implications. Journal of the Neurological Sciences 27:1

Partanen J, Lang H 1982 EMG dynamics in polymyositis. Journal of the Neurological Sciences 57:221

Patten B M, Hert A, Lovelace R 1972 Multiple sclerosis associated with defects in neuromuscular transmission. Journal of Neurology, Neurosurgery and Psychiatry 32:12

Payan J 1978 The blanket principle: a technical note. Muscle and Nerve 1:423

Pearson C M 1964 The periodic paralyses. Brain 87:341

Perkoff G T, Dioso M M, Blisch V, Klinkerfuss G 1967 A spectrum of myopathy associated with alcoholism. 1 Clinical and laboratory features. Annals of Internal Medicine 67:481

Petajan J H, Thurman D J 1981 EMG and histochemical findings in neurogenic atrophy with electrode localisation. Journal of Neurology, Neurosurgery and Psychiatry 44:1050

Petersén I, Kugelberg E 1949 Duration and form of action potentials in the normal human muscle. Journal of Neurology, Neurosurgery and Psychiatry 12:124

Pickett J B, Schnidley J W 1980 Sputtering positive potentials in the EMG: An artefact resembling positive waves. Neurology (Minneapolis) 30:215

Pickett J, Berg B, Chaplin E, Brunstetter-Shafer M A 1976 Syndrome of botulism in infancy: Clinical and electrophysiologic study. New England Journal of Medicine 295:770

Pinelli P, Buchthal F 1953 Muscle action potentials in myopathies with special regard to progressive muscular dystrophy. Neurology (Minneapolis) 3:347

Pittinger G, Adamson R 1972 Antibiotic blockade of neuromuscular function. Annual Review of Pharmacology 12:169

Polgar J, Bradley W G, Upton A R M, Anderson J, Howat J M L, Petito F, Roberts D F, Scopa J 1972 The early detection of dystrophia myotonica. Brain 95:761

Polgar J, Johnson M A. Weightman D, Appelton D 1973 Data on fibre size in thirty-six human muscles. An autopsy study. Journal of the Neurological Sciences 19:307

Pollak V 1971 The waveshape of action potentials recorded with different types of electromyographic needles. Medical Biological Engineering 9:657

Preswick G 1965 The myasthenic syndromes and their reactions. Proceedings of the Australian Association of Neurologists 3:61

Price T M L, Allott E H 1958 The stiff-man syndrome. British Medical Journal 1:682

Prineas J W, Hall R, Barwick D D, Watson A J 1968 Myopathy associated with pigmentation following adrenalectomy for Cushing's syndrome. Quarterly Journal of Medicine 37:63

Pryse-Phillips W, Johnson G J, Larsen B 1982 Incomplete manifestations of myotonic dystrophy in a large kinship in Labrador. Annals of Neurology 11:582

Purves D, Sakmann B 1974 Membrane properties underlying spontaneous activity of denervated muscle fibres. Journal of Physiology 239:125

Puvanendran K, Cheah J S, Naganathan N, Wong P K 1979 Thyrotoxic myopathy. A clinical and quantitative analytic electromyographic study. Journal of the Neurological Sciences 42:441

Radu H, Ionasescu V 1972 Nemaline (neuro-)myopathy: rodlike bodies and type 1 fibre atrophy in a case of congenital hypotonia with denervation. Journal of the Neurological Sciences 17:53

Radu H, Killyen I, Ionasescu V, Radu A 1977 Myotubular (centrinuclear) (neuro-)myopathy. European Neurology 15:285

Ramsay I D 1965 Electromyography in thyrotoxicosis. Quarterly Journal of Medicine 34:225

Rao S N, Katiyar B C, Nair K R P, Misra S 1980 Neuromuscular status in hypothyroidism. Acta Neurologica Scandinavica 61:167

Rathjen R, Simons D G, Peterson C R 1968 Computer analysis of the duration of motor unit potentials. Archives of Physical Medicine and Rehabilitation 49:524

Richardson A T 1956 Clinical and electromyographical aspects of polymyositis. Proceedings of the Royal Society of Medicine 49:111

Ricker K, Hertel G, Langsheid K, Stodieck G 1977 Myotonia not aggravated by cooling: force and relaxation of the adductor pollicis in normal subjects and in myotonia as compared to paramyotonia. Journal of Neurology 216:9

Ricker K, Haas A, Rüdel R, Bohlen R, Mertens H G 1980 Successful treatment of paramyotonia congenita (Eulenberg): muscle stiffness and weakness prevented by tocainide. Journal of Neurology, Neurosurgery and Psychiatry 43:268

Roohi F, List T, Lovelace R E 1981 Slow motor nerve conduction in myotonic dystrophy. Electromyography and Clinical Neurophysiology 21:97

Rosenfalck P, Buchthal F 1962 Studies on the fibrillation potentials of denervated human muscle. Electroencephalography and Clinical Neurophysiology (suppl) 22:130

Rossouw J E, Keeton R G, Hewlett R H 1976 Chronic proximal muscular weakness in alcoholics. South African Medical Journal 50:2095

Roth G 1982 The origin of fasciculations. Annals of Neurology 12:542

Rowland L P, Aranow H, Hoefer P F A 1961 Observations on the curare test in the differential diagnosis of myasthenia gravis. In: Viets H R (ed) Myasthenia gravis. Thomas, Springfield

Rubenstein A E, Wainapel S F 1977 Acute hypokalemic myopathy in alcoholism. Archives of Neurology 34:553

Rüdel R, Lehmann-Horn F, Ricker K, Kuther G 1984 Hypokalemic periodic paralysis: in vitro investigation of muscle fibre membrane parameters. Muscle and Nerve 7:110

Rüdel R, Lehmann-Horn F 1985 Membrane changes in cells from myotonia patients. Physiology Reviews 65: 310–365

Sacco G, Buchthal F, Rosenfalk P 1962 Motor unit potentials at different ages. Archives of Neurology 6:366

Salick A I, Pearson C M 1967 The electrical silence of myo-oedema. Neurology (Minneapolis) 17:899

Sanders D B, Howard J F, Johns T R 1979 Single fibre electromyography in myasthenia gravis. Neurology 29:68

Sanders D B, Kim Y I, Howard J F 1980 Eaton–Lambert syndrome: A clinical and electrophysiological study of a patient treated with 4-aminopyridine. Journal of Neurology Neurosurgery and Psychiatry 43: 978–985

Sanderson K V, Adey W R 1952 Electromyographic and endocrine studies in chronic thyrotoxic myopathy. Journal of Neurology, Neurosurgery and Psychiatry 15:200

Sandstedt P E R, Henriksson K G, Larsson L E 1982 Quantitative electromyography in polymyositis and dermatomyositis. A long-term study. Acta Neurologica Scandinavica 65:110

Satoyoshi E 1978 A syndrome of progressive muscle spasms, alopecia and diarrhoea. Neurology 28:258

Schiller H H, Schwartz M S, Friman G 1977 Disturbed neuromuscular transmission in viral infection. New England Journal of Medicine 296:884

Schiller H H, Stålberg E 1978 Human botulism studied with single fibre electromyography. Archives of Neurology 35:346

Schimrigk K 1978 Combination of electromyographic and histological examination of skeletal muscle with an aspiration biopsy needle. European Neurology 17:333

Schwartz M S, Stålberg E, Schiller H H, Thiele B 1976 The reinnervated motor unit in man. A single fibre EMG multi-electrode investigation. Journal of the Neurological Sciences 27:303

Schwartz M S, Moosa A, Dubowitz V 1977 Correlation of single fibre EMG and muscle histochemistry using an open biopsy recording technique. Journal of the Neurological Sciences 31:369

Schwartz M S, Stålberg E, Swash M 1980 Pattern of segmental motor involvement in syringomyelia: a single fibre EMG study. Journal of Neurology, Neurosurgery and Psychiatry 43:150

Seaba P J, Walker D D 1983 Fundamentals of electronics and instrumentation. In: Kimura J Electrodiagnosis in disease of nerve and muscle. Davis, Philadelphia

Segura R P, Saghal V 1981 Hemiplegic atrophy: electrophysiological and morphological studies. Muscle and Nerve 4:246

Shahani M, Astur F D, Dastoor D H, Mondekar V P, Bharucha E P, Nair K G, Shah J C 1979 Neuropathies in tetanus. Journal of the Neurological Sciences 43:173

Sherrington C S 1926 Remarks on some aspects of reflex inhibition. Proceedings of the Royal Society B 97:303

Shields R W 1984 Single fibre electromyography in the differential diagnosis of myopathic limb girdle syndromes and chronic spinal muscular atrophy. Muscle and Nerve 7:265

Shy G M, Engel W K, Somers J E, Wanko T 1963 Nemaline myopathy: a new congenital myopathy. Brain 86:793

Sica R E P, McComas A J, Ferreira J C D 1978 Evaluation of an automatic method for analysing the electromyogram. Canadian Journal of the Neurological Sciences 5:275

Simpson J A 1962 Recent studies on the physiology of the human spinal cord and its disturbance in poliomyelitis. Proceedings of the 8th Symposium of the European Association for Poliomyelitis. Masson, Paris

Simpson J A 1966 Control of muscle in health and disease. In: Andrew B L (ed) Control and innervation of skeletal muscle. Livingstone, Edinburgh

Simpson J A, Lenman J A R 1959 The effects of frequency of stimulation in neuromuscular disease. Electroencephalography and Clinical Neurophysiology 11:604

Singh N, Lovelace R E 1979 Quantitive electromyography using on line computer. Acta Neurologica Scandinavica 60 (suppl) 73:309

Skaria J, Katiyar B C, Srivastava T P, Dube B 1975 Myopathy and neuropathy associated with osteomalacia. Acta Neurologica Scandinavica 51:37

Slomic A, Rosenfalck A, Buchthal F 1968 Electrical and mechanical responses in normal and myasthenic muscle. Brain Research 10:1

Smith H L, Amick L D, Jonson W W 1966 Detection of subclinical and carrier state in Duchenne muscular dystrophy. Journal of Paediatrics 69:67

Smith J W, Thesleff S 1976 Spontaneous activity in denervated mouse diaphragm muscle. Journal of Physiology 257:171

Somers J E, Winer N 1966 Reversible myopathy and myotonia following administration of a hypocholesterolemic agent. Neurology (Minneapolis) 16:761

Spielholz N I, Sell G H, Gold J, Rusk H A, Greens S K

1972 Electrophysiological studies in patients with spinal cord lesions. Archives of Physical Medicine and Rehabilitation 53:558

Stålberg E 1966 Propagation velocity in human muscle fibres in situ. Acta Physiologica Scandinavica 70 (suppl) 287:1

Stålberg E 1977 Electrogenesis in human dystrophic muscle. In: Pathogenesis of human muscular dystrophies. Proceedings of the Fifth International Conference of the Muscular Dystrophy Association. Excerpta Medica, Amsterdam

Stålberg E 1980a Macro EMG, a new recording technique. Journal of Neurology, Neurosurgery and Psychiatry 43:475

Stålberg E 1980b Clinical electrophysiology in myasthenia gravis. Journal of Neurology, Neurosurgery and Psychiatry 43:622

Stålberg E 1982 Electrophysiological studies of reinnervation in ALS. In: Rowland L (ed) Human motor neurone diseases. Raven Press, New York, p 49

Stålberg E 1983 Macro EMG. Muscle and Nerve 6:619

Stålberg E, Trontelj J V 1970 Demonstration of axon reflexes in human motor nerve fibres. Journal of Neurology, Neurosurgery and Psychiatry 33:571

Stålberg E, Eksedt J, Broman A 1971 The electromyographic jitter in normal human muscles. Electroencephalography and Clinical Neurophysiology 31:429

Stålberg E, Thiele B 1972 Transmission block in terminal nerve twigs: a single fibre electromyographic finding in man. Journal of Neurology, Neurosurgery and Psychiatry 35:52

Stålberg E, Ekstedt J 1973 Single fibre EMG and the microphysiology of the motor unit in normal and diseased muscle. In: Desmedt J E (ed) New developments in electromyography and clinical neurophysiology. Karger, Basel

Stålberg E, Hansson O 1973 Single fibre EMG in juvenile myasthenia gravis. Neuropadiatrie 4:20

Stålberg E, Ekstedt J, Broman A 1974 Neuromuscular transmission in myasthenia gravis studied with single fibre electromyography. Journal of Neurology, Neurosurgery and Psychiatry 37:540

Stålberg E, Schwartz M S, Trontelj J V 1975 Single fibre electromyography in various processes affecting the anterior horn cell. Journal of the Neurological Sciences 24:403

Stålberg E, Trontelj J, Schwartz M S 1976 Single muscle fibre recording of the jitter phenomenon in patients with myasthenia gravis and in members of their families. Annals of the New York Academy of Sciences 274:189

Stålberg E, Trontelj J V 1979 Single fibre electromyography. Mirvalle Press, Old Woking, Surrey

Stålberg E, Antoni L 1980 Electrophysiological cross section of the motor unit. Journal of Neurology, Neurosurgery and Psychiatry 43:469

Stålberg E, Antoni L 1981 Microprocessors in the analysis of the motor unit and the neuromuscular transmission. In: Yamaguchi N, Fujisawa K (eds) Recent advances in EEG and EMG data processing. Elsevier/North-Holland Biomedical Press, Amsterdam, p 295

Stålberg E, Sanders D 1981 Electrophysiological tests of neuromuscular transmission. In: Stålberg E, Young R R (eds) Clinical neurophysiology. Butterworth, London

Stålberg E, Trontelj J V 1982 Abnormal discharges generated within the motor unit as observed with single-fibre electromyography. In: Culp W J, Ochoa J (eds) Abnormal nerves and muscles as impulse generators. Oxford University Press

Stålberg E, Fawcett P R W 1982 Macro EMG in healthy subjects of different ages. Journal of Neurology, Neurosurgery and Psychiatry 45:870

Stålberg E, Fawcett P R W 1984 Electrophysiological methods for the study of the motor unit in spinal muscular atrophy. In: Gamstorp I, Sarnat H B (eds) Progressive spinal muscular atrophies. Raven Press, New York

Stohr M, Heckl R 1977 Das stiff-man syndrome. Archiv für Psychiatrie und Nervenkrankheiten. 223:171

Streib E W, Wilbourn A J, Mitsumoto H 1979 Spontaneous electrical muscle activity in polymyositis and dermatomyositis. Muscle and Nerve 2:14

Swank R L, Price J C 1943 Fascicular muscle twitchings in amyotrophic lateral sclerosis. Archives of Neurology and Psychiatry 49:22

Swash M 1980 Vulnerability of lower brachial myotomes in motor neurone disease. Journal of the Neurological Sciences 47:59

Swift T R, Ignacio O J, Dyken P R 1975 Neonatal dystrophia myotonica: Electrophysiological studies. American Journal of Diseases of Childhood 129:374

Swift T R, Leshner R T, Gross J A 1980 Arm–diaphragm synkinesis. Neurology 30:339

Takamori M, Gutmann L, Crosby T W, Martin J D 1972 Myasthenic syndromes in hypothyroidism. Electrophysiological study of neuromuscular transmission and muscle contraction in two patients. Archives of Neurology 26:326

Tanzi F, Tagletti V, Zucca G, Arrigo A, Moglia A, Sandrini G, Cinquini G 1979 Computerised EMG analysis. Electromyography and Clinical Neurophysiology 19:495

Taylor A 1962 The significance of grouping of motor unit activity. Journal of Physiology 162:259

Taylor R G, Layzer R B, Davis H S, Fowler W M 1972 Continuous muscle fibre activity in the Schwartz-Jampel syndrome. Electroencephalography and Clinical Neurophysiology 33:497

Taylor R G, Kewalramani L S, Fowler W M 1974 Electromyographic findings in lower extremities of patients with high spinal cord injury. Archives of Physical Medicine and Rehabilitation 55:16

Thage O, Trojaborg W, Buchthal F 1963 Electromyographic findings in polyneuropathy. Neurology (Minneapolis) 13:273

Thesleff S 1963 Spontaneous electrical activity in denervated rat skeletal muscle. In: Gutmann E, Hnik P (eds) The effect of use and disuse on neuromuscular functions. Czechoslovak Academy of Sciences, Prague

Thesleff S 1982 Fibrillation in denervated mammalian skeletal muscle. In: Culp W J, Ochoa J (eds) Abnormal nerves and muscles as impulse generators. Oxford University Press

Thesleff S, Ward M R 1975 Studies on the mechanism of fibrillation potentials in denervated muscle. Journal of Physiology 244:313

Thiele B, Stålberg E 1974 The bimodal jitter: a single fibre electromyographic finding. Journal of Neurology, Neurosurgery and Psychiatry 37:403

Thiele B, Stålberg E 1975 Single Fibre EMG findings in polyneuropathies of different aetiology. Journal of Neurology, Neurosurgery and Psychiatry 38:881

Thiele B, Böhle A 1978 Anzahl der Spike-Komponenten im Motor-Unit Potential. EEG-EMG 9:125

Trojaborg W, Buchthal F 1965 Malignant and benign fasciculations. Acta Neurologica Scandinavica 41 (suppl) 13:251

Trojaborg W, Franzen E, Andersen I 1969 Peripheral neuropathy associated with carcinoma of the lung. Brain 92:71

Van Alphen H A, Lammers H J, Walder H A D 1962 On remarkable reaction of motor neurons of lumbosacral region after traumatic cervical transection in man. Neurochirugie 8:328

Van Den Bosch J 1963 Investigation of the carrier state in the Duchenne type dystrophy. In: Proceedings of the 2nd Symposium on Research in Muscular Dystrophy. Pitman, London

Venables G S, Bates D, Shaw D A 1978 Hypothyroidism with true myotonia. Journal of Neurology, Neurosurgery and Psychiatry 41:1013

Vicale C T 1949 The diagnostic features of a muscular syndrome resulting from hyperparathyroidism. Osteomalacia owing to renal tubular acidosis, and perhaps to related disorders of calcium metabolism. Transactions of the American Neurological Association 74:143

Vincent A, Cull-Candy S G, Newsom Davis J, Trautman A, Molinar P C, Polak R L 1981 Congenital myasthenia: end-plate acetylcholine receptors and electrophysiology in five cases. Muscle and Nerve 4:306

Wagner A, Kopeć J, Szimdt Salkowska E 1979 Normal values obtained by automated system in analysis of electromyogram. Electromyography and Clinical Neurophysiology 19:343

Wallis W E, VanPoznak A, Plum F 1970 Generalised muscular stiffness fasciculations and myokymia of peripheral nerve origin. Archives of Neurology 22:430

Walton J N, Adams R D 1958 Polymyositis. Livingstone, Edinburgh

Warmolts J R, Mendell J R 1980 Neurotonia: impulse-induced repetitive discharges in motor nerves in peripheral neuropathy. Annals of Neurology 7:245

Warren W R, Gutmann L, Cody R C, Flowers P, Segal A T 1977 Stapedius reflex decay in myasthenia gravis. Archives of Neurology 34:496

Weddell G, Feinstein B, Pattle R E 1944 The electrical activity of voluntary muscle in man under normal and pathological conditions. Brain 67:178

Weiderholt W C 1970 'End-plate noise' in electromyography. Neurology (Minneapolis) 20:214

Welander L 1951 Myopathia distalis tarda hereditaria. Acta Medica Scandinavica 141 (suppl) 265:1

Welch L K, Appenzeller O, Bicknell J M 1972 Peripheral neuropathy with myokymia — sustained muscular contraction and continuous motor unit activity. Neurology (Minneapolis) 22:161

Werk E E, Sholiton L J, Monell R J 1961 The stiff-man syndrome and hyperthyroidism. American Journal of Medicine 31:647

Wiechers D O 1977 Mechanically provoked insertional activity before and after nerve section in rats. Archives of Physical Medicine and Rehabilitation 58:402

Williams R S 1959 Triamcinolone myopathy. Lancet 1:698

Willison R G 1968 Quantitative electromyography: the detection of carriers of Duchenne dystrophy. Proceedings of the 2nd International Congress of Neurogenetics, Montreal

Wilson J, Walton J N 1959 Some muscular manifestations of hypothyroidism. Journal of Neurology, Neurosurgery and Psychiatry 22:320

Yates D A H 1963 The estimation of mean potential duration in endocrine myopathy. Journal of Neurology, Neurosurgery and Psychiatry 26:458

Yee R D, Cogan D G, Zee D S, Baloh R W, Hornubia V 1976 Rapid eye movements in myasthenia gravis. Archives of Ophthalmology 94:1465

Young J I, Rowley W F 1982 Physiological alterations of motor units in hemiplegia. Journal of the Neurological Sciences 54:401

Zellweger H, Ionasescu V 1973 Early onset of myotonic dystrophy in infants. American Journal of Diseases of Childhood 125:601

Zellweger H, Pavone L, Biondi A, Cimino V, Gullotta F, Hart M, Ionasescu V, Mollica F, Schieken R 1980 Autosomal recessive generalised myotonia. Muscle and Nerve 3:176

Studies in nerve conduction

INTRODUCTION

Primary disorders of the peripheral nerves constitute a large and important cause of neuromuscular dysfunction in patients of all ages. Following the introduction of motor and sensory nerve conduction measurement by Hodes et al (1948) and Dawson & Scott (1949) respectively, the techniques have become well-established clinical tools for the investigation of peripheral nerve function in humans, enabling disorders of these structures to be differentiated from primary diseases of the anterior horn cell, neuromuscular junction and muscle. While the basic concepts of the two techniques have changed little since their introduction, marked advances in instrumentation over the years have led to their widespread use for the provision of objective data on peripheral nerve function.

Since the first and subsequent editions of this book a number of excellent texts dedicated to the description of nerve conduction techniques and their findings in different disorders have been published (Goodgold & Eberstein 1983, Ludin 1980, Kimura 1983). Accordingly the emphasis of this chapter has been changed to reflect the place of nerve conduction and related techniques in the investigation of patients presenting with more generalised disorders of the neuromuscular system. Specific nerve lesions or nerve injuries have been omitted, and the reader should refer to the above-mentioned texts for expert guidance on these topics.

TECHNIQUE

Apparatus

The last few years have seen quite radical changes in the design of equipment used for nerve conduction measurement and electromyography (EMG). The increasing use of microprocessors has resulted in major alterations in the mode of operation, with the incorporation of various forms of keyboards in some instruments. The ability to link the basic EMG machine to a small computer has considerably extended the scope of investigations which can be performed, and has made available features such as rapid and sophisticated signal analysis and data storage.

Factors concerning the technical requirements of EMG equipment are described in detail in the report of the committee on EMG instrumentation (Guld et al 1983).

Stimulation

There are two basic types of stimulator: (1) constant-voltage stimulator, which should be capable of delivering up to 250 V: this form of stimulation is satisfactory in most situations, but may be inadequate when electrode and/or skin impedances increase; (2) constant current stimulator, which should provide a current output of up to 100 mA (Guld et al 1983). The latter is preferable as the current remains relatively constant despite minor changes in impedance, which may be detected if current output is simultaneously monitored (Buchthal & Rosenfalck 1966). It is essential that the stimulator is isolated in order to reduce stimulus artefact and this is most conveniently achieved using a shielded isolation transformer (Guld 1960).

The most common form of stimulus is a rectangular pulse, the duration of which may be varied between 0.05 and 1.0 ms. Stimulation is achieved by outflow of current at the cathode (−ve pole) which depolarises the underlying nerve, while at the anode (+ pole) hyperpolarisation of the nerve occurs. The cathode must always be placed nearer to the recording electrodes to avoid the possibility of anodal conduction block. A wide range of stimulus frequencies (0.5–100 Hz) should be available, but for nerve conduction studies a frequency of 1 Hz is usually employed and is well tolerated by the patient.

The optimal site for stimulation of the nerve at each location may found using a submaximal stimulus (usually 3–5 mA at 0.1 ms) and moving the stimulating electrode until a maximal response for that stimulus is obtained. Theoretically, larger-diameter nerve fibres have lower stimulus thresholds than smaller fibres, but in practice the location of nerve fibres in the nerve trunk also influences the order of excitation, with a tendency for those closer to the stimulating electrode to be excited before more distant fibres (McComas et al 1971).

For the purposes of conduction velocity measurement it is essential that the nerve is stimulated supramaximally in order that all the nerve fibres capable of contributing to the response are activated at each stimulus site. This is achieved by increasing the stimulus strength until the evoked muscle or sensory responses are maximal, following which the stimulus is further increased by about 25%. Too high a stimulus intensity, however, may result in spread of the effective stimulus point away from the stimulating cathode towards the recording electrode (Wiederholt 1970), giving erroneously short latencies.

Stimulating electrodes. Peripheral nerves may be stimulated using either surface or near-nerve needle electrodes, both of which have their advantages and disadvantages. Surface electrodes are more convenient, less time-consuming and non-invasive, but provide a less precise stimulus point and generally require higher stimulus intensities which may be uncomfortable. With near-nerve needle electrodes the stimulus point may be more accurately localised and a much lower stimulus strength is needed. They may also be used when the nerve to be stimulated lies deeply (e.g. the sciatic) or when skin resistance is high due to hyperkeratosis. On the other hand, insertion of the needle may cause discomfort and there is a slight risk of injuring the nerve by direct puncture which may produce unpleasant persisting paraesthesiae. Use of needle electrodes also requires more time.

A convenient type of bipolar surface electrode which may be used to stimulate nerve trunks consists of saline-soaked felt pads of 3–5 mm diameter in contact with silver discs mounted 2.5 cm apart in a perspex holder, which may be either hand-held or strapped to the skin. Henriksen (1956) has shown that the effective stimulus point is the centre of the circular electrode. Various kinds of ring electrodes may be used to evoke sensory potentials by stimulation of digital nerves. Dawson (1956) recommends silver strip electrodes 2–4 mm wide covered in salinated lint, although pipe-cleaners soaked in saline perform equally well.

Recording

Recording electrodes. As for stimulation, surface or needle electrodes may be used to record both motor and sensory responses. In the case of motor conduction, surface electrodes are preferable as they avoid the need for needle puncture and pick up from a wider and more representative area of the muscle. The needle electrode records from a restricted region within the muscle and it is possible that the recorded activity may not arise from motor units supplied by the fastest-conducting motor fibres. There is also a tendency for the shape of the response to vary because of slight needle displacements caused by the accompanying mechanical twitch. Needle electrodes have the one advantage of being more selective, enabling the motor response to be isolated to a single muscle. Surface electrodes usually consist of 0.5–1 cm silver discs which are covered with electrode paste and attached to the skin with adhesive tape.

For recording evoked nerve potentials, saline-soaked felt pads of 0.5–1 cm diameter set in silver cups mounted in a perspex holder with a fixed interelectrode distance of 2.5–3 cm are suitable, and may be conveniently applied in line with the underlying nerve trunk. In this situation Gilliatt et al (1965) showed that the interelectrode distance significantly affects the amplitude and duration of the potential. It is therefore important that each laboratory should standardise on one type of recording electrode. Buchthal & Rosenfalck (1966) prefer needle electrodes which consist of stainless steel needles insulated with Teflon to within a short distance of the tip. The active recording electrode is inserted through the skin and positioned as closely as possible to the underlying nerve, while the reference electrode is inserted subcutaneously 2–4 cm perpendicularly to the nerve at the same level as the active electrode. With this arrangement a unipolar recording of the nerve action potential is obtained which gives rather shorter latency values than those obtained by bipolar recording.

Signal averaging

The size of sensory action potentials from normal and pathological nerves may be of the order of 5 μV or less and as a result may not easily be distinguished from noise. Considerable improvement in the signal–to–noise ratio may be obtained using the process of signal averaging, which allows the extraction of these small signals from the background noise. The method is based on the principle that stimulus-linked events will enhance as successive traces summate algebraically, while randomly occurring activity will cancel out. Improvement of the signal–to–noise ratio is a function of the square root of the number of sweeps averaged. Signals as low as 0.03 μV may be detected by averaging 1000 sweeps or more (Singh et al 1974), but such large numbers of stimuli may be unpleasant for the patient, and usually 16–128 sweeps are satisfactory.

METHODS

General

Ideally, the patient and machine should be placed in a screened environment to reduce extraneous electrical interference to a minimum, but satisfactory recordings can often be obtained without these precautions. However, adequate earthing of the patient is essential, using a plate or strap-type electrode placed where possible between the stimulating and recording electrodes to minimise stimulus artefact.

Motor conduction

Motor conduction velocity may be most satisfactorily measured in the median, ulnar, radial, peroneal and posterior tibial nerves which are accessible for stimulation at two or more points along their course. When indicated, the velocity may also be determined in the musculocutaneous, femoral and sciatic nerves. Normally, a small distal muscle supplied by the nerve under study is chosen to record the evoked compound muscle response or 'M response'. The M response represents the summated electrical activity generated by all the motor units following a supramaximal stimulus of the motor nerve.

Placement of the recording electrodes is crucial: it is essential that the active electrode is situated over the region of the end-plate zone in order to identify accurately the onset of the muscle action potential which will have an initial negative deflection. The reference electrode should be placed over the tendon of insertion. Failure to record from the end-plate zone will result in the inclusion of extra time taken for the much slower action-potential conduction in the muscle fibres, and will give an erroneously prolonged terminal latency; this situation may be recognised by an initial positive deflection of the response. A relatively high gain (e.g. 0.2 or 0.5 mV/division) should be used to identify the onset of the potential, while other characteristics of the response including amplitude, duration and shape may be assessed at a gain which allows the display of the whole signal (Fig. 31.1).

With the above recording arrangement the M response is generally biphasic with initial negative and terminal positive phases. The motor terminal latency is measured between the stimulus delivered to the nerve at the most distal point and onset of the muscle potential, and is accounted for by conduction in the tapering nerve trunk and progressively smaller nerve branches, invasion of the nerve terminals and finally transmission across the synapse at the neuromuscular junction. The amplitude, which is usually measured from baseline to negative peak (or peak-to-peak), provides a measure of the volume of active muscle tissue. Duration of the response may be determined between the onset of the negative deflection and final return to baseline of the positive deflection, or be simply defined as the duration of the negative phase. Both the amplitude and duration are influenced by the synchronicity of impulse

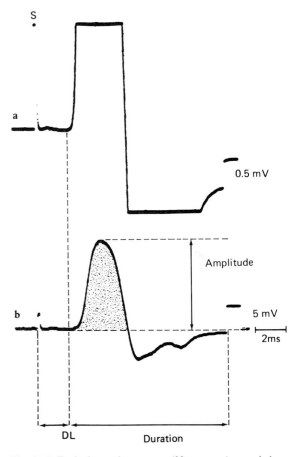

Fig. 31.1 Evoked muscle response (M response) recorded from abductor pollicis brevis in a normal adult: a. an amplifier gain of 0.5 mV/div. and sweep of 2 mV/div. are used for latency measurement; b. measurement of the M response, baseline to negative peak amplitude (or peak-to-peak amplitude) is performed with a gain of 5 mV/div. Estimation of the area of the negative peak requires the use of a computer

conduction in the population of motor axons. A more accurate measurement of the bulk of active muscle tissue may be obtained by estimating the area of the M response, which is now possible with some of the present computer-based systems.

Motor conduction velocity is determined by recording the M response following supramaximal stimulation of the motor nerve at two or more proximal sites. Differences in latency between the onset of these separate responses are determined and the velocities are calculated by dividing the distances between stimulus points by the appro-

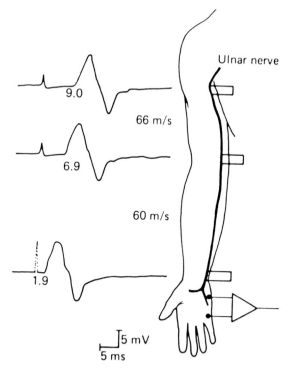

Ulnar nerve

9.0

66 m/s

6.9

60 m/s

1.9

]5 mV
5 ms

Fig. 31.2 Sequence of evoked M responses recorded in hypothenar muscles following stimulation of ulnar nerve at wrist, elbow and axilla, for calculation of the motor conduction velocity in forearm and arm segments in a normal adult. Latencies to onset of the M response at each stimulus site shown, together with the calculated conduction velocities in the intervening segments

priate latency differences (Fig. 31.2). It should be stressed that this procedure gives the maximum motor conduction velocity because the onset of the M response probably represents activity derived from the largest and fastest conducting motor fibres.

Upper limb nerves. For median and ulnar nerves the active recording electrode is placed over the belly of abductor pollicis brevis and abductor digiti minimi respectively, with the reference electrode over the tendon of insertion at the base of the appropriate digit. The nerves may be stimulated at the wrist, elbow, axilla and Erb's point, and the conduction velocity measured over each intervening segment. Spread of the stimulus from median to ulnar nerve, and vice versa when stimulating at the wrist and axilla, may give rise to misleading responses when recording from the

small muscles of the hand. The shape of the muscle response, however, is helpful in avoiding any error of interpretation (Mavor & Libman 1962). Other errors may arise from the anomalous innervation of the intrinsic muscles of the hand (Gassel 1964).

Motor conduction in the radial nerve may be determined by stimulating the nerve above the clavicle and in the mid-arm (Gassel & Diamantopoulos 1964), or in the axilla and 6 cm proximal to the lateral epicondyle of the humerus (Trojaborg & Sindrup 1969), recording the muscle response from brachioradialis or other forearm muscles innervated by the radial nerve.

Lower limb nerves. Conduction velocities in fibres supplying the small muscles of the foot may be tested in the distribution of the common peroneal and posterior tibial nerves. The distal stimulus is applied to the deep peroneal or posterior tibial nerve at the ankle, and the proximal stimulus at the head of the fibula or in the lower popliteal fossa respectively. The muscle action potential is usually recorded from the extensor digitorum brevis or abductor hallucis (Mavor & Atcheson 1966). Conduction rate in the sciatic nerve can also be estimated (Gassel & Trojaborg 1964) using needle electrodes placed deeply in the gluteal region to provide the proximal stimulus.

The F response

Supramaximal stimulation of a peripheral motor nerve, as well as producing a direct M response, often results in a small-amplitude late response of variable latency, amplitude and configuration, which Magladery & McDougal (1950) separated from the H reflex and called the 'F wave' (Fig. 31.3). It is best obtained from the distal muscles of the hand and foot and, in contrast to the latency of the M response, that of the F response decreases as the stimulus is applied more proximally, indicating a centripetal conduction of the impulse before distal transmission.

Despite early controversy surrounding its origins, there can now be little doubt that the F response is produced by recurrent discharges of a few antidromically excited motor neurones

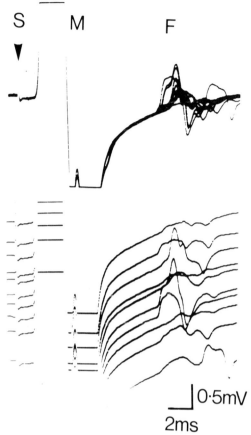

Fig. 31.3 Recordings from abductor pollicis brevis following supramaximal stimulation of the median nerve at the wrist in a normal adult. Note the initial large M response followed by small F responses which show variation of latency and configuration

if not all — of the late responses are recurrent discharges.

Not all motor neurones appear to respond to the antidromic stimulus and, in those that do, the production of an F response is a relatively uncommon event (Schiller & Stålberg 1978, Yates & Brown 1979). On the basis of the amplitude ratio of the F response and M response, it has been estimated that about 1% of the motor neurone pool participates in the production of each F response (Kimura et al 1984). Using the collision technique, Kimura et al (1984) have suggested that F responses occur in both fast- and slow-conducting axons, and hence are generated by a relatively wide spectrum of motor neurone sizes. Fisher (1985) challenges this view and feels that there is selective activation of larger motor neurones with faster-conducting axons. Certainly, the conduction velocities calculated using the earliest F response latencies and the direct M response latencies obtained at two sites of stimulation are almost identical, suggesting that they represent conduction in the same fastest conducting axons.

Generation of the recurrent discharge depends upon a variety of factors, including the ability of the antidromic impulse to depolarise the initial segment of the axon hillock and the time required for repolarisation of the same segment before reinvasion by the soma-dendritic spike (Schiller & Stålberg 1978). This latter critical phase is influenced principally by the balance of excitatory and inhibitory postsynaptic potentials on individual anterior horn cells. Despite this, the chances of an F response occurring with each supramaximal stimulus to the nerve trunk are relatively high, with a frequency of between 50% to 95% in the ulnar nerve in different normal individuals (Peioglou-Harmoussi et al 1985a).

Over recent years, the F response has proved to be of considerable value in the investigation of peripheral nerve disorders, and in particular the examination of conduction in the proximal nerve segment which is inaccessible to conventional nerve conduction techniques. Kimura (1974) first described the method for calculating the conduction velocity in the proximal portion of the nerve using F response latencies, but a number of assumptions upon which the method is based have been questioned by Young & Shahani (1978). The

(Dawson & Merton 1956). The F response can be elicited in a deafferented limb (Mayer & Feldman 1967), and single motor unit studies (Thorne 1965, Trontelj & Trontelj 1973, Schiller & Stålberg 1978) have shown it to occur only when preceded by an identical direct motor unit response. Moreover, on single-fibre EMG the variation in latency of the recurrent responses recorded from single muscle fibres is only slightly greater than that of the direct response from the same fibres (Trontelj 1973), and quite markedly less than that seen in a reflex response (Trontelj et al 1973). Although, with surface recording techniques, reflex components cannot be excluded completely, particularly in the presence of spasticity, it can be assumed that in the resting state and following supramaximal stimulation, most —

latter authors prefer to use the shortest F response latency obtained following stimulation of the nerve at its most distal site to provide a measure of the F response conduction time. This is the time taken for retrograde propagation of the impulse to the cord, turnabout at the cell body and finally orthodromic conduction to the muscle. This latency value is then compared with a nomogram relating F response latency to arm length or height of the individual.

Opinions vary with regard to the number of F responses required to obtain the 'correct' minimal latency value. Lachman et al (1980) suggest that 10 responses are sufficient, while Panayiotopoulos et al (1977) state that at least 20 responses are necessary in order to establish the shortest latency. Even with this sample size, the shortest latency may not be derived from the fastest-conducting axon (Peioglou-Harmoussi et al 1985b). Fisher (1982) suggests that calculation of the mean latency of 10 responses is more reproducible than minimal latency. We feel that a sample of 20 is a satisfactory compromise and is generally well tolerated by most patients. The minimal and maximal latencies are determined for comparison with control data corrected for age and height (Peioglou-Harmoussi et al 1985b).

Increases in F response latency have been found in both axonal and demyelinating types of peripheral neuropathy and have proved more sensitive than maximal motor and sensory conduction velocity measurement in the demonstration of abnormal nerve function (Shahani & Sumner 1981). F response abnormalities have also been reported in cervical and lumbar radiculopathies (Eisen et al 1977a,b).

Other F response parameters. In addition to latency, a number of other characteristics of the F response including frequency, presence and frequency of identical responses, amplitude, duration, and shape have been examined (Shahani & Sumner 1981, Peioglou-Harmoussi et al 1985a,b).

Spectrum of motor axonal velocities

In conventional conduction studies, measurement of the latency to the onset of the evoked muscle action potential results in the conduction velocity being calculated for the fastest-conducting motor fibres. It is possible, in some conditions, that selective involvement of motor axons may occur according to their size, and therefore techniques have been devised to estimate the range of conduction velocities in different sizes of α-fibres within normal and diseased nerves (Thomas et al 1959, Hopf 1963).

These techniques employ the collision principle, and require two independently variable stimuli applied to the nerve at two points — one proximal, the other distal. In the method of Thomas et al (1959), a supramaximal stimulus applied at the proximal site is preceded at a set interval by a gradually increasing distal stimulus. Initially, at low stimulus intensities, low-threshold fast-conducting axons will be excited distally, and the antidromically propagated action potentials will collide with the orthodromic impulses generated at the proximal site in the same axons. Further increases in stimulus intensity lead to occlusion in progressively smaller axons until the process is complete. In the Hopf technique, supramaximal stimuli are applied at both sites and the time interval between the two stimuli is progressively decreased from a point at which there is no interaction to one at which complete blocking occurs. By these means, conduction in the slowest fibres may be assessed as a percentage of the maximal conduction velocity. Thomas et al (1959) found that the majority of motor fibres have conduction velocities within 15–20% of the maximum, although the slowest fibres may conduct at rates of 35–40% below the maximum.

Gilliatt et al (1976) have slightly modified the technique of Thomas et al (1959), stimulating at two sites in the proximal part of the limb instead of one, the conduction velocity being calculated by subtraction in the usual way. The theoretical considerations upon which these methods are based are not entirely beyond dispute, but they do give a reflection of the spectrum of fibre velocities and, by implication, fibre size.

More recently, a further modified version of the collision technique has been proposed which employs, in sequence, a proximal stimulus, distal stimulus and then a second proximal stimulus (Davis et al 1985). As the time interval between the first proximal and the distal stimuli is increased, so an increasing proportion of the axon responses from the second proximal shock are blocked, with a resulting progressive decline in the evoked muscle response. The spectrum of conduction velocities obtained with this technique is smaller than that seen with the other methods.

Sensory nerve conduction

Sensory conduction may be determined in various cutaneous nerves and, consequently, the responses receive no contribution from muscle afferent fibres. The radial, median and ulnar nerves are usually studied in the upper limb, while in the lower limb the sural, medial plantar and superficial peroneal nerves are most suitable.

Characteristics of the sensory potential and measurement of the latency for calculation of the conduction velocity depend on the method for recording. With bipolar surface recording, the volume-conducted response has a triphasic appearance, with a small positive deflection preceding the larger negative depolarisation and a final positive deflection (Fig. 31.4). Gilliatt et al (1965) suggest that the latency should be measured to the onset of the negative deflection, as this represents the arrival of the action potentials in the fastest-conducting fibres at the first electrode.

In the case of monopolar needle recordings, the sensory potential may be biphasic or triphasic with an initial positive deflection (Buchthal & Rosenfalck 1966). Occasionally in normal subjects, and more frequently in pathological nerves, the main component may be followed by much smaller deflections which represent the activity from slower-conducting fibres. Although, theoretically, the latency should be measured to the point where the negative deflection crosses the baseline (Buchthal & Rosenfalck 1966), the initial positive peak is usually taken because it is more easily defined. Gilliatt et al (1965) observed that an accurate estimate of the conduction velocity can be obtained in the segment between the stimulating cathode and active recording electrode, provided that the stimulus is not more than 25% supramaximal. The velocity may also be calculated by the subtraction method, after recording the potential at two sites along the nerve. The size of the potential decreases with increasing distance away from the stimulating site due to dispersion of the action potentials of individual fibres with differing conduction velocities.

The amplitude of the sensory potential recorded with needle electrodes is much larger than the surface-recorded potential, but with both techniques the amplitude is rather variable and, particularly in the case of needle electrodes, sensitive to electrode position.

In the upper limb, conduction in the median, ulnar and radial nerves may be performed with both orthodromic and antidromic techniques (Fig. 31.5). The digital nerve branches of the median and ulnar nerves are stimulated with ring electrodes placed over the first interphalangeal joint, while the recording is made over the mixed nerve trunk at the wrist or elbow (Dawson 1956). Reversal of this stimulation and recording arrangement produces a larger response (Sears 1959), probably because the nerve branches are more superficial. The response also has no initial positive component, and occasionally may be contaminated by volume conduction of simultaneously evoked muscle potentials. The radial nerve is accessible for stimulation and recording at several sites along its course, but usually the cutaneous superficial branch is examined either orthodromically or antidromically in the distal forearm segment (Downie & Scott 1967).

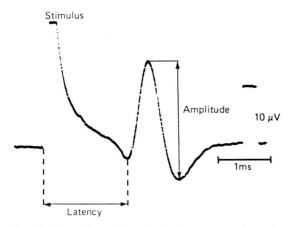

Fig. 31.4 Recording of the orthodromic sensory action potential from the median nerve at the wrist following stimulation of digit I. Latency is measured between stimulus artefact and initial positive peak; amplitude is measured between negative and positive peaks

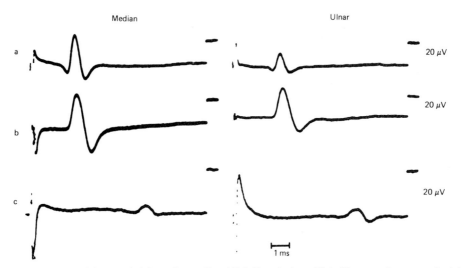

Fig. 31.5 Sensory action potentials recorded from the median (digit I) and ulnar (digit V) nerves in a normal adult: a. stimulus to digit, recording at wrist; b. stimulus to wrist, recording from digit; c. stimulus to digit, recording at elbow. S = stimulus. Calibration: 20 μV, 1 ms

In the lower limb, the medial plantar nerve may be stimulated with ring electrodes applied over the first toe, recording the response over the posterior tibial nerve trunk in the region of the medial malleolus (Mavor & Atcheson 1966, Guiloff & Sherratt 1977). Examination of the sural (Di Benedetto 1970, Burke et al 1974) and superficial peroneal nerves (Di Benedetto 1970) is best achieved antidromically, but because the potentials are often buried in noise, averaging techniques are usually necessary for their retrieval. The above authors have found the use of surface recording electrodes to be quite satisfactory, but Behse & Buchthal (1977) prefer needle recording electrodes and have reported their extensive findings on all of these nerves using this technique.

Di Benedetto (1970) and Burke et al (1974) suggested that measurement of the sensory action potential in the sural nerve may be a more sensitive index of peripheral neuropathy than the sensory potentials in the upper limbs. However, Guiloff & Sherratt (1977) found that changes in the medial plantar sensory action potential was an even more sensitive test of peripheral nerve damage.

Compound nerve action potential

When the median or ulnar nerve is stimulated at the wrist, the compound action potential elicited above the elbow is formed by orthodromic conduction in sensory fibres and antidromic conduction in motor fibres (Fig. 31.6). Dawson (1956) showed that the sensory fibres have a lower threshold and faster conduction rate than motor fibres. In some pathological situations, e.g. severe anterior horn cell disease, it is likely that the residual evoked potential seen at the elbow originates in sensory fibres only. Conduction within the brachial plexus may be assessed by recording potentials above the clavicle from the upper part of the plexus following stimulation of the median, ulnar or radial nerves at the wrist or elbow. This arrangement is particularly employed during cervical and cortical somatosensory potential recordings in order to ensure the integrity of the peripheral nerve pathway.

Conduction velocity distributions

Recently, two methods have been reported for estimating the nerve-fibre conduction-velocity distributions by computer analysis of the compound action potential recorded from nerve trunks. Barker et al (1979) base their technique on analysis of the dispersion components present in two compound action potentials recorded from the same site following stimulation at two points

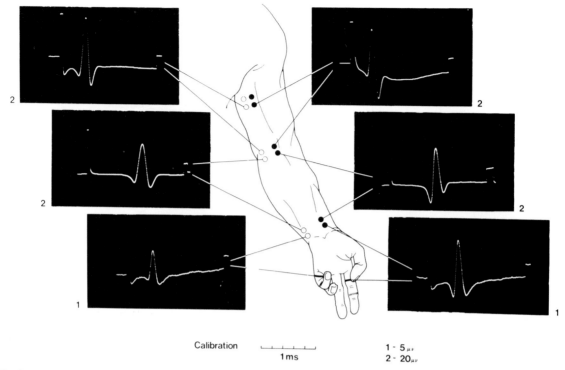

Calibration   1 ms

1 - 5 μν
2 - 20 μν

Fig. 31.6 Normal evoked potentials in the median and ulnar nerves. In each case the stimulus was applied distally and the response was recorded proximally. In the digit to wrist segment the response is purely sensory, while in the other segments the response is derived from sensory and motor fibres, giving the compound nerve action potential

along the nerve. Cummins and colleagues (Cummins et al 1979a,b) have developed a model of the compound action potential in terms of constituent single-fibre action potentials. They have applied this to the study of two compound action potentials separated by a known distance along the nerve, from which they are able to derive an estimate of the distribution of fibre conduction velocities. Both these techniques are extremely complex, requiring sophisticated analysis, and as yet their application in pathological situations is limited (Barker 1981, Cummins et al 1981).

Sources of errors

Problems of measurement and possible sources of errors in the estimation of nerve conduction velocities have been discussed by Mavor & Libman (1962), Gassel (1964), Simpson (1964) and Kimura (1984),

Errors in the measurement of conduction velocity may derive from both technical and biological causes. A number of the former have already been mentioned, including the use of differing stimulus strengths or amplifier gains at the different stimulus sites. It is important to ensure that the oscilloscope sweep is triggering correctly and to check for inaccuracies of the latency calibration.

Measurement of the distance between the two points of stimulation on the surface can be only an approximation of the true length of the underlying nerve, accounting for one of the most significant sources of error. Nevertheless, comparison of surface and true nerve measurement in cadavers has shown a close correlation between the two (Carpendale 1956). This relationship is less certain when the course of the nerve is non-linear, e.g. around the elbow and through the brachial plexus. In the latter situation, measurement of the distance by obstetric calipers may be more accurate than with a surface tape (Jebsen 1967, London 1975). The error of measurement is more significant for shorter distances and care should be taken to ensure that as long a segment as possible — usually more than 10 cm — is examined. In some circumstances, however, inclusion of a long section of normally conducting nerve may conceal the presence of a minor localised conduction defect and estimation of conduction through the affected small segment may be necessary to reveal such a lesion.

Anatomical variations of nerves may also give rise to confusion if their presence is not appreciated. Communication between the median and ulnar nerves in the forearm occurs in 15–31% of the normal population (Buchthal et al 1974, Gutmann 1977), which may lead to simultaneous activation of ulnar-supplied muscles, the volume-conducted potentials of which may interfere with the response from median-innervated muscles. This is particularly apparent in the pres-

ence of a carpal tunnel syndrome (Iyer & Fenichel 1976). The same effect may be seen simply with distant spread of responses arising from more proximally situated muscles (Gassel 1964).

NORMAL FINDINGS

General

Because of variations in technique, it is highly desirable that each laboratory obtains its own control values for each nerve and segment of nerve. Tables 31.1 and 31.2 give a representative sample of results obtained by different authors and show the considerable variation from segment to segment and the wide range of values even within one segment in normal nerves. Several studies have shown conduction to be slower in more distal than proximal segments for both motor and sensory nerves (Gilliatt & Thomas 1960, Trojaborg 1964, Kaeser 1975, Peioglou-

Table 31.1 Normal values for motor conduction velocity in different nerves

Nerve and segment	No. of examinations	Conduction velocity (m/s) mean	Conduction velocity (m/s) range	Distal latency ms mean	Reference
Median					
Er-A	21	65.1	57.1–76.2	3.9	Ginzburg et al 1978
A-E	15	71.1	60.3–86.4	3.3	Mavor & Libman 1962
A-E (R)	58	69	(SD 6.5)		Peioglou-Harmoussi et al 1985a
E-W (R)	58	58	(SD 4.5)	3.5 (SD 0.35)	Peioglou-Harmoussi et al 1985a
E-W	145	58.8		3.5	Mulder et al 1961
Ulnar					
Er-A	22	63.0	55.0–73.2	3.5	Ginzburg et al 1978
Er-above E	30	58.9	50.0–67.7		London 1975
A-E	47	63.8			Trojaborg 1977
A-E (R)	64	68	(SD 6.8)		Peioglou-Harmoussi et al 1985a
E-W (R)	64	57	(SD 5.1)	2.7 (SD 0.32)	Peioglou-Harmoussi et al 1985a
E-W	225	59.9		2.7	Mulder et al 1961
Radial					
A-E	9	70.0	(SD 4.9)	2.5 (to brachioradialis)	Trojaborg & Sindrup (1969)
Sciatic	29	56.0	(SD 5.5)	5.4 (to soleus)	Gassel & Trojaborg 1964
Common peroneal	41	50.2	30.0–60.0	5.0	Mulder et al 1961
	172	50.1	(SD 7.2)		Johnson & Olsen 1960
Posterior tibial	12	48.7	(SD 3.5)	5.0	Mavor & Atcheson 1966
	30	43.2	(SD 4.9)		Thomas et al 1959

Er = Erb's point; A = axilla; E = elbow; W = wrist; (R) = right;
SD = standard deviation

Table 31.2 Normal values for sensory conduction velocity in different nerves

Nerve and segment	No. of examinations	Age (years)	Conduction velocity (m/s)	Amplitude (μV)	Reference
Median					
digit II to wrist (S)	76	10–72	56.2 (SD 6.8)	18.6 (SD 8.8)	Fawcett et al 1982
digit II to wrist (N)	13	18–25	50.2 (SD 5.2)	—	Buchthal & Rosenfalck 1966
wrist to elbow (N)	10	70–88	44.1 (SD 3.6)	—	Rosenfalck 1966
	9	18–25	63.9 (SD 5.1)	—	
Ulnar					
digit V to wrist (S)	59	19–76	55.1 (SD 5.7)	15.4 (SD 7.1)	Fawcett et al 1982
digit V to wrist (N)	9	18–25	51.9 (SD 5.6)	—	Buchthal & Rosenfalck 1966
	10	70–89	50.2 (SD 3.7)	—	
wrist to elbow (N)	9	18–25	63.9 (SD 5.1)	—	
Radial					
digit I to wrist (S)	23	16–28	58 (SD 6.0)	13 (SD 7.5)	Trojaborg & Sindrup 1969
wrist to elbow (S)	19	16–28	64 (SD 6.0)	31 (SD 11.7)	Sindrup 1969
Superficial peroneal					
big toe to above (N)	19	15–25	46.1 (SD 4.1)	1.2	Behse & Buchthal 1971
extensor retinaculum	17	40–65	42.2 (SD 6.3)	0.5	
Posterior tibial					
big toe to (S)	11	20–29	34.9 (SD 2.6)	3.0 (SD 2.3)	Guiloff & Sherratt 1977
medial malleolus	13	50–59	33.5 (SD 3.8)	1.7 (SD 0.6)	
big toe to (N)	23	15–30	46.1 (SD 3.5)	—	Behse & Buchthal 1971
medial malleolus	10	40–65	43.4 (SD 3.8)	—	
Sural					
calf to lateral (S)	26	21–40	46.2 (SD 3.7)	16.4 (SD 5.5)	Burke et al 1974
malleolus	23	41–60	46.4 (SD 3.7)	13.6 (SD 7.5)	Fawcett et al 1982
	34	17–52	49.5 (SD 4.3)	34.3 (SD 9.9)	
dorsum of foot to (N)	16	15–30	51.2 (SD 4.5)	—	Behse & Buchthal 1971
lateral malleolus	15	40–65	48.3 (SD 5.3)	—	

S = Surface recording electrodes; N = needle recording electrodes

Harmoussi et al 1985b). Conduction velocity is directly related to fibre diameter by a factor of about 6 ms/μm (Hursch 1939), and therefore part of the distal slowing can be attributed to progressive tapering of axons (Magladery & McDougal 1950). A slight but significant decline in limb temperature distally may also be a contributory factor. Velocities are faster in the shorter upper-limb than longer lower-limb nerves, while a general inverse relationship between conduction velocity and height has been established in an adult control population (Campbell et al 1981).

Variations due to age

Various studies (Thomas & Lambert 1960, Gamstorp 1963, Baer & Johnson 1965, Gamstorp & Shelburne 1965) have shown that conduction velocity in motor fibres at birth is only about one half of that in adults. After an initial rapid increase in the first year, the velocity more gradually approaches that of adults by three to five years, with further more complex patterns of changes in velocity occuring in later childhood and adolescence (Lang et al 1985). The rate of increase in conduction velocity varies in different nerves, and appears to depend upon maturation of the axon, the process of myelination and the actual length of the nerve (Lang et al 1985).

Slowing of conduction in motor fibres with increasing age in adult life has been demonstrated by several authors (Norris et al 1953, Mulder et al 1961). Buchthal & Rosenfalck (1966) observed a significant decrease in sensory conduction velocity in upper arm and forearm segments and also an increase in distal latency with advancing age; in addition, they, and more recently

Andersen (1985), have noted a reduction of the amplitude and increase in duration of the sensory evoked response.

Effects of temperature

Studies by Henriksen (1956) and Johnson & Olsen (1960) in motor fibres, and by Buchthal & Rosenfalck (1966) in the larger sensory fibres, show that conduction rate slows with cooling by a factor of 2–2.4 ms/°C. Cooling also results in prolongation of the terminal motor latency (Fig. 31.7), and less well-appreciated changes in the muscle and nerve action potential, the amplitude and duration of which increase as the temperature falls (Denys 1977, Bolton et al 1981). In order to minimise the effect of temperature, the laboratory should be warm and the skin temperature should be maintained at about 34 °C either by prior immersion in warm water or with a heating lamp. Particular

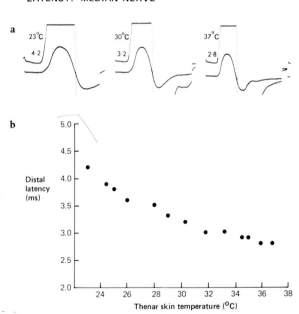

EFFECT OF TEMPERATURE ON DISTAL MOTOR LATENCY. MEDIAN NERVE

a

23°C 4·2

30°C 3·2

37°C 2·8

b

Distal latency (ms)

5.0
4.5
4.0
3.5
3.0
2.5
2.0

24 26 28 30 32 34 36 38

Thenar skin temperature (°C)

Fig. 31.7 Relationship between temperature and the distal latency, amplitude and duration of the M response recorded from the thenar muscles following stimulation of the median nerve at the wrist in a normal adult. Note (in b) the progressive increase in latency as the overlying skin temperature falls from 37 °C to 23 °C. Associated with this (a) there is an increase in both the amplitude and duration of the M response

care is required if the course of a progressive or recovering neuropathy is being monitored by repeated measurements in the same patient at different times, when accurate temperature control is essential.

ABNORMAL NERVE CONDUCTION

General considerations

The last two decades have seen considerable advances in our understanding of the major factors which determine impulse conduction in myelinated nerve fibres, and the ways in which pathological changes may influence this foremost of nerve functions (Rasminsky & Sears 1972, Bostock & Sears 1978, Waxman 1980, McDonald 1980, Sumner 1980). A number of studies have compared structural and electrophysiological changes in the nerve in various forms of neuropathy (Lambert & Dyck 1975, Behse & Buchthal 1977, Buchthal & Behse 1977, Behse et al 1977, Bolton et al 1979b), and while comparison of morphological aspects based on short segments of nerve with conduction characteristics obtained over a much longer segment may lead to inconsistencies, much valuable information has resulted from this type of study. Gilliatt (1966) has suggested that peripheral neuropathies can be separated into two groups according to the nerve conduction findings, which can be correlated pathologically with primary axonal degeneration and segmental demyelination. Although most neuropathies can be categorised in this manner, it has become increasingly clear that a combination of both these features may be present in most neuropathies (Thomas 1971), reflecting a close functional relationship between axons and Schwann cells. Nevertheless, one or other process may predominate, and in broad terms relatively distinctive patterns of changes in clinical nerve conduction may be observed.

Axonal degeneration

Axonal disruption following direct nerve section results in Wallerian degeneration of the distal nerve portion. The earliest detectable change in motor nerves is failure of neuromuscular transmission (Miledi & Slater 1970), with little or no significant slowing of conduction in the motor fibres distal to the interruption for several days, after which conduction fails abruptly (Gilliatt & Taylor 1959, Gilliatt & Hjorth 1972). In many conditions, axonal degeneration occurs in a centripetal fashion, producing a 'dying-back' neuropathy (Cavanagh 1964), suggesting that the 'sick' parent cell body is unable to sustain the most distal portions of the long axon. In some hexacarbon-induced neuropathies, abnormalities appear to occur simultaneously at numerous sites along the distal part of the axon, giving rise to the term distal axonopathy (Spencer & Schaumburg 1979).

Nerve conduction in axonal neuropathies is usually only minimally slowed, but is accompanied by a reduction in the size of either the evoked muscle response or nerve action potential, proportionate to the loss of functioning axons. In experimental acrylamide neuropathy, a 20% reduction in the maximum motor conduction velocity may occur, which has been attributed to selective loss of the largest and . fastest-conducting axons (Fullerton & Barnes 1966, Hopkins & Gilliatt 1971). More usually a wider spectrum of fibre sizes is involved by the degenerative process (Walsh & McLeod 1970, Behse & Buchthal 1977), and a sufficient number of large-diameter axons remain, so that the maximum velocity is little affected. With increasing severity of the neuropathy the velocity may decline further, but not to the degree seen with demyelination, and the evoked nerve or muscle potential may be lost.

One consequence of the dying-back process is that conduction slowing may be first detected in the most distal portions of the nerves, when velocity in more proximal segments is normal (Casey & Le Quesne 1972). Because of the relatively minor changes in conduction and wide range of evoked response amplitudes in normal nerves and muscle, measurement of maximal conduction velocity is a rather insensitive method for identifying axonal neuropathies, particularly in the early stages. Determination of F-response latency may improve the diagnostic yield (Shahani & Sumner 1981), while EMG examination of the muscle for evidence of denervation is an essential part of the investigation. Serial studies may reveal a progressive decline in velocity and response amplitude, even though the values remain within the normal range.

Demyelinating disorders

Disorders of the myelin sheath resulting in either paranodal or segmental demyelination produce much more dramatic changes in conduction than are seen in axonal neuropathies. Such changes may take the form either of marked slowing of conduction, usually by more than 30% of their normal value to as low as 7 m/s, or of conduction block. Terminal latencies are often strikingly prolonged, sometimes up to 35 ms, and the duration of the evoked response is often increased, particularly following proximal stimulation. Conduction block may be recognised by a reduction in the amplitude of the evoked response elicited from proximal sites. Lewis & Sumner (1982) recommend that the proximal response should be 50% or less of the amplitude following more distal stimulation in order to differentiate conduction block from the effects of impulse dispersion in variably affected nerve fibres, which may result in phase cancellation of responses from individual motor units.

The pathophysiological mechanisms relating conduction slowing or block and demyelination have been reviewed in detail by McDonald (1980). Loss or thinning of myelin in the region of nodes of Ranvier or internodal segments leads to a reduction in resistive and increase in capacitive properties across the nerve fibre. This has the effect of reducing the longitudinal electrotonic flow of current preceding the active action potential, thereby delaying excitation at the next node or, if severe enough, resulting in failure of excitation and block of conduction. Experimental studies have revealed that segmental demyelination may, in certain circumstances, be associated with continuous rather than saltatory conduction through an affected segment, in which case conduction is markedly slowed (Bostock & Sears 1978). Whether this occurs in diseased human nerve is not known.

In addition to slowing of impulse propagation, demyelination renders the nerve fibre even more sensitive to changes in temperature. Rasminsky (1973) has shown that even slight increases of temperature within the physiological range can result in block of impulse conduction through demyelinated segments. The refractory period is also prolonged (Lehmann et al 1971), leading to a reduction in the capacity of the fibre to transmit repetitive trains of stimuli causing intermittent failure of conduction.

DISEASES OF THE ANTERIOR HORN CELL

Degeneration of the anterior horn cell occurs in a number of disorders including poliomyelitis, spinal muscular atrophy in its various forms, motor neurone disease (MND) and syringomyelia. Muscle atrophy, in e.g. motor neurone disease and syringomyelia, may often begin in a focal manner and, while the clinical findings may point to a central lesion, patients are seen occasionally in whom it is not possible to exclude a disturbance of the peripheral nerves on clinical grounds. It is therefore important to know whether diseases involving the anterior horn cell have an effect on peripheral nerve function, other than the consequential loss of motor axons.

Henriksen (1956) found only minor degrees of slowing amounting to no more than 10% in patients with poliomyelitis, provided that allowance was made for the lower temperature in the paretic limb. Similarly, Lambert & Mulder (1957), Lambert (1962), Willison (1962) and Ertekin (1967) found maximal motor conduction velocity was within the normal range in most patients with motor neurone disease. Mild slowing of conduction was seen in those cases with severe muscular atrophy with correspondingly small M-response amplitudes, consistent with the loss of the fastest-conducting axons (Lambert & Mulder 1957, Hansen & Ballantyne 1978).

Using the Hopf technique, Miglietta (1968) and Chaco (1970) found that the range of conduction velocities in MND was narrowed, suggesting perhaps an early loss of the slower-conducting and therefore smaller axons. Hausmanowa-Petrusewicz & Kopec (1973) observed the same phenomenon in very severe cases, but in early cases the spectrum of velocities was normal, while it was increased due to slowing of the minimum conduction velocity value in an intermediate group. Ingram et al (1985) also found abnormal

conduction velocity distributions in most cases, initially with slowing of conduction in some fibres, progressing eventually to involve all fibres in advanced patients. None of these studies has shown any evidence of preferential involvement of a particular class of anterior horn cell by the disease process in MND.

Recent F-response studies in patients with MND (Peioglou-Harmoussi 1983) have shown occasional increases in minimum latency and more often maximum latency of 20 F responses in median and ulnar nerves. This suggests either impaired conduction in surviving axons, or because the longest-latency response was more frequently abnormal, that changes in central excitability might result in F responses occurring in a population of neurones with slower conduction velocities than is usually seen in control subjects. The presence of an excessive degree of segmental demyelination and remyelination of peripheral nerves in MND (Dayan et al 1969, Hanyu et al 1982) might acccount for the delayed F responses. Peioglou-Harmoussi (1983) also noted a decline in the frequency of F responses, particularly in later stages when the muscles were markedly atrophic. Nevertheless, the frequency with which individual F responses occurred was increased, probably as a result of enhanced excitability in the remaining motor neurone pool due to upper motor neurone involvement. The amplitude of the F response is generally slightly increased, reflecting an increase in size of surviving motor units following collateral reinnervation (Argyropoulos et al 1978, Peioglou-Harmoussi 1983).

Several studies have shown normal sensory potentials and mixed nerve action potentials in motor neurone disease (Willison 1962, Fincham & Van Allen 1964, Ertekin 1967) and this finding will help to exclude a peripheral nerve lesion in patients presenting with muscle wasting. Others (Brown & Jaatoul 1974, Stålberg 1982, Peioglou-Harmoussi 1983) have demonstrated a reduction in sensory potential amplitudes and slowing of sensory conduction in some patients, which suggests that the degenerative process may not be restricted to the motor system.

Motor conduction velocity is normal in most patients with juvenile and adult onset spinal muscular atrophy (SMA) (Gardner-Medwin et al 1967, Meadows et al 1969, Buchthal & Olsen

1970, O'Sullivan & McLeod 1978, Harding & Thomas 1980a). Excluding cases with the distal form of SMA, the amplitude of the response evoked from intrinsic hand and foot muscles is usually within normal limits (personal observation), consistent with the predominant involvement of proximal muscle groups. Sensory conduction velocities and action-potential amplitudes are also usually normal (O'Sullivan & McLeod 1978, Harding & Thomas 1980a), although Swift (1984) has observed abnormal sensory conduction in some juvenile-onset cases. Nevertheless, the generally normal findings help to distinguish the distal form of SMA from the axonal variant of peroneal muscular atrophy (HMSN type II).

Motor conduction in infantile SMA (SMA types I, II) may be normal or slightly reduced according to the degree of muscle wasting (Hausmanowa-Petrusewicz et al 1975). Swift (1984) has also noted impaired sensory conduction in some of the infantile-onset group.

In syringomyelia, several studies have reported normal motor and sensory conduction velocities (Fincham & Cape 1968, Schwartz et al 1980, Peioglou-Harmoussi 1983), except when there is marked muscular atrophy and loss of larger neurones. Patients are at risk of developing ulnar nerve lesions at the elbow in relation to a Charcot arthropathy of the joint (Peioglou-Harmoussi et al 1986). Delayed F responses have been observed in upper limb nerves in which conduction was normal in distal segments (Peioglou-Harmoussi et al 1986), suggesting either minor traumatic damage to the peripheral nerves, or abnormalities of the intraspinal portion of the motor nerve fibres and anterior horn cells. Normal sensory findings help to confirm that the characteristic sensory impairment seen in these individuals is due to a lesion in the sensory pathways which is proximal to the dorsal root ganglion.

PRIMARY MUSCLE DISEASES

Motor and sensory conduction is usually normal in patients with primary diseases of muscle, particularly in the Duchenne, Becker, limb-girdle and facioscapulohumeral forms of muscular dystrophy (Sica & McComas 1971, Panayiotopoulos & Scarpalezos 1977, Hilton-Brown & Stålberg 1983, personal observations). Conduction is also normal in hereditary distal myopathy (Sumner et al 1971), helping to distinguish this rare disorder from the more common hereditary motor and sensory neuropathies.

Reduction in motor conduction velocity has been reported in some patients with myotonic dystrophy (Mongia & Lundervold 1975, Olson et al 1978, Panayotopoulos 1978). Using the Hopf technique, Rossi et al (1983) were able to show slowing of both maximal and minimal velocities, implying that the whole spectrum of fibres was affected. There was no evidence of preferential involvement of smaller motor neurones supplying type I motor units which might have been expected from the histopathological findings of selective atrophy of type I muscle fibres (Brooke & Engel 1969). Abnormal peripheral sensory conduction has also been demonstrated by somatosensory evoked potential studies (Mongia & Lundervold 1975, Bartel et al 1984). These findings suggest the peripheral nerve abnormality may be part of the more generalised disturbance of cellular function seen in this disorder.

While nerve conduction studies have been reported as normal in the vast majority of patients with mitochondrial myopathy, slight reductions in the motor and sensory velocities have occasionally been found, consistent with an axonal neuropathy (Spiro et al 1970, Berenberg et al 1977, Bertorini et al 1978, Markesbery 1979). More marked slowing of conduction has been described in other cases (Shy et al 1966, Drachman 1968, Peyronnard et al 1979) indicating a demyelinating neuropathy. The latter authors suggest that the mitochondrial abnormality may also impair Schwann cell function, leading to a disturbance of myelin formation and axon maintenance. In a recent study, Yiannikas & McLeod (1985) found neurophysiological evidence of a peripheral neuropathy in 45% of 20 cases of mitochondrial myopathy, suggesting more frequent involvement of the peripheral nerves than has been suspected. It should be noted, however, that in some cases of familial mitochondrial myopathy there is an increased incidence of diabetes mellitus (Mechler et al 1981) which may account for the peripheral neuropathy (Fawcett et al 1982).

A decrease in motor conduction velocity was reported in one patient with myopathic carnitine deficiency which was associated with an abnormal accumulation of lipid droplets in Schwann cells (Markesbery et al 1974).

PERIPHERAL NEUROPATHIES

General considerations

The presentation of peripheral nerve disorders varies according to the nature and distribution of the abnormalities within the nerves. The principal clinical patterns seen include isolated lesions in individual nerves (mononeuropathy), isolated lesions in two or more separate nerves (mononeuropathy multiplex), or diffuse involvement of the peripheral nerves (polyneuropathy).

Compressive lesions of individual nerves, e.g. the median nerve within the carpal tunnel and the ulnar nerve at the elbow, are common and may occur in isolation or complicating a more generalised disturbance of the peripheral nerves. Predominant involvement of the nerve roots is seen in some cases of acquired inflammatory neuropathy (see below) and in cervical and lumbar spondylosis. Isolated lesions in nerve trunks, referred to above, may be associated with axonal degeneration, e.g. in the neuropathy of polyarteritis nodosa and in some cases of diabetes mellitus. Rarely, focal demyelination sufficient to produce conduction block may present in this manner. Thus, by appropriate assessment of nerve conduction velocity and nerve and muscle response characteristics in different peripheral nerves, the examiner may not only identify the presence of abnormal peripheral nerve function, but may also provide information which is of primary diagnostic value.

Axonal neuropathies

Axonal degeneration represents the main pathological change in a large proportion of peripheral neuropathies. Included in this group are the neuropathies associated with diabetes mellitus, uraemia, chronic alcoholism, carcinoma, primary amyloidosis, porphyria, malnutrition and vitamin deficiency, toxic chemicals and drugs, including some used in anticancer therapy. The axon is primarily affected in the type II variant of HMSN, and in Friedreich's ataxia.

Demyelinating neuropathies

Segmental demyelination occurs as the principal pathological change in a number of neuropathies, including acute or subacute inflammatory polyradiculoneuropathy or the Guillain–Barré syndrome, chronic inflammatory polyneuropathy, the hypertrophic form of Charcot–Marie–Tooth disease (HMSN type I) and the neuropathies of Dejerine–Sottas disease, Refsum's disease, metachromatic leukodystrophy, Krabbe's leukodystrophy, hereditary neuropathies with liability to pressure palsy, some cases of diabetic and myeloma neuropathy and the neuropathies associated with para-proteinaemia and leprosy.

The electrophysiological changes in some of these specific neuropathies are described in more detail below.

Diabetic neuropathy may present in various forms, with consequently different patterns of nerve conduction abnormalities. Several studies have revealed slowing of motor and sensory conduction in those with and, to a lesser extent, those without clinical evidence of neuropathy (Downie & Newell 1961, Lawrence & Locke 1961, Mulder et al 1977, Gilliatt & Willison 1962, Behse et al 1977), the changes being more marked in the lower-limb nerves. Some patients have a mononeuropathy of either the median, ulnar or common peroneal nerves at common sites of compression, with local slowing of conduction in the affected segment (Mulder et al 1961, Gilliatt & Willison 1962), conduction in the remaining nerves being normal or borderline.

Slowing of motor conduction in the lower limbs and delayed F-response latencies (Dyck et al 1985) have been reported to be the earliest changes, while Lamontagne & Buchthal (1970) found abnormalities of the sensory potentials and the presence of fibrillation potentials in distal muscles to be sensitive indicators of a subclinical neuropathy. These latter findings reflect axonal degeneration (Thomas & Lascelles, 1966, Behse et al 1977, Hansen & Ballantyne 1977) which may be particularly marked in chronic cases, leading to loss of the evoked potentials. Nevertheless, slowing of conduction is mainly accounted for by segmental demyelination and remyelination (Thomas & Lascelles 1966, Chopra et al 1969, Behse et al 1977).

Uraemic polyneuropathy. Peripheral nerve abnormalities are a well-recognised complication of chronic renal failure, usually taking the form of a mixed sensorimotor neuropathy. Moderate slowing of motor and sensory conduction occurs in both proximal and distal nerve segments of upper and lower limbs (Neilsen 1973a). Conduction changes may precede clinical symptoms (Preswick & Jeremy 1964, Jennekens et al 1971, Neilsen 1973b), while the degree of slowing is correlated with a reducing creatinine clearance and the duration of renal failure (Jennekens et al 1971, Neilsen 1973b).

Improved nerve conduction may lag behind clinical improvement following the institution of haemodialysis (Konatey-Ahulu 1965, Tenckhoff 1965, Neilsen 1974b), whereas renal transplantation usually results in considerable amelioration of both clinical and electrophysiological findings (Neilsen 1974a). Neilsen (1974a) found significant increases in conduction within weeks of transplantation, and suggests that this rapid change may reflect a restoration of the normal axon membrane potential, although early remyelination could not be excluded. A secondary, more protracted, phase of recovery was thought to be due to axonal regeneration, correlating with the main histological findings of axonal damage with secondary segmental demyelination (Dyck et al 1971a, Thomas et al 1971).

Recently, the creation of forearm and antebrachial arteriovenous fistulas have been reported to be associated with localised neuropathies of the median nerve at the wrist or forearm and ulnar nerve at the elbow (Warren & Otieno 1975, Harding & Le Fanu 1977, Bolton et al 1979a, Hamilton et al 1980, Knezevic & Mastaglia 1984).

The mechanism(s) by which these lesions are produced is uncertain, but ischaemia due to shunting of the blood away from forearm tissues distal to the fistula and increased venous pressure leading to venous congestion and oedema have been proposed. It is also possible that aneurysmal dilatation of forearm veins may lead to localised nerve compression, particularly at the usual sites of entrapment beneath tendons or fascial bands (Knezevic & Mastaglia 1984).

Alcoholic polyneuropathy. Mild to moderate slowing of motor and sensory conduction (Mawdsley & Mayer 1965, Walsh & McLeod 1970, Behse & Buchthal 1977) and increased F-response latencies (Lefebvre-D'Amour et al 1979) have been demonstrated in alcoholic patients with and without clinical features of peripheral nerve disease. Changes are present in upper and lower limb nerves, but tend to be more pronounced in the lower extremities and in the most distal portions of the nerves (Casey & Le Quesne 1972). Histological findings in sural nerve biopsies (Walsh & McLeod 1970, Behse & Buchthal 1977) indicate axonal degeneration of large and small fibres, which accounts for the main electrophysiological abnormality of a reduction in the sensory potential amplitude with only slight slowing of the maximal conduction velocity. Behse & Buchthal (1977) were unable to find any evidence of vitamin deficiency in their patients and concluded that the neuropathy was the result of a direct neurotoxic effect of alcohol.

Paraneoplastic neuropathy. Several studies have shown impairment of sensory and motor conduction in a small proportion of patients with various underlying neoplasms (Moody 1965, Trojaborg et al 1969, Walsh 1971, Campbell & Paty 1974). Generally only mild slowing of conduction was seen, a reduction in the amplitude of the sensory response (Walsh 1971, Campbell & Paty 1974) or the presence of fibrillation potentials (Trojaborg et al 1969) being the main changes. These features suggested principally axonal degeneration, with secondary segmental demyelination occurring only at a late stage (Campbell & Paty 1974). In patients with primary sensory neuropathy, first described by Denny-

Brown (1948), the sensory action potentials are absent and the motor velocities are generally normal (Horwich et al 1977).

A study on patients with bronchial carcinoma (Lenman et al 1981) showed only a slight but significant impairment of motor conduction velocity in the group as a whole, whereas rather more marked abnormalities of sensory conduction were found. EMG changes of fibrillations or positive sharp waves were recorded in just under half the patients and tended to be more pronounced in distal muscles, suggesting a 'dying back' process. A slight but significant improve ment in conduction was observed in a group of patients who had undergone successful treatment of their carcinoma.

Amyloid neuropathy. The neuropathy associ- ated with primary systemic amyloidosis and inherited amyloidosis has been reported to be axonal in nature. Nerve conduction studies in the vast majority showed only minimal slowing of motor conduction and small or more usually absent sensory responses, while EMG revealed fibrillation activity in distal lower limb muscles (Kelly et al 1979).

Myeloma neuropathy. Nerve conduction velocities in patients with myeloma neuropathy in the absence of amyloid showed moderate slowing of mainly motor conduction, consistent with an axonal sensorimtor neuropathy (Kelly et al 1981). In patients with the sclerotic variety of myeloma, motor conduction was moderately to severely slowed, the evoked muscle responses were mark- edly reduced and the EMG showed fibrillation activity. The sensory velocities were moderately slowed and the responses small or absent, indi- cating a mixture of axonal degeneration and demyelination (Kelly et al 1981).

Neuropathy associated with parapro- teinaemia. Some patients with benign IgM and IgG paraproteinaemia develop a chronic, slowly progressive sensorimotor neuropathy with moderate to marked slowing of motor conduction and absent sensory action potentials in the majority of cases, indicating demyelination (Swash et al 1979, Dalakas & Engel 1981, Smith et al 1983).

Drug-induced and toxic neuropathies. Numerous drugs have been implicated as the cause of peripheral neuropathy, and the reader is referred to Chapter 29 which deals with this topic. In most drug-induced neuropathies in which nerve conduction studies have been performed, mild to moderate slowing of motor and sensory conduc- tion have been observed, consistent with axonal damage, e.g. neuropathies caused by nitrofuran- toin (Toole et al 1968), metronidazole (Bradley et al 1977a), misonidazole (Mamoli et al 1979), disul- firam (Bradley & Hewer 1966), vincristine (Bradley et al 1970, Casey et al 1973) and phenytoin (Lovelace & Horowitz 1968, Eisen et al 1974, Chokroverty & Sayeed 1975). The neur- opathy associated with dapsone appears to be purely motor, with normal or slightly reduced motor conduction together with EMG changes of denervation and normal sensory action potentials (Gutmann et al 1976).

In contrast to the above drug-induced neur- opathies, that produced by perhexiline maleate is associated with moderate to severe slowing of motor conduction and reduction or loss of sensory evoked potentials (Bousser et al 1976, Said 1978), indicative of demyelination.

Nearly all neuropathies associated with exogenous chemical toxins such as heavy metals, solvents, organophosphates etc. are axonal in nature (Cohen 1970) and are accompanied by minor changes in motor and sensory conduction. An important exception to this general finding is seen in the neuropathy induced by n-hexane which is a constituent of many adhesive agents. 'Glue- sniffing' has become an all-too-common habit in many countries and accounts for an increasing number of young people presenting with neur- opathy. Nerve biopsy studies have revealed striking focal axonal swellings and accumulation of neurofilaments, together with thinning of the overlying myelin and widening of the nodes of Ranvier (Korobkin et al 1975). Motor conduction has been found to be moderately slowed consistent with the abnormal myelination.

The Guillain–Barré syndrome

The pattern of nerve conduction changes may show considerable variation in patients presenting with this disorder, and the findings in any one patient may differ according to the time interval between the onset of the neuropathy and the neurophysiological examination (Albers et al 1985). Usually there is slowing of motor conduction to about 60–70% of normal in one or more nerves. Proximal and distal segments may be affected to roughly the same extent (Kimura & Butzer 1975, King & Ashby 1976) although in some patients slowing may be patchy (Isch et al 1964) or most pronounced in common sites of nerve compression such as the carpal or cubital tunnel (Lambert & Mulder 1964, Eisen & Humphreys 1974). Prolonged distal motor latencies in the presence of normal or only slightly reduced conduction velocities may be the only abnormality in a proportion of patients. Figure 31.8 shows the motor and sensory conduction findings in a patient with Guillain–Barré syndrome of recent onset.

Although slowing may be present early in the illness, it may not be apparent until after the condition has reached its peak. A number of studies (Lambert & Mulder 1964, McQuillen 1971, Eisen & Humphrreys 1974, Albers et al 1985) have shown normal motor conduction in distal segments in about 10–20% of cases. However, using the F-response conduction technique to examine velocity over the proximal segments including the roots, Kimura & Butzer (1975) and King & Ashby (1976) showed significant slowing restricted to this segment in some patients. Ambler et al (1985) also found delayed or absent F responses to be the most sensitive parameter for detecting abnormal conduction in the early stages of the disease.

Evidence of conduction block is frequently seen in the acquired inflammatory demyelinating neuropathies and, together with multifocal conduction slowing, helps to distinguish this group from the familial demyelinating neuropathies (Lewis & Sumner 1982). In some cases with the chronic form of the disorder, the clinical presentation may be in the pattern of a mononeuropathy multiplex due to the multifocal nature of the conduction block. In the acute form Ambler et al (1985) observed a reduction in M-response amplitude following proximal stimulation in a large proportion of cases, which they attributed

to conduction block and/or temporal dispersion. Mills & Murray (1985), employing the recently introduced technique of direct percutaneous spinal cord stimulation, reported conduction block in the most proximal nerve segments in two cases of Guillain–Barré syndrome. Although the electrophysiological finding of reduced conduction velocity correlates well with the predominantly demyelinating nature of the defect (Arnason 1984), a significant proportion of patients may demonstrate fibrillations and positive sharp waves in the EMG, indicating axonal damage.

Sensory nerve conduction changes tend to be less marked and more variable than the motor findings, being normal or only slightly altered in distal nerve segments in milder cases. The distribution of affected nerves is often unusual for a polyneuropathy, with abnormal median and ulnar nerve responses but normal or relatively spared radial and sural nerve responses (see Albers et al 1985 and Fig. 31.8). Abnormalities of the cervical and cortical evoked sensory responses have been reported in the early phase of the disease, suggesting defective conduction in proximal segments despite normal peripheral sensory function. In severe cases, however, distal sensory conduction may be slowed and the responses lost (Bannister & Sears 1962, Eisen & Humphreys 1974, Raman & Taori 1976).

The electrophysiological features may have predictive value, because those patients with no conduction abnormalities tend to recover rapidly within about four weeks (Eisen & Humphreys 1974), whereas those with only slowing of conduction generally take longer. Recovery in the presence of axonal degeneration is more protracted and often incomplete, pronounced residual deficits being more common (Eisen & Humphreys 1974, Raman & Taori 1976). It is important that the latter factor is taken into account when new forms of therapy, e.g. plasmapheresis, are being assessed in this disorder

Neuropathy associated with leprosy

Peripheral nerve involvement is a characteristic feature of leprosy. Electrophysiological changes may be apparent in clinically normal nerves (McLeod et al 1975), or restricted to the enlarged

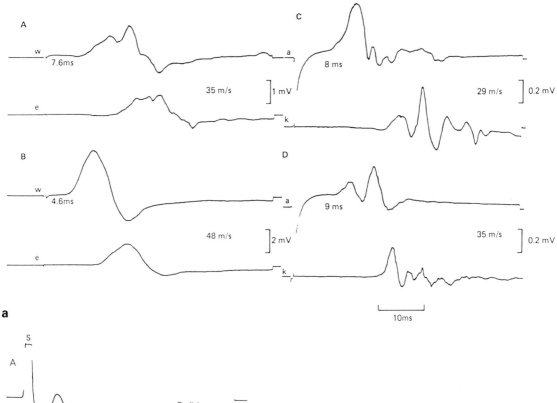

Fig. 31.8 Motor and sensory conduction findings in a 67-year-old woman with the Guillain-Barré syndrome: a. Motor findings in A, median, B, ulnar, C, common peroneal, D, posterior tibial nerves (upper — distal stimulus, lower — proximal stimulus); note the small and dispersed M responses, particularly following proximal stimulation. The large drop in amplitude of the proximal ulnar response suggests conduction block in addition to velocity dispersion. b. Sensory recordings in A, radial, B, median, C, ulnar nerves; the radial response is relatively well preserved in contrast to the absence of responses in the median and ulnar nerves

segments (Swift et al 1973). Slowing of sensory conduction velocity has been found to occur in both tuberculoid and lepromatous leprosy, and velocity measurement in the superficial radial nerve has been proposed as a sensitive index of peripheral nerve involvement (Sebille 1978). Slowing of motor conduction velocities also occurs (Hackett et al 1968), and these conduction findings correlate with the principal pathological changes of segmental demyelination (Shetty et al 1977).

Hereditary motor and sensory neuropathies (HMSN)

Types I and II (Charcot–Marie–Tooth disease, peroneal muscular atrophy). Early studies of motor conduction velocity in this disorder revealed considerable slowing to about half the normal value or less (Gilliatt & Thomas 1957, Amick & Lemmi 1963, Dyck et al 1963). However, later reports on patients with a similar clinical picture showed some to have normal or only slightly reduced motor conduction velocities (Earl & Johnson 1963). This was confirmed by Dyck & Lambert (1968), who separated two main groups on the basis of clinical, genetic, electrophysiological and histological findings — a hypertrophic group with slowed conduction, and a neuronal group with virtually normal conduction. Thomas & Calne (1974) also found that their patients displayed a bimodal distribution of the median motor conduction velocity with a cut-off point at about 40 m/s. By contrast, others have observed a wide spectrum of motor conduction velocity (Salisachs 1974, Brust et al 1978) or have found evidence of an intermediate group (Bradley et al 1977b). However, Buchthal & Behse (1977), in a combined study of sensory conduction and biopsy findings in the sural nerve, supported the presence of two main groups, the hypertrophic and neuronal types, with no evidence of an intermediary type. More recently, Harding & Thomas (1980b) in a large series of 228 patients found clear evidence of two genetically distinct forms based on whether motor conduction in the median nerve was above or below 38 m/s. The hypertrophic and neuronal groups are now termed hereditary motor and sensory neuropathy (HMSN) types I and II respectively (Thomas et al 1974, Dyck 1975). In most cases in both groups the pattern of inheritance is autosomal dominant, although sporadic cases occur and occasionally families with an autosomal recessive pattern are seen (Harding & Thomas 1980b,c). Motor conduction in patients with the recessive type I was shown to be significantly slower than in those with the dominantly inherited type (Harding & Thomas 1980c). Sensory action potential amplitudes are abnormal in all cases, being absent or significantly reduced, even if the velocity in some of the type II patients is normal (Buchthal & Behse 1977, Harding & Thomas 1980b). This latter finding is of considerable importance for the differentiation of HMSN from distal spinal muscular atrophy, in which sensory conduction and the sensory action potentials are normal (Harding & Thomas 1980a). Fig. 31.9 shows an example of a motor conduction study in a patient with type I HMSN.

Measurement of the conduction velocity may help to identify clinically normal carriers in a family (Dyck et al 1963) and can also be of prog-

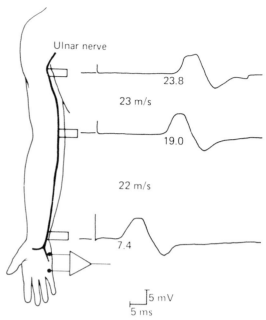

Fig. 31.9 Motor conduction study in the median nerve in a patient with HMSN type I. The distal latency is increased and there is marked slowing of conduction in distal and more proximal segments. Despite this, the M response is relatively compact at each stimulus site, indicating that minimal temporal dispersion of individual nerve fibre conduction velocities has occurred, and that the surviving nerve fibres are affected to a similar degree by the demyelinating process

nostic value as the neuropathy seems to progress more rapidly in the hypertrophic than the neuronal variety.

Type III (Dejerine–Sottas' disease). Motor conduction is markedly slowed in this form of hypertrophic neuropathy with values ranging from 3 m/s to 22 m/s (Dyck & Lambert 1968, Thomas & Lascelles 1967, Dyck et al 1971b).

Type IV (Refsum's disease). Extreme slowing of motor conduction has also been reported in Refsum's disease: after the patient had been on an appropriate diet to reduce the phytanic acid level, conduction showed a significant improvement, from a pre-treatment value of 7 m/s to 19 m/s one year later (Eldjarn 1966).

Friedreich's ataxia

Involvement of the peripheral nerves in this condition has been confirmed by the finding of slightly reduced motor conduction velocities and either very small or absent sensory action potentials (Preswick 1968, McLeod 1971, Dunn 1973, Oh & Halsey 1973, Salisachs et al 1975, Bouchard et al 1979). The conduction velocities show no significant change with age (Dunn 1973, Salisachs et al 1975, Peyronnard et al 1976), and large myelinated cutaneous fibres appear to be preferentially affected (Dyck 1984).

Metachromatic leukodystrophy (sulphatide lipidosis)

Peripheral nerve involvement is a well-described and generally early feature of the infantile and the less common adult forms of this disorder. The universal finding of quite markedly slowed conduction velocities reflects the presence of demyelination (Fullerton 1964, Yudell et al 1967, Pilz & Hopf 1972), and abnormal nerve conduction studies provide a useful screening test when the diagnosis is suspected, definite confirmation then being given by nerve biopsy.

Globoid leukodystrophy (Krabbe)

As in metachromatic leukodystrophy, slowing of conduction in peripheral nerves has also been demonstrated in this disorder (Hogan et al 1969).

REFERENCES

Albers J W, Donofrio P D, McGonagle T K 1985 Sequential electrodiagnostic abnormalities in acute inflammatory demyelinating polyradiculopathy. Muscle and Nerve 8: 528–539

Ambler Z, Stålberg E, Fink R, Rydin E 1985 Electrodiagnosis in early stages of Guillain–Barré syndrome. Electroencephalography and Clinical Neurophysiology 61: S19

Amick L D, Lemmi H 1963 Electromyographic studies in peroneal muscular atrophy. Archives of Neurology 9: 273–284

Andersen K 1985 Surface recording of orthodromic sensory nerve action potentials in median and ulnar nerves in normal subjects. Muscle and Nerve 8: 402–408

Argyropoulos C J, Panayiotopoulos C P, Scarpalezos S 1978 F- and M-wave conduction velocity in amyotrophic lateral sclerosis. Muscle and Nerve 1: 479–485

Arnason B G W 1984 Acute inflammatory demyelinating polyradiculoneuropathies. In: Dyck P J, Thomas P K, Lambert E H, Bunge R (eds) Peripheral neuropathy, vol 2, 2nd edn. W B Saunders, Philadelphia, p 2050

Baer R D, Johnson E W 1965 Motor nerve conduction velocities in normal children. Archives of Physical Medicine and Rehabilitation 46: 698–705

Bannister R G, Sears T A 1962 The changes in nerve conduction in acute idiopathic polyneuritis. Journal of Neurology, Neurosurgery and Psychiatry 25: 321–328

Barker A T 1981 Nerve conduction velocity distributions: an iterative method using two compound action potentials recorded from the same site. In: Dorfman L J, Cummins K L, Leifer L J (eds) Conduction velocity distributions: a population approach to electrophysiology of nerve. Liss, New York, p 137

Barker A T, Brown B H, Fressdon I L 1979 Determination of the distribution of conduction velocities in peripheral nerve trunks. IEEE Transactions of Biomedical Engineering 26: 76–81

Bartel P R, Lotz B P, van der Meyden C H 1984 Short-latency somatosensory evoked potentials in dystrophia myotonica. Journal of Neurology, Neurosurgery and Psychiatry 47: 524–529

Behse F, Buchthal F 1971 Normal sensory conduction in the nerves of the leg in man. Journal of Neurology, Neurosurgery and Psychiatry 34: 404–414

Behse F, Buchthal F 1977 Alcoholic neuropathy: clinical, electrophysiological and biopsy findings. Annals of Neurology 2: 95–110

Behse F, Buchthal F, Carlsen F 1977 Nerve biopsy and conduction studies in diabetic neuropathy. Journal of Neurology, Neurosurgery and Psychiatry 40: 1072–1082

Berenberg R A, Pellock J M, DiMauro S et al 1977 Lumping or splitting? 'Ophthalmoplegia-Plus' or Kearns–Sayre syndrome? Annals of Neurology 1: 37–54

Bertorini T, King Engel W, Di Chiro G, Dalakas M 1978 Leukoencephalopathy in oculocraniosomatic neuromuscular disease with ragged-red fibres. Archives of Neurology 35: 643–647

Bolton C F, Driedger A A, Lindsay R M 1979a Ischaemic neuropathy in uraemic patients caused by bovine arteriovenous shunt. Journal of Neurology, Neurosurgery and Psychiatry 42: 810–814

Bolton C F, Gilbert J J, Girvin J P, Hahn A 1979b Nerve and muscle biopsy: Electrophysiology and morphology in polyneuropathy. Neurology 29: 354–362

Bolton C F, Sawa G M, Carter K 1981 The effects of temperature on human compound action potentials. Journal of Neurology, Neurosurgery and Psychiatry 44: 407–413

Bostock H, Sears T A 1978 The internodal axon membrane: Electrical excitability and continuous conduction in segmental demyelination. Journal of Physiology 280: 273–301

Bouchard J P, Barbeau R, Bouchard R, Bouchard R W 1979 Electromyography and nerve conduction studies in Friedreich's ataxia and autosomal recessive spastic ataxia of Charlevoix-Saguenay (ARSACS). The Canadian Journal of Neurological Sciences 6: 185–189

Bousser M G, Bouche P, Brochard C, Herreman G 1976 Neuropathies périphériques au maléate de perhexiline. A propos de 7 observations. Coeur Médicale Internal 15: 181–188

Bradley W G, Hewer R L 1966 Peripheral neuropathy due to disulfiram. British Medical Journal 2: 449–450

Bradley W G, Lassman L P, Pearce G W, Walton J N 1970 The neuropathy of vincristine in man. Clinical, electrophysiological and pathological studies. Journal of the Neurological Sciences 10: 107–131

Bradley W G, Karlsson I J, Rasool C G 1977a Metronidazole neuropathy. British Medical Journal 2: 610

Bradley W G, Madrid R, Davis C J F 1977b The peroneal muscular atrophy syndrome. Clinical, genetic, electrophysiological and nerve biopsy studies. Part 3. Clinical, electrophysiological and pathological correlations. Journal of the Neurological Sciences 32: 123–136

Brooke M H, Engel W K 1969 The histographic analysis of human muscle biopsies with regard to fibre types. Neurology (Minneapolis) 19: 221–233

Brown W F, Jaatoul N 1974 Amyotrophic lateral sclerosis: Electrophysiologic study (number of motor units and rate of decay of motor units). Archives of Neurology 30: 242–284

Brust J C M, Lovelace R E, Devi S 1978 Clinical and electrophysiological features of C.M.T. syndrome. Acta Neurologica Scandinavica 58:(supp. 68) 1–42

Buchthal F, Rosenfalck A 1966 Evoked action potential and conduction velocity in human sensory nerves. Brain Research 3: 1–22

Buchthal F, Olsen P Z 1970 Electromyography and muscle biopsy in infantile spinal muscular atrophy. Brain 93: 15–30

Buchthal F, Rosenfalck A, Trojaborg W 1974 Electrophysiological findings in entrapment of the median nerve at the wrist and elbow. Journal of Neurology, Neurosurgery and Psychiatry 37: 340–360

Buchthal F, Behse F 1977 Peroneal muscular atrophy (PMA) and related disorders. 1. Clinical manifestations as related to biopsy findings, nerve conduction and electromyography. Brain 100: 41–66

Burke D, Skuse N F, Lethlean A K 1974 Sensory conduction of the sural nerve in polyneuropathy. Journal of Neurology, Neurosurgery and Psychiatry 37: 647–652

Campbell M J, Paty D W 1974 Carcinomatous neuromyopathy: 1. Electrophysiological studies. An electrophysiological and immunological study of patients with carcinoma of the lung. Journal of Neurology, Neurosurgery and Psychiatry 37: 131–141

Campbell W W, Ward L C, Swift T R 1981 Nerve conduction velocity varies inversely with height. Muscle and Nerve 4: 520–523

Carpendale M T F 1956 Conduction time in the terminal portion of the motor fibres of the ulnar, median and peroneal nerves in healthy subjects and in patients with neuropathy. M.S. (Physical Medicine) thesis, University of Minnesota

Casey E B, Le Quesne P M 1972 Electrophysiological evidence for a distal lesion in alcoholic neuropathy. Journal of Neurology, Neurosurgery and Psychiatry 35: 624–630

Casey E B, Jelliffe A M, Le Quesne P M, Millett Y L 1973 Vincristine neuropathy: clinical and electrophysiological observations. Brain 96: 69–86

Cavanagh J B 1964 The significance of the 'dying-back' process in experimental and human neurological disease. International Review of Experimental Pathology 3: 219–267

Chaco J 1970 Conduction velocity of motor nerve fibres in progressive spinal atrophy. Acta Neurologica Scandinavica 46: 119–122

Chokroverty S, Sayeed Z A 1975 Motor conduction study in patients on diphenylhydantoin therapy. Journal of Neurology, Neurosurgery and Psychiatry 38: 1235–1239

Chopra J S, Hurwitz L J, Montgomery D A D 1969 The pathogenesis of sural nerve changes in diabetes mellitus. Brain 92: 391–418

Cohen M M 1970 Toxic neuropathy. In: Vinken P J, Bruyn G W (eds) Handbook of clinical neurology, vol 7. North Holland, Amsterdam, p 510

Cummins K L, Perkel D H, Dorfman L J 1979a Nerve fibre conduction-velocity distributions. I. Estimation based on the single-fibre and compound action potentials. Electroencephalography and Clinical Neurophysiology 46: 634–646

Cummins K L, Dorfman L J, Perkel D H 1979b Nerve fibre conduction-velocity distributions. II. Estimation based on two compound action potentials. Electroencephalography and Clinical Neurophysiology 46: 647–658

Cummins K L, Dorfman L J, Perkel D H 1981 Nerve conduction velocity distributions: a method for estimation based upon two compound action potentials. In: Dorfman L J, Cummins K L, Leifer L J (eds) Conduction velocity distributions: a population approach to electrophysiology of nerve. Liss, New York, p 181

Dalakas M C, Engel W K 1981 Polyneuropathy with monoclonal gamopathy: studies of 11 patients. Annals of Neurology 10: 45–52

Davis G R, Ingram D A, Schwartz M S, Swash M 1985 Use of modified collision technique for determination of the normal motor nerve conduction velocity distribution. Electroencephalography and Clinical Neurophysiology 61:S124

Dawson G D 1956 The relative excitability and conduction velocity of sensory and motor nerve fibres in man. Journal of Physiology 131: 436–451

Dawson G D, Scott J W 1949 The recording of nerve action potentials through the skin in man. Journal of Neurology, Neurosurgery and Psychiatry 12: 259–267

Dawson G D, Merton P A 1956 'Recurrent' discharges from motor neurones. (Abstract) 20th International Congress of Physiology, Bruxelles, p 221–222

Dayan A D, Graveson G S, Illis L S, Robinson P K 1969 Schwann cell damage in motoneuron disease. Neurology (Minneapolis) 19: 639–653

Denny-Brown D 1948 Primary sensory neuropathy with muscular changes associated with carcinoma. Journal of Neurology, Neurosurgery and Psychiatry 11: 73–87

Denys E H 1977 The effect of temperature on the compound action potential in neuromuscular disease and normal controls. Electroencephalography and Clinical Neurophysiology 43:598

Di Benedetto M 1970 Sensory nerve conduction in the lower extremities. Archives of Physical Medicine 51: 253–258

Downie A W, Newell D J 1961 Sensory nerve conduction in patients with diabetes mellitus and controls. Neurology (Minneapolis) 14: 839–843

Downie A W, Scott T R 1967 An improved technique for radial nerve conduction studies. Journal of Neurology, Neurosurgery and Psychiatry 30: 332–336

Drachman D A 1968 Ophthalmoplegia plus. The neurodegenerative disorders associated with progressive external ophthalmoplegia. Archives of Neurology 18: 654–674

Dunn H G 1973 Nerve conduction studies in children with Friedreich's ataxia and ataxia-telangiectasia. Developmental Medicine and Child Neurology 15: 324–337

Dyck P J 1975 Inherited neuronal degeneration and atrophy affecting peripheral motor, sensory and autonomic neurones. In: Dyck P J, Thomas P K, Lambert E H (eds) Peripheral neuropathy, vol 2. Saunders, Philadelphia, p 825

Dyck P J 1984 Neuronal atrophy and degeneration predominantly affecting peripheral sensory and autonomic neurons. In: Dyck P J, Thomas P K, Lambert E H, Bunge R (eds) Peripheral neuropathy, vol 2, 2nd. edn. Saunders, Philadelphia, p 1557

Dyck P J, Lambert E H, Mulder D W 1963 Charcot–Marie–Tooth disease: nerve conduction and clinical studies in a large kinship. Neurology (Minneapolis) 13: 1–11

Dyck P J, Lambert E H 1968 Lower motor and primary sensory neuron diseases with peroneal muscular atrophy. 1. Neurologic, genetic, and electrophysiologic findings in hereditary polyneuropathies. Archives of Neurology 18: 603–618

Dyck P J, Johnson W J, Lambert E H, O'Brien P C 1971a Uraemic polyneuropathy — segmental demyelination secondary to axonal degeneration. Mayo Clinic Proceedings 46: 400–429

Dyck P J, Lambert E H, Sanders K, O'Brien P C 1971b Severe hypomyelination and marked abnormality of conduction in Dejerine–Sottas hypertrophic neuropathy: myelin thickness and compound action potential of sural nerve in vitro. Mayo Clinic Proceedings 46:432

Dyck P J, Karnes J L, Daube J, O'Brien P, Service F J 1985 Clinical and neuropathological criteria for the diagnosis and staging diabetic polyneuropathy. Brain 108: 861–880

Earl W C, Johnson E W 1963 Motor nerve conduction velocity in CMT disease. Archives of Physical Medicine 44: 247–252

Eisen A, Humphreys P 1974 The Guillain–Barré syndrome. A clinical and electrodiagnostic study. Archives of Neurology 30: 438–443

Eisen A, Woods J F, Sherwin A L 1974 Peripheral nerve function in long term therapy with diphenylhydantoin. Neurology (Minneapolis) 24: 411–417

Eisen A, Schomer D Melmed C 1977a The application of 'F' wave measurements in the differentiation of proximal and distal upper limb entrapments. Neurology (Minneapolis) 27: 662–668

Eisen A, Schomer D, Melmed C 1977b An electrophysiological method for examining lumbar root compression. Canadian Journal of Neurological Sciences 4: 117–123

Eldjarn L, Try K, Stokke O, Munthe-Kaas A W, Refsum S, Steinberg D, Avigan J, Mize C 1966 Dietary effects on serum-phytanic-acid levels and on clinical manifestations in heredopathia atactica polyneuritiformis. Lancet 1: 691–693

Ertekin C 1967 Sensory and motor conduction in motor neurone disease. Acta Neurologica Scandinavica 43: 499–512

Fawcett P R W, Mastaglia F L, Mechler F 1982 Electrophysiological findings including single fibre EMG in a family with mitochondrial myopathy. Journal of the Neurological Sciences 53: 397–410

Fincham R W, Van Allen M W 1964 Sensory nerve conduction in amyotrophic lateral sclerosis. Neurology (Minneapolis) 14: 31–33

Fincham R W, Cape C A 1968 Sensory nerve conduction in syringomyelia. Neurology (Minneapolis) 18: 200–201

Fisher M A 1982 F response latency determination. Muscle and Nerve 5:730–734

Fisher M A 1985 F waves. Muscle and Nerve 8: 71–72

Fullerton P M 1964 Peripheral nerve conduction in metachromatic leucodystrophy (sulphatide lipidosis). Journal of Neurology, Neurosurgery and Psychiatry 27: 100–105

Fullerton P M, Barnes J M 1966 Peripheral neuropathy in rats produced by acrylamide. British Journal of Industrial Medicine 23: 210–105

Gamstorp I 1963 Normal conduction velocity of ulnar, median and peroneal nerves in infancy, childhood and adolescence. Acta Paediatrica Scandinavica (suppl) 146: 68–76

Gamstorp I, Shelburne S A 1965 Peripheral sensory conduction in ulnar and median nerves of normal infants. Acta Paediatrica Scandinavica 54: 309–314

Gardner-Medwin D, Hudgson P, Walton J N 1967 Benign spinal muscular atrophy arising in childhood and adolescence. Journal of the Neurological Sciences 5: 121–158

Gassel M M 1964 Sources of error in motor nerve conduction studies. Neurology (Minneapolis) 14: 825–835

Gassel M M, Diamontopoulos E 1964 Pattern of conduction times in the distribution of the radial nerve. Neurology (Minneapolis) 14: 222–231

Gassel M M, Trojaborg W 1964 Clinical and electrophysiological study of the pattern of conduction times in the sciatic nerve. Journal of Neurology, Neurosurgery and Psychiatry 27: 351–357

Gilliatt R W 1966 Applied electrophysiology in nerve and muscle disease. Proceedings of the Royal Society of Medicine 59:989

Gilliatt R W, Thomas P K 1957 Extreme slowing of nerve conduction in peroneal muscular atrophy. Annals of Physical Medicine 4: 104–106

Gilliatt R W, Taylor J C 1959 Electrical changes following section of the facial nerve. Proceedings of the Royal Society of Medicine 52: 1080–1083

Gilliatt R W, Thomas P K 1960 Changes in nerve conduction with ulnar nerve lesions at the elbow. Journal of Neurology, Neurosurgery and Psychiatry 23: 312–320

Gilliatt R W, Willison R G 1962 Peripheral nerve conduction in diabetic neuropathy. Journal of Neurology, Neurosurgery and Psychiatry 25: 11–18

Gilliatt R W, Melville I D, Velate A S, Willison R G 1965 A study of normal nerve action potentials using an averaging technique (barrier grid storage tube). Journal of Neurology, Neurosurgery and Psychiatry 28: 191–200

Gilliatt R W, Hjorth R J 1972 Nerve conduction during Wallerian degeneration in the baboon. Journal of Neurology, Neurosurgery and Psychiatry 35: 335–341

Gilliatt R W, Hopf H C, Rudge P, Baraitser M 1976 Axonal velocities of motor units in the hand and foot muscles of the baboon. Journal of the Neurological Sciences 29: 249–258

Ginzburg M, Lee M, Ginzburg J, Alba A 1978 Median and ulnar nerve conduction determinations in the Erb's point–axilla segment in normal subjects. Journal of Neurology, Neurosurgery and Psychiatry 41: 444–448

Goodgold J, Eberstein A 1983 Electrodiagnosis of

neuromuscular diseases, 3rd edn. Williams and Wilkins, Baltimore

Guiloff R J, Sherratt R M 1977 Sensory conduction in the medial plantar nerve. Journal of Neurology, Neurosurgery and Psychiatry 40: 1168–1181

Guld C E 1960 Use of screened power transformers and output transformers to reduce stimulus artefacts. In: Medical electronics. Thomas, Springfield, Illinois

Guld C E, Rosenfalck A, Willison R G, 1983 Report of the committee on EMG instrumentation. In: Recommendations for the practice of clinical neurophysiology. Elsevier, Amsterdam, p 83

Gutmann L 1977 Median–ulnar nerve communications and carpal tunnel syndrome. Journal of Neurology, Neurosurgery and Psychiatry 40: 982–986

Gutmann L, Martin J D, Welton W 1976 Dapsone motor neuropathy — an axonal disease. Neurology 26: 514–516

Hamilton D V, Evans D B, Henderson R G 1980 Ulnar nerve lesion as complication of Cimino–Brescia arteriovenous fistula. Lancet 2: 1137–1138

Hackett E R, Shipley D, Livengood R 1968 Motor nerve conduction velocity studies of ulnar nerve in patients with leprosy. International Journal of Leprosy 36: 282–287

Hansen S, Ballantyne J P 1977 Axonal dysfunction in the neuropathy of diabetes mellitus: quantitative electrophysiological study. Journal of Neurology, Neurosurgery and Psychiatry 40: 555–564

Hansen S, Ballantyne J P 1978 A quantitative electrophysiological study of M.N.D. Journal of Neurology, Neurosurgery and Psychiatry 41: 773–783

Hanyu N, Oguchi K, Yanagisawa N, Tsukagoshi H 1982 Degeneration and regeneration of ventral root motor fibres in amyotrophic lateral sclerosis. Journal of the Neurological Sciences 55: 99–115

Harding A E, Le Fanu J 1977 Carpal tunnel syndrome related to antebrachial Cimino–Brescia fistula. Journal of Neurology, Neurosurgery and Psychiatry 40: 511–513

Harding A E, Thomas P K 1980a Distal spinal muscular atrophy: a report of 34 cases and review of the literature. Journal of the Neurological Sciences 45: 337–348

Harding A E, Thomas P K 1980b The clinical features of hereditary motor and sensory neuropathy types I and II. Brain 103: 259–280

Harding A E, Thomas P K 1980c Autosomal recessive forms of hereditary motor and sensory neuropathy. Journal of Neurology, Neurosurgery and Psychiatry 43: 669–678

Hausmanowa-Petrusewicz I, Kopec J 1973 Motor nerve conduction velocity in anterior horn lesions. In: Desmedt J E (ed) New developments in electromyography and clinical neurophysiology, vol 2. Karger, Basel, p 298–305

Hausmanowa-Petrusewicz I, Fidzianska A, Dobosz I, Drac H, Ryniewicz B 1975 The foetal character of the lesion in the acute form of Werdnig–Hoffmann disease. In: Bradley W G, Gardner-Medwin D, Walton J (eds) Recent advances in myology. Excerpta Medica, Amsterdam, p 546

Henriksen J D 1956 Conduction velocities of motor nerves in normal subjects and patients with neuromuscular disorders. M.S. (Physical Medicine) thesis, University of Minnesota

Hilton-Brown P, Stålberg E 1983 The motor unit in muscular dystrophy, single fibre EMG and scanning EMG study. Journal of Neurology, Neurosurgery and Psychiatry 46: 981–995

Hodes R, Larrabee M G, German W 1948 The human electromyogram in response to nerve stimulation and the conduction velocity of motor axons. Archives of Neurology and Psychiatry 60: 340–365

Hogan G R, Guttman L, Chou S M 1969 The peripheral neuropathy of Krabbe's (globoid) leukodystrophy. Neurology (Minneapolis) 19: 1094–1100

Hopf H C 1963 Electromyographic study on so-called mononeuritis. Archives of Neurology and Psychiatry 9: 307–312

Hopkins A P, Gilliatt R W 1971 Motor and sensory nerve conduction in the baboon: Normal values and changes during acrylamide neuropathy. Journal of Neurology, Neurosurgery and Psychiatry 34: 415–426

Horwich M S, Cho L, Porro R S, Posner J B 1977 Subacute sensory neuropathy: a remote effect of carcinoma. Annals of Neurology 2: 7–19

Hursch J B 1939 Conduction velocity and diameter of nerve fibres. American Journal of Physiology 127: 131–139

Ingram D A, Davis G R, Schwartz M S, Swash M 1985 Motor nerve refractory period and conduction velocity distributions in motor neurone disease. Electroencephalography and Clinical Neurophysiology 61:S30

Isch F, Isch-Treussard C, Buchheit F, Delgado V, Kircher J P 1964 Measurement of conduction velocity of motor nerve fibres in polyneuritis and polyradiculitis. (Abstract) Electroencephalography and Clinical Neurophysiology 16: 416

Iyer V, Fenichel G M 1976 Normal median nerve proximal latency in carpal tunnel syndrome: a. due to co-existing Martin–Gruber anastomosis. Journal of Neurology, Neurosurgery and Psychiatry 39: 449–452

Jebsen R H 1967 Motor conduction velocities in the median and ulnar nerves. Archives of Physical Medicine and Rehabilitation 48: 185–194

Jennekens F G I, Dorhout Mees E J, van der Most van Spijk D 1971 Clinical aspects of uraemic polyneuropathy. Nephron 8: 414–426

Johnson E W, Olsen K J 1960 Clinical value of motor nerve conduction velocity determination. Journal of the American Medical Association 172: 2030

Kaeser H E, 1975 Nerve conduction velocity measurements. In: Vinken P, Bruyn G W (eds) Handbook of clinical neurology, vol 7. North-Holland, Amsterdam, p 116

Kelly J J, Kyle R A, O'Brien P C, Dyck P J 1979 The natural history of peripheral neuropathy in primary systemic amyloidosis. Annals of Neurology 6: 1–7

Kelly J J, Kyle R A, Miles J M, O'Brien P C, Dyck P J 1981 The spectrum of peripheral neuropathy in myeloma. Neurology (New York) 31: 24–31

Kimura J 1974 'F' wave velocity in the central segment of the median and ulnar nerve. A study in normal subjects and in patients with Charcot–Marie–Tooth disease. Neurology (Minneapolis) 24: 539–546

Kimura J 1983 Electrodiagnosis in diseases of nerve and muscle: Principles and practice. F A Davis, Philadelphia

Kimura J 1984 Principles and pitfalls of nerve conduction studies. Annals of Neurology 16: 415–429

Kimura J, Butzer J F 1975 'F' wave conduction velocity in Guillain–Barré syndrome. Assessment of nerve segment between axilla and spinal cord. Archives of Neurology 32: 524–529

Kimura J, Yanagisawa H, Yamada T, Mitsudome A, Sasaki H, Kimura A 1984 Is the F wave elicited in a select group of motoneurons? Muscle and Nerve 7: 392–399

King D, Ashby P 1976 Conduction velocity in the proximal

segments of a motor nerve in the Guillain–Barré syndrome. Journal of Neurology, Neurosurgery and Psychiatry 39: 538–544

Knezevic W, Mastaglia F L 1984 Neuropathy associated with Brescia–Cimino arteriovenous fistulas. Archives of Neurology 41: 1184–1186

Konatey-Ahulu F I D, Baillod R, Compty C M, Heron J R, Shaldon S, Thomas P K 1965 Effect of periodic dialysis on the peripheral neuropathy of end-stage renal failure. British Medical Journal 2: 1212–1215

Korobkin R, Asbury A K, Sumner A J, Neilsen S L 1975 Glue-sniffing neuropathy. Archives of Neurology 32: 158–162

Lachman T, Shahani, B T, Young R R 1980 Late responses and aids to diagnosis in peripheral neuropathy. Journal of Neurology, Neurosurgery and Psychiatry 43: 156–162

Lambert E H 1962 Diagnostic value of electrical stimulation of motor nerves. Electroencephalography and Clinical Neurophysiology (suppl) 22: 9–16

Lambert E H, Mulder D W 1957 Electromyographic studies in amyotrophic lateral sclerosis. Proceedings of the Staff Meetings of the Mayo Clinic 32: 441–447

Lambert E H, Mulder D W 1964 Nerve conduction in the Guillain–Barré syndrome. Electroencephalography and Clinical Neurophysiology 17: 86

Lambert E H, Dyck P J 1975 Compound action potentials of sural nerve in vitro in peripheral neuropathy. In: Dyck P J, Thomas P K, Lambert E H (eds) Peripheral neuropathy, vol 1. Saunders, Philadelphia, p 241

Lamontagne A, Buchthal F 1970 Electrophysiological studies in diabetic neuropathy. Journal of Neurology, Neurosurgery and Psychiatry 33: 442–452

Lang A H, Puusa A, Hynninen P, Kuusela V, Jantti V, Sillanpaa M 1985 Evolution of nerve conduction velocity in later childhood and adolescence. Muscle and Nerve 8: 38–43

Lawrence D G, Locke S 1961 Motor nerve conduction velocity in diabetes. Archives of Neurology 5: 483–489

Lefebvre-d'Amour M, Shahani B T, Young R R, Bird K T 1979 Importance of studying sural conduction and late responses in the evaluation of alcoholic subjects. Neurology (Minneapolis) 29: 1600–1609

Lehmann H J, Lehmann G, Tackmann W 1971 Refraktarperiode und Ubermittlung von Serienimpulsen ii N.tibialis des Meeerschweinchens bei experimenteller allergischer Neuritis. Zeitschrift Neurol. 199: 67–85

Lenman J A R, Fleming A M, Robertson M A H, Abbott R J, Clee M D, Ferguson I F, Wright D S 1981 Peripheral nerve function in patients with bronchial carcinoma. Comparison with matched controls and effects of treatment. Journal of Neurology, Neurosurgery, and Psychiatry 44: 54–61

Lewis R A, Sumner A J 1982 The electrodiagnostic distinctions between chronic familial and acquired demyelinative neuropathies. Neurology (New York) 32: 592–596

London G W 1975 Normal ulnar nerve conduction velocity across the thoracic outlet: comparison of two measuring techniques. Journal of Neurology, Neurosurgery and Psychiatry 38: 756–760

Lovelace R E, Horowitz S J 1968 Peripheral neuropathy in long term diphenylhydantoin therapy. Archives of Neurology 18: 69–77

Ludin H P 1980 Electromyography in practice. Georg Thieme Verlag, Stuttgart

McComas A J, Fawcett P R W, Campbell M J, Sica R E P 1971 Electrophysiological estimation of the number of motor units within a human muscle. Journal of Neurology, Neurosurgery and Psychiatry 34: 132–139

McDonald W I 1980 Physiological consequences of demyelination. In: Sumner A J (ed) The physiology of peripheral nerve disease. Saunders, Philadelphia, P 265

McLeod J G 1971 An electrophysiological and histological study in patients with Friedreich's ataxia. Journal of the Neurological Sciences 12: 333–349

McLeod J G, Hargrave J C, Walsh J C, Booth G C, Gye R S, Barron A 1975 Nerve conduction studies in leprosy. International Journal of Leprosy 43: 21–31

McQuillen M P 1971 Idiopathic polyneuritis: serial studies of nerve and immune functions. Journal of Neurology, Neurosurgery and Psychiatry 34: 607–615

Magladery J W, McDougal D D Jr 1950 Electrophysiological study of nerve and reflex activity in man. 1. Identification of certain reflexes in the electromyogram and the conduction velocity of peripheral nerve fibres. Bulletin of the Johns Hopkins Hospital 86: 265–290

Mamoli B, Wessely P, Kogelnik H D, Muller M, Rathkolb O 1979 Electroneurographic investigation of misonidazole polyneuropathy. European Neurology 18: 405

Markesbery W R 1979 Lactic acidemia, mitochondrial myopathy, and basal ganglion calcification. Neurology 29: 1057–1061

Markesbery W R, McQuillen M P, Procopis P G, Harrison A R, Engel A G 1974 Muscle carnitine deficiency. Association with lipid myopathy, vacuolar neuropathy and vacuolated leukocytes. Archives of Neurology 31: 320–324

Mavor H, Libman I 1962 Motor nerve conduction velocity measurement as a diagnostic tool. Neurology (Minneapolis) 12: 733–744

Mavor H, Atcheson J B 1966 Posterior tibial nerve conduction. Archives of Neurology 14: 661–669

Mawdsley C, Mayer R F 1965 Nerve conduction in alcoholic polyneuropathy. Brain 88: 335–356

Mayer R F, Feldman R G 1967 Observations on the nature of the 'F' wave in man. Neurology (Minneapolis) 17: 147–156

Meadows J C, Marsden C D, Harriman D G F 1969 Chronic spinal muscular atrophy in adults, Part 1. The Kugelberg–Welander syndrome. Journal of the Neurological Sciences 9: 527–550

Mechler F, Fawcett P R W, Mastaglia F L, Hudgson P 1981 Mitochondrial myopathy. A study of clinically affected and asymptomatic members of a six-generation family. Journal of the Neurological Sciences 50: 191–200

Miglietta O 1968 Motor nerve fibres in amyotrophic lateral sclerosis. American Journal of Physical Medicine 47: 118–124

Miledi R, Slater C R 1970 On the degeneration of rat neuromuscular junctions after nerve section. Journal of Physiology 207: 507–528

Mills K R, Murray N M F 1985 Conduction in proximal nerve segments in demyelinating neuropathy. Electroencephalography and Clinical Neurophysiology 61: S70

Mongia S K, Lundervold A 1975 Electrophysiological abnormalities in cases of dystrophia myotonica. European Neurology 13: 360–376

Moody J 1965 Electrophysiological investigations into the neurological complications of carcinoma. Brain 88: 1023–1036

Mulder D W, Lambert E H, Bastron J A, Sprague R G 1961 The neuropathies associated with diabetes mellitus. Neurology (Minneapolis) 11: 275–284

Neilsen V K 1973a The peripheral nerve function in chronic renal failure. V. Sensory and motor conduction velocity. Acta Medica Scandinavica 194: 445–454

Neilsen V K 1973b The peripheral nerve function in chronic renal failure. VI. The relation between sensory and motor nerve conduction and kidney function, azotaemia, age, sex and clinical neuropathy. Acta Medica Scandinavica 194: 455–462

Neilsen V K 1974a The peripheral nerve function in chronic renal failure. IX. Recovery after renal transplantation. Electrophysiological aspects (sensory and motor conduction). Acta Medica Scandinavica 195: 171–180

Neilsen V K 1974b The peripheral nerve function in chronic renal failure (a survey). Acts Medica Scandinavica (Suppl) 573

Norris A H, Shock N W, Wagman I H 1953 Age changes in the maximum conduction velocity of motor fibres in human ulnar nerves. Journal of Applied Physiology 5: 589–593

Oh S J, Halsey J H 1973 Abnormality in nerve potentials in Friedreich's ataxia. Neurology (Minneapolis) 23: 52–54

Olson N D, Jou M F, Quast J E, Nuttal Q 1978 Peripheral neuropathy in myotonic dystrophy. Archives of Neurology 35: 741–745

O'Sullivan D J, McLeod J G 1978 Distal chronic spinal muscular atrophy involving the hands. Journal of Neurology, Neurosurgery and Psychiatry 41: 653–658

Panayiotopoulos C P 1978 F-wave conduction velocity in the deep peroneal nerve: Charcot–Marie–Tooth disease and dystrophia myotonica. Muscle and Nerve 1: 37–44

Panayiotopoulos C P, Scarpalezos S 1977 'F' wave studies on the deep peroneal nerve. Part 2–1. Chronic renal failure. 2. Limb-girdle muscular dystrophy. Journal of the Neurological Sciences 31: 331–341

Panayiotopoulos C P, Scarpalezos S, Nastas P E 1977 F-wave studies on the deep peroneal nerve. Part 1. control subjects. Journal of the Neurological Sciences 31: 319–329

Peioglou-Harmoussi S 1983 Studies in F-response behaviour. PhD thesis, University of Newcastle upon Tyne

Peioglou-Harmoussi S, Fawcett P R W, Howel D, Barwick D D 1985a F-responses: a study of frequency, shape and amplitude characteristics in healthy control subjects. Journal of Neurology, Neurosurgery and Psychiatry 48: 1159–1164

Peioglou-Harmoussi S, Howel D, Fawcett P R W, Barwick D D 1985b F-response behaviour in a control population. Journal of Neurology, Neurosurgery and Psychiatry 48: 1152–1158

Peioglou-Harmoussi S, Fawcett P R W, Howel D, Barwick D D 1986 F-responses in syringomyelia. Journal of the Neurological Sciences 75: 293–304

Peyronnard J M, Bouchard J P, Lapointe L, Lamontagne A, Lemieux B, Barbeau A 1976 Nerve conduction studies and electromyography in Friedreich's ataxia. Canadian Journal of Neurological Sciences 3: 313–318

Peyronnard J-M, Charron L, Bellavance A, Marchand L 1979 Neuropathy and mitochondrial myopathy. Annals of Neurology 7: 262–268

Pilz H, Hopf H C, 1972 A preclinical case of late adult metachromatic leukodystrophy? Manifestation only with lipid abnormalities in urine, enzyme deficiency, and decrease of nerve conduction velocity. Journal of Neurology, Neurosurgery and Psychiatry 35: 360–364

Preswick G 1968 The peripheral neuropathy of Friedreich's ataxia. Electroencephalography and Clinical Neurophysiology 25: 399

Preswick G, Jeremy D 1964 Subclinical polyneuropathy in renal insufficiency. Lancet 2: 731

Raman P T, Taori G M 1976 Prognostic significance of electrodiagnostic studies in the Guillain–Barré syndrome. Journal of Neurology, Neurosurgery and Psychiatry 39: 163–170

Rasminsky M 1973 The effects of temperature on conduction in demyelinated single nerve fibres. Archives of Neurology 28: 287–292

Rasminsky M, Sears T A 1972 Internodal conduction in undissected demyelinated nerve fibres. Journal of Physiology 227: 323–350

Rossi B, Sartucci F, Stefanini A, Pucci G, Bianchi F 1983 Measurement of motor conduction velocity with Hopf's technique in myotonic dystrophy. Journal of Neurology, Neurosurgery and Psychiatry 46: 93–95

Said G 1978 Perhexiline neuropathy: a clinico-pathological study. Annals of Neurology 3: 252–266

Salisachs P 1974 Wide spectrum of motor conduction velocity in Charcot–Marie–Tooth disease. An anatomic-physiological interpretation. Journal of the Neurological Sciences 23: 25–31

Salisachs P, Codina M, Pradas J 1975 Motor conduction velocity in patients with Friedreich's ataxia. Journal of the Neurological Sciences 24: 331–337

Schiller H H, Stålberg E 1978 'F' responses studied with single fibre E.M.G. in normal subjects and spastic patients. Journal of Neurology, Neurosurgery and Psychiatry 41: 45–53

Schwartz M, Stålberg E, Swash M 1980 Pattern of segmental motor involvement in syringomyelia: a single fibre EMG study. Journal of Neurology, Neurosurgery and Psychiatry 43: 150–155

Sears T A 1959 Action potentials evoked in digital nerves by stimulation of the mechano receptors in the human finger. Journal of Physiology 148: 30–31P

Sebille A 1978 Respective importance of different nerve conduction velocities in leprosy. Journal of the Neurological Sciences 38: 89–95

Shahani B T, Sumner A J 1981 Electrophysiological studies in peripheral neuropathy: early detection and monitoring. In: Stålberg E, Young R R (eds) Clinical neurophysiology. Butterworth, London, p 117

Shetty V P, Mehta L N, Antia A H, Irani P F 1977 Teased fibre study of early nerve lesions in leprosy and in contacts with electrophysiological correlates. Journal of Neurology, Neurosurgery and Psychiatry 40: 708–711

Shy G M, Gonatas N K, Perez M 1966 Two childhood myopathies with abnormal mitochondria. I. Megaconial myopathy. II. Pleoconial myopathy. Brain 89: 133–158

Sica R E P, McComas A J 1971 An electrophysiological investigation of limb-girdle and facioscapulohumeral dystrophy. Journal of Neurology, Neurosurgery and Psychiatry 34: 269–474

Simpson J A 1964 Fact and fallacy in measurement of conduction velocity in motor nerves. Journal of Neurology, Neurosurgery and Psychiatry 27: 381–385

Singh N, Behse F, Buchthal F 1974 Electrophysiological study of peroneal palsy. Journal of Neurology, Neurosurgery and Psychiatry 37: 1202–1213

Smith I S, Kahn S N, Lacey B W, King R H M, Eames R A, Whybrew D J, Thomas P K 1983 Chronic demyelinating neuropathy associated with benign IgM paraproteinaemia. Brain 106: 169–195

Spencer P S, Schaumburg H H 1979 Neurotoxic chemicals as probes of cellular mechanisms of neuromuscular disease. In: Aguayo A J, Karpati G Current topics in nerve and muscle research. Excerpta Medica, Amsterdam, p 274

Spiro A J, Moore C L, Prineas J W, Strasberg P M, Rapin I 1970 A cytochrome-related inherited disorder of the nervous system and muscle. Archives of Neurology 23: 103–112

Stålberg E 1982 Electrophysiological studies of reinnervation in ALS. In: Rowland L P (ed) Advances in neurology, Human motor neuron disease, Raven Press, New York, p 47

Sumner A J 1980 Axonal polyneuropathies. In: Sumner A J (ed) The physiology of peripheral nerve disease. Saunders, Philadelphia, p 340

Sumner D, Crawford M A, Harriman D G F 1971 Distal muscular dystrophy in an English family. Brain 94: 51–60

Swash M, Perrin J, Schwartz M S 1979 Significance of immunoglobulin deposition in peripheral nerve in neuropathies associated with paraproteinaemia. Journal of Neurology, Neurosurgery and Psychiatry 42: 179–183

Swift T R 1984 Commentary: Electrophysiology of progressive spinal muscular atrophy. In: Gamstorp I, Sarnat H B (eds) Progressive spinal muscular atrophies. Raven Press, New York, p 135

Swift T R, Hackett D E, Shipley D E, Miner K M 1973 The peroneal and tibial nerves in lepromatous leprosy — clinical and electrophysiological observations. International Journal of Leprosy 41: 25–34

Tenckhoff H A, Boen F S T, Jebsen R H, Spiegler J H 1965 Polyneuropathy in chronic renal insufficiency. Journal of the American Medical Association 192:1121

Thomas J E, Lambert E H 1960 Ulnar nerve conduction velocity and 'H' reflex in infants and children. Journal of Applied Physiology 15: 1–9

Thomas P K 1971 The morphological basis for alterations in nerve conduction in peripheral neuropathy. Proceedings of the Royal Society of Medicine 64: 295–298

Thomas P K, Sears T A, Gilliatt R W 1959 The range of conduction velocity in normal motor nerve fibres to the small muscles of the hand and foot. Journal of Neurology, Neurosurgery and Psychiatry 22: 175–181

Thomas P K, Lascelles R G 1966 The pathology of diabetic neuropathy. Quarterly Journal of Medicine 35: 489–509

Thomas P K, Lascelles R G, 1967 Hypertrophic neuropathy. Quarterly Journal of Medicine 35: 489–509

Thomas P K, Hollinrake K, Lascelles R G, O'Sullivan D J, Baillod R A, Moorhead J F, Mackenzie J C 1971 The polyneuropathy of chronic renal failure. Brain 94: 761–780

Thomas P K, Calne D B 1974 Motor nerve conduction velocity in peroneal muscular atrophy: evidence for genetic heterogeneity. Journal of Neurology, Neurosurgery and Psychiatry 37: 68–75

Thomas P K, Calne D B, Stewart G 1974 Hereditary motor and sensory polyneuropathy (peroneal muscular atrophy). Annals of Human Genetics (London) 38: 111–153

Thorne J 1965 Central responses to electrical activation of the peripheral nerves supplying the intrinsic hand muscles. Journal of Neurology, Neurosurgery and Psychiatry 28: 482–495

Toole J F, Gergen J A, Hayes D M, Felts J H 1968 Neural effects of nitrofurantoin. Archives of Neurology 18: 180–187

Trojaborg W 1964 Motor nerve conduction velocities in normal subjects with particular reference to the conduction in proximal and distal segments of median and ulnar nerves. Electroencephalography and Clinical Neurophysiology 17: 314–321

Trojaborg W, Sindrup E H 1969 Motor and sensory conduction in different segments of the radial nerve in normal subjects. Journal of Neurology, Neurosurgery and Psychiatry 32: 354–359

Trojaborg W, Frantzen E, Andersen I 1969 Peripheral neuropathy and myopathy associated with carcinoma of the lung. Brain 92: 71–82

Trontelj J V 1973 A study of the F-responses by single fibre electromyography. In: Desmedt J E (ed) New developments in electromyography and clinical neurophysiology. Karger, Basel, p 318–322

Trontelj J V, Trontelj M 1973 'F' responses of human facial muscles. A single motor neurone study. Journal of the Neurological Sciences 20: 211–222

Trontelj J V, Trontelj M, Stålberg E 1973 The jitter of single human muscle fibre responses in certain reflexes. Electroencephalography and Clinical Neurophysiology 34: 825

Walsh J C 1971 Neuropathy associated with lymphoma. Journal of Neurology, Neurosurgery and Psychiatry 34: 42–50

Walsh J C, McLeod J G 1970 Alcoholic neuropathy. An electrophysiological and histological study. Journal of the Neurological Sciences 10: 457–469

Warren D J, Otieno L S 1975 Carpal tunnel syndrome in patients on intermittent haemodialysis. Postgraduate Medical Journal 51: 450–452

Waxman S G 1980 Determinants of conduction velocity in myelinated nerve fibres. Muscle and Nerve 3: 141–150

Weiderholt W R 1970 Stimulus intensity and site of excitation in human median nerve sensory fibres. Journal of Neurology, Neurosurgery and Psychiatry 33: 438–441

Willison R G 1962 Electrodiagnosis in motor neurone disease. Proceedings of the Royal Society of Medicine 55:1024

Yates S K, Brown W F 1979 Characteristics of the F response: a single motor unit study. Journal of Neurology, Neurosurgery and Psychiatry 42: 161–170

Yiannikas C, McLeod J G 1985 Peripheral neuropathy associated with mitochondrial myopathy. Electroencephalography and Clinical Neurophysiology 61:S20

Young R R, Shahani B T 1978 Clinical value and limitations of 'F' wave determination. Muscle and Nerve 1: 248–249

Yudell A, Gomez M R, Lambert E H, Dockerty M B 1967 The neuropathy of sulfatide lipidosis (metachromatic leukodystrophy). Neurology (Minneapolis) 17: 103–111

Integration and analysis of the electromyogram and the study of reflexes

INTRODUCTION

The recognition of different patterns of muscle fibre activity and motor unit (MU) recruitment by means of concentric needle electrode electromyography (CNEMG) has a ready clinical application and, together with nerve conduction measurement, provides the greater part of the work carried out in many EMG laboratories. Methods for the quantitative analysis of the EMG have been relatively slow to develop; while they have provided much information that is of physiological interest, their clinical application has so far been limited although, when carried out in association with CNEMG, they may lead to an increased diagnostic yield. Important exceptions are the measurement either by visual analysis or data processing techniques of action potential duration during weak voluntary contraction and techniques involving the use of single-fibre electrodes (SFEMG). These are now widely employed and have been dealt with fully, together with CNEMG and nerve conduction velocity measurement in earlier sections.

An important field of study has been the relationship which exists between the force output of a muscle and the EMG. Applications of this include the study of the relative activity of different muscles in kinesiology, in association with conditions where there may be inappropriate activity or inactivity in particular muscle groups and also in the study of fatigue and of MU recruitment. Several techniques have proved helpful in clinical diagnosis and also in assessing the progress of a disease process. Particular applications have been helpful in estimating the number of MU in a muscle both in health and disease. A limitation of all these methods is that only certain muscles can be examined and these are not always the muscles about which information is required.

The Fourier analysis of the EMG has proved to be of some clinical value as the power spectrum of a muscle at different frequencies may be altered in neuromuscular disease and in fatigue. The method is relatively non-invasive as information can be obtained using surface electrodes and, with suitable microprocessors, can be rapidly employed. The refractory period of the muscle and nerve is of physiological interest as it is dependent on the properties of the muscle membrane or the axon; a number of studies have shown that important changes in the refractory period can be detected both in muscle disease and in disease of peripheral nerve.

The study of muscle action potentials after electrical or mechanical stimulation of muscle has provided a means of examining reflex action and of measuring the excitability of the motor neurone pool as well as conduction along the afferent and efferent pathways. Early work concentrated mainly on reflexes involving the peripheral nerves such as the H reflex (Hoffman 1918) but at present much interest attaches to the cranial nerves and brain stem.

In this chapter consideration is given first to methods of EMG analysis, particularly those associated with the integration and analysis of the EMG, and the recording of muscle tension. In the later sections the electrophysiological study of reflexes will be reviewed.

INTEGRATION OF THE EMG

Methods and normal findings

In the electromyographic examination with either surface or concentric needle electrodes (CNEMG) the number of motor units seen to be recruited increases as the force of the contraction of the muscle under study is increased. There is a corresponding increase in the amplitude of the interference pattern as is seen clearly if this is photographed and the height of the envelope potential is measured. In an early experiment it was shown that this relationship was approximately linear. The EMG was recorded through surface electrodes over the biceps muscle and the mean voltage was measured on a meter while the subject held weights of differing magnitude to produce isometric contractions of differing force (Bayer & Flechtenmayer 1950).

A more elaborate method for integrating the EMG is to record it on an oscilloscope or pen recorder after full wave rectification. This type of analogue display is useful in kinesiology and in the assessment of patients with hyper- or hypoactivity of particular muscle groups.

Lippold (1952) studied the relationship between mean voltage and tension by visual inspection of the photographed record, measuring the area of the action potentials with a planimeter. Later, this technique was automated by the use of an integrator which gave out pulses at a frequency proportional to the mean voltage after full wave rectification (Bates & Cooper 1955). With present-day equipment the EMG can be processed to give either an analogue output for visual display or a digital output for data processing.

The EMG before integration can be recorded either with surface or needle electrodes and both methods have been used in different laboratories. The results with the two methods are not always comparable and, in principle, surface electrodes have an advantage in that they sample a larger portion of the muscle.

When the relationship between voltage and tension is studied, the two parameters can be expressed graphically and the regression equation for the slope of the voltage–tension curve obtained by computation. A method which avoids the necessity for computing voltage–tension curves is to apply the voltage representing tension to the X plates of an oscilloscope and the rectified mean voltage of the EMG to the Y plates. If this is done through a series of graded contractions the voltage–tension curve is obtained automatically (Simpson & Sanderson 1965, Zuniga & Simons 1969, Stephens & Taylor 1972, 1973). Technical considerations in the recording and integration of EMG signals have been discussed by Zuniga et al and McLeod (1973).

Lippold (1952) studied the relationship between the integrated EMG recorded through surface electrodes over the calf muscle and the isometric tension of graded voluntary contractions, and found a linear relationship between the two. As the force of a contraction depends on the number of motor units which are taking part and their frequency of activation, it is reasonable to conclude that the integrated EMG gives an index of the number and activity of the motor units participating. During an isotonic contraction the relationship is more complex in that, if a muscle is allowed to shorten, there is still a linear relationship between integrated activity and tension provided that the velocity of shortening is not allowed to change. Likewise, if a muscle is allowed to shorten at a constant tension, then the integrated electrical activity is proportional to the velocity of shortening (Bigland & Lippold 1954a,b).

The question of the strict linearity of the voltage–tension relationship is still not completely resolved. Many have found a linear relationship (Inman et al 1952, Lenman 1959a,b, Simpson & Sanderson 1965, Stephens & Taylor 1972) but Zuniga & Simons (1969), working with the biceps brachii, found a curvilinear relationship between EMG and tension, recording progressively increasing values of electrical activity with increasing tension. Similarly, Kuroda et al (1970), studying the movement of extension of the knee and recording from the rectus femoris, found the relationship between force and EMG to be linear throughout the greater part of the force range, but when the tension approached that of maximum voluntary contraction there was a steep increase in electrical activity. Fuglsang-Frederikson et al (1984), using needle electrodes, found a curvilinear relationship between voltage and tension but a linear relationship when tension was plotted against the square root of integrated mean voltage. Possible reasons for this non-linearity include the possibility that there may be increased synchronisation at high values of tension where fatigue may also be a modifying factor. When movement at a joint such as the elbow is studied, the situation may be further complicated by the action of other forearm flexors apart from the muscle from which recordings are made. Stephens & Taylor (1973) however found a strictly linear relationship between integrated electrical activity and tension when recording from the first dorsal interosseus muscle.

Discharge frequency and motor unit recruitment during graded muscular contraction

How far the integrated EMG reflects the number of fibres taking part, and how far it is a measure of their frequency of activation, is a question which bears closely on how the force of a voluntary contraction is graded. The frequency of nerve impulse transmission in motor nerves has a range of approximately 5–100 Hz (Adrian & Bronk 1929) but it is doubtful whether the higher frequencies often occur, at least in the limb muscles. If a muscle is stimulated through its motor nerve, at different rates, the tension developed by the muscle increases in linear fashion with stimulus frequency, until a frequency of the order of 50 Hz is attained. With higher frequencies there is relatively little increase in tension (Adrian & Bronk 1929). Marsden et al (1971) monitored action potentials from an aberrant unit supplied by the median nerve in adductor pollicis when the ulnar nerve was blocked, and recorded potentials which had a peak frequency of 150 Hz at maximum effort. Because of the difficulty in recording single-unit discharge at high frequencies, due to interference from other units within the take-up area of the recording electrode, most studies have been carried out using fine wire electrodes with a very small recording surface, or on paretic muscle with a reduced number of units. In general there is agreement that firing frequencies of greater than 50 Hz are seldom seen, except in short bursts at maximum effort where rates of the order of 100 Hz may be recorded briefly (Lindsley 1935, Seyffarth 1941a,b, Bigland & Lippold 1954a,b, Norris & Gasteiger 1955). However in certain muscles which subserve rapid movements, such as the external ocular muscles, action potential frequencies of up to 200 Hz have been recorded (Bjork & Kugelberg 1953).

Bigland & Lippold (1954b) studied the rate of firing of single units in the small hand muscles. When a single-unit potential was observed through different grades of contraction it was seen that, although discharge frequency increased as did tension, it did so through a restricted range and not in a linear movement. Frequencies above 50 Hz were never observed and frequencies of

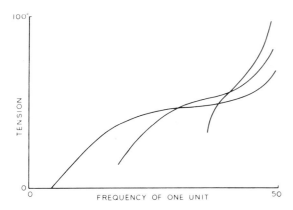

Fig. 32.1 Scheme illustrating possible mode of behaviour of individual motor units during voluntary contraction of a muscle. A particular unit starts firing when the tension in a muscle reaches a certain level, its frequency increasing with tension over a comparatively small range, except at low and high tensions (from Bigland & Lippold 1954b)

40–50 Hz occurred only during very strong contractions. It was often found that a particular unit would always start firing at a definite tension and ceased to fire when a certain level of tension was reached (Fig. 32.1). When a unit appeared in this manner during a limited part of the range of contraction, its discharge rate often remained relatively constant. When the average frequency of all the units observed at different tensions was plotted against the force of contraction, it was seen that the relationship between frequency and tension was given by an S-shaped curve. Broadly similar findings were reported by Norris & Gasteiger (1955) in gastrocnemius and rectus femoris. They were able to record units which fired at rates of 100 Hz during brief bursts at maximum effort and, in addition, a small number of large motor units which appeared only during powerful contractions and fired at a rate of less than 5 Hz.

It might be concluded that an important, if not the major, factor in grading the force of a muscular contraction is the recruitment and dropping out of motor units as the tension rises and falls, variations in the frequency of motor unit discharge serving to provide fine adjustments of muscular tension. However, it is evident from studies of motor unit recruitment and firing frequency at different tensions that the majority of motor units are recruited at relatively low

tension, nearly half reaching activation before the tension attains 20% of maximum and relatively little recruitment occurring at tensions greater than 50% of maximum. In general, the discharge frequency of single units increases with the force of contraction, although the relationship between the firing rate of single units and force is dependent on the rate of increasing or decreasing voluntary force. It would appear, therefore, that the contribution of motor unit recruitment to the increase in voluntary force is greatest at low levels of tension, at higher levels changes in firing frequency becoming increasingly important (Milner-Brown et al 1973a,b, Tanji & Kato 1973a,b). It is of interest that, in these studies, motor unit recruitment is seen to occur in an orderly manner, larger units tending to be recruited at higher tensions. This is consistent with the size principle (Henneman et al 1965) according to which the smallest motor neurones have the lowest threshold of excitation. Further evidence that this principle applies to human muscle is provided by the observation of Freund et al (1973), that the conduction velocity of nerve fibres innervating high threshold units is faster than that of fibres innervating low threshold units.

Milner-Brown & Stein (1975) have reviewed the studies which have been carried out to explain the theoretical basis for a relation between EMG and muscular force. These, in general, suggest that electrical activity should increase with the square root of the tension rather than linearly, which would give a change in slope in the opposite direction to that observed by workers who have found a non-linear relationship experimentally. To try to clarify the relationship between surface EMG and muscular force, and to discover how this depends on motor unit activity, these authors have studied the recruitment of motor units in the first dorsal interosseous muscle, using an averaging technique to determine the waveform contributed by each motor unit to the surface EMG. By this means they found that the amplitude of the waveform of the surface EMG contributed by a single unit tended to increase according to the threshold force at which the unit was recruited, but not in a linear manner, the increase being proportional to the square root of the threshold force. Recruitment of motor units, however, was found to be less important at higher levels where firing frequency contributed predominantly to tension. The non-linear effect on the surface EMG of motor unit recruitment could be compensated for if the tension increment derived from increased firing frequency were also non-linear: it is likely that this may, indeed, be the case because the firing rates of some units may be high enough to give rise to a fused tetanus. The observed linear relationship between EMG and tension may, therefore, depend on a balance between non-linear summation of EMG potentials and contractile responses at higher levels of tension.

Fatigue

Early EMG studies on fatigue showed that during a fatiguing contraction there was slowing of the rhythmic activity of the EMG (Piper 1912) and increase in the amplitude of the potentials (Cobb & Forbes 1923).

These observations have been confirmed repeatedly but understanding of the mechanisms underlying fatigue remains incomplete and methods for its quantitative measurement have been slow to develop. In myasthenia gravis, where there is

abnormal fatiguability of muscle, there may be a decline in amplitude of the action potentials which may be evoked by repetitive stimulation through its nerve (Harvey & Masland 1941). A similar fatigue of evoked potentials has been observed in some forms of neurogenic atrophy, particularly poliomyelitis (Hodes 1948) and motor neurone disease (Mulder et al 1959, Simpson & Lenman 1959). In healthy mammalian muscle, exhaustion at the motor end-plate occurs less readily and is probably only one aspect of fatigue which is less important than exhaustion of the contractile substance of the fibre (Brown & Burns 1949, Merton 1954, Naess & Storm-Mathison 1955).

In 1956, Edwards & Lippold suggested that, if a voluntary contraction is maintained for a period at a constant tension, it might be expected that more motor units would be recruited as the tension developed by the fatigued muscle fibres declined. This would alter the proportionality which has been shown to exist between electrical activity and tension. They measured the tension of the calf muscles at the same time as the integrated EMG throughout a range of tensions before and after a prolonged fatiguing contraction. They found that after fatigue the relationship between

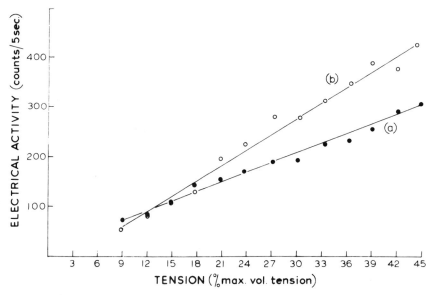

Fig. 32.2 Comparison of relation between integrated electrical activity and tension in soleus muscle (a) before and (b) after a 4-minute fatiguing contraction. Tension values are given as a percentage of maximum voluntary tension; electrical activity in counts of integrator pulse/5 s (from Edwards & Lippold 1956)

voltage and tension remains linear but the slope of the curve alters so that a given tension is associated with more electrical activity (Fig. 32.2). Similar observations have been made on the human biceps and triceps (Lenman 1959b) and also with isotonic contractions (Scherrer et al 1954). In addition to recruitment of motor units, other factors may participate in the increased electrical activity, such as synchronisation of motor unit discharges and the shift towards lower frequencies which occurs in the power spectrum of fatigued muscle (Lindström & Petersén 1981) (Fig. 32.2).

The observations are consistent with the view that the fatigue of a muscular contraction, at least during its later stages, is largely due to exhaustion of the contractile substance of the muscle fibres, although other factors, including neuromuscular block (Stephens & Taylor 1972) and a reduction in central drive (Bigland-Ritchie et al 1975), may operate earlier.

Muscle training

If fatigue is associated with recruitment of motor units to maintain a given tension, one would expect the reverse situation with fully trained muscle. This should apply in some degree, whether the effects of training were due to hypertrophy of the muscle fibres or to a neuromuscular adaptation leading to reorganisation and more efficient use of the available motor units (Lenman 1959a). This possibility is supported by several sets of observations.

Stepanov (1959) recorded the EMG through surface electrodes from the muscles of athletes during training in heavy weight lifting. It was found that both the mean amplitude and the frequency of the action potentials decreased as training proceeded. De Vries (1968) has used the slope of the voltage–tension curve to measure what he terms efficiency of electrical activity (EEA). In subjects of differing strength, the slope of the voltage–tension curve corresponded to less electrical activity for a given muscle tension in strong, as opposed to weak, individuals; this change in slope, the reverse of that which occurs in fatigued muscle, became more pronounced as

the strength of the muscle was increased by training. After immobilisation in a plaster cast the reverse effect occurred, so that more electrical activity corresponded to a given tension.

Muscle weakness

In 1959 Lenman found that in a group of patients with myopathy due either to muscular dystrophy or polymyositis, the voltage–tension relationship showed a change in slope compared with controls comparable to that seen in fatigued muscle, which suggests that the ability of dystrophic motor units to develop tension is impaired (Lenman 1959b, Fig. 32.3). In peripheral nerve disease, on the other hand, the slope of the voltage–tension curves did not differ significantly from that of healthy subjects. Results in patients with weakness resulting from old poliomyelitis differed from those in other patients with neurogenic weakness. Here the slope of the curves showed a shift in the direction of reduced efficiency; in addition, the absolute values obtained for mean voltage were considerably higher than those obtained from healthy subjects, a finding which was previously reported by Knowlton et al (1956). It is likely that these curves reflect the alterations in motor unit structure which follow recovery from poliomyelitis, in particular the increase in size of the motor units. Histologically, many of the collateral sprouts which gave rise to this increase are immature and poorly differentiated (Wohlfart 1959) and this may have a significant bearing on the efficiency of the enlarged units (Fig. 32.3).

In spastic weakness in hemiparetic patients there is also an increase in slope of the voltage–tension curve and a possible explanation of this is that the force generated by the muscle fibres may be reduced because of low rates of motor unit firing (Tang & Rymer 1981). In morning stiffness resulting from rheumatoid arthritis there is also a tendency for the curves to increase in slope after relatively minor exertion, in keeping with abnormal fatiguability (Lenman & Potter 1966).

As an aid to the diagnosis of muscular dystrophy, although the general features of the relationship have for the most part been confirmed

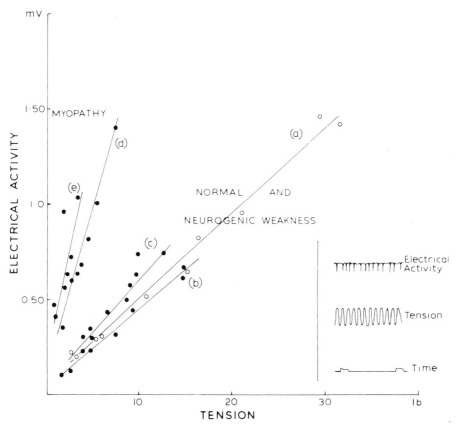

Fig. 32.3 Regression lines for relationship between mean voltage and isometric tension of biceps muscle of healthy subject and patients with neurogenic and myopathic weakness: a. healthy subjects; b. peripheral neuritis; c. motor neurone disease; d. polymyositis; e. muscular dystrophy. Insert shows specimen of ink writer recording from subject (a) in which time (seconds), tenson (amplitude of sine wave) and integrated electrical activity (number of pulses) are recorded simultaneously (Lenman 1959b)

by other workers, the test does not appear to be sufficiently sensitive, e.g. to identify clinically healthy carriers of muscular dystrophy (Gardner-Medwin 1968). Its main clinical usefulness at present would appear to be the possibility of providing a non-invasive technique to study the progress of the disease (Simpson & Sanderson 1965).

Fuglsang-Frederikson and his colleagues have studied the clinical usefulness of a modified technique. Using concentric needle electrodes they found a curvilinear relationship between voltage and tension but the ratio was linear when tension was plotted against the square root of the voltage. Using this method they found an increase in slope of the voltage–tension curve in 44% of their patients with myopathy and 64% of their patients with neurogenic disorders. For identifying abnormality this method therefore showed a fairly high

diagnostic yield but it did not serve to differentiate myopathy from neuropathy (Fuglsang-Frederikson et al 1984).

INTERFERENCE PATTERN ANALYSIS

In Chapter 30 the quantitative examination of individual motor unit potentials is described. This is a highly informative technique but, as it can be carried out only at low levels of contraction, it gives no information concerning the interference pattern. A number of different techniques have been developed for this purpose.

Frequency analysis

The frequency spectrum of the EMG as shown by Fourier analysis is dependent on both the mean duration of the motor units and the number of polyphasic units. Early studies (Richardson 1951, Walton 1952) involved the use of tuned circuits which enabled the frequency analysis to be displayed on the oscilloscope simultaneously with the interference pattern. Using this method the dominant frequency in limb muscles of normal subjects was found to be 100–200 Hz tailing off to zero at 800 Hz. In patients with myopathy the dominant frequency might exceed 400 Hz (Fig. 32.4) (Walton 1952). In patients with weakness due to motor neurone disease or following poliomyelitis, the shift in frequency may be towards the lower end of the spectrum (Fex & Krakau 1957). This method, particularly when combined with the loudspeaker, proved helpful in the clinical examination of patients but is not sufficiently sensitive to assist in the identification of disease where diagnosis is difficult, such as the recognition of patients with milder forms of dystrophy or suspected carriers.

Larsson (1968, 1975) made use of an analyser, developed by Kaiser & Petersen (1963), which employs four octave band filters with centre frequencies of 50, 200, 800 and 1600 Hz. It also includes a facility for statistical analysis and comparison of the values with control data. In patients with neuropathy, and using this method, long-standing cases showed a shift towards the low frequency end of the spectrum. New cases tended to show a shift towards the higher frequencies.

Recent interest has focused on the Fourier analysis applied to the EMG obtained through surface electrodes and its interpretation by means of mathematical models and computer stimulation techniques (Lindström 1985). Surface electrode spectra appear to be highly reproducible and to be closely dependent on the propagation velocity of muscle fibres as well as the frequency and the number of polyphasic units. The propagation velocity is slowed in fatigue (Stålberg 1966) and this is reflected in a shift towards the low-frequency end of the spectrum in fatigued muscle. In polyneuropathy there is a shift towards the low-frequency end of the spectrum and a shift towards the high frequencies occurs both in dystrophia myotonica and spinal muscular atrophy. These analyses are complex but non-invasive and with

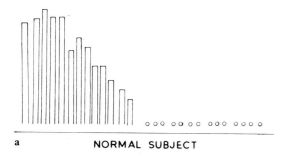

a   NORMAL SUBJECT

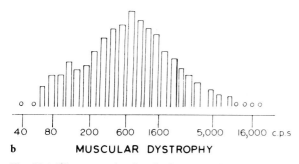

40   80   200   600   1600   5,000   16,000 c.p.s

b   MUSCULAR DYSTROPHY

Fig. 32.4 Histograms showing the frequency distribution of the electromyogram represented on the screen of an oscilloscope by means of an audio-frequency spectrometer: a. healthy subject; b. patient with faciosapulohumeral dystrophy showing a shift towards the high frequency end of the spectrum (adapted from Walton 1952)

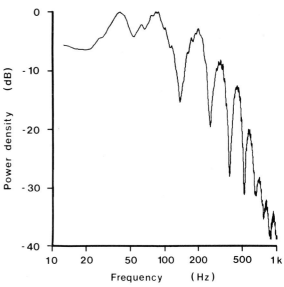

Fig. 32.5 Power spectrum of a myoelectric (EMG) signal with a predominant single motor unit contribution led off with a bipolar surface electrode from biceps brachii muscle. On the high-frequency side of the spectrum are seen multiple so-called 'dips' which are caused by the electrode arrangement. From the position of these dips, propagation velocity of the action potentials can be calculated (from Lindström & Petersén 1981)

the increasing availability of microprocessors may become more widely used (Lindström & Petersén 1981, Lindström 1985) (Fig. 32.5).

Spike analysis

Counting the number of spikes in the interference pattern during a voluntary quantitative contraction is a method which has been widely applied in the analysis of the interference pattern. Two parameters have been found to be particularly useful, namely, the total number of spikes related to a fixed reference level and the total number of changes in phase which occur regardless of any fixed crossing point. The first are known as zero crossings, the second as spikes (turns). These have been found to be related both to the force of a muscular contraction and the mean voltage of the EMG (Bergström 1959, Close et al 1960). More recently, attempts have been made to develop an index which correlates with muscular dystrophy, including other factors such as amplitude and the mean duration of the deflections (Van den Bosch 1963, Gardner-Medwin 1968, Moosa & Brown 1972).

A difficulty with any form of spike counting is to reach an objective definition of the size of potential change to be regarded as a spike. Willison (1964) therefore counted as spikes all changes in phase of greater than 100 μV. Later, with a computer program, spikes were counted automatically as one set of pulses (Fig. 32.6) and turns defined as changes in voltage regardless of phase and without reference to any base line. Each turn's pulse represented an increment of 100 μV. From these data the voltage between turns, i.e. the total voltage, in a given time could be derived (Fitch 1967).

This analysis was originally applied when the muscle contracted against a standard load. With this method it was found that in muscular dystrophy there is a marked increase in turns per unit time compared with controls and, if the spike count is not affected, the interval between spikes may be reduced. In neuropathies, on the other hand, the number of turns may be unaffected but the mean amplitude increased (Willison 1964, 1968, 1971, Dowling et al 1968, Hayward & Willison 1977).

In a recent study Fuglsang-Frederikson & Månsson (1975) found that muscles of different strength may not give comparable results and that this can be corrected if contractions of a predetermined power in relation to a maximum

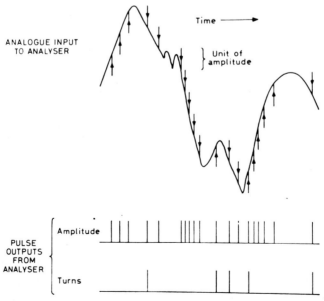

Fig. 32.6 Analysis of a typical waveform to show pulses derived from the analyser, each of which represents increments of voltage and changes of phase (from Fitch 1967)

contraction are used. A further useful parameter which can be derived is the ratio between number of turns and mean amplitude which can be obtained without using any predetermined force. This is particularly useful in the examination of children who may have difficulty in maintaining a sustained contraction at a given tension (Smyth & Willison 1982) and Fuglsang-Frederikson et al (1984) have found this ratio to be the most sensitive index for differentiating between patients with myopathy and controls.

Many studies have now confirmed that automatic spike counting, as described above, is a highly useful technique for the recognition of myopathic disorders as well as other forms of neuromuscular disease. In a recent study Yu & Murray (1984) found it to be less sensitive than single-fibre EMG (SFEMG) in patients with neuropathy but more helpful than SFEMG in the identification of cases of myopathy.

REFRACTORY PERIOD

The refractory period of a nerve or muscle depends on the recovery time of the fibre membrane after it has been depolarised. For a short interval after a stimulus the fibre will not respond to a second stimulus, however powerful; this is the absolute refractory period. The relative refractory period follows, in which a second stimulus of sufficient magnitude is effective. Finally, there may be a supernormal phase in which the tissue is hyperexcitable. The refractory period of nerve is shorter than that of muscle. In human peripheral nerve the absolute refractory period is 0.6–0.7 ms (Gilliatt & Willison 1963), whereas in healthy human muscle it ranges from 2.2 to 4.6 ms (Farmer et al 1960). While the refractory period is defined as the shortest interval between two effective stimuli, the shortest time between two evoked potentials is known as the irresponsive period (Lucas 1910). The irresponsive period may differ from the refractory period, and one explanation of this may be that the conduction velocity in a fibre may be reduced during the relative refractory period. This reduction in conduction velocity has been demonstrated in human nerve (Buchthal & Rosenfalck

1966) and in frog muscle (Buchthal & Engbaek 1963) but has not been shown to be present in human muscle.

The refractory period of muscle fibres is of interest because it gives information regarding the membrane properties of individual fibres. In the human subject study of the refractory period is limited by the fact that fibres do not have the same refractory period and, even when small electrodes are used to stimulate and record from a muscle, it is not possible to measure the refractory period of single fibres. In man, by the use of fine electrodes to stimulate small bundles of muscle fibres, it was found that the average refractory period is reduced in dystrophic muscle and lengthened in partially denervated muscle (Farmer et al 1959). An important observation was that the average refractory period of muscle fibres is frequently shorter than normal in clinically unaffected carriers of muscular dystrophy (Caruso & Buchthal 1965).

Measurements of the refractory period in peripheral nerve suggest that in certain types of peripheral neuropathy, such as may occur in association with diabetes, alcoholism and uraemia, the refractory period may be increased when nerve conduction velocity remains normal (Lowitzsch & Hopf 1975). Lithium has been found to give rise to a marginal lengthening of refractory period, and a marked increase has been recorded in patients who have taken rubidium (Betts et al 1978). Measurement of refractory period in motor nerves is not readily carried out by direct measurement, but methods have been described which use collision techniques (Hopf & Lowitzsch 1975, Kimura et al 1978) and Kopec et al (1978) have developed a subtraction technique by which the refractory period of the distal motor nerve branches and the muscle fibres can be determined.

PROPAGATION VELOCITY

The technical arrangements used to determine refractory period in human muscle may also be used to measure the propagation velocity along the muscle fibre. The stimulus is applied through a bipolar electrode in the distal end of the muscle, as far from the innervation zone as possible, and evoked potentials are recorded from three concentric electrodes inserted for a short distance proximally into the fibre bundle. With this method a mean propagation velocity of 4.1 ± 0.13 m/s has been found in the biceps brachii following electrical stimulation, compared with 4.7 ± 0.1 m/s with voluntary activation (Buchthal et al 1955). In denervated muscles a 50–80% reduction in conduction velocity has been found (Buchthal & Rosenfalck 1958) but in dystrophic muscle normal values have been obtained (Farmer et al 1959).

A different method was adopted by Stålberg (1966). This makes use of a concentric multielectrode which contains 14 platinum wires, the tips of which are exposed through an opening in the shaft of the electrode to form a row of adjacent recording points. When this electrode is aligned close to a muscle fibre the action potential can be recorded at different points, separated by a known distance, along the same fibre. Using this method to record the propagation velocity of voluntary evoked potentials, a mean propagation velocity of 3.37 ± 0.67 m/s was recorded in biceps brachii. In fatigue the propagation velocity is relatively slow, which may explain the shift which occurs in the frequency analysis (Lindström & Petersén 1981).

CONTRACTION TIME

The duration of a muscle contraction is lengthened in a wide variety of conditions including myxoedema (Chaney 1924), muscular dystrophy (Botelho et al 1960, Buchthal & Schmalbruch 1969) and weakness of neurogenic origin (Buchthal et al 1971a,b). In Duchenne dystrophy all the phases of the twitch may be prolonged (McComas & Thomas 1968) and histochemically there may be a preponderance of slow-twitch fibres. Likewise, there is a preponderance of fibres rich in mitochondrial enzymes in weakness of neurogenic origin (Buchthal et al 1971a,b).

Fetal muscle tends to be composed mainly of slow-twitch fibres which become differentiated into slow and fast units as maturation progresses and they are incorporated into fast and slow motor units. In muscular dystrophy, maturation may be slow and incomplete (Vrbová et al 1978) and

denervated muscle assumes some of the features of fetal muscle, including a slow contraction time.

Differentiation between fast and slow units can be recognised clinically by a preponderance of large units with a high threshold and rapid contraction or, alternatively, small units with a low threshold of excitation and a slow contraction. According to the size principle (Henneman 1957, Henneman et al 1965) the excitability of motor units is dependent on their size, small units having a lower threshold twitch time and conduction velocity in comparison with large. To differentiate slow and fast units requires a method which can record twitch tension of motor units and single or small groups of muscle fibres, and several methods to do this have been developed (Buchthal & Schmalbruch 1969, Milner-Brown et al 1973a,b). Tokizane & Shumazu (1964) put forward the hypothesis that the variability of spike frequency is greater when there is a preponderance of fast units and they described a population of fast or K units with marked variation in frequency and tonic or T units with little variation in frequency. Others, however, have not been able to differentiate two distinct populations of units in this way (Das Gupta 1963, Freund et al 1973, Rosenfalck & Andreassen 1980).

ESTIMATION OF MOTOR UNIT POPULATION

A different approach to the quantitative analysis of the EMG is to estimate the number of functioning motor units in a muscle compared with that in a control population. Measurement of the twitch at the same time enables one not only to measure the degree of partial denervation from the motor unit count but also to assess the capability of the muscle to compensate functionally.

McComas et al (1971a) described a method to estimate the number of functioning units in extensor digitorum brevis (EDB). The method is illustrated in Fig. 32.7. The EDB is stimulated through electrodes over the deep peroneal nerve and recording is by means of three silver strip electrodes — the stigmatic over EDB, a reference electrode on the sole of the foot and an earth electrode between the stigmatic and reference elec-

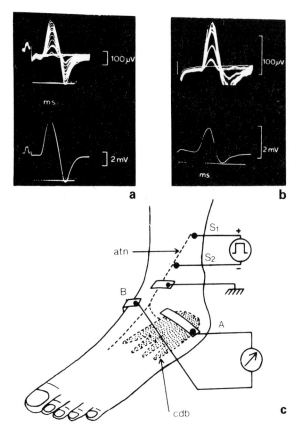

Fig. 32.7 Action potentials in extensor digitorum brevis evoked stimulation of deep peroneal nerve in (a) control subject and (b) a 16-year-old boy with Duchenne dystrophy. The recording arrangements are illustrated in c (from McComas et al 1971a)

trodes. With gradually increasing stimuli the evoked potentials increase by discrete increments, each of which may be considered to represent the recruitment of an additional unit. The number of motor units can be taken as the amplitude of the potential obtained by supramaximal stimulation divided by the mean amplitude of the increments, a figure which is obtained by measuring the respective amplitudes of the first group of increments recorded.

Using this method, McComas et al (1971b) studied a group of patients with disorders of innervation measuring both numbers of units and twitch tension. In the patients studied there was a marked reduction in numbers of motor units which, however, had a higher amplitude compared with controls. There was little change in twitch

tension until the motor unit count had fallen to about 10% of normal. These changes could be accounted for on the basis that the surviving units were enlarged as a result of collateral sprouting from surviving units.

In Duchenne dystrophy and also in dystrophia myotonica, facioscapulohumeral and limb-girdle dystrophy there was also a significant reduction in the motor unit count, an observation which raised the possibility that the primary disturbance in muscular dystrophy might be in the motor neurones (McComas et al 1971c, Sica & McComas 1971). Ballantyne & Hansen (1974a,b,c) used a digital computer to measure not only the change in amplitude produced by each increment of stimulus but also the latency, duration and area of the potentials comprising the summated response (Fig. 3.8). The motor unit potentials were each stored in digital form in a separate computer memory trace or template. If the second template contained the summated potentials of the first and second evoked responses, and the third template that of the first, second and third evoked responses, subtraction of the first template potential from the second would yield the second evoked response in isolation; similarly, subtraction of the third template from the second would yield the third evoked response in isolation. In this way the configuration of any of the stored motor unit potentials could be derived by template subtraction (Fig. 32.8). If the motor unit potential (MUP) derived from supramaximal stimulation were stored in the final template of the series, the number of motor unit potentials in the EDB could be calculated from the formula

$$MUC = n \times \frac{A(M)}{A(n)}$$

where MUC = motor unit count
   A(M) = area of supramaximal evoked MUP
   A(n) = area of compound muscle action potential containing n MUPs.

In healthy subjects this method gave motor unit counts broadly similar to those obtained by the amplitude summation technique. Reduced motor unit counts were found in myotonic muscular dystrophy but in patients with Duchenne, limb-

Normal (MCG, 53 years)

TEMPLATE

UNIT

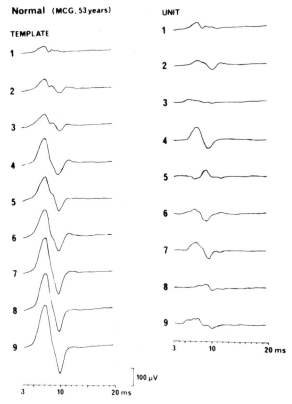

Fig. 32.8 Computer printout of templates and units obtained by template subtraction (from Ballantyne & Hansen 1974a,b,c)

girdle or facioscapulohumeral muscular dystrophy and with myasthenia gravis, motor unit counts within the normal range were obtained. The authors also used this method of measuring motor unit loss from a muscle as a means of evaluating the relative preponderance of axonal degeneration and segmental demyelination in different varieties of peripheral neuropathy (Ballantyne & Hansen 1974a, b, c, Hansen & Ballantyne 1977).

Other workers have stressed the technical problems which may affect the accuracy of motor unit estimation. Thus Panayiotopoulos et al (1974), who obtained similar motor unit counts in patients with Duchenne dystrophy and controls by the amplitude summation method, commented that the noise level of the recording system may obscure low-amplitude potential changes and they used enlarged superimposed photographs to identify incremental responses. Milner-Brown & Brown (1976) found that fluctuation in response

and overlapping firing levels of motor axons may lead to over-estimation of the number of motor units. In addition, they pointed out that the presence of large motor units with a high threshold of excitation may signify that the motor units that give rise to the potentials, from which the mean motor unit action potential is derived, may not always be representative of the motor unit population in the muscle.

THE STUDY OF REFLEXES

Introduction

The phasic reflex may be tested clinically by applying stretch or vibration to a muscle spindle primary ending to produce the familiar tendon jerk. The tonic stretch reflex normally is seen only when excitability is increased by reinforcement (Jendrassik's manoeuvre), or when a vibrator is applied to a muscle or tendon — the tonic vibration reflex (TVR). The third type of reflex studied in clinical practice belongs to the exteroceptive group of nociceptive responses, which result from cutaneous stimulations: particularly useful are the abdominal, plantar and blink reflexes.

Many of these reflexes can be precisely recorded electrophysiologically using the EMG or a tension recorder to register the response to an electrical or mechanical stimulus. The time course of the reflex is useful when studying the integrity of the reflex arc. In order to examine suprasegmental influences on the reflex, measurement of the effect of conditioning stimuli and factors such as habituation and sensitisation can be undertaken. The deep tendon reflex can be simply measured by an arrangement whereby the impact of a hammer triggers the sweep of an oscilloscope with a device for recording muscle contraction. This technique has been useful when studying the jaw jerk and the ankle jerk in patients with thyroid disease, where a prolonged relaxation time occurs (Ord 1884, Chaney 1924, Lambert et al 1951).

This section will discuss reflexes that can be elicited by electrical or mechanical stimulation: electrical stimulation of group Ia afferents of the appropriate peripheral nerve will evoke an H reflex; a tap on the chin will elicit the jaw jerk.

Tonic stretch reflexes, as distinct from phasic reflexes, can be studied by the application of manual stretch to a muscle while action potentials are recorded from surface or intramuscular electrodes, and this method was previously used to study changes in muscle evoked by passive stretch in patients with spasticity, rigidity or torsion dystonia. The application of vibration provides a controlled stimulus which will activate dynamic stretch receptors in muscle spindles and evoke the tonic stretch reflex.

The cutaneous reflex which has proved most useful for quantitative study is the blink reflex (see p. 1127).

The H reflex

If the posterior tibial nerve is stimulated in the popliteal fossa, an evoked muscle action potential may be recorded from the triceps surae muscle. If a weak stimulating pulse is employed, a second action potential has a relatively low threshold, requiring a smaller stimulus to evoke it than the first and disappearing as the stimulus increases (Fig. 32.9). The latency of this second potential is long enough to suggest that it represents a spinal reflex. This is supported by the fact that the latency is increased if the stimulus site is moved distally. This late potential, first described by Hoffman (1918), is called the H wave. The first potential attributable to direct stimulation of the muscle through its nerve is known as the M wave.

The reflex nature of the H wave was established by Magladery and his associates. They stimulated the posterior tibial nerve in the popliteal fossa, recording spinal root potentials from intrathecally placed electrodes. When these electrodes were placed close to the cord at L1, the time interval between anterior and posterior root potentials was only 1.5 ms. Allowing for the conduction time in the afferent and efferent arcs of the reflex, this is sufficient time for passage through a single cord synapse. With increasing strength of stimulus an antidromic potential was recorded on the anterior roots, which, with strong stimuli, occluded the anterior root potential (Magladery et al 1951). Conduction velocity studies showed that the afferent arc of the reflex is subserved by low-threshold, rapidly conducting group I fibres, and

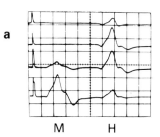

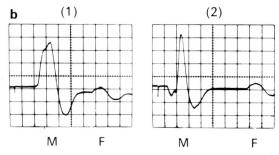

Fig. 32.9 a. H wave evoked from triceps surae muscle following stimulation of medial popliteal nerve with stimuli of increasing intensity (uppermost trace, weakest stimulus). When stimulus is adequate to evoke direct muscle response (M wave), amplitude of H wave is diminished. b. F wave evoked from abductor digiti minimi following stimulation of ulnar nerve at elbow (1), and at wrist (2). Latency of F wave diminishes as stimulation cathode is moved proximally. Squares on horizontal axis of graticule represent 5 ms; on vertical axis 2 mV

it seems that the H reflex represents the electrical equivalent of the ankle jerk elicited by stimulation proximal to the muscle spindle. The monosynaptic character of the ankle jerk has been shown by Lloyd (1943).

Under normal circumstances the H reflex can be elicited only from the calf muscles (Magladery & McDougal 1950) and until recently it was the only spinal monosynaptic reflex that could be elicited readily by electrical stimulation. Schimscheimer et al (1985) have, however, obtained flexor carpi radialis H reflexes in 143 normal subjects and patients with lesions of the sixth and seventh cervical roots.

The H wave has been widely studied as a measure of motor neurone excitability. If it is elicited by paired stimuli there is a period of up to several seconds after the conditioning stimulus when the excitability to the test stimulus is altered (Magladery et al 1952). The shape of the recovery curve depends on a variety of factors, among them the strength of the conditioning stimulus. If a stimulus of slightly above threshold is employed, the test reflex may be evoked during the 10 ms following the conditioning stimulus ('early facilitation'). After that, until about 80 ms after the conditioning stimulus, the reflex cannot be obtained. From 100 to 300 ms after the conditioning stimulus, the H wave builds up to reach a maximum at about 250 ms, 'the second facilitation'. There is then a second period of depression when the H reflex following the test stimulus is again reduced in size. This late depression is most marked at about 600 ms. Thereafter the test response gradually returns to normal (Fig. 32.10).

Magladery et al (1952) found that, in patients with upper motor neurone lesions, the shape of the recovery curve was altered in that, throughout the cycle, the H wave was more readily elicited by the test stimulus. In subsequent studies, the increased excitability associated with spasticity was confirmed (Takamori 1967) and increased excitability was also demonstrated in Parkinson's disease (Matsuoka et al 1966, Olsen & Diamantopoulos 1967, Yap 1967). In spinal shock the recovery cycle of the H reflex is depressed (Diamantopoulos & Olsen 1966) and this is also

the case in patients with the Holmes–Adie syndrome (McComas & Payan 1966). In a study of evolving hemiplegia, Garcia-Mullin & Mayer (1972) found that the level of neurone excitability, judged by the H/M ratio and the H wave recovery cycle, may be depressed in acute hemiplegia but enhanced in chronic hemiplegia, when the H reflex may also be elicited in the upper limbs. McLeod & Walsh (1972), using paired stimuli of near-threshold intensity in patients with Parkinson's disease, found that the initial unresponsive period was significantly shorter in patients than in controls, but lengthened after treatment with levodopa.

A major difficulty in the use of the H reflex as a measure of motor neurone excitability is the variability of the response and its liability to be influenced by peripheral factors. Thus it is facilitated by active contraction or by passive stretch of the muscle, and depressed by contraction of the antagonist (Mayer & Mawdsley 1965). It may show post-tetanic facilitation (Hagbarth 1962) and is abolished by vibration applied to the muscle or to its tendon (Hagbarth & Eklund 1966). Clearly, if the recovery curve is to have any meaning, it must be recorded using a technique that will avoid peripheral modifying factors as far as possible.

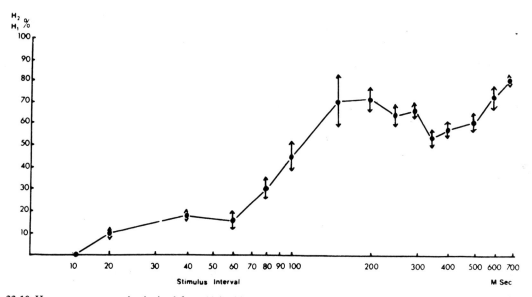

Fig. 32.10 H-wave recovery cycle obtained from 10 healthy adults. Ratio of test stimulus to conditioning H reflex stimulus, plotted against stimulus intervals. Conditioning and test stimuli of equal magnitude, stimulus strength selected to give maximum H response. Vertical bars represent standard error of means

McLeod & Van Der Meulen (1967) studied the significance of these factors in the cat by comparing the recovery curve of the H reflex with that of the monosynaptic reflex recorded from the ventral root, before and after section of the posterior tibial nerve. There was no difference in the duration of the unresponsive period but the first and second periods of facilitation were reduced after section. The unresponsive period is, therefore, a valid measurement of the excitability of the motor neurone pool, but the two periods of facilitation may be related to spindle activation determined by the reflex muscle contraction. Taborikova & Sax (1969) reduced the influence of peripheral factors in the human subject by using a sub-threshold conditioning stimulus which is too small to elicit an H response. With this technique a full-sized H reflex is obtained following the test stimulus, at stimulus intervals of up to 25 ms. This is followed by successive stages of early depression, intercurrent facilitation, late depression and then a gradual recovery. They suggest that the depression of the H reflex, after the test stimulus, can be accounted for by depletion of transmitter output following the conditioning stimulus. The intercurrent facilitation which occurs after a latent period of 50–300 ms could be explained by a long-loop reflex acting through brain-stem and cerebellar pathways. For a review of the methodology for eliciting an H reflex the reader is referred to the recommendations of Hugon et al (1973).

The amplitude of the H reflex may have some significance as representing the proportion of the motor neurone pool which can be excited. Unfortunately, the size of the reflex depends on many variables, such as site of electrode placement, stimulus strength and state of relaxation of the muscle. Angel & Hofman (1963) have suggested that these variables will affect the H and M waves equally and they have studied the ratio of the largest obtainable H wave divided by the largest obtainable M wave. They found this ratio to be higher than normal in spastic limbs, but to be little affected in parkinsonian rigidity. McComas & Payan (1966) found that the ratio was reduced in patients with the Holmes-Adie syndrome. Matthews (1966) studied the effect of relaxant drugs on this ratio in spastic patients but found that diazepam, while it reduced the size of the

ankle jerk, had little effect on that of the H reflex. Taborikova & Sax (1969) have commented that estimation of the size of the motor neurone pool from the ratio of the H and M waves is inaccurate. One possible reason is that a stimulus capable of evoking an H wave without evoking an M wave may be too weak to excite a maximum Ia volley. They describe a method whereby a stimulus large enough to evoke a maximal M wave is given after a previous stimulus has evoked a large H wave. If the second stimulus is given at an interval after the first, so that the M wave occurs when the muscle fibres are still refractory following the H wave, the M wave will be reduced in size in proportion to that fraction of the muscle fibres which was activated by the H reflex.

Studies on the effect of reinforcement on the H reflex have not yielded wholly consistent results. Sommer (1940) observed that, while the Jendrassik manoeuvre augments the ankle jerk, it may have little effect on the H reflex, and argued that reinforcement must proceed through motor nerves acting on spindles. These observations were confirmed by Buller & Dornhorst (1957) and by Paillard (1959) but Landau & Clare (1964) found it possible to augment the H reflex by reinforcement, provided that the H reflex is submaximal. Others have found the situation variable (Mayer & Mawdsley 1965, McComas & Payan 1966) and it remains uncertain to what extent the Jendrassik manoeuvre depends on fusimotor activity, and how far on excitation of α-neurones in the motor neurone pool.

If the H reflex is elicited by stimulation of the posterior tibial nerve during a voluntary contraction, it may be facilitated (Corrie & Hardin 1964, Takamori 1967). If the median nerve is excited during a voluntary contraction, two late responses can be recorded in the abductor pollicis brevis. One occurs about 2–3 ms after the F wave and the second has a latency of between 48 and 60 ms. These two potentials have been termed V_1 and V_2; V_1 has the characteristics of a potentiated H reflex. The origin of V_2 is unknown, but it may represent a polysynaptic reflex. If V_1 is elicited in patients with hemiparesis, it has been found that the potentiation produced by a voluntary contraction is less than that in healthy subjects; it has been suggested that a background facilitatory mechanism, which is normally present, is reduced (Sica et al 1971).

It is possible to measure the conduction velocity of both the afferent and efferent segments of the H reflex arc, but results have differed in different laboratories (Diamantopoulos & Gassel 1965, Mayer & Mawdsley 1965). In healthy adults, the latency varies between 26 and 32 ms. In peripheral neuropathy this latency may be substantially prolonged (Mayer & Mawdsley 1965).

The F wave

In contrast to the H reflex, the F wave can be recorded easily from most skeletal muscles. If the ulnar or median nerve is stimulated, and evoked potentials are then recorded from the hand muscles, the M wave may be followed by a late response, of relatively high threshold, with a latency of up to 30 ms. Increasing the strength of the stimulus increases the size of the response up to a certain level, but it is not blocked by supramaximal stimuli. If the stimulating electrode is moved distally, the latency increases. This late response appears irregularly, shows occasional variations in latency and has been designated the F wave (Magladery & McDougal 1950).

The F wave can be recorded from patients with tabes dorsalis, the Holmes–Adie syndrome and patients with congenital sensory neuropathy, associated with loss of reflexes. It does not show post-tetanic potentiation and, after a conditioning stimulus, there is no consistent long-lasting depression (Thorne 1965).

The nature of the F wave has been a matter of dispute since Magladery & McDougal (1950) suggested that it was a polysynaptic reflex. Dawson & Merton (1956) and Thorne (1965) considered that the F wave was due to a small recurrent discharge of a few motor neurones, produced by an antidromic volley reaching the neuronal perikaryon via motor fibres. Following section of all the dorsal roots derived from a baboon forelimb, McLeod & Wray (1966) obtained a response with the characteristics of an F wave from the small muscles of the hand.

Mayer & Feldman (1967) found that an F response could still be obtained from a patient with a chronic deafferented upper limb. Single-

fibre electrode studies have confirmed the recurrent nature of the F response in man, because it can be recorded only from single fibres after a preceding M response and the jitter is too short to be compatible with synaptic transmission (Trontelj 1973). As in the H reflex, there is a distinct relationship between the minimal F-wave latency and the height of the subject (Young & Shahani 1978). There are nomograms for normal minimal latencies plotted for different heights. F waves have been used in the diagnosis of mild, and even subclinical, neuropathies (Shahani & Young 1980).

THE TONIC VIBRATION REFLEX (TVR)

A tendon tap evokes a reflex contraction. This is a phasic reflex as distinct from the tonic stretch reflex, which gives rise to muscle tone in the clinical sense.

Sustained tonic stretch reflex activity is normally seen only when excitability is increased by mental or physical activation (reinforcement), or when a vibrator is applied to muscle or tendon. This stimulus activates repetitively the primary and secondary endings in muscle spindles, thus exposing the spinal cord to Group Ia and II afferent fibre discharge. The Ia afferents synapse not only directly with motor neurones, but also with facilitatory interneurones. These polysynaptic group Ia pathways are under suprasegmental control and have a role in the generation of the TVR (Hultborn & Wigstrom 1980, Burke 1980, Delwaide 1984).

Although vibration induces a tonic reflex contraction, it depresses tendon jerks and H reflexes simultaneously (Hagbarth & Eklund 1966, Lance et al 1966). This may be a result of spinal presynaptic inhibition (Gillies et al 1969).

A small vibrator oscillating at about 150 Hz can be strapped to muscle tendons. The response, which is often difficult to correlate quantitatively with the intensity or frequency of stimulation, is then measured by recording mechanical tension and muscle electrical activity. The TVR then slowly develops, increasing to a plateau over 15–30 s: the tonic contraction will persist for as long as vibration is maintained (Eklund 1971).

Vibration-induced tonic contraction can be potentiated by a preceding tetanic stimulation — lengthening the muscle or cooling the subject. Suppression of the TVR is observed when the subject is warmed or after administration of sedatives (Lance et al 1966).

Hemiplegic and spinal cord spastic subjects have a TVR which is lower in amplitude and more abrupt in onset and cessation than in normal subjects (Hagbarth & Eklund 1968, Burke et al 1972).

Attempts have been made to assist movement patterns in hemiplegics, using myoelectric-potential-activated vibrators (Hedberg et al 1967). In patients with Parkinson's disease, with rigidity, the TVR is normal and it is reduced or absent in patients with cerebellar disease (Hagbarth & Eklund 1968).

The blink reflex

Overend (1896) described a clinically useful cranial reflex, which may occur as a result not only of corneal stimulations, but also of a tap to the glabella. Electrical stimulation of the supra-orbital nerve provides a standardised stimulus to permit quantitative study of this reflex. The blink reflex has two components comprising an initial response; Rl, with a latency of 10–15 ms (the difference in latency between right and left responses not exceeding 1.5 ms), and a more prolonged late response, R2, with a more variable latency of 25–40 ms (latency difference of up to 8 ms) (Kugelberg 1952, Rushworth 1962).

When the reflex is elicited by an electrical stimulus, the R2 will be recorded bilaterally, the R1 appearing only on the ipsilateral side. The afferent arc of the reflex is the sensory route of the trigeminal nerve; the efferent is through the facial nerve. There is clinical evidence that the R1 is conducted through the pons and relayed in the area of the principal sensory nucleus of the fifth nerve (Kimura 1970, Namerow & Etamadi 1970) (Fig. 32.11).

The R2 component innervation descends along the spinal trigeminal tract to make connections via medullary polysynaptic pathways with both facial nuclei in the pons (Kimura & Lyon 1972). The physiological nature of the R1 remains in dispute.

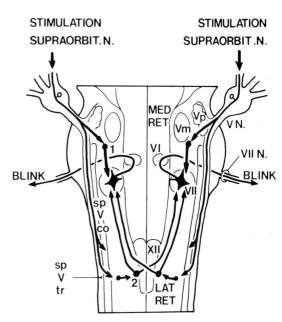

Fig. 32.11 Diagram with presumed location of bulbar interneurones subserving the two components of the blink reflex, R_1 and R_2. Vm = trigeminal motor nucleus; Vp = trigeminal principal sensory nucleus; Sp Vtr = spinal trigeminal tract Sp V co = spinal trigeminal complex, VI = abducens nucleus; VII N = facial nerve; XII = hypoglossal nucleus; MED RET = medial reticular formation; LAT RET = lateral reticular formation (from Ongerboer de Visser & Kuypers 1978)

Many authors believe it to be a monosynaptic stretch reflex (Brown & Rushworth 1973, Moldaver 1973, Messina 1975), whereas others state that it is exteroceptive, cutaneous and oligosynaptic in nature (Penders & Delwaide 1971, Shahani & Young 1973, Trontelj & Trontelj 1973).

Abnormalities of the blink reflex may occur in peripheral lesions affecting the trigeminal and facial nerves or their central connections, and in the presence of disturbances of suprasegmental function. In lesions of the trigeminal nerve, the first component may be small or absent, or have a prolonged latency (Fig. 32.12) (Ferguson 1978, Ongerboer de Visser & Kuypers 1978). In patients with Bell's palsy, conventional methods (distal conduction studies, facial EMG and studies of threshold for stimulation of the nerve or muscle with chronaxie, rheobase and strength duration curves) are useful mainly in the detection of changes produced by Wallerian degeneration and

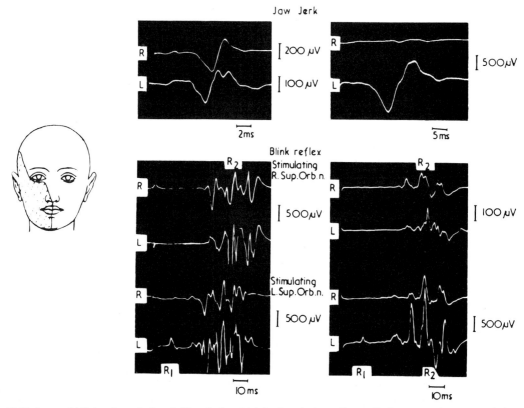

Fig. 32.12 Jaw and blink reflexes before (left) and after (right) trigeminal ganglion radio frequency thermocoagulation. Diagram of the face indicates minimal hypaesthesia of right maxillary and mandibular divisions. Note absent early blink response (R1) when stimulating the right supraorbital nerve, and absent jaw jerk after operation (from Ferguson 1978)

cannot localise proximal facial nerve segment lesions (Shahani & Young 1977). The blink reflex reflects conduction along the entire facial nerve. Kimura et al (1976) found serial testing a useful guide to determining a recovery pattern.

Significant prolongation of latency in both components of the blink reflex is observed in peripheral neuropathies of the segmental demyelinating type, including the Guillain–Barré syndrome (Shahani & Young 1977). Patients with cerebellopontine angle tumours may show either absence or prolongation of latency of the R1 (Eisen & Danon 1974, Rossi et al 1979, Ferguson 1981, Ongerboer de Visser 1983).

In multiple sclerosis, the latency of the R1 may be prolonged (Kimura 1975), but the reflex is not as clinically helpful as visual or auditory evoked potentials (Rodnitzky & Kimura 1978). In coma caused by supratentorial lesions, the R2 may be lost but the R1 is generally retained, unless the

brain stem is affected, whereas in sleep the R2 can be evoked if strong enough stimuli are used (Lyon et al 1972).

The habituation of the second component of the blink reflex, which usually occurs in healthy subjects, is frequently modified in diseases of the central nervous system. In Parkinson's disease, the R2 consistently fails to habituate (Penders & Delwaide 1971), a feature also seen in dementia (Gregoric 1973, Ferguson et al 1978). Conversely, in Huntington's chorea, habituation may occur abnormally rapidly (Esteban & Gimenez-Roldan 1975). Penders & Delwaide (1971) described a useful habituation index to indicate the stimulus frequency at which the blink reflex fails to habituate. Patients with blepharospasm have recently been shown to have normal blink reflex R1 and R2 latencies, yet an increase in amplitude and duration. The excitability cycle of recovery in the R2 component, after a conditioning stimulus, was enhanced in these patients. All these features suggest intact facial reflexes but an abnormal excitatory drive, perhaps from basal ganglia, to facial motor neurones (Berardelli et al 1985).

The jaw jerk

Jaw reflexes can be obtained by using a reflex hammer containing an inertia-triggered micro-switch (Ferguson 1978, Ongerboer de Visser & Goor 1974). At the moment of tap on the patient's chin, the hammer triggers the oscilloscope sweep, thus recording evoked potentials from the masseter muscles, with either surface or coaxial needle electrodes. The reflex is of limited clinical application, except when exaggerated, where it is indicative of a suprasegmental lesion above the fifth nerve nucleus.

The reflex is of physiological interest in that early animal work suggested that the afferent and efferent fibres shared a common pathway in the motor root of the fifth cranial nerve (Szentagothai 1948, McIntyre 1951). McIntyre & Robinson (1959) believed that this arrangement also existed in man. However, two studies of patients who have undergone surgery for trigeminal neuralgia

showed that an abnormal jaw jerk could be obtained in a patient with no clinical or EMG evidence of motor root involvement (Fig. 32.12). It was concluded that normal jaw reflexes can change into abnormal responses, after destructive lesions of the trigeminal sensory root, suggesting that proprioceptive afferent fibres from masseter muscle spindles run along the mandibular sensory division and not the trigeminal motor root (Ferguson 1978, Ongerboer de Visser 1982).

The jaw jerk can always be demonstrated electrically, except in very elderly subjects, where it may be absent bilaterally. The latency varies from 6 to 9 ms. A difference of more than 0.5 ms between the two sides or a consistent unilateral absence can be taken as abnormal. It may be abnormal in the presence of trigeminal nerve lesions (Ongerboer de Visser & Goor 1974).

The central pathway studies in cats (Corbin & Harrison 1940, Szentagothai 1948, Jerge 1962) and in patients with midbrain lesions (Dehen et al 1976) suggest that afferent impulses are relayed to the trigeminal mesencephalic nucleus and that then via collateral connections, they link with the efferent side of the reflex — the trigeminal motor nerve nucleus and nerve.

REFERENCES

Adrian E D, Bronk D W 1929 The discharge of impulses in motor nerve fibres, Part II. Journal of Physiology 67:119

Angel R W, Hoffman W W 1963 The H reflex in normal, spastic and rigid subjects. Archives of Neurology 8:591

Ballantyne J P, Hansen S 1974a A new method for estimation of the number of motor units in a muscle. 1. Control subjects and patients with myasthenia gravis. Journal of Neurology, Neurosurgery and Psychiatry 37:907

Ballantyne J P, Hansen S 1974b Computer method for the analysis of evoked motor unit potentials. 1. Control subjects and patients with myasthenia gravis. Journal of Neurology, Neurosurgery and Psychiatry 37:1187

Ballantyne J P, Hansen S 1974c A new method for the estimation of the number of motor units in a muscle. 2. Duchenne, limb-girdle and facioscapulohumeral, and myotonic muscular dystrophies. Journal of Neurology, Neurosurgery and Psychiatry 37:1195

Bates J A V, Cooper J D 1955 Simple technique for making EEG audible. Electroencephalography and Clinical Electrophysiology 7: 137–139

Bayer H, Flechtenmayter C 1950 Ermüding und Aktionspannung bei der isometrischen Muskelkontraktion des Menschen. Arbeitsphysiologie 14:261

Berardelli A, Rothwell J C, Day B L, Marsden C D 1985 Pathophysiology of blepharospasm and oromandibular dystonia. Brain 108:609

Bergström, R M, 1959 The relation between the number of impulses and the integrated electrical activity in the electromyogram. Acta Physiologica Scandinavica 45:97

Betts R P, Paschalis C, Jarratt J A, Jenner F A 1978 Nerve fibre refractory period in patients treated with rubidium and lithium. Journal of Neurology, Neurosurgery and Psychiatry 41:791

Bigland B, Lippold O C J 1954a The relation between force, velocity and integrated electrical activity in human muscles. Journal of Physiology 123:214

Bigland B, Lippold O C J 1954b Motor unit activity in voluntary contraction of human muscle. Journal of Physiology 125:322

Bigland-Ritchie B, Hosking G P, Jones D A 1975 The site of fatigue in sustained maximal contractions of the quadriceps muscle. Journal of Physiology 250:45P

Bjork A, Kugelberg E 1953 Motor unit activity in human extraocular muscles. Electroencephalography and Clinical Neurophysiology 5:271

Botelho S Y, Beckett S B, Bendler E 1960 Mechanical and electrical responses of intact thenar muscles to indirect stimuli. Neurology (Minneapolis) 10:601

Brown G L, Burns B D 1949 Fatigue and neuromuscular block in mammalian skeletal muscle. Proceedings of the Royal Society of London (Series B) 36:182

Brown W F, Rushworth G 1973 Method for counting motor

units in thenar muscles and changes in motor unit count with ageing. In: Desmedt J E New developments in electromyography and clinical neurophysiology, vol. 3. Karger, Basel, p 660

Buchthal F, Guld C, Rosenfalck P 1955 The innervation and propagation velocity in human muscle. Acta Physiologica Scandinavica 35:174

Buchthal F, Rosenfalck P 1958 Rate of impulse conduction in denervated human muscles. Electroencephalography and Clinical Neurophysiology 10:521

Buchthal F, Engbaek L 1963 Refractory period and conduction velocity of the striated muscle fibre. Acta Physiologica Scandinavica 59:199

Buchthal F, Rosenfalck P 1966 Spontaneous electrical activity of human muscle. Electroencephalography and Clinical Neurophysiology 20:321

Buchthal F, Schmalbruch H 1969 Spectrum of contraction times of different fibre bundles in the brachial biceps and triceps muscles of man. Nature 222:89

Buchthal F, Schmalbruch H, Kamieniecka Z 1971a Contraction times and fibre types in neurogenic paresis. Neurology (Minneapolis) 21:58

Buchthal F, Schmalbruch H, Kamieniecka Z 1971b Contraction times and fibre types in patients with progressive muscular dystrophy. Neurology (Minneapolis) 21:131

Buller A J, Dornhorst A C 1957 The reinforcement of tendon reflexes. Lancet 2:1260

Burke D, 1980 Muscle spindle activity induced by vibration in man; implications for the tonic stretch reflex. In: Desmedt J E (ed) Progress in clinical neurophysiology, vol. 8. Karger, Basel, p 243

Burke D, Andrews C J, Lance J W 1972 Tonic vibration in spasticity, Parkinson's disease and normal subjects. Journal of Neurology, Neurosurgery and Psychiatry 35:477

Caruso G, Buchthal F 1965 Refractory period of muscle and electromyographic findings in relatives of patients with muscular dystrophy. Brain 88:29

Chaney W C 1924 Tendon reflexes in myxoedema: A valuable aid in diagnosis. Journal of the American Medical Association 82:2013

Close J R, Nickel E D, Todd F N 1960 Motor-unit action potential counts. Their significance in isometric and isotonic contractions. Journal of Bone and Joint Surgery (America) 42-A:1207

Cobb S, Forbes A 1923 Electromyographic studies of muscular fatigue in man. American Journal of Physiology 65:234

Corbin B K, Harrison F 1940 Function of mesencephalic root of the fifth cranial nerve. Journal of Neurophysiology 3:423

Corrie W S, Hardin W B Jr 1964 Post-tetanic potentiation of H reflex in normal man. Archives of Neurology 11:317

Das Gupta A 1963 The possibility of selective involvement of motor units in muscular dystrophy. In: Research in muscular dystrophy. Proceedings of Second Symposium on Current Research in Muscular Dystrophy. Pitman, London, p 256

Dawson G D, Merton P A 1956 'Recurrent' discharges from motoneurones. XX International Congress on Physiology. Abstracts of Communications, Brussels, p 221

Dehen H, Willer J C, Bathien N 1976 Blink reflex in hemiplegia. Electroencephalography and Clinical Neurophysiology 40(4):393

Delwaide P T 1984 In: Shahani B T (ed) Electromyography

in CNS disorders: Central EMG. Butterworth, London, p 77

De Vries H A 1968 'Efficiency of Electrical Activity' as a physiological measure of the functional state of muscle tissue. American Journal of Physical Medicine 47:10

Diamantopoulos E, Gassel M M 1965 Electrically induced monosynaptic reflexes in man. Journal of Neurology, Neurosurgery and Psychiatry 28:496

Diamantopoulos E, Zander Olsen P 1966 Motoneurone excitability in patients with abnormal reflex activity. In: Granit R (ed) Muscular afferents and motor control. Proceedings of the First Nobel Symposium, Stockholm. Almqvist and Wiksell, Stockholm

Dowling M H, Fitch P, Willison R G 1968 A special purpose digital computer (Biomac 500) used in the analysis of the human electromyogram. Electroencephalography and Clinical Neurophysiology 25:570

Edwards R G, Lippold, O C J 1956 The relationship between force and integrated electrical activity in fatigue muscle. Journal of Physiology 132:677

Eisen A, Danon J 1974 The orbicularis oculi reflex in acoustic neuromas: A clinical and electrodiagnostic evaluation. Neurology 24:306

Eklund G 1971 Some physical properties of muscle vibrators used to elicit tonic proprioceptive reflexes in man. Acta Social Medical Uppsala 76:271

Esteban A, Gimenez-Roldan S 1975 Blink reflexes in Huntington's chorea and Parkinson's disease. Acta Neurologica Scandinavica 52:145

Farmer T W, Buchthal F, Rosenfalck P 1959 Refractory and irresponsive periods of muscle in progressive muscular dystrophy and paresis due to lower motor neurone involvement. Neurology (Minneapolis) 9:747

Farmer T W, Buchthal F, Rosenfalck P 1960 Refractory period of human muscle after the passage of a propagated action potential. Electroencephalography and Clinical Neurophysiology 12:455

Ferguson I T, Lenman J A R, Johnston B B 1978 Habituation of the orbicularis oculi reflex in dementia and dyskinetic states. Journal of Neurology, Neurosurgery and Psychiatry 41:824

Ferguson I T 1978 Electrical study of jaw and orbicularis oculi reflexes after trigeminal nerve surgery. Journal of Neurology, Neurosurgery and Psychiatry 41:819

Ferguson I T 1981 An electrophysiological study of brain stem reflexes. M.D. Thesis, University of Dundee

Fex J, Krakau C E T 1957 Some experiences with Walton's frequency analysis of the electromyogram. Journal of Neurology, Neurosurgery and Psychiatry 20:178

Fitch P 1967 An analyser for use in human electromyography. Electronic Engineering 39:240

Freund H J, Dietz V, Wita C W, Kapp H 1973 Discharge characteristics of single motor units in normal subjects and patients with supraspinal motor disturbances. In: Desmedt J E New developments in electromyography and clinical neurophysiology, vol. 3. Karger, Basel, p 242

Fuglsang-Frederiksen A, Månsson A 1975 Analysis of electrical activity of normal muscle in man at different degrees of voluntary effort. Journal of Neurology, Neurosurgery and Psychiatry 38:683

Fuglsang-Frederiksen A, Lo Monaco M, Dahl K 1984 Integrated electrical activity and number of zero crossings during a gradual increase in muscle force in patients with neuromuscular diseases. Electroencephalography and Clinical Neurophysiology 58(3):211

Garcia-Mullin R, Mayer R F 1972 H reflexes in acute and chronic hemiplegia. Brain 95:559

Gardner-Medwin D 1968 Studies of the carrier state in the Duchenne type of muscular dystrophy. 2. Quantitative electromyography as a method of carrier detection. Journal of Neurology, Neurosurgery and Psychiatry 31:124

Gilliatt R W, Willison R G 1963 The refractory and supernormal periods of the human median nerve. Journal of Neurology, Neurosurgery and Psychiatry 26:136

Gillies J D, Lance J W, Neilson P D, Tassinari C A 1969 Presynaptic inhibition of the monosynaptic reflex by vibration. Journal of Physiology 205: 329–339

Gregoric M 1973 Habituation of the blink reflex. In: Desmedt J E New developments in electromyography and clinical neurophysiology, vol. 3. Karger, Basel, p 673

Hagbarth K E 1962 Post-tetanic potentiation of myotatic reflexes in man. Journal of Neurology, Neurosurgery and Psychiatry 21:1

Hagbarth K E, Eklund G 1966 Motor effects of vibratory muscle stimuli in man. In: Granit R (ed) Muscular afferents and motor control. Proceedings of the First Nobel Symposium Stockholm. Almquist and Wiksell, Stockholm, p 177

Hagbarth K E, Eklund G 1968 The effects of muscle vibration in spasticity, rigidity and cerebellar disorders. Journal of Neurology, Neurosurgery and Psychiatry 31:207

Hansen S, Ballantyne J P 1977 Axonal degeneration in the neuropathy of diabetes mellitus: a quantitative electromyographic study. Journal of Neurology, Neurosurgery and Psychiatry 40:555

Harvey A M Masland R L 1941 The electromyogram in myasthenia gravis. Bulletin of the Johns Hopkins Hospital 69:1

Hayward M, Willison R G 1977 Automatic analysis of the electromyogram in patients with chronic partial denervation. Journal of the Neurological Sciences 33:415

Hedberg A, Oldberg B, Tové P A 1967 EMG-controlled muscle vibrators to aid mobility in spastic paresis. In: Jacobson B (ed) International conference on medical and biological engineering. Almquist and Wiksell, Stockholm, p 197

Henneman E 1957 Relations between size of neurones and their susceptibility to discharge. Science 126:1345

Henneman E, Sonjen G, Carpenter D O 1965 Functional significance of cell size in spinal motoneurones. Journal of Neurophysiology 28:560

Hodes R 1948 Electromyographic study of neuromuscular transmission in human poliomyelitis. Archives of Neurology and Psychiatry 60:457

Hoffman P 1918 Über die Beziehungen der Sehnenreflex sur willkürlichen Bewegung und zum Tonus. Zeitschrift fur Biologie 68:351

Hopf H C, Lowitzsch K, 1975 Relative refractory period of motor nerves. In: Kunze K, Desmedt J E (eds) Studies on neuromuscular diseases. Proceedings of an International Symposium, Giesson 1973. Karger, Basel, p 264

Hugon M, Delwaide P, Pierrot-Deseilligny E, Desmedt J E 1973 A discussion of the methodology of the triceps sural T- and H-reflexes. In: Desmedt J E (ed) New developments in electromyography and clinical neurophysiology, vol. 3. Karger, Basel, p 773

Hultborn H, Wigstrom H 1980 Motor response with long latency and maintained duration evoked by activity in Ia afferents. In: Desmedt J E (ed) Progress in clinical neurophysiology, vol. 8. Karger, Basel, p 99

Inman V T, Ralston H J, Saunders J B.de C M, Feinstein B, Wright E W 1952 Relation of human electromyogram to muscular tension. Electroencephalography and Clinical Neurophysiology 4:187

Jerge C R J 1962 Organisation and function of the trigeminal mesencephalic nucleus. Journal of Neurophysiology 26:379

Kaiser E, Petersén I 1963 Frequency analysis of muscle action potentials during tetanic contraction. Electromyography 3:5

Kimura J 1970 Alteration of the orbicularis oculi reflex by pontine lesions: Study in multiple sclerosis. Archives of Neurology (Chicago) 22:156

Kimura J 1975 Electrically elicited blink reflex in diagnosis of multiple sclerosis (review of 260 patients over a seven year period). Brain 98:413

Kimura J, Lyon L W 1972 Orbicularis oculi reflex in the Wallenberg syndrome: alteration of the late reflex by lesions of the spinal tract and nucleus of the trigeminal nerve. Journal of Neurology, Neurosurgery and Psychiatry 35:228

Kimura J, Giron L T, Young S M 1976 An electrophysiological study of Bell's palsy. Archives of Otolaryngology 100:140

Kimura J, Yamada T, Rodnitzky R L 1978 Refractory period of human motor nerve fibres. Journal of Neurology, Neurosurgery and Psychiatry 41:784

Knowlton G C, Hines T F, Keever K W, Bennett R L 1956 Relation between electromyographic voltage and load. Journal of Applied Physiology 9:473

Kopec J, Delbeke J, McComas A J 1978 Refractory period studies in a human neuromuscular preparation. Journal of Neurology, Neurosurgery and Psychiatry 41:54

Kugelberg E 1952 Facial reflexes. Brain 75:385

Kuroda V, Klissouras V, Milsum J H 1970 Electrical and mechanical activities and fatigue in human isometric contraction. Journal of Applied Physiology 29:358

Lambert E H, Underdahl L O, Beckett S, Mederos L O 1951 A study of ankle jerk in myxodema. Journal of Clinical Endocrinology 11:1186

Lance J W, De Gail P, Neilson P D 1966 Tonic and phasic spinal cord mechanisms in man. Journal of Neurology, Neurosurgery and Psychiatry 29:535

Landau W M, Clare M H 1964 Fusimotor function Part IV. Reinforcement of the H-reflex in normal subjects. Archives of Neurology 10:117

Larsson L E 1968 Frequency analysis of the EMG in neuromuscular disorders. Electroencephalography and Clinical Neurophysiology 24:89

Larsson L E 1975 On the relation between the EMG frequency spectrum and the duration of symptoms in lesions of the peripheral motor neurone. Electroencephalography and Clinical Neurophysiology 38(1):69

Lenman J A R 1959a A clinical and experimental study of the effects of exercise on motor weakness in neurological disease. Journal of Neurology, Neurosurgery and Psychiatry 22:182

Lenman J A R 1959b Quantitative electromyographic changes associated with muscular weakness. Journal of Neurology, Neurosurgery and Psychiatry 22:306

Lenman J A R, Potter J L 1966 Electromyographic measurement of fatigue in rheumatoid arthritis and neuromuscular disease. Annals of the Rheumatic Diseases (London) 25:76

Lindsley D B 1935 Electrical activity of human motor units

during voluntarty contraction. American Journal of Physiology 114:90

Lindström L 1985 Spectral analysis of EMG. In: Struppler A, Weindl A (eds) Electromyography and evoked potentials. Springer-Verlag, Berlin, p 103

Lindström L, Petersén I 1981 Power spectra of myoelectric signals: motor unit activity and muscle fatigue. In: Stålberg E, Young R R (eds) Neurology I; Clinical neurophysiology. Butterworth, London, p 66

Lippold O C J 1952 The relation between integrated action potentials in a human muscle and its isometric tension. Journal of Physiology 117:492

Lloyd D P C 1943 Conduction and synaptic transmission of the reflex response to stretch in spinal cats. Journal of Neurophysiology 6:317

Lowitzsch K, Hopf H C 1975 Propagation of compound action potentials of the mixed peripheral nerves in man at high stimulus frequencies. In: Kunze K, Desmedt J E (eds) Studies on neuromuscular diseases. Proceedings of an International Symposium, Giessen, 1973. Karger, Basel

Lucas K 1910 On the refractory period of muscle and nerve. Journal of Physiology 39:331

Lyon L W, Kimura J, McCormick W F 1972 Orbicularis oculi reflex in coma: clinical electrophysiological and pathological correlations. Journal of Neurology, Neurosurgery and Psychiatry 35:582

McComas A J, Payan J 1966 Motoneurone excitability in the Holmes-Adie syndrome. In: Andrew B L (ed) Control and innervation of skeletal muscle. Livingstone, Edinburgh, p 182

McComas A J Thomas H C 1968 A study of muscle twitch in the Duchenne type muscular dystrophy. Journal of the Neurological Sciences 7:309

McComas A J, Fawcett P R W, Campbell M J, Sica R E P 1971a Electrophysiological estimation of the number of motor units within a human muscle. Journal of Neurology, Neurosurgery and Psychiatry 34:121

McComas A J, Sica R E P, Campbell M J, Upton A R M 1971b Functional compensation in partially degenerated muscles. Journal of Neurology, Neurosurgery and Psychiatry 34:453

McComas A J, Campbell M J, Sica R E P 1971c Electrophysiological study of dystrophia myotonica. Journal of Neurology, Neurosurgery and Psychiatry 34:132

McIntyre A K 1951 Afferent limb of the myotatic reflex arc. Nature 168:168

McIntyre A K, Robinson R G 1959 Pathway for the jaw jerk in man. Brain 82:468

McLeod J G, Wray S H 1966 An experimental study of the F wave in the baboon. Journal of Neurology, Neurosurgery and Psychiatry 29:196

McLeod W D 1973 EMG instrumentation in biochemical studies: amplifiers recorders and integrators. In: Desmedt J E (ed) New developments in electromyography and clinical neurophysiology, vol. 2. Karger, Basel, pp 511

McLeod J G, Van der Meulen J P 1967 Effects of cerebellar ablation on the H reflex of the cat. Archives of Neurology 16:421

McLeod J G Walsh J C 1972 H reflex studies in patients with Parkinson's disease. Journal of Neurology, Neurosurgery and Psychiatry 35:77

Magladery J W, McDougal D B 1950 Electrophysiological studies of nerve and reflex activity in normal man. Bulletin of the Johns Hopkins Hospital 86:265

Magladery J W, Porter W E, Park A M, Teasdall R D 1951 Electrophysiological studies of nerve and reflex activity in normal man. Bulletin of the Johns Hopkins Hospital 88:499

Magladery J W, Teasdall R D, Park A M, Languth H W 1952 Electrophysiological studies of reflex activity in patients with lesions of the nervous system. Bulletin of the Johns Hopkins Hospital 91:219

Marsden C D, Meadows J C, Merton P A 1971 Isolated single motor units in human muscle and their rate of discharge during maximal voluntary effort. Journal of Physiology 217:12

Matsuoka S, Waltz J M, Terada C, Ikeda T, Cooper I S 1966 A computer technique for evaluation of recovery cycle of the H reflex in abnormal movement disorders. Electroencephalography and Clinical Neurophysiology 21:496

Matthews W B 1966 Ratio of maximum H reflex to minimum M response as a measure of spasticity. Journal of Neurology, Neurosurgery and Psychiatry 29:201

Mayer R F, Mawdsley C 1965 Studies in man and cat of the significance of the H reflex. Journal of Neurology, Neurosurgery and Psychiatry 28:201

Mayer R F, Feldman R G 1967 Observations on the nature of the F wave in man. Neurology 17:147

Merton P A 1954 Voluntary strength and fatigue. Journal of Physiology 123:553

Messina C 1975 On the nature and meaning of the blink reflex early response. Electromyography and Clinical Neurophysiology 15(2):119

Milner-Brown H S, Stein R B, Yemm R 1973a The orderly recruitment of human motor units during voluntary isometric contractions. Journal of Physiology, 230:359

Milner-Brown H S, Stein R B Yemm R 1973b Changes in firing rate of human motor units during linearly changing voluntary contractions. Journal of Physiology 230:371

Milner-Brown H S, Stein R B 1975 The relation between the surface electromyogram and muscular force. Journal of Physiology 246:549

Milner-Brown H S, Brown W F 1976 New methods of estimating the number of motor units in a muscle. Journal of Neurology, Neurosurgery and Psychiatry 39:258

Moldaver J 1973 In: Desmedt J E (ed) New developments in electromyography and clinical neurophysiology, vol. 3. Karger, Basel, p 658

Moosa A, Brown B H 1972 Quantitative electromyography: a new analogue technique for detecting changes in action potential duration. Journal of Neurology, Neurosurgery and Psychiatry 35:216

Mulder D W, Lambert E H, Eaton L M 1959 Myasthenic syndrome in patients with amyotrophic lateral sclerosis. Neurology (Minneapolis) 9:627

Naess K, Storm-Mathison A 1955 Fatigue of sustained tetanic contractions. Acta Physiologica Scandinavica 34:351

Namerow N S, Etamadi A 1970 The orbicularis oculi reflex in multiple sclerosis. Neurology (Minneapolis) 20:1200

Norris F H Jr, Gasteiger E L 1955 Action potentials of single motor units in normal muscle. Electroencephalography and Clinical Neurophysiology 7:115

Olsen P Zander, Diamantopoulos E 1967 Excitability of spinal motor neurones in normal subjects and patients with spasticity, Parkinsonian rigidity and cerebellar hypotonia. Journal of Neurology, Neurosurgery and Psychiatry 30:325

Ongerboer de Visser B W 1982 Pathway of jaw jerk in man. Neurology (New York) 32:563

Ongerboer de Visser B W 1983 Anatomical and functional organisation of reflexes involving the trigeminal system in man: Jaw reflex, blink reflex, corneal reflex and exteroceptive suppression. In: Desmedt J E (ed) Motor control mechanisms in health and disease. Raven Press, New York, p 727

Ongerboer de Visser B W, Goor C 1974 Electromyographic and reflex study in idiopathic and symptomatic trigeminal neuralgias: latency of the jaw and blink reflexes. Journal of Neurology, Neurosurgery and Psychiatry 37:1225

Ongerboer de Visser B W, Kuypers H G J M 1978 Late blink reflex changes in lateral medullary lesions. Brain 101:285

Ord W M 1884 On some disorders of nutrition related with affections of the nervous system. British Medical Journal 2:205

Overend W 1896 Preliminary note on a new cranial reflex. Lancet 1:619

Paillard J 1959 Functional organisation of afferent innervation of muscle studies in man by monosynaptic testing. American Journal of Physical Medicine 38:239

Panayiotopoulos C P, Scarpalezos S, Papapetropoulos Th 1974 Electrophysiological estimation of motor units in Duchenne muscular dystrophy. Journal of the Neurological Sciences 23:89

Penders C A, Delwaide P L 1971 Blink reflex studies in patients with Parkinsonism before and during therapy. Journal of Neurology, Neurosurgery and Psychiatry 34:674

Piper H 1912 Elektrophysiologie menschlicher Muskeln. Julius Springer, Berlin

Richardson A T 1951 Newer concepts of electrodiagnosis. St. Thomas's Hospital Reports 7:164

Rodnitzky R L, Kimura J 1978 The effect of induced hyperthermia on the blink reflex in multiple sclerosis. Neurology (Minneapolis) 28:431

Rosenfalck A, Andreassen S 1980 Impaired regulation of force and firing pattern of single motor units in patients with spasticity. Journal of Neurology, Neurosurgery and Psychiatry, 43(10):907–16

Rossi R, Buonaguidi A, Muratorio A, Tusin G 1979 Blink reflexes in posterior fossa lesions. Journal of Neurology, Neurosurgery and Psychiatry 42:465

Rushworth G 1962 Observation on blink reflexes. Journal of Neurology, Neurosurgery and Psychiatry 25:93

Scherrer J, Samson M, Soula C 1954 Étude électromyographique de la fatigue musculaire normale. Journale de Physiologie 46:517

Schimsheimer R T, Ongerboer de Visser B W, Kemp B 1985 The flexor carpi radialis H reflex in lesions of the sixth and seventh cervical nerve roots. Journal of Neurology, Neurosurgery and Psychiatry 48:445

Seyffarth H 1941a The behaviour of motor units in healthy and paretic muscles in man. I. Acta Psychiatrica et Neurologia 16:79

Seyffarth H 1941b The behaviour of motor units in healthy and paretic muscles in Man. II. Acta Psychiatrica et Neurologica 16:261

Shahani B T, Young R R 1973 In: Desmedt J E (ed) New developments in electromyography and clinical neurophysiology vol 3. Karger, Basel, p 641

Shahani B T, Young R R 1977 Blink, H and tendon vibration reflexes. In: J Goodgold, Aberstein A (eds) Electrodiagnosis of neuromuscular diseases, 2nd edn. Williams and Wilkins, Baltimore 11, 245

Shahani B T, Young R R 1980 Studies of reflex activity from a clinical viewpoint. In: Aminoff M J (ed) Electrodiagnosis in clinical neurology. Churchill Livingstone, Edinburgh

Sica R E P, McComas A J 1971 An electrophysiological investigation of limb girdle and facioscapulohumeral dystrophy. Journal of Neurology, Neurosurgery and Psychiatry 34:469

Sica R E P, McComas A J, Upton A R M 1971 Impaired potentiation of H reflexes in patients with upper motor neurone lesions. Journal of Neurology, Neurosurgery and Psychiatry 34:712

Simpson J A, Lenman J A R 1959 The effect of frequency of stimulation in neuromuscular disease. Electroencephalography and Clinical Neurophysiology 11:604

Simpson J A, Sanderson I D 1965 Experimental studies of the effect of 'Laevadosin' in muscular dystrophy. In: Research in muscular dystrophy. Proceedings of the Third Symposium on Current Research in Muscular Dystrophy. Pitman, London, p 342

Smyth D P, Willison R G 1982 Quantitative electromyography in babies and young children with no evidence of neuromuscular disease. Journal of the Neurological Sciences 56 (2–3): 209–17

Sommer J 1940 Periphere Bahnung von Muskeleigenreflexen als Wesen des JendrasssiksenPhänomens. Deutsche Zeitschrift fur Nervenheilkunde 150:249

Stålberg E 1966 Propagation velocity in human muscle fibres in situ. Acta Physiologica Scandinavica 70 (Suppl):287

Stepanov A S 1959 Electromyogram changes produced by training in weight lifting. Fiziologicheskii Zhurnal (Moscow) 45:129

Stephens J A, Taylor A 1972 Fatigue of maintained voluntary muscle contraction in man. Journal of Physiology 220:1

Stephens J A, Taylor A 1973 The relationship between integrated electrical activity and force in normal and fatiguing human voluntary muscle contractions. In: Desmedt J E (ed) New developments in electromyography and clinical neurophysiology, vol. 1. Karger, Basel, p 623

Szentagothai J 1948 Anatomical considerations of monosynaptic reflex arcs. Journal of Neurophysiology 11:445

Taborikova H, Sax D S 1969 Conditioning of the H-reflexes by a preceding subthreshold H-reflex stimulus. Brain 92:203

Takamori M 1967 H reflex study in upper motoneuron diseases. Neurology (Minneapolis) 17:32

Tang A, Rymer W Z 1981 Abnormal force — EMG relations in paretic limbs of hemiparetic human subjects. Journal of Neurology, Neurosurgery and Psychiatry 44(8): 690–8

Tanji J, Kato M 1973a Recruitment of motor units in voluntary contraction of a finger muscle in man. Experimental Neurology 40:759

Tanji J, Kato M 1973b Firing rate of individual motor units in voluntary contraction of abductor digiti minimi muscle in man. Experimental Neurology 40:771

Thorne J 1965 Central responses to electrical activation of the peripheral nerves supplying intrinsic hand muscles. Journal of Neurology, Neurosurgery and Psychiatry 28:482

Tokizane T, Shimazu H 1964 Functional differentiation of human skeletal muscle. Corticalisation and spinalization of movement. Charles C. Thomas, Springfield, Illinois

Trontelj J V 1973 A study of the F response by single fibre electromyography. In: Desmedt J E (ed) New developments in electromyography and clinical neurophysiology, vol. 3. Karger, Basel, p 318

Trontelj M A, and Trontelj J V 1973 First component of human blink reflex studied on single facial motoneurones. Brain Research 53:214

Van den Bosch J 1963 Investigations of the carrier state in the Duchenne type dystrophy. In:Research in muscular dystrophy. Proceedings of the Second Symposium on Current Research in Muscular Dystrophy. Pitman, London, p 23

Vrbová E, Gordon T, Jones R 1978 Nerve-muscle interaction. Chapman and Hall, London

Walton J N 1952 The electromyogram in myopathy: analysis with the audio frequency spectrometer. Journal of Neurology, Neurosurgery and Psychiatry 15:219

Willison R G 1964 Analysis of electrical activity in healthy and dystrophic muscle in man. Journal of Neurology, Neurosurgery and Psychiatry 22:320

Willison R G 1968 Problems of detecting carriers of Duchenne muscular dystrophy by quantative electromyography. In: Research in muscular dystrophy. Proceedings of the fourth Symposium on Current Research in Muscular Dystrophy. Pitman, London, p 433

Willison R G 1971 Quantitative electromyography. In: Licht S (ed) Electrodiagnosis and electromyography, 3rd edn. Elizabeth Licht, New Haven, Connecticut

Wohlfart E 1959 Clinical considerations on innervation of skeletal muscle.

Yap C-B 1967 Spinal segmental and long loop reflexes in spinal motoneurone excitability in spasticity and rigidity. Brain 80:887

Young R R, Shahani B T 1978 Clinical value and limitations of F-wave determination. Muscle and Nerve 1:248

Yu Y L, Murray N M 1984 A comparison of concentric needle electromyography, quantitative EMG and single fibre EMG in the diagnosis of neuromuscular diseases. Electroencephalography and Clinical Neurophysiology 58(3):220

Zuniga N E, Simons D G 1969 Non linear relationship between averaged electromyogram potential and muscle tension in normal subjects. Archives of Physical Medicine and Rehabilitation 50:613

Zuniga E N, Truong X T, Simons D G 1969 Effects of skin electrode position on averaged electromyographic potentials. Archives of Physical Medicine and Rehabilitation 51:261

Index

Polymyositis
(See p 1160 After
Protozoal
Disorders)